AUNDERS
ELSEVIER

1830 Westline Industrial Drive
. Louis, Missouri 63146

TRAUMA NURSING: From Resuscitation Through Rehabilitation ISBN: 978-1-4160-3772-9

Notice

Knowledge and best practice in this field are constantly changing. As new research and experience broaden our knowledge, changes in practice, treatment, and drug therapy may become necessary or appropriate. Readers are advised to check the most current information provided (i) on procedures featured or (ii) by the manufacturer of each product to be administered, to verify the recommended dose or formula, the method and duration of administration, and contraindications. It is the responsibility of the practitioner, relying on their own experience and knowledge of the patient, to make diagnoses, to determine dosages and the best treatment for each individual patient, and to take all appropriate safety precautions. To the fullest extent of the law, neither the Publisher nor the Authors assume any liability for any injury and/or damage to persons or property arising out of or related to any use of the material contained in this book.

The Publisher

International Standard Book Number: 978-1-4160-3772-9

Executive Publisher: Tom Wilhelm
Managing Editor: Maureen Iannuzzi
Publishing Services Manager: Deborah L. Vogel
Project Manager: Pat Costigan
Book Designer: Paula Catalano
Marketing Manager: John Lewellan

Printed in the United States of America

Last digit is the print number: 9 8 7 6 5 4 3 2 1

TRAUMA NURSING

From Resuscitation Through Rehabilitation

Fourth Edition

KAREN A. McQUILLAN, RN, MS, CCRN, CNRN
Clinical Nurse Specialist
R Adams Cowley Shock Trauma Center
University of Maryland Medical Center
Baltimore, Maryland

MARY BETH FLYNN MAKIC, RN, PhD, CNS, CCNS, CCRN
Research Nurse Scientist and Assistant Professor, Adjoint
University of Colorado Hospital and University of Colorado at Denver,
College of Nursing
Aurora, Colorado

EILEEN WHALEN, RN, BSN, MHA
Vice President
Trauma, Emergency Medicine and Perioperative Services
University Medical Center
Tucson, Arizona
Past president of the Society of Trauma Nurses

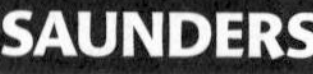

SAUNDERS

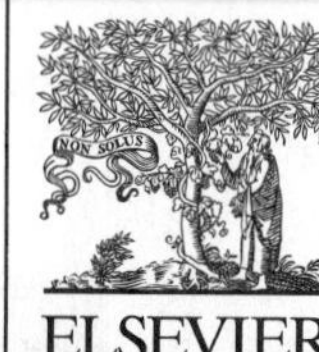

ELSEVIER

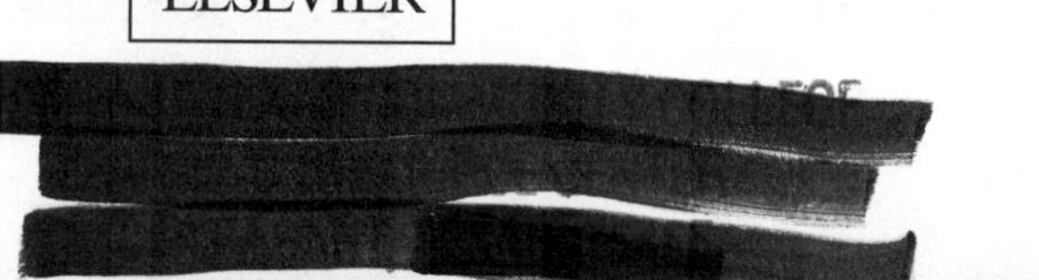

To my friends and colleagues at the R Adams Cowley Shock Trauma Center who taught me so much about the art and science of trauma care. Their tireless efforts to provide the best possible care to trauma patients and their families are truly an inspiration.
Special thanks to my family for all of their love and support.

Karen A. McQuillan

To my trauma colleagues and patients who taught me the importance of excellence in trauma care.
To my parents, husband, and children, whose unconditional love and support are ever present in my life.

Mary Beth Flynn Makic

Over the last twenty five years I have devoted my professional career to the advancement of trauma systems. Never in my darkest hour did I ever believe I or my family would need to call on the resources of a trauma system. Now, as a survivor, I am humbled by the urgent need to transfer knowledge and improve systems of care globally. Let this text awaken your sense of wonder and rekindle your commitment to quality trauma care.

Eileen Whalen

CONTRIBUTORS

Marilyn C. Algire, RN, MSN, MPH
Infection Control Practitioner
University of Maryland Medical Center
Baltimore, Maryland
15, Infection and Infection Control

Mary Beachley, MS, RN, CEN
Director, Office of Hospital Programs
Maryland Institute for Emergency Medical Services Systems
Baltimore, Maryland
1, Evolution of the Trauma Cycle

Janet M. Beebe, MS, CRNP-A
Nurse Practitioner
Bowie Internal Medicine Associates
Bowie, Maryland
33, Substance Abuse and Trauma Care

John Bleicher, RN
Trauma Coordinator
St. Patrick Hospital and Health Sciences Center
Missoula, Montana
8, Rural Trauma

Pamela J. Bolton, RN, MS, ACNP, CCNS, CCRN, PCCN
Acute Care Nurse Practitioner
Good Samaritan Hospital
Harrison, Ohio
13, Shock and Multiple Organ Dysfunction Syndrome

Sharon A. Boswell, RN, MS, ACNP
Nurse Practitioner
R Adams Cowley Shock Trauma Center
University of Maryland Medical System
Baltimore, Maryland
14, Initial Management of Traumatic Shock

T. Catherine Bower, RN, BSN
Acute Pain Management Nurse Coordinator
The James L. Kernan Hospital
Baltimore, Maryland
18, Analgesia, Sedation, and Neuromuscular Blockade in the Trauma Patient

Karen J. Brasel, MD, MPH, FACS
Associate Professor
Medical College of Wisconsin
Milwaukee, Wisconsin
12, Mechanism of Injury

Patricia B. Casper, RN, CRNP
Nurse Practitioner
R Adams Cowley Shock Trauma Center
University of Maryland Medical System
Baltimore, Maryland
15, Infection and Infection Control

Franki L. Chabalewski, RN, MS
Professional Services Coordinator
UNOS (United Network for Organ Sharing)
Richmond, Virginia
34, The Organ and Tissue Donor

Will Chapleau, EMT-P, RN, TNS
Manager, ATLS Program
American College of Surgeons
Chicago, Illinois
7, Prehospital Care of the Trauma Patient

Martha A. Conlon, RN, BSN, MAS
The Johns Hopkins Hospital
Baltimore, Maryland
22, Ocular Injuries

Cheryl Edwards, RN, MSN, CCRN, CPTC
Procurement Coordinator
New England Organ Bank at the Yale University
Division of Transplantation and Immunology
Waterbury, Connecticut
34, The Organ and Tissue Donor

Mary Kate FitzPatrick, RN, MSN, CRNP
Clinical Director, Nursing Operations
Hospital of the University of Pennsylvania, Nursing Administration
Philadelphia, Pennsylvania
3, Performance Improvement and Patient Safety in Trauma Care

Carolyn J. Fowler, PhD, MPH
Assistant Professor
The Johns Hopkins Bloomberg School of Public Health
Center for Injury Research and Policy
The Johns Hopkins School of Nursing
Director, Injury Prevention Program
Baltimore County Department of Health
Baltimore, Maryland
6, Injury Prevention

P. Milo Frawley, RN, MS, ACNP
Nurse Practitioner
R Adams Cowley Shock Trauma Center
University of Maryland Medical Center
Baltimore, Maryland
24, Thoracic Trauma

Kurt Haspert, RN, BSN, CARN
Nurse Consultant–Addictions
R Adams Cowley Shock Trauma Center
University of Maryland Medical Center
Baltimore, Maryland
33, Substance Abuse and Trauma Care

Robert W. Heilig, JD, MPA
Consultant
Robert W. Heilig & Associates
Nogales, Arizona
5, Legal Concerns in Trauma Nursing

Mary C. Hirsh, RN, BSN, CARN
Nurse Consultant–Addictions
R Adams Cowley Shock Trauma Center
University of Maryland Medical Center
Baltimore, Maryland
33, Substance Abuse and Trauma Care

Kimmith M. Jones, RN, MS
Advanced Practice Nurse
Critical Care and Emergency Services
Sinai Hospital of Baltimore
Baltimore, Maryland
25, Abdominal Injuries

Manjari Joshi, MD
Associate Professor of Medicine
R Adams Cowley Shock Trauma Center
University of Maryland Medical System
Baltimore, Maryland
15, Infection and Infection Control

Daniel G. Judkins, RN, MS, MPH
Trauma Outreach Educator and Injury Coordinator
University Medical Center
Tucson, Arizona
8, Rural Trauma
9, Mass Casualty Incidents

Catherine J. Klein, PhD, RD, CNSD
Director, Bionutrition Research Program
Children's National Medical Center
Washington, DC
17, Metabolic and Nutritional Management of the Trauma Patient

Jorie Klein, RN
Director, Trauma Services
Parkland Health and Hospital System
Dallas, Texas
12, Mechanism of Injury

Rifat Latifi, MD, FACS
Director, UMC Telemedicine Services
Associate Director, Arizona Telemedicine Program
University Medical Center
University of Arizona
Tucson, Arizona
8, Rural Trauma

Mary Beth Flynn Makic, RN, PhD, CNS, CCNS, CCRN
Research Nurse Scientist and Associate Professor, Adjoint
University of Colorado Hospital and University of Colorado at Denver, College of Nursing
Aurora, Colorado
16, Wound Healing and Soft Tissue Injuries
32, Burn Injuries

MAJ Elizabeth A. Mann, RN, MS, CCRN, AN
Clinical Head Nurse
Institute of Surgical Research, US Army
San Antonio, Texas
32, Burn Injuries

Ruby J. Martinez, RN, PhD, APRN-BC
Associate Professor Emeritus
University of Colorado Hospital and University of Colorado at Denver, College of Nursing
Nurse Manager, Adult In-Patient
Denver Health Medical Center
Denver, Colorado
19, Psychosocial Impact of Trauma

Janet McMaster, RN, MHSA
Trauma Performance Improvement Coordinator
Hospital of the University of Pennsylvania
Philadelphia, Pennsylvania
3, Performance Improvement and Patient Safety in Trauma Care

Karen A. McQuillan, RN, MS, CCRN, CNRN
Clinical Nurse Specialist
R Adams Cowley Shock Trauma Center
University of Maryland Medical System
Baltimore, Maryland
16, Wound Healing and Soft Tissue Injuries
20, Traumatic Brain Injuries
21, Maxillofacial Trauma

Patricia A. Moloney-Harmon, RN, MS, CCRN
Advanced Practice Nurse/Clinical Nurse Specialist, Children's Services
Sinai Hospital of Baltimore
Baltimore, Maryland
29, Pediatric Trauma

Ellen Plummer, DL, MJ, RN, CCRN
Senior Partner, Trauma Resuscitation Unit
R Adams Cowley Shock Trauma Center
University of Maryland Medical Center
Baltimore, Maryland
30, Trauma in the Elderly

Joan M. Pryor-McCann, PhD, RN, CNS
Associate Professor of Nursing
Otterbein College
Westerville, Ohio
4, Ethics in Trauma Nursing

Stephanie Raine, RN, MA
Professional Services Coordinator
UNOS (United Network for Organ Sharing)
Richmond, Virginia
34, The Organ and Tissue Donor

Jameson P. Reuter, PharmD
Clinical Specialist Critical Care
Union Memorial Hospital
Annapolis, Maryland
18, Analgesia, Sedation, and Neuromuscular Blockade in the Trauma Patient

Tammy A. Russo-McCourt, RN, BSN, CCRN
Clinical Specialist
Intensive Care On-line Network (ICON)
Hampstead, Maryland
23, Spinal Cord Injuries

Thomas M. Scalea, MD
Physician in Chief
R Adams Cowley Shock Trauma Center
University of Maryland Medical System
Baltimore Maryland
14, Initial Management of Traumatic Shock

Suzanne Frey Sherwood, RN, MS
Full Partner, Trauma Resuscitation Unit
R Adams Cowley Shock Trauma Center
University of Maryland Medical Center
Faculty, University of Maryland School of Nursing
Baltimore, Maryland
21, Maxillofacial Trauma

Lynn Gerber Smith, MS, RN
Full Partner
R Adams Cowley Shock Trauma Center
University of Maryland Medical System
Baltimore, Maryland
28, The Pregnant Trauma Patient

Kara A. Snyder, RN, MS, CCRN, CCNS
Clinical Nurse Specialist, Critical Care/Trauma
University Medical Center
Tucson, Arizona
26, Genitourinary Injuries and Renal Management

Gena Stiver Stanek, RN, MS, CCRN
Clinical Nurse Specialist
R Adams Cowley Shock Trauma Center
University of Maryland Medical System
Baltimore, Maryland
17, Metabolic and Nutritional Management of the Trauma Patient

Valerie Summerlin, RN, MS, CNAA, BC
Vice President of Patient Care Services
The James L. Kernan Hospital (Kernan Orthopaedics and Rehabilitation)
Baltimore, Maryland
11, Rehabilitiation of the Trauma Patient

Sheryl L. Szczensiak, BSN
Assistant Nurse Manager, Emergency Department
Cedars-Sinai Medical Center
Los Angeles, California
31, Trauma in the Bariatric Patient

Paul A. Thurman, RN, BSN, CCRN, CNRN
Full Partner
R Adams Cowley Shock Trauma Center
University of Maryland Medical System
Baltimore, Maryland
20, Traumatic Brain Injuries

Thomas C. Vary, PhD
Distinguished Professor of Cellular and Molecular Physiology
Pennsylvania State University College of Medicine
Hershey, Pennsylvania
13, Shock and Multiple Organ Dysfunction Syndrome

Victoria R. Veronese, RN, BSN
Patient Care Manager, Surgical/Trauma ICU
University Medical Center
Tucson, Arizona
26, Genitourinary Injuries and Renal Management

Kathryn Truter Von Rueden, RN, MS, FCCM
Assistant Professor
University of Maryland School of Nursing
Clinical Nurse Specialist
R Adams Cowley Shock Trauma Center
University of Maryland Medical Center
Baltimore, Maryland
10, Nursing Practice Through the Cycle of Trauma
13, Shock and Multiple Organ Dysfunction Syndrome

Colleen R. Walsh, RN, MSN, ONC, CS, ACNP
Faculty, Graduate Nursing
University of Southern Indiana
Evansville, Indiana
27, Musculoskeletal Injuries

Frank G. Walter, MD, FACEP, FACMT, FAACT
Associate Professor of Emergency Medicine
Chief, Division of Toxicology
Director of Clinical Toxicology
University of Arizona College of Medicine
Tucson, Arizona
9, Mass Casualty Incidents

John A. Weigelt, MD, DVM, FACS
Department of Surgery
Medical College of Wisconsin
Milwaukee, Wisconsin
12, Mechanism of Injury

Christopher Welsh, MD
Associate Professor, Psychiatry, Alcohol and Drug Abuse
University of Maryland Medical Center
Baltimore, Maryland
33, Substance Abuse and Trauma Care

Eileen Whalen, RN, BSN, MHA
Vice President
Trauma, Emergency Medicine and Perioperative Services
University Medical Center
Tucson, Arizona
2, Economic and Administrative Issues in Trauma Care

REVIEWERS

Bizhan Aarabi, MD, FRCSC, FACS
University of Maryland School of Medicine
Baltimore, Maryland

Pamela Bourg, RN, MS
St. Anthony Central Hospital Trauma Program
Denver, Colorado

Sandy Brannan, MSN, RN
Lamar University
Beaumont, Texas

William C. Chiu, MD, FACS, FCCM
R Adams Cowley Shock Trauma Center
University of Maryland Medical Center
Baltimore, Maryland

James Cushman, MD, FACS
University of Maryland School of Medicine
Baltimore, Maryland

Christine R. Duran, APRN, BC, ND, CNS, CCTN
Solid Organ Transplant Unit
University of Colorado Hospital
Denver, Colorado

Laura R. Favand, RN, MS, CEN
US Army Nurse Corps, 67th Forward Surgical Team
Miesau, Germany

Joyce Foresman-Capuzzi, BSN, RN, CEN, CPN, CTRN, EMT-P
Temple University Health System
Philadelphia, Pennsylvania

Michael A. Frace, MSN, RN, RRT
Summit Healthcare Regional Medical Center
Show Low, Arizona

Alice A. Gervasini, PhD, RN
Massachusetts General Hospital
Harvard Medical School
Boston, Massachusetts

Robbi Lynn Hartsock, RN, MSN, PCNP
R Adams Cowley Shock Trauma Center
University of Maryland Medical Center
Baltimore, Maryland

H. Bebe Hoff, RN, MS, CNS
University of Colorado Hospital
Denver, Colorado

Heidi Hotz, RN
Cedars-Sinai Medical Center
Los Angeles, CA

Dianne Husbands, BA, RN, BScN, MN
St. Joseph's Healthcare
Hamilton, Ontario, Canada

Nicholas T. Iliss, MD
Johns Hopkins Hospital
Baltimore, Maryland

Karen Johnson, RN, PhD
University of Maryland School of Nursing
Baltimore, Maryland

Daniel G. Judkins, RN, MS, MPH
University Medical Center
Tucson, AZ

Michelle J. Klosterman, RN
Adams County Regional Medical Center
Seaman, Ohio

Karen LeDuc, MS, RN, CPN, CNS
The Children's Hospital
Regis University
University of Colorado
University of Northern Colorado
Denver, Colorado

Erica McHugh, RN, MSN
Denver Health Medical Center
Denver, Colorado

Hugh E. Mighty, MD, FACOG, MBA
Department of Obstetrics, Gynecology and Reproductive Services
University of Maryland Medical Center
Baltimore, Maryland

Nancy C. Molter, RN, MN, PhD
Choctaw Management Services Enterprises
U.S. Army Institute of Surgical Research
Fort Sam Houston, Texas

Robert K. Montgomery, RN, ND, CNS
University of Colorado Health Sciences Center
Denver, Colorado

Jo-Anne O'Brien, RN, MScN, ENC(C)
The Ottawa Hospital
Ottawa, Ontario, Canada

James O'Connor, MD, FACS
University of Maryland School of Medicine
Baltimore, Maryland

Mehrnaz Pajoumand, PharmD
R Adams Cowley Shock Trauma Center
University of Maryland Medical Center
Baltimore, Maryland

Bari Platter, MS, RN, CNS
University of Colorado Hospital
Denver, Colorado

Andrew N. Pollak, MD, FAAOS, FACS
University of Maryland School of Medicine
Baltimore, Maryland

Peggy Plylar, MS, RN, CRRN, CNS
University of Colorado Hospital
Denver, Colorado

Ronald Rabinowitz, MD, FACP
Division of Infectious Disease
Department of Medicine
R Adams Cowley Shock Trauma Center
University of Maryland Medical Center
Baltimore, Maryland

Eduardo Rodriguez, MD, DDS
Plastic Surgery/Oral Surgery
R Adams Cowley Shock Trauma Center
University of Maryland Medical Center
Baltimore, Maryland

Kathryn Schroeter, PhD, RN, CNOR
Medical College of Wisconsin
Marquette University
Milwaukee, Wisconsin

Susan Seiboldt, MSN, RN
Carl Sandburg College
Galesburg, Illinois

Carol A. Soderstrom, MD, FACS
University of Maryland School of Medicine
Baltimore, Maryland

Deborah M. Stein, MD, MPH, FACS
R Adams Cowley Shock Trauma Center
University of Maryland Medical Center
Baltimore, Maryland

Roderick Wold, RN, ND
Airlife Denver
Swedish Medical Center
Englewood, Colorado

Michele K. Ziglar, RN, MSN
Shands at the University of Florida
Gainesville, Florida

FOREWORD

The initial edition of this text published in 1988 and was the first comprehensive textbook to provide a holistic framework for trauma nursing using the concept of the cycle of trauma care. This framework described trauma care from the initial interventions for prevention through the prehospital, resuscitation, critical care, intermediate care, and rehabilitation phases. It focused in-depth on the pathophysiologic approach to trauma nursing practice that combined both current science and the caring aspects of nursing. Elizabeth Scanlon, RN, MS, then Director of Nursing at the R Adams Cowley Shock Trauma Center (RACSTC), sponsored the writing of the textbook. She supported her clinical nurse specialists in their efforts to collate into one text the knowledge learned from their research, from their experiences treating trauma patients at the RACSTC and other trauma centers, and from lessons learned in the Vietnam War. Virginia Cardona, RN, MS, one of the clinical nurse specialists at RACSTC, had served in the Vietnam War and was the lead editor for the first and second editions of *Trauma Nursing: From Resuscitation Through Rehabilitation.*

This edition has been updated to reflect the most current medical and nursing research effecting changes in the dynamic specialty of trauma care. In addition to ongoing research, there have been several major events in recent years that accelerated the accumulation of new knowledge and skills related to trauma care. The terrorist attacks of 2001, the hurricanes on the gulf coast, and the wars in Iraq and Afghanistan, along with the ongoing increase in violence and high-risk behaviors in our society, are examples of the events that have influenced trauma nursing.

These events have presented us with new challenges and opportunities to improve organized trauma systems, trauma centers, and the clinical care provided to the injured population. At the same time, we are faced with healthcare provider shortages that are requiring new approaches to the provision of care. For example, responsibilities for care have shifted and new roles have developed to address the complex and timely treatment interventions needed by trauma patients. In addition, the development of new, more complex diagnostic technologies and electronic health information systems require additional knowledge and skills for trauma nurses.

Opportunities for advancing the trauma specialty include more interagency cooperation and planning for large-scale mass casualty events. Collaboration among trauma centers is essential to plan for events that require evacuation and interhospital transfers of critically injured patients. Another major opportunity is to continue to raise public and government awareness of the need for trauma centers and organized trauma systems.

There is still much work to do in organizing trauma systems and trauma centers. To that end, trauma nurses continue to play an important role in developing systems of care as well as providing holistic care to trauma patients. Roles have expanded for nurses in many trauma care arenas. Nurses hold positions in local and state government agencies responsible for designing and regulating trauma systems. Trauma center roles for nurses include senior executives, program managers, trauma program coordinators, acute care nurse practitioners, trauma nurse researchers, clinical nurse specialists, case managers, trauma-prevention coordinators, and direct care providers in all units providing care to trauma patients.

The updated edition of this textbook will continue to provide trauma nurses with the evidence-based content to refresh and build on the specialty knowledge of trauma nursing. I am honored to be asked to write the foreword for this comprehensive trauma nursing textbook and to be included among the authors for the second, third, and fourth editions. I have had many opportunities over my years in trauma nursing to function in a variety of roles, including direct care provider, educator, and trauma system manager. Each role has been very rewarding and has influenced my professional and personal growth. This new edition of the textbook provides trauma nurses a comprehensive resource with current information to assist in their continued learning and the transfer of knowledge into practice.

Mary Beachley, MS, RN, CEN
Director, Office of Hospital Programs
Maryland Institute for Emergency Medical Services Systems
Baltimore, Maryland

PREFACE

Research developments and practice changes in the dynamic field of trauma care necessitate a fourth edition of the highly acclaimed text, *Trauma Nursing: From Resuscitation Through Rehabilitation.* Like the first three editions of this text, the fourth edition provides a comprehensive description of the art and science of trauma nursing. It builds on the strengths of the previous editions while updating content, expanding on specific topics, and introducing relevant new material.

Trauma Nursing: From Resuscitation Through Rehabilitation employs a unique cycle of trauma framework. This format provides the reader with an easy-to-follow organization of material describing evaluation and management of the trauma patient through the continuum of trauma care, including prevention and prehospital considerations; resuscitation; and the operative, critical, intermediate, and rehabilitation phases of care. Evidence-based information about issues that affect trauma care systems, injury pathophysiology, and currently recommended assessment and care of the trauma patient are described for each phase of the trauma cycle.

This edition of *Trauma Nursing: From Resuscitation Through Rehabilitation* has three new chapters—Mass Casualty Incidents, Trauma in Rural Areas, and Trauma in the Bariatric Patient—reflecting the greater emphasis on these issues in the current health care environment and the essential roles that nurses have in these areas of trauma care. Content on soft tissue injuries and wound healing has been combined into one chapter to reduce redundancy.

The text is divided into four major parts:

Part I, General Concepts in Trauma Nursing, covers healthcare concerns that affect trauma care facilities and trauma systems, ultimately affecting patient care. These concerns include economic and administrative considerations, quality improvement, ethics, and legal issues. Injury prevention, mass casualty incidents, trauma in rural settings, prehospital care, and rehabilitation of trauma patients are also discussed.

Part II, Clinical Management Concepts, addresses specific issues that affect all trauma patients regardless of their injuries. These topics include mechanism of injury; pathophysiology and management of traumatic shock; psychosocial adaptations of the patient and family; infection; wound healing and soft tissue injuries; metabolic and nutrition management; and management of pain, sedation, and neuromuscular blockade.

Part III, Single System Injuries, describes the pathophysiology, assessment, and state-of-the-art treatment of specific types of systemic injuries throughout each of the phases of trauma care.

Part IV, Unique Patient Populations, reviews the special trauma care considerations and needs of unique patient groups such as pregnant women, children, the elderly, bariatric individuals, burned patients, those with a history of substance abuse, and organ donors.

This text, authored by content experts from around the country, will serve as an excellent evidenced-based reference for the novice and the experienced nurse caring for trauma patients in a variety of settings. Clinicians, advanced practitioners, researchers, administrators, managers, educators, and students will find this text a useful and comprehensive reference for trauma-related issues. It is our hope that knowledge gained using this resource will enhance your ability to achieve optimal outcomes for your patients as they progress through the cycle of trauma care.

Karen A. McQuillan, RN, MS, CCRN, CNRN
Mary Beth Flynn Makic, RN, PhD, CNS, CCNS, CCRN
Eileen Whalen, RN, BSN, MHA

ACKNOWLEDGMENTS

We wish to thank the following authors, whose contributions to the first, second, and third editions made this textbook such a successful endeavor:

Sharon L. Atwell
Judith K. Bobb
Virginia D. Cardona
Howard R. Champion
Warren T. Chave
Donna York Clark
Linda S. Cook
Christine Cottingham
Margareta K. Cuccia
Sandra L. Deli
Patricia C. Epifanio
Jocelyn A. Farrar
Pamela Phillips Gaul
Robbi Lynn Hartsock
Erkan Hassan
Karen Klender Heist
Benny Hooper
Nancy J. Hoyt
Patricia D. Hurn
Connie A. Jastremski
Connie Joy
James W. Karesh
Marguerite T. Littleton Kearney
Paula M. Kelly
Barbara J. Keyes
Karen M. Kleeman
Melva Kravitz
Steven Linberg
Susan M. Luff
Marcia S. Mabee
Mary E. Mancini
Janet A. Marvin
Paula J. Bastnagel Mason
Roy L. Mason
Patricia E. McCabe
Paul McClelland
Anne F. McCormack
Gerri Spielman McGinnis
Barbara McLean
Carolyn Milligan
Pamela H. Mitchell
Jean M. Montonye
Mary Murphy-Rutter
Donna A. Nayduch
Bradley C. Robertson
Lisa Robinson
Elizabeth Scanlan
Ann M. Scanlon
Barbara E. Schott
Ellen K. Shair
Navin Singh
Sarah C. Smith
Julie Mull Strange
Peggy Trimble
Beth A. Vanderheyden
Susan W. Veise-Berry
Neil Warres
JoAnne D. Whitney
Margaret Widner-Kolberg
Charles E. Wiles III
Joyce S. Willens

CONTENTS

PART I

General Concepts in Trauma Nursing

1

EVOLUTION OF THE TRAUMA CYCLE

Mary Beachley

Incidents of trauma occur in epidemic proportions in our society today; however, this is not a new phenomenon. Traumatic injury has been recognized as a part of the human experience since early civilization. Anthropologic studies of the bony remains of Neanderthal humans have shown that members of this group sustained a great deal of trauma during their lifetimes.[1] Disfigured skeletal structures and long-term bony calcification are evidence that the trauma they experienced was a result of their relatively dangerous lifestyle. Many injuries were sustained as a result of constant exposure to the raw elements of nature, including frequent encounters with wild animals.

Although the concept of traumatic injury as a recognized societal affliction has remained unchanged since the time of the Neanderthals, the incidence, magnitude, cause, mechanism, and treatment of traumatic injury *have* changed. Human interaction with the environment at given points throughout our life span and the effects of a variety of forces—industrialization, societal influences (including belief systems), and educational orientation and level—have influenced the ways in which injury occurs in our society today. Currently, traumatic injury is a major public health problem in the United States and the world, and the incidence of traumatic injury is predicted to increase worldwide in the twenty-first century.

TRAUMA SYSTEMS DEVELOPMENT

Trauma is one of the major challenges in emergency, critical care, intermediate care, acute care, and rehabilitation nursing practices today. To recognize and develop a keen appreciation for trauma nursing as a specialty field, one must not only examine state-of-the-art practices but also review the historic events that led to the creation of a systems approach to care and to the development of the clinical knowledge base that has formed the foundation for this distinct area of clinical nursing practice.

The term *trauma* is used to describe a variety of injuries, and the concept of trauma embodies several associated terms—*shock, injury, accident, accidental injury, fatality,* and *casualty.* These terms are sometimes used synonymously and may be used interchangeably throughout this book, although use of the term *accidental* is avoided when possible because it implies that an event is unexpected or unavoidable. Over the years a deeper understanding of the underlying causes of traumatic injury has led to the belief that most unintentional events are predictable and therefore preventable.

MAGNITUDE OF THE PROBLEM

In the United States, unintentional injury is the most common cause of death for individuals aged 4 to 44 years.[2] The National Safety Council reported that unintentional injury continues to be the fifth leading cause of death for all ages, exceeded only by heart disease, cancer, stroke, and chronic lower respiratory diseases.[2] The primary causes of unintentional injury are as follows:

- Motor vehicle crashes
- Falls
- Poisonings
- Drowning
- Burns[2]

Although ranked fifth as the cause of death for all age groups, injury is the leading killer of one of our nation's most valued resources—young people. Children and youths between ages 5 and 24 years have a greater chance of dying from unintentional injury than from any other cause, and more than three of four individuals in this age group who die from injury are male.[2]

In 2003, nonfatal injuries that affect millions of Americans caused about 1 out of 12 people to seek medical care and 2.8 million to require hospitalization.[2] The economic impact of both fatal and nonfatal unintentional injuries was estimated to be $574.8 billion in 2004.[2]

The Centers for Disease Control and Prevention (CDC) reports that trauma is estimated to cause more than 161,000 deaths in the United States annually.[3] According to the National Highway Traffic Safety Administration's (NHTSA) National Center for Statistics and Analysis for 2005, 43,443 people were killed in motor vehicle crashes. This translates into one person killed in a vehicular crash every 12 minutes.[4] This report ranks motor vehicle crashes as the leading cause of death for people aged 4 to 34 years.

In contrast, the fatality rate per 100 million vehicle miles of travel decreased from 1.73 reported in 1995 to 1.47 in 2005.[3] The NHTSA report credits an 82% rate of safety belt use nationwide and a reduction in the rate of alcohol involvement in fatal crashes (39% in 2005, down from 42% in 1995) as significant factors in lowering the fatality rate. Motor vehicle crashes remain an economic burden from loss of life, disabilities from injury, and costs of property damage. The economic cost alone of motor vehicle crashes was reported to be $230.6 billion in 2000.[4]

The CDC's National Center for Injury Prevention and Control cites falls as the most common cause of nonfatal unintentional injury for people aged 35 through 65+ years.[3] Falls are the main cause of unintentional injury deaths for people 78 years old and older and the second cause of unintentional injury death for people aged 65 to 74 years.[2] Falls and motor vehicle incidents are the leading cause of nonfatal injuries treated in hospital emergency departments (EDs). About 8 million people were treated in EDs for fall-related injuries in 2003.[2]

The age-adjusted unintentional injury death rate declined by 59% per 100,000 people from 1912 to 2004.[2] During this same period, the nation's population tripled. The decrease in motor vehicle–related deaths during the past 86 years is in part due to the development of emergency medical systems, trauma care systems, advances in surgical and critical care, and improvements in road design, enhanced vehicle safety features, and increased use of driver and passenger restraints.

About 35% of all visits to EDs in the United States were injury related in 2003.[2] The substantial economic impact of both fatal and nonfatal unintentional injuries amounted to $574.8 billion in 2003.[2] This cost is described as equivalent to the following:

- 72 cents of every dollar paid in federal personal income taxes or
- 50 cents of every dollar spent on food in the United States[2]

All citizens are burdened by this cost, whether out of pocket, through higher prices for goods and services, or through higher taxes and user fees.

In addition to the human loss and disability resulting from trauma, the economic cost also must be addressed. The National Safety Council defines a disabling injury as one that results in some degree of permanent impairment. This includes injuries that render a person unable to effectively perform regular duties or activities for a full day beyond the day of the injury. Cost estimates therefore include the following:

- Wage loss
- Medical expenses
- Insurance administration costs
- Property damages in motor vehicle crashes
- Fire losses
- Indirect work loss (Indirect loss from work injuries is the money value of the time lost by noninjured workers, including time spent filling out reports or giving first aid to injured workers and time lost as a result of production slowdown.)

Despite an alarmingly high incidence of unintentional injury over the years, the significance of this problem has not always been recognized by the public. The first sign that this issue had reached the level of national politics appeared in 1960 when John F. Kennedy, during his presidential campaign, issued a statement acknowledging that "traffic accidents constitute one of the greatest, perhaps the greatest, of the nation's public problems."[5] Since that time, attention has been directed toward raising public awareness about this sizable problem. Concurrent efforts have been made to identify fundamental elements that would render the nation's health care delivery system more responsive to the needs of those who have sustained traumatic injury. Over the years, greater effort has been focused on injury prevention. However, this area still requires further funding and research.

THE MILITARY EXPERIENCE

Before the 1960s, advances in caring for the critically injured were made primarily by the military. Injuries sustained by military personnel and civilians during war were the primary focus of studies on traumatic injury and shock. These study findings became the initial source for information regarding the treatment of traumatic injuries.

In 1916, during World War I, the U.S. National Research Council of the National Academy of Sciences formed a Committee on Physiology, whose Subcommittee on Traumatic Shock began to collect, review, and analyze objective data regarding the physiology of circulation and its relationship to the various models that had been defined for the study of shock.[6] This was the first coordinated prospective study organized for the purpose of obtaining a better understanding of the body's responses to severe trauma. The information from these studies was discussed at formal meetings and conferences, which resulted in a more widespread dissemination of knowledge about shock resulting from traumatic injury. Although by the mid nineteenth century the term *shock* began to be applied to the clinical state of individuals who had sustained severe trauma, the nature of clinical shock remained a mystery.[6]

During World War II, the care of patients who had undergone trauma and the understanding of the nature of shock improved significantly. This was due largely to the prompt application of information obtained by the Medical Board for the Study of the Treatment of the Severely Wounded. This 22-member board was appointed on September 3, 1943, by the Theater Commander, Lt. General Jacob B. Devers, and was made up of medical officers, nurses, technicians, and support personnel who worked as a research team.[6] This team responded to any medical request from the field and compiled casualty data during an 8-month period in Italy. The data from observations of 186 military casualties comprised the first volume of the historic series by the Medical Department of the United States Army. It was titled *Surgery in World War II: The Physiologic Effects of Wounds.*[7] The information obtained by the board was disseminated not only in the field hospitals that were treating and studying the wounded but also throughout the front line and in base hospitals. The study results were impressive and led to a change in policy regarding the treatment of hypovolemic shock. Resuscitation practices improved as hemodynamic alterations became better understood and knowledge about posttraumatic renal failure, an often fatal complication of severe shock, emerged.

A similar but more extensive program was established during the Korean War (1950-1953) and later during the Vietnam War (1957-1975). The research efforts put forth during World War II by the Medical Board for the Study of the Treatment of the Severely Wounded continued and was strengthened by a newly established Surgical Research Team. This was made possible in part by the support services that had been made available from stateside organizations and institutions in the form of high-tech equipment sent to the combat zone. The emergence of the research team represented a significant achievement for military medicine during the twentieth century. Research findings of the team contributed to further refinement of care delivered to trauma patients during the Korean War. Through these efforts, progress was made in the clarification of the hemodynamic disturbances that occur with different forms of traumatic injury, and extensive knowledge was gained about organ function and the metabolic disturbances in shock and acute circulatory failure.

The pressing demands of surgery during war, coupled with the advances in medical care that occurred during the previous century, contributed in part to the improved trauma care outcomes that were realized during the Vietnam War. Improvements in field resuscitation, increased efficiency of transportation, and aggressive treatment of war casualties proved to be major factors contributing to life-saving endeavors. The death rates of war casualties reaching designated facilities decreased from 8% in World War I, to 4.5% in World War II, to 2.5% during the Korean War, to less than 2% in the Vietnam War.[8]

Experience in caring for battlefield injuries sustained during the wars in Iraq and Afghanistan also offers new knowledge and expertise that can help to improve treatment outcomes for the injured. For example, a large number of military personnel have been exposed to blasts causing significant injuries, particularly affecting the brain. This has prompted investigations into how to best care for victims of blast injuries and development of evidence-based *Guidelines for Field Management of Combat-Related Head Trauma.*[9] Further knowledge about the effectiveness and risks of agents such as factor VIIa used to stop bleeding are also being realized. These and other revelations made during wartime can be considered to assist in determining the best trauma care for those injured and cared for on and off the battlefield.

The Military Influence

Over time, it became clear that our national health care delivery system needed changes on the basis of what had been learned during wartime about the significance of time in saving lives and about the physiologic responses to injury. The need for an effective system to care for the severely injured was just as pressing in the civilian sector as in the military arena. As had been demonstrated consistently during wartime, rapid evacuation of the seriously injured from the battlefield to advanced treatment stations (mobile army surgical hospital units), which were equipped with necessary supplies and staffed with highly skilled personnel, saved lives. Although long overdue, the principles on which this system was designed have since been found to be easily transferable to and as effective in civilian life.

The modern era of a civilian systems approach, which focused on more efficient emergency health care for the injured, began in 1966 with the publication of a document by the National Academy of Sciences, National Research Council. This document, *Accidental Death and Disability—The Neglected Disease of Modern Society,* was a far-sighted approach to the development of an effective emergency medical services (EMS) system throughout our nation. It was the product of a 3-year study conducted by a committee on trauma, shock, and anesthesia in conjunction with special task forces from the Division of Medical Sciences, the National Academy of Sciences, and the National Research Council. The results were compiled after representatives from health care organizations reviewed the status of initial emergency care provided after "accidental" injury. The study groups reviewed a broad spectrum of factors, including ambulance services, voice communication systems, hospital EDs, and intensive care units, while incorporating research results in shock, trauma, and resuscitation. On the basis of identified deficiencies, the general areas of consideration recommended by the committee and outlined in the published document[10] included the following:

- "Accident" prevention
- Emergency first aid and medical care
    - Ambulance services
    - Communications
    - EDs
    - Interrelationships between the ED and the intensive care unit
- Development of trauma registries
- Hospital trauma committees
- Convalescence, disability, and rehabilitation
- Medicolegal problems
- Autopsy of the victim
- Care of casualties under conditions of natural disaster
- Research in trauma

The national effort for establishing an improved emergency health care system and much of the basic framework on which the nation's EMS system has subsequently been built were presented in this document. This classic "white paper" represented the first major government report acknowledging that significant numbers of people were killed or disabled as a result of unintentional injuries in the civilian population, which was costing the nation billions of dollars each year. Contributing significantly to the high mortality and morbidity rates were the inefficiencies in the nation's emergency health care delivery system. Unskilled health care personnel working with inadequate transportation and communication system policies and guidelines were taking the injured to facilities that were not sufficiently prepared to treat them. It became apparent that the problems of initial care and management of injured persons were similar in kind, although different in magnitude and scope, to those encountered by the military during periods of war. The time was right for the application of new knowledge and skills in caring for the injured.

Early Pioneering Efforts

During the late 1960s and early 1970s, the need for a systematic approach to the care of the seriously injured patient became apparent. The initial efforts to design and develop emergency medical clinical delivery systems were based on the care requirements of specific types of injury (e.g., trauma, burns, and spinal cord injuries).[10] The conceptual design of a systems approach required that effective medical and surgical treatment regimens be applied in situations other than the traditional in-hospital setting. This necessitated the reorganization of existing health care structures, the implementation of new technologies, and the development of educational programs so that clinical treatment modalities proven effective in the hospital environment could be applied and tested in the prehospital and interhospital phases. Physician-supervised educational programs and extrahospital emergency care programs began to emerge, with emergency medical technicians-ambulance (EMT-A) and advanced life support emergency medical technicians-paramedic (EMT-P) assuming key roles.[11]

In several parts of the country, hospitals were categorized regionally, and those with demonstrated expertise were designated as trauma, burn, or spinal cord injury centers. In Illinois, for example, the regionalization of emergency care for multiple and critical injuries was initiated and developed statewide in 1971. As the Illinois trauma program began to develop and mature, a program of patient transfer and burn center care also was initiated for the four burn units and major burn center (Cook County Hospital) in Chicago, which used a patient distribution program and central bed registry.[12] In 1972, in collaboration with the Illinois trauma program, representatives from the Midwest Regional Spinal Cord Injury Care Systems at Northwestern Memorial Hospital and the Rehabilitation Institute of Chicago (McGaw Medical Center, Northwestern University) formulated a macroregional catchment program for acute spinal cord injuries.[13] In 1973, the shock-trauma program of the University of Maryland, supported by the Maryland state government, was expanded statewide and became the Maryland Institute for Emergency Medicine (MIEM).[14]

These pioneering efforts were significant because they represented working models for further regional trauma/EMS systems development. The apparent successes resulting from these system designs became the catalysts for a more intense national effort to plan and implement improved trauma/EMS systems. In Maryland, the overall age-adjusted death rate and adverse effects from injuries has been declining steadily since the implementation and maturation of the statewide emergency medical and trauma care systems. The rate declined from 29.8 in 1988 to 26.5 in 2003.[15] In comparison, the national figures for the same years were 35 and 36.1, respectively.[15]

Federal Support of Trauma/EMS Systems

Federal support of EMS started during the early 1970s, when congressional hearings were held to promote development of a comprehensive EMS law. In 1973, the Emergency Medical Services Systems (EMSS) Act was passed, which contained guidelines and specific technical measures that supported a nationally coordinated and comprehensive system of emergency health care accessible to all citizens. The identification of fundamental elements of the EMS system deemed necessary for the comprehensive care of the critically ill and injured was accomplished with this mandate. Included in the EMSS Act were 15 requirements (Box 1-1) that would assist EMS system project planners and health care professionals in establishing comprehensive, area-wide, and regional EMS programs.[16]

The 1973 EMSS Act, with its subsequent changes in 1976, is considered one of the most important factors influencing the development of EMS systems throughout this country. This act focused on improving the nation's emergency death and disability statistics by mandating that the emergency medical care programs that were federally funded by the Department of Health and Human Services (DHHS) must plan and implement a systems approach on a regional basis for emergency response and immediate care provisions. Although many emergency medical conditions had been

BOX 1-1 Emergency Medical Systems Act 1973 Requirements

- Provision of manpower
- Training of personnel
- Communications
- Transportation
- Facilities
- Critical care units
- Use of public safety agencies
- Consumer participation
- Accessibility to care
- Transfer of patients
- Standard medical record keeping
- Consumer information and education
- Independent review and evaluation
- Disaster linkage
- Mutual aid agreements

identified, it was determined that the seven critical target patient care areas for regional EMS systems planning were major trauma, burns, spinal cord injuries, poisonings, acute cardiac conditions, high-risk infants and mothers, and behavioral emergencies. In-depth knowledge of the incidence, epidemiology, and clinical aspects of these categories is essential for appreciating a systems approach to regional planning and delivery of care. Much of this information, specifically that related to multiple traumas, spinal cord injuries, and burns, is explored in greater detail in this book.

The federal government withdrew from its lead role in EMS development in 1981 with the passage of the *Reconciliation Act*, which integrated the EMS program into the Health Prevention Block Grants and gave responsibility back to the states for direction and development of EMS. The General Accounting Office (GAO) report of 1986[17] disclosed the effect of this transition of EMS system programs from federal to state leadership under the block grant program, which concluded the following about a major sector of the United States (more than 50%):

- It lacked the usage and access to the universal phone access number 911.
- It lacked access to and use of advanced life support ambulance services in rural areas.
- It did not have any formal developed trauma care systems at all.

Senators Alan Cranston and Edward M. Kennedy first introduced legislation to address the recommendations of the 1986 GAO report in the 100th Congress in January 1987.

President Bush finally signed this legislation into law as Public Law 101-590 on November 16, 1990. This legislation, titled the *Trauma Care Systems Planning and Development Act of 1990,* is significant because it provided federal assistance for the development of emergency/trauma care systems throughout the United States. This Act amended the Public Health Services Act by adding a new title, Title XII. The act authorized the Department of Health and Human Services (DHHS), through the Health Resources and Services Administration (HRSA), to make grants to states for trauma systems planning and development. The major provisions of this act included the following[18]:

1. *A council on trauma care systems.* The purpose of the council is to report needs of the trauma care system and how states are responding to such needs. This council has 12 public members, including two nurse positions (one critical care position and one emergency medical training position).
2. *A clearinghouse on trauma care and EMS.* This is to be established by contract to serve as a collection, compilation, and dissemination point for information relating to all aspects of emergency medical services and trauma care.
3. *Programs for improving trauma care in rural areas.* Grants will be authorized for public and private nonprofit entities for research and demonstration projects that will improve the availability and quality of emergency medical/trauma care in rural areas.
4. *Formula grants with respect to modification of state plans.* Most of the appropriated funds (80%) will be allotted by formula for each state and territory. Beginning in the second fiscal year that states receive funds, they must make a matching nonfederal contribution (in cash or in kind) in specified ratios.
5. *State plans and modifications.* Each state must submit to the Secretary of Health and Human Services the trauma care component of the state's EMS plan. The funds allotted for each state may be used only to make such modifications to the state plan as are necessary to ensure access to the highest quality of trauma care.
6. *Trauma care standards and a model trauma care plan.* Each state must adopt standards for designating trauma centers and for triage, transfer, and transportation policies. In addition, the Secretary must develop in the first year of this act a model trauma care plan that may be adopted for guidance by the states.
7. *Data and reporting requirements.* Each state must report annually to the Secretary the number of severely injured patients; the cause of injury and contributing factors; the nature and severity of the injury; monitoring data sufficient to evaluate the diagnoses, treatment, and outcomes of such trauma patients in each trauma center; and expenditures.
8. *Technical assistance and supplies and services in lieu of grant funds.* The Secretary shall provide technical assistance with respect to planning, development, and operation of any program carried out with the allotted funds, at no charge to the state.
9. *Waiver.* Under certain limited conditions, the Secretary may allow a state to use a percentage of allotted funds to reimburse designated trauma centers for uncompensated care.

The Trauma Systems Planning and Development Act was first funded with $5 million in fiscal year 1992 and for the following 4 years; however, in 1995 the 104th Congress rescinded most of the funding and did not provide any funding for fiscal year 1996. Senate Bill 1745 was passed in 1998, reauthorizing a number of public health programs, including the *Trauma Systems Planning and Development Act.* This legislation authorized the program through fiscal year 2002 and provided $6 million in funding for states to plan and develop organized systems of trauma care. This program provided grant funding to states to implement trauma systems and developed partnerships with stakeholders to promote trauma system development nationally. The program was closed out in March 2006 because no funds were appropriated (zeroed out) by the DHHS. This occurred because no funding was approved in the *Education and Related Agencies Appropriations Act 2006* passed by Congress in December 2005.

As mandated by the Trauma Systems Planning and Development Act, a model trauma care plan was developed and published by HRSA as a template for states to use to design a local trauma system. This plan contained mandatory components necessary to meet the needs of all injured patients who require the services of an acute care facility. The plan stressed two important concepts:

1. The need for a trauma care system to be integrated into the overall EMS system
2. The incorporation of existing EMS resources[19]

The plan classified the components as "administrative" and "operational and clinical."

The administrative component included leadership, system development, legislation, and finance. The operational and clinical component included public information/education and prevention initiatives, human resources, prehospital care, EMS medical direction, triage, transport, definitive care facilities, interfacility transfer, medical rehabilitation, and evaluation.[18] As a result of the 2002 appropriations for a division of trauma and EMS within the HRSA, a revision and update to the *Model Trauma System Plan* was published and released in February 2006.[20] The revised document, *Model Trauma System Planning and Evaluation*, used a public health framework to address what a trauma system does, whereas the earlier *Model Trauma System Plan* addressed the components necessary for a trauma system.[20] The new *Model Trauma System Planning and Evaluation* document contains a self-assessment for trauma system planning, development, and evaluation that can assist a state or region to perform an objective trauma system assessment and to define its system-specific health status benchmarks and performance indicators.[20]

Trauma/EMS System Development

As EMS systems have developed, the design seems to represent a composite of individual and unique systems of care for particular patient groups (e.g., multiple trauma, spinal cord injuries, burns). Although it is necessary for these systems to utilize common EMS components such as transportation, communications, and specialty skilled prehospital health team members, the care, resources, and facilities must be specifically designed for each patient group. EMS system components must be adapted to address and accommodate specific clinical needs if accurate and effective planning is to occur. The key EMS components for the trauma patient population are facilities categorization and trauma center designation (Table 1-1). For trauma patients, the establishment of triage and transfer protocols is critical to ensure that immediate intervention is consistent and decision(s) regarding transfer to a designated trauma facility for definitive care are facilitated. Thus it is of utmost importance that regional trauma/EMS systems plan and develop clinically sound trauma care programs on a geographic basis. Because of the complex requirements, the care of the trauma patient has provided an excellent model from which to design a basic health care delivery system. This has since been expanded to include other types of emergency medical conditions.[21]

TABLE 1-1 Key Components of a Clinical Emergency Medical Services System

Trauma	Facilities categorization Trauma center designation Transfer agreements and triage protocols
Cardiac Emergency	Patient access (911) Citizen cardiopulmonary resuscitation (CPR) Advanced cardiac life support (ACLS) paramedic response
Poisonings	Information specialists Toxicologic information and treatment protocols Telephone-directed home care and physician consultation

From Boyd DR, Edlich RF, Micik S: *Systems approach to emergency medical care,* Norwalk, Conn, 1983, Appleton-Century-Crofts.

The clinical significance of the systems approach in developing a regional trauma/EMS system was clearly identified by the Division of Emergency Medical Services of the DHHS and reflected in their program guidelines.[21] In congressional testimony, representatives of this agency described the unique clinical requirements of the patient with multiple trauma, the need for a regionalized system of care, and the key EMS system components crucial to a successful and efficient trauma care program (i.e., facilities, critical care units, and transfer of patients). Although it was believed that a trauma/EMS system must respond adequately to all declared emergency calls within its designated geographic region, which included nonemergency cases (80%), truly emergent cases (15%), and critical cases (5%),[20] emphasis was placed on the need to identify effectively the critical patient whose chance of survival desperately depended on a competent trauma care delivery system. It was toward increasing the chance of survival for these critical patients that conceptual system planning and initial program development were directed.

In 1987, the American College of Emergency Physicians' (ACEP) Trauma Committee published *Guidelines for Trauma Care Systems.*[22] The ACEP guidelines state "trauma care represents a continuum that is best provided by an integrated system extending from prevention through rehabilitation and requiring close cooperation among specialists in each phase of care."

Facilities Categorization

In the 1976 report "Optimal Hospital Resources for Care of the Seriously Injured,"[23] the Task Force of the Committee on Trauma of the American College of Surgeons called for hospitals to commit personnel and facility resources to caring for seriously injured patients. The original proposal, presented in the 1966 landmark document *Accidental Death and Disability: The Neglected Disease of Modern Society,* suggested that the categorization of facilities should be based on the individual institution's capacity to handle a broad spectrum of emergency conditions.[9] This plan—the implementation of a variety of categorization schemes—proved to be unsuccessful, and a more detailed set of guidelines was provided by the Task Force of the Committee on Trauma of the American College of Surgeons in 1979. This revised document, *Hospital Resources for Optimal Care of the Injured Patient,* replaced the 1976 report.[23] Emphasis was placed on special problems of geography, population density, availability of community and regional resources and personnel, and the pervasive demands for cost-effectiveness, with the most significant element being commitment, institutional and personal. Institutional commitment was defined as the immediate availability of capable personnel and accessibility to sophisticated equipment, laboratory and radiologic facilities, operating rooms, and intensive care units. The personal commitment of hospital trustees, administrators, physicians, nurses, and other health care professionals also was imperative because the responsibility for providing optimal hospital resources for the care of the seriously injured patient rests with these individuals.

Trauma Center Designation

In the 1979 report,[24] optimal standards for categorization of trauma care facilities were expanded and refined. Three distinct levels of trauma care services were identified, with functional responsibilities, capabilities, and comparable nomenclature outlined for each level. These were intended to serve as a guide for assessing an institution's potential for trauma center designation.

In the 1999 and 2006 editions of the American College of Surgeons' Committee on Trauma report, *Resources for the Optimal Care of the Injured Patient,*[25,26] the emphasis was on the trauma system rather than a single trauma center. For optimal trauma care, a community must develop an all-encompassing systems approach to provide the appropriate level of trauma care. This system of care involves a lead-governing agency for development and oversight, a prehospital emergency care system, and a network of hospitals that provide a spectrum of care to all injured patients. Each hospital within the definitive care network is identified as Level I, II, III, or IV, depending on the depth of resources.[25,26]

A *Level I* trauma care facility is a tertiary teaching hospital that takes a lead role in education, research, and system planning in a regional trauma care system. Level I trauma centers are usually located in metropolitan areas. A Level I institution must make a firm commitment to furnish the personnel, facilities, and equipment necessary to provide total care for every aspect of injury through the phases of care from prevention through rehabilitation.[26]

A *Level II* trauma care facility is most likely a tertiary institution that may or may not be an academic center. A Level II trauma center should provide initial definitive trauma care for all levels of injury severity; however, because of limited resources it may not be able to provide the same comprehensive care as a Level I trauma center.[26] The role of the Level II trauma center in a regional trauma system varies depending on its location and proximity to a Level I trauma center. If the Level II center were located in a population-dense area with a short ambulance transport time to the closest Level I trauma center, the Level II would supplement the clinical activity and expertise of the Level I center. It is expected that the Level I and Level II trauma centers would work together to optimize resources in the region to provide the appropriate level of care for all injured patients. When the Level II trauma center is located in a more rural setting or is the only tertiary hospital in a region, it serves as the lead trauma facility for that region.[26]

A *Level III* trauma facility is most often a community hospital in an area that lacks Level I and Level II hospital facilities. It must make a strong commitment to the optimal care of the trauma patient. Clear and concise transfer protocols are essential. These centers must have the capability to resuscitate and manage the initial definitive care of most injured patients. However, timely transfer of injured patients to higher-level trauma centers must be provided when a patient's needs exceed the resources of the Level III center.[26]

An additional *Level IV* is generally a small hospital or clinic in a rural or remote area. This center is part of a regional trauma care network and will have transfer agreements with Level I and II centers. The Level IV center provides timely resuscitation and transfer of most injured patients and is the de facto primary care provider.[26]

Many other hospitals, both large and small, that have ED capabilities but have made no official commitment to an organized approach to the care of the seriously injured patient are encouraged to upgrade their trauma care. This type of institution is an implied fourth level of trauma care and requires strict treatment protocols and transfer agreements with higher-level facilities.

The intent of the guidelines outlined in *Resources for the Optimal Care of the Injured Patient* is to encourage each hospital to constantly monitor its capabilities as a trauma care facility and continue to strive to upgrade its resources. Ideally, if the guidelines are actualized, the severity of injury should be matched equally with appropriate facility resources and personnel expertise. Health care professionals working within a hospital who have an interest in trauma care, are educated and skilled in managing the special problems of trauma patients, and assume a well-defined role on a trauma team organized especially to provide optimal care will produce more favorable patient outcomes than those who view trauma care as another general service.

Although there is a distinct difference between the categorization of hospital emergency and critical care capabilities and the more formal process of selecting and designating certain facilities for specialty clinical services, the categorization of all hospitals within a particular trauma/EMS region is beneficial for two reasons:

- First, categorization allows assessment of the hospital's general ED capabilities to care for seriously injured

patients and of its overall critical care capabilities for specific patient groups. This is considered an integral part of the planning activity helpful in documenting the existing resources and in identifying deficits that may ultimately lead to appropriate improvements in trauma/EMS systems. This information is considered when decisions are made concerning the official designation of specialty care centers.
- Second, once designated, these specialty referral centers are held accountable for maintaining their capabilities.

Transfer Agreements and Triage Protocols

The relationship of a regional trauma/EMS system to the overall EMS system is an important consideration when a comprehensive systems approach to trauma care is planned. EMS and trauma/EMS systems involve a complex series of events that must be coordinated effectively to provide a consistent mechanism for efficient health care delivery. Clinical research has provided a deeper understanding of the natural course of traumatic disease and has demonstrated that time is of the essence in treating these diseases. A standard mortality curve clearly shows that if a medical emergency is measured against time, death will eventually result if effective emergency care is not initiated promptly. The time constraints that exist for the seriously injured patient have served as the impetus for creating more effective care systems in an attempt to reduce mortality and morbidity rates.

Experience has shown that the outcome of traumatic injury is more favorable if resuscitation and stabilization efforts are initiated early and sustained. Although the time of patient death varies depending on the magnitude and variety of the traumatic pathology, a prompt trauma/EMS system response, provision of initial basic field care, use of a sophisticated communications system, and rapid and safe transport of the patient will save valuable time, and death may be prevented. Each phase of EMS activity has a critical effect on mortality. Every single act can save time. Rescue squads and first responders are prepared to perform basic life support skills in the field. In many parts of the country, more sophisticated and advanced measures are being taken by EMT-Ps in caring for critically injured patients both during extrication efforts and during transport within the EMS system.[27]

The EMS process begins when notification is received by EMS system operators that an injury incident has occurred; an ambulance team is dispatched to the scene. The patient's condition is assessed, and resuscitation and stabilization efforts are initiated in the field. Level of educational preparation and certification dictates the interventions and skill levels of the ambulance team members and field personnel. A sophisticated communications system allows the field personnel to contact authorized personnel at an appropriate trauma center for instructions concerning triage and treatment and provides the receiving hospital with an estimated time of patient arrival. Measures are then taken to transfer the patient to the most appropriate facility. This decision must be guided not only by the patient's condition and injury type but also by the geographic dynamics of that area. Thus each regional trauma/EMS system must be organized in such a way as to accommodate the unique needs of the area. Because there are distinct differences between urban and rural areas, three sociogeographic regional trauma/EMS models have been proposed that can be incorporated into the planning of trauma/EMS systems throughout the country[9]:

- Urban-suburban model
- Rural-metropolitan model
- Wilderness-metropolitan model

When these sociogeographic models were developed, population density, trauma care resources, and geography were considered.[10] Although some absolute examples of these models exist within regional trauma/EMS systems, most systems include more than one type model, as seen in Maryland, Oregon, Pennsylvania, Virginia, and San Diego County, California. Generally, attempts are made to centralize designated trauma or specialty care facilities within regional trauma/EMS systems to facilitate timely and efficient primary triage or secondary transfer of patients, if needed. Protocols for field identification, triage, resuscitation, and transportation to designated trauma centers have been adopted and have become operational in many communities. These protocols not only facilitate consistency within the trauma/EMS system but also ensure that injured patients are taken to hospitals capable of continuing and expanding life support measures initiated in the field. A sophisticated systems approach to triage, communication, and transport is of little avail if clinical expertise of the highest quality does not await the injured patient's arrival.

The trauma facility notified of a pending admission has the responsibility of alerting the in-house trauma team, whose members will report to the designated resuscitation area to prepare for the patient's arrival. Staff specialists and expert clinicians, equipment, supplies, and ancillary support systems must be immediately available if the complex problems of the seriously injured patient are to be properly managed in a timely fashion. Effective resuscitation and stabilization efforts are based on the implementation of a predetermined series of activities performed simultaneously by appropriate trauma team members. Once the patient is stabilized, priorities are established for definitive care. Depending on the type, magnitude, and severity of the patient's injuries, subsequent treatment may include additional diagnostic studies, surgical intervention, intensive, intermediate or acute care management, or long-term rehabilitation.

In summary, the trauma/EMS system by design must provide immediate and appropriate care at the scene of an incident, safe and efficient transportation to the appropriate trauma center, definitive diagnostic and surgical interventions, critical care management, acute care, and rehabilitation services. This broad scope of capabilities may be available within the respective geographic region. If not, the trauma/EMS system must respond by transferring patients out of that region to a distant trauma care facility where their specific needs can be met. It has become apparent that all EMS systems throughout the country need a stratified, or graded, echelon system of trauma/EMS care so that flexibility within the emergency health care system is guaranteed. To support an effective trauma care system, integration of and cooperation among all hospitals treating injured persons in a region are crucial. An inclusive systems approach can minimize geographic and geopolitic constraints, allowing efficient and effective use of resources to provide optimal trauma care to all injured persons served in the region.[25-28]

The challenge for future trauma system development and maturation will depend on society's commitment of resources. The health care system must justify these resources by ensuring that the benefits and ultimate cost savings for such expenditures are recognized. Outcomes of the trauma system's performance must have data-driven multidisciplinary evaluation that looks not only at mortality rates but also includes functional patient outcomes and the efficient use of resources to achieve the optimal outcome.[29] A major effort to facilitate trauma systems outcome evaluation was initiated by Dr. Mullins and Dr. Mann, who organized and directed the Skamania Conference in July 1998.[30] They invited trauma care experts from all regions of the United States to attend this 2-day conference for the following purposes:

1. Reviewing currently available data that have been used to evaluate the effectiveness of trauma systems
2. Assessing the strengths and usefulness of prior trauma system effectiveness studies
3. Defining the characteristics of a valid assessment of trauma system effectiveness
4. Identifying the direction, format, and goals for future research[30]

The Skamania Conference was supported by two federal agencies, the National Center for Injury Prevention and the NHTSA. A supplement to the *Journal of Trauma: Injury Infection and Critical Care* published in September 1999 focused on the Skamania Conference and outcomes research for trauma systems.[30] A recent nationwide study was conducted by researchers at the Johns Hopkins Bloomberg School of Public Health and the University of Washington School of Medicine, Harborview Injury Prevention and Research Center to determine the effect of trauma center care on patient mortality rates.[31] This National Study on the Costs and Outcomes of Trauma compared the mortality outcomes of 5191 adult patients who received care at either one of 18 Level I trauma centers or were treated at one of 51 nontrauma centers. The characteristics of each hospital were analyzed, such as the number of patients treated and the types of specialty services available. After adjusting for difference in case mix including factors such as severity of injury, patient age, and preexisting medical conditions, the researchers found a 25% overall decrease in the risk of death after care in a trauma center compared with those patients treated in a nontrauma center.[31] This landmark study continues to provide evidence to support that trauma centers make a significant difference in saving lives of injured patients.

THE EVOLUTION OF TRAUMA NURSING

HISTORIC BACKGROUND

Nurses have long been challenged by the complexity of the health care needs of seriously injured patients and their families. Because wars have been responsible for producing traumatic injuries in epidemic proportions, military nurses have gained experience in caring for the wounded. The beginnings of trauma nursing in the United States occurred during the Revolutionary War, when women were hired by George Washington to provide care to the wounded.[32] The first organized nursing effort focusing on battlefield injuries was pioneered during the Crimean War (1854), when Florence Nightingale, Lady Superintendent-in-Chief of female nursing in the English General Military Hospitals, led a group of women in caring for war casualties.[33] For approximately 2 years, this group of nurses provided makeshift hospital facilities; bathed and dressed wounds; and painstakingly sought proper sanitation, hygiene, and control of infection. In October 1861, Nightingale was asked by the U.S. Secretary of War for advice on setting up military hospitals for the Union army, and her suggestions were widely adopted throughout the course of the Civil War (1861-1865).[34] Clara Barton, the first woman clerk of the U.S. Patent Office, served as a nurse caring for wounded men on the battlefield after the outbreak of the Civil War in 1861 and later during the Franco-Prussian War (1869). In 1881, after her return to the United States, Barton organized the American Red Cross, a volunteer society that was modeled after the International Red Cross (established in 1863 by Jean Henri Dunant).[35]

In subsequent wars, nurses cared for the wounded on and off the battlefield, seeking new ways to manage the devastating injuries resulting from the ever-increasing power of weaponry. Under the most adverse circumstances, combat nurses worked to help salvage mutilated extremities, tried to replace massive losses of blood, and attempted to administer appropriate medications, when available, to those with severe clinical complications. All actions were taken to prolong life; even if initial efforts proved to be successful, death as a result of infection after a complicated clinical course was always a possibility.[36]

Enormous problems existed for nurses who cared for the wounded. They found that the scars of battle extended far beyond those from burns, bayonets, or bullets. The psychologic implications for nursing care were just as pervasive as the physical demands; the mind and spirit were scarred as well. While caring for the wounded, nurses came to understand the long-term effects and difficulties their patients faced as a result of war.

Violetta Thurstan, an English military nurse who served in World War I, writes the following in her *Textbook of War Nursing:*

> Since the war, times and seasons have lost their meaning. Sometimes half one's life seems to have been crushed into a space of a very few hours, sometimes each day is so drawn out

> that it is an eternity in itself. August 1914, seems a dim, faraway epoch and those who played their part in the early days are veterans now. In many ways nursing was more interesting in the early days of the war, when everything had to be improvised or adapted, than later on when the excitement and the first rush were over, organisation brought to an undreamt-of pitch of perfection, and all necessaries amply and even lavishly supplied.... Who shall say how many lives and limbs were saved by the nurses' ready inventiveness and clever fingers?
>
> There was of course another side to this, the tragedy which no one who worked at that period will ever be able to forget, of seeing precious lives ebbing away for the want of some necessary that might have saved them if only it had been there.[36]

The knowledge gained from the experiences of the frontline nurses has provided valuable information in helping to understand trauma in civilian life.[36-39] Military nurses continue to contribute to the advancement and the development of innovative improvements to trauma nursing care. The changing war theaters and fighting tactics as seen in Vietnam, Desert Storm, Somalia, Afghanistan, and Iraq continue to provide not only treatment challenges; they offer an ever-changing opportunity to address new and improved treatment protocols for trauma care.

CHANGES WITHIN THE HOSPITAL SETTING

During the 1970s, because of improved access to EMS, expanded educational preparation of emergency medical technicians, development of sophisticated communication systems (including telemetry), and use of more efficient means of transportation (including air evacuation), more viable patients were being brought to hospital facilities. During this same 10- to 15-year period of improved prehospital care, however, commensurate changes were not necessarily being made in the hospital. Reports indicated that basic errors in assessment and treatment of seriously injured patients were occurring with alarming regularity.[39-44] These errors, coupled with inadequate preplanning on the part of the hospital and poor mobilization and organization of hospital resources, often resulted in unnecessary death. The task of overcoming these unfavorable statistics presented a tremendous challenge to nurses, physicians, other health care professionals, and hospital officials.

EVOLUTION OF THE TRAUMA RESUSCITATION TEAM

In the late 1960s and 1970s, categorization of hospital facilities had been one strategy demanded by the federal government in an attempt to ensure that patients were taken to institutions capable of caring for their injuries. Unfortunately, in most parts of the country this change was occurring very slowly, if at all. However, a few facilities throughout the country began to make tremendous advances in caring for seriously injured trauma patients. Because these institutions cared for a large number of injured patients, they developed a staff of physicians and nurses proficient in caring for complex injuries. Statistical trends began to indicate that mortality and morbidity rates were substantially lower in these designated hospitals, which had more qualified and experienced personnel and more extensive facilities.[45] The success of the nurses and physicians depended on a number of factors, including the implementation of an interdisciplinary team approach to care, which facilitated the coordination of resuscitation efforts, evaluation, and definitive management plans. The success of the trauma team depended not only on the knowledge base and skill level of each physician and nurse, but also on the consistency and repetition of their practices as a team. Proven in both military and civilian settings, a dedicated trauma team approach is the most effective and efficient means to care for the critically injured trauma patient. The predetermined delegation of specialized role responsibilities to each nurse and physician team member fosters the efficient organization of talents, which decreases the time between the patient's arrival and the onset of definitive care. Thus, the hospital's trauma team effort to save lives continues to best support the life-sustaining activities initiated during the prehospital phase of care.

The development of rapid and more efficient transport systems was instrumental in reducing the precious time interval between the onset of injury and the patient's arrival at the hospital. This time factor underlies many of the principles on which the initial care of the trauma patient was based. A firmer understanding of the volume requirements for circulatory resuscitation on the part of nurse and physician team members also had a significant impact on the team's approach to care. Success during the resuscitation phase of care increased the number of patients who then needed to be monitored closely and managed in an environment that provided continuity of intense nursing supervision and care. The extent of the patient's injuries, compounded by the potential for postresuscitation complications (e.g., respiratory insufficiency, renal failure, sepsis, coagulopathy), necessitated a new phase of trauma care that required critical care medical and nursing management.[44]

TRAUMA NURSING

The critical care phase has provided unique challenges for nurses as new concepts of physiology and biochemistry have been applied. Concurrently, new assessment techniques and management therapies have been introduced, which contributed to the advances made in the care of the seriously injured trauma patient. With the advent of technologic advances affecting physiologic monitoring and diagnostic procedures and improvements in medical treatments, trauma nursing began a new frontier. One of the natural outcomes of this rapidly expanding technology was the nurse's increasing responsibility for making complex decisions that directly affect the treatment outcome.

The introduction of innovative diagnostic methods and tools contributed to greater efficiency in the clinical evaluation and treatment process; some of these included the following:

- Recognizing the strengths of peritoneal lavage as a diagnostic tool, sparing many trauma patients unnecessary operative procedures

- Development of the computed tomographic (CT) scanner, which allowed precise diagnosis of intracranial injuries and provided more exact diagnoses for vertebral, acetabular, mediastinal, and some abdominal injuries
- Advances in angiography provided a mechanism for precise diagnosis of vessel injuries in the chest, pelvis, and extremities. Once bleeding vessels could be visualized, this technology also offered the opportunity to use interventional radiologic technology to embolize vessels and halt blood loss by use of a nonoperative approach. Advances in technology continue to aid in more accurate, timely diagnosis and treatment of injuries
- Use of ultrasound to detect abdominal injury, spiral CT, and magnetic resonance imaging during the resuscitation phase

Because of the complex care required by the critically injured patient, many trauma specialty fields within medicine began to emerge. These specialty services included the following:

- Traumatology
- Neurosurgery
- Orthopedic surgery
- Thoracic surgery
- Plastic surgery
- Oral surgery
- Critical care
- Infectious disease medicine

With this trend came the potential for these specialists to care for the patient by focusing on the area of their expertise in partial or complete isolation from the patient's other health care problems. The unfavorable consequences of this fragmented approach to care became obvious. Because they provided bedside care on a 24-hour basis, nurses were in a position to facilitate the coordination of multidisciplinary patient care activities. They appropriately began to take measures to incorporate a comprehensive approach to planning care for the critical trauma patient.

The role of the trauma nurse expanded as problem-solving and decision-making responsibilities increased, leading to a new era in collegial relationships. Nurses who cared for trauma patients in the ED, operating room, postanesthesia care unit, intensive care unit, intermediate care unit, and acute care unit needed to develop special knowledge and skills to provide optimal care for trauma patients. As the trauma nursing theory and specialty practice was being developed, advanced practice roles emerged for nurses.

The trauma coordinator and trauma clinical specialist roles were created in the late 1970s along with the early hospital trauma program development. Because of financial pressures from hospital cost-containment efforts in the 1980s, the role of the trauma nurse case manager was developed to manage the hospital stay and discharge of trauma patients. The goal of this role is to move the trauma patient through the hospital care phase as quickly as possible to avoid denied hospital days by the insurance companies and Medicare. In the 1990s, as financial pressures on hospitals continued, the nurse case manager role in some trauma centers evolved to the use of acute care trauma nurse practitioners as active care providers and case managers for trauma patients within the hospital and for continuing follow-up care after discharge. Current advances in trauma nursing include development and use of evidence-based treatment algorithms to guide care and provide nursing autonomy in making and implementing treatment decisions. In addition, nurses in collaboration with other members of the health care team identify and incorporate generic best practice guidelines for patients (e.g., hyperglycemia management, peptic ulcer disease prophylaxis, and ventilator-associated pneumonia prevention) and apply them when appropriate in the care of trauma patients to contribute to better outcomes.

Trauma Rehabilitation Nursing

During previous decades, as advances in the care of the seriously injured patient were made and incorporated into the resuscitation and critical care phases, more lives were saved, and the importance of another phase of trauma care was recognized: the rehabilitation phase. As trauma patients emerged from intensive care settings, it became apparent that their medical and nursing care needed to take a new focus. Intensive care stays shortened for most patients throughout the recent decade. For the trauma patient, this early move to the intermediate care or medical-surgical unit requires the nurses on these units to deal with the complex acute care needs of these patients as well as their rehabilitation needs. The trauma patient's rehabilitation needs must be identified early in the acute phase of care. Appropriate care that addressed these rehabilitation needs is initiated while the patient is in the intensive care unit and continues through the hospital stay. A discharge plan for continuing rehabilitation in an inpatient or outpatient rehabilitation program is created. Attention also is placed on assisting patients as they prepare for reintegration into their homes, jobs, and social groups. The nursing care during this intermediate or rehabilitation phase requires the acquisition of new knowledge and skills in areas such as patient-family teaching, cognitive retraining, occupational and physical therapy, and discharge planning.

When appropriate interventions are used to manage the critically injured patient from injury through reentry into society, a number of desirable outcomes are met. These include the following:

- Enhanced clinical outcomes with reduced disability and mortality rates
- Promotion of personal autonomy, which fosters patient independence
- Possibly shorten inpatient length of stays

Rehabilitation is a process whereby the patient and family collaborate with nurses, physicians, and other specialists to identify mutual goals and plans to assist the trauma patient in achieving an optimal level of recovery. A multidisciplinary rehabilitation system can provide all trauma patients with the opportunity to achieve maximal physical, social, psychologic, and vocational recovery by striving to overcome functional limitations. Limitations may involve numerous functions such as the following:

- Communication
- Self-care
- Mobility
- Hygiene
- Vocation
- Family role
- Coping abilities

In an effort to provide empiric data for effective rehabilitation, several studies were conducted on patients with severe lower extremity fractures. These studies have shown that a patient's ability to return to maximal function is complex and involves factors other than the functional disability, such as the physical, social, and economic environments.[46-48]

Trauma Nursing—The Focus of Care

In response to changes in incidence, magnitude, and severity of injuries, the complexity of the therapeutic needs of the trauma patient population, and ultimately the demands on the entire health care system, the specialty field of trauma nursing has carved its niche in the health care arena. Influenced by a rapidly expanding body of knowledge focusing on how the human system responds to traumatic injury and which factors may make a difference in improving care, trauma nursing has expanded beyond traditional practice. The effects of stress and adaptability on the course of illness, factors traditionally recognized by nurses, have become more readily valued as critical variables in the trauma patient's recovery. This is supportive of the holistic approach to patient care—attention on the whole individual, which is easily contrasted with a fragmented approach that focuses on specific pieces of information without acknowledging that these pieces are woven in an intricate fashion into the human fabric. The emphasis of trauma nursing addresses best meeting the needs of the injured patient, which can be encompassed in five spheres:

- Support of vital life functions
- Support for physiologic adaptation
- Promotion of safety and security
- Support for psychologic and social adaptation
- Support of spirituality

Holistic care of the trauma patient requires continuity in the delivery of expert nursing care that addresses all five spheres of patients' care needs. Several significant factors must be considered if this continuity is to be accomplished.

The Human Response to Traumatic Injury

The impact of trauma on the individual can be viewed from various angles, including physiologic, psychologic, spiritual, and socioeconomic perspectives. The biologic makeup provides the human species with miraculous capabilities for maintaining itself in a relative state of homeostasis. As insults such as infectious agents, foreign bodies, and/or traumatic injuries are imposed on the human system, various physiologic components are activated in an attempt to counteract the insult and its effects. The human system has the function of maintaining a sense of equilibrium or balance; this function or process is often referred to as the "natural healing power" of the human species. This healing energy exists within all of us in some form to varying degrees. The biologic response of the individual to insults such as traumatic injury is in part dependent on the human organism's natural ability to adjust or adapt physiologically. The "how and to what degree" the individual is able to adapt can be determined by observing behavioral responses and by monitoring certain physiologic parameters. These findings can often be translated by nurses and used as measurable tools to guide therapy and predict outcomes.

The human organism cannot, however, be viewed simply from a biologic perspective. To do so would defy the laws of nature. No organism can be understood completely by studying only one aspect of it without acknowledging the effects of others on the composition of the entire system. This is not to say that scientific studies cannot be organized so that separate bodies of knowledge are identified and developed according to established processes. However, the scientific exploration of one human parameter in isolation, without considering the effects on the total human configuration, results in fragmented, useless information.

In keeping with this theme, the individual human response to traumatic injury also must be examined from the physical, psychologic, spiritual, and socioeconomic perspectives. To provide efficient and effective nursing care that encompasses all realms of human response, the trauma nurse must use a systematic means of assessing and monitoring the patient to elicit care needs in all five spheres. Part of the challenge for trauma nurses is to identify negative adaptation responses, behaviors, and attitudes and to help the patient adapt more positively.

Trauma patients face other hazards in addition to the physiologic effects of injury. They also must face the effects of traumatic insult on their thought patterns and attitudes. These effects may be worsened by deprived sensory systems, a situation that frequently occurs in an intensive care setting, from a prolonged hospital stay, when sedative or analgesics are in use, or in the presence of neurologic injury. In making compensatory adjustments, the mind may create illusions, hallucinations, and visions. When the patient is unable to cope with or to adapt independently to increasing tension, the trauma nurse must apply energies to provide emotional, psychologic, and physical support until the patient regains enough energy to resume independent functioning. This requires that the nurse formulate a plan of action based on open communication, especially important in the emotional atmosphere of an acute care environment. Thus, at the first available opportunity, the nurse encourages the trauma patient to communicate fears, frustrations, and anxieties about the traumatic incident, the injuries sustained, the medical and nursing management regimen, and the future course of events. Obtaining information about religious orientation, culture, beliefs, and values and the patient's sense of belonging or connectedness with family, friends, and community assesses the patient's spiritual orientation.

After comprehensive assessment, the nurse must choose appropriate nursing actions to enhance the forces of adaptation by redirecting the dynamic processes in a positive direction. The nurse can offer assistance to the patient in developing a new future on the basis of assessment of the past and appraisal of realistic goals or limitations in the present. Ideally, the trauma nurse's support and understanding will help the patient to accept the limitations caused by the traumatic injury.

In developing a comprehensive plan of care, the trauma nurse also is alert to socioeconomic dynamics. Trauma has an impact on the social groups of which the patient is a member. In addition to the family system, these groups include work and church groups, as well as clubs and other social affiliations, all of which have an effect on the individual trauma patient. To enable the trauma nurse to assist the injured patient effectively in adapting, the reactions and expectations of family members and friends must be considered. Generally, the way in which injury and disability are viewed depends on a variety of factors:

- Type of injury
- Previous personal experience with illness or injury
- Norms and values of the individual and particular social groups
- Perceived expectations for social reintegration

Understanding the social dynamics unique to each patient's situation assists the nurse in identifying appropriate resources within the hospital and community that will help in planning the patient's discharge. Understanding social dynamics is critical to the following:

- The nurse's management of the patient's care plan
- Facilitation of hospital discharge to rehabilitation services
- Follow-up during the recovery phase of care

End-of-life care for trauma patients who have sustained critical injuries and are not predicted to survive is a critical component to providing compassion and comfort to the dying patient and the patient's family. Nurses need to collaborate with physicians and other members of the trauma team to plan for palliative care that is appropriate for the patient and family. A recent study by Jacobs et al.[49] has established that there is a need for quality end-of-life care in trauma.

The effect of an injured family member on the entire family structure must not be overlooked. Considered an important and essential component in the nursing care plan, the family must receive attention and support from the trauma nurse. It is important that the trauma nurse establish a firm base of knowledge about the family and develop skill in interacting with the patient's family members. The nature and severity of the impact of trauma on members of the family will vary as a function of the following:

- The type of traumatic injury
- The phase or point at which the family is observed
- The family structure
- The role of the injured person in the family (e.g., mother, daughter, grandfather)
- The point at which the traumatic injury occurs during The course of the individual's life
- The point at which it occurs in the life of the family

The family's response to a sudden traumatic injury that represents a crisis event is dynamic and interactive. To understand the family system and its individual members, the nurse must assess the crisis response of all family members and others who have significant relationships with the patient.[50,51] Family function may be affected in different ways when sudden traumatic injury is sustained by a family member. As the impact of traumatic injury on the patient is considered from the biologic, psychologic, spiritual, and socioeconomic perspectives, so may the impact on the family structure.

The biologic functions of a family unit include the nurturing and physical care of a family member: feeding, cleaning, and tending to the injury or illness. This may include identifying, preventing, and attempting to cure health threats and determining when advice or assistance from others outside the family unit is necessary. Trauma nurses should identify themselves as supportive resources to family members so that open lines of communication are established, thereby fostering the sharing of valuable information between the patient's family and the trauma health care team.

The development and maintenance of the patient's self-image and self-esteem are among the psychologic functions of the family system. This is accomplished through emotional communication patterns, which involve the expression of fear, anger, anxiety, frustration, joy, excitement, and contentment. The conditions under which these emotional expressions are permitted, not permitted, or controlled also must be identified within the family and the context of the culture with which the family identifies.

Included among the family's social functions are the tasks of defining group membership and group boundaries and establishing norms for relationships within the group and outside the group. The family is also considered within the context of the formal or informal societal structure and is viewed as a wage-earning, product-consuming, help-giving, tax-paying unit within our socioeconomic system.

Each of the functions described represents an important component for assessing how well the family unit is fulfilling biologic, psychologic, emotional, and social functions.[51] The trauma nurse must be alert to the patterns of family system functions and incorporate the unique characteristics of patient-family lifestyles into the comprehensive plan of care.

Nurses' Role in Prevention

An examination of the impact that trauma has made on the community raises issues that must be addressed. In most communities, unintentional injuries are taken for granted. Perhaps a major problem relates to the knowledge, or lack thereof, that communities have about injury and the effects not only on the individual and family but also on the community as a whole. The cost of trauma to the community must be seen in health care costs and in the monetary expenditure resulting from reduced worker hours. As responsible members of the health care community, nurses find themselves more often taking on responsibility for disseminating information about the nation's trauma problem. Health care professionals and consumers need to be alert to the causes of injuries and how they can be prevented.

As with many health care problems, the cause of injury cannot be reduced to a single factor but must be viewed within the context of a broad spectrum of related factors. The predominant factor is human error. In 1990, 78% of vehicular crashes resulting in fatal or nonfatal injuries were caused by improper driving practices. A much smaller percentage was caused by vehicle defects or poor road conditions. Exceeding the posted speed limit or driving at an unsafe speed were the most common errors reported in injuries of all severities in rural areas and in fatal injuries in urban areas. Right-of-way violations predominated in the occurrence of urban motor vehicle injuries.[2] Alcohol is a factor in approximately 41% of fatal motor vehicle crashes,[2] and illegal drugs and many legally prescribed medications can slow reaction time, thus contributing to the occurrence of injury.

The home and community can be dangerous places as well. In 2003, unintentional injuries that occurred in the home and community resulted in 54,400 deaths and 15 million disabling injuries. With an injury total of this magnitude, it is estimated that 1 of 19 U.S. citizens was disabled one or more days by injuries received in home mishaps.[2] Falls, poisonings, fires, criminal violence (including child abuse, domestic violence, and injuries from bullets and bombs), and sporting injuries, although representing a smaller proportion of the total number of trauma-related deaths or cases requiring hospitalization each year, should be cause for public concern and raise interest in effective prevention strategies.

Many injuries are both predictable and preventable in the same way that many impairments are treatable and the resulting disabilities preventable. The development of effective trauma prevention programs provides countless opportunities for addressing the trauma problem as it currently exists in our society. Likewise, the ample availability of rehabilitation programs can create a proliferation of opportunities for thousands of trauma patients. Yet despite these common truths, a passive societal posture seems to prevail. It has been described as a "pervasive fatalistic attitude that equates impairment with disability and concludes that accidents just happen and nothing can be done to prevent them."[52]

Consumer involvement is imperative in gaining legislative support for issues pertaining to health, safety, and the prevention of unintentional injury. Unfortunately, the beneficial economic impact of trauma prevention has not always been adequately and effectively translated into compelling public policy. An example of this is the motorcycle helmet laws. Some states have repealed motorcycle helmet laws as a result of public challenges. The NHTSA reported a 13% rise in motorcycle fatalities from 4,028 in 2004 to 4,553 in 2005 and noted that almost half of the people who died were not wearing a helmet.[52] Trauma nurses have spoken out and should continue to do so as they assume a leadership role in influencing issues of injury prevention and control, refusing to accept the grim statistics regarding trauma in our society.

A considerable number of current active prevention programs have been initiated and maintained by trauma nurses throughout the country—courageous testimony to the energy, interest, and accountability exemplified by nurses on behalf of the public. Although a complete list of such programs is not available and a program-specific description and an in-depth discussion are beyond the scope of this chapter, it is important to note that trauma nurse-activists are addressing the following issues:

- Alcohol and drug abuse and their implications for every injury mechanism and etiology
- Highway safety issues, including safety belt use, child restraint, and helmet laws
- Domestic violence issues, including child abuse, firearms, and environmental influences[53,54]

Most important, trauma nurses continue to voice the strong belief that, in matters pertaining to trauma care, those who have assumed an intricate role in meeting the complex needs of the trauma patient population should play a key role in shaping policy.

Trauma Nursing Today

When the evolution of the trauma nursing specialty is studied, several significant developments and events of the past three decades must be considered (Table 1-2). A review of pertinent factual information in congressional testimony, technical reports, and the literature has established a historic perspective of the development of trauma/emergency medical services systems. The proliferation of designated trauma care facilities and the increasing regularity of formal meetings and

TABLE 1-2 **Milestones of Trauma Nursing**

1961	First shock trauma nurses. Elizabeth Scanlan, RN, and Jane Tarrant, RN, pioneered the nurse's role in the first two-bed shock/trauma research center with R. Adams Cowley, MD, at University of Maryland Hospital, Baltimore, Maryland.
1963	National Research Center awarded a first-of-a-kind grant to the University of Maryland in Baltimore to establish a center for the study of trauma.
1966	Cook County Hospital in Chicago opened a trauma unit with Robert Freeark, MD, as medical director and Norma Shoemaker, RN, as nursing supervisor.
1966	*Accidental Death and Disability: The Neglected Disease of Modern Society* (white paper on trauma) published, citing needs of trauma population. This led to federal funding of trauma centers.
1971	First trauma nurse coordinators hired for Level I trauma centers in Illinois. David Boyd, MD, hired Theresa Romano, RN, to direct the education and training of nurses working in the designated trauma centers in Illinois.
1973	Federal contracts awarded to Texas Women's University, University of Cincinnati, and University of Washington to begin graduate nursing programs in burns. These programs were the model for the first graduate trauma nursing programs.
1975	Maryland state EMS system established trauma nurse coordinator position for training, designation, and evaluation.
1982	ATLS for nurses (pilot program) taught in conjunction with physician course. Nursing track was developed by MIEMSS Field Nursing, Baltimore.
1983	Trauma nurse network organized to provide communication link for trauma nurses.
1986	TNCC course, Emergency Nurses Association.
1987	First national census forum on Development of Trauma Nurse Coordinator Role, Washington, DC.
1989	Society of Trauma Nurses formed.
1993	The Society of Trauma Nurses publishes the inaugural issue of the *Journal of Trauma Nursing.*
2000	Society of Trauma Nurses collaborates with the American College of Surgeons COT and ATLS Committees to provide the Advanced Trauma Care for Nurses course.
2005	*Society of Trauma Nurses Journal* "The evolution of trauma nursing and the Society of Trauma Nurses: a noble history." Mary Beachley, October 2005.
2006	Formal collaboration between the Society of Trauma Nurses (STN) and the Eastern Association for the Surgery of Trauma (EAST) to join the EAST's Annual Scientific Assembly meeting and hold concurrent STN meetings.

conferences joining major organizations and professionals together are measures of the progress in recognizing trauma patients as a unique population requiring specialty services. These professional gatherings are indicative of the need for increased coordination. Clearly defined responsibilities are needed if each group—nurses, physicians, paramedics, and other allied health care professionals—is to deliver effective and efficient care.

In the past 40 years, achievements and advances in the development and implementation of regional trauma care systems have been monumental and drastically surpass all efforts made during the preceding century. The technologic advances, the unquestioned recognition of need, and the impetus from many concerned individuals and professional groups have contributed to the development and implementation of trauma care systems. These factors have resulted in support from local, state, and federal governments for regional planning and implementation of efficient trauma care services. It is essential that nurses become involved in this regional trauma EMS planning, implementation, and evaluation locally, nationally, and internationally.

Many of the goals of the white paper *Accidental Death and Disability—The Neglected Disease of Modern Society*[10] have been attained or at least movement toward them has begun. The development and designation of trauma centers may be viewed as a natural evolution as a result of the dramatically increasing magnitude of the trauma problem and the demands of the trauma patient population on the entire health care system. Likewise, the demanding clinical needs of critically injured trauma patients, coupled with trauma nursing crossing established boundaries within the traditional nursing educational structure, have led to the natural evolution of trauma nursing as a specialty field within the larger emergency health care system.

As with all systems that change over time, trauma nursing continues to advance toward a higher level of organization. As trauma patient care requirements have become more complex, nurses have emerged as coordinators capable of integrating the actions of other health care professionals. This process has allowed the integration of the total care regimen, including all trauma specialty fields, which potentiates the process of unified action. Several expanded roles have been established as a means of meeting the special care needs and complexities of trauma patients and their families, among them the trauma nurse coordinator, trauma nurse practitioner, and trauma case manager.[55-59]

This book presents a working body of knowledge based on principles from nursing models and from the theoretic frameworks of medicine, psychology, physical science, education, and behavioral and social sciences. Perhaps it is this broad spectrum of required knowledge that has attracted nurses to accept the challenge of contributing the integral components of a multidimensional and holistic focus in caring for the trauma patient. The nature of severe injuries resulting in multisystem disruptions requires the trauma nurse to comprehend extensive scientific data; to synthesize care in life-threatening emergencies; and to lead, assist, and support the patient and family on the long journey toward recovery. Daily, this group of caregivers is bombarded with uncharted pathophysiologic phenomena and unceasing psychologic and emotional crises. For the nurse to function efficiently in this situation, high levels of energy and stamina are required. To do this, each nurse must take responsibility for periodically examining his or her stress levels while constantly being alert to the stress levels of others. This fosters an atmosphere of caring, not only for the patients and families but also for one another.

The Trauma Cycle—Conceptual Development

In closely examining the cycle of events that occur throughout the many phases of trauma care—from the time of injury; through the resuscitative, operative, critical, intermediate, acute (medical-surgical unit), and rehabilitation phases of care; to the return to home and community—a wealth of information can be derived and added to the existing body of knowledge and skills of trauma nursing. This process of continued growth and development will determine the future direction of trauma nursing practice.

Although a traumatic injury occurs within a very short time frame, it has long-term effects. Trauma can therefore be viewed as a disease process with far-reaching consequences. Many of the changes that occur during and after a traumatic incident are a direct result of the individual's ability to adapt to the injured state. For this reason, this book is organized with the subject content presented in the context of time and space.

We believe that it is beneficial to look at the individual's traumatic incident and subsequent care as it occurs in a cyclic pattern. What happens to an individual when an injury occurs will be described in blocks of time, or phases, within the trauma cycle. This method takes into account what circumstances existed before the injury, which may or may not have precipitated the incident; what occurs at the exact time of the incident, with consideration of the biomechanics of the injury and the circumstances that may have contributed to its nature and extent; and what changes occur after a traumatic injury. This exploration of events will begin with time representing the resuscitation phase and will continue through the operative, critical care, and intermediate and rehabilitation phases to the time at which the individual is integrated into the community. At any time during this cyclic pattern, valuable information can be learned that will assist the skilled nurse in assessing and planning, implementing, and evaluating a special plan of care for the trauma patient and his or her family.

Reflected throughout the book is the view that the care of the trauma patient is not performed on a linear continuum with a beginning and an end but instead throughout a cyclic process. The trauma cycle represents a series of changes that leads back to its starting point; the patient enters the emergency health care system from the community and at some point re-enters the community. As the individual returns to the community, the cycle is completed, yet the potential always exists for the cycle to be repeated. Accordingly, prevention is a concept that must receive prime consideration when caring for patients throughout the process.

On the basis of the strong belief that prevention is better than cure, increased emphasis will be placed not only on the prevention of traumatic injury but also on the prevention of complications, disability, and maladaptive adjustments on the part of the patient and family once a traumatic injury has occurred. The trauma sequel represents a complete cycle of phenomena and operations—changes that lead toward the restoration of a state of well-being. Helping the patient and family return to a healthy state is the goal of the trauma nurse—and the target of all interventions.

References

1. Trinkaus E, Zimmerman MR: Trauma among the Shanidar Neanderthals, *Am J Phys Anthropol* 57:61-76, 1982.
2. National Safety Council: *Injury facts,* Chicago, 2005-2006, National Safety Council.
3. National Center for Injury Prevention and Control: *Injury fact book 2001-2002,* Atlanta, GA, 2001, Centers for Disease Control and Prevention: http://www.cdc.gov/ncipc/fact_book.htm. Accessed March 21, 2006.
4. National Highway Traffic Safety Administration's National Center for Statistics and Analysis: *Traffic safety facts 2005,* DOT HS 810 623, Washington, DC, 2005, NHTSA.
5. U.S. Department of Health, Education, and Welfare: *Report of the Secretary's Advisory Committee on Traffic Safety,* Washington, DC, 1968, U.S. Government Printing Office.
6. Simeone FA: Studies of trauma and shock in man: William S. Stone's role in the military effort (1983 William S. Stone Lecture), *J Trauma* 24:181-187, 1984.
7. Board for the Study of the Severely Wounded, Medical Department, United States Army: In Beecher HR, editor: *Surgery in World War II: the physiologic effects of wounds,* Washington, DC, 1952, U.S. Government Printing Office.
8. Heaton LD: Army medical service activities in Vietnam, *Milit Med* 131:646, 1966.
9. Brain Trauma Foundation: *Guidelines for field management of combat-related head trauma,* New York, 2005, Brain Trauma Foundation.
10. U.S. Department of Health, Education and Welfare: *Accidental death and disability: the neglected disease of modern society,* Rockville, Md, 1996, Division of Medical Sciences, National Academy of Sciences, National Research Council.
11. Boyd D, Edlich RF, Micik SH: *Systems approach to emergency medical care,* Norwalk, Conn, 1983, Appleton-Century-Crofts.
12. Ogilivie RB: *Special message on health care,* Springfield, Ill, 1971, State of Illinois Printing Office.
13. Meyer P, Rosen HB, Hall W: Fracture dislocations of the cervical spine: transportation assessment, and immediate management, *Am Acad Orthop Surg* 25:171-183, 1976.
14. Cowley RA: Trauma center—a new concept for the delivery of critical care, *J Med Soc N J* 74:979-986, 1977.
15. Maryland Department of Health and Mental Hygiene: *Maryland vital statistics annual report,* Rockville, Md, 2004, Maryland Department of Health and Mental Hygiene.

16. U.S. Congress: *Emergency medical services systems act,* Public Law 93-154, Pub No SB2 410, Washington, DC, 1973, U.S. Government Printing Office.
17. U.S. General Accounting Office: *States assume leadership role in providing emergency medical services,* Publication No. GAO/HRD-86-132, Washington, DC, 1986, U.S. Government Printing Office.
18. U.S. Congress: *Trauma care systems planning and development act of 1990,* Public Law 101-590, 104 Stat 2915, Washington, DC, 1990, U.S. Government Printing Office.
19. U.S. Department of Health and Human Services, Health Resources and Services Administration: *Model trauma care system plan,* Rockville, Md, 1992, Bureau of Health Services Resources, Division of Trauma and Emergency Medical Services.
20. U. S. Department of Health and Human Services, Health Resources and Services Administration: *Model trauma system planning and evaluation,* Rockville, Md, 2006, DHHS.
21. Division of Emergency Medical Services, Health Services Administration, Bureau of Medical Services Administration: *Emergency medical services systems program guidelines,* DHHS Publication No, (HSA) 75-2013, Washington, DC, 1975, DHHS.
22. American College of Emergency Physicians' Trauma Committee: Guidelines for trauma care systems, *Ann Emerg Med* 16:459-463, 1987.
23. Committee on Trauma of the American College of Surgeons: Optimal hospital resources for care of the severely injured, *Bull Am Coll Surg* 61:15-22, 1976.
24. Committee on Trauma of the American College of Surgeons: Hospital resources for optimal care of the injured patient, *Bull Am Coll Surg* 64:43-48, 1979.
25. American College of Surgeons' Committee on Trauma: *Resources for the optimal care of the injured patient,* Chicago, 1999, American College of Surgeons.
26. American College of Surgeons' Committee on Trauma: *Resources for the optimal care of the injured patient,* Chicago, 2006, American College of Surgeons.
27. U.S. Department of Transportation and National Highway Traffic Safety Administration: *Emergency medical technician: basic national standard curriculum,* Washington, DC, 1994, U.S. Government Printing Office.
28. Miller T, Levy D: The effect of regional trauma care systems on costs, *Arch Surgery* 130:188-193, 1995.
29. U.S. Department of Health and Human Services, Public Health Services, Centers for Disease Control and Prevention, Trauma Care Systems Panel: *Injury control.* Presented as a position paper at the Third National Injury Control Conference, Washington, DC, April 1992, pp. 377-426.
30. Skamania Symposium: Trauma systems supplement, *J Trauma* 47:3, 1999.
31. MacKenzie EJ, Rivara FP, Jurkovich GJ et al: A national evaluation of the effect of trauma-center care on mortality, *N Engl J Med* 354:366-378, 2006.
32. Beachley M: The evolution of trauma nursing and the society of trauma nurses: a noble history, *J Trauma Nursing* 12:105-115, 2006.
33. Nightingale F: *Notes on nursing: what it is and what it is not,* New York, 1969, Dover.
34. Huxley EJ: *Florence Nightingale,* New York, 1975, Putnam.
35. *History of American Red Cross nursing,* chapters 1 and 2, New York, 1922, Macmillan.
36. Thurstan V: Active science. In Thurstan V, editor: *A textbook of war nursing,* London, 1917, GP Putnam.
37. Mays ET: *Clinical evaluation of the critically ill,* Springfield, Ill, 1975, Charles C Thomas.
38. Oakes AR: Trauma: twentieth-century epidemic, *Heart Lung* 8:918-922, 1979.
39. Von Wagoner FH: Died in hospital: a three year study of deaths following trauma, *J Trauma* 1:401-408, 1961.
40. Gertner HR Jr, Baker SP, Rutherford RB et al: Evaluation of the management of vehicular fatalities secondary to abdominal injury, *J Trauma* 12:425-431, 1972.
41. Foley FW, Harris LS, Pilcher DB: Abdominal injuries in automobile accidents: review of care of fatally injured patients, *J Trauma* 17:611-615, 1977.
42. Houtchens BA: Major trauma in the rural mountain West, *J Am Coll Emerg Phys* 6:343-350, 1977.
43. Frey CF, Huelke DF, Gikas PW: Resuscitation and survival in motor vehicle accidents, *J Trauma* 9:292-310, 1969.
44. Allgöwer M, Border JR: Advances in the care of the multiple trauma patient: introduction, *World J Surg* 7:1-3, 1983.
45. Committee on Trauma Research Commission on Life Sciences, National Research Council and the Institute of Medicine: *Injury in America: a continuing public health problem,* Washington, DC, 1985, National Academy Press.
46. MacKenzie EJ, Cushing BM, Jurkovich GJ et al: Physical impairment and functional outcomes six months after severe lower extremity fractures, *J Trauma* 4:528-538, 1993.
47. Mackenzie EJ: Return to work following injury: the role of economic, social, and job-related factors, *Am J Public Health* 11:1630-1637, 1998.
48. McCarthy ML, McAndrew MP, MacKenzie EJ et al: Correlation between the measures of impairment, according to the modified system of the American Medical Association, and function, *J Bone Joint Surg* 80-87:1034-1042, 1998.
49. Jacobs LM, Jacobs BB, Burns, KJ: A plan to improve end-of-life care for trauma victims and their families, *J Trauma Nurs* 12: 73-76, 2005
50. Leske JS: Treatment for family members in crisis after critical injury, *AACN Clin Issues* 9:129-139, 1998.
51. Tuck D, Kerns R: *Health, illness and families: a life span prospective,* New York, 1985, Wiley.
52. National Highway Traffic Safety Administration: *Rise in motorcycle and pedestrian deaths lead to increase in overall highway fatality rate in 2005:* http://www.nhtsa.dot.gov/portal/site/nhtsa/template. Accessed January 31, 2007
53. Ségal E: Straight Talk on Prevention (STOP) Program, *Maryland EMS Newsl* 17:1-2, 1991.
54. Dearing-Stuck B: Trauma prevention. In Cardona G, editor: *Trauma nursing,* Oradell, NJ, 1985, Medical Economics Press.
55. Beachley M, Snow S, Trimble P: Developing trauma care systems: the trauma nurse coordinator, *JONA* 18:34-42, 1988.
56. Spisso J, O'Callaghan C, McKennan M et al: Improved quality of care and reduction of house staff workload using trauma nurse practitioners, *J Trauma* 30:660-663, 1990.
57. Gantt D, Price J, Pollock D: The status of the trauma coordinator position: a national survey, *J Trauma* 40:816-819, 1966.
58. Keough V, Jennrich J, Holm K et al: A collaborative program for advanced practice in trauma/critical care nursing, *Crit Care Nurse* 16:120-127, 1996.
59. Daleiden A: The CNS as trauma case manager: a new frontier, *Clin Nurse Specialist* 7:295-298, 1993.

2

ECONOMIC AND ADMINISTRATIVE ISSUES IN TRAUMA CARE

Eileen Whalen

Trauma exerts financial stresses on patients, hospitals, and society. According to 2001 data, for all age groups, unintentional injuries continue to be the fifth leading cause of death, exceeded only by heart disease, cancer, stroke, and lower respiratory tract diseases.[1] Injury is the leading cause of death in people aged 1 to 34 years.[1] In 2002, approximately 23.7 million people, or 1 out of 12, were treated for an injury. About 2.7 million people were hospitalized for injuries.[1] Injuries that occurred in 2000 cost the U.S. health care system $80.2 billion in medical care costs: $1.1 billion for fatal injuries, $33.7 billion for hospitalized injuries, and $45.4 billion for nonhospitalized injuries, with 70% ($31.8 billion) of the nonhospitalized costs attributable to injuries treated in emergency departments (EDs). Injuries requiring hospitalization are more expensive to treat in the short term, and frequently these patients require long-term rehabilitation, compounding lifetime costs.[2] In 2003, the financial impact of fatal and nonfatal unintentional injuries totaled $602.7 billion. This dollar amount equates to $2,100 per capita or about $5,700 per household.[1]

The economic burden of injury can be determined knowing the incidence, medical costs, productivity losses (i.e., wage and household work losses), and total costs (i.e., the sum of medical costs and the dollar value of productivity losses). Burden is further defined by medical expenditures to prevent illness and injury. The economic burden of injury is now being calculated, as the costs associated with health care continue to rise and increase the strain on public and private sector payers.[2] The combined economic burden of medical treatment plus the lost productivity for injuries that occurred in 2000 totals more than $326 billion: $142 billion for fatal injuries, $58.7 billion for hospitalized injuries, and approximately $125.3 billion for nonhospitalized injuries.[2] The adverse effects of trauma are more likely to occur at younger ages relative to the adverse effects of smoking and other preventable diseases, and productivity losses are likely to be the dominant cost associated with injury.[2] It is imperative to include these costs to accurately quantify the burden of injury.

Much has been published regarding the efficacy of trauma care systems in reducing death and disability since publication of the 1966 white paper by the National Academy of Sciences, identifying trauma as the "neglected disease of modern society."[3] The financial burden placed on the trauma system and trauma centers continues to be a deterrent to expansion of comprehensive trauma systems. An in-depth understanding of the economic issues that surround the provision of high-quality trauma care is essential to continuing development of trauma systems and to proactively implement changes that will increase the ability to provide the needed care.

As part of the health care system, trauma systems and trauma centers are facing the same turbulent economic times as the rest of the health care arena. Trauma care is both labor and resource intensive, and the financing of health care overall is shrinking. In addition, the care provided to many of the victims of trauma is uncompensated care, either self-pay or no funding. These economic forces, joined with the high cost of providing care to the injured, are conspiring to further compromise the delivery of high-quality trauma care in the United States. This chapter focuses on the economic and administrative issues that surround trauma care delivery.

THE FINANCING OF TRAUMA CARE

In 1966, the National Academy of Sciences and the National Research Council published a landmark report, *Accidental Death and Disability: The Neglected Disease of Modern Society.*[3] This report created the recognition that trauma is a disease and that improvements in care of the injured could make a difference in the survival rates of trauma victims. It also prompted the development of organized trauma systems.

The emerging trauma system concept involved the tenets of treating the patient within the "golden hour"[4] and getting the "right patient to the right place at the right time."[5] Federal funding for the development of trauma systems was made available by the Highway Safety Act of 1966[6] and the Emergency Medical Services Act of 1973.[7] Supported by guidelines developed by the American College of Surgeons (ACS) Committee on Trauma, the American College of Emergency Physicians, and the American Association for the Surgery of Trauma, trauma centers and systems began to develop.

In 1979, West et al.[8] produced the seminal study comparing preventable deaths in a trauma system with those in a geographic area without trauma centers. Despite the evidence

that a systematic approach to care was best, the monies to support such systems were not forthcoming. A follow-up report by the National Academy of Sciences in 1985 concluded that insufficient progress had been made in injury control since the original study 20 years earlier.[9] The legislative response was the Trauma Care Systems Planning and Development Act of 1990, which awarded state grants for the implementation of statewide trauma systems.[10] This act directed the U.S. Department of Health and Human Services Resources and Services Administration (HRSA) to develop the 1992 *Model Trauma Care System Plan*. This plan focused on an inclusive system of trauma care involving not only the trauma centers but all health care facilities based on availability of trauma resources.[11] In 1995, Bazzoli et al.[12] released the second national assessment of trauma care systems, which revealed very little progress in states' ability to meet all criteria for successful implementation of trauma systems. This study was replicated in 1998 by Bass et al.[13] and again in 2003 by the HRSA,[14] indicating that states are making improvements toward this goal. This latter assessment by the HRSA indicated that the more comprehensive a state's trauma system development is, the more prepared the state was to provide medical care in the face of all kinds of incidents. The tragic events of September 11, 2001, and the aftermath of Hurricane Katrina prompted great attention and reassessment of the strengths and weaknesses of emergency medical systems and trauma care systems. These events have also led to additional public funding under the auspices of Homeland Security to shore up necessary education and resources to states for response to disaster and multicasualty events.

Although funding to states for the development of trauma systems is key to future success, little attention has been paid to the economic burden to the trauma centers, which form the nuclei of the trauma systems. Trauma centers are under intense financial pressure. Unfortunately, an understanding of the importance of trauma centers has not been widely adopted by the general public or our elected officials. No direct federal funding support to trauma centers or physicians performing trauma care exists despite the extraordinary costs involved in providing this vital care. The United States faces increased risk of terrorist attacks and natural disasters, yet we continue to fail in providing this necessary infusion of dollars to support the cost of care. In 2004, 32 trauma centers were reportedly threatening closure or actually closed.[15]

According to Daily et al.,[16] in 1992 one of the most important factors in prompting closure of trauma centers was unfavorable payer mix because of the provision of uncompensated care and underreimbursement by public programs (commonly Medicare). Subsequent studies by the National Foundation for Trauma Care in 2004 and 2006 indicate that trauma center closures were not only due to uninsured/underinsured patients but more important to lack of physician commitment, negative effect on physicians' private practice, physician malpractice costs, physician call pay, availability of specialists, and extra operating costs.[15] Hospital-physician relationship is a primary contributing factor in the decision to close or downgrade trauma service coverage. The primary services affected are general surgery, neurosurgery, orthopedics, and plastic surgery. Contributing services were cited as hand, ear-nose-throat, and maxillofacial surgery. When asked if the impact of closure of trauma services was positive, the response from chief operating officers (COOs) was that it improved the "bottom line" and contributed to happier physicians and specialists. When asked about negative outcomes, the same COOs reported adverse publicity, loss of prestige within a community, public opposition, loss of administrative and physician leadership, and increased risk of exposure and litigation.[15]

A component of this physician problem is the physician reimbursement system, the Resource Based Relative Value Scale (RBRVS) implemented by the Health Care Financing Administration (now the Centers for Medicare and Medicaid Services [CMS]) in 1992. This system was developed in an attempt to reform Medicare's physician reimbursement policy. The payment system lumps together fees paid to physicians. Despite the active participation of surgeons on the RBRVS review boards, the scales still undervalue their efforts expended on critically injured patients.[17] The general surgeon is the surgeon most often in house 24 hours a day, yet only 12% to 13% of blunt trauma patients have a general surgery operation. Trauma surgeons frequently perform multiple procedures and services to the same patient on the same day, so their charges for many services are denied. Additionally, instead of overbilling by unbundling charges, which was a common fear by Medicare, surgeons typically underbill out of ignorance.[17] Uniformly, surgeons have never received any education on billing and coding processes, nor do many practice plans provide these valuable resources to busy productive surgeons. It is unrealistic for surgeons to understand the complexity of Medicare regulations, and trauma centers may be wise to provide coder/biller specialists to surgeons to assist in maximizing reimbursement efforts. In a study from the Department of Surgery in Louisville, published in 2005, the authors demonstrated that the reimbursement to direct cost ratio was 2- and 35-fold greater for the trauma centers serving commercial and government insured patients than for the professional fees of the trauma/critical care surgeons. The addition of local and/or federal funding for uninsured patients paid to the institution allowed the trauma center to cover direct cost with no profit margin. In contrast, for every dollar in direct cost generated by the trauma/critical care surgeon caring for uninsured patients, the physicians were able to recover 55 cents or a loss of 45 cents per direct cost dollar spent.[18] Trauma centers have been very successful over the years in negotiating contracts with commercial carriers, better than many physician practice plans. Additionally they have been very aggressive in charge capture and revenue cycle enhancements. Trauma/critical care surgeons should be encouraged to get involved with efforts to maximize reimbursement, such as properly coding interventions by capturing E and M codes on the floor and in the ED and appropriately billing for line insertions and other procedures at nights and on weekends. It is important for the trauma surgeon to understand the collection processes and champion reform in areas regarding reimbursement.

Although rural trauma centers have been affected by the same issues as urban centers, their financial outcomes appear to be better. The net reimbursement for rural trauma is higher because of injury patterns, lower severity of injury, and favorable payer mix. Rogers et al.[19] reported that more fee-for-service patients were admitted to their rural center in 1995. Patients' lower severity of injury demands less resource utilization. The authors stressed that specific policies and measures had been implemented to reduce the costs of caring for trauma patients.

The problems of reimbursement have increased with prospective payment plans, lower payments from the government (Medicare and Medicaid), and increasing numbers of uninsured patients. This inadequate reimbursement threatens the organization of trauma care. Although Level I facilities have enjoyed a high level of physician support because of their teaching resources, financial pressures are particularly acute for teaching hospitals as managed care plans become dominant players in evolving patient referral patterns. Additionally the impact of reduction of residency work hours to 80 per week compounded by a shortage of surgical residents and fellows has profoundly affected Level I centers. One of the consequences has been excessive work hours by faculty physicians and inability to focus on research and teaching missions. These same physicians are typically the ones expected to lead national, statewide, and regional trauma system development.

The impact of lower Medicare and Medicaid payments coupled with managed care has been profound at all trauma centers but disproportionately so at Level I centers.[16] In the past, before statewide trauma systems, most critically injured patients were referred to the "university hospital" because it was believed that resources were available at the Level 1 center that were not reliably available in a community hospital. With the advent of statewide trauma systems and the proliferation of Level II and III centers in some areas of the country where reimbursement is favorable, Level I centers have been faced with a paradoxic loss of market share. Overdesignation of trauma centers is rarely addressed because it is a political problem. Many markets, such as San Diego, Denver, Salt Lake City, Portland, Phoenix, and Los Angeles, to name a few, have struggled with this phenomenon. Many of the urban Level I centers may be disadvantaged in competitive markets because it is often seen by patients and referring physicians as a repository for uninsured patients. This has threatened their teaching and research missions and their financial bottom line.[16]

This concern was further underscored by Selzer et al.[20] in a review of 553 trauma patients admitted to a public urban Level I center during a 6-month period. Data related to cost, payment, source of reimbursement, and profit and loss margins were compared with and without government funding. Without Disproportionate Share Hospital (DSH) funds, a net loss of more than $2.1 million was realized. The greatest gap was from Medicaid, self-pay, and prisoner groups. The addition of DSH funds provided a positive return of more than $600,000.

It is clear that trauma centers are in financial trouble for many reasons, the major ones being the cost of uncompensated care, the high operating cost of caring for the critically injured, and inadequate reimbursement from government medical assistance programs.

STRATEGIES FOR ECONOMIC SOLUTIONS

Financial support is essential for ensuring trauma system integrity to develop, maintain, and improve the trauma system over time. The system in any state must have facilities at a constant state of readiness, so long-term financial and community support is required. State legislatures have identified various ways to ensure continuing trauma system funding in addition to general fund appropriations.

Many states have stepped up in their legislative attempts to address the funding short fall for trauma care. Examples include the following:

- Motor vehicle fees, fines, and penalties
- Court fees, fines, and penalties (not motor vehicle–related)
- 911 system surcharges
- Intoxication offense fees
- Controlled substance act or weapons violation fees
- Taxes on sales of tobacco
- Tribal gaming[11]

States have formulated their own individual formulas for directing earmarked monies to the trauma centers. In every state where general fund money exists for trauma and emergency care, there is state law to support trauma systems and the designation of trauma centers. In most instances this reimbursement is tied to formal designation as a trauma center by a lead agency.

Some trauma centers have been successful lobbying their own legislative constituency for special earmarks to support operational expenses associated with trauma care. For example, many academic institutes have lobbied their congressional representatives for special requests in the form of legislative earmarks to expand hospital facilities to meet their trauma mission.

In 2002, the Universal Billing-1992 (UB-92) revenue codes for trauma patients came about largely as a result of successful lobbying by the National Foundation for Trauma Care (NFTC). The NFTC, with the help of many other groups, successfully petitioned the American Hospital Association's National Uniform Billing Committee to initiate two new codes. The first of the two codes consists of designating a new patient type, "trauma center," which assists hospitals, government agencies, and insurance databases to identify trauma patients. This code is used to identify both outpatient and inpatient trauma victims. The code facilitates the electronic transmission of data for billing instruments to identify trauma patients for contract purposes. This code also allows trauma centers a mechanism to identify trauma patients and accurately report costs associated with the trauma population.[15]

The second code allows trauma centers the opportunity to reflect the extraordinary costs related to trauma readiness. The 68X revenue code "trauma response" is separate and distinct from ED codes. This allows trauma centers to charge for ED services and to add a charge to cover the added costs of overhead for trauma center participation, specifically in-house coverage of specialists, staff dedicated to trauma care, operating room teams, additional support staff for ancillary departments such as radiology and laboratory, trauma registry, and performance improvement functions, as well as specialized equipment. It is important for each trauma center to establish trauma response fees and other UB-92 charges and to identify direct costs associated with the provision of trauma care. The UB-92 code for trauma critical care has been in place but is rarely used. This code is a little more labor intensive for hospitals. UB-92 208 is an accommodation code, and the trauma patient does not have to be in a specialized unit per se but must meet the definition of a trauma patient (by state lead agency or the ACS). Trauma critical care is a service, not a place. UB-92 208 must be used in lieu of other codes for general critical care and surgical critical care. The care must be rendered by a team that meets standards for trauma care (as defined by the institution).[15]

Trauma centers have experienced success in reimbursement from the commercial payer sector and auto insurance. Since 2003, Medicare has recognized 68X to be fiscal intermediaries. In addition, use of the 68X and UB-92 charges has led to successful receipt of "outlier" payments from the CMS, which increases Medicare's reimbursement for high-intensity trauma patients.

Many trauma centers have improved reimbursement by adding extra charges for the cost of taking high-acuity patients directly to the surgical suite. Although these charges are not part of UB-92, they are added to an institution's chargemaster. Ancillary services may add surcharges to cover the unscheduled, highly intensive costs associated with trauma care. These are less uniformly used by trauma centers. These charges often come under great scrutiny and are frequently challenged by payers.[15] CMS has recently released the 2007 outpatient prospective payment system final rule, which compared with previous years' is favorable for trauma centers. Additional payment will be made when trauma response team activation occurs acknowledging that hospitals incur additional costs when critical care includes trauma activation.[21]

Trauma centers must constantly strive to control operational expenses by benchmarking costs, charges, and resources. Aggressive payer strategies and realistic managed care contracts help profitability. In a recent study based on trauma registry data in Florida, treatment at a trauma center resulted in an 18% reduction in mortality. Mean costs for care in a trauma center versus a nontrauma center were $11,910 and $6,019, respectively. When the mean cost difference was divided by the reduction in mortality rates, the authors assigned a cost of $34,887 per life saved. They concluded that triage to a Florida trauma center is associated with less risk of death and cost/life saved is favorable compared with other expenditures for health care.[22]

Hospitals have been successful implementing cost reduction strategies while reducing variability in care and outcomes. The literature is replete with examples of physician-directed initiatives to control costs.[23,24] Physician efforts on cost containment focus on decreased resource utilization and reduction in length of stay. The introduction of patient care guidelines for specific injuries or patient populations has been effective in reducing length of stay and comorbidities. Controlling supply chain variables has been highly effective in decreasing costs.

Costs Associated with Trauma Care

The managed care focus has forced hospitals to evaluate their delivery of care systems and processes throughout the continuum of care. In performing this review, many organizations developed cost-effective methods for delivering trauma care. Trauma centers have become very savvy in their ability to define the costs associated with trauma care. To understand these costs, three categories must be defined: fixed costs, variable costs, and marginal costs.

Fixed costs do not vary with input into the system. We often think of these costs as overhead (e.g., costs to turn on the lights, for heating or air conditioning, and to pay salaries and the mortgage).

Variable costs do vary with input. These costs are influenced by tests ordered, medications administered, length of stay, and treatments prescribed. This is the component of cost over which we have the most control. Most studies on cost reduction and increased efficiency focus on decreasing the variable costs.

The incremental marginal costs are associated with putting one more patient through the system. Marginal costs are usually negligible in health care unless caring for the patient creates an increase in fixed costs, such as requiring overtime.

Trauma Program Resource Allocation

Personnel Resources

Costs associated with trauma care include several factors, most of which fall in the category of either personnel (concerned with individual workers) or nonlabor (related to supplies and capital equipment). A trauma program is complicated by the need for service to be available at all times, 24 hours a day, 7 days a week. A trauma program affects every department in the hospital in some way, from prehospital care to rehabilitation, including every support service. The most expensive allocation of any trauma program is the professional and ancillary personnel required to staff it. Staffing of the program depends on the level of service provided. In many Level I or II trauma centers, nursing and ancillary services are staffed 24 hours a day to meet the demands of existing programs such as emergency services, cardiac surgery, labor and delivery, and critical care. This may not be true of centers desiring to increase their level of service or of rural centers.

Each trauma program requires, at minimum, a trauma program manager (TPM) and a trauma medical director. The TPM at a Level I or II facility is typically a masters-prepared nurse working in a full-time capacity. In high-volume Level I and II centers, it is necessary to budget additional support to the TPM, such as case managers, additional trauma coordinators, nurse practitioners, physician assistants, injury prevention coordinators, clinical nurse specialists, educators, trauma registry analysts, and billers and coders. It is important to understand the additional requirements of a Level I or II center as they relate to performance improvement (PI), professional education, public education, injury prevention activities, and research. For PI activities at a busy Level I or II center, depending on volume, one to three trauma registrars may be needed to manage data-reporting requirements. Many organizations use existing resources in their nursing or professional education departments to meet the educational demands of the trauma program. In some instances, these resources do not exist and must be added. However the functions are assigned, it must be realized that trauma care has unique requirements for professional education, which must be considered during planning and budgeting. Level I trauma centers have taken a lead role in trauma outreach and injury prevention, fully integrating activities within existing community special interest groups and programs.

Depending on trauma patient volume, the TPM in a Level III or IV center may perform other duties, such as working as the nurse manager of the ED or critical care area. Because the hospital's commitment to public education, professional education, outreach, research, and injury prevention is substantially less or nonexistent at this level, the staff requirement can be adjusted accordingly.

The trauma medical director must be a general surgeon regardless of the level of service provided. His or her time commitment to the program varies according to the level of service, that is, Level I versus Level IV. The number and variety of compensation programs for surgeons and specialists are as varied as the number of trauma centers. Administrators should be aware that it is customary to pay an annual administrative fee to a medical director and compensate the surgeons providing call. Contracts for service must comply with all antikickback statutes or inurement standards required by state and federal laws. In most Level I centers, the trauma surgeons are covering emergency general surgery and surgical critical care. The requirements for surgical subspecialists such as orthopedics, neurosurgery, emergency medicine, and anesthesia must be considered. Level II and III facilities are typically covered with private practice physicians rotating call. These scenarios vary, again depending on the culture of the organization and the resources at hand.

Supplies and Equipment

Most trauma centers allocate costs for clinical supplies related to patient care through the department where the service is rendered. Budgeting supplies for an entire fiscal year requires an understanding of how to project trends in supply use, census, and inflation.

Capital Equipment

As in any hospital budget, capital equipment is defined by the dollar amount of the purchase. Priorities in capital expenses are set on the basis of several factors. Equipment that will contribute to the revenue of the hospital will most likely receive high priority in the budget process. Ideally, the costs of the equipment and the anticipated annual operating costs will be either less than or, at minimum, balanced against the revenue. Equipment needed for patient safety and quality care is also given high priority in budgeting although no revenue is anticipated directly from its use. Trauma program capital equipment is often allocated to the department where it will be housed or for which it will be charged, such as the operating room, radiology, or critical care areas.

Professional Education

Each trauma center is committed to some level of participation in professional education. The standards for professional education are rigorous, and meeting them can be costly. The standards span the continuum of trauma care, encompassing prehospital providers, nurses, physicians, and ancillary personnel. Many hospitals provide paid educational days, free continuing education opportunities within the organization, tuition reimbursement, and advanced training in specialty areas or certification within professional groups. Each trauma center must be cognizant of the educational requirements for the level of service they seek to provide and must develop a written plan as to how the requirements will be met. Inherent in the plan should be a commitment to funding commensurate with the level of care the hospital will provide.

Trauma education is multidisciplinary in keeping with the fundamental idea of a team approach. The PI program should set priorities for continuing educational offerings. Funding of professional education within the trauma center is an objective measurement of institutional commitment to the trauma program and the system as a whole.

Injury Prevention

Trauma centers play an important role in reducing the occurrence of injury by providing or participating in injury prevention activities. Data from the trauma registry can be used to identify the patterns, frequency, and risks of injury. In many states, regional trauma committees aggregate data to prioritize needs. The development and maintenance of injury prevention programs can be costly, so the ability to work collaboratively within a region, optimizing the integration of existing community coalitions, is critical for success.

Injury prevention activities do not happen just from the kindness of volunteers in the trauma center. Every trauma center, regardless of resources, has a commitment to injury prevention. Anticipating the cost of fulfilling this commitment is imperative when writing the injury prevention portion of the trauma center strategic plan. The plan must be evaluated periodically and changed as the type and frequency of traumatic events change in the community and during the maturation of the trauma program.

Research

Ideally, all trauma centers will participate in research activities as their resources and patient population allow. Traditionally, the requirement to conduct research to advance knowledge in trauma care and trauma systems has distinguished a Level I trauma center from other trauma centers. Research requires funding, and the administration of Level I centers should contribute to the effort with financial support of facilities and personnel. The level of funding dedicated to research activities is another objective measurement of institutional commitment to the trauma program.

Expanded Roles for Nursing

The trauma nurse practitioner (TNP) is a vital role in the acute care arena, serving as a midlevel practitioner who provides high-quality care within cost-containment constraints.[25] TNPs have a variety of responsibilities as a part of the trauma team. Their major role is direct patient care along with facilitating collaboration, coordination, and communication between the trauma surgeon and other subspecialty services. More specifically, the TNP's responsibilities include care of the trauma patient from the resuscitation bay to the intensive care unit and to the floor through discharge and clinic follow-up.

As the number of residency programs in the specialties decreases, the TNP can fulfill some of the responsibilities formerly performed by less-well-prepared residents. With the advent of resident hour restrictions, the TNP provides the consistency on the trauma service and commonly manages the stable in-house trauma patients. The TNP plays a key role in medication reconciliation, patient progression (timely discharge), patient and family education about the injury process, and discharge care. The TNP also has a key role in patient safety initiatives and patient satisfaction. It is the TNP who ensures that appropriate services are consulted such as pain management, dietary, and therapies to enhance multidisciplinary patient care delivery. The TNP typically manages the postinjury trauma clinics. The successful implementation of this role has afforded the opportunity to allow trauma surgeons and house staff to prioritize and maximize their time in the resuscitative phase and emergency surgery. If multiple trauma patients arrive simultaneously, the TNP can assist with the resuscitation. The TNP can be a very valuable member of the trauma team and reduce the overall costs to the trauma center.

The hallmark study published in the *Journal of Trauma* in 1990 demonstrated the value of TNPs on the trauma team. Spisso et al.[26] retrospectively examined the use of nurse practitioners in a tertiary care center. Outcomes were measured for 12 months before and after implementation of the TNP role. The findings demonstrated the value of the TNP, including decreased length of stay for trauma patients, increased documentation of quality of care, decrease in patient complaints, and documented time savings for house staff.[26]

Administrative Issues in Trauma Care

The successful management of any area of health care requires skill, talent, and creative leadership. Knowledge of current health care issues, such as changes in reimbursement practices, legal and political implications of such changes, and personnel management, is essential in administration. A clear understanding of social and political motivating factors is critical to every health care administrator. Health care is a business, requiring managers to provide a businesslike approach in their decisions, keeping cost containment as a goal while still maintaining optimal provision of care. Innovative approaches to management are greatly valued, and leaders in trauma care have been at the forefront of ensuring quality patient outcomes while responding thoughtfully to institutional and national fiscal concerns.

Trauma center administrators are faced with significant pressures today. The demand for hospital care is rising, both outpatient and inpatient. At the same time, total margins in hospitals are down 22% since 1997.[27] Growing government (Medicare and Medicaid) shortfalls relative to costs put many hospitals' financial health at risk. Shortages in the workforce for selected key caregiving positions further drive up costs. As our nation faces increased risk of natural and human-provoked disasters, our health care system has become disproportionately reliant on trauma centers to provide required resources and services. According to the Institute of Medicine report on emergency care, three fourths of hospitals report difficulty finding specialists to take emergency and trauma calls.[28] Many institutions have had to relax bylaws, forcing physician participation in on-call panels, which further burdens the trauma centers. At any given time in any community, the only hospital to have specialty call available (including general surgery and orthopedics, which was traditionally available in most urban hospitals) is the trauma center. Because many systems have no provisions for trauma centers to divert, trauma centers are seeing a higher number of minor injuries because the necessary specialist is no longer on call to the community hospital. Additionally, the requirements of the Emergency Medical Treatment and Active Labor Act have become onerous to trauma centers because by virtue of the resources available, the trauma centers are almost always in the position to provide a higher level of care.

At the same time the ability of trauma centers to provide the depth of call coverage in many specialties has diminished. The increased burden of call pay is crippling many institutions. Well over half of the EDs across our nation reported they were at capacity in 2005 and, as a result, were forced to divert ambulances and patients to other facilities. The issue is more problematic at teaching hospitals (Level I trauma centers), of which 79% reported that their ED was at or over capacity.[29] Patients wait hours to be seen by the emergency physician and then, once admission to the hospital is required, they wait hours or days for an inpatient bed to become available.[28] Overcrowding is a topic all to itself, and an in-depth discussion is beyond the scope of this chapter, but it is integral to the crises trauma centers are facing today.

Physicians and nurses today are increasingly unwilling to work in understaffed stressful conditions when lives are at risk. The issue is compounded by an aging workforce, which makes fewer surgeons available for ED coverage. A growing shortage of surgical specialists threatens access to emergency services. The number of surgeons trained has remained stable but has been outpaced by our U.S. population growth. The elderly make up a disproportionate share of the surgical population. The "graying of America" places higher demand on the supply of specialists.[29] About half the residency matches of all general surgery residents go on to pursue fellowships and subspecialization. The result over time is that many surgeons no longer feel qualified to manage the range of problems associated with emergency and certainly trauma call.

Hospitals today are faced with burdening responsibilities of patient safety and public reporting of data to participate in federal funding. Although there is no question that this is the right thing to do for patients, the burden of cost to implement, to educate practitioners, and to provide tools to successfully operationalize change falls to the hospitals.

The Role of Administration in a Trauma Care Delivery System

Health care is in transition, and trauma care is no exception. Historically the direction of trauma care has been toward the development of trauma centers, using a rational approach based on the concept of centralization, of tertiary care.[30] Since the inception of organized trauma care, care has been provided in regional systems driven by the most severely injured trauma patients, requiring treatment at a designated trauma center.[11] The paradigm has shifted to an inclusive model of trauma care. Emphasis has changed, recognizing that few individual facilities can provide all resources to all comers in all situations. Trauma systems are designed to match each trauma care provider or facility's resources to the needs of the injured patient. The trauma center is an integral player in a trauma system that encompasses all phases of care from hospital discharge through rehabilitation and re-entry into society. Trauma systems must be fully integrated into emergency medical services (EMS) systems and attempt to meet the needs of all injured patients regardless of the severity of injury.[11]

Given the inclusive model of trauma care systems, administrators of trauma centers can no longer focus on the trauma center only. Trauma center administrators must be involved in multiple components of the trauma system to ensure the efficacy of the system and thereby the success of their own centers within the system. The administrative components of a trauma system consist of leadership, authority, planning and development, legislation, and finances.[11] These components are essential for the success of a trauma system and are fundamental to the success of a trauma center as well.

The model trauma plan mentioned earlier in this chapter describes the leadership role in a trauma care system from multiple perspectives. On a statewide level, there needs to be a lead agency with the authority to provide overall system development. This typically falls to the state department of health, with some notable exceptions. In California, individual counties or groups of counties have developed trauma systems that are based on authority granted by state statute. In Pennsylvania, the state agency has delegated the authority for system development and management to the Pennsylvania Trauma Foundation. In Florida and Massachusetts, state and regionally based agencies share authority for the development and operation of trauma systems.[12,13]

Typically, the lead agency is responsible for establishing standards for system performance. The lead agency serves as the arbitrator to ensure integration of the trauma system and the EMS system and make certain of cooperation across state lines with no thought to geographic boundaries. The lead agency must have established authority that is based on enabling legislation and, ideally, legislation that provides funding for the system. Key provisions of enabling legislation include plan development, integration of trauma and EMS systems, adoption of standards for trauma care, organization of data collection systems, system evaluation, confidentiality protection for performance improvement activities, and authorization for funding.[11,30]

On a local level, many states (e.g., Montana, Mississippi, Oregon, and North Dakota) have developed a regional trauma committee structure typically led by a Level I or Level II trauma center. These committees are developed geographically on the basis of regional referral patterns. They function to develop treatment and transfer guidelines, conduct PI activities, share collective resources to develop public and professional education programs, and coordinate injury prevention activities. These committees are integrated with local EMS functions and serve as the conduit for communication among providers for local, state, and national changes. Many regional committees report to a state trauma advisory committee, the functions and membership of which are set by statute.

Because system development and continuous changes occur at the regional or state committee level, it is imperative that senior administrators of the trauma center actively participate on these committees. Decisions regarding catchment areas, trauma center standards, funding of indigent care, and changes in legislation can dramatically affect the survival of an individual trauma center. The administrator's participation at local and state lead agency meetings is a major strength to a program and an obvious measurable indication of the institution's commitment to the trauma system.

State and local trauma care committees are commonly composed of members appointed by professional associations, such as the state hospital association or medical association. To this end, it is essential that senior administrators not delegate this responsibility if they are invited to represent their own peer group.

Administrative Components of a Trauma Program

The success of any organization largely depends on the planning and vision of the leaders. Trauma programs must be planned strategically to ensure their initial success and maturation within the regional system and the institution. In the late 1970s and early 1980s and to some degree today, the administration of the trauma program within an institution was delegated largely to the TPM and the medical director. These two individuals ensured the quality of care, monitored adherence to regulatory standards, and facilitated public and professional education. Strategic planning for the program was never considered, and administrators were rarely involved with its maturation. The program manager was a middle-level manager responsible for a product line within the organization. The institution as a whole did not share in the planning, evaluation, or accountability of the program.

In today's health care environment, it is essential that the administration of any trauma program be integrally involved with the trauma program strategic plan. This plan should be determined by available resources, community needs, and socioeconomic factors and driven by consensus of the medical staff and administration, including nursing. The plan should be motivated by outcome measurements common to the organization and fully integrated with areas of excellence already established within the institutional culture. The hospital board of trustees or directors must be fully committed to the trauma program and provide necessary support. The planning process should be influenced by available data and should involve key clinical leaders and medical staff visionaries. The process should begin with an assessment of community needs, followed by an analysis of the appropriate trauma center standards to begin the determination of resources available within the organization. Hospitals must decide where their organization best fits within the regional trauma system and determine what level of service is appropriate for their organization. An assessment of current capabilities compared with the required standards will give the management team the opportunity to identify deficiencies and create opportunities for improvement. Once a decision is made as to what level of service will be provided, educational forums should be executed to convey accurate information to all key players. Financial barriers must be addressed. Medical staff commitment must be assessed. Strengths and weaknesses must be analyzed realistically, and threats to the organization must be addressed, whether they are real or perceived. A work plan should be developed to address the deficiencies and a budget prepared to commit resources in a way that will guarantee the success of the trauma program. This level of planning and decision making requires administrative leadership and will not be successful if delegated to a well-meaning trauma nurse coordinator.

The trauma center strategic plan should be reassessed and refined at various stages during the life span of the trauma center. Certainly before and after an accreditation process an evaluation should occur, and it should be repeated subsequently in 3- to 5-year increments. As the program matures, the performance improvement process should guide the evolution of the plan.

The administrative structure of a trauma program defines institutional support and organizational commitment. The structure must include an accountable administrator, a medical director, and program manager. The medical director and program manager must be given the power and authority to administer the trauma program. The program must be positioned strategically within the organizational structure so that it may interact with equal authority with other departments that provide patient care services.[3] There should be written resolutions by the administration/board and medical staff supporting the trauma program. Typically a management council or executive planning committee meets on a regular interval to manage the administrative policy, marketing, and overall health of the program. This committee determines the resources necessary to adhere to regulatory demands and to support the fiscal wellness of the program. The peer review committees of the trauma program deal with clinical performance improvement issues and should have direct reporting linkage to the hospital executive committee or quality councils. Without strong administrative leadership and vision, the planning and implementation of a trauma program within an organization and subsequently within a region will be jeopardized.

Trauma Center Accreditation

Trauma accreditation systems have been developed to meet the unique needs of trauma systems and trauma centers within the systems. The regulatory entity in a region or state will design a system to determine whether trauma hospitals are meeting the criteria written in their trauma systems plan. Typically, states either adopt the current standards published by the Committee on Trauma of the ACS or, through a committee process, write their own standards based on the college's criteria. These standards are customized to meet the unique needs of the individual state on the basis of available resources. Only the regulatory entity has the legal authority to designate a trauma hospital. Enabling legislation discussed previously in this chapter is the basis of this authority.

Trauma center accreditation usually occurs in one of two ways. The first is through the verification and consultation program of the ACS. The program may be conducted in a two-part process. Members of the Committee on Trauma conduct a consultation visit at the request of the hospital, community, or state authority. The purpose of the consultation is to assess current trauma care and to prepare the facility for a subsequent verification visit.[3] The consultation visit is typically conducted by a team of two general surgeons and results in a written list of recommendations for program improvement on the basis of the latest version of the *Resources for Optimal Care of the Injured Patient.*[31] Through trauma center verification the college verifies that a hospital is performing as a trauma center and meets established criteria.[3] The college's process of verification is one method used by states to ensure that trauma centers are meeting the standards specified in the state trauma plan.

The other method of verifying trauma centers' compliance with written standards is the use of independent reviewers hired by the regulatory agency to verify that the trauma care provided meets the standards as written. Typically this process uses a multidisciplinary team approach. The teams are composed of an experienced trauma surgeon, a trauma nurse, a trauma center administrator, an EMS administrator, and possibly a neurosurgeon, orthopedic surgeon, or emergency medicine specialist, depending on the needs of the regulatory agency. The team is asked to substantiate for the regulatory agency that the hospital is in compliance with the approved trauma center standards for the region.

Regardless of the approach, there are cost implications, both direct and indirect, associated with the trauma center accreditation process that need to be considered by the trauma center. Because of the political and fiscal implications to the trauma center, administration must be intricately involved in the planning for the site review and must participate on the day of the verification visit. It is important that managers at all levels have an understanding of the trauma center standards so that the implications for their own departments are clear.

After successful completion of the accreditation process, most regulatory authorities will formally designate trauma hospitals for a period of time. Typically, if the hospital substantially meets the criteria, it is awarded a 3-year contract for service. This period varies depending on the maturity of the trauma system. Trauma center accreditation processes usually contain an appeal method to allow the hospital the right to resolve disagreements.

Summary

The financial aspects of trauma care are extremely complex. On the public policy side is the continued lack of recognition of the tremendous economic burden that injury, unintentional or intentional, has on the public welfare of this country. On the hospital practitioner side is the tremendous financial burden of providing high-quality care to these patients. Addressing these problems requires a multipronged approach.

Lobbying for improved reimbursement from government programs that provide coverage for health care is of continued importance. As the population ages, more Medicare dollars will be spent on health care. Active lobbying of local and state legislatures is also necessary to ensure support of trauma systems. Letters and testimony can influence the process of legislating changes in reimbursement laws.

As practitioners of trauma care, we must assume our responsibility in controlling the costs of care. Examining the costs of providing trauma care is the first step in identifying changes that can be made. Improving the cost efficiency of diagnostic and therapeutic procedures and changing the delivery of care can make a significant difference in the viability of the trauma service. Practitioners must learn more about health economics, a discipline concerned with determining the best way of using available health care resources to maximize the health of the community.

Because administration is an interpersonal process, it relies greatly on managers to influence, motivate, catalyze, and facilitate activities that lead to fulfillment of the organization's mission. The challenge of trauma care provides an unparalleled opportunity for innovative managers to effect system changes. Although the challenges presented to the administrator are constantly changing and evolving, the astute individual uses this opportunity to design innovative systems that support quality outcomes. The successful trauma program relies on aggressive administrative leadership and planning processes that are evaluated constantly and changed to respond to the needs of the community and institution and the unique needs of the trauma program.

References

1. National Safety Council: *Injury facts, 2004 edition.* Itasca, IL, 2004, National Safety Council.
2. Finkelstein EA, Corso PS, Miller TR: *The incidence and economic burden of injuries in the United States,* New York, 2006, Oxford University Press.
3. U.S. Department of Health, Education, and Welfare: *Accidental death and disability: the neglected disease of modern society,* Rockville, MD, 1966, Division of Medical Sciences, National Academy of Sciences, National Research Council.
4. Cowley RA: Trauma center: a new concept for the delivery of critical care, *J Med Soc N J* 74:979-986, 1977.
5. Taylor B: Seen by the right people with the right patient in the right facility: close encounters of the Cowley kind: an inclusive journal interview with R. Adams Cowley, MD, Director of the Maryland Institute for Emergency Medical Services, State of Maryland, *MD State Med J* 27:35-49, 1978.
6. Highway Safety Act of 1966 (PL89-564. September 9, 1966).
7. Emergency Medical Services System Act of 1973 (PL 93-154, November 16, 1973).
8. West JG, Trunkey DD, Lim RC: Systems of trauma care: a study of two counties, *Arch Surg* 114:455-460, 1979.

9. Committee on Trauma Research, Commission on Life Services, National Research Council, Institute of Medicine: *Injury in America: a continuing public health problem*, Washington, DC, 1985, National Academy Press.
10. Trauma Systems Planning and Development Act of 1990 (PL 101-590, 1990).
11. Health Resources and Services Administration: *Model trauma system planning and evaluation,* Washington, DC, 2006, US Department of Health and Human Services Program Support Center, Visual Communications Branch.
12. Bazzoli GJ, Madura KJ, Cooper GF et al: Progress in the development of trauma systems in the United States: results of a national survey, *JAMA* 273:395-401, 1995.
13. Bass RR, Gainer PS, Carlini AR: Update on trauma system development in the United States, *J Trauma*, 47:S15-S21, 1999.
14. Health Resources and Services Administration, Trauma-EMS Systems Program: *National assessment of state trauma system development, emergency medical services resources, and disaster readiness for mass casualty events,* Rockville, MD, 2003, Health Resources and Services Administration.
15. National Foundation for Trauma Care: *Trauma funding imperils access to trauma care*, Las Cruces, NM, 2006, National Foundation for Trauma Care.
16. Daily JT, Teter H, Cowley RA: Trauma center closures: a national assessment. *J Trauma* 33:539-547, 1992.
17. Reed RL, Luchette F, Davis KA et al: Medicare's bundling of trauma care codes violates relative value principles, *J Trauma* 57:1164-1172, 2004.
18. Rodriguez JL, Christmas AB, Franklin GA et al: Trauma/critical care surgeon: a specialist gasping for air, *J Trauma* 59:1-7, 2005.
19. Rogers FB, Shackford SR, Osler TM et al: Rural trauma: the challenge for the next decade, *J Trauma* 47:802, 1999.
20. Selzer D, Gomez D, Jacobson L et al: Public hospital-based Level I trauma centers: financial survival in the new millennium, *J Trauma* 51:301-307, 2001.
21. Centers for Medicaid and Medicare Services: Outpatient Prospective Payment System and Physician Fee Schedule, *http://www.cms.hhs.gov.* Accessed February 1, 2007.
22. Durham R, Pracht E, Orban B et al: Evaluation of a mature trauma system, *J Trauma* 243:775-785, 2006.
23. Taheri PA, Wahl EL, Butz DA et al: Trauma service cost: the real story, *J Trauma* 227:720-725, 1998.
24. Taheri PA, Butz DA, Griffes LC et al: Physician impact on the total cost of trauma care, *J Trauma* 231:432-435, 2000.
25. Cupuro PA, Alperovich CG: Letters to the editor, *J Trauma* 43:988, 1997.
26. Spisso J, O'Callaghan C, McKennan M et al: Improved quality of care and reduction in house staff workload using trauma nurse practitioners, *J Trauma* 30:660-665, 1990.
27. American Hospital Association: *The state of America's hospitals—taking the pulse, findings from the 2006 AHA survey of hospital leaders,* Chicago, IL, 2006, American Hospital Association.
28. Institute of Medicine of the National Academies: *The future of emergency care in the United States health system:* http://www.nap.edu. Accessed December 19, 2006.
29. American College of Surgeons: *A growing crisis in patient access to emergency medical surgical care,* Chicago, IL, 2006, American College of Surgeons.
30. Cales RH, Heilig RW: *Trauma care systems: a guide to planning, implementation operation and evaluation,* Rockville, MD, 1986, Aspen Publishers.
31. American College of Surgeons' Committee on Trauma: *Resources for the optimal care of the injured patient,* Chicago, IL, 2006, American College of Surgeons.

3

Performance Improvement and Patient Safety in Trauma Care

Mary Kate FitzPatrick, Janet McMaster

Historical Perspective of Performance Improvement in Trauma Care

A universal condition of trauma center designation is that specified injury data must be collected, analyzed, and maintained. In addition, the data must be monitored routinely by the trauma program in an effort to improve performance. The standards published by the American College of Surgeons (ACS) Committee on Trauma in *Resources for Optimal Care of the Injured Patient* are the foundation for performance review in trauma centers.[1] These standards have continued to evolve and were most recently updated in 2006.

The terms and principles related to quality have gone through many changes in recent times. "Quality assurance," "quality improvement," "continuous quality improvement," "total quality management," and "performance improvement" are all approaches to quality review that have been used in the past.[2] A major conceptual shift in these approaches has been the movement from a punitive quality assurance model to the more accepted system/process review. In addition, performance improvement in health care settings is being more closely integrated with patient safety. The health care industry continues to evolve its methodology for quality review, and the days of the "ABCs" of morbidity and mortality (*a*ccuse, *b*lame, and *c*riticize) are fading. This system/process performance improvement model is focused on outcomes, benchmarking, and performance of the system as a whole and moves away from emphasis on reviewing an individual's practice as a root cause. There must, however, also be a structured physician peer review process to evaluate clinical competency. Traditionally, hospital performance improvement and quality improvement have been service-line or unit specific. Depending on the institution, specific performance or quality committees would develop and implement projects, quite often following The Joint Commission (formerly known as the Joint Commission on Accreditation of Healthcare Organizations [JCAHO]) format, the performance improvement cycle (Figure 3-1). In the trauma care arena, there are standards that outline the basic type of performance review that trauma centers need to complete. Included in these standards are recommendations for performance indicators (including definitions) that should be monitored over time. Because of the strict standards set forth by trauma center accrediting agencies, often it is the trauma program that leads performance improvement efforts in hospitals.

Health care practitioners struggle to understand and operationalize the concepts of what we now call performance improvement. The popular literature on quality, which includes the works of pioneers such as Juran and Deming, is focused on industrial settings. W. E. Deming, considered one of the leading figures in the movement to measure quality in industry, developed theories that are widely published. His work has been applied to multiple venues outside the traditional business world, including health care. *Out of the Crisis* (1986),[3] considered one of Deming's major works, provides anecdotes and examples of how to put his theories into practice.

A particular challenge to health care practitioners is determining how to apply techniques and principles designed for more "constant" industrial environments to the unpredictable and dynamic practice of medicine. One example of a methodology that was initially developed for manufacturing and that has been applied to health care is Six Sigma. This is a structured format that uses reliable and valid data and statistics to improve performance by identifying and eliminating variations or "defects" in processes.[4] The current environment in health care has presented additional challenges in the quest to operationalize performance improvement. Human and financial resources are lean and patient demographics are changing. To our advantage, however, are modern technologic advancements and the power of computerization in the maintenance and analysis of patient data.

Patient Safety

The Joint Commission oversees the development and annual updating of the National Patient Safety Goals and Requirements. This process is overseen by an expert panel that includes a multidisciplinary team including patient safety experts, nurses, physicians, pharmacists, risk managers, and other professionals who have hands-on experience in addressing patient safety issues in a wide variety of health care settings. Trauma programs, with mature performance

HOW DO WE DO PERFORMANCE IMPROVEMENT?

PLAN Identify an opportunity for improvement, measure current performance, set goals and develop an improvement plan.

DO Implement improvement plan by identifying resources and piloting the solution.

CHECK Measure performance again to see if the plan worked.

ACT Standardize the process and monitor to sustain improvement.

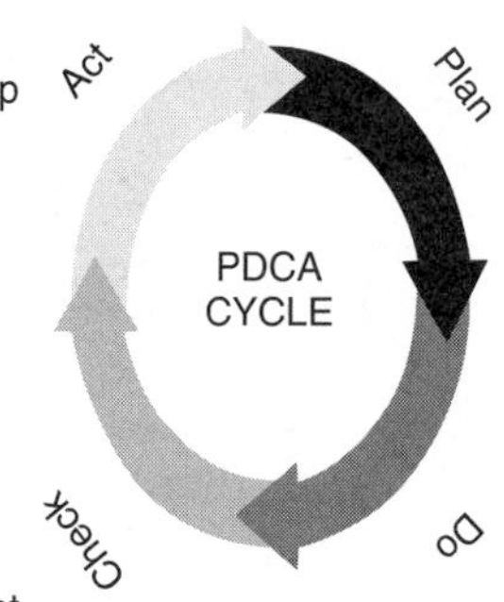

FIGURE 3-1. Performance improvement cycle. (From The Joint Commission: *Joint Commission accreditation manual,* Oakbrook Terrace, Ill, 1998, The Joint Commission.)

improvement programs, have traditionally provided a model approach to monitoring potentially high-risk events and ensuring a review of cases where defined risk criteria are present. The ACS in the 2006 edition of *Resources for Optimal Care of the Injured Patient,* has recognized that performance improvement and patient safety are intricately linked and should be approached in unison. The patient safety process is focused on the environment in which care is given and the performance improvement process is directed at the care provided. The boundaries between these two often cross over and in many cases are indistinguishable.

A number of topics central to the delivery of trauma care provide excellent examples of practical links between patient safety and performance improvement. Some of the past patient safety goals set forth by The Joint Commission, such as patient identification, right site surgery, medication safety, and communications/handoffs are particularly relevant to trauma care delivery. Each of these presents unique challenges to the trauma program. Given the rapidity of the initial evaluation, the routine need for urgent surgery, and the issues related to workforce shortages, all these Joint Commission safety goals are reasonable focus points in the trauma performance improvement program.[5]

Another approach that has become very important in hospital care delivery is the concept of rapid response teams. These teams are designed to be deployed early to assist patients in distress (precardiac/respiratory arrest) and to avoid a full-arrest response. The concept is to activate an in-house emergency response team early when a patient is in trouble to potentially avoid a code situation. Some institutions have implemented rapid response/readiness teams modeled after trauma resuscitation teams. Utilizing strategies used by trauma performance improvement programs to monitor team effectiveness is a likely model to evaluate the effectiveness of rapid response teams. From a number of perspectives, closer integration of clinical effectiveness, trauma performance improvement, and patient safety initiatives throughout an institution has the potential to evaluate/affect care on a larger scale.

TRAUMA PERFORMANCE IMPROVEMENT PLAN

Trauma programs should establish a written trauma performance improvement plan that addresses basic operational details and contains an overview of the process. This plan should be the result of a multidisciplinary effort and should be a dynamic document that is reevaluated periodically and updated to encompass key changes within the hospital trauma system and trauma care standards. The trauma performance improvement plan should clearly integrate with the hospital performance improvement plan. There should be descriptions on how outcomes are shared with the hospital structure, for example, through linkages to the department of surgery, the medical executive committee, or the even the board of directors. Recommended distribution of the plan might include hospital quality improvement staff, nursing leadership, physician leadership from medical divisions involved in trauma care, and trauma program staff. This plan could be used as part of the orientation process for new hospital leadership who will be responsible for trauma patient care. The performance improvement plan should include the following:

- Overview of the process—issue identification
- Personnel involved and their roles
- Performance improvement forums/committees
- Link to hospital/system performance improvement
- Performance indicators (dynamic)/patient safety goals
- Data maintenance methods
- Guidelines for determining peer review judgment decisions (accountability)
- Performance improvement reports/provider profiles
- Performance improvement loop closure (reevaluation)
- Provision for protection of confidentiality

The performance improvement plan should consider state, regional, and national standards related to trauma care. The ACS document titled *Trauma Performance Improvement, A How to Handbook* provides practitioners with an operational manual for establishing and maintaining a trauma performance improvement program.[6] In addition, programs such as the Society of Trauma Nurses Trauma Outcomes Performance Improvement Course "T.O.P.I.C." assist practitioners with developing a comprehensive trauma performance improvement plan and provides practical approaches to operationalizing performance improvement in all levels of trauma centers.[7]

INTEGRATION OF TRAUMA PERFORMANCE IMPROVEMENT WITH INSTITUTION AND SYSTEM PERFORMANCE IMPROVEMENT

Trauma programs lead the way in many institutions in terms of the depth, scope, and sophistication of performance improvement reviews. It is important that trauma programs be integrated into the overall hospital or system quality structure. Many health care organizations have adopted service-line teams to oversee performance improvement–related projects. Trauma crosses over and affects many service lines of the hospital structure, including nursing, emergency medicine, neurosurgery, anesthesia, orthopedics, rehabilitation services, radiology, laboratory services, perioperative care, critical care, nutrition, and the blood bank. It is challenging to devise a single initiative that coordinates the activities of the multiple service lines through which care is provided to trauma patients. There must be some means of overseeing continuing projects and determining areas of overlap, mutual benefit, and level of impact. For example, many hospitals collect intensive care unit (ICU) data; these data could be stratified to look at trends specifically within the trauma patient group. Conversely, data maintained by the trauma program may be stratified by phases of care and reported through the hospital performance improvement structure. Analysis of various levels of data from hospital departments can generate specific institutional projects. Projects that have the highest return on investment should be selected. Projects that target key areas or have strong potential to affect outcomes, patient satisfaction, or cost should be prioritized.

Health care organizations are required by The Joint Commission to respond to sentinel events, defined as unexpected occurrences involving death or serious physical or psychologic injury, or any event that carries a significant chance of a serious adverse outcome. Appropriate responses include the following:

- Conducting a thorough and credible root cause analysis, focusing on systems and processes, not individual performance
- Implementing improvements to reduce risk
- Monitoring the effectiveness of those improvements

The trauma performance improvement program must have a mechanism in place to report any identified sentinel events to the hospital department or committee responsible for Joint Commission compliance.

Two useful techniques for analyzing unexpected outcomes are (1) FMECA (*f*ailure *m*ode, *e*ffect, and *c*riticality *a*nalysis), which is a systematic way to examine a process for possible ways that failure can occur, usually initiated by a "near miss" incident, and (2) root cause analysis, which looks for the cause of variation after a sentinel event or unexpected outcome has taken place.[8,9] Regardless of the analysis technique used, benchmarking with other similar centers provides meaningful perspective for trauma programs.

Patient/Issue Identification

Identifying patients for trauma performance improvement review can be challenging. In hospitals without a designated trauma service, patients can be admitted to any one of a number of surgical or medical services. To help identify patients admitted with injury-related diagnoses, hospital information systems can produce reports with diagnoses, injury codes, and reasons for admission. The emergency department log or the admission log can be used to identify trauma patients. Often this is done by using an indicator assigned by emergency department admissions staff or through customized admission reports using primary or secondary diagnosis or physician name. The trauma program needs to have validation steps in place to ensure that all appropriate injured patients are captured by the registry on the basis of established inclusion criteria.

Information for performance improvement review comes from many sources. Prehospital records, including fire, rescue, or ambulance records, and flight records from air ambulances, can provide information about the scene conditions, treatment rendered, and length of time at the scene. The patient's medical record is the main source for identifying performance improvement issues. The emergency department and trauma resuscitation documents should be designed to capture the timing and sequence of the resuscitation easily because this is key to evaluating care. Parts of the medical record that provide important performance improvement information may include the following:

- Physician documentation on progress notes or consultation records
- Perioperative records, including anesthesia notes and postanesthesia care notes
- Nurses' notes
- Radiology and laboratory reports
- Physical and occupational therapy notes
- Social work, pastoral care, or case management notes
- Transfer records for patients referred from another facility

Because many hospitals have converted to electronic records, it will become essential for the person responsible for performance improvement to have access to the entire medical record, including electronically stored documents/information.

In addition to review of the medical record, it is helpful to have a mechanism for health care providers in all areas of the hospital, on all shifts, to provide referrals to the performance improvement process. They can report issues by a confidential, dedicated phone "hotline" or through issue identification forms, which can be submitted confidentially. Significant issues that affect patient care should also be reported to risk management through appropriate institutional channels. Ideally, communication with risk management is two way. Issues reported to the hospital-wide incident/quality reporting system can be channeled to the trauma program for further action and follow-up. Audiovisual recording of trauma resuscitations can identify opportunities for improvement that may not be evident through medical record review. Examples are provider compliance with standard precautions, evaluation of overall team interactions, and the monitoring of proper technique during procedures such as urinary catheter placement.

Other departments in the hospital may be a source of information regarding performance improvement issues.

Infectious disease reports can identify patients with complications such as urinary tract infections or pneumonia, supporting or validating trauma performance improvement data. Postdischarge records are a source of information regarding outcomes because they may identify missed injuries, delayed diagnoses, readmissions, or patient satisfaction issues. It is important that there are processes to identify and report performance improvement issues in the trauma outpatient arena. Postdischarge information can be obtained from outpatient records, feedback from rehabilitation facilities, follow-up from home care agencies, or autopsy reports. The medical examiner or coroner can often provide additional valuable data at mortality review forums. This can be achieved through direct participation of medical examiner staff or through the retrospective review of written or verbal autopsy reports.

Trauma Performance Improvement Process: Levels of Review

There are many ways to structure a review of clinical care. Having both concurrent and retrospective features is ideal. Key steps should be established and should be modified on the basis of the specific features of the trauma program (size, volume, resources, etc.). Key elements in the performance improvement process are diagrammed in Figure 3-2.

Data collection for performance improvement can occur concurrently with abstraction of data while care is being provided **(primary review).** The person in charge of concurrent review, usually a nurse (typically the trauma coordinator/program manager, trauma performance improvement coordinator, trauma case manager, or trauma advanced practitioners), or trained trauma registrar, uses various mechanisms to identify and follow up on issues as they occur. Patient care rounds, chart reviews, and direct staff and patient interaction are among the sources of data for concurrent review. The major advantages of concurrent review are that it allows (1) changes to occur in the patient's plan of care, which can influence outcome immediately, and (2) prompt feedback to providers regarding quality-of-care issues. One disadvantage is that it precludes an overview of the entirety of the case with all patient data from dictated radiology reports, discharge information, and postdischarge follow-up. Retrospective review occurs after the patient has been discharged, with data abstracted from medical records, registry reports, and so on **(secondary review).** During secondary review, decisions are made to determine where in the performance process the case/issues should go next. This could include closing the case (no action needed), referral to other service for review and comment, referral to an established performance improvement committee for in-depth review, and analysis by the peer review judgment determination process **(tertiary review).**

Retrospective review provides a comprehensive assessment of overall care and affords the opportunity to see trends in data and to compile statistics on groups of patients for analysis. The limitations of performing only retrospective reviews are (1) feedback to individual providers is delayed, (2) incidents must be reconstructed from memory, and most important, (3) patient care cannot be affected in "real time." A mature, comprehensive performance improvement program will have components of both concurrent and retrospective reviews.

Performance Improvement Forums

Case Selection Guidelines for Tertiary Review

Criteria for determining which cases need to be discussed at a trauma performance improvement committee (tertiary review) must be established. These will vary on the basis of volume and on local and state standards related to trauma performance improvement. Many institutions may review only cases that meet criteria for submission to the state and regional trauma registry (e.g., *International Classification of Diseases, Clinical Modification* [ICD-CM] 800 to 959.9, deaths, ICU admissions, hospital length of stay [LOS] more than 48 to 72 hours, pediatrics). Depending on resources available, an institution may opt to review only clinical sentinel events, cases with unexpected outcomes, and those that involve preventable or potentially preventable occurrences as calculated through the trauma registry system and Trauma Injury Severity Score (TRISS) analysis. Other issues can be reviewed as aggregate data, and focused audits should be performed when data trends reflect significant fluctuations. Review of systems issues should be included in performance improvement committees. Appropriate hospital or system staff should be included in the forums when system issues will be discussed.

Ensuring attendance at performance improvement forums can be difficult. To facilitate attendance, a set calendar of meetings should be established on a routine day and time that are convenient for team members with consideration of their clinical responsibilities. It may be helpful to incorporate trauma performance improvement committees into existing hospital and departmental forums, such as departmental morbidity and mortality conferences. There should be records of attendance (ACS standard for participation in multidisciplinary peer review forums), and confidential files should be kept on the topics, patients, and participants at performance improvement forums. Preparation before meetings should include compiling a roster of cases to be presented, obtaining/accessing the on-line medical records (when possible), and gathering the performance improvement case files. The guidelines for reaching peer review decisions and summary trauma registry data on individual cases should be available at performance improvement committee meetings. Using technology to enhance interactivity can be beneficial. Projecting patient case summaries to a screen viewable to participants during performance improvement meetings is one method that has been used to improve team participation in performance improvement discussions.

A key component of the performance improvement process is the provision of a peer review forum to discuss individual cases, trends in data, and comparative data related to system

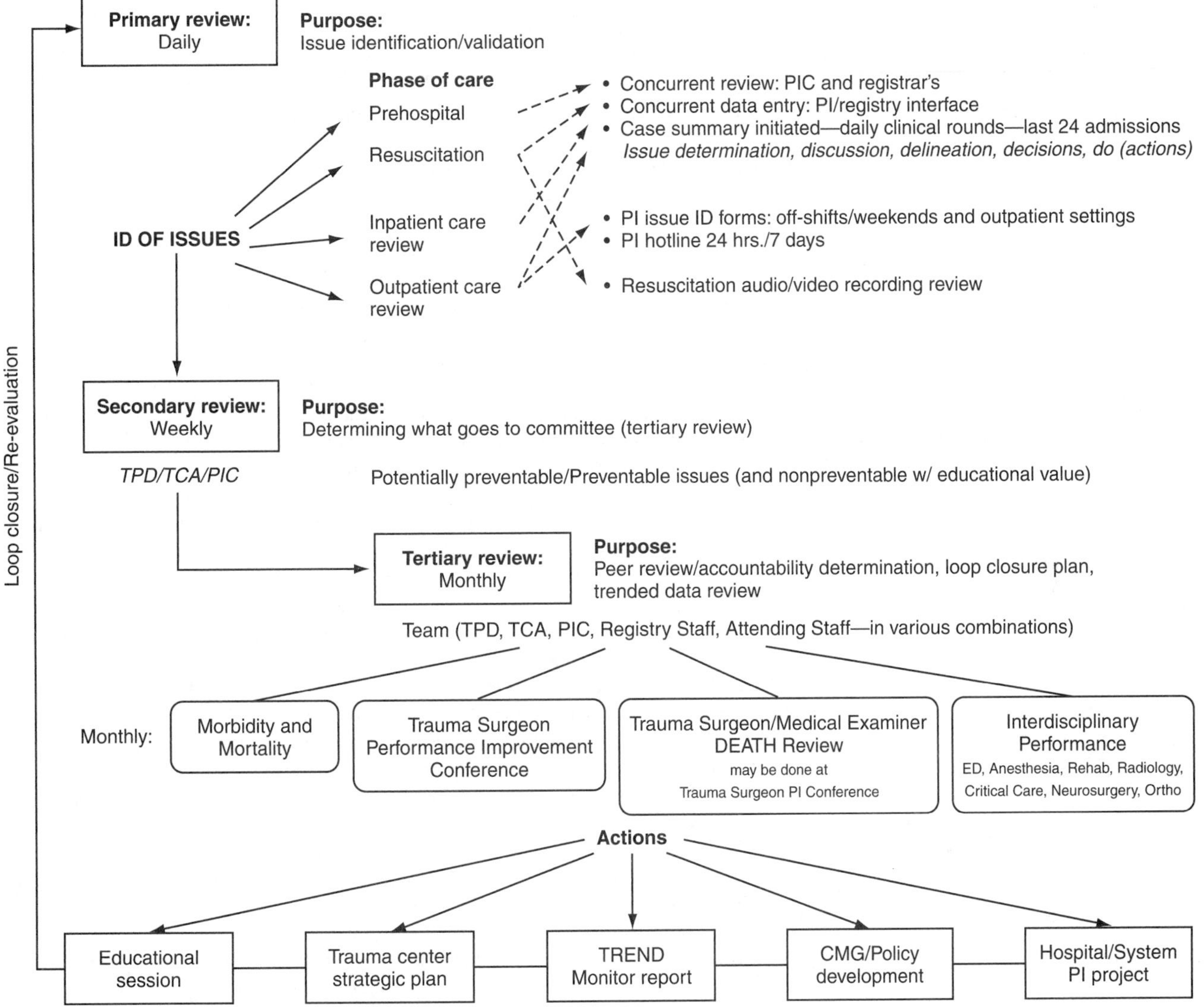

FIGURE 3-2. Trauma performance improvement process: levels of review. *PIC,* Performance improvement coordinator; *PI,* performance improvement; *ID,* identification; *TPD,* trauma program director; *TCA,* trauma clinical administrator; *CMG,* case mix group.

performance. Peer review forums should involve key trauma program/hospital staff (Table 3-1). Hospital/medical staff bylaws may dictate attendance at physician peer review sessions. These should be considered when determining the structure for peer review forums. Performance improvement committees can be structured in a variety of ways depending on the resources available, the volume of cases, and the local, state, and regional rules related to performance improvement reviews.

There are many options for designing the forum(s) in which trauma performance improvement issues will be reviewed. Surgeons taking trauma call could meet at a designated forum along with the trauma coordinator/program manager, trauma director, and registry staff, for example. In addition, there should be (based on the 2006 ACS standards) an interdisciplinary forum to review cases in which multiple services were involved or cases in which a single subspecialty was involved (e.g., neurosurgery, orthopedics, emergency medicine) but trauma surgeons or general surgeons taking trauma call were not involved. Finally, decisions must be made regarding how death cases should be reviewed and how to capture information from personnel such as the coroner or medical examiner.[10] Some programs will evaluate mortality and morbidity cases in a single forum; other may choose to have separate meeting where deaths are reviewed.

Trauma performance improvement discussions can occur in forums with an emphasis on education. However, the practice of peer review should be confined to peer review–protected forums based on local confidentiality rules and medical staff bylaws. Multidisciplinary trauma conferences (morbidity and mortality conferences, resuscitation audiovisual review forum, and journal clubs) may have elements of performance improvement review. The performance improvement aspects should be documented and filed appropriately.

TABLE 3-1 **Performance Improvement Roles of Trauma Program Staff in a Level I Trauma Program**

Personnel	Role in Performance Improvement
Trauma Performance Improvement Coordinator RN or Trauma Coordinator/Program Manager	• Identifies issues concurrently • Creates case file • Selects cases for performance improvement committees • Validates registry data • Reports on clinical management guideline compliance • Monitors trends in performance improvement reports/provider profile development • Tracks loop closure/resolution • Maintains performance improvement data
Trauma Performance Improvement Medical Director	• Selects cases for performance improvement committees • Moderates performance improvement committee meetings • Performs chart review • Analyzes performance improvement trended data/provider profiles • Coordinates generation of correspondence for performance improvement follow-up • Leads peer review judgment discussions with trauma director
Trauma Program Manager/Coordinator	• Analyzes trended performance improvement reports • Participates in peer review judgment discussions • Manages follow-up on performance improvement system issues • Oversees development and implementation of performance improvement/registry plans • Provides backup coverage for performance improvement coordinator • Validates trauma registry data • Facilitates interdisciplinary performance improvement team • Oversees clinical management guideline process: development implementation and surveillance • Directs loop closure—practice/policy changes/educational changes • Links to hospital/system performance improvement structures
Trauma Program Director	• Facilitates the performance improvement committee discussions • Moderates peer review decision/judgment determinations • Directs development of performance improvement plan with trauma program manager • Performs chart reviews • Facilitates interdisciplinary performance improvement team • Directs evidence-based clinical management guideline development • Directs "loop closure"—practice/policy/educational changes • Links to hospital performance improvement system
Trauma Registry Staff	• Performs concurrent data abstraction and maintenance of trauma registry database • Prepares performance improvement summaries from the trauma registry to facilitate data validation • Participates in performance improvement committee meetings • Oversees emergency medical services documentation and autopsy report retrieval • Prepares monthly standing registry reports
Trauma Surgeons/Fellows and Interdisciplinary Liaisons	• Participate in performance improvement committee meetings • Participate in peer review decisions/judgments • Perform chart reviews
Trauma Advanced Practitioners	• Participate in issue identification • Assist with maintenance of performance improvement data systems • Conduct focused audits of select performance issues • Provide surveillance of compliance with clinical practice management guidelines

PERFORMANCE INDICATORS: AUDIT FILTERS, OCCURRENCES, AND COMPLICATIONS

Performance improvement indicators are screens or triggers that are designed to activate review of potential risk-associated clinical or system occurrences. The ACS published trauma audit filters that became the national standard for trauma programs. The utility of current audit filters has not been determined definitively. Research has been done on whether the commonly used trauma audit filters have consistent links to improved outcome.[11] Literature suggests that, although some have found existing audit filters to be useful, others have found them labor intensive and costly.[12] In the 2006 ACS document, *Optimal Resources for Care of the Injured Patient,* the use of audit filters is downplayed. Trauma programs should focus their resources and time on institution-specific filters that provide the most meaningful measures of patient outcome. This is an area that clearly requires continual review and analysis.

There are national recommendations regarding the types of clinical complications (now commonly referred to as "occurrences") that a trauma performance improvement system should monitor. The ACS provides a list of occurrences and definitions for performance improvement tracking. Many states and regions have developed their own list of occurrences based on the ACS standards. Establishing universal definitions for these performance indicators is very important. To assess or compare trauma clinical care at a state or national level, there must be conformity in the definitions of occurrences tracked. This conformity ensures that incidence rates of a given occurrence are truly comparable (e.g., what one institution calls pneumonia is consistent with what another institution classifies as pneumonia).

The comprehensiveness of the performance improvement program will depend on many factors: center maturation, volume, resources, and local and state requirements. The utility of reviewing certain trauma performance indicators for trauma has been studied.[13,14] Trauma programs should strive to routinely review the occurrences and filters used to monitor quality outcomes. One approach to analysis of performance indicators is a rate-based method (frequency of occurrence/denominator of total cases). The stage of the trauma program in its evolution and development will affect an institution's ability to review rate-based indicators. Performance indicators that prove to be ineffective measures of outcome (through rate-based measurements or other types of trending) should not be prioritized. One way to approach performance indicator review is to group indicators into categories such as "nondiscretionary" and "discretionary." Nondiscretionary indicators are mandated through local and state trauma rules. It often is these nondiscretionary audit filters that programs prioritize. Discretionary indicators may be the institution-specific audit filters and occurrences. There are opportunities in terms of continued research studies for reviewing the use of audit filters and determining a definitive link between certain trauma performance indicators and desired patient outcomes. In summary, those indicators that best capture desired clinical outcomes should be the focus of the performance improvement process.

A key component of reviewing performance indicators is a systematic approach to determining peer review judgments. Having the multidisciplinary peer review committee consider a set of specific conditions and then basing the decision on preventability on responses to the conditions posed is a useful approach. The following are examples of questions that the team can consider to facilitate consensus on final peer review judgment:

- Were accepted protocols and policies followed?
- Were clinical management guidelines adhered to?
- Was the case managed in accordance with advanced trauma life support (ATLS) guidelines?
- If the occurrence involves a resident or student, was there evidence of adequate supervision?
- Was the system response optimal? Examples of system shortfalls include prolonged prehospital time, communications problems, failure of the paging system, delays in internal response, blood bank delays, and equipment malfunctions.
- Did the patient have preexisting medical conditions that contributed to the occurrence (e.g., diabetes, cardiac condition, or age extreme)?
- Was the occurrence evident before hospitalization (e.g., hypothermia, arrhythmia, or urinary tract infection)?

Example: A 35-year-old man was involved in a front-end motor vehicle crash. His medical history was unremarkable. He was the unrestrained driver of a compact car; the airbag deployed on impact. Pneumothorax and evidence of blood in the abdomen were detected by sonography. The patient was taken to the operating room for exploratory laparotomy. A review of the resuscitation videotape clearly shows a break in sterile technique during the insertion of the indwelling urinary catheter by the trauma resident. On hospital day 3, the patient's temperature is elevated, and it is determined that he has a urinary tract infection (Table 3-2).

TABLE 3-2 **Performance Improvement: Analysis of an Early Urinary Tract Infection**

Determinants of Preventability	Responses	Discussion	Determination
Were accepted policies/procedures followed?	No	Proper technique for insertion of indwelling urinary catheter was not followed	
Were clinical management guidelines adhered to?	NA		
Was management done as per ATLS guidelines?	Yes	Indwelling urinary catheter required for this patient	
If complication involves a resident or student, was there evidence of adequate supervision?	No		
Was the system response optimal?	Yes		
Did the patient have preexisting medical conditions that contributed to the occurrence?	No		
Was the occurrence/complication evident before hospitalization?	No		
Determination			**Error in technique** **Supervision deficiency**

TABLE 3-3 American College of Surgeons Effect Occurrence Grade

Occurrence Grade	Effect
Grade I	Alteration from ideal postoperative course, or Non–life-threatening, or No lasting disability, or Requires only bedside care, or Does not extend hospital stay
Grade II	Potentially life-threatening, or No residual disability, or Requires invasive procedure
Grade III	Residual disability, or Organ loss, or Persistent threat to life
Grade IV	Death

Used with permission from Performance Improvement Subcommittee of the American College of Surgeons Committee on Trauma. *Trauma Performance Improvement Reference Manual,* Chicago, 2002, American College of Surgeons.

One tool to assist with objective analysis of occurrences and complications is the use of the ACS grading system, which applies a numerical value to the impact of a surgical complication on a patient's overall outcome (Table 3-3). Applying this method, the complication of the urinary tract infection in the above example would be assigned a grade I.

OUTCOMES

Evaluation of outcomes is an essential component of performance improvement in a trauma center. Outcomes can include quality-of-life indicators, measured by patient satisfaction surveys, and functional outcomes, measured by functional independence measure (FIM) or by collecting information regarding a patient's ability to return to work or preinjury activities. Hospitals and insurance providers are interested in financial outcomes, measured by costs, readmissions, denied days, hospital LOS, and ICU LOS. Other outcome measures include death, occurrences/complications, delayed diagnoses, and missed injuries.

DEATHS

One starting point for evaluating care is the use of the TRISS to review cases ending in the death of the patient. In short, the TRISS method is based on the following:

- Physiologic parameters, including respiratory rate (RR), Glasgow Coma Scale (GCS) score, and systolic blood pressure (BP)
- Age (younger than 15 years, 15 to 55 years, older than 55 years)
- Mechanism of injury (blunt or penetrating)
- Anatomic scoring of injuries by the Injury Severity Score (ISS)

Based on these parameters, the probability of a patient's survival is calculated, and the outcome is expressed as unexpected death or unexpected survivor. TRISS is useful in identifying unexpected outcomes, and it offers a standardized way to compare outcomes with those in other trauma centers, other states, and other populations. However, it has some limitations that reduce its usefulness in performance improvement review. Because TRISS depends on physiologic parameters on admission, patients who arrive intubated, without a recorded RR, are excluded from analysis. Similarly, intubated patients lack the verbal component of the GCS, which excludes them from analysis.[15] Additionally, patients who arrive dead may have no injuries recorded; therefore, no ISS can be calculated. These patients are excluded from TRISS analysis until final anatomic diagnoses are determined from autopsy results. Another weakness of TRISS analysis is that it is based on the ISS. The ISS was initially developed as a way to standardize severity of injuries for patients who were involved in motor vehicle crashes and had injuries to multiple body areas. The ISS is less accurate at classifying patients with multiple injuries to one body region, a disadvantage when calculating scores for patients with penetrating injuries.

Over the years, investigators have evaluated TRISS and tried to improve the method of evaluating trauma care objectively.[16-19] Some of the more recent innovations based on ICD-9-CM coding have the advantage of being more cost efficient to calculate because they are based on injuries identified by medical record coders rather than specialized trauma registrars. Several factors should be considered when staffing models for the trauma registry are determined. For example, training for medical record coders emphasizes coding to capture diagnosis-related groups (DRGs); if this staff will have responsibilities for trauma registry coding, there must be specific training to optimize injury severity coding.

Scoring systems can also be used to describe outcomes such as morbidity and LOS, not just mortality. Another proposed method, the New Injury Severity Score (NISS), enhances ISS by including all the most serious injuries, not just the most serious in one body area.[20-22] These new methods need to be tested on a large scale before they become widely accepted, although recent studies have compared their validity and their potential to enhance a trauma center's ability to predict mortality.[23] No one method can replace a critical evaluation of patient care in a multidisciplinary forum using a framework for reaching peer review judgments. In this setting, the reviewers make determinations of whether the deaths and morbidities are nonpreventable, preventable, or potentially preventable. The purpose of determining preventability in the case of an unexpected outcome is not to place blame but to provide an honest appraisal of what went wrong to prevent future errors and to enhance patient safety.[24,25] Questions that need to be asked to determine preventability include the following:

- Was the death an expected outcome based on TRISS? (Despite its limitations, TRISS is widely used to predict outcomes and it provides a starting point for review.)
- Are the patient's injuries considered nonsurvivable (i.e., ISS = 75)?[26]
  - *Head:* Crush injury of skull or brain or massive destruction or penetration of brainstem
  - *Thorax:* Major laceration, perforation, or puncture of ventricle
  - *Spine:* Complete spinal cord injury with quadriplegia at C3 or higher
  - *Abdomen and pelvis:* Hepatic avulsion, grade VI
- Were standard procedures and protocols followed? Did patient care follow guidelines, such as in ATLS or hospital-specific protocols? Keep in mind that guidelines do not replace clinical judgment, and there are situations when deviation from the guidelines is appropriate. If this is the case, the reason must be clearly documented.
- Was the care appropriate? Provider errors that could contribute to a patient's death include missed injuries, delayed diagnosis of injuries, technical errors, errors in judgment, and errors in management.
- Was system response optimal? Examples of system issues include prehospital transport time, communication problems, failure of the paging system, internal response issues, blood bank delays, equipment malfunctions, delays in final reading of radiographs, or unavailability of operating room staff.
- Did the patient have preexisting medical conditions that contributed to the outcome? Preexisting conditions that contribute to a higher mortality rate include cirrhosis, coagulopathy, cardiac disease, renal disease, and malignancy.[22,27]

NONPREVENTABLE DEATHS

If the response to all these questions is *yes*, the death can be considered nonpreventable. However, even though the patient's injuries are considered nonsurvivable and the death nonpreventable, the remainder of the care should still be evaluated to identify areas for improvement.

Example: A 24-year-old man arrived at the trauma center within 10 minutes after being stabbed in the chest. The trauma team had prenotification of his arrival and was in the trauma bay. The patient's initial SBP was 60 and his GCS score was 8. He was intubated and resuscitated with intravenous (IV) fluids and packed red blood cells, which were readily available. A chest tube drained an initial 1000 ml of bright red blood, which was administered by autotransfusion. The patient's subsequent SBP was 90, and he was taken to the operating room within 18 minutes after arrival. Thoracotomy revealed that he had exsanguinated from a laceration of the right ventricle and could not be resuscitated (Table 3-4).

PREVENTABLE DEATHS

If the responses to the previous questions, regarding TRISS, standard protocols, appropriate care, system response, and preexisting conditions, are *no*, the death can be considered preventable. This indicates that the patient's injuries were considered relatively minor and survivable, but there were errors in judgment or management or technical errors that directly caused the patient's death.

Example: A 28-year-old man was transported to the emergency department by rescue services after falling from a curb. He was reportedly unconscious at the scene but was awake and responsive on arrival, with stable vital signs and a minor head laceration. Because he was apparently intoxicated and agitated, he was medicated with a sedative to calm him and placed in a room to "sleep it off." After a few hours, he was found to be unresponsive. A computed tomography (CT) scan was requested, but there was a delay in obtaining the scan because of a change of shift and personnel. Finally the CT scan showed a large epidural hematoma, and the neurosurgeons, who had left for the day, had to be called back to perform an emergency craniotomy. Despite their efforts, the patient did not recover, and he continued to be unresponsive until his death a few weeks later (Table 3-5).

POTENTIALLY PREVENTABLE DEATHS

The categorization of potentially preventable death requires an unbiased, critical review by the peer review committee. Determining that a death was potentially preventable indicates that the injuries and preexisting conditions were serious but the patient had the potential to survive if all other conditions were

TABLE 3-4 **Performance Improvement: Analysis of a Nonpreventable Death**

Determinants of Preventability	Responses	Discussion	Determination
Was the death an expected outcome on the basis of TRISS?	Yes	Expected death	
Are the patient's injuries considered nonsurvivable?	Yes	Probability of survival 0.004	
Were standard procedures and protocols followed?	Yes		
Was the care provided appropriate?	Yes		
Was the system response optimal?	Yes		
Was the outcome affected by the patient's preexisting conditions?	Unknown		
DETERMINATION			**Nonpreventable**

TABLE 3-5 **Performance Improvement: Analysis of a Preventable Death**

Determinants of Preventability	Responses	Discussion	Determination
Was the death an expected outcome on the basis of TRISS?	No	Unexpected death by TRISS	
Are the patient's injuries considered nonsurvivable?	No	Probability of survival 0.924	
Were standard procedures and protocols followed?	No	Incomplete evaluation of potential head-injured patient with impaired neurologic evaluation	
Was the care provided appropriate?	No	Inadequate monitoring of potentially head-injured patient Administration of sedatives Delay in diagnosis	
Was the system response optimal?	No	Delay in CT scan, delay in neurosurgery response	
Was the outcome affected by the patient's preexisting conditions?	No	Intoxication affected his evaluation but should not have affected his outcome	
DETERMINATION			**Preventable**

optimal. Errors in technique, errors in management, delays in care, or deviations from standard of care may have contributed to the patient's death.

Example: After a fall from a height, an elderly woman was admitted with a combination of injuries, including pelvic fractures, evidence of closed-head and intra-abdominal injuries, and lower extremity fractures. Her initial vital signs were stable, but she quickly became hemodynamically unstable, requiring massive resuscitation with crystalloids and blood for hemorrhagic shock. During resuscitation, cardiac arrhythmia and ventricular fibrillation developed, and the patient could not be resuscitated. Review of her trauma flow sheet revealed that her admission temperature was 34° C (93.2° F), yet fluids and blood products were administered without the use of warming devices (Table 3-6).

Missed Injuries

Missed injuries and delayed diagnoses can be a significant cause of morbidity or mortality. Diagnoses not made during the initial assessment or during the tertiary survey/subsequent evaluations during hospitalization can be labeled "delayed." Injuries not diagnosed until after the patient's discharge can be categorized as "missed." Approximately 10% to 15% of all patients with multiple injuries will have a delayed or missed diagnosis.[28,29] Some missed injuries are unavoidable. Circumstances that contribute to missed or delayed diagnosis of injuries include the inability to assess patients thoroughly for pain because of hemodynamic instability or shock, decreased level of consciousness from head injury or alcohol intoxication, intubation, spinal cord injury, or the use of chemical paralytics. It may not be possible to examine patients with closed-head injuries for pain, and extremity injuries may show up much later during rehabilitation. Nurses can play a role in revealing injuries by reporting swelling, bruising, or signs of discomfort when moving patients. Some missed injuries may be prevented if the health care providers maintain a high level of suspicion. For example, patterns related to mechanism of injury should be appreciated. A person who has fallen from a height, landed on a hard surface, and sustained bilateral calcaneal fractures could also have fractures of the knees, hip, or thoracic spine, caused by the force transmitted up the skeletal

TABLE 3-6 **Performance Improvement: Analysis of a Potentially Preventable Death**

Determinants of Preventability	Responses	Discussion	Determination
Was the death an expected outcome based on TRISS?	N/A	Unable to calculate TRISS, intubated before arrival	
Are the patient's injuries considered nonsurvivable?	No	Injuries potentially survivable	
Were standard procedures and protocols followed?	No	Institutional guidelines to prevent hypothermia were not followed	
Was the care provided appropriate?	No		
Was the system response optimal?	Yes		
Was the outcome affected by the patient's preexisting conditions?	No		
DETERMINATION			**Potentially preventable**

system. Additionally, at the end of a fall, the victim usually has outstretched hands, causing bilateral Colles' fractures of the wrists ("Don Juan" or "lover" syndrome).[30]

Unrestrained drivers or front seat passengers involved in motor vehicle crashes who sustain a posterior dislocation of the hip should also be evaluated for knee injury, caused when the knee hits the dashboard. Lower right-sided rib fractures can be associated with liver lacerations. Lower left-sided rib fractures can be associated with splenic lacerations. Fractures of the neck of the fibula can cause a stretch injury of the peroneal nerve.

Provider-related issues that may contribute to missed or delayed diagnosis of injuries include failure to appreciate signs of injury, failure to complete a thorough physical examination, or failure to read x-ray films correctly. It is beneficial to have a system in which "rereads" by a radiologist are communicated to the trauma team directly so that a delay in diagnosis does not lead to further delay in care. Data regarding missed injuries or delayed diagnosis of injuries can be gathered from the patient's medical records, radiology reports, readmission data, outpatient records, and follow-up from rehabilitation hospitals. Autopsy reports may identify injuries that remained undiagnosed during the patient's hospitalization.

ACCOUNTABILITY

Most performance improvement issues are related to inadequacies in the system. Most complications are related to patient disease and are thought to be unavoidable. It is occasionally necessary to assign to a specific provider the responsibility for an error in management or technique, a missed or delayed diagnosis of an injury, failure to follow standard protocols or guidelines, or a complication. If the patient was being managed by a group of physicians rather than a specific provider, the responsibility should be assigned to the "team." If a patient has an unrecognized esophageal intubation, then the provider who was in charge of intubating and confirming airway placement is responsible, and the error in technique is assigned to the specific provider. If a patient has upper gastrointestinal bleeding after a long ICU stay and if on review it is determined that the patient had never received appropriate stress ulcer prophylaxis, who was responsible is not as clear cut. The team of physicians responsible for that patient's care, whether it is the critical care service or the trauma service, is responsible, and the failure to follow guidelines is assigned to the appropriate team.

The issue of supervision should also be addressed in academic centers that provide learning experiences for students, residents, and fellows. Ultimate responsibility for the care of patients must be linked to a supervising attending physician, and means of monitoring this role in the performance improvement process should be considered.

Resources for Optimal Care of the Injured Patient stresses the critical importance of an evaluation of provider-specific mortality rates, complication rates, compliance with continuing education, resource utilization, and participation in guidelines and protocols. The performance improvement program will be required to demonstrate that there is a systematic mechanism in place to collect objective data regarding trauma physician's performance and to provide feedback to individual providers. Sample reports are displayed in Table 3-7.

CORRECTIVE ACTION PLAN

Once system- or provider-related issues are identified, corrective actions should be taken, with the goal of improving patient care, not merely to be punitive. Possible actions include the following:

- Collection of data for a period of time to determine whether the variation represents a trend or an isolated occurrence
- Change in or better enforcement of policy or procedure
- Development of clinical management guidelines
- Presentation of the issue as a topic in an educational setting
- Physician/provider counseling
- Mandatory continuing education
- Probation or suspension of staff members who have varied from accepted standards of care
- Notification of risk management

REEVALUATION (LOOP CLOSURE)

As mentioned previously, the performance improvement process can be viewed as a cycle, as per Joint Commission guidelines. One very important activity in closing a performance improvement case is to ensure that the recommended actions are implemented and that the actions have the desired effect of improving patient care, or "closing the loop." Strategies to ensure resolution include a "tickler" file or a field in a database to indicate unresolved issues. This continuous reevaluation of the outcome guarantees that the performance improvement process remains dynamic and responsive to the changing environment in medicine.

RECORDKEEPING

Each state has regulations regarding the confidentiality of performance improvement or peer review documents, but some guidelines regarding recordkeeping are universal. Patient identification should be limited to numbers or initials. Full names should be avoided if possible. Providers should be identified by a number rather than by name, and the list matching providers to numbers should remain confidential. Reports that are distributed at performance improvement meetings should be clearly marked "confidential" or "for peer review only" and include a statement on peer review from the appropriate state statute. Any handouts for review at performance improvement meetings should be counted and then accounted for at the close of the meeting. Extras should be destroyed. Issues discussed at performance improvement forums must not be made public, and documents must not be published and distributed to others. Documentation must be limited to objective statement of the facts. As long as the information is not made public or distributed to others, it is usually protected from legal discovery.

TABLE 3-7 **Trauma Surgeon Provider Profile CY 2005**

Provider: #6

Individual Provider Data						Data Categories		CY 2005 Group Data
CY 2000	**CY 2001**	**CY 2002**	**CY 2003**	**CY 2004**	**CY 2005**	**Clinical Care**	**Group Mean**	**Group Total**
						Total No. of patient contacts		
						% Blunt		
						% Penetrating		
						# Patients eligible for state registry submission		
						# Patient's with ISS >16		
						Mean ISS for all patients all providers		
						Operations—trauma		
						Operations—ESS		
						Deaths		
						Total deaths		
						**Preventable		
						**Potentially preventable		
						**Nonpreventable		
						Peer judgment not valued		
						Unexpected TRISS deaths		
						Unexpected TRISS survivors		
						Complications		
						Provider specific:		
						Attendance		
						Performance improvement (PI) meetings:		
CY 2000	CY 2001	CY 2002	CY 2003	CY 2004	CY 2005	*Continuing medical education (CME)		
						Total:		
						Pediatric:		

Source: Trauma Registry/Trauma PI Database/Credentialing Database.
Group mean = 8 trauma attending surgeons on service CY 2005.
* = Transition to calendar year tracking for CME in 2001.
** = As determined by peer review judgment.

Attendants at performance improvement forums must have a professional or legitimate reason to be present.

It is important that performance improvement documents remain separate from medical records and not referenced in the patient chart because medical records can be requested in a subpoena. Performance improvement documents kept on file must be maintained in a secure manner, for example, in locked cabinets. If data are stored in a computer, the files must be password protected with access limited to those with a legitimate reason to view the documents. It is tempting to use the convenience and speed of e-mail or fax to communicate performance improvement information, but this practice should be discouraged unless strict guidelines regarding confidentiality are maintained.

There must be institution-specific, written guidelines regarding the handling of audiovisual recordings of trauma resuscitations. These should be stored in limited-access files/areas. They should be viewed only by those who have a professional reason to view a trauma resuscitation. There must be a specific time frame in which the recordings must be erased or destroyed. Having the hospital legal department review the procedures of the performance improvement program to ensure compliance with approved state regulations regarding confidentiality of peer review documents is paramount. Other documents generated from the performance improvement process must be stored in a secure manner. Many centers generate files for select cases reviewed in the performance improvement process.

Typical contents found in a performance improvement file may include the following:

- Case summary
- Registry data, including TRISS data
- Issue identification forms
- All correspondence sent and received
- Supporting documents related to follow-up and closure
- Autopsy reports, if applicable

PRACTICE MANAGEMENT GUIDELINES

Standardizing (where appropriate) the approach to the care of injured patients has become an important goal of trauma programs. One strategy used to standardize aspects of trauma care is the use of practice management guidelines. The Eastern Association for the Surgery of Trauma has published evidence-based templates of practice management guidelines for injured patients, which have been modified and adopted by trauma programs across the country.

There are key steps that are recommended in developing practice management guidelines successfully (Table 3-8). One important step is to link them to the trauma performance improvement program. Practice management guidelines should be evidence based (e.g., review of literature on clinical outcomes related to specific approaches). The trauma performance improvement program should guide development of practice guidelines through analysis of trends in practice patterns and patient outcomes. When guidelines that affect several disciplines are developed, input should be collected from the staff members who will be affected by the change. For example, a change in the procedure for clearing a trauma patient's cervical spine should be reviewed by representatives of radiology, neurosurgery, trauma, nursing, physical medicine, and rehabilitation services. A key element of a successful clinical management guideline program is education of all involved in implementing the guideline. Operational issues that could arise as a result of a new guideline should be determined during the planning stage, not after implementation.

Surveillance is probably the most critical element of a successful practice management guideline program. There must be an identified mechanism to track and report compliance with guidelines. Measures to enhance compliance should be investigated, for example, inserting computerized prompts into physician order entry systems or providing pocket guides that remind providers of guidelines. Several surveillance models can be used: the trauma coordinator, registry staff who are performing concurrent abstraction, advanced practice nurses or trauma nurse clinicians or case managers, or if one is in place, a trauma performance improvement coordinator.[31]

TABLE 3-8 Steps in the Development of Clinical Management Guidelines

- Monitor current performance.
- Collect input from multiple disciplines.
- Review published literature on the topic.
- Educate staff members affected by the guideline about the upcoming change.
- Implement the new guideline.
- Maintain surveillance and routine reporting of compliance.

REGISTRY: PERFORMANCE IMPROVEMENT INTEGRATION

A requirement of *Resources for Optimal Care of the Injured Patient* is that data be maintained on injured patients who are evaluated and managed at the trauma center. Based on local protocols and state statutes, data requirements may differ slightly. The trauma registry is a fundamental component of the center or trauma system. Only through the collection and analysis of data can the center and system develop and improve. Nationally, the ACS and more recently the Heath Resources Services Administration (HRSA) has partnered to create a national trauma registry data dictionary that serves as the foundation of the National Trauma Databank (NTDB). The ACS directs the NTDB, which contains more than 1.5 million records from trauma centers in the United States and Puerto Rico. The goal of the NTDB is to inform the medical community, the public, and decision makers about a wide variety of issues that characterize the current state of care for injured persons.

Many commercial trauma registry software packages are available. The type of registry package selected should be based on the desired features sought. Some key elements to consider when choosing a trauma registry package include database networking possibilities, report writing capabilities, compatibility/interface capability with other standard hospital information systems (e.g., radiology, laboratory, hospital registration systems), and compatibility with popular commercial personal computer platforms such as Microsoft Windows.

There should be a close interface between the trauma registry and the trauma performance improvement programs. The data collected by the trauma registry provide the foundation for trauma performance improvement activities. Depending on the program's size, resources, and organizational structure, there may be overlapping roles and responsibilities for a single team member related to the registry and performance improvement functions. In this era of lean program resources, reducing duplicate abstraction and streamlining information flow should be the goal. Hospitals should investigate the possibility of interfacing existing hospital data sources to minimize duplicate data entry and to better use personnel. An important consideration in trauma registry program design is ensuring there are processes to validate data accuracy/productivity.

Key systems for the trauma program to access would include the hospital admission database, the radiology system, laboratory system, operating room scheduling and tracking system, and computerized portions of the medical record. It is also suggested that, when feasible, trauma registry staff be integrated into the overall trauma administrative team. This is difficult when the trauma registry is housed in medical records or another location physically separate from the trauma program office and staff. Measures to incorporate the registry staff and to validate the accuracy of abstraction need to be determined. The registrar role in the trauma performance improvement program will enhance the overall process. Having the registrar(s) participate in performance improvement forums serves several purposes: It strengthens the issue identification process, allows for validation of the information entered into the registry, and can enhance registrar job satisfaction and sense of contribution. Registrars strengthen performance improvement discussions by providing insight into the coding of injuries, a unique understanding of the scoring methodologies commonly used in trauma care, and explanation of the criteria for audit filter and occurrence (complication) capture. The registry staff can be instrumental in the generation of reports that are essential to the performance improvement process. In addition, the registry staff can provide guidance on customization of the registry database for tracking performance improvement–related data. In terms of day-to-day operations, the movement toward concurrent data collection presents opportunities to strengthen the integration of registry and performance improvement programs.[32]

With the implementation of the NTDB, there is now a powerful set of national data that is available to fuel research, prevention, and system development initiatives. Technologic advancements and the new and rapidly expanding field of health information management have helped facilitate the development of the NTDB.

TECHNOLOGY

Computerization can enhance the performance improvement process. Records can be stored in a database program and then manipulated in other spreadsheet programs. Most spreadsheet programs can display the data in graphs or charts for presentation, demonstrating trends over time or comparing performance by provider. Merging the information in the performance improvement database with templates in word processing programs allows for the generation of correspondence that can be sent as feedback to referring physicians, requests for medical records from transferring institutions, requests for follow-up information from rehabilitation facilities, or as a referral of patient cases to other physicians for review. Creative approaches such as using an LCD projector or plasma technology to display data or case summaries during performance improvement meetings enables the team to make additions, corrections, or deletions to case minutes; encourages participation; and makes the meetings interesting and interactive.

LOOKING TO THE FUTURE

Technology advancements will continue to lead to challenges in the future. Traditionally, *CPR* has stood for cardiopulmonary resuscitation. This acronym now takes on an additional meaning in the age of information technology advances: **c**omputer-based **p**atient **r**ecord. The advent of full or partial electronic medical records has already minimized issues of storage and retrieval of paper records. In addition, computerized records can eliminate legibility issues and perhaps decrease duplicative data entry within hospital systems. Furthermore, technology advancements will allow for easier communication of data between departments and interfaces between existing hospital systems. There are systems that allow information to be electronically downloaded into the trauma registry database for laboratory, radiology, and patient registration. Other technology improvements to look for in the future (in use in some places now) include the following:

- Voice recognition charting documentation
- Web links for interhospital/agency data transfer
- Handheld/portable technology for prehospital and hospital data collection
- Remote ICU monitoring systems such as VISICU
- Clinical decision support systems

The elements of and format for trauma performance improvement reviews continue to evolve. As technology continues to develop, efforts need to be directed at the continued enhancement/growth of the NTDB that will guide policy and practice patterns for injury care on a larger scale than has been possible before. This has required a standard data collection format and the involvement of other data sources (e.g., law enforcement, coroners) in addition to the trauma centers. Much emphasis has been given to development of benchmarking trauma clinical outcomes. The University Health Consortium (UHC) has been studying a subset of the nation's trauma centers for comparing clinical outcomes. This process is still in development and only compares the outcomes from university-based/affiliated trauma centers. Although focusing on the clinical mission, UHC supports research and education. As an idea-generating and information-disseminating enterprise, UHC assists members to pool resources, create economies of scale, improve clinical and operating efficiencies, and influence the direction and delivery of health care.[33]

The issue of limited health care dollars is another factor that must be considered as trauma performance improvement continues its evolution. Using data to streamline and improve care effectiveness while maintaining positive outcomes will be a priority for trauma care clinicians in the new millennium. Continuing to link the hospital clinical effectiveness and quality improvement efforts with patient safety initiatives and the trauma performance improvement process will lead to better coordinated hospital efforts geared at minimizing untoward patient events/outcomes.

The NTDB, in its short existence, has already enhanced the ability to perform more meaningful trauma benchmarking. Including data from hospitals with 24-hour emergency departments (nontrauma centers that treat injured patients) would provide yet another very powerful source of injury information, which could then guide public health and safety initiatives to prevent injury, the ultimate in loop closure.

REFERENCES

1. American College of Surgeons, Committee on Trauma: *Resources for optimal care of the injured patient,* Chicago, 2006 American College of Surgeons.
2. Wright JE: The history of the surgical audit, *J Qual Clin Pract* 15:81-88, 1995.
3. Deming WE: *Out of the crisis,* Cambridge, Mass, 1986, MIT-CAES.
4. http://healthcare.isixsigma.com/st/data/. Accessed November 8, 2006.
5. McMaster J: Update on the National Patient Safety Goals—changes for 2006, *J Trauma Nurs* 12(3):83-85, 2005.
6. American College of Surgeons, Committee on Trauma: *Trauma performance improvement, a how to handbook,* Chicago, 2002, American College of Surgeons.
7. Trauma Outcomes Performance Improvement Course, T.O.P.I.C. Presented at Annual Meeting of Society of Trauma Nurses, March 24-25, 2003, Las Vegas, Nevada.
8. http://www.jointcommission.org/SentinelEvents/se_glossary.htm. Accessed November 1, 2006.
9. Day S, Dalto J, Fox J et al: Failure mode and effects analysis as a performance improvement tool in trauma, *J Trauma Nurs* 13(3):111-117, 2006.
10. Nayduch D, FitzPatrick MK: The application of forensic findings to the trauma quality management process, *J Trauma Nurs* 6(4):98-102, 1999.
11. Cryer HG, Hiatt JR, Fleming AW et al: Continuous use of standard process audit filters has limited value in an established trauma system, *J Trauma* 41(3):389-395, 1996.
12. Rhodes M, Sacco W, Smith S: Cost effectiveness of trauma quality assurance audit filters, *J Trauma* 30:724-727, 1990.
13. Nayduch D, Moylan J, Snyder BL et al: American College of Surgeons audit filters: an analysis of outcome in a statewide trauma system, *J Trauma* 37:565-575, 1994.
14. Hoyt DB, Hollingsworth-Fridlund P, Fortlage D et al: An evaluation of provider-related and disease-related morbidity in a level I university trauma service: directions for quality improvement, *J Trauma* 33:586-601, 1992.
15. Offner P, Jurkovich G, Gurney J et al: Revision of TRISS for intubated patients, *J Trauma* 32:32-35, 1992.
16. Baker SP, O'Neill B, Haddon W et al: The Injury Severity Score: a method for describing patients with multiple injuries and evaluating emergency care, *J Trauma* 14:187-196, 1974.
17. Champion HR, Sacco WJ, Cornazzo AK et al: A revision of the trauma score, *J Trauma* 29:623-676, 1989.
18. Sacco WJ, Copes W, Staz C et al: Status of trauma patient management as measured by survival/death outcomes: looking toward the 21st century, *J Trauma* 36:297-298, 1994.
19. Rutledge R, Osler T, Emery S et al: The end of the Injury Severity Score (ISS) and the trauma and injury severity score tool (TRISS): ICISS, an international classification of diseases, the ninth revision-based prediction tool, outperforms both ISS and TRISS as predictors of trauma patient survival, hospital charges, and length of stay, *J Trauma* 44:41-49, 1998.
20. Al West T, Rivara F, Cummings P et al: Harborview assessment for risk of mortality: an improved measure of injury severity on the basis of ICD-9-CM, *J Trauma* 49(3):530-541, 2000.
21. Hoyt DB: Is it time for a new injury score [commentary]? *Lancet* 44:580-582, 1998.
22. Boyd CR, Tolson MA, Copes W: Evaluating trauma care: the TRISS method, *J Trauma* 27:370-378, 1987.
23. Hannan, EL, Waller CH, Farrell LS et al: A comparison among the abilities of various injury severity measures to predict mortality with and without accompanying physiologic information, *J Trauma* 58(2):244-251, 2005.
24. Gruen RL, Jurkovich GJ, McIntyre LK et al: Patterns of errors contributing to trauma mortality: lessons learned from 2,594 deaths, *Ann Surg* 244 (3):371-380, 2006.
25. Pierluissi E, Fischer MA, Campbell AR et al: Discussion of medical errors in morbidity and mortality conferences, *JAMA* 290(21):2838-2842, 2003.
26. Morris JA, Mackenzie EJ, Edelstein SL: The effect of preexisting conditions on mortality in trauma patients, *JAMA* 14: 1942-1946, 1990.
27. Milzman D, Boulanger B, Rodriguez A et al: Pre-existing disease in trauma patients: a predictor of fate independent of age and injury severity score, *J Trauma* 32:236-244, 1992.
28. Sommers M: Missed injuries: a case of trauma hide and seek, *AACN Clin Issues* 6:187-195, 1995.
29. Enderson BL, Reath DB, Meadors J et al: The tertiary trauma survey: a prospective study of missed injuries, *J Trauma* 30:666-669, 1990.
30. Musculoskeletal colloquialisms: How did we come up with these names? http://radiographics.rsnajnls.org/cgi/content/abstract/24/4/1009. Accessed November 8, 2006.
31. Frankel HL, FitzPatrick MK, Gaskell L et al: Strategies to improve compliance with evidence-based clinical management guidelines, *J Am Coll Surg* 189(6):533-538, 1999.
32. FitzPatrick MK, Heliger L, McMaster J et al: Integration of concurrent trauma registry and performance improvement programs, *J Trauma Nurs* 7(4):92-97, 2000.
33. University Health Consortium: *Trauma clinical and operational benchmarking, executive summary* (2000): www.uhc.edu. Accessed November 8, 2006.

4

Ethics in Trauma Nursing

Joan M. Pryor-McCann

Many ethical questions confront nurses in their everyday practice. Trauma nurses, however, face a unique set of problems that make the resolution of ethical issues more difficult than in other nursing settings. For example, patients admitted to trauma units often have not chosen to be admitted there. Usually these persons have experienced a medical emergency requiring immediate health care intervention and admission. A trauma-induced hospital visit differs markedly from an elective surgery hospital admission or even an admission in which the patient walks into the emergency unit under his or her own power. If a voluntarily admitted patient has a cardiac arrest, the nurse can reasonably infer that the patient sought and wanted care, but in the event of a cardiac arrest in a nonvoluntarily admitted trauma patient, this inference cannot be made.

Not only is it unknown whether the trauma patient wants care, but often the trauma nurse cannot ascertain what the patient's wishes are regarding particular treatment options. For example, the trauma patient's decision-making ability is commonly incapacitated by an altered level of consciousness or is impaired by severe pain, anxiety, anger, or drugs. Sometimes such alterations are amenable to reversal with short-term treatment, and direction for care can then be obtained from the patient. More often than not, however, crucial life-or-death decisions must be made immediately, before these conditions can be reversed, in which case temporary alterations in decision-making ability are as problematic as any long-term ones. Community health nurses or hospital floor nurses are generally familiar with their patients' wishes and those of their families, but the trauma nurse is often not, and gaining speedy access to such information can be difficult or impossible.

At the same time, experienced trauma nurses are all too familiar with the practical implications of their ethical decisions. For example, they are keenly aware that if they place an 80-year-old patient with chronic obstructive pulmonary disease (COPD) on a ventilator, that person may never be able to be weaned from the machine. They also know that many people survive initial trauma but are unable to obtain or afford quality rehabilitative care.

The trauma setting is fast paced compared with other health care settings. Trauma settings require quick decision making and allow very little time for information gathering, deliberation, or weighing alternatives. This, of course, is part of the reason emergency care guidelines for particular health care interventions are necessary in such settings. Yet whereas trauma nurses usually have clearly delineated procedures to follow during the resuscitation phase, similar guidelines for making crucial ethical decisions are more difficult to find. Frequently treatment decisions involve both issues. The decision whether to code a patient, for example, is both an ethical decision and a health care decision.

This chapter attempts to provide the trauma nurse with some guidance for making ethical decisions. Knowledge of nursing's code of ethics and knowledge of moral principles and theories will help trauma nurses resolve troublesome ethical issues that arise in this setting. It is vitally important that trauma nurses become familiar with these aspects of ethics so they can make sound ethical decisions in their practice.

The Difference Between Ethics and Law

Some nurses believe that when their legal obligation is clear their ethical obligation is also clear. Some nurses even claim that their legal obligation always coincides with or determines their ethical obligation. In other words, these nurses hold that when a nurse knows that a physician's orders call for a code to be initiated, this fact alone ends any deliberation about whether it is ethical to code the patient in question. Although this may sometimes be true, it is certainly not always true. Several crucial distinctions must be made between ethical and legal decisions.

First of all, ethics and law are not the same thing. The former deals with moral behavior and the latter deals with legal behavior. Admittedly, ethical choices are often reduced by pressures of the moment to worries about legal risk, but compliance with the law does not guarantee ethical behavior, nor is it an excuse for ignoring the ethical aspects of a decision.[1] For example, slavery was once legal in parts of the United States, but even at that time many persons questioned its morality, and most of us would agree today that slavery is ethically unacceptable. Similarly, abortion is now a legal alternative for pregnant women, but many persons question the morality of abortion. Laws themselves are not necessarily ethically sound. In fact, laws themselves are properly the subjects of ethical appraisal and evaluation. Therefore, the assumption that if nurses do their legal duty and follow physician's orders they will also be performing their ethical duty is not necessarily correct.

Another difference between law and ethics is evident in the fact that existing laws do not always give direction for particular ethical problems. The law often lags behind current ethical questions. For example, it took years for legislatures to enact statutes accepting brain death criteria as part of the legal definition of biologic death, yet nurses were faced with ethical decisions about the care of such patients long before these laws were enacted. Currently, the legal status of living wills (one kind of advance directive) is another issue that remains unresolved in some states, but ethical questions about the care of people who express their wishes in living wills must be addressed now in practice. Ethics, then, is broader and more inclusive than law, and the nurse is not always able to gain direction for current ethical difficulties by consulting the law.

On the other hand, law is not irrelevant to ethics. Difficult ethical decisions can often be clarified by referring to the reasoning used by courts and legal scholars on the issue in question or related issues. This is true because legal reasoning reflects our society's perceptions on a subject and because the law has its roots in public acceptance and its adherence to fair and reasonable procedures for decisions on issues. Some ethicists also claim that knowledge of one's legal obligations, although not decisive for answering ethical questions, is necessary for discerning one's ethical obligation.[2] Such obligations are often taken to be limited by the risks of legal liability or financial loss that an agent might incur as a result of a particular choice. For example, should nurses consider the legal risks they would be taking if they do not act consistently with their legal obligation to follow a physician's orders to code a patient? This is certainly not the only information they should consider, but it is information that is clearly relevant to whether they should code their patients.

So, legal risks are relevant data to consider when making moral decisions, but more analysis of a case is needed before moral decisions can be reached. To approach such situations properly, nurses need more knowledge. Compliance with the law is not enough to guarantee morally correct decisions, so many nurses look for guidance to the ethical code proposed by their professional association. The next section discusses this document for nurses.

THE CODE OF ETHICS FOR NURSES

In 1950 the American Nurses' Association (ANA) adopted a code of ethics to guide professional nursing practice.[3] This document codifies nursing's traditional involvement with the obligations that health care workers owe to those under their care.[4] After several revisions, the code is now known as the *Code of Ethics for Nurses With Interpretive Statements.*[5] (Hereafter it is referred to as the *Code of Ethics for Nurses,* or simply the *Code.*) The *Code* serves as a public declaration of the standards and values by which all professional nurses are expected to practice. The *Code* has "performative force" because of its influence on nursing licensure, institutional accreditation, and curricula and its use in court cases as the document representing accepted professional values and standards.[6]

Professional codes of ethics are always mixtures of creed and commandments (beliefs and rules). The belief aspects of the *Code of Ethics for Nurses* can be found in the preface, and the rule aspects are delineated in the nine provision statements and the interpretations that follow them. Although the ethical codes of some health professions have been criticized as paternalistic and limited, the nursing code has garnered much praise for its comprehensiveness and the emphasis it places on the autonomy of the patient.[7] In addition, the *Code* provides protection for patients by explicitly prohibiting behaviors that Jameton and others have called "the dark side of nursing," such as the labeling, stereotyping, or stigmatizing of patients by word or deed.[8] Every professional nurse should familiarize herself with the *Code of Ethics for Nurses* because its ideals are those deemed by the profession as essential for ethical nursing practice.

Besides giving guidance about the ethical approach nurses must have toward patients, the *Code* provides support for individual nurses to take care of themselves. For example, Rushton[9] notes that the most recent revision of the *Code* "adds a bold new provision" that supports nurses, namely, Provision 5. It reads as follows: "The nurse owes the same self-regarding duties to self as to others, including the responsibility to preserve integrity and safety, to maintain competence and to continue personal and professional growth." This has been interpreted as acknowledging "the importance of caring for oneself in order to care for others" and seems consistent with the push of many professional organizations for better work environments for nurses.

The *Code of Ethics for Nurses* also serves to inform the public that nurses acknowledge their unique position of care and assures the public of the standards and values by which all nurses are expected to function.[6] Duties such as supporting patient autonomy and being a patient advocate are mentioned explicitly in the code. The preface states that the *Code* reflects all the approaches for addressing ethics, including ethical theories, ethical principles, and cultivating virtues. It also states that the *Code* "is the profession's nonnegotiable ethical standard." According to the ANA and state boards of nursing, all nurses in all nursing situations in the United States must adhere to the *Code.* This is true regardless of whether the nurse is a member of the ANA.

But, as impressive and important as the *Code* is, it cannot provide a specific answer to all the ethical questions that arise in nursing practice. Like other professional codes, the *Code of Ethics for Nurses* provides general guidelines that must be applied in specific situations. Making this deductive shift from the general to the specific is especially difficult in trauma settings, where treatment decisions often have to be made quite rapidly, where patients may be either upset or unresponsive, and where adequate information about the patient and the patient's life situation is lacking.

For example, Section 1.4 of the *Code of Ethics for Nurses* states, "Patients have the moral and legal right to determine what will be done with their own person... to accept, refuse or terminate treatment...." How should a trauma nurse respond to a very anxious and despondent battered woman who insists, "Don't you dare treat me. I just want to die"? Does this patient's statement constitute a refusal of treatment? Should the trauma nurse abide by this woman's expressed wishes? Can a trauma nurse always get permission to render necessary life-saving treatment? If the patient ends up in the trauma unit after a suicide attempt, does the suicide victim have the right to refuse emergency life-saving treatment? Clearly the *Code for Nurses* does not address these complex questions in which the nurse's obligations and duties conflict and a resolution is not immediately apparent.

The same section of the *Code* states, "Patients have the moral and legal right…to be given accurate, complete and understandable information…." But should a trauma nurse tell a mother that her baby has just died if the nurse knows that the mother has stated that she will stop any life-saving treatment for herself if her baby dies? This is a case where there is a conflict of nursing obligations. The nurse has both the obligation to tell the truth and the obligation to do good for her patient. The *Code of Ethics for Nurses* expects nurses to fulfill both these obligations, but it is unclear in the preceding case whether the nurse can actually fulfill both in this situation. The *Code* does not completely address what the nurse should do when such conflicts arise.

Trauma nurses also must make decisions about triaging patients and distributing scarce resources. The *Code of Ethics for Nurses* simply does not provide much direction for these essential activities. In fact, Provision 1 of the *Code* states that "The nurse … practices … unrestricted by considerations of social or economic status, personal attributes, or the nature of the health problems." Taken at face value, this requirement of basic respect for persons seems to undermine the very practice of nursing itself. Currently it is unquestionably understood that prognosis and illness are valid considerations for triage decisions, but obviously little guidance is provided by the *Code of Ethics for Nurses* about how this process should be carried out.

Admittedly, no professional ethical code could capture all the myriad of ethical questions that arise within the scope of that profession's practice. The limits of the *Code of Ethics for Nurses* illustrate that strict adherence to it is not enough to guarantee ethical behavior on the part of professional nurses. Even adherence to published professional position papers and standards of care are not enough. To evaluate thorny ethical issues such as those involved in the situations discussed, the nurse needs to explore both moral principles and ethical theories.

ETHICS

Ethics can be defined as the philosophic study of moral conduct, whereas morals or morality is understood philosophically as dealing with what is right and what is wrong in a practical sense.[10] In this chapter, as in common usage, the terms *ethics* and *morals* are used interchangeably. Likewise, theories about ethics are sometimes referred to as moral theories or as ethical theories. In addition, the morality of an action is explored by looking at the ethical or moral justifications for the action. Ethics, then, involves a systematic appraisal of moral situations by using moral principles and ethical theories to justify resolution of the question: "What, all things considered, ought to be done in this situation?"[11]

Ethics is a human enterprise that requires a person to look at one's own obligations and provide justification for one's own actions. Nursing ethics requires nurses to look at their professional obligations and explore how these obligations coincide with or are justified by general ethical principles and theories.

Trauma nurses deal with a myriad of ethical issues in their everyday practice. Some of these issues are clear and easily answered by referring to the *Code of Ethics for Nurses;* however, many issues are ambiguous and difficult to answer. An ethical dilemma occurs either when there is no obvious answer to the issue at hand or the available alternative actions are each somewhat morally justifiable or are all morally undesirable. Olesinski and Stannard[12] conclude that the overall nature of the ethical dilemmas confronted by critical care and emergency department nurses lies in the disparity between actual and ideal nursing practice. Gaul[13] clarified the nature of such ethical dilemmas by analyzing responses of 270 nurses from 39 different states. She identified what she called the "four major causes of ethical suffering" in these nurses. These include situations in which (1) the patient's interests conflict with the treatment plan, (2) the nurse's responsibility to the family conflicts with those owed to the patient, (3) the nurse has opposing moral responsibilities, or (4) the nurse experiences a sense of powerlessness and lack of control over the elements of the ethical dilemma. The *Code of Ethics for Nurses* cannot and should not be expected to resolve all these kinds of cases. Each one has numerous facets and considerations to take into account. Despite the complexity and uniqueness of each individual case, however, there are some commonalties on which the nurse can and should base his or her ethical decisions. These are the general moral principles that provide the foundation for ethical nursing practice.

MORAL PRINCIPLES

Ethicists discuss the basic moral principles that affect nursing practice. One of the principles is that of *beneficence,* which requires that the nurse "ought to do good for and prevent or avoid doing harm to" the patient.[14] This latter obligation, that of avoiding harm, is called *nonmaleficence,* and in general ethics it is usually considered more binding than the duty to do good.[14] However, given the nurse's specialized education and training, coupled with the reasonable expectation by the public that nurses can resolve or ameliorate many health care problems, professional nurses do have responsibilities of beneficence and nonmaleficence to their patients. Sometimes a nurse cannot avoid causing some harm to a patient while properly performing his or her professional responsibilities. For example, nurses give injections or deliver other types of painful treatments such as debriding burn wounds or inserting a nasogastric tube. These treatments are considered ethically acceptable only if the harm is minimized as much as possible and the benefit to be gained is worth the pain. One great difficulty with the principle of beneficence involves determining just what constitutes good or worthwhile gain for a particular patient. For example, is it beneficent to withhold food and water from a patient who has no likely chance of recovering from a terrible head injury and remains comatose? Withholding food clearly does constitute some harm, but does the good of allowing nature to take its course and letting the patient die outweigh the harm of not feeding him or her? Some nurses and ethicists reason that it does, whereas others claim that it does not. How should this issue be resolved? Investigating other moral principles will provide some guidance.

Autonomy is another moral principle that has gained prominence in health care settings as patients' rights and informed consent issues have arisen.[15] *Autonomy* refers to the freedom to rule oneself. It includes the right of informed consent, the right to accept or refuse treatment, and the right to confidentiality. The principle of beneficence often conflicts with the principle of autonomy. For example, when a patient chooses not to have a recommended treatment needed to save his life, the nurse must decide whether to override the patient's decision to do the beneficent thing and administer the treatment or abide by the patient's refusal. Which principle should have the most weight for the trauma nurse in such a situation, the principle of autonomy or the principle of beneficence? Most ethicists today agree that autonomy has more weight in moral decision making than beneficence, but despite this, nurses often take a paternalistic stance vis-à-vis their patients.

Benjamin and Curtis[16] point out how difficult it is to justify taking any paternalistic actions toward adults. They list three criteria that must be met to decide ethically to carry out any paternalistic action:

1. *The autonomy condition:* when the patient is, under the circumstances, irretrievably ignorant of relevant information or the patient's capacity for rational reflection is significantly impaired.
2. *The harm condition:* when the patient is likely to be significantly harmed unless interfered with.
3. *The ratification condition:* when it is reasonable to assume that if the patient regained greater knowledge or recovery of his or her capacity for rational reflection at a later time, the patient would ratify the decision to interfere by consenting to it.

These are strong criteria, and they require much justification to warrant any overriding of a patient's autonomy. Often trauma nurses restrain patients against their wishes for safety reasons or out of legal or medical concerns. In cases in which patients are awake and alert enough to make decisions and refuse to be restrained, if the nurse continues with the restraining, he or she clearly is choosing to override the patient's own autonomous wishes. The more difficult case is one in which the patient is refusing, but the nurse has reason to think that his or her capacity to decide is impaired. The criteria listed above require more than this to justify overriding the patient's wishes such as knowing that the harm is significant and that there is reason to assume that the patient would authorize the restraining if he or she could reason better. If these conditions are met, the restraining is justified. Use of placebos also can be contrary to a patient's autonomy rights, and yet some health care workers continue to try to justify the use of placebos solely on the basis of beneficence.

Most ethicists agree that the autonomy rights of a patient override the professional's beneficence obligations in usual cases.[17-20] For example, the moral and constitutional legitimacy for withholding or withdrawing life-sustaining treatment at the request of the patient appears well settled in the United States.[21] Even when a patient is in a coma and the question is whether to continue nutrients and water, many think the issue is resolved if a living will made by the patient requests such withdrawal. This is because most regard living wills as akin to the patient exercising his or her autonomy, and they agree that such autonomy should be respected. Unfortunately, many people do not have a living will or the document itself may be unclear on this issue. In such cases the nurse is in a difficult position in trying to determine what action beneficence requires because the patient's autonomous wishes are unclear. In such cases decisions regarding whether to withdraw certain forms of treatment often fall to the family, to a legal guardian, or to the person the patient designated as the decision maker through another type of advanced directive (i.e., a durable power of attorney for health care).

Ozuna[22] encourages nurses to be knowledgeable about aspects of the patient that the family may be most interested in such as whether the patient can experience pain or suffering or whether the patient is capable of responding meaningfully to stimuli. Sharing such information with families repeatedly and with compassion helps them to accept the realities of the patient's current status. Unfortunately, sometimes this precise information cannot be determined by current technology, in which case the nurse is unable to meet the family needs and is left with ambiguity about how to maximize the beneficent interests of the patient.

Another ethical principle is *justice,* which requires that nurses treat all their patients fairly. This does not necessarily mean that every patient is treated exactly alike, but rather that equals are treated equally and that those who are unequal should be treated differently according to their differences.[23,24] This means that patients with similar health care problems deserve the same care and those who have different needs should be attended to according to those needs. It also means that the nurse should take into consideration a patient's cultural and religious preferences. However, when one looks at the way the general principle of justice functions in mainstream ethics, a possible problem does arise for the nurse.

General ethics requires everyone to be fair to everyone. When justice is limited in scope to a particular nurse's patients, duty to those patients may conflict with general ethical duty to everyone at large. This issue rears its head vociferously when scarcity of resources comes into play. Consider a case in which a trauma nurse is to receive a large number of patients from a disaster site. Does the nurse owe a duty to the patients he or she already has, to the ones he or she might get, or to both?[25] What if the duties seem to conflict? This difficult issue will occur more and more as health care resources become increasingly scarce. Can the trauma nurse justify using current resources on patients who have a lower chance of recovery rather than saving those resources for potential patients who will have a better chance to recover? What if the latter patients never arrive? The answers to these questions remain unclear, especially when one acknowledges the special obligation nurses have to patients already in their care.[26] Furthermore, if the public decides that nurses have obligations of justice to persons not included in the nurses' current patient load, this would have profound implications for the principle of fairness in future health care decisions. It is unclear whether the nurse could ethically function under such a requirement because of the traditional nursing commitment of special duties owed to current patients. These issues are only part of the conundrum of gray areas currently under consideration in the arena of public and professional ethics.

Finally, the moral principle of *fidelity* may shed some light on the appropriate actions of a nurse in promise-making situations. Fidelity involves being faithful to one's promises. What are the promises nurses implicitly make to patients in their care? Minimally, nurses promise that they will do no harm to that person, and it is hoped that they will do as much good for their patients as they can. This includes the promise that the nurse is capable of delivering the care the patient needs (i.e., that the nurse is competent). Note that these promises are made implicitly to patients already under the nurse's care. However, the principle of fidelity does not provide very clear directions for what obligations (if any) the nurse owes to any potential or future patients.

What is clear is that if a nurse makes an individual promise to a patient, then he or she has an obligation to follow through on it. The proper content of any promise a nurse should make to a patient, however, is still a gray area. Should a nurse remain faithful to a promise not to code a patient even if a physician has ordered such a procedure? What if this nurse needs her job to feed her five children and has reason to believe that if she resists the order she could be fired? Considerations about the nurse's own risks in making certain choices seem relevant to the moral weight of her promise, but to what extent should they prevail? Should the trauma nurse withhold pain medication from a patient because of persistent low blood pressure readings, despite the nurse's explicit promise to try to relieve the patient's pain? These complex questions are not entirely resolvable using only moral principles as guidelines. A review of ethical theories will help to clarify the nurse's obligations in these complex cases.

MORAL THEORIES

Moral or ethical theories are more general than rules and principles and provide the most basic foundation for ethical decision making, especially when rules or principles conflict. Theories set priorities on which rules or principles override others in specific instances.[27] There are two major types of moral theories: teleologic and deontologic.

The term *teleology* is derived from the Greek word *telos,* meaning "goal" or "end." Teleologic moral theories are consequentialist theories because they hold that the rightness or wrongness of an act is determined solely by the consequences the act produces or is foreseen to produce. All consequentialist theories are alike in that they require that a moral agent's actions maximize good; however, they differ in what they consider good to be. Such theories view no particular act as morally wrong in and of itself; only the consequences determine the morality of any action. Thus a particular act can be right in one situation and wrong in another situation as long as the consequences of the act differ in terms of the amount of good they produce.[11]

The term *deontology* is rooted in the Greek word *deon,* meaning "duty." Deontologic theories deny what consequentialist theories affirm. Deontologic theories claim that the morality of an act is determined by more than the consequences of that action. The moral status of an act is a result of other relevant factors such as the nature of the act itself. Using this type of theory to evaluate the morality of actions involves looking at established rules and principles that govern human conduct such as the Ten Commandments, the *Code of Ethics for Nurses,* or other procedures for determining formal duties.[10]

Although there are many different kinds of consequentialist or deontologic theories, the most familiar ones are utilitarian consequentialism and Kantian deontology. These two kinds of theories illustrate the reasoning often offered in discussions of ethical questions facing trauma nurses.

UTILITARIANISM

Classic utilitarianism has its roots in the early nineteenth-century works of Jeremy Bentham and John Stuart Mill. Despite the variations in their particular theories, both held that actions are to be judged by the amount of happiness or unhappiness that results from the action and that no one person's happiness or unhappiness counts any more than another's. Each person's welfare is equally weighted in the utilitarian calculus.

The power of utilitarianism lies in two important points. First, promoting the "most good overall" has strong intuitive appeal. It certainly seems like a laudable thing to do and may be the very best that one can hope to accomplish in the complex cases that face trauma nurses. Second, utilitarianism offers an objective way (in theory) to determine the answer to any and every ethical dilemma. One merely assesses the consequences of the various alternatives and chooses the one that leads to the greatest happiness. In effect, utilitarianism does away with every ethical dilemma, and all cases have a decisive, determinative best way to proceed.

Despite the obvious advantages of utilitarianism, there remain some grave difficulties for nurses who accept this as their sole theory of morality. Beneficence, autonomy, justice, and fidelity are accepted principles that apply to nursing practice. These principles cannot be accommodated in their appropriate weight for proper ethical decision making of nurses in a utilitarian framework. This is because utilitarianism gives no moral status to any principle beyond that it accords to the principle of utility (i.e., maximizing overall good).[10]

Here is an example showing the type of difficulty that a nurse might face by accepting utilitarianism as the appropriate ethical theory to guide his or her actions. Suppose a wealthy, famous patient was admitted to the trauma unit from the scene of a car crash and imagine that all the currently available nursing resources were lavished on this patient while other needy patients went unattended. Such an action would clearly seem to be unethical and violate the basic principle of fairness. However, if this patient subsequently gave a huge donation to the trauma center, which resulted in equipment being available for a greater number of patients than those left unserved originally, the actions of the nursing staff would be judged as right according to utilitarian standards. This is because a greater good resulted from the lavishing of resources on this one patient than would have occurred if the nurses had not done that. Surely this is an unacceptable outcome of moral decision making. Nurses do believe that unfair treatment of patients is morally wrong, just as the *Code of Ethics for Nurses* claims. Thus utilitarianism falls short of capturing some of the basic moral principles that nurses incorporate into their professional practice in this case. It does not have the theoretic flexibility to allow for the special duties that nurses believe they owe to their patients.

However, utilitarianism does have some insights to offer nurses considering ethical questions. It does seem that consequences should have some bearing on ethical decisions. Although it is apparent that nurses cannot consider consequences as the only relevant moral factor, it remains to be determined just how much weight should be given to consequences by the nurse. An exploration of deontology will shed some light on this difficult question.

DEONTOLOGY

Immanuel Kant,[28] an eighteenth-century philosopher, believed that morality consisted of following absolute rules no matter what the consequences. His primary test of whether a rule should be followed was to apply the categorical imperative of universality to the considered action. Whether an action was moral did not depend on the desire of the agent or the consequences of the action but rather on whether one's duty was to perform the action as determined by his moral test, better known as the *categorical imperative*. The appeal of Kantian ethics remains for persons who believe that acting on principle rather than because of good results is an important ethical insight. Kant also places a high value on autonomy and respect and can accommodate the special duties that nurses are thought to owe their patients. However, Kant's exploration of several applications of his categorical imperative in assessing the morality of lying, stealing, and suicide have been studied intensely and nearly uniformly rejected by later ethicists. For example, Kant concluded that stealing and suicide are always wrong and one must always tell the truth in all circumstances. Most contemporary deontologists think Kant went too far in concluding that morality requires absolute rules that do not take into account any consequences of actions. His theory is also limited in that it cannot adjudicate cases in which more than one duty applies but no alternative action can maximize both. Conflicts-of-duty situations are common in nursing practice, but Kant's ethics offer no way to resolve them. Several ethicists have tried to remain faithful to the spirit of Kantian ethics while trying to accommodate these common-sensical, well-established aspects of morality.

W. D. Ross[10] proposes a theory that provides some guidance in this regard. He claims that duties originate from the social relationships one finds oneself in and that eventually these duties are coalesced by humans into general duties. Ross claims that general duties have prima facie status and are overridable only in very particular circumstances. Furthermore, any overriding of a prima facie principle requires its own justification. He lists fidelity, reparation, gratitude, justice, beneficence, and nonmaleficence as prima facie duties owed to others. Ross does not prioritize these duties but says that some apply more stringently than others and all can be overridden at times. Presumably, circumstances and possible consequences play a role in defining the proper kind of justification for overriding a general principle. Thus Ross's theory manages to support some of the special duties of a nurse while allowing for mitigating circumstances such as the consequences of the act to be considered. Unfortunately, however, Ross's theory gives little direction about the way that justification is to proceed. He offers no rules or procedures to use in weighing the stringency of application of a particular principle in a specific moral situation nor any ways to justify one principle being applicable over another; thus his theory is incomplete in that it provides little guidance for deciding difficult cases.

W. K. Frankena,[29] another modern deontologist, posits a theory in which the principles of beneficence and justice are considered to be the most basic of all moral principles. Thus, for Frankena, in cases in which there is a conflict between one of these primary principles and autonomy or fidelity, the right moral action will be the one that maximizes the basic principle. For example, in a nursing situation in which justice and autonomy conflict, justice prevails; or when beneficence and fidelity conflict, beneficence triumphs. However, a major problem persists, for how is a case of conflict between beneficence and justice to be decided? Some of the cases discussed previously involving scarcity of resources and duties owed to very ill patients with questionable prognoses have this exact issue at their heart. If two patients have equal need to go to the intensive care unit (ICU) but there is only one ICU bed available, how does one decide which patient to send? Frankena's theory does not provide specific guidance for these difficult yet pressing cases.

As can be seen, both the utilitarian and deontologic theories have their own unique contributions to moral reasoning and their own sets of difficulties. In fact, no moral theory is without some problems. All moral theories fall short of some common-sensical and well-accepted portion of ethical judgment. This does not necessarily mean that any one of the moral theories is itself in error because it could also be the case that more than one moral theory is needed to deal with new and complex issues in health care settings. It should be noted, however, that each theory provides the nurse with some very important ethical insights and therefore can offer guidance for the nurse dealing with difficult ethical problems.

THE ETHICS OF CARING

Some nursing ethicists and theorists, such as Gadow,[30] Benner et al,[31] Bishop and Scudder,[32] Watson and Ray,[33] and others,[6] have described the ethic of nursing as the "ethic of caring." Gaul, Olesinski, and others opt for Gilligan's term, calling the ethical theory of nursing practice the "ethic of care."[13,34] Although definitions vary, *care* and *caring* are associated most often with the principle of beneficence. Some say care and caring are the same thing as beneficence. Others believe that the nurse's obligation to care for patients (to be caring) is merely supported by the principle of beneficence. As discussed previously, this emphasis on beneficence has its problems. Paternalism has often clouded the moral ideal of "doing good," and the ethic of care or caring is vulnerable to this difficulty. Perhaps this is why advocacy is so often linked by nursing scholars to the ethic of care or caring. But Winslow[35] and Trandel-Korenchuk[36] point out several complex difficulties inherent in the concept of advocacy. Much of the difficulty lies in the need to clarify exactly what advocacy requires. For example, is advocacy *doing* for a patient, *assisting* a patient, *defending* a patient, or some combination of these actions? Other problems involve clarifying *what* is to be advocated; that is, should the nurse advocate the patient's actual wishes or rather what is in the best interest of the patient? Furthermore, who is to define what constitutes the "best interest" of the patient? Should it be the patient, his or her family, the most expert health care professional, or someone else? How do the rules change with patients of different ages, competencies, or levels of consciousness?

Gadow[30] describes a model of "existential advocacy" that she claims avoids paternalism while maintaining the nurse as an involved, caring participant in the patient's decision-making process, but aspects of her model remain controversial.[35] For example, Gadow states that, as advocates, nurses should answer patients directly if asked their opinions about treatment options. Yet many question whether nurses can ever recommend a course of action for patients without interfering with the patients' autonomy by inadvertently manipulating or coercing them. Others question Gadow's claim that nurses gain ethical knowledge about where the boundary between benefit and harm lies for patients based on the nurse's special role as the touching, ministering caregiver.[30]

Bandman and Bandman[6] point out that the caring ethic has its roots in both the history of philosophy and the contemporary work of Carol Gilligan,[37] and Gaul notes that current literature in philosophy, feminist studies, and nursing have devoted much attention to the ethic of care.[13] However, Bishop and Scudder[32] claim that nursing's caring ethic belongs primarily to nursing's own history and practice.[22] Whatever the basis of the caring ethic, it offers important insights for nurses who seek to practice ethically. For example, the caring ethic describes the orientation nurses should have toward their patients; it demands empathy and compassion. It provides a basis for explaining the special duties that nurses owe their patients, such as beneficence and advocacy. Many authors regard the ethic of caring as a virtue theory of ethics because it deals primarily with the required moral excellence of nurses' character, demanding that nurses be caring toward their patients.[13,34] However, difficulties arise when one attempts (as Gadow[30] and Gilligan[37] do) to use the ethic of caring as a theory of moral obligation, that is, a theory that determines what actions are morally permissible, impermissible, or required. One difficulty is that the ethic of caring seems to be based on feelings, values, and intuition in such a way that the charge of pernicious relativism and subjectivism is hard to defend.

Gastmans and colleagues have attempted to give a fuller account of the morality of nursing practice.[34] They claim that moral nursing practice requires three components: a caring relationship between nurse and patient, an episode of caring behavior toward the patient that integrates the virtue of care with expert activity, and the goal of "good care" as the aim for the nursing activity. The "virtue of care" requires the acceptance of a "caring attitude" by the nurse and the performance of caring behaviors inspired by this attitude. This affective involvement of the nurse in the well-being of the patient is distinguished from other kinds of feelings such as those that may occur when attracted to certain personal features of a person. The former kind of affection is required for moral nursing practice, whereas the latter is not. It is not clear whether this amended version of the ethic of caring avoids the problems of relativism and subjectivism mentioned earlier. But even if it does, Gastmans and colleagues point out another limitation of their theory and one that would seem to plague any other ethic of caring theory. It involves the scope of the theory. Ethic of care theories require a relationship between the nurse and the patient, so they can only be used to justify the ethical nature of direct patient contact types of nursing practice. Gastmans and colleagues agree that other kinds of nursing practice that do not involve a relationship between patient and nurse may have moral significance, but they admit that their ethic of caring cannot provide any support, explanation, or guidance for such areas of practice.[34] This limitation might not be a problem for a caring ethical theory if no other sorts of nursing had moral significance, but that seems not to be the case.

McDaniel,[38] for example, claims that the work of nurse managers has a moral component. She holds that nurse managers are required ethically to create work environments that provide opportunities for nurses to engage in discussions about ethical concerns, that support nurses in their quest to provide ethical nursing care, and that develop policies and procedures that sustain nurses' ethical care with patients. Likewise, Aroskar[39] and Corley[40] claim that nurse managers have a moral responsibility to support collegial and collaborative relationships within nursing and between nursing and medicine because research has shown that positive patient outcomes and compassionate nursing care are dependent on such relationships. The ethic of care cannot provide any direct support for these claims, yet most nurses agree that nurse managers have moral obligations of this sort.

As has been shown, although the ethical theories and principles discussed thus far offer some direction regarding the moral dimensions of nursing practice, none is without significant limitations. Although ethical decision making requires a process that considers all the relevant moral factors, it is not endless, nor is it arbitrary. How should a nurse decide important ethical questions? How should a nurse judge between the ethical insights offered by the various moral theories and principles to act responsibly? The next section provides some direction in this regard.

Ethical Decision-Making Approaches

DeGrazia,[41] Baker,[42] and others[13] have pointed out various problems with using a foundationalist approach to ethical decision making. In this approach, a specific ethical theory or principle is used as the first premise in a deductive logical argument, and the pertinent facts about the ethical case are used as the second one. The ethically correct action is then deduced from these two premises. This method of ethical decision making has been criticized as not being sensitive enough to the complexity of the facts involved in ethical cases and for assuming a specific cultural value perspective. In addition, this approach is not very comprehensive. It gives little direction for new or unusual cases, yet these are just the sorts of cases that trauma nurses deal with all the time.

Callahan,[43] Curtin,[44] Degrazia,[41] and others support a more "coherentist" approach to ethical justification. A Harvard philosopher named John Rawls[45] has proposed such an approach in his theory of justice. He calls it "wide reflective equilibrium." Degrazia tests what he calls "specified principles" using the process of wide reflective equilibrium; and Gaul, following Arras,[13,45] also suggests using wide reflective equilibrium to decide ethical questions, but in combination with a case-based method called *casuistry.* The wide reflective equilibrium process can help nurses clarify their own moral framework by comparing and contrasting three important ethical databases—their own beliefs, values, and considered moral judgments—to moral principles and ethical theories. It is the preferred decision-making process for nurses to use when making ethically supportable choices in health care settings. The usefulness of this process is well illustrated by Benjamin and Curtis[16] in their book on nursing ethics when they discuss the justification process that led to the acceptance of using brain death criteria as a definitive way of establishing a person's death.

When beginning the reflective equilibrium process, the nurse should clarify the pertinent facts of the case at hand, the ethical question it presents, and the possible alternative actions that are available. Minimally, the facts include the patient's medical status, prognosis, stated wishes (if any), and current mental status. There may be more than one ethical issue involved in the case, but often there is only one clear dilemma—for example, whether to code a patient. Finally, the nurse should list the alternative actions available, such as calling a code, not calling a code, beginning some but not all code actions, or discussing the patient's code status with the patient, family, or physician. Then, while considering each alternative in turn, the nurse should clarify his or her own moral judgments about the alternative by exploring background beliefs and considered moral reasoning and then cross-referencing these with known and accepted moral principles and theories. Such deliberation might proceed something like this:

Considering the first alternative (i.e., calling a code), the nurse should initially identify his or her values and beliefs about the morality of calling a code on the patient in question. If the nurse has concerns about calling a code on this patient, it is likely that he or she has some moral compunction against taking this action. However, this alone is not enough to ensure that the nurse's moral judgment in this case is ethically sound. The nurse must then examine that judgment for validity by comparing it with accepted moral beliefs, principles, and theories. The nurse might find that some people question the rightness of coding the kind of patient in question, whereas others do not. The nurse should then further consider the action of calling a code.

In reflecting on the principle of beneficence, the nurse should consider his or her obligation not to harm the patient and his or her responsibility to do good. The nurse therefore needs to clarify whether calling a code is good in this situation and whether the harm that might be incurred by conducting a code is ethically warranted. If the nurse thinks that death is a more desirable end in this case than coding the patient, he or she needs to test the initial judgment by looking for further verification from the moral theories of utilitarianism and deontology.

Utilitarianism might confirm the nurse's tentative conclusion that coding the patient is wrong if the good of not coding outweighs the bad of coding. Things to consider are the consequences for the patient, the outcomes for society in terms of resource use and other payoffs, and the possible legal, financial, and other results that such a decision may cause for the nurse, physician, family, and hospital. In utilitarianism the possible legal difficulties for the health care team count in this assessment just as much as the actual outcome for the patient. Depending on the good or bad consequences that might occur for the nurse, patient, and others, utilitarianism might lead to the conclusion that the coding of the patient in question is the right moral action or the wrong moral action.

Given the status of the principle of beneficence in their systems, the deontologic theories of Frankena and Ross would support the coding of a patient if it was in the patient's best interests to survive. However, these theories could also support the decision to not code the patient if it was in the patient's best interest to end the patient's suffering and this was only possible by dying. Thus the difficulty here lies in determining what is in the patient's best interest, and this is often very difficult to do. If the patient's autonomous wishes about coding are known, given the status of autonomy in deontologic frameworks, it is likely that those wishes would prevail. When a patient's wishes are not known, there is still some disagreement about who should decide whether a code should be called in any particular case. Clearly the expertise of the physician is relevant to such a decision, but in most cases the decision cannot be made definitively on a purely medical basis. At this point in the analysis, the coding of the patient would be considered an ethically supportable action if the patient desired it or if the patient's best interests demanded it. On the other hand, it would not be morally supportable to call the code if the patient did not want such action or if the patient's best interests boded against such action. After conducting this inquiry concerning the first of the possible alternative actions, the nurse should go on to do a similar analysis of all the other possible actions available to resolve the ethical issue in question.

Obviously this type of analysis is very thorough and as such gives much credence to the decisions made. It is the preferable approach when the nurse has the time for prolonged deliberation. However, this process is time consuming, and it is not feasible in situations that require quick decision making.

Kenneth Iserson[46] has suggested another approach to ethical decisions when a rapid appraisal is needed, such as in many emergency and trauma situations. He claims that one should begin by asking whether the ethical problem at hand is similar in type to any other ethical problem for which one has already worked out a rule about how to proceed. If so, he suggests that the individual follow that rule, not because it is necessarily correct but rather because it is more likely than not to be an ethically acceptable action, given that the individual has used it before and discussed it with others. In addition to Iserson's guidelines, the rule should be an ethically comfortable stance for the nurse, and the nurse should already have clarified the facts, the moral question, and the alternative actions available in the situation. If the rule is ethically unacceptable for the nurse or if the nurse has no rule for this type of situation, then any option that would buy time for further deliberation without excessive risk to the patient must be considered. If there is such an option, the nurse should take it. If there is no available option, then the nurse should perform three quick moral assessment tests on the alternative action under consideration:

1. *Impartiality test:* The nurse asks whether he or she would be willing to have this action performed if the nurse were in the patient's place.
2. *Universalizability test:* The nurse asks whether he or she would be willing to have this action performed in all relevantly similar circumstances.
3. *Interpersonal justifiability test:* The nurse asks whether he or she is able to provide good reasons to justify his or her actions to others.[46]

The first test is not infallible, but it is a good way to correct one obvious source of moral error, that of partiality or self-interested bias. The second test is also designed to eliminate a moral decision difficulty, shortsightedness. It enables the nurse to evaluate the action by considering whether it should be followed as a general practice in all similar circumstances. This is important because, although one may approve of the action in the particular situation, it may not be an acceptable practice to follow in similar circumstances. Moral rules are supposed to apply generally, and it is this that the nurse is assessing with this test. The final test requires that the nurse has reasons for proceeding in the way decided on and, further, that others would approve of the reasons for this action. This ensures that the nurse has considered the decision thoughtfully and that his or her reasons are sound and not idiosyncratic.

All ethical stands should be reviewed periodically for relevance and credence. Sometimes this process results in rule adjustments, whereas at other times it merely confirms the nurse's preexisting stance. Whatever way it goes, the review process will help to clarify and reinforce sound ethical decision making on the part of the nurse. Schroeter and Taylor[26] identify several strategies that nurses in critical care environments can use to address the ethical issues that they confront in practice. Becoming familiar with typical issues and with new issues that arise is an important first step. Three new issues that deserve particular attention here are: the practice of family presence during invasive procedures and cardiopulmonary resuscitation (CPR), non–heart-beating organ donation (NHBOD), and end-of-life care for trauma patients. Each of these is discussed in the next section.

NEW ISSUES IN TRAUMA CARE

FAMILY PRESENCE

Family presence during invasive procedures and CPR is an issue that trauma nurses need to consider from a practical and ethical perspective when caring for trauma patients. According to Clark et al.,[47] family presence is usually defined as "the presence of family in the patient care area, in a location that affords visual or physical contact with the patient during invasive procedures or resuscitation events." Nurses have been at the forefront in supporting family presence for nearly 15 years. For example, in 1993, the Emergency Nurses Association adopted a resolution supporting family presence and developed a position paper on the practice the following year. Since then the American Association of Critical Care Nurses have also recommended the practice. Other health care groups such as the American Heart Association, the National Association of Social Workers, and the National Association of Emergency Medical Technicians have developed recommendations incorporating the practice. More recently, the American Academy of Pediatrics and the American College of Emergency Physicians expressed support for the parental option of being with the child during medical procedures. However, policies supporting family presence in these situations at trauma centers are less common. The reasons for this are somewhat unclear, although the obvious intensity of the trauma setting and the emotionally charged atmosphere of the trauma situation are sometimes cited as contributing factors.

Family presence must be handled on an individual basis and should be offered in appropriate circumstances but should not be demanded or expected. According to Clark et al.,[47] research shows that approximately 30% of families report not wanting to be present during invasive procedures or CPR, and their right to refuse being present must be honored. Although initially nurses and physicians often voice concerns about having families present in such circumstances, the literature shows that when they have had an experience with family presence during invasive procedures or CPR, they generally form a positive view toward the practice. Studies affirm that family presence does not interrupt care, negatively affect providers' performance, or increase litigation rates. "For patients, family presence may provide comfort, increased feelings of safety, and lessen fear."[48]

Several things need to be in place to allow for family presence during invasive procedures or CPR. For example, a clear policy should be written about family presence and the staff needs to be educated about the practice. It is also important to have a designated person to provide support to the family before, during, and after the procedure or resuscitation. This could be the chaplain or social worker, although in some institutions advance practice nurses function in this capacity. Family members who are angry, violent, intoxicated, or under the influence of drugs should not be allowed in the room where invasive procedures or CPR is being done for the safety of the patient and health care personnel. The trauma nurse needs to use good judgment and sound ethical reasoning to maximize the benefits of family presence while minimizing the possible harm that could occur if the family members themselves seem like they might harm the patient or staff.

Donation After Cardiac Death

Donation after cardiac death (DCD), previously known as NHBOD, is a newer option that conscious dying patients and the nurses and families of unconscious dying patients might face after trauma events. DCD involves the taking of organs after cessation of the patient's heartbeat, whereas since the 1980s most cadaveric organ donations are taken from brain-dead patients.

Many trauma centers, including the prestigious R Adams Cowley Shock Trauma Center at the University of Maryland Medical Center, have instituted policies supporting the practice of DCD. The reasons are quite clear. Since 1981 (after brain death criteria were included in the Determination of Death Act) 25% of organ donations come from live donors, whereas 75% come from cadaveric donors, mainly brain-dead donors. However, although more than 30,000 Americans had an organ transplant in 2005, more than 19 die every day waiting for an organ transplant, and there are more than 92,000 people in the United States still waiting for an organ donor. It is estimated that the practice of DCD could increase the donor pool by 25%, greatly improving the odds of getting a viable organ for many thousands of people. In addition, many non–brain-dead trauma patients and their families might wish to donate organs, and DCD provides an opportunity for them to do so. The possibility of organ donation may also bring some comfort to patients and families at a time when a situation seems to have no good associated with it.[49]

A well-accepted ethical rule about organ donation is the so called "dead donor" rule. It holds that no life-sustaining organs can be removed from a person's body until a reliable determination is made that the person is dead. This rule clearly stipulates that persons cannot be killed for their organs or by the removal of their organs. Furthermore, vital organs can only be removed from dead patients, and living patients cannot have their death hastened to remove organs. The practice of DCD is considered by some to violate this nearly universally accepted dead-donor rule. Even those who agree that it does not, believe that at least the procedures involved in the harvesting of organs from cardiac death donors must be carefully developed to avoid the possibility of violating this nearly universally accepted ethical rule.[49-51]

This issue surfaces because organ retrieval from a DCD donor must occur within a few minutes after circulation has ceased to minimize warm ischemia, whereas organ donation from a heart-beating cadaver (i.e., someone who is brain dead) can be delayed for hours if need be. Therefore, removal of life support from the potential DCD donor must occur in or near the operating room (OR) just as is true for heart-beating brain-dead donors, but in the former case the family may want to remain with the patient until he or she dies (i.e., until the heart stops beating and respirations cease), whereas they are not usually present with the brain-dead donor when the "life support" measures are removed. Although family members may want to remain with the patient until death is pronounced, if this event is occurring in the OR environment, it is not always allowed because there are concerns for the safety of the family members in the OR as family members may become faint or possibly contaminated with blood or body fluids. Many hospitals are using a room very close to the OR so that the families can be with their loved one as cardiac and respiratory death occurs. Another ethical concern is that of maintaining a standard of care for the dying patient no matter where the death is occurring (i.e., a patient being taken off of life support in the OR should receive the same care as the patient who is being "allowed to die" in the intensive care unit). The problem is that in the sterile environment of the OR it is difficult to maintain the same patient and family comfort measures. These are some other reasons why the issue of DCD is being examined from an ethical perspective.

There are two types of DCD: controlled and uncontrolled. The controlled scenario involves a patient who is ventilator dependent and has a poor prognosis but is not brain dead. The decision is made by the patient (if conscious) or the family to remove the ventilator and not initiate CPR. Sometimes medications such as heparin and phentolamine mesylate (Regitine) are given before the ventilator is withdrawn to ensure better organ perfusion and better organ viability. The ventilator is withdrawn and the team waits for the patient's heart to stop beating. Cardiac death is pronounced 2 to 5 minutes after asystole, and the dead person's organs are rapidly removed before they deteriorate. If the patient's heart does not stop beating within a predetermined time frame, the organ procurement is cancelled and the patient returns to the unit to die. Uncontrolled DCD takes place when a person dies suddenly and cannot be resuscitated. The patient is pronounced dead and cold preservation fluid is instilled through a femoral catheter until organ procurement permission is sought from next of kin. Organs are removed if permission is obtained.

Certain ethical safeguards are important to have in place in the case of DCD. First of all, the decision to withdraw life support must be made before and independently from the decision for organ donation. Second, the decision of where to withdraw life support requires informed consent and it is preferable that familiar staff are allowed to remain with the patient and his or her family. Third, the family should be allowed to remain with the patient until the patient's heart stops beating and organ retrieval begins. Fourth, the physicians involved in pronouncing death cannot be involved in organ retrieval. And fifth, no payment can be given to the donor or family and no financial burden should be borne by them for the organ retrieval.

Even when these safeguards are in place, there remain areas of ethical concern about the practice of DCD. For example, should the nonbeneficent practice of premortem cannulation and the injection of agents given solely to optimally preserve organ function be permitted? Disagreement remains about the time, place, and required observations for determination of death. Because the DCD donor is not brain dead, questions about whether sentience remains when organs are being procured persist. In addition, questions about whether circulatory and respiratory functions of the DCD donor have been irreversibly lost when the donor is pronounced dead are still being asked.[50,52]

Despite the persistence of such ethical questions, the demand for organs is increasing. So in 2003, the Department of Health and Human Services launched the "Organ Donation Breakthrough Collaborative" to bring together donation professionals and hospital leaders to identify and share best practices to maximize donation rates from potential donors who die in their facilities.[53] Health care institutions in major cities throughout the United States are collaboratively developing protocols for DCD. Some of these protocols have been put into place and have increased the donor pool by 16% over 2003 numbers. However, studies still need to be done to determine whether those DCD protocols safeguard patient's rights and ethical rules while increasing the organ donation pool. This is an area that deserves continued scrutiny by both ethicists and practitioners.

END-OF-LIFE CARE

For nearly 20 years there has been an increased emphasis on improving the care of dying persons and their families in American hospitals. But as Ahrens et al.[54] point out, "...instances of withholding or withdrawing life-sustaining or prolonged treatments are increasing. Most deaths are somehow 'negotiated,' underscoring the need to study and improve end-of-life care." Jacob et al.[55] note, however, that "End of life care for trauma patients is unique...." Some of the challenges for trauma end-of-life care include "unfamiliarity with patient's wishes and values, the critical nature of the injury, the overwhelming feelings of guilt that families often experience, the suddenness and acuity of the crisis, and the need to make life-and-death decisions...."[55] Currently, trauma nurses work within their own systems and use their own ethical resources to resolve end-of-life care ethical issues, but soon specific directions for end-of-life care will be available from the American Trauma Society (ATS).

In 2003, the ATS began a process that culminated in a plan to develop a best-practice model specifically for dying trauma patients and their families. The product being developed is called the Trauma End-of-Life Optimum Support project or TELOS. It aims to standardize the care of dying trauma patients and their families from the time of injury through to death. It will focus on six clinical domains: decision making, communication, physical care, psychologic care, spiritual care, and culturally sensitive social care. *Telos* is a Greek word meaning "end" or "purpose" and was chosen intentionally to underscore the philosophic foundations of this project. The TELOS developers conclude that dying trauma patients should have end-of-life care that is "right" in the sense of medically appropriate and "good" in the sense of morally appropriate. These guidelines should go a long way to support the health care team in end-of-life care trauma situations. Besides a best-practice model, by 2008 the TELOS product will also include educational programs to guide implementation, evaluation tools to determine end-of-life care outcomes, and references for practitioners about cutting-edge end-of-life care for trauma patients and their families.[55]

But for now, decisions about when to institute end-of-life care and what that care should involve are difficult in trauma settings. Although generally physicians write the orders for treatment withdrawal on dying patients, it is the nurses who most often attend to the end-of-life care needs of those patients and their families. The literature confirms that critical care nurses are concerned about providing dying patients with the best care possible at the end of their lives and this undoubtedly includes nurses working in trauma settings. Providing the patient's family with a peaceful, dignified bedside scene as the family member is dying is vitally important. This involves giving the patient adequate pain and antianxiety medication, which can include the use of morphine for the discomfort related to shortness of breath. Families also need to be encouraged to talk with their loved one, whatever the patient's level of consciousness. Often they feel comforted by assisting with their love one's physical care. Talking with families about their concerns, providing them with timely information about what to expect, and allowing flexible visiting hours also helps them to deal with the death. Such accommodations are within the purview of the trauma nurse to institute. Sometimes, however, families can create barriers for the nurse trying to provide good end-of-life care for patients.

In a 2000 study by Kirchhoff and Beckstrand,[56] critical care nurses identified that six of the top ten obstacles they encounter when trying to provide good end-of-life care were due to patient families. Multiple calls from family and friends to the nurse rather than appointing a designated family contact was the top barrier noted. Also families that do not understand what "life-saving" measures mean or who do not accept the patient's prognosis can create conflicts for the nurse trying to give good end-of-life care. Sometimes families are angry or are fighting among themselves about whether to continue life-saving measures. Physicians can also create problems for nurses trying to provide end-of-life care to dying patients, especially when they are overly optimistic about the patient surviving or do not communicate with other physicians or family members.

This study also identified things that help the nurse provide good end-of-life care. Agreement among physicians about what care should be given was ranked as first. Others included having the family accept that the patient is dying, having time to prepare the family for the death, allowing the family adequate time alone with the patient, and being able to provide a peaceful, dignified bedside scene for the family after death were the highest ranked helpful factors.[56] The better a trauma setting is able to support nurses to carry out these activities for dying patients and their families, the better the end-of-life care for those patients will be.

SUMMARY

Trauma nurses will encounter new ethical issues as technology and practice changes occur. They should discuss new issues with resource persons such as ethicists, ethics committee members, administrators, and peers. Nurses also need to keep abreast of the literature on familiar and new ethical issues and seek out the opinions of other health care professionals, especially physicians, on these issues. Nurses can form groups to support each other in ethically ambiguous situations and to help brainstorm about the means to deal with such issues. Trauma nurses should know and understand the policies of their institutions regarding such things as brain death criteria, donation after cardiac death, and the status of living wills and durable power of health care attorney documents. If nurses have questions about these policies, it is their duty to seek clarification and to bring problems to the appropriate person. In addition, departmental processes should be put into place to address common ethical problems and to acknowledge the suffering that nurses experience in such situations.[26] Although there is no way to eliminate or totally resolve all ethical questions in practice, having a structure in place to assist the staff nurses in dealing with ethical dilemmas will go a long way toward resolving the ethical difficulties that nurses face.

In addition, trauma nurses themselves will be more prepared to deal with ethical problems if they are knowledgeable about the nursing profession's code of ethics, general moral principles, ethical theories (including the ethic of caring), and ethical decision-making processes. Armed with these guideposts, nurses have at their fingertips the tools they need to make sound ethical decisions in nursing practice.

REFERENCES

1. Capron AM: Legal setting of emergency medicine. In Iserson KV, Arthur B, Sanders MD, editors: *Ethics in emergency medicine,* ed 2, Tucson, 1995, Galen Press.
2. Buchanan AE: What is ethics? In Iserson KV, Arthur B, Sanders MD, editors: *Ethics in emergency medicine,* ed 2, Tucson, 1995, Galen Press.
3. Veins DC: A history of nursing's code of ethics, *Nurs Outlook* 37(1):45-49, 1989.
4. Yeaworth RC: The ANA code: a comparative perspective, *J Nurs Scholarship* 17(3):94-98, 1985.
5. American Nurses' Association: *Code of ethics for nurses with interpretive statements,* Kansas City, Mo, 2001, American Nurses' Association.
6. Bandman E, Bandman B: *Nursing ethics through the life span,* ed 4, Norwalk, Conn, 2002, Prentice Hall.
7. Post S, editor: *Encyclopedia of bioethics,* 3rd rev ed, Tappan, NJ, 2003, Macmillan.
8. Corley MC, Goren S: The dark side of nursing: impact of stigmatizing responses on patients, *Sch Inq Nurs Pract* 12(2): 99-122, 1998.
9. Rushton CH: ANA code of ethics for nurses revision adds bold new provision, *AACN Newsletter* 22(8):5, 17, 2005.

10. Feldman F: *Introductory ethics,* Englewood Cliffs, NJ, 1978, Prentice-Hall.
11. Rachels J: *The elements of moral philosophy,* ed 3, Burr Ridge, Ill, 1998, McGraw-Hill.
12. Olesinski N, Stannard D: Commentary on casuistry, care, compassion and ethics, *AACN Nurs Scopes Crit Care* July-Sept, 1996.
13. Gaul AL: Casuistry, care, compassion, and ethics data analysis, *Adv Nurs Sci* 17(3):47-57, 1995.
14. Mitchell C, Achtenberg B: *Study guide for code gray film,* Boston, 1984, Fanlight Productions.
15. Fry ST: Ethical principles in nursing education and practice: a missing link in the unification issue, *Nurs Health Care* 3(9):363-368, 1982.
16. Benjamin M, Curtis J: *Ethics in nursing,* ed 3, New York, 1991, Oxford University Press.
17. Davis AJ, Aroskar MA, Liaschenko J: *Ethical dilemmas and nursing practice,* ed 4, Englewood Cliffs, NJ, 1997, Prentice Hall.
18. Jameton A: *Nursing practice: the ethical issues,* Englewood Cliffs, NJ, 1984, Prentice Hall.
19. Thompson JE, Thompson HO: *Bioethical decision-making of nurses,* New York, 1995, Appleton-Century-Crofts.
20. Veatch RM: *Medical ethics,* ed 2, Boston, 1997, Jones & Bartlett.
21. Gostin LO: Deciding life and death in the courtroom, *JAMA* 278(18):1523-1528, 1997.
22. Ozuna J: Persistent vegetative state: important considerations for the neuroscience nurse, *J Neurosci Nurs* 28(3):199-203, 1998.
23. Beauchamp TL, Walters L, editors: *Contemporary issues in bioethics,* ed 6, Belmont, Calif, 2002, Wadsworth.
24. Beauchamp T, Childress JF: *Principles of biomedical ethics,* ed 5, New York, 2001, Oxford University Press.
25. Reverly S: An historical perspective. In Mitchell C, Achtenberg B, editors: *Study guide for code gray film,* pp 20-21, Boston, 1984, Fanlight Productions.
26. Schroeter K, Taylor GJ: Ethical considerations in organ donation for critical care nurses, *Crit Care Nurse* 19(2):60-69, 1999.
27. Bandman EL, Bandman B: Ethical aspects of nursing. In Flynn JB, Heffron PB, editors: *Nursing from concept to practice,* ed 2, Norwalk, Conn, 1988, Appleton & Lange.
28. Kant I: *Fundamental principles of the metaphysics of morals,* New York, 1949, Liberal Arts.
29. Frankena WK: *Ethics,* ed 2, Englewood Cliffs, NJ, 1988, Prentice Hall.
30. Gadow S: Ethical dimensions. In Beare PG, Myers JL, editors: *Principles and practice of adult health nursing,* St. Louis, 1998, Elsevier.
31. Benner P, Tanner CA, Chesla CA: *Expertise in nursing practice: caring clinical judgement and ethics*, New York, 1996, Springer.
32. Bishop AH, Scudder JR: *The practical, moral, and personal sense of nursing,* Albany, 1990, State University of New York Press.
33. Watson J, Ray MA, editors: *The ethics of care and the ethics of cure: synthesis in chronicity*, Publication No. 15-2237, New York, 1988, National League for Nursing.
34. Gastmans C, Dierckx de Casterle B, Schotsmans P et al: Nursing considered as moral practice: a philosophical ethical interpretation of nursing, *Kennedy Inst Ethics J* 8(1):43-69, 1998.
35. Winslow GR: From loyalty to advocacy: a new metaphor for nursing, *Hastings Cent Rep* June 1984.
36. Trandel-Korenchuk D, Trandel-Korenchuk K: Nursing advocacy of patients' rights: myth or reality? *NLN Publ* 20-2294:111-120, June 1990.
37. Gilligan C: *In a different voice,* Cambridge, Mass, 1982, Harvard University Press.
38. McDaniel C: Ethical environments: reports of practicing nurses, *Nurs Clin North Am* 33(2):363-371, 1998.
39. Aroskar MA: Ethical working relationships in patient care: challenges and possibilities, *Nurs Clin North Am* 33(2): 313-324, 1998.
40. Corley MC: Ethical dimensions of nurse-physician relations in critical care, *Nurs Clin North Am* 33(2):325-337, 1998.
41. DeGrazia D: Moving forward in bioethical theory: theories, cases and specified principalism, *J Med Philos* 17(8):511-539, 1992.
42. Baker R: A theory of international bioethics: multiculturalism, post-modernism, and the bankruptcy of fundamentalism, *Kennedy Inst Ethics J* 8(3):201-231, 1998.
43. Callahan JC, editor: *Ethical issues in professional life,* New York, 1988, Oxford University Press.
44. Curtin LL: Nursing ethics: theories and pragmatics, *Nurs Forum* 17:4-11, 1978.
45. Rawls J: *A theory of justice,* rev ed, Cambridge, Mass, 1999, Belknap Press.
46. Iserson KV: An approach to ethical problems in emergency medicine. In Iserson KV, Arthur B, Sanders MD, editors: *Ethics in emergency medicine,* ed 2, Tucson, 1995, Galen Press.
47. Clark AP, Meyers TA, Eichhorn DJ, et al: Family presence during cardiopulmonary resuscitation and invasive procedures, *Crit Care Nurs Clin North Am* 1(4):569-575, 2001.
48. Emergency Nurses Association: *Position statement: family presence at the bedside during invasive procedures and cardiopulmonary resuscitation,* Des Plaines, Ill, 2005, Emergency Nurses Association.
49. Truog RD, Robinson WM: Role of brain death and the dead-donor rule in the ethics of organ transplantation, *Crit Care Med* 31(9):2391-2396, 2003.
50. Bell MD: Non-heart beating organ donation: old procurement strategy—new ethical problems, *J Med Ethics* 29:176-181, 2003.
51. Snell GI, Levey B J, Williams TJ: Non-heart beating organ donation, *Intern Med J* 24:501-50, 2004.
52. Zamperetti N, Bellomo R, Ronco C: Defining death in non-heart beating organ donors, *J Med Ethics* 29:182-185, 2003.
53. U.S, Department of Health and Human Services: New high set for organ transplants, news release, March 29, 2005.
54. Ahrens T, Yance V, Kollef M: Improving family communications at the end of life: implications for length of stay in the intensive care unit and resource use, *Am J Crit Care* 7(12):317-324, 2003.
55. Jacob LM, Jacobs BB, Burns KJ: A plan to improve end-of-life care for trauma victims and their families, *J Trauma Nurs* 12(3):73-76, 2005.
56. Kirchhoff KT, Beckstrand RL: Critical care nurses' perceptions of obstacles and helpful behaviors in providing end of life care to dying patients, *Am J Crit Care* 9(2):96-105, 2000.

5

LEGAL CONCERNS IN TRAUMA NURSING

Robert W. Heilig

Trauma nursing has undergone a rapid evolution, as is evident by the nursing, medical, and scientific content of this book. Before the 1950s any nursing book that dealt with the law could do so in the context of ethical or administrative considerations only. Up to that time, the law for nurses was subordinate to the law for physicians, as was the nurse's role in patient care.

The legal notion of independent judgment by nurses was established during the late 1950s and early 1960s.[1,2] Today the nurse in a trauma setting performs highly skilled functions in the care of patients, including the coordination and delivery of services, the monitoring of complex physiologic data, the diagnosis of psychologic and physical states, and the operation of sophisticated life-saving equipment. The performance of such functions mandates the regular exercise of independent judgment without the supervision of a physician.[3]

This increased sophistication and the added authority bring additional responsibility. This in turn requires that the nurse have greater knowledge of medical, scientific, and especially legal issues. Trauma nursing takes place against the backdrop of a legal system growing increasingly complex and vigilant of professionals.

The purpose of this chapter is to provide trauma nurses with a survey of the primary legal issues that affect their professional lives. Its main themes are the patient's right to control over his or her body and life and the nurse's obligation to act reasonably and prudently according to current standards of nursing care. This chapter does not substitute for the advice of an attorney. It will provide nurses with a working knowledge of those subject areas in which they or their patients have specific rights and responsibilities.

SOURCES OF LAW

U.S. law is divisible into four main areas: common law, statutory law, administrative law, and constitutional law. These divisions correspond to the three branches of government at the federal and state level: judicial, legislative, and executive. Constitutional law deals with those rights and protections granted by our Constitution.

Common law, sometimes referred to as *case law,* results from decisions of the courts. The judiciary, including juries, is given the responsibility to seek the facts in particular cases and controversies and to apply the law to reach a decision. *Statutory law* derives from acts passed by legislatures. The legislatures (Congress at the federal level and legislative bodies at the state level) are empowered to pass laws dealing with subjects for whom the respective constitutions have granted them authority. *Administrative law* stems from the rule-making process and results in regulations promulgated by the executive branch. The president of the United States and the governors of individual states preside over the operation of executive or regulatory agencies that have been given specific authority to make rules by acts of the legislatures. All three branches of federal and state government are restricted by the "higher" law of the Constitution of the United States. Constitutional law, in particular the first 10 amendments (the Bill of Rights), set forth many of the rights of patients and nurses (as employees). Actions that are contrary to its provisions cannot be incorporated into common, statutory, or administrative law. State governments are also restricted by any additional provisions contained in the constitutions of the individual states.

Each of these sources of law influences the legal issues discussed in this chapter. These issues are constantly undergoing change as the law evolves. The methods by which the law is created and the manner in which it changes are discussed in the following section.

COMMON LAW

Common law is the term used to describe the body of principles that arises from court decisions. More generally, it is known as *case law* and consists of the accumulation of judicial opinions prepared by judges at the trial and appellate levels from lawsuits initiated by parties (litigants) to a controversy. Common law traces its roots back to eleventh-century England. The underlying principle of the common law is *stare decisis,* which means the law will provide continuity by deciding cases consistent with the precedents set by earlier cases. This means only that controversies between two litigants that are the same factually and that raise the same legal issues will be decided the same way. This continuity is dependent on there being no changes in statutory law and no changes in public policy. Because both evolve as society changes, common law also evolves. The reliance on precedent in judicial decrees generally guarantees controlled change in the common law on which the public can rely.

Over the years judges have recognized the existence of a number of rights that are necessary for the orderly operation of society. Many of these have been embodied in the law of torts. For nursing, the area of common law that is most relevant is *tort law,* which is more commonly known as negligence (malpractice), assault and battery (unauthorized and unprivileged contact between two people), and the judicially recognized right to privacy.

Torts are civil (as opposed to criminal) "wrongs" committed by one person against another. Typically these wrongs can be "righted" through an action brought before a judge or jury. For example, hundreds of years ago courts established the individual's right to be free of the negligent acts of another that cause harm, and it established the right to the remedy to this harm (i.e., monetary compensation to the injured party). Whereas civil law speaks to the relations between people, criminal law speaks to actions prohibited by society as a whole. Legal actions under civil law are between private parties; actions under criminal law are brought by the government (society) against individuals (or corporations).

Statutory Law

Statutes are the acts of Congress and state legislatures that regulate the lives of the people. Unlike common law, statutory law does not change through time and evolution but rather by the deliberate acts of the legislatures to create, amend, or repeal statutes. Statutory law deals with such diverse topics as taxation, interstate commerce, and the regulation of professions, which is pertinent to nursing.

Trauma nursing, like all nursing, is affected by state laws that define the minimum standards required of a licensed nurse. These laws, generally called *Nurse Practice Acts,* exist to protect citizens from untrained or incompetent persons who offer to practice nursing.[4,5] They regulate nursing by defining the types of acts that licensed practical nurses and registered nurses can perform and by providing a mechanism to exclude from the profession those who are incompetent.

Trauma nursing is also affected by statutes dealing with brain death and by laws requiring that nurses report incidents of child or spousal abuse, abuse of the elderly, and certain criminal acts. Other legislative acts prescribe the manner in which criminal evidence must be handled for it to be admissible in a criminal action. These statutes have been the subject of many judicial proceedings over the past 40 years, so the law relative to the handling of criminal evidence is grounded in common law and statutory law.

Administrative Law

Administrative law is created when a regulatory agency is empowered by the legislature through a statute to make rules to control the actions of a class of individuals. These rules and regulations are the clarification of statutes passed by the legislature or Congress and must be consistent with the intent of the legislature.

Administrative law is a relatively modern form of law unique to the United States. Rules and regulations can be and are changed by the administrative agencies that administer them as the circumstances underlying them change. The administrative procedure statutes of the state and federal governments control the process for developing and changing regulations. This means that regulatory agencies are empowered to make rules and to change them only after the class of individuals affected has had the opportunity to comment on the changes. The purpose of these requirements is to ensure that regulations reflect the reality of, for example, nursing practice and that they not be unreasonable. Furthermore, the rules cannot be made in an arbitrary or capricious manner. Regulations change not exclusively as a result of societal evolution and not solely by the act of a legislative body. Rather, they are the result of statutory changes and changes in the work of the people regulated.

Trauma nursing is affected by administrative law through the state boards of nursing. They exist as a result of the legislature empowering the boards to regulate nursing through Nurse Practice Acts.[4] These boards establish and enforce the rules that define requirements for licensure, but they also are empowered to further define allowable nursing acts and the education requirements for nurses. State boards of nursing decide cases involving violations of the professional standards of care embodied in these regulations or set forth in the enabling legislation. The board of nursing can discipline nurses if they violate the standards established for practice. While fundamentally the same, these standards do vary slightly from state to state, and the reader is encouraged to investigate the particulars of the state in which he or she is licensed. Some of the bases for disciplinary action common to all states include fraud in obtaining or in using a nursing license, conviction of a felony or other crime involving moral turpitude (acts involving abusive behavior, dishonesty, or immodesty), knowingly failing to file a required record or report, knowingly filing a false record or report, and drug or alcohol addiction or other physical or mental condition rendering the individual nurse incapable of acting as a nurse. The grounds for disciplinary action also may include refusing to provide, withholding of, denial of, or discrimination in providing nursing services to patients who have tested positive for the human immunodeficiency virus.[4] A nurse's license is likely to be suspended or revoked for a serious violation of the standards of practice or for repeated violations.

Another area of law that may significantly affect trauma nurses is local ordinances. In many regions the trauma system is controlled locally. That is, a county may be empowered to designate and adopt rules regulating trauma centers. These local rules (ordinances) frequently contain reporting and educational requirements for nurses.

Law affects the lives of all professionals. The types of laws and the manner in which they come into being have been briefly explained. What remains is to relate these concepts to the specific aspects of trauma nursing practice.

Legal Issues of Trauma Nursing

The issues of law that affect trauma nursing derive from the three sources of law and the actions of the corresponding branches of government. The general legal concepts discussed in the following sections contain both the pertinent elements of the law and their relevance to nursing actions. Many of these concepts are interwoven with ethical considerations discussed in Chapter 4.

Consent to Treatment

The nature of trauma practice requires that nurses touch patients and administer therapeutic care. The law, on the other hand, has as a basic principle the right of the individual to determine who shall touch him or her and in what manner and that the competent individual can refuse to be treated. Violation of this right of the individual is a violation of common law.[6]

Every human of adult years and sound mind has a right to determine what shall be done with his or her own body. A professional who provides treatment without the patient's consent commits an assault for which he or she is liable in damages.[7] About this right the law is quite rigid, and failure to obtain consent for a treatment may subject the professional to a lawsuit.

Three elements must be present if consent is to be valid: (1) capacity, (2) information, and (3) voluntariness. *Capacity* refers to the right of the patient to give consent. Minors and incompetent adults, legally, lack the capacity to give consent. *Information* refers to the sufficiency of the patient's understanding of what is being consented to. If the descriptions of treatments given on consent forms or made verbally fail to state clearly what is to be done in a way the patient can understand, then consent is not valid. *Voluntariness* refers to lack of coercion. Consent obtained by trick or by threat is not valid.

The requirement to obtain consent applies to all treatments done to a patient. Specific consent for invasive procedures must be obtained by the person performing the procedure, generally the physician. Nurses frequently are involved in witnessing consent for such procedures. Although the nurse is not directly responsible for the performance of these procedures and the particulars of such consent, it is prudent to be aware of them. For nursing practice separate from physician practice, the reasonable act for the nurse is to inform the patient of any touching to be performed and the reason for the touching and to obtain the patient's consent.

Violations of common law for obtaining valid consent require that the patient shows that the treatment caused some harm and that the treatment would not have been permitted if the possibility of this harm were known. This is true even if there is no lack of care in administering the treatment. It is therefore *critical* to obtain consent to stay within the law. Note that harm does not necessarily equate to injury, and nonconsensual contact, even if beneficial to the health of the patient, is not permitted under the law.

Informed Consent

Over the years, the concept of consent has been refined so that it is now referred to generally as *informed consent.* The adjective *informed* is not superfluous in this concept. It exists because the courts mandate that consent can be given only if the patient is knowledgeable about the effects of the treatment and has made an affirmative decision to receive the treatment.

Hospitals and trauma centers all require patients to sign a consent to treatment form upon admission. Nurses should look on this form as constituting consent by the patient to be taken care of in the facility and not as consent to all procedures, treatments, and therapies. Each time the patient is to be touched, the action involved should be explained, and either verbal or written agreement or some action demonstrating willingness to participate in the treatment should be received from the patient. Consent forms that specifically list the procedures to be performed and the risks or consequences are gaining increasing favor under the law. Note, however, that a signed consent form obtained from a patient who does not understand its contents is not valid consent.

The general rule of consent is that the patient should be told everything that is to be done each time something is to be done to or for the patient and that the patient should agree to the treatment or procedure. The patient should be informed of the nature of the treatment, its benefits and risks, and any reasonable alternatives. Furthermore, the explanation should be couched in terms *understandable* to patients because courts tend to favor what the "reasonable patient would expect to know to make an informed decision regarding consent for treatment" as opposed to the prior practice of relying on what a "reasonable practitioner" would tell the patient.

Of course, not all patients are capable of giving consent. The law has permitted exceptions to the requirement of informed consent.

Emergency Doctrine

The first such exception is one that has great application in trauma care. When a patient is unconscious or otherwise incapable of giving consent, treatment may proceed under the *emergency doctrine,* which implies consent.[8] This implication frees the nurse from liability for violation of common law. *Implied consent* means that the patient would have consented to the treatment required to maintain his or her health had that patient been able because the alternative would have been death or serious disability.[8] The law assumes that the patient would act reasonably, and the maintenance of bodily integrity is a reasonable act. Note, however, that the emergency doctrine's implication of consent terminates as soon as the patient's disabling condition (e.g., unconsciousness) abates.

Competency to Give Consent

A second exception to the informed consent rule relates to competency. Consent is legally valid only if it is given by someone who is recognized as being of "adult years and sound mind."[7] This means that someone not of legal age or who is judged to be in some way incompetent cannot give the consent that would constitute a valid defense to a lawsuit for battery. A parent or legal guardian must give consent for the treatment of a minor. Even in an emergency, an attempt to contact a parent or guardian must be made and some notation that the parent or guardian was unavailable should be made in the chart. A listing of the steps taken to find the parent will be critical in the event a lawsuit is filed.

There are further considerations to this exception to the informed consent rule. A minor is generally considered to be anyone under the age of 18 years. In some states an individual under the age of 18 years who is married, has a child, or is otherwise emancipated from his or her parents is considered an adult for purposes of giving consent to medical treatment.[9] Additionally, some states permit a minor to consent to emergency medical treatment without a parent's consent.[9] Most hospitals have written policies and procedures that specifically deal with many of these circumstances. A second consideration, and one that bears some watching, is consent by the state as legal guardian. The majority of the states protect parents from criminal liability for denying life-saving medical care to their children on religious grounds. Although uncommon, the state may consent to the treatment of a minor after the parents have refused consent. The reason some states consent to the life-saving treatment when the parents will not is to protect the child's rights. This will most likely occur when the parents' religious beliefs preclude the use of blood transfusions or other medical interventions. This type of consent is not common and is given only under extreme circumstances because the states are typically loath to interfere in the parent-child relationship. The consent, when given by the state, is effective in the same way as described previously.

Some patients, although not minors, may not be competent to give consent. The concept of being of sound mind is the second half of the competency equation. Any person who is not competent because of some mental disability (e.g., lack of mental capacity or senility) or physical disability or disease that renders the individual incapable of making reasoned judgments should be under the control of a guardian.[9] Another common cause of incompetency is the injury that caused the patient to be brought to the hospital or the sequelae from trauma. Examples are shock, severe pain, severe emotional distress, head injuries, and the presence of mind-altering drugs (legal and illegal).[10] In cases where there is no guardian, one may have to be appointed by the court. Consent for this type of patient is obtained in the same manner as for minors, with the guardian substituting for the parent. Consent is implied by law for such patients when emergency medical treatment is required.[9] Where there is no guardian and no durable power of attorney relative to medical care (a document by which a person grants a designated individual the authority to make health care decisions in the event of the person's incapacity to make decisions), state law may provide that the consent of a spouse, adult child, adult sibling, adult grandchild, or a grandparent be substituted.[9,11]

Issues of consent must be considered before each treatment or procedure is commenced, whether in the resuscitation, operative, critical care, intermediate, or rehabilitative phase. It is important that the nurse be knowledgeable about consents obtained because the patient's nurse is the consistent coordinator of care.

Refusal of Treatment

One of the reasons that consent should be obtained separately for each treatment or procedure is that the patient has the right to control all touching of the body not only through consent but also through refusal of treatment. The nurse needs to be aware of the consent obtained by the physician or other practitioner so that a patient's subsequent refusal of treatment can be identified. The withdrawal of consent or any other refusal of treatment must be documented properly in the chart and, because it is often against medical advice, should be witnessed by several people. Again, hospital policy should dictate how this must be documented and by whom. Readers are encouraged to investigate and become familiar with the policies regarding these issues at their institutions. Any treatment or procedure done after a patient refuses treatment is a violation of that patient's legal rights and may become the subject of a successful lawsuit, even if the treatment has beneficial results.

Assault and Battery: Failed Consent

Assault and *battery* are common law torts that protect the individual from the threat of contact and from unpermitted contact, respectively. (Some torts have legal parallels in the criminal statutes. Although we will not address these here, the reader needs to be aware that some issues can arise as civil and criminal issues. The notorious O. J. Simpson case is an example of this. Simpson was found not guilty in the criminal case but guilty of many of the same charges in the civil case.) They are intentional torts, distinguished from negligent torts. The legal elements of battery are that the person committing the action intends to cause a harmful or offensive contact and that the act is unpermitted and unprivileged. Assault is similar except actual contact is not required; only the immediate apprehension of a harmful or offensive contact is needed. The good intentions of the nurse do not justify action constituting assault or battery.[12] The nurse may have the patient's best interests in mind, but if the contact is not consensual, a lawsuit may follow.

In a nursing context, failure to obtain informed consent followed by the performance of a procedure is battery. Continued treatment after the patient's refusal of treatment is also battery. Although this may seem bizarre in the face of successful treatment or the saving of the patient's life, a patient's deeply held belief may make the contact sufficiently offensive to take the matter to court.

Mandatory Reporting

Mandatory reporting requirements exist in the law to identify actions that society abhors. The general rule stated earlier is that the facts of a patient's injuries and treatments are confidential and protected by the right to privacy. That right is superseded by mandatory reporting requirements because public policy dictates that these reportable actions are illegal.

Reporting laws require that hospitals, physicians, and nurses notify the appropriate state agency when certain incidents occur. They also protect the individual reporting the incident from liability for an inaccurate report unless a false report was made with knowledge of its falsity. There is a flip side to this protection from liability: If a nurse or physician fails to report an incident and a further injury occurs from the same proscribed action, that health care provider may be held liable for the failure to report it.[13]

The trauma or emergency nurse must see whether the trauma was the result of an act proscribed by law. Examples include child, elder, and spousal abuse. Many states have reporting requirements when such abuse is identified. When injuries resulting from abuse are discovered, the nurse must take two actions: (1) notify the physician in charge of the patient's case and any other person identified by hospital policy, and (2) make sure a report is filed with the appropriate agency. Failure to follow these two steps in the reporting of an abuse may subject the nurse to liability even though all internal policies have been followed.

Additional examples of incidents with mandatory reporting requirements are abuse in nursing facilities; attempted suicide; and injuries resulting from violence, illegal abortions, animal bites, and motor vehicle crashes. As noted earlier, most hospitals have extensive policies and procedures in place regarding these issues.

Negligence/Malpractice

The main theme of the common law that pervades the legal issues discussed thus far is that of reasonableness. Patients expect that their injuries and conditions will be explained to them in a manner that they can reasonably be expected to understand. A patient incapable of giving consent because of injuries will consent to the course of life-saving treatment because it is reasonable to do so, or so the law presumes. The patient has the right to have reasonable expectations of privacy protected by the nurse.

The issue of law discussed in this section also focuses principally on this notion of reasonableness. Suits for malpractice, or professional negligence, are actions brought by patients against nurses because the nurse is seen by the patient as not having exercised reasonable care in the treatment of the patient's injuries.

The law of negligence, simply stated, is the breach of a duty owed by the nurse to the patient that results in injury to the patient. Four elements are identified in the law:

- A duty of care
- Breach of this duty
- A causal connection between the flawed conduct (act or failure to act) and injury
- Injury or damage suffered by the patient[12]

The crux of the action for negligence is that the nurse did not provide reasonable care and an injury resulted.

When applied to professionals, *negligence* is referred to as *malpractice.* The law measures the professional's duty of care differently than the duty of care owed by nonprofessionals. This one distinction separates ordinary negligence from malpractice. It is mentioned here because, although it is generally accepted that nurses exercise independent professional judgment and should be treated as professionals, not all states allow nurses to be sued for malpractice. Such states hold nurses to the standard of negligence only.[14]

In daily life, individuals must act with reasonable caution so as not to cause harm to others. Drivers are expected to exercise reasonable care. Failure to do so (such as when a car runs a red light, strikes a pedestrian, and breaks his leg) is a failure to use reasonable care. It is negligence because (1) the driver had a duty to drive carefully, (2) the driver breached that duty by running the red light, (3) the pedestrian was struck by the car, and (4) the pedestrian suffered a broken leg.

Establishing the Nurse's Liability

The nurse has the duty to provide competent care to patients. If that care is provided in a less than competent manner and the patient is injured as a result, malpractice has occurred. The critical definition is of the duty of care and its measurement by the law. The causal connection between the nurse's conduct and the injury must then be established and damages assessed.

Duty of care in negligence is defined as what the reasonably prudent person would do in the same or similar circumstances. This is a fiction recognized by the law because there is no person or group of people identifiable as the "reasonably prudent person." It is not what the average person does, but what the law thinks the average person should have done. Due care requires that people not engage in conduct that involves unreasonable danger to others. Critical to the understanding of this duty is that it is conduct being evaluated, not state of mind.[12]

In states that do not have malpractice standards for nurses, the duty of nursing care is based on what the reasonably prudent person (not nurse) would do.[14] The specialized training and knowledge of the nurse are not considered when the standard of care is measured in negligence suits in these states.

Malpractice differs from negligence for precisely this reason. The knowledge and training of the nursing profession define the standard for malpractice. This means that nursing as a profession establishes certain minimum qualifications of education through, for example, the licensure requirements of the boards of nursing. All nurses must meet such professional standards to be considered "reasonably prudent nurses." An action that falls below these minimum qualifications and causes injury is malpractice. In addition, specially qualified nurses (e.g., critical care registered nurses) must maintain educational and practice requirements set down by the boards and, in addition, may be held to a standard for all such specialty qualified nurses on a national basis.[15] These requirements form the basis for the duty of care required of such a certified nurse over and above the qualifications of all nurses. As the number of speciality certifications increase, so do the standards of care.

A description of emergency nursing, which shares many traits with trauma nursing, helps to illustrate these qualifications. Emergency nursing practice is the nursing care of individuals of all ages with perceived physical or emotional alterations that are undiagnosed and may require prompt intervention. Emergency nursing care is unscheduled and most commonly occurs in a specific care setting, such as an emergency department, a mobile unit, or a suicide prevention center. Thus the nursing care is episodic, primary, and acute in nature.

The scope of emergency nursing practice encompasses nursing activities directed toward health problems of various levels of complexity. A rapidly changing physiologic or psychologic status that may be life threatening requires assessment of the severity of the health problem, definitive intervention, continuous reassessment, and supportive care to significant others. The level of physiologic or psychologic complexity may require life support measures, appropriate health education, and referral. The scope of emergency nursing practice encompasses not only nursing activities directed toward health problems presented by the individuals but also knowledge of and the observance of legal aspects, such as reporting an incident to governmental agencies (e.g., police or public health departments) when a situation calls for such action. Emergency nursing practice is affected by the brevity of patient interaction with the nurse, the stressful climate created by lack of control over the number of individuals seeking emergency care, and the limited time frame in which to evaluate the effectiveness of intervention.

In emergency settings, nurses have assumed an increasingly independent, professional role. With this change comes the added burden of legal responsibility for their actions. One particular legal problem that may confront the nurse in the field occurs when an injured victim is treated on the scene with physician support provided only through radio communication. If the physician orders treatment that will be harmful to the patient, the nurse can be held responsible (and the trauma center vicariously) if the orders are followed and the nurse knew or should have known that the harm would occur.[16] This is a dilemma for the nurse at the scene. If the prescribed treatment fails, the physician may be subject to a malpractice action. However, the increased knowledge and ability of nurses exposes them to liability if their compliance with the physician's orders results in an injury.

Standards of reasonable nursing care are required of nurses at all stages of the patient's treatment. This is particularly true in managing the discharge process. A patient being prepared for discharge must be thoroughly educated in, for example, wound care and the use of pharmaceuticals. Reasonable care mandates that the patient be given oral and written instructions explaining how to perform the daily tasks that will promote recovery. Where appropriate, the patient must have demonstrated the ability to perform these tasks. It is also important to provide clear instruction on when the patient should return for a follow-up visit with health care personnel at the trauma center or with his or her personal provider. Symptoms that warrant emergency care or an appointment to return to the trauma center should be explained. In all cases the patient's understanding of the instructions must be demonstrated clearly to the nurse. The patient's support system, whether it is family, home health care providers, or a rehabilitation facility, must be prepared to care for the patient.

Elements of a Malpractice Suit

In a patient's suit for malpractice, what constitutes due care is established through the testimony of expert witnesses. An expert is qualified in court through educational credentials and experience and is then permitted to state an opinion about what is or is not proper care. No one other than a duly qualified expert is permitted to give opinions about what is the duty of care in a court of law. This expert will, in all likelihood, be a nurse who will give testimony about what constitutes proper care for nursing. Physician experts also may be called to differentiate between the duties of physicians and nurses' practice, especially where a nurse is claimed to have exceeded the limits of nursing practice.

As with duty of care, the proximate cause of the injury is established in court by the expert witness. The patient's experts can be expected to state that the injury was a result of the nurse's failure to follow proper practice protocols. The nurse's experts will, of course, state that the injury occurred in a different way. Although this creates a "battle of the experts," this process has been deemed necessary by the judiciary because the knowledge of professional practice is not within the common knowledge of laypersons serving as jurors.

Expert witnesses are needed in proving the nexus, or connection, between the care and the injury because the patient, as the plaintiff, has the burden of proof to show that malpractice occurred. The plaintiff, through the expert, must convince the jury by a preponderance of evidence (51%). There is an exception to the rule that only experts can prove the causal nexus between action and injury; it is rarely applied but bears noting. Some injuries are considered to be of a type that most likely does not happen in the absence of malpractice. This narrow class of injuries shifts the burden of proof to the defendant without the need for expert testimony for the patient. The legal concept is *res ipsa loquitur,* which translated literally is "it speaks for itself."[8] An example might be a patient who goes to the operating room to have a fractured arm repaired and returns to his or her room with serious burns on the hip. The concept says that the burns could not have occurred except through negligence during the operation. The nurse, as a defendant in these cases, must prove that the injury did not occur from the treatment.

Once the first three elements of malpractice are established, damages must be proved for the nurse to be liable to the patient. Damages are characterized as either compensatory or punitive. *Compensatory* damages are the monies necessary to make the patient "whole." They include the medical expenses associated with the injury, past and future; lost earnings and earning potential; pain and suffering; and loss of consortium (inability to function as a spouse). The injury is viewed as a continuum beginning at the time of injury and extending until cured. If the elapsed time between these points is short, damages are assessed for only that brief time. If, however, the resulting injury is permanent, damages are estimated for the patient's estimated life span. Damages awarded to pay for pain and suffering are usually the largest part of the award. Many state legislatures have acted to place a cap on the amount of these types of awards. Damages awarded are to pay for what the patient must endure as a result of the nurse's breach of the professional duty of care.

Punitive damages are monies awarded in excess of compensatory damages to punish the nurse for his or her conduct. Because there is this element of punishment, punitive damages are rarely awarded and then only in cases involving "gross negligence," where the nurse acted maliciously or in reckless disregard of the patient's life. Many states either limit or prohibit punitive damages in medical negligence cases.

Respondeat Superior and Vicarious Liability

The law of malpractice does not view the nurse's actions in isolation. A trauma nurse is generally an employee of a hospital (trauma center). The employer-employee relationship is established when the employer has the ability to control and direct the performance and duties of the employee. The nurse's actions, by this definition, are considered to be those of an employee if they are within the scope of employment.

If all the conditions of an employer-employee relationship are satisfied, the negligence of the nurse will be imputed to the hospital as well. This is the doctrine of *respondeat superior*.[8] *Respondeat superior* applies only to employees, not independent contractors. Courts recognize that a hospital employs nurses to work for it rather than merely providing a place where nurses can act of their own volition. This means that the trauma center is liable for the negligence of its nurses who are operating within the scope of their employment.

The only complication in the application of respondeat superior occurs when, for example, the nurse is assisting a surgeon who is not a "house officer" (employee of the hospital). A surgeon employed and paid by the trauma center is an employee of that center in the same way the nurse is. Respondeat superior applies equally to both because they share the same "master," the trauma center. The difficulty arises when the surgeon is not an employee of the hospital but is reimbursed by fees charged directly to the patient. In states that apply this distinction to a lawsuit, the doctrine of the "borrowed servant" applies. This rule states that the negligence of the nurse is imputed to the surgeon even though the surgeon does not employ the nurse. Furthermore, the liability of the surgeon for the nurse's negligence accrues only if the negligence occurred when the surgeon exercised control over the nurse's actions. The accepted rule in states that apply the borrowed servant doctrine is to hold the hospital liable for the nurse's negligence and to hold the surgeon jointly liable. Vicarious liability does not extend to the nurse supervisor for the malpractice of subordinates because a true employer-employee relationship does not exist. The supervisor is an employee of the trauma center, as is the staff nurse. Nurse supervisors can be held liable, however, if acts of commission or omission in supervising (negligent supervision) cause a patient's injury.

Although the discussion of vicarious liability and respondeat superior has centered on the nurse's malpractice, these concepts apply equally to the other torts previously discussed. Like malpractice, they occur during the course of the nurse's duties and are therefore imputed to the employer.

Good Samaritan Rule

As with many of the legal issues discussed in this chapter, there is an exception to the law of malpractice where a negligent nurse may not be held liable. The trauma nurse who becomes involved in the care of the victim of a car crash or of a violent crime during off-duty hours may not be liable for negligent acts. When an off-duty nurse happens to be at an incident scene, there is an ethical and moral, if not legal, duty to stop and render assistance. To encourage professionals to help injured victims, the legislatures of all states have passed statutes that grant nurses (and generally all medical professionals) immunity from liability for negligent acts. These statutes, named after the biblical Good Samaritan, state that health care professionals who stop and aid injured victims without compensation for that help will not be liable for their acts, even if they are negligent.[5,17]

There is also, however, an exception to the Good Samaritan rule. The law will not exempt the nurse from acts that constitute gross negligence, acts that manifest a reckless disregard for the life of the patient.[18] The rule is that if the care was rendered in good faith and an emergency existed, the nurse will be free from liability. The nurse who is a member of an emergency team sent to the scene of an incident is not covered by the Good Samaritan rule. The professional duty of care is required of this type of nurse.

Law of Death and the Dying Patient

The laws relating to such issues as brain death, the Anatomic Gift Act, living wills, and the withholding or withdrawal of treatment and do-not-resuscitate orders are highly complex areas. Because these areas are so complex and can vary significantly from state to state, they are out of the scope of this chapter. (See the ethics chapter.) If you, as a nurse, have reason to believe that you will be involved with any of these issues, you should seek out your hospital's guidelines/protocols that address these issues.

Physical Evidence and Chain of Custody

Chain of custody of physical evidence is particularly applicable in cases in which the injury resulted from a violent crime such as a shooting or a rape, although it also has application in civil matters. Chain of custody consists of two parts: a documentation component and a handling component. The first mandates meticulous recording of all evidence discovered (or samples taken), where it came from, when, and to whom it was given. Receipts should be maintained as each piece of physical evidence or sample is given by the nurse to, for example, a laboratory technician. These receipts should list what was given, who gave it, to whom it was given, and the date and time of the transfer of possession.

The handling component speaks to the need for purity in a sample and the need to keep physical evidence in its original condition. Potential contaminants should be kept away from tissue samples. A weapon, such as a gun, should not be handled unless it is absolutely necessary so that fingerprints are retained. If a patient is suspected of firing a weapon, the person's hands should not be washed and should be placed in paper bags until tests for gunpowder residue have been completed. If possible, when removing clothing from victims, care should be taken not to tear or cut through holes made by penetrating objects, such as bullets or knives. After removal, clothing should be stored in well-labeled paper bags and given to the appropriate authorities using the same chain of custody documentation described previously.

Protection of Patients' Property

When a patient is brought into a trauma center, the trauma nurse is engaged in many activities that may involve resuscitation and preparation for surgery. The protection of a patient's property can be forgotten easily. Although this may seem a relatively mundane concern in comparison with resuscitation, surgery, or critical care, property loss and damage frequently result in monetary claims against the hospital. The law underlying the responsibility to protect the patient's personal possessions is a bailment.

The patient entrusts the trauma center through the trauma nurse to hold property and clothing until it is reclaimed at a later time. Property should be marked and secured so that it can be returned to the patient upon request or discharge or, upon death, to the family. The patient is the only person authorized to determine its disposition. Proper documentation is therefore necessary.

Emergency Treatment and Labor Act

Perhaps the most complicated area of law facing nurses in trauma care is the Emergency Medical Treatment and Labor Act (EMTALA).[19] This law, passed in 1986, was originally known as the Consolidated Omnibus Budget Reconciliation Act. Today these acts are known more commonly as the antidumping laws or EMTALA.

Under EMTALA, Medicare-participating hospitals (most hospitals receive some federal monies) are required to provide a "medical screening exam" and, if necessary, stabilizing treatment to all individuals who "come to the hospital" and request evaluation or treatment for a medical condition. The definitions of "medical screening exam" and "come to the hospital" have been the subject of numerous hearings.[20]

On November 10, 1999, the Health Care Financing Administration (HCFA, now known as the Centers for Medicare and Medicaid Services) and the Office of the Inspector General (OIG) of the Department of Health and Human Services issued a final special advisory bulletin on the antidumping statute.[21] After reviewing numerous comments, HCFA/OIG issued an advisory bulletin stating that their purpose was "to provide clear and meaningful advice with regard to the application of the antidumping law."[21] The advisory bulletin, in and of itself, does not have the force of law, but HCFA surveyors, OIG attorneys, and others involved in the enforcement of the law rely heavily on the document's recommendations.

A major purpose of the advisory bulletin was to address issues created by managed care. The managed care phenomenon was still in its formative stages when the law was passed in 1986. Issues related to managed care specifically addressed by the HCFA/OIG document include delay in treatment while obtaining authorization and dual staffing arrangements.

Furthermore, there are specific guidelines regarding the reporting of known or suspected violations of the law. A nurse could be found to have violated the act if she or he knew a patient's transfer was a clear violation of the act and did not report the violation. This has become known as the "snitch rule."[22] This obligates nurses at both the transporting and receiving hospitals to report suspected violations of the law.

American Health Insurance Portability and Accountability Act

The American Health Insurance Portability and Accountability Act of 1996 (commonly referred to as HIPAA) is a set of rules to be followed by hospitals, physicians, and other health care providers.[23] Although HIPAA was enacted on August 21, 1996, and the regulations became effective on April 14, 2001, full compliance with them by "covered entities"—which includes all health care providers—was not required until April 14, 2003. HIPAA regulations cover almost every aspect of a health care provider's business. These regulations provide the following:

1. Establish how providers may internally use patients' personal health information and when they may disclose it externally to others
2. Establish new rights for patients to access their own health information, to ask for amendment of that information if it is inaccurate or incomplete, to request an accounting of disclosure of their health information
3. Require providers to have vast policies and procedures to support compliance and to take other administrative actions to comply with the regulations[23]

Because HIPAA is a relatively new law, its precise impact is not yet known. Anyone working in health care since HIPAA's implementation cannot have missed the tremendous amount of retraining required of all covered entities. Hospital emergency departments and trauma departments have been significantly affected by HIPAA. The age-old practice of having a patient status board at the nurse's station has been changed. Hallway discussion of patients has ceased. With the advent of electronic medical records, a whole new realm of privacy issues arose. How do you make the patient's record accessible to those who are providing direct medical care but restrict the patient's information from all others, even though they have access to electronic medical records? How many times has a trauma nurse received a phone call from a friend saying, "A friend of mine was just in a car accident. Can you tell me how he's doing?" To answer this question is very clearly a violation of HIPAA. Hospitals have been forced to not only develop comprehensive HIPAA compliance guidelines; they must put teeth into these policies. In many facilities, answering the caller's question would mean immediate termination.

To attempt to discuss the entire scope and implications of this law are outside the purview of this chapter. Virtually every professional medical journal has published articles on the impact of HIPAA. Every hospital has developed an extensive set of policies and procedures relating to HIPAA compliance. Persons reading this chapter should refer to the facility's HIPAA manuals, to professional journals, and to the federal government's comprehensive website (www.hhs.gov/ocr/hipaa/) for answers to further questions.[24]

Discussion

Given the obligation of advising nurses with a single phrase, an attorney would most likely say, "Act reasonably." Although this phrase is fundamentally true, it provides the nurse with only a general framework for guarding patients' rights and for protection from professional liability. Handling the day-to-day legal dilemmas of trauma nursing requires both this framework of reasonableness and specific knowledge of common points of law as applied to the patient-oriented situation in question.

Acting reasonably means that patients should be consulted at all possible times so that they are aware of the nature and rationale of nursing interventions. This will promote the patient's cooperation in recovery, which is critical to the nurse's protection against subsequent legal actions.

Acting reasonably means knowing and following standing orders and protocols for the assessment and care of the patient at the time of arrival in the emergency department. These protocols ensure that medically appropriate assessment and triage are performed even in the absence of a physician. Clearly, standing orders do not take the place of nursing judgment and are not to be followed blindly when additional injury to the patient may result. Objective self-assessment is also inherent in reasonable practice. Tasks and procedures for which the nurse is inadequately trained should not be done without seeking help from a senior nursing colleague, supervisor, or physician.

There is no complete protection from malpractice litigation, and recent trends suggest that nurses suffer expanded susceptibility to lawsuits. However, liability can be limited through a number of actions. Because nurses are often in a position in which they possess exclusive patient information, the importance of proper documentation and communication of this information takes on great significance. It must be stressed that the entire medical record plays a crucial role as evidence in determining the standard of care provided by the nurse. It also can be used by the nurse during a lawsuit to help recall the details of actions taken in the patient's care long ago. Documentation must be accurate and complete, describing the patient's changing condition, nursing diagnoses, plans and actions, and reports to physicians and other professionals. Effective verbal and written communication provides continuity among nurses and between nurse and physician.

Incident reporting is a specific type of nondiscoverable documentation excluded from the medical record that is reasonable in the eyes of the law. A well-written incident report states facts rather than conclusions without supporting observations. An incident may also be reported verbally. Hospital policies detail the steps to follow in reporting an incident such as a patient fall or the injection of the wrong drug or an incorrect dosage. The policies should include how an incident report is prepared and who is responsible for its disposition. Incident reports are important to the hospital as indicators of areas of potential liability. As employees, nurses are required to report incidents promptly and thoroughly.

Maintaining current and adequate levels of malpractice insurance is another prudent and protective action. Hospitals may provide malpractice insurance for their nurses. Nurses should be aware of the extent of this coverage and any exclusionary clauses present in the insurance agreements that leave them open to personal liability for adverse judgments. Nurses must be aware of the relevant periods covered by the policies. There are two types of malpractice insurance. The first covers claims made during the period of coverage. The second covers claims resulting from occurrences during the period of coverage, even if the claim is made after the policy's expiration date.

Being aware of new medical and scientific issues through continuing education is also important. Nursing supervisors and administrators must be responsive to the need for nurses to remain current on hospital policies and changes in state laws that affect their practice.

These reasonable acts, coupled with adherence to the standards of quality nursing care, will generally reduce the trauma nurse's risk of being found liable for negligence or malpractice. Although such acts may not always keep the nurse out of court, they will significantly reduce the chance of an adverse judgment in a lawsuit.

SUMMARY

The legal issues of this chapter identify areas of exposure of the trauma nurse to liability. They also speak of responsibilities that nurses have to society, to the hospital where they are employed, and to themselves. In the future, trauma nurses' actions will be subject to increasing scrutiny. There may be changes so that emergency and critical care nurses are granted a different license endorsement to practice based on higher educational and experience requirements. Higher standards of professional conduct will, in turn, be expected. Trauma nurses as expert witnesses will become more commonplace as their professionalism is more widely recognized by the law. By offering the court the benefit of years of special training, skill, and education, trauma nurses may perform a valuable service in advocating for the nursing specialty and bringing about changes in the law that reflect the realities and expertise of trauma nursing practice.

As has been noted throughout this chapter, there are or should be many hospital policies and procedures relating the subjects discussed here. Without a doubt, nurses can reduce their risk of legal liability if they follow hospital protocols. Failure to be aware of or follow existing policy may place the nurse out on a legal limb by himself or herself. It is incumbent on nurses to make themselves aware of hospital policies and procedures that relate to their areas of work.

Central to U.S. jurisprudence and the legal issues presented in this chapter is the right to control one's own life and to expect others to act in a reasonable fashion. Trauma patients, despite their incapacitation, are accorded these rights by the laws of the United States and of the individual states. Trauma nurses must operate within this framework to be legally effective.

The law need not be viewed as the nurse's adversary. A rapport can be established easily in which nurses maintain respect for the rights of patients while exercising their judgment about types of treatment and quality of care. Knowledge of the law and legal responsibilities can enhance the nurse's relationship with patients.

REFERENCES

1. *Goff v. Doctors General Hospital*, 333 P2d 29 (Cal App 1958).
2. *Darling v. Charleston Community Hospital*, 33 Ill 2d 326, 211 NE 2d 253 (1965), *cert denied*, 383 U.S. 946 (1966).
3. Louisell DH, Williams H: *Medical malpractice*, p. 16A-2, New York, 1985, Matthew Bender.
4. Health Occupations Article, *Annotated code of Maryland*, sec 8.
5. West's Annotated California Code Business and Professions, sec 2725, 2727.5.
6. *Nancy Beth Cruzan v. Missouri*, 497 U.S. 261, 269 (1990).
7. *Schloendorf v. Society of New York Hospital*, 211 NY 125, 105 NE 92 (1914).
8. Restatement (Second) of torts, sec. 892 (D).
9. Health General Article, *Annotated code of Maryland*, sec 5, 20-102, 107.
10. *Anonymous v. State*, 17 App Div 2d 495, 236 NYS 2d 88 (1963).
11. Arizona revised Statutes, sec. 14-5101.
12. Prosser WL: *Handbook of the law of torts*, ed 5, pp 28-34, St. Paul, Minn, 1984, West-Wadsworth Publishing.
13. *Landeros v. Flood*, 551 P2d 389, Cal Sup Ct (1976).
14. Morris WO: The negligent nurse: the physician and the hospital, *Baylor Law Rev* 33:109, 1981.
15. Rocereto LR, Maleski CM: *The legal dimensions of nursing practice*, New York, 1982, Springer.
16. Connors JP: Nursing errors. In Mackauf SH: *Hospital liability*, pp 33-66, New York, 1985, Law Journal Seminars Press.
17. Courts and judicial proceedings article, *Annotated code of Maryland*, sec 5-309.
18. *Black's law dictionary*, ed 8 (rev), St. Paul, Minn, 2004, West-Wadsworth Publishing.
19. 41 W.S.C. 1395 dd, codified at 42CFR 489.24.
20. First Supreme Court decision on patient dumping, *Law Watch* 99:9, March 2, 1999.
21. HCFA/OIG issue final special advisory bulletin on patient dumping, *Law Watch* 99:54, November 23, 1999.
22. 42 CFR 489.20 (m); 42 CFR 489.24 (d).
23. Public Health Law 104-191, 42 W.S.C 1301 codified at 45 CFR Parts 160 and 164.
24. U.S. Department of Health and Human Services: *Medical privacy—National standards to protect the privacy of personal health information:* www.hhs.gov/ocr/hipaa/privacy.html. Accessed February 1, 2007.

6

INJURY PREVENTION

Carolyn J. Fowler

Injury is the most underrecognized public health problem facing the nation today. Overall, injuries (unintentional injuries, homicides, and suicides combined) account for 7% of all deaths in the United States each year[1,2] and were responsible for 167,184 deaths in 2004.[1] Between ages 1 and 45 years, unintentional injury alone (without the contribution of homicide and suicide) is the leading cause of death[2,3] and the fifth leading cause of death across all ages in the United States (Table 6-1).[4] Among adolescents and young adults (ages 15 to 24 years), three of every four deaths in 2003 were injury related.[1,5] Injury (unintentional injury, homicide, and suicide combined) is the leading cause of premature death for young people and thus is the leading cause of years of potential life lost before the age of 75 years.[6] The societal cost of injury is enormous. Health care charges for the treatment of injury represent only a portion of the total financial burden. Other costs include those associated with loss of income, productivity, and property. Social costs are harder to measure but include pain, suffering, reduced quality of life, lost human potential, and disrupted families. For the year 2000 alone, the estimated total lifetime cost resulting from injury in the United States was estimated at $406 billion.[7]

Injury is perceived to be a condition that affects young people disproportionately, yet trauma continues to be a major health problem throughout life. Despite the obvious importance of injury as a cause of premature death, the highest injury-related death rates are experienced by the elderly—a sector of the population that is expected to increase from 12.4% (in 2000) to 20.4% by the year 2040.[8] Similarly, our oldest citizens (those older than 75 years) experience death rates nearly three times those of the general population; this group is expected to increase from 5% to 9% of the population in the next three decades.[8] Nonfatal injuries in the elderly are also a major concern. For many older adults, a hip fracture may begin a downward spiral of immobility-related morbidity, an end to independent living in the community, and shortened life span. Indeed, half of all elders who are hospitalized for a hip fracture are unable to return home or live independently after the injury.[9] Unless we are able to reduce death and injury rates among people older than 65 years, it is estimated that by the year 2030 this group will sustain more than one third of all injury-related deaths and hospitalizations. The social impact of this cannot be overstated.

Injury can be prevented or controlled at three levels. Primary prevention involves preventing the event, such as the car crash, that has the potential to cause injury. Secondary prevention involves preventing an injury or minimizing its severity during that crash. Tertiary prevention is optimization of outcome through medical treatment and rehabilitation. Trauma nurses will be most familiar with tertiary prevention and to a lesser extent with secondary prevention. Development of emergency medical services and systems and expert trauma management has improved—and will continue to improve—the outcomes of injured patients. However, these advances will never be enough to reduce the toll of injury-related death significantly. Why? The majority of deaths from traumatic injury occur early. It is estimated that, because of the severity of the injuries, half of all trauma deaths cannot be prevented with even the best medical management.[10] For those who survive their injuries, the sequelae may be profound and, in some cases, increase that individual's chance of reinjury.[10] Achieving a significant reduction in trauma-related mortality and morbidity therefore must include attention to primary prevention. Indeed, the American Trauma Society website carries the message *that when prevention succeeds, trauma is conquered.*[11]

At some time, all trauma nurses will ask, "Could this have been prevented?" Why then has injury prevention received so little attention in trauma training programs and trauma services? Trauma, it seems, is so endemic in our society that we fail to realize the enormity of its financial and social costs or our potential as a society to reduce its toll. In 1988, Dr. William Foege, former director of the Centers for Disease Control and Prevention, called injury "the principal public health problem in America today."[12] One year later, Surgeon General C. Everett Koop testified that "if some infectious disease came along that affected children [in the proportion that injuries do], there would be a huge public outcry and we would be told to spare no expense to find a cure and to be quick about it."[13] Much progress has been achieved in the ensuing years, but the commitment of the public, and of the health care profession, to injury prevention is still woefully inadequate—a symptom of society's "general tendency to underinvest in programs designed to prevent social problems."[14] Why? Three answers come to mind: (1) injury is underrecognized and, as such, grossly underfunded and understudied relative to other health problems of similar magnitude; (2) injury prevention is relatively young as a field

TABLE 6-1 The Ten Leading Causes of Death—United States, 2004

	Age Groups (years)				
Rank	<1	1-4	5-9	10-14	15-24
1	Congenital anomalies 5,622	***Unintentional injury 1,641***	***Unintentional injury 1,126***	***Unintentional injury 1,540***	***Unintentional injury 15,449***
2	Short gestation 4,642	Congenital anomalies 569	Malignant neoplasms 526	Malignant neoplasms 493	***Homicide 5,085***
3	Sudden infant death syndrome 2,246	Malignant neoplasms 399	Congenital anomalies 205	***Suicide 283***	***Suicide 4,316***
4	Maternal pregnancy complications 1,715	***Homicide 377***	***Homicide 122***	***Homicide 207***	Malignant neoplasms 1,709
5	***Unintentional injury 1,052***	Heart disease 187	Heart disease 83	Congenital anomalies 184	Heart disease 1,038
6	Placenta cord membranes 1,042	Influenza and pneumonia 119	Chronic low respiratory disease 46	Heart disease 162	Congenital anomalies 483
7	Respiratory distress 875	Septicemia 84	Benign neoplasms 41	Chronic low respiratory disease 74	Cerebrovascular 211
8	Bacterial sepsis 827	Perinatal period 61	Septicemia 38	Influenza and pneumonia 49	HIV 191
9	Neonatal hemorrhage 616	Benign neoplasms 53	Cerebrovascular 34	Benign neoplasms 43	Influenza and pneumonia 185
10	Circulatory system disease 593	Chronic low respiratory disease 48	Influenza and pneumonia 33	Cerebrovascular 43	Chronic low respiratory disease 179

Produced by Office of Statistics and Programming, National Center for Injury Prevention and Control, Centers for Disease Control and Prevention. Accessed February 2007.
Trauma-related diagnoses in bold italic.
HIV, Human immunodeficiency virus.

of scientific inquiry and professional practice; and (3) training in injury prevention methods is lacking.

Trauma nurses know all too well how a few seconds can alter the course of a healthy young person's life forever. They have witnessed the effects of alcohol and other substance abuse and access to lethal weapons as risk factors for injury; they recognize predictable trauma case histories; they know that certain days, times, and weather conditions are associated with increased caseload. Fortunately, many have also witnessed the protective effects of interventions such as seatbelts, helmets, and improved vehicle design. Clearly, trauma nurses possess the awareness and many of the attributes needed by injury preventionists and can make valuable contributions to injury prevention. The goal of this chapter, therefore, is to enable the trauma nurse to think about injury in a critical and systematic way. Traumatic injury is approached as a health problem to be solved. A public health problem-solving paradigm[15] and two related conceptual frameworks for problem diagnosis and decision making are introduced.

An Overview of Injury Prevention

Although traumatic injury has been a problem throughout the ages, injury prevention is a relatively new field of scientific inquiry. Historically, injuries (often called *accidents*) have been viewed as the result of human error, fate, or bad luck. Injury prevention efforts reflected and inadvertently supported this belief by encouraging people to adopt safe and responsible behaviors or by blaming the victims for the events that led to their injuries or deaths. Most attempts at injury prevention focused on training individuals to be more careful, a preoccupation with what Leon Robertson called "[a] basic cultural theme... that sufficient education will resolve almost any problem."[16] The concept that injury, like disease, is the product of the interaction of a human host and an agent within the environment, and can therefore be examined by epidemiologic methods, first appeared in the public health literature in 1949,[17] more than a century after epidemiologists knew that explaining the development of epidemics as the consequence of individual behaviors was inaccurate

25-34	35-44	45-54	55-64	65+	All Ages
Unintentional injury 13,032	***Unintentional injury 16,471***	Malignant neoplasms 49,520	Malignant neoplasms 96,956	Heart disease 533,302	Heart disease 652,486
Suicide 5,074	Malignant neoplasms 14,723	Heart disease 37,556	Heart disease 63,613	Malignant neoplasms 385,847	Malignant neoplasms 553,888
Homicide 4,495	Heart disease 12,925	***Unintentional injury 16,942***	Chronic low respiratory disease 11,754	Cerebrovascular 130,538	Cerebrovascular 150,074
Malignant neoplasms 3,633	***Suicide 6,638***	Liver disease 7,496	Diabetes mellitus 10,780	Chronic low respiratory disease 105,197	Chronic low respiratory disease 121,987
Heart disease 3,163	HIV 4,826	***Suicide 6,906***	Cerebrovascular 9,966	Alzheimer's disease 65,313	***Unintentional injury 112,012***
HIV 1,468	***Homicide 2,984***	Cerebrovascular 6,181	***Unintentional injury 9,651***	Diabetes mellitus 53,956	Diabetes mellitus 73,138
Diabetes mellitus 599	Liver disease 2,799	Diabetes mellitus 5,567	Liver disease 6,569	Influenza and pneumonia 52,760	Alzheimer's disease 65,965
Cerebrovascular 567	Cerebrovascular 2,361	HIV 4,422	***Suicide 4,011***	Nephritis 35,105	Influenza and pneumonia 59,664
Congenital anomalies 420	Diabetes mellitus 2,026	Chronic low respiratory disease 3,511	Nephritis 3,963	***Unintentional injury 35,020***	Nephritis 42,480
Septicemia 328	Influenza and pneumonia 891	Septicemia 2,251	Septicemia 3,745	Septicemia 25,644	Septicemia 33,373

and ineffective for the development of preventive strategies. This and later developments in injury control are discussed in a comprehensive article by Julian Waller.[18] Dr. Waller, a pioneer of the injury field, is one of many who advocated for the removal of the term "accident" from discussions of injury.[19] This was promoted to draw attention to the fact that injuries do not exhibit the randomness conveyed by the term "accident," and that injuries can be explained by using scientific methods common to public health.[20]

The late Dr. William Haddon, considered by many to be the father of injury epidemiology, refined the understanding of the role of energy as the agent of injury. Haddon's work formed the well-known definition of injury published by the National Committee for Injury Prevention and Control in 1989: "Injury is any unintentional or intentional damage to the body resulting from acute exposure to thermal, mechanical, electrical, or chemical energy or from the absence of such essentials as heat or oxygen."[21] A more recent definition from the World Health Organization adds ionizing radiation to the exposure list and includes the important clarification that energy "interacts with the body in amounts or at rates that exceed the threshold of human tolerance."[22]

For an energy transfer (or energy deprivation) to occur, a human host and the agent of injury must interact within an environment. Interaction of host, agent, and environmental factors produces both the injury and the eventual outcome from that injury. This pivotal work of identifying the agent of injury and the vehicle (or carrier of the energy) and refining the relationships of host, agent, and environment in producing injury and its outcomes resulted in the development of the Haddon Phase-Factor Matrix.[23] This tool is still an important and frequently used conceptual framework in injury epidemiology; it is explained in detail later. Despite these contributions, and later efforts to reject "accident proneness" as an explanation for childhood injuries,[24] the tendency to look at human behavior as the root of the injury problem and to focus prevention efforts on changing those behaviors is still pervasive. Individual knowledge, attitudes, beliefs, and behaviors are very important factors in injury prevention, as is the role of education and health behavior change; but to develop effective, sustainable injury prevention strategies, we must expand our field of vision beyond the individual. In short, we must subject injury problems to thorough scrutiny before we act.

IDENTIFYING AND DEFINING THE INJURY PROBLEM

The focus of trauma management is on the individual and his or her unique combination of injuries. The focus of injury prevention is much broader. Injury is a health problem of populations and, as such, must be identified on more than a case-by-case basis. Thereafter, it may be grouped and defined in several ways. Knowing how a problem was identified and how it has been defined is critical at all levels of injury prevention. For example, a trauma nurse interested in an area of tertiary prevention, such as optimizing functional outcome after severe head injury, may decide to review articles about management protocols and patient outcomes. The patients in Study I may seem to do much better than those in Study II. The nurse may decide to further investigate or even consider implementing the management protocols used by Study I. However, to implement these protocols would be unwise; essential preliminary information has been ignored. We cannot begin to compare differences in outcome unless we understand the differences in input. How are the hospitals and the patient populations in Studies I and II similar and different? What were the criteria used to determine the severity of injury in the study? Were penetrating head injuries included or excluded? Were all deaths reported, or only those that occurred after admission and within a defined time frame after injury? What was the average time to admission? If Study I included many cases that were transfers from other centers, early deaths in the transfer population are essentially excluded, thus reducing the total case fatality rate. What was the average age of the patients? What were the causes of the head injuries in the two studies? Were the patients comparable in terms of total injury severity? These considerations apply throughout all levels of prevention. For example, studying the protective effect of bicycle helmets or child passenger restraints in populations receiving trauma care fails to reveal those persons who are protected so effectively that they do not require any medical management. The issue of assessing exposure remains a great challenge to the injury prevention community. It is therefore important not only to gather information about the injury problem but also to be familiar with the source of that information and how the injury population of interest was defined.

Even more important to trauma professionals is the awareness that the quality of the trauma team's documentation influences the quality and value of sources of injury data. Hospital records and death certificates are important sources of data. Health professionals must realize that the information they document in the trauma facility will find its way into aggregate data sets that are used for research and policy development. For example, our national injury fatality data are based on vital statistics data. These, of course, are derived from information reported on death certificates. Other important research data sets such as the Fatal Analysis Reporting System of the National Highway Traffic Safety Administration also use vital statistics data. Data errors or omissions originating in the hospital can therefore affect the ultimate quality of our national data. Even more important is the fact that injury coding and classification systems use data contained in patients' records. Illegible, ambiguous, inaccurate, contradictory, or missing information compromises our ability to develop and maintain accurate data systems. An elderly patient who succumbs to pneumonia after sustaining a hip fracture will appear as a "natural death" in vital statistics data if the initiating event, the fall, is not clearly documented in medical records and on the death certificate. Information from emergency medical providers, such as the circumstances of a car crash or the use of restraints, will be lost if not documented. Careful and thorough reporting of information available on the etiology, clinical course, and outcome of the injury is in itself a contribution to injury prevention.

Definition of the injury problem of interest is a critical and often ignored step that must precede attempts to survey, measure, investigate, or prevent injuries. An injury problem can be defined in many different ways, and it is important that all stakeholders involved in the prevention initiative understand and agree on the working definition before action is taken. Although an injury problem definition may include clinical variables, such as severity, it may be a purely social or political definition such as *injuries occurring in the uninsured.* The following section presents examples of variables used in defining injury problems.

Most commonly, injuries are reported by severity: fatal, severe, moderate, minor. Surrogates for actual injury severity (e.g., hospital admissions, emergency department visits, ambulatory care visits, length of stay) are also common in the injury literature. Trauma nurses are familiar with identifying injuries by body region (head injury, spinal cord injury, maxillofacial injury, lower extremity injury) or by the nature of injury (burns, penetrating injuries, blunt force injury, etc.). Injury can also be defined using statements of the population at risk: the pediatric population, the elderly, adolescents, pregnant women, construction workers, urban populations, rural populations, minority groups, and gender groups. The setting or circumstances in which injury occurs may also be used to define the injuries of interest. Sport and recreational injuries, injuries in school or day care, occupational injuries, injuries occurring in nursing homes, injuries occurring between intimate partners, and injuries in the home are examples of such definitions.

An important way of classifying injury is by intent: unintentional or intentional. Unintentional injury, sometimes referred to in lay terms as "accidental" injury, includes motor vehicle and other transportation injury, drowning, fire and burn injury, falls, sport and recreational injury, and other unintentional injuries, such as a needlestick injury. Intentional injuries are the result of intended actions. This does not necessarily mean that the result was intended. For example, one person may strike another intentionally without intending to kill that person. Of course, there are many intentional injuries for which the outcome as well as the action was intended. Intentional injuries may be inflicted on another, or they may be self-inflicted, such as completed suicide, attempted suicide, and other self-destructive behaviors, such as self-mutilation. This latter category, assaults and homicides, receives much public attention. Although this is entirely appropriate and necessary, because firearm injuries have become the leading cause of death in some groups and areas of the nation, many health care providers may be surprised to realize that in the United States firearm suicides outnumber firearm homicides (16,750 and 11,624, respectively, in 2004)[25] or that, overall, intentional injuries are far less common than unintentional injuries.[2,4,5]

For some types of injuries, intent is hard to determine. Examples are carbon monoxide poisoning, drowning, and drug intoxication. When confronted with a person who has died as a result of a drug overdose, there is a possibility that this is an unintended overdose. It could also be a suicide or even homicide, if the supplier contaminated the supplied substance intentionally. Many factors are considered when determining the manner of death ("accidental," suicide, homicide, or undetermined). For almost all injury deaths, whether early or late, determining manner of death is the responsibility of the medical examiner or coroner. The criteria used to do this vary slightly by jurisdiction and must therefore be understood by those wishing to identify categories of deaths, especially if deaths in several jurisdictions are to be compared.

One of the problems with identifying and defining deaths by intent is that it may break out, and therefore diminish, the apparent magnitude of deaths from the same mechanism. Reporting injuries and deaths by using a matrix approach that places primary emphasis on the cause (or mechanism) of injury and only secondary emphasis on intent is a recent development in the injury field, one with great value for injury prevention policy development.[2] For example, in 2004 firearms accounted for 67% of homicides and 52% of suicides but fewer than 1% of unintentional injury deaths.[1] The social burden of firearms is most apparent when the primary focus is on the proportion of all injury deaths that are the result of firearm injury. In 2004, firearms accounted for 17.7% of all injury deaths, second only to motor vehicles at 27%.[1]

The role of alcohol is an example of a problem that is magnified as one looks beyond individual mechanisms of injury. In 2001 there were 75,766 alcohol-attributable deaths in the United States.[25] Of these deaths, 40,005 (or 53%) could be considered injury related. The relationship between alcohol consumption and motor vehicle crashes is well described in the scientific literature and kept in the public eye by the tireless efforts of the country's most successful grassroots advocacy organization, MADD (Mothers Against Drunk Driving).[26] Less well known by the public is the association between alcohol consumption and numerous other types of injury such as boating and drowning deaths, violence, domestic violence, and recreational injury.[27,28] Trauma has been called a "symptom of alcoholism,"[29] an opinion supported by numerous investigators.[27,30,31] Alcohol intoxication on initial admission is also associated with a 2.5-fold increase in the likelihood that the patient will be readmitted for trauma in the future.[30] Although alcohol involvement in trauma has decreased by approximately 25% in the past decade, conservative estimates still implicate alcohol and illicit drugs in 19% of the estimated 2.2 million trauma patients hospitalized each year.[28] A study of seriously injured patients in a trauma center found that a high percentage of patients were at risk for a current psychoactive substance use disorder and that this group's prevalence of current alcohol dependence was nearly three times higher than estimates for U.S. residents aged 15 to 54 years.[31] Detecting and managing alcohol-related problems in trauma patients poses an enormous challenge to the trauma care system.

Defining the injury problem is a difficult step in program development, but injury prevention programs developed without adequate definition will flounder. If we pursue a medical analogy, problem definition is the beginning of the diagnostic process. A 70-year-old woman has come to the emergency department with a hip fracture after a fall. Fall-related hip fractures in elderly women are a common and well-identified injury problem. But fall-related hip fractures occur in very different circumstances. A broad definition of the problem may be useful when the total burden of fall-related hip fractures in elderly women is measured, but it is inadequate as the basis for an intervention. Yes, we wish to prevent falls in the elderly, but in relation to what?

- Group (age range, gender, community-dwelling, patients with existing disabilities such as visual impairment, frequent fallers)
- Region (the country, the state, a community, a residential facility)
- Environments (individual homes, nursing homes, recreational facilities, the street, the workplace, unfamiliar environments)
- Circumstances (ice, rain, on stairs, when getting up at night, in the shower, when taking certain medications, during dementia transitions)
- Severity (any fall, any injury, any fracture, hip fracture, traumatic brain injury)
- Consequences (injury requiring hospitalization, disabling injury, injury that requires that the person be placed in an elder care facility, falls that cause elders to restrict their activities from fear of subsequent falls)
- Other social considerations (falls in the uninsured, falls in patients of a certain health maintenance organization, falls in persons with a history of falls, falls that result in litigation)

Careful definition of the problem is the foundation for all future analyses. It may help to ask this question: "What is the specific problem I need to solve—and why?" If the answer is not clear, an intervention cannot be focused adequately. Definitions of injury problems may also evolve over time as our knowledge, awareness, and social practices change. The area of child passenger safety is one such example. At one time the problem definition for deaths and injuries to child motor vehicle occupants might have been that child passengers were unrestrained in cars. An early study by another pioneer of the injury prevention field, Professor Susan Baker, defined a specific problem: disproportionately high injury and death rates in infant passengers. Her work laid the foundation for the development of rear-facing infant seats.[32] Next came the realization that children needed special restraints, but the public's awareness of this fact was low. Attention was given, appropriately, to building public awareness, passing child restraint laws, and making child safety seats available. As safety seat usage rates increased, so did awareness of a new problem: restraint misuse. It was not enough that people knew they should restrain the child in a safety seat, that they purchased a seat, or that they used it all the time. New problems were defined: car seat–vehicle incompatibility, high levels of incorrect use, the problem of rear-facing infant seats placed in front of an air bag. Most recently, there is growing realization that our almost exclusive attention to the youngest children (0 to 4 years of age) and our nonspecific "Buckle Up" message for older children has left the 4- to 8-year-olds inadequately protected in vehicles.[33] National attention is now focused on increasing booster seat use in children in the 40- to 80-pound weight range (4- to 8-year-olds), who cannot be restrained adequately by adult seat belts.[34]

Evolving problem definitions require similar evolvement of injury prevention initiatives. For example, on July 1, 2002, 24 years after the first statewide child passenger safety law was passed in Tennessee, Washington State's *Anton Skeen Law* (HB 2675) took effect.[35] This bill, signed into law during the 2000 legislative session, was the first state law in the United States to require booster seat use. By November 2006, 38 states and the District of Columbia had enacted some form of booster seat law.[36] Members of first responder, trauma, and emergency medical communities played active advocacy roles to help ensure passage of the *Anton Skeen Law* and are still, as noted by former U.S. Transportation Secretary Norman Mineta on February 14, 2006, "doing their part to address the consequences of this country's failure to put children in booster seats."[37] There remains much work to be done to increase compliance with the laws, revise other child passenger safety laws and prevention initiatives of yesterday, and limit exemptions and close gaps to keep pace with the changing understanding of what is required to best protect this age group of children in motor vehicles. The critical lesson here is that problem definitions are not universally relevant. Time invested in this problem definition stage of the problem-solving process will reduce subsequent frustration and enhance the potential for success.

MEASURING THE INJURY PROBLEM

Once identified and defined, the injury problem should be measured. Measurement is important for several reasons, including resource procurement and allocation, intervention planning and delivery, and evaluation. The choice of measurement criteria is influenced by data availability, time, and needs. When an injury problem is presented, the nurse begins with some triage questions:

What is the magnitude of this injury?

- Incidence (the number of new cases of an injury that occur during a specified period of time in a population at risk for that injury)[38]
- Prevalence (the number of affected persons with a particular injury present in the population at a specified time divided by the number of persons in the population at that time)[38]

What is the severity of the injury?

- High case fatality (such as firearm injuries or suicide attempts)
- Low case fatality (such as playground injuries) in high numbers
- High morbidity (such as traumatic brain injury, spinal cord injury, severe lower extremity injury, hip fracture in the elderly, and burn)

How preventable is the injury?

- Do we have proven interventions that can be used to prevent this injury (e.g., bicycle helmets, seat belts, product modification)?
- Are there distinct clusters of injuries (clustering of injuries suggests that specific environmental risk factors are present)?

What are the costs of this injury?

- Direct costs such as financial costs of medical care (both acute and long term) and other nonmedical goods and services related to the injury (e.g., "costs for home modifications, vocational rehabilitation, administrative costs for health and indemnity insurance")[39]
- Indirect morbidity costs (i.e., "the value of foregone productivity due to injury-related illness and disability") and mortality costs (i.e., "the value of foregone productivity due to death at an early age")[39]
- Additional costs such as those associated with property damage; police and fire services; legal fees related to compensation; and social costs such as pain, suffering, quality of life, lost human potential, and disrupted families[39]

Is some group disproportionately affected (e.g., young, urban African-American men; elderly women; children in custody; health care workers)?

What is the public's interest in this injury problem (e.g., will the public support stronger child passenger safety laws; are they aware that firearms are used more frequently in suicides than in homicides; do they care whether a child's playground is safe and well maintained)?

What are the consequences of not acting to prevent this problem (e.g., with a rapidly aging population, can we afford to ignore the problem of injuries in the elderly)?

Answering these questions adequately often involves significant training and effort. A complete discussion of measurement methods is beyond the scope of this chapter. Nevertheless, much time, money, effort, and expertise is devoted to measuring the burden of injury, and there are many valuable data resources available to those interested in determining the magnitude of an injury problem. A list of such resources is included at the end of this chapter.

Even without extensive resources, it is possible to work through the checklist (above), as one might work through a triage situation, to guide decision making about optimal use of resources. When, for example, a high-profile injury death triggers public interest and demands that action be taken, should we respond with a prevention initiative? Is this one of many similar deaths and injuries? If so, we may use the heightened awareness to generate support for prevention initiatives. If this turns out to be a relatively rare but emerging injury problem, we would be wise to invest our resources in learning more about the injury through data collection and surveillance before we intervene. If, however, this is a truly rare event, can we justify allocating any resources to this problem at the expense of other more significant problems?

Measurement is important to determine the extent of the injury problem, but it is also critical to our ability to evaluate the effectiveness of interventions or any shifts in injury patterns that may be occurring as a result of interventions. Careful measurement of the injury problem is a wise investment.

Identifying Key Determinants

Having identified, defined, and measured the injury problem, one must begin the diagnostic process required to determine the causal factors associated with the problem. Injuries do not occur in a vacuum. To prevent injuries or reduce their severity, one must understand the circumstances in which they happen. As with infectious and chronic diseases, the six basic questions of epidemiology apply: *what* is happening to *whom*, *when*, *where*, *why*, and *how*? These supposedly simple questions are problematic because what we see when we examine a situation is a function of where and how we look. If, for example, we are convinced that teenage drivers are fundamentally unsafe, we may assume on hearing of a single-vehicle crash in which a teenage boy died that the crash was the result of human error—another tragic example of teenage risk taking. But what if we were to visit the crash site and find that the road was narrow, winding, and lined with trees? What if we were to look at police crash records or newspaper reports and find that several other single-vehicle crashes involving drivers of different ages had occurred in this location? What if several other similar crashes had occurred, but drivers of small vehicles were the only ones to die? Most injuries occur within environments that humans have made; understanding the contribution of environmental factors is therefore essential.

Typically, numerous factors interact to produce an injury and its outcome. In focusing prevention efforts on the most obvious factor, usually human behavior, we ignore other critical factors that may in fact be more modifiable than human behavior. The history of efforts to prevent child pedestrian injury is one such example. The road environment is complex; navigating it safely requires significant cognitive ability not present in children before age 9 years.[40,41] Although this has been understood for nearly 40 years, when a 5-year-old child is killed or injured as a pedestrian, it is not uncommon to read the phrase "pedestrian error" on the police report. Even when an unsupervised child runs into a road at 10 PM, the incident is frequently called "accidental." Over the years, most pedestrian safety programs have focused on persuading or training children to be safer pedestrians and have shown little success. But, why should an exclusively child-focused approach work? If we pause to look beyond the victim, we will see numerous other factors that contribute to these injuries: design of the road, traffic speed, traffic density, signage, visibility, the size and design of the vehicle, driver training, driver awareness and behavior (including substance use), supervision of children, the presence of distractions (e.g., dogs, balls, other children), the child's level of exposure to the traffic environment, the level of traffic enforcement, and the legal and social consequences of hitting a child pedestrian. Individually, each of these factors may influence the child's risk of injury. Together, their interaction produces a set of circumstances that either supports or discourages the likelihood of pedestrian injury. Examining the presence and interactions of these factors in a systematic way is an important problem-solving step.

Factors that are important precursors of a public health problem, and therefore possible targets for prevention initiatives, may be referred to as *key determinants*.[15] Key determinants may be numerous. It is important therefore to use an organizational framework to examine these multiple factors and their interactions in a logical manner. Usually organization of key determinants begins by grouping factors. The organizational framework used most commonly in injury problem solving is the Haddon Phase-Factor Matrix. As shown in Table 6-2, the Haddon Matrix is a 3 × 4 table. The four *factors* of the matrix are human (individual) factors, agent (and carrier) factors, physical environmental factors, and social environmental factors.[42] Identifying these factors and assessing their relative importance is crucial to the development of effective prevention strategies. A second important concept is that, although the energy transfer occurs quickly, it is only one part of a dynamic process. Haddon described three *phases* representing stages in a time continuum that begins before the injury occurs and ends with the outcome. These phases are known as the *pre-event*, the *event*, and the *postevent* phase.[42] The interaction of factors in the *pre-event phase* determines whether an event (such as a car crash) that has the potential to cause injury will occur. Factors interacting in the *event phase* influence whether an injury will result from this event and what the type and severity of that injury will be. Finally, the interactions in the *postevent phase* determine the consequences (short- and long-term outcomes) of the injury.

The Haddon Matrix can be used in several ways. Most commonly, it is used to think about the factors involved in an injury problem. Becoming familiar with the literature on the injury problem of interest, before filling out the matrix, will help identify possible risk factors that may otherwise be ignored. Not only does the Haddon Matrix help us to think *out of the box* (the *blame the victim box*), but it also helps us

TABLE 6-2 **The Haddon Phase-Factor Matrix (Completed for Motor Vehicle Crashes)**

Factors→ ↓Phases	Human (Individual Factors)	Agent and Vehicle	Environment-Physical	Environment-Social
Pre-event	Age,* gender,* visual acuity, alcohol or other substance use, fatigue, distraction, cell phone use, risk-taking behavior, driving skill and experience, reaction time, exposure (frequency of travel)	Vehicle design (road-holding ability, rollover risk, braking capacity) and maintenance Condition of tires Visibility (e.g., daytime running lights)	Design and maintenance of roadway, traffic density and flow, condition of road surface (wet, icy, oil slick, etc.), weather, visibility, traffic control (signals, lights, signage), animals and other obstacles in roadway	Speed limits, licensing laws and restrictions, impaired driving laws, motor vehicle occupant restraint laws (for all ages), regulations limiting driving hours for truck drivers, regulations limiting cell phone use, vehicle maintenance regulations, road rage.
Event	Restraint use, age-related health status, preexisting conditions such as osteoporosis Position in vehicle	Speed, size, and crash tolerance of vehicle Type of restraint systems (seat belts, airbags, child safety seats) Interior surface hazards (e.g., protruding handles)	Roadway design: median dividers, guardrails, break-away poles, roadside hazards (e.g., trees, parked vehicles)	Enforcement of speed limits and restraint laws Policy/regulation mandating vehicle safety design standards Social norm of "safety sells" influencing consumer's choice of motor vehicle
Post-event	Age* and preexisting comorbidities that may influence clinical course	Integrity of fuel system Vehicle design–related barriers to extrication	Urban/rural location, distance from emergency medical services, barriers to extrication and emergency management	Good Samaritan laws Bystander assistance Planning and delivery of emergency medical services Quality of trauma care and rehabilitation Insurance and compensation practices Psychosocial support structure Job retraining

*Note: Age and gender are not modifiable variables and so appear in this matrix as surrogates for longer descriptive phrases such as "age-related developmental level" or to indicate the need to consider risk factors that may be associated with age or gender. Elderly drivers may have cognitive, visual, or other physical limitations; others will not. Elderly women may have osteoporosis and reduced bone density; others will not.

identify what we need to find out about the problem. For example, do we have reliable data on restraint use? Do we know how many of the children who do not wear bicycle helmets already own a helmet? The value of the Haddon Matrix is that it illustrates the multifactorial etiology of injury. A potential problem it creates, however, is that one may feel lost in a maze of causal factors. Faced with so much information, some preventionists complain that it is difficult to know what to target. To overcome this problem, it is necessary to take another step. Look at all the factors listed in the matrix and ask which of these factors is controllable? For example, we cannot change an elderly woman's age but we may be able to enhance her general health status, her muscle tone, or her balance. Next, look at the list of modifiable factors and consider which of these changes is the most likely to be accomplished. For example, which is the most likely to be accomplished: teaching 16-year-old drivers to drive safely or limiting their crash exposure through graduated licensing programs? Look at this final list to determine whether altering the variable would change the outcome significantly. For example, emergency medical services (EMS) response time is modifiable, but some injury mechanisms, such as firearm injury and drowning, result in such severe injuries that enhanced EMS alone does not have the potential to reduce the death toll significantly. This process forms the basis of causal thinking, which is critical to intervention and evaluation planning and is discussed in the next section.

Identifying Potential Intervention Strategies

Once the problem is diagnosed and the factor(s) to be targeted with intervention(s) identified (the change targets), the mechanism that will be used to achieve the desired change must be identified. The danger at this point is a "knee-jerk" response when selecting an intervention. The easiest, most obvious, most affordable, or most acceptable strategy is seldom the most effective. As is the case when treatment modalities for injured patients are selected, knowledge of the range of potential injury prevention strategies is critical when prevention options are chosen. Another legacy of Dr. William Haddon is his list of ten injury control strategies that can be applied to all types of injury.[42-44] These strategies address the control of hazards with the potential to cause injury, but each targets a different point along a continuum between creation of the hazard and the final outcome. These strategies, with examples of their application, are presented in Table 6-3.

The Haddon strategies describe the countermeasures that must be put in place to prevent the occurrence of injury, reduce its severity, or achieve the best possible outcome from the injury. In essence, they describe an *end* we wish to achieve. The *means* we take to achieve that end may vary. For example, when faced with the problem of young children being poisoned when they ingest multivitamins containing iron, we may decide to implement Haddon strategy two: *reduce the amount of the hazard.* We eliminate strategy one: *prevent creation of the hazard* as an option because iron-containing vitamins exist for valid health reasons and we cannot justify not producing them. Because a major group of users of these products, pregnant and lactating women, are also likely to have children of ages at high risk for ingestions, we must accept that exposure to the hazard (iron-containing vitamins) is probable. The strongest possible (most upstream) intervention possible is therefore necessary. Strategy two is much more upstream than the now widely used strategy six: *placing a barrier between the child and the hazard* with child-proof closures or use of safe storage such as locked cabinets. It also addresses the dose-response nature of iron-ingestion poisoning. Having selected *reducing the amount of the hazard* as our strategy, we must identify means to that end. An educational approach might be to educate mothers (and grandparents) of young children to buy small containers of the medication. A technologic solution might be to manufacture vitamins with lower unit doses so that a child would have to ingest greater quantities of the pills before reaching a toxic dose. A regulatory approach might be to mandate warning labels on containers or limited dose dispensing of the vitamins or to restrict their over-the-counter distribution. Often, we combine approaches for maximum effect. For example, we may limit over-the-counter availability of the vitamins, require that they be dispensed in a child-resistant container, and provide educational materials about the risk of iron-containing vitamins to those who purchase them.

In general, we aim to intervene as early in the causal chain as possible. An analogy used in the injury prevention community is finding multiple people drowning in a river. Do we focus our efforts downstream on pulling them out of the water one by one and attempting resuscitation, or do we walk upstream to find out why they are all falling (or being pushed) into the river? In the acute-care setting, the trauma nurse is the rescuer downstream. Nurses who embrace (directly or indirectly) a primary prevention role move upstream to deal with the factors that led to the trauma epidemic. Fortunately for injury prevention, some trauma professionals have found it possible to do both. Indeed, for accreditation purposes, some trauma services are required to demonstrate involvement in prevention.[45] Comprehensive prevention requires work at all levels of the continuum. Investing all our efforts and resources downstream will never be enough to control the injury epidemic. Furthermore, if we fail to monitor activities and trends *upstream*, we cannot equip ourselves to deal with future consequences *downstream.*

Perhaps the greatest challenge to identifying effective primary prevention strategies is preoccupation with the individual: the *blame the victim, train the victim* paradigm. It has been said that "no mass disorder afflicting mankind was ever brought under control or eliminated by attempts at treating the individual."[46] Injury is, indeed, a *mass disorder* requiring urgent preventive action. To *control* this problem we must move beyond talking to individuals about safety and embrace the wide range of intervention options available to us.

TABLE 6-3 **The Haddon Strategies Applied**

	Haddon Strategy	Example Applications
1	Prevent creation of the hazard	Do not manufacture three-wheeled all-terrain vehicles, certain types of ammunition, and certain poisons Ban human pyramids
2	Reduce amount of the hazard	Limit pills per container Decrease water temperature in homes Limit contact drills in football
3	Prevent release of the hazard	Provide handrails for the elderly Improve braking capability of vehicles Reduce alcohol use by drivers
4	Alter release of the hazard	Blister-package pills Use child safety seats and seat belts to control deceleration forces Use release bindings on skis
5	Separate person and hazard in time and space	Construct bike and pedestrian paths Remove trees near roadways Evacuate hurricane paths
6	Place barrier between the person and the hazard	Use bike helmets Use childproof closures Use four-sided pool fencing Use protective goggles Ensure insulation of electrical cords
7	Modify basic qualities of the hazard	Use breakaway poles near roadways, energy-absorbing surfacing, shatterproof glass in windshields
8	Strengthen resistance to the hazard	Prevent osteoporosis Promote muscle conditioning in athletes Apply earthquake and hurricane building codes
9	Begin to counter damage done	Provide early detection: smoke detectors, roadside phones, early warning systems, emergency response systems
10	Stabilize, repair damage, and rehabilitate	Provide treatment, rehabilitation, vocational and self-care retraining Modify environment for disabled

Adapted from Baker SP, O'Neill B, Ginsburg MJ et al: *The injury fact book*, 2nd edition, New York, 1992, Oxford University Press, and Haddon W Jr: The basic strategies for preventing damage from hazards of all kinds, *Hazard Prev* 16:8-12, 1980.

Intervention strategies fall into four main categories—sometimes called the Four E's:

1. Education (and behavior change)
2. Engineering (and technology)
3. Enforcement (and legislation)
4. Economic approaches (incentives and disincentives)

Each of these approaches is described below.

Education encompasses a wide range of strategies that range from one-on-one education to initiatives that educate society and eventually influence social norms. Health education and health promotion, although criticized by some in the past as ineffective, have much to offer the field if used strategically. We must, however, move beyond a preoccupation with reaching individuals with brochures, fliers, posters, and overcrowded informational displays. Effective prevention frequently requires modification of the nature of the hazard or of the physical or social environment, which is usually the purview of *engineering* or *enforcement*. This has led to suggestions that we should focus on engineering solutions rather than educational approaches. In reality, there is no place for either/or; we need both.[47] Little is accomplished in our society without the commitment and involvement of groups of people. Mobilization of this valuable resource—be it parents, health care providers, legislators, law enforcement agencies, the media, product manufacturers, or funding agencies—requires the ability to influence knowledge, attitudes, beliefs, and behaviors. The behavioral sciences can also help us identify barriers to change and those factors that predispose, enable, or reinforce change, whether at the individual or national level. Trauma nurses who wish to present educational programs are encouraged to identify, and consider as a resource, professional health educators and behavioral scientists in their organizations and communities. They may also choose to review a recent textbook by Gielen et al. on behavioral approaches to injury and violence prevention.[48]

Engineering involves *engineering out the hazard* (such as designing safer products and safer roadways) or using engineering and technology to protect the person in an energy-transfer situation (helmets, restraint systems, crumple zones in cars, automatic sprinkler systems). After injury has occurred, engineering approaches include the development of technology to enhance early warning and emergency response and, of course, the technology associated with management, rehabilitation, and reintegration of the injured person into society. Many of the injury hazards in today's world are the result of products or environments that we have created with technology. It is not surprising therefore that technology is an important part of the solution. Engineering interventions to prevent injury are so pervasive in our society, however, that we may not notice them, take them for granted, and forget how relatively recent these achievements are. The fact that *safety sells*, so evident in current motor vehicle advertising campaigns, is a very recent development in our society and the result of years of injury prevention and consumer advocacy. Indeed, each step forward in road design, product modification, product labeling, policy and legislation, and changed social norms about injury has been hard won.

Enforcement is an oversimplified term for a wide-ranging area that involves the development and enforcement of law, regulation, and policy. Federal, state, and local laws and regulation have been used to advance injury prevention in numerous and varied ways.[49] For example, laws and regulations have been used to establish and fund federal safety programs; create a mandate for EMS systems development; mandate hospital reporting of external cause of injury codes in 26 states; require the use of seat belts, child safety seats, booster seats, bicycle helmets, and other safety equipment; establish graduated driver's licensing, speed limits, and traffic control regulations; regulate the manufacture and distribution of consumer products; set safety standards for schools, school buses, child care facilities, health care settings, and the workplace; control high-risk behaviors such as drunk driving; establish building codes; set standards for vehicle design and performance; and create trauma registries and other data systems. Tort law or private litigation has been used successfully to protect the public from unsafe products.[49] This has been achieved in several ways, including seeking compensation for victims of negligence and deterring, through liability, negligent practices by companies.[50,51]

Despite numerous successes, gaps in some existing laws compromise both coverage and effectiveness.[49] Additionally, the effect of any law, regulation, or policy is closely linked to its enforcement. Challenges to enforcement are not limited to inadequate law enforcement resources. Those responsible for enforcing a law or policy must believe in the law, their ability to enforce it, and the utility of that enforcement. Building support for enforcement may be as important as creating public support for the law, if it is to be implemented. Many injury prevention laws encounter powerful opponents and are challenged or overturned. Achieving passage of and defending injury prevention legislation usually requires compelling data and extensive and prolonged advocacy efforts. In 1981, Lawrence Berger suggested that six conditions be met when the implementation of injury legislation is contemplated. These are that one "be thoroughly convinced that the bill addresses a strikingly important issue. One should have evidence that the bill's action can be effective; support from judges and police officers that the law can be enforced expeditiously; economic estimates that excessive costs will not be involved; legal counsel confirming the constitutionality and compatibility of the proposed law with existing legislation and ordinances; and broad-based support from constituents."[52] Clearly, writing, passing, and implementing injury prevention laws is not the sole responsibility of lawyers, legislators, and the law enforcement community.[53] Elizabeth McLoughlin, a tireless injury prevention activist, has documented many of the lessons learned in California's prolonged efforts to achieve legislation requiring the use of helmets by motorcyclists.[54] One valuable advocacy lesson, which she continues to develop and apply in other areas of injury prevention, is the power of using "the authentic voice of survivors and family members who have been affected" in support of legislation.[54,55] Because of their expertise and personal experience of caring for trauma victims, trauma nurses can make valuable contributions when they join efforts to develop and advocate the passage and implementation of injury prevention laws.

Economic incentives—or, in many cases, disincentives—are used to persuade people or organizations to adopt safe practices or behaviors. Examples include fines for traffic offenses, increased insurance premiums, withholding of federal funds, and financial penalties imposed by courts on the manufacturers of unsafe products. Positive incentives include lowered insurance premiums for safe drivers or those buying safer vehicles and incentives to corporations that provide safe working environments.

To be effective, interventions must target the risk factors. The relationship between the chosen intervention and the risk factor we hope to change must be stated explicitly. For example, if an identified risk factor for adolescent bicycle crash–related head injury in your community is that teens do not own helmets, helmet distribution would be a logical intervention choice. Helmet distribution would not be a logical choice if the identified risk factor is teenagers' refusal to wear helmets, even if they have them.

The Haddon Matrix (described previously) can be used in a second way to assist in the identification of possible interventions. This is accomplished by thinking about what interventions might be used to address risk factors present in different cells of the matrix. Pre-event phase interventions attempt to reduce the number of events with the potential to cause injury: prevent car and bike crashes, falls, house fires, ingestion of poisons, assaults, and so on. Examples of such interventions would be graduated licensing programs for teenage drivers, limiting the number of hours driven without rest by truck drivers, enforcing speed limits, legislation that penalizes people caught driving while intoxicated, putting traffic-calming measures in place in areas with many pedestrians, mandating use of safety harnesses for construction workers, enforcing building standards in nursing homes, and closing beaches when there are strong currents. Event phase interventions attempt to reduce the number and severity of injuries that occur in these events. Examples include seat belts and air bags, enhanced vehicle crashworthiness, bicycle helmets and handlebar design, bulletproof vests for police officers, smoke detectors and automatic sprinkler systems, controlling access to lethal weapons, prevention of osteoporosis, and physical conditioning of athletes. Postevent phase interventions attempt to prevent complications and optimize outcome. Those most familiar to the trauma nurse include emergency medical management, medical care, and rehabilitation. Others include improving the integrity of vehicle gas tanks to reduce the chances of postcrash fires, early detection and notification of injury, preventing entrapment, improving health insurance status and social support structures (to optimize rehabilitation), and job retraining.

Injury prevention also uses active and passive strategies. An *active* strategy is one that requires a person to act each time he or she, or the person he or she hopes to protect, is to be protected. A *passive* strategy will afford protection without action on the part of the person to be protected. All intervention strategies lie on a continuum from entirely active to entirely passive. Seat belts, for example, are not entirely active. They require that a person fasten the seat belt each time he or she gets into the vehicle but, once fastened, the belt will protect the person for the duration of the trip. Figure 6-1[56] illustrates the relationship between the type of strategy and the likelihood of prevention effectiveness.

An inverse relationship is observed: prevention effectiveness increases as the need for action decreases. For this reason, whenever possible, injury prevention specialists will try to implement an intervention that is passive. In most cases, achieving passive strategies—such as modification of an unsafe product or environment—requires that some infrastructure be established. This infrastructure might be public support for a law or policy, designated funds for road improvement, legal or financial penalties for the manufacture of products that lead to injury, or an energetic advocacy effort.

Trauma nurses who feel uncomfortable with the idea of engineering or law and policy approaches may find it helpful to realize that they can contribute to these efforts in other ways. Increasingly, injury prevention efforts include comprehensive or multicomponent approaches and interdisciplinary collaborations. The *spectrum of prevention* (Table 6-4)[57,58] is a tool that has been used to encourage comprehensive programs that move beyond a purely educational approach. The six levels of the spectrum represent areas in which prevention initiatives can be implemented. The critical concept, however, is that the levels are synergistic; prevention effectiveness may be enhanced by creating strong linkages between the components. Level 3, *educating providers*, is of particular relevance to trauma nurses. Cohen and Swift[57] emphasize that "providers have influence within their fields of expertise and opportunities to transmit information, skills and motivation to clients, and colleagues. It is essential, therefore, that they receive education to improve their own understanding of prevention." They go on to comment that certain professionals (such as trauma nurses) "can be highly effective advocates for policy changes related to their job experience." When used with the Haddon Matrix, the spectrum can suggest systematic approaches to an injury problem.

Possible intervention strategies can be identified in many ways. The injury prevention literature is a rich source of information. Several injury prevention texts[9,21,43,49,59-61] devote chapters to different types of approaches. The excellent website of the Injury Control Resource Information Network at the University of Pittsburgh (www.injurycontrol.com/icrin), which can be searched by topic area, provides extensive links to other sites. Through it, the trauma nurse can access the Center for Injury Prevention and Control of the Centers for Disease Control and Prevention (CDC), CDC-funded injury control research centers, federal agencies, and a wealth of injury prevention resources. A valuable source of information on best practices for child and adolescent injury prevention can be accessed on the website of the Harborview Injury Prevention and Research Center (http://depts.washington.edu/hiprc/practices/index.html). Readers are encouraged to browse the websites listed in Box 6-1 for further information about injury and injury prevention.

The range of possible interventions and access to information about them expand constantly. The main challenge to identifying intervention options is not a lack of information; it is failure to consider this information-gathering step an important part of the problem-solving process.

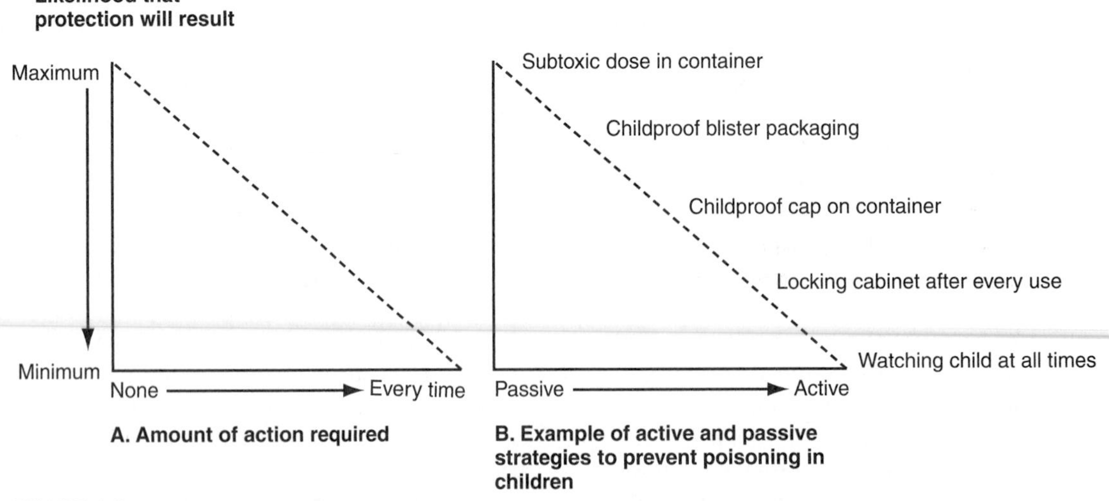

FIGURE 6-1 The relationship between the amount of action required and the likelihood that protection will result. *(Modified from Baker SP: Childhood injuries: the community approach to prevention,* J Public Health Policy *2:235-246, 1981.)*

TABLE 6-4 The Spectrum of Prevention

Influencing Policy and Legislation
Developing strategies to change laws and policies
Changing Organizational Practices
Adopting regulations and shaping norms
Fostering Coalitions and Networks
Convening groups and individuals for greater impact
Educating Providers
Informing providers who influence others
Promoting Community Education
Reaching groups with information and resources
Strengthening Individual Knowledge and Skills
Enhancing individual capacity

Adapted from Cohen L, Swift S: The spectrum of prevention: developing a comprehensive approach to injury prevention, *Inj Prev* 5:203-207, 1999, and from Prevention Institute: [Prevention] tools and frameworks: www.preventioninstitute.org/tools.html.

SELECTING A STRATEGY TO IMPLEMENT

At first, the range of potential strategies may be intimidating. Recognizing the importance of technologic or regulatory strategies may cause a nurse comfortable with one-on-one patient encounters to feel inadequate. Even injury prevention specialists feel at times that the obstacles to achieving such interventions are insurmountable, causing some to retreat to easier, more familiar, or more immediate interventions. The Revised Intervention Decision Matrix[62] is a simple tool designed to identify intervention options and choose among them (Table 6-5). It can also identify long-term goals and intervention options that support each other.

Eight elements of the Intervention Decision Matrix are used as decision criteria for selecting an intervention:

Effectiveness
Feasibility
Cost feasibility
Sustainability
Political will
Social will
Potential for unintended risks
Potential for unintended benefits

Effectiveness refers to the likelihood that the intervention will do what it is intended to do. Specifically, will the intervention reduce the number and/or severity of injuries? As discussed previously, a passive injury prevention strategy is more likely to be effective than an active strategy.

Feasibility refers to the likelihood that an intervention will happen. Is it technically possible, practical, achievable, and viable? Are safer products and technical solutions possible and available? Do they work? This is not a recommendation to choose low-risk and easily achieved interventions, for these are seldom effective. Rather, it cautions the enthusiastic preventionist to avoid trying to change the essentially unchangeable, such as the road-crossing abilities of 4-year-old pedestrians. Some of our most effective interventions have taken numerous years to achieve. Through the efforts of others, what was not feasible 10 years ago is feasible today.

Cost feasibility refers to the affordability of an intervention. At a time of limited resources, cost considerations are an important factor in intervention selection. The danger is that cost becomes the only consideration, to the detriment of effectiveness. Selecting an intervention with low effectiveness because it is the least expensive alternative squanders all resources. No matter how "affordable" an intervention appears to be, if it yields very low injury prevention returns, the cost per protected person will be enormous.

Sustainability refers to the potential for continued effect. It can be thought of in two ways:

1. Will the effect persist after the intervention is completed? For example, will driving in excess of the speed limit return to pre-enforcement levels when the police leave the site?
2. Will the intervention become institutionalized? For example, will it become the social norm that people wear seat belts? Will a community assume responsibility for the maintenance of a newly renovated playground?

Political will can also be viewed in two ways:

1. Is the intervention ethical? Is it equitable? Does it violate human rights? Is it unreasonably intrusive? These, of course, are critical issues that must be weighed carefully when any intervention is considered.
2. What is the prevailing political mood about this intervention? For example, it is often easier to pass legislation that requires protection of children than that protecting adults. Many areas of injury control are impeded by the fact that the political process creates barriers to interventions that compelling scientific evidence and, in many cases, public opinion support. An intervention that has low political acceptability faces a major obstacle and alerts us to the need for awareness building. But, and this is important to remember, political obstacles of this type are not insurmountable.

Social will is the key to building constituent support and challenging political barriers. Low social will indicates the need to generate support for the initiative. This may be achieved in various ways but requires that the factors contributing to the low social will be assessed. People may be unaware of the problem, unconcerned about it, resistant to change, afraid of the cost or inconvenience of interventions, or too busy to care. Each reason requires a different remedial approach. The key issue is that with time social will, and ultimately political will, may be changed. If, however, low social will is a barrier to prevention, understanding and addressing the causes of this should be a priority. Attempting to implement interventions in settings where social will is low is like swimming against the current. Coalitions and informal networks that bring together diverse sectors of the community may help build social support for prevention initiatives.[53] As often-quoted social anthropologist Dr. Margaret Mead once

BOX 6-1 Sources of Injury and Injury-Prevention Information

The following resources are included so that readers can find additional information about injury and injury prevention. This list is by no means exhaustive. Many of these resources have good search engines and extensive links to other sites.

General

Agency for Healthcare Research and Quality: www.ahrq.gov
American Association for the Surgery of Trauma: www.aast.org
American Public Health Association Injury Control and Emergency Health Services Section: www.icehs.org
American Society of Safety Engineers: www.asse.org
Association for the Advancement of Automotive Medicine: www.carcrash.org
Association of American Medical Colleges: www.aamc.org
Consumer Product Safety Commission: www.cpsc.gov
Core Competencies for Injury and Violence Prevention: www.injuryed.org (developed by the SAVIR-STIPDA Joint Committee on Infrastructure Development: http://www.injuryed.org/docs/Core%20Competencies.doc)
Department of Veterans' Affairs: www.va.gov
National Training Initiative for Injury and Violence Prevention: http://www.injuryed.org/
North Carolina Institute for Public Health: http://www.sph.unc.edu/nciph/
The Prevention Institute: www.preventioninstitute.org
State and Territorial Injury Prevention Directors: http://www.stipda.org/
The Trauma Foundation at San Francisco General Hospital: www.traumaf.org

Data Sources

These sites link to numerous other data sites.

Administration for Children and Families, federal and state reporting systems: http://www.acf.hhs.gov/programs/cb/systems/index.htm
Bureau of Justice Statistics: http://www.ojp.usdoj.gov/bjs/
Bureau of Transportation Statistics: www.bts.gov
Census Bureau database and extracts: www.census.gov
Fedworld: www.fedworld.gov
Injury Control Resource Information Network: www.injurycontrol.com/icrin/
Injury Databases and Published Statistics: www.injurycontrol.com/icrin/stats.htm
National Center for Health Statistics: http://www.cdc.gov/nchs/
National Center for Injury Prevention and Control, scientific data and injury statistics (WISQARS™): www.cdc.gov/ncipc/osp/data.htm
National Data Archive on Child Abuse and Neglect: www.ndacan.cornell.edu
State Injury Profiles (maps and tables of injury deaths and death rates for all states in the nation): www.cdc.gov/ncipc/stateprofiles/index.htm

Children

ABC's of Raising Healthy Kids: Steps to Staying Safe and Healthy: http://www.cdc.gov/women/owh/kids/abc.htm
American Academy of Pediatrics: www.aap.org
American Academy of Pediatrics: Car Safety Seats and Transportation Safety: http://www.aap.org/healthtopics/carseatsafety.cfm
Archives of Pediatrics and Adolescent Medicine: http://archpedi.ama-assn.org/
Bicycle Helmet Safety Institute: www.bhsi.org
Bicycle Related Injury: www.cdc.gov/ncipc/bike/
Booster Seat Coalition (Washington state): http://depts.washington.edu/booster
Children's Hospital of Philadelphia Trauma Link: http://www.chop.edu/consumer/jsp/division/generic.jsp?id=71016
The Children's Hospital of Philadelphia, Partners for Child Passenger Safety: http://www.chop.edu/consumer/jsp/division/generic.jsp?id=77974
Children's Hospital of Pittsburgh–Injury Prevention: http://www.chp.edu/besafe/index.php
Children's Safety Network: http://www.childrenssafetynetwork.org/
Emergency Medical Services for Children: http://bolivia.hrsa.gov/emsc/index.aspx
Injury Free Coalition for Kids: www.injuryfree.org
International Society for Child and Adolescent Injury Prevention: http://www.iscaip.net/
The Journal of Injury Prevention: http://ip.bmj.com/
Juvenile Products Manufacturers' Association: www.jpma.org
KidsandCars.org: http://www.kidsandcars.org/
National Coalition for School Bus Safety: www.ncsbs.org
National Network for Child Care: http://www.nncc.org/
National Safe Kids Campaign: www.safekids.org

BOX 6-1 Sources of Injury and Injury-Prevention Information—cont'd

National Transportation Safety Board's Child Passenger Safety: www.ntsb.gov/Surface/Highway/childseat.htm
National Trauma Data Bank: http://www.facs.org/trauma/ntdb.html
Prevent Child Abuse America: http://www.preventchildabuse.org/index.shtml
Safety Belt Safe USA: www.carseat.org

Domestic Violence/Family Violence/Relationship Violence
Center for the Study and Prevention of Violence: www.colorado.edu/cspv/index.html
Center for Violence Prevention and Control, University of Minnesota: http://www1.umn.edu/cvpc/
Family Violence Prevention Fund: http://endabuse.org/
National Domestic Violence Hotline: www.ndvh.org
Relationship Violence Warning Signs and Resources: http://ub-counseling.buffalo.edu/warnings

Elderly
The American Association for Retired Persons: www.aarp.org
Fall Prevention Center of Excellence: http://www.stopfalls.org/index.shtml
Injury Prevention Web, Elder Safety: www.injurypreventionweb.org/links/links-elder.htm
US Consumer Product Safety Commission, Safety for Older Consumers, Home Safety Checklist for Seniors: http://www.cpsc.gov/cpscpub/pubs/701.html

Firearms
Johns Hopkins Center for Gun Policy and Research: http://www.jhsph.edu/gunpolicy/
The Million Mom March Foundation: www.millionmommarch.com
Trauma.Org, Firearms and Gun Control Internet Resources: http://www.trauma.org/index.php/main/article/372/

Fires
Fire Prevention in the Home: http://seniors.tcnet.org/articles/article04.html
National Fire Protection Association: http://www.nfpa.org/index.asp
US Fire Administration: http://www.usfa.dhs.gov/

Government Agencies
CDC Injury Topics and Fact Sheets: www.cdc.gov/ncipc/cmprfact.htm
CDC National Center for Injury Prevention and Control: www.cdc.gov/ncipc/ncipchm.htm
CDC National Center for Injury Prevention and Control Fact Book: http://www.cdc.gov/ncipc/fact_book/factbook.htm
CDC WISQARS™: http://www.cdc.gov/ncipc/wisqars/default.htm
CDC Wonder Compressed Mortality: http://wonder.cdc.gov/mortSql.html
Consumer Product Safety Commission: www.cpsc.gov
Department of Justice, Office of Justice Programs: www.ojp.usdoj.gov
Department of Veterans' Affairs: www.va.gov/
Food and Drug Administration: www.fda.gov
Indian Health Services: http://www.ihs.gov/
Insurance Institute for Highway Safety: www.iihs.org
Morbidity and Mortality Weekly Report: http://www.cdc.gov/mmwr/
National Center for Biotechnical Information: http://www.ncbi.nlm.nih.gov/
National Center for Injury Prevention and Control: www.cdc.gov/ncipc
National Highway Traffic Safety Administration: www.nhtsa.dot.gov
National Institutes of Health: www.nih.gov
National Institute on Alcohol Abuse and Alcoholism: www.niaaa.nih.gov
National Institute on Drug Abuse: www.nida.nih.gov
National Institute of Mental Health: www.nimh.nih.gov
National Institute for Occupational Safety and Health: http://www.cdc.gov/niosh/homepage.html
National Library of Medicine: www.nlm.nih.gov
Occupational Safety and Health Administration: www.osha.gov

Injury Centers (Selected)
Alberta Centre for Injury Control and Research: http://www.acicr.ualberta.ca/
California Department of Health Services, Epidemiology and Prevention for Injury Control Branch: http://www.dhs.ca.gov/epic/
The Center for Injury Research and Prevention: http://stokes.chop.edu/programs/injury/
Center for Rural Emergency Medicine at West Virginia University: http://www.hsc.wvu.edu/crem/
Emory Center for Injury Control: http://www.sph.emory.edu/center_cic.php
Harborview Injury Prevention and Research Center: http://depts.washington.edu/hiprc/

Continued

BOX 6-1 Sources of Injury and Injury-Prevention Information—cont'd

Home Safety Council: http://www.homesafetycouncil.org/index.aspx
The Interdisciplinary Pediatric Injury Control Research Center: www.traumalink.chop.edu
The Johns Hopkins Center for Injury Research and Policy: http://www.jhsph.edu/InjuryCenter/
Kentucky Injury Prevention and Research Center: www.kiprc.uky.edu
Marshfield Clinic, Farm Medicine, Rural Health and Safety: http://www.marshfieldclinic.org/nfmc/pages/default.aspx
Marshfield Clinic, Research Foundation, National Children's Center for Rural and Agricultural Health and Safety: http://www.marshfieldclinic.org/nfmc/pages/default.aspx?page=nccrahs_welcome
Prevention Institute: http://www.preventioninstitute.org/
The San Francisco Injury Center: http://www.surgery.ucsf.edu/sfic/
World Health Organization, Department of Injuries and Violence Prevention: http://www.who.int/violence_injury_prevention/en/

Motor Vehicle Crashes

CRDL: CARE (Crash Analysis and Reporting Environment) Research and Development Laboratory: http://care.cs.ua.edu/
Institute of Transportation Engineers: www.ite.org
Insurance Institute for Highway Safety: www.iihs.org

Poisoning

American Association of Poison Control Centers: www.aapcc.org
Canadian Network of Toxicology Centres: www.uoguelph.ca/cntc
National Capital Poison Center: www.poison.org

Playgrounds

HealthyKids.com: www.healthykids.com
The National Program for Playground Safety: www.uni.edu/playground
National Recreation and Parks Association: http://www.nrpa.org/

Specific Injury Prevention Areas

American Association of Suicidology: http://www.suicidology.org/
American Association for the Surgery of Trauma: www.aast.org
American Burn Association: www.ameriburn.org/
American Trauma Society: www.amtrauma.org
Brain Injury Association of America: www.biausa.org
Centre for Neuro Skills: www.neuroskills.com/
Foundation for Aquatic Injury Prevention: www.aquaticisf.org
Foundation for Spinal Cord Injury Prevention, Care, and Cure: http://fscip.org
Institute for Preventative Sports Medicine: http://www.ipsm.org/
National Rehabilitation Information Center Home Page: http://www.naric.com/
National Resource Center for Traumatic Brain Injury: www.neuro.pmr.vcu.edu
Ski and Snowboard Injuries: www.ski-injury.com
Spinal Research: www.spinal-research.org
Suicide Prevention Resource Center: http://www.sprc.org/featured_resources/ps/index.asp

School Violence Prevention

CDC Healthy Schools—Healthy Youth!: http://www.cdc.gov/HealthyYouth/index.htm
Center for the Prevention of School Violence: http://www.ncdjjdp.org/cpsv/
HRSA—Stop Bullying Now: http://www.stopbullyingnow.hrsa.gov/index.asp?area=main
Office of Safe and Drug Free Schools: http://www.ed.gov/about/offices/list/osdfs/index.html

Workplace Violence Prevention

Violence in the Workplace: www.cdc.gov/niosh/violcont.html

said, "Never doubt that a small group of thoughtful, committed citizens can change the world. Indeed, it is the only thing that ever has."

Potential for unintended risks must be considered because an important principle in injury control is—as in medicine—first, do no harm. Some interventions with the potential to protect may also have the potential to cause harm. One well-publicized example was the airbag-related deaths of approximately 70 children that led, in part, to the development of second-generation or "smart" airbags.[63] High school driver education courses that increased the driving exposure of 16-year-olds led to increases in motor vehicle crash involvement and death rates in this group. When courses were discontinued[64] or driving curfews imposed,[65,66] crashes were reduced substantially. In April 2000, the American Academy of Pediatrics issued a policy statement (RE9940) discouraging swimming programs for children under the age of 4 years. Many potentially harmful

TABLE 6-5 **The Revised Intervention Decision Matrix**

Intervention Decision Criteria	**Intervention Option 1**	**Intervention Option 2**	**Intervention Option 3**
Effectiveness			
Feasibility			
Cost feasibility			
Sustainability			
Ethical acceptability ("Fatal cell" must be high to proceed)			
Political will			
Social will			
Potential for unintended benefits			
Potential for unintended risks* (LOW risk = HIGH priority)			
Final priority rating			

1. Compare intervention options by ranking each cell against the criterion as "high, medium, or low priority." Decisions should be evidence based. 2. Which option is strongest? Effectiveness and sustainability are critically important. 3. Ethical acceptability is a critical variable. Any intervention option that is not highly ethically acceptable should not be considered.

unintended consequences of early training were noted in the discussion, such as the fact that early lessons did not translate into higher levels of swimming proficiency, removal of a child's fear of water may inadvertently encourage an unsupervised child to enter the water, parents of trained children may develop a false sense of confidence in their child's ability, the lack of an established relationship between safety training and observed safety skills, and the potentially tragic consequences of even a brief lapse in supervision.[67]

PLANNING THE IMPLEMENTATION

A familiar saying, *those who fail to plan, plan to fail*, is wise counsel to anyone implementing injury prevention programs. Time invested in implementation planning will save time, resources, and frustration. Ideally, implementation and evaluation (discussed below) should be planned together. A prudent first step is to review factors that are key to successful implementation of education, engineering, and enforcement strategies. These factors are summarized in Table 6-6, compiled from a comprehensive discussion of injury prevention by Sleet and Gielen.[68]

Next it is time to plan the implementation. Before taking any intervention actions, one should consider and document the following:

1. The project goal
2. Project objectives
3. Action steps (sometimes called process objectives)
4. The intended audience for each step
5. The methods/strategies to be used for each step
6. The indicators of success for each step
7. Evaluation methods for each step (discussed below)
8. A project time line
9. A person (or group) responsible for each action step
10. The resources (financial or other) necessary to achieve the objectives

The *project goal* is a statement of your project's destination. Ideally, it should be specific and measurable within a reasonable time frame. It is not always practical to define outcomes as reductions in deaths and injuries. Although reducing the burden of injury is our ultimate goal, it may be wiser to define a more attainable goal such as "*to reduce within the next 12 months the number of vehicles that run red lights in Hazard City by 25%.*"

Project objectives are the map to your destination. They provide a set of outcomes that will need to be reached if the project goal is to be achieved. Remember two words—DOTS and SMART—as you write objectives. The DOTS criteria (**D**iscreet, **O**utcome-focused, **T**ime-framed, and **S**pecific) are described below:

- "Discreet" means that each desired outcome should have its own objective. Writing "*increase overtime funding and levels of enforcement at high-risk intersections*" combines two objectives. This is a problem because the two desired outcomes pose different intervention challenges.
- "Outcome-focused" implies that something will change and that the change will be measurable. For example, "*funds will be obtained to cover the cost of 100 hours of overtime enforcement activity.*"
- "Time-framed" means that the stated objective should include a date by which the outcome will be achieved. *By October 1, 2008, funds will be obtained to cover the cost of 100 hours of overtime enforcement activity.* Typically, program objectives are short-term objectives (see below).

TABLE 6-6 Key Factors for Successful Implementation of Injury Prevention Strategies

For successful implementation of education and behavior strategies, the target group must:	Be exposed to the appropriate information Understand and believe the information Have the resources and skills to make the proposed change(s) Derive benefit (or perceive a benefit) from the change Be reinforced to maintain the change over time
For successful implementation of engineering and technology solutions, the technology must:	Be effective and reliable Be acceptable to the public and compatible with the environment Result in products that dominate in the marketplace Be easily understood and properly used by the public
For successful implementation of legislation and law enforcement strategies:	The legislation must be widely known and understood The public must accept the legislation and its enforcement provisions The probability, or perceived probability, of being caught if one breaks the law must be high The punishment must be perceived to be swift and severe

Compiled from Sleet D, Gielen A: Injury prevention. In Gorin SS, Arnold J, editors: *Health promotion handbook,* St. Louis, 1998, Mosby.

- "Specific" refers to how, and to what extent, the outcome will be achieved. *By October 1, 2008, X dollars will be obtained through a grant from the Magnanimous Foundation to cover the cost of 100 hours of overtime enforcement activity.*

The SMART criteria (**S**hort-term, **M**easurable, **A**chievable, **R**elevant/realistic, and **T**ime-framed) are described below:

- "Short-term": ideally, objectives should be able to be accomplished in weeks rather than months or years. Many planners prefer to split large long-term objectives into several smaller and shorter-term objectives.
- "Measurable": specific enough that a change can be measured
- "Achievable": select objectives that can be accomplished. Large, overly ambitious objectives increase the likelihood of program failure.
- "Relevant/realistic": to the program's goal. If one hopes to encourage an adolescent to adopt a lasting behavior change, a simple public service announcement is not a relevant or realistic intervention choice.
- "Time-framed": described above

Action steps (sometimes called process objectives) are the actions one takes to achieve the program objectives. These may include securing letters of support for a grant application, ordering incentive items, convening an advisory group that includes members of partner agencies, developing educational materials, organizing media events, gathering data to identify hazardous intersections, and conducting training of field workers.

The *intended audience for individual action steps* (sometimes called the target group) is not necessarily the same as that stated in the program goals and objectives. Organizing a media event will involve one group of people, planning enforcement schedules another, targeting repeat offenders yet another. Being specific about the group involved in each step conserves resources and helps identify the partners you will need to involve in program implementation.

The *methods/strategies to be used for each step* represent the bottom line: how will this happen? Writing down each step may seem unnecessary but it protects from errors of omission. Additionally, it provides the basis for a realistic estimate of time and resources needed to complete the project.

The *indicators of success for each step* determine how you will know the process objective (action step) has been achieved. This is what you hope to find when you evaluate this part of the process. For example, what will indicate to you that the activity has increased law enforcement's willingness to do enforcement?

Evaluation methods identified for each step are the key to good program management and evaluation throughout the life of the program. Evaluation methods are used to determine/measure to what extent an indicator has been achieved. For example, if our desired indicator is that we will increase bicycle helmet use rates by 25%, our evaluation methods could include observational surveys or self-report. The choice of evaluation method influences the strength of evidence produced, but many methods are quick and affordable. The benefits of evaluation are discussed later.

A *project time line* is most useful if it is written down using real dates instead of week markers, such as *Weeks 12 to 16*. This alerts project staff to potential conflicts, such as meetings scheduled for public holidays, a training session planned for the week of Thanksgiving, and so on.

A *lead person (or group) should be designated as responsible for each step*. This enhances resource management, project monitoring, and staff accountability.

The resources (financial or other) necessary to achieve the objectives. It is important to consider the resources required to implement a program. Money is a valuable resource but fortunately, given that injury prevention is a significantly underfunded area, not the only important resource. Strategic partnerships for prevention can prove important *resource mobilizers,* both in terms of financial resources and nonfinancial resources, such as time, space, in-kind contributions, volunteer expertise, and so forth. Partnerships, however, require investment of resources (notably time and leadership) to be productive. In summary, implementation planning will help to do the following:

1. Eliminate planning gaps
2. Keep you focused and on track
3. Manage resources wisely
4. Make objectives attainable

PROGRAM EVALUATION

Evaluation is a valuable part of any injury prevention program. Contrary to popular opinion, evaluation is not a personal judgment of the program staff, nor is it used to trick unsuspecting programs into revealing their flaws, nor is it to be undertaken only if funding absolutely depends on it. Evaluation is a tool that, if used well, can build better programs. Evaluations may be simple or complex depending on one's needs, resources, training, and professional perspective. Real-world program evaluations need not be exhaustive or complex to provide valuable information about the program and should be considered prevention partners rather than adversaries. There are only four categories of information that evaluation can reveal about the program: good things that you have already identified, good things that you had not identified (a bonus), bad things that you have identified, and bad things that you had not yet identified. Fear of discovery in this latter category deters many from doing evaluation, yet most of us would like to know as early as possible if we had a malignant tumor. In the same way that early detection and management of a malignancy may enhance the chances for a good outcome, early detection and management of program problems enhances the chance of a good outcome. Evaluation is therefore an excellent management tool if it is integrated into the program from the very beginning.

There are many practical reasons to do evaluation, and to do it throughout the life of the program[69,70]:

1. To determine whether the planned program objectives are adequately defined and measurable

When planning an evaluation, it is essential to clearly define the program goals and objectives to be measured (discussed later). Early evaluation planning will identify overly broad or vague intervention objectives that put programs at risk of failure.

2. To identify the program preferences of your intended audience and program partners

Once the desired intervention has been identified (e.g., building community support to modify an unsafe playground near the hospital), evaluation can help you determine which approaches are most likely to be acceptable and productive.

3. To ensure that program materials and program messengers are suitable for and acceptable to the recipients

This is one of the most important reasons to evaluate programs. So many programs produce materials that are entirely unsuitable for the people who will receive them. Common problems include a reading level that is too high; too much information; vague information (e.g., all children should buckle up); culturally inappropriate language, pictures, or messages; cluttered or overcrowded materials; and incorrect idiom for the age group. This extends beyond written materials. For example, program presenters must have credibility with the target audience, and a program venue in a community where few people own cars must be easily accessible by public transportation during the hours the program will be offered.

4. To determine whether what you plan to do is feasible

Many programs flounder because they are too ambitious. Others fail because planning occurred in a vacuum. Many factors can affect your ability to deliver the program. Potential barriers to implementation should be assessed carefully and the program plans modified accordingly. Successful programs tend to be focused and well defined. Start with small, achievable programs and build your experience, credibility, and support base.

5. To monitor whether program activities are happening as planned

No matter how well conceived a program is, it cannot be effective if it does not happen. For example, are the activities happening, are people attending events, are coalition members delivering the information necessary for drafting the proposed legislation? These important questions must be answered: Is it happening? If not, why? How can it be improved? Did that work?

6. To have an early warning system for unintended consequences of your intervention

As discussed previously, interventions to prevent injuries may have side effects. These unintended consequences may be positive or negative. It is important to identify both. Negative consequences are critical because they may increase risk of injury to certain members of the population or create a new risk entirely. Positive effects may help support the current intervention or similar initiatives in the future.

7. To determine whether program objectives are being met and you are progressing toward the stated goal

If, for example, your program objective is to achieve passage of legislation, there are several interim objectives that will need to be accomplished during the process. Each should be considered an outcome to be measured. In your journey toward legislation, these outcomes are the mileposts that will let you know whether you are moving in the right direction and whether you are covering enough miles each day to get to your destination on time. For example, did the bill get to the house committee on time? Missed preliminary deadlines may mean a year's delay, lost social support momentum, or an end to funding.

8. To provide baseline data for future projects

Injury prevention gains are often achieved incrementally; seat belt or bicycle helmet use rates that were successes 5 years ago are only starting points for new initiatives. Information we gather about our target community for a current project may help identify future priorities or approaches. If planned and conducted carefully, evaluation and needs assessment form part of the same information cycle, thus conserving valuable resources.

9. To determine whether the intervention is effective

This is the most well known reason to do evaluation, and one frequently tied to program funding. Did the program work? Did it make a difference? Can we demonstrate an association between our program and the observed changes?

10. To identify factors that may limit the effectiveness of such interventions

Many factors may limit the effectiveness of apparently successful interventions. Failure to sustain the intervention effect is an important factor. Programs that demonstrate short-term successes such as increased bicycle helmet use or the presence of a working smoke detector may find that, over time, these gains are lost. Educational and enforcement campaigns that are intensive but of short duration should, if at all possible, include a long-term evaluation component. Other factors that may limit effectiveness may include decreased funding for overtime needed to enforce a law, the emergence of cheaper and unsafe alternatives to safe products, or challenges to policy and law.

11. To justify resource allocation and qualify for funding in the future

Increasingly, prevention programs are required to demonstrate the benefits that result from investment of resources. Assessments of the cost-effectiveness and cost-benefit of programs may be used to determine whether a program is fiscally responsible and whether it should be funded or continued.[71] It can also be used to determine, in times of multiple priorities and resource limitation, where and how prevention dollars should be invested. Cost-effectiveness analysis examines the relationship between program costs and program outcomes when those outcomes (e.g., lives saved) are not measured in dollars.[72] Cost-benefit analysis expresses the relationship between program costs and program benefits in dollars (e.g., X dollars invested in prevention results in Y dollars saved).[72] Although the nurse may never be asked to conduct such an analysis, one practical step toward such an evaluation should always be taken. This is the monitoring and documentation of resources obtained and expended during the program. Monitoring the budget is only part of this task. As mentioned previously, resources invested may be more than money: volunteer time, in-kind services, discounted prices on safety equipment, use of personal vehicles, and so forth.[49] All should be considered when program cost is calculated.

12. To develop your own experience and self-efficacy in conducting evaluations

When asked why they do evaluations, many people answer "because we must to get funded." This illustrates the lack of confidence people have in their ability to conduct evaluations and, more important, their failure to realize what evaluation can do for them. Even a simple evaluation can provide valuable information about the program. The hardest evaluation is the first.

13. To promote the viability and commitment of your program team

At some time, every trauma nurse will experience the frustration that results when, having invested considerable time and energy in an activity, she or he receives no feedback about the outcome. Unlike the immediate reward that may be apparent when a trauma nurse helps save a life in the clinical setting, it has been said that the rewards for prevention are more "ethereal."[73] Stephen Teret, a prominent injury preventionist, notes that "if the preventionist is highly successful, the individual who was spared injury... may never even know that he or she was at risk."[73] Given the absence of immediate feedback, evaluation can help prevent burnout by demonstrating to those involved in the project the early, tangible outcomes that result from their actions. In its role as a management tool, evaluation also enhances the likelihood that a program will be focused, well organized, and implemented. This in itself promotes the viability of the team.

14. To prevent—through dissemination of negative findings—replication of ineffective programs

The worst program outcome is not a program that fails but a program that fails in silence. News of successful interventions are published and reported in many ways; not so negative findings. If an intervention fails, the program team should have access to enough information from the evaluation to determine, at least in part, why. This information can help the team—and others considering implementation of similar programs—to overcome these problems in the future.

15. To contribute to the body of knowledge about the effectiveness of interventions to prevent injury

Trauma nurses will be familiar with the term *evidence-based medicine*.[74] Although growing, the body of knowledge about the effectiveness of interventions to prevent injury is limited. Evaluations of intervention effectiveness therefore enhance our ability to practice *evidence-based prevention*.

16. To increase community support[56,75]

This may seem to be a peripheral reason to evaluate, but it has several program benefits. Evidence of early program successes may decrease resistance to the initiative; releasing information to stakeholders may increase their awareness of, support of, and trust in the project; and coalitions that are kept involved and informed are more likely to function effectively. A well-integrated program evaluation can enhance the overall *health* of the program.

Evaluation can be divided into four distinct stages:

1. Formative
2. Process
3. Impact (short-term outcomes)
4. Outcome (longer-term outcomes)

Formative evaluation is pilot testing (of intervention components) or troubleshooting (when something changes or goes wrong). It is done for quality assurance and to ensure that program materials are suitable for the target audience. Examples of formative evaluation questions might include the following:

- When is the best time to offer training sessions?
- Do teenage mothers understand the educational materials that are available for new mothers?
- How is our community different from community X?
- Do kids prefer yellow or green helmets?
- Is this instructor suitable for this audience?
- How difficult is it to install a rear-facing infant seat correctly?

Formative evaluation is very affordable and should be done during program planning and when any situation (e.g., the trainer) changes.

Process evaluation is used to determine whether the intervention activities are happening as planned. Ideally, it should be done throughout the life of the program. Examples of process evaluation questions include the following:

- How many people attended the health fair?
- What percentage of coalition members attend all meetings?
- How many bicycle helmets were distributed?
- Have we identified a sponsor for the proposed legislation?

Process evaluation is an early warning system for things that may go wrong. Use the information to enhance the implementation.

Impact (or short-term outcomes) evaluation measures the short-term impact the program has on the participants. It is determining whether the intervention had any effect on the audience. Where possible, it should be done after each encounter with the target group. Examples of short-term outcomes evaluation questions are listed below:

- How many people left the car seat check with correctly installed seats for each child?
- [After the presentation] did parents' awareness of their child's need to ride in a booster seat increase?
- Did the audience's knowledge of risk factors for falls increase?
- Did vehicle speed decrease during the enforcement period?

Outcome evaluation or longer-term outcomes evaluation assesses whether the program made a measurable difference: did it work? Examples of outcome evaluation questions include those listed below:

- To what extent have injuries to 4- to 8-year-old motor vehicle occupants decreased?
- By what percentage have bicycle helmet use rates increased?
- Have resources for youth programs increased as a result of this advocacy effort?
- Have we reduced the number of crashes associated with running red lights?

Repeat evaluations may be necessary to demonstrate that the intervention effect is real, sustained, and generalizable. Unfortunately, because of the cost involved, few interventions are evaluated this rigorously.

The choice of evaluation design will influence the strength of the conclusions and the value of information available to the program team and others. Poor quality data, the wrong data, or the wrong conclusions will undermine the evaluation. Pick the strongest design you can afford and, when in doubt, discuss your plans with an expert. Ideally, the program should be evaluated by an outside investigator, but few projects have funds available to hire an evaluation consultant for more than a few hours. These suggestions are offered to make evaluation more affordable:

- If you are able to contract an evaluation expert, do so during the design phase of the intervention. No matter how skilled a statistician the evaluator is, she or he will be unable to produce good answers from bad data.
- Try to establish relationships with local universities, colleges, or research organizations. These may provide lower-cost or in-kind technical assistance.
- Decide what your evaluation objectives are. What do you need to know and why? The evaluation should meet the needs of your project.
- Establish a database for formative and process evaluation data at the beginning of the project. In this way, resources are conserved as program management and evaluation activities merge.
- Never underestimate the power of information. Look at the data regularly. They are collected to inform and improve program implementation. Discuss any concerns with someone you trust who is experienced in your area.
- Recognize that needs assessment and evaluation form part of the same cycle. Time invested in careful

planning will conserve valuable resources now and in the future.

It is beyond the scope of this chapter to describe evaluation methods in more detail. Readers are encouraged to read the referenced resources for additional information. Evaluation is much more than an inconvenient requirement imposed by funding agencies. It is a critical component of successful injury prevention programs and a valuable prevention partner.

Challenges to Implementation

As many injury researchers search for new and innovative solutions to complex injury problems, we should not forget that, for some problems, we have effective solutions. Bicycle helmets work,[76] occupant restraints work,[77,78] regulating water heater temperature works,[79] modification of household and infant products works, child-resistant packaging works,[80] graduated licensing works,[81] and many other interventions and approaches work. Why then are there so many injuries from causes for which we have solutions? The answer is warehousing—not delivering the interventions to the population at risk. In some cases, we plan to deliver the intervention—the product leaves the warehouse—but it is not delivered intact or in time.

Implementation of effective injury prevention strategies may be our greatest challenge. No matter how well conceived and planned a program is, it will not be effective if it does not happen, if it is implemented inadequately, or the intervention time frame is too short. Prevention program planners with limited resources are advised to look at the literature (and Web sites listed in this chapter) and select proven interventions whose implementation is well documented. So many resources are wasted as the same mistakes are made again and again. When considering an intervention, the nurse who reads or hears about a similar program should not hesitate to contact the people running the program. A phone call or e-mail correspondence can yield valuable, practical information not readily available elsewhere.

Fractionation of effort is a major impediment to program implementation. Essentially it is as if we were to hire a team of people to build a house, each with responsibility for a different piece of the project but without any team planning or communication before, during, or after the project. If, in fact, this house were ever built, it is likely that it would be flawed, over budget, and behind schedule. It is not uncommon to find several groups or organizations within a community working on aspects of the same injury problem in isolation from each other. Institutional and organizational mandates, real or imagined traditional roles, and interagency politics may reinforce this fractionation. To optimize resource utilization and the chances for success, fractionation of effort must be challenged. Coalitions and collaborative initiatives are energizing prevention efforts in many areas of injury control. If well managed, coalitions can increase the visibility of the issue, funding opportunities, and the skill base of the participants. Readers interested in coalitions are encouraged to visit the Web site of the Prevention Institute, www.preventioninstitute.org, for more information on coalition building for injury control.

It is important that the trauma nurse be aware of several modifiable barriers to implementation of effective programs. These include the following:

1. Inadequate or absent evaluation
2. Overly broad problem definition
3. Incomplete problem diagnosis
4. Unrealistic goals
5. Poorly defined program objectives
6. Working in a vacuum
7. Turf wars
8. Planning and implementation gaps
9. Cruise control and tunnel vision
10. Burnout

Reference has been made to each of these previously. Of all 10 problem areas, the first one, *inadequate or absent evaluation,* is the most important. To understand why, the reader is encouraged to re-read problems 2 through 10 and ask whether *evaluation throughout the life of the program could have prevented, or reduced the severity of, this problem.* The answer to all nine is *yes.* Investing limited resources, energy, and expectations in poorly designed and implemented programs will lead to failure, frustration, and burnout. Even well-planned prevention efforts may take years to bear fruit, and they face numerous challenges along the way. Persistence and patience, combined with a continued sense of urgency, are notable attributes of successful preventionists. Get to know your opponents as well as your supporters. Start small and build your prevention skills; nothing breeds success like success.

Battling obstacles to effective prevention programs may be demoralizing at times but not nearly as demoralizing as watching again and again as young lives are lost to injuries that could have been prevented. Adopting a problem-solving approach to injury control does not guarantee program success, but it will assist readers to think about injury problems—and the trauma nurse's role in injury prevention—critically, systematically, and creatively.

References

1. Centers for Disease Control and Prevention, National Centers for Injury Prevention and Control: *Web-based injury statistics query and reporting system (WISQARS)* (2004): www.cdc.gov/ncipc/wisqars. Accessed March 13, 2007.
2. National Center for Health Statistics: *Deaths/mortality 2004* (preliminary data: http://www.cdc.gov/nchs/fastats/deaths.htm. Accessed March 13, 2007.
3. Centers for Disease Control and Prevention, National Center for Health Statistics: *Fact sheet: data on injuries*: http://www.cdc.gov/nchs/data/factsheets/injury.pdf. Accessed March 13, 2007.

4. Centers for Disease Control and Prevention, National Centers for Injury Prevention and Control: *10 Leading causes of death report, United States* 2004, all races, both sexes: www.cdc.gov/ncipc/wisqars. Accessed March 13, 2007.
5. Centers for Disease Control and Prevention, National Center for Health Statistics: 2003 Mortality data. *Natl Vital Stat Rep* 54:22, 2006. Available from http://www.cdc.gov/nchs/data/nvsr/nvsr54/nvsr54_13.pdf. Accessed March 13, 2007.
6. Centers for Disease Control and Prevention, National Centers for Injury Prevention and Control: *Years of potential life lost (YPLL) before age 75, United States* 2004, all races, both sexes, all deaths: www.cdc.gov/ncipc/wisqars. Accessed March 13, 2007.
7. Finkelstein EA, Corso PS, Miller TR: *Incidence and economic burden of injuries in the United States,* 2006, Oxford University Press, 2006. Data cited as part an Economic Cost of Injury Fact Sheet. Available from: http://www.cdc.gov/ncipc/factsheets/CostBook/Economic_Burden_of_Injury.htm. Accessed March 13, 2007.
8. http://www.census.gov/ipc/www/usinterimproj/natprojtab02a.pdf. Accessed March 13, 2007.
9. National Center for Injury Prevention and Control: *Working to prevent and control injury in the United States: fact book for the year 2000,* Atlanta, Centers for Disease Control and Prevention.
10. Mackenzie EJ, Fowler CJ: Epidemiology of injury. In Mattox KL, Feliciano DV, Moore EE, editors. *Trauma,* 5 ed, New York, 2004, McGraw-Hill.
11. http://www.amtrauma.org/injuryprevention/injuryprev.html. Accessed March 13, 2007.
12. Institute of Medicine: *The future of public health,* Washington, DC, 1988, National Academy Press.
13. Koop CE: Surgeon General's statement before the subcommittee on children, family, drugs, and alcoholism, U.S. Senate, February 9, 1989.
14. Institute of Medicine: *Reducing the burden of injury: advancing prevention and treatment,* Washington, DC, 1999, National Academy Press.
15. Guyer B: A problem solving paradigm for public health. In Armenian H, Shapiro S, editors: *Epidemiology and health services research,* New York, 1997, Oxford University Press.
16. Robertson LS: *Injuries: causes, control strategies, and public policy,* Lexington, MA, 1983, Lexington Books.
17. Gordon JE: The epidemiology of accidents, *Am J Public Health* 39:504-515, 1949.
18. Waller JA: Reflections on a half century of injury control, *Am J Public Health* 84(4):664-670, 1994.
19. Waller JA, Klein D: Society, energy, and injury—inevitable triad. In *Research directions towards the reduction of injury in the young and old,* DHEW Publication No. NIH 73-124, Bethesda, MD, 1973, National Institute of Child Health and Human Development.
20. Grossman DC: The history of injury control and the epidemiology of child and adolescent injuries, *Future Child* 10(1):23-52, 2000.
21. National Committee for Injury Prevention and Control: *Injury prevention: meeting the challenge,* New York, 1989, Oxord University Press.
22. World Health Organization: *Violence and injury prevention:* http://www.emro.who.int/vip. Accessed March 13, 2007.
23. Haddon W Jr: The changing approach to epidemiology, prevention, and amelioration of trauma: the transition to approaches etiologically rather than descriptively based, *Am J Public Health* 58:1431, 1968.
24. Langley J: The "accident-prone" child—the perpetration of a myth, *Aust Pediatr J* 18:243-246, 1982.
25. Stahre MA, Brewer RD, Naimi TS, et al. Alcohol-attributable deaths and years of potential life lost—United States, 2001, *MMWR Morbid Mortal Wkly Rep* 53(37):866-870, 2004.
26. Hamilton WJ: Mothers against drunk driving—MADD in the USA, *Inj Prev* 6:90-91, 2000.
27. Smith GS, Branas CC, Miller TR: Fatal nontraffic injuries involving alcohol: a metaanalysis. *Ann Emerg Med* 33(6):659-668, 1999.
28. Li G: Epidemiology of substance abuse among trauma patients, *Trauma Q* 14:353-364, 2000.
29. Clark DE, McCarthy E, Robinson E: Trauma as a symptom of alcoholism, *Ann Emerg Med* 14(3):274, 1985.
30. Rivara FP, Koepsell TD, Jurkovich GJ et al: The effects of alcohol abuse on readmission for trauma, *JAMA* 270(16):1962-1964, 1993.
31. Soderstrom CA, Smith GS, Dischinger PC et al: Psychoactive substance use disorders among seriously injured trauma center patients, *JAMA* 274:1043-1048, 1997.
32. Baker SP: Motor vehicle occupant deaths in young children, *Pediatrics* 64:860-861, 1979.
33. Winston FK, Durbin DD: Buckle up! is not enough: enhancing protection of the restrained child, *JAMA* 281(22):2070-2072, 1999.
34. National Highway Traffic Safety Administration: *Strengthening child safety laws* (DOT HS 810 728W) (2007): http://www.nhtsa.dot.gov/people/injury/TSFLaws/PDFs/810728W.pdf. Accessed March 13, 2007.
35. Office of the Governor [of Washington State]: *Locke signs bill to strengthen seat belt law for safety* (2000): http://access.wa.gov:80/news/article.asp?name=n0003195.htm. Accessed March 13, 2007.
36. National Highway Traffic Safety Administration: *State booster seat use requirements* (2007): http://www.nhtsa.dot.gov/people/injury/childps/BoosterSeatLaws_OverviewMaps07.pdf. Accessed March 13, 2007.
37. National Highway Traffic Safety Administration: DOT 24 06 (press release): http://www.nhtsa.dot.gov/portal/site/nhtsa/template.MAXIMIZE/menuitem.9f8c7d6359e0e9bbbf30811060008a0c/?javax.portlet.tpst=4670b93a0b088a006bc1d6b760008a0c_ws_MX&javax.portlet.prp_4670b93a0b088a006bc1d6b760008a0c_viewID=detail_view&javax.portlet.begCacheTok=com.vignette.cachetoken&javax.portlet.endCacheTok=com.vignette.cachetoken&itemID=87d1dee1f8879010VgnVCM1000002c567798RCRD&viewType=standard&overrideViewName=PressRelease&printable=true. Accessed March 16, 2007.
38. Gordis L: *Epidemiology,* Philadelphia, 1996, W. B. Saunders.
39. Institute of Medicine: *Reducing the burden of injury: advancing prevention and treatment,* Washington, DC, 1999, National Academy Press.
40. Sandels S: Young children in traffic, *Br J Educ Psych* 40:111-115, 1970.
41. Vinje MP: Children as pedestrians: abilities and limitations, *Accident Analysis Prev* 13(3):225-240, 1981.
42. Haddon W Jr: Advances in the epidemiology of injuries as a basis for public policy, *Public Health Rep* 95:411-421, 1980.
43. Baker SP, O'Neill B, Ginsburg MJ, et al: *The injury fact book,* 2nd edition, New York, 1992, Oxford University Press.
44. Haddon W Jr: The basic strategies for preventing damage from hazards of all kinds, *Hazard Prev* 16:8-12, 1980.

45. Committee on Trauma, American College of Surgeons: *Resources for optimal care of the injured patient,* Chicago, 2006, American College of Surgeons.
46. Albee GW: Psychopathology, prevention and the just society, *J Primary Prev* 4:5-40, 1983.
47. Shield J: Have we become so accustomed to being passive that we've forgotten how to be active, *Inj Prev* 3:243-244, 1997.
48. Gielen AC, Sleet DA, DiClemente RJ, editors: *Injury and violence prevention: behavioral science theories, methods, and applications,* San Francisco, 2006, Jossey-Bass.
49. Christoffel T, Gallagher SS: *Injury prevention and public health: practical knowledge, skills and strategies,* 2nd edition, New York, 2006, Jones & Bartlett.
50. Teret SP: Injury control and product liability, *J Public Health Policy* 2:49-57, 1981.
51. Teret SP: Litigating for the public's health, *Am J Public Health* 76:1027-1029, 1986.
52. Berger LR: Childhood injuries: recognition and prevention, *Curr Prob Pediatr* 12:24, 1981.
53. Christoffel T: The misuse of law as a barrier to injury prevention, *J Public Health Policy* 10:444, 1989.
54. McLoughlin E: The almost successful California experience: what we and others can learn from it. In Bergman AB, editor: *Political approaches to injury control at the state level,* pp 57-67, Seattle, 1992, University of Washington Press.
55. Trauma Foundation. *Channeling grief into policy change: survivor advocacy for injury prevention,* Injury Prevention Network Newsletter 13, San Francisco, 2000, San Francisco General Hospital.
56. Baker SP: Childhood injuries: the community approach to prevention, *J Public Health Policy* 2:235-246, 1981.
57. Cohen L, Swift S: The spectrum of prevention: developing a comprehensive approach to injury prevention. *Inj Prev* 5:203-207, 1999.
58. Prevention Institute. [Prevention] tools and frameworks: www.preventioninstitute.org/tools.html. Accessed March 16, 2007.
59. Committee on Injury and Poison Prevention: *Injury prevention and control for children and youth,* 3rd edition, Elk Grove Village, IL, 1997, American Academy of Pediatrics.
60. Doll LS, Bonzo SE, Mercy JA, et al, editors: *Handbook of injury and violence prevention,* 2007, Secaucus, NJ, Springer.
61. Liller KD, editor: *Injury prevention for children and adolescents: research, practice and advocacy,* 2006, Washington, DC, American Public Health Association.
62. Fowler CJ, Dannenberg AL: *The revised intervention decision matrix,* Baltimore, 1995 (rev 1998, 2000. 2003), Johns Hopkins Center for Injury Research and Policy.
63. Centers for Disease Control and Prevention: Notice to readers: warning on interaction between air bags and rear-facing child restraints, *MMWR Morb Mortal Wkly Rep* 42:280-282, 1993.
64. Robertson LS, Zador PL: Driver education and fatal crash involvement of teenaged drivers, *Am J Public Health* 68: 959-965, 1978.
65. Robertson LS: Crash involvement of teenaged drivers when driver education is eliminated from high school, *Am J Public Health* 70:599-603, 1980.
66. Preusser DF, Williams AF, Zador PL, et al: The effect of curfew laws on motor vehicle crashes, *Law Policy* 6:115-128, 1984.
67. American Academy of Pediatrics Committee on Sports Medicine and Fitness and Committee on Injury and Poison Prevention: Swimming programs for infants and toddlers (RE9940), *Pediatrics* 105(4):868-870, 2000.
68. Sleet DA, Gielen AC: Injury prevention. In Gorin SS, Arnold J, editors: *Health promotion handbook,* St. Louis, 1998, Mosby.
69. Dannenberg AL, Fowler CJ: Evaluation of interventions to prevent injuries: an overview, *Inj Prev* 4:141-147, 1998.
70. Thompson NJ, McClintock HO: *Demonstrating your program's worth: a primer on evaluation for programs to prevent unintentional injury,* Atlanta, 2000, National Center for Injury Prevention and Control.
71. Miller TR, Levy DT: Cost outcome analysis in injury prevention and control: a primer on methods, *Inj Prev* 3:288-293, 1997.
72. Patton MQ: *Utilization focused evaluation,* 3rd edition, Thousand Oaks, CA, 1997, SAGE Publications.
73. Teret SP: Postponing appointments: in praise of preventionists, *Johns Hopkins Public Health* Spring:5, 1999.
74. Gray JAM: *Evidence-based health care: how to make health policy and management decisions,* London, 1997, Churchill Livingstone.
75. Capwell EM, Butterfoss F, Francisco VT: Why evaluate? *Health Promotion Pract* 1:15-20, 2000.
76. Rivara FP, Thompson DC, Thompson RS et al: The Seattle children's bicycle helmet campaign: changes in helmet use and head injury admissions, *Pediatrics* 93:567-569, 1991.
77. Evans L: The effectiveness of safety belts in preventing fatalities, *Accident Anal Prev* 18:229-241, 1986.
78. National Highway Traffic Safety Administration: *The effect of a standard seat belt use law:* http://www.nhtsa.dot.gov/people/injury/airbags/seatbelt/effect.htm. Accessed March 16, 2007.
79. Erdmann TC, Feldman KW, Rivara FP, et al: Tap water burn prevention: the effect of legislation, *Pediatrics* 88:572-577, 1991.
80. Walton WW: An evaluation of the poison prevention packaging act, *Pediatrics* 69:363-370, 1982.
81. Foss RD, Evenson KR: Effectiveness of graduated driver licensing in reducing motor vehicle crashes, *Am J Prev Med* 16(1 Suppl):47-56, 1999.

7

PREHOSPITAL CARE OF THE TRAUMA PATIENT

Will Chapleau

Although prehospital care is not typically a nursing activity, two critical points make it an important component of this text and trauma nurse training programs. First, trauma nurses are often members of critical care transport teams both on traditional ground ambulance crews and on aero medical services. These critical care transport teams are most often involved in transferring patients from one facility to another but they can also be involved in direct field response. Second, it's important for trauma nurses to have knowledge of what care is performed during the prehospital phase of the trauma cycle. It is essential to ensure optimal communication between prehospital personnel and the in-hospital trauma team so that appropriate preparations can be made in advance of the patient's arrival. This chapter defines prehospital care, describes its components, and explains the connection between the prehospital and intrahospital operations in trauma care.

THE PREHOSPITAL CARE TEAM

Trauma directly affects approximately 60 million people per year in the United States. In 2003, 164,002 died of those injuries.[1] The significance of this problem has led to the development of specialized systems to respond to the injured, with the goal of decreasing mortality and morbidity. Teamwork is an essential determinant in the outcome of trauma care, for there are few individual successes and even fewer individual failures.[2] Each member of the team is dependent on the others.

Effective teamwork among health care providers must begin in the prehospital setting for the patient who has sustained injury to achieve optimal outcomes. "Prehospital" describes the phase when health care providers attend to the needs of patients outside the hospital. Other authors or texts may use the phrase "out of hospital" to describe the same subject.

Traumatic injury can generate chaos. This chaos may envelop all participants at the scene of the incident, including those injured, family members, and bystanders. There is a need to bring order to the situation. In many locations, dialing 911 is the method to access help from prehospital providers and public safety personnel for assistance in managing the situation.

ACCESS TO EMERGENCY MEDICAL SYSTEMS

The three-digit number 911 was set aside by Congress in the late 1960s to provide a simple method for accessing assistance from public safety personnel. Currently 911 systems exist in approximately two thirds of the United States. Calls to 911 are received by emergency dispatchers, who are trained in emergency medical dispatch or priority medical dispatch.[3] Many of these "trained" dispatchers have also completed emergency medical dispatch programs based on curriculum provided by the U.S. Department of Transportation (USDOT). Dispatchers are a critical component of the prehospital care team. A 911 communications center receives requests for help, determines the type of resources to deploy, and documents all activity related to a particular incident. The simplest 911 systems route calls to the appropriate central dispatch center. Enhanced 911 centers are able to display the address of the caller on monitors to speed the dispatch of assistance to the callers. By federal mandate, even cellular calls can provide location. Minimally, 911 calls will go to the 911 center servicing the area where the phone is located. The latest enhancements to this system can pinpoint the location of the caller to within a few feet. Internet-based phones initially presented a problem in that the location of the phone could not be determined at 911 centers. Here again, federal regulation has mandated that these phones report their location into the system as well. Some of the providers have come online, but Internet-based phone users should check with their 911 centers and service providers to determine whether the phone location can be retrieved.

Determining the most desirable use of prehospital resources—police, fire, paramedic unit, or air medical helicopter—is a complex process. Each prehospital system has protocols fine-tuned to the available resources for the area that guide the dispatcher's decision making. The dispatcher will solicit key initial information such as the type and location of the incident and the number of individuals involved.[4] This information will direct the dispatcher to activate the appropriate team members to facilitate the delivery of care and restore order to potentially life-changing situations. The dispatcher will also give prearrival instructions to the caller.

The types of available prehospital care resources vary from region to region. Contrary to public perception, in many parts of the United States prehospital care is provided by volunteer personnel. Some emergency medical systems (EMS) programs are fire based, whereas others are private or third-party service agencies. Currently in the United States there are about 891,000 EMS professionals transporting 16.2 million patients annually.[5] Department of Labor statistics for 2004 showed that 4 of 10 emergency medical technicians (EMTs) and paramedics work for private ambulance services, 3 of 10 work for local government agencies, and 2 of 10 are employed by hospital-based services.[6] Currently there are four levels of trained prehospital care providers in the United States: emergency medical responder (formally known as first responders), EMT, advanced emergency medical technician (AEMT) (formally known as EMT-Intermediate), and paramedic. Table 7-1 describes the training required and level of care that can be provided by each level prehospital provider.[7]

Other EMS team members include nurses trained to communicate with prehospital care providers over telemetry radio or cell phone. The training and recognition of these nurses varies from state to state, yet these professionals are educated to guide prehospital care providers through established treatment protocols. Although physicians are responsible for the medications and treatments in the protocols, nurses work together with prehospital personnel to evaluate patients' needs and choose the best treatment options.

Critical care transport specialists receive additional training to support the challenging needs of patients in critical condition requiring transport. These critically ill patients may require transport from the scene or transfer from one facility to another offering a higher level or specialty type of care. Flight nurses and flight paramedics receive specific training in air transport. Many flight programs use critical care transport training programs as the basic training level.

TABLE 7-1 Prehospital Care Providers: Required Training and Primary Role

Team Member	Training and Primary Role in Trauma Scene Response
Medical first responder	Trained first responders act as a bridge until transport-trained EMTs and/or paramedics arrive on the scene. Typically require 40 hours of training. Medical first responders may or may not be certified or licensed in the state in which they work.
Emergency medical technician (EMT)	Basic level of emergency responder trained to complete basic assessments, initiate oxygen therapy, and provide advanced first aid. 110 hours or more of training. Certified or licensed.
Advanced emergency medical technician (AEMT)	EMTs trained in additional ALS skills, such as insertion of IVs, intubation, or administration of a limited amount of specific medications. Up to 400 hours of training. Licensed or certified.
Paramedic	Advanced-level emergency responder trained to complete advanced assessments, initiate IV therapy, administer drugs, and institute airway management, including endotracheal intubation; practices as a physician extender; all practice directed by standing orders and protocols or by online physician order. More than 1,000 hours of training. Licensed or certified.
Emergency communications radio nurse (ECRN)	Specially trained RN who provides online consultation to prehospital personnel; participates in destination choices. Licensed provider.
Flight nurse	Specially trained RN with broad experience in emergency and critical care nursing. Routinely an expanded practice role. Provides patient care in a helicopter or fixed-wing aircraft. Performs advanced assessments and interventions including but not limited to endotracheal intubation, RSI intubation, central line placement, chest tube placement, and pharmacologic intervention. Practice directed by a physician medical director and authorized program-based protocols. Licensed provider.
Flight paramedic	Specially trained paramedic with broad experience in prehospital care and transport. Most flight nurses and flight paramedics receive the same flight-specific training. Many perform similar skills, including advanced assessments and intervention such as endotracheal intubation, RSI intubation, central line placement, and chest tube placement. Practice directed by a physician medical director and authorized program-based protocols. In some areas practice may be limited by state-defined paramedic scope of practice. Licensed in some states, certified in others.
Flight physician	Physician serving as an air medical team member. Level of experience varies from intern to well-seasoned, board-certified physician specialist. Licensed provider.
Medical director	Multifaceted role, varies system to system. Provides medical direction in policy and procedure formation and on-line advice to responding teams. Most agencies involved in prehospital response have assigned physicians for this role. Ensures quality care delivery.

ALS, Advanced life support; *RSI*, rapid sequence intubation.

INCIDENT COMMAND

In the early 1970s the incident command system (ICS) was adopted by fire and police services in the United States.[8] The purpose of the ICS was to formalize job descriptions of prehospital care providers and ensure effective, clear, concise communications between providers in mass casualty situations. The intention was to create a mechanism that brings order to chaos.

The ICS is a field management tool that is flexible enough to be exercised in a variety of incidents (e.g., a building fire or a roadside crash). It is organized around five major activities: command, operations, planning/intelligence, logistics, and finance/administration (Table 7-2). This system requires the designation of an incident commander (IC) who is responsible for all functions required at the response. The IC may choose to delegate authority to others during the incident; however, this does not relieve the IC from overall responsibility. The ICS incorporates the principle of unified command, which allows all agencies that have jurisdictional or functional responsibility (e.g., state-based highway patrol and a local fire agency responding to a multiple-vehicle crash on a state road) to jointly develop a common set of incident objectives and strategies. Unified command ensures that no single agency loses authority or accountability[9] (Figure 7-1).

The ICS provides more than organization; it is a common language used in emergency response systems. For some incidents, only a small number of the ICS elements may be necessary. If the incident enlarges, the ICS system has the capability to incorporate many more individuals to meet the needs of the incident. The objective is to have clear goals and job descriptions for all involved—a universal response to aid those who are injured.

THE NATIONAL INCIDENT MANAGEMENT SYSTEM

On February 28, 2003, President Bush issued a Homeland Security directive instructing the Secretary of Homeland Security to develop and administer a National Incident Management System (NIMS). The NIMS is a comprehensive, national approach to incident management designed to be applicable across a full spectrum of events regardless of size, complexity, or cause. This national system identifies common terminology, architecture, planning, interface, and training, ensuring that all participants in an incident know their roles and how their roles fit into the overall plan. The common terminology and language ensures that communications and resourcing are best supported. The NIMS was authorized on March 1, 2004, and all emergency management agencies were mandated to adopt the system. Further, enforcement of compliance was ensured by tying all federal emergency response grants to NIMS compliance. Any emergency responder should receive training in NIMS and any agency receiving federal grants will have to show NIMS compliance. NIMS activities are coordinated through the NIMS Integration Center available on the Federal Emergency Management Administration website.[10]

COMMUNICATIONS

Communication is the cornerstone to an effectively run prehospital response and it is essential for a successful EMS system.[11] Effective communication systems are all encompassing; they include information sharing with the public, EMS units, fire, police, air operations, and medical directors. The tools used for effective communication include mobile data terminals (MDT), two-way radios, cellular/digital/satellite phones, and pagers.

Radios are a mainstay of EMS communications. In this era of high technology, every agency and municipality involved in EMS response has internal and external radio communication capabilities. Like telephone numbers, radio frequencies are dedicated to certain agencies by the Federal Communications Commission and, unlike traditional phone lines, can be designated for specific activities. For example, a certain frequency may be designated as a tactical frequency, and all responders from agencies participating in an extrication will be directed to that frequency, but medical operations may use another frequency. Radio channels are divided into bands and frequencies. Table 7-3 outlines the available radio frequencies and the pros and cons associated with their use.

It is essential that people who are active in an EMS system have a clear understanding of the communications equipment available to them and the ability to troubleshoot technical and tactical challenges. Communication is the key element to the success of the EMS team and a critical tool in the safety of the operations. Communications can also be the weak link that precipitates failure.

TABLE 7-2 Incident Command System: Function Overview

Functions	Responsibilities
Command	Coordinates all activity; a command is present for all incidents
Operations	Directs activity (resources, machinery, personnel) required to meet incident goals
Planning/intelligence	Collects, evaluates, and displays incident information; maintains status of resources; prepares incident action plan and incident-related information
Logistics	Provides adequate services and support to meet needs of incident resources
Finance/administration	Tracks incident-related costs, including personnel and equipment

Modified from State of California, Office of Emergency Services: *Standardized emergency management system field course module 2—principles and features of ICS,* Sacramento,1995, Office of Emergency Services.

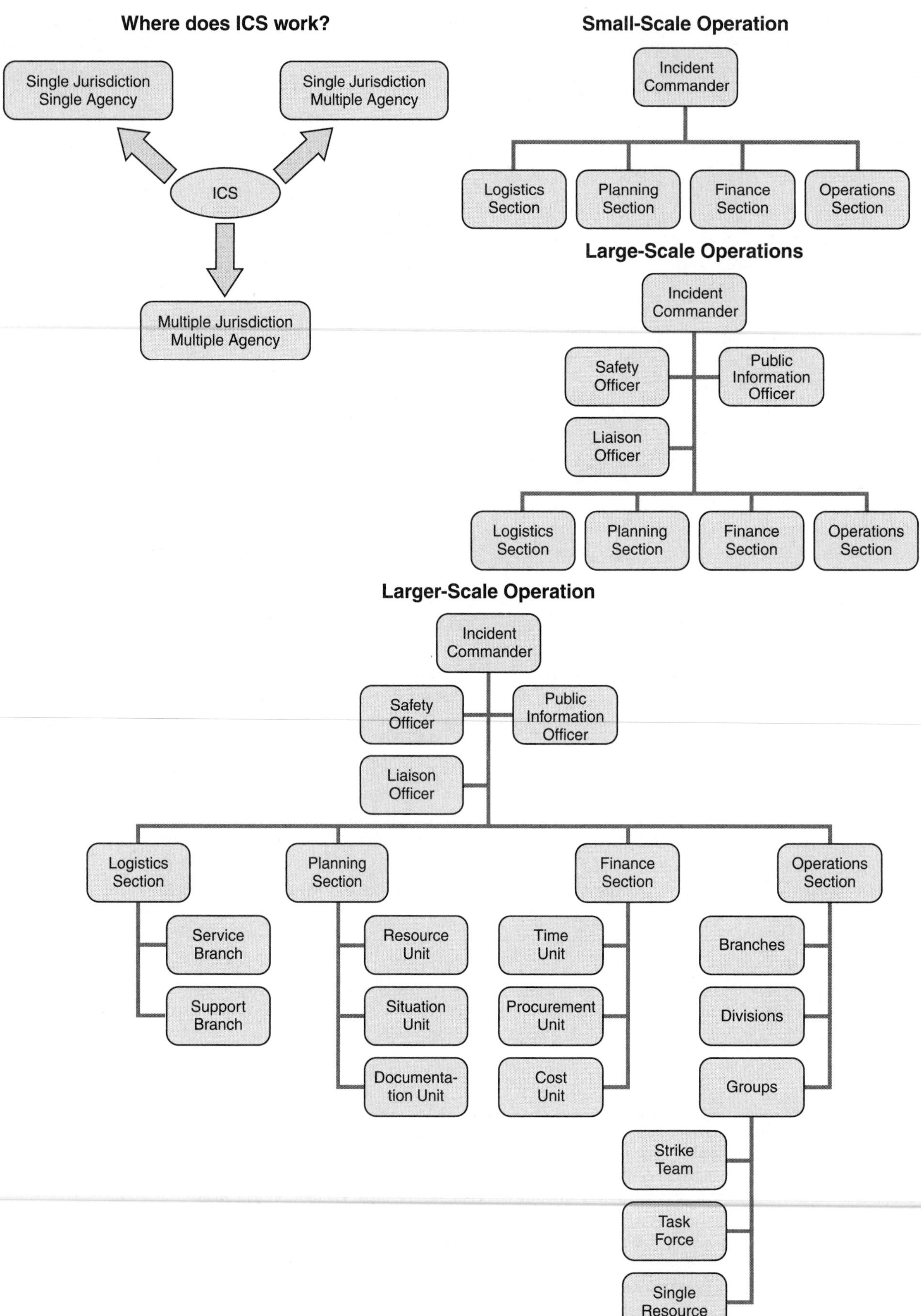

FIGURE 7-1 Where does ICS work? *(From Prehospital Trauma Life Support Committee of the National Association of Emergency Medical Technicians in Cooperation with the Committee on Trauma of the American College of Surgeons:* Prehospital trauma life support, *6th Edition, p 84, St. Louis, 2007, Mosby Elsevier.)*

TABLE 7-3 **Pros and Cons of Tools Used for Communication**

Communication Tool	Pros	Cons
Radio Channel Frequencies and Bands		
Very high frequency (VHF)	Long range	Often disrupted
VHF—low band	Effective in wide areas	Difficult to use in metropolitan areas
	Possible to transmit and receive on the same frequency	Commonly monitored by civilians
VHF—high band	Less easily disrupted	Difficult to transmit within structures
	Possible to transmit and receive on same frequency	Commonly monitored by civilians
	Usable in metropolitan areas	
	Covers large area	
	Cost-effective	
Ultra high frequency (UHF)	Least susceptible to interference	Cost increases because of repeaters and equipment required
	Possible to transmit and receive simultaneously	Commonly monitored by civilians
	Possible to add repeaters or relays to extend service area	
800 megahertz band	Suited for metropolitan use	Shorter range of service
	Possibility of sharing frequencies among agencies	Unable to transmit telemetry
	Can be integrated with computerized dispatch systems	Cost may increase because of equipment required
	Less commonly monitored by civilians	
Cellular/digital/satellite phones	Costs are decreasing	Unable to monitor multiple-agency transmission
	User-friendly	
	Allows one-on-one communication	Cannot be used for air-to-ground communications
	Option in some radio dead zones	Cell sites may be overwhelmed in a disaster
	Relatively private	
Mobile data terminals (MDT)	Allows readable, secure text information	Costly
	Recallable	Mandates close proximity to unit
Pagers	Cost-effective	One-way or two-way transmission of information
	User-friendly	

THE TRAUMA SCENE

The goal of prehospital response is to deliver high-quality care to the patient and maintain the safety of the responders. A specific incident triggers the prehospital provider response. For example, when a pedestrian is struck by a motor vehicle, many people react: the people directly involved, the bystanders, and those who stop to help. Someone at the scene of the incident initates the EMS response.

ACTIVATION OF THE EMS RESPONSE

The EMS response is usually initiated by a civilian who calls 911. The caller describes the incident to the EMS dispatcher. From the description of the incident, the dispatcher gleans many important facts: the number of victims, the exact location of the incident, the general age of the victim(s), and the mechanism of injury including the estimated kinetic energy involved (e.g., derived from the estimated speed of the vehicle). This information is relayed to the prehospital care provider team before their arrival at the scene so that they arrive with expectations regarding the types of injuries they may encounter.

The prehospital/EMS provider's response is activated by the dispatch service. Most EMS systems require that providers adhere to time limits (i.e., response time and time at the scene). Acceptable response times in urban and suburban settings range from 4 to 8 minutes (measured from the time dispatch takes the call until the arrival of the first responder), whereas response times in rural areas may be much longer. As a result of varying geography, population, roadways, and resources, acceptable response times will vary from area to area.

SAFETY AT THE SCENE

Regardless of the level of responder, the first arriving prehospital care provider assesses the scene for safety. A primary goal during all EMS response is to do no further harm to victims and to maintain the safety and well-being of all responders involved. Safety requires constant attention. Safe practices are one of the most critical components of an emergency response system's success because unsafe practices breed further injuries.

It is critical to eliminate the potential for additional injuries. The scene must be evaluated for fire sources, potential explosions, continued gunfire, "hot" electrical wires, unruly crowds, and other hazards. First responders alter traffic patterns to limit risk of further incident and call for additional resources as indicated. If the incident involves a vehicle, it must be determined whether the vehicle is secure. Is the vehicle at risk of rolling down an embankment? If the vehicle struck a tree, is that tree strong enough to serve as a brace? If the vehicle is not secure, it must be secured with cribbing (wood blocks or air bags) to ensure stability.

Hazardous materials (HAZMAT) (substances capable of posing unreasonable risk to health, safety, or property) present a significant threat to prehospital operations. The presence of HAZMAT can elevate an incident that affects one individual to a catastrophic event affecting an entire metropolitan area. It is the responsibility of the emergency response team to suspect HAZMAT when responding to incidents involving trucks, railcars, industrial buildings, or unmarked containers and to take appropriate precautions (Figure 7-2).

The approach to a HAZMAT scene is one of caution and investigation. Fire and other public safety personnel should enter the scene in a coordinated fashion. Responding teams should ascertain the name and chemical number of the material if possible. This information may be collected from the truck's "bill of lading" and material safety data sheet or perhaps other documents accompanying the driver. If this information is available, the prehospital care provider may obtain more information about the material from the USDOT or the Chemical Transportation Emergency Center (CHEMTREC).[12] CHEMTREC, a public service of the Chemical Manufacturers Association, supports a 24-hour telephone number (800-262-8200) allowing access to databases that assist in identifying hazardous zones and decontamination priorities. Another source for HAZMAT advice is the regional poison control center.

"Hazardous material" is not a misnomer. Such a substance can add more hazard and risk to the rescue, extrication, and transport of an injured individual. If the victim has had contact with a hazardous substance, a specific course of action is advocated (Table 7-4) to minimize the physiologic effects and to protect medical personnel in the prehospital and in-hospital phases of care. The objectives of scene safety are to keep the patient and crew safe and to complete the job at hand. Once the scene has been secured, patient care may begin.

Any professional working in prehospital care should have formal training regarding HAZMAT. This ensures that each responder can recognize scenes that have hazardous substances to prevent contamination of response personnel. There are multiple levels of HAZMAT training available, and the response objective of the prehospital personnel will determine the most appropriate level to complete.

Awareness training is the initial HAZMAT training level and all prehospital care providers should have this level of training. This level of training provides the knowledge necessary to prevent prehospital care providers from getting into scenes with HAZMAT and creating further exposures and injuries. The next level of training is the operations level, which is completed by providers who isolate the hazard. HAZMAT technicians are trained to the level of being able to attempt to stop or neutralize the release of the hazard. Finally, the highest level of HAZMAT training is the specialist level, in

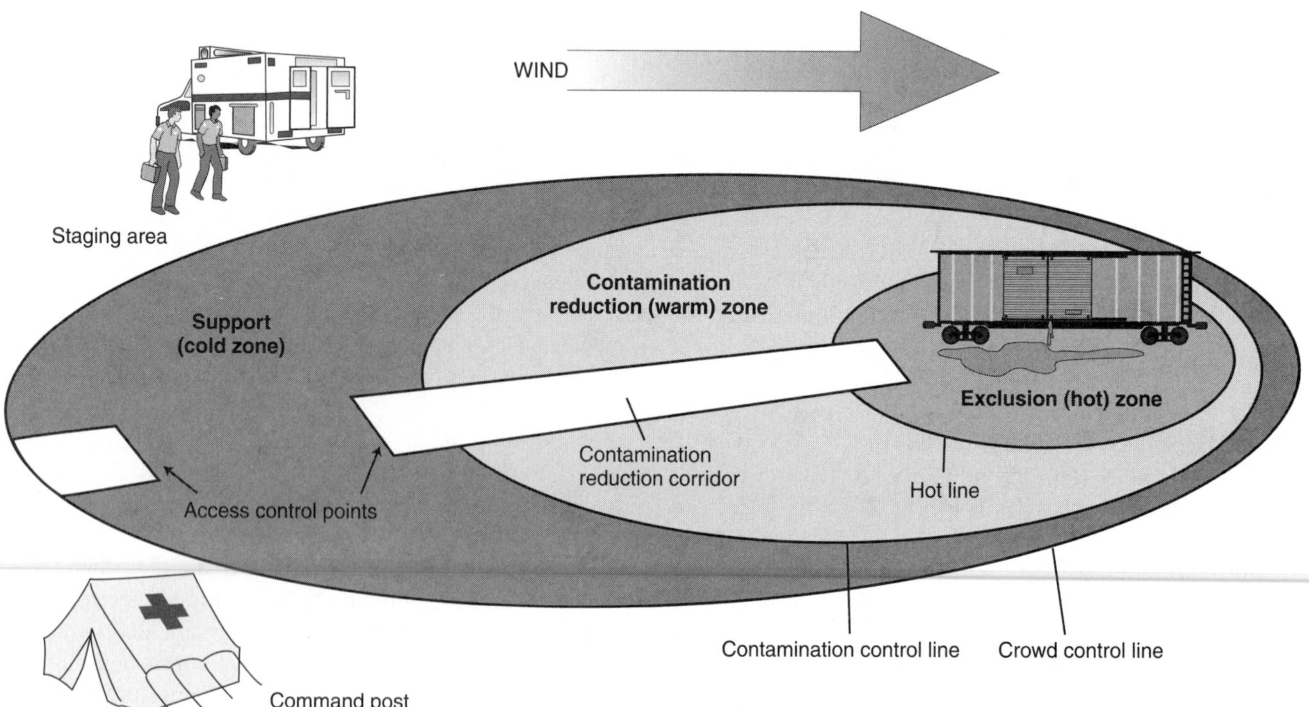

FIGURE 7-2 The scene of a WMD or HAZMAT incident is generally divided into hot, warm, and cold zones. *(From Chapleau W:* Emergency first responder, *p 351, St. Louis, 2007, Mosby.)*

TABLE 7-4 Interaction With Hazardous Materials

Set up safety zones for HAZMAT response as outlined in the incident command system guidelines.
Protect rescuers by applying nonporous personal protective clothing and goggles.
Move the victim to safe area upwind with fresh air.
Support the patient's ventilatory efforts; apply oxygen if indicated.
Initiate cardiopulmonary resuscitation if indicated; follow triage guidelines.
If toxic material contacts skin or eye, vigorously flush areas with water (contain runoff if possible).
Remove contaminated clothing and footwear.
Isolate contaminated items.

which training focuses on providing the skills for command and control of HAZMAT operations.

INITIAL CARE OF THE TRAUMA VICTIM

First responders are often police officers or fire/rescue personnel (EMTs) trained in basic life support (BLS); in some cases responders trained in advanced life support (ALS) (e.g., paramedics) are not part of the first responder team.[13] BLS care involves basic life-saving techniques. An ABC approach to assessing and caring for the patient is applied. Initially, the victim's airway must be assessed and opened with chin lift or jaw thrust. In trauma cases the jaw thrust is the maneuver of choice. The goal is to ensure airway patency while maintaining cervical spine immobility. Breathing is assessed and ventilatory assistance is provided if needed. Circulation is then assessed and cardiopulmonary resuscitation (CPR) and bleeding control are administered when necessary.

Paramedics are trained in more extensive patient evaluation techniques and are capable of performing advanced patient care procedures. Recent trends in paramedic education stress the importance of rapid assessment and the performance of only those interventions required to maintain survival en route to a trauma center. The "load and go" mantra of the 1960s has been revised to allow airway control, proper immobilization, and then rapid transport. Additional procedures such as placement of intravenous lines and splinting are done en route to the facility. Chapter 14, Initial Management of Traumatic Shock, has more information on resuscitation guided by evidence of improved outcomes.

EXTRICATION

Extrication is the removal of a trapped victim. A person may be pinned by an automobile, a motorcycle, a fallen object, or roadside obstructions—the possibilities are infinite. A basic principle of extrication is that a few designated prehospital care providers should remove the entrapped victim rather than having all providers enter the area of entrapment.[14] Although all activities are time critical, the safety of responders and the injured is paramount. Work zones are defined and access is restricted to the specialists in extrication. Medical personnel may be staged away from the victim to await delivery of the patient or until they are invited into the area when it is safe for them to approach.

Once the area in which the victims are trapped is determined to be safe to approach, the locations of the injured are determined. If any are in imminent danger, they are removed in the safest, most efficacious manner. The goal is to cause no further harm. All efforts are made to protect the victim's airway and spine during this extrication process.

Extrication becomes complicated when the patient cannot be removed by routine maneuvers. An example is an unrestrained driver involved in a head-on high-speed collision whose lower extremities are entangled in the pedals and flooring of the car. Removal of this traumatically injured person requires more than lifting: It requires specialized tools and expertise in extrication. Rescue specialists are trained to recognize and secure hazards, determine the nature of entrapment, and make use of available tools to effect extrication of the entrapped patient.

In most municipalities in the United States the experts in extrication are fire department personnel, with additional special rescue capabilities provided by law enforcement. Although equipment may vary, fire department personnel have expertise and training in extrication. As noted in earlier discussion, fire services should be a resource in all EMS plans. These services are often mobilized by the 911 dispatcher seconds after the call is received.

Rescue personnel assess the scene for safety and determine the techniques and tools required to accomplish removing the victim. Then the extrication process begins. The rescuers can access the victim through the vehicle's doors (if they are operable), by breaking glass and entering through window openings, or by using tools to cut or pry the vehicle apart. The extrication team will use the tools that most effectively and efficiently accomplish the job. The choice depends on the mechanism of injury, vehicle, and location. Different situations require different tools. Tools used in extrication are listed in Table 7-5.[15]

TABLE 7-5 Extrication Tools

Tool Type	Function
Hand tool	Any common hand tool such as a hammer or screwdriver
Portapower	Hand-driven hydraulic cylinder/hand-powered spreader and cutter
Sawzall	Hand saw that cuts through metal and glass
Torch	Cuts through rebar or other metal debris; mostly seen in building collapse situations
Saw	Cuts through sheet metal, wood, or other material
Spreader/ cutter	Pries open vehicle doors and hinges Cuts sheet metal and pillars
Ram	Pries open doors and peels back roofs

TREATMENT

Once access to the victims has been gained, the rescuers will rapidly triage them. As outlined in *Flight Nursing: Principles and Practices,* the care delivered should include the following[14]:

1. Establish an airway with cervical spine precautions.
2. Provide artificial ventilation with oxygenation. Oxygen use *may* be deferred if nearby petroleum-based products present the possibility of ignition or fire.
3. Control external hemorrhage.
4. Initiate CPR as indicated. (CPR may be ineffective, depending on patient position and location.)

PREHOSPITAL TRAUMA CARE: HOW MUCH AND WHEN?

The priorities of assessment and treatment are based on the ABCs—airway, breathing, and circulation.

AIRWAY

Evaluation of the airway begins with an assessment of patency. The provider looks at the chest movement, listens, and feels to determine whether the patient can move air through the passageway. If the answer is yes, the provider moves on to the next phase of evaluation. If the answer is no, immediate further evaluation and intervention are warranted.

When airway patency is in question, the jaw thrust is the initial maneuver used in an attempt to quickly open the airway. Airway adjuncts such as nasopharyngeal or endotracheal tubes may be needed to support airway integrity (Table 7-6). Intervention will be dictated by the ability to maintain airway patency, protocols for airway management, and the level of skill the prehospital provider has in use of artificial airways.[16]

Burn patients have great potential for development of complete airway obstruction.[17] This obstruction is caused by inflammation of airway tissue from exposure to steam heat, inhaled gas, or fire. As resuscitation fluids are administered, the risk for airway edema and obstruction increases. The prehospital care provider must assess the burn patient's airway carefully. This evaluation should include but not be limited to assessing for the presence of carbonaceous sputum, a reddened or enlarged tongue, hoarseness of voice, difficulty swallowing, and a "tightening throat" as described by the patient. All these symptoms are indications of airway edema and, if they are not managed early, could result in complete airway obstruction. Early endotracheal intubation is recommended for the severely burned and for patients with burns involving their airways or the circumference of the neck or chest.

Most trauma patients are suspect for spinal injury and should be treated accordingly. This treatment includes maintaining in-line stabilization of the cervical spine and placing the victim on a long backboard with a stiff cervical collar and adequate strapping.[13] If further airway intervention is required, consistent alignment of the cervical spine must be maintained. Recommended airway interventions may include nasotracheal intubation in the absence of maxillofacial trauma because of the reduced neck movement with this procedure. In many areas of the United States, rapid-sequence intubation (RSI) is the airway intervention of choice for cervical spine–injured patients.[18] Actual or potential spinal cord injury directs many of the airway choices of the prehospital provider.

In most incident responses ALS providers are secondary responders and will receive the patient from firefighters, EMTs, or other BLS providers. The paramedics begin their care by confirming the primary survey. The objective of the

TABLE 7-6 **Airway Adjuncts**

Adjunct	Uses	Contraindications/Risks
Suctioning	Removes debris or blood from the upper respiratory tract	
Nasopharyngeal airway	Maintains open nasopharyngeal airway in a stuporous or comatose patient	Head/facial trauma particularly if presence of a basilar skull fracture is suspected; risk for placement into the brain with basilar skull fracture
Oropharyngeal airway	Prevents tongue from obstructing airway; used only in unconscious patients	Placement may be difficult or impossible if patient's jaw is clenched; may induce gagging and vomiting
Laryngeal mask airway	Provides unsecured airway; easy to position for placement; limited use in prehospital setting at present; used only with unconscious patients	May cause aspiration
Endotracheal intubation	Provides secure airway, avenue for artificial ventilation; high degree of skill required for placement	Risk for esophageal intubation
Rapid sequence intubation	Delivery of sedative and paralytic agents to facilitate orotracheal intubation	Failure of intubation; removal of patient's ventilatory drive
Needle cricothyroidotomy	Short-term, rapid airway security; high training competency requirements for placement	Penetration of the airway; difficult to find landmarks in bloody or edematous patients
Surgical cricothyroidotomy	Used in emergency situations when endotracheal intubation cannot be performed	High training requirements for placement

primary survey is to identify any life-threatening issues and address them immediately.

Initially, unless contraindicated, less-invasive airway adjuncts (oropharyngeal or nasopharyngeal) may be tried to maintain airway patency in the patient unable to do so spontaneously. Additionally, the use of the laryngeal mask airway, which has been widely used in Europe for years, is an option when intubation is not possible. Keep in mind when using any of these adjuncts that they do not offer the protection against aspiration that intubation affords.[14] If these prove unsuccessful, endotracheal intubation may or may not be an option. The presence of trismus precludes direct laryngoscopy. In most states the paramedic scope of practice does not include the use of sedatives or neuromuscular blocking agents to facilitate intubation. If intubation is impossible or unsuccessful, bag-valve-mask ventilation is the only option available.

In states where paramedic care does include paralytic and sedative administration or where air medical services include nurse or physician team members, RSI may be used to accomplish definitive airway control. RSI has become the standard of care in air medical prehospital practice to secure airway control for severely injured patients.[19,20] RSI is the consecutive administration of a sedative and a neuromuscular blocking agent to induce paralysis and unconsciousness for the purpose of fostering laryngoscopy followed by endotracheal intubation.[21] A sample RSI protocol is presented in Box 7-1 and drugs commonly used to assist with intubation are listed in Table 7-7. Prehospital providers ensure that an intravenous line is established to allow drug administration so that the RSI process can begin. In most scenarios a cardiac monitor with pulse oximetry is applied. Within minutes, the RSI agents are administered and the airway secured. Recent review of the literature on prehospital intubation has called into question this practice. At the very least, care should be taken to ensure that ventilation is provided regardless of whether intubation is accomplished, and prehospital care providers should be aware of the effects of delays in transport.[22]

At times, intubation is not possible. This may be due to patient condition, position, or anatomy. However, the critical need for airway stabilization remains. Advanced providers in some EMS systems and most air medical crews would proceed to more advanced interventions. These advanced airway adjuncts include insertion of a needle cricothyroidotomy or a surgical cricothyroidotomy.

BREATHING

Evaluation of the patient's breathing includes: assessment of his or her responsiveness, respiratory rate, chest excursion, chest symmetry, skin color, and oxygen saturation levels. Not all prehospital care providers have access to pulse oximeters as an assessment tool.

Once an initial assessment has been completed, oxygen is administered. As outlined earlier, the environment must be evaluated and all risks associated with oxygen administration must be ruled out before its application. In most trauma cases high-flow oxygen delivered by a nonrebreather mask is administered. In patients with insufficient ventilation, bag-valve-mask ventilation or intubation to allow mechanical ventilation may be necessary to enable adequate oxygen delivery to the alveoli.

Research has demonstrated that hyperventilation can cause cerebral ischemia in patients with severe traumatic brain injury and significant hypoxia in animals subjected to hemorrhagic hypovolemia, which could influence poor outcomes from resuscitation. Studies have shown the importance of ventilating patients in the range of 12 to 20 breaths per minute to ensure adequate respiratory gas exchange and prevention of hypoxia.[23] In the field, where ventilators are usually not available, the rate of manual ventilation can often be driven by caffeine or epinephrine rather than the patient's need. In the past, providers might have assumed "more is better" and that breathing faster might help and certainly could not harm. As stated, research has suggested quite the opposite. Hyperventilation may contribute to hypoxia. In a study by Pepe et al.,[23] eight swine were ventilated by using a fractional concentration of oxygen in inspired gas (FIO_2) of 0.28 with a tidal volume of 12 ml/kg at a rate of 12 breaths per minute and hemorrhaged to a systolic blood pressure (SBP) of less than 65 mm Hg. Respiratory rates were then changed every 10 minutes to 6, 20, 30, and then back to 6. At 6 breaths per minute, the pH was greater than 7.25, and the oxygen saturation in arterial blood was greater than 99%. The mean SBP increased from 65 to 84 mm Hg. The time-averaged coronary perfusion pressure increased from 50 to 60 mm Hg, and the cardiac output increased from 2.4 to 2.8 L/min. At 20 and 30 breaths per minute, the SBP decreased to 73 and 66 mm Hg, respectively, coronary perfusion pressure decreased to 47 and 42 mm Hg, respectively, cardiac output decreased to 2.5 and 2.4 mm Hg, respectively, and the partial arterial oxygen tension and the partial pressure of carbon dioxide in arterial blood decreased (less than 30 mm Hg) ($P < .05$). When the rate was returned to 6 breaths per minute, the measurements recovered. It is suggested that hyperventilation causes increased intrathoracic pressure, created by "air trapping" or "auto-PEEP" (positive end-expiratory pressure), which impedes venous return to the heart in the same manner as a tension pneumothorax.[23] In the presence of hypovolemia, hyperventilation can have adverse effects on hemodynamic status and respiratory gas exchange.

Alteration in breathing and ineffective oxygen delivery may be caused by a loss of chest wall or pleural space integrity as a result of thoracic injury. Chapter 24 provides a more extensive discussion about thoracic injuries. Chest wall or pleural space injuries may require some prehospital intervention, such as needle thoracostomy or chest tube placement.

Tension pneumothorax occurs when thoracic trauma allows air to enter the pleural space but provides no escape,

BOX 7-1 Sample Protocol for Rapid-Sequence Intubation

1. Ensure availability of required equipment.
   a. Oxygen supply
   b. Bag-valve-mask of appropriate size and type
   c. Nonrebreathing mask
   d. Laryngoscope with blades
   e. Endotracheal tubes
   f. Surgical and alternative airway equipment
   g. RSI medications
   h. Materials or devices to secure endotracheal tube after placement
   i. Suction equipment
2. Ensure that at least one (but preferably two) patent intravenous line is present.
3. Preoxygenate the patient with a nonrebreathing mask or bag-valve-mask with 100% oxygen. Preoxygenation for 3 to 4 minutes is preferred.
4. Apply cardiac and pulse oximetry monitors.
5. If the patient is conscious, strongly consider the use of sedative agents.
6. Consider the administration of sedative agents and lidocaine in the presence of potential or confirmed traumatic brain injury.
7. After administration of paralytic agents, use the Sellick (cricoid pressure) maneuver to decrease the potential for aspiration.
8. Confirm tube placement immediately after intubation. Continuous cardiac and pulse oximeter monitoring is required during and after RSI. Reconfirm tube placement periodically throughout transport and each time the patient is moved.
9. Use repeat doses of paralytic agents as needed to maintain paralysis.

Procedure

1. Assemble the required equipment.
2. Ensure the patency of the intravenous lines.
3. Preoxygenate the patient with 100% oxygen for approximately 3 to 4 minutes if possible.
4. Place the patient on cardiac and pulse oximeter monitors.
5. Administer a sedative, such as midazolam, if appropriate.
6. In the presence of confirmed or potential TBI, administer lidocaine (1.5 mg/kg) 2 to 3 minutes before administration of a paralytic agent.
7. For pediatric patients, administer atropine (0.01-0.02 mg/kg) 1 to 3 minutes before administration of paralytic agent to minimize the vagal response to intubation.
8. Administer a short-acting paralytic agent intravenously, such as succinylcholine. Paralysis and relaxation should occur within 30 seconds.
   a. Adult: 1 to 2 mg/kg
   b. Pediatric: 1 to 2 mg/kg
9. Insert an endotracheal tube. If initial attempts are unsuccessful, precede repeat attempts with preoxygenation.
10. Confirm endotracheal tube placement.
11. If repeated attempts to achieve endotracheal intubation fail, consider placement of an alternative or surgical airway.
12. Use dose of long-acting paralytic agent, such as vecuronium, to continue paralysis.
    a. Initial dose: 0.1 mg/kg IV push
    b. Subsequent doses: 0.01 mg/kg every 30 to 45 minutes

Note: Requirements vary with individual patients.
From Prehospital Trauma Life Support Committee of the National Association of Emergency Medical Technicians in Cooperation with the Committee on Trauma of the American College of Surgeons: *Prehospital trauma life support,* 6th edition, p 130, St. Louis, 2007, Mosby Elsevier.)

creating increasing pressure within the thorax. This injury may be caused by blunt or penetrating mechanisms of injury. Signs and symptoms of a tension pneumothorax include respiratory distress, tracheal deviation away from the affected side, neck vein distention (if patient is euvolemic), absent or decreased breath sounds on the affected side, hyperresonance to percussion, and shock. A diagnostic and interventional maneuver for tension pneumothorax is needle decompression (needle thoracostomy).[24] A 14- or 16-gauge angiocatheter (2½ inches or greater) or a long spinal needle is placed at the second or third intercostal space at the midclavicular line on the affected side. When a tension pneumothorax is present, as the needle enters the pleural space a rush of air, ease in ventilatory pressure, and/or a rise in blood pressure may be noted. Each of these occurrences indicates a release of pressure from the pleural space, which enables more effective gas exchange.

Chest tube insertion in the prehospital setting has been a topic of discussion for many years. Debate continues as to whether chest tubes should be placed in the field.[25,26] In some areas of the country prehospital chest tube insertion is performed by specially trained transport teams, which in most cases include nurses or physicians.

TABLE 7-7 **Common Drugs Used for Pharmacologically Assisted Intubation**

Drug	Dose (Adult)	Dose (Pediatric)	Indications	Complications/Side Effects
Pretreatment				
Oxygen	High flow Assist ventilation as needed to achieve oxygen saturation of 100% if possible	High flow Assist ventilation as needed to achieve oxygen saturation of 100% if possible	All patients undergoing pharmacologically assisted intubation	—
Lidocaine	1.5 mg/kg	1.5 mg/kg IV	Brain injury	Seizure
Atropine	—	0.01-0.02 mg/kg IV	Pediatric intubation, prevention of bradycardia and excess secretions	Tachycardia
Induction of Sedation				
Midazolam (Versed)	0.1-0.15 mg/kg up to 0.3 mg/kg IV	0.1-0.15 mg/kg up to 0.3 mg/kg IV	Sedation	Respiratory depression/apnea, hypotension
Fentanyl (Sublimaze)	2-3 mcg/kg IV	1-3 mcg/kg IV	Sedation	Respiratory depression/apnea, hypotension, bradycardia
Etomidate	0.2-0.3 mg/kg IV	Not approved for patients <10 years of age	Sedation, induced anesthesia	Apnea, hypotension, vomiting
Chemical Paralysis				
Succinylcholine	1-2 mg/kg	1-2 mg/kg	Muscle relaxation and paralysis (short duration)	Hyperkalemia, muscle fasciculations
Vecuronium	0.1 mg/kg	0.1 mg/kg	Muscle relaxation and paralysis (intermediate duration)	Hypotension
Pancuronium (Pavulon)	0.04-0.1 mg/kg	0.04-0.1 mg/kg	Muscle relaxation and paralysis (long duration)	Tachycardia, hypertension, salivation

From Prehospital Trauma Life Committee of the National Association of Emergency Medical Technicians in cooperation with the Committee on Trauma of the American College of Surgeons. *PHTLS: Prehospital trauma life support,* ed 6 St. Louis, 2007, Mosby.

Another significant thoracic injury that requires prehospital intervention is the open pneumothorax, or sucking chest wound. An open pneumothorax allows communication of outside atmospheric pressure with pleural space pressure. Signs and symptoms of an open pneumothorax include respiratory distress, subcutaneous air and decreased or absent breath sounds on the affected side, tracheal deviation, and hemodynamic decompensation.[27] Prehospital interventions for a patient with an open pneumothorax include airway management, oxygen administration, application of a three-sided dressing, and possibly insertion of a chest tube. All these interventions must be performed rapidly and can be accomplished during transport to the receiving center.

CIRCULATION

Prehospital evaluation of circulation is accomplished by assessing the patient's level of consciousness, the presence or absence of gross bleeding, skin color, capillary refill, pulse (rate and quality), blood pressure, and cardiac monitor tracing.

Initial intervention includes application of direct pressure to areas of active bleeding. Once bleeding is slowed, initiation of volume replacement is a priority. Intravenous access with multiple large-bore catheters should be accomplished as long as obtaining access does not slow transport. Over the past few years the emphasis for fluid resuscitation has been on administering fluid in a manner that supports circulation without disrupting blood clots or washing away the red blood cells. Current protocols for managing uncontrolled hemorrhage in the field call for infusing intravenous crystalloid solutions to maintain systolic blood pressure in the 80 to 90 mm Hg range or a mean arterial pressure of 60 to 65 mm Hg. In the case of controlled hemorrhage in the adult patient in class II, III, or IV shock, when there is no suspicion of internal uncontrolled bleeding, 1 to 2 L of warm crystalloid solution can be infused. In the pediatric population advanced trauma life support guidelines direct prehospital administration of 20 ml/kg as a fluid bolus.[13] These changes in prehospital fluid resuscitation have come about as a result of research that has challenged the practice of early rapid administration of crystalloids by demonstrating worse outcomes in victims of penetrating trauma who received early prehospital fluid resuscitation compared with similar patients who did not receive aggressive fluid resuscitation in the prehospital phase.[28,29]

After airway, breathing, and circulation have been established, the prehospital care provider evaluates the patient for other injuries that may compromise life or limb. The team begins the secondary survey, which is a head-to-toe assessment of the patient. The objective of the secondary survey is to identify all potentially life-threatening or complicating factors. The secondary survey is often done during transport to the receiving hospital. At times this survey may not be completed before arrival and should not delay transport.

Traumatic Brain Injury

Annually approximately 1.6 million people experience traumatic brain injury (TBI).[30] The impact of these injuries is significant to both the individual and society. It is critical to initiate appropriate care for the patient with TBI as soon after the injury as possible. The Brain Trauma Foundation describes prehospital care as "the first critical link in providing appropriate care for individuals with severe brain injury."[30]

It has been established that episodes of hypoxemia and hypotension in the prehospital setting are commonly associated with poor outcomes from TBI.[30] Focusing on adequate oxygenation and hemodynamic stability in the field is critical for these patients. In its recent publication, *Guidelines for Prehospital Management of Traumatic Brain Injury,* the Brain Trauma Foundation recommends the following[30]:

- All patients should have blood pressure and oxygenation reassessed as frequently as possible and continuously, if possible.
- Adult or pediatric patients with Glasgow Coma Scale (GCS) score less than 9, unable to maintain a sufficient airway or hypoxemic despite administration of supplemental oxygen, should have an airway established by the most appropriate means available.
- Routine use of paralytics to assist in endotracheal intubation is not recommended in adult patients transported by ground in an urban setting who are spontaneously breathing and maintaining oxygen saturation above 90% on supplemental oxygen.
- If endotracheal intubation is performed, tube placement should be confirmed by end-tidal CO_2 ($ETCO_2$) determination and lung auscultation.
- Once an airway is established, normal breathing rates should be maintained ($ETCO_2$ 35 to 40 mm Hg) and hyperventilation (ETCO2 less than 35 mm Hg) should be avoided. However, hyperventilation may be used as a temporizing measure to treat adult or pediatric patients with evidence of cerebral herniation or acute neurologic deterioration. Utilize hyperventilation (20 breaths/min for adults, 25 breaths/min for a child, 30 breaths/min for an infant younger than 1 year) with the goal of maintaining an $ETCO_2$ of 30 to 35 mm Hg and discontinue when signs of herniation are alleviated.
- All patients with suspected TBI should have their oxygen saturations maintained at greater than 90%.
- Systolic blood pressure should be monitored and maintained at greater than 90 mm Hg in adults and those pediatric patients older than 10 years, greater than 70 mm Hg + 2 times age in years for those ages 1 to 10, greater than 70 mm Hg for those ages 1 to 12 months, and greater than 60 mm Hg for infants 0 to 28 days old.
- Isotonic fluids should be used to treat hypotension in patients with TBI. In adult patients with GCS score less than 8, hypertonic fluids may be used as a treatment option for resuscitation.

Rapid recognition and correction of airway, breathing, and circulation compromise and transport to a definitive care facility are essential for the brain-injured patient to have the greatest chance for optimal recovery.

Orthopedic Injuries

Orthopedic injuries are not the primary focus of the prehospital caregiver. Once the primary assessment and interventions are completed, the focus is on moving the patient to the most appropriate trauma receiving center. Although pelvic injuries and femur fractures constitute life-threatening injuries that will receive attention in the primary survey, most orthopedic injuries will be addressed in the secondary survey.

Extremities may be epvaluated while en route to the trauma center. If extremities have obvious fractures, pulses are evaluated serially. If pulses are present, extremities are splinted in the position they are found. If no pulses are present, the extremity is positioned anatomically and the pulses reassessed. The presence or absence of the pulse will dictate further intervention. The goal of all prehospital care related to orthopedic injuries is to preserve circulation and neurovascular integrity and do no further harm. Adjuncts available to aid the prehospital provider in caring for orthopedic injuries are described in Table 7-8.

Transport of the Trauma Patient

Transport Modalities

Once safe access to the injured patient has been accomplished, the focus of the team is on delivery of the injured to the appropriate receiving center. How is the patient to be

TABLE 7-8 **Orthopedic Adjuncts**

Device	Indication	Comments
Splint	Maintain placement Decrease pain	Wide variety available (e.g., cardboard, metal, pneumatic and plastic)
Traction	Splints apply traction to reinstate positioning for adequate blood flow	Include Hare traction and Sager splints
Pneumatic trousers	Pelvic fracture Provide tamponade effect	Rapid removal in hospital may result in severe drop in blood pressure

transported? The options are by ground, by air, or by water. Factors to consider include the following:

- The number of patients
- Condition and acuity level of the patients, type of injuries
- The care required of the patients en route
- The scope of practice of the transporting prehospital care providers
- Potential patient difficulties (e.g., airway management in a combative child)
- Available modes for patient transportation and ability for these transport vehicles to access the patient
- Weather conditions
- Time of day and traffic patterns
- Trauma plan and protocols of the municipality
- Location of the nearest appropriate trauma center
- Other available resources

The ground options include transport by a BLS ambulance and crew or transport by an ALS ambulance and crew. In most areas of the country, the BLS crew's scope of practice allows delivery of first aid and administration of oxygen and CPR during transport. BLS providers can also place nasal and oropharyngeal airways and apply and maintain splints. If the patient requires any advanced intervention, including intubation or intravenous fluid administration, an ALS scope of practice is required and the patient should be transported by an ALS ambulance and crew.

If the incident has required activation of an air ambulance, whether because of the number of patients, the location of the patient, or the acuity of care required, it is important to note the reason. Helicopters and crews have diverse capabilities and skills depending on classification and training.

The widespread availability of air transport with highly trained medical team members gives many EMS responders an important tool in the care of the trauma patient. Like any intervention, air transport has inherent risks and benefits and should be used appropriately. In many areas of the country, a medical helicopter is activated by paramedics or first responders based on pre-established launch criteria; therefore, the vehicle and advanced medical team members are available soon after the arrival of paramedics and secondary responders. If it is determined that the helicopter and its team are not needed at the scene, the request can be canceled. Air medical transport should be considered for critically injured patients in situations that require prolonged extrication, extended ground transport to the appropriate trauma center, or protracted manual transport out of a remote area.[31] The National Association of Emergency Medical Services Physicians developed guidelines to promote effective and consistent use of air medical services (Table 7-9).

When air medical resources are used, one of the most significant considerations is the ability to land the aircraft near enough to the patient to allow rapid and uncomplicated access but distant enough to prevent the patient and caregivers from being affected by the noise and rotor wash of the helicopter. When an air medical helicopter is landed at an injury scene, there are many things to consider in preparing the landing zone (LZ). General guidelines for selecting an LZ are described below; however, it is important to confirm these with local operators before initiating practices. Select a landing site that is at least twice the overall length and width of the aircraft, with a firm level surface, usually 75 feet by 75 feet. The slope of the ground should be less than 10 to 15 degrees to prohibit anyone from walking uphill into a spinning blade and to avert rotor blades from dipping and making contact with the ground. An LZ must also have approach and departure paths that are clear of obstructions (wires, trees, towers, etc.) and that allow flight into the wind. Finally, the LZ must have a coordinator, someone with the ability to immediately communicate to the pilot and crew regarding pertinent issues.

Each area of the United States has a different method of determining how air providers are classified and how the scope of practice is defined. For example, in California air medical providers are defined under Title 22 of the state Code of Regulation.[32] In this document a rescue helicopter is defined as "an aircraft whose usual function is not prehospital emergency patient transport but may be utilized, in compliance with local EMS policy, for prehospital emergency patient transport." An air ambulance is described as "any aircraft specially constructed, modified or equipped and used for the primary purpose of responding to emergency calls and transporting critically ill or injured patients whose medical flight crew has at a minimum two attendants certified or licensed in advanced life support." The state of California has additional classifications: ALS rescue aircraft, BLS aircraft, and auxiliary rescue aircraft. These types of aircraft carry different crews who meet specific requirements and have specific medical care capabilities. In this chapter air medical transport is discussed by using the Commission of Accreditation of Medical Transport Systems requirements that define the scope of care and type of caregiver.[33]

In situations where air medical transport is used, the entire team participates in preparing the patient for transport. Injured patients are transported on a long backboard with a cervical collar in place. The patient is secured with safety belts to prohibit movement and maintain stability in flight or during ground transport. In all transport situations everyone involved has a specific responsibility, which keeps things running smoothly and precludes oversight of critical activities. In most air transport team role delineations, one individual is responsible for the essential role of patient airway management. The same crew member responsible for maintaining the airway directs movement to be sure that any artificial airway (e.g., endotracheal tube) is not dislodged. In helicopter operations, one crew member is specifically responsible for directing others' activity around the aircraft to ensure safety and to limit confusion during loading or off-loading.

Operational safety is a vital focus in all air medical activities. The most critical phases of flight are takeoff and landing. During these times the entire crew focuses their attention

TABLE 7-9 Clinical Indicators and Operational Situations in Which Air Medical Transport Should Be Considered

I. Specific clinical indicators
  a. Spinal cord or spinal column injury
  b. Partial or total amputation of an extremity (excluding digits)
  c. Two or more long bone fractures or a major pelvic fracture
  d. Crushing injuries to the trunk or head
  e. Major burns
  f. Patients younger than age 12 or older than age 55 years
  g. Patients with near-drowning injuries, with or without existing hypothermia
  h. Adult patients with any of the following vital sign abnormalities:
    1. Systolic blood pressure less than 90 mm Hg
    2. Respiratory rate less than 10 or greater than 35 breaths/min
    3. Heart rate less than 60 or greater than 120 beats/min
  i. Patient unresponsive to verbal stimuli
  j. Any head injury producing lateralizing signs
II. Operational situations
  a. Mechanism of injury
    1. Vehicle rollover with unbelted passengers
    2. Vehicle striking pedestrian at more than10 mph
    3. Falls from more than 15 feet
    4. Motorcycle victim ejected at more than 20 mph
    5. Multiple victims
  b. Difficult access situations
    1. Wilderness rescue
    2. Ambulance access or exit impeded at the scene by road conditions, weather, or traffic
  c. Time and distance factors
    1. Transportation time to the trauma center more than 15 minutes by ground ambulance
    2. Transport time to local hospital by ground longer than transport time to trauma center by helicopter
    3. Patient extrication time more than 20 minutes
    4. Use of local ground ambulance leaves local community without ground ambulance coverage

Modified from National Association of Emergency Medical Services Physicians: Air medical dispatch: guidelines for scene response, *Prehosp Disaster Med* 7:75-78, 1992.

outside the aircraft, looking for wires, flying debris, or anything else that would interfere with a safe, unobstructed flight path. In most air medical operations, takeoffs and landings are considered "sterile cockpit" times. This means that only mission safety–specific discussions are held by the crew via the intercabin communication system or radio. During this time air medical crews will not routinely give information over the radio or respond to calls. This "sterile cockpit" heightens awareness and directs attention.

During this entire time the patient's heart rate, blood pressure, oxygen saturation, and (in many cases) end-tidal CO_2 levels are monitored. Other interventions are performed as directed by the patient condition and clinical protocol. In some areas of the United States, blood is transfused in the prehospital setting. The crew focuses on the patient and safety simultaneously.

A critical component of the transport phase is making hospital contact. The goal is to give the receiving hospital as much information as possible to allow adequate preparation for the delivery of the critically injured person. Time is of the essence, and the succinct delivery of information may be the difference between life and death.

WHERE TO DELIVER THE PATIENT

In most areas of the United States, critically injured patients are delivered to dedicated trauma centers. The objective of a trauma system is to have necessary resources immediately available to best meet the needs of the injured patient.

In *Resources for Optimal Care of the Injured Patient: 2006*,[34] the American College of Surgeons states that the care of the trauma patient requires an organized, systematic approach with preset plans and protocols that ensure rapid access to care by dedicated and expert personnel at specialized facilities. Trauma care requires a significant commitment of personnel and resources. The goal for designated trauma centers is to be ready for any type of injured patient at any time. Trauma centers are classified by the American College of Surgeons as Level I, II, III, or IV. For specific delineation of trauma center standards the reader is referred to the most recent edition of the *Resources for Optimal Care of the Injured Patient* published by the American College of Surgeons Committee on Trauma.[34] A decision scheme recommended for use in field triage when deciding if a patient requires transport to a trauma center is described in Figure 7-3.

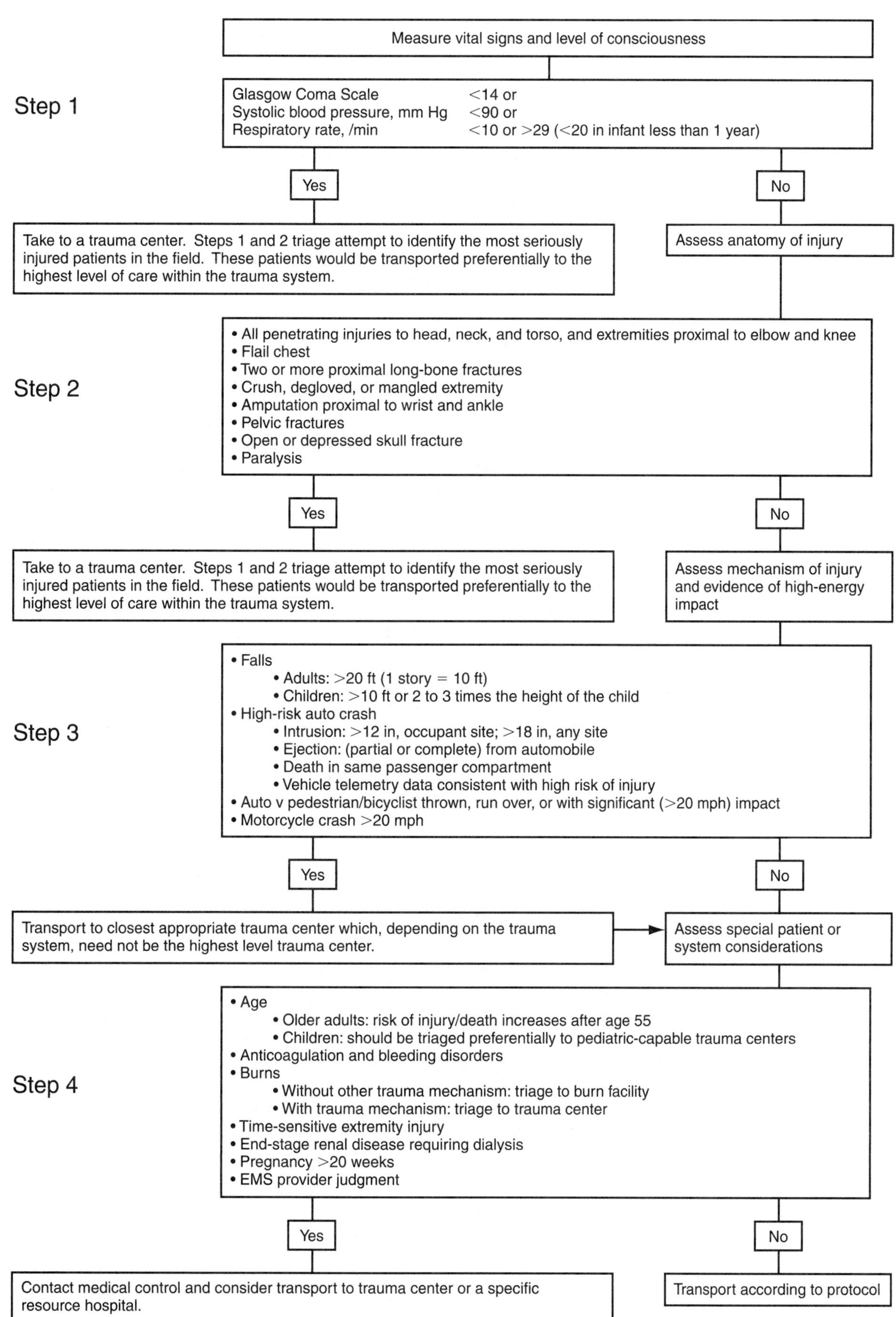

FIGURE 7-3 Field triage decision scheme. *(Used with permission from American College of Surgeons Committee on Trauma:* Resources for optimal care of the injured patient: 2006, *p 22, Chicago, 2006, American College of Surgeons.)*

The effectiveness of trauma center care was well documented in a study published in *The New England Journal of Medicine* in January 2006.[35] In this study the mortality outcome of patients treated in 18 hospitals with a Level I trauma center were compared with those of patients treated in 51 hospitals without a trauma center. Results showed that "the in-hospital mortality rate was significantly lower at trauma centers than at non–trauma centers (7.6% vs. 9.5%; relative risk, 0.80; 95% confidence interval, 0.66 to 0.98), as was the 1-year mortality rate (10.4% vs. 13.8%; relative risk, 0.75; 95% confidence interval, 0.60 to 0.95)."[35]

In systems where the receiving hospital is not a trauma center, it is necessary for the accepting hospital to have policies and practices in place to foster the rapid transfer and transport of an injured patient whose needs outweigh the capabilities of that hospital to an appropriate trauma care facility. In situations where an air ambulance is used, determination of a safe LZ must be considered. Most trauma centers have helipads designated to receive these patients. Each state has different regulations regarding landing of emergency medical helicopters; it is critical to evaluate these rules and procedures before using this service.

At the discretion of the air medical program, the aircraft may be unloaded "hot" (with engines/rotor blades turning) or only when "cold" (after the blades have stopped turning and engines are shut down). Regional differences and program philosophies influence this choice. Some believe "hot" off-loading saves critical minutes; others counter that "cold" off-loading is safer because it limits movement of staff and equipment under moving rotor blades.[36,37]

Transfer of Care to Receiving Facilities

In all situations the transporting crew transfers the care of the injured individual soon after arrival at the receiving hospital. The members of this crew deliver information and the patient. Essential information includes the mechanism of injury, extrication time, condition of the patient on arrival, treatment rendered, and the patient's response to therapy. It is the responsibility of the crew delivering the patient to verify before leaving the facility that the accepting team has a clear understanding of the patient's recent event, vital signs, and all other assessment and intervention data. The exact time of transfer has been the subject of debate. A guiding principle is a team focus on delivering the best care to the patient, which is facilitated by communication and interaction.

Transport Documentation

All events, assessments, and interventions must be documented accurately and descriptively. The patient care record must be clear, objective, and succinct, containing an accurate accounting of the care provided and the circumstances of the transport. In general, documentation must be legible and free of unrecognized or dangerous abbreviations. It is recommended that documentation be completed as soon as possible after the conclusion of patient care. Most EMS and air medical systems have documentation forms in a checklist format to ensure that all significant areas are addressed. If there are nonapplicable areas, the caregiver draws lines through them to prevent late additions by others. Documentation marks the close of the prehospital phase of patient care. It is critical that it is a true reflection of events.

Summary

Effective delivery of care in the prehospital environment is essential to enhance the outcomes of the 60 million people injured each year. As discussed in this chapter, success is affected by the cohesiveness of the multidisciplinary prehospital team, communication flow, and appropriate care delivery.

The prehospital environment is different from other health care settings. In no other practice area is safety of the provider such an essential component in minute-by-minute decision making. At times the scene it is without lights, electricity, or other adjuncts and support systems of which in-hospital providers are easily assured. Nurses have a strong role in this arena as caregivers and team members. It is appropriate that nurses participate in a system that ensures the injured patient receives the best possible care in the field.

The definition of appropriate prehospital care must be critically evaluated. There are many practice approaches that lack a strong research base, which has led to regional practice variations. Included in these differences are scope of practice requirements, airway management techniques, and fluid resuscitation, to name just a few. Additional research and continued refinement of prehospital care is necessary to improve the ultimate outcome of those injured.

References

1. Office of Statistics and Programming, National Center for Injury Prevention and Control, Centers for Disease Control and Prevention: 2003 WISQARS report: NCHS vital statistics system for numbers of deaths, bureau of census for population estimates. Atlanta, 2003, Centers for Disease Control and Prevention.
2. Patruras JL: The EMS call. In Pons P and Cason D, editors: *Paramedic field care: a complaint-based approach*, St. Louis, 1997, Mosby, pp. 27-34.
3. Dernocouer K: Safety and the field/dispatch connection, *Emerg Med Serv* 27:23-24, 1998.
4. Clawson J: *Emergency medical dispatch priority card system*, Salt Lake City, 1979, Salt Lake City Fire Department.
5. Centers for Disease Control and Prevention: GAO Report on Emergency Medical Services, Oct. 2004. *J Emerg Manage* 2004.
6. U.S. Department of Labor Statistics: (2004) http://www.dol.gov/. Accessed April 29, 2007.
7 Chapleau W, Burba M, Pons P et al: *The paramedic*, New York, McGraw-Hill. In press, pp. 17-18.
8. Johnson JC: Multiple casualty incidents and disasters. In Pons P and Cason D, editors: *Paramedic field care: a complaint-based approach*, St. Louis, 1997, Mosby, pp 629-642.

9. State of California, Office of Emergency Services: *Standardized emergency management system field course module 2—principles and features of ICS*, Sacramento, 1995, Office of Emergency Services.
10. National Incident Management System Integration Center: http://www.fema.gov/emergency/nims/index.shtm. Accessed April 29, 2007.
11. Chapleau W, Pons P: *Emergency medical technician, making the difference*, St. Louis, 2007, Elsevier/Mosby.
12. Chapleau W: *Emergency first responder, making the difference*, St. Louis, 2004, Elsevier/Mosby.
13. National Association of Emergency Medical Technicians: *Prehospital trauma life support: basic and advanced*, ed 6, St Louis, 2006, Mosby.
14. Holleran RS: Extrication and scene management. In National Flight Nursing Association: *Flight nursing: principles and practice*, ed 2, St. Louis, 1996, Mosby, pp. 37-48.
15. Stewart C, Conover K, Terry M: General principles of rescue. In Pons P and Cason D, editors: *Paramedic field care: a complaint-based approach*, St. Louis, 1997, Mosby, pp. 616-627.
16. Walls RM, editor: *Advanced emergency airway management*, Dallas, 1997, American College of Emergency Physicians.
17. American Burn Association: *Advanced burn life support provider's manual*, Lincoln, Neb, 1996, American Burn Association.
18. Adnet F, Lapostolle F, Ricard-Hibon A et al: Intubating trauma patients before reaching hospital—revisited, *Crit Care* 5:290–291, 2001.
19. Mageau AP: Airway management/oxygen therapy. In Krupa D, editor: *Flight nursing core curriculum*, Park Ridge, IL, 1997, National Flight Nurses Association, pp. 69-75.
20. Sing RF, Rotundo MF, Zonies DH et al: Rapid sequence induction for intubation by an aeromedical transport team, *Am J Emerg Med* 16:598-602, 1998.
21. York D: Rapid sequence induction for intubation. In Proehl J, editor: *Emergency nursing procedures*, ed 2, Philadelphia, 1999, W. B. Saunders, pp. 26-30.
22. Hoyt D: Prehospital care: do no harm? *Ann Surg* 237:161-162, 2003.
23. Pepe PE, Raedler C, Lurie KG et al: Emergency ventilatory management in hemorrhagic states: elemental of detrimental? *J Trauma* 54:1048-1057, 2003.
24. Patrick VC: Emergency needle thoracentesis. In Proehl J, editor: *Emergency nursing procedures*, ed 2, Philadelphia, 1999, W. B. Saunders pp. 130-132.
25. Barton ED, Epperson M, Hoyt D et al: Prehospital needle aspiration and tube thoracostomy in trauma victims: a six year experience with aeromedical crews, *J Emerg Med* 13:155-63, 1995.
26. York D, Dudek L, Larson R et al: A comparison study of chest tube thoracostomy: air medical crew and in-hospital trauma services, *Air Med J* 12:227-229, 1993.
27. Bravo AM: Trauma and burns. In: Johns Hopkins Hospital Department of Pediatrics, Barone M, editor: *The Harriet Lane handbook*, ed 15, St. Louis, 2000, Mosby, pp. 73-75.
28. Bickell WH, Wall MJ, Pete PE: Immediate versus delayed fluid resuscitation for hypotensive patients with penetrating torso injuries, *N Engl J Med* 331:1105-1109, 1994.
29. Demetriades D, Chan L, Cornwall E et al: Paramedic vs. private transportation of trauma patients: effect on outcome, *Arch Surg* 131:133-138, 1996.
30. Brain Trauma Foundation Writing Team: Guidelines for prehospital management of traumatic brain injury, ed 2, *Prehospital Emerg Care* 12(Suppl):1-53, 2007.
31. National Association of Emergency Medical Services Physicians: Air medical dispatch: guidelines for scene response, *Prehosp Disaster Med* 7:75-76, 1992.
32. State of California: California code of regulation, Title 22, Div 9, 2000.
33. Commission on Accreditation of Medical Transport Systems: *Accreditation standards of CAMTS:* http://www.airaasi.com/camts.html. Accessed April 29, 2007.
34. American College of Surgeons' Committee on Trauma: *Resources for optimal care of the injured patient: 2006*, Chicago, 2006, American College of Surgeons.
35. MacKenzie EJ, Rivara FP, Jurkovich GJ et al: A national evaluation of the effect of trauma-center care on mortality, *N Engl J Med* 354:366-78, 2006.
36. Deimling D, deJarnett R, Rouse M et al: Helicopter loading time study: hot versus cold, *Air Med J* 18:145-148, 1999.
37. Criddle LM: The hot loaded patient: review and analysis of 1 year experience, *Air Med J* 18:140-144, 1999.

8

RURAL TRAUMA

Daniel G. Judkins, John Bleicher, Rifat Latifi

Two 19-year-olds are driving home from a party at a Forest Service campground 10 miles outside a town of about 1000 residents. It's 3 AM on a chilly, damp spring morning. Neither occupant is restrained. The driver is traveling at an unsafe speed and misses a curve on the winding gravel road, overcorrects, and rolls his pickup truck multiple times, ejecting both himself and his passenger.

Three hours later, a man driving up the road to park at the campground and go for a run spots the vehicle in the trees about 50 feet away. He finds the two victims another 50 feet from the vehicle. Both are alive but obviously critically injured. There is no cell phone service in the area, so he covers each victim (one with a blanket and the other with spare clothing) and drives back to town to call for help. Twenty minutes later, a Basic Life Support ambulance crew arrives to stabilize and transport the victims. One has a compromised airway, both are hypothermic and have multisystem injuries with a Glasgow Coma Scale score less than 8.

They are initially taken to a small, nondesignated hospital (the hospital would be considered a Level IV facility by the American College of Surgeons [ACS]) that has a radiograph machine but no computed tomography (CT). They are met by two registered nurses (RNs) and a physician assistant (PA). Here they will be stabilized and prepared for transport to the nearest regional trauma center, which is 75 miles away. One will be flown by helicopter and the other will be transported by ground ambulance, with one of the two RNs providing care along with the Basic Emergency Medical Technicians (EMTs). The RN is a recent graduate who has no trauma training and has never taken care of a patient in the back of an ambulance.

DEFINITION OF RURAL/FRONTIER

Defining the term *rural* is actually complicated. Three agencies of the federal government all define it differently. Variables in definitions include the size of the area, whether the area constitutes a county, proximity to an urban area, percentage of residents who commute to an urban area, topography, distances, and available resources. One example of a workable definition is, "A rural trauma region would be an area in which the population served is less than 2500, has a population density of less than 50 persons per square mile, has only basic life support prehospital care, has prehospital transport times that exceed 30 minutes on average, and is lacking in subspecialty coverage for specific injuries (such as a neurosurgeon to manage the patient with head injuries)."[1]

Most agree on a definition of a frontier area: "An area with extremely low population density, usually fewer than 6 people per square mile."[2] A more complex definition, in the form of a matrix including population density plus distance in time and miles to service/market, has been formulated by the National Clearinghouse for Frontier Communities.[3] Northern plains and Rocky Mountain states, along with Alaska, have vast frontier areas. In Montana, one third of the residents live in seven counties. The average population density of the other 49 counties is 2.7 persons per square mile.[4]

UNIQUE NATURE OF RURAL TRAUMA

Obviously, life is very different in rural areas than it is in urban areas. But what urban dwellers usually fail to understand is how different trauma is in the less-populated regions of the world. The people themselves are different. Rural residents tend to be older with more preexisting medical conditions that make recovery from trauma more difficult. Many of these medical conditions are poorly managed, at times because of poverty (rural areas being generally less well off financially than urban ones), and sometimes because of problems with access to care. Overall, rural residents are almost 50% more likely to die of trauma than their urban peers.[1] The rural death rate from motor vehicle crashes (MVCs) is almost twice the urban rate.[1] Of the other 10 most frequent causes of traumatic death, rural rates are higher than urban rates in all but one. Nearly 60% of all trauma deaths occur in rural areas, despite the fact that only 20% of the nation's population live in these areas. Rural patients who survive longer than 24 hours post-event before dying are older, less severely injured, have more comorbidities and are more likely to die of multiple organ system failure compared with urban patients. Once again looking at Montana, more than 50% of people who die of trauma in that state never make it to the hospital for treatment, usually due to a delay in discovery.[5]

Not only are the people different, but the traumatic events they deal with are different as well. More than 90% of rural trauma is blunt and unintentional.[6] The majority of critical cases cared for by rural facilities are MVCs, predominately single-vehicle rollovers with ejection. Occupational hazards abound. Farming, ranching, logging, mining, and recreational guiding have high injury rates, and these injuries occur far from facilities providing definitive care. Rural people tend to recreate outdoors, often leading to serious injuries. The incidence of significant injuries from skiing, snowboarding, river recreation, and riding horses, snowmobiles, jet skis, and all-terrain vehicles is on the rise. Time to definitive care is almost always an issue when people are injured participating in these activities. Rural trauma providers sometimes talk about the "golden day" rather than the "golden hour" to reaching definitive care.

Prehospital Care

Most rural ambulance services are staffed by volunteers. These civic-minded individuals deal with extremely challenging calls with very little financial or educational support. Call volumes are low and effective performance improvement (PI) programs commonly do not exist, so even those who are most motivated are challenged to provide quality care. Communities typically struggle just to keep an ambulance or two in service and may have limited resources left to invest in quality monitoring and improvement measures.

Staffing Issues

Many rural EMTs actually have to pay to volunteer. Their initial provider course (110 to 120 hours) is usually free, but they are rarely compensated for the hours spent in class or studying away from the classroom. There is rarely compensation for required continuing education. In fact, many EMTs must travel on their own time and pay course or conference fees and travel expenses to receive quality continuing education (CE). Most also have to travel, sometimes great distances, to take certification exams.

The typical rural scenario has volunteers on-call with pagers and/or radios from their homes or workplaces. When a call comes in, they travel to the facility where the ambulance is housed, wait for a partner or two, and then respond to the scene. The time when staffing is most problematic is during the day, Monday through Friday. This is because most volunteers are at their regular jobs during these hours and may not be able to leave, especially when a single ambulance call can take hours to complete.

There are rarely financial incentives to stay involved with the local service. Some are paid a minimal stipend for time actually spent on calls. Even fewer are covered by insurance or have a pension plan. This is a greater problem today than in the past as the rural population ages. Fewer volunteers are signing up to take the places vacated by those leaving the services. It is not uncommon for there to be no one to answer the call.

Barriers to Providing Quality Care

Not only is access to education an issue, but the quality of the education provided can also be problematic in rural areas, especially the farther one gets from the larger communities. Because of the costs of travel, community agencies tend to become self-reliant and provide most of their own education for their volunteers. The lack of involvement by knowledgeable outsiders with current information can lead to stagnation in the messages delivered.

Clearly, the biggest barrier to providing quality care is low call volume. In many rural and frontier services, individual EMTs may have only a couple trauma calls per year. This is especially problematic when these providers have to manage multiple-patient incidents, such as a high-speed, head-on collision between two vehicles on a rural highway causing injuries to four or more individuals. This problem of low call volume is compounded by immature to nonexistent PI programs. Rural EMTs may deliver the patient to the emergency department (ED) and stay to help with resuscitation, but then they go home or back to work. It is very difficult for them, especially in this time when facilities must protect patient confidentiality, to get helpful follow-up information. They may never learn that they missed a life-threatening injury, thereby missing an opportunity to improve their assessments and treatments for their next patient. One might think this should be the responsibility of the service medical director. In a perfect world, every service would have an involved physician leading the team. This is actually a rarity in rural communities. Many rural physicians are already overextended, and many do not possess the knowledge or expertise to mentor EMTs. The combination of limited feedback from facilities and little service involvement by physicians not only results in knowledge deficits for EMTs but is a big reason why many choose not to continue participation after years of service. The sense of isolation can be profound.

A number of system issues unique to the rural/frontier environment become barriers to providing quality care. First, dispatchers frequently lack proper training and protocols, and information passed along to the responding units is often incomplete or inaccurate. Second, locating the patient(s) can be very difficult, especially at night. Many rural residents live on unnamed roads, have unnumbered residences, or both. An ambulance may be dispatched to "the old McClellan place, a brown trailer, up highway 12." Not only is no actual address given, but the color of the trailer is useless at night. And, the McClellan family may have lived in that trailer for 20 years but has not lived there for the past 5 years. A different family lives there now, but in many parts of rural America the "address" of that home is the name of the family that lived in it for the longest period. Imagine the frustration of the well-intentioned EMT who moved to that community within the last 2 years! The third major barrier is lack of radio communications. Owing to topography, long distances, and insufficient placement of transmission towers, EMTs often cannot communicate with the hospital. They can receive no assistance from medical control, and they cannot alert the facility that they are bringing a critical trauma patient.

Nurse and Physician Education

One of the greatest challenges facing rural systems is providing quality CE to nurses and physicians. They typically are unable to meet their own needs, because frequently neither the nurses nor the physicians have the time or expertise in trauma care to develop educational modules that fulfill local needs. Plus, the distance between facilities makes it very difficult for outsiders to assist on a regular basis. New technologies, such as web and video links, are being used to solve some of the problems, but many needs remain unmet.

Financial Constraints

Most rural facilities are struggling financially. Education budgets are commonly cut (or eliminated altogether) when facilities endure financial crises. It is difficult for staff members to travel to larger communities for classes or conferences, because these trips usually involve an overnight stay. This is expensive and takes nurses from their families and jobs. It is even difficult for rural facilities to get nurses to attend classes when providers from larger communities come in to provide them. First, when budgets are tight, administrators will not make CE mandatory. Staff must attend on their own time without compensation from the facility. Second, rural facilities are commonly understaffed, so it can be difficult to release nurses to attend classes because they are needed to care for patients. This dilemma could be solved by using traveling nurses, but this can challenge already tight budgets. Educators from regional trauma centers often must present the same class twice in a single community in order for most of the interested nurses to attend. This places a significant burden on the trauma center staff, as they may serve 20 to 30 facilities within their region.

It can also be difficult for rural physicians to leave their practices to attend conferences or Advanced Trauma Life Support (ATLS). The same financial considerations that affect nurses also affect physicians. Furthermore, leaving town can create difficulties in maintaining medical coverage for local citizens. Hiring locum tenens physicians to cover is an option, but is expensive.

Meeting Unique Needs

Rural practitioners work in a unique environment, and their educational needs are similarly unique. They often benefit when standard courses are adapted to meet their needs. Further complicating the picture is the fact that different facilities have different needs. One center may encounter chronic delays in getting patients transferred to definitive care, whereas another may be admitting patients who should be transferred. Unfortunately, PI programs specific to trauma are usually immature in rural facilities, and the providers might not even recognize the existence of patient care or system dilemmas.

Using grant monies and telemedicine has helped solve many of these rural trauma education problems. State and national groups are working to improve access to quality education. Much of the burden will continue to be borne by the regional trauma centers, which must accept responsibility for assisting the smaller facilities in their respective regions.

Limitations on Hospital Resources

The overall financial performance of the nation's rural hospitals has improved; however, small rural hospitals (those having 50 beds or less) continue to be at risk of financial instability and closure. Representing about half of all rural hospitals, small hospitals as a group report substantial negative operating margins and are highly dependent on Medicare as a source of payment. Medicare pays for almost 50% of all hospital discharges in rural areas, compared with 37% for urban hospitals.[7] Rural hospitals typically have lower Medicare margins than urban hospitals. Rural hospitals tend to provide relatively more outpatient and postacute care, and relatively less inpatient care. Therefore, low Medicare payments (relative to costs) for outpatient services are not as easily compensated by inpatient payments. Also, the ratio of total Medicaid days to total days has a significant contribution to hospitals' financial performance, because hospitals with a higher proportion of Medicaid patients will get additional payment through the Medicaid disproportionate hospital share (DSH) payments system. Rural hospitals are in a disadvantaged position to receive DSH payments because most Medicaid patients are located in the large metropolitan areas and inner cities. Our empirical findings suggest that rural hospitals generate less revenue per bed than urban hospitals.[7]

One of the main reasons rural facilities are struggling is difficulty in managing costs. Between 1990 and 1999, rural hospitals' cost increases have consistently been one to two percentage points higher than those of urban hospitals, and the cumulative change in cost per case was nearly 30% for rural hospitals and just 14% for urban hospitals.[8] Though much of this cost differential can be linked to economies of scale, a large part appears to have been caused by smaller reductions in length of stay.[8]

This financial picture is one of many reasons it can be difficult to recruit and retain nurses and physicians in rural areas, causing major challenges in caring for trauma patients. Though many physicians love the rural lifestyle and work environment, many others feel more at home in cities with larger hospitals, more resources, and less sense of professional isolation. Many rural physicians who receive trauma patients in their facilities have never taken ATLS. It can be very difficult for them to attend courses and conferences because of travel costs and the stress of leaving their practices uncovered. Recruitment and retention can be problematic, even if a physician or nurse wants to accept a position, if there are few employment opportunities for his or her spouse or good educational opportunities for children.

Rural practitioners must be the proverbial jack-of-all-trades, working with nursing home patients at the start of the day, later moving to obstetrics to deliver a baby, then going to the ED for trauma resuscitation. Rural nurses, even recent graduates, must at times care for critically injured patients without benefit of trauma training or in-services. Because of weather, distances, and delay in discovery, it is common for their patients to arrive many hours after their traumatic event. Their diagnostic equipment is rarely state-of-the-art, and supplies can be limited, especially in multiple-patient events. It is a challenging work environment.

Improving Rural Trauma Care

Prehospital

The report of the Institute of Medicine (IOM) of the National Academies Committee on the Future of Emergency Care in the U.S. Health System offers the following conclusion: "Much progress has been made in the improvement of the nation's (emergency medical services [EMS]) capabilities. But in some important ways, the delivery of those services has declined.... (T)he committee's overall conclusion... is that today the system is more fragmented than ever, and the lack of effective coordination and accountability stand in the way of further progress and improved quality of care."[9] So, how can we move toward a more integrated and accountable system that is affordable and sustainable and meets the needs of our communities? The recommendations that follow are from both the IOM report and from the National Highway Traffic Safety Association (NHTSA) "EMS Agenda for the Future."[10]

Both groups feel that an important step in addressing the lack of coordination and accountability in emergency and trauma systems is establishment of a lead federal agency for emergency and trauma care. Responsibility is currently scattered among several agencies, including Health and Human Services (HHS), Homeland Security, and the Department of Transportation. The IOM feels this agency should be housed in HHS and should have primary responsibility for trauma and emergency care from dispatch through hospital resuscitation. Each state should have a paid EMS Medical Director, and the American Board of Emergency Medicine should create a subspecialty certification in EMS. HHS should also convene a panel to develop evidence-based indicators of emergency care system performance, and the lead agency should have accountability for their implementation. There must be better coordination within EMS, as well as improved coordination between EMS and public health agencies, especially in disaster preparedness.

In order for EMS to meet the ever-increasing demands on its resources, the payment structure must be changed. Especially in rural areas, where a higher percentage of patients transported are elderly, Medicare is an important payor. Payment for transports is marginal at best, but this is only part of the problem. EMS agencies spend a lot of money maintaining readiness, and current payment schemes do not reimburse for these expenses. Both the IOM and NHTSA recommend including readiness costs and permitting payment to EMS agencies without transport.

One of the goals of EMS trauma care is getting the patient to the right facility in the right amount of time. This can be very problematic in rural/frontier areas, as EMTs often must decide whether to transport a patient (or patients) to a closer but less prepared facility, or to take more time to transport directly to a designated trauma center. Under the current "system," hospital staff commonly do not know the capabilities of the EMS agencies in their areas, and the EMTs do not know the overall capabilities of the facilities, let alone their ability to accept patients at any given time. Clearly, there must be more precise categorization of EMS agencies and hospitals so more informed decisions can be made. Once this categorization is complete, the next step would be development of evidence-based protocols for movement of patients throughout the system based on patient acuity and facility capability and capacity.

The education and training requirements for both basic and advanced EMTs vary not only from state to state, but sometimes within individual communities. Different agencies may offer courses of varying length and with uneven standards for completion. Standardization of curriculum, scope of practice, and state licensing standards is a goal that would improve patient care and increase the professional standing of EMS personnel.

As discussed earlier, communication in rural areas is commonly problematic. As stated in the IOM report, "hospitals, trauma centers, EMS agencies, public safety departments, emergency management offices and public health agencies should develop integrated and interoperable communications and data systems... HHS should fully involve prehospital EMS leadership in discussions about the design, deployment and financing of the National Health Information Infrastructure."[9]

The number of air medical helicopters operating in the United States has tripled in the last 15 years. Many operate independently. There are safety and operational concerns as some of these programs operate outside the realm of local systems with no involvement in system-wide PI. Less than 50% of air medical transport agencies are accredited by the Commission on Accreditation of Medical Transport Systems (CAMTS). Many programs suffer from a lack of involved, qualified medical direction. States should assume regulatory oversight of medical air services, including communications, dispatch, and transport protocols.

EMS has lagged behind other public safety entities in disaster planning and operations. EMS must be placed on the same level as these other entities, because few other system components will be able to function effectively if EMS fails. Per the IOM report, "Congress should substantially increase funding for EMS-related disaster preparedness through dedicated funding streams ... the professional training, continuing education and credentialing and certification programs for all relevant EMS professional categories should incorporate disaster preparedness training into their curricula and require the maintenance of these skills."[9]

A model EMS system must recognize the unique needs of pediatric patients. The pediatric patient should always be considered when developing prehospital protocols, planning for disasters, creating performance improvement programs, and in the structure of any agencies that have jurisdiction over EMS services. All providers should receive specialty pediatric training and should have all necessary pediatric-specific equipment. Large gaps in the research arena relative to pediatric emergency care must be filled. Programs such as Emergency Medical Services for Children (EMS-C) that support quality care for children and injury prevention programs must be funded, and all hospitals and EMS agencies that care for injured children should have a staff member responsible for quality oversight in this area.

Both the IOM and NHTSA recognize a critical need for research in EMS, and nowhere is this more needed than in rural/frontier areas. An analysis of current needs should be undertaken, followed by formulation of a strategy to organize and fund research. The emphasis of this research should be on systems and outcomes. Towards this end, the IOM recommends that Congress establish 10 demonstration sites, appropriating $88 million over 5 years, to determine "which strategies work best under which conditions."[9] It is imperative that rural providers be active in establishment of this project to ensure some of these sites are in rural/frontier areas.

Our nation needs an emergency care system that is coordinated, regionalized, and accountable. Nowhere is the need greater than in rural/frontier areas. The results of efforts to establish effective, sustainable trauma systems in rural states have been largely disappointing. These efforts, though at times successful, have been plagued by intermittent funding, political/financial turf battles, complaints about rigid federal constraints and the difficulties of conducting research on patient outcomes.

In 1990 Congress allocated federal funding in support of the Trauma Care Systems and Development Act, with the goal of developing a Model Trauma Systems plan. The plan was developed under the direction of staff at the Health Resources and Services Administrations with input from a coalition of trauma systems experts.[10] In 1993 Bazzoli et al. conducted a survey of trauma system administrators to evaluate trauma systems status. "We found that, although many states had made progress by 1993, most had a long way to go to develop comprehensive trauma systems."[11] During this period when federal funding for trauma system development was sporadic, efforts were complicated by a national decline in health care reimbursement that put financial pressures on states, communities, and hospitals, especially in poorer rural areas. Much of the hard-earned momentum from the early 1990s was lost as financially strapped urban facilities relinquished their trauma center designations.

One of the primary functions of a statewide trauma system is to oversee the initiation of standardized protocols designed to ensure the timely triage and transfer of severely injured patients to facilities with appropriate therapeutic resources.[12] Many rural states have no trauma system or designation of facilities. States without trauma systems typically do not have protocols governing either the initial triage or subsequent transfer of patients, or the means by which they are transported. They lack oversight, regional or statewide PI, and educational support for local providers.

Some rural states have established *inclusive* systems, "designed to care for all injured patients and involve all acute care facilities to the extent that their resources allow, as opposed to *exclusive* systems, in which care is formally organized only at a relatively few high-level centers that deliver definitive care."[13] No data exist to support which system is best suited for urban versus rural environments. Those who advocate for inclusive systems feel that, because of the vast distances separating tertiary care facilities, efforts must be made to improve trauma care in all facilities, no matter how small.

Certain components of trauma systems have proven to be of value, yet no study has been able to prove or disprove the hypothesis that a statewide system leads to better outcomes for patients injured in rural/frontier environments. Nor are there data to support which type of system (inclusive vs exclusive) should be established by those states choosing to build one. Additional research is needed to address these issues.

There are many challenges in improving rural trauma care.[14]

Hospital Trauma Care

Rural hospitals should assess their resources and capabilities for providing trauma care. All rural hospitals that provide emergency services will receive trauma cases. Some rural areas may operate a clinic program that provides some level of emergency services, even without inpatient hospital services. Larger towns in rural areas may feature a hospital with an ED that has higher capabilities for providing trauma care. A useful approach to self-assessment of rural trauma care capability is to apply the trauma center criteria developed by the ACS[15] or state trauma center criteria.

The ACS criteria include four levels of trauma centers. Some states have additional levels in their trauma care plan. A small rural hospital without surgeon coverage may assess itself using the ACS "Level IV Trauma Center" criteria. These criteria list both "essential" requirements and "desirable" characteristics of such a program. Larger rural hospitals with around-the-clock on-call coverage for emergency medicine, anesthesia, surgery, and orthopedics may use the "Level III Trauma Center" criteria. Self-identified deficiencies become the roadmap for improvement. The hospital may elect to pursue official verification of a Level III or IV trauma center status by the ACS or official designation at these levels by the appropriate state agency (if available).

Hospital Staffing

Staffing the hospital with appropriate personnel is key to providing good trauma care in the rural area. Recruitment and retention of skilled nursing and medical staff is often the most challenging step. The jack-of-all-trades rural nurse may be suddenly pulled from other duties to help when the occasional serious trauma patient arrives, and then must instantly function as a skilled trauma nurse during the resuscitation phase. At one moment the rural nurse is a generalist and at the next must function as a trauma specialist under intense circumstances. The patient's life depends on it. Rural hospitals need nurses who are well rounded, experienced, flexible, creative, energetic, and have a commitment to continual improvement in critical areas such a trauma. In an era of nurse shortages, finding and keeping such nurses at a rural hospital demands great effort. The hospital should consider carefully an attractive pay and benefits package that is likely to succeed in this effort. The provision of resources for excellent CE will be an essential part of the package.

Attracting medical staff may be even more challenging. The smallest rural hospitals must work hard to have even one or a few good generalist doctors on the staff. Some rural hospitals may have 24-hour physician staffing for the ED. Frequently this is a combination of interested local physicians and itinerant doctors who come and go. Maintaining quality is a challenge. Rural EDs should insist that such physicians maintain their ATLS certification as a first quality assurance step. Rural hospitals in larger towns may have a more developed medical staff, including some specialties. The most important for trauma care are the general surgeon and the orthopedic surgeon. To maintain 24-hour coverage by these two specialties, there typically must be two or three or more of each such specialty on the staff.

A contingency staffing plan should be developed to supplement regular on-duty staff in the event that one or more critical trauma cases demand additional help. The rural hospital should maintain a staff call-back plan for nurses, doctors, technicians, and others that can be rapidly implemented when the need arises.

Trauma Education for Rural Providers

Rural nurses who may be called upon to care for trauma patients need regular CE in trauma. The less often a nurse participates in trauma resuscitation, the greater the need for CE. Many such rural nurses will find themselves doing trauma resuscitation less than once a week. Because the more you do something, the better you get, a low volume of trauma cases demands more education. The rural hospital should provide a program of regular CE in trauma. A minimally acceptable trauma education standard should be established. This should include sending the rural nurses to the Advanced Trauma Care for Nurses (ATCN) or Trauma Nurse Core Course. In addition, a minimum level of annual trauma-related CE could be mandated. This would vary from hospital to hospital. Box 8-1 shows an example of a simple trauma nursing CE program for a small rural hospital. Setting such a standard for trauma CE should be a local decision, made in view of local circumstances and resources.

The rural hospital should take maximum advantage of rural trauma outreach education programs, often conducted by the regional Level I trauma center and sometimes by helicopter EMS programs. By working cooperatively with the regional trauma center, the smaller rural hospital can obtain expert trauma education while reducing costs and duplication of effort. The jointly coordinated trauma education program should be planned in advance to best schedule expert trauma resources. Other sources of trauma education may be the "Critical Access Hospital" program for rural hospitals, programs from the state health department or university rural health service, online or teleconferenced trauma education, and courses offered by state-regional-county EMS councils or state or regional trauma systems councils or boards. The nurse in charge of providing trauma CE at the rural hospital should seek out all such sources, develop relationships, and frequently ask for trauma outreach programs.

Some rural hospitals may have the advantage of a relationship with a regional Level I or II trauma center that offers a program for rural nurses to spend a shift or two at the larger trauma center observing the trauma team in action and interacting with the trauma nurses there. This may involve clinical time in trauma resuscitation, in the trauma critical care unit, and possibly even ride-alongs with an urban ambulance service, fire department, or helicopter program. Staffing at the rural hospital will usually be strained to let even one nurse off the regular work schedule to participate in such a program, but the rewards will likely be worth it.

BOX 8-1 Sample Rural Trauma Nursing Continuing Education Program

- Complete Advanced Trauma Care for Nurses (ATCN) or Trauma Nurse Core Course (TNCC) within 1 year of hire; then maintain every 4 years.
- Receive 8 hours of annual trauma-related continuing education.
- Demonstrate trauma competencies annually through local assessment testing. (Possible competencies could include blood warming, chest drainage set-up, assisting with special procedures, and preparing for a trauma patient transfer.)
- Attend at least one regional trauma conference every other year.
- Log a shift as an "observer" at the regional Level I or II trauma center every 2 years (if program is available).
- Participate twice yearly in a mock trauma resuscitation drill, with evaluation.
- Participate in local hospital trauma quality improvement program.

The rural hospital may find it useful to schedule joint trauma CE with the local EMS personnel. Relationships are often close, extending even to the local EMS personnel staying and helping in the ED when they deliver a critical trauma case. These relationships can be further strengthened, plus the hospital can take advantage of economy of scale, by providing joint rural hospital nurse/local EMS provider trauma education opportunities.

Trauma CE for rural physicians should include, at minimum, the expectation that the physician take the ATLS course and attend the every-4-year refresher course. This can be made a requirement through contracts or medical staff credentialing processes and will often have to be supported through funding provided by the hospital. Local rural physicians should request and expect the trauma surgeon staff at the regional Level I trauma center to provide additional trauma education opportunities. Mid-level providers, such as nurse practitioners and PAs, may also be able to attend ATLS courses and available medical trauma CE programs. They can also participate with the local nurses and EMS personnel in other local trauma CE opportunities.

A good way to know what trauma education is needed for rural trauma personnel is to conduct a formal trauma education needs assessment. This can be as simple as a brief written questionnaire to be completed by trauma staff (nurses, mid-level providers, physicians, even local EMS personnel) that asks specific and open-ended questions about perceived needs and wants for trauma education.

A formal annual plan for trauma CE should be developed at every rural hospital. Such a plan maximizes the likelihood that such CE will actually occur, and it helps set the expectation that staff participate in the program. The annual plan should be developed with input from staff, from the education needs assessment, and from actual trauma case follow-up and quality assessment. Box 8-2 shows a typical annual plan for trauma education presentations.

Build a small local trauma resources library for the rural hospital ED. It could include this book, the "STN Electronic Library of Trauma Lectures,"[16] the trauma center standards book by the ACS,[15] a standard medical trauma textbook, an ATLS Provider manual,[17] an ATCN provider manual,[18] a Basic Trauma Life Support[19] or Prehospital Trauma Life Support[20] text, the latest book of evidence-based brain injury guidelines from the Brain Trauma Foundation (*Guidelines for the Management of Severe Traumatic Brain Injury*),[21] a set of local trauma care policies and guidelines, selected CD- or DVD-based individualized computer learning programs on trauma topics, and a list of useful trauma websites containing reliable trauma clinical guidelines (such as that operated by the Eastern Association for the Surgery of Trauma at www.east.org). Encourage the staff to use these resources regularly. When a clinical question is brought up, suggest that the answer may be found in these references, and proceed to look up the answer.

Equipment and Resources

No matter how small the space in the rural ED, appropriate equipment must be on hand to properly care for a severely injured patient during the early resuscitation phase. Excellent lists of minimum equipment can be found in the 1997 version of the trauma center criteria published by the ACS[22] and/or in documents created by the state trauma center designation authority. In general, all equipment and supplies needed in a typical ED should be supplemented with several trauma-specific items (Box 8-3).

The rural hospital should assess its capacity to keep an appropriate blood supply on hand. This should include at least several units of universal-donor packed cells and a laboratory technician on-call program to ensure rapid availability of the blood for transfusion to the trauma patient.

Many rural hospitals now have CT scanners. This can certainly be useful for certain trauma patients. Personnel, however, must recognize that doing CT scans on a critical trauma patient should not delay the patient's transfer to a higher level of care.

BOX 8-2 Typical Rural Hospital Annual Plan for Trauma Continuing Education Presentations

- Trauma assessment: primary survey, secondary survey, and reassessment
- Bleeding, shock, and resuscitation priorities
- Brain injury: assessment and initial management
- How to transfer a trauma patient to the Level 1 trauma center, including helicopter landing safety
- Major chest injuries
- Trauma care for special populations: pediatrics and geriatrics
- Extremity trauma
- Mock trauma resuscitation drill (several times yearly)

BOX 8-3 Trauma Equipment Needed in the Rural Emergency Department

- A method to warm blood rapidly
- A cabinet for maintaining warm intravenous solutions and blankets
- Equipment for rewarming a hypothermic patient
- Equipment to establish and maintain a patent airway, including endotracheal and tracheal tubes in all sizes (i.e., appropriate options to fit a large to small adult, child, and infant)
- Emergency cricothyrotomy tray
- Medications needed for rapid-sequence intubation and chemical paralysis
- Chest tube insertion tray, and chest drainage system with autotransfusion capability
- Supplies for spinal immobilization and fracture splinting

An appropriate landing zone for an EMS helicopter is extremely important. Staff should be trained and should drill regularly on safety procedures regarding helicopter landings.

The ED should have a computer with Internet search capability. This can be extremely useful for rapid access to treatment guidelines for uncommon types of trauma cases and other reference and continuing education needs. A digital camera can be useful. Selected clinical photos can be sent as e-mail attachments to the trauma surgeon at the trauma center where the patient is being transferred.

Team Organization

An organized team response plan should be designed for the rural hospital. The structure of the plan will depend on the size of the hospital and its staff and local circumstances and resources. A minimum of three or four persons will be needed for any complex trauma resuscitation. Personnel roles should be planned to cover airway maintenance, spinal immobilization, vital signs monitoring, vascular line insertion, and special procedures, such as chest tube insertion. The medical technician from the laboratory and the x-ray technician will likely be needed. If a respiratory therapist or anesthetist is available, their services will be needed. The plan should include contingency staffing to rapidly secure additional nursing and medical staff if required. Once the plan is developed, staff should be educated in the various roles, and mock trauma resuscitation drills should be conducted to practice role functions and fine-tune the process. Attention should be given to working relationships between the lead nurse and the physician. Efforts should be directed to developing a team approach.

A useful resource for developing the rural hospital trauma team is the "Rural Trauma Team Development Course" offered by the Trauma Division of the ACS.[23] This course can be offered, in conjunction with the regional trauma center, for several rural hospitals simultaneously.

Trauma System Integration

How does the rural hospital fit into the regional trauma care plan? The hospital and its nurses should get involved in regional system planning groups and committees to ensure a good understanding of how the trauma system works in the region, to represent the unique needs of the rural hospital, and to develop smooth working relationships with others in the system. This is also a good way to speak up and obtain additional trauma resources that may be limited at the rural hospital. Face-to-face meetings with the key trauma care providers at the regional Level I or II trauma centers (trauma surgeons, trauma manager, trauma outreach educator) will facilitate communication and smooth working relationships during intense situations when caring for a critical trauma patient, such as when consulting on immediate diagnostic and treatment needs, arranging for patient transport, and getting the patient accepted for transfer to the trauma center. Rural hospitals and EMS agencies must maintain a place at the table to represent local needs and concerns during trauma system planning and the development of EMS treatment and transfer protocols. Those who remain uninvolved are easily overlooked and may be left out of the regional trauma care plan.

Trauma Patient Assessment and Treatment in a Rural Hospital

The goal of assessment immediately on patient arrival is to find any life-threatening conditions. On another level, the goal is to establish whether the patient is suffering from serious trauma. Determining what injuries are present will be easy when assessment proceeds according to the standard approach using the primary and secondary survey. The primary survey should begin immediately on patient arrival and usually takes only a minute or two (unless interrupted by the need to treat life-threatening conditions). The standard **A-B-C-D-E** assessment approach should be used:

- **A**irway with C-spine control
- **B**reathing and oxygenation
- **C**irculation and shock status
- **D**isability/neurologic status
- **E**xpose the patient while maintaining **E**nvironmental controls to prevent hypothermia

When a life-threatening condition is discovered during this primary survey assessment, someone must immediately intervene to treat that threat (resuscitation).

After the primary survey is completed, a brief head-to-toe search for injuries should be conducted as the secondary survey. The patient must be completely undressed to accomplish this properly, and attention should be given to areas of the anatomy that may be overlooked (posterior surface of the body, ear-nose-mouth, axillary area, perineum/vagina/rectum, and distal extremities). The secondary survey may be supplemented by judicious use of diagnostic testing, as long as this does not in any way delay the patient's transfer to a higher level of trauma care. This may include x-rays, CT scans, and laboratory tests. Few laboratory tests are urgent in the early phases of trauma care, save arterial blood gas analysis (to evaluate oxygenation, CO_2 levels, and base deficit as a measure of shock), type and crossmatch if blood may be given urgently, and lactic acid levels. Few rural hospitals are currently able to obtain lactic acid levels rapidly, but this test would be useful to assess shock status, if available.

By this point in the assessment and resuscitation process, hopefully only a very short period after patient arrival at the rural hospital (minutes, not hours), the trauma team should be closing in on making a decision about whether to keep the patient at the current facility or to transfer the patient to a higher level trauma center. The rural hospital nurses and physicians, as a team, should carefully self-assess capacity and capability for providing trauma care locally at various acuity levels. This should result in a rational plan for what types of trauma patients, specific injuries, and various severity levels can be reasonably and safely cared for locally, and which require transfer to a higher-level trauma center. In addition, this plan should include a contingency for what to do when the patient requires transfer but such transfer is delayed or not possible due to various factors, such as unavailability of a means of transport, adverse weather conditions, or lack of an accepting higher-level trauma center.

A well-developed plan for effecting a trauma transfer should be developed in cooperation with transport agencies and high-level trauma centers that may be available for accepting patients. Box 8-4 shows key features of such a plan.

The rural hospital and EMS agencies should develop prehospital trauma triage criteria that specify which trauma patients, under which circumstances, should be directly transported to the regional Level I or II trauma center, bypassing the smaller rural hospital. This plan should include circumstances under which prehospital personnel can request rendezvous with a medical helicopter at the rural facility or other appropriate location.

Detailed plans should be developed in advance if there is the possibility that a local nurse from the rural hospital will be needed to accompany the patient during a ground ambulance transport to a distant trauma center. Who will this nurse be? What will be the required orientation or training and special skills needed for the accompanying nurse? Who will be paying this nurse (hospital or EMS agency)? What special equipment or medications will be needed during transport? Will blood be taken for possible transfusion during transport? What medical orders or protocols will be used during the trip? What are the plans for radio or cell phone contact with the local sending physician during transport? These are all questions that should be answered in the established plan.

Certain conditions may affect the mode-of-transport decision for trauma transfers. Weather is a particular concern in many areas. Adverse weather conditions may force the use of a lengthy ground ambulance transport instead of a helicopter, or even delay or prevent the transfer entirely. Distance, terrain, and special traffic conditions may also affect this decision. Finally, the EMS helicopter may not be available, or may even be delayed or turned back while heading toward the rural hospital. Many small communities may have only one ambulance or ambulance crew available, and its use in a time-consuming long-distance trauma case transfer may adversely affect the availability of local EMS response to other calls for help.

Rural Hospital Trauma Quality Improvement

All rural hospitals should have an active trauma quality improvement plan. All trauma cases should be logged or tracked. This can be as simple as flagging such cases in the ED log or maintaining a simple computerized trauma register. With low case volume, maintaining such a computerized register program is not as complex at the rural hospital as it is in the larger-volume trauma center. This process all starts with carefully defining the trauma population and who is entered into the log. Trauma is usually defined on the basis of some severity measure. Such a case definition may be available from the state or regional trauma system planning organization. With

BOX 8-4 Elements of a Plan for Transferring a Trauma Patient From a Rural Hospital

- Contact phone numbers, particularly special phone lines for trauma transfers
- Names of attending trauma surgeons at the regional Level I and II trauma centers
- Names and contact information of key persons at the receiving trauma center who should be called if the system breaks down or is not working well
- How to conduct communication between the local doctor and accepting doctor
- How to get immediate treatment and decision advice and consultation
- How to conduct communication between the transferring nurse and accepting nurse
- A list of regional trauma centers offering special services (pediatrics, burns, reimplantation, and specialized neurologic care)
- Ground and air transport services and their contact phone numbers
- A clear plan for who will take responsibility for arranging the transport (sending rural hospital or receiving trauma center)
- Plans for possible use of a sending-hospital nurse to provide trauma care during ground ambulance transports, if needed
- A list of issues that may affect transport decisions (e.g., patient weight prohibits flying in helicopter, violent or out-of-control behavior, pneumothorax, need for specific types of critical care during transport)
- A summary of steps to ensure Health Insurance Portability and Accountability Act compliance during transfer
- Landing zone preparation and safety issues
- Procedures for "patient packaging" for transport that are favored by the transport agency to be used
- Local hospital equipment or supplies needed during the transport, particularly blood products
- Specifications for copying and transmitting patient registration information, medical records, laboratory and radiology test results, and copies of x-rays and CT scans to the receiving hospital and the transport agency
- Information for family members who cannot accompany the patient during transfer: directions to the receiving trauma center, its address and parking information, relevant telephone numbers
- Cell phone numbers of family members who will be traveling (also shared with receiving facility)
- Methods for obtaining follow-up information and patient outcomes from the receiving trauma center, as well as feedback that could help improve the quality of trauma care at the rural facility

only a few such cases a month, the typical small rural hospital can easily identify and enter data on these cases into a register program without the need to hire special staff; a clerical employee with nurse supervision can do much of the work, or an ED nurse can accomplish this. The software can be a special trauma registry program used by the other trauma centers in the state, or something as simple as a locally designed spreadsheet with a minimum number of data elements.

Plans should include a method for obtaining follow-up and outcome information on all trauma cases transferred from the rural hospital to a higher-level trauma center. A method to track any quality issues or concerns on a specific trauma case should be in place. Customized local trauma "audit filters" or other quality indicators should be developed that may be useful in flagging possible quality concerns. Some possible rural hospital trauma audit filters are shown in Box 8-5.

The trauma committee at the rural hospital should conduct an interdisciplinary review of select trauma cases, particularly those where a quality concern has been raised or that trigger a local trauma audit filter. The group should assess the quality of care provided, make plans for improvement of any quality problems, see that those plans are implemented, and later reassess the situation to evaluate whether the problem has been corrected. Whenever possible, the rural hospital trauma committee should conduct its trauma quality improvement program cooperatively with the regional trauma center, thereby benefiting from their expertise. At some rural hospitals, representatives attend the quality improvement committee at the regional trauma center. If a system trauma quality improvement forum exists, such as through the county or regional EMS or trauma council, or in conjunction with the regional top level trauma center, the rural hospital should routinely participate in such trauma quality improvement efforts.

Rural Injury Prevention Programs

As a vital part of any rural community, the local hospital should take an active role in local injury prevention projects. This could easily be done in partnership with the local ambulance agency, fire department, school system, or public health department. A local injury prevention program that is linked with the regional trauma center's program or national injury prevention groups often works well. Some national injury prevention organizations with proven programs are Safe Kids, the American Trauma Society, and *Think First!* Nurses who take the lead in such programs should be recognized and rewarded for their community mindedness and leadership. All the general approaches to doing good injury prevention outlined in Chapter 6 of this book also apply to rural communities.

BOX 8-5 Sample Rural Hospital Trauma Quality Audit Filters

- Helicopter not immediately available for trauma transfer
- Inadequate or delayed medical staff response
- Transport crew delayed while procedures are completed (diagnostics or record-keeping)
- Transfer initiated more than 1 hour after arrival
- Significant "missed" injuries (based on feedback from receiving trauma center)
- Trauma patient transferred to the trauma center turns out to have minor injuries and is discharged from that center's emergency department

TRAUMA TELEMEDICINE

An exciting technology is now becoming available to help deal with many of the challenges of providing good trauma care in remote and rural environments.[24] Recent technologic advances in telemedicine and telepresence, and progress in building more robust trauma care systems, should lead to a reduction in the urban-rural quality disparity. Already several well-developed trauma telemedicine systems have been established,[25,26] and other applications of telemedicine technology to trauma care have been made successfully.[27-36] Such systems will likely proliferate in the early twenty-first century since they offer an easy-to-use solution to the lack of trauma care resources in remote locations.

Several systems have already successfully used simple approaches to trauma telemedicine technology. A simple digital camera can be used to capture photos of patients, specific injuries, x-rays, and crash scenes. Such still digital images can be easily transmitted to the trauma center as e-mail attachments.[28,29,35] Digital transfer of radiology images is already in wide use by rural hospitals, allowing the rapid transfer of an x-ray or CT image to a radiologist at a remote location, who returns an interpretation of those films within a short time. The radiologist may be located at the regional trauma center, other urban hospital, or even on the other side of the world—in India or Australia, for instance.

Fully evolved, live, two-way video systems connecting a trauma center with its referral rural ED remain uncommon. Two programs have clearly established their feasibility and effectiveness. The established programs in Burlington, Vermont,[25] and Tucson, Arizona,[26] can serve as models for further development of trauma telemedicine systems to serve additional rural populations. Such systems are likely to proliferate and might even be an expectation or requirement of the Level I regional trauma center of the future.

The initial results of the program in Vermont indicated a positive impact on the quality of care provided in the small rural EDs where this technology was used.[25] The University of Vermont and its teaching hospital, Fletcher Allen Health Care (a Level I trauma center), joined to install telemedicine units in multiple locations at the hospital in Burlington and in three of the trauma surgeons' homes. The trauma center initially partnered with four small community hospitals in rural areas (one in Vermont and three in New York). Three of the smaller hospitals used a portable telemedicine cart that could be positioned at the trauma patient's bedside in the ED. The fourth small hospital mounted the system permanently on a shelf in the ED. The rural locations also installed a second ceiling-mounted camera and microphone.

The infrastructure of the telemedicine network uses integrated services delivery network (ISDN) lines, which is actually a digital phone service provided by the phone company. The system is capable of handling 384 kilobits per second (kbps) using three ISDN lines per call. These lines connect the cameras and personal computer-based workstations at either end. The trauma surgeon at the trauma center in Burlington is able to control the cameras at the remote locations, panning, zooming, and tilting, to get the best view of the patient. The trauma surgeons are not credentialed on the medical staffs of the rural hospitals.

Specific criteria were used to select which trauma cases should use the system. Initial results demonstrated that there were 26 teletrauma consults in the first 10 months, starting in April 2000. Almost all of the cases involved blunt trauma. Of the 26 patients, 19 were subsequently transferred to the trauma center. Six (23%) remained at the local hospital. One died before a transfer occurred, but the trauma surgeon guided the rural physician through an emergency room thoracotomy for a ruptured aorta. In two cases, the teletrauma system was felt to be instrumental in saving the patient's life. In one case the rural surgeon, initially reluctant to perform a cricothyrotomy since he had not done one in 20 years, was able to successfully obtain the surgical airway with step-by-step guidance from the trauma surgeon in Burlington.[25]

The teletrauma program based in Tucson, Arizona,[26] has also demonstrated its utility in improving the quality of rural trauma care. The system started as a 2-year pilot study beginning in 2004, with one remote hospital in Douglas, Arizona, on the United States–Mexican border, partnering with the University of Arizona (UA) and the University Medical Center in Tucson (a Level I trauma center). In 2006, three additional rural hospitals were added, with plans for five more to come online in early 2007. This teletrauma program uses T1 lines installed at each rural hospital to connect with the Arizona Telemedicine Program system in Tucson, where a dedicated server then directs the communication to a trauma telemedicine room located adjacent to the offices of the trauma surgeons at the UA and the University Medical Center. Personal computer workstations are located at both the UA and on a mobile cart at each of the rural hospitals. The mobile cart system allows the direct transmission of video, audio, and live vital signs, including pulse oximetry, from the bedside of the trauma patient. The software system used is by VitalNet, Inc. In addition, video and audio of the trauma surgeon at the UA are transmitted to the mobile cart at the rural hospital, so that the surgeon is visible and audible to the physician, nurse, and patient. Several sets of headphones are used at the rural location to allow for private communication between the UA trauma surgeon and the rural doctor. If needed, the headphones can also be placed on the patient to allow for direct communication between the rural trauma patient and the trauma surgeon in Tucson. The trauma surgeon can control the pan, tilt, and zoom of the video camera in the rural ED. Each Tucson trauma surgeon was appointed to the medical staffs of the rural hospitals on a consulting or courtesy basis.

Initial results from the Tucson-based system demonstrated that of the first 26 cases, the teletrauma system was judged to be lifesaving in five cases (24%) and instrumental in avoiding an unnecessary and expensive helicopter trauma transfer in another five cases (24%) by keeping the patient at the local hospital.[36] An unexpected use of the system involved follow-up care of trauma patients who were ultimately discharged back to their home community after receiving care at the Tucson trauma center. In one case, an extensive and complicated post-surgical abdominal wound (Figure 8-1) was managed by weekly telepresence visits with the Tucson trauma surgeon. The patient went to his local ED in Douglas, Arizona, for a scheduled weekly virtual visit with the trauma surgeon in Tucson, resulting in successful wound healing without the otherwise necessary 240-mile weekly round trips by the

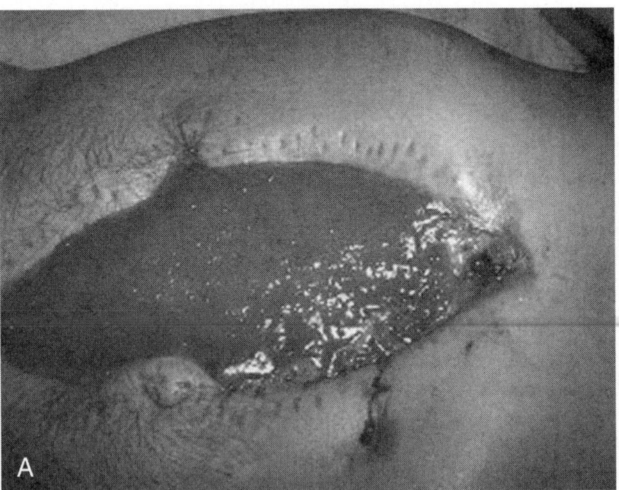

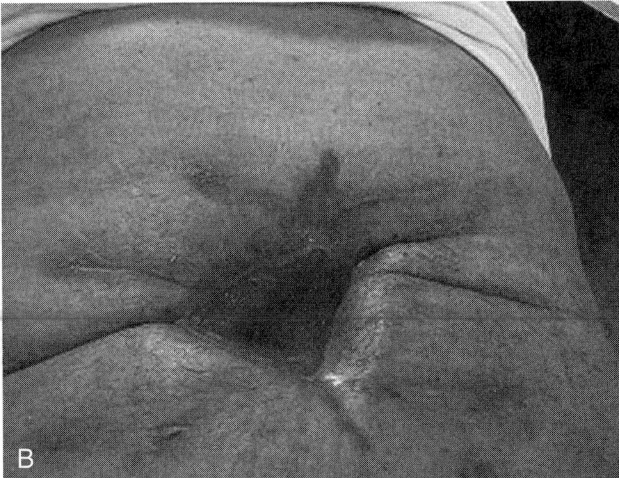

FIGURE 8-1 **A,** Complicated abdominal wound. **B,** Postdischarge follow-up management of this wound was done via the trauma telemedicine system.

patient. Staff in the rural ED quickly accepted the system as a vital component for providing trauma care in their remote location. Once the system is in place and staff become accustomed to its use, other possibilities present themselves.

In addition to the rural hospital/trauma center telemedicine system, another approach to trauma telemedicine has recently been implemented in Tucson. Called the Tucson "ER-Link" project,[26] it is a system that uses two-way video to connect ambulances in the field with the trauma center. This involves installation of a video camera in Tucson Fire Department ambulances, which allows transmission of audio and images directly to the trauma center through a system of wireless Internet connections throughout the city of Tucson. Launched late in 2006, the system was initially used only for trauma cases. It was a grant-funded project administered through the City of Tucson Transportation Department, in cooperation with the Tucson Fire Department and the University Medical Center. Plans call for several enhancements to the project beyond the initial phase. One will be integrating the existing city-wide traffic-control video camera system, currently used to make traffic control decisions, into the "ER-Link" network so that those at the trauma center can view active car crash scenes and even zoom in for closer views. Also planned is installation of external cameras on the tops of ambulances to allow viewing of crash scenes (already successfully tested), expansion of the wireless network to the outer margins of the city, and eventually expanding the wireless system into certain rural areas. Already, rural Santa Cruz County, Arizona, which is located on the Mexican border south of Tucson, has installed a wireless network along Interstate 19 as part of a Homeland Security emergency communications network. Along with a planned wireless network in one small town in southern Pima County near the same highway, this provides the infrastructure that could be used for rural EMS vehicle-to-trauma center live video connections for a nearly 60-mile stretch of rural highway. Both ground ambulances and EMS helicopters flying along this corridor would be able to connect into the system for instant communication with the trauma center. This could enhance the level of communications needed to provide improved medical oversight to the prehospital personnel, as well as allow the trauma center team a better preview of the details of incoming cases. "A picture is worth a thousand words" and may serve to heighten the awareness of personnel at the trauma center about the condition of an incoming trauma patient.

Based on these extraordinary initial successes, the State of Arizona's Department of Health Services initiated a grant-funded program in 2006 that will, when fully implemented, link the state burn center with multiple other hospitals that agree to provide the initial 48 hours of burn care in the event of a widespread disaster involving a large number of burn victims.[37] Using a trauma telemedicine system, Maricopa Medical Center in Phoenix, the state's only full burn center (the hospital is also a Level I trauma center), would then be able to supervise and direct the initial burn care being provided at a number of hospitals distributed throughout the state in the event of a major burn disaster event. This plan significantly extends the capacity and expertise of a single burn center. This sort of approach, enabled by teletrauma systems, can be applied to the trauma care system in general, thus improving the trauma system infrastructure and making it more capable of handling surges during disasters and Homeland Security emergencies.

Other potential future uses of the instant wireless transfer of information to the trauma center include systems that could be automatically activated when a car crashes. Most new cars now include sophisticated event data recorders, or "black boxes," that record many data elements during a car crash (vehicle speed, throttle speed, deceleration over time, brake position, number of occupied seats, whether a seatbelt was in use by each passenger, weight of each passenger, and airbag deployment).[38,39] Such data can be used to instantly calculate survival probability.[40] Coupled with global positioning system (GPS) location data and a cell phone or satellite-based communication system (similar to the On-Star system currently available as an option in many new cars), this information could be instantly transmitted to both 911 dispatch centers as well as the regional top-level trauma center. This would alert EMS and the trauma center staff to the crash and provide useful information, such as number of victims, speed, and crash severity.

Setting up such regional trauma telemedicine systems[41,42] takes careful planning, the faith and courage to try a cutting-edge approach to improving trauma care, and financial support. For instance, the costs for each rural location in the Southern Arizona system were about $42,000, not counting indirect costs such as staff education and the services of a local part-time teletrauma coordinator (usually a nurse). Grant funds significantly reduced the actual costs for each hospital to join the system.

To start a full trauma telemedicine system linking rural hospitals with the regional trauma center, a thorough business plan[43] should be developed by the lead agency. The business plan used to launch the Tucson trauma telemedicine program included a number of sections, as outlined in Box 8-6. Based on the business plan, a commitment by the lead organization should follow. With the use of knowledgeable consultants, available communications technology can then be thoroughly explored (satellite-based, microwave relay systems, T1 lines, Internet-based). Significant funding will be required and may be available through various grant-fund sources. A commitment to the concept by the trauma center surgeons is required. Then a program of outreach to the rural hospitals will be needed to discuss the program capabilities with their chief executive officer, chief nursing officer, ED nurse manager, ED physicians and other medical staff members, and the information technology officer. Plans for many system elements must be made, including medical staff privileges, how to initiate a trauma consult using the system, registration and medical records issues, staff training on the use of the system, contracts, finances, and local publicity. A plan must be made and implemented for the

BOX 8-6 Business Plan for Trauma Telemedicine Program, Organizational Elements

- Executive summary
- Vision
- Products/services
  - Product/service description
  - Technology
- Market analysis
  - Overall market
  - Market segments
  - Target market and customers
  - Customer needs
  - Opportunities
  - Threats and risks
- Marketing and sales
  - Marketing strategy
  - Promotion and incentives
  - Publicity
- Operations
  - Steps to product/service delivery
  - How a trauma telemedicine consult works
  - Management team
  - Personnel plan
  - Trauma surgeon staffing
  - System downtime
  - Support staffing
  - Facilities
  - Other management considerations
  - Telemedicine program infrastructure
  - Medical staff credentials
  - Medical records
  - Project database
  - Contracts
- Finance
  - Costs
  - Revenues
  - Grant-funding opportunities

collection of data and a way to evaluate program effectiveness. This all clearly requires significant resources and trauma center support staff energy and commitment.

SUMMARY

Providing quality trauma care in rural areas presents many challenges. Many of the barriers encountered, such as delay in discovery, insufficient resources, limited educational opportunities, and a paucity of relevant research, may be difficult to overcome. But progress is being made. Educational opportunities are expanding, aided in large part by advances in telecommunications technology. Rural trauma systems are being established. Rural providers are working hard to make certain their unique needs are recognized by national trauma organizations. Thoughtful planning and implementation of trauma systems in rural areas can improve outcomes.

REFERENCES

1. Rogers FB, Shackford SR, Osler TM et al: Rural trauma: the challenge for the next decade, *J Trauma* 47(4):802-821, 1999.
2. *Office of Community and Rural Health Rural Health Data Book.* Available online at www.doh.wa.gov/hsqa/ocrh/. Accessed October 26, 2006.
3. *National Clearinghouse for Frontier Communities.* Available online at www.frontierus.org. Accessed October 26, 2006.
4. *Montana Department of Commerce Census 2000 Census and Economic Education Center.* Available on-line at http://ceic.mt.gov/urban_rural.asp. Accessed October 6, 2006.
5. *Traffic Safety Problem Identification FY 2002.* Annual Report from the Traffic Safety Bureau, Transportation Planning Division of the Montana Department of Transportation. Available at www.mdt.state.mt.us. Accessed October 6, 2006.
6. Rinker CF: Rural Trauma. In Mattox KL, Feliciano DV, More EE, editors: *Trauma,* ed 4, New York, 2000, McGraw-Hill.
7. Younis MZ: Comparison study of urban and small rural hospitals financial and economic performance. *Online Journal of Rural Nursing and Health Care 2003.* Available online at http://www.rno.org/journal.issues/Vol-3/issue-1/Younis.htm.
8. *Report to the Congress: Medicare in Rural America,* June 12, 2001. Statement of Glenn M. Hackbarth, J.D., Chairman, Medicare Payment Advisory Commission before the Subcommittee on Health Committee on Ways and Means, U.S. House of Representatives.
9. Institute of Medicine of the National Academies Committee on the Future of Emergency Care in the U.S. Health System: *Emergency Medical Services at the Crossroads,* released June 14, 2006. The report series was sponsored by the Josiah Macy Jr. Foundation; the U.S. Department of Health and Human Services Health Resources and Services Administration, Agency for Healthcare Research and Quality, and Centers for Disease Control and Prevention; and the U.S. Department of Transportation's National Highway Traffic Safety Administration.
10. Mullins RJ: A historical perspective of trauma system development in the United States, *J Trauma* 47(3):S8-S14, 1999.
11. Bazzoli GJ, Madura KJ, Cooper GF et al: Progress in the development of trauma systems in the United States: results of a national survey, *JAMA* 273(5):395-401, 1995.
12. Mann NC, Hedges JR, Mullins RJ et al: Rural hospital transfer patterns before and after implementation of a statewide trauma system, *Acad Emerg Med* 4(8):764-771, 1997.
13. Position paper on trauma care systems. Third National Injury Control Conference April 22-25, 1991, Denver, Colo, *J Trauma* 32(2):127-129, 1992.
14. *EMS Agenda for the Future.* The National Highway Traffic Safety Administration (NHTSA), the Health Resources and Services Administration, together with the National Association of State Emergency Medical Services Directors and the National Association of EMS Physicians, submitted April 16, 1996.
15. Committee on Trauma. *Resources for Optimal Care of the Injured Patient 2006,* Chicago, 2006, American College of Surgeons.
16. *The Electronic Library of Trauma Lectures,* Santa Fe, NM, Society of Trauma Nurses, 2004.
17. Committee on Trauma. *Advanced Trauma Life Support for Doctors: Student Course Manual,* ed 7, Chicago, 2004, American College of Surgeons.

18. Hotz HA, Henn R, Lush S et al, editors: *Advanced Trauma Care for Nurses Provider Manual,* Santa Fe, NM, 2003, Society of Trauma Nurses.
19. Campbell JE, editor: *Basic Trauma Life Support for Paramedics and Other Advanced Providers*, ed 5, Upper Saddle River, NJ, 2004, Brady.
20. McSwain ME, Frame S, Salomone JP, editors. *PHTLS: Basic and Advanced Prehospital Trauma Life Support*, ed 5, St. Louis, 2003, Mosby.
21. Brain Trauma Foundation, American Association of Neurological Surgeons, Congress of Neurological Surgeons, AANS/CNS Joint Section on Neurotrauma and Critical Care: Guidelines for the management of severe traumatic brain injury, ed 3, *J Neurotrauma* 24(Suppl 1):S1-S106, 2007.
22. Committee on Trauma: *Resources for Optimal Care of the Injured Patient 1997.* Chicago, 1997, American College of Surgeons.
23. *Rural Trauma.* Available at www.facs.org/trauma/ruraltrauma. Accessed January 16, 2007.
24. Ricci MA, Caputo M, Amour J et al: Telemedicine reduces discrepancies in rural trauma care, *Telemed J E Health* 9(1):3-11, 2003.
25. Rogers FB, Ricci M, Caputo M et al: The use of telemedicine for real-time video consultation between trauma center and community hospital in a rural setting improves early trauma care. Preliminary results, *J Trauma* 51(6):1037-1041, 2001.
26. Latifi R, Ong CA, Peck KA et al: Telepresence and telemedicine in trauma and emergency care management. In Latifi R, editor: *Establishing Telemedicine in Developing Countries: From Inception to Implementation*, Amsterdam, 2004, IOS Press.
27. Maull K: The Friendship airport disaster exercise: pioneering effort in trauma telemedicine, *Eur J Med Res* 7(suppl):48, 2002.
28. Krupinski E, Gonzales M, Gonzales C et al: Evaluation of digital camera for acquiring radiographic images for telemedicine applications, *Telemed J E Health* 6(3):297-302, 2000.
29. Corr P, Couper I, Beningfield SJ et al: A simple telemedicine system using a digital camera, *J Telemed Telecare* 6(4):233-236, 2000.
30. Lambrecht CJ: Telemedicine in trauma care: description of 100 trauma teleconsults, *Telemed J* 3(4):265-268, 1997.
31. Tachakra S, Lynch M, Newson R et al: A comparison of telemedicine with face-to-face consultations for trauma management, *J Telemed Telecare* 6 (suppl 1):S178-S181, 2000.
32. Wirthlin DJ, Buradagunta S, Edwards RA et al: Telemedicine in vascular surgery: feasibility of digital imaging for remote management of wounds, *J Vasc Surg* 27(6):1089-1099, 1998.
33. Schopp LH, Johnston BR, Merveille OC: Multidimensional telecare strategies for rural residents with brain injury, *J Telemed Telecare* 6(suppl 1):S146-S149, 2000.
34. Tachakra S, Jaye P, Bak J et al: Supervising trauma support by telemedicine, *J Telemed Telecare* 6(suppl 1):S7-S11, 2000.
35. Chiao L, Sharapov S, Sargsyan AE et al: Ocular examination for trauma: clinical ultrasound aboard the international space station, *J Trauma* 58(5):885-889, 2005.
36. Latifi R, Judkins D, Ziemba M et al: *A New Model for Rural Trauma and Emergency Management: Southern Arizona Teletrauma and Telepresence Program,* a research abstract presented at the 2006 AHSC Frontiers in Biomedical Research Poster Forum at the University of Arizona, Tucson, December 1, 2006.
37. *Burn Care Network Project*, Office of Emergency Preparedness, Arizona Department of Health Services, 2006.
38. Chidester A, Hinch J, Mercer TC et al: *Recording Automotive Crash Event Data.* Presented at the International Symposium on Transportation Recorders, May 3-5, 1999, Arlington, Va. Available online at www.nhtsa.dot.gov/cars/problems/studies/record/chidester.htm. Accessed December 20, 2006.
39. Niehoff P, Gabler HC, Brophy J et al: *Evaluation of Event Data Recorders in Full Systems Crash Tests.* Available online at www.nrd.nhtsa.dot.gov/pdf/nrd-01/esv/esv19/Other/Print%2009.pdf.
40. Champion H, Augenstein B, Cushing KH et al: *Reducing Highway Deaths and Disabilities with Automatic Wireless Transmission of Serious Injury Probability Ratings from Crash Recorders to Emergency Medical Services Providers.* Presented at the International Symposium on Transportation Recorders, May 3-5, 1999, Arlington, Va. Available online at www.nhtsa.dot.gov/cars/problems/studies/acns/champion.htm. Accessed December 20, 2006.
41. Aucar J, Granchi T, Liscum K et al: Is regionalization of trauma care using telemedicine feasible and desirable? *Am J Surg* 180(6):535-539, 2000.
42. Boulanger B, Kearney P, Ochoa J et al: Telemedicine: a solution to the follow-up of rural trauma patients? *J Am Coll Surg* 192(4):447-452, 2001.
43. Judkins D, et al: *Business Plan and Operational Protocols to Ensure Sustainability and Acceptance of Teletrauma Program.* Congress of International Society for Telemedicine and E-Health and the 2nd Conselho Brasileiro de Telemedicine e Telessaude, Brazil, October 19, 2005.

9

MASS CASUALTY INCIDENTS

Daniel G. Judkins, Frank G. Walter

The timing of traumatic incidents is usually erratic. There are slow times with few or no trauma patients, then several traumatic events may occur nearly at once, with each producing more than one patient. Some incidents may produce a larger than usual number of injured persons. Calls for emergency medical services (EMS) trauma response and trauma case arrivals at the hospital occur in this same episodic manner. When the number of injury incidents, or the scope of a single incident, is much larger than usual (a large-scale trauma incident), multiple casualties can result and trauma care systems must rapidly expand capacity to handle the high number of cases.

The question for any trauma care system becomes not *if* such a large-scale trauma incident will occur, but *when*, and *what* will be its cause and characteristics. Preparing for an abnormally large surge of trauma cases is an essential part of providing quality trauma care in any system.

Various terms are used to refer to large-scale injury incidents. Most have no precise, universally accepted definition. However, the definitions in Box 9-1 provide the reader with an idea of the generally accepted meaning for various terms frequently associated with large-scale trauma incidents. Contingency planning for trauma care under any of these scenarios becomes more challenging as the scope of the event enlarges.

The medical response to any large-scale trauma incident will depend on many factors, including the nature or cause of the incident. Events that cause disasters can be categorized as natural or man-made (Table 9-1). The majority of large-scale disasters worldwide have inflicted physical injuries and deaths. There are several notable examples in which the disaster event inflicted harm simply by exposure to a toxic substance or infectious organisms rather than by direct force. These include the 1984 Bhopal, India, chemical release; the 1986 Chernobyl nuclear power plant incident; the 1995 Tokyo sarin gas attack; the 2002 Moscow theater anesthetic gas incident; and the 2003 severe acute respiratory syndrome (SARS) epidemic. Exposure to excessive thermal energy can cause burn injuries and deaths, such as happened in the 1996 disco fire in Manila, Philippines. The lack of essential agents, such as food, has led to several large-scale famines, and insufficient oxygen has caused death in the case of mass drownings (e.g ., the 2004 Indian Ocean tsunami). Many disasters, however, produce physical injuries by direct exposure to kinetic energy (e.g., blunt, penetrating, and blast). An analysis of "significant terrorist events" for a 5-year period (1999-2003) shows that only two of 128 incidents (1.5%) were not caused by direct exposure to kinetic energy, usually a gunshot or explosion; 69% (89/128) were a result of a bombing or explosion.[1]

Because the potential remains for natural and man-made events that can precipitate disaster, and because such disasters can occur at any time, trauma systems must remain prepared. Disaster preparedness, therefore, should focus on trauma system preparedness for extreme casualty surges.

BOX 9-1 Definitions of Terminology Related to Mass Casualty Incidents

Mass casualty incident (MCI): A trauma event in which the needs of numerous injured individuals overwhelm the capability of the trauma center or trauma system.* For example, at a small rural hospital, the arrival of two or more seriously injured patients may be referred to as an MCI, whereas at a larger trauma center the term may apply to an incident producing even more trauma patients, perhaps 5, 10, or more.

Disaster: A sudden natural or man-made event that results in destruction, damage, injuries, or deaths. (See Table 9-1 for examples of events that can cause disaster.)

Weapons-of-mass destruction (WMD) event: Event involving weapons of extraordinary destructive power.

CBRNE: Chemical, biological, radiological, nuclear, or explosive incident. (This term is now used in favor of the older "NBC," which stood for nuclear, biologic, or chemical.)

*Farmer JC, Jimenez EJ, Talmor DS et al: *Fundamentals of Disaster Management*, Des Plaines, Ill, 2003, Society of Critical Care Medicine.

TABLE 9-1 **Types of Disasters**

Natural	Man-Made
Flood	Fire
Severe thunderstorm, hail, lightning	Firearm multiple assault
Tornado	Accidental explosion
Hurricane or typhoon	Explosive device (intentional)
Blizzard, ice storm, river ice jam, iceberg	Riot
Avalanche	Crowd stampede
Weather-caused transportation crash event (fog, sand storm)	Electrical power failure
Volcano eruption	Structure collapse (building, bridge, mine)
Earthquake	Dam collapse
Tsunami/tidal wave	Transportation event (airplane, railroad, motor vehicle, boat)
Fire (large urban or wildfire)	Toxic chemical release
Landslide	Radiological/nuclear release
Meteorite/asteroid/comet	War/military
Epidemic	Despotism/genocide
Famine, drought	Weapons of mass destruction (chemical, biological, radiological, nuclear, explosive)

Adapted from Dallas CE, Coule PL, James JJ et al, editors: *Basic Disaster Life Support Provider Manual, Version 2.5.* 2004, American Medical Association.

INITIAL RESPONSE

Initial response to a multicasualty incident (MCI) includes discovery of the event and casualties; calls for help; EMS response to the scene; and search, rescue, triage, prehospital treatment, and transport of victims. Hospital facilities, particularly trauma-designated facilities, that may receive patients also begin immediate preparation for an influx of wounded as an initial response to the event.

AT THE SCENE

After the incident is first discovered, EMS and law enforcement groups will be dispatched. As additional details indicate the size of the event, more response units may be requested and dispatched. First-arriving units will assess the scene, making first impressions about the size and scope of the event, and the presence of ongoing safety hazards. One method of approaching the scene assessment uses the familiar ABCDEF mnemonic, as described in Box 9-2.[2]

Organizing Scene Efforts

One useful scheme to organize initial efforts is called the RED survey.[3] *RED* stands for *R*apid *E*valuation of *D*isaster. Step 1 of the RED survey is the incident survey (again based on ABCDE) as described in Box 9-3. Part of step 1 is "D = DISASTER,"[3] which is another approach aimed at organizing the management of the disaster scene. The mnemonic *DISASTER* is described in Box 9-4.

Step 2, the Casualty Survey, is synonymous with the customary trauma primary survey, in which the provider identifies immediate life threats. This also forms the basis for MCI triage. In a disaster, one addition to the "D" (disability) step of the clinical primary survey, is to consider differential diagnoses that are commonly caused by the type of MCI that occurred.

Step 3 is the provision of immediate life-saving interventions, such as open and maintain airway, assist ventilation, stop bleeding, needle thoracostomy, pericardiocentesis, and antidote administration.

BOX 9-2 **Mnemonic for Sizing Up the Scene of a Mass Casualty Incident**

A Anticipate victims and injuries. What types of injuries can you expect given the nature of the incident?
B Breathing. Is this possibly a toxic environment? Assess for toxic releases.
C Cars/crowds. Look for safety hazards associated with traffic and large crowds of people.
D Disability. What further threatens victims and rescuers? Search for additional hazards, such as unstable buildings and adverse weather.
E Electricity. Look for potential for electrocution from a damaged electrical supply.
F Fuel/fire. Are there spilled fuels or other causes of potential fire, such as natural gas leaks?

Adapted from Augustine J: *The ABCs of Size-Up. Emergency Medical Services* (EMSResponder.com). Available online at http://publicsafety.com/article/article.jsp?id=2727&siteSection=2 2007. Accessed July 6, 2007.

BOX 9-3 Incident Survey of the Rapid Evaluation of Disaster

A Aware of all hazards
B Barrier. *Barrier* and *Contain* refer to efforts to prevent the enlargement of the disaster scene.
C Contain
D DISASTER (see Box 9-4 for more details)
E Enter the scene (all done before starting patient care)

American Medical Association. *Advanced Disaster Life Support Provider Manual* (Version 2.0), 2004:1-4 to 1-5.

BOX 9-4 Mnemonic Aimed at Organizing the Management of the Disaster Scene

D Detect the reason for the disaster
I Incident Command
S Scene security and safety
A Assess hazards
S Support (What resources are needed?)
T Triage and treatment
E Evacuation (transport)
R Recovery (long-term implications, costs, impact)

American Medical Association: *Advanced Disaster Life Support Provider Manual* (Version 2.0), 2004:1-19.

Scene Safety

Assessing scene dangers should be the first priority of responding units. If first responders are themselves injured, the problem of trying to provide care for numerous injured patients is compounded. In their zeal to help the injured, initial care providers often push past obvious hazards; a great deal of discipline and frequent practice drills are required to overcome this natural but dangerous impulse. Hazards may include oncoming traffic, structural instability, adverse weather, criminal or terrorist activity, the presence of hazardous materials (HAZMAT), and many other dangers. These hazards must be properly contained, controlled, or otherwise appropriately mitigated to pave the way for effective rescue and treatment of the victims.

Triage

As safety hazards are controlled and casualties are located, the next priority becomes triage. The casualties must be rapidly sorted into severity categories. Discipline and practice are again needed to thwart the impulse to begin immediate resource-intensive treatment of the first serious cases identified. Those performing triage must press on to continue to count and triage the injured, refusing to be sidetracked from this goal by stopping to provide treatment. As additional personnel arrive, they can begin early treatment of the most seriously injured. The discipline and determination to perform the triage task effectively may be one of the most difficult aspects of MCI management.

A widely used scheme for multicasualty triage is the START protocol (Simple Triage and Rapid Treatment).[4] This method (Figure 9-1) effectively categorizes casualties as immediate (red), delayed (yellow), minor (green), or dead/dying (black). Those with impairment to breathing, circulation, and consciousness are categorized as immediate. These are the critical cases that require treatment without delay. The delayed cases may have serious injury, such as fractures or bleeding without shock, but will likely survive some delay in initiation of treatment. The minor cases are often referred to as the "walking wounded." They should be asked to assemble in an identified area nearby, to be treated when more resources become available. A pediatric modification of this triage method is known as "JumpSTART."[5] Although similar to the START triage method, JumpSTART includes pediatric-specific steps, such as defining respiratory rates differently than in the adult approach.

Another useful triage scheme is the MASS Triage model (M = Move, A = Assess, S = Sort, S = Send) with its associated "*ID-me!*" mnemonic for triage severity categories (I = Immediate, D = Delayed, M = Minimal, E = Expectant).[3]

Incident Command

As triage continues, additional arriving personnel should establish an incident command center. Usually a senior official of the EMS agency with jurisdiction will take control of this effort. The Incident Command System (ICS)[6] is an effective method of bringing organization and control to the complex effort of providing initial care at the disaster scene. An overall incident commander takes control of the entire scene response and all associated major decisions. Assisting the incident commander are any number of possible staff, such as those in charge of:

- Planning—Evaluate information received; develop action plans and strategy
- Finance—Oversee monetary aspects of personnel, staff injuries, and overall event management
- Logistics—Ensure adequate supplies, equipment, water, food
- Operations—Manage scene control, rescue, triage, decontamination, treatment, ambulances, helicopters, other transport, communications, and medical support

One issue common to many large-scale disaster events is the organization and control of medical personnel on the scene. Often responding from many different agencies, EMS personnel can be numerous. In addition, nurses and physicians may respond to the scene. With large numbers of personnel present who do not usually work with each other, disorganization and a chaotic work environment are major risks. An additional factor often contributing to scene disorganization is the frequent lack of radio communication resources with common interagency operational frequencies. Responding personnel should yield to the direction of the ICS.

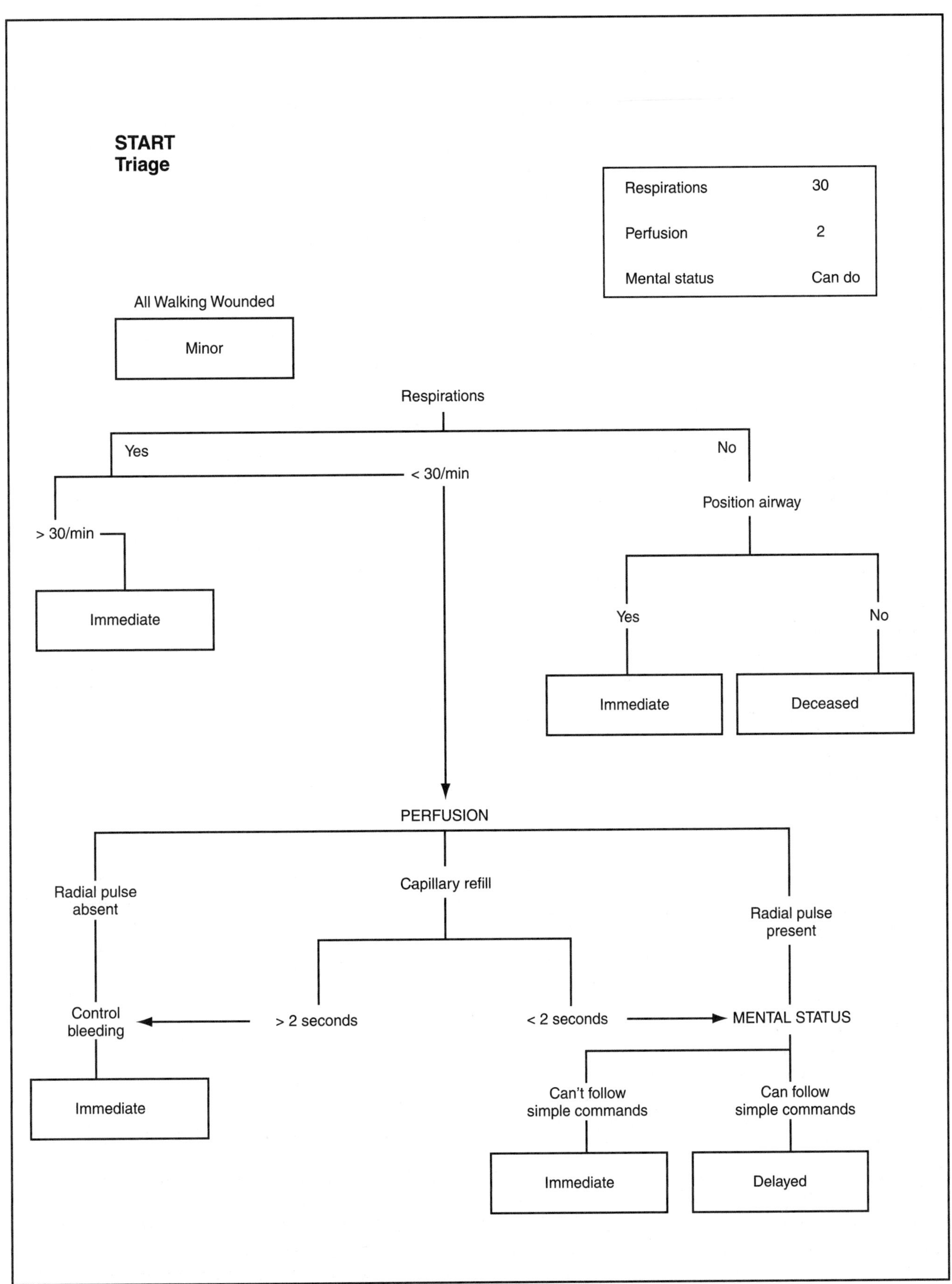

FIGURE 9-1. START algorithm. *Used with permission from Young K:* Simple triage and rapid treatment, START, 1999. *Office of Education and Certification, MIEMSS. Available online at http://miemss.umaryland.edu/Start.pdf.*

At the Hospital

News of the incident often arrives at the hospital first through EMS radio communications to the emergency department (ED), although sometimes word is received through the media. Many systems provide for automatic early hospital notification of large-scale incidents through central dispatch systems. Monitoring EMS communications is crucial. Getting accurate details helps the hospital to implement its disaster response appropriately, ramping up capacity rapidly while guarding against overresponse. The ED should immediately relay all news to the on-duty hospital clinical nursing supervisor and the hospital administrator on call.

First Decisions

First decisions are made based on an assessment of the probable impact of the incident on the hospital. These decisions are usually made by the nursing clinical supervisor and the administrator on call. Such decisions are usually made in close collaboration with on-duty ED and trauma personnel. Does the hospital need to be protected from dangers? Will increased capacity be needed? What are the likely medical needs of the casualties? How many casualties can be expected to arrive? What personnel need immediate notification? Should the hospital incident command center be opened now? Should the disaster plan be implemented, and to what extent? Should off-duty personnel be called in?

Hospital Security. Protecting the hospital from dangers, to ensure that it is able to continue operations, is always the first priority in any emergency situation. It is the same concept as ensuring scene safety for EMS personnel at the disaster site. Sometimes the walking wounded and citizens concerned about their loved ones or their own safety will quickly arrive at the hospital. If they arrive in large numbers, they will contribute to chaos and interfere with the hospital's capacity to respond to the disaster. Some multicasualty incidents may involve HAZMAT. Steps must be taken immediately to prevent the inadvertent introduction of such materials into the hospital. Care must be taken when dealing with a possible terrorist event that all persons brought to the hospital are carefully evaluated outside of the hospital to ensure that they do not have explosives, weapons, or HAZMAT hidden on their person. Therefore, the first decision after notification should be whether to secure the hospital via a lock-down procedure. When in lock-down, all entries should be locked using a preplanned and frequently practiced procedure. Admittance to the hospital should be through defined areas carefully controlled by security. When doing this, provision should be made for identification of and rapid admittance to the hospital of arriving off-duty hospital staff.

Implementing the Disaster Plan. The next priority is launching the disaster plan in a measured manner. Quick attempts should be made to clarify the details of the incident, given that early information about such an incident is often inaccurate. But the decision must be made quickly. A disaster plan that has incremental steps built in facilitates expanding the scale of the response rapidly while guarding against overreaction.

Hospital Incident Command System. The hospital command center should be opened and an incident commander identified. One good example of an administrative organization for hospital disaster response is the hospital incident command system (HICS) developed by the California Emergency Medical Services Authority.[7] The HICS plan calls for a hospital incident commander (IC) to be in charge of all disaster decisions. The IC will be assisted by several section chiefs, typically including the operations chief, the planning section chief, the logistics chief, and the finance/administration section chief. In addition, support for administrative decision making will be provided by a public information officer, a safety officer, and a liaison officer. Additional managers and unit leaders may be organized under the section chiefs, as the scope of the incident demands. The details of a typical HICS organizational chart can be found in Figure 9-2.

The HICS is outlined in great detail in the *Hospital Incident Command System Guidebook,*[7] which is available online for download. All appropriate hospital leaders and key medical staff members should be thoroughly trained on the HICS system. Many such personnel will not want to devote the time necessary to this training. As a result, HICS education and practice exercises should be of the highest quality, providing realistic scenarios that demand that the participants think critically and thoroughly explore the implications of the various HICS roles. Practice drills and exercises with realistic scenarios should be conducted on a regular and frequent basis (such as quarterly). These approaches will demonstrate the relevance of the HICS education and enhance administrative commitment to devoting the time necessary to training. The "Introduction to ICS for Healthcare/Hospitals" (IS 100 HC) course and the "Applying ICS to Healthcare Organizations" (IS 200) course are available online.[6]

Several key trauma and emergency nurses, as well as hospital personnel who are expert in the function of local/regional EMS and trauma systems, should also participate in the HICS training and practice. The key liaison person responsible for integration of the hospital incident command structure with the local/regional unified command at the community emergency operations center should be a senior hospital leader with extensive knowledge of local EMS and trauma system function.

The preestablished hospital command center should be located in an area likely to remain accessible during a disaster, large enough to accommodate the command staff, and stocked with all needed supplies and equipment. Communications equipment is particularly critical, including multiple telephone lines, radio communications, and computer systems. The command center should be able to view multiple television channels simultaneously, project video, and have communication tools available to support decision making such a white boards, charts, and flip charts. Regional maps,

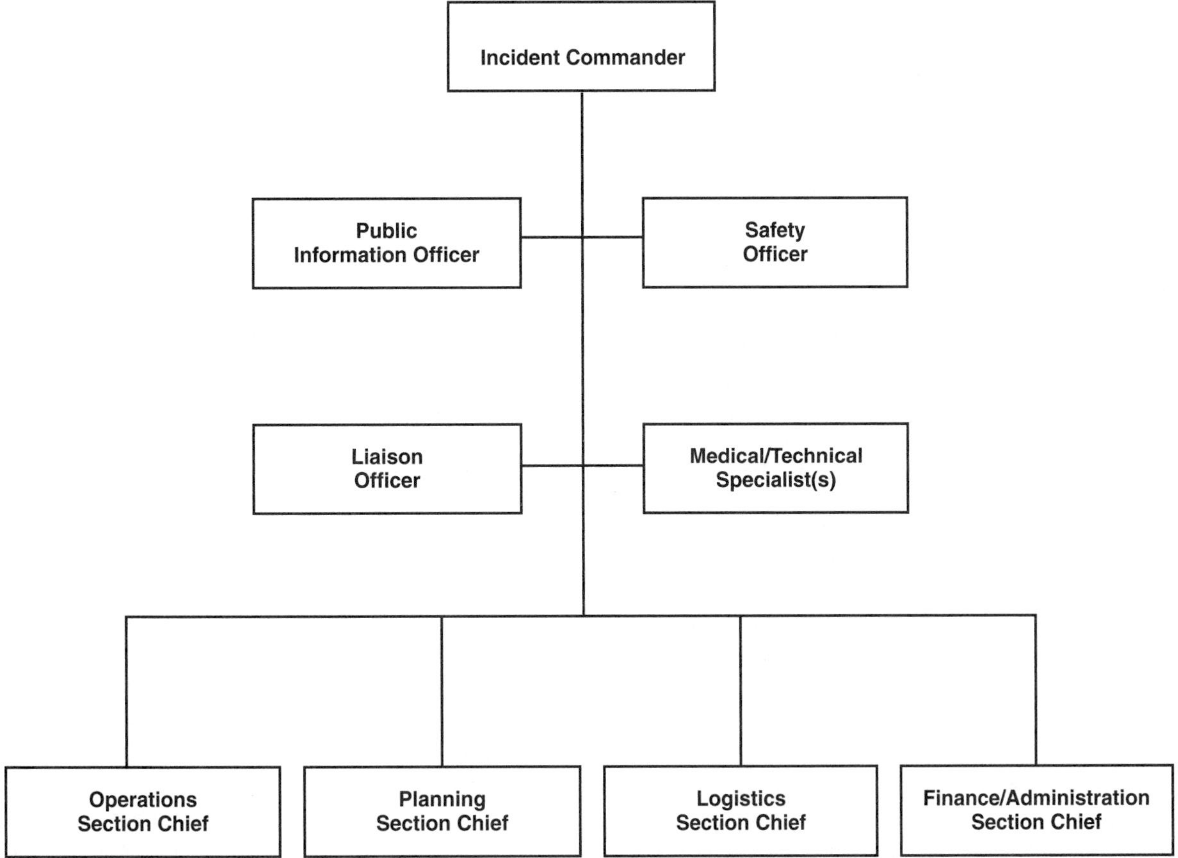

FIGURE 9-2. Hospital Incident Command System Organizational Chart. *Adapted from Skivington S, DeAtley C, Saruwatari M et al:* Hospital Incident Command System Guidebook. *California Emergency Medical Services Authority, 2006. Available online at http://www.emsa.ca.gov/hics/hics guidebook and glossary.pdf.*

hospital architectural plans, copies of hospital and community disaster plans, personnel and supply inventories, job action sheets, and other disaster supplies and equipment should be on hand. Frequent HICS practice exercises should take place involving the hospital command center so that all HICS leaders are familiar with its capabilities.

Decontamination

If HAZMAT are involved in the incident, hospital decontamination facilities should be immediately activated. These facilities should be outside the hospital, to prevent contamination and closure of the ED or hospital. This can only be accomplished through careful preplanning and frequent drilling. If patients are properly decontaminated at the scene, procedures at the hospital arrival area may be limited to a rapid reassessment and a determination that the patients are ready to move to the triage area. If solid or liquid contamination is adherent to patients, then they should be decontaminated before proceeding to triage. Special provision must be made for critical cases that may need simultaneous decontamination and immediate intervention for life threats without placing the resuscitation personnel in jeopardy. Again, this requires pre-event practice and drill by the trauma resuscitation personnel.

An organized approach to handling HAZMAT cases is facilitated by use of another modification to the familiar ABCDE approach, using the Poisoning Treatment Paradigm™ A^2BCDE (Box 9-5).[8] Absorption is altered by decontamination, removal of adherent material, and dilution. Certain antidotes alter catabolism, which is the process of the body breaking down chemicals. Sometimes the toxic material

BOX 9-5 Poisoning Treatment Paradigm™

A Alter absorption
A Administer antidote
B Basics
C Change catabolism
D Distribute differently
E Enhance elimination

Bronstein AC: Medical management of hazmat victims. In Walter FG, editor: *Advanced HAZMAT Life Support Provider Manual*, ed 3, Tucson, AZ, 2003, Arizona Board of Regents for the University of Arizona.

can be distributed differently in the body so that it creates a less harmful effect, such as displacing carbon monoxide from hemoglobin by providing high-flow oxygen. The elimination from the body of some materials can be enhanced by administering oxygen, providing dialysis, or forcing diuresis.

Triage

A triage receiving area should then be opened rapidly. Often outside the ED at the ambulance area, it must be large enough to handle the expected surge of arrivals. Preassembled triage supplies should be distributed to personnel assigned to the triage function. Those performing this function should be experienced in triage and trauma (trauma or emergency nurses, emergency medicine physicians, or trauma surgeons).[9,10] Minimal record-keeping is facilitated by brief disaster tags or forms and help from scribes or medical records personnel. Communication between the triage area and patient-receiving areas for red, yellow, and green cases should be established (perhaps via portable radio). A communication link between triage and the hospital incident command center is also essential. Such a communication link can facilitate, for example, the transfer of logs documenting patient arrivals and dispositions from the triage area to the hospital incident command center.

Trauma Resuscitation Surge

Quick preparations should be made for handling the expected surge of seriously injured victims. The key to increasing surge capacity is to develop well-rehearsed plans using two general approaches: expanding physical capacity of the resuscitation area and decreasing the case throughput time.

How to Develop Trauma Resuscitation Surge Capacity: A 10-Step Plan

1. **Rapidly discharge existing trauma resuscitation case load.** Sort existing cases in trauma resuscitation by identifying those who can be delayed (yellow) and those who are minor (green). Send the green and yellow cases to their ultimate destination (e.g., home, an inpatient unit, or a separate holding area such as a clinical decision unit). Finish up existing serious (red) trauma cases rapidly by making decisions now and performing needed damage-control[11-13] surgery immediately. These patients can also then be sent to their ultimate destination.
2. **Rapidly discharge existing general ED patients.** This will open up additional space and health care staff that can be used for trauma resuscitation. Consider sending minor existing ED cases home with minimal treatment and instructions for later follow-up after providing necessary but simplified treatment (e.g., medication, temporary splint). Some work has been published on approaches for ED admission avoidance in the event of nondisaster routine ED overcrowding. Principles from these efforts might be applicable in large-scale trauma incident situations.[14] ED patients who still remain can be rapidly sent to general nursing inpatient units.[15,16]
3. **Increase nursing and support staffing.** Decide on the number and type of additional nursing staff that will be needed for trauma resuscitation duties. Nurses from the ED and other units throughout the hospital need to be called upon to provide staff for the resuscitation area. Increase support staff as needed (e.g., housekeepers, materials management personnel, laboratory technicians, radiologists, and social workers). This can be coordinated by the hospital clinical supervisor.
4. **Make orientation of nursing personnel new to the trauma resuscitation area and disaster procedure more efficient.** This may be accomplished by presenting nurses with a very simplified role instruction card (Box 9-6).
5. **Increase physician staffing.** Have additional doctors report to a specified area, such as the triage area, to be teamed with a nurse and to receive an incoming trauma patient for resuscitation.
6. **Use staffing efficiently.** Do this by reducing superfluous personnel per case. For instance, assign one doctor and one nurse to each immediate/serious trauma case (red triage category), and send each delayed (yellow triage category) case to a designated area, where each doctor/nurse team can evaluate and treat several cases simultaneously. Minor trauma (green category) cases can be sent to a large but minimally staffed holding area.
7. **Increase resuscitation space.** Convert ED beds near the trauma resuscitation area into trauma beds for immediate cases. Make use of any adjacent large, open spaces such as waiting rooms and, when weather permits, outdoor protected spaces. Ideal alternate treatment areas may include the post–anesthesia care unit and special procedure rooms, such as the catheterization lab and endoscopy units, which are typically well equipped with supplies, medical gases, and monitoring systems. (One trauma center [Scottsdale Healthcare Osborne, Scottsdale, Arizona] has installed multiple medical gas outlets (oxygen and suction) in their ED waiting rooms and hallways to be used during disaster trauma surges.)
8. **Increase supplies and equipment.** Have additional general trauma supply carts, airway supplies, IVs, and procedure trays brought immediately to the resuscitation area from the supply department. The supply department should begin rapid turnaround of used sterile procedure trays.
9. **Decrease time-consuming diagnostics and procedures that can be safely deferred.** Defer all diagnostics and interventions for conditions that are not life-threatening (e.g., postpone x-rays until later for simple extremity fractures with good distal circulation and defer suturing of lacerations that are not bleeding excessively). Suspend all elective

Box 9-6 Simple Trauma Resuscitation Nursing Role Card

1. You will be assigned one serious trauma case, coming in from the triage area located at the ED ambulance receiving area. Report there now to receive your case.
2. At the triage area, you will be teamed with one physician for this case.
3. You will be directed to a location in or near the ED trauma resuscitation area. Take your patient there.
4. Perform a rapid trauma assessment, looking for life threats (airway, breathing, circulation/bleeding/shock/lack of limb perfusion, disability neurologic/brain/spinal cord) and immediately notify the physician of these problems and assist to resolve the issue.
5. Airway supplies are located in Room 123, shelf A. Procedure trays are located on shelf B, and additional medical supplies are located on shelf C.
5. Limit diagnostic tests to what is absolutely essential for making immediate clinical decisions.
6. Your goal is immediate treatment of life threats and moving your patient rapidly out of the trauma resuscitation area. Contact the lead trauma resuscitation nurse (pager 1001) for help with getting your patient to the operating room, intensive care unit, inpatient unit, or essential diagnostic area.
7. Make abbreviated clinical notes on the one-page disaster medical record.
8. Work very fast.
9. Report back to the triage area for another patient when you finish with the first.

surgery and elective scheduled procedures until the situation is stabilized.[16]

10. **Decrease resuscitation throughput time** (time of arrival to discharge from resuscitation area). Focus on life-threatening problems only and making decisions rapidly. Decide "yes" or "no" on immediate surgery. Get patients moved to their ultimate destinations rapidly so that additional incoming cases can be accommodated. All receiving units must also work to ensure there are no delays in receiving cases from trauma resuscitation. Assign one experienced doctor and one senior nurse to the role of expediting trauma resuscitation throughput for all cases. This nurse-physician team should continually round through the resuscitation area and communicate with receiving units and institutions, to encourage rapid decision making and removal of barriers to throughput.

SUSTAINED RESPONSE

After the initial response, large-scale events may require sustained efforts extending from hours to days to manage large numbers of casualties. Management of the effort must shift gears from the initial response and now focus on how the effort will be maintained for an extended period.

AT THE SCENE

Safety and Scene Security

Continued reassessment of safety concerns must remain a priority. Building instability and collapse potential must be carefully assessed and reevaluated. Other types of disaster scenes also call for continued vigilance for possible hazards (e.g., earthquake aftershocks, fire flare-ups, delayed release of toxic chemicals, secondary explosive devices designed to injure rescuers). To keep the rescue effort well organized, security must be established at the scene. Unauthorized persons should be kept away for their own safety. Eager volunteers should be required to follow directions. Over-eager rescuers who persist in ignoring efforts to properly organize the work effort and who ignore safety issues may have to be removed from the scene.

Evacuations

Evacuation of the disaster area may be required because of ongoing or developing safety concerns. Many logistical issues will have to be considered carefully by the incident management team, including the safety of the rescue team while carrying out the evacuation.

Treatment Area

In certain large-scale events, logistical issues such as obtaining transport vehicles may delay transport of some of the injured. A treatment area should then be established, located back a safe distance from the disaster site. An additional reason for establishing a treatment area is to obviate the need for transport of less serious cases to already overloaded hospitals. The number of victims and the anticipated length of time that this area will be needed will dictate how extensive the area must be. Physicians, nurses, and others will be needed for ongoing staffing. Appropriate medical supplies and equipment will be needed in addition to shelter, power, water, sanitation, and food.

Handling the Walking Wounded

Those triaged to the minor or green category may need to be held until a suitable means of transport becomes available. These people may be appropriately transported in buses or similar nonmedical vehicles. Sufficient personnel will have to be dedicated to the effort of keeping this group of disaster victims together and monitoring them for clinical deterioration. Issues of pain relief and hydration, as well as dealing with stress and mental health, will arise.

Keeping Track of Cases Handled

Minimal record-keeping, such as through a disaster tagging system, should be used. A master list of victims identified and treated should be developed. The disaster tags or master list or database should record major injuries identified, vital signs, significant treatment administered, when such patients leave the disaster scene, for what destination, and by what means of transport.

Staging Area for Ground Transport

At scenes that require multiple ambulances and other patient transport vehicles, a transport staging area should be established. Arriving vehicles go to this area and wait for a transport assignment. Someone must be in charge of the organization of this area, reporting to the logistics chief at the incident command post. A log of arrivals and departures should be kept.

Helicopter Landing Zone

If helicopters will be used, a safe and secure landing zone should be established and personnel assigned to coordinate safe landing and takeoff. The area will need adequate security, a lack of obstacles such as tall buildings and power lines, and dust and debris control. Radio communications with the aircraft should be established. Helicopters may be used to transport priority cases to trauma centers.

Transport Destination Decisions

It is critically important that injured patients being transported away from the scene of an MCI are sent to the appropriate hospital. *Immediate* (red) cases should be transported first, and they should go to area trauma centers. If multiple trauma centers are available close by, cases should be distributed among them according to their capacity and capability. *Delayed* (yellow) cases also may be transported to trauma centers, provided that they are not already at maximum capacity with the immediate cases. If they are at capacity, consideration should be given to sending them to other capable hospitals. The *minor* (green) cases should be transported last, or at least in such a manner that their transport does not interfere with that of the immediate and delayed cases. They can go to general hospitals and to more distant facilities. All of this should be done in a manner consistent with predeveloped regional disaster plans or normal trauma system operating procedures. Some systems have a centralized medical control capability, which can assist with these decisions during a disaster. The need to base these decisions on trauma center or hospital capacity and capability implies a means of two-way communication between the scene and hospital incident command centers. Good communications about patient distribution between the decision makers at the scene and the leading trauma centers in the area will help to ensure that each patient gets the best care under the circumstances. As much as possible, care should be taken to avoid overloading a trauma center with too many immediate cases, as patient care will suffer as a result. Likewise, the trauma center should not be overloaded with less-serious cases, distracting them from what they are uniquely good at doing—resuscitating seriously injured patients.

Other Logistics Issues

Some incident scenes will require specialized equipment, such as heavy equipment (e.g., bulldozers, cranes), special extrication equipment, rescue dogs, audio and video detection devices, and specific antidotes. In addition, adequate general medical supplies and equipment will be needed (e.g., backboards, oxygen, IVs, bandages). Provisions for water, food, shelter, and rest areas will be required for an on going effort. Fresh personnel will be needed if the rescue effort extends beyond many hours.

The Incident Command Post

Numerous jurisdiction issues will arise when an MCI involves multiple fire and EMS agencies, law enforcement agencies, local political entities, the military, and national emergency management agencies. The incident commander must be adept at leadership, organization, negotiation, diplomacy, and political action. The commander must rapidly build a management team, with each team member in charge of various aspects of the incident. If the rescue effort extends beyond 8 to 10 hours, plans should call for another person to relieve the initial incident commander.

The command post should be located in a safe area a distance from the actual rescue scene, but close enough to aid in good communications. A temporary shelter may be needed, and communications equipment will be required (e.g., telephones, radios, and computers.)

AT THE HOSPITAL

The Hospital Incident Command System[7]

Early in the first hour of the large-scale trauma event, the incident command center may have been established. If the event is large in scope and will be ongoing for some time, the command center will continue its operations, expanding in scope to match the demands of the event.

Second-Level Triage

Initial hospital triage of incoming disaster victims using the START or similar triage system was discussed under "Initial Response" on page 125. But there is another type of triage, a second-level triage, which will be required. This involves the effective sorting and prioritization of patients to scarce resources within the hospital. Which patients should go first to the operating rooms, to diagnostic studies (e.g., computerized tomography scans, angiography), and to limited ICU beds? Which patients will use ventilators and other medical equipment that are limited in availability? An effective approach must be used for allocating these high-demand hospital resources. This will involve central decision making by a key medical leader.

Surgery

Scheduled elective surgery cases should be immediately suspended and those in progress finished as quickly as possible. Trauma surgeons, general surgeons, anesthesiologists, operating room (OR) staff, and operating rooms will likely be in short supply during a surge of immediate trauma cases. Using a thoughtful secondary triage approach as outlined above, leaders must decide which critical operative cases go to the OR first and which will be delayed. The focus should be on meeting the needs of those in critical need of immediate surgery, and such surgery should be performed on a damage control[11-13] basis where possible. Every effort should be taken to hasten operating room throughput.

Critical Care

Immediately after the disaster plan is implemented at the hospital, robust efforts to discharge existing cases from the critical care units should be initiated.[16] Disaster cases going to the intensive care units should also undergo secondary triage, with the effort focused on identifying those cases most in need of critical care resources. Resources required for patient survivability must be kept in mind.

Other Concerns

Continuous attention will be needed to manage discharges from the hospital. This effort will need to occur on an ongoing basis to make room for new arrivals. Charge nurses working in collaboration with physicians need to facilitate this process and keep the centralized nursing coordinator informed of actual and pending discharges.

Communicating with off-duty staff and reorganizing the work schedule will be a challenge, and in some circumstances may have to rely on messages sent through mass media. In a community-wide disaster, staff will have concerns about their families and even their pets and animals.[17] Adequate staff rest during a sustained disaster response will have to be provided. Stress reactions in various forms may occur and should be dealt with in appropriate ways.

Attention must also focus on maintaining the physical integrity of the hospital facility and its infrastructure and supply chain. Water, food, medical gases, fuel, sewer, heating/air conditioning, and medical supplies and equipment inventories can be affected immediately by the disaster or may rapidly become depleted if the disaster event extends beyond hours to days.

This can create a major issue in maintaining the functional capabilities of the facility.

If the hospital facility becomes physically threatened by the disaster event or if necessary support services are cut off, the decision to evacuate patients from the hospital to an alternate location may become necessary. This will require thorough and detailed planning and advance practice exercises. The experience of one hospital in North Dakota in grappling with this decision provides a good review of the issues involved.[18]

Lessons Learned

Cumulative experience from many recent large-scale trauma events,[19,20] such as the 2004 Indian Ocean tsunami,[10] the 2004 Madrid terrorist bombings,[21,22] the 2005 Hurricane Katrina disaster,[23,24] and a large number of terrorist bombings in Israel,[25] provides several lessons learned about disaster management. These general principles include:

1. Have a well-developed and well-rehearsed disaster plan.
2. Understand that communications issues frequently arise.
3. Keep the hospital facility secure from external threats, and have a plan for hospital evacuation if it becomes necessary.
4. Ensure everyone knows who is in charge.
5. Implement effective triage upon patient arrival at the hospital using personnel with good triage experience.
6. Lubricate "throughput" of arriving casualties through the hospital system.
7. Focus on those cases with survivable injuries most in need of care to deal with life threats.
8. Expect to encounter blast injuries frequently.
9. Avoid overtriage of the minor injured to top-level trauma centers, and undertriage of the severely injured to the closest hospital, which may not be a higher-level trauma center.
10. Plan for dealing with overworked and overstressed hospital staff, their concerns about family, and possible postevent mental health issues.

Government Involvement

Sustained major disaster events will require response and support from various government agencies. In the United States, requests for such support must always be routed through the state governor. Some communities may have functioning emergency operations centers operated by a coalition of local government agencies. Officials at this center can facilitate communications with the state governor. In other countries, alternate paths may be defined. State and national resources usually follow declarations of emergency by the governor. In the United States, various federal agencies and systems may become involved, including the National Guard and other military units, federal Disaster Medical Assistance Teams (DMATS),[26] the National Disaster Medical System (NDMS),[27] the National Incident Management System (NIMS),[28], the Federal Emergency Management Agency (FEMA),[29] and the

Department of Homeland Security.[30] National pharmaceutical stockpiles[31] (medications, poison antidotes, and vaccines), stockpiles of special medical equipment (ventilators), and other national resources may also need to be accessed.

DISASTER PREPAREDNESS

PLANNING, PRACTICE, AND DRILL

Things often do not go well in a disaster response if the hospitals and trauma centers, trauma care providers, and the trauma system have not become engaged in the planning process.[32,33] The blasé attitude of noninvolvement and "I'm too busy" by trauma personnel must yield to active involvement. Klein and Weigett it noted this attitude some time ago: "Working at a level I trauma center, we shared an attitude of complacency about disaster drills. We had a disaster plan, the available manpower, the experience, and the knowledge, and we felt confident that we could handle a local disaster. The knowledge we gained through three aircraft disasters proved to us that most of our preconceptions were wrong."[34] Trauma care personnel should take an active and major role in the development and regular practice of the disaster plan.

SPECIAL ISSUES BEYOND GENERAL TRAUMA CARE

Most trauma care providers are accomplished in the clinical care of patients with blunt and penetrating trauma. Most patients cared for in an MCI or disaster situation are these same kinds of patients. But there are some special types of trauma and associated clinical syndromes that the general trauma care provider may need to deal with, depending on the nature of the disaster. These include blast and compression injuries, contamination with HAZMAT, bioterrorism-related illnesses, and nuclear or radiation exposures.

Blast Injuries

Explosions and bombings are increasingly used as part of terrorist acts. Patients injured in blasts frequently sustain blunt injuries (e.g., pressure injuries from the blast effect), penetrating injuries from flying shrapnel and other debris, and burns. Blasts are increasingly a result of improvised explosive devices (IEDs), such as car and truck bombs, letter bombs, pipe bombs, and backpack or satchel bombs.[35-37]

Injuries from blasts are often categorized as primary, secondary, tertiary, and quaternary. Primary injuries are from the overpressurization wave and affect mainly air-filled structures such as the lungs, gastrointestinal tract, and middle ear. "Blast lung" can be fatal, and the key signs are apnea, bradycardia, hypotension, and a characteristic "butterfly" pattern on the chest x-ray, as well as hypoxia, cough, hemoptysis, and chest pain. Treatment is similar to that of pulmonary contusion. Ruptured tympanic membrane and bowel perforation are also common. Secondary blast injuries are both penetrating and blunt from flying debris and bomb fragments. Tertiary injuries are those sustained by the victim being thrown by the blast wind. Quaternary injuries include all other explosion-related injuries such as burns, crush injuries, and exacerbation of preexisting conditions. Blasts occurring in enclosed spaces may produce more severe injuries and enhance the likelihood that hot gases, toxins, or poisons were inhaled. Air embolism is common. Communication with the patient may be difficult due to hearing loss.[38-40]

Crush Injuries and Compartment Syndrome

Crush syndrome includes injuries that result from a body part being subjected to prolonged force or pressure. For example, a body part may be trapped in a collapsed building causing prolonged pressure on a fascial enclosed muscle compartment. Compartment syndrome results from excessive intracompartment pressure that impairs perfusion to the affected muscle leading to muscle tissue edema and ischemia. Once the pressure on the compartment is released, reperfusion injury with release of toxic superoxide radicals can occur. Muscle tissue ischemia and breakdown and reperfusion injury can cause multiple electrolyte abnormalities, lactic acidosis, arrhythmias, renal damage, and coagulopathy. The reader is referred to Chapter 27 for a more in-depth explanation of this complication. The patient sustaining crush injury may also be hypothermic and dehydrated. The greatest danger is immediately after the release of the crushed limb from entrapment. Treatment includes aggressive fluid resuscitation and diuresis. Dialysis may be required for renal insufficiency. Compartment pressure monitoring is indicated to detect compartment syndrome, and, if present, fasciotomy may be required.[35]

HAZMAT Preparedness

Trauma care providers should become familiar with the basics of dealing with injured patients contaminated with HAZMAT. This can be the result of a traffic crash when HAZMAT are being transported or an inadvertent release of chemicals during construction and other activities. Terrorism using hazardous chemicals could also occur, and this could be combined with a standard explosive attack.

Protection of health care providers and hospitals must be a priority in such an event. Plans and drills should emphasize early detection, immediate security action to "lock down" the hospital, thorough decontamination, and provision of lifesaving trauma care to victims not yet fully decontaminated, with clinicians in appropriate personal protective equipment (PPE). Clinicians should be adept at diagnosis of the key "toxidromes," toxic syndromes resulting from the various classifications of hazardous chemicals (Table 9-2).[41] Antidotes for major chemical agents should be on hand and personnel should be familiar with their use.[42] This requires frequent review and drilling as such antidotes are not often used in routine emergency and trauma care practice. Select individuals at all emergency departments and trauma resuscitation units should attend intensive training in this area. Multiple online resources are available for training, such as the Centers for Disease Control and Prevention websites

TABLE 9-2 **Toxidromes**

Type of Toxin	Examples of Agents
Irritant gases	Ammonia, formaldehyde, hydrogen chloride, sulfur dioxide, chlorine, phosgene, nitrogen dioxide
Asphyxiants	Carbon dioxide, methane, propane, isobutyl nitrite, carbon monoxide, hydrogen sulfide, hydrogen azide
Cholinergics	Organophosphate and carbamate pesticides
	Organophosphate nerve agents: Sarin (GB), Soman (GD), Tabun (GA), VX
Corrosives	Strong acids (hydrochloric, nitric, and sulfuric)
	Strong bases (ammonium, sodium, and potassium hydroxides)
	Hydrocarbon and halogenated hydrocarbons (propane, gasoline, toluene, and chloroform)

and such courses as the 2-day Advanced HAZMAT Life Support (AHLS) course or the shorter AHLS Toxic Terrorism course.[43] The National Poison Center should be contacted at 1-800-222-1222 to obtain expert consultation.

Bioterrorism Preparedness

Trauma and emergency clinicians should be familiar with the key bioterrorism syndromes and knowledgeable about the primary bioterror agents that may be used. It is possible, though less likely, that bioterror agents could be dispersed at the same time as a more traditional terror event, such as an explosion. Clinician suspicion and routine syndromal surveillance are the best approaches to early detection of an outbreak in the absence of an overt or advertised attack. Care providers should review the different characteristics of smallpox (*Variola major*) versus chickenpox (*Varicella*) lesions, as well as be familiar with the typical appearance of the anthrax (*Bacillus anthracis*) skin lesion. Other clinical signs of both of these diseases should be studied. In addition, other clinical syndromes should be reviewed, including those related to infection with plague (*Yersinia pestis*), tularemia (*Francisella tularensis*), and certain viruses, including the viral hemorrhagic fevers (e.g., hantavirus pulmonary syndrome, dengue fever). Finally, clinicians should know the signs of poisoning by the botulism toxin produced by *Clostridium botulinum*.[44]

Protection of care providers, isolation to prevent spread of infection, antibiotics and other medical treatment, and use of vaccines must all be considered in responding to a bioterror outbreak. Quick clinical references (such as those readily available from Centers for Disease Control and Prevention websites) should be at hand in emergency care facilities.

Nuclear-Radiologic Incidents

Ionizing radiation can produce tissue damage. Ionizing radiation is electromagnetic energy or energetic particles emitted from a radioactive source. There are five basic types of such radiation: alpha, beta, neutron, gamma, and x-ray. Alpha particles do not penetrate deeply and are stopped by clothing or skin. They are a hazard only if taken internally. Beta particles are usually high-energy electrons and can penetrate a bit deeper into tissue. Neutron particles penetrate deeply into or through tissues. Gamma rays and x-rays are electromagnetic radiation that also penetrate deeply or through tissues. Appropriate shielding (lead, concrete, depleted uranium or adequate distance) can significantly diminish but not completely stop gamma and x-rays. A patient can be exposed via external radiation, contamination with radioactive particles, or ingestion/inhalation of radioactive particles into the body.[45] A victim can be exposed to a nearby radioactive source or become a victim of a "dirty bomb" (a conventional explosive device designed to spread radioactive particles) or a nuclear explosion.

Radiation produces cellular damage resulting in tissue breakdown. The patient may experience a local radiation injury (skin burn, blisters, hair loss, and localized necrosis), or the more serious acute radiation sickness (ARS). Initial signs of ARS include nausea, vomiting, diarrhea, and headache. Very high dose exposure will result in rapid loss of consciousness and later shock. Infection and bleeding may occur in serious cases due to decreased production of white blood cells and platelets (hematopoietic syndrome).[45] A useful mnemonic for remembering the initial signs of severe ARS is the Three Ps: *P*oop, *P*uke, and *P*ass Out (with no closed head injury).

Contamination of staff and the facility with radioactive particulate matter must be prevented through proper and thorough decontamination procedures and the use of appropriate barriers. Various antidotes may have some effect on internally contaminated patients. Other treatment includes supportive and symptomatic treatment, as well as efforts to enhance elimination in internal contamination cases. Clinicians should review the principles of nuclear and radiologic incident response and patient care. Many online resources are available, such as Radiation Event Medical Management at http://www.remm.nim.gov[46] and Introduction to Radiological Preparedness at http://emilms.fema.gov/IS331-REP/index.htm.[47]

Trauma Systems and Disaster Events

Since the majority of multicasualty and disaster events involve physical injury, trauma care providers at all levels, as well as those managing trauma care systems, should be integrally involved in planning for disasters. This includes involvement in frequent practice and drills. Disaster response is not the sole business of first responders and emergency medical services. Definitive care will be provided to the majority of the serious victims by hospital-based trauma care providers. Involvement of trauma care providers in preparedness is essential.

REFERENCES

1. U.S. State Department: *Significant Terrorist Incidents, 1961-2003: A Brief Chronology.* Available online at www.state.gov/r/pa/ho/pubs/fs/5902.htm. Accessed July 2, 2007.
2. Augustine J: The ABCs of scene size-up, *Emerg Med Serv* 35(1):34, 36, 2006.
3. American Medical Association: *Advanced Disaster Life Support Provider Manual Version 2.0,* 2004.
4. Hoag Memorial Presbyterian Hospital and Newport Beach Fire Department: Available online at http://www.start-triage.com. Accessed May 29, 2007.
5. Romig L: *The Jump Start pediatric MCI Triage Tool and Other Pediatric Disaster and Emergency Medicine Resources.* Available online at http://www.jumpstarttriage.com. Accessed May 29, 2007.
6. National Incident Management System: *Incident Command Systems (ICS) National Training Curriculum.* Available online at www.nimsonline.com/. Accessed May 29, 2007.
7. California Emergency Medical Services Authority: *Hospital Incident Command System Guidebook, 2006.* Available online at http://www.emsa.ca.gov/hics/hics.asp. Accessed May 29, 2007.
8. Bronstein A: Medical management of hazmat victims. In Walter FG, editor: *Advanced HAZMAT Life Support Provider Manual,* ed 3, Tucson, Ariz, 2003, Board of Regents for the University of Arizona.
9. Ashkenazi I, Kessel B, Khashan T et al: Precision of in-hospital triage in mass-casualty incidents after terror attacks, *Prehosp Disaster Med* 21(1):20-23, 2006.
10. Leiba A, Ashkenasi I, Nakash G et al: Response of Thai hospitals to the tsunami disaster, *Prehosp Disaster Med* 21(1):s32-s37, 2006.
11. McArthur BJ: Damage control surgery for the patient who has experienced multiple traumatic injuries, *AORN J* 84(6): 991-1000, 2006.
12 Lee JS, Peitzman AB: Damage-control laparotomy, *Curr Opin Crit Care* 12(4):346-350, 2006.
13. Sutton E, Bochicchio GV, Bochicchio K et al: Long term impact of damage control surgery: a preliminary prospective study, *J Trauma* 61(4):831-835, 2006.
14. Hughes G: Rapid assessment teams and early discharge of the elderly from ED; vulnerable in the current financial climate? *Emerg Med J* 18:435-441, 2007.
15. Almogy G, Belzberg H, Mintz Y et al: Suicide bombing attacks: update and modifications to the protocol, *Ann Surg* 239(3):295-303, 2004.
16. Avidan V, Hersch M, Spira RM et al: Civilian hospital response to a mass casualty event: the role of the intensive care unit, *J Trauma* 62(5):1234-1239, 2007.
17. Conklin R (personal communication, July 26, 2002), in reference to the Rodeo-Chideski fire of 2002 and operations at Navapache Regional Medical Center, Showlow, Arizona.
18. Reed MK: Disaster preparedness pays off, *J Nurs Admin* 28(6): 25-31, 1998.
19. Hirshberg A: Multiple casualty incidents: lessons from the front line, *Ann Surg* 239(3):322-324, 2004.
20. Frykberg ER: Principles of mass casualty management following terrorist disasters, *Ann Surg* 239(3):319-321, 2004.
21. de Ceballos JP, Turégano-Fuentes F, Perez-Diaz D et al: 11 March 2004. The terrorist bomb explosions in Madrid, Spain—an analysis of the logistics, injuries sustained and clinical management of casualties treated at the closest hospital, *Crit Care* 9(1):104-111, 2005.
22. Frykberg ER: Commentary: terrorist bombings in Madrid, *Crit Care* 9(1):20-22, 2005.
23. Centers for Disease Control and Prevention: Surveillance for illness and injury after Hurricane Katrina—New Orleans, Louisiana, September 8-25, 2005. *MMWR* 54:1018-1021, 2005.
24. Sariego J: A year after Hurricane Katrina: lessons learned at one coastal trauma center, *Arch Surg* 142:203-205, 2007.
25. Einav S, Feigenberg Z, Weissman C et al: Evacuation priorities in mass casualty terror-related events: implications for contingency planning, *Ann Surg* 239(3):304-310, 2004.
26. Michael GE: *United States Disaster Medical Assistance Teams, 2006.* Available online at http://www.dmat.org/. Accessed May 29, 2007.
27. United States Department of Health and Human Services: *National Disaster Medical System.* Available online at http://www.oep-ndms.dhhs.gov/. Accessed May 29, 2007.
28. United States Department of Homeland Security: *Federal Emergency Management Agency. National Integration Center Incident Management Systems Division.* Available online at http://www.fema.gov/emergency/nims/index.shtm. Accessed May 29, 2007.
29. United States Department of Homeland Security: *Federal Emergency Management Agency.* Available online at http://www.fema.gov/. Accessed May 29, 2007.
30. United States Department of Homeland Security: *United States Department of Homeland Security.* Available online at http://www.dhs.gov/index.shtm. Accessed May 29, 2007.
31. Department of Health and Human Resources, Centers for Disease Control and Prevention: *Strategic National Stockpile. April 14, 2005.* Available online at http://www.bt.cdc.gov/stockpile/. Accessed May 29, 2007.
32. Ciraulo DL, Barie PS, Briggs SM et al: An update on the surgeons' scope and depth of practice to all hazards emergency response, *J Trauma* 60(6):1267-1274, 2006.
33. Lennquist S: Management of major accidents and disasters: an important responsibility for trauma surgeons, *J Trauma* 62(6):1321-1329, 2007.
34. Klein JS, Weigelt JA: Disaster management. Lessons learned, *Surg Clin North Am* 71(2):257-266, 1991.
35. Centers for Disease Control: *Bombings: Injury Patterns and Care. A One-Hour On-Line Learning Program.* Available online at www.bt.cdc.gov/masscasualties/explosions.asp. Accessed June 6, 2007.
36. Frykberg ER: Medical management of disasters and mass casualties from terrorist bombings: how can we cope? *J Trauma* 53(2):201-212, 2002.
37. Kapur GB, Hutson HR, Davis MA et al: The United States twenty-year experience with bombing incidents: implications for terrorism preparedness and medical response, *J Trauma* 59(6):1436-1444, 2005.
38. Centers for Disease Control and Prevention: *Explosions and Blast Injuries: A Primer for Clinicians. A One-Hour On-Line Learning Program.* Available online at www.bt.cdc.gov/masscasualties/ppt/bombings. Accessed June 6, 2007.
39. Ciraulo DL, Frykberg ER: The surgeon and acts of civilian terrorism: blast injuries, *J Am Col Surg* 203(6):942-950, 2006.
40. DePalma RG: Blast injuries. *N Engl J Med* 352(13):1335-1342, 2005.
41. Walter FG, Klien R, Thomas RG: Toxidromes and toxicodynamics. In Walter FG, editor: *Advanced HAZMAT Life Support for Toxic Terrorism: Chemical, Biological, Radiological and Nuclear Casualties,* Tucson, Ariz, 2003, Arizona Board of Regents for the University of Arizona.

42. Hall AH, Walter FG, Phillips, SD et al: Antidotes in detail. In Walter FG, editor: *Advanced HAZMAT Life Support for Toxic Terrorism: Chemical, Biological, Radiological and Nuclear Casualties.* Tucson, Ariz, 2003, Arizona Board of Regents for the University of Arizona.
43. The University of Arizona: *Advanced Hazmat Life Support (AHLS) Course. 2007.* Available online at www.ahls.org. Accessed July 1, 2007.
44. Darling RG, Mothershead JL, Eitzen E: Bioterrorism. In Walter FG, editor: *Advanced HAZMAT Life Support for Toxic Terrorism: Chemical, Biological, Radiological and Nuclear Casualties.* Tucson, Ariz, 2003, Arizona Board of Regents for the University of Arizona.
45. Edsall K: Radiological and nuclear incidents and terrorism. In Walter FG, editor: *Advanced HAZMAT Life Support for Toxic Terrorism: Chemical, Biological, Radiological and Nuclear Casualties.* Tucson, Ariz, 2003, Arizona Board of Regents for the University of Arizona.
46. U.S. Department of Health and Human Services: Radiation event medical management: guidance for diagnosis & treatment for health care providers. Available online at http://www.remm.nlm.gov. Accessed June 16, 2007.
47. Federal Emergency Management Agency: *Introduction to Radiological Preparedness. An On-line Course.* Available online at http://emilms.fema.gov/IS331-REP/index.htm. Accessed June 6, 2007.

10

NURSING PRACTICE THROUGH THE CYCLE OF TRAUMA

Kathryn Truter Von Rueden

Because of the uniqueness and complexity of patients with multiple injuries, trauma nursing has evolved as a highly specialized field that has spawned a specialty professional organization, the Society of Trauma Nurses, a journal, and certifications.[1] One of the most challenging aspects of caring for trauma patients is the development of a plan of care that addresses the patient's needs in a logical, organized fashion to ensure continuity and coordination of all care disciplines. Formulation of such a plan requires incorporation of the five components of the nursing process: assessment, diagnosis, planning, implementation, and evaluation. In addition, nursing management is inextricably intertwined with and reflective of the plans of other trauma team members as the overall plan of care is developed and implemented throughout the cycle of trauma care.

The coordination of patient care requires individuals with a wide range and breadth of knowledge and skills. Trauma nurses must have an understanding of the significant impact that traumatic injury has on the patient, the patient's family, and society. They must be adept at sophisticated monitoring and at caring for the intense physiologic needs, and they must be able to respond to the psychologic and social demands of the patient. They also must be able to assist the family in coping with the stress and emotional devastation that accompany a sudden traumatic event. Patient and family recovery is heavily dependent on the skills of the nurses as caregivers, communicators, collaborators, and coordinators throughout the cycle of trauma.

TRAUMA NURSING PRACTICE

A philosophy of trauma nursing encompasses beliefs about the trauma patient's care from prevention through reintegration into the community. Nurses caring for these patients are challenged to help the patient attain his or her highest level of cognitive, psychosocial, and physiologic functioning following traumatic injury.

Nurses caring for patients throughout the cycle of trauma must possess a strong pathophysiologic knowledge base. This is needed to assess the patient and to plan and direct care in each of the phases of recovery and rehabilitation. In the resuscitation and critical care phases, it is advantageous for the trauma nurse to have significant experience in emergency and critical care nursing before caring for patients whose injuries may involve many body systems and whose psychologic responses are often complex.

During the initial phase of care immediately after injury and during stabilization of the patient, the focus includes both nursing care and delegated medical care to restore basic physiologic functioning. As patients enter the rehabilitative phase, the restoration of cognitive and psychosocial functioning takes on more significance as patients learn ways to live with residual impairments from their injuries and become reintegrated into society. Trauma nurses have an essential role in injury prevention through the educational process by providing information to the public and to people of all ages.

Throughout the cycle of trauma care, specialized expertise is required to provide quality care and to achieve optimal outcomes for this complex patient population. Credentialing of trauma nurses is a way to ensure accountability in practice and competence in performance. Competency-based orientation and periodically required cognitive and psychomotor certifications are a means to this end. In addition, annual competency verification updates staff on new or revised procedures and complex or high-risk procedures, and provides trauma center designation-required educational content.

PROFILE OF THE TRAUMA PATIENT

Several characteristics of the multiply injured contribute to the complexity of this unique patient population:

- Traumatic injuries occur suddenly. Unlike a patient who is hospitalized for elective surgery, the trauma patient and family have no warning. The injury is an unexpected, severe interruption of normal life. There is no time to plan or prepare; one must simply cope with the injury once it occurs.
- Drug and alcohol abuse commonly plays a causative role in injury. The multiply injured patient whose history includes substance abuse is typically more difficult to initially assess and later to manage effectively. Often

family members' feelings of guilt because of their inability to convince the patient to seek help for a drug or alcohol problem may affect the ability to cope effectively with the family member's injury.

- Because of the severity and complexity of injury, many trauma patients require long-term rehabilitative care. Systemic sequelae and physical handicaps also may result. Learning to adequately cope, adapt, and adjust, both physically and psychologically, can be a lengthy process.
- Psychological sequelae are common in multiply injured patients. Many experience posttraumatic stress syndrome and grieving after the injury. Depending on the individual's existing support systems and coping mechanisms, adaptation to severe injuries may be difficult.
- Trauma continues to be primarily a disease of the young. Their inexperience with life crises, developmental stage, and level of maturity creates special needs that must be considered when planning effective interventions. In 1996, the average age of the multiply injured patient was reported to be between 15 and 34 years.[2] More recently, the 2005 National Trauma Data Bank Report database shows that 21% of trauma patients are in the 14- to 24-year range, and 30% are in the 25- to 44-year range.[3]
- The average age of trauma patients and the number of elderly trauma patients is increasing and will continue to do so with the "graying of America." In 1995 unintentional injury was the third leading cause of death in patients ages 45 to 65 and the seventh leading cause of death in patients age 65 and older.[4] In 2004, more than 500,000 patients older than age 65 were hospitalized for nonfatal traumatic injuries, and more than 50% of these were transportation related.[5] This population has unique needs that necessitate alterations in the typical approaches to resuscitation, critical care, and rehabilitative practices.
- Many critically injured patients who do not survive are potential subjects of a medical examiner's investigation when their injuries are a result of violence or unintentional injury. Therefore legal implications must be considered as the plan of care and all documentation may be subjected to scrutiny by staff, hospital administrators, criminal investigators, attorneys, and patients' families.
- Serious injuries are often subtle. Many injuries are obvious, and they often mask others that may be even more life threatening. Nursing assessment is of greater significance when the occurrence of subtle injuries is considered because the diagnosis may be delayed.
- The multiply injured patient has tremendous potential for developing complications during hospitalization. The nurse is largely responsible for the prevention, early detection, and for minimizing the consequences of such complications.
- Initial injuries or their required treatments create additional problems that greatly influence care planning for multiply injured patients. Many are immobilized because of orthopedic or neurologic injury. Communication is often difficult if an endotracheal tube or a tracheostomy tube is necessary for ventilatory support. The risk of developing infection is high due to the nature of traumatic injuries; multiple invasive procedures; lines, tubes, and drains; and exposure to the numerous trauma team members who provide care for them.
- Because multiple injuries affect several body systems, implementation of standard and accepted methods of treatment for each injury may be difficult or contraindicated. For example, severe brain injury may prohibit or limit routine repositioning and chest physiotherapy treatments required by a patient with thoracic injuries or respiratory failure. Alternative methods of treatment that do not compromise the patient's existing injuries must be explored.
- The treatment of critically injured patients often imposes serious economic burdens on their families. The cost of critical care and rehabilitative care can be staggering.

These characteristics and the necessarily complex treatment modes make planning and providing care for the multiply injured patient a difficult and challenging task.

Implementation of a philosophy of care that focuses on a well-communicated and organized approach to the delivery of trauma care and health care provider expertise is essential. The Committee on Trauma (COT) of the American College of Surgeons (ACS) suggests the following for that approach[6]:

1. Rapid identification of the injury followed by easy access to the emergency medical system (EMS)
2. A central emergency dispatching system such as 911
3. Appropriately trained and appropriate level of EMS provider available to respond to the scene, that is, basic versus advanced life support
4. Prehospital triage protocols that authorize the EMS providers to make triage decisions *before* the patient is taken to a hospital
5. A communication system that allows direct conversation between the prehospital providers, trauma center personnel, and the physicians who provide medical direction
6. A designated trauma center with immediate availability of specialized surgeons, anesthesia providers, nurses, and emergency resuscitative equipment and radiologic capabilities
7. A trauma system that coordinates care among all levels of trauma centers and an interfacility transfer process that allows for prompt transfer of the patient to a higher level of care
8. Access to rehabilitative services in both the acute and long-term phases of recovery

Crucial Considerations Throughout the Cycle of Trauma

Patient Advocacy

The role of the trauma nurse as a patient advocate is critical in many situations during the cycle of trauma care. An advocate can be described as one who defends or who pleads the cause for or in the behalf of another. Nursing advocacy is the act of defending, supporting, or recommending a best course of action in the care of trauma patients. A trauma patient may be frightened, cognitively impaired, paralyzed, sedated, or in pain. These conditions alter the patient's ability to ask questions and participate actively in decision making. Such conditions also may contribute to a communication deficit, increasing the potential for care to become disjointed among the many involved services and personnel.

Nurses caring for trauma patients, from resuscitation through rehabilitation, are in the ideal position to advocate for the patient. Examples of advocacy behaviors include ensuring sterile technique is maintained during procedures, providing relief from pain and anxiety through administration of medication or by using nonpharmacologic strategies, coordinating family conferences, communicating the desires of the family or patient to other members of the health care team, and assuring that the patient's dignity is maintained and respected throughout the cycle of trauma care.

Family Centered Care

Beginning on the first day of a patient's admission, the bedside nurse and, if appropriate, the advanced practice nurse must assess the family members for their knowledge of the patient's injuries and their ability to interpret and accept what has been communicated to them. Coping mechanisms and support systems that they use to deal with crisis should also be identified and documented. Research suggests that families of patients with gunshot wounds may feel more stress and have fewer coping strategies than families of patients in motor vehicle crashes; thus, interventions need to be customized to meet the needs of the specific family.[7] All family information, assessment data, and the planned interventions and strategies to assist them are documented for all caregivers to refer to in the patient record. This fosters a consistent approach to the care of family members.

Families in crisis often latch on to a single piece of information, and unless it is clear to all those caring for the patient what the family has been told, family members may receive mixed messages. On initial contact with the family members, a spokesperson is identified so that all communication relating to the patient's condition can be relayed to that one person to avoid the possibility of varied interpretations by several different family members. To prevent inaccurate or inconsistent information from being delivered to the family, regular communication by the primary or coordinating nurse or physician with the spokesperson is important.

The initial approach with the family often sets the tone for the entire hospital stay of the patient. Joy[8] suggests the following guidelines for communicating with the family in crisis:

1. Recognize that the traumatic event affects everyone associated with the injured person, including the family, neighbors, friends, coworkers, and community associates.
2. Acknowledge that family members in crisis may each express their reactions in unique ways. These include crying, fighting among themselves, being disruptive, showing anger or guilt, or being silent.
3. Overcome language barriers by obtaining appropriate interpreters to allow the family to be fully informed and fully heard.
4. Avoid using medical jargon when speaking to family members unless they are health care providers who have a full understanding of the terminology. Technical words provide little information to the family and serve more to confuse and frighten them.
5. Acknowledge the family's concerns related to the financial impact and potential legal ramifications related to the traumatic event. Offer them the appropriate resources to answer their questions.
6. Be an attentive listener. Attempt to secure a quiet place to talk with the family so that other things happening in the clinical setting do not distract from the discussion.

Recent research supports the presence of family members at the bedside with appropriate preparation and support during invasive procedures or resuscitation.[9] Family presence during these times can be beneficial to both the patient and the family in coping with the psychologic effects of critical illness and injury. Early assessment and appropriate nursing interventions such as providing information, active listening, facilitating flexibility in visiting, and family caregiver conferences are key to effective family-centered care and management of families of trauma victims.[10]

Visiting Considerations

Family visits are a vital part of the overall plan of care and can influence patient outcome. Visiting by family members and others should be encouraged during all phases of the cycle of trauma care. Patient and family needs are important considerations in the nurse's individualization of visiting practices. Flexible visiting policies that include the family, friends, children, and even pets have been implemented successfully in a number of institutions.[10-13] Visits provide the nurse with an opportunity to assess the family's understanding and perception of their loved one's injuries and to provide information. Families who are restricted from visiting a critically ill member often suffer fear, anxiety, hopelessness, and helplessness. These may be displayed as hostility and anger toward the staff in an attempt to appear in control of the situation.

The Dying Patient

Caring for a dying patient in any phase of the cycle of trauma can be stressful, difficult, and even painful for nurses. The role of the trauma nurse is broad, encompassing a clinical component, ensuring that dignity is afforded to the patient, as well as assisting the family with coping and decision making, either directly or by helping to provide appropriate resources for them.

Occasionally, conflicting opinions among the medical staff, nurse, and family regarding the continuation of aggressive treatment arise. In these situations the nurse must assume the role of coordinator and patient advocate. The nurse's roles include: working with all team members; involving appropriate resources such as the chaplain or ethics committee to assist in decision making and emotional support of the family and the health care team; participating in development of a final plan of care that is implemented consistently; and documenting the decisions in the patient's medical record.[14,15]

Traumatic injury, especially severe head injury, often creates the potential for organ donation. Trauma patients are frequently young, with many healthy organs suitable for donation. The potential organ donor patient requires a specialized plan that involves physiologic management, and the family requires intense emotional support. Nurses are in a position to aid family decision making regarding requests for organ donation. Specific education addressing the care of patients who are potential organ donors and supporting a family decision to consent is an especially important aspect of the orientation for critical care trauma nurses.

Once the patient has been identified as a potential donor, the local organ/tissue procurement organization is contacted. These groups often assume responsibility for many aspects of care of the family and patient. The staff are highly trained experts, skilled and sensitive in requesting the gift of organ donations from grieving families and in providing specific guidelines for patient management in preparation for organ donation.

The dying patient, whether eligible as an organ donor or not, has the right to an individualized plan of care that integrates "caring" as the most vital component. The transition from life to death is a voyage that requires the company and quiet reassurance of another. The potential exists, in these moments, for the exchange of many human gifts and values that otherwise go unnoticed.

Collaborative Practice

When planning and implementing care for the multiply injured patient, collaborative practice among health care professionals is crucial to integrate care regimens into a comprehensive approach. This concept is a common theme in current medical and nursing literature. It describes the ideal working relationship between the physician, nurse, and personnel from other disciplines, resulting in higher quality care and improved patient outcomes.

Collaborative practice can significantly affect morbidity and mortality of the critically ill.[16] Critical care units with the most effective, high-quality care have highly coordinated systems for patient management. Excluding other variables, investigators have concluded that the *process* of care is essential to reduce morbidity and mortality. Inherent in the process is the positive interaction and collaboration of physicians, nurses, and other health care professionals in achieving optimal results and the adherence to established protocols and procedures to guide their care.[17] Hope for the survival of the multiple trauma patient rests with the collaborative efforts of the paramedics, trauma nurses, physicians, technicians, and therapists who constitute the trauma team and who work together to resuscitate, stabilize, diagnose, and treat the severely injured patient.

Quality care of trauma patients implies minimal errors and complications and maximal efficiency and continuity. Quality care can only be provided by a team that accurately and consistently communicates, beginning with the field providers and subsequently with the nurses and physicians who follow the patient from admission throughout the resuscitative and operative phases. Strategies that can improve collaboration and communication between health care providers as well as improved patient outcomes include use of formal, written guidelines and protocols, multidisciplinary rounds, and the addition of nurse practitioners to the health care team.[18] The incorporation of nurse practitioners into the trauma care team has significantly increased over the past decade and the role has become an essential one in many trauma centers.[19] In 2005 the Society of Trauma Nurses released a position paper on the role of the nurse practitioner in trauma.[20]

Responsibility for collaborative practice applies to all members of the trauma team throughout the cycle of trauma, from prehospital to rehabilitative care, working together to achieve the common goal—providing the best possible trauma care. Without collaborative practice, this goal and optimal patient outcomes cannot be realized.

Strategies to Plan and Provide Quality Care and Patient Safety

A specialized plan of care is clearly a necessity for the multitrauma patient. Regardless of the facility (a designated trauma center versus a community or large university hospital), mechanisms to address the severely injured trauma patient's multiple needs must exist.

Highly specialized trauma care requires numerous strategies for the planning and provision of care. Policies and protocols specifically addressing the care of trauma patients should be developed and based on current, evidence-based literature. It is imperative that the established protocols, policies, standards, and procedures be reviewed on a consistent basis and updated to reflect and incorporate new modes of therapy, technology, and recent research findings. As well, policies, procedures, protocols, and guidelines need to be consistent with the standards and guidelines set forth by organizations such as the American College of Surgeons' Committee on Trauma (ACSCOT), the Eastern Association for the Surgery of Trauma, the Society of Trauma Nurses, the American Association of Critical Care Nurses, and the Society of Critical Care Medicine.

From these guidelines, standards of trauma nursing practice can be developed to facilitate the implementation of these policies and protocols. These standards should reflect an aim for the highest levels of care, yet they must be realistic and based on the resources available to implement them. Adherence to standards, protocols, procedures, and guidelines, and comparison against benchmarks also form the basis for evaluation of nursing care and the effect of best practice on patient outcomes. It is important to note that if the standardized guidelines and procedures promulgated by the preceding organizations are used, they must be flexible and tailored to meet the individual patient needs and adapt to changing pathophysiologic status. For example, a procedure outlining the proper use of the hypothermia/hyperthermia blanket must include special precautions in relation to aspects of the trauma patient's care, such as its use in spinal cord–injured patients whose thermoregulation mechanisms may be significantly impaired.

Care Delivery Models

A system of nursing care delivery capable of providing highly specialized care and ensuring continuity of care through the cycle of trauma is paramount. Primary nursing, and the more recently espoused relationship-based care model[21] are examples of care delivery systems that facilitate the coordination of specialized care across the continuum of trauma care. The nurse is central to the goal-directed coordination of the many care providers who are involved in the management of a trauma patient's care. Other systems of care delivery may be equally effective, as long as they ensure nursing accountability for patient and family-centered care, interdisciplinary goal-directed care, and for communication and coordination within the trauma team.

One member of the trauma team should be in charge of coordinating this care, and the primary nurse who cares for the patient on a consistent basis is ideal for orchestrating this process. Ensuring that treatment plans and interventions from the various disciplines are congruent with the overall plan of care is the primary function of this role. The trauma nurse's level of assessment skills, accountability, and educational preparation combine to make the primary nurse's role an excellent one to assume this level of complicated care coordination.

To further ensure collaboration and continuity of trauma patient care, a case-management system is implemented in most trauma centers and is generally a requirement for trauma center verification or designation. Typically the trauma case manager is a master's-prepared clinical nurse specialist or trauma nurse coordinator. The case manager is responsible for the daily review and coordination of multidisciplinary services, efficient use of resources, patient disposition through the system, and arrangement of follow-up care. The trauma case manager role is absolutely essential in trauma centers where a strong primary nursing system is not in place.

The Plan of Care

The written plan of care is a vital component of the trauma patient's care. The Joint Commission (formerly the Joint Commission on Accreditation of Healthcare Organizations [JCAHO]) requires a documented plan of care that addresses physiologic, psychologic, and environmental factors.[22] The care plan for the trauma patient satisfies this regulatory requirement and serves as the link between injury and readaptation—the basis from which all care is delivered. This plan should be developed by, familiar to, and used by *all* members of the trauma team. It must be succinct and reflect changes in care as they become necessary. The plan also should be evaluated and revised at regular intervals, dictated by patient acuity and specific goals or outcomes. Ideally a consistent "relief nurse" should assume this responsibility in the absence of the primary or coordinating nurse.

Clinical Pathways, Protocols and Guidelines

In the past two decades, clinical pathways, protocols, and practice guidelines have been developed to save time, to ensure consistent, evidence-based quality care for trauma patients, and to allow measurement of quality outcomes. Standardization of practice is increasingly advocated by thought leaders in the area of trauma care.[23,24]

Consistent incorporation of evidence-based protocols for high-volume diagnoses and care processes into daily management of patients has been shown to reduce complications and mortality.[25] In addition to utilization of multidisciplinary protocols, critical care units and hospitals with lower than predicted critical care unit and hospital mortality use daily interdisciplinary rounds to enhance communication, monitor adherence to guidelines and protocols, regularly report outcome data, and incorporate findings into clinical performance improvement initiatives.

Clinical pathways prescribe day-to-day multidisciplinary activities, such as interventions, consultations, diagnostic testing, and patient and family education for trauma patients with common physiologic alterations or those with similar injuries. Developed and agreed on by a multidisciplinary group, pathways concretely direct the efforts of all services. These are beneficial when planning care for the trauma patient and may be used throughout the phases. Many trauma patients exhibit similar responses to specific injuries; therefore, standardized pathways and guidelines addressing these responses have several advantages. They conserve valuable time and promote continuity and consistency of care.

The reluctance of some physicians and nurses to use standardized plans or protocols usually stems from the concern that patient individuality will be lost. For this reason, pathways, guidelines, and protocols must have flexibility to be adaptable to the patient's changing physiology or psychosocial needs.

Computerization of the medical record facilitates utilization of standardized clinical decision support and management plans, affords individual patient customization, and allows monitoring of patient outcomes related to compliance with protocols and guidelines.

Plans of care, protocols, or guidelines that are successful in driving evidence-based care and achieving superior outcomes should have the following characteristics:

- Based on physiologic priorities
- Provide an organized, logical approach to trauma patient care
- Identify specific goals or outcomes and interventions
- Developed and used by the multidisciplinary trauma team
- Have utility throughout the cycle of trauma care

Evidence-Based Practices

Patient care that is driven by research-based protocols and guidelines enhances patient outcomes, allows measurement of outcomes by reducing practitioner preferences, and increases the cost-effectiveness of care and resource use. For example, protocols for suctioning, tracheostomy care, tracheostomy changes, head of bed elevation, and oral care should be integrated into the pulmonary care regimen for all patients.[26] Prone positioning, institution of kinetic therapy, and early mobilization are other examples of evidence-based interventions that can reduce the risk of nosocomial pneumonia and improve oxygenation and ventilation.[27,28]

The use of specialty beds and mattress overlays has become common practice in the care of the multiply injured patient. When prescribed appropriately, they can enhance the patient's recovery process. The placement of a patient on one of these beds should be a collaborative nursing and medical decision based on specific criteria. Identification of risk factors for development of respiratory failure or nosocomial pneumonia[29] and guidelines for placing patients on these beds prevent unnecessary or inappropriate use and expenditures. For instance, kinetic therapy beds have proven to be efficacious in reducing the incidence of nosocomial pneumonia and other immobility-related complications when instituted within 72 hours of admission and rotated for 15 hours per day.[27] Prone positioning and beds to facilitate prone positioning can improve both oxygenation and ventilation in critically ill trauma patients with acute respiratory failure.[28] The use of air-fluidized or low-air-loss beds reduces the risk of pressure sore development and enhances healing of large wounds. These are appropriate for patients who are at high risk for skin breakdown as determined by a risk assessment such as the Braden scale.[30]

The belief that rehabilitation begins on admission has long been accepted, but it is particularly relevant when planning care for the trauma patient. At the time the patient enters the critical care phase, rehabilitation needs are addressed according to protocol to minimize the impact of immobility on all systems and lessen the possibility of delayed recovery. Attempts to reduce musculoskeletal alterations begin in the critical care phase. Early splinting of extremities when appropriate, active and passive range of motion exercises, and frequent repositioning aid in prevention of serious contractures and other musculoskeletal problems arising from immobilization. Literature also supports the application of pneumatic leg compression devices early after hospital admission to deter the development of deep vein thrombosis related to injury and immobility.[31]

In the past decade, the use of evidence-based initiatives has included protocols called "bundles." These have been embraced and championed by interdisciplinary organizations, such as the Institute for Health Care Improvement and professional health care organizations such as the American Association of Critical Care Nurses, Society of Critical Care Medicine, Society of Trauma Nurses, and Emergency Nurses Association. For example the 100,000 Lives Campaign[32] includes a "ventilator bundle" to prevent ventilator-acquired pneumonia and guidelines for rapid response teams, preventing adverse drug events, preventing surgical site infections, and preventing central line infections. Similarly, a "sepsis bundle" (from the Surviving Sepsis Campaign[33]) is an evidence-based approach to early detection and aggressive management of infection and sepsis.

Nurses managing patients throughout the phases of trauma are responsible for continually and critically analyzing their practice to ensure that the most recent and best evidence is incorporated into care of the trauma patient, and that practices are not based on outdated information and traditions.[34,35]

Impact of Pharmaceutical and Technologic Advances

Nursing care during the resuscitation, critical care, and acute care phases has become increasingly specialized and complex. Pharmacologic and technologic advances continue to improve the care of critically ill trauma patients. As new drugs and devices become available and are incorporated into patient care, nurses are challenged to maintain a high level of expertise and keep abreast of the indications for use, desired physiologic effects, side effects or complications, and other related implications. For example, administration of new therapeutic agents, such as drotrecogin alfa[36] and recombinant factor VIIa,[37,38] are increasingly common in the trauma population and have significant nursing implications associated with their administration. The clinical pharmacist, as a trauma team member, is an invaluable resource to the nurses and physicians, not only as new pharmacologic agents are introduced but also in the routine management of the patient receiving multiple medications.

The use of sophisticated technology in trauma care requires a high level of expertise and competence. Nurses and other staff members must be properly educated and credentialed before assuming the responsibilities of caring for patients supported by sophisticated life-support devices. Extracorporeal lung assistance and continuous renal replacement therapy are examples of therapies in which the nurse must monitor the device's function and the patient's response and manipulate multiple variables (e.g., gas flow rates, blood flow rates, and fluid and electrolyte replacement) accordingly. In addition, advances in ventilatory support technologies for traumatically injured patients, such as airway pressure release ventilation, that are directed toward preventing acute lung injury or aiding the management of acute respiratory disease syndrome (ARDS)[26,39] demand increasing collaborative, interdisciplinary education programs as well as collaborative care.

A system of equipment evaluation and control is important. For example, it is advantageous to have all units use the same monitoring system or emergency equipment so that the entire staff can become familiar with and secure in its use. Evaluation, acquisition, and integration of new technology are important aspects of trauma/critical care nursing. Participation in the technology assessment and value analysis process, developing specific criteria for use and establishing outcome measures, and planning the integration and education processes are important aspects of the nurse's role.[40]

When using highly technical equipment, computer systems, and other devices, the trauma nurse should know that an important role is humane caring. Naisbitt's theory[41] of "high tech, high touch" is relevant to the trauma patient's care and should be incorporated in the plan of care. This formula describes the way we have responded to technology. Whenever new technology is introduced into society, there must be a counterbalancing human response—that is, high touch—or the technology is rejected. High technology is inherent and ever-expanding in the trauma/critical care field.

Naisbitt acknowledges that there is no way to keep humans from devising new tools, but we must take care not to use these tools as the sole solution. Particularly in this age of increased technology use, health care providers have a personal responsibility to provide humane care, recognizing the need for human touch.[41] As the need for more high-touch care increases, ensuring consistent patient care is essential to providing holistic care and optimizing patient outcomes. In addition, consideration of the care environment is important to minimize the untoward effects of high-tech resuscitation and critical care areas. Strategies to promote physical and psychologic healing for the patient and family include reducing extraneous noises, using dim and indirect lighting, using soft colors, hanging pictures and photographs, and playing music of the patient's choice.[42]

Clinical Research

Because of the complexity of traumatic injury, the interdisciplinary approach to trauma care is a rapidly evolving field, and efforts are continuously made to encourage trauma practitioners to conduct research to increase the scientific basis of nursing and medical care. Studies of the characteristics of the trauma population and multiple therapeutic interventions should continue to refine the process and improve outcomes of trauma care.

The multitrauma patient may suddenly become the vehicle for a number of simultaneous medical and nursing research endeavors that can improve care and clinical operations. In addition to the organization's formal institutional human subject review committee, a trauma center should have an established multidisciplinary committee for reviewing all proposed research studies and existing protocols to protect the patient (and family), yet facilitate both nursing and medical research projects. Exploring the trauma patient's responses to injury and the effectiveness of specific treatments is vital to developing evidence-based patient management; therefore, conducting and implementing research is an essential component of high-quality patient care, as long as established protocols for scientific investigations are followed.

Phase I: Field Stabilization and Resuscitation

The ultimate goal in the prehospital phase is to stabilize and transport the multiply injured patient to the appropriate level trauma center via the safest and most rapid transport mode.[43] Accomplishing this requires collaboration that begins at the scene where the patient is injured. An effective EMS system provides a means for specially trained paramedics to communicate with trauma physicians at the receiving hospital and a centralized communications center to assist in planning the appropriate mode of transport for that patient. Conditions at the scene also may require calls for additional personnel to help with extrication or additional law enforcement officers to assist with crowd control or to direct traffic to prevent further injuries. In addition to the indispensable role of the paramedic, the role of the nurse and physician in the field can be of great value, as the concept of "go teams" (physicians and nurses who go from the hospital to the scene) has illustrated. In addition, flight nurses (and physicians in some programs) who staff hospital-based helicopter programs are in widespread use across the country. The three priorities for the prehospital providers at arrival on the scene are (1) scene assessment, (2) evaluation of individual patients, and (3) recognition of possible multiple patient involvement and mass casualty incidents.[43]

Assessment and Diagnosis

The Prehospital Trauma Life Support (PHTLS), Advanced Trauma Life Support (ATLS), and Advanced Cardiac Life Support (ACLS) guidelines for initial assessment provide a standardized approach to care in the prehospital setting.[43-45] In the field or at the scene of any injury, the priorities and primary survey are based on ABCDE (airway, breathing, circulation, disability, exposure).

Establishing an airway at the scene can be difficult. The injured individual may be trapped inside a vehicle with a steering wheel crushed against the chest or may have been ejected from the vehicle, resulting in serious head and facial injuries with severe bleeding causing airway obstruction. EMS personnel suspect the trauma patient of having a cervical spine injury until proved otherwise, and an airway should be established with this possibility in mind.

Immediately following attention to the ABCs, neurologic status and disability should be assessed. The baseline neurologic status (level of consciousness and pupillary size and reaction) of the trauma patient is so critical that it must be included as part of the primary assessment.[43] Exposing the patient by removal of clothing is important to identifying all injuries. However, only the amount of clothing necessary is removed to protect the patient from the environment, particularly in colder climates. Once the primary survey has been completed, a secondary survey is performed to establish the presence of further injuries.

External evidence of trauma alerts the caregiver to the possibility of internal injury. These signs may be easily overlooked in the presence of obvious hemorrhage or other significant wounds. Abrasions, contusions, and pain on movement can be observed at the scene and may lead to early recognition of occult injuries. Back and neck pain may suggest spinal injury. Abrasions and contusions of the chest and abdomen may herald occult internal injuries and concomitant head injury. Deformity and pain suggest extremity injury. All patients should be managed as though they have sustained serious injuries until a thorough examination can be made at an appropriate trauma center. If the patient is unresponsive, spinal, thoracic, and abdominal injuries are assumed present until proven otherwise. In this phase the mechanism of injury is always considered when assessing for signs of obvious or occult injury. It is essential that EMS personnel provide as much information as possible about how the injury occurred and relate specific assessment findings to the receiving facility.

Developing and Implementing the Plan

Assessment, diagnosis, and initiation of planned interventions are nearly simultaneous activities. As quickly as alterations in the ABCs are identified, treatment is instituted. A primary objective of care in the field is to prevent further injury. Care in extricating and transporting patients to avoid further damage in spinal cord injuries cannot be overemphasized. Attention to limb position and to the handling and splinting of fractures may decrease the possibility of neurovascular damage or fat emboli. Further contamination of open wounds must be avoided to decrease the incidence of overwhelming infection at a later stage.

In the prehospital phase, effective triage is vital to ensuring that the patient is sent to the most appropriate facility based on the injuries present. Specific guidelines for making these decisions must be in place and rigorously followed. Triage protocols are defined within each jurisdiction or state EMS system. Once the appropriate level of trauma center is identified, decisions about the mode of transport are made. Transporting the patient from the scene to the hospital requires selection of the method best suited to avoid or reduce complications.

The communication system used during the prehospital phase must be clear, accurate, rapid, and cost effective. Depending on the EMS system, biomedical telemetry systems, radio transmitters, standard or cellular telephones, or telemedicine may be used. When communicating assessment findings to the receiving hospital, it is imperative that a common language and approach be used, such as a specific trauma injury scoring system or the Glasgow Coma Scale. When the patient arrives at the hospital, a more detailed account of the mechanism of injury, assessment findings, and treatment administered at the scene is given to the hospital's trauma team.

Documentation from the field is crucial to the plan of care. EMS records should include information on patient status, vital signs, mechanism of injury, therapy received, and present medical history (if relevant). Any relevant social history (e.g., involvement of other family members) is also documented. Injury data include time of injury, geographic location, and any other pertinent data. These prehospital written records become part of the patient's permanent medical record and are kept because the data from them are essential in completing data requirements for trauma registries and databases. In addition, most trauma center verification or designation standards also require that the prehospital sheets be present in the medical record. Recently, the Centers for Disease Control and Prevention (CDC) and National Highway Traffic Safety Administration (NHTSA), together with several agencies throughout the country, developed a standard prehospital dataset and a dataset dictionary, available online with data entry systems.[46]

Evaluation

During the prehospital phase, ongoing evaluation of the treatment and transport plans is imperative. Continuous assessment of the patient's condition is vital to detect any signs of deterioration that may necessitate a change in plans. If the patient's condition worsens, transport to the *closest* hospital for stabilization with subsequent transfer to an appropriate level trauma center may be required. If delays in the planned transport mode occur, alternate transport might be necessary to save time and the patient's life. Changes in the patient's condition also must be relayed to the receiving facility to allow alternate orders for treatment to be issued. In situations in which EMS personnel require assistance in treatment or triage decisions, the existence of some means for consultation with a trauma physician is essential. This dedicated radio or telephone allows field personnel to communicate directly with a trauma physician as vital decisions are made.

After the patient has reached the trauma facility, it is important that the trauma team reviews the prehospital care. Any identified concerns from the prehospital phase of care (e.g., esophageal intubation, inappropriate triage or treatment decisions) should be communicated back to the prehospital jurisdictional leadership or appropriate persons. This is essential for improving quality in the trauma system as a whole. EMS representatives are key stakeholders in trauma center System Performanace Improvement Committees.

In summary, an effective plan of care for the injured victim begins at the scene of the injury. In the 1970s, Dr. R. Adams Cowley, father of the "golden hour" concept, found that multiple trauma patients who received definitive care within 60 minutes of their injuries had the best chance for recovery.[47] Rapid assessment, treatment, and transport, and clear communication during this phase will impact all subsequent stages of the patient's care.

PHASE II: IN-HOSPITAL RESUSCITATION AND OPERATIVE PHASE

Because the patient often arrives at the receiving facility from the scene with little of the golden hour remaining, immediate life-saving measures are required. A coordinated, collaborative, unified approach is the cornerstone of trauma patient care in the resuscitation area. Philosophically, all trauma patients are in critical condition until proven otherwise. Advanced preparation to allow immediate access to equipment, supplies, and personnel is essential. This is made possible by prehospital providers' notification of the patient's pending arrival at the trauma center.

PREPARATION AND INITIAL CONTACT

The resuscitation nurse plays a vital role prior to the patient's arrival. Requisite equipment for treating all injury priorities is established by ASCOT in the ATLS manual.[44] This equipment should be readily accessible and located in the area where the trauma patient arrives. In some institutions proximity of the resuscitation area to the operating room (OR) may be such that the trauma resuscitation area must be able to support major surgical procedures in emergency situations. The design of some small resuscitation areas and emergency departments makes this a challenge, but every second lost as a result of disorganization decreases the patient's chance of survival. Receiving prior notice of a patient's arrival allows preparation of routine equipment and supplies and acquisition of any unusual equipment required for specific injuries. Preassembled sterile instrument trays should be readily available to save valuable time.

Members of the trauma team are notified prior to patient arrival and must be present when the patient is admitted. In major trauma centers this team usually consists of an attending (trauma surgeon or emergency medicine physician), a trauma fellow, one or two emergency medicine or surgery residents, one or two nurses, a respiratory therapist, anesthesia personnel, and a patient care technician. Response times and presence of these individuals is dictated and monitored by the trauma center verification or designation process. Preparation also includes donning of appropriate protective attire (goggles/face shield, mask, gloves, and water-impervious cover gown) before the patient's arrival.[48] These CDC guidelines and Occupational Safety and Health Administration (OSHA) requirements are considered to be the minimal personal protection by ASCOT for all health care providers who may be in contact with the patient's body substances.[44] Each member of the team is assigned a specific role during the resuscitation, which is determined before the patient arrives.

Some patients may be initially treated and stabilized in a hospital that does not provide a full complement of trauma services. These patients are subsequently transferred to a higher level trauma center. Before transfer, these patients may require aggressive management to achieve hemodynamic stability and adequate tissue oxygenation while preventing further deterioration. Of great importance is the documentation and communication of events prior to transfer. When the referring facility communicates with the receiving hospital, the report should include the data shown in Table 10-1.

ASSESSMENT

The resuscitation nurse plays a vital role in the quick assessment and stabilization of patients at admission. After the notification of a pending admission, the resuscitation area is inspected to ensure all required supplies are available; the bedside monitor, suction apparatus, and overhead lights turned on; and intravenous (IV) lines primed with the appropriate fluids. Additional equipment is prepared based on specific information obtained from the field personnel. Trauma patients who arrive at the trauma facility by helicopter should be met by some members of the trauma team—ideally the resuscitation nurse and a person trained in emergency airway techniques. The comprehensive plan of care for the hospital phase is initiated on the helipad by performing a rapid primary survey to ensure that the ABCs are intact. If the patient is conscious, the nurse may also obtain a brief initial history at this time.

While assessing the patient, therapeutic communication is a priority. The nurse meeting the patient at the helipad, at the ambulance entrance, or in the emergency department establishes verbal communication and continues the exchange throughout this phase of care. Although ensuring the basic ABCs is the highest priority, the nurse needs to talk calmly to the patient, providing support and reassurance to help reduce fear and anxiety. The trauma patient is often frightened and confused and may be experiencing pain or hypoxia. Although the emphasis during this phase is on assessment and stabilization of the patient's physical condition, the patient's emotional state also must be considered. Psychologic support to calm the patient, prepare him or her for what is ahead, and establish trust is important during this stage.

On arrival in the resuscitation area from the helipad or ambulance entrance, the nurse and paramedic provide the trauma team with a succinct report of the assessment and clinical findings. The initial assessment and resuscitation activities are protocol driven and should be well ingrained in the minds of all team members. Throughout the resuscitation

TABLE 10-1 Example of Report Form Used to Provide Patient Information to Receiving Hospital from Transferring Facility

Transferring Hospital: ______________________________

Name ______________________________ Direct Family Contact ______________

Age ______________________________ Name ______________

Date/Time of Injury ______________________________ Phone # ______________

Mechanism of Injury ______________________________

Injuries ______________________________

Allergies ______________________________

Medications ______________________________

Substance Abuse ______________________________

Presenting Symptoms ______________________________

Isolation History ______________________________

Vital Signs: ______________________________

Diagnostic Tests:

Labs ______________________________

(include blood alcohol and lactate)

X-rays ______________________________ CT Scans: ______________

Angiography ______________________________

Operative Procedure: ______________________________ __/__/__

______________________________ __/__/__

______________________________ __/__/__

______________________________ __/__/__

Estimated Blood Loss: ______________

Systems Report:

Neuro TBI: Exam: ______________________________

Treatment: ______________________________

FFP: ______________ Vitamin K: ______________

Pre-existing Meds: ______________________________

(Aspirin, Coumadin, etc.)

Spine: Steroids Given: ______________ Dose: ______________

Collar: ______________ Vasopressors: ______________

Motor: ______________ Sensation: ______________

Pulmonary ______________________________

Cardiac ______________________________

Gastrointestinal ______________________________

Genitourinary ______________________________

Extremities ______________________________

Skin ______________________________

Temperature ______________

Peripheral IVs ______________________________

Central Lines ______________________________

Volume In ______________ Crystalloids ______________ Colloids ______________

Intubation ______________________________ Ventilator Settings: ______________

Pulse Oximetry ______________________________

Arterial Blood Gases ______________ Backboard Time: On______

Medications ______________________________

Pain: ______________ Antibiotics: ______________

Tetanus: ______________ Other vaccines given: ______________

Pneumovax: ______________

DVT Prophylaxis ___ Heparin ___ Lovenox ___ Filter ___ SCD

Oro/nasogastric Tube

Foley ______________ Urine Output ______________ Since When ______________

Ortho ___ Splints ___ Binder

Soft Tissue Cultures: Blood Wound

When: ______________ ______________

Results: ______________ ______________

Family Social: ______________________________

What Information Was Given to the Family: ______________________________

REMINDER: PLEASE SEND THE CTS, ALL X-RAY FILMS, LABS WITH THE PATIENT BEING TRANSFERRED

TBI, traumatic brain injury; *DVT*, deep vein thrombosis; *SCD*, sequential compression device.

Courtesy of RA Cowley Shock Trauma Center, University of Maryland Medical Center, Baltimore, MD.

and stabilization phase, the physician team leader and admitting nurse coordinate procedures, not only to carry out the established protocols for treatment but also to individualize care when appropriate. Specialists are consulted when appropriate; sedation and occasionally pharmacologic paralytic agents and intubation may be required to allow a thorough medical examination and establish treatment priorities.

Documentation is critical during this phase of care and includes information that is crucial to the plan of care. Vital signs and hemodynamic stability must be monitored continuously to detect subtle changes in the patient's condition. Particular attention must be paid to intake and output. Intravascular volume administration and massive fluid resuscitation may predispose the patient to severe pulmonary dysfunction and coagulopathies within a few hours.[49] Continuous monitoring following the collection of baseline data is done to detect changes in the patient's condition as early as possible. Recording vital signs and electrocardiographic changes as often as every 5 minutes may be necessary.

The team approach is the most important factor during both the assessment and treatment of the patient. Following established protocols, the trauma nurse and physician approach the assessment of the patient in a systematic, organized fashion.

The assessment must be done quickly and efficiently. Priority-based trauma protocols provide the framework for detecting and treating life-threatening injuries. The first priorities focus on the traditional ABCs of airway, breathing, and circulation, and are expanded to include D for neurologic disability and E for exposing all injuries and for environmental control (thermoregulation). Secondary priorities identify less evident but still life-threatening respiratory or cardiovascular dysfunctions. Third priorities are to detect and evaluate more subtle injuries that may contribute to morbidity and mortality but that are not necessarily life threatening.

History

The resuscitation nurse obtains as accurate a database as possible if the patient is alert. In addition to physical symptoms, initial information includes allergies, significant medical history, current medications, age, religion, and weight. A brief history can be accomplished rapidly by an "AMPLE" history: A, allergies; M, medications currently being taken; P, past illnesses; L, last meal; E, events preceding the injury.[44]

Information regarding these aspects of the patient's medical background is important for the trauma team to know before initiating treatment. It is often impossible to obtain such a history when families are not available and the patient is comatose. The belongings of the patient are examined for medic-alert cards delineating allergies or medical problems, or prescription medications that might give a clue to underlying medical conditions. The Patient Self-Determination Act (1990)[50] requires that the hospital also seek information regarding any advanced directives that the patient may have made. This information, in addition to the resources of the social worker and pastoral care, are valuable to the trauma team in making ethical decisions regarding treatment.

Diagnosis

The resuscitation nurse must be aware of the actual or suspected medical diagnoses to begin the plan and the care. Establishing the patient's database helps to guide patient care by organizing facts concerning the patient history, causes and the nature of injury, and the degree of trauma sustained. The data collected can provide a basis for both medical and nursing care.

Prehospital events and care information are important components of the patient database. This information provides an understanding of the mechanisms of injury, the initial physical findings, and other clues important to the management of the patient. Evaluation of a critical patient's status and the ultimate medical and nursing management are dependent on analysis of vital signs, fluid resuscitation, and other critical data entered in the trauma database. Establishing and maintaining an accurate database are key responsibilities of the resuscitation nurse. Accuracy of diagnosis, therapeutic medical and nursing plans of care, and patient outcomes depend on this function.

Diagnostic Studies

The multiply injured patient may require several diagnostic studies before accurate medical diagnoses can be made. The nurse plays a vital role in preparing the patient and in coordinating these studies. Portable radiography equipment should be readily available in the trauma resuscitation area. Access to a Picture Archiving and Communications System (PACS), digital radiographic scanning, and online transmission of radiographic images (teleradiology) can increase real-time interpretation and reduce diagnostic delays and errors. Other initial bedside diagnostic studies may include focused assessment sonography for trauma (FAST), which provides rapid, accurate, and noninvasive assessment of intraabdominal fluid[44]; diagnostic peritoneal lavage (DPL); and 12-lead electrocardiogram (ECG). Appropriate laboratory tests are drawn and typically include type and cross-match or screening for blood, blood gases, metabolic panel with a serum lactate, toxicology, and alcohol screens. Many centers utilize point of care bedside laboratory studies to expedite access to laboratory test data.

New technology for whole-body radiographs is available in the resuscitation area or emergency department of some larger trauma centers. One such device is the Statscan Critical Imaging System, a low-dose digital x-ray machine. This device provides a head-to-toe radiographic image of good quality in less than 15 seconds to allow rapid evaluation of the presence and severity of fractures without repositioning a patient to place the radiographic plates or film. After these initial measures and a secondary survey, thorough radiographic studies are initiated.

Additional studies, such as computerized tomography (CT), angiography, or magnetic resonance imaging (MRI) must be done in other areas of the hospital. Transporting the patient in a safe and timely manner is the responsibility of the trauma resuscitation nurse. During transport, patient care should be maintained at the same level as that provided in the resuscitation unit. This is a team effort that may require a trauma physician, nurse, and respiratory therapist. A multipurpose cart, transport bag, or box equipped with the supplies required for resuscitating and monitoring patients during transport or in the area where the studies are performed can be developed for this purpose. Portable monitoring equipment (ECG, pulse oximetry, end-tidal CO_2, and pressure monitors) should be available and used during transport when appropriate. Blood products may also be transported safely with the use of an insulated container.

Developing and Implementing the Plan

Appropriate patient management consists of the rapid assessment and treatment of life-threatening pathology. Logical sequential treatment priorities are established on the basis of overall patient assessment. Patient management consists of a rapid initial evaluation, resuscitation of vital functions, more detailed secondary and tertiary assessments, and, finally, the initiation of definitive care. Prevention of irreversible tissue hypoxia is the essence of trauma resuscitation. Treatment of life-threatening respiratory and cardiovascular instability, brain injury, and spinal cord injury before definitive diagnosis is often essential in the management of the multiply injured patient. The time taken to establish a firm diagnosis before life-saving measures are instituted may mean the difference between life and death. End points of resuscitation may include stabilization of vital signs, with normalization, or trend to normalization of serum lactate, base deficit, intestinal pH (pHi), central venous oximetry ($ScvO_2$) or other markers of hypoperfusion and hypoxia.[51]

Stabilization of Life-Threatening Conditions

The immediate objective in this phase of care is the stabilization of life-threatening conditions. The concept of "treatment prior to final diagnoses" is based on establishment of an airway, adequate ventilation, circulation, and perfusion and includes control of hemorrhage and initiation of fluid resuscitation.

A chest tube may need to be inserted rapidly to relieve a tension pneumothorax or hemothorax. The amount of chest drainage is monitored closely to assist in determining blood replacement needs and the need for surgical intervention. In a life-threatening emergency, uncross-matched O-negative blood for females of child-bearing age, O-positive blood for males, or type-specific blood may be administered until laboratory results and cross-matching have been completed. Immediate and rapid access to blood is imperative. Large centers have separate blood refrigerators; however, a system for access and guidelines for massive transfusion and a rapid access plan is necessary.

Trauma resuscitation nurses use the principles and techniques of Advanced Trauma Care for Nurses (ATNC)[52] and ATLS.[44] In most trauma centers, nurses do not intubate or insert central venous lines; however, they prepare equipment for and assist with these procedures in addition to understanding their priority in resuscitative care. Trauma nurses must be familiar with and adept at setting up and performing an autotransfusion. Critical thinking and advanced proactive management are essential in the resuscitation phase. After the patient is stabilized and emergency procedures are complete, a more thorough secondary survey can be done. For example, FAST or peritoneal lavage may be performed to determine the need for abdominal surgery, or obvious or suspected fractures are immobilized with splints if these are not already in place.

Relief of pain is important and carefully managed. Consideration needs to be given to the administration of medication, such as sedatives or opioids, that can make accurate neurologic assessment difficult and may cause hypotension in an underresuscitated patient. On the other hand, if a patient arrives in a combative or severely restless state that hinders airway control and thorough examination, anesthetic or paralyzing agents may need to be used. Anesthesia providers often must be involved in managing these patients, and in some trauma centers, a pain service or clinical pharmacist is available for rapid access to drugs and to aid in pain management plans. These roles also provide resources to verify medication appropriateness and dosages so that patient safety goals are met.

Achieving and maintaining a euthermic body temperature in trauma patients has long been considered a mainstay of nursing care, particularly as a mechanism to improve hemostasis.[49] Infusion of warmed fluids and use of warming lights and blankets are standard. However, recent research in traumatic brain injury populations provides evidence that intracranial pressure is significantly decreased at brain temperatures below 37° C (98.6° F) and is further reduced at temperatures 35° to 36° C. (95° F to 96.8° F).[53] In addition, the 2005 ACLS guidelines reference the research related to the protective effect of hypothermia on the brain and other organs during and following cardiac arrest. The most recent recommendation is *not* to actively rewarm patients who are hemodynamically stable and develop a mild hypothermia (greater than 33° C [91.5° F]) after cardiac arrest resuscitation.[45] The guidelines also provide specific rewarming strategies based on the level of hypothermia.

Cardiac Arrest

Most patients who arrest during the resuscitation phase following traumatic injury do so secondary to profound intravascular volume depletion.[44] An arrest caused by hypovolemia requires massive volume infusion with red blood cells and closed chest compressions or, in some instances, manual compression of the ventricles via open thoracotomy. Resuscitative thoracotomy is indicated in only a few specific patients or situations. It may be lifesaving for patients with penetrating cardiac, thoracic, or exsanguinating abdominal vascular injuries who arrest in the resuscitation unit or immediately before arrival. Very rarely is resuscitative thoracotomy successful in blunt trauma.[45] Due to risk of blood exposure in this procedure, trauma centers may develop a protocol/guideline for blunt chest trauma thoracotomies. The nurse on the trauma team must ensure the accessibility of the necessary equipment for open or closed cardiopulmonary resuscitation and assist the trauma surgeon accordingly.

The potential for sudden cardiac arrest remains through the critical care phase and even into the intermediate and rehabilitation phases, although the etiology of cardiac arrest differs through the phases of the trauma cycle. In the critical care phase, cardiac arrest may result from overwhelming sepsis, arrhythmias secondary to myocardial damage, multiple organ failure, respiratory failure, tension pneumothorax, or pulmonary embolus. In the intermediate and rehabilitative phases, a pulmonary embolus or complications from long-term care may precipitate an arrest.

Communication With the Family During the Resuscitation Phase

The initial communication with the patient's family occurs during the resuscitation phase of care. Family members are generally in a state of crisis, having had no time to prepare for the suddenness of an injury to their loved one. Ideally, the trauma nurse and physician together provide information concerning the patient's injuries and condition. The initial patient and family histories are obtained. The nurse thereafter serves as a liaison to the patient's family, keeping them updated on their family member's condition as often as time will allow. Social service and pastoral care personnel are valuable and collaborative resources for both the nurse and the families in these situations.

Psychologic Support. Psychological support for the patient is also a priority throughout this early phase of trauma care. Patients are in as much a state of crisis as their family members. Even though the total systems approach to trauma is used to guide treatment, it is essential to recognize that the total system being dealt with is a human being. The patient has had no time to anticipate the injury. Attempts to cope with this fact are often worsened by pain or hypoxia. The rapid sequence of unfamiliar activities, beginning with rescue, impairs the patient's ability to perceive events realistically.

For full recovery, the patient's emotional state must be acknowledged and addressed from the beginning. The nurse should introduce himself or herself and provide the patient with a brief description of the surroundings and an explanation of procedures as they are performed. These explanations should be short and concise and may need to be repeated. Patients in the resuscitation phase feel powerless. They have little control and a significant amount of fear of the unknown. Keeping them informed aids in reducing these feelings.

Spiritual Considerations. The spiritual component is also vital to the multiply injured patient's plan of care. The nurse must consider the patient's spiritual practices as soon as that information is available. These practices are important to ensure support for the patient and family, and they may have a significant impact on the plan of care. For example, if the patient is critically injured and death is imminent, the need for a priest to administer the sacrament of the sick to a Catholic patient must be addressed. Often it is the nurse who calls a priest, especially if the family has not yet arrived in the emergency area. If the patient is identified as a Jehovah's Witness, the treatment plan typically requires modification, particularly during the resuscitation and critical care phases. Each trauma facility should have a clear policy covering the withholding or administration of blood for these patients.

Evaluation and Transition

Nursing management during the initial resuscitation phase is first directed by established protocols and priorities of care. The overall assessment of the patient by the physician and nurse will guide the plan of care as it evolves. Throughout this phase the nurse must continuously anticipate and assess changes in the patient's condition, prepare equipment, assist the trauma team with procedures aimed at stabilization, and evaluate the appropriateness and effectiveness of medical and nursing interventions. As the patient's condition stabilizes or changes, the plan of care is reevaluated and altered to accommodate the changing profile. Determination of the patient's readiness to move into another phase is a collaborative decision. Clear communication is essential. Using a standardized communication handoff, required by the Joint Commission for all patient handoffs,[54] the resuscitation nurse shares pertinent information regarding injuries, diagnostic test results, interventions, treatments, psychosocial issues, and the plan of care with the next care providers to facilitate transition to the next phase.

Perioperative Phase

After the initial resuscitation, many traumatic injuries require surgical intervention; some are emergent while other procedures may be done hours or days after admission. The perioperative nurse assumes responsibility at this time as the patient advocate and ensures coordination of care. Many aspects of the role of the OR nurse include the traditional responsibilities of any perioperative nurse. However, in addition to these, the operative needs of the multiply injured patient make the nurse's role more complex and demanding.

ORs in major trauma centers require fully staffed teams around the clock and the ready availability of at least one suite for direct admissions into the OR. In other facilities the OR team must be prepared to react promptly when the trauma patient arrives. Trauma patients may require repeated surgical procedures to treat their injuries successfully. Rooms must be available for these elective procedures without sacrificing availability of rooms for emergent cases.

Assessment

The role of the perioperative nurse, which traditionally includes a preoperative assessment and interview of the patient, may be drastically altered during the resuscitation phase for any of the following reasons:

1. The patient may be comatose or unable to communicate effectively if an endotracheal tube or a tracheostomy is in place.
2. The emergency care necessitated by the instability of the patient may render him or her inaccessible to the operative nurse until arrival in the operating room.
3. The patient may have required induction of anesthesia immediately on arrival in the resuscitation area to allow implementation of resuscitative and diagnostic measures.
4. If the patient is awake, the physiologic and psychological impact of injury may be so overwhelming as to preclude any assimilation of information given.

In these situations the priorities for the trauma nurse in the perioperative phase include the following: ascertaining the urgency of the need for surgical intervention, arranging for the availability of a room, preparing the necessary equipment for the procedures to be performed, and coordinating the participation of the various specialty surgical teams who will be operating on the patient. Any data collection needed is obtained from the resuscitation trauma nurse or physician. The OR nurse must obtain a detailed summary of what occurred during resuscitation. As the patient progresses past the critical care phase, elective surgical procedures may be necessary to restore maximal function. In these cases the OR nurse plays a vital role in establishing trust and providing the appropriate patient education.

Diagnosis

From a medical standpoint the trauma patient who arrives in the operating room is far different from the patient undergoing elective surgery. The latter has been diagnosed preoperatively, and surgical intervention has been prescribed to correct the disorder. The multiply injured trauma patient, on the other hand, often arrives in the operating room without a specific diagnosis. FAST may have identified the presence of a hemoperitoneum, but the specific organs injured will not be known until an exploratory laparotomy is performed. The perioperative nurse needs to ensure that all instruments and equipment that may be needed are accessible for unexpected findings or alterations in the planned surgical procedure. In collaboration with the surgical teams and anesthesiologist, continuous assessment of the patient's hemodynamic stability is a priority.

Developing and Implementing a Plan

The circulating trauma nurse plays a major role as coordinator. Multiply injured patients often require procedures performed by several different specialty teams, either simultaneously or sequentially. Coordination between the teams is essential. Equipment for multiple teams and procedures needs to be readily available and properly placed for easy access. The nurse must be able to set up equipment that might be needed to repair injuries that were totally unsuspected until surgical exploration identified them. The OR nurse and the surgical services that will be performing the procedures generally determine the order of surgical procedures based on time and priority of surgical intervention. If conflict arises, the attending trauma surgeon makes the decision about which procedure has priority. A patient who has a hemoperitoneum, an open ankle fracture, a deep chin laceration, loose teeth, and multiple facial fractures might be treated in the following manner: One team of surgeons will perform the exploratory laparotomy, while the oral surgeon extracts teeth and applies arch bars. On completion of these procedures, the orthopedic surgeon may set the ankle, while the plastic surgeon closes the laceration of the chin.

Because of the need for multiple surgical procedures, the patient may be on the OR table for many hours. Trauma patients are at risk for developing venous thromboembolism; therefore, early initiation of prevention strategies is important, for example, application of external pneumatic compression devices to uninjured lower extremities.[31] The effects of prolonged positioning on the OR table and administration of anesthesia must be addressed. Skin breakdown can occur even before the patient leaves the surgical suite if vulnerable areas have not been adequately protected. Decreased circulation from high OR table surface to skin pressure, blood loss and hypoperfusion, hypothermia, and prolonged administration of anesthesia all contribute to this preventable problem.

Blood and blood products must be readily available to the trauma ORs. Many trauma centers have established separate refrigerators in the OR area for the storage of blood and blood products. To prevent severe hypothermia, all blood and intravenous fluids should be warmed by whatever equipment the individual facility has chosen for that purpose.

The anesthesia providers have additional responsibilities when the trauma patient undergoes anesthesia for emergency surgery versus when elective surgery is performed. These patients must be monitored carefully and constantly. Often their past medical history is unknown, including medications or inherited diseases that increase the risks of general anesthesia. Assessment of hemodynamic and pulmonary status, maintenance of multiple intravenous catheters, administration of appropriate medications, blood, blood products, and fluids, and preparation for sudden, unexpected deterioration of the patient are responsibilities that make the trauma anesthesia provider unique.

Communication with the Family. Another primary responsibility of the perioperative trauma nurse is communicating with the family. Every attempt should be made to keep the family informed both before and during the surgical procedures. Before surgery the information conveyed to the family includes suspected injuries, planned surgical procedures, estimated time the patient will be in surgery, and potential for death. When operative procedures are prolonged, consistent communication with family members is paramount to help to alleviate fear of the unknown. Typically information that is provided intraoperatively includes an update on the current status of the patient, what the family can expect postoperatively, the surgeon's name, necessary phone numbers to obtain information postoperatively, and reiteration of the time estimate for completion of surgical procedures. After the procedure the trauma surgeon should explain which operative procedures were performed, the stability and prognosis of the patient, and the unit to which the patient will be admitted.

Comfortable waiting areas for families should be available as close to the OR floor as possible. Beverages and access to a telephone make their wait less unpleasant. Often during this phase, the family members are at a loss to know what they can do to help. The nurse can suggest that they and their friends donate blood to help replace the blood that was given to their loved one. This may provide them a purpose during this time of waiting and uncertainty.

Evaluation and Transition. After surgery the patient must be reassessed and prepared for transport to the postanesthesia care unit (PACU) or critical care unit. A brief communication with the receiving unit nurse is required before transport to allow the nurses in the next phase to prepare for the admission. The initial communication with the receiving unit should, however, occur soon after the patient's arrival in the OR. Periodic updates related to the patient's condition or disposition status assist other units to prepare for the patient's arrival. Often critical care units need to alter current patient assignments and obtain specific supplies and equipment to accommodate the needs of a postoperative trauma patient.

On arrival in the PACU or the critical care unit, again a standardized, thorough report to the receiving unit nurse is essential. An accurate report of the resuscitation efforts, surgical procedures performed, vital sign trends, fluid balance, estimated blood loss, and medications and anesthesia administered ensures continuity of care. A survey of vascular access sites, fluids and medications being infused, and drainage tubes by both the OR nurse or anesthesia provider and the receiving trauma nurse in the PACU or critical care unit is imperative.

Severely injured patients often require additional surgeries to treat injuries or complications that may have developed after primary surgery. Many of these occur while the patient still requires critical care and maximal technologic support. The perioperative nurse and anesthesia provider, in conjunction with the critical care nurse and respiratory therapist, are responsible for ensuring that the patient is safely transported.

PHASE III: CRITICAL CARE

The critical care phase for the patient with multiple system injuries requires the skills and collaboration of a variety of health care professionals. Because of the wide spectrum of physiologic, psychological, and sociologic derangements encountered after severe traumatic injury, coordination of the health care team is integral to management of trauma patients in the critical care phase. The efforts of the health care team must be synchronized to provide optimal care, to minimize the physiologic and psychologic stress of the injuries, and to provide cost-effective care with appropriate resource use. It is essential that one physician and nurse be designated to coordinate the many disciplines involved in the critical care phase. Depending on the trauma care management model embraced by the institution, the physician coordinator may be the admitting trauma surgeon or a critical care intensivist. When multiple services are involved, coordination by a critical care intensivist has been shown to provide more efficient, cost-effective care delivery with improved patient outcomes.[55] Similarly, the nurse coordinator may be an advanced practice nurse such as the trauma coordinator, trauma case manager, clinical nurse specialist, or acute care nurse practitioner; in other models the coordinating nurse may be a staff-level primary coordinating nurse. Regardless of the title, the nurse designated to coordinate the patient's care has the responsibility to remain abreast of the status and progress of the patient, activities and plan of care of the multidisciplinary team, flow of information between team members, and interactions with the family members.

ASSESSMENT

Just as the resuscitation area nurse prepares for the emergency admission of a multitrauma patient, the critical care nurse must identify and anticipate the many needs of the patient and prepare for arrival in the critical care unit (CCU). The resuscitation nurse, the anesthesia provider, or the PACU nurse gives the CCU nurse a thorough standardized report, including the physical aspects of the patient's injuries, interventions, current status, family information, and any special equipment that will be needed. For example, monitoring, ventilatory, warming, and emergency equipment should be available and checked for proper functioning before the patient's arrival. Anticipation of physiologic derangements is necessary to prepare for the admission of a potentially unstable hypotensive, bleeding, hypothermic patient. The scope and fundamental principles of critical care assessment of trauma patients are similar to those for other critically ill populations.

General Considerations

Admission of the severely injured patient to the CCU directly from the OR is usually preferable because it enhances the continuity of care and avoids an additional transport that might put the critically ill patient at risk. In addition, a CCU typically has more readily available support services and resources than a PACU. If a PACU is used, continuity in the plan of care and family contact is essential. On admission to the critical care area, the patient is immediately connected to monitoring equipment and placed on a ventilator. Infusions of IV fluids or blood products are noted, and the site for each is identified immediately. The position and patency of drains; the condition of wound dressings; and the location, type, and status of skeletal traction are established. An important method to improve patient safety, reduce errors, and capture appropriate admission orders is to utilize computerized or preprinted physician order sets. If not initiated in the resuscitation phase, implementing standardized orders for mechanical ventilation and weaning, electrolyte replacement, brain injury or spinal cord injury management, as examples, ensures that critical patient care needs are addressed in a timely manner.

After establishing that vital physiologic functions are intact, the CCU nurse continues receiving a detailed report from the previous care providers (Box 10-1) and conducts a thorough assessment. This information is documented to provide a baseline for assessing changes in patient status and family interactions and to guide initial interventions during the critical care phase.

A total systems assessment is conducted and documented completely, system by system, in the nursing record at least once every 24 hours. Use of a standardized assessment form or computer documentation system decreases time needed for recording. Frequent reassessment and documentation of changes are ongoing responsibilities. Most often the nurse at the bedside identifies changes in the patient's condition that warrant notification of the medical team for corresponding changes in treatment.

BOX 10-1 Information Required From Anesthesia, Operating Room, or Resuscitation Area Personnel Upon Patient Transfer to Inpatient Unit

- Admitting trauma surgeon
- Mechanism of injury
- List of injuries
- Diagnostic tests completed and results
- Test results still pending
- Resuscitation area interventions
- Hypotensive or hypoxic episodes before or during admission
- Surgical procedures, findings, and complications
- Type of anesthesia and medications administered
- Current infusions
- Type and volume of blood products received
- Estimated blood loss
- Fluid balance
- Drains, intravenous catheters
- Most recent vital signs and trends
- Management plans
- Family information
  - Notification
  - Name of spokesperson
  - What they have been told about the patient's injuries
  - If they have seen the patient
  - How they can be reached

Nearly constant evaluation of the multiply injured critical care patient is vital during this phase for many reasons. The body responds to the stress of trauma with many physiologic and emotional changes. The trauma patient's condition may deteriorate and fail to achieve physiologic stability as a result of systemic inflammatory response syndrome (SIRS) from the initial injuries, due to sequelae of massive fluid resuscitation, or from injuries that may have been missed on admission. Possible life-threatening complications that often occur in this phase demand early detection for prevention or treatment to increase chances of survival. Ongoing assessment data act as validating criteria for accurate diagnoses and interventions. The patient's tolerance of and response to prescribed medical and nursing therapies must be monitored.

Throughout the phase of critical care, one of the major values of ongoing assessment is the early detection of actual or potential sequelae of injuries and complications. For example, the patient with a severe pulmonary contusion may go on to develop acute lung injury or acute respiratory distress syndrome (ARDS); early recognition of this condition allows early therapeutic intervention. A primary objective in the early detection of complications following traumatic injury is anticipation by the nurse of potential complications that are associated with specific injuries, surgical procedures, and volume resuscitation. During assessment the nurse must keep in mind the injuries that the patient has sustained and the complications commonly associated with them.

Diagnostic Studies

A tertiary survey should be considered early in the critical care phase, or in whichever phase follows resuscitation or perioperative phases. The tertiary survey includes a complete head-to-toe assessment and reevaluation of previous radiologic, laboratory, or other diagnostic studies. The benefit to the patient is in the discovery of injuries that may have been missed due to urgent resuscitation efforts, management of life-threatening injuries, and distracting pain. In some organizations, the advanced practice nurse may assume responsibility for initiating the tertiary survey.[56]

Critically ill trauma patients typically require multiple and frequent diagnostic studies. Although most often appropriate, periodic evaluation of practice protocols is important to ensure cost-effective care and resource use. Opportunities to reduce the number of diagnostic procedures a patient is subjected to without affecting the quality of care delivered should be explored. Examples include scrutiny of the need for complete blood laboratory panels versus individual tests, routine chest radiographs after over-the-wire central venous catheter change, or follow-up CT scans.

During the critical care phase, serial laboratory studies have a role in the evaluation of the patient's status and are used with other data to alter the treatment plan. Protocols for obtaining these tests ensure that appropriate monitoring takes place. Protocols include the types of tests and their frequency, the type of container to be used for each test sample, and where they are to be sent for analysis or if they should be done using bedside technology.

Blood samples for serial hematocrit, hemoglobin, coagulation profile, serum lactate level, electrolytes, and arterial and venous blood gases should be drawn based on clinical protocols or pathways reflecting the patient's condition. Routine complete panels often are not necessary, and laboratory diagnostic studies that do not trigger an intervention should be avoided. Although laboratory studies provide needed data for assessment, the volume of blood drawn must be minimized. Unnecessary blood sampling affects the patient, resource consumption, and costs.

Multiple trauma patients who are hemodynamically compromised and require a high level of ventilatory support may be too unstable to risk an unnecessary transport for diagnostic studies in areas outside the CCU. Interruption of traction devices also may be detrimental to a patient. In these cases, bedside studies may be necessary. These studies (e.g., evoked potentials, electroencephalogram) are often time consuming and involve large pieces of equipment. The nurse caring for the patient should coordinate proper timing of the tests so they do not interfere with other needed treatments or the patient's rest or sleep schedule. While a test is being done, monitoring of the patient must not be interrupted. Care should be scheduled so that necessary treatments may be completed just before or immediately after a test.

Psychosocial

The ongoing evaluation of a trauma patient's psychologic adjustment to injury is as important as ongoing physical assessment. It is a vital component of holistic care. The psychologic response to trauma may fluctuate dramatically as adjustment to the injuries occurs. One moment the patient may demonstrate signs of adjustment to the injury; the next he or she may succumb to depression or anger and lash out or not cooperate with treatment.

Trauma patients' psychologic responses may be unpredictable. A 40-year-old patient with paraplegia secondary to a thoracic spine injury may adjust better than a 16-year-old boy whose severely fractured femur will keep him from fulfilling his life's dream of playing professional football. A continuous psychologic assessment will enable the primary nurse to plan interventions that will help a trauma patient deal with the injuries more effectively. Knowledge of the patient's support systems, or lack thereof, how the patient usually responds to stressful situations, and the patient's previous coping mechanisms will enable the nurse to develop a more individualized plan of care. The trauma nurse plays a key role in facilitating patient and family access to resources that can provide support.

Developing and Implementing the Plan

During the critical care phase the concept of collaborative practice, begun in the resuscitation phase, becomes even more important. Many different medical services may be involved in the care of the multiply injured (e.g., orthopedics, neurosurgery, plastic surgery, infectious disease, and critical care). Respiratory therapists, physical therapists, nutritionists, and others who have daily contact with the patient assume integral roles in the care plan. The primary nurse, patient care coordinator, or case manager is the individual with a global view of all the services involved; therefore, the nurse's role as coordinator is of great significance. The trauma patient is dependent on the nurse at this stage of care. The patient looks to the nurse as the coordinator, decision maker, and advocate. It is beyond the scope of this chapter to address all nursing care concerns during the critical care phase. In caring for trauma patients, however, there are particular aspects of critical care nursing practice that have special relevance to this phase of care.

Interdisciplinary Approach

All aspects of the plan of care for the critically ill trauma patient involve multiple disciplines. Coordination of these disciplines to ensure common patient goals is uniquely the responsibility of the primary care nurse. Daily interdisciplinary rounds facilitate sharing of information and objectives, reviewing variances in protocols, clinical pathways, and developing or revising short- and long-term plans; the primary coordinating nurse or designee must be part of these interactions and decisions. Interdisciplinary collaboration and integration of interdisciplinary protocols, guidelines or clinical pathways, management guidelines, and protocols facilitates the coordination of disciplines and promotes achievement of positive patient outcomes.[17,23-25] Interdisciplinary daily rounding with input from various care providers and services is critical for care management.

In very complex cases, holding interdisciplinary conferences every 2 to 3 weeks allows all disciplines to discuss their perspectives and agree on priorities and specific long-term goals. This plan should be documented for reference by all the disciplines. Subsequent conferences focus on evaluation of progress and revising the plan. Participants in caregiver conferences include representatives from all the specialty areas and services involved in the patient's care.

Emergency Procedures

The multitrauma patient has the potential for developing sudden life-threatening complications. Critical care trauma nurses require the cognitive and psychomotor capabilities to deal with emergent situations. The need for emergency equipment is unpredictable; thus, accessibility is essential. Up-to-date emergency equipment in good working condition must be available at all times. Seconds count: patients' lives may depend on the anticipation of critical events and the readiness of emergency equipment. Nursing orientation programs and skills updates need to include competency-based education and training on emergency equipment and supplies, such as internal and external temporary pacemakers, surgical trays for opening a patient's chest or abdomen, and intracranial pressure monitors.

Bedside operative procedures may be necessary, and the critical care nurse should be prepared to facilitate these. The nurse coordinates the efforts, ensures the presence of appropriate personnel (e.g., an anesthesia provider and OR nurses), obtains necessary equipment, provides continued high-level care and monitoring, serves as the patient's advocate, and maintains communication with the family.

Documentation

The physiologic monitoring that occurs in the CCU generates a large amount of data that, together with the clinical picture of the patient, provides the basis on which to prescribe treatment. Identifying trends from these data is crucial to detecting subtle changes in patients' conditions and to altering therapy accordingly. To identify these trends in a timely and objective manner, documentation must be thorough and must allow for visual examination of various categories of data in relation to other sets of data. For example, whether a computer or a flow sheet is used, it is important to be able to look at all parameters, interventions, and the patient's response to interventions (e.g., vital signs, oxygen delivery and uptake, intake and output, medications, and neurologic status) simultaneously over a given time in the patient's course of treatment.

Electronic records are very useful for documenting physiologic data. Automatic physiologic monitoring capabilities, IV drug calculation programs, and recording of laboratory data are helpful adjuncts to the development of specialized and individualized plans of care. The computer allows data gathered by various disciplines involved in trauma patient care to be accessed and used by care providers at any given time and from various locations.

Transporting Critical Care Patients

Effective diagnostic procedures and therapies for the multitrauma patient often depend on information obtained through special tests, such as CT or nuclear medicine studies. An already compromised, critically injured patient may have to undergo the additional stress of transport to other areas of the hospital. When the patient is multiply injured or unstable, the potential problems and the nurse's responsibilities increase in direct proportion to the number and severity of life-threatening injuries already present. To ensure patient safety before, during, and after the transfer, the trauma nurse must use advanced planning to coordinate care requirements, personnel, backup equipment, and supplies. The level of patient monitoring and care should not change during transport.

Once the risks have been weighed against the necessity of the test, the nurse assumes responsibility for the coordination of the transport. Patient needs during transport are many and include respiratory support, medications (routine and emergency medications and premedications for diagnostic tests) that must be given while out of the unit, IV fluids, and adequate monitoring.

During any transport the nurse has the responsibility to protect and preserve all IV and monitoring catheters, cables, and drains. Unintentional dislodgment of these may pose significant risks to the patient and in some cases may be life threatening.

The number and type of personnel accompanying the patient must also be decided. A transport policy should provide guidelines for these decisions. If it is necessary to transport blood with an unstable trauma patient, an insulated container with a temperature indicator to monitor the temperature range of the blood should be used. Any equipment specific to the individual patient also must be taken. The nurse must be aware of the nearest emergency equipment cart en route and at the destination.

After all plans have been made, a final checklist ensures that all aspects have been covered and often alerts the nurse to facts that may affect the procedure for which the patient is being transported. For example, a patient with a Hoffman device in place may need that device adjusted before transport to enable the patient to fit into the CT scanner, and some very large patients may not fit into the CT scanner. If such factors are overlooked, they may cause cancellation of the test at the last minute after the patient has already undergone the risk of transportation.

Evaluation and Transition

The evaluation component of the nursing process is ongoing during the critical care phase. During the initial postoperative or critical care period, emphasis is on physiologic stabilization as the body attempts to regain homeostasis following the stressor of traumatic injury. Just as assessment is continuous and appropriate interventions are based on the assessment, the evaluation of the patient's response is also a continuous process to allow timely alterations in interventions. During this phase, adjustments in the plan of care are based on the patient's response to therapy, development of complications, or emergence of SIRS. The coordinating nurse and physician have the responsibility to monitor and reevaluate the patient's status.

As the patient's condition stabilizes, assessment again becomes a critical factor to prepare him or her for transfer to a less critical care environment. Evaluation in the critical care phase entails assessment of the patient's physiologic readiness for transfer to a lower level of care. The basis of the decision to transfer the patient from the critical care unit should be specific criteria to ensure that the resources are available in the intermediate care (IMC) unit or acute care unit to meet the needs of the patient.[57]

Planning for transfer and discharge begins early in the critical care phase. Often the need for a rehabilitation facility or long-term ventilator unit is evident early in this phase. Collaborative discussions and plans with the family, discharge planner, case manager, and other health care providers should take place to identify the suitable and desired facility and expedite transfer when the patient is healed sufficiently.

The transition from critical care to a less-intensive care unit may be difficult for the patient and family, who have for days or months depended on the critical care primary nurses and formed strong relationships and trust. Early planning for transfer will assist the patient and family to make the transition. Discussions related to patient readiness and characteristics of the new unit or facility, written material with information regarding the next phase of care, structured education programs and daily routines or schedules similar to those in the intermediate, acute care, or rehabilitation setting help the patient and family to prepare. Ideally this takes place as far in advance as possible and may serve as a motivator for the patient.[58]

Notifying and communicating with the receiving unit nurses in advance, identifying the next primary care nurse, reviewing the plan of care and personal details with him or her, and introducing the patient to the nurse facilitates the transition, maintains continuity of care and meets the JCAHO National Patient Safety Goal related to a formal and standardized handoff.[54] Particularly in cases of long-term stays on the CCU, the predesignation of a primary coordinating nurse is useful to ease the transition. The nurse on the IMC unit can begin to establish a trusting relationship by visiting the patient and family before transfer from the CCU. These pretransfer visits also serve as early assessment opportunities and may elucidate special needs of the patient or family. The patient and family also need to be prepared for the necessity of a move to another unit related to other patient acuity changes or the need for the CCU to emergently accept new admissions.

PHASE IV: INTERMEDIATE AND ACUTE CARE

Many trauma patients do not require critical care and are admitted directly to the immediate or acute care unit from the resuscitation unit, emergency department, or PACU. These patients and their families have unique physical and psychological needs that should not be minimized because the patient is not injured severely enough to require critical care.

An integrated approach to care continues to be a vital concept as the patient progresses to an IMC level. Many health team members continue to be involved in assessing the patient's progress and in planning and implementing different aspects of care. The roles of the coordinating nurse and physician are significant in this phase to maintain continuity of patient care. Many of the concepts previously presented in the critical care phase continue to apply to nursing care of trauma patients in the intermediate phase.

ASSESSMENT

Physical

Patients admitted to the IMC unit from the resuscitation unit or PACU may not be considered "critically ill"; however, they still require very close observation, especially during the first 72 hours. Initially, undiagnosed injuries may become evident and require rapid interventions on the part of the nurse and physician team. In addition, IMC units are admitting more acutely ill patients from the critical care area as a result of improved resource use and the need for critical care beds.[57,58] Complications, commonly related to immobility, infection, and sepsis, may develop within this time. Astute assessment of vital signs, sensorium, physical signs and symptoms, laboratory values, and ECG changes allows early identification of problems and interventions, which may substantially reduce patient morbidity.

The immediate or acute care phase still requires a high level of vigilance because physiologic and psychologic complications may occur. Ongoing assessment is vital. The nurse performs and documents a complete systems assessment once every shift. Any unexpected physiologic changes must be reported promptly to the appropriate individual, be it the physician, nurse practitioner, or physician assistant. During this phase the trauma patient often appears to be doing well. Seemingly insignificant changes noted during the assessment have the potential of being overlooked or viewed as unimportant when, in fact, they may be signaling the onset of complications. A high index of suspicion alerts the nurse to subtle changes in physiologic status and more intensive investigation of the cause of the change. Complications after traumatic injury may occur unexpectedly and on a delayed basis in the postcritical phase. Dislodgment of a deep vein thrombus with embolization to the pulmonary vasculature is a far too common example.

Psychologic

Trauma patients may exhibit significant psychologic changes from their baseline personality. The changes may be related to the psychologic effect of the injuries or to latent effects of mild brain injury. Distinguishing between these is essential to implement appropriate strategies to aid the rehabilitation process. During the critical phase, a predominant concern is whether the patient will live or die. Once the patient recognizes that the immediate crisis is over and he or she is going to live, the emotional trauma manifested by psychosocial problems may begin to surface. For example, the patient may exhibit disproportionate sick-role behavior or have difficulty in expressing grief. Anger, blaming, and withdrawal are also signs of altered or ineffective coping. This reaction frequently occurs when the patient realizes that the incurred injuries require a long period of rehabilitation for complete recovery.

These are just a few examples of psychological problems that may surface during this phase. Continuous assessment for symptoms that signal the actual or potential presence of altered coping mechanisms facilitates institution of preventive measures and interventions. The families of these trauma patients experience similar shock and disbelief. The nurse must assess the family's ability to cope with the crisis of sudden injury.

Rehabilitative

During the intermediate care phase a more vigorous assessment of rehabilitation needs takes place. Anticipating and assessing for potential complications that may prolong rehabilitation is essential. The patient whose tibial fracture heals well with external fixation but who develops footdrop as a result of inconsistent splinting, range-of-motion therapy, and exercise is at risk for prolonged hospitalization, additional rehabilitation, and possibly additional surgery to correct the problem. Early in this phase of trauma care, the coordinating nurse, case manager, discharge planner, or trauma coordinator evaluates the patient for the need for extensive rehabilitation at a specialty center. Assessment of patient and family requirements for a rehabilitation facility and assessment of available rehabilitation centers is important to determine which facility is most appropriate to meet the needs of the patient and family. Early identification of rehabilitation needs is essential to facilitate referral and timely placement in a rehabilitation facility.

Developing and Implementing a Plan

One of the most effective means of planning care in the intermediate phase is the patient-centered multidisciplinary conference. Conferences include all the disciplines involved with the trauma patient's recovery. In addition to medicine and nursing, representatives from speech, occupational, and physical therapy should be involved. Needs assessments are presented, outcomes are established, and a specific plan is determined. As a plan is established, the patient is included in mutual goal setting. A flexible plan allows the patient to take an active part in identifying long- and short-term goals and in outlining how these goals will be reached. Monitoring patient progress toward achievement of desired goals and outcomes is the responsibility of the coordinating nurse. Subsequent conferences should focus on evaluation of progress and identification of additional strategies to expedite the patient's recovery and discharge.

Active Patient Involvement

As the patient recovers from his or her physical injuries, the plan of care focuses on maintaining physiologic stability, preventing complications, and facilitating emotional recovery. Interventions become more consistent but continue to be outcome driven. Outcomes are often more predictable during this phase and should be documented on a timeline. The patient must be included and given responsibility for a more active role in planning and participating in care. A primary objective in the intermediate phase is to move the trauma patient from a dependent role to a more independent one, striving toward regaining optimal function. Interventions that aid the patient and family in adapting to the residual effects of the injuries and functioning independently are a priority.

Even an immobilized patient needs to be involved in making choices about his or her care. Initially, patient involvement may be limited to the opportunity to make simple choices, such as deciding when to bathe. Or, for example, if there are three activities of daily living that must be relearned, which one is personally important to the patient to learn first? Allowing the patient some choices in care and collaboratively developing schedules provide the patient with some control and encourage him or her to assume a more active role and strive toward independence.

Rehabilitation Needs

The familiar statement "rehabilitation begins on admission" takes on greater relevancy when formulating the plan of care for the trauma patient, especially the multiply injured patient. During the resuscitation, operative, and critical care phases, rehabilitation needs are addressed; however, the emphasis of patient care is clearly on achieving physiologic stability. In the phase of intermediate care, the rehabilitative focus assumes greater significance. The patient learns to take increasing responsibility for his or her care and activities of daily living. Often specific plans are required for the patient to relearn activities of daily living. This is especially true of patients with neurological dysfunction related to injuries or the long-term effects of paralytic agents used in the critical care phase. The overall long-term plan for rehabilitation needs is developed during this phase of care.

Preparation for transfer to a rehabilitation facility requires collaborative planning and communication with the multidisciplinary team, the patient, the family, and the receiving center. Early discussions and planning for rehabilitation and long-term follow-up are important during the acute and intermediate care phases to assist the patient and the family to prepare for the emotional, physical, and financial stressors that may be encountered.[59] All must be involved in the decision making process and informed of the timeline and potential date of transfer to facilitate patient preparation and a timely, smooth transition.

Family Involvement

During this phase, family members begin to be less concerned about the physiologic problems of the patient and start to focus more on what needs to be accomplished before discharge can occur. They begin to want to be involved with the patient's care. They no longer ask, "Will the patient live?" but now ask, "How long will it be before the patient can go home?"

In this stage family involvement in patient teaching is important. Many patients continue to require dressing changes, pin care, or tracheostomy and airway care after their discharge. After teaching family members a procedure, part of the learning process includes return demonstrations and reinforcing the teaching by having the families administer care during their visits. This not only allows the nurse to evaluate how well the family member performs the care but also gives the family member confidence in the new skills and a sense of self-satisfaction from actually assisting in the patient's care. This also may increase the patient's feelings of acceptance by family members, especially if disfiguring injuries are present.

The family-centered conference is an integral component of this phase. The family should be made aware of the goals that have been formulated and the plan of care that has been developed to meet these goals. The need for family members' involvement in the development and implementation of the plan is emphasized, and appropriate resources should be mobilized to assist them in this role. The family may be faced with helping to find or choose an appropriate rehabilitative facility for the patient. The coordinating nurse, or an advanced practice nurse, with the assistance of the family service or social service counselors, can assist the family by providing them with information to make this decision. The specific type of rehabilitation needed by the patient may require placement in a facility far from home. This can be a difficult decision for the family if they are not helped to understand the importance of proper rehabilitation center placement. Financial counselors, visiting nurse associations, and self-help groups are resources commonly needed by the family and patient to aid the transition from acute care to a rehabilitation center or home.

Unique Considerations During the Intermediate Care Phase

Adjustment to Injury

Patients experience interrelated physical, cognitive, and personal responses to their traumatic injuries. The nurse needs to appreciate the full extent of the cognitive and personal aspects of the patient's physical recovery. Understanding the wide range of responses to trauma allows the nurse to "harness the patient's natural healing ability and promote optimal recovery."[60]

When these responses are identified as maladaptive, a specific, consistent care plan that mobilizes all resources must be developed. As the patient physically feels better, attempts to manipulate health care personnel may be made, often resulting in a delayed progression toward discharge, especially if leaving the security of the hospital environment is frightening. Depression may occur as the sequelae of the injuries are recognized by the patient. This can lead to resistance or noncompliance with the therapeutic regimen or delayed progression through the grief process.

Difficulties coping with alterations in body image often surface during this stage. It is important to recognize behavior patterns that may signal that the patient is having problems preserving or adjusting to his or her body image after traumatic injury. If it is identified early, therapy to assist the patient in dealing with changes in body image can be planned and implemented. Family service counselors or a psychiatric liaison nurse are valuable participants of the health care team when patients begin to elicit maladaptive responses to their injuries. A visit by a former trauma patient with a similar injury may prove beneficial.

Immobilization

Even though many multitrauma patients are immobilized intentionally by orthopedic devices, pharmacologic agents, or personal protective devices, the side effects of immobilization linger and assume greater significance during the intermediate phase of care. By the time the patient reaches this stage of care, he or she may already have been immobilized for a significant time, and complications of immobility may be apparent. Some of these include muscular and cardiac deconditioning; ventilation and perfusion abnormalities; orthostatic abnormalities; alterations in ingestion, digestion, and elimination; and development of deep vein thrombus with embolization. The prevention and treatment of complications from immobility are priorities in the plan of care.

Early and aggressive mobilization is beneficial and necessary to prevent sequelae from immobility. Some techniques of fracture management, such as the use of intermedullary rods, plates, screws, or external fixator devices, allow earlier mobilization of patients with multiple fractures. However, even patients in traction may be mobilized if creative methods for maintaining the traction are used. For example, hanging the traction rope and weights over a straight-backed chair may maintain sufficient tibial traction so that the patient may sit up in a chair several times a day. The patient with turning restrictions who needs chest physiotherapy to prevent or treat atelectasis can still be treated if the nurse works with the physician to select the safest way to position the patient. Prophylaxis against deep vein thrombus is imperative, even when mobilizing patients, using external pneumatic compression devices or plantar plexus pulsation devices and low-dose or low-molecular-weight heparin.[31]

Evaluation and Transition

As in previous phases, nursing and medical interventions need to be evaluated continuously for effectiveness. Overall evaluation is directed at the patient's progression toward discharge to home or a rehabilitation center. Discharge needs to be a predicted and planned event, so that when it does occur, the patient and family members look forward to it and feel comfortable rather than frightened or insecure.

Phase V: Rehabilitation

It is difficult to address rehabilitation as a separate phase from the others because, as previously discussed, it begins on admission and continues throughout the patient's acute care hospitalization. Once physiologic stability is achieved, emphasis of care progresses to recovery and adaptation. The primary nursing objectives in the rehabilitation phase are to assist the patient in overcoming disabilities or adapting to his or her environment within the confines of permanent disabilities resulting from trauma. This involves dealing with the total psychosocial and physical needs regardless of whether the disabilities are temporary or permanent. The family is an integral part of the care in reorientation, teaching, and discharge planning and in helping to reintegrate the patient into the family system and the community. Nurses have a pivotal role in recruiting and mobilizing patient and family resources. The nurse in the rehabilitation phase can also be viewed as the coordinator of care. Ensuring coordination of the activities of multiple disciplines, continuing medical or surgical interventions, and the day-to-day interactions with health-care providers, families, and the patient is critical to achieving optimal outcomes during this phase.[61]

Assessment

As previously discussed, rehabilitation begins on admission. Even during resuscitation and operative phases of care, assessment for and prevention of potential problems that prolong the period of rehabilitation must occur. For example, improper positioning on the OR table for extensive and multiple surgical procedures may cause skin breakdown even before the patient reaches the critical care area or IMC unit. During the critical care phase, assessment is crucial to recognizing conditions that may ultimately lead to prolonged rehabilitation. For example, a patient receiving continuous sedation and narcotic infusions to manage pain, anxiety, and facilitate mechanical ventilation may need bilateral foot splints to prevent footdrop, a preventable complication that can prolong and complicate rehabilitative efforts.

Assessment continues to be a mainstay of nursing care in the rehabilitation phase. Assessment in this phase includes determining the patient's psychologic response to injury, evaluating the patient's potential level of function, ascertaining the availability of support mechanisms to assist the patient in injury adjustment and eventual reintegration into society, and coordinating the various community resources and health disciplines that facilitate a smooth rehabilitative process.

The patient's and family's economic situations must be assessed early during acute care so that, by the time the patient is ready for rehabilitation treatment, a plan can be developed that places the lowest economic burden on those involved. Insurance coverage and the patient's and family's economic resources are vital considerations when determining which rehabilitation center will be best for the patient. The center not only must meet the patient's physical needs but also be economically feasible.

Developing and Implementing a Plan

If rehabilitative needs have been assessed as the patient moved through the initial and intermediate phases of care, a well-developed plan should be in place (with the ultimate goal of returning the patient to an optimal level of functioning) by the time the patient moves into the rehabilitative phase. During this phase a goal is for the patient to regain control—to become the decision maker with the support of the health care team. The care plan in this phase would allow for resumption of normal cycles of activity, rest, and increased interaction with family and friends. Mutual goal setting, providing an atmosphere so that the patient can work toward community reentry, and ensuring that he or she remains medically stable are essential components of the plan. Each patient uniquely adapts to traumatic injury; thus, planning care requires creativity and persistence.

The patient must be and must perceive himself or herself as an integral part of the rehabilitation process. The plan should address physical, psychologic, and teaching needs of both patient and family. Family members may need assistance from social service counselors if they begin to feel they will be unable to cope with an injured family member's care or disability once they return home. During the rehabilitation phase, encouraging family members to participate as much as possible in the plan of care is important and will help them to effectively deal with the reality of residual disabilities.

A consistent, planned approach is the essential component of the care plan during this phase. All members of the health care team must be working toward the same defined goals on an outcome-oriented timeline and each should be aware of other members' roles as they strive to achieve these goals. The roles of physical therapists, speech therapists, and occupational therapists are vital to the care plan and must be included in its development and evaluation. Thorough discharge planning is crucial.

During the rehabilitation phase, the patient may exhibit a cycle of progression/regression. The patient may be fully cooperative and demonstrate consistent progress for a day or a period of several weeks, only suddenly to become uncooperative, depressed, and unwilling to comply with the care plan he or she helped develop. These periods of setback are not uncommon as the patient struggles to adapt to the injury and the lifestyle changes it has imposed.

Evaluation

Consistent weekly evaluation of the plan of care or rehabilitation critical pathway is vital during this phase. Assessment of patient response to interventions that address physical and psychological needs may indicate a need to alter those interventions to meet the set goals effectively. The nurse's role as coordinator of the health care team takes on even more importance during the rehabilitation phase because more team members and outside resources become involved actively in the care plan.

The rehabilitation phase continues when the patient is discharged to home or to a rehabilitation center. The process is not complete until the patient is reintegrated successfully into the community. Reintegration is actually the final phase, and all resources that are available to assist the patient toward the goal should be used. Rehabilitation is an integral part of trauma nursing care and significantly affects the patient's potential for maximal recovery.

Postdischarge Phase

Assessment of the trauma patient does not end at hospital discharge; rehabilitation also includes caring for the patient's physical and psychologic status after leaving the hospital. This process must take into account the patient's family as well.

Trauma patients, especially those requiring extended care, often develop significant support systems and "significant other" relationships while hospitalized. If these relationships are interrupted suddenly, patients often face additional readjustment problems in their homes. As demonstrated by war victims whose injuries have resulted in body image changes (such as amputation), trauma patients often display a facade of total acceptance of their injury while hospitalized, but after discharge they experience severe depression or loss of motivation when they reenter society. As long as their environment includes patients with similar injuries, they often do well psychologically. When they return home, however, they begin to feel "different" from the healthy, so-called normal people who surround them.

Postdischarge patient assessment can occur by several means: return clinic visits, home visits from a visiting nurse association or public health home referral, or home visits from trauma nurses who cared for the patient (if the facility provides for this). Assessment factors critical to the evaluation of the patient, such as coping mechanisms, response to family and friends, and general mood and affect, should be identified in a nursing discharge summary or a visiting nurse referral form. Severely injured trauma patients may never fully recover and return to their preinjury physical or cognitive level of functioning. These patients and their families may require considerable psychological, emotional, and financial support. This appears to be particularly of concern for the ever-growing population of traumatically injured, hospitalized patients who are older than age 65.[62] Identification and availability of community resources, support groups, charitable organizations, and the like is an important focus of nursing care throughout the cycles of trauma and especially in the postdischarge phase.[59]

Phase VI: Prevention

The trauma nurse has an essential role in all levels of injury prevention—primary, secondary, and tertiary. In addition, designing and implementing effective public education programs is a required standard in most trauma center verification or designation processes.

Programs that are data driven from the hospital-based or statewide trauma registry ensure that the message delivered to the community focuses on the most common mechanisms of injury for that population and age group. For example, in an urban community where pedestrian injuries as a result of drivers running red lights are a major cause of injury, safety campaigns focused on farm injuries will have no impact. Similarly, red-light–running awareness programs in a rural community with no traffic lights are equally ineffective.

There are numerous national, state, and local organizations whose primary mission is injury prevention and public education. These include the American Trauma Society, SAFE KIDS, the NHTSA, Emergency Medical Services for Children (EMSC), and the CDC's Injury Control Division. These organizations are only a few of the many that work collaboratively to reduce the incidence and consequences of traumatic injuries, as well as educate the lay public on the causes of injury and methods to prevent it.[63] Underlying all injury prevention efforts is the belief that trauma is no accident; therefore, the use of the word *accident* is discouraged because it implies random and unpreventable injury.

Summary

The trauma patient is unique because of the nature of injuries, the suddenness of the traumatic event, and the multiplicity of health care professionals required to organize and implement an effective plan of care from the scene of injury through reintegration into the community. The hope for survival and the physical and emotional recovery of the trauma patient depends on the collaborative efforts of the trauma nurses, physicians, therapists, and others who constitute the trauma team.

Three essential components are necessary to ensure high-quality care and the best possible outcomes for multiply injured patients: collaborative practice; use of evidence-based protocols, procedures, and plans of care; and the often indefinable art of nursing and medicine.

Coordination of care by a primary nurse, nurse practitioner, trauma coordinator, or other advanced practice nurse is an effective model for delivering efficient and high-quality care to the trauma patient through collaborative practice. "Best practice, best care" for the multiply injured, to maximize resources, minimize and reduce complications, and optimize continuity and outcomes, is provided by a physician-nurse team that follows the patient from admission and resuscitation through hospital discharge, and then periodically follows the patient and family in the rehabilitation and postdischarge phases. The multidisciplinary approach to trauma care ensures the ready availability of needed experts. Inherent in this approach is the significant involvement of numerous services and individuals. The strength of the multidisciplinary approach is the expertise that each group brings to the care of the patient. Essential are a coordinating physician and a coordinating nurse as key links to continuity and early collaborative care planning.

Florence Nightingale described the role of the nurse as having "charge of somebody's health," on the knowledge of "how to put the body in such a state to be free of disease or recover from disease."[64] The nurse who coordinates the plan of care for the multiply injured patient exemplifies this historical definition.

Finally, in addition to the science of providing quality trauma care, the art of trauma care is an essential component through all the phases. For it is this art, the undefined humanistic element, the finely developed "sixth sense" of experienced trauma nurses and physicians, that often determines whether a multiply injured patient lives or dies. The multiply injured patient is truly complex and challenging. Through collaborative teamwork, quality care can be planned and delivered from resuscitation to reintegration into society.

REFERENCES

1. Beachley M: Evolution of trauma nursing and the Society of Trauma Nurses: a noble history, *J Trauma Nurs* 12(4): 105-115, 2005.
2. Jacobs BB, Jacobs LM: Epidemiology of trauma. In Feliciano DV, Moore EE, Mattox KL, editors: *Trauma,* ed 3, Stamford, Conn, 1996, Appleton and Lange, pp. 15-30.
3. American College of Surgeons: *National Trauma Data Bank Report 2005.* Available online at www.ntdb.org. Accessed January 19, 2006.
4. Davis JW, Kaups KL: Base deficit in the elderly: a marker of severe injury and death, *J Trauma* 45(5):873-877, 1998.
5. National Center for Injury Prevention and Control: *WISQARS Nonfatal Injuries: Nonfatal Injury Reports.* Available online at http://webappa.cdc.gov/sasweb/ncipc/nfirates.html. Accessed January 20, 2006.
6. American College of Surgeons' Committee on Trauma: *Resources for Optimal Care of the Injured Patient.* Chicago, 2006, The College.
7. Leske JS: Comparisons of family stresses, strengths and outcomes after trauma and surgery, *AACN Clin Issues* 14(1):33-41, 2003.
8. Sister Agnes Mary Joy: Psychosocial complications. In Mattox KL, editor: *Complications of trauma,* New York, 1994, Churchill Livingstone, pp. 313-328.
9. Halm MA: Family presence during resuscitation: a critical review of the literature, *Am J Crit Care* 14(6):494-511, 2005.
10. Henneman EA, Cardin S: Family-centered critical care: a practical approach to making it happen, *Crit Care Nurs* 22(6):12-19, 2002.
11. Gonzales CE, Carroll D, Elliott J et al: Visiting preferences of patients in the intensive care unit and in a complex care medical unit, *Am J Crit Care* 13(3):194-201, 2004.
12. Pierce B: Children visiting in the adult ICU: a facilitated approach, *Crit Care Nurse* 18(2):85-90, 1998.
13. Proulx D: Animal-assisted therapy, *Crit Care Nurse* 18(2):80-84, 1998.
14. Daly B: End of life decision-making, organ donation and critical care nurses, *Crit Care Nurse* 26(2):78-86, 2006.
15. Beckstrand RL, Kirchhoff KT: Providing end-of-life care to patients: critical care nurses' perceived obstacles and supportive behaviors, *Am J Crit Care* 14(5):395-403, 2005.
16. Baggs J, Schmitt M, Mushlin A et al: Association between nurse-physician collaboration and patient outcomes in three intensive care units, *Crit Care Med* 27(9):1991-1998, 1999.
17. Malila FM, Von Rueden KT: The impact of collaboration on outcomes, *J Clin Syst Manage* 4:10-12, 2002.
18. Vazirani S, Hays RD, Shapiro MF et al: Effect of a multidisciplinary intervention on communication and collaboration among physicians and nurses, *Am J Crit Care* 14(1):71-77, 2005.
19. Martin KD, Molitor-Kirsch S, Elgart H et al: Trauma advanced practice nurses: implementing the role, *J Trauma Nurs* 11(2):67-74, 2004.
20. Society of Trauma Nurses: Position statement on the role of the nurse practitioner in trauma, *J Trauma Nurs* 12(3): 71-72, 2005.
21. Koloroutis M: *Relationship-Based Care: A Model for Transforming Practice.* Minneapolis, 2004, Creative HealthCare Management, Inc.
22. Joint Commission on Accreditation of Healthcare Organizations: *Comprehensive Accreditation Manual for Hospitals,* Oakbrook Terrace, IL, 2005, The Commission.
23. Rhodes M: Practice management guidelines for trauma care: presidential address, Seventh Scientific Assembly of the Eastern Association for the Surgery of Trauma, *J Trauma* 37(4):635-644, 1994.
24. Maier RV, Bankey P, McKinley B et al: Inflammation and the host response to injury, a large-scale collaborative project: patient-oriented research core—Standard operating procedures for clinical care, *J Trauma* 59(3):762-763, 2005.
25. Zimmerman JE, Alzola C, Von Rueden KT: The use of benchmarking to identify top performing critical care units and assess their policies and practices, *J Crit Care* 18(2):76-86, 2003.
26. Huggins S: Reducing morbidity of acute respiratory distress syndrome in hospitalized patients: preventing nosocomial infections or aspiration, *Topics in Advanced Practice Nursing eJournal* 6(2), 2006. Posted 07/05/06.
27. Ahrens T, Kollef M, Stewart J et al: Effect of kinetic therapy on pulmonary complications, *Am J Crit Care* 13(5):376-383, 2004.
28. Murray TA, Patterson LA: Prone positioning of trauma patients with acute respiratory distress syndrome and open abdominal incisions, *Crit Care Nurse* 22(3):52-56, 2002.
29. Harris J, Joshi M, Morton P et al: Risk factors for nosocomial pneumonia in critically ill trauma patients, *AACN Clin Issues* 11(2):198-231, 2000.
30. Bergstrom N, Braden B, Laguzza A et al: The Braden scale for predicting pressure sore risk, *Nurs Res* 36(4):205-210, 1987.
31. Geerts WH, Pineo GF, Heit JA et al: Prevention of venous thromboembolism: the Seventh ACCP Conference on Antithrombotic and Thrombolytic Therapy, *Chest* 126(3 suppl):338S-400S, 2004.
32. Institute for Healthcare Improvement: *100,000 Lives Campaign.* Available online at www.ihi.org. Accessed January 3, 2006.
33. Dellinger RP, Carlet JM, Masur H et al: Surviving Sepsis Campaign guidelines for management of severe sepsis and septic shock, *Crit Care Med* 32(3):858-873, 2004.
34. Bridges N, Jarquin-Valdivia AA: Use of the Trendelenburg position as the resuscitation position: to T or not to T? *Am J Crit Care* 14(5):364-368, 2005.
35. Schwenker D, Ferrin M, Gift A: A survey of endotracheal suctioning with instillation of normal saline, *Am J Crit Care* 7(4):255-260, 1998.
36. Dahlberg Z, Dimitriou R, Chalidis B et al: Coagulopathy and the role of recombinant human activated protein C in sepsis and following polytrauma, *Expert Opin Drug Saf* 5(1):67-82, 2006. Erratum in *Expert Opin Drug Saf* 5(2):345, 2006.
37. Stein DM, Dutton RP: Uses of recombinant factor VIIa in trauma, *Curr Opin Crit Care* 10(6):520-528, 2004.
38. Harrison TD, Laskosky J, Jazaeri O et al: "Low-dose" recombinant activated factor VII results in less blood and blood product use in traumatic hemorrhage, *J Trauma* 59(1):150-154, 2005.
39. Habashi N, Andrews P: Ventilator strategies for posttraumatic acute respiratory distress syndrome: airway pressure release ventilation and the role of spontaneous breathing in critically ill patients, *Curr Opin Crit Care* 10(6):549-557, 2004.
40. Ackerman MH: A primer in technology assessment, *AACN Advanced Crit Care* 17(2):111-115, 2006.
41. Naisbitt J: *Megatrends: ten new directions transforming our lives,* New York, 1982, Warner Books, pp. 39-53.

42. Hamilton DK, editor: *ICU 2010. ICU Design for the Future, A Critical Care Design Symposium.* Houston, 2000, Center for Innovation in Health Facilities.
43. McSwain NE, Frame S, Salomone JP, editors: *Prehospital Trauma Life Support,* ed 5, St. Louis, 2003, Mosby, Inc.
44. American College of Surgeons' Committee on Trauma: *Advanced Trauma Life Support,* ed 7, Chicago, 2004, The College.
45. 2005 American Heart Association guidelines for cardiopulmonary resuscitation and emergency cardiovascular care, *Circulation* 112(24)(suppl I), 2005.
46. National EMS Information System (NEMSIS) NHTSA, Pre-Hospital Care Data Base. Available online at http://www.nemsis.org. Accessed November 17, 2006.
47. Cowley RA: Trauma center: a new concept for the delivery of critical care, *J Med Soc N J* 74(11):979-986, 1977.
48. Occupational Safety and Health Administration, U.S. Department of Labor: *Intro to 29 CFR 1910.1030, Occupational Exposure to Bloodborne Pathogens,* Washington, DC, March 5, 1992, Government Printing Office.
49. Lapointe LA, Von Rueden KT: Coagulopathies in trauma patients. *AACN Clin Issues* 13(2):192-203, 2002.
50. US Congress: *Patient Self-Determination Act,* Washington, DC, 1990, Government Printing Office.
51. Tisherman SA, Barie P, Bokhari F et al: *Clinical Practice Guideline: Endpoints of Resuscitation. Eastern Association for the Surgery of Trauma 2003.* Available on-line at www.east.org. Accessed February 24, 2006.
52. *Advanced Trauma Care for Nurses: Instructor Course Manual.* Springfield, IL, 2006, Society of Trauma Nurses.
53. Tokutomi T: Optimal temperature for the management of severe traumatic brain injury: effect of hypothermia on intracranial pressure, systemic and intracranial hemodynamics, and metabolism, *Neurosurgery* 52(1):102-112, 2003.
54. Joint Commission on Accreditation of Healthcare Organizations: *2006 Critical Access Hospitals and Hospital National Patient Safety Goals.* Available online at www.jointcommission.org/Patient Safety/National Patient Safety Goals/06-npsg. Accessed January 3, 2006.
55. Hanson C, Deutschman C, Anderson H et al: Effects of an organized critical care service on outcomes and resource utilization: a cohort study, *Crit Care Med* 27(2):270-274, 1999.
56. Howard J, Sundararajan R, Thomas S et al: Reducing missed injuries at a level II trauma center, *J Trauma Nurs* 13(3):89-95, 2006.
57. Nasraway SA, Cohen IL, Dennis RC et al: Guidelines on admission and discharge for adult intermediate care units. American College of Critical Care Medicine of the Society of Critical Care Medicine. *Crit Care Med* 26(3):607-610, 1998.
58. Chaboyer W, James H, Kendall: Transitional care after the intensive care unit, *Crit Care Nurse* 25(3):16-28, 2005.
59. DePalma JA, Fedorka P, Simko LC: Quality of life experienced by severely injured trauma survivors, *AACN Clin Issues* 14(1):54-63, 2003.
60. Fontaine DK: Physical, personal, and cognitive responses to trauma, *Crit Care Nurs Clin North Am* 1(1):11-22, 1989.
61. Pryor J: Co-ordination of patient care in inpatient rehabilitation, *Clin Rehabil* 17(3):341-346, 2003.
62. Richmond TS, Thompson HJ, Kaunder D et al: A feasibility study of methodological issues and short term outcomes in seriously injured older adults, *Am J Crit Care* 15:158-165, 2006.
63. Berube JE: The Department of Transportation should take a leading role in traumatic brain injury research and prevention initiatives, *J Head Trauma Rehabil* 20(3): 279-281, 2005.
64. Nightingale F: *Notes on nursing: what it is and what it is not,* New York, 1860, Harrison and Sons.

11

REHABILITATION OF THE TRAUMA PATIENT

Valerie Summerlin

The evolution of the specialty of trauma during the past 30 years has been accompanied by great strides in medical technology. Emergency services and trauma care have become highly sophisticated, creating the ability to save the lives of even the most severely injured people. The introduction of rapid transport from the scene of injury, often involving air evacuation, to designated trauma centers offering expert care has resulted in a new population of injured people who probably would have died several decades ago.

Highly effective emergency and critical care services have created a demand for services that restore quality of life to people who have survived severe injury. The result is the specialty practice of trauma rehabilitation. Needs continue to be identified and services designed to complete the cycle of trauma care.

Trauma rehabilitation begins the instant health care services are provided to a trauma patient. At first the focus is on preventing further injuries by thorough assessment and stabilization. As the patient's condition stabilizes, the focus changes to restoring and maximizing function. Rehabilitation attempts to meet the patient's physical, intellectual, and psychosocial needs at each point throughout the trauma cycle.

An understanding of the philosophy of rehabilitation is essential for all nurses engaged in the trauma cycle of care, from those in emergency departments and critical and intermediate care units to those in rehabilitation hospitals, subacute units, long-term acute care (LTAC)/chronic care hospitals, skilled nursing facilities or transition teams, and in-home care agencies. Nurses must think as rehabilitation professionals throughout the trauma cycle to support the patient and family system toward optimal return to function.

DEFINITION OF REHABILITATION

Rehabilitation is "the process by which physical, sensory, and mental capacities are restored or developed in (and for) people with disabling conditions, reversing what has been called the disabling process, and therefore called the enabling process."[1] This is achieved both through functional changes in the individual and through changes in the physical and social environments that surround them.[1]

Among the many factors that affect patient outcome, the one most influential is the patient's motivation. It is the role of the rehabilitation professional to support trauma patients until they assume full responsibility for themselves.[2,3] For example, depression following a spinal cord or brain injury may hinder self-motivation and prevent the patient from setting his or her own recovery goals.

HISTORY OF TRAUMA REHABILITATION

The focus of rehabilitation following trauma has changed through its development. In its early stages, rehabilitation was referred to as "physical medicine," primarily referring to restoration of motor skills and adaptation by compensation following physical disability.[4] Most early benefits in rehabilitation were seen in patients with acute diseases, such as polio, and in veterans, many of whom sustained disabling spinal cord injuries or lower extremity amputations. Other forms of rehabilitation, such as for psychiatric problems; substance abuse; traumatic brain injury; stroke; behavioral and learning disability; and developmental disorders, received far less attention and treatment. Therefore most of the early rehabilitation programs were oriented to the treatment of the physically disabled. Today an emphasis on motor recovery continues within rehabilitation.

Vocational rehabilitation emerged as a need after the success of individual adaptation to a physical disability. Vocational rehabilitation programs initially involved evaluation of the patient's physical capacity followed by vocational testing, training, and placement. Subsequently, emphasis was placed on neuropsychological assessment to identify cognitive factors related to work performance. The complex interrelationship among physical, cognitive, and psychosocial rehabilitation remains underappreciated by professionals, patients, families, society, legislators, and third-party payers.

During the 1980s greater attention was given to the development of rehabilitation programs for people recovering from severe brain injury. More than any other disabled population, brain-injured survivors require treatment from professionals in all disciplines working with them on cognitive, physical, and psychosocial issues. For example, it is difficult for a physical therapist to treat a gait disorder and ignore impaired attention and memory. It is impossible for a speech pathologist to help a person overcome a severe dysarthria while ignoring motor control problems that prohibit the person's use of an augmentative communication system. The brain-injury rehabilitation model expanded rehabilitation from its limited focus on physical and vocational disability to include cognitive, behavioral, and psychosocial disability.

The knowledge gained and techniques learned from the treatment of psychiatric disorders, including substance abuse, have also been integrated into trauma rehabilitation. Substance abuse is becoming more common as a coexisting factor among the injured, requiring addiction treatment to be more available in the rehabilitation process. Also, patients with brain and spinal cord injury who have preexisting learning disabilities will require special consideration during their recovery process. Improvements in rehabilitation programming better meet the needs of all trauma patients. There is heightened sensitivity among health care professionals to identify all the rehabilitation needs of the trauma patient.

There has been a proliferation of rehabilitation services and settings in response to the demand for rehabilitation, yet access to these services remains inconsistent, particularly in the community reintegration phase. Appropriate services are not conveniently available to all trauma patients because of poor understanding of what specialized services are required, decreased appreciation for recovery potential, and lack of funding. Infrequently, disabled patients must go out of state for specialized rehabilitation programs. This does not support continuity from the trauma center to a rehabilitative environment. It is important that the full continuum of services be available within the patient's community if possible.

The Balanced Budget Act of 1997 (BBA) deeply affected health care delivery in the United States. This Act contained numerous cost-saving measures for rehabilitation hospitals, home health agencies, skilled nursing facilities, and outpatient programs. The payment method was restructured and reduced reimbursement, particularly Medicare reimbursement, for rehabilitation services.[5] A dramatic impact has already been experienced by health care providers.[6,7] In response, numerous rehabilitation providers have eliminated staff, sold their practices, or closed their programs. Without funding to support rehabilitation services, the availability of care will decline significantly. The government's goal is to eliminate overuse and abuse of services.

TRAUMA POPULATIONS THAT REQUIRE REHABILITATION

Most trauma patients require some rehabilitation services. Services may be as basic as the emergency department staff providing patient and family education about postconcussive symptoms and the availability of follow-up services for a patient with a mild brain injury. Provision of this rehabilitative teaching can avoid unnecessary patient suffering. More severely injured persons require specialized rehabilitation services based on their diagnosis. Patterns of services have been established for many disabilities. The most common specialized rehabilitation programs in trauma are for spinal cord injury, brain injury, orthopedic and soft tissue injury, and multiple trauma. Pediatric and adult rehabilitation are distinct subspecialties. Each group benefits from different rehabilitation program components, including unique facilities, equipment, mix of professionals, and approaches to treatment. The Commission on Accreditation of Rehabilitation Facilities (CARF) provides standards for comprehensive integrated inpatient rehabilitation programs, spinal cord system of care, brain injury, home- and community-based rehabilitation, health enhancement, medical rehabilitation case management, outpatient medical rehabilitation, pediatric family-centered rehabilitation, occupational rehabilitation, and stroke specialty programs. These standards have evolved and been refined over 40 years with input from providers, consumers and purchasers of services.[8] These standards define the expected input, processes, and outcomes of rehabilitation programs.

Spinal cord injury programs place a strong emphasis on patient/caregiver education, offering a comprehensive program addressing issues such as coping with spinal cord injury, sexuality, attendant/caregiver issues, skin/nutrition, parent and child care issues, travel issues with mobility and home accessibility, bowel and bladder management, and health and wellness. A CARF-accredited spinal cord system of care program maintains expertise to provide services in both its inpatient and outpatient components.[8] This specialized system of care provides or formally links with key components of care that address lifelong needs of the persons served.[8] Advances in computer technology, electrical muscle stimulation, management strategies for neuropathic pain, and research in nerve cell growth are shaping the future of spinal cord injury rehabilitation. (See Chapter 23 for additional information.)

Patients with head trauma benefit from programs specializing in brain injury that focus on reaching the best possible patient outcomes. These outcomes will drive the treatment plan and delivery for each individual patient.[9] The goal for patients in such a program is to reduce disabilities while obtaining the maximum independence and best quality of life in the least restrictive setting. The pace and the extent of a patient's recovery from a brain injury can vary considerably, even between patients with similar injuries, depending on whether proper physical and cognitive rehabilitation was provided.[9] In patients with traumatic brain injury, two different scoring systems are used that can help determine needs for rehabilitation services: the Glasgow Coma Scale[10,11] which quantifies level of consciousness and severity of brain injury, and the Rancho Los Amigos Scale,[10,12] which levels patients based on their cognitive deficits and behavioral characteristics. (For more information on these scoring systems, see Chapter 20.)

Recovery from a brain injury is a long, unique, complex process, and rehabilitation is just one phase in the continuum of care. The acute phase is often followed by outpatient rehabilitation or home care. The rehabilitation program used depends on the degree of deficit resulting from the injury.[10] Patients in coma require multisensory stimulation and prevention of physical complications caused by immobility. Confused patients or those displaying inappropriate behavior need specific behavioral modification and therapeutic behavioral approaches, taking into consideration the safety of the patient. Patients with mild brain injury who have persistent problems, such as difficulty concentrating or poor memory, may find outpatient rehabilitation or therapy sufficient. All health care team members should address improvement in cognitive function and social awareness. The physical effects of brain injury are as varied as the cognitive deficits. (See Chapter 20 for information specific to the brain-injured patient.)

The patient education component of brain injury rehabilitation is also unique. Because of the patient's cognitive and behavioral deficits, most of the teaching about the injury, its effects, and management of problems is provided to the patient's family and support systems. As the patient recovers enough insight to learn and use the information, more teaching is provided. This is also true in the provision of psychosocial support.

Patients with orthopedic or soft tissue injuries and those with multiple-system trauma need a rehabilitation program with both medical and surgical emphasis. Complex injuries may require an extended time for recovery because of multiple surgeries. Attention is given to prevention of infection and other complications during tissue healing. Amputees may require the use of prosthetic or adaptive devices. Psychosocial support addresses changes in body image, loss of independence and control, and lower self-esteem. Health education commonly emphasizes the patient's physical needs and should expand to address psychosocial issues.

Components of Rehabilitation

Although certain trauma populations require a specialized rehabilitation program for the best outcome, several components are common to all programs regardless of the setting. Two key elements to maximizing the patient's potential are the integrated team approach and the development of an individualized rehabilitation plan.

Rehabilitation Team

Not unlike other specialties in health care, trauma rehabilitation requires an integrated team approach. The concept of a team as a group of specialists working toward a common goal is simplistic, yet it is implemented quite literally in the rehabilitation setting. Also inherent in this team philosophy is congruency in goals, consistency in approach, and communication among all team members.[13] Most teams treat a specific group of patients exclusively. Members of the interdisciplinary team constantly ensure that everyone on the team is aware of the plan of care for each person served. Exchange of information is fostered between team members, and the established plan is implemented.[8] Decisions about the plan are made in collaboration with the persons served and communicated to all members of the team.

Early rehabilitation teams were multidisciplinary, with each specialty having separate goals and approaches. This method offered the benefit of input from many specialties to the patient's plan of care, but each discipline had individual goals. Fragmentation of care became a major problem.

The use of an interdisciplinary team avoids fragmentation. Each member of the team focuses on a particular area of expertise and blends with the expertise of other team members. In an interdisciplinary approach, patient goals are developed by the team rather than by each discipline. An example of this is the cooperative effort of behavior modification strategies used to manage a brain-injured patient's agitation. Consistent approaches to patient behavior may include reducing external stimuli, avoiding patient fatigue, and providing treatment in a quiet area.

A growing approach in team dynamics, the transdisciplinary team,[14] is similar to the interdisciplinary team in the method in which mutual goals are formed. Team members often include family and patients. Team members bring their special expertise to the group. The distinguishing characteristic in this model is that each member is responsible for sharing observations about all aspects of the patient's rehabilitation, particularly when the team meets to review progress. An observer of the team would find it more difficult to determine each member's primary discipline based on his or her verbal input during a team conference. Disciplines may approach therapeutic treatments collectively rather than individually. Physical and occupational therapists may have joint therapy sessions with the patient to establish the most appropriate custom wheelchair for proper positioning. A speech pathologist, occupational therapist, and rehabilitation nurse may schedule a mealtime session with the dysphagic patient to assess and establish team approaches to feeding.

Each team specialist has the responsibility to address the overall functional goals for the patient. It takes mature professionals to let go of the traditional territory associated with each discipline, allowing team members to make observations across disciplines while understanding the perspectives of fellow team members.

Composition of the Team

The team is composed of those who have input into the rehabilitation plan, including the patient, family members, and care providers. The team can number just a few or consist of a large group of specialists. Rehabilitation for specific injuries requires a complement of appropriate specialists who are able to meet the comprehensive needs of the patient. In some cases the mix of team members reflects more physical rehabilitation emphasis in the early phases (e.g., a comatose patient on a ventilator). Often the cognitive and psychosocial components of rehabilitation are implemented further along in the cycle. By the time the patient is in the reintegration phase, the physical impairments may have been largely resolved, leaving the team focused primarily on psychosocial adaptation after injury.

All members of the team are equally essential to the patient's success. Some disciplines, such as nursing, case management, and social services, remain involved with the patient throughout the continuum of care, but the focus of their involvement may change. Other primary team members are involved for limited periods during the initial critical care phase, working with the patient more extensively through the intermediate and rehabilitation phases. For example, physical, occupational, and speech therapists are intensively active during the intermediate and acute care periods and throughout rehabilitation hospitalization.

The most important member of the rehabilitation team is the patient. It is the responsibility of the professionals on the team to help the patient understand his or her active role in rehabilitation. In many outpatient rehabilitative settings, patients are referred to as "clients," reflecting the cooperative investment between the injured person and the rehabilitation professionals. As the patient moves through the trauma care cycle, he or she sheds the patient role and returns to a status of self-responsibility.[15]

Team Leadership

To ensure that the most appropriate and individualized team is organized, a team leader assumes a holistic view of the patient's rehabilitative process and anticipated outcome. The team leader defines a realistic expected outcome for each patient. In addition, the team leader, either directly or indirectly, determines which specialists will be needed on the team. The form of leadership used by a team may vary. Models of team leadership include the physician-led team, the multidisciplinary team, the rehabilitation coordinator role, and the case manager role.

Early team models were based on physician leadership. The physician ordered rehabilitation therapies and progress reports from the therapists to establish patient goals. The advantage of this model was consistency of goals for all members. But by limiting the input and influence of a variety of disciplines, this structure can yield goals based only on the physician's perspective. In the early years of trauma rehabilitation, most rehabilitation goals were related to mobility and self-care achievements, often neglecting cognitive, linguistic, and psychosocial needs. This scope of rehabilitation reflected the priorities the physician chose for the patient's outcome. Many of the physicians attending to trauma patients had limited knowledge of and experience in the specialty of rehabilitation. Currently, in all CARF-accredited rehabilitation programs, the medical director of the program is board certified in his or her specialty area and has completed a formal residency in physical medicine and rehabilitation, a fellowship in rehabilitation for a minimum of 1 year, or has a minimum of 2 years' experience as a collaborative team member providing rehabilitation services in a comprehensive inpatient rehabilitation program.[8]

Rehabilitation Nurse. As a member of the integrated disciplinary team, the goal of the rehabilitation nurse, as identified by the Association of Rehabilitation Nurses, is to assist individuals with disability and/or chronic illness to attain and maintain maximum function.[16] The rehabilitation nurse, in addition to providing hands-on nursing care, is responsible for coordinating the educational activities. The rehabilitation nurse is teacher, caregiver, collaborator, and client advocate.[16]

Case Manager. The role of case manager was introduced when managed care sought to save costs by streamlining care. Managed care initiated the use of external case managers—that is, clinicians, who do not provide direct care but who review and manage catastrophic cases with high costs to insurance companies and are employed or contracted by the insurer.[17] Many of these cases involve traumatic injuries. Facility-based case management has become the standard of practice for many rehabilitation programs.

Most case managers are registered nurses, but there are other models that combine the social worker and case management role together. They monitor and coordinate a rehabilitation plan that is clinically advantageous to the patient but also extends the patient's health care funding to the best use of coverage and clinical benefit as projected over the long-term course of recovery. Some case managers, often those employed by third-party payers, follow the care during the patient's lifetime, spanning multiple clinical settings.[17] Case managers working for medical care providers do not follow the patient on a long-term basis; however, they do consider the future impact of health care decisions.

The case manager's role is to coordinate and facilitate access to timely and appropriate health care services and ensure continuity throughout the recovery continuum. The case manager is a valuable resource to help ensure that the patient receives the health services and benefits needed to make the best recovery possible. The case manager keeps the patient served, and the family and the insurance company informed about the treatment and progress toward rehabilitation goals. They act as advisor, mentor, and advocate throughout recovery and return to work. Some organizations also include the role of discharge planner in the case manager role.

It is important in all aspects of rehabilitation care to encourage patients and families to become informed and active members of the health care team. Initiatives nationwide are promoting this concept as the health care industry focuses on patient safety. During the recovery phase it is important to keep the family involved and, as the patient is able to participate, the case manager, along with the team, will need to bring the patient into the decision-making process.

Rehabilitation Plan

Rehabilitation Potential

Thorough assessment and evaluation of the patient's rehabilitation potential are the first steps following trauma. Although it is difficult to predict a final outcome after trauma, there are parameters that help to determine the amount and rate of a patient's potential progress. These factors represent the patient's strengths and weaknesses in the areas of physical, cognitive, and psychosocial functioning.[2,18] Other factors that influence rehabilitation potential are the patient's age, length of time since injury, premorbid health, support systems, secondary complications, and availability of resources.

Physical Factors. For some disabilities there are well-established outcomes. These outcomes are changing as technology advances. Perhaps in the future there will be fewer physical limits because medical technology will be able to replace, rebuild, or stimulate regrowth of injured areas of the body. For example, there is an extensive body of research focused on promising interventions for repair of the injured spinal cord, such as cell transplant to bridge the area of injury and neurotropic agents to stimulate neuronal regrowth. Although a complete discussion of these interventions is outside the scope of this chapter, it is important that rehabilitation professionals maintain their awareness of current research so that their patients can benefit when new products and/or initiatives become available.

Concurrent diagnoses also influence rehabilitation outcome. Many trauma patients have multiple injuries, preexisting conditions, or complications of trauma that significantly impact their potential to recover. As the population ages, the incidence of trauma in the elderly will constitute a prominent proportion of trauma patients.[19] Individuals are physically active well into their 80s and beyond, and thus are subject to the risks of an active adult lifestyle. The effects of normal aging and a higher likelihood of concurrent medical conditions, such as diabetes, osteoporosis, and multiple injuries, complicate healing and make rehabilitation of the elderly more difficult.[20]

Cognitive and Psychosocial Factors. If physical impairment were the only factor determining rehabilitation potential, two patients with similar injuries would have comparable outcomes. Cognitive and psychosocial factors influence rehabilitation outcome as well. Cognitive factors include the patient's ability to learn new things, solve problems, and make appropriate judgments and decisions; educational level; readiness to learn; prior experiences; and many other complex factors.[21] Psychosocial factors, including income, family support, lifestyle, mood, relationships, personality, and coping ability, all affect the patient's potential. Today, with the culturally and economically diverse backgrounds of our patients, health care providers' responsibilities include working with interpreters and understanding the culture and financial needs of the patient to determine best interventions and expected outcomes.

Evaluating Rehabilitation Potential. Each professional working with a trauma patient needs to evaluate the patient's rehabilitation potential. The clinician first defines the rehabilitation outcome that is typically expected for others with the same injury as the patient. The outcome can be further analyzed by assigning a probability factor or percentage of predicted success to the estimated outcome. For example a patient who has had a traumatic below-the-knee amputation may have excellent potential to return to work and be independent in activities of daily living with the use of a prosthesis. However, when the evaluator considers that the patient is 53 years old, developmentally disabled, lives alone, and has sustained multiple infections and required numerous stump revisions, the potential for independent living and return to work becomes significantly lower. Recognizing these probability factors provides rehabilitation professionals with a clearer picture that the patient either will need significantly greater resources or may not be able to reach the standard desirable outcome. The focus of the integrated team is to work with the patient to achieve the most independent level of care no matter where the patient will be discharged. Maximizing independence optimizes quality of life.

Rehabilitation potential should not be a question of yes or no or good or poor. The important point is that the rehabilitation assessment summarizes the positive aspects that will support rehabilitative efforts and considers strategies to work with or around the negative aspects to prevent failure. Nearly every patient has some potential for improvement, but the potential must be weighed against what is both cost effective and a reasonable expectation for patient success.

From a quality-of-care perspective, an individual's expected outcome and rate of recovery dictate the type of rehabilitation program that is best for the patient. Cost-benefit analysis is a critical element in the formulation of rehabilitation program recommendations following the evaluation of potential. The ability of the rehabilitation industry to measure its success and failure with clinical and functional outcomes will greatly influence future decisions.

Realistic goals are set for the patient, and an estimated time for achievement is established. If these goals are individualized and sensitive to the patient's strengths and weaknesses, any patient should have good potential to achieve his or her unique rehabilitation goals.

Goal Development

The development of long-term and short-term patient goals is a collaborative process. The goals are adjusted based on the patient's progress and should reflect the uniqueness of the patient. Long-term goals reflect a phase of the patient's recovery after hospitalization. Short-term goals are the achievable steps toward the overall long-term goal. Goals should be functional, such as dressing or transferring, and directed toward overcoming the impairment. Goals can also be developed for the family to demonstrate knowledge about a concept or mastery of an intervention. For example, teaching about range-of-motion techniques can be done with the goal that the family will be able to perform this intervention for the patient in a persistent vegetative state after a severe brain injury. Increased range of motion alone is not a functional goal. However, the resulting improved positioning when seated in a chair benefits the patient's quality of life and avoids complications by increasing stimulation, improving hygiene, reducing spasticity, and preventing decubiti and contractures.

To establish a functional goal, the team considers the most realistic and appropriate outcomes for an individual patient. Ambulating for 20 feet is a measurable goal. The ability to get to and from the bathroom focuses on function and is measurable. All goals should be measurable and reproducible. The appropriateness of specific goals should be meaningful to the patient's functional independence.

For successful rehabilitation, mutuality of goals between the patient and the rehabilitation specialists is essential.[15] Mutuality is a concept defined as a unified acceptance and agreement by both parties of what will be achieved. It should be based on the patient's value system, not that of the professional. Often a trauma patient begins treatment with a fairly passive position in the plan of care. The patient usually agrees to follow the regimen or to allow treatments to be conducted without much thought or question. As the crisis period subsides, the patient becomes more interested and actively involved in decision making.

The assumption that a compliant patient is an ideal patient is misleading. Even the term *compliance* suggests that the decision and plan are created and enforced by outside sources. It is the patient, not the staff, who has the ultimate responsibility for outcome. The patient should be included as an equal partner in the decision-making process. Values play a major role in the functional goals set by both the staff and the patient. A conflict in values should be recognized openly, and mutual goals should be sought. Education in culture and values clarification is helpful to staff members working in rehabilitation to prepare for resolution of these conflicts.

Implementation of the Plan

Individualized strategies are developed for the achievement of functional goals.[8] Any strategy to be used should be understood by all team members to avoid incongruent techniques that could erode functional gains. Strategies used to achieve restoration of function are different from those used to compensate for disability.

Therapy implementation has traditionally been provided through one-on-one sessions. In recent years therapists have used other approaches, including group treatment and cotreatment by professionals from two disciplines working with one patient. This frequently occurs in the rehabilitation or reintegration phases of the trauma care cycle.

In the first option, functional goal groups are created, such as social skills, mobility, and self-care skills. Patients with common goals are gathered together to follow a specific program to achieve that goal with the benefit of group dynamics and peer feedback. The use of group technique improves application of rehabilitation strategies in the real world. Society revolves around interactions with others in one-on-one, small-group, and large-group situations. To approximate society, various interactive strategies are used. This prepares the injured patient to function in society, builds coping skills, and allows the patient to test his or her adaptation to injury in a supportive group setting. It is appropriate for the rehabilitation nurse to participate in this therapy and, in some situations, to direct it.

Cotreatment sessions allow several specialists to work with one patient at the same time. An example might be a daily mealtime session with the occupational therapist, speech pathologist, and nurse or nurse extender to improve a dysphagic patient's ability to feed himself or herself. The team members become more integrated because they focus on functional, rather than discipline-specific, goals. The interactive nature of cotreatment enhances the evaluation and treatment process, resulting in an outcome that is more effective than can be gained through individual sessions with each of the component disciplines.

Reimbursement and state discipline practice standards continue to affect clinical practice in rehabilitation. Many funding sources, both government and private, require authorization for special treatment sessions or impose specific guidelines for their use. Discipline practice standards, which are state specific, also impact the interventions practiced by therapists. These standards impact both reimbursement and how the hours of treatment are computed to meet the rehabilitation criteria for an inpatient stay. Payers may have specific guidelines for the staff-to-patient ratio for authorized group therapy treatment. Payment for any rehabilitation treatment option is best supported and measured by outcome data systems.

Rehabilitation Outcome

One of the most important components of rehabilitation is the accurate, comprehensive measurement of patient outcome.[18,22] Literally hundreds of outcome scales exist. All CARF-accredited rehabilitation programs are required to collect outcome data relevant to their own program(s). One measurement system used by many for documenting the severity of patient disability and outcomes of medical rehabilitation is the Uniform Data System for Medical Rehabilitation (UDSMR). Some of their products include Functional Independence Measurement (FIM) System, Functional Independence System for Children (WeeFIM II) System, and UDS-PRO System. The FIM system is an outcomes management tool for measuring and managing the effectiveness of medical rehabilitation services and programs.[23] This tool measures the functional ability of an individual for 18 items across the motor, cognitive, and self-care domains. The FIM tool is used for skilled nursing and long-term care, as well as acute care hospitals.[23] UDSMR maintains separate databases for each provider group. The WeeFIM II System measures and documents functional performance in children and adolescents with other acquired or congenital disabilities in a consistent manner.[24] It is used in inpatient, outpatient, and community-based settings. The UDS-PRO System tool is a software database that combines patient-assessment functionality with reimbursement.[25] Currently, there are approximately 870 inpatient rehabilitation facilities out of 1250 facilities nationwide using the UDS-PRO product according to Justin Foster, marketing specialist for UDSMR. Specific measurement systems have improved for comparison of outcomes in similar settings, but they remain lacking in sensitivity for comparison outcomes across varied rehabilitation settings, including acute rehabilitation, subacute care, LTAC, skilled nursing facilities, home care, and outpatient programs.

What constitutes a quality outcome? Functional gains that are not retained over time initially may give the appearance of an inflated outcome. An example of good outcome measurement includes measures of function done at the time of admission to and discharge from a rehabilitation program, followed by measures at 3 months, 6 months, and 1 year after discharge. Postdischarge interval measurements are used to document functions that have been sustained. Exorbitant expenditures to achieve a slightly higher outcome may not be the wisest use of the patient's financial resources. Clinical and functional outcome measures related to rehabilitation costs are most influential to support funding for rehabilitation.

The Joint Commission on Accreditation of Healthcare Organizations (JCAHO) introduced in February 1997 the ORYX initiative, which integrated outcomes and other performance measurement data into the accreditation process. In July 2002, JCAHO-accredited hospitals began collecting data on "standardized" or core performance measures.[26] In 2004, JCAHO and the Center for Medicare and Medicaid (CMS) announced that they were working together to standardize common hospital measures. These measures were only for acute care hospitals. Currently, all accredited rehabilitation programs are required to continue to collect noncore measures from an approved list.

One of the most widely used outcome data systems associated with rehabilitation is the UDSMR.[27] This and other standard functional measures can be applied easily at varying intervals before, during, and after discharge. The UDSMR uses its credentialing process to ensure that clinicians fully understand how to rate their patients. To date, the UDSMR has credentialed nearly 150,000 clinicians.[27] The UDS-PRO System joins information from the Inpatient Rehabilitation Facilities Patient Assessment (IRF-PAI) and the Case Mix Index Group (CMG) and transmits these data to both the Centers for Medicare and Medicaid Services and the UDSMR.[27] IRF-PAI includes real-time reporting and contains regional and national benchmarks. It also provides rehabilitation facilities with their Presumptive Eligibility Estimation Report (PEER), which is their estimated conformity with CMS's mandate that at least 75% of admissions fall within specific diagnostic groups.[27] IRVEN (Inpatient Rehabilitation Validation and Entry) is a computerized data entry system for Inpatient Rehabilitation Facilities (IRF).[28] IRVEN also offers users the ability to collect IRF-PAI information in a database and create a file in the CMS standard format that can be transmitted to the IRF-PAI National database.[28]

The rehabilitation industry has been affected by the Health Care Financing Administration's (HCFA) initiation of the medical prospective payment system (PPS). The Balanced Budget Refinement Act (BBRA) of 1999 authorized the implementation of a per-discharge PPS for IRFs. The PPS replaced the Tax Equity and Fiscal Responsibility Act (TEFRA) payment system. This represented a major change in how providers are reimbursed by Medicare for the services provided. The amount of reimbursement is now based on patient acuity, which is determined by a new patient classification system. The new IRF PPS classifies patients into distinct diagnostic groups based on clinical characteristics and expected resource needs. The CMS revised the criteria for classifying hospitals as inpatient rehabilitation facilities known as the "75% rule." These criteria went into effect on July 1, 2004, and were to be phased in gradually. The criteria focused on medical necessity and functional capability and required the inpatient rehabilitation hospitals to have at least a certain percentage of their admissions fall into the 13 categories. Separate payments are calculated for each group, including the application of case and facility level adjustments. As long as the required percentage of patients met the categories, designation hospitals could still admit other rehabilitation patients who did not meet the criteria for these categories. Under these criteria, total joint replacements no longer qualified for inpatient rehabilitation. These patients could still be admitted, but the admissions to the IRF must meet the required percentage first. IRFs have struggled with this over the past several years. The American Medical Rehabilitation Professional Association (AMRPA) lobbied to successfully change this Act. In May 2006, CMS revised the IRF PPS phase-in instructions in legislation called The Deficit Reduction Act of 2005, which extended the phase-in of the IRF compliance percentage. It calls for a freeze of the 75% percent rule at the current 50% compliance for 2 years. An advisory council was developed to review issues with the 75% rule.

Availability of Rehabilitation for the Trauma Patient

Available rehabilitation options have become widely divergent. Traditional medical inpatient rehabilitation is now just one of many types of programs. Because the complex needs of trauma patients have been recognized, a full range of rehabilitation programs and services have been developed. One of the confusing aspects of understanding what types of rehabilitation options exist is defining the difference between rehabilitation programs and rehabilitation services. It is also necessary to recognize when each option is most appropriate for meeting the patient's rehabilitation goals. CARF offers a guide for the consumer on selecting a rehabilitation provider. This guide includes questions around performance, service delivery, quality, and the satisfaction of the people served.

Programs and Services

A rehabilitation service is a single component in a rehabilitation program. An example is physical therapy services on an outpatient basis for a posttraumatic amputee needing prosthetic gait training. In this example the patient may not require other therapy or rehabilitative services, so the single service of physical therapy meets the patient's needs. Counseling or occupational therapy also would be available within the program.

In comparison, a rehabilitation program is much more than the cumulative effect of multiple rehabilitation services. It is the coordination and synergy of multiple disciplines. A program can exist in an inpatient, outpatient, or residential (home care) setting if the services are coordinated and if the approach is a team effort.

A successful rehabilitation program allows for cooperation and communication by the entire team assigned to the patient. An inpatient setting that provides nursing and medical care of the patient and offers physical, occupational, and other therapies does not automatically become a rehabilitation program. When multiple disciplines integrate their efforts toward mutual functional goals and carryover occurs from therapy to nursing care, the essence of a true rehabilitation program is being offered to the patient.

Discharge planning for the trauma patient involves understanding whether he or she requires a single service or a comprehensive program. Fragmentation of care is one of the primary risks for failure of rehabilitative efforts. The match of patients' needs and goals to appropriate programs or services maximizes outcomes. When evaluating rehabilitation programs, it is important to determine whether there is adequate coordination of services to provide integration rather than fragmentation of goals.

Severely injured patients in the late rehabilitative phase and reintegration phase of the trauma cycle could appropriately have their follow-up needs met by a single rehabilitation service. This depends on the complexity of injury, psychosocial supports, and intellectual ability of the patient and family to carry out the plan. Discharge planners should take into consideration that a highly motivated patient or family support system can provide a great deal of care coordination for home-based rehabilitation services. Each case must be evaluated on individual need.

Centers of Excellence

Certain rehabilitation programs have elevated themselves to distinction through continual research in the specialty of rehabilitation and application of that research to practice. Often these facilities are known for a subspecialty in rehabilitation, such as spinal cord injury, brain injury, or burn rehabilitation. Some of them are known regionally, whereas others have a national reputation. Patients with extremely complex or unique injuries may require a facility of this level of expertise. Referral is determined by agreement among the referring medical acute care treatment team, a payer representative (often a case manager), the family, and the patient. Use of these facilities by patients from outside the local region or state has decreased because the specialty of rehabilitation has grown and managed care has put tighter controls on health care spending.

Influence of Managed Care

The availability of resources continues to be influenced by managed care. Managed care is defined as a group of "systems and techniques used to control the use of health care service."[29] Managed care is a broad term and encompasses many different types of organizations, payment mechanisms, review mechanisms, and collaborations.[29] A payer selects preferred rehabilitation providers to deliver services for the patient population at different points in the cycle. These preferred provider arrangements sometimes limit alternatives for the patient. However, the coordination of services by managed care often is greatly improved. Case management, discussed earlier in this chapter, can be a component of a managed care system. Acute care trauma nurses may find themselves providing referral documentation to utilization review nurses, case managers, and other payer representatives to plan transfer to a rehabilitation facility.

Current and Future Rehabilitation Alternatives

The future of rehabilitation delivery promises a full spectrum of programs and services ranging from acute inpatient rehabilitation, LTAC, subacute, and skilled nursing facilities to care provided in outpatient and residential settings. With an increased availability of cost-effective alternatives and continued pressure to cut health care costs for rehabilitation, the number of patients served by acute inpatient programs is expected to decrease significantly in the next decade.

The following sections describe rehabilitation program options that may be provided to the trauma population. It is not an all-inclusive list; rather, it is an attempt to demonstrate the variety of programming available throughout the country. Not all these options are cost effectively accessible to all patients, particularly in rural areas.

Inpatient Rehabilitation

Inpatient rehabilitation may be provided in a hospital, hospital-based, skilled nursing facility, LTAC hospital, acute hospital (Canada), or hospital with transitional rehabilitation beds (Canada).[8] A CARF-accredited facility means it has passed an in-depth review of its services. It is an assurance that it meets the CARF guidelines for service and quality.

Subacute rehabilitation, an alternative to "acute rehabilitation," experienced a boom in the 1990s. This alternative setting meets the needs of patients who are not able to tolerate the daily intensity of an acute inpatient rehabilitation program and those who are making slower progress but still require the coordinated services of an interdisciplinary team. Subacute rehabilitation is provided in a variety of bed-licensing arrangements, including acute hospitals, long-term or chronic hospitals, and skilled nursing facilities. In addition, many long-term care facilities provide therapy services to patients needing rehabilitation. One of the critical factors that differentiates subacute rehabilitation in a skilled nursing facility from long-term care is that the subacute patient requires an active rehabilitation program by a coordinated team, rather than a residential placement that utilizes rehabilitation services that are focused on maintaining the patient's current quality of life. With the implementation of the new PPS, there has been a decrease in the number of subacute programs available.

Transitional living programs focus specifically on community reintegration. The patient lives in a structured home environment, usually with 4 to 10 other patients. Social and behavioral adaptation skills are an important focus, in addition to the adjustment to physical disabilities in a home and community setting. The home environment is typically paired with a modified work or school setting in either the same or a nearby location. Some states provide transitional living as a step toward community living. It is not a long-term residential placement, as the name indicates.

Structured living, on the other hand, is an extended placement that provides life skills and rehabilitation support services. It may also be called a group home or nonmedical residential rehabilitation.

Outpatient Rehabilitation

An outpatient medical rehabilitation program provides a wide range of therapeutic services and approaches by a coordinated team in both individual and group sessions. Outpatient settings are not limited to freestanding outpatient rehabilitation centers. Acute hospitals, day hospital programs, private practice settings, and other community settings also offer outpatient rehabilitation programs. The patients require minimal medical and nursing care and are functionally independent enough to live at home and commute to their rehabilitation program. Depending on the intensity of need, patients are seen on a daily or intermittent basis. CARF has accreditation criteria to ensure consistency of outpatient medical rehabilitation programs.[8]

Work hardening commonly is associated with an outpatient medical rehabilitation program and provides physical and cognitive strengthening of the patient's functional abilities. The program simulates components of the patient's actual or potential work functions, gradually increasing the complexity and repetition of tasks until patients are prepared to return to a work setting.

Patients in day treatment programs demonstrate significantly higher functional independence than those in inpatient rehabilitation settings. The focus of the day treatment program is to address a specialized aspect of reintegration, such as social behavior, cognitive rehabilitation, and prevocational training. Day hospitals provide nursing, medical, and therapy services to a patient in a day care setting to improve the level of patient function.

Vocational programs may provide highly specialized services, including in-depth patient evaluation, work assessment, trial work settings, work hardening, supervised and assisted work settings, and training for new employment skills. A sheltered workshop is a supervised and structured work setting used for either short-term rehabilitation or job placement, depending on the rehabilitation potential of the patient.

Home-Based Rehabilitation

Home-based rehabilitation programs are possible if there is full coordination of the therapeutic services involved; however, they are usually not the most cost-effective option. The patient lives and participates in the program at home. The patient does not have to be independent and can require up to 24-hour-a-day nursing care. Home-based programs are an especially desirable approach if mandated by third-party payers, if the family is committed to the patient being at home, and if inpatient and outpatient programs are not readily available. It is also a good alternative if the patient's nursing care needs preclude the patient from benefiting from a more aggressive inpatient rehabilitation setting, or if a transportation problem interferes with outpatient rehabilitation.

A high level of family input and involvement is characteristic of home-based programs. However, these programs may lack adequate social and behavioral rehabilitation because of isolation from the patient's peer group. A combination of home-based and outpatient programs is an effective option, especially when an inpatient program would be inappropriate. Home-based rehabilitation often is not a cost-effective option and is not used as frequently as other alternatives. Often the payer may require that the patient be homebound and unable to participate in rehabilitation through any other alternative. Some families opt to pay privately for services at home.

With such a variety of rehabilitation settings, careful consideration is necessary to match the patient's needs to services and programs. Rehabilitation providers must clearly distinguish between the types of programs offered so that the most appropriate setting can be identified.

What factors really determine placement? In theory the patient's needs are matched to program goals. In reality the factors of local program availability and funding play major roles in decision making. Within the limitations of funding, discharge decisions are driven primarily by the patient's medical stability, types and intensity of services needed, functional ability, and social and psychologic considerations.

Focus of Rehabilitation Throughout the Cycle

Rehabilitation is the motivation that moves the patient through the entire cycle, although it often is referred to as a specific period within the cycle. Maximized patient function is the common goal of all health care providers.[13] As the patient proceeds through the cycle, the focus of rehabilitation shifts. After the initial crisis of injury, the patient is medically stabilized. At this early stage, the severely injured patient depends on family and professionals to anticipate complications and plan for future progress. Later the patient takes on a much more active role in the rehabilitation team, eventually determining all individual goals.

No clear distinction or key event marks the patient's departure from one phase and entry into the next. Depending on the complexity of the injury, complications, and the psychosocial system into which the patient tries to reintegrate, movement through the cycle may be at varying paces and intensities. Patients may need to return to earlier phases in the cycle during the course of recovery. Most rehabilitation protocols are diagnosis specific.

RESUSCITATION PHASE

Beginning at the injury scene through resuscitation and immediate stabilization, the rehabilitation goal during the resuscitation phase is to prevent further injury and secondary complications. Delay in treatment, unidentified injuries, and unintended harm caused by emergency procedures can impose additional impairment, resulting in a lengthened and complicated recovery. Decreased functional recovery may be a consequence of preventable complications during the resuscitation phase.

Life-threatening injury is the greatest concern in an emergency setting; however, the long-term effects of non-life-threatening injury may be the most disabling to the patient. For example, in a patient with multisystem injuries, such as multiple fractures, a pneumothorax, and abdominal bleeding, a brachial plexopathy may be undiagnosed. When the other injuries are resolved, loss of motor function and chronic pain from the brachial plexopathy may persist and interfere with the patient's productive return to work and home life. The severity of injury must be considered in context. A minor injury may have severe consequences. This is not to say that stabilizing the most life-threatening injury is not the priority. Rather, it implies that the emergency practitioner needs to be aware of all the patient's injuries, the potential complications associated with the patient's condition, and the possible lifelong consequences of all injuries and related complications. This awareness by emergency professionals can foster prevention of further injury and appropriate follow-up.

Another rehabilitation goal during the resuscitation phase is to establish a baseline assessment of the patient's adjustment to the injury. Coping is an individualized process that depends on the perspective of the patient and family. People respond to injury in terms of the perceived loss or potential loss of function. A construction worker may be more devastated by the loss of a limb than a computer data processor because a source of income is threatened. A teenage girl may be more concerned about a facial laceration than internal injuries. Generalizations cannot be made, but a perceptive emergency practitioner can anticipate these priorities. Those who have initial contact with the family or with the patient, if appropriate, should note the initial reaction to suspected diagnoses. Documentation of such responses provides valuable insights into patient and family values and the impact each injury potentially has on the patient. Early assessment of social history provides another indicator of the type of psychosocial and rehabilitative support the patient has and will need in the future. Even in this early resuscitation phase, this information can become the basis for an individualized rehabilitation plan.

CRITICAL CARE AND INTERMEDIATE CARE PHASES

The critical and intermediate care phases of rehabilitation include the period of medical stabilization, which may occur in critical care, intensive care, progressive or intermediate care, and other medical-surgical care units. During this period the focus is on acute treatment of injuries, including surgery, multiple procedures, medications, and other complex care. Even though most emphasis is placed on medically treating the patient, the necessary rehabilitation focus for this phase is the prevention of complications. The critical care nurse should blend technical treatment expertise with application of rehabilitation fundamentals, such as positioning for proper body alignment, providing psychosocial support and patient education, and minimizing the complications of immobility.[30,31]

Prevention of physical complications can avert interruption or delay of progress toward functional recovery, and it also can prevent additional cost for care of the patient.[32] Although it is only one of many complications, decreased mobility is common in severely traumatized patients. All body systems are at risk for complications from immobility.[13,33] Specific nursing measures for minimizing complications related to immobility include positioning to prevent pressure sores and contractures and ensuring proper nutrition for healing and prevention of skin breakdown. Nurses need to work collaboratively with other members of the health care team to prevent complications from immobilization.

Regardless of how complex the trauma, the nurse initiates mobilization techniques and compensatory strategies to prevent complications. The trauma nurse benefits from a thorough understanding of normal body mobilization and physiology of body systems. Many prevention techniques are based on approximating normal body function. For example, many new surgical treatments for serious fractures promote early weight bearing and ambulation. The trend is to eliminate the need for unnecessary immobilization and to promote a normalization of activity even through the critical care and intermediate phases of trauma.

In addition to physical complications, immobility has a number of psychosocial effects. Sensory deprivation, loss of control, and changes in body image and self-esteem are all problems related to immobility. Both the physical and psychosocial effects of immobility could alter the patient's ability to adapt and to recover from the injury.

Support from the trauma nurse as a caregiver prevents or reduces psychologic overreactions of the patient. The nurse can use empathy and receptive listening to allow the patient to ventilate stress. Supporting communication and visitation by family and significant others helps to prevent social isolation. Encouragement of independence in daily activities, care-related decision making, and making choices whenever possible promotes improved feelings of self-determination, self-esteem, and self-worth, which increase the patient's motivation to progress toward recovery. The trauma nurse and other clinicians need to be sensitive to the personal, social, and situational factors that may alter the effectiveness of coping strategies for both the patient and their families.[34]

Patient and family education occurs throughout the critical care and intermediate phases. The nurse, a readily accessible member of the trauma team, may be overwhelmed with questions from the patient and family. An understanding of their readiness to learn helps the nurse recognize the purpose behind these questions. In the early phases of trauma care, many families and patients are not ready to learn fully about the injuries and the consequences. They are more specifically searching for comfort and support. This is evidenced in the case of a family that asserts several weeks later that "no one ever told me this" in regard to information that was shared weeks earlier in response to questions. When the families and patients are under stress, they are not able to use their maximal learning potential.

Readiness for learning includes the right environment and motivation for learning and the ability to retain the presented material. When a family asks a question to find support and comfort, the technical answer often is lost, whereas the feeling of comfort is retained. With this in mind, the trauma nurse prepares to teach, repeat, and review important information to validate that learning has taken place. The trauma nurse can be a key resource to the patient and family to prepare them for the cycle of care ahead and the prospective outcomes associated with the patient's type of injury.[31]

Choosing the rehabilitation specialties that should be active on the care team depends on the diagnosis and effects of injury. During the critical care and intermediate phases, the trauma nurse coordinates closely with the clinical specialties working with an individual patient and makes appropriate recommendations to the physician for rehabilitation referrals.

Physical therapists, occupational therapists, speech and language pathologists, and respiratory therapists are among the first rehabilitation specialists to evaluate and treat the patient. Largely focused on physical aspects of disability, they may begin treatment in the critical care unit. Until the patient is medically stable enough to be seen in the therapy department or treatment area, they provide bedside interventions.

Physical therapists encourage patient mobility and prevent contractures through range-of-motion exercises, positioning techniques, and active exercise programs. Results of musculoskeletal evaluation suggest specific needs for movement and positioning in daily care. Physical therapists may also begin early transfer to a chair and weight-bearing activity.

Respiratory therapists or, in some instances, physical therapists, work on mobilization of respiratory secretions by percussion, vibration, and postural drainage. Physiologic monitoring of respiratory status through blood gas analysis, pulse oximetry monitoring, and pulmonary function testing provides measures of treatment benefit and need for further therapy.

An occupational therapist can assess the patient's ability to perform activities of daily living while the patient is still bedridden. Assessment findings can be used to establish functional goals focusing on the patient's ability to perform self-care activities, which promotes improved self-esteem and a sense of control. For those who are severely neurologically impaired, the occupational therapist may focus on maintaining upper extremity position and mobility, which will allow functional use of limbs or muscle groups. Splinting of the extremities may be used for therapeutic positioning. The occupational therapist may also suggest specific adaptive equipment and techniques to be implemented by the nursing staff.

A speech pathologist is an appropriate early rehabilitation referral for trauma patients with brain injury, high cervical spinal cord injury, and facial injury. Any patient with an artificial airway, such as a tracheal or endotracheal tube, may also benefit from a speech or communication specialist. A speech pathologist can offer various techniques to promote stimulation from coma, cognitive rehabilitation, communication through alternative methods and devices, and improvement of perceptual deficits.

Dysphagia is a specific area of disability that may need to be evaluated and treated in the intermediate phase because the patient becomes ready for oral intake. The speech pathologist may use video fluoroscopy to assess the exact nature of a swallowing problem. Treatment of swallowing disorders often includes consultation by a speech pathologist, an occupational therapist, a rehabilitation nurse, and a respiratory therapist.

An early referral to a physiatrist, a physician specialized in rehabilitation medicine, expedites the implementation of rehabilitation care during the critical or intermediate care phase. In some settings a rehabilitation clinical nurse specialist, nurse practitioner, or nurse case manager can begin to plan and implement the rehabilitation process. Early assessment by rehabilitation specialists permits a projection of rehabilitation potential and an active plan for maximal recovery.

Rehabilitation may be a new concept for the patient and family. They may not realize that acute medical stabilization is just the beginning of recovery. Preparation for transfer to a rehabilitation program includes education about potential patient functional goals, identification and selection of appropriate programs, and support during the upheaval of the transfer process.

Transfer from the atmosphere of the intensive care unit, where the patient is given total care, or an intermediate care unit, where the patient is still provided significant support with daily care, to a rehabilitation unit that fosters independence can be a shock to the patient and family. There comes a point in the patient's acute hospital stay when the emphasis of care should begin to change, and the patient should be encouraged to be independent. Implementing strategies to promote independence as early as possible better prepares the patient for the process of rehabilitation.

Rehabilitation Phase

A great deal of rehabilitation effort and expertise is necessary during the rehabilitation phase, especially for severely injured patients. However, this phase is only one facet of the continuing rehabilitation that occurs throughout the trauma cycle. If rehabilitation were ignored in the other phases, functional outcomes could be severely decreased.

Most rehabilitation occurs in an inpatient setting, such as a rehabilitation unit of an acute care hospital or a freestanding rehabilitation facility. Depending on the type and severity of the disability, the frequency and type of medical monitoring and nursing care required, insurance coverage, family support systems, and patient motivation, a subacute, LTAC or skilled nursing home setting, or an outpatient or home-based rehabilitation program could be appropriate if a comprehensive team approach is provided.

Key themes throughout the rehabilitation phase are restoration, compensation, and adaptation. The rehabilitation team evaluates each individual case for (1) the ability to recover normal function, (2) appropriate areas to replace normal function with other strategies (compensation), and (3) areas in which the patient must change his or her lifestyle, roles, and expectations to adapt to disability. This evaluation results in a rehabilitation plan, with setting of both long-term and short-term goals. Depending on the patient's progress, these goals may need periodic adjustment. These goals are reviewed weekly by the rehabilitation team and may be reported as frequently as daily to the patient's managed care organization.

Active rehabilitation includes learning new skills, practicing them, and testing skills in the environment. The average length of stay (ALOS) years ago would have been months depending on the type of injury the patient had sustained. Today, the ALOS is contingent on diagnosis with comorbidities and the focus is on moving the patient to the next level of care. Not all patients are completely independent when discharged from an acute rehabilitation program. They may be transferred to another level of care, such as a skilled nursing facility or outpatient setting, to continue their rehabilitation. This is why the rehabilitative process takes weeks to months to complete. Some patients may be in and out of rehabilitation programs for years, learning and further improving skills with each admission. Few people have the capacity for learning all that is necessary to adapt to injury at one time. Many goals spill over into the reintegration phase. Progress with each short-term goal may vary.

As medical stability and functional independence increase, the patient asserts his or her rights for self-determination. This issue is extremely frustrating at times to the trauma team, whose values may conflict with those of the patient they have worked so hard to help. For example, a patient who had sustained a C4-5 spinal cord injury with resulting quadriplegia was transferred to a rehabilitation hospital from an acute care setting. The acute care staff had made every effort to maintain function of all body systems. Specifically, the patient's upper extremity range of motion was outstanding. About 8 weeks after transfer, the rehabilitation hospital provided the acute trauma nurses with a progress report on the patient. He was taking notably more control of his life and responsibility for his own actions. But the presence of upper extremity contractures was a shock to the acute care staff. At first the acute care staff blamed the rehabilitation staff for neglect. Later they began to understand that this severely injured young man chose to maintain only enough range of motion to scratch his nose for comfort. He did not share the rehabilitation team's goal of self-feeding. His goal was control of his comfort and reserving his energy for activities other than self-feeding.[35]

The patient's values guide the course of rehabilitation. The challenge is understanding when a traumatized patient is ready to be released from the sick role and considered competent and sufficiently informed to make self-determining judgments. The trauma rehabilitation nurse strives to provide as many options as possible for maximizing function, but the injured person makes the ultimate decision.

Reintegration Phase

Community reintegration strategies usually begin during the rehabilitation phase. One strategy is the use of a therapeutic leave of absence from an inpatient setting, which allows the patient and family to test the adapted function in the real world. This strategy is also used in modified reintegration settings that blend home care and outpatient programs. Of all areas in trauma rehabilitation, the reintegration process is the most limited in alternatives because of limited reimbursement avenues.

Reintegration is the process of applying therapeutic adaptation and compensation to the patient's premorbid lifestyle. A difficult question facing rehabilitation specialists is, when does rehabilitation end and lifelong health management begin? Trauma patients stay in the health care system for extended periods. Functional gains are achieved even years after injury. Rehabilitation programs strive for maximized patient potential. Who determines when a patient has reached his or her potential?

Issues in Trauma Rehabilitation

Funding for Rehabilitation

The most challenging issue after trauma is the lack of funding for patients needing rehabilitation programs and services. The prospect of paying out of pocket for rehabilitation is extremely lofty for the average person. Because of inadequate private funding and limited federal and state reimbursement systems, many trauma patients never receive the rehabilitation that is appropriate for their disability. This is particularly true of rehabilitation during the reintegration phase of the cycle. Emergency and life-saving services are provided to many people who are not able to return to a fully functional role in society.

Experts in the field of rehabilitation continue to provide data to third-party payers to increase funds available for care of the injured. Insurers are using the expertise of rehabilitation nurses as case managers to enhance the cost-effectiveness and appropriateness of rehabilitation admissions. An administrative waiver, in which a third-party payer agrees to a cost-effective plan of care not specifically covered by the patient's policy, is an alternative that can sometimes be negotiated on a case-by-case basis. Health care consumers continue to pressure the managed care industry for expanded benefits.

With the implementation of the Balanced Budget Act of 1997, HCFA replaced cost-based reimbursement with a PPS for rehabilitation hospitals, skilled nursing facilities, and community-based settings.[5] PPS manages cost by using a national standard for payment for similar services, adjusted by clinical need and geographic costs. Based on rate implementation to date, overall the reimbursement is lower than received in the cost-based system. Phase-in of PPS rates began for skilled nursing facilities in July 1998.

Managed care administration of medical assistance funds has occurred for various populations in most states. Implementation of state-funded managed care related to rehabilitation and long-term care remains in its infancy. It is unclear at this time how state funding for rehabilitation and catastrophic care will be funded under a managed care design.

Every avenue of rehabilitation funding is under pressure to reduce costs. Over the next few years we are likely to see the environment for rehabilitation continue to evolve due to the Balanced Budget Act. The resulting reimbursement systems will determine which service alternatives will survive. However, expectation for successful outcomes will remain high. There will be a great deal of pressure on the field of rehabilitation to reinvent itself to some degree if it is to remain financially viable.

Acceptance of the Trauma-Disabled Person in Society

Long-term disability in such a young population leads to an ever-increasing percentage of people whose lives have been altered by trauma. The media have helped to enlighten society about physical disability. Disabled parking, curb ramps, and other accessibility-related standards, such as those defined in the Americans with Disabilities Act of 1990, are accepted and expected in daily life.[36] Adaptations in the workplace are becoming more visible. Physically challenged persons are depicted as role models in sports, business, and other areas of success. Society has accepted the physically challenged more readily.

Unfortunately, not much progress has been made regarding awareness of the cognitive and psychosocial ramifications of injury. Cognitive and behavioral disabilities caused by head injury and injury-related psychologic traumas are poorly understood by the public. People who do not comprehend the nature of the problem and the needs of the cognitively and behaviorally disabled become anxious and reject them. There is an attempt to label people with behavior problems as mentally retarded, crazy, or rude. Mental illness has a long history of poor acceptance in society. As the mentally disabled population grows, more people will have contact with these individuals in work, home, and community settings. Efforts at public education and sensitization enhance the true reintegration of intellectually and behaviorally disabled people. This process is necessary for trauma-disabled people to return to a contributing role in society. However, it is unrealistic to think that all catastrophically injured people will return to the community, whether because of limited function or societal resistance.

Trauma Prevention

Issues related to rehabilitation would not exist if the initial trauma were prevented. The Centers for Disease Control and Prevention (CDC) recognizes that injuries continue to occur despite our best efforts at prevention and seeks to improve the outcomes of those who experience severe injuries. The CDC also seeks to improve acute injury care practices.[37] Prevention focuses on violence prevention and unintentional injury prevention. Violence prevention focuses on child maltreatment, intimate partner violence, sexual violence, suicide, and youth violence.[38] Unintentional injury prevention focuses on child passenger safety, fall prevention of the elderly, fire deaths, fireworks injury, impaired driving, older adult drivers, playground injuries, teen drivers, and water-related injuries.[38] The list of possible trauma prevention initiatives is endless.

Trauma prevention is an educational process. As awareness of trauma increases, so will legitimate public support for those actions that can prevent the injuries from occurring. It is the responsibility of all health care professionals to support education through individual, family, and community teaching; media exposure; community interest groups; churches; schools; and other settings in the community. The public also expects health care professionals to act as role models of healthier and safer living.

Total prevention of traumatic injury is a worthy challenge to professionals and our society. It is a reasonable goal for society to work toward reduced incidence and severity of injury and disability in the immediate future.

Summary

Role of the Trauma Rehabilitation Nurse

Rehabilitation of the trauma patient presents many exciting and expanding opportunities for nurses. New roles for rehabilitation experts will benefit from nursing's holistic approach to the physical, cognitive, and psychosocial components of rehabilitation programming. Rehabilitation liaison and discharge planning roles in trauma centers effectively link the intermediate and rehabilitation phases of care.[1] Clinical nurse specialists and nurse practitioners support early initiation of rehabilitation techniques by awareness of the benefits of rehabilitation. In the rehabilitation and reintegration phases, nurses also contribute through their roles as rehabilitation coordinators and case managers.[21,39,40] In addition to clinical practice, many nurses have blended rehabilitation specialization with administration, public relations, business, and research to provide a wealth of expertise and skill to health-related companies and insurers. Nurses are also effective in program development, management, marketing, and consulting roles.

Regardless of the trauma rehabilitation nurse's specific function, it is essential that all members of the profession involve themselves in the issues that rehabilitation will face in the future. Active participation in professional and disability-related organizations such as the Association of Rehabilitation Nurses, the American Congress of Rehabilitation Medicine, the American Association of Spinal Cord Injury Nurses, the Case Management Society of America, the National Association of Rehabilitation Professionals in the Private Sector, the American Spinal Cord Injury Association, and the Brain Injury Association and their local networks offers an opportunity for nurses to work creatively and constructively toward improved legislation and guidelines for practice, community awareness, and community support for the disabled population. Involvement in rehabilitation issues may occur on an individual basis or through activities by the employing facility or organization. Nurses in clinical practice who have direct interaction with patients and families have the vital role of educating those most directly affected about rehabilitation issues. Through this comprehensive effort, issues can be resolved.

A wealth of personal and professional growth is available to nurses in trauma rehabilitation. The specialty continues to work through its new stages of development and welcomes creative ideas and expertise. For the person who longs to create an advanced practice role in nursing, trauma rehabilitation may offer this opportunity.

FUTURE RESEARCH

A great deal of research still needs to be conducted on the phases of rehabilitation after traumatic injury. Trauma rehabilitation has borrowed therapeutic approaches from many other specialties, such as stroke and neurologic disease rehabilitation, psychiatry, and normal and abnormal child development. The areas in which clinical research can be conducted over the next decade are unlimited. The National Center for the Dissemination of Disability Research (NCDDR) funds research for eight key areas of impact.[41] These research areas include emphasis on health and function of the disabled, application of technology, community reintegration and employment, and public education. Advocates for the injured are lobbying for a significant increase in federal funds for clinical research.

It is the responsibility of every rehabilitation practitioner and facility to closely examine and study the cost-effectiveness and benefits of treatments and practices. Many health care professionals assume that more care is better care. Future research could be directed toward identifying minimal standards that still result in high-quality outcomes. In the years to come, federally mandated clinical outcome tools may provide a base of information across rehabilitation settings, perhaps initiating research and practice guidelines for the best alternatives in rehabilitation. Other studies may consider how often a specific treatment is needed. For example, what level of staff member is most cost effective for each aspect of clinical care? The implementation of evidence-based practice in the rehabilitation arena will produce innovation and additional research.

Because outcome measurement for trauma rehabilitation is still developing, adequate data are not yet available to evaluate the long-term and lifelong needs of the traumatized population. Studies of the effects of aging and lifestyle on people who have experienced a catastrophic illness will also help the rehabilitation profession provide appropriate education, adaptation, and follow-up for lifelong support.

Clinical research focuses not only on how to improve trauma care but on how to improve recovery from some of the most catastrophic injuries such as brain and spinal cord injuries. Physiologic studies of central nervous system tissue support the theory that nerve cells are able to regenerate. Electrical stimulation of muscle groups supports the use of previously ineffective limbs. There are studies in the area of cognitive research to test different programs on people to see if their memories show any signs of improvement. The goal is to fund effective ways to manage and improve memory problems following a brain injury or in old age. There are also studies using the Lokomat (a robotic gait trainer) to study ways to enhance locomotion after neurologic injury. Advances in technology, such as computer software, hardware, and telecommunication, have made the application of distance communication to rehabilitation a reality. This has allowed assessments and follow-up services to be performed without traveling to a remote rehabilitation facility. It also provides online education opportunities for the clinicians as well as patients and families. The potential for improved recovery is positive. To this end, the field of trauma rehabilitation and its patient population benefit from the research, education, expert clinical practice, and leadership of professional rehabilitation nurses.

REFERENCES

1. Brandt E, Pope E: Enabling America: *Assessing the Role of Rehabilitation Science and Engineering,* Washington, DC, 1997, National Economic Press.
2. Brillhart B: Studying the quality of life and life satisfaction among persons with spinal cord injury, *Rehabil Nurs* 29(4): 122-126, 2004.

3. Krause JS: Prediction of long-term survival of persons with SCI: an 11-year prospective study. In Eisenberg MG, Glueckauf RL, editors: *Empirical Approaches to Psychosocial Aspects of Disability,* New York, 1991, Springer.
4. Stryker R: *Rehabilitation Aspects of Acute and Chronic Nursing Care,* ed 2, Philadelphia, 1996, WB Saunders.
5. Silversmith J: The impact of the 1997 Balanced Budget Act on Medicare, *Minn Med* 83(12):42-49, 2000.
6. The impact of the Balanced Budget Act of 1997 on Medicare in the USA: the fallout continues, *Int J Health Care Quality Assurance Leadership Health Serv* 15(6):249-254, 2002.
7. American Hospital Association: *Summary of the Medicare Prescription Drug, Improvement and Modernization Act of 2003 (P.L. 108-173) Dec. 18, 2003.* Available online at www.aha.org/aha/content/2003/pdf/MedicareRxSummary031218.pdf. Accessed December 28, 2006.
8. Commission on Accreditation of Rehabilitation Facilities: *Medical Rehabilitation Standards Manual.* Tucson, Ariz, 2006, The Commission on Accreditation of Rehabilitation Facilities.
9. *Brain Injury Recovery.* Available online at http://www.brain.injury.com/recovery/html. Accessed May 6, 2006.
10. *Coma Levels.* Available online at http://www.waiting.com/levelsofcoma.html. Accessed May 26, 2006.
11. *Glasgow Coma Score: Trauma Scoring.* Available online at http://www.trauma.org/scores/gcs.html. Accessed December 28, 2006.
12. *The Expanded Rancho Levels of Cognitive Function.* Available online at http://www.rancho.org/patient_education/cognitive_description.pdf. Accessed December 28, 2006.
13. Dean-Baar S, editor: The purpose and function of the rehabilitation team. In Mumma CM, editor: *Rehabilitation Nursing: Concepts in Practice, A Core Curriculum,* ed 6, Evanston, Ill, 2005, Rehabilitation Nursing Foundation.
14. Stepans MB, Thompson CL, Buchanan ML: The role of the nurse on a transdisciplinary early intervention assessment team, *Public Health Nursing* 19(4):238, 2002.
15. Chan F, Berven NL, Thomas KR, editors: *Counseling Theories and Techniques for Rehabilitation Health Professionals,* New York, 2004, Springer.
16. *Rehabilitation Nursing.* Available online at http://www.rehabnurse.org/profresources/staffnurse.html. Accessed May 6, 2006.
17. Powell S: *Case Management: A Practical Guide to Success in Managed Care,* Philadelphia, 2000, Lippincott Williams & Wilkins.
18. Rondinelli RD, Murphy JR, Wilson DH et al: Predictors of functional outcome and resource utilization in inpatient rehabilitation, *Arch Phys Med Rehabil* 72(7):447-453, 1991.
19. Taylor MD, Tracy JK, Meyer W et al: Trauma in the elderly: intensive care unit resource use and outcome, *J Trauma* 53(3):407-414, 2002.
20. Weatherall M: Rehabilitation of elderly patients with multiple fractures secondary to falls, *Disability Rehab* 15(1):38-40, 1993.
21. Lambert J: Meeting the emotional needs of a patient, *Rehabil Nurs* 24(4):141-142, 1999.
22. Faraci P, Leiter P, Weeks DK: Trends in lengths of stay, charges, and functional outcomes: implications for the rehabilitation industry, *J Rehabil Admin* 20(2):137-151,1996.
23. *Uniform Data System for Medical Rehabilitation.* Available online at http://www.udsmr.org/fim2_about php. Accessed December 28, 2006.
24. *WeeFIMII System.* Available online at http://www.udsmr.org/Wee_about.php. Accessed December 28, 2006.
25. UDS-PRO System. Available online at http://www.udsmr.org/pro_about.php. Accessed December 28, 2006.
26. The Joint Commission on Accreditation of Healthcare Organizations: *Facts About ORYX® for Hospitals Core Measures.* Available online at http://www.jcaho.org/accredited+organziations/hospitals/oryx/oryx+facts.htm. Accessed February 26, 2006.
27. *Uniform Data System for Medical Rehabilitation (UDSMR).* Available online at www.udsmr.org/. Accessed February 26, 2006.
28. *IRVEN.* Available online at http://www.cms.hhs.gov/InpatientRehabFacPPS/06_Software.asp. Accessed December 29, 2006.
29. *Glossary of Terms in Managed Care.* Available online at http://www.pohly.com/terms_in.html. Accessed December 28, 2006.
30. Sherburne E: A rehabilitation protocol for the neuroscience intensive care unit, *J Neurosci Nurs* 18(3):140-145, 1986.
31. Deering-Stuck B, Brunner SL: Rehabilitation of trauma patients. In Cardona VD: *Trauma Nursing,* Oradell, NJ, 1985, Medical Economics Books.
32. Deutsch PM, Sawyer HW, editors: *A Guide to Rehabilitation,* White Plains, NY, 2005, AHAB Press.
33. Cuccurullo SJ, editor: *Physical Medicine and Rehabilitation Board Review,* New York, 2004, Demos Medical Publishing, LLC.
34. Aldwin C, Yancura L: *Coping and Health: A Comparison of the Stress and Trauma Literature.* Available online at http://www.med.ucdavis.edu/faculty/aldwin/Coping.pdf. Accessed December 29, 2006.
35. Ridley B: Tom's story: a quadriplegic who refused rehabilitation, *Rehabil Nurs* 14(5):250-253, 1989.
36. *The Americans with Disabilities Act of 1990.* Available online at http://www.usdoj.gov/crt/ada/adahom1.htm. Accessed December 29, 2006.
37. *Acute Injury Care.* Available online at http://www.cdc.gov/ncipc/dir/AcuteInjuryCare/htm. Accessed January 10, 2008.
38. *CDC Injury Fact Book.* Available online at http://www.cdc.gov/ncipc/fact_book/factbook.htm. Accessed January 10, 2008.
39. *Rehabilitation Nurses Make a Difference.* Available online at http://www.rehabnurse.org/about/definition. Accessed December 28, 2006.
40. Association of Rehabilitation Nursing: *Role Description of Case Managers.* Available online at http://rehabnurse.org/profresource/casemgr.html. Accessed December 28, 2006.
41. *The National Center for the Dissemination of Disability Research (NCDDR).* Available online at www.ncddr.org. Accessed December 29, 2006.

PART II

CLINICAL MANAGEMENT CONCEPTS

12

MECHANISM OF INJURY

John Weigelt, Karen J. Brasel, Jorie Klein

In *Webster's Dictionary*, *trauma* is defined as "an injury or wound to a living body caused by the application of external violence." Injury is a public health problem of vast proportions. In 1999 injury was the leading cause of death for persons ages 1 to 34 and was the fifth leading cause of death overall.[1] There were 29 million nonfatal injuries from all causes in 2005 for a rate of 9,871 per 100,000.[2] Some 93% of these injuries were unintentional.

Mortality is the most common way to assess the impact of injury. In 2004 there were 167,184 injury deaths in the United States, for a rate of 57 per 100,000. The most common cause of injury death was motor vehicle crashes, with a total of 44,933 deaths and a rate of 15.30 per 100,000.[2] Among people age 65 and older, falls are the most common cause of injury death and nonfatal injuries.[1]

Another way to measure the impact of injury to our society is to examine the years of potential life lost.[3] Unintentional injury accounts for more than 2 million years of potential life lost before the age of 65, compared with 1.8 million for cancer and 1.4 million for cardiovascular disease. Suicide and homicide each account for more than a half million years of potential life lost.

A final method to evaluate the effect injury has on society is to estimate the cost of injury, done by the National Safety Council.[4] These estimates of the costs of unintentional injury emphasize the value of preventive initiatives that reduce unintentional injury rates. Their estimates are provided as averages. In 2005, the economic cost of a death was $1,150,000; for a nonfatal disabling injury it was $52,900 and for a nondisabling injury it was $7500. These figures do not include long-term costs for the disabling injuries. An estimate in 1995 dollars places the total injury costs at $260 billion.[1] However you assess impact, injury remains a major drain on our society.

Injury results from acute exposure to different types of energy, such as kinetic (as conveyed by crashes, falls, and bullets), chemical, thermal, electrical, or ionizing radiation. Injury also results from a lack of essential agents, such as oxygen (e.g., drowning) and heat (e.g., frostbite). The injury occurs because of the body's inability to tolerate exposure to the excessive acute energy. Wounds vary depending on the injuring agent. For example, damage from a gunshot blast is dependent on the missile's mass and velocity; degree of burn varies with temperature and duration of contact; injuries from deceleration depend on the victim's body mass, rate of deceleration, and area over which the energy is dissipated. Effects of an injury are also dependent on personal and environmental factors, such as age, sex, nutrition, underlying disease processes, and geographic region (rural versus urban). These factors help define populations at risk for various types and severities of injuries.

RISK FACTORS

Risks of injury from different causes vary by age, sex, race, income, and environment. Factors such as substance abuse, geographic region, and temporal variation can also affect risk for injury. Identification of characteristics inherent in different populations and subgroups at risk for injury allows prevention measures to be focused on high-risk groups.

One way of subdividing injury groups is according to intentional and unintentional events. For example, ingestion of a toxic substance can be intentional, as in a suicide attempt, or unintentional. The mechanism of injury is the same, but the events leading to the injury differ.

AGE

Death rates from injuries are highest in patients age 75 or older.[5] A factor contributing to this high death rate in the elderly may be presence of associated medical conditions.[5,6] The in-hospital fatality rate for this group is 15% to 30% compared with 4% to 8% in younger patients.[5] In patients with rib fractures, the mortality rate for patients older than age 55 is twice that for those younger than age 55.[7,8]

The highest injury rate occurs in persons between the ages of 15 and 34[1] because of their participation in high-risk activities. Poor judgment associated with the use of alcohol and drugs also contributes to the high injury rate. The lowest injury rate is for children ages 5 to 14.[1] The highest homicide rate occurs among people ages 15 to 24.[1] Suicide rates for both sexes show little variation with age. The incidence of domestic violence is highest among women between ages 16 and 24.[9]

Specific injury mechanisms and risk of injury also vary by age. The elderly suffer a disproportionate number of falls, as well as pedestrian-related injuries.[10,11] They are more likely to suffer significant injury with minimal energy transfer.[10] Assault among elderly patients is recognized as a health care problem. During 2001, more than 30,000 persons age 60 and older were treated in U.S. emergency departments for nonfatal assault injuries.[12] This is a rate of 72 per 100,000 population. Rates were highest among the 60- to 69-year age group. Although not well recognized, some of these assaults probably represent elder maltreatment.[13]

Gender

Injury rates are highest for 15- to 24-year-old males.[1] The mortality risk for males is 4.6 times that for females, possibly because of male involvement in hazardous activities. The unintentional injury death rate for males peaks between ages 15 and 24. It is the third most common cause of death for males and females in the 45- to 54-year age group.[1] The rate of homicide is among the top three causes of death for males ages 10 to 34.[1] In females, the death rate peaks at ages 15 to 19 for unintentional injury and at 20 to 24 for homicide. Women in their late 40s have the highest suicide rate. Nonfatal injury rates for men and women do not differ significantly, suggesting that injuries to males are more severe than those to females.[1]

Domestic violence is more often directed against females than males.[14] In 1996, 75% of the approximately 1,800 homicides perpetrated by an intimate partner involved a female victim. An intimate partner is responsible for 28.5% of homicides in women ages 18 to 24 compared with only 2.5% of male victims.[9] In addition to those hospitalized as a direct result of intentional injury, intimate partner violence is much more prevalent in patients admitted for unintentional injury than in the general population. It is related to alcohol use disorders in both the perpetrator and the victim.[15]

Race and Income

Injury death rates vary according to race and socioeconomic level. In a depressed economy the suicide and homicide rates increase and the number of motor vehicle crashes (MVCs) decreases.[16] Native Americans (Indians, Eskimos, and Aleuts) have the highest death rate from unintentional injury regardless of income. In 1999, this was estimated to be 61 per 100,000 population.[1] African Americans have the highest homicide rate. Caucasians and Native Americans have the highest suicide rate. Asian Americans (Chinese, Japanese, Koreans, Hawaiians, Filipinos, Guamanians) have the lowest death rates from unintentional injuries, homicide, and suicide. The unintentional injury rate is higher in low-income areas than in the wealthiest areas. An inverse relationship exists between income levels and death rates for African Americans and Caucasians; that is, the higher the income, the lower the death rate. This relationship is maintained for domestic violence.[17]

Alcohol

Alcohol not only contributes to injury-producing events, such as MVCs, it also can increase the severity of injury.[18] Alcohol is a major factor in many motor vehicle, home, industrial, and recreational injuries and in crime, suicide, and family abuse.[19] Unhealthy alcohol use is believed to occur in 4% to 30% of the population.[20] Alcohol abuse occurs in 5% and alcohol dependence in 4% of the population. Recent evidence suggests that alcohol interventions in a trauma center may reduce the risk of injury recurrence.[21] A brief intervention regarding alcohol consumption resulted in fewer arrests in the subsequent 3 years for driving under the influence of alcohol.[22] The value of these brief interventions for patients with acute alcohol intoxication has been endorsed by the American College of Surgeons Committee on Trauma in their trauma center verification program since 2006.[23]

Rural versus Urban

Patterns of injury differ between rural and urban environments. A major difference is a higher intentional injury rate in large urban areas. Homicide is highest in cities. Suicide is 80% greater in rural areas than in metropolitan areas. Clearly the physical environment has an important influence on injury rate.[24] Overall mortality rates from injury are higher in rural communities compared with urban communities. When considering MVCs, the higher mortality might be related to road characteristics, lower use of seatbelts, reduced density of traffic enforcement officials, slower detection of crashes, and distance to the closest trauma center. In rural settings, agricultural equipment is another source of injury, especially among children. Cuttings and machinery injuries are also common causes of injury in rural environments.[25] Falls are a common unintentional injury in rural and urban communities. Urban and rural environments share poisoning as a common unintentional injury. However, urban poisonings are commonly medications and household chemicals, whereas rural poisonings are usually related to agricultural products.

Initial Assessment and History

In the initial evaluation of the trauma patient, a careful history of the events leading to the injury must be obtained. The practitioner must attend to urgent therapeutic needs along with the usual diagnostic evaluation.[26] Obtaining an accurate history—especially asking about the mechanism of injury—can help identify likely injuries and thereby reduce morbidity and mortality.

Answers to questions about the circumstances of the impact are helpful when assessing potential injuries sustained in a motor vehicle–related crash (such as automobile, motorcycle, and pedestrian injuries). At the site of the incident, prehospital care personnel should quickly survey the scene, noting the appearance of the vehicle(s) involved and the damage sustained to the passenger compartment. It is important to know the speed the vehicle involved was traveling, the point of impact, and the type of impact (single-vehicle, high-speed, front-end, rear-end, or T-bone intersection collision). In a MVC with a combined speed of 30 miles per hour, near-side lateral impact crashes have the highest risk of injury, followed by far-side lateral impact and frontal crashes.[27] The evaluating team should determine whether the patient was the driver or the passenger, whether safety devices (safety belt, child safety seat, and airbag) were used, and where the victim was found at the scene. Death of an occupant in the vehicle should alert the team to potential energy forces within the collision. Patients from a vehicle in which an occupant has died and individuals who are ejected from a vehicle have a higher morbidity and mortality and warrant a thorough evaluation for injury.

Frontal-impact collisions that cause a bent steering wheel or column, knee imprints in the dashboard, or a broken windshield are associated with head injuries, hemopneumothoraces, injuries to the spleen or liver, and dislocation of the patella.[28,29] Femur fractures with or without posterior fracture-dislocation of the ipsilateral hip must be considered. Deceleration injuries such as aortic rupture and small bowel injury must be ruled out.

Side-impact collisions produce contralateral neck sprains, cervical fractures, head injuries, lacerations to the soft tissues, lateral rib fractures or flail chest, abdominal injuries, and pelvic and acetabular fractures. Although the mechanism is not as classic as frontal deceleration, aortic injuries often result from side-impact collisions. The risk is significantly higher for near-side rather than far-side impact.[30]

Rear-impact collisions result in hyperextension neck injuries, and there may be rebound frontal-impact injuries. Ejection from the vehicle produces a multitude of injuries, such as penetrating impalement wounds, head injuries, cervical fractures, and road burns. Ejection increases not only the risk of injury, but the risk of serious injury.[27,31]

Motorcycle crashes produce single or multiple impacts. The evaluating team must determine the type of collision (direct impact with stable object or impact with another vehicle), rate of speed, where the victim was found in relation to the cycle, and if protective devices were worn (helmet, gloves, and boots). Head injuries, long-bone fractures, pelvic fractures, and soft tissue injuries are common.

Pedestrians hit by vehicles may have many injuries. The prehospital team should identify (or estimate) how fast the vehicle involved was traveling, the type of vehicle, the point of impact, and whether the victim was thrown or dragged. Waddell's triad (Figure 12-1) occurs when a pedestrian is struck by a car.[32] Age influences both type and severity of injuries.[33] When the victim is a child, injuries are caused by three events: (1) the bumper and hood impact the femur and/or chest, (2) the victim is thrown upon impact, and (3) the contralateral skull is injured by the force of impact upon hitting the ground. One of the resulting injuries is often missed in the initial evaluation. Adult pedestrians receive a lateral impact from contact with the bumper and hood, injuring the lower and upper leg, because adults try to protect themselves by turning sideways (Figure 12-1). Fractures to this area are recognized, but ligament damage in the other knee is often overlooked.

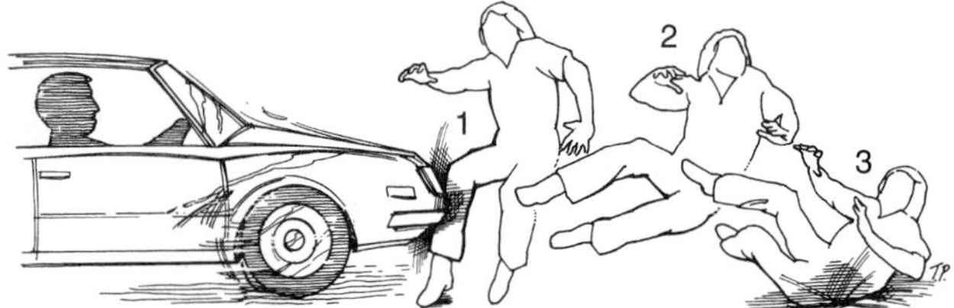

FIGURE 12-1 Waddell's triad in adult pedestrians. Impact *(1)* with the bumper or hood and lateral rotation *(2)* produces injury to the upper and/or lower leg *(3)*.

Penetrating trauma refers to any injury produced when a foreign object passes through the tissue. Energy is dissipated through the tissue, producing the injury. Injuries from penetrating trauma are more predictable than those caused by blunt trauma. It is important to identify the type of weapon (caliber of gun, length of knife blade), stance of the assailant, distance from the assailant to victim, and potential number of wounds.

It is not always possible and is sometimes impractical to obtain a detailed history, but information can be obtained from family members, paramedics, firefighters, police officers, onlookers, or eyewitnesses. Priority is obviously given to managing life-threatening injuries, including those that cause inadequate ventilation, hypoxia, or bleeding. After the patient is resuscitated and stabilized, the trauma practitioner should begin a detailed review of the patient's history, physical findings, and laboratory results to direct further investigations.

A quick, thorough physical examination must be performed during or immediately after resuscitation. It is important to systematically examine the undressed patient to avoid overlooking injuries. Injuries are easier to detect in patients with penetrating trauma than in those with blunt injury, because surface injury may or may not be present with blunt injury. Failure to diagnose the patient's injuries correctly is associated with a high mortality rate.[28] An index of suspicion for associated injuries based on the mechanism of injury must be maintained.

Some body areas do not lend themselves easily to physical examination, such as the cranium, vertebral column, and bony thorax. Injury may exist without classic signs, but the mechanism of injury may raise suspicion enough to warrant further diagnostic examinations. Examples include computed tomography (CT) for diagnosis of brain injury, CT or angiography for blunt chest injury and possible aortic injury, and plain radiography, CT, and magnetic resonance imaging for spinal column evaluation.[34] Specific protocols to evaluate certain types of injury may help identify injuries while conserving resources. All tests must be performed without placing the patient at risk of further injury. The patient is reexamined continually to identify changing physical findings.

Complete assessment of the trauma patient is aided by knowing the cause of injury. MVCs are the most common cause of injury, followed by falls. Other causes of injury are pedestrian collision, drowning, fire, burn, explosion, poisoning, firearm, assault, aspiration, machinery, and sports activity. In some cases the cause can be related to an expected pattern of injury. For example, distinct injury patterns may be found with sports-related trauma associated with sudden deceleration (diving, falling), excessive forces (twisting, hyperextension, hyperflexion), or changes in momentum (boxing). Because of repeated blows to the head in boxing, cumulative brain damage may occur, with resultant neurologic damage depending on the affected area. Spinal cord injuries can occur while participating in gymnastics or playing football. Head injuries can occur while playing football or horseback riding. Skiing can produce fractures, and knee injuries are common with skiing and football. This information plus the events preceding the incident can provide clues to the practitioner regarding the patterns of injuries, expected severity of injury, and possible occult or missed injuries.[28] Common areas where injuries are missed include the extremities (hand and foot), upper extremities (forearm and upper arm), and skin (scalp lacerations). Repetitive examinations and review of information after admission will detect missed injuries in 10% of patients.[35,36]

MECHANISM OF INJURY

The mechanics of injury are related to the type of injuring force and subsequent tissue response. A thorough understanding of these two facets of injury helps in determining the extent and nature of damage. Injury occurs when the force deforms tissues beyond their failure limits. This can result in anatomic and physiologic damage. Anatomic damage, such as skeletal fractures, will usually heal, and function will return. Physiologic damage, such as central nervous system injury, may be permanent despite the healing process. The mechanism of injury can help explain the type of injury, predict eventual outcome, and identify common injury combinations. Knowledge of this information improves trauma patient management.

BIOMECHANICS

The principles of mechanics are used to investigate the mechanisms of physical and physiologic responses to force. The injuring force can be penetrating or nonpenetrating. The resultant injury depends on the energy delivered and area of contact. Penetrating injury usually involves a concentration of injury to a small body area; nonpenetrating injury distributes energy over a larger area. Injury can occur by slow deformation of tissue; however, the predominant force is usually fast and violent, such as the impact of the head against a windshield or a bullet's penetration into an extremity.

The field of biomechanics involves a variety of disciplines, including engineering, physiology, medicine, biology, and anatomy.[37] Knowledge of injury mechanisms allows the appropriate biomechanical measurements to be made to characterize injuries. Many approaches are used in this field of inquiry, and research is best conducted with representatives of as many of the disciplines as possible. For example, the Crash Injury Research and Engineering Network (CIREN) program uses a multidisciplinary approach to explain the injuries that result from car crashes and direct biomechanical research to improve car safety.[38]

INJURY CONCEPTS

Among the factors that influence injury are velocity of collision, object shape, and tissue rigidity. Body tissue has inertial resistance as well as tensile, elastic, and compressive strength. *Tensile strength* equals the amount of tension a tissue can withstand and its ability to resist stretching forces. *Elasticity* is the ability of a tissue to resume its original shape and size after being stretched. *Compressive strength* refers to the tissue's ability to resist squeezing forces or inward pressure. Whenever the force exceeds maximum tissue strength, a fracture or tear occurs.[39]

Force is a physical factor that changes the motion of a body either at rest or already in motion. It is calculated by the following equation:

$$\text{Force} = \text{Mass} \times \text{Acceleration}$$

The more slowly the force is applied, the more slowly energy is released, with less subsequent tissue deformation. If the same force is dissipated over a large surface area, the tissue disruption is further reduced. The forces most often applied are acceleration, deceleration, shearing, and compression. *Acceleration* is a change in the rate of velocity or speed of a moving body. As velocity increases, so does tissue damage. *Deceleration* is a decrease in the velocity of a moving object. *Shearing forces* occur across a plane, with structures slipping relative to each other. *Compressive resistance* is the ability of an object or structure to resist squeezing forces or inward pressure.[39]

Viscoelastic properties of tissue help absorb energy and protect vital organs from the effects of impact. If the energy transmitted to the tissue remains below the limit of injury, the energy will be absorbed without causing injury.[40] This phenomenon is used to protect against injury by using energy-absorbing structures and padding. These protective objects do not prevent deformation of tissues but can extend the duration and reduce the force of impact below the limit of injury.

When the tissues are deformed beyond the recoverable limit, injury occurs. Tissue or structure deformation can be measured according to changes in shape, commonly defined as a change in length divided by the initial length. Another term for this change is *strain.* Two major types of strain are tensile and shear. A third type is compressive, which is less common and is responsible for crushing injuries. Tensile and shear strain applied to an artery is illustrated in Figure 12-2. Stretching of the artery along its longitudinal axis increases its length and tissue strain. If the strain or increase in length is too great, the tissue will break. An "all or none" phenomenon is not present, so the artery may completely or partially break. A similar result can be produced by a force applied at 90 degrees to the long axis of the artery. This shear strain occurs when the

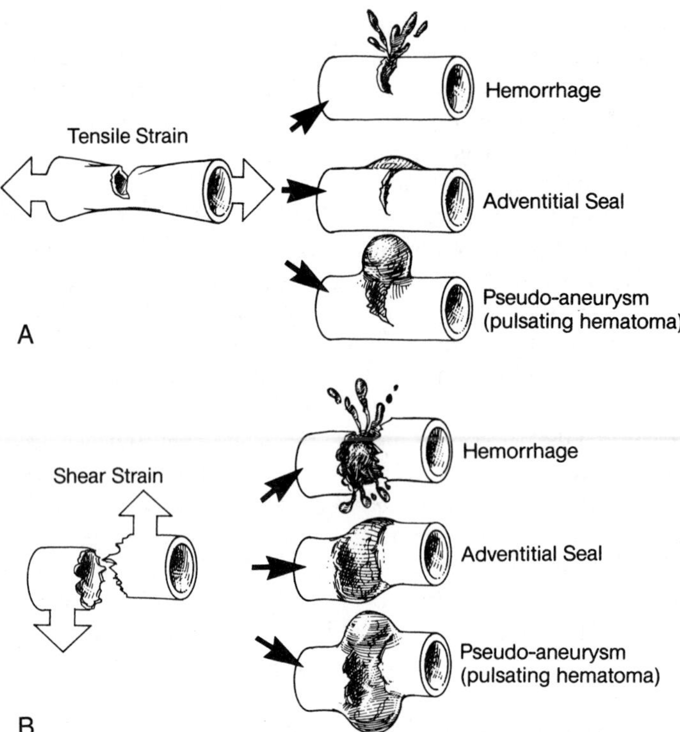

FIGURE 12-2 **A**, As the artery is stretched along its longitudinal axis, its length and amount of tissue strain increase. An increase in length that exceeds tensile strength causes the artery to break. The injury can result in a complete tear or can produce lower degrees of damage if the strain is less. **B**, Shear strain occurs when the force is applied 90 degrees to the longitudinal axis. Varying degrees of injury can occur with different levels of force. *(Modified from Committee on Trauma Research, National Research Council and the Institute of Medicine:* Injury in America, *Washington, DC, 1985, National Academy Press.)*

movement of tissue in opposite directions exceeds recoverable limits. Other examples of tensile strain injuries are femur and rib fractures. Shear strain injuries include hepatic vein laceration from differential movements of hepatic lobes and brain injury from movement of the brain within the skull. Compressive or deformation strain is a factor in contusion injury. This type of injury often leaves the surface of the tissue undamaged (Figure 12-3).

Another factor in strain injury is the loading or strain rate.[41] Tissue response depends on both strain and rate of strain application. Bony injuries can be used to demonstrate this principle. Compact bone will fail at lower strain values if the strain applied is at a rapid rate. The same strain applied more slowly will not cause tissue failure. In general, the viscous tolerance of a tissue is proportional to the product of loading rate and amount of compression. A tissue's tolerance to compression decreases as the rate of loading increases.

Our overall knowledge regarding injury mechanisms for specific organ systems continues to improve. The CIREN has been instrumental in enhancing our knowledge regarding injuries in MVCs.[38] The mission of this program is to improve the prevention, treatment, and rehabilitation of MVC injuries, thereby reducing deaths, disabilities, and human and economic costs. CIREN is sponsored by the National Highway Traffic Safety Administration and uses a multidisciplinary approach to investigate crashes. Information from this program demonstrates that proper seat belt restraint reduces head injury from frontal crashes, but not lateral crashes.[42] Also, belts do not prevent abdominal injuries in lateral crashes, and contact intrusion injuries

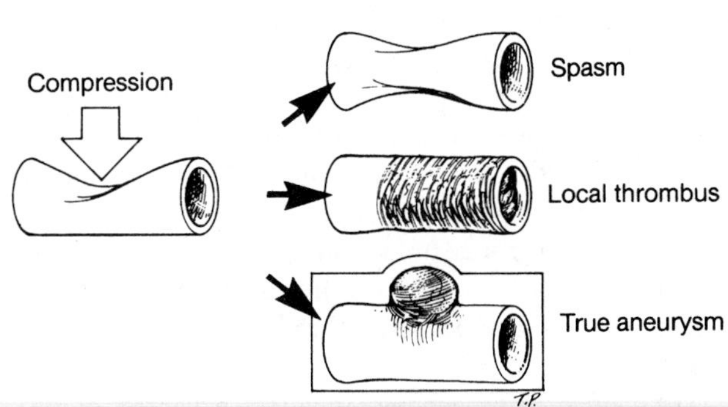

FIGURE 12-3 A crushing force can be applied over an artery, causing damage to the arterial wall. Little or no damage occurs to the overlying skin. The compression produces stretching and shear forces in the arterial wall, which cause injuries similar to those produced by a pure tensile or shear force. *(Modified from Committee on Trauma Research, National Research Council and the Institute of Medicine:* Injury in America, *Washington, DC, 1985, National Academy Press.)*

commonly cause brain, liver, and lung injuries. Many engineering changes in vehicle design can be traced to findings made by CIREN investigations.

Impact biomechanics is an important aspect of injury mechanisms, especially for MVCs. Impact biomechanics has four principal areas of study: (1) understanding the mechanism of injury, (2) establishing levels of human tolerance to impact, (3) soliciting the mechanical response to injury, and (4) designing more human-like test dummies and other surrogates.[43] The following discussion covers trauma caused by blunt, thermal, and penetrating mechanisms and the various organ responses to these forces.

BLUNT INJURY

Blunt trauma is caused by a combination of forces: deceleration, acceleration, shearing, crushing, and compression. Multiple injuries are common. Blunt trauma is often more life-threatening than penetrating trauma because the extent of injuries is less obvious and their diagnosis is difficult.

Results from laboratory, radiographic, and invasive and noninvasive studies, along with physical examination findings, aid in the diagnostic process. Knowledge of tissue properties can help decide what diagnostic studies are needed. Explosion injuries can occur in air-filled organs such as the bowel and lung. The forces are transmitted in all directions; if pressure is not released, tissues will break or burst. Solid organs that have sustained crush injuries may display little external evidence of injury.

Common causes of blunt-force injury include MVCs, falls, aggravated assaults, and contact sports. The automobile is responsible for at least 50% of these nonpenetrating injuries. Direct impact causes the greatest injury and occurs when there is direct contact between the body surface and the injuring agent. Indirect forces are transmitted internally, with dissipation of energy to the internal structures. The extent of injury from indirect forces depends on the transference of energy from an object to the body. Injury occurs as a result of energy released and the tendency for tissue to be displaced on impact.

Acceleration-deceleration forces are a common cause of blunt injury. An example is injury to the thoracic aorta. Rapid deceleration in MVCs can cause major vessels to undergo stretching and bowing. Thoracic deceleration leads to nonphysiologic stretching of localized aortic regions. Shearing is produced when stretching forces exceed the elasticity of vessels. Shearing damage is seen in the vessel walls, causing them to tear, dissect, rupture, or form an aneurysm.[44] The aorta is fixed by the left subclavian artery and the ligamentum arteriosum. Movement of the aorta above and below this fixation point produces a shearing force, causing injury (Figure 12-4). Although aortic injuries are most commonly seen after

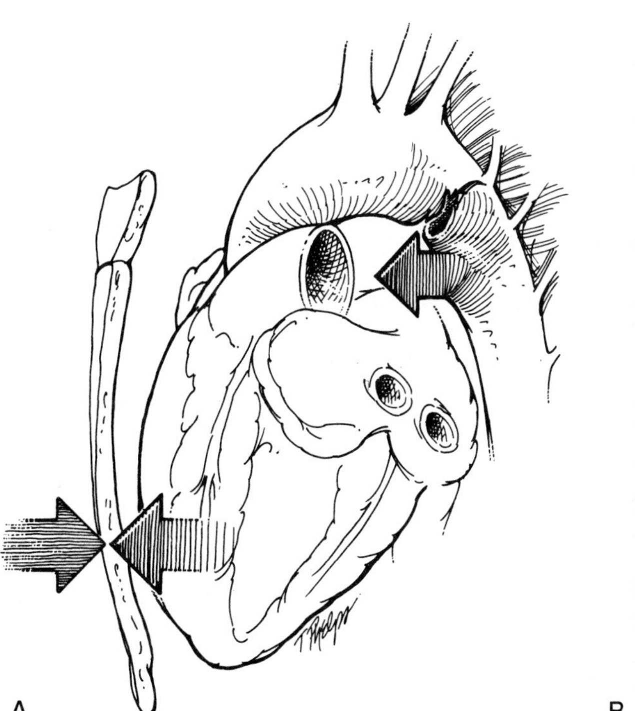

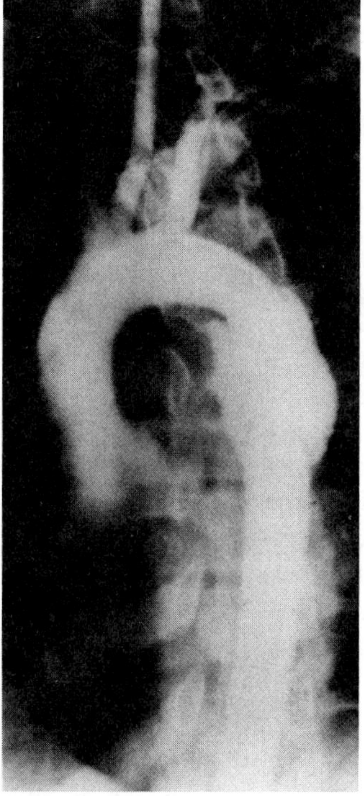

FIGURE 12-4 **A,** As the chest wall decelerates, the heart and aorta are still in motion. The aorta continues to move anteriorly after the chest wall has stopped, causing shear forces to be focused on the aorta at its point of attachment to the posterior chest wall. If the forces exceed tissue strength, an aortic laceration occurs. **B,** The aortogram reveals an aortic injury after a deceleration injury, with the dye column interrupted just beyond the aortic isthmus. Proper management dictates surgical repair as soon as possible.

frontal MVCs, side-impact acceleration-deceleration also occurs, as side-impact collisions are responsible for up to 30% of aortic injuries.[45] The lowest rate of aortic injury in MVCs is associated with use of three-point restraint belts and an air bag.[46] Similar deceleration occurs in falls from heights greater than 12 feet, and in pedestrians struck and thrown significant distance.[44]

Previous attempts to define the patient population at risk for aortic injury have not identified many factors beyond a sudden, violent deceleration. This potential for significant deceleration obtained from the history is key in making the diagnosis of this injury, as the physical examination is often unrevealing. Visible chest wall injury is present in less than 50% of patients with blunt aortic injury. In addition, a normal chest radiograph on hospital admission is not uncommon among patients with a blunt thoracic aortic injury.[47]

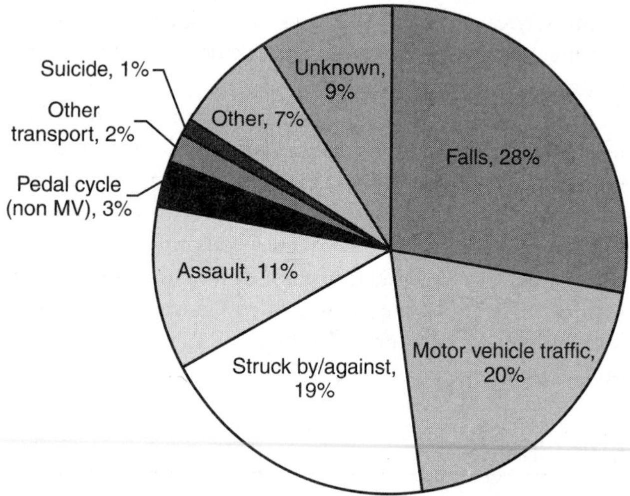

FIGURE 12-5 (Modified from Langlois JA, Rutland-Brown W, Thomas KE: Traumatic brain injury in the United States: emergency department visits, hospitalizations, and deaths. Atlanta, 2004, Centers for Disease Control and Prevention, National Center for Injury Prevention and Control.)

BRAIN INJURIES

The Centers for Disease Control and Prevention (CDC) estimates that at least 5.3 million Americans or about 2% of the U.S. population currently have a long-term or lifelong need for help to perform activities of daily living secondary to an injury to their brain.[48] Traumatic brain injury (TBI) ranges from mild, when there is a brief change in mental status or consciousness, to severe, when the individual has an extended period of unconsciousness or amnesia after the injury. Approximately 75% of TBIs that occur yearly are concussions or a mild form of TBI.[49]

One review suggests approximately 1.4 million people sustain a TBI each year in the United States. A number of outcomes are possible for these patients. It is estimated that 50,000 die, 235,000 require hospitalization, and 1.1 million are treated as outpatients.[50]

Falls are the most common cause of brain injury followed by motor vehicle crashes (Figure 12-5). Primary brain injury is produced by the initial impact. The impact can cause skull fracture, brain contusions, hematomas outside or within the brain, lacerations of the brain as it moves across the inner surfaces of the skull, and diffuse axonal injury, which is felt to be secondary to shear forces applied to the various nerve fibers within the brain. Secondary brain injury can increase the severity of brain injury. It is caused by a number of physiologic vascular and biochemical effects. These events can occur secondary to brain swelling with increased intracranial pressure, hypoxemia, systemic hypotension, electrolyte changes, and a number of other factors.[51] The value of preventing secondary brain injury is suggested by outcome data that show aggressive control of factors known to exacerbate secondary TBI, such as intracranial pressure, in the brain-injured patient lowers mortality.[52] (The reader is referred to Chapter 20 for more extensive information of this topic.)

A confounding problem with brain injuries is their high incidence in the elderly who may be taking anticoagulants. An elevated coagulation profile secondary to warfarin in the head-injured patient will worsen the outcome. Early reversal of anticoagulation with fresh frozen plasma improves outcomes.[53]

SPINAL CORD INJURIES

The soft tissue and bony supports of the spinal cord are insufficient to tolerate violent forces. Spinal injuries are most prevalent in the cervical region where the vertebrae are small, a high degree of flexibility is conferred, and there is less strength in stabilizing structures (i.e., bones, ligaments, muscles). Mechanisms of injury involved with spinal cord damage include penetration, axial loading, flexion, extension, rotation, lateral bending, and distraction [54,55]

Axial loading injury occurs when the force is applied upward or downward to the spinal column with no posterior or lateral bending of the spine. A burst fracture of the vertebral body or disk extrusion results. This type of injury is common in MVCs when a person's head is thrown upward and strikes the roof of the car.

In a flexion injury, the force causes extreme forward movement of the spine. Flexion injury can occur with only a small amount of force. A vertebral body is thrown forward, and the cord is compressed. The wedging force placed on an adjacent vertebra crushes it and drives fragments of bone into the spinal canal. Posterior longitudinal or articular ligaments are torn, displacing the fracture forward into the lower vertebra. Flexion with rotation produces a more severe injury.

In hyperextension injuries the spine is bent back sharply. A downward force causes compression of the vertebral bodies. Fracture of the pedicles or lamina can be seen, depending on the direction and intensity of the force.[54] Posterior dislocation of the upper vertebrae on the lower occurs, further complicating the injury. These injuries can squeeze the spinal cord, supplying the main stress in the center of the cord, resulting in the syndrome of acute central cervical cord injury. In this syndrome, there is greater motor impairment of the upper limbs compared with the lower because the motor nerve fibers supplying the lower limbs are more peripherally situated and suffer less damage.

Hangings are associated with distraction injury to the cervical spine, a separation of the spinal column with cord stretching.[55] The axis pedicle fractures seen in MVCs are often called hangman's fractures but actually have a different mechanism. The hangman's fracture is caused by severe hyperextension and distraction between C1 and C2. The fracture seen in patients after an MVC or fall is caused by extension, axial compression, flexion, and disk disruption. Neurologic involvement is not common. Whiplash injury is another form of cervical spinal column injury that has three components that may cause injury. These include extension, downward loading, and rebound.[56]

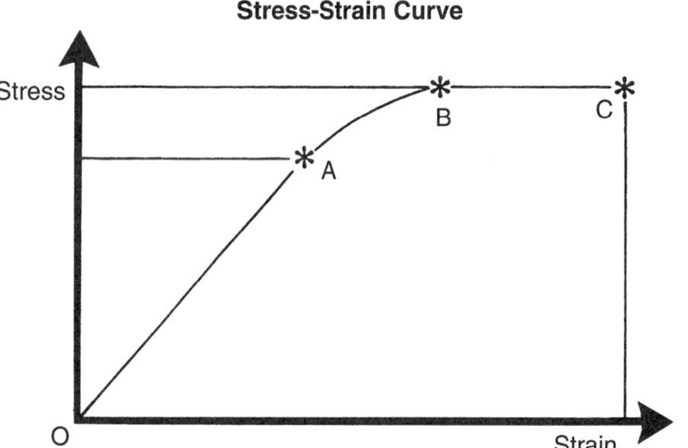

FIGURE 12-6 Stress-strain curve. Strain increases proportionately with stress to point A. From point A to point B, the strain is greater than the stress. Point A is called the *yield point,* or *limit of proportionality,* and point B represents the *ultimate tensile strength.* Point C is the *break point,* or *breaking strain,* of the material. At point C, the material remains permanently deformed and does not recover its original shape.

FRACTURES

Some basic definitions used to describe fracture biomechanics are helpful in understanding possible injuries. Force and strain have already been discussed and defined. Stress is defined as the internal resistance to deformation or the internal force generated from the application of a load.[41]

Stress = Load/Area on which the load acts

Stress cannot be measured directly. It is measured in force per unit area and expressed as pounds per square inch (psi) or kilograms per square centimeter (kg/cm^2). Other terms for force include *pound force, kilogram force,* and *dynes.*

Both extrinsic and intrinsic factors are important determinants of whether a bone will fracture when stress is applied. Extrinsic factors include magnitude, duration, direction, and rate of force application. Intrinsic factors are properties of bone that determine its susceptibility to fracture. These include energy-absorbing capacity, modulus of elasticity (Young's modulus), fatigue, strength, and density.[39] Energy-absorbing capacity is related to the strain characteristics of the bone. Stress-strain curves (Figure 12-6), or Young's modulus, measure elasticity. Fatigue failure occurs when a material is subjected to repeated stresses that are below its breaking point but the cumulative stress results in failure. Bone strength is directly related to its density. As bone density is reduced by osteoporosis, the stress required to fracture the bone decreases.

Fractures can be classified by their mechanism of injury. Fractures caused by direct trauma are tapping, crush, low-velocity penetrating, and high-velocity penetrating. Tapping injuries occur from blows to bony areas (e.g., kicks to the shin, hit with a nightstick). Little energy is absorbed by soft tissue. Crush and high-velocity injuries produce multiple comminuted areas as well as soft tissue damage. Indirect trauma also can produce fractures. Traction injuries usually involve tendons pulling pieces of bone away at their attachments, such as external rotation injuries of the ankle. Angulation fractures are explained by tension and compression stress. As a lever is angulated, the convex surface is under tension stress and the concave surface is under compression stress. The convex surface fails first, giving rise to a transverse fracture. Rotational fractures are rare because it is difficult to apply a true rotation force to a bone. Compression fractures do occur and are explained by vector analysis. If a homogeneous cylinder is loaded axially until it fails, the fracture will appear at an angle of almost 45 degrees (Figure 12-7). Because bones are not homogeneous, most axial loading produces T- or Y-shaped fractures at the lower end of the bone. Combinations of forces usually produce oblique or curved fracture lines.

Fractures in the thoracolumbar spine can present interesting clinical findings.[57] Wedge or compression fractures are the most common fractures in this area of the spine.

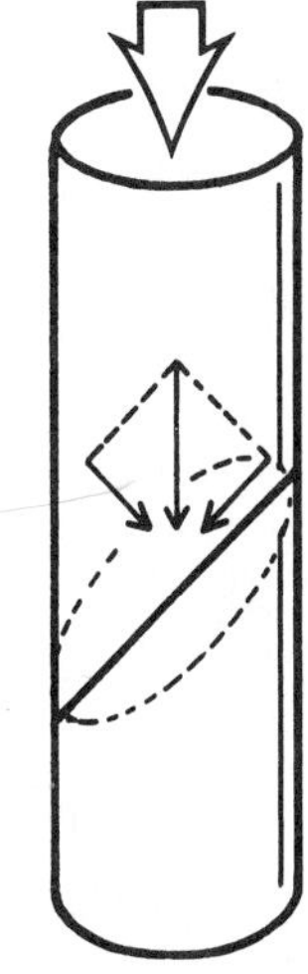

FIGURE 12-7 Vertical forces applied to a homogeneous cylinder will cause the structure to fail at an angle of 45 degrees to the long axis of the cylinder. The forces can be resolved into two forces, with the maximum shear force at 45 degrees to the long axis.

They result from acute flexion forces. The injury can occur after a fall with the feet landing first. An associated injury is a calcaneal fracture. Burst fractures are produced when forces are applied perpendicularly to the spinal column. Spinous process fractures occur from direct force to the flexed spine or a violent muscle pull.

Pelvic fractures can be simple to manage or may be complex and produce life-threatening hemorrhage.[58] Associated injuries to the lower genitourinary tract, rectum, pelvic vasculature, and pelvic nerves all increase the morbidity and mortality of pelvic fractures. Most pelvic fractures have a low mortality, but mortality may approach 50% when there is an open fracture with injury to major vascular structures or bowel. Traction fractures of the ischial tuberosity and anterior iliac spine represent stable simple pelvic injuries.[58]A shear fracture of the ilium is found in the motorcycle rider who is thrown forward and catches the iliac crest on the handlebars. Straddle fractures result from direct trauma to the perineum. Urethral injury is always possible in these patients, especially males. Patients with blood at the penile meatus, perineal or scrotal hematoma, or a nonpalpable prostate gland by rectal examination should not have a Foley catheter placed until a urethral injury is excluded by urethrogram.[59] Anterior-posterior compression fractures with complete disruption of the sacroiliac joints posteriorly have been associated with massive exsanguinating hemorrhage (Figure 12-8). This is related to disruption of arterial and venous structures immediately anterior to the sacroiliac joints.

Acetabular fractures happen when the hip is flexed and abducted during an MVC. The knee hits the dashboard during the forward body acceleration, and the femur is driven through the acetabulum.[60] If the thigh is crossed at impact, a posterior dislocation of the hip is produced.[61] The presence of these injuries should suggest the need for evaluation of the ipsilateral knee. An anterior dislocation of the hip is found when a posterior force is applied to an abducted, externally rotated thigh. Leg deformity in posterior and anterior hip dislocation is diagnostic (Figure 12-9).

Tibial fractures are commonly divided into low- and high-energy fractures.[62] Most indirect fractures are caused by a torsional force and result in little soft tissue damage. Direct fractures occur as a motor vehicle strikes the lower extremity and are usually high-energy fractures. A crushing injury to the leg usually causes bony injury with additional compromise of soft tissue, the vasculature, and even nerves. As many as 30% of patients with tibial injuries will have multiple injuries complicating their fracture management. Other orthopedic injuries commonly associated with tibial shaft fractures include ipsilateral fibula fracture and ligamentous injury of the knee.[62]

Abdominal Injuries

The liver, spleen, and small bowel are the most common organs injured after blunt trauma.[63] The mechanisms of blunt visceral injury include crushing, shearing, and bursting

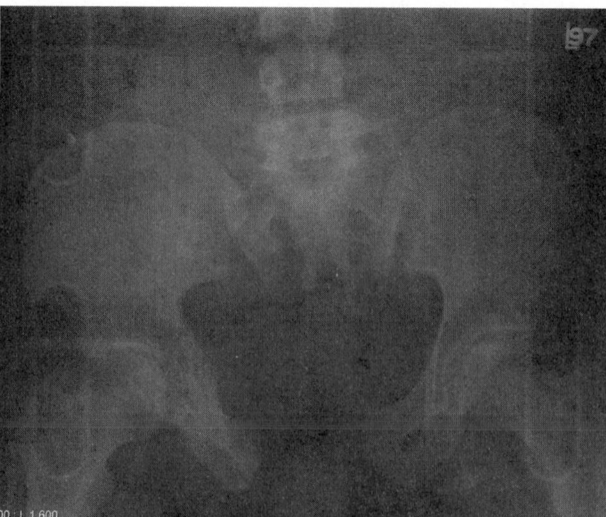

FIGURE 12-8 Pelvic ring is disrupted through bilateral sacroiliac joints posteriorly and symphysis pubis anteriorly. This injury was associated with massive blood loss and profound shock.

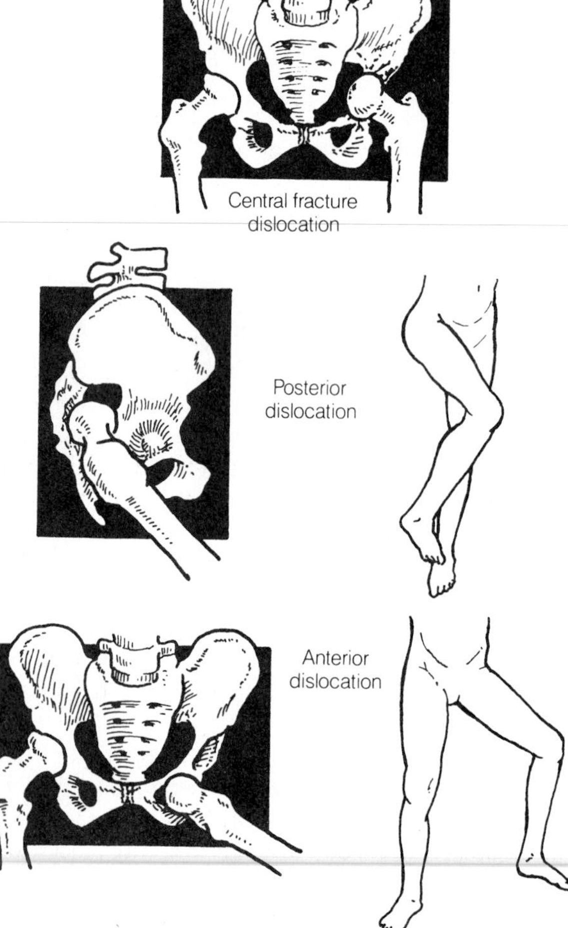

FIGURE 12-9 Three types of hip dislocation. *(From Hughes JL: Initial management of fractures and joint injuries. In Zuidema GD, Ballinger RB, Rutherford RB, editors:* Management of Trauma, *Philadelphia, 1985, WB Saunders.)*

forces.[64] In low-velocity, high-compression injuries, the mechanism is most likely due to organ motion and shearing forces.[65] In high-velocity, low-compression mechanisms, the likely cause is bursting. A crushing injury is represented by a midbody laceration of the pancreas. This can occur when the force is applied anterior to posterior, causing the pancreas to be crushed against the vertebral body. As pancreatic injuries can be relatively asymptomatic, knowledge of the mechanism and appreciation of an abdominal seatbelt bruise are key to early diagnosis.[66]

A shearing injury can result from acceleration-deceleration forces acting on the hepatic small bowel mesentery or renal vessels. In both cases the momentum of the organ mass applies the force to the organ's vascular pedicle, causing injury. The apparent weight of the liver (actual weight, 1.8 kg) during a 36 km/hr impact would be 18 kg; a 72 km/hr impact, 72 kg; and a 108 km/hr impact, 162 kg. It is easy to understand how vessels attaching this organ to its blood supply could be stretched and torn. Impact velocities for hepatic injuries up to 8 m/sec do not produce hepatic injury.[67] Significant hepatic contusion occurs at velocities above 12 m/sec. At 20 m/sec, deep lacerations and transections are produced.[68] Understanding these mechanisms of injury is useful in selecting patients for diagnostic studies.[69]

The intestines are susceptible to a bursting injury if they are compressed in a closed loop formation, resulting in failure of the wall strength. These patients may not be symptomatic on initial examination, and CT scanning helps with diagnosis.[70]

As mentioned, associated factors influence the risk of abdominal injury in an MVC. Patients older than age 75 are more likely to suffer abdominal injury at lower speeds and in the absence of other injuries. The probability of abdominal injury increases significantly at velocities above 20 km/hr and reaches 5.0% at approximately 30 km/hr.[69] However, these abdominal injuries are not usually isolated. In the absence of injury to the head, spine, legs, or chest, intraabdominal injury is unlikely regardless of crash velocity.[68]

Cerebrovascular Injuries

Blunt cerebrovascular injury occurs as a result of a direct blow, hyperflexion, or hyperextension.[71] Hyperflexion may trap the carotid artery between the mandible and the spine, while hyperextension may stretch it over the lateral masses of C3 and C4. The carotid also may be trapped between an improperly worn seatbelt and the spine or suffer a direct blow. All can lead to intimal tears, dissection, and thrombosis.[72] Vertebral artery injuries may be caused by cervical fractures or dislocations.[73]

The incidence of blunt cerebrovascular injuries, both carotid and vertebral, is increasing. This is likely not due to an actual increase in the incidence of the disease but an increase in our awareness and the resultant screening that is performed. Screening for blunt cerebrovascular disease is based on identification of a high-risk group, using mechanistic criteria, physical exam findings, and associated injuries. These include hyperflexion and hyperextension mechanisms, neck hematoma or seatbelt mark, cervical bruit, lateralizing neurologic signs, abnormal Glasgow Coma Scale score without findings on head CT, or associated cervical spine fracture.[72,74] As with aortic injury, screening based on mechanism alone is key. Significant neurologic deficit, including devastating hemispheric stroke, may be the first sign of injury.[73]

Causative Agents in Blunt Trauma

Motor Vehicle Crashes

Automobile crashes cause approximately 45,000 deaths annually.[1] Some factors affecting the risk of occupant injury or death are amount of highway travel, road characteristics, speed, vehicle size, and restraint use.[39] Road characteristics, speed, vehicle size, and restraint use can also affect the mechanism of injury.

Highway design can change the injury pattern. Crashes are reduced by separating opposing streams of traffic, eliminating intersections, removing obstacles from roadsides, using breakaway barriers, and surfacing roads with materials that decrease skidding. Successful examples of these changes include a death rate on interstate highways in 1979 of 1.6 per hundred million vehicle miles (mvm), whereas on rural, two-way roads it was 4.8 per hundred mvm.[39] Fatal collisions occur when roadside objects are struck within 40 feet of the road, emphasizing that road design should include a wide shoulder space free of obstacles.[39]

Speed is also an important determinant of the likelihood and severity of injury. The energy dissipated increases with the square of the change in velocity. Speed limits have recently been increased from 55 to 65 miles per hour (mph). There was a 14% increase in fatalities on rural interstate highways that raised the speed limit by 10 mph.[75]

Vehicle size and design also change injury patterns. Small cars are involved in more crashes per mile and are associated with more deaths and injuries per crash than larger cars. The importance of vehicle mismatch as a cause of injury in passenger vehicles is now recognized and has prompted an increase in registered light truck vehicles and sport utility vehicles (SUVs).[76] The simple approach of making cars larger is not viable, because approximately 40% of occupant deaths occur in single-vehicle crashes. Changing vehicle design, especially interior design, can improve the safety of the occupants. Crash testing is commonly used to evaluate vehicle safety. While improvements in vehicle design have made cars safer, the benefits of crash testing may or may not be valid.[77] Incorporating design changes used in automobile racing would increase the likelihood of escaping a vehicular crash without injury, but many changes would not be accepted by current car users.[78]

Before a collision the occupant is moving at the same speed as the vehicle. During the collision the vehicle and occupant decelerate to a speed of zero, but not necessarily at the same rate. The deceleration forces are transmitted to the body according to the following relationship[79]:

$$\text{Gravity} = \text{mph}^2/30 \times \text{Stopping distance (ft)}$$

Three collisions actually happen. The first is the car impacting another object. The second collision is the occupant's body with the interior of the car. A third collision may occur when internal tissues impact against rigid body structures. An example is the fracture of ribs by the steering wheel from the second collision and lung perforation by the ribs from the third collision (Figure 12-10).

Unrestrained occupants are injured by contact with the steering wheel, instrument panel, or other car interior structures or by ejection. The most significant cause of death is ejection from the vehicle, which is fatal in 27% of cases.[80] Other causes of mortality are impact with front or rear doors (18%), the steering assembly (16%), and the instrument panel (13%).[78]

Restraint systems allow occupants to decelerate with their vehicles rather than more abruptly when thrown against unyielding structures inside or outside the vehicles.[46,80,81] Injuries are reduced by preventing ejection of the occupant during crashes, prolonging deceleration time, and reducing severity of impact by the occupant against the car interior. The interior design of the vehicle can make a difference in injury mechanisms. A stiff armrest is more damaging than a soft armrest for lateral impacts. Stiff armrests produce an injury with an Abbreviated Injury Scale (AIS) score of 4 compared with an AIS of 2 when a soft armrest is in place.[82] Collapsible steering columns and high–impact-resistant windshields can also help decrease injury from the second collision.

Properly worn restraints decrease the number of fatalities and severity of injury.[83] Lap belts decrease the likelihood of ejection but not of impact with the vehicle interior. A three-point shoulder lap belt is the most effective restraint.[80] The harness belt reduces the impact of the second

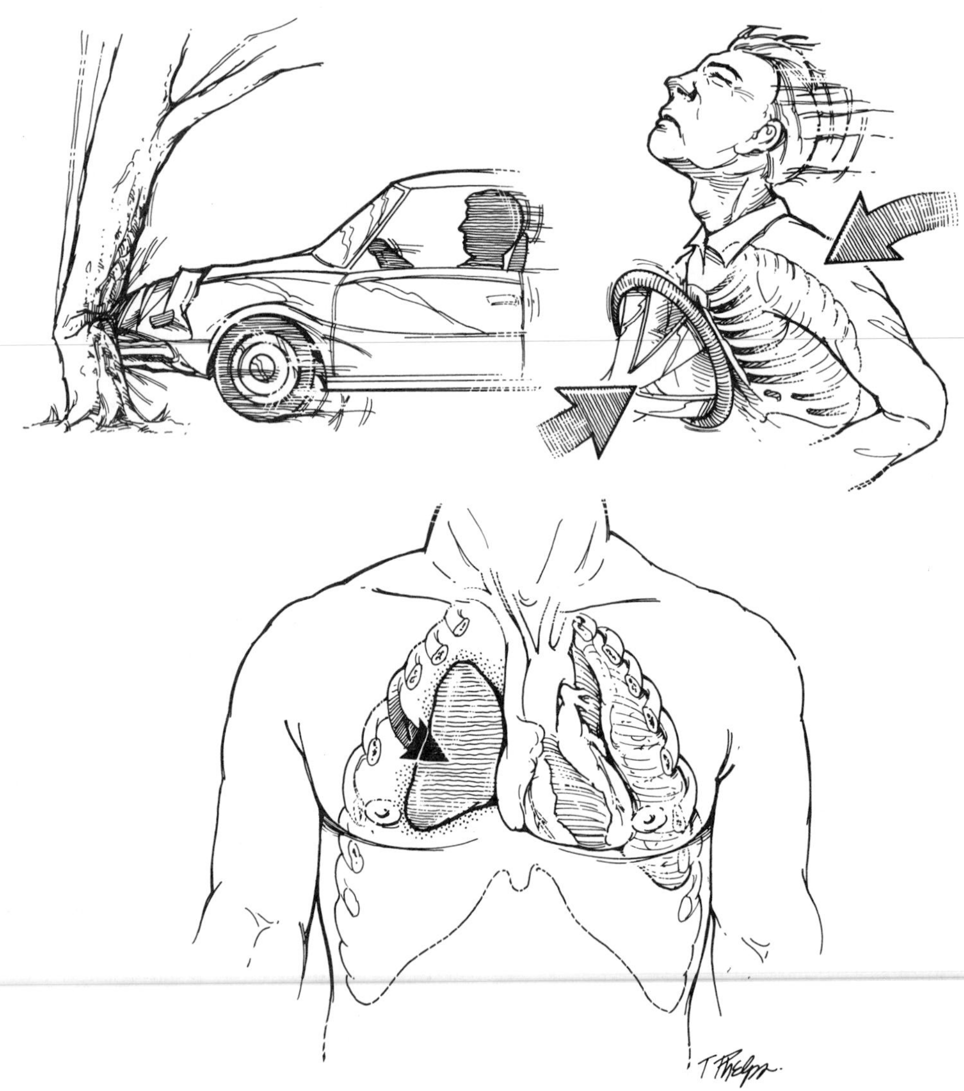

FIGURE 12-10 The three collisions of a head-on motor vehicle crash: the car hits an object, and the occupant's body impacts on some surface within the motor vehicle. The result is collision between internal tissues and the rigid body surface structures.

collision and thus reduces head and facial injuries, intraabdominal solid viscus injuries, and long-bone fractures.[81] One study found that the use of seatbelts would have prevented 40% of deaths and lap belt/shoulder harnesses would have prevented another 13%.[81] However, crash victims who were restrained had an increase in the incidence of abdominal hollow viscus injury.[84] This could be a result of a sudden increase in intraluminal pressure or shearing of relatively fixed ligaments and mesenteric attachments by the deceleration forces against the restraining device. These are the same forces that may cause an intraabdominal aortic injury.[65] Patients with Chance fractures (vertebral body fracture extending through the pedicles of the spinous process, usually in the lumbar region) are commonly rear-seat passengers who are using only a lap belt. This type of restraint use is also found among patients who suffer a hollow viscus injury.[65,84]

Seat belts do reduce injury morbidity and mortality, but they can be misplaced intentionally or unintentionally and actually produce injury. Examples of intentional misuse include placing small children in a harness designed for an adult. Neck, chest, and abdominal injuries have been reported in association with improper use of seat belts.[85,86] Use of seat belts by pregnant women is always a concern. Proper application of a seat belt is associated with a decrease in maternal and fetal injury.[87]

Airbags are an adjunct to seatbelts as a passive restraint system.[46,88] Airbags alone are not effective in reducing injury. They must be used with an active restraint system such as the seatbelt. As with any restraint device, airbags can also cause injury when improperly used. These injuries range from the mild to lethal.[89-91] Most injuries are minor (abrasions and fractures of extremities). In fatal injuries, car occupants have been in unusual positions or improperly restrained when the air bag is activated.

Other motorized vehicles can present different mechanisms of injury. One type of transportation that is of concern is the all-terrain vehicle (ATV), which is essentially a motorcycle.[92] Injuries with an ATV are produced by two mechanisms: The rider strikes an unseen wire or branch or the rider flips the motorcycle while turning or avoiding an obstacle. It is not uncommon for the vehicle to strike the rider after it flips. Younger age is associated with increased injury severity.[93] Few regulations concerning these vehicles are in force, although strong warnings from the manufacturers have been issued in response to consumer action.[94]

Snowmobile injuries cause more than 200 deaths per year in the United States.[95] Most of these injuries appear related to human factors. These include inexperience, use of alcohol, excessive speed, driver recklessness, and poor adherence to manufacturer recommendations. Ejection from these vehicles, resulting in injuries to the head and extremity fractures, is common. Children younger than age 17 account for 12% of the snowmobile injuries. Extremity injuries are the most common site of injury. Head and neck injuries account for 67% of deaths.[96]

Personal watercraft injuries have increased fourfold since 1990.[97,98] Human error is again a common theme. Proper supervision and training is recommended, as well as the use of personal flotation devices when using watercraft. Alcohol use has also been linked to personal watercraft injuries, and safety initiatives have been developed.

Falls: Vertical Deceleration Injuries

Falls are the second leading cause of death as a result of trauma in the United States.[1] In falls the relationship between physical forces of deceleration and biomechanical factors of the organism determines the type and severity of injury. Energy of a body in motion is expressed by kinetic energy *(KE)*, which is a function of the body mass *(m)* and its velocity *(v)* expressed as $KE = mv^2$. Mass, acceleration, and deceleration of the body in addition to the duration and area of application of the force are important when determining extent of injury sustained as the result of a fall.[99] Although the distance of a fall is often used to identify patients likely to have sustained major injury, it correlates poorly with injury severity.[100] Other factors can be related to the energy sustained in a fall.

Duration of force application relates to whether the force is applied slowly or rapidly. The following formula describes the kinematics of vertical deceleration:

$$W = KE \times k/TA$$

Wounding *(W)* is directly related to the kinetic energy of the body modified inversely by the time of deceleration *(T)* and area through which the energy is dissipated *(A)*.[99] The *k* is a constant for a tissue type or an organism. The velocity at impact for a fall of 1 second over a distance of 16 feet is 32.2 ft/sec, or 21.9 mph. If duration is increased to 6 seconds and distance to 580 feet, the velocity at impact is 193.2 ft/sec, or 131.7 mph. The velocity at impact can be used as a measure of the kinetic energy of the body, which is related to the severity of tissue injury.

Tissue elasticity and viscosity must be considered as biomechanical factors of vertical deceleration. Elasticity is the tissue's ability to resist stretching and resume its previous shape. If the tissue remains distorted, it is said to be *plastic.* Viscosity is the tissue's resistance to change in shape when there are changes in motion. The body's ability to withstand deceleration forces is a combination of these two tissue properties.[99]

Tissue disruption at impact is caused by the motion of the tissues. The body's ability to withstand this force increases if there is uniform motion of all tissues. Increasing stopping distance or time of deceleration and enlarging the area of energy dissipation can minimize the injury. These concepts are emphasized in a report of a woman who fell 50 feet and landed at a speed of 37 mph on her back and side, depressing the earth 4 inches. She had no loss of consciousness or signs of injury.[101] The magnitude of injury increases as tissue cohesion is overcome. Forces transmitted at impact include compression, stretching, and shearing, which can occur singly or in combination.

Skeletal injuries, especially of the lower extremities, are common with vertical deceleration. Spinal column fractures are extremely common especially among individuals older than age 15.[102] Torsion injury frequently occurs and results from the force being transmitted to the feet and up the legs to the pelvis and supporting structures of bone, muscle, and cartilage (Figure 12-11).[101]

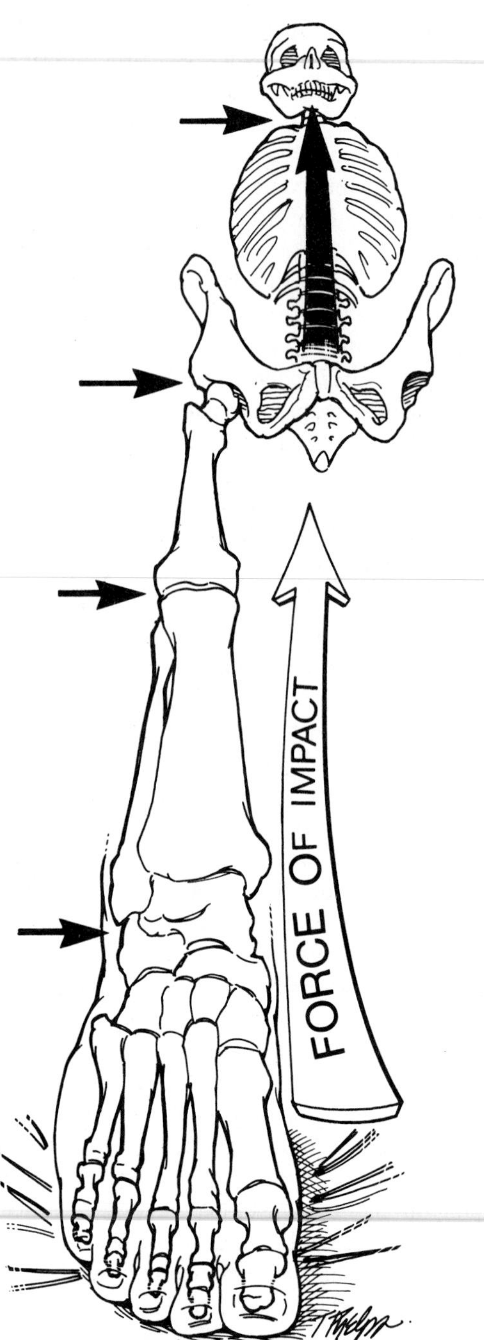

FIGURE 12-11 Forces resulting from a fall are transmitted up to the spine through the long leg bones and pelvis.

PENETRATING TRAUMA

Penetrating trauma refers to injury produced by foreign objects penetrating the tissue. The severity of injury is related to the structures damaged. The mechanism of injury with penetrating trauma is the energy created and dissipated by the object into the surrounding areas.[103] Evaluation of injury is often difficult and dependent on the type and characteristics of the injuring agent, energy dissipation, tissue characteristics, and distance from weapon to target (Figure 12-12).

The extent of injury is proportional to the amount of kinetic energy *(KE)* that is lost by the missile[104]:

$$KE = \text{Mass} \times (V1^2 - V2^2)/2$$

*V*1 is impact velocity, and *V*2 is exit or remaining velocity. It should be noted that doubling the mass only doubles the energy, whereas doubling the velocity quadruples the energy. Rotational energy is also a factor, because most missiles are

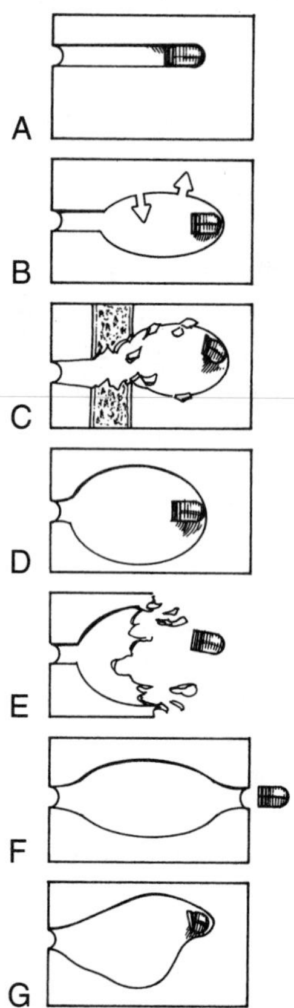

FIGURE 12-12 Patterns of injury in animal tissue secondary to variations in the ballistics of the missile and tissue characteristics. **A,** Low velocity, no cavitation, entrance and exit small. **B,** Higher velocity, formation of cavity, arrows show direction and magnitude of acceleration of tissue. **C,** Velocity as in **B,** but deformation of bullet and creation of secondary missiles after penetrating bone. **D,** Very high velocity, large cavity, and small entrance. Exit may be small. **E,** Very high velocity, thin target, large and ragged exit. **F,** Velocity, caliber, and thickness of tissue such that cavitation occurs deep inside and entrance and exit are small. **G,** Asymmetric cavitation as bullet begins to deform and tumble. *(Modified from Swan KG, Swan RC, editors:* Gunshot Wounds: Pathophysiology and Management, *Littleton, Mass, 1980, PSG Publishing.)*

shot from barrels that are rifled, causing the bullet to spin. Total kinetic energy can be estimated by adding velocity and rotational energy. Velocity at impact depends on three factors: muzzle velocity, distance of weapon from target, and influence of air friction on the missile.

Low-velocity weapons at a range less than 50 yards and high-velocity weapons at less than 100 yards have impact velocities that equal muzzle velocities. To penetrate skin, a missile must have an impact velocity of 150 ft/sec; a velocity of 195 ft/sec is required to break bone. Increase in mass can affect total energy (magnum shells will usually increase energy by 20% to 60%).

The amount of kinetic energy lost by the missile is directly related to the tissue damage. The energy lost by the missile is transferred to the tissue. Factors that increase the amount of kinetic energy transferred effectively increase tissue destruction. As the missile penetrates, a tract is created that temporarily displaces tissue forward and laterally. This tissue acceleration creates a temporary cavity as tissues are stretched and compressed, a process called *cavitation.* Cavitation is directly proportional to the amount of kinetic energy transmitted to the tissue.[104] It commonly occurs with missiles traveling 1000 ft/sec or greater. The size of this cavity may be many times the diameter of the bullet. This phenomenon produces damage to structures outside the direct missile path and is commonly referred to as *blast effect.* The effect that cavitation has on wounding potential was illustrated by a wounding study that attempted to control the size of the temporary cavity.[103] The average tissue destruction was reduced by one third if the cavity size was limited by an external envelope.

The velocity of a missile determines the extent of cavitation and tissue deformation. Low-velocity missiles localize injury to a small radius from the center of the tract and have little disruptive effect. A low-velocity missile travels less than 1000 ft/sec, or 305 m/sec.[104] Low-velocity bullets cause little cavitation and blast effect. They essentially only push the tissue aside.

High-velocity missile injuries are more serious because of the greater amount of energy lost and cavitation produced. High-velocity missiles travel at more than 3000 ft/sec, or 914 m/sec.[105] Damage from high-velocity missiles is dependent on three factors: density and compressibility of tissue injured, missile velocity, and the primary missile's fragmentation.

High-velocity bullets compress and accelerate tissue away from the bullet, causing a cavity around the bullet and its entire tract. The cavity enlarges as the bullet transfers its kinetic energy to the tissue. A negative pressure is created behind the missile, drawing foreign material in to contaminate the wound. The diameter of the cavity might be 30 to 40 times the diameter of the bullet. This area is often devitalized and requires debridement. The cavity collapses and tissue recoils until all energy is dissipated. Tissue cohesiveness and elasticity resist expansion of the cavity. More cohesive and elastic tissues experience less damage. Dense tissue absorbs more kinetic energy, causing greater damage. This retarding factor can be related to tissue specific gravity. The higher the specific gravity, the more energy imparted and the greater the damage[103] (Table 12-1).

In injuries from high-velocity missiles, the exit wound through narrow structures or tissue such as an extremity will be larger than the entrance wound because all energy is not dissipated at the exit point. Cavitation, along with yawing and tumbling, is still occurring. Through dense broad tissue, the exit wound is small because energy is dissipated and cavitation is complete. If bullet fragmentation occurs, there may be no exit wound. The need for debridement can be extensive with high-velocity missile damage. Amputation and mortality rates are high.[105] High-velocity missile injuries to the head are destructive because the cranial vault is fixed and not able to yield to the expanding temporary cavity created by the missile.

After velocity, missile yaw is the second most important factor in tissue destruction. As a bullet's velocity increases, it becomes unstable in flight and may yaw or tumble. *Yawing* is the deviation or deflection of the nose of the bullet from a straight path. The bullet strikes the body at an angle. With greater angles of yaw, the bullet is slowed and more kinetic energy is lost to the tissue. *Tumbling* is the action of forward rotation around the center of mass, a somersault action of the missile that can create massive injury.[106] Yawing and tumbling increase the area of the missile as it hits the target. Impact increases these motions, which increases the amount of energy released by the bullet, producing more damage.

Various types of bullets are made to alter (in most cases, increase) the amount of energy transmitted. A bullet that passes through tissue without deforming transfers little energy and causes less damage than the bullet that slows down or stops in the tissue. One way to increase the energy transferred is to allow the missile to alter shape on impact. Bullets with hollow points mushroom on impact and yield great amounts of kinetic energy. Soft-nosed and flat-nosed bullets have similar effects.[104]

Muzzle blast is another mechanism of injury for penetrating trauma. *Muzzle blast* refers to the cloud of hot gas and burning powder at the muzzle immediately after firing.[103] This is a factor when the gun is in contact with the skin or at close range (within 3 feet). The gas and powder enter the cavity and cause internal explosion by creating a

TABLE 12-1 **Specific Gravity of Tissues**

Tissue	Specific Gravity
Rib	1.11
Skin	1.09
Muscle	1.04 to 1.02
Liver	1.02 to 1.01
Fat	0.8
Lung	0.5 to 0.4

burn. Cavitation is caused by combustion of powder and the forceful expansion of gases. This is common with a shotgun wound but is not seen with handguns because the amount of gas released is less and the wound is too small for it to enter. As the gas is trapped between skin and bone, a stellate tear results from the ballooning of skin out from the bone. This injury does not occur if subcutaneous tissue is present, because of tissue cohesiveness and elasticity.

Shotgun Injuries

Shotguns are short-range, low-velocity weapons that use multiple lead pellets encased in a larger shell for ammunition. Each pellet is considered a missile; there can be 9 to 200 small pellets, depending on the size of pellet and gauge of the gun.[107] A brief description of the mechanism of shotgun injuries, including the weapon, ammunition, and ballistics, is important in understanding the clinical findings in patients sustaining wounds from these weapons. Gauge designates the bore of the gun. Common gauges include 10, 12, 16, 20, 28, and .410.

The shotgun shell is made up of the primer, powder, wad, and shot, in that order. Shotgun powder is fast burning and creates a low chamber pressure. Common shot sizes range from size 2 through 9 and have a respective pellet diameter of 0.15 to 0.08 inches. Ninety no. 2 shot pellets equal 585 no. 9 shot pellets in weight. Larger shot sizes include buckshot and BBs. Buckshot sizes are designated as 4, 3, 2, 1, 0, and 00. Each 00 buckshot is 0.328 inches in diameter. There are also single projectiles, called "slugs" or "pumpkin balls."[108] The plastic or paper wad separates the pellets from the gunpowder. This wad of unsterile material increases the potential of infection in a shotgun wound. The wad is expelled with the pellets but loses momentum and drops about 6 feet from the barrel. The pellets leave the barrel close together and separate as they move away from the barrel.

Wounding capacity is the function of mass and projectile velocity. Considering only ballistics, the shotgun is inferior to a single-projectile, high-velocity rifle such as the M-16. The average muzzle velocity of a shotgun is between 1100 and 1350 ft/sec. Rifle slugs have a muzzle velocity approaching 1850 ft/sec. The M-16, with a bullet weighing 55 g, has a muzzle velocity of 3200 ft/sec. The kinetic energy of the M-16 at the muzzle is 1248 foot-pounds (ft-lb). A no. 6 shotgun pellet, 0.11 inches in diameter, has striking forces of 7.21 ft-lb per pellet at the muzzle and 3.88 ft-lb per pellet at 20 yards. A 12-gauge shotgun with 225 to 428 pellets in the load theoretically has 1694 ft-lb at the muzzle. Therefore, at point-blank or very close range, a shotgun injury has the potential for creating extensive tissue damage, similar to a high-velocity missile injury.

The shot pattern is of clinical importance. The major factor affecting the nature of the shotgun wound is the range from the target at which the gun is discharged. Most significant wounds occur in a range up to 15 yards. At less than 6 feet a tight, dense pattern is produced with extensive damage from the muzzle blast and mass of pellets. At 3 to 6 feet, the single entrance wound is 1.5 to 2 inches in diameter with scalloping at the edges.[109] There is extensive contamination from shotgun wadding, clothing, skin, hair, and powder entering the wound. At greater distances, a pellet does less damage because of the loss of velocity and energy.

If a 12-gauge shotgun loaded with no. 6 shot (275 pellets) were fired accurately at a distance of 40 yards into the center of a 6-foot, 160-pound person, approximately 200 of the pellets would strike within a 30-inch diameter. This would be between the mid-thigh and the shoulders, across the trunk, and extending approximately 9 inches on either side. If the shot were absolutely evenly distributed, there would be approximately 2 inches between each pellet. At a range of 10 yards, this wound would be only 7 inches in diameter. Type 1 is a penetrating wound at a range of more than 7 yards. Type 2 is a perforating wound at a range of 3 to 7 yards. Type 3 is a massive point-blank wound inflicted at a range of less than 3 yards.[110]

Low-Velocity Penetrating Wounds

Other types of penetrating wounds, such as stab wounds and impalements, are low-velocity wounds. These wounds are usually obvious, yet the patient must be undressed and inspected for entrance and exit wounds. If the offending agent remains in place, its trajectory can be traced and underlying trauma predicted. If removed, the gender of the assailant can be helpful in estimating the trajectory: males tend to stab with an upward thrust and females with a downward thrust. This assessment should not be considered absolute, because intentional injuries often follow no pattern.

Stab wounds are low velocity and therefore low energy; the injuries produced depend on the location of penetration. Little damage occurs to tissue except in the locale of the injury. It must be remembered that multiple body cavities can be penetrated by a single wound. In particular, the thoracic and abdominal cavities can be injured by a wound whose entrance is located over one or the other cavity. Lower chest wounds, from the nipples to the costochondral margin, are frequently found to injure abdominal contents because the diaphragmatic excursion extends superiorly up to the nipple line or fifth intercostal space during exhalation (Figure 12-13).

Impalement injuries usually result from a forceful collision between the object and patient during MVCs or falls or from falling objects. The spectacular nature of these injuries should not preclude proper management. The impaled object should be left in place until definite surgical therapy is available.[111] Removal of these foreign bodies can remove the vascular control, causing exsanguinating hemorrhage. Another concern with these injuries is bacterial and foreign-body contamination. Care should be taken to remove all foreign material from these wounds; occasionally, extensive wound debridement is required.

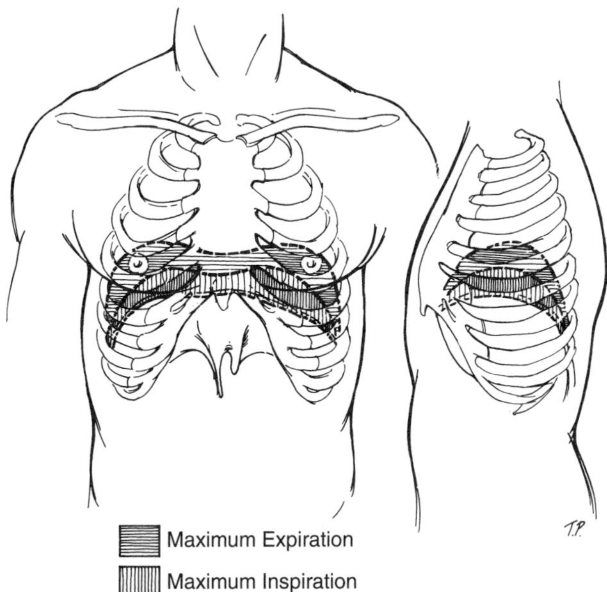

FIGURE 12-13 Diaphragmatic excursion during inspiration and expiration and its possible effect on penetrating injuries to the lower chest and upper abdomen.

Smoke Inhalation and Pulmonary Burns

Inhalation injuries occur when the respiratory tract is exposed to the products of combustion. The type and severity of injury are determined by the type of gases inhaled, their concentration, and the duration of exposure. Thermal injury to the respiratory tree is uncommon because the heat-exchanging efficiency of the respiratory tract is so high that even superheated air is cooled before it gets below the larynx.[112] Steam inhalation can produce thermal injury of the lower respiratory tract because steam has 4000 times the heat capacity of air. The presence of these injuries should be suspected if certain circumstances are present: (1) fire in a closed space, (2) unconsciousness or inebriation associated with smoke exposure, (3) fires involving plastics, (4) presence of carbonaceous sputum, and (5) steam explosions.[113]

The most immediate concern in a patient exposed to a fire is carbon monoxide (CO) intoxication. This is the most frequent immediate cause of death. Carbon monoxide has an affinity for hemoglobin 210 times that of oxygen.[114] The signs and symptoms of CO intoxication are related to blood carboxyhemoglobin (COHb) concentration (Table 12-2).

Inhalation of toxic constituents of smoke may damage alveolar epithelium and capillary endothelium. This results in increased permeability of the alveolar-capillary membrane, which can produce noncardiac pulmonary edema and hypoxemia.[113] These toxic products also reduce bacterial clearance and mucociliary transport. Combustion of many common construction materials produces a large number of toxic byproducts capable of this type of injury (Table 12-3).

TABLE 12-2 **Signs and Symptoms Caused by Various Concentrations of Carboxyhemoglobin**

Blood Saturation (% COHb)	Signs and Symptoms
0.3 to 10	None
10 to 20	Tightness across forehead, headache
20 to 30	Throbbing headache, abnormal fine manual dexterity
30 to 50	Severe headache, syncope, nausea and vomiting
60 to 70	Coma, convulsions, death

Explosive Blasts

Explosive blasts are a result of detonated explosives being converted to large volumes of gases.[115] The pressure created ruptures the casing, and resultant fragments become high-velocity projectiles. The blast shock wave created by the remaining energy has three components: positive phase, negative phase, and mass movement of air. The blast shock wave's velocity is as high as 3000 m/sec (10,000 ft/sec), which decreases to the speed of sound within a variable distance.[115] This is dependent on the composition and amount of explosive used. The positive-pressure phase is the maximum pressure reached by the blast wave and is greatest next to the immediate explosion. Pressure falls as the wave moves away from the explosion source. The negative-pressure phase follows immediately and lasts 10 times as long. An equal volume of air is displaced along with the expanding gas and travels behind the blast wave. The mass movement of air can actually cause disruption of tissue, traumatic amputation, and evisceration.[115]

Blast injuries in water are more severe than in air because the blast wave travels farther and more rapidly in water as a result of its greater density. Explosions in closed areas are more damaging than those in open spaces because of the toxic gases and smoke that are inhaled. Posttraumatic pulmonary

TABLE 12-3 **Common Toxic Products of Combustion**

Substance	Toxic Products of Combustion
Polyvinyl chloride	Hydrogen chloride, phosgene, chloride
Wood, cotton, paper	Acrolein, acetaldehyde, acetic acid, formaldehyde, formic acid
Petroleum products	Acrolein, acetic acid, formic acid
Nitrocellulose	Oxides of nitrogen, acetic acid, formic acid
Polyurethane	Isocyanate, hydrogen cyanide
Polyfluorocarbons (Teflon)	Octafluoroisobutylene
Melamine resins	Ammonia, hydrogen cyanide

insufficiency results and is reflected in blood gases with low Pao_2 and increased $Paco_2$.[116]

Damage occurs most often at tissue-air interfaces. Damage in the lung is in the alveolar wall, with resultant hemorrhage and edema. The abdominal organs will show damage to the visceral wall, and the trauma may cause perforation.[115] These types of injuries are rare if the explosion occurs in the open and the victim is not close to the detonation point. In a study by Guy and colleagues, animals exposed to a thoracic blast of 100 psi demonstrated transient apnea, bradycardia, and hypotension.[117] The same blast applied to the abdomen produced no acute changes in cardiopulmonary parameters. The ear is the most sensitive organ to explosions; eardrums will rupture at about 7 psi.[115,117] Burns also can be seen if a fireball effect is present. Penetrating injuries can occur if projectiles are released.

TERRORISM

It has been suggested that terrorism is a medical issue.[118] Conventional weapons, such as bombs, produce blast injury, burns, smoke inhalation, as well as blunt and penetrating injuries. Over a 20-year period (1983 to 2002), 36,110 bombing incidents have been recorded.[119] These caused nearly 6,000 injuries and 699 deaths. Government installations were a common target. Bombs remain a common form of terrorism that must be considered in any disaster preparedness plan. A planned response is essential for optimal outcomes.[120,121] The threat of nuclear, biologic, and chemical (NBC) weapons also cannot be ignored.[122,123] Acute radiation syndrome can be divided into the hematopoietic, gastrointestinal, cerebrovascular, and cutaneous syndromes. Dose values that predict each syndrome are known, as well as fatal exposure levels. The latter would be important in a triage approach to a major radiation disaster.[124] Chemical emergencies can be a result of terrorism or from unintentional exposures, especially from an industrial source. Major chemical exposures are classified into asphyxiants, cholinesterase inhibitors, respiratory tract irritants, and vesicants.[125] Symptoms are used to distinguish the various types. These agents will often allow large numbers of people to be exposed and to survive to reach medical care. This can overwhelm resources. Most patients have minimal symptoms and require little medical intervention except to provide psychologic support in the aftermath.

Any NBC agent can be used as an instrument of mass destruction, and they represent new challenges to our medical system.[126] These challenges include identifying the causative agent as a first step, understanding the mechanisms of injury, and developing systems to deal with the effects. In some cases our medical capabilities will be limited to control attempts because no treatment is known (e.g., Ebola virus). In others, early recognition and administration of treatments can be life saving (e.g., Sarin gas). Responses to chemical and biologic agents are different (Table 12-4).

TABLE 12-4 Differences in Chemical and Biologic Agents That Could Be Used for Terrorism

	Chemical	Biologic
Onset	Rapid, minutes to hours	Delayed, days to weeks
Patient Location	Downwind from release point	Widely spread through geographic region
First Responder	Paramedics, police, firefighters	ED nurses and physicians, ID physicians
Decontamination	Critical	Not necessary
Treatment	Chemical antidotes	Vaccines, antibiotics
Patient Isolation	None after decontamination	Absolute with communicable diseases

ED, Emergency department; *ID,* infectious disease.
Modified from Henderson DA: The looming threat of bioterrorism, *Science* 283:1279-1282, 1999. Reprinted with permission from AAAS.

Biologic weapons are especially frightening. The number of agents that can be used is large and some are especially frightening.[127] Most agents appear easy to obtain, easy to apply, and difficult to detect early enough to intervene successfully if at all. Smallpox is a viral agent that has drawn much attention because of its ability to be disseminated easily and the high attack and mortality rate. The recent anthrax outbreak in the United States is an example of what a biologic agent is capable of doing.[128]

INJURY SCORING

An objective system for measuring severity of injury is helpful in triaging patients, allocating and evaluating medical resources, assessing quality of medical care, conducting institutional auditing, and evaluating morbidity and mortality.[129] These systems help stratify patients with similar mechanisms into severity categories, which can enhance the value of comparative studies. A number of severity indices are available; however, each has its problems and limitations.

A commonly used system is the Injury Severity Score (ISS), which was developed by Baker and associates.[129] This system uses an AIS and is best applied to patients with blunt injuries. The AIS was first published in 1971 as a single comprehensive scale for injuries related to MVCs. The most recent edition is the AIS-90.[130] The system divides the body into seven regions and uses a severity code for each injury. One is a minor injury and six is a fatal injury. Mortality increases with the AIS grade, and the increase is not linear but quadratic. The top three AIS scores correlate with an increased risk of death. To calculate the ISS, the AIS scores from the three most severely injured body regions are used to define a number score that relates to severity of injury. Because the association of the AIS score to mortality is quadratic, the ISS is defined as the sum of the squares of the highest AIS grade in each of the three most severely injured areas. A problem with the ISS is that it is a retrospective tool. This score can only be calculated once all injuries are known. Additionally, the mix of injuries can affect mortality calculations, which is a recognized weakness of ISS.[131]

While the ISS has held much weight in injury scoring, its value has been challenged in a number of different ways. There is a concern that physiologic data should be incorporated into severity scoring.[132,133] In some reports the physiologic score is championed over an anatomic score.[134] The Trauma and Injury Severity Score (TRISS) method is based on regression equations, which consider patient age, severity of anatomic injury (ISS), and physiologic status of the patient (TS). TRISS also can be used to compare populations of trauma patients while controlling for severity mix. A weakness of TRISS is an underestimation of the outcome of patients with multiple injuries in one anatomic area.[135]

This problem is answered with a number of systems, including the New Injury Severity Score (NISS), A Severity Characterization of Trauma (ASCOT), and ICD-9-Based Illness Severity Score (ICISS).[135-137] ASCOT was developed to improve on TRISS. ASCOT works for penetrating and blunt mechanisms, as well as with different age groups. The ICISS emerged as another prediction tool.[138]

The ICISS was developed to predict survival, length of stay, and hospital charges. It has subsequently been compared with TRISS and found to be superior in predictive power.[139] It is clear that the perfect scoring system is still elusive. It is probably more important to identify the need for severity scoring and use the tool that best fits the stated need. One must remember that all were developed and use administrative databases, which can lead to inaccuracies in their ability to predict outcome.[140]

The most recent development related to injury scoring and outcome measurement after any mechanism of injury is to measure quality of life and functional outcome.[141,142] The Short Form 36 (SF36) and Quality of Well-Being Scale are commonly used.[143-145] Functional outcomes have been especially useful to assess recovery from injury mechanisms that produce orthopedic injuries.[146,147] Their application outside of orthopedic injuries is proving to be useful.[148,149]

SUMMARY

With injury as our fourth leading cause of death and one of the United States' most expensive health problems, a thorough understanding of the circumstances that result in injury is necessary for all health care personnel. Mechanism of injury helps to identify the type, extent, and pattern of injury and even relates to potential complications and outcome. Mechanism of injury affords the practitioner an opportunity to suspect certain injuries in addition to the obvious ones, thereby improving delivery of patient care. Prevention of injury is also aided by knowing the mechanism of injury. Active involvement of the trauma practitioner in organizations and programs aimed at injury prevention should be sought so their firsthand knowledge can be used to educate the public in injury prevention. This knowledge must be used if successful programs are to be developed that will prevent injury and improve on the currently dismal statistics of injury in the United States.

REFERENCES

1. *CDC Activity Report 2001.* Available online at http://www.cdc.gov/ncipc/pub- res/unintentional activity. Accessed February 2007, from Centers for Disease Control and Prevention.
2. *WISQARS Injury Mortality Report.* Available online at http://webappa.cdc.gov. Accessed February 2007.
3. National Center for Injury Prevention and Control: *Years of Potential Life Lost Report.* Available online at http://webappa.cdc.gov/cgi-bin/broker.exe. Accessed February 2007.
4. *Estimating the Costs of Unintentional Injuries, 2005.* Available online at http://www.nsc.org/lrs/statinfo/estcost.htm. Accessed February 2007
5. Kuhne CA, Ruchholtz S, Kaiser GM et al: Mortality in severely injured elderly trauma patients—when does age become a risk factor? *World J Surg* 29(11):1476-1482, 2005.
6. Morris JA Jr, MacKenzie EJ, Edelstein SL: The effect of preexisting conditions on mortality in trauma patients, *JAMA* 263(14):1942-1948, 1990.
7. Brasel KJ, Guse CE, Layde P et al: Rib fractures: relationship with pneumonia and mortality, *Crit Care Med* 34(6):1642-1646, 2006.
8. Bulger EM, Arneson MA, Mock CN et al: Rib fractures in the elderly, *J Trauma* 48(6):1040-1046, 2000.
9. Sisley A, Jacobs LM, Poole G et al: Violence in America: a public health crisis—domestic violence, *J Trauma* 46(6):1105-1113, 1999.
10. Helling TS, Watkins M, Evans LL et al: Low falls: an underappreciated mechanism of injury, *J Trauma* 46(3):453-456, 1999.
11. Schwartz SW, Rosenberg DM, Wang CP et al: Demographic difference in injuries among the elderly: an analysis of emergency department visits, *J Trauma* 58(2):347-352, 2005.
12. Mitchell RA, Hasbrouck L, Ingram ME et al: Public health and aging: Nonfatal physical assault-related injuries among persons aged >60 years treated in hospital emergency departments, US 2001, *MMWR* 52(34):812-816, 2003.
13. Krug EG, Dahlberg LL, Mercy JA et al: *World Report on Violence and Health.* Geneva, Switzerland, 2002, WHO.
14. Tjaden P, Thoennes N: *Extent, Nature, and Consequences of Intimate Partner Violence: Findings from the National Violence Against Women Survey.* Washington (DC): Department of Justice (US); 2000a. Publication No. NCJ 181867. Available online at www.ojp.usdoj.gov/nij/pubs-sum/181867.htm. Accessed February 2007.
15. Weinsheimer RL, Schermer CR, Malcoe LH et al: Severe intimate partner violence and alcohol use among female trauma patients, *J Trauma* 58(1):22-29, 2005.
16. Cinat ME, Wilson SE, Lush S et al: Significant correlation of trauma epidemiology with the economic conditions of a community, *Arch Surg* 139(12):1350-1355, 2004.
17. *Intimate Partner Violence: Fact Sheet.* Available online at http://www.cdc.gov/ncipc/factsheets/ipvfacts.htm. Accessed

February 2007 from National Center for Injury Prevention and Control.
18. Moore EE: Alcohol and trauma: the perfect storm, *J Trauma* 59(3):S53-S56, 2003.
19. Maier RV: Controlling alcohol problems among hospitalized trauma patients, *J Trauma* 59 (3):S1-S2, 2005.
20. Hungerford DW: Interventions in trauma centers for substance use disorders: new insights on an old malady, *J Trauma* 59(3):S10-S17, 2005.
21. Gentilello LM, Ebel BE, Wickizer TM et al: Alcohol interventions for trauma patients treated in emergency department and hospitals: a cost benefit analysis, *Ann Surg* 241(4):541-550, 2005.
22. Schermer CR, Moyers TB, Miller WR et al: Trauma center brief interventions for alcohol disorders decrease subsequent driving under the influence arrests, *J Trauma* 60(1):29-34, 2006.
23. American College of Surgeon's Committee on Trauma: *Resources for Optimal Care of the Injured Patient.* Chicago, 2006, American College of Surgeons.
24. Peek-Asa C, Zwerling C, Stallones L: Acute traumatic injuries in rural populations, *Am J Public Health* 94(10):1689-1693, 2004.
25. Nordstrom DL, Zwerling C, Stromquist AM et al: Epidemiology of unintentional adult injury in a rural population, *J Trauma* 51(4):758-766, 2001.
26. May M: Initial assessment. In Nwariaku F, Thal E (editors): *Parkland Trauma Handbook,* London, 1999, Mosby.
27. Augenstein J, Perdeck E, Stratton J, et al. Characteristics of crashes that increase the risk of serious injuries, *Annu Proc Assoc Adv Automot Med* 47:561-576, 2003.
28. Feliciano DV: Patterns of injury. In Feliciano DV, Moore EE, Mattox KL (editors): *Trauma,* ed 4, Stamford, CT, 1999, Appleton & Lange.
29. American College of Surgeon's Committee on Trauma. Initial assessment. In *Advanced Trauma Life Support Course Manual,* Chicago, 2004, American College of Surgeons.
30. Franklyn M, Fitzharris M, Fildes B et al: A preliminary analysis of aortic injuries in lateral impacts, *Traffic Inj Prev* 4(3):263-269, 2003.
31. Gongora E, Acost JA, Wang DS et al: Analysis of motor vehicle ejection victims admitted to a level I trauma center, *J Trauma* 51(5):854-859, 2001.
32. Rewers A, Hedegaard H, Lezotte D et al: Childhood femur fractures, associated injuries, and sociodemographic risk factors: a population-based study, *Pediatrics* 115(5):543-552, 2005.
33. Demetriades D, Murray J, Martin M et al: Pedestrians injured by automobiles: relationship of age to injury type and severity, *J Am Coll Surg* 199(3):382-387, 2004.
34. Brown CVR, Antevil JL, Sise MJ et al: Spiral computed tomography for the diagnosis of cervical, thoracic, and lumbar spine fractures: its time has come, *J Trauma* 58(5):890-896, 2005.
35. Houshian S, Larson MS, Holm C: Missed injuries in a level I trauma center, *J Trauma* 52(4):715-719, 2002.
36. Hoff WS, Sicontris CP, Lee SY, et al: Formalized radiology rounds: the final component of the tertiary survey, *J Trauma* 56(2):291-295, 2004.
37. Bonnie RJ, Fulco CE, Liverman CT: Prevention research. In Bonnie RJ, Fulco CE, Liverman CT, editors: *Reducing the Burden of Injury,* Washington, DC, 1999, National Academy Press.
38. Crash Injury Resource and Engineering Network. Available online at http://www-nrd.nhtsa.dot.gov/departments/nrd-50/ciren/CIREN.html. Accessed February 2007.
39. Foege WH, Baker SP, Davis JH et al: Injury biomechanics research and the prevention of impact injury. In Grossblatt N, editor: *Injury in America,* Washington, DC, 1985, National Academy Press.
40. Hyde AS: How we break and tear the stuff we are made of. In *Crash Injuries: How and Why They Happen,* Key Biscayne, Fla, 1992, HAI.
41. Hipp JA, Hayes WC: Biomechanics of fractures. In Browner BD, Jupiter JB, Levine AM, Trafton PG, editors: *Skeletal Trauma, Basic Science, Management, Reconstruction,* Philadelphia, 2003, Elsevier Science.
42. Siegel JH, Mason-Gonzalez S, Dischinger P et al: Safety belt restraints and compartment intrusions in frontal and lateral motor vehicle crashes: mechanisms of injuries, complications and acute care costs, *J Trauma* 5(34):736-759, 1993.
43. King AI, Yang KH: Research in biomechanics of occupant protection, *J Trauma* 38(4):570-576, 1995.
44. Swan KG Jr, Swan BC, Swan KG: Decelerational thoracic injury, *J Trauma* 51(5):970-974, 2001.
45. Nagy K, Fabian T, Rodman G et al: Guidelines for the diagnosis and management of blunt aortic injury: an EAST practice management guidelines work group, *J Trauma* 48(6):1128-1143, 2000.
46. Brasel KJ, Quickel R, Yoganandan N et al: Seat belts are more effective than airbags in reducing thoracic aortic injury in frontal motor vehicle crashes, *J Trauma* 53(2):309-313, 2002.
47. Cook AD, Klein JS, Rogers FB et al: Chest radiographs of limited utility in the diagnosis of blunt traumatic aortic laceration, *J Trauma* 50(5):843-847, 2001.
48. National Center for Injury Prevention and Control. *Overview.* Available online at http://www.cdc.gov/ncipc/tbi/Overview.htm. Accessed February 2007.
49. Centers for Disease Control and Prevention (CDC), National Center for Injury Prevention and Control. *Report to Congress on Mild Traumatic Brain Injury in the United States: Steps to Prevent a Serious Public Health Problem,* Atlanta, Ga, Centers for Disease Control and Prevention, 2003.
50. Langlois JA, Rutland-Brown W, Thomas KE: *Traumatic Brain Injury in the United States: Emergency Department Visits, Hospitalizations, and Deaths,* Atlanta, Ga, Centers for Disease Control and Prevention, National Center for Injury Prevention and Control, 2004.
51. Vincent JL, Berre J: Primer on medical management of severe brain injury, *Crit Care Med* 33(6):1392-1399, 2005.
52. Bulger EM, Nathens AB, Rivara FP et al: Management of severe head injury: institutional variations in care and effect on outcome, *Crit Care Med* 30(8):1870-1876, 2002.
53. Ivascu FA, Howells GA, Junn FS, et al: Rapid warfarin reversal in anticoagulated patients with traumatic intracranial hemorrhage reduces hemorrhage progression and mortality, *J Trauma* 59(5):1131-1139, 2005.
54. Viano DC: Causes and control of spinal cord injury in automotive crashes, *World J Surg* 16(3):410-419, 1992.
55. Hecht AC, Silcox III DH, Whitesides Jr TE: Injuries of the cervicocranium. In Browner BD, Jupiter JB, Levine AM et al, editors: *Skeletal Trauma, Basic Science, Management, Reconstruction,* Philadelphia, 2003, Elsevier Science.

56. Viano DC, Olsen S: The effectiveness of active head restraint in preventing whiplash, *J Trauma* 51(5):959-969, 2001.
57. Prevost MA, McGuire RA, Garfin SR et al: Thoracic and upper lumber spine injuries. In Browner BD, Jupiter JB, Levine AM et al, editors: *Skeletal Trauma, Basic Science, Management, Reconstruction*, Philadelphia, 2003, Elsevier Science.
58. Starr AJ, Malekzadeh AS: Fractures of the pelvic ring. In Bucholz RW, Heckman JD, Court-Brown CM, editors: *Rockwood and Green's Fractures in Adults,* ed 6, Philadelphia, 2006, Lippincott Williams and Williams.
59. Durkin A, Sagi HC, Durham R et al: Contemporary management of pelvic fractures, *Am J Surg* 192(2):211-223, 2006.
60. Reilly MC: Fractures of the acetabulum. In Bucholz RW, Heckman JD, Court-Brown CM, editors: *Rockwood and Green's Fractures in Adults,* ed 6, Philadelphia, 2006, Lippincott Williams and Wilkins.
61. Dakin GJ, Eberhardt AW, Alonso JE et al: Acetabular fracture patterns: associations with motor vehicle crash information, *J Trauma* 47(6):1063-1071, 1999.
62. Trafton PG: Tibia shaft fractures. In Bucholz RW, Heckman JD, Court-Brown CM, editors: *Rockwood and Green's Fractures in Adults,* ed 6, Philadelphia, 2006, Lippincott Williams and Wilkins.
63. Fabian TC, Croce MA: Abdominal trauma. In Mattox KL, Feliciano DV, Moore EE, editors, *Trauma,* ed 4, New York, 1999, McGraw Hill.
64. Miller MA: The biomechanics of lower abdominal steering-wheel loading, *J Trauma* 31(9):1301-1309, 1991.
65. Diebel LN: Stomach and small bowel. In Moore EE, Feliciano DV, Mattox KL, editors: *Trauma,* ed 5, New York, 2004, McGraw Hill.
66. Cirillo RL, Koniaris LG: Detecting blunt pancreatic injuries, *J Gastrointest Surg* 6(4):587-598, 2002.
67. Cheynel N, Serre T, Arnoux PJ et al: Biomechanic study of the human liver in frontal deceleration, *J Trauma* 61(4):855-861, 2006.
68. Lau VK, Viano DC: Influence of impact velocity on the severity of nonpenetrating hepatic injury, *J Trauma* 21(2):115-123, 1981.
69. Brasel KJ, Nirula R: What mechanism justifies abdominal evaluation in motor vehicle crashes? *J Trauma* 59(5):1057-1061, 2005.
70. Stafford RE, McGonigal MD, Weigelt JA et al: Oral contrast solution and computed tomography for blunt abdominal trauma, *Arch Surg* 134(6):622-627, 1999.
71. Rozycki GS, Tremblay L, Feliciano DV et al: A prospective study for the detection of vascular injury in adult and pediatric patients with cervicothoracic seat belt signs, *J Trauma* 52(4):618-624, 2002.
72. Biffl WL, Egglin T, Benedetto B et al: Sixteen-slice computed tomographic angiography is a reliable noninvasive screening test for clinically significant blunt cerebrovascular injuries, *J Trauma* 60(4):745-51; discussion, 751-752, 2006.
73. Cothren CC, Moore EE, Biffl WL et al: Cervical spine fracture patterns predictive of blunt vertebral artery injury, *J Trauma* 55(5):811-813, 2003.
74. Miller PR, Fabian TC, Croce MA et al: Prospective screening for blunt cerebrovascular injuries: analysis of diagnostic modalities and outcomes, *Ann Surg* 236(3):386-395, 2002.
75. Report to Congress, 1998. *The Effect of Increased Speed Limits in the Post NMSL Era.* Available online at www-nrd.nhtsa.dot.gov. Accessed February 2007.
76. Acierno S, Kaufman R, Rivara FP et al: Vehicle mismatch: injury patterns and severity, *Accid Anal Prev* 36(5):761-772, 2004.
77. Nirula R, Mock CN, Nathens AB et al: The new car assessment program: does it predict the relative safety of vehicles in actual crashes? *J Trauma* 57(4):779-786, 2004.
78. Dolan WD, Gifford RW, Smith RJ et al: Automobile-related injuries, *JAMA* 249(23):3216-3221, 1983.
79. Rouhana SW, Lau IV, Ridella SA: Influence of velocity and forced compression on the severity of abdominal injury in blunt, non-penetrating lateral impact, *J Trauma* 25(6):490-500, 1985.
80. Newman RJ: A prospective evaluation of the protective effect of car seatbelts, *J Trauma* 26(6):561-564, 1986.
81. Wild BR, Kenwright J, Rastogi S: Effects of seat belts on injuries to front and rear seat passengers, *Br Med J* 290(6482):1621-1623, 1985.
82. Viano DC, Andrzejak DV: Biomechanics of abdominal injuries by armrest loading, *J Trauma* 34(1):105-115, 1993.
83. Kerwin AJ, Griffen MM, Tepas JJ, et al: The burden of noncompliance with seat belt use on a trauma center, *J Trauma* 60(3): 489-493, 2006.
84. Denis R, Allard M, Atlas H et al: Changing trends with abdominal injury in seatbelt wearers, *J Trauma* 23(11):1007-1008, 1983.
85. Anderson PA, Rivara FP, Maier RV et al: The epidemiology of seatbelt-associated injuries, *J Trauma* 31(1):60-67, 1991.
86. Huelke DF, Mackay CM, Morris A: Vertebral column injuries and lap-shoulder belts, *J Trauma* 38(4):547-556, 1995.
87. Tyroch AH, Kaups KL, Rohan J et al: Pregnant women and car restraints: beliefs and practices, *J Trauma* 46(2):241-245, 1999.
88. http://www.safercar.gov/airbags/index.html. Accessed February 2007 from National Highway Traffic Safety Administration.
89. Maxeiner H, Hahn M. Airbag-induced lethal cervical trauma, *J Trauma* 42(6):1148-1151, 1997.
90. Duma SM, Kress TA, Porta DJ et al: Airbag-induced eye injuries: a report of 25 cases, *J Trauma* 41(1):114-119, 1996.
91. Perdikis G, Schmitt T, Chait D et al: Blunt laryngeal fracture: another airbag injury, *J Trauma* 48(3):544-546, 2000.
92. Acosta JA, Rodriguez P: Morbidity associated with four wheel all terrain vehicles and comparison with that of motorcycles, *J Trauma* 55(2):282-284, 2003.
93. Smith LM, Pittman MA, Marr AB et al: Unsafe at any age: a retrospective review of all-terrain vehicle injuries in two level I trauma centers from 1995-2003, *J Trauma* 58(4):783-788, 2005.
94. ATV Safety Institute. Available online at http://www.atvsafety.org/. Accessed February 2007.
95. Pierz JJ: Snowmobile injuries in North America, *Clin Orthop Relat Res* 409:29-36, 2003.
96. Rice MR, Alvanos L, Kenney B: Snowmobile injuries and deaths in children: a review of national injury data and state legislation, *Pediatrics* 105(3, Part 1 of 2):615-619, 2000.
97. Shatz, DV, Kirton OC, McKenney MG et al: Personal watercraft crash injuries: an emerging problem, *J Trauma* 44(1):198-201, 1998.
98. Branche CM, Conn JM, Annest JL: Personal watercraft-related injuries: a growing public health concern, *JAMA* 278(8):663-665, 1997.
99. Maull KI, Whitley RE, Cardea JA: Vertical deceleration injuries, *Surg Gynecol Obstet* 153(2):233-236, 1981.

100. Goodacre S, Than M, Goyder EC et al: Can the distance fallen predict serious injury after a fall from height? *J Trauma* 46(6):1055-1058, 1999.
101. DeHaven H: Mechanical analysis of survival in falls from heights of fifty to one hundred and fifty feet, *War Med* 2:586, 1942.
102. Demetriades D, Murray J, Brown C et al: High level falls: type and severity of injuries and survival outcome by age, *J Trauma* 58(2):342-345, 2005.
103. Ordog GJ, Wasserberger J, Balasubramanium S: Wound ballistics: theory and practice, *Ann Emerg Med* 13(12):1113-1122, 1984.
104. McSwain NE: Ballistics. In Ivatury RR, Cayten GC editors: *Textbook of Penetrating Trauma,* Philadelphia, 1996, Williams and Wilkins.
105. Janzon B, Seeman T: Muscle devitalization in high-energy missile wounds, and its dependence on energy transfer, *J Trauma* 25(2):138-144, 1985.
106. Fackler ML: Gunshot wounds, *Ann Emerg Med* 28(2):194-203, 1996.
107. Ordog GJ, Wasserberger J, Balasubramanium S: Shotgun wound ballistics, *J Trauma* 28(5):624-631, 1988.
108. Gestring ML, Geller ER, Akkad N et al: Shotgun slug injuries: case report and literature review, *J Trauma* 40(4):650-653, 1996.
109. Deitch EA, Grimes WR: Experience with 112 shotgun wounds of the extremities, *J Trauma* 24(7):600-603, 1984.
110. Flint LM, Cryer HM, Howard DA et al: Approaches to the management of shotgun injuries, *J Trauma* 24(5):415-419, 1984.
111. Cartwright AJ, Taams KO, Unsworth-White MJ et al: Suicidal nonfatal impalement injury of the thorax, *Ann Thorac Surg* 72(4):1364-1366, 2001.
112. Fein A, Leff A, Hopewell PC: Pathophysiology and management of the complications resulting from fire and the inhaled products of combustion: review of the literature, *Crit Care Med* 8(2):94-98, 1980.
113. Demling RH: *Pulmonary Problems*, 2004. Available online at http://www.burnsurgery.org/. Accessed February 2007.
114. Demling RH: Smoke inhalation injury, *New Horiz* 1(3):422-434, 1993.
115. DePalma RG, Burris DG, Champion HR et al: Blast injuries, *N Engl J Med* 352(13):1335-1342, 2005.
116. Singer P, Cohen JD, Stein MD: Conventional terrorism and critical care, *Crit Care Med* 33(1):S61-S65, 2005.
117. Guy RJ, Kirkman E, Watkins PE et al: Physiologic responses to primary blast, *J Trauma* 45(6):983-987, 1998.
118. Cole LA: The specter of biologic weapons, *Sci Am* 275(6):1-14, 1996.
119. Kapur GB, Hutson HR, Davis MA et al: The United States twenty year experience with bombing incidents: implications for terrorism preparedness and medical response, *J Trauma* 59(6):1436-1444, 2005.
120. Feeney JM, Goldberg R, Blumenthal JA et al: September 11, 2001, revisited: a review of the data, *Arch Surg* 140(11): 1068-1073, 2005.
121. Johannigman JA: Disaster preparedness: it's all about me, *Crit Care Med* 33(1):S22-S28, 2005.
122. Schecter WP, Fry DE: The surgeon and acts of civilian terrorism: chemical agents, *J Am Coll Surg*, 200(1):128-135, 2005.
123. Fry DE, Schecter WP, Hartshorne MF: The surgeon and acts of civilian terrorism: radiation exposure and injury, *J Am Coll Surg* 202(1):146-154, 2006.
124. Waselenko JK, MacVittie TJ, Blakely WF et al: Medical management of the acute radiation syndrome: recommendations of the Strategic National Stockpile Radiation Working Group, *Ann Intern Med* 140(12):1037-1051, 2004.
125. Kales SN, Christiani DC: Acute chemical emergencies, *N Engl J Med* 350(8):800-808, 2004.
126. Bravata DM, McDonald KM, Smith WM et al: Systematic review: surveillance systems for early detection of bioterrorism-related diseases, *Ann Intern Med* 140(11):913-922, 2004.
127. Inglesby TV, Dennis DT, Henderson DA et al: Plague as a biological weapon: medical and public health management, *JAMA* 283(17):2281-2290, 2000.
128. Inglesby TV, O'Toole T, Henderson DA et al: Anthrax as a biologic weapon, 2002, updated recommendations for management, *JAMA* 287(17):2236-2252, 2002.
129. Wisner DH: History and current status of trauma scoring systems, *Arch Surg* 127(1):111-117, 1992.
130. Offner P: *Trauma Scoring Systems,* 2002. Available online at http://www.emedicine.com/med/topic3214.htm. Accessed February 2007.
131. Kilgo PD, Meredith JW, Hensberry R et al: A note on the disjointed nature of the injury severity score, *J Trauma* 57(3):479-487, 2004.
132. Hannan EL, Waller CH, Farrell LS et al: A comparison among the abilities of various injury severity measures to predict mortality with and without accompanying physiologic information, *J Trauma* 58(2):244-251, 2005.
133. Guzzo JI, Bochicchio GV, Napolitano LM et al: Prediction of outcomes in trauma: anatomic or physiologic parameters, *J Am Coll Surg* 201(6):891-897, 2005.
134. Kuhls DA, Malone DI, McCarter RJ et al: Predictors of mortality in adult trauma patients: the physiologic trauma score is equivalent to the trauma and injury severity score, *J Am Coll Surg* 194(6):695-704, 2002.
135. Champion HR, Copes WS, Sacco WJ et al: Improved Predictions from a Severity Characterization of Trauma (ASCOT) over Trauma and Injury Severity Score (TRISS): results of an independent evaluation, *J Trauma* 40(1):42-49, 1996.
136. Osler TM, Baker SP, Long W: A modification of the injury severity score that both improves accuracy and simplifies scoring, *J Trauma* 16(11):882-885, 1976.
137. Rutledge R, Osler T: The ICD-9-based illness severity score: a new model that outperforms both DRG and APR-DRG as predictors of survival and resource utilization, *J Trauma* 45(4):791-799, 1998.
138. Osler T, Rutledge R, Dies J et al: ICISS: an International Classification of Disease 9-based injury severity score, *J Trauma* 41(3):380-386, 1996.
139. Hannan EL, Szpulski Farrell L, Bessey PQ et al: Predictors of mortality in adult patients with blunt injuries in New York state: a comparison of the Trauma and Injury Severity Score (TRISS) and the International Classification of Disease, Ninth Revision-Based Injury Severity Score (ICISS), *J Trauma* 47(1):8-13, 1999.
140. Hunt JP, Baker CC, Fakhry SM et al: Accuracy of administrative data in trauma, *Surgery* 126(2):191-197, 1999.
141. Brenneman FD, Wright JG, Kennedy ED et al: Outcomes research in surgery, *World J Surg* 23(12):1220-1223, 1999.
142. Wright JG: Outcomes research: what to measure, *World J Surg* 23(12):1224-1226, 1999.

143. Kaplan RM, Ganiats TG, Sieber WJ et al: The Quality of Well-Being Scale: critical similarities and differences with SF-36, *Int J Qual Health Care* 10(6):509-520, 1998.
144. Michaels AJ, Michaels CE, Smith JS et al: Outcome from injury: general health, work status, and satisfaction 12 months after trauma, *J Trauma* 48(5):841-850, 2000.
145. Holbrook TL, Hoyt DB, Coimbra R et al: Long-term posttraumatic stress disorder persists after major trauma in adolescents: new data on risk factors and functional outcome, *J Trauma* 58(4):764-771, 2005.
146. MacKenzie EJ, Cushing BM, Jurkovich GJ et al: Physical impairment and functional outcomes six months after severe lower extremity fractures, *J Trauma* 34(4):528-539, 1993.
147. Butcher JL, MacKenzie EJ, Cushing B et al: Long-term outcomes after lower extremity trauma, *J Trauma* 41(1):4-9, 1996.
148. Kiely JM, Brasel KJ, Weidner K et al: Predicting quality of life six months after traumatic injury, *J Trauma* 61(4):791-798, 2006.
149. Michaels AJ, Michaels CE, Moon CH et al: Posttraumatic stress disorder after injury: impact on general health outcome and early risk assessment, *J Trauma* 47(3):460-467, 1999.

13

Shock and Multiple Organ Dysfunction Syndrome

Kathryn Truter Von Rueden, Pamela J. Bolton, Thomas C. Vary

Shock is the hemodynamic manifestation of cellular metabolic insufficiency resulting from either inadequate cellular perfusion, a basic biochemical inability to properly utilize oxygen and other nutrients, or an inappropriate or amplified stimulation of cellular signaling cascades. A state of hyperinflammation, hypoperfusion, and hypermetabolism may influence the critically injured patient's initial presentation. The common denominator in shock is a decreased utilization of oxygen by the tissues. Prolonged deficits in oxygen utilization lead to tissue injury and multiple organ dysfunction syndrome (MODS), which may progress to organ failure and death.

Categories of Shock

Shock can be classified based on the physiologic etiology of the underperfusion of tissues. The three categories of shock are cardiogenic, distributive, and hypovolemic. The causes of shock states and clinical presentation specific to each type of shock are discussed.

Cardiogenic

In cardiogenic shock (cardiac pump failure), the underlying pathogenesis is related primarily to the failure of the left ventricle to adequately pump blood to the systemic circulation. Cardiogenic shock results with a loss of approximately 40% of the heart's pumping ability. Heart failure, acute myocardial infarction, acute arrhythmias, papillary muscle rupture, ventricular septal rupture, end-stage valvular disease, severe pulmonary hypertension, massive pulmonary embolism, cardiac tamponade, tension pneumothorax, or MODS may cause cardiac pump failure. Tamponade, pulmonary embolus, and tension pneumothorax are obstructive mechanisms that impede venous return, inhibit pulmonary vascular blood flow, impair the Frank-Starling mechanism, and reduce cardiac output causing cardiogenic shock.

As the cardiac output diminishes, tissue perfusion becomes compromised. The major compensatory mechanism is an increase in heart rate and vascular tone in order to maintain essential organ perfusion (e.g., brain, heart, lungs). Cardiogenic shock is a combination of failure to mobilize venous volume, a loss of myocardial contractility, and a compensatory vasoconstriction response, which promotes a systemic shunt mechanism. The combination of failures creates venous volume overload with relative arterial hypovolemia as blood flow is redirected to the central organs.

Clinical Presentation. Signs and symptoms of shock states related to cardiac pump failure include hypotension, increased systemic vascular resistance (SVR), tachycardia, decreased stroke volume index (SVI), decreased urine output (UO) and increased ventricular volumes measured by central venous pressure (CVP), right atrial pressure (RAP), and pulmonary artery occlusion pressure (PAOP). Refer to Table 13-1 for formulas and normal values of hemodynamic parameters. Assessment features include alteration in mentation, crackles (rales), increased respiratory rate, decreased bowel sounds, and pale, cool skin.

Distributive

Shock may also occur when vascular tone is lost, resulting in massive vasodilation. The etiology may be neurogenic, anaphylactic, septic (infectious), or from acute adrenal insufficiency. In neurogenic shock, depression of the central nervous system diminishes sympathetic outflow, causing a loss of vasomotor control. The loss of a vasomotor response leads to vasodilation and pooling of blood in both the arterial and venous circulatory systems. Inadequate venous return (preload) decreases myocardial end-diastolic fiber stretch, reduces the stroke volume, and ultimately impairs tissue perfusion. Neurogenic shock may be induced by deep general or spinal anesthesia; brain injury, particularly in the medulla near the vasomotor center; or spinal cord injury (usually complete lesions at or above the T6 region). Bradycardia associated with neurogenic shock is due to sympathetic denervation in the cervical or high thoracic spine. The loss of sympathetic innervation results in an unopposed vagal-induced bradycardia.

Loss of local vascular tone is also the underlying pathophysiologic mechanism of anaphylactic shock. The body reacts to a foreign substance by activating the immune

TABLE 13-1 **Hemodynamic Parameters**

Parameter	Formula	Normal Values
CO	Heart rate × stroke volume	4-8 L/min
CI	CO/Body surface area	2.5-4 L/min/m^2
SVI	CI/Heart rate	33-47 ml/beat/m^2
RAP	Direct measurement	0-8 mm Hg
PAOP	Direct measurement	8-12 mm Hg
RVEDVI	$\frac{\text{Stroke volume}}{\text{RV ejection fraction}}$	60-100 ml/m^2
SVRI	$\frac{(\text{MAP} - \text{RAP}) \times 80}{\text{CI}}$	1360-2200 dyne/sec/cm^{-5}/m^2
PVRI	$\frac{(\text{MPAP} - \text{PAOP}) \times 80}{\text{CI}}$	<425 dyne/sec/cm^{-5}/m^2
LVSWI	SVI (MAP − PAOP) × 0.0136	40-70 gm−m/m^2/beat
RVSWI	SVI (PAP − RAP) × 0.0136	5-10 gm−m/m^2/beat

CI, Cardiac index; *CO,* cardiac output; *LVSWI,* left ventricular stroke work index; *MAP,* mean arterial pressure; *MPAP,* mean pulmonary artery pressure; *PAOP,* pulmonary artery occlusion pressure; *PVRI,* pulmonary vascular resistance index; *RAP,* right atrial pressure; *RVEDVI,* right ventricular end-diastolic volume index; *RVSWI,* right ventricular stroke work index; *SVI,* stroke volume index; *SVRI,* systemic vascular resistance index.

system against an antigen. The inflammatory response to the antigen-antibody reaction directly alters the endothelial lining of the blood vessels, increasing vascular permeability. The antigen-antibody reaction also induces the release of histamine or histamine-like substances, which possess vasodilator properties. Histamines increase vascular capacity through venodilation, reduce arterial pressure by dilating arterioles, and increase capillary permeability, promoting a rapid shift of fluids into the interstitial spaces. Both neurogenic and anaphylactic shock can be acutely treated by infusion of intravenous fluids to restore a euvolemic state and administration of sympathomimetic drugs to promote vasoconstriction, increase venous return, and enhance myocardial contractility.

Septic shock is triggered by an overwhelming inflammatory response to infection. It is characterized by fever, elevated white blood cell count, loss of vascular endothelial integrity, hypotension despite intravascular volume administration, and an increase in oxygen requirements[1] (Table 13-2). Cardiac output is elevated due to increased heart rate and vasodilation. Septic shock is discussed in detail later in this chapter.

Acute adrenal insufficiency triggers distributive shock states through a lack of activation of essential catecholamines and hormones from the adrenal gland. During stress the adrenal medulla releases catecholamines such as epinephrine, norepinephrine, and dopamine, activating a sympathetic response (i.e., vasoconstriction, tachycardia). The adrenal cortex is also stimulated during stress, releasing cortisol, which promotes glyconeogenesis, and, at high levels, cortisol suppresses the inflammatory response. Aldosterone is also stimulated by the adrenal cortex; activating aldosterone increases preload. Adrenal insufficiency results in a lack of adrenal gland activity with resultant vasodilatation, hypovolemia, and lack of glucose for cellular metabolism.[2]

TABLE 13-2 **Definitions of Systemic Inflammatory Response Syndrome (SIRS) and Sepsis[1]**

SIRS

Response to a variety of severe clinical insults having two or more of the following conditions:
- Temperature above 38° C or below 36° C
- Heart rate greater than 90 beats/min
- Respiratory rate above 20 breaths/min or Pa_{CO_2} less than 32 torr
- WBC greater than 12,000 cells/mm^3, less than 4,000 cells/mm^3, or greater than 10% immature (band) forms

Infection

Inflammatory response to the presence of microorganisms or the invasion of a normally sterile host by microorganisms.

Sepsis

Systemic response to infection, manifested by two or more of the SIRS criteria as a consequence of infection.

Severe Sepsis

Sepsis associated with organ dysfunction, hypoperfusion, or hypotension; hypoperfusion and perfusion abnormalities may include, but are not limited to, lactic acidosis, oliguria, and an acute alteration in mental status.

Septic Shock

Sepsis with hypotension despite adequate resuscitation with fluids, with the presence of perfusion abnormalities that may include, but are not limited to, lactic acidosis, oliguria, and an acute alteration in mental status; patients receiving inotropic or vasopressor agents may not be hypotensive when perfusion abnormalities are measured.

Hypotension

Systolic blood pressure of less than 90 mm Hg or a reduction of more than 40 mm Hg from baseline in the absence of other causes for hypotension.

MODS

Presence of altered organ function in an acutely ill patient; homeostasis cannot be maintained without intervention.

SIRS, Systemic inflammatory response syndrome; MODS, multiple organ dysfunction syndrome; WBC, white blood cells.

Clinical Presentation. Signs of distributive shock include hypotension, decreased UO, decreased SVR, and decreased SVI. The relative hypovolemia in distributive shock decreases right and left ventricular end-diastolic ventricular volumes (preload), which are usually reflected by low CVP, RAP, and PAOP. Cardiac output may be initially elevated due to the significant reduction in afterload (vasodilation). Patients with septic and anaphylactic shock typically have tachycardia, whereas those in neurogenic shock usually present with bradycardia.

Hypovolemic Shock

Hypovolemic shock is caused by a reduction in intravascular volume. Depletion of the effective circulating blood volume subsequently decreases stroke volume and cardiac output and therefore oxygen delivery. Inadequate intravascular volume and a hypovolemic shock state can occur in a number of conditions.

Most often hypovolemic shock is associated with hemorrhage and a 15% to 30% blood loss.[2,3] Examples of clinical conditions that may cause nonhemorrhagic hypovolemic shock include burns, intestinal disorders, and some traumatic injuries. Severe burn injury may create loss of fluids and electrolytes through denuded areas, resulting in enormous ongoing loss of plasma volume and hemoconcentration. Intestinal obstruction, ischemic bowel, and intestinal injuries may cause sequestration of fluid in the peritoneal cavity, leading to a significant decrease in circulating volume, preload, and stroke volume. The increased peritoneal volume may also cause abdominal compartment syndrome, further decreasing distal arterial blood flow and decreasing venous return. Nonhemorrhagic trauma may induce hypovolemic shock. Severe contusion or crushing damage to soft tissues often sequesters blood and plasma in the interstitial space of the injured tissues. The net effect is diminished intravascular blood volume, decreasing venous return, and stroke volume. Hypotension may not become evident until at least 30% or more of the patient blood volume is lost or the patient's position is changed for diagnostic procedures, such as upright chest radiographs. The delay in hypotension occurs because of physiologic mechanisms that are normally able to compensate for moderate intravascular volume loss. The end result is a fall in cardiac output, intravascular volume, and oxygen delivery that are present in hypovolemic shock.

Hemorrhagic hypovolemic shock affects the patient in two ways: through a loss of circulating volume and a decrease in oxygen-carrying capacity. In addition to the loss of circulating volume, the acute decrease in red blood cells reduces both oncotic pressure and oxygen-carrying capacity. The oxygen transport deficit superimposed on the circulatory volume loss presents the characteristic features of hemorrhagic hypovolemia: significant base deficit and lactic acidosis. The initial compensatory response is a profound tachycardia combined with a compensatory systemic shunt as long as central and local sympathetic tone are intact (Figure 13-1). The vasoconstrictor response may significantly and urgently place the nonessential organs (e.g., intestines, kidney, skin) at risk of severe underperfusion.

Clinical Presentation. Signs of hypovolemic shock include altered level of consciousness; reduced UO; tachycardia; hypotension; increased SVR; decreased SVI; decreased right and left ventricular end-diastolic volumes reflected by low CVP, RAP, and PAOP; and increased negative base excess related to tissue hypoperfusion and resulting anaerobic metabolism. Severe base deficit and lactic acidosis are seen with hypovolemic shock.

Common Shock Pathways

Regardless of the pathology, when tissue perfusion is inadequate to meet the tissue metabolic demands, a shock state can ensue. Hypoperfusion promotes a response heralded by a compensatory increase in circulating catecholamines, which augments oxygen delivery. The additional availability of oxygen supports an increase in cellular extraction of oxygen to meet higher metabolic requirements.[3-5] The response to increased circulating catecholamines causes an increase in venous return and thus preload; arteriole vasoconstriction (raising afterload); increased heart rate; and enhanced myocardial contractility. Combined, these compensatory mechanisms also alter the myocardial balance of systole to diastole and increase myocardial oxygen demand and requirement for high-energy phosphate bonds.

The shock episode can be divided into three major phases: compensatory, progressive, and irreversible. In the compensatory phase, tissue perfusion is altered, but organ function is maintained through compensatory mechanisms. An intact neuroendocrine compensatory response is essential to survival. Stress hormones are released to preserve intravascular volume and perfusion of essential organs, shunting blood away from nonessential organs. The increase in sympathetic discharge requires intact receptor sites, adequate neurotransmitters, functional thyroid hormones, and responsive fibers. As fibers respond, heart rate increases, arterioles and venules constrict at the nonessential tissue level, and perfusion pressure to essential organs is maintained. For a time the patient is able to maintain function of essential organs. During the progressive phase, there is a decreased response to the compensatory mechanisms, and arterial perfusion cannot be maintained to essential organs. In the decompensated, irreversible stage, the patient becomes increasingly refractory to therapy.

The common underlying mechanisms of shock are oxygen deficiency, cellular hypoxia, ischemia, and anoxia. Oxygen deficit promotes a response heralded by increased circulating catecholamines, resulting in a compensatory increase in oxygen delivery (hallmarked by increasing heart rate and vasoconstriction of both arterial and venous beds) and an increased cellular extraction of oxygen. If the shock state is prolonged, the patient may suffer insurmountable cellular hypoxia, which can cause organ failure and death.

As a result of injury, prolonged hypoxic and hypoperfused states, or sepsis, complex inflammatory pathways are stimulated. These pathways, when overactivated or unregulated, may result in catastrophic consequences. Humoral and chemical mediators change the vascular structures and metabolic pathways to such a degree that capillary blood flow and oxygen delivery mechanisms may be significantly impaired and a profound metabolic acidosis ensues. Even if oxyhemoglobin is available in the arterial bed, metabolic dysfunction, altered capillary flow, and intracellular dysfunction may prevent the extraction of oxygen, leading to organ dysfunction and eventually organ failure.[5]

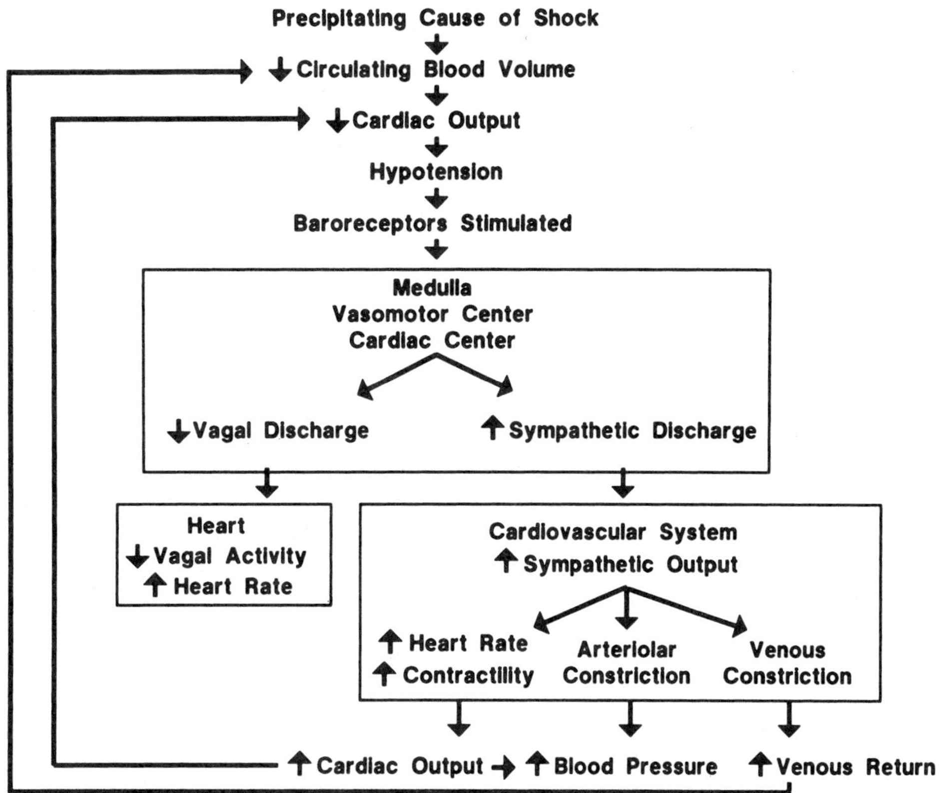

FIGURE 13-1 Compensatory mechanisms for the restoration of circulatory blood volume.

The hypothalamic-pituitary-adrenal axis is activated during critical illness, trauma, and infection/sepsis. Effective neuroendocrine functioning is vital for a patient to adapt to the stress of illness and maintain normal cellular homeostasis. In critical illness, there is an alteration in the normal corticosteroid response, which results in the patient's inability to increase cortisol production.[2] This is also seen during sepsis as inflammatory cytokines, such as tumor necrosis factor, promote corticosteroid resistance and suppress cortisol-releasing hormone leading to adrenal insufficiency.[2]

Early recognition of the cause of shock is essential to appropriately treat and successfully reverse the disorder. Prompt and adequate resuscitative interventions are vital to protect, preserve, or restore organ function and to maintain cellular hemostasis.

Compensatory Responses to Hemorrhage

Hemorrhage, regardless of its cause, results in a compensatory response designed to stabilize a life-threatening situation. Blood loss of less than 10% may occur without any significant effect on blood pressure or cardiac index. Blood loss of greater than 10% initiates a powerful response designed to maintain perfusion of vital organs until the circulating volume and oxygen delivery are restored either by replacement of blood and fluid during resuscitation or through a redistribution of fluid volumes in the body. When more than 10% to 15% of the total blood volume is lost, cardiac index diminishes as a result of decreased venous return. Venous return is a major determinant of preload (stretch of ventricular fibers). A proportional relationship exists between preload (ventricular filling) and stroke volume. A reduction in preload reduces stroke volume. Failure to maintain cardiac index leads to decreased arterial pressure, which causes an increase in sympathetic discharge. The sympathetic stimulation increases the heart rate and promotes vasoconstriction, which may further limit ventricular filling and ejection. Hemorrhagic loss of more than 40% of the total blood volume precipitates a profound decrease in the cardiac index and blood pressure and renders the compensatory mechanisms ineffective (see Figure 13-1).

Circulatory Reflexes Related to Hypovolemia

The circulatory reflexes triggered by all forms of shock, particularly acute hemorrhage, are designed to restore arterial pressure and blood flow to normal to prevent organ damage. An integrated response to intravascular volume losses greater than 10% of the total blood volume is initiated by the baroreceptors, which respond to the fall in blood pressure. Hypotension stimulates the vasomotor center, increasing sympathetic outflow. The carotid artery chemoreceptors respond to decreases in the blood pH and a rise in carbon dioxide (CO_2) and the metabolic acid, H^+ ion concentration. Activation of the carotid body chemoreceptors stimulates the vasomotor center and normally inhibits the autonomic nervous system (ANS) (Figure 13-2).[4] The net effect of the baroreceptor response is an increased sympathetic discharge by the medullary vasomotor center, which is carried over the sympathetic efferent fibers to the heart, systemic arterioles, and adrenals. Increased sympathetic discharge has a positive inotropic effect on the myocardium that augments contractility. Improved myocardial performance results from the direct release of catecholamines at the cardiac sympathetic nerve endings in the proximity of myocardial β_1-adrenergic receptors and by vasomotor center inhibition of vagal parasympathetic outflow. This change in the balance between the sympathetic and parasympathetic pathways increases atrial pacemaker activity and reduces atrioventricular conduction time, resulting in an increased heart rate. An increase in heart rate is a compensatory response mediated by sympathetic nervous system (SNS) stimulation; however, a heart rate greater than 120 beats/min may limit ventricular filling and decrease stroke volume.

Increased arteriolar constriction, via the α_1-adrenergic receptors, results in a systemic shunt, which redistributes blood flow away from nonessential organs with low oxygen requirements, such as skin and skeletal muscle. If the cause of the hypovolemia is not corrected, blood flow to the visceral organs will eventually be diminished. Despite a reduced blood volume, venous constriction in response to the sympathetic stimulation tends to enhance venous return and prevent pooling of the blood in the venous circulation. Because the venous system has a capacitance of up to 60% of the circulating volume, venoconstriction can markedly increase venous return, ensuring adequate blood volume for maintenance of myocardial preload. Hemodynamic compensation by stimulation of the sympathetic nervous system is extremely efficient if the shock state is not allowed to continue for a long period and blood and fluid losses do not persist.

Fluid Shifts

To compensate for the reduced circulating blood volume, fluids shift from extravascular to intravascular spaces. The fluid shift occurs as a direct result of the decreased intracapillary hydrostatic pressure associated with the loss of blood volume. Normally, the balance between hydrostatic pressure that promotes filtration, and the plasma oncotic pressure, which fosters reabsorption, favors a small net loss of fluid into the interstitial space. In a shock state, the reduction of blood pressure decreases the capillary hydrostatic pressure, decreasing filtration. The net effect is an increased movement of fluid volume into the capillaries. Decreased venous pressure and arteriolar vasoconstriction

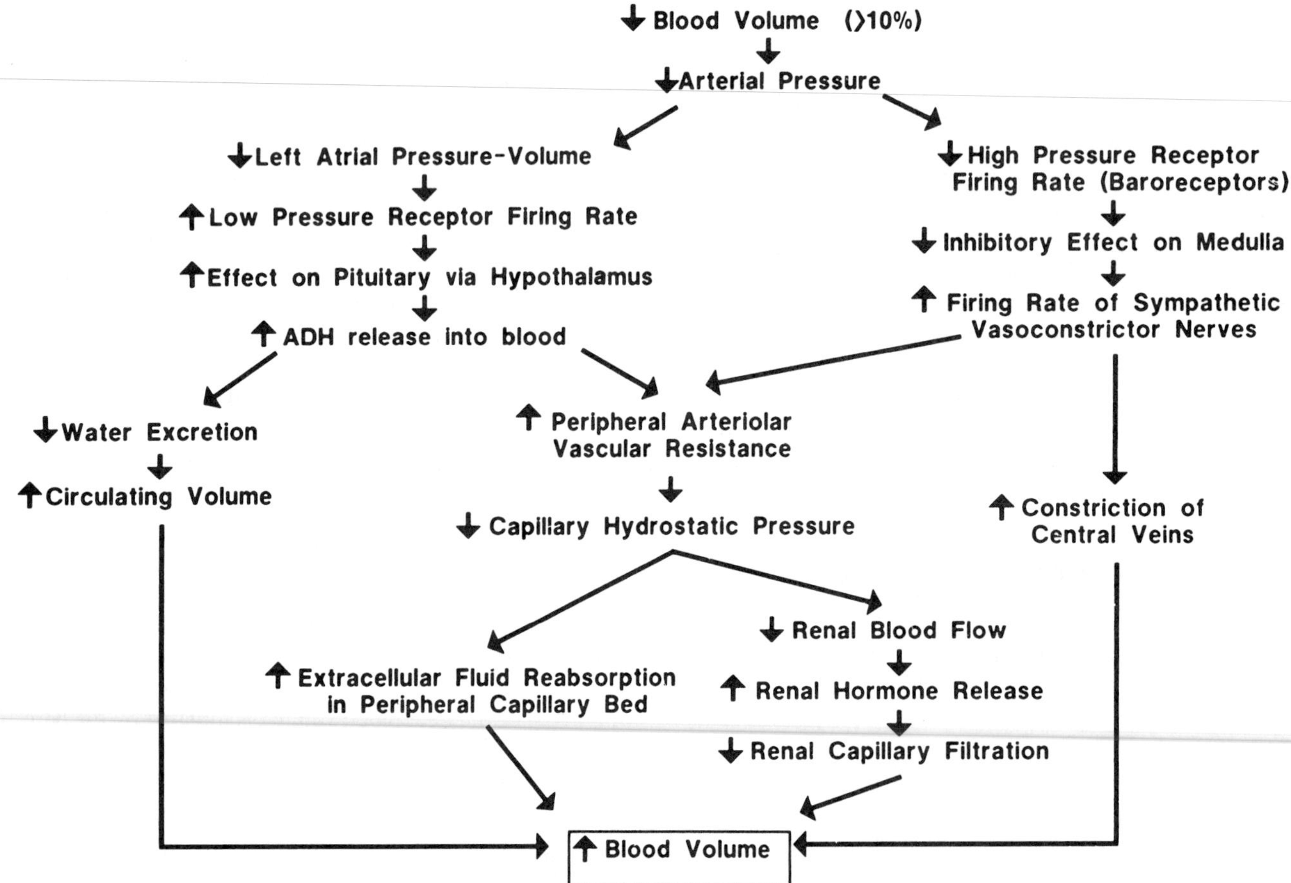

FIGURE 13-2 Compensatory mechanisms after loss of greater than 10% of blood volume.

are separate factors contributing to the reduced capillary hydrostatic pressure and fluid movement into the vascular compartment.

In hemorrhagic shock, the loss of red cells may cause a significant decrease in oncotic pressure. Coupled with an inflammatory process that alters vascular tone and endothelial permeability, there may be a significant loss of volume into the interstitial space, further exacerbating arterial hypovolemia. "Relative" hypovolemia that is treated aggressively with volume resuscitation therefore may also result in a significant increase in the extravascular volume. Compensatory redirection of blood flow from the splanchnic circulation to the heart and brain reduces blood flow to the kidneys in hypovolemic states. Decreased renal perfusion initiates efferent renal arteriolar vasoconstriction through the stimulation of the juxtaglomerular apparatus (a renal baroreceptor). Renin is subsequently released and is converted to angiotensin I and II by the endothelial cells of the lung and liver, respectively. Angiotensin II, a potent vasoconstrictor, raises arterial pressure and stimulates aldosterone secretion by the adrenal cortex. Aldosterone increases blood volume by increasing sodium reabsorption and water reabsorption in the renal tubules. Responses to hypovolemia can occur within seconds, as occurs with increased sympathetic discharge, or can require days, as with kidney-mediated changes in water and salt excretion. All the compensatory mechanisms initially result in increased circulating blood volume in an attempt to increase stroke volume and oxygen delivery.

Limits of Compensation

Prolonged hypovolemia (loss of more than 10% of blood volume without timely intervention) or hypovolemic shock can exhaust compensatory mechanisms so that the circulatory system cannot be maintained or restored to normal (Figure 13-3). The most important factor in patient survival is arresting the hemorrhage or cause of hypovolemia. If the hemorrhage is not stopped or volume replacement is insufficient, myocardial performance deteriorates. When the arterial pressure falls low enough, coronary blood flow decreases below that required for adequate delivery of oxygen to the myocardium. Myocardial ischemia secondary to inadequate coronary perfusion pressures reduces cardiac index, further lowering arterial pressure. The end result is deterioration of heart function.

A positive-feedback cycle develops, and the initial hypovolemia leads to dire consequences. As cardiac index diminishes, cerebral perfusion is also reduced and the patient becomes increasingly obtunded. Eventually blood flow to the vasomotor center of the medulla is so compromised that the vasomotor center becomes progressively less active and finally fails. The systemic vasculature is no longer able to maintain its vascular tone; vasodilation and vascular collapse ensue. During this stage, the vascular beds behave as passive distensible

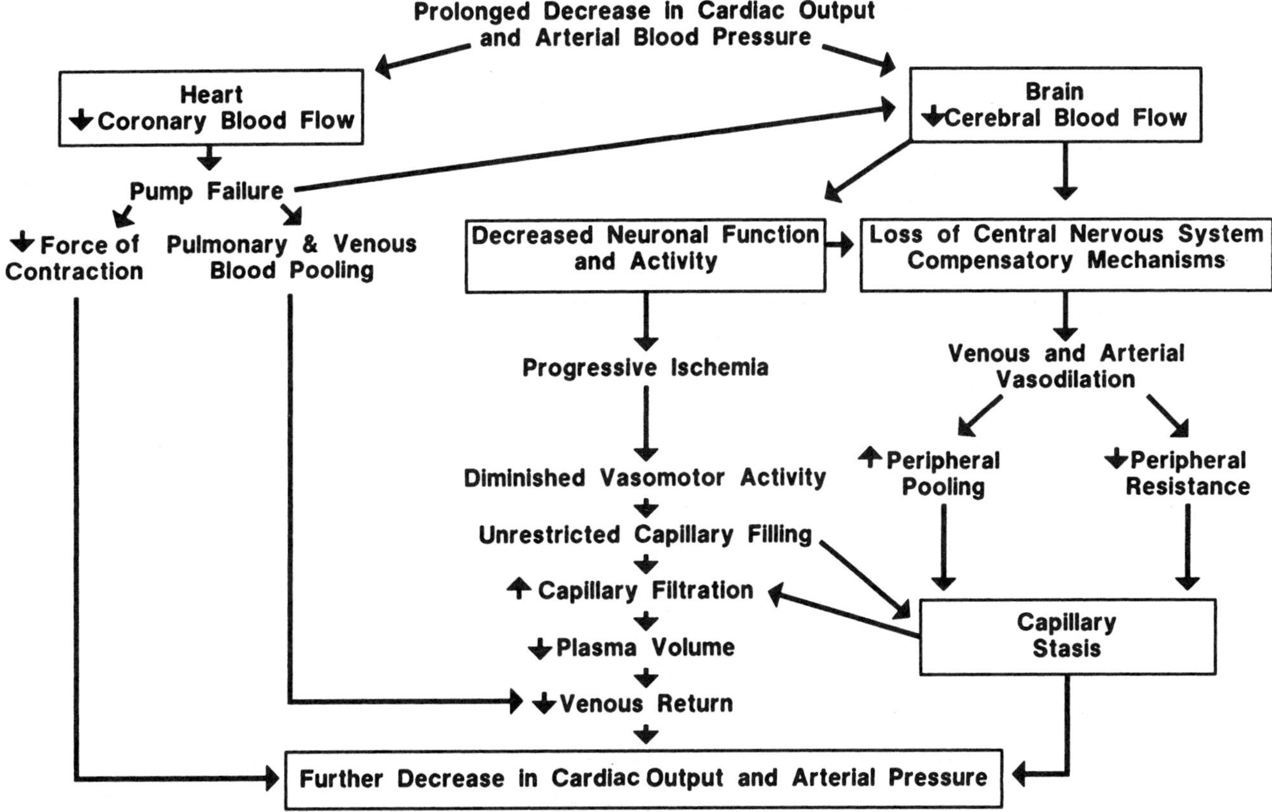

FIGURE 13-3 Negative effects of prolonged hypovolemic shock.

tubes and no longer exhibit active adjustment to circulatory changes. Arterial vasodilation can lead to reduced blood flow to capillary beds in critical organs, whereas venous dilation causes blood to pool in the veins, decreasing venous return and further reducing cardiac output. Eventually, this sluggish blood flow in the periphery leads to changes in the capillaries that increase permeability, and large volumes of fluid move out of the vascular spaces, further lowering blood volume. Unless this cycle and these conditions are reversed rapidly, survival of the patient is doubtful. Irreversible shock occurs when damage to the cells is sufficient to depress metabolic and structural functions. At this point, widespread cellular necrosis occurs in most tissues, leading to organ failure and death.

TABLE 13-3 **Oxygen Delivery Parameters**

Parameter	Formula	Normal Values
Cao_2	$(Hb \times 1.37 \times Sao_2) + (0.003 \times Pao_2)$	20 ml O_2/dl
Cvo_2	$(Hb \times 1.37 \times Svo_2) + (0.003 \times Pvo_2)$	15 ml O_2/dl
Dao_2I	$CI \times Cao_2 \times 10$	500-600 ml $O_2/min/m^2$
Dvo_2I	$CI \times Cvo_2 \times 10$	375-450 ml $O_2/min/m^2$

Cao_2, Arterial oxygen content; *CI*, cardiac index; *Cvo_2*, venous oxygen content; *Dao_2I*, arterial oxygen delivery index; *Dvo_2I*, venous oxygen delivery index; *Hb*, hemoglobin.

Oxygen Consumption

Normal cell function is dependent on the delivery of adequate oxygen and other substrates to ensure adequate adenosine triphosphate (ATP) production by the mitochondria. Delivery of oxygen (DaO_2) is dependent on the oxygen content in the arterial blood (CaO_2) and blood flow through the tissue beds provided by the cardiac output (CO). The hemoglobin content and oxygen saturation of hemoglobin in the arterial blood (SaO_2) and the partial pressure of oxygen in arterial blood (PaO_2) determine CaO_2. Hemoglobin and SaO_2 are major determinants of CaO_2 because only a very small percentage of the total oxygen content of the blood is present in a dissolved state as measured by PaO_2. Table 13-3 summarizes the variables used for clinical evaluation of the adequacy of oxygen transport.

Oxygen consumption index (VO_2I) is an indicator of oxygen utilization by the tissues. VO_2I is affected by the adequacy of oxygen delivery and cellular ability to extract oxygen. In an afebrile, resting patient, VO_2I averages 140 ml $O_2/min/m^2$ (3.5 ml O_2/min/kg or 250 ml O_2/min). The normal stress response to trauma, surgery, or early sepsis is associated with an increase in oxygen consumption of 15% to 35%.[6-8] In a critically ill, hyperdynamic patient, cellular failures of oxidative metabolism may occur even with increased perfusion and oxygen delivery (Figure 13-4). Table 13-4 summarizes the variables used for clinical evaluation of the adequacy of oxygen utilization.

In the absence of metabolic failure, a mismatch between oxygen delivery and tissue demand is caused by reduced oxygen delivery in low perfusion syndromes.[4,8] Such a condition

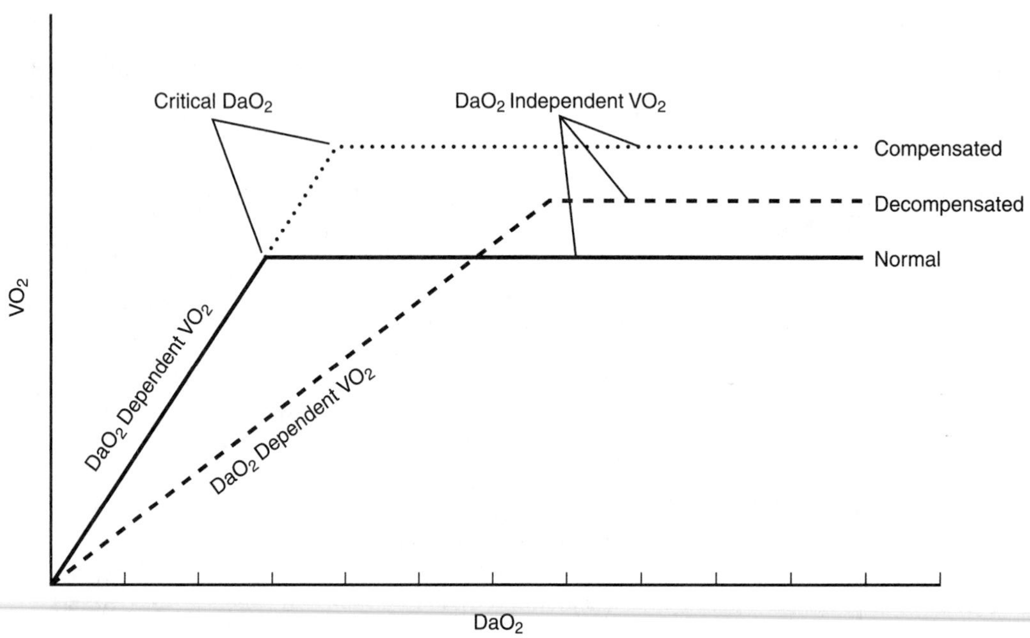

FIGURE 13-4 The relationship of oxygen delivery (Dao_2) and consumption (Vo_2), showing oxygen consumption as dependent on oxygen delivery and cellular extraction of oxygen up to a critical level where consumption becomes independent of oxygen delivery and is sustained by cellular oxygen uptake. Under normal oxygen demand conditions, increased Dao_2 is associated with a rise in Vo_2 *(solid line)*. In compensated SIRS/MODS, Dao_2 is increased to meet high oxygen demands and is associated with a rise in Vo_2 *(dotted line)*. In decompensated SIRS/MODS, Vo_2 is insufficient to meet high oxygen demands because of altered cellular oxygen extraction, despite an increase in Dao_2 *(dashed line)*.

TABLE 13-4 Oxygen Utilization Parameters

Parameter	Formula	Normal Values
Svo_2	Direct measurement	60%-80%
Pvo_2	Direct measurement	35-45 mm Hg
O_2 extraction	Cao_2-Cvo_2	3-5 ml O_2/dl
OER	Cao_2-Cvo_2/Cao_2	22%-30%
Vo_2I	(Cao_2-Cvo_2) × CI × 10	120-170 ml/min/m^2
pHa	Direct measurement	7.35-7.45
BE/BD	Direct measurement	−2 to +2
Lactate	Direct measurement	0.5-2.2 mmol/l

BE/BD, Base excess/base deficit; *OER,* oxygen extraction ratio; *pHa,* arterial pH; *Vo_2I,* oxygen consumption index; for all other abbreviations see Tables 13-1 and 13-2.

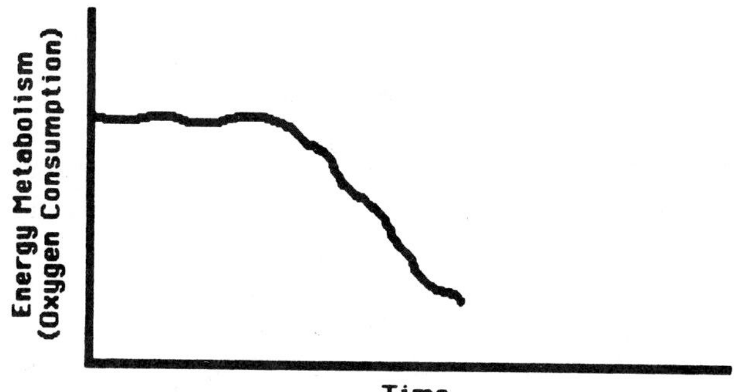

FIGURE 13-5 Oxygen consumption falls in hemorrhagic shock as the supply of oxygen to the body is reduced subsequent to the fall in circulating blood volume.

is caused by hypovolemic or cardiogenic shock, or underperfusion of localized tissue beds as a consequence of compensatory shunting of blood flow away from less essential organs and tissues. The loss of perfusion and systemic pressure causes a reduction in oxygen delivery and thus cellular VO_2 (Figure 13-5).

Oxygen availability is the most important determinant of viable oxidative energy metabolism. Cellular oxygen consumption is influenced by the availability of oxygen delivered via the microcirculation and extraction of oxygen from the capillaries to meet cellular oxygen requirements. A reduction in oxygen delivery results in several characteristic changes. A decline in blood flow results in a greater extraction of arterial oxygen in an attempt to maintain oxygen consumption. Furthermore, a compensatory increase in sympathetic stimulation results in augmented stroke volume and/or heart rate as a mechanism to increase oxygen delivery. Inadequate oxygen delivery, cellular extraction, and consumption result in cellular conversion to anaerobic metabolism for energy substrate production that causes a concomitant increase in production and release of lactate. The ability of the body to maintain a normal lactate level is an indicator of adequate resuscitation. Adversely, the higher the lactate or the longer it takes for lactate clearance, the higher the patient mortality.[9-11] Therefore, lactate provides an objective, global measure to determine adequacy of tissue perfusion.

Cell Function

Maintenance of normal cellular structure and function depends on the cell's ability to synthesize large amounts of energy. The energy requirements of different cells and organs vary depending on their functions. Continuous demands for energy are dictated by cellular and subcellular membrane ion pumps necessary to maintain the internal cellular environment; by the rate of protein synthesis, especially in cells with a high rate of protein turnover; and by mechanical work such as muscle contraction in cardiac and skeletal muscle (Figure 13-6). The energy reserves of the cell are limited, and the demand for energy is generally derived from the continual catabolism of various fuels, particularly glucose and fatty acids. The energy derived from metabolism of these fuels is stored in the form of ATP. ATP is synthesized by the phosphorylation of adenosine

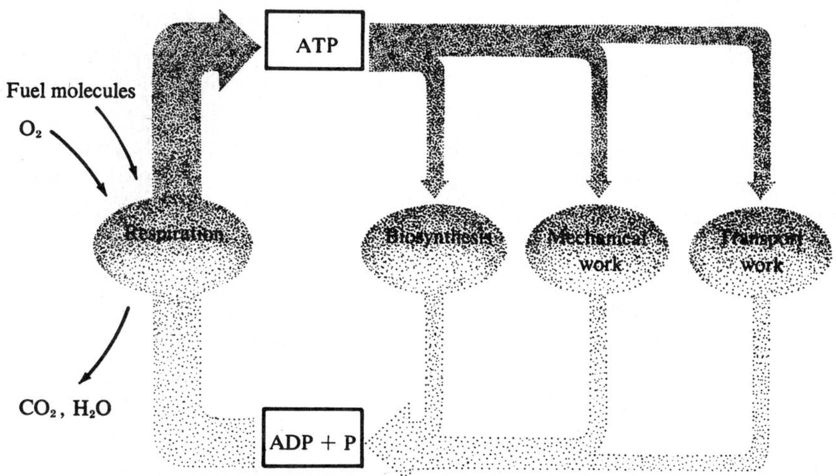

FIGURE 13-6 Relationship between energy production and energy use in maintenance of normal cell function. *(From Lehninger AL:* Bio-energetics, *ed 2, Menlo Park, Calif, 1971, Benjamin.)*

diphosphate (ADP) via three processes: oxidative phosphorylation using the mitochondrial electron-transport chain; substrate phosphorylation; and conversion of creatine phosphate to creatine, with the synthesis of ATP and ADP catalyzed by the enzyme creatine phosphokinase. Oxidative phosphorylation is by far the most important pathway for ATP synthesis and if interrupted by mutations or deficiencies of the proteins necessary for this process, ATP production will be severely impaired.[12]

In well-oxygenated tissues, the rates of oxidative phosphorylation and oxygen consumption are coupled tightly to the rate of ATP use. Mitochondrial ATP synthesis depends on a continuous supply of oxygen and substrates. Tissues cannot store oxygen; hence, effective perfusion is necessary to provide sufficient delivery of oxygen for maintenance of adequate ATP production. Thus, any condition that compromises oxygen delivery to the tissues would tend to alter the mitochondrial capability to synthesize ATP via oxidative phosphorylation. Oxygen deficiency and the ensuing anaerobic metabolic effect put the cell at risk for swelling, rupture, and death.

SYSTEMIC INFLAMMATORY RESPONSE SYNDROME

PATHOPHYSIOLOGY

Systemic inflammatory response syndrome (SIRS) is a sustained, intravascular inflammation resulting from an uncontrolled patient response to multiple stimuli that continually evoke a series of cascades. The response to a noxious stimulus (e.g., trauma, pancreatitis, or aspiration) evokes a cascade of inflammatory mediator responses that in turn stimulate a secondary mediator response. Inflammatory mediators are designed to heal wounds and combat pathologic invaders through a controlled inflammatory response. However, a continuously stimulated inflammatory response may result in a sustained inflammation, known as SIRS. Overwhelming SIRS occurs when the inflammatory responders are continuously activated and upregulated. These cascades create an imbalance in tissue perfusion and cellular oxygen supply and demand, which results in the hallmark oxygen extraction deficit (tissue hypoxia).

Persistent inflammation is fueled by the ongoing disruption of aerobic cellular cycles, which oxidize metabolic fuels to produce ATP. In the presence of SIRS, proportional use of oxygen further decreases as cellular signaling produces metabolic failure when the cells lose their ability to extract oxygen. With failure to produce these energy processes (ATP), the cells become dysfunctional and no longer maintain homeostasis. The cytokine cellular signal stimulates the immune-coagulation-inflammatory axis, which further perpetuates the hypermetabolic, hyperdynamic, and humoral response. More than 200 mediators are known to be involved with this response. Monocytes and macrophages are involved in the generation and release of the inflammatory cytokines, which are responsible for the clinical manifestations of SIRS. The major cytokines involved in SIRS include interleukin-1 (IL-1), tumor necrosis factor-α (TNF-α), IL-6, eicosanoids, and platelet-activating factor.[13] The effects of these cytokines are far-reaching and diverse. Cellular and systemic effects include alteration in vascular permeability, cellular metabolism modifications, adhesion of molecules, chemotaxis, activation of the coagulation cascade, and the production of other cytokines.[14] Changes in either cellular metabolism or vascular permeability can profoundly affect the delicate balance between oxygen delivery and extraction. The decrease in vascular resistance requires a profound increase in cardiac index in order to sustain oxygen delivery and cellular oxygen uptake. Increased vascular permeability also reduces effective arterial volume and widens capillary-cell diffusion distance, further contributing to cellular ischemia. The resulting hypotension represents both the compensatory response, attempting to increase oxygen delivery to tissue, and a pathologic response, vasodilation caused by cascading mediators, procoagulation, and platelet aggregation.

As ischemia becomes more severe, inflammation continues at the cellular level and organ dysfunction ensues. Cells increase lactate production from anaerobic metabolism of pyruvate, the ATP ionic gradient fails, and cells begin to lyse, further contributing to the stimulating signal of the SIRS cascade. Hypermetabolic demand coupled with an acute deficit in oxygen extraction and metabolic failure initiates MODS.

CELLULAR SIGNALING, SIRS, SEPSIS, AND MODS

Historically, infection has been considered the primary cause of SIRS and MODS. However, the precipitating inflammatory response may be independent of infection. The presence of a bacterial invasion identifies a septic nidus and is termed *sepsis,* however; approximately 70% of patients will have clinical signs of sepsis without an apparent bacterial invader.[13] In fact, any severe insult may stimulate the host-defense mechanisms implicated in the evolution of SIRS and MODS.

Activation of the body's host-defense mechanisms precipitates a widespread inflammatory response that is not organism specific. The innate immune system provides a first-line defense against pathogens and activates a humoral-mediated response. Systemic inflammatory response syndrome results from the effects of cytokines such as TNF-α, interleukins, and from a overwhelming proinflammatory response.[14] The evolution of an uncontrolled inflammatory response and the concomitant MODS is now recognized as a defect in cellular signaling.[15,16]

Cytokines

The first line of defense in resisting bacterial invasion is the macrophage. In addition to their phagocytic and bactericidal functions, macrophages rapidly release cytokines that activate secondary mediators of the immune system and alter the host metabolism after an inflammatory insult. Cytokines communicate messages between cells. They promote proinflammatory effects, pyogenesis and upregulation of acute-phase proteins, and an antiinflammatory response. They affect both the innate and specific (acquired) immune systems. The overlapping stimulatory and inhibitory functions among the various cytokines regulate the host's response to injury, promoting control of the invading insult and tissue repair.[17] Prolonged or exaggerated elaboration of cytokines can have deleterious effects, perpetuating SIRS and contributing to MODS. TNF, IL-1, and IL-6 have received the most attention as mediators of the inflammatory response.

TNF, primarily produced by macrophages, initiates a process that can lead to tissue injury and shock. It elicits dose-responsive hypotension, vasodilation, pyrexia, hypermetabolism, and hyperglycemia followed by hypoglycemia.[14,18,19] The major effect is on the vascular endothelium, promoting adhesion of leukocytes and stimulating further cytokine secretion. In addition, TNF is a part of the acute-phase response in which there is an alteration in the plasma protein concentrations, including increased C-reactive protein lipogenesis, lipolysis, and a decrease in albumin.[15,16] Chronic exposure to low plasma concentrations of TNF induces the wasting diathesis observed in various disease states. Evidence also implicates TNF in accelerating apoptosis, or programmed cell death.[20-22] Although programmed cell death is a homeostatic process, its acceleration via specific cell signaling accounts for the progression from SIRS to multiple organ dysfunction.

IL-1 is an additional macrophage-derived cytokine with potent biologic effects. IL-1 is pyrogenic, accelerates the basal metabolic rate, increases oxygen consumption, augments skeletal muscle catabolism and consequently releases amino acids, reduces vascular smooth muscle reactivity, and increases the induction of IL-6 synthesis.[23,24]

IL-6 contributes to proinflammatory effects in the cascade; it is a potent pyrogenic, accelerates apoptosis acceleration, and impacts hepatic acute-phase protein production.[23,25] IL-6 levels are significantly elevated in infected patients with SIRS and correlate with mortality in some shock states.[4,26] Trauma patients appear to have initial elevation, then inhibition, of TNF and a primary elevation of IL-6.[26,27] Another inflammatory cytokine, IL-8, is associated with increased lactic acid, development of disseminated intravascular coagulation (DIC), severe hypoxemia, and higher mortality in patients with severe sepsis and septic shock.[24] IL-10, an anti-inflammatory cytokine, correlates with survival after severe trauma.[27]

Complement Activation

Bacterial infection induces a complex interaction of humoral and cellular responses. The humoral response induces a primary sequence of relatively nonspecific immunologic reactions. The early responding cytokines and the acute-phase proteins such as C-reactive protein bind to antibody proteins on the cell walls of the offending organisms. Stimulation of the complement system elicits the generation of complement split products, collectively known as *anaphylatoxins.* Three of the most notable are C3a, C3b, and C5a. Both C5a and C3b possess chemotactic properties for neutrophils, macrophages, and monocytes. They serve to attract these cells to areas of inflammation, enhance their adhesiveness, and promote aggregation.[28] All three cell types protect against bacterial invasion by virtue of their ability to engulf bacteria via phagocytosis. Nevertheless, large-scale infiltration and activation of neutrophils, which occur with sepsis and trauma, can be detrimental to tissues rather than protective of them. Activated neutrophils release oxygen free radicals (superoxide, peroxide, and the hydroxyl radical) during phagocytosis. These toxic oxygen products normally serve a protective function by virtue of their bactericidal nature. However, if generated in sizable amounts, oxygen free radicals destroy cell membrane integrity, which ultimately leads to widespread tissue injury and impairment of organ function.

C3a induces leukocyte production of superoxides and causes extensive mast cell degranulation, which results in the liberation of histamine.[28] Histamine relaxes cell-to-cell junctions, permitting the extravasation of fluid into the interstitial spaces. It is for this reason that C3a has been implicated in the genesis of permeability edema, which may contribute to organ dysfunction.[4]

These events facilitate bacterial ingestion by the defending white cells, which promote changes in the bacterial cell structure as well as the external environment, fostering bacterial death and lysis. Stimulation of the complement cascade has an indirect capability of triggering the activation of other enzyme cascades. These include fibrinolysis and coagulation systems, as well as the generation of prostaglandins and leukotrienes from granulocytes. These substances behave as mediators, which modulate tissue injury during sepsis and MODS. Both IL-1 and IL-2 amplify host-defense responses by stimulation of lymphocyte propagation. Moreover, these immune responses effect blast transformation and proliferation of leukocytes and promote their migration and adherence to the invading organisms and to nonviable or damaged tissues.[28] Consequently the release of leukocyte proteases is increased, which completes the destruction of the bacteria and necrotic tissue, thereby facilitating their removal. Leukotrienes synthesized from white blood cells during this process also stimulate cellular immunity and alter the balance among suppressor, helper, and killer lymphocytes.[29]

Although cellular responses are aimed primarily at defense, sepsis and SIRS may produce an overstimulation of some of these protective mechanisms. Certain cells appear to make an abundance of substances that are postulated to intensify tissue malperfusion and injury. In a process termed "malignant inflammation," neutrophils, macrophages, lymphocytes, and perhaps platelets liberate vasoactive mediators, which may amplify the pathogenesis of the septic process as well as organ failure.

Margination of neutrophils along vascular endothelium likely leads to damage of the cells lining the blood vessels, exposure of plasma to the underlying collagen, and activation of the coagulation cascade via Hageman factor (factor

XII in the intrinsic pathway). Activated neutrophils may also cause Hageman factor formation. Hageman factor then triggers the synthesis of the vasoactive kinins. The most commonly formed is bradykinin, a potent vasodilator that also increases capillary permeability. Changes in capillary permeability and vasodilation have a role in local tissue injury and malperfusion further contributing to organ dysfunction. Activated neutrophils extrude a variety of proteases, including elastase, cathepsin G, and collagenase. These proteases degrade extracellular matrices if produced in surplus and combined with free radical production damage surrounding tissues.[28]

Neutrophils, macrophages, and monocytes all are known to synthesize metabolic products of arachidonic acid catabolism. The arachidonic acid derivatives, lipid mediators called *eicosanoids,* include the leukotrienes, prostaglandins, and thromboxane; all have been implicated in modulating the physiologic response to sepsis.

Lipid Mediators

Leukotrienes. Collectively identified as slow-reacting substances of anaphylaxis, leukotrienes (LT) LTC_4, LTD_4, and LTE_4 possess the ability to alter tissue permeability, produce bronchoconstriction, and trigger vasoconstriction in some vascular beds.[27] The exact role of leukotrienes in sepsis remains unclear. They appear to participate in regional alterations in microvascular perfusion in addition to the exacerbation of tissue edema, particularly in the lung.[30,31] Inflammation and tissue ischemia can induce generation of LTB_4, a potent chemotactic agent for leukocytes. Once formed, it fosters neutrophil aggregation with release of granular constituents.[31,32] Consequently, more neutrophils are attracted to the area. The aggregation of substantial numbers of cells promotes increased free radical production and perpetuates eicosanoid synthesis. Additionally, leukocyte clumping in the microvasculature can cause mechanical obstruction to blood flow.

Thromboxane. Thromboxane (TX), known to be elevated in trauma and sepsis, is manufactured by white blood cells and platelets, as well as by other vascular and parenchymal tissues.[29,31] An extremely potent vasoconstrictor, TXA_2 has the additional ability to aggregate both platelets and neutrophils. Once platelets aggregate, they release thromboxane, which also enhances leukocyte aggregation, thus creating a vicious cycle. Aggregation of white cells and platelets may subsequently aggravate sluggish tissue blood flow. Vasoconstriction may permit regions of malperfusion, intensifying tissue hypoxia. Thromboxane plays a significant role in microvascular thrombosis because it increases vascular resistance and tissue ischemia.[29,31]

Prostaglandin. The metabolism of arachidonic acid yields prostaglandin. Prostaglandin is further metabolized into TXA_2, prostaglandin E_2 (PGE_2), or prostaglandin I_2 (PGI_2). PGI_2 regulates the vasomotor tone and inhibits platelet aggregation, whereas PGE_2 contributes more to the antiinflammatory response in sepsis, inhibiting the cytokine response.[29,31] Prostaglandins decrease afterload, cause significant hypotension, dilate the coronary arteries, and have antiproteolytic properties.

Free Radicals. Nitric oxide (NO) is a potent free radical. In the presence of oxygen and the enzyme NO synthase (NOS), NO is produced by conversion of L-arginine to NO and citrulline. At normal production levels, NO acts as a messenger and performs as an antioxidant. At higher circulating levels, NO may become cytotoxic.[33] NO is one of the compounds implicated as a mediator of the sepsis-induced loss of vascular tone. Its potential involvement stems from its multifactorial role governing interactions among platelets, leukocytes, and vascular endothelium and as an endogenous vasodilator. Besides its effects on vascular tone, NO is involved in other processes considered beneficial to the septic patient. These include inactivation of oxygen free radicals, prevention of microvascular thrombi, inhibition of platelet aggregation and leukocyte adhesion, bronchodilation, and protection of myocardium from ischemic damage.[34] Nitrate and nitrite are the inactive and stable end products of NO production. Plasma concentrations of nitrate and nitrite are elevated in septic patients.

Cellular products of gram-negative (endotoxin) and gram-positive bacteria generate inducible nitric oxide (iNOS) through a cytokine-mediated process. NO formed by endothelial iNOS is an important regulator of tissue blood flow and plays an essential role in cardiovascular function. Inhibition of the NOS pathway, for example by glucocorticoids, would be anticipated to raise blood pressure and systemic vascular resistance in septic patients. However, in studies using an NOS inhibitor, cardiac index is reduced, heart rate decreases, and pulmonary vascular resistance increases. These changes are detrimental to the patient in hypodynamic septic shock, because inhibition of NOS may aggravate tissue hypoperfusion.[34] Thus indiscriminate inhibition of NO production may cause more harm than good. Selective inhibition of iNOS to limit the deleterious effects of NO may provide a better therapeutic approach.

Patients with persistent inflammation present initially with an overwhelming inflammatory cascade response. The most common cause of inflammatory stimulation is the local release of bacteria or other toxic mediators. Central to the patient's ability to combat a bacterial insult is the immune response. The immune system limits the spread of the pathogen, augments the flux of immune cells, and modulates the host's metabolism to enhance the environment necessary for the destruction of bacteria. These changes are mediated by the factors secreted by cells of the immune system. Complement system fragments are pivotal in the synthesis of cellular and humoral mediators associated with sepsis and MODS. Severe bacterial invasion results in an excessive release of the mediators eliciting a shock state in which inadequate tissue perfusion may lead to organ damage. Further stimulation and generation of cytokines increases the inflammatory response. The cytokines directly affect the organs and act through secondary mediators. The secondary mediators promote both proinflammatory and antiinflammatory responses, adhesion of molecules on the endothelial cells, and migration of these molecules into the extravascular space, causing additional microvascular and tissue injury. The endothelial injury activates the extrinsic pathway and may lead to consumptive coagulopathy and fibrin deposition. White cell and red cell clotting, along with alterations in vascular tone, contribute to the cardiovascular manifestations and systemic deficits noted in inflammatory shock states, such as SIRS and septic shock.

Clinical Evaluation of Sepsis and Hypovolemic Shock

Patients with sepsis and hypovolemic shock, specifically hemorrhagic shock, may develop MODS, which continues to be a common cause of death in severely injured trauma patients. The continuum of the inflammatory response and the introduction of a bacterial nidus presents in a significant pattern. Despite advances in therapy and aggressive interventions, mortality from septic shock continues to be high.

Patterns of Response

Hyperdynamic Septic State

Sepsis is characterized by increased oxygen requirements, which must be met with augmented oxygen delivery. Elevated cardiac index and minute ventilation are required to sustain increased oxygen delivery. Mechanisms that augment cardiac index include an increase in heart rate and vasodilation. The combination of an increased cardiac index with decreased vascular resistance characterizes the hyperdynamic cardiovascular state associated with sepsis. This hyperdynamic state is necessary to meet the high cellular energy demands required to defend against the insult and maintain normal organ function.[34] Although cardiac function is normally maintained, patients may present with myocardial dysfunction. Survival depends on the patient's ability to mount a hyperdynamic response.

Research illustrates that decreased ejection fraction, ventricular dilation, and weakened contractile response to volume loading are common characteristics of the impaired cardiac function in septic patients.[35,36] It has been suggested that the etiology of this depressed function is related to myocardial edema, alterations in sarcolemmal or intracellular calcium homeostasis, and disruption of β–adrenergic signal transduction, and is less likely due to myocardial ischemia.[36] A number of cytokines, such as prostanoids, platelet-activating factor, TNF, IL-1, and IL-2, as well as NO have been proposed to contribute to the cardiac depression seen in these patients.[22] As cardiac index and ejection fraction fall, the body attempts to compensate for reduced blood flow to the peripheral tissues by increasing oxygen extraction, leading to a widening of the arteriovenous oxygen content gradient. Hypotension and acidosis may occur if the cardiac depression is severe enough to limit oxygen delivery to the tissues or there is a cellular extraction deficit. In the septic state, the increased cardiac index appears to support cell function for a time; however, transition from a high to low cardiac output state contributes to the perpetuation of sepsis-related SIRS, maldistribution of flow, and hypoperfusion of tissue beds, and thus progression to MODS.

In addition to myocardial depression, sepsis-related mediator release induces reduced systemic vascular resistance. In a large number of patients, hypotension is unresponsive to treatment with vasopressive agents or fluid resuscitation. There may be a downregulation of alpha-adrenergic receptors secondary to the high levels of circulating catecholamines. At the microvascular level, disturbances in endothelial function give rise to increased permeability of capillaries and maldistribution of blood flow, reducing tissue perfusion and potentially causing parenchymal cell damage. Subsequent fluid extravasation widens the capillary-cell diffusion gradient and further limits cellular oxygen extraction. Both vasodilation, caused by mediators such as histamine, kinins, and prostaglandins, and vasoconstriction (e.g., as a result of thromboxane and TNF release) contribute to maldistribution of perfusion. The combined result is profound oxygen deficiency and cellular dysfunction.

Anoxia, Hypoxia, and Ischemia

Differentiation of anoxia, hypoxia, and ischemia is important. Although all three conditions result in diminished oxygen delivery to the tissues, the consequences of each condition with regard to energy metabolism are different. In the strictest sense, anoxia is defined as an absence of oxygen where blood flow is either normal or increased. In hypoxia, the arterial oxygen content is decreased, but blood flow is maintained at normal values. Primarily, inadequate hemoglobin or SaO_2 and PaO_2 reduce oxygen transport. Ischemia is caused by decreased blood flow, which results in inadequate oxygen delivery. Ischemia differs from anoxia and hypoxia in that oxygen content is normal but blood flow is curtailed. An ischemic condition may exist when (1) blood flow falls below that required to meet the normal energy needs at rest, (2) blood flow fails to augment oxygen delivery in response to an increased oxidative demand, or (3) capillary perfusion is altered by humoral and chemical substances. Reduced blood flow also results in hypoperfused capillary beds and leads to accumulation of potentially harmful metabolic products in the surrounding tissues.[5,6] These metabolic products, such as lactate or long-chain fatty acyl esters, are toxic to the cell and promote further damage. Therefore, ischemia may be a more detrimental insult than hypoxia or anoxia alone. The toxic metabolic byproducts encourage surrounding cell failure, and when reperfusion through previously shunted capillary beds does occur, these products are "washed out," causing damage even to distant tissues.

PHYSIOLOGIC MONITORING

Monitoring alterations in cardiac function, oxygen delivery, and metabolic response has become a standard by which to evaluate the physiologic response and effectiveness of management of posttraumatic shock and sepsis. Traditional end points for medical management of shock—that is, return of arterial blood pressure, heart rate, and urine output to normal—are inadequate. Hypoperfusion may be masked by normal vital signs in compensated shock states.[4,5,37] Specific methods for monitoring tissue oxygenation may provide a more focused perspective on peripheral perfusion and resolution of oxygen debt.

Oxygen Delivery and Debt

In the initial presentation of traumatic shock, both the delivery of oxygen and the oxygen extraction are affected. Hemorrhagic hypovolemia profoundly decreases DaO_2, and oxygen extraction dramatically increases in an attempt to meet oxidative requirements. Oxygen debt, the difference between cellular oxygen requirement and the actual cellular oxygen consumption, may result. Perfusion and oxygen uptake must be restored to prevent or reverse ischemia and to prevent cell death (Figure 13-7). If it is not, organ function may become unrecoverable. Clinical evidence of oxygen deficit includes a reduction of oxygen consumption, rising serum lactate concentration and base deficit, and derangement of other metabolic indicators. Early evidence suggested increasing oxygen delivery to supranormal levels during resuscitation from traumatic shock was superior as a means of repaying the oxygen deficit.[38] Recent research has shown conflicting results. Supranormal oxygen delivery was defined as achieving predetermined goals of a cardiac index greater than 4.5 L/min/m^2, oxygen delivery index greater than 600 L/min/m^2, and oxygen consumption index greater than 170 L/min/m^2. This approach may actually contribute to increased mortality. All patients do not benefit from a supranormal resuscitation; rather, survival is more dependent on the patient's ability to respond to therapy or mount a response to the insult.[5,38-40]

In sepsis, current evidence supports use of early goal-directed therapy.[41] Rapid initiation of a protocol that included administration of fluids, inotropes, vasoactive agents and/or red blood cells to achieve preestablished desired end points for central venous pressure, mean arterial pressure, and central venous oxygen saturation resulted in a 16% reduction of in-hospital mortality in patients admitted with sepsis/SIRS.[41]

EVALUATION OF OXYGEN UTILIZATION

Monitoring tissue oxygen consumption is an essential aspect of the clinical evaluation and management of critically ill trauma patients and is described in detail in Chapter 14. Formulas, normal values, and clinical parameters used to assess oxygen delivery and utilization are summarized in Tables 13-1, 13-3, and 13-4.

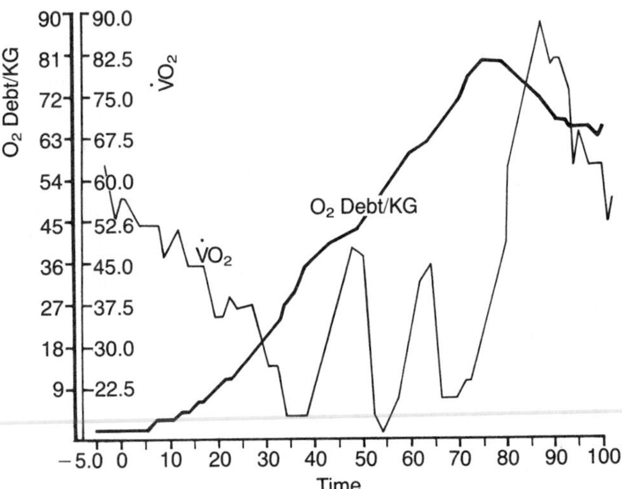

FIGURE 13-7 As oxygen consumption falls, the oxygen debt gradually accumulates. With resuscitation, oxygen consumption exceeds the baseline demands, and the oxygen debt is gradually repaid.

Global Oxygenation Monitoring

Mixed Venous Blood Gases. Oxygen availability is the most important determinant of viable oxidative energy metabolism. Cellular oxygen consumption is influenced by the availability of oxygen delivered via the microcirculation and extraction of oxygen from the capillaries to meet cellular oxygen requirements. Most organ systems use less than 50% of the available arterial oxygen. The exception is the myocardium, which extracts nearly 80% of the available oxygen in a single pass.

A reduction in oxygen delivery results in several characteristic changes. A decline in blood flow results in a greater extraction of arterial oxygen. Mixed venous blood gases from the pulmonary artery (SvO_2) and central venous oxygen saturation ($ScvO_2$) measurements from a triple-lumen catheter may be used to evaluate the oxyhemoglobin reservoir after cellular uptake of dissolved oxygen and subsequent release of oxygen from hemoglobin to keep the dissolved oxygen relatively constant. These are global indicators of oxygen consumption at the cellular level. Use of central venous oxygen saturation as a measure of global tissue oxygen supply-demand balance appears to be a valuable therapeutic guide in early resuscitation of sepsis.[34,41]

Lactic Acid. In most forms of shock, plasma lactate concentration correlates with the quantity of anaerobic metabolism and hypoperfusion. During shock, when tissue oxygenation is reduced, mitochondrial respiration shifts to anaerobic metabolism. The cellular fuel, pyruvate, rather than being converted into acetyl coenzyme A and subsequently entering into the tricarboxylic acid cycle, is metabolized to lactate. The continued hydrolysis of ATP by cellular processes produces excessive protons, yielding a metabolic acid. Increasing oxygen delivery is a means to reverse the anaerobic processes, which is evidenced by normalization of elevated plasma lactate concentrations (greater than 2 mmol/L). Patients who are unable to normalize their lactate level within 24 to 48 hours have an increased mortality.[9-11] Lactate levels may remain elevated in septic patients secondary to reduced hepatic uptake and renal elimination.[42] Sequential lactate measurements are useful as an indicator of cellular stress, response to resuscitation, and prognosis in trauma patients.[9,11,42-44]

Base Deficit. Base deficit is an indirect, calculated measure of tissue acidosis. The measurement of base deficit is related to the amount of base in millimoles required to titrate a liter of whole blood to a pH of 7.40. Base deficit correlates with the response to resuscitation and is a reasonable predictor of survival.[11] However, an increased base deficit has no predictive value in the presence of a normal lactate level.[45]

Regional Oxygen Monitoring

As discussed, blood flow and perfusion are not uniformly distributed to all organs. Investigators suggest that it is advantageous to identify and monitor those tissue beds that are significantly at risk for hypoperfusion in shock. Following stabilization, regional variables have been shown to be important predictors of mortality when compared to global oxygen-monitoring parameters.[44]

Optical Spectroscopy. Optical spectroscopy examines the chemical characteristics of substances by measuring the alterations of light in various parts of the spectrum. This technology may be used to assess tissue and cellular oxygenation.[42] It measures the oxygen saturation of hemoglobin in the microcirculatory blood, the cellular mitochondrial energy state, and the oxygen pressure in the plasma. Although this technology is noninvasive, at this time quantitative measurements are unattainable, making clinical inferences difficult.[42]

Orthogonal Polarization Spectral Imaging. Orthogonal polarization spectral (OPS) imaging provides quantitative measurements of diameter, flow velocity, and functional capillary density for various tissue beds and provides valuable information on the adequacy of microvascular perfusion.[42,45] The technology has been incorporated into a small probe that is placed on the tissue to be imaged. (e.g., sublingual vascular bed). In sepsis, it can distinguish between normal, slow, and hyperdynamic flow patterns.[45] In hemorrhagic shock, OPS data from the sublingual tissue bed have been extrapolated to reflect perfusion changes in internal organs such as the intestine and liver.[42] This noninvasive technology has the potential to provide valuable information for assessment of microcirculatory flow patterns.

Intramucosal pHi. Reduced splanchnic perfusion is an early response to hypoperfusion in shock.[46] Tonometry, used to evaluate perfusion of the gastric or intestinal mucosal bed, serves as a measure of splanchnic perfusion and may allow early detection of systemic hypoperfusion.[46] Evaluation of gut perfusion via measurement of gastric mucosal pH (pHi) is based on the assumption that gastric mucosal bicarbonate equals serum bicarbonate. Intramucosal measurement of hydrogen ions may be measured with saline or air tonometry and used to calculate pHi. Reduced blood flow to the gastrointestinal mucosa causes anaerobic metabolism in these tissue beds and thus, a decrease in pHi. Early identification of altered perfusion provides an opportunity to optimize resuscitation efforts and more rapidly reverse oxygen debt accumulation.

For some patient populations, gastric pHi may be predictive of outcome; however, parameters have not proved to be consistently predictive.[44,46] In addition, gastric arterial CO_2 gradient and pHi are more difficult to interpret in patients with sepsis, as an alteration in these values may not reflect global tissue oxygenation.[46] Thus, clinical interpretation of the values and use as a guide during resuscitative efforts are difficult.

Local Oxygen Monitoring

Near infrared spectroscopy (NIRS) provides a noninvasive method for monitoring oxidized cytochrome aa_3. Cytochrome aa_3, when oxygenated, changes its absorption spectra and has been shown to measure local tissue blood flow and oxygen utilization at the cellular level. Lower tissue oxygen saturation values may indicate the need for further resuscitation.[6] The advantages of NIRS are that it is noninvasive and demonstrates potential as a method of monitoring regional oxygenation in a number of tissues during shock.[6]

Hemodynamic Monitoring

The management of multi-injured trauma patients may be guided, in part, by parameters measured by a pulmonary artery catheter (PAC), which evaluates cardiac output, RAP, pulmonary artery pressures, and PAOP, and provides intermittent or continuous measurement of mixed venous blood gases and pH. An assumption underlying PAC data interpretation is that changes indicative of left ventricular function will be reflected by the right-sided heart catheter. In a cardiac failure patient, without preexisting pulmonary disease, this assumption typically is true. However, the information is influenced by changes in the compliance of the right and left sides of the heart, intrathoracic pressures, the compliance of the pulmonary vasculature, and cardiac valve integrity. The PAOP provides an estimation of left ventricular preload; however, it also may be beneficial in evaluating right ventricular ejection fraction and end-diastolic volume to assess the adequacy of preload. In the previously healthy trauma patient, the importance of evaluating the right side of the heart is at least as significant as assessment of left ventricular function.[47,48] Evaluation of end-diastolic volume as it relates to the Frank-Starling mechanism (i.e., increasing initial myocardial fiber length to enhance contractile force and stroke volume) is an established principle that may aid in the resuscitation of trauma and septic patients. Careful interpretation of elevated PAOP, RAP, and pulmonary artery pressures is warranted in the presence of a high cardiac index, arterial hypotension, or hypoperfusion as evidenced by metabolic indicators of tissue hypoxia and oxygen debt accumulation (e.g., high lactate level). Since PAC-derived parameters are affected by ventricular compliance, pulmonary vascular vasoconstriction, and airway pressure, PAOP and RAP may not be reliable indicators of end-diastolic volume and preload.[47,49,50] Other traditional markers of adequate resuscitation, such as blood pressure, heart rate, and urine output, are also unreliable as indicators of intravascular and end-diastolic volumes.[49,51]

Earlier studies noted a high incidence of right ventricular dysfunction in the trauma and shock population. This is possibly related to increased right ventricular stress and volume overload secondary to acute pulmonary hypertension.[50,52] An associated elevation of PAOP more likely is due to pulmonary hypertension and the inability of the right ventricle to adjust contractile tension to volume and resistance loads, causing a leftward shift of the intraventricular septum and reducing left ventricular compliance. Right ventricular end-diastolic volume index, therefore, may be a more appropriate indicator of ventricular preload than traditional PAOP.[48,50] A specialty volumetric PAC can be used to calculate right ventricular end-diastolic index.

Initially the trauma patient in hemorrhagic hypovolemic shock displays symptoms of tachycardia, hypotension, base deficit, low PAOP and RAP, low stroke volume index, and poor tissue perfusion (e.g., decreased capillary refill time, low urine output, change in mentation). After appropriate volume resuscitation, the patient will generally improve and metabolic indicators of oxygen debt accumulation normalize. Subsets of trauma patients do not improve or have a secondary nidus that triggers SIRS. These patients develop cellular hypoxia and organ dysfunction as a result of humoral mediator and oxygen free radical release, capillary endothelial changes, reduction in ATP production, and mitochondrial dysfunction. Their clinical presentation subsequently includes an increasing cardiac index, reduced systemic vascular resistance, tachycardia, normal to low RAP and PAOP, and metabolic acidosis. As shock or SIRS progresses, cardiac index continues to be elevated; RAP, PA pressures, and PAOP increase; and severe metabolic acidosis ensues.

Recently, arterial-based technologies for monitoring cardiac output have become available and are known as *arterial pressure cardiac output* (APCO). These technologies use arterial pressure or pulse waveforms to determine stroke volume. Arterial pressure–based stroke volume is derived from the aortic pulse pressure, the difference between systolic pressure and diastolic pressure.[53] Aortic pulse pressure is proportional to SV. CO is determined by arterial pulsations (heart rate) multiplied by the SV. One such device has the capability to compensate for changes in the patient's vascular tone through internal waveform analysis. The APCO technology provides alternative parameters to assess fluid status. These include systolic pressure variation (SPV), stroke volume variation (SVV), and pulse pressure variation (PPV). These parameters provide an objective assessment of the patient's response to fluid resuscitation. The end users of this technology must be alert to factors that alter the pressure waveforms and subsequently produce unreliable values.

Other methods for evaluating cardiac output, ventricular function, and intravascular volume are available. These include esophageal Doppler, impedance cardiography, and echocardiography; however, their use is less common than other devices in the trauma population and further research is warranted.

Metabolic Changes Associated with Impaired Oxygen Delivery

Reduction in oxygen availability leaves intermediates in the electron-transport chain in a more reduced state. Phosphorylation of ADP via oxidative phosphorylation ceases despite reduced ATP and increased ADP concentrations (Figure 13-8). Creatine phosphate concentrations decline by 80% to 90% within minutes, followed by a slower decline in ATP.[54,55]

This imbalance between energy production and energy utilization results in altered adenine nucleotide metabolism. Initially, high-energy phosphates stored as creatine phosphate are utilized to maintain cellular ATP concentrations near normal. However, the amount of high-energy phosphates the cell can store is limited, and creatine phosphate concentrations are depleted within 5 minutes of the onset of ischemia. After the depletion of creatine phosphate, ATP concentrations begin to fall. The reduction in ATP concentrations is accompanied by a rise in ADP and AMP. As the duration of ischemia is increased, this alteration becomes more pronounced. In addition, there is a fall in the sum of the adenine nucleotides (ATP + ADP + AMP). The concen-

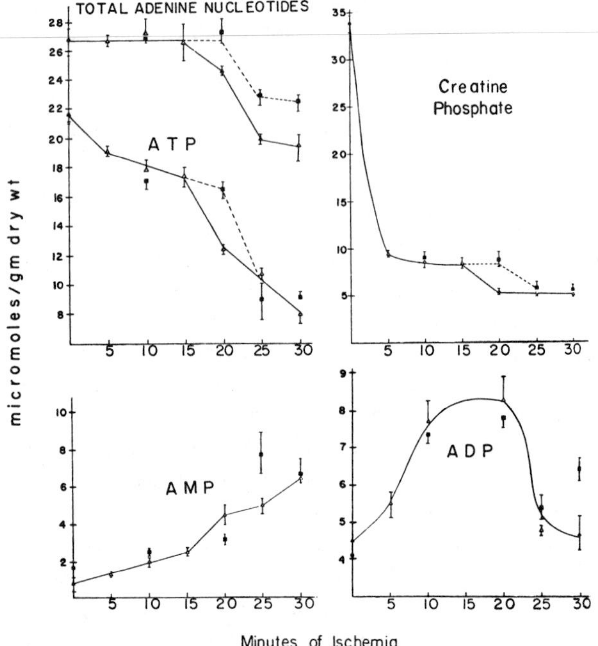

FIGURE 13-8 Effect of ischemia on tissue adenine nucleotide and creatine phosphate concentrations. Hearts were perfused with Krebs-Henseleit solution, supplemented with either glucose *(triangles)* or glucose plus acetate *(squares)* for a 15-minute equilibration period. The hearts were then exposed to a period of severe global ischemia and rapidly frozen. *(From Vary TC, Angelakos ET, Schaffer SW: Relationship between adenine nucleotide metabolism and irreversible tissue damage in isolated perfused rat heart,* Circ Res *45[2]:220, 1979.)*

tration of adenine nucleotides may be of importance in maintaining cell viability, as well as in the ability of the cell to recover normal function after restoration of normal blood flow (Figure 13-9).[54,55]

During ischemia, the breakdown of ATP for cellular metabolic needs leads to relatively high cellular concentrations of hypoxanthine and xanthine. Reoxygenation of the ischemic area presents oxygen to the large pools of substrate or the enzyme xanthine oxidase, which is felt to be contained in the capillary endothelium. As a result, the capillary endothelium of the compromised tissues is showered with superoxide free radicals. Once the initial xanthine oxidase–mediated capillary injury has occurred, complement activation can attract leukocytes to the affected area, resulting in cellular death. The monitoring of xanthine oxidase may be used as an indicator of tissue oxygenation in the future.

Simple oxygen deficiency does not itself cause irreversible tissue damage. If the oxygen supply is restored within several minutes, both ATP synthesis and tissue function return to normal. However, if the reduction in oxygen supply is continued, the tissue becomes irreversibly damaged (Figure 13-10). Because ATP functions as the energy source, much attention has been focused on the role of ATP in reperfusion. Reperfusion and restoration of oxygen delivery to ischemic tissue result in the rapid resynthesis of creatine phosphate, but ATP concentrations may remain depressed.

Although a relationship between survival and oxygen deficit has been demonstrated,[56,57] perhaps a finer relationship can be drawn between oxygen deficit and morphologic and functional injury to cells. It appears that as ischemia worsens cellular perfusion, there is intracellular accumulation of lactic acid and hydrogen ions. Eventually changes in

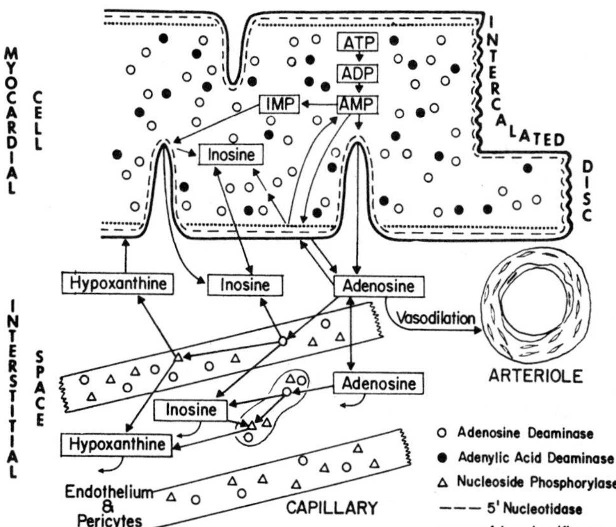

FIGURE 13-9 Formation, fate, and site of action of adenosine. The distribution of the different enzymes involved in the metabolism of adenosine is illustrated by the different symbols defined at the right of the diagram. *(From Rubio R, Wiedmeier T, Berne RM: Nucleoside phosphorylase: localization and role in myocardial distribution of purines,* Am J Physiol *222[3]:554, 1972.)*

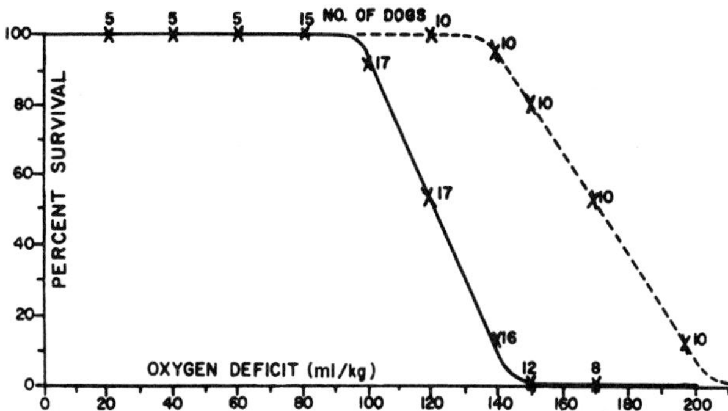

FIGURE 13-10 The total oxygen deficit has been shown to be an excellent quantitative predictor of survival after hemorrhagic shock in the dog model. The *solid line* shows the survival rate for control animals at various oxygen deficits; the *dashed line* shows the survival rate for digitalized animals. *(From Crowell JW, Smith EE: Oxygen deficit and irreversible hemorrhagic shock, Am J Physiol 206:313, 1964.)*

cell membrane and function occur, followed by influx of sodium and potassium extrusion. This causes increased activity of sodium-potassium ATPase. As discussed earlier, there is a decreased production of ATP during ischemia. Consequently, the balance of the intracellular environment is disrupted, leading to intracellular swelling. Mitochondria and cell organelles are disrupted, which ultimately results in cell death.

Nutrient Substrate Flux in Trauma and Sepsis

There is a fine balance between anabolism, the building up of energy stores, and catabolism, the breakdown of these energy stores. The adaptive ability of the body to use alternative fuels instead of glucose is of fundamental importance to the survival of the individual. This is because certain cells, such as erythrocytes and cells of the renal medulla and central nervous system, have an absolute requirement for glucose, amounting to approximately 180 g/day. Less than half this demand can be supplied simply by the breakdown of glycogen to glucose in the liver. However, the liver and, to some extent, the kidneys synthesize glucose from different carbon sources via the process of gluconeogenesis. Glucose is synthesized from glycerol, lactate, pyruvate, and certain amino acids. Glycerol is obtained from adipose tissue after the breakdown of triglycerides. Lactate and pyruvate are derived primarily from skeletal muscle tissue secondary to the breakdown of skeletal muscle glycogen. Amino acids are derived from protein degradation, particularly in skeletal muscle.

When reduced oxygen supply limits oxidative energy production, ATP produced glycolytically via substrate phosphorylation is increased. In cardiac muscle, the maximal rate of glycolytically produced ATP represents only about 25% of the normal energy requirements. In ischemia, there is a transient increase in glycolysis that results primarily from the breakdown of glycogen. However, if flow is reduced to a low enough level, the transient increase in glycolysis is succeeded by an inhibition of glycolysis to a rate about 10% the rate observed in anoxia. The mechanism responsible for this difference between ischemia and anoxia appears to be related to the buildup of metabolic products in ischemia.[54,55] ATP production through glycolysis becomes restricted by the accumulation of metabolic products, particularly lactate, which are not removed from the ischemic tissue during poor perfusion.

Although oxygen can become rate limiting for energy production, a reduction in blood flow also decreases the delivery of carbon substrates for oxidative metabolism. In anoxia, the tissues are oxygen deficient, but flow is fast enough to remove metabolic products and prevent glycolytic inhibition. Under these conditions, glycolysis is maximally stimulated. However, when flow is reduced, glycolysis becomes inhibited. This suggests that glycolytic inhibition during ischemia is more dependent on flow than on oxygen availability.[2] Oxidation of fatty acids is inhibited in proportion to decreased availability and is not flow dependent other than to the extent that flow affects oxygen delivery.

CATABOLISM

Physiologic monitoring of the septic patient has demonstrated that the normal balance between anabolic and catabolic processes is altered in the direction of catabolic metabolism.[58-60] This results in pathologic alterations in glucose, fatty acid, and amino acid (protein) metabolism, often manifested clinically by mild hyperglycemia, a rise in serum triglycerides, and changes in plasma amino acid and acute-phase protein concentrations. The degree of metabolic dysfunction reflects the extent of organ dysfunction induced by invading organisms or traumatic injury. The pattern of alterations in the plasma concentrations of these fuels is superimposed over changes in the plasma concentration of hormones and cytokines.[61] Both trauma and sepsis initiate a pattern of physiologic and metabolic adaptation characterized initially by an increase in protein metabolism.[62,63] The interwoven network of responses to inflammation is designed to limit the extent of damage elicited by the initial insult. Virtually every organ system of the body becomes affected and displays recognizable metabolic alterations.

HORMONAL CHANGES

Typically, sepsis is characterized by a fall in the thyroid hormone T_3, whereas the other stress hormones (cortisol, epinephrine, and glucagon) are elevated. Glucagon concentrations rise to extraordinarily high levels. Although the rise in glucagon is accompanied by a rise in immunoassayable insulin, the insulin/glucagon ratio is reversed compared with its value in the postabsorptive state. This reversal of the insulin/glucagon ratio may be responsible in part for the accelerated rate of glucose production by the liver in sepsis. Both insulin and glucagon have immediate and delayed effects on hepatic glucose metabolism.

Catecholamines also stimulate both glycogenolysis and gluconeogenesis. The levels of plasma catecholamines, epinephrine, and norepinephrine have been demonstrated to rise progressively with increasing severity of injury.[61-64] Both epinephrine and norepinephrine rise to levels considered high enough to produce metabolic changes. In this regard, plasma epinephrine concentrations are more important for stimulating hyperglycemia than is the severity of the injury.

The stimulation of hepatic output of glucose by epinephrine involves the breakdown of glucagon with the release of glucose. However, changes in the hormonal milieu are not solely responsible for enhanced gluconeogenesis in sepsis. Unlike other pathologic conditions, such as starvation or diabetes, in sepsis, gluconeogenesis is not suppressed by the infusion of glucose.[59,65] This lack of response to glucose has been proposed to occur as a result of enhanced and continual delivery of gluconeogenic precursors, namely lactate, alanine, glycine, serine, and glycerol, from peripheral tissues.[59]

Insulin Resistance

Abnormally high serum glucose is commonly observed after traumatic injury, burn, shock, or sepsis despite normal or accentuated insulin secretion. The primary sites of insulin resistance are in systemic tissues, particularly skeletal muscle and adipose tissue, where insulin stimulates glucose uptake. Evidence suggests that the insulin concentration is the same or increased in sepsis as no anti-insulin antibodies have been detected. At the receptor level, alterations in receptor affinity or receptor number also would decrease the biologic response for a given plasma insulin concentration. However, the sensitivity of the receptor to circulating insulin appears to be normal.[65-68] The septic process seems to inhibit the initial steps in the signal transduction pathway for insulin.

With regard to the potential mediators responsible for the sepsis-induced insulin resistance, evidence indicates a potential link between TNF and insulin resistance. First, plasma concentrations of TNF-alpha are increased after infection.[68,69] Second, TNF blocks the action of insulin through its ability to inhibit insulin receptor tyrosine kinase activity.[70-72] Third, obesity-induced insulin resistance is prevented in mice lacking a functional TNF response.[73] Fourth, inhibition of TNF secretion improves insulin action limiting skeletal muscle catabolism and lactate production after infection.[74]

Regulation of Glucose Metabolism

Variations in carbohydrate metabolism after severe trauma and during sepsis include hyperglycemia, increased gluconeogenesis, elevated blood lactate, and insulin resistance. Hyperglycemia and hyperlactatemia are frequent manifestations of the human metabolic response to sepsis and are implicated in the clinical development of the process.[9,62,69] Sepsis-induced hyperlactatemia with concomitant acidosis is most easily explained when the septic shock episode is associated with tissue ischemia secondary to hypoperfusion. Under these circumstances, augmenting oxygen delivery by increasing volume resuscitation and cardiac index reduces the lactate production.[39-41,75,76]

In contrast to the hypodynamic septic state, the hemodynamically stable, hyperdynamic, and hypermetabolic phase of sepsis is characterized by an elevated cardiac index and augmented oxygen consumption, maintenance of normal high-energy phosphate contents in skeletal muscle, and normal lactate/pyruvate ratios.[77] Enhancing oxygen delivery does not decrease plasma lactate concentration in these patients.[78,79] The failure of plasma lactate concentrations to abate after increasing oxygen delivery indicates that metabolic abnormalities other than inadequate oxygen delivery are responsible for the elevation of serum lactate.[59] Thus, hyperlactatemia results from altered control of glucose metabolic pathways rather than a deficit in oxygen availability in the hyperdynamic septic patient.

Lactate Metabolism

The plasma lactate concentration represents a balance between the rate of lactate production and its utilization. The liver and kidney are primarily responsible for uptake and utilization of lactate, whereas systemic tissues such as skeletal muscle represent the major sites of lactate production. Lactate that diffuses into the bloodstream is carried to the liver, where it is taken up and either oxidized or converted into glucose. Release of lactate from skeletal muscle, its transport and removal from the blood, and its subsequent synthesis into glucose by the liver represents an interorgan physiologic pathway.[59] An imbalance in metabolism will lead to changes in the plasma concentration. The increased lactate production by skeletal muscle provides the necessary gluconeogenic precursors for maintenance of sustained rates of gluconeogenesis in sepsis.[77,80] Lactate production exceeds its use, accounting for elevated plasma lactate concentrations in sepsis.

Pyruvate Dehydrogenase Complex. Impaired glucose oxidation in conjunction with normal or increased lactate, alanine, or pyruvate production suggests a specific inhibition of the pyruvate dehydrogenase (PDH) reaction in sepsis. The PDH complex catalyzes the mitochondrial decarboxylation of pyruvate into acetyl CoA, which is a key participant in glucose homeostasis[77,80] (Figure 13-11). Mediators responsible for the inhibition of PDH complex during sepsis remain unclear. TNF is implicated as playing a pivotal role in mediating some of the adverse metabolic responses to sepsis. Reduction of TNF secretion prevents inhibition of the PDH complex and attenuates hyperlactatemia.[74,80]

Hyperlactatemia in Sepsis. Altered lactate metabolism plays an important role in the development and clinical complications of sepsis. Hyperlactatemia is a prognostic indictor of organ failure and mortality in critically ill septic patients.[9,10,75,81] Sepsis-induced hyperlactatemia can be easily explained when tissue ischemia exists. In the hyperdynamic, hypermetabolic state of sepsis, oxygen consumption and oxygen delivery are increased, with adequate tissue perfusion and maintenance of normal high-energy phosphate concentrations. Hyperlactatemia is present under conditions in which tissue oxygen delivery is elevated. The ratio of lactate to pyruvate is unchanged, suggesting that the increased plasma lactate does not result from inadequate oxygen delivery. Increased plasma lactate concentrations in sepsis result from either an increased production of lactate or altered metabolism of lactate, or both. As previously discussed, the liver is the major organ responsible for lactate clearance by the body. Lactate taken up by the liver is synthesized to glucose by the pathway of gluconeogenesis. Although the rate of glucose production by the liver is increased in sepsis, the rate of lactate delivery may exceed the capacity for gluconeogenesis. The sepsis-induced increases in plasma lactate probably result from a combination of metabolic abnormalities. Sepsis-induced alterations of skeletal muscle carbohydrate metabolism include increased glucose uptake, accelerated lactate production, and decreased glucose oxidation in muscle.

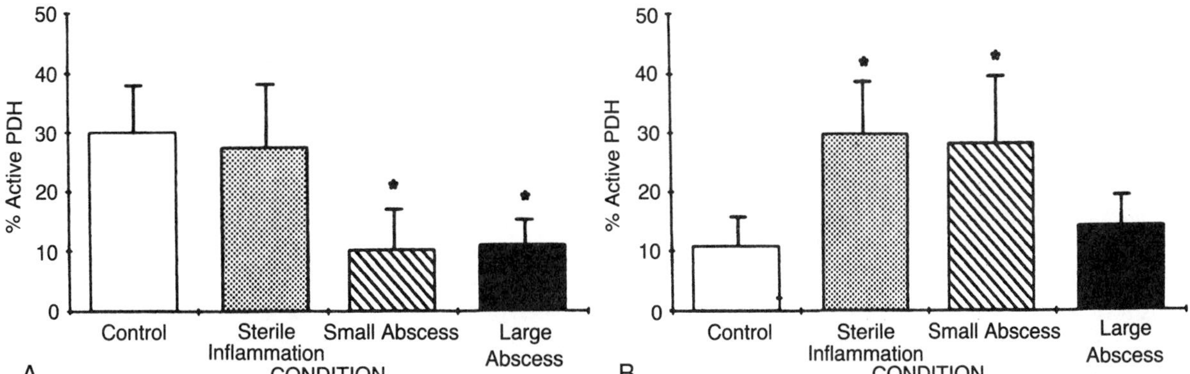

FIGURE 13-11 Effect of sepsis on activity of pyruvate dehydrogenase complex in skeletal muscle (**A**) and liver (**B**). Skeletal muscle and liver samples were frozen in situ 5 days after intraabdominal introduction of a rat fecal agar pellet. Four groups of animals were used: control (no pellet); sterile inflammation (no bacterial inoculation); small septic abscess (*Bacteroides fragilis* 10^8/ml + *Escherichia coli* 10^6/ml; 0.8 ml pellet); and large septic abscess (*B. fragilis* 10^8/ml + *E. coli* 10^2/ml; 1.5 ml pellet). Extracts of frozen tissue were assayed for active and total pyruvate dehydrogenase (PDH) activity in duplicate. Results are presented as a percentage of total PDH complex existing in active form. Values shown are means ± SE for 10 to 14 animals.
* $P < 0.005$ versus control, Scheffe's analysis for all contrasts. *(From Vary TC, Siegel JH, Nakatani T et al: Effect of sepsis on activity of pyruvate dehydrogenase complex in skeletal muscle and liver,* Am J Physiol *250[6 Pt 1]:E636, 1986.)*

Altered Skeletal Muscle Protein Metabolism

In addition to its role in locomotion and respiration, skeletal muscle, by virtue of its mass in relation to body weight, represents the major reservoir of amino acids (Figure 13-12). Some of these amino acids are important substrates for gluconeogenesis in liver. A hallmark of the septic response is the rapid erosion of lean body mass. The imbalance in protein metabolism leading to loss of lean body mass is manifested by excretion of urea, resulting in a significant negative nitrogen balance. The septic condition initiates a severe catabolic response.[58-60] Positive nitrogen balance in septic patients cannot be achieved through aggressive nutritional support alone. Nitrogen and body protein losses may occur over the course of a septic episode (see Chapter 17). Because skeletal muscle comprises approximately 45% of body weight, the sepsis-induced whole-body negative nitrogen balance reflects increases in net catabolism in this tissue. Mobilization of amino acids from skeletal muscle results from an increase in proteolysis or a decrease in protein synthesis. The relative contribution of protein synthesis and proteolysis to the overall net catabolic state in muscle varies depending on the severity of the septic insult. In this regard, protein synthesis is reduced to the same extent regardless of the severity of the septic insult, whereas protein degradation continues to accelerate as the septic episode worsens. The persistent loss of large amounts of protein in sepsis leads to organ system dysfunction and eventually organ failure. Clinical implications of continued loss of skeletal muscle protein in septic patients include poor wound healing, loss of muscle strength, diminished muscle activity, and, if severe enough, death.

Increased net proteolysis results in the release of amino acids from structural protein stores, particularly in skeletal muscle. The protein economy of the whole body can be estimated by monitoring the nitrogen balance. This catabolic phase is an intrinsic response to trauma and sepsis, with the amount of muscle loss exceeding that simply because of bed rest. The catabolic phase can abate within a few days of injury, followed by the restoration of positive nitrogen balance and lean body mass. In the septic hyperdynamic state, the catabolic phase may continue, even when nutritional support is provided.

Mediators of Proteolysis. A certain amount of muscle catabolism in the trauma patient can be attributed to direct injury to the muscle, with subsequent repair of the damaged tissues. However, enhanced catabolism also occurs in the septic patient with no overt signs of direct tissue trauma. The metabolic milieu of the septic host is complex. The catabolism of muscle is probably the net result of interactions between multiple mediators and regulatory pathways. The potential mediators of muscle catabolism and negative nitrogen balance in sepsis can be broadly divided into two categories: hormones and cytokines. Altered responsiveness to both stress hormones (glucocorticoids, glucagon, and epinephrine) and anabolic hormones (insulin, growth hormone, and insulin-like growth factors) have been implicated in causing the sepsis-induced metabolic derangement in protein turnover. Cortisol is a major determinant of the catabolic response.[61,82]

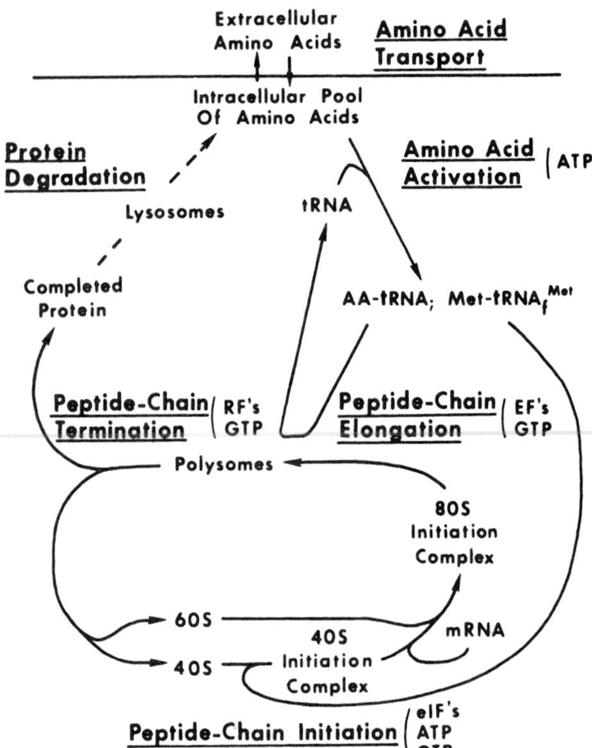

FIGURE 13-12 Pathway of skeletal muscle protein turnover. The figure schematically depicts the major steps involved in protein synthesis and in protein degradation. *ATP,* Adenosine triphosphate; *GTP,* guanosine triphosphate; *tRNA,* transfer RNA; *AA-tRNA,* aminoacyl-transfer RNA; *Met-tRNAf*^{Met}, the initiator methionyl-transfer RNA; *eIF's,* eukaryotic initiation factors; *mRNA,* messenger RNA; *EFs,* elongation factors; *RFs,* releasing factors; *40S* and *60S,* small and large ribosomal subunits, respectively. *(From Jefferson LS: Role of insulin in the regulation of protein synthesis,* Diabetes *29[6]:488, 1980.)*

Insulin conserves muscle protein by both stimulating protein synthesis and inhibiting protein degradation.[83] However, in sepsis the breakdown of muscle protein is increased despite increased insulin concentration.[84] Furthermore, animal studies have shown both a decreased sensitivity and maximal response to the inhibitory effects of insulin on protein degradation in sepsis.[59,74,84] These observations also suggest that additional factors resulting from the septic episode accelerate muscle catabolism or that injury renders the muscle resistant to insulin action.

As discussed previously in this chapter, cytokines are released by activated macrophages or lymphocytes in response to infection or trauma, and serum concentrations of inflammatory cytokines (TNF, IL-1, IL-6) are elevated.[23] The association of enhanced plasma cytokine concentrations with accelerated muscle catabolism has led to the hypothesis that cytokines are proximal mediators of the septic insult and important regulators of protein metabolism in skeletal muscle.[84,85]

Acute-Phase Protein Metabolism. Trauma and sepsis increase the hepatic synthesis and secretion of a number of proteins referred to as acute-phase proteins. The acute-phase proteins include C-reactive protein, fibrinogen, ceruloplasmin, and alpha$_1$-antitrypsin. Many of these acute-phase proteins are linked to the patient's ability to resist or control infection. The functions of these proteins include complement activation and opsonization needed for bacterial killing (C-reactive protein); coagulation, surface structure and support lattice formations needed for leukocyte entrapment of foreign material (fibrinogen); superoxide scavenging (ceruloplasmin); and inactivation of excess proteases needed to prevent damage to viable cells (alpha$_1$-antitrypsin). A differential pattern in the plasma acute-phase protein profile has been demonstrated in trauma and septic patients[86] (Figure 13-13). The presence of sepsis, whether clinically evident or not, modifies the posttraumatic acute-phase protein response to favor the increase of some acute-phase proteins while effecting a decrease in the concentration of other proteins that may not be as critical for survival.

Lipid Metabolism

Dependence on Fatty Acid Metabolism. The metabolic course of the traumatized or septic patient shows that fatty acids become the preferred fuel for oxidative metabolism. This conclusion is based on analysis of respiratory quotients and indirect calorimetry studies.[86,87] Fatty acids are stored as triglycerides in adipose tissues. Sepsis accelerates the breakdown of triglycerides in adipose tissue with the net result being the release of fatty acids into plasma at a rate that exceeds their oxidation. For tissues that use fatty acids for oxidative fuels, the rate of oxidation of fatty acids is proportional to plasma fatty acid concentrations. Thus, large increases in availability of fatty acids lead to a greater reliance on fatty acids as energy sources.[88] The accelerated fatty acid oxidation is manifested by a fall in respiratory quotient in septic patients.

Fatty acids released continually into the bloodstream are delivered to the liver. After removal from the plasma, fatty acids may undergo either oxidation for energy and ketone body production or esterification to triglycerides (Figure 13-14). A significant proportion of fatty acids taken up by the liver are reesterified, leading to accelerated hepatic triglyceride formation.[86,88] Acetyl-CoA synthesis catalyzes the activation of fatty acids to fatty acetyl-CoA esters, which are further metabolized in either anabolic (triglyceride formation) or catabolic (oxidation) pathways. Endotoxin and the proinflammatory cytokines TNF and IL-1 enhance fatty acid synthesis and reesterification. A large increase in hepatic triglycerides can ensue if the rate of excretion of triglycerides is not accelerated to the same extent as triglyceride formation. Indeed, elevated hepatic and serum triglyceride levels are a characteristic feature of sepsis.

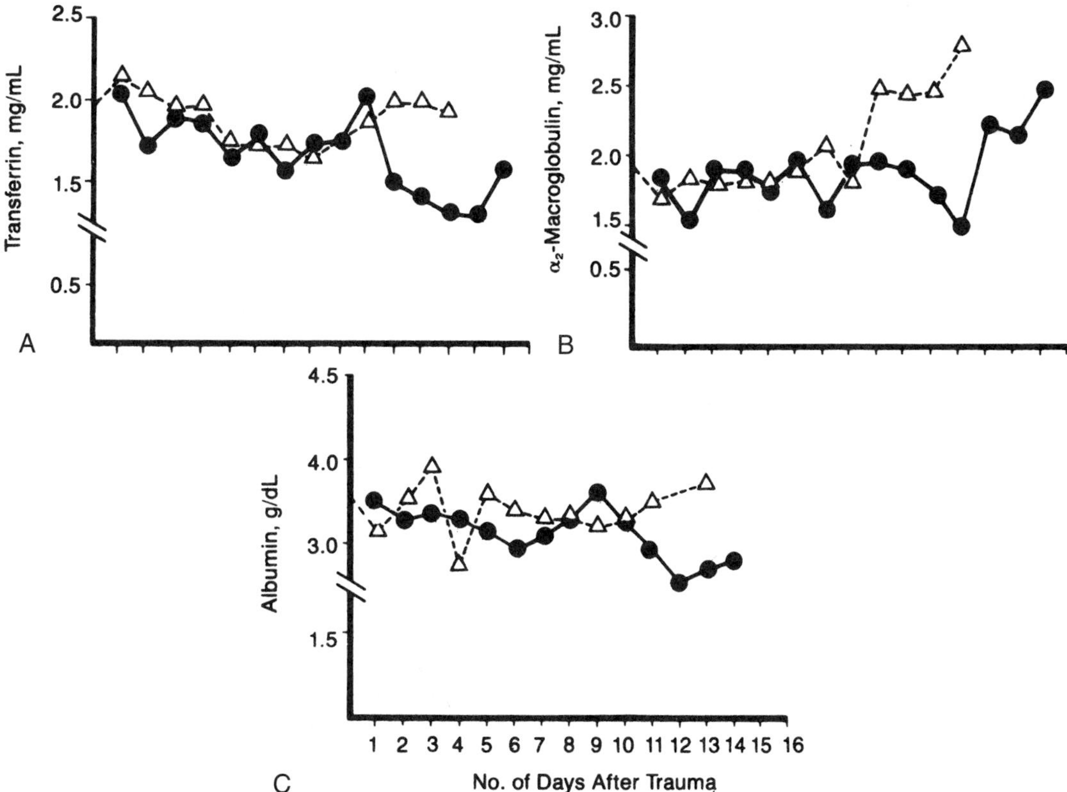

FIGURE 13-13 Plasma acute-phase protein concentrations after trauma in 16 patients *(open triangles)* and trauma complicated by sepsis in 10 patients *(solid circles)*. Mean values for transferrin (**A**), α_2-macroglobulin (**B**), and albumin (**C**), in patients with sepsis developing after trauma are compared with nonseptic trauma patients. Most changes occur only after patients become clinically septic between 5 and 7 days. *(From Sganga G, Siegel JH, Brown G et al: Reprioritization of hepatic plasma protein release in trauma and sepsis,* Arch Surg *120[2]:192, 1985.)*

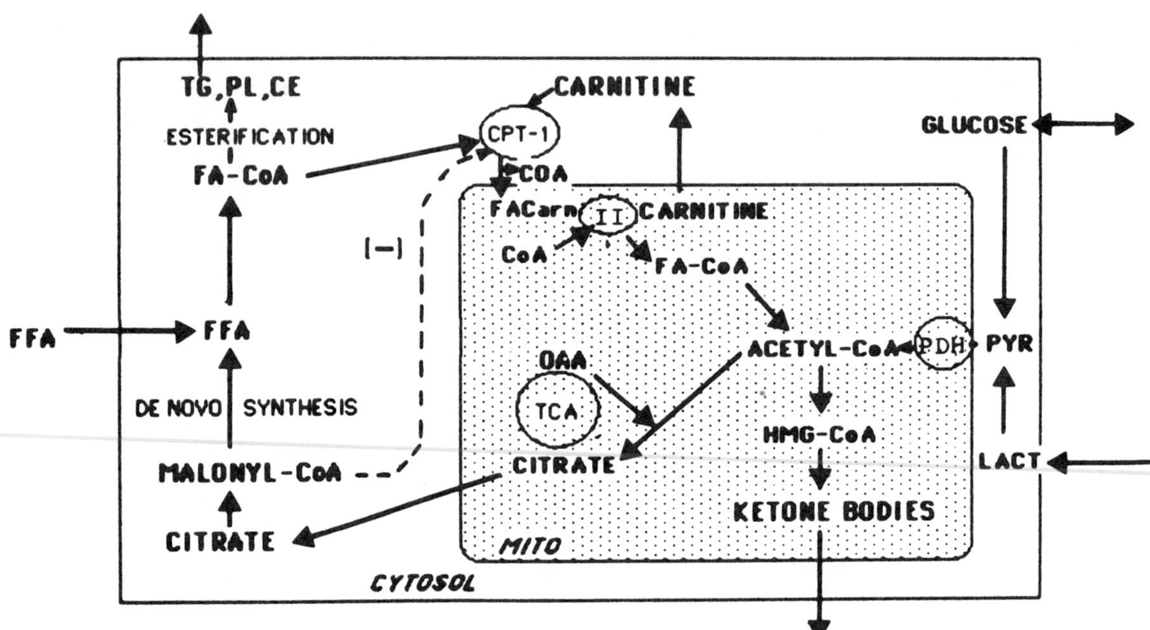

FIGURE 13-14 Relationships of hepatic fatty acid oxidation, ketogenesis, and fatty acid synthesis (---). Malonyl-CoA inhibition of carnitine:acyl-CoA transferase I. Carnitine:acyl-CoA transferases are bound to the inner mitochondrial membrane in vivo, but for clarity the reactions are shown away from membrane. *FFA,* Long-chain fatty acids; *FA-CoA,* long-chain fatty acyl-CoA; *FACarn,* long-chain fatty acyl-carnitine; *CoA,* coenzyme A; *OAA,* oxaloacetate; *PYR,* pyruvate; *LACT,* lactate; *TCA,* citric acid cycle; *TG,* triglycerides; *PL,* phospholipids; *CPT-I,* carnitine:acyl-CoA transferase I; *II,* carnitine:acyl-CoA transferase II; *PDH,* pyruvate dehydrogenase complex; *MITO,* mitochondria. *(From Vary TC, Siegel JH, Nakatani T et al: A biochemical basis for depressed ketogenesis in sepsis,* J Trauma *26[5]:420, 1986.)*

In addition to an increase in hepatic triglyceride synthesis, the systemic triglyceride disposal mechanisms may be impaired. The activity of lipoprotein lipase, the enzyme responsible for clearance of plasma triglycerides, is reduced in both adipose tissue and muscle from septic animals.[89] Concomitant with the lowered lipoprotein lipase activity, plasma triglyceride concentrations are increased. TNF is responsible for lowering lipoprotein lipase activity by reducing lipoprotein lipase synthesis in sepsis.

Reduced Ketone Bodies. The normal response of the liver to increased delivery of fatty acids is the synthesis of ketone bodies (3-L-hydroxybutyrate and acetoacetate). In addition, reversal of the insulin/glucagon ratio enhances the ketogenic capacity of the liver. In sepsis there is a rise in the glucagon/insulin ratio, but the hepatic and plasma ketone body concentrations are lower than expected. The lack of elevated plasma ketones does not indicate a lack of fatty acid oxidation, because these patients have respiratory quotients of 0.75, indicative of fat oxidation. Changes in hepatic fatty acid metabolism prevent or reverse maximal rates of ketogenesis in sepsis.[90,91] The failure to effect elevations in plasma ketone bodies in septic patients may be an additional factor influencing the markedly increased rates of proteolysis in septic patients.

Lipogenesis in Sepsis. Ketogenesis may be inhibited during sepsis, but lipogenesis appears to be accelerated. In septic patients receiving only glucose in excess of 800 cal/m^2, the respiratory quotient rises above 1.0, indicative of net lipogenesis.[86] The capacity to synthesize lipids is increased, suggesting an increased flow of acetyl groups toward fatty acid synthesis and away from ketone body function. These observations support the concept of a reciprocal relationship between lipogenesis and ketogenesis, thus preventing both fatty acids and ketone bodies from being synthesized simultaneously, which would result in an energy-wasting futile cycle.

Metabolic Dysfunction During MODS

Successful resuscitation with restoration of adequate tissue perfusion may improve the patient's well-being in the hours immediately following the trauma episode. However, some combination of inflammatory stimuli, cellular signaling, and ischemia-reperfusion injuries change the stabilized early postresuscitation presentation of many trauma patients. Early stratification of an at-risk group may be essential to treatment and prevention. Investigators note that obese trauma patients have an increased risk of postinjury organ dysfunction.[92-94] Others score the predictability of developing MODS based on the number and severity of organ involvement.[95] Consistently, significant organ dysfunction is present by 24 hours after injury in the majority of patients who develop multiple organ failure.[96]

Multiple Etiologic Factors

All basic research, as well as clinical practice, supports the hypothesis that the pathogenesis of MODS relates to prolonged systemic inflammatory activation. Immediately after traumatic injury and resuscitation, patients progress into a mild, host-beneficial SIRS.[97] The primary factors associated with the development of severe SIRS, MODS, and organ failure have been well documented and include Injury Severity Score, blood transfusion, coagulopathies, and infectious processes.[97-100]

Bacteria in the intestine can lead to infection through translocation of organisms after disruption of the intestinal mucosa due to tissue ischemia. Changes in the intestinal flora coupled with impairment of the normal barrier function of the gastrointestinal tract allow the bowel to serve as a reservoir for pathogens. Bacteria or their products (such as endotoxins) can enter the portal and systemic circulations and initiate a septic process or perpetuate an ongoing septic process. Gut-derived bacteria or endotoxins may be contributors to the development of MODS in the patient without evidence of an infectious source. In the presence of bacterial translocation, decontamination of the gut with selective suppression of lumina flora would be expected to reduce both nosocomial infections and mortality. Although a decline in infection rates has been noted, significant reductions in the incidence and mortality associated with sepsis and MODS have not been achieved.[97-101]

The precise mechanisms involved in the failure of organ systems as a consequence of sepsis remain unknown; in those patients who die, the process of organ dysfunction appears metabolic in origin. Sepsis alters the dynamic flux of metabolic substrates among skeletal muscle, gut, kidney, and liver. In the process that culminates in the clinical syndrome of organ failure, instead of the metabolic response to injury abating, hypermetabolism persists. Hypermetabolism represents a phase of altered metabolic regulation that becomes pathologic as the organ failure phase begins. The metabolic dysfunction may be related to either altered hormonal environment, generation of host inflammatory or immunologic mediators, or enhanced substrate fluxes overloading an already damaged organ system. Most likely, all three mechanisms are necessary for the manifestation of multiple organ failure in the critically ill patient. This metabolic dysfunction is associated with the development of profound anergy, lymphopenia, inadequate wound healing, and, if left uncorrected, death. The metabolic adaptations in the posttraumatic or septic state are unique and are sometimes different from the physiologic responses in fasting, exercise, starvation, diabetes, and other pathologic conditions. As described, two early manifestations of organ dysfunction in sepsis are a massive excretion of urea and alterations in glucose kinetics resulting in increased rates of glucose appearance. The degree of metabolic dysfunction is indicative of the extent of organ dysfunction induced by the invading organism or inflammatory response to traumatic injury.

Organ Interrelationships in MODS

Organ and system dysfunction is the sum of individual cellular failures. Thus, there exists a wide spectrum of metabolic and functional abnormalities within any given organ system. Organ dysfunction occurs only when enough cells of that particular organ system fail. Failure of an individual organ affects all organs because of the interdependence of all organ systems and homeostatic mechanisms of the whole individual. For example, hypovolemia or severe myocardial depression causes hypoperfusion and decreased oxygen delivery to previously healthy tissues of other organ systems, which subsequently causes dysfunction and perhaps failure of those organ systems.

After severe trauma, respiratory dysfunction is a common complication necessitating mechanical ventilatory support. In addition, there may be renal, hepatic, gastrointestinal, cardiovascular, neurologic, hematologic, immunologic and/or metabolic dysfunction progressing to failure. In the absence of severe traumatic injury, individual organ dysfunction or failure is more easily managed, and the likelihood of effective treatment may be high. However, in the presence of posttraumatic SIRS, or whenever two or more of these systems are failing, the mortality from MODS increases. There is a relationship between the number of organ systems involved and the likelihood of death. One organ system failure is associated with 20% mortality. The mortality rate increases up to 54% with two dysfunctional organs and may be up to 70% as four or more organs fail.[102,103] The combination of respiratory failure with renal failure, metabolic failure, or cardiac failure is associated with poor prognosis, particularly in the presence of sepsis.

Clinical Progression

The classic MODS syndrome in trauma patients is described by a pattern of injury, acute respiratory distress syndrome (ARDS), hypermetabolism with circulatory instability, followed by impairment in renal, hepatic, gut, hematology, endocrine, and central nervous systems.[37,95] The onset of MODS begins, as does SIRS, with a low-grade fever, tachycardia, and dyspnea, with appearance of infiltrates on chest radiographs but normal liver and renal function tests. Dyspnea progresses until endotracheal intubation and mechanical ventilatory assistance are required. Initial compensatory mechanisms promote hemodynamic stabilization, often associated with a cardiac index over 5 L/min/m^2 and a systemic vascular resistance of less than 600 dyne-sec/cm^{-5}. VO_2 may be greater than 180 ml/min/m^2.[19,40,44,104] Hyperglycemia is prevalent in the absence of diabetes mellitus or pancreatitis, and hyperlactatemia and increased urea nitrogen excretion (more than 5 g/day) are observed, consistent with the hypermetabolic state.

After 7 to 10 days, bilirubin begins to rise progressively, approaches 10 mg/dl, heralding the onset of hepatic dysfunction. Accompanying the increased bilirubin, serum creatinine begins to rise. The hyperdynamic cardiovascular state and hypermetabolism become more pronounced. Bacteremia associated with enteric organisms, positive culture of pathogens, usually gram-negative, from bronchial aspirate, urine, and wounds is not uncommon. Poor peripheral perfusion and metabolic dysfunction causes impaired wound healing. Compromised cutaneous perfusion also increases risk for development of skin breakdown at pressure points. Positive inotropic support and intravascular volume administration are increasingly required to maintain preload, myocardial contractility, and DaO_2. Between days 14 and 21, compensatory mechanisms begin to fail, and hemodynamic instability ensues despite aggressive intervention. Renal dysfunction worsens and dialysis may be required. By day 21 survivability is doubtful, and death often ensues within 21 to 28 days after the initial insult.[95,105]

Microbial factors alone do not dictate the host response to traumatic injury. SIRS with progression to MODS can occur without an initial bacterial infection[1] (see Table 13-2). A number of years ago, this observation led to modification of the definition of sepsis. Clinicians previously used the term *sepsis* to refer to the "septic-like" clinical presentation and systemic manifestations of the response to injury even when bacteria could not be cultured. The clinical signs of sepsis, such as fever, tachycardia, tachypnea, and leukocytosis were, in fact, those of SIRS.

Simple SIRS/sepsis may progress to severe SIRS/sepsis with the presence of acute organ dysfunction, hypotension, or hypoperfusion, and eventually to shock, as hypotension persists despite adequate fluid resuscitation. MODS is the failure of cell and organ function associated with acute illness in which normal homeostasis cannot be maintained. MODS may be a direct result of a well-defined insult or a multiplicity of interacting pathophysiologic events.

MANAGEMENT CONSIDERATIONS

Temporizing and resuscitative efforts are designed to reestablish effective tissue perfusion and halt oxygen deficit. The magnitude of oxygen deficit is directly related to survival and most likely also related to the extent of multiple organ dysfunction and failure that follows a shock episode. Significant tissue ischemia may occur before arrival at the trauma center. The rate and magnitude of accumulation influence the development of cellular dysfunction and lethal metabolic injury. Rapid correction of hypoperfusion is essential (see Chapter 14). Although trauma-related resuscitation end points are controversial and definitive evidence supporting use of target end points is still lacking, most experts use a combination of base deficit, lactate, and other regional or global tissue perfusion indicators.[44,48,105-107]

Paramount to the immediate resuscitative effort in the trauma population is the control of hemorrhage. Although the mainstay of resuscitation is intravascular volume administration, the amount and types of fluid used and the optimal hemoglobin concentration are not definitive in the literature. Persistent or refractory hypotension may require vasoconstrictive agents to maintain arterial pressure and cardiac index. A variety of vasoactive pharmacologic agents have been studied. To date, no vasoactive drug has been identified as the superior choice for the treatment of hypotension.[108-111] It is clear that low-dose dopamine does not provide renal protection or prevent the development of acute renal failure and should be dropped from practice.[109-112]

Guidelines are available outlining the recommendations for the treatment of severe sepsis or septic shock.[36,113,114] A summary of treatment includes early goal-directed therapy, glycemic control, appropriate antimicrobial therapy, inotropic therapy in the presence of low cardiac output, source control, recombinant human activated protein C for severe sepsis associated with high risk of death, corticosteroids in the presence of septic shock with persistent hypotension despite fluid resuscitation and vasopressors, and low tidal volume mechanical ventilation.

Activated protein C (Drotrecogin Alpha) is a natural anticoagulant that has antiinflammatory, profibrinolytic, and thrombotic benefits in severely septic patients.[13,115] Protein C is a vitamin K–dependent anticoagulation protease that circulates in the blood in an inactive state and prevents microcirculatory clotting. Protein C binds with thrombomodulin and the endothelial protein C receptor. Once activated, this protease preserves perfusion by decreasing vascular clotting. In sepsis, low levels of protein C, activation of the coagulation cascade, and decreased fibrinolysis contribute to the microcirculatory clotting in vital organ systems. In patients with severe sepsis, use of activated protein C is associated with a 19% relative risk reduction in mortality and improvement of cardiovascular and pulmonary dysfunction.[115] Consideration must be given to patients with a high risk of bleeding, as this is the major adverse effect of the drug.[13,115]

Hyperglycemia, unrelated to diabetes, is frequent during critical illness and is perceived by the clinician as part of the systemic metabolic response to stress. Patients with hyperglycemia during acute illness present with an increased risk for fluid and electrolyte disturbances, nosocomial infections, and impairments of host defenses characterized by diminished polymorphonuclear leukocyte mobilization, chemotaxis, and phagocytic activity. This suggests that hyperglycemia contributes to perpetuate the systemic proinflammatory response. These complications negatively affect outcomes among various patient populations, including trauma patients presenting with hyperglycemia, higher rates of infection, increased length of hospital stay, resource utilization, and mortality.[116] Insulin resistance and hyperglycemia that accompany critical illness and the severity of this "diabetes of stress" are reflected in risk for death. Compared with nondiabetic survivors, nondiabetic nonsurvivors had longer periods with glucose levels greater than 144 mg/dl.[117] In addition, patients with a mean blood glucose concentration greater than 144 mg/dl had higher mortality.

In the past, clinicians tolerated hyperglycemia in critically ill patients. However, the initial observations by Van den Berghe provided evidence that intensive insulin treatment for some critically ill populations (nontrauma patients) with the goal of maintaining blood glucose levels between 80 and 110 mg/dl significantly reduced morbidity and mortality without significant risk of hypoglycemia.[118,119] Intensive insulin therapy has been shown to reduce intensive care unit length of stay, organ dysfunction, and in-hospital mortality, with the greatest reduction involving deaths resulting from multiple-organ failure with a septic focus.[120]

The mechanisms by which insulin treatment reduces mortality are not yet well understood. Beneficial effects of intensive insulin therapy in critically ill patients are dependent on metabolic and nonmetabolic molecular pathways.[121] Insulin acts by two major molecular pathways: reduction of the inflammation process induced by free fatty acid excess in tissues and decrease of reactive oxygen species production induced by hyperglycemia. Insulin prevents microcirculation alteration and subsequent cellular hypoxia by reducing inducible NO synthase expression and activity in the endothelium.

The clinical benefits of glycemic control are present whether or not patients had previously diagnosed diabetes, and they seem independent of severity and type of critical illness. The incidence of nosocomial infections, including intravascular device-related bloodstream and surgical site infections, is lower in patients receiving strict glucose control in comparison with those who are not.[122] Patients who receive intensive insulin therapy are less likely to require prolonged use of antibiotics than patients who do not receive this therapy. Strict glucose regulation results in modulation of cytokine production, causing a shift toward a more antiinflammatory pattern.[123] This shift in the cytokine balance may account for the decrease in infection-related complications and mortality.

Several reports have indicated abnormalities in protein turnover prevent ambulation and recovery in critically ill patients, leading to longer length of stay and complications associated with prolonged bed rest. High doses of insulin reverse the sepsis-induced stimulation of protein catabolism,[124] whereas a short-term low-dose insulin regimen is inefficient in influencing mild hyperglycemia and protein catabolism in critically ill medical patients.[125]

Also, strict glycemic control with intensive insulin therapy prevented or reversed ultrastructural and functional abnormalities of hepatocyte mitochondria. Maintenance or restoration of mitochondrial function is another therapeutic target, in addition to optimization of cardiac output, systemic oxygen delivery, and regional blood flow, that might improve outcome for critically ill patients.[126]

Patients in the intensive care unit exhibit lower glutamine concentrations. Glutamine supplementation has beneficial effects on the clinical outcome of critically ill and surgical patients, which may be explained by glutamine's influences on the inflammatory response, oxidative stress, cell protection, and the gut barrier. In addition, glutamine may improve glucose metabolism by reducing insulin resistance. Asymmetric dimethylarginine is a byproduct of normal protein metabolism that inhibits NO production. It has been shown to be a strong and independent predictor of mortality in critically ill patients with clinical evidence of organ dysfunction. Insulin modulates asymmetric dimethylarginine concentration, which may partly explain the beneficial effects seen in critically ill patients receiving intensive insulin therapy.[127]

Euglycemia is best achieved, and hypoglycemia attenuated, through use of a protocolized approach to treatment of hyperglycemia among critical care patients.[128-131] Precise management protocols for hyperglycemia due to acute illness have been evaluated in clinical practice. A nurse-driven insulin infusion protocol in postoperative cardiothoracic surgical intensive care patients with or without diabetes led to lower mortality.[129] Implementation of such a protocol provided more rapid and effective glucose control in critically ill surgical patients compared with physician management. The relation of hyperglycemia and mortality is pronounced in critically ill trauma patients, as well as SICU patients admitted for other reasons.[116,131] Serum glucose measurement frequency of 1 to 2 hours in these populations is critical to achieving and maintaining tight control. Development of continuous blood glucose monitoring has begun and will soon be incorporated into routine practice in the same way that continuous electrocardiographic monitoring and pulse oximetry are standards of care in the intensive care unit.

SUMMARY

Severe multiple trauma that overwhelms the numerous compensatory mechanisms designed to stabilize a life-threatening situation results in a complex series of pathophysiologic processes. Subsequent hemorrhagic shock and sepsis result in cellular dysfunction and are reflected in altered hemodynamic and metabolic statuses. The diagnosis and effective treatment of posttrauma shock states is guided by an understanding of these pathophysiologic events and the risk of sequential or multiple organ dysfunction and failure. Although SIRS and MODS may have many causes in the patient with traumatic injuries, two of the most common are hypovolemia and sepsis. Of the two, the pathophysiology of hypovolemia is best understood and, as a consequence, more readily managed. Significant advances have been made in the understanding of the pathophysiology of SIRS and MODS; however, much remains to be elucidated. Despite aggressive management of septic shock, mortality remains high. Newer therapies are focused on the metabolic inflammatory processes. Studies investigating endotoxin modulation and therapies directed at neutrophil adhesion molecules, among others, are currently under way. These laboratory and clinical investigations will continue to broaden our knowledge of the complex processes involved in inflammation, sepsis, and MODS and contribute to exploration of more effective prevention and management strategies.

REFERENCES

1. Levy MM, Fink MP, Marshall JC: 2001 SCCM/ESICM/ACCP/ATX/SIS International sepsis definitions conference, *Crit Care Med* 31(4):1250-1256, 2003.
2. Johnson K, Renn C: The HPA axis in critical illness, *AACN Clin Issues Adv Prac in Acute Crit Care* 17(1):39-49, 2006.
3. Kelley DM: Hypovolemic shock: an overview, *Crit Care Nurs Q* 28(1):2-19, 2005.

4. Harbrecht BG, Alarcon LH, Peitzman AB: Management of shock. In Moore EE, Feliciano DV, Mattox KL, editors: *Trauma*, New York, 2004, McGraw Hill.
5. Hameed SM, Aird WC, Cohn SM: Oxygen delivery, *Crit Care Med* 31(12):S658-S667, 2003.
6. Huang YT: Monitoring oxygen delivery in the critically ill, *Chest* 128(5 Suppl 2):554S-560S, 2005.
7. Cuthbertson DP: Post-shock metabolic response, *Lancet* 1:433-436, 1942.
8. Shoemaker WC, Lim L, Boyd DR: Sequential hemodynamic events after trauma to the unanesthetized patient, *Surg Gynecol Obstet* 132(4):1033-1038, 1971.
9. Nguyen BH, Rivers EP, Knoblich BP et al: Early lactate clearance is associated with improved outcome in severe sepsis and septic shock, *Crit Care Med* 32(8):1637-1642, 2004.
10. Shapiro NK, Howell MD, Talmor D et al: Serum lactate as a predictor of mortality in emergency department patients with infection, *Ann Emerg Med* 45(5):524-528, 2005.
11. Husain FA, Martin MJ, Mullenix PS et al: Serum lactate and base deficit as predictors of mortality and morbidity, *Am J Surg* 185(5):485-491, 2003.
12. Clay AS, Behnia M, Brown KK: Mitochrondrial disease: a pulmonary and critical-care medicine perspective, *Chest* 120(2):634-648, 2001.
13. Kleinpell R: Advances in treating patients with severe sepsis: role of drotrecogin alfa (activated), *Crit Care Nurse* 23(3): 16-29, 2003.
14. Sommers MS: The cellular basis of septic shock, *Crit Care Nurse Clin North Am* 15(1):13-25, 2003.
15. Cone JB: Inflammation, *Am J Surg* 182(6):558-562, 2001.
16. Szabo G, Romics L, Frendl G: Liver in sepsis and systemic inflammatory response syndrome, *Clin Liver Dis* 6(4): 1045-1066, 2002.
17. Workman ML: The cellular basis of bacterial infections, *Crit Care Nurse Clin North Am* 15(1):1-11, 2003.
18. Sommer MS, Bolton PJ: Multisystem. In Alspach JG, editor: *Core Curriculum for Critical Care Nursing*, St. Louis, 2006, Saunders.
19. Balk RA: Optimum treatment of severe sepsis and septic shock: evidence in support of the recommendations, *Dis Mon* 50(4):168-213, 2004.
20. Hotchkiss RC, Tinsley KW, Swanson PE et al: Endothelial cell apoptosis in sepsis, *Crit Care Med* 30(5):S225-228, 2002.
21. Freitas ID, Fernandez-Somoza M, Sekler EE et al: Serum levels of the apoptosis-associated molecules, tumor necrosis factor alpha necrosis factor type I receptor and Fas/FasL, in sepsis, *Chest* 125(6):2238-2246, 2004.
22. Lu X, Hamilton JA, Shen J et al: Role of tumor necrosis factor alpha in myocardial dysfunction and apoptosis during hindlimb ischemia and reperfusion, *Crit Care Med* 34(2): 484-491, 2006.
23. Giannoudis PV, Smith RM, Banks RE et al: Stimulation of inflammatory markers after blunt trauma, *Br J Surg* 85(7): 986-990, 1998.
24. Balk RA, Ely EW, Goyette RE: *Sepsis Handbook*, ed 2. Thomson Advanced Therapeutics Communications and Vanderbilt University School of Medicine, 2004, 24-32.
25. Reinhart K, Bayer O, Brunkhorst F et al: Markers of endothelial damage in organ dysfunction and sepsis, *Crit Care Med* 30(5):S302-S312, 2002.
26. Perl M, Gebhar F, Braumulle S et al: The pulmonary and hepatic immune microenvironment and its contribution to the early systemic inflammation following blunt chest trauma, *Crit Care Med* 34(4):1152-1159, 2006.
27. Majetschak M, Borgermann J, Waydhas C et al: Whole blood tumor necrosis factor-alpha and its relation to systemic concentrations of interleukin 4, interleukin 10, and transforming growth factor-beta-1 in multiply injured blunt trauma victims, *Crit Care Med* 28(6):1847-1853, 2000.
28. Molina H: Complement and immunity, *Rheum Dis Clin North Am* 30(1):1-18, 2004.
29. Cook JA: Eicosanoids, *Crit Care Med* 33(12):S480-491, 2005.
30. Knoller J, Schoenfeld W, Joka T et al: Generation of leukotrienes in polytraumatic patients with adult respiratory distress syndrome, *Prog Clin Biol Res* 236:311-316, 1987.
31. Bugler EM, Maier RV: Lipid mediators in the pathophysiology of critical illness, *Crit Care Med* 28(4 Suppl): N27-N36, 2000.
32. Smith MJH, Ford-Hutchinson AW, Bray MA: Leukotriene B: a potential mediator of inflammation, *J Pharm Pharmacol* 32(7):517-518, 1980.
33. Liaudet L, Soriano FG, Szabo C: Biology of nitric oxide signaling, *Crit Care Med* 28(4 Suppl): N37-N52, 2000.
34. Giantomasso DD, May CN, Bellomo R: Vital organ blood flow during hyperdynamic sepsis, *Chest* 124(3):1053-1059, 2003.
35. Hollenberg SM, Ahrens TS, Annane D: Practice parameters for hemodynamic support of sepsis in adult patients: 2004 update, *Crit Care Med* 32(9):1928-1948, 2004.
36. Nguyen HB, Rivers EP, Abrahamian FM et al: Severe sepsis and septic shock: review of the literature and emergency department management guidelines, *Ann Emerg Med* 48(1):28-54, 2006.
37. McKinley MG: Shock and sepsis. In Sole ML, Klein DG, Moseley MJ, editors: *Introduction to Critical Care Nursing*, St. Louis, 2005, Elsevier Saunders.
38. Bishop MH, Shoemaker WC, Appel PL et al: Relationship between supranormal circulatory values, time delays, and outcomes in severely traumatized patients, *Crit Care Med* 21(1):56-63, 1993.
39. Bishop MH, Shoemaker WC, Appel PL et al: Prospective, randomized trial of survivor values of cardiac index, oxygen delivery, and oxygen consumption as resuscitation endpoints in severe trauma, *J Trauma* 38(5):780-787, 1995.
40. Vincent J: The international sepsis forum's frontiers in sepsis: high cardiac output should be maintained in severe sepsis, *Crit Care* 7(4):276-278, 2003.
41. Rivers E, Nguyen B, Havstad S, et al: Early goal-directed therapy in the treatment of severe sepsis and septic shock, *N Engl J Med* 345(19):1368-1378, 2001.
42. Koch T, Geiger S, Ragaller MJ: Monitoring of organ dysfunction in sepsis/systemic inflammatory response syndrome: novel strategies, *J Am Soc Nephrology* 12(17):S53-S59, 2001.
43. Martin MJ, FitzSullivan E, Salim A et al: Discordance between lactate and base deficit in the surgical intensive care unit: which one do you trust? *Am J Surg* 191(5):625-630, 2006.
44. Poeze M, Solberg BC, Greve JW et al: Monitoring global volume-related hemodynamic or regional variables after initial resuscitation: what is a better predictor of outcome in critically ill septic patients? *Crit Care Med* 33(11): 2494-2500, 2005.
45. Boerma EC, Mathura KR, van der Voort PH et al: Quantifying bedside-derived imaging of microcirculatory abnormalities in septic patients: a prospective validation study, *Crit Care* 9(6):601-606, 2005.

46. Hameed SM, Cohn SM: Gastric tonometry: the role of gastric pH measurement in the management of trauma, *Chest* 123(5):475S-481S, 2003.
47. Chang MC, Mondy JS III, Meredith JW et al: Redefining cardiovascular performance during shock resuscitation: ventricular stroke work, power, and the pressure-volume diagram, *J Trauma* 45(3):470-478, 1998.
48. Tisherman SA, Barie P, Bokhari F, et al: Clinical practice guidelines: endpoints of resuscitation, *J Trauma* 54(4):898-912, 2004.
49. Calvin JE, Driedger AA, Sibbald WJ: Does the pulmonary capillary wedge pressure predict left ventricular preload in critically ill patients, *Crit Care Med* 9(6):437-443, 1981.
50. Chang MC, Meredith JW: Cardiac preload, splanchnic perfusion, and their relationship during resuscitation in trauma patients, *J Trauma* 42(4):577-584, 1997.
51. Deitch E, Dayal S: Intensive care unit management of the trauma patient, *Crit Care Med* 34(9):2294-2301, 2006.
52. Diebel LN, Wilson RF, Tagett MG et al: End-diastolic volume: a better indicator of preload in the critically ill, *Arch Surg* 127(7):817-821, 1992.
53. Headley JM: Arterial pressure-based technologies: a new trend in cardiac output monitoring, *Crit Care Nurs Clin North Am* 18(2):179-187, 2006.
54. Reibel DK, Rovetto MJ: Myocardial ATP synthesis and mechanical function following oxygen deficiency, *Am J Physiol* 234(5):H620-H624, 1978.
55. Neely JR, Vary TC, Liedtke AJ: Substrate delivery in ischemic myocardium. In Tillsmanns H, Kubler W, Zebe H, editors: *Microcirculation of the Heart,* Berlin, 1982, Springer-Verlag.
56. Crowell JW, Smith EE: Oxygen deficit and irreversible hemorrhagic shock, *Am J Physiol* 206:313-316, 1964.
57. Kern JW, Shoemaker WC: Meta-analysis of hemodynamic optimization in high-risk patients, *Crit Care Med* 30(8): 1686-1692, 2002.
58. Liddell MJ, Daniel AM, McClean LD et al: Role of stress hormones in the catabolic metabolism of shock, *Surg Gynecol Obstet* 149(6):822, 1979.
59. Vary TC: Inter-organ protein a carbohydrate relationships during sepsis: necessary evils or uncanny coincidences? *Curr Opin Clin Nutr Metab Care* 2(3):235-242, 1999.
60. Zoico E, Roubenoff R: Role of cytokines in protein metabolism and muscle function, *Nutrition Rev* 60(2),39-51, 2002.
61. Burchard K: A review of the adrenal cortex and severe inflammation: quest of the "eucorticoid" state, *J Trauma* 51(4):800-814, 2001.
62. Wilmore DW: Metabolic response to severe surgical illness: an overview, *World J Surg* 24(6):705-711, 2000.
63. Vary TC: Regulation of skeletal muscle protein turnover during sepsis, *Curr Opin Clin Nutr Metab Care* 1(2):217-224, 1998.
64. Desborough JP: The stress response to trauma and surgery, *Br J Anaesth* 85(1):109-117, 2001.
65. Black PR, Brooks DC, Bessey PQ et al: Mechanism of insulin resistance following injury, *Ann Surg* 196(4):420-425, 1982.
66. Vary TC, Drnevich D, Jurasinski CV et al: Mechanisms regulating skeletal muscle glucose metabolism in sepsis, *Shock* 3(6):403-410, 1995.
67. Fan J, Li Y, Wojnar M et al: Endotoxin-induces alterations in insulin-stimulated phosphorylation of insulin receptor, 1RS-1, and MAP kinase in skeletal muscle, *Shock* 3(6):164-170, 1996.
68. Chang H, Bristrian B: The role of cytokines in the catabolic consequences of infection and injury, *J Parenter Enteral Nutr* 22(3):156-166, 1998.
69. Carlson GL: Insulin resistance in sepsis, *Br J Surg* 90(3): 259-260, 2003.
70. Kroder G, Bossenmaier B, Kellerer M et al: Tumor necrosis factor-alpha and hyperglycemia-induced insulin resistance: evidence for different mechanisms and different effects on insulin signaling, *J Clin Invest* 97(6):1471-1477, 1996
71. Peraldi P, Hotamisligil G, Buurman W et al: Tumor necrosis factor (TNF)-alpha inhibits insulin signaling through stimulation of the p55 receptor and activation of sphingomyelinase, *J Biol Chem* 271(22):13018-13022, 1996.
72. Peraldi P, Spiegelman B: TNF-alpha and insulin resistance: summary and future prospects, *Mol Cell Biochem* 182(1-2): 169-175, 1998.
73. Uysal T, Wiesbrock S, Marino M et al: Protection from obesity-induced insulin resistance in mice lacking TNF-alpha function, *Nature* 389(6651):610-614, 1997.
74. Vary TC, Dardevet D, Obled C et al: Modulation of skeletal muscle lactate metabolism during sepsis by insulin or insulin-like growth factor-I: effects of pentoxifylline, *Shock* 7(6):432-438, 1997.
75. Mizock BA: Lactic acidosis in critical illness, *Crit Care Med* 20(6):80-93, 1992.
76. Dunham CM, Siegel JH, Weireter L et al: Oxygen debt and metabolic acidemia as quantitative predictors of mortality and the severity of the ischemic insult in hemorrhagic shock, *Crit Care Med* 19(2):231-243, 1991
77. Vary TC, Hazen SA, Maish III G et al: TNF binding protein prevents hyperlactatemia and inactivation of PDH complex in skeletal muscle during sepsis, *J Surg Res* 80(1):44-51, 1998.
78. Yu M, Burchell S, Takiguchi S et al: The relationship of oxygen consumption measured by indirect calorimetry to oxygen delivery in critically ill patients, *J Trauma* 41(1):32-40, 1996.
79. Weil MH, Afifi AA: Experimental and clinical studies on lactate and pyruvate as indicators of the severity of acute circulatory failure, *Circulation* 41(6):989-1001, 1970.
80. Vary TC, Hazen SA, Maish III G et al: TNF binding protein prevents hyperlactatemia and inactivation of PDH complex in skeletal muscle during sepsis, *J Surg Res* 80(1):44-51, 1998.
81. Vary TC, Siegel JH, Rivkind A: Clinical and therapeutic significance of metabolic patterns of lactic acidosis, *Perspect Crit Care* 1:85-132, 1988.
82. Michie HR: Metabolism of sepsis and multiple organ failure, *World J Surg* 20(4):460-464, 1996.
83. Jefferson LS: Role of insulin in the regulation of protein synthesis, *Diabetes* 29(6):487-490, 1980.
84. Vary TC, Dardevet D, Grizard J et al: Pentoxifylline improves insulin action limiting skeletal muscle catabolism after infection, *J Endocrinol* 163(1):15-24, 1999.
85. Cooney RA, Pantaloni A, Sarson Y et al: *A pilot study on the metabolic effects of IL-1ra in patients with severe sepsis.* 4th International Congress on Immune Consequences of Trauma, Shock and Sepsis, Bologne, Italy, 1997, Mondozzi Editore S.P.A.
86. Sganga G, Siegel JH, Brown G et al: Reprioritization of hepatic plasma protein release in trauma and sepsis, *Arch Surg* 120(2):187-199, 1985.
87. Sganga G, Siegel JH, Coleman B et al: The physiologic meaning of respiratory index in various types of critical illness, *Circ Shock* 17(3):179-193, 1985.

88. Wolfe RR: Substrate utilization/insulin resistance in sepsis/trauma, *Baillieres Clin Endocrinol Metab* 11(4):645-657, 1997.
89. Memon RA, Fuller J, Moser AH et al: In vivo regulation of acyl-CoA synthetase mRNA and activity by endotoxin and cytokines, *Am J Physiol* 275(1 Pt 1):E64-72, 1998.
90. Scholl RA, Lang CH, Bagby GJ: Hypertriglyceridemia and its relation to tissue lipoprotein lipase activity in endotoxemic *Escherichia coli* bacteremic, and polymicrobial septic rats, *J Surg Res* 37(5):394-401, 1984.
91. Wannemacher RW, Pace JG, Beall FA et al: Role of liver in regulation of ketone body production during sepsis, *J Clin Invest* 64(6):1565-1572, 1979.
92. Byrnes M, McDaniel MD, Moore MB et al: The effect of obesity on outcomes among injured patients, *J Trauma* 58(2):232-237, 2005.
93. Brown C, Neville A, Rhee P et al: The impact of obesity on the outcomes of 1,153 critically injured blunt trauma patients, *J Trauma* 59(5):1048-1051, 2005.
94. Ciesla DJ, Moore EE, Johnson, JL et al: Obesity increases risk of organ failure after severe trauma, *J Am Coll Surg* 203(4):539-545, 2006.
95. Vincent JL, de Mendonca A, Cantraine F et al: Use of SOFA score to assess the incidence of organ dysfunction/failure in intensive care units: results of a multicenter, prospective study, *Crit Care Med* 26(11):1793-1800, 1998.
96. Cryer HG, Leong K, McArthur DL et al: Multiple organ failure: by the time you predict it, it's already there, *J Trauma* 46(4):597-606, 1999.
97. Hoover L, Bochicchio GV, Napolitano LM, et al: Systemic inflammatory response syndrome and nosocomial infection in trauma, *J Trauma* 61(2):310-306, 2006.
98. Barie PS, Hydo LJ: Epidemiology of multiple organ dysfunction syndrome in critical surgical illness, *Surg Infec* 1(3):173-185, 2000.
99. Johnson D, Mayers I: Multiple organ dysfunction syndrome: A narrative review, *Can J Anesth* 48:502-509, 2001.
100. Lee CC, Marill KA, Carter WA et al: A current concept of trauma-induced multiorgan failure, *Ann Emerg Med* 38(2):170-176, 2001.
101. Dhainaut J, Shorr AF, Macias WL et al: Dynamic evolution of coagulopathy in the first day of severe sepsis: relationship with mortality and organ failure, *Crit Care Med* 33(2):341-348, 2005.
102. Martin GS, Mannino DM, Eaton S, et al: The epidemiology of sepsis in the United States from 1979 through 2000, *N Engl J Med* 348(16):1546-1554, 2003.
103. Angus D, Linde-Zwirble WT, Lidicker J et al: Epidemiology of severe sepsis in the United States: analysis of incidence, outcome, and associated costs of care, *Crit Care Med* 29(7):1303-1310, 2001.
104. Von Rueden KT, Dunham CM: Evaluation and management of oxygen delivery and consumption in multiple organ dysfunction syndrome. In Secor V, editor: *Multiple Organ Dysfunction and Failure: Pathophysiology and Clinical Implications,* ed 2, St. Louis, 1996, Mosby.
105. Third European Consensus Conference in Intensive Care Medicine: Tissue hypoxia: how to detect, how to correct, how to prevent, *Am J Respir Crit Care Med* 154(5):1573-1578, 1996.
106. Bakker J, Gris P, Coffernils M et al: Serial blood lactate levels can predict the development of multiple organ failure following septic shock, *Am J Surg* 171(2):221-226, 1996.
107. Friedman G, Berlot G, Kahn RJ et al: Combined measurements of blood lactate concentrations and gastric intramucosal pH in patients with severe sepsis, *Crit Care Med* 23(7):1184-1193, 1995.
108. Bracco D: Pharmacologic support of the failing circulation: practice, education, evidence, and future directions, *Crit Care Med* 34(3):890-892, 2006.
109. Sakr Y, Reinhart K, Vincent JL et al: Does dopamine administration in shock influence outcome? Results of the Sepsis Occurrence in Acutely Ill Patients (SOAP) study, *Crit Care Med* 34(3):589-597, 2006.
110. Bellomo R., Chapman M, Finfer S et al: Low-dose dopamine in patients with early renal dysfunction: a placebo-controlled randomized trial, *Lancet* 356:2139-2143, 2000.
111. Beale RJ, Hollenberg SM, Vincent J et al: Vasopressor and inotropic support in septic shock: an evidence-based review, *Crit Care Med* 32(11):S455-S465, 2004.
112. Venkataraman R, Kellum JA: Prevention of acute renal failure, *Chest* 131(1):300-308, 2007.
113. Dellinger RP, Levy MM, Carlet JM et al: Surviving Sepsis Campaign: International guidelines for management of severe sepsis and septic shock: 2008, *Crit Care Med* 36(1):296-327, 2008.
114. Hurtado FJ: The role of bundles in sepsis care, *Crit Care Clin* 22(3):521-529, 2006.
115. Bernard GR, Vincent JL, Laterre PF et al: Efficacy and safety of recombinant human activated protein C for severe sepsis, *N Engl J Med* 344(10):699-709, 2001.
116. Sung J, Bochicchio GM, Joshi M et al: Admission hyperglycemia predictive of outcome in critically ill trauma patients. *J Trauma* 59(1):80-83, 2005.
117. Rady MY, Johnson DJ, Patel BM et al: Influence of individual characteristics on outcome of glycemic control in intensive care unit patients with or without diabetes mellitus, *Mayo Clinic Proc* 80(12):1558-1567, 2005.
118. Van den Berghe G, Wouters P, Weekers F: Intensive insulin therapy in critically ill patients, *N Engl J Med* 345(19): 1359-1367, 2001.
119. Van den Berghe G: Role of intravenous insulin therapy in critically ill patients, *Endocr Pract* 10 Suppl 2:17-20, 2004.
120. Krinsley JS: Effect of an intensive glucose management protocol on the mortality of critically ill adult patients, *Mayo Clin Proc* 79(8):992-1000, 2004.
121. der Voort PH, Feenstra R, Bakker AJ et al: Intravenous glucose intake independently related to intensive care unit and hospital mortality: an argument for glucose toxicity in critically ill patients, *Clin Endocrinol* 64(2):141-145, 2006.
122. Grey NJ, Perdrizet G: Reduction of nosocomial infections in the surgical intensive care unit by strict glycemic control, *Endocr Pract* 10 Suppl 2:46-52, 2004.
123. Pickkers P, Hoedemaekers A, Netea MG et al: Hypothesis: normalisation of cytokine dysbalance explains the favourable effects of strict glucose regulation in the critically ill, *Netherlands J Med* 62(5):143-150, 2004.
124. Jurasinski C, Gray K, Vary TC: Modulation of skeletal muscle protein synthesis by amino acids and insulin during sepsis, *Metabolism* 44(9):1130-1138, 1995.
125. Holzinger U, Zauner A, Nimmerrichter P et al: Metabolic inefficacy of a short-term low-dose insulin regimen in critically ill patients: a randomized, placebo-controlled trial, *Wiener Klin Woch* 116(17-18):603-607, 2004.

126. Vanhorebeek I, De Vos R, Mesotten D et al: Protection of hepatocyte mitochondrial ultrastructure and function by strict blood glucose control with insulin in critically ill patients, *Lancet* 365(9453):53-59, 2005
127. Siroen MP, van Leeuwen PA, Nijveldt R et al: Modulation of asymmetric dimethylarginine in critically ill patients receiving intensive insulin treatment: a possible explanation of reduced morbidity and mortality? *Crit Care Med* 33(3):504-510, 2005.
128. Conner TM, Flesner-Gurley KR, Barner JC: Hyperglycemia in the hospital setting: the case for improved control among non-diabetics, *Ann Pharmacother* 39(3):492-501, 2005.
129. Dilkhush D, Lannigan J, Pedroff T et al: Insulin infusion protocol for critical care units, *Am J Health System Pharm* 62(21):2260-2264, 2005.
130. Lonergan T, Le Compte A, Willacy M, et al: A simple insulin-nutrition protocol for tight glycemic control in critical illness: development and protocol comparison, *Diabetes Tech Ther* 8(2):191-206, 2006.
131. Taylor BE, Schallom ME, Sona CS, et al: Efficacy and safety of an insulin infusion protocol in a surgical ICU, *J Am Coll Surg* 202(1):1-9, 2006.

14

Initial Management of Traumatic Shock

Sharon A. Boswell, Thomas M. Scalea

Rapid recognition of shock is the cornerstone of the early evaluation and treatment of severely injured patients. Sometimes shock is obvious, and even the unsophisticated clinician clearly recognizes the patient in extremis from blood loss. Frequently, however, the findings are substantially more subtle, necessitating increased levels of clinical sophistication and experience to recognize shock, particularly when the victim is able to compensate for blood loss. Shock represents an uncoupling of normal physiologic functioning. Compensatory mechanisms initially strive to maintain homeostasis. This compensation can be robust, particularly in young patients, and patients with substantial blood loss or severe injuries can appear relatively stable initially.[1]

The importance of early recognition of shock cannot be overemphasized. When untreated or treated very late, shock produces acute organ dysfunction that almost always leads to death, often within 24 hours.[2] Late recognition of shock, even if not accompanied by classic signs, produces a profound hypoperfusion insult, with the accumulation of a significant oxygen debt. Patients may survive for the short term but then develop sequential organ failure several days later.[2] Despite an increased understanding of injury and resuscitation, we have yet to significantly alter the mortality associated with multiple organ failure.

Although the term *traumatic shock* may seem redundant, it actually describes a distinct clinical entity. Shock following injury is multifactorial. Hemodynamic alterations from blood loss can be compounded by mediator release from injured soft tissue. Both of these can be further compounded by cardiovascular dysfunction resulting from blunt cardiac injury or cardiac tamponade. Hypoxia from pulmonary contusion may limit oxygen delivery and worsen cardiac function. Thus traumatic shock can include aspects of other types of shock or be exacerbated by associated organ dysfunction.

Oxygen Transport

Central to the understanding of the concept of shock is the principle of oxygen transport (Table 14-1). The vast majority of oxygen (98% to 99%) exists in the body bound to hemoglobin. A small portion is freely dissolved in plasma. Thus oxygen content is a function of hemoglobin and oxygen saturation. Cardiac output delivers oxygen to the periphery. The cells then unload the amount of oxygen they need, and the unneeded portion is returned to the heart via the venous circulation. The oxygen extraction ratio is approximately 25%.

A number of physiologic variables can alter this relationship. After injury, loss of circulating blood volume (via hemorrhage or loss of serum into the soft tissue) decreases cardiac preload impeding cardiac output. Increased needs in the periphery create a state in which the body must compensate by increasing oxygen delivery. This can be accomplished in a number of ways. Cardiac output, a function of the stroke volume of the heart and the heart rate, can increase. Stroke volume is a function of preload, afterload, and contractility. Thus an increase in myocardial contractility or heart rate can increase cardiac output. An increase in vascular resistance (afterload), which initially maintains blood pressure, also limits cardiovascular performance. Alternatively, the cells can unload more oxygen in the periphery, thus maintaining oxygen consumption. Both methods can be used simultaneously.

The ability of the cell to unload oxygen can be affected by a number of factors. The oxyhemoglobin dissociation curve governs the principles of oxygen affinity to the hemoglobin molecule (Figure 14-1). Some conditions such as alkalosis, hypothermia, or a loss of 2,3-diphosphoglycerate (2,3-DPG) increase oxygen's affinity for hemoglobin, thus impeding the body's ability to unload oxygen at the cellular level. Conversely, acidosis, hyperthermia, and increases in 2,3-DPG, shift the curve in the opposite direction, allowing for increased peripheral oxygen unloading. These relationships can be dynamic, particularly in a patient with complicated diagnoses.

At some point, oxygen demand can exceed oxygen supply. As compensation fails, the cells must shift to anaerobic metabolism to generate the high-energy phosphate compounds needed for cellular metabolism.[3] Anaerobic metabolism is an extremely inefficient means of generating adenosine triphosphate (ATP)—approximately 5% as efficient as aerobic metabolism using the Krebs cycle.[4] In addition, lactate is a byproduct of anaerobic metabolism. Lactate may depress cardiac function and limit oxygen delivery. As acidosis worsens, so does cardiac performance, and ultimately death ensues.

TABLE 14-1 **Oxygen Transport**

Variables	Abbreviation	Units	Calculation	Normal Value
Hb saturation	Sao_2	%	Direct measurement	95-99
Arterial oxygen content	Cao_2	ml O_2/dl	$Cao_2 = (Hb \times 1.39 \times Sao_2) + (.003 \times Pao_2)$	16-22
Venous oxygen content	Cvo_2	ml O_2/dl	$Cvo_2 = (Hb \times 1.39 \times Svo_2) + (.003 \times Pvo_2)$	12-17
Oxygen delivery	Do_2 I	ml/min/m^2	$Do_2 = Cao_2 \times CI \times 10$	520-720
Oxygen consumption	Vo_2 I	ml/min/m^2	$Vo_2 = C(a\text{-}v)O_2 \times CI \times 10$	100-180

Modified from Shoemaker WC: Relation of oxygen transport patterns to the pathophysiology and therapy of shock states, *Intensive Care Med* 13:234, 1987.
CI, Cardiac index; *Hb,* hemoglobin.

Shock can then be defined as the hemodynamic manifestations of any state in which oxygen demand exceeds oxygen supply or utilization regardless of the underlying cause. Thus all shock can be defined as inadequate cardiovascular performance. Given the nature of injury, we attempt to estimate peripheral oxygen delivery through the use of blood pressure or target organ function. Although this practice has the advantage of being quick and readily available in the clinical arena, these parameters are at best nonspecific and in some cases can lead to faulty decision making. Some patients who are hypotensive may not be in shock. Conversely, many patients who are not hypotensive may be in shock. Recognizing this possibility and knowing when it is necessary to obtain more data are key to optimizing care, particularly in patients with complex diagnoses.

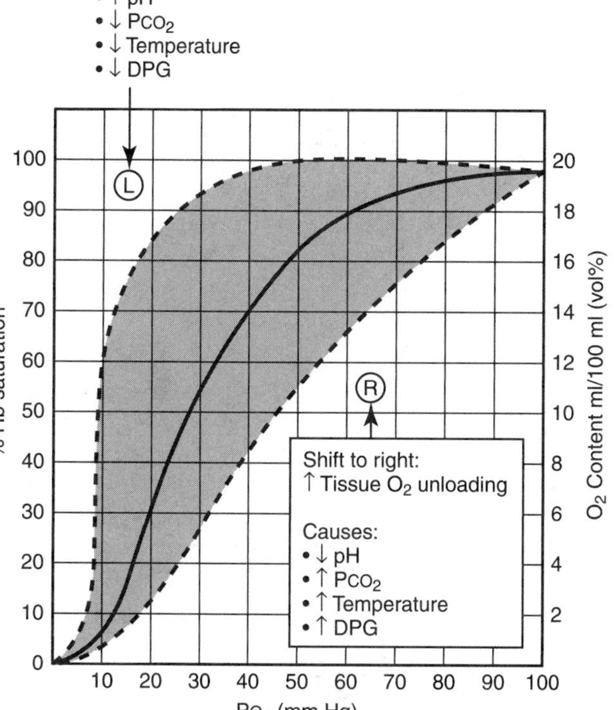

FIGURE 14-1 Oxyhemoglobin dissociation curve.
(From Moms MT: Adult respiratory distress syndrome. In Secour VH, editor: Multiple organ dysfunction & failure, *ed 2, St. Louis, 1996, Mosby, 174.)*

PATHOPHYSIOLOGY OF SHOCK

PHYSIOLOGY OF BLOOD LOSS

Blood loss is the most common cause of inadequate cardiovascular performance after injury.[5] It can be accompanied by intravascular volume loss from extravasation of plasma into body cavities (e.g., peritoneal cavity) or the interstitium of injured tissues further depressing cardiovascular performance. Fluid losses may also occur through open wounds. Initial attempts to compensate for blood loss are multifactorial. Catecholamine-mediated systemic vasoconstriction is primarily responsible for the increase in systemic vascular resistance seen in many shock states. This allows for the shunting of blood flow away from nonessential organs. Blood is initially directed away from the skin and skeletal muscle, maintaining flow to the more central vascular beds. Ultimately, as blood loss continues, the only core organs protected are the most essential—the heart and brain. Under normal conditions, the perfusion pressure and degree of smooth muscle tone in the supplying vessels determine regional blood flow to any individual organ. As organisms bleed, autoregulatory mechanisms attempt to maintain a steady-state pressure flow to these vital organs. Thus tissue hypoxia will initially be more marked in tissues and organs in which autoregulatory compensation fails.

Tachycardia, a narrowing of pulse pressure, and loss of capillary refill are thought to be the first measurable signs of blood volume loss (Table 14-2). Presentation of these clinically measurable parameters indicates that initial mechanisms thought to provide compensation for inadequate intravascular volume are activated. As blood loss continues, there may be a stepwise change in these and other parameters. When blood loss approximates 40% to 50% of total circulating blood volume (>2 L in a 70-kg man), compensation fails and patients develop bradycardia, obtundation, and cardiac arrest.[6] This stepwise change in vital signs allows for estimation of the amount of blood loss and can be used to direct care. For instance, patients who are stable (i.e., normotensive and not tachycardic) could be presumed to have a minor injury and have suffered less than a 15% loss in circulating blood volume.

TABLE 14-2 **Estimated Fluids and Blood Losses Based on Patient's Initial Presentation**

	Class I	Class II	Class III	Class IV
Blood loss (ml)	Up to 750	750-1500	1500-2000	>2000
Blood loss (% blood volume)	Up to 15%	15%-30%	30%-40%	>40%
Pulse rate	<100	>100	>120	>140
Blood pressure	Normal	Normal	Decreased	Decreased
Pulse pressure (mm Hg)	Normal or increased	Decreased	Decreased	Decreased
Respiratory rate	14-20	20-30	30-40	>35
Urine output (ml/hr)	>30	20-30	5-15	Negligible
CNS/mental status	Slightly anxious	Mildly anxious	Anxious, confused	Confused, lethargic
Fluid replacement (3:1 rule)	Crystalloid	Crystalloid	Crystalloid and blood	Crystalloid and blood

Used with permission from American College of Surgeons, Committee on Trauma. *Advanced Trauma Life Support for Doctors, Student Course Manual,* ed 7, Chicago, 2004, American College of Surgeons.
For a 70-kg man.
CNS, Central nervous system.
The guidelines in Table 14-2 are based on the "3-for-1" rule. This rule derives from the empiric observation that most patients in hemorrhagic shock require as much as 300 ml of electrolyte solution for each 100 ml of blood loss. Applied blindly, these guidelines can result in excessive or inadequate fluid administration. For example, a patient with a crush injury to the extremity may have hypotension out of proportion to his or her blood loss and require fluids in excess of the 3:1 guidelines. In contrast, a patient whose ongoing blood loss is being replaced by blood transfusion requires less than 3:1. The use of bolus therapy with careful monitoring of the patient's response can moderate these extremes.

Those who are initially somewhat hypotensive or tachycardic and who respond to initial resuscitation may then be classified as "stabilizable." Although they must be presumed to have suffered a significant blood loss, they are generally able to undergo diagnostic evaluation to precisely identify the source of blood loss. Some of these patients may even be managed nonoperatively. Patients who present in extremis and do not respond to initial resuscitation must be presumed to have serious ongoing blood loss. Their initial evaluation should be tailored to minimize time, and hemorrhage must be arrested immediately.

Unfortunately, vital signs are often imprecise and may incorrectly classify patients with marginally compensated shock as stable. Tissue oxygen extraction, as measured by either mixed venous or central venous oxygen saturation, is much more specific and correlates reliably with blood loss (Figure 14-2). This has been demonstrated in controlled laboratory models of both anesthetized and unanesthetized canine hemorrhage.[7] It has also been investigated in humans who presented to an emergency department with mechanisms of injury suggestive of acute blood loss but who initially seemed to be hemodynamically stable.[8] Forty percent of these stable patients had central venous oxygen desaturation, although their blood pressure and pulse rate were similar to those of patients with normal central venous oxygen saturations. Central venous oxygen desaturation was used to reliably predict major blood loss, such as large hemothoraces or hemorrhage from pelvic fractures.

Urine output has been reported to be a reliable indicator of the depth of shock.[6] Patients who are oliguric should be presumed to be underresuscitated. Patients who are nonoliguric are generally deemed stable. However, work from the authors' laboratory seems to refute those conclusions.[9] In a porcine model of nonhypotensive shock, animals that lost 15% of their total circulating volume behaved as expected by becoming oliguric. They held on to both salt and water, as evidenced by low urine sodium concentrations. In contrast, animals bled more severely—losing 21%, 27%, and 35% of the total circulating blood volume—all developed an acute salt-wasting nephropathy and acute tubular insufficiency. These animals had high urine-sodium

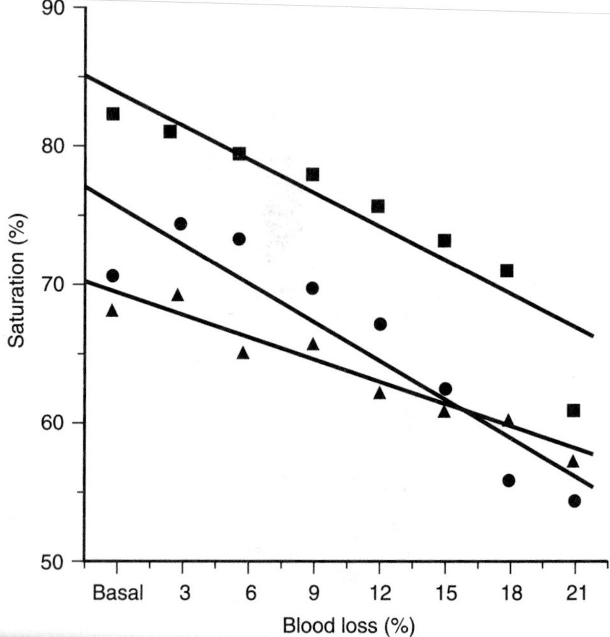

FIGURE 14-2 Relationship between venous oxygen saturation and blood loss in awake and anesthetized dogs. Squares represent mixed venous oxygen saturation (anesthetized); circles represent central venous oxygen saturation (awake); and triangles represent mixed venous oxygen saturation (awake). *(Modified from Scalea TM, Holman M, Fuortes M et al: Central venous blood oxygen saturation: an early, accurate measurement of volume during hemorrhage,* J Trauma *28:728, 1988.)*

concentrations, and their urine output was not different from that of control animals.

Other factors may alter cardiac performance and perfusion parameters after blood loss. One is mechanism of injury. Patients who have sustained blunt trauma respond differently than those with penetrating injuries. Penetrating trauma approximates a pure blood loss situation. A tissue crush injury that accompanies blunt trauma, however, can stimulate a cascade that, even acutely, liberates vasoactive mediators that can affect hemodynamic performance. Patients with this type of injury may develop a high cardiac output/low vascular resistance state similar to sepsis. Ethanol use, which is commonly associated with trauma, has been shown to modulate plasma norepinephrine concentrations after injury, blunting the vascular response and moderating the effect of adrenergic stimuli.[10] Street drugs such as cocaine may also affect cardiovascular performance. Animals pretreated with cocaine and then subjected to blood loss had a blunted response to hemorrhage compared with control animals.[11]

Some vascular beds may respond differently than others. Global parameters such as mixed venous oxygen saturation reflect a mixing of blood from all vascular beds. Identification of the most responsive vascular beds could allow earlier diagnosis of blood loss. The mesenteric circulation is exquisitely sensitive to falls in preload.[12] Blood flow to the gut is reduced primarily via vasoconstriction caused by elevated renin angiotensin activity. This is opposed to the renal circulation, in which hemorrhagic hypotension may activate renal vasodilatory signals via local release of prostaglandins and nitric oxide. Monitoring of mesenteric circulation could potentially provide early warning signals to critical but non-hemodynamically significant hemorrhage. The adequacy of flow can be measured via intracellular pH. Indirect measurement of this parameter via gastric tonometry catheters has been demonstrated to predict adequacy of resuscitation in the general class of intensive care unit (ICU) patients.[13] Unpublished work from the authors' laboratory has demonstrated that gastric tonometry is an extremely sensitive indicator of blood loss that changes before other vital signs. In addition, the authors have demonstrated that reduction in gastrointestinal oxygen delivery is accompanied by oxygen supply dependency.

Neurogenic Shock

Efferent sympathetic neurons in the thoracic and cervical spinal cord are dependent on descending input from the hypothalamus and brainstem for vasomotor control. Brainstem damage or spinal cord injury at or above the T6 level may then produce neurogenic shock. In this type of shock, loss of vasoconstrictor-sympathetic activity leads to vascular collapse. With loss of vasomotor control, even previously adequate blood volume becomes incapable of filling the now dilated capacitance vessels. Bradycardia and hypotension are common. However, unlike hemorrhagic shock, neurogenic shock is characterized by a slow pulse rate and warm, dry skin. This is a relative hypovolemia resulting from decreases in peripheral vascular and cardiac sympathetic activity. Hemodynamic patterns can be variable. Decreases in systemic vascular resistance, central venous pressure, and pulmonary capillary wedge pressure are nearly universal. Cardiac output, on the other hand, may be low, normal, or elevated. The loss of vascular resistance allows unimpeded forward flow from the heart. These salutary effects on cardiac performance may be counterbalanced, however, by the negative effect of inadequate preload from the vasodilation. Refer to Chapter 23 for information on management of neurogenic shock.

The hemodynamics of neurogenic shock may be further complicated by differences in mechanism of injury. A spinal cord injury may be accompanied by blood loss, which can exacerbate any of the hemodynamic consequences. The lack of sympathetic response may also mask the signs of acute blood loss. Soderstrom et al demonstrated that nearly 70% of patients with cervical spine injury and blunt trauma are hypotensive from their spinal cord injury, not concomitant blood loss.[14] In contradistinction, a series of patients with penetrating spinal cord injuries found that neurogenic shock explained hypotension in approximately 20% of patients.[15] This underscores the need to completely evaluate all patients regardless of the obvious nature of one particular injury.

Cardiogenic Shock

The most frequent cause of cardiogenic shock is acute myocardial infarction.[5] This can accompany injury, particularly in elderly patients. Cardiogenic shock occurs when 35% to 40% of the left ventricular muscle mass is damaged.[16] The resulting impairment in left ventricular function produces elevated end-systolic volumes and filling pressures. This in turn limits diastolic filling. Cardiac output falls and produces often profound hypotension. Coronary perfusion is thereby decreased, potentially extending the area of ischemia. This ischemia further drops cardiac output and creates an ever-widening cyclic process, which will result in patient death unless truncated early.

Patients with acute cardiac failure after injury are a special subset of patients and present many challenges. Peripheral oxygen delivery needs must be met to maintain aerobic metabolism. Inotropic support may be necessary to support the failing heart. Cardiac protection with beta blockade, afterload reduction, and conservative fluid administration will help preserve myocardium but will limit forward flow. Despite all interventions, cardiogenic shock in this setting is often a lethal state.[17]

Septic Shock

Pure septic shock resulting from infection is unusual immediately after acute trauma. The only exception may occur in patients with grossly contaminated wounds. Significant soft tissue infection is seen in patients with multiple long-bone fractures, and these patients occasionally present with septic shock several hours after injury. The mediator release stimulated by significant soft tissue injury, especially when accompanied by gross contamination or dead muscle, often presents in a manner similar to septic shock.

Septic shock is most commonly characterized by vasodilation, and the resulting hemodynamics are generally related to unopposed forward cardiac flow. Septic shock is not a pure hypovolemic state. It is better described as maldistribution of blood flow. The vasodilation, with resultant arteriolar and venous dilation, lowers cardiac preload as well as afterload. Although many patients present with warm, seemingly well-perfused extremities and high cardiac output, those with septic shock may actually exhibit high, normal, or low cardiac output states. Relative myocardial failure can come as a result of inadequate cardiac preload or direct myocardial depression from circulating mediators. In fact, a subset of patients, usually the elderly, who are septic can present with high systemic vascular resistances and low cardiac outputs in a manner similar to that of cardiogenic shock. This form of septic shock carries an extremely poor prognosis.

The initial decrease in blood pressure seen with all forms of septic shock is multifactorial. An infectious process leads to the release of vasoactive mediators such as histamine and bradykinin. These vasoactive agents ultimately cause pooling of peripheral blood and extravasation of plasma into the interstitium. The acute capillary leak and peripheral pooling decrease venous return, with resultant decrease in cardiac output and blood pressure. Compensation for this aberrant ventricular filling is mediated initially through increases in sympathoadrenal stimuli. Ultimately, however, myocardial dysfunction will override this attempt at compensation.

Initially the availability of substrates (particularly oxygen and glucose) is increased to support metabolic need as demands rise. However, as peripheral perfusion decreases, substrate delivery may be inadequate and anaerobic metabolism ensues. In addition, visceral redistribution of flow creates a state of relative mitochondrial failure. Even with increased peripheral oxygen delivery, the ability of the cell and the mitochondria to upload and use oxygen decreases.

Injury Demographics

Last year nearly 40,000,000 people were seen in our nation's emergency departments as a result of unintentional injury. More than 2 million of them required hospitalization. In 2004 the number of deaths from unintentional injury increased for the seventh consecutive year, to 167,184.[18] Experts expect this trend to continue.

Patients die in a trimodal distribution after injury. The vast majority of deaths occur at the scene from immediately life-threatening airway compromise, brain injury, and/or exsanguinating hemorrhage. In fact, there is little that trauma care can do to improve these patients' survival other than implement trauma prevention strategies. An additional 20% of trauma deaths occur in the early phase, generally from exsanguinating hemorrhage.[19] It is this group of patients in whom prehospital and emergency department decision making can potentially have an effect. The last group of patients die later from multiple organ failure. The cause of multiple organ dysfunction and subsequent failure usually originates from a systemic inflammatory response initiated by injury or sepsis. This group represents approximately 10% of trauma deaths.[19] Some of these deaths may be prevented by limiting shock and using optimal resuscitation strategies. The exact percentage of lives that can be saved by altering trauma care, although not insignificant, remains unknown.

Blunt Trauma

Blunt trauma is the most common mechanism of injury in the United States.[20] The mechanics of blunt injury involve a compression or crushing mechanism via energy transmission and direct injury. If compressive, shearing, or stretching forces exceed the tolerance limit of a tissue or an organ, the tissues are disrupted. This may result in injury to the solid viscera, such as the liver or spleen, or rupture of the hollow viscera, such as the gastrointestinal tract.

Injury can also result from movement of the organs within the body. Some organs are rigidly fixed, whereas others are more mobile. Injuries are particularly common in areas where the organ transitions from being mobile to immobile because the part not rigidly fixed is free to move with a great degree of velocity.

The most common cause of death and disability from unintentional injuries worldwide is the motor vehicle crash. In 2003 the number of deaths from motor vehicle-related incidences in the United States alone rose to more than 43,000, and nearly 21,000,000 people suffered some disabling injury.[18] The injury patterns seen with motor vehicle crashes are difficult to predict because a number of factors contribute to them. Certainly the speed of the vehicle and the surface that it strikes are important in determining the vectors of energy. The use of restraint systems such as seat belts and air bags also influences both the severity of injury and the type of injury seen. A high-speed, head-on collision into a bridge abutment with an unrestrained driver at the wheel is far different from the car traveling at 20 mph that strikes a tree with a glancing blow with a driver protected by a seat belt and an air bag. Both are motor vehicle crashes, but the injury patterns will be substantially different.

Falls are the second leading cause of unintentional death in the United States and were responsible for more than 7,500,000 emergency department visits in 2002. They continue to account for more than 20% of all injury-related hospital admissions.[18] Falls from a height can produce a unique pattern of injury. The degree of injury is a function of the distance of the fall, the surface on which the victim lands, and whether the fall is broken by objects during flight. The center of gravity in adults resides in the pelvis, whereas in young children the center of gravity is in the head. Therefore children who fall a great distance often land on their head and thus are likely to suffer severe traumatic brain injury.

Adults, on the other hand, often right themselves as they fall and land on their feet. The force is then transmitted up the axial skeleton into the spine. Lower extremity, pelvic, and thoracolumbar spinal fractures are common, as well as injuries to the retroperitoneal viscera. Brain injury and intraabdominal injury, however, are relatively rare.

Pedestrians struck by cars may likewise have unique patterns of injury. Pedestrians are completely unprotected, so all the force is applied directly to the portion of the body that is struck. Additional injury can be caused if victims are thrown through the air and strike a second object. Motorcyclists or bicyclists are also poorly protected, except for the protection afforded by helmets. Their risk of injuries is compounded by the fact that vehicles such as motorcycles can travel at great rates of speed.

Penetrating Trauma

Penetrating trauma differs from blunt trauma in that it does not cause a diffuse pattern of injury. In the case of stabbings the wounding blade directly injures tissues as it passes through the body. Because the penetrating object produces a hole in the skin no larger than the blade, external examination of the size of the wound may grossly underestimate the degree of internal damage. In addition, the trajectory of the blade is not apparent by external examination. Any stab wound located in the lower chest, pelvis, flank, or back must be presumed to have a transabdominal trajectory and accompanying injury until proven otherwise.

Gunshots injure in several ways. Bullets may injure organs directly. Secondary missiles can be formed as bullets shatter bone and the bony fragments then disperse. In addition, the bullet produces a concussive zone of injury from energy transmission as it travels through the body. High-energy missiles can cause a significant amount of injury somewhat distant from their direct path. Some bullets are designed to expand or break apart as they enter the victim. These tend to cause more tissue destruction.

Entrance and exit wounds can approximate missile trajectory. Plain radiographs help to localize the foreign body, allowing prediction of vascular structures at risk for injury. Unfortunately, however, bullets often do not travel in a straight line. Thus all structures in any proximity to the presumed trajectory must be considered injured until proven otherwise.

Diagnosis and Treatment of Shock

The early diagnosis of shock is based on the ability to identify problems with peripheral perfusion. As the patient moves from the prehospital phase through resuscitation and into critical care, the ability to diagnose shock increases as more sophisticated diagnostic and monitoring tools become readily available. Although the prehospital providers are now utilizing more technologically advanced diagnostic equipment, they have only relatively rudimentary tools, in addition to their clinical acumen, to use in the identification of shock. Thus it can be reasonably assumed that they will not be as accurate or specific in diagnosing shock as clinicians in an intensive care unit (ICU), whose arsenal includes invasive hemodynamic monitoring devices as well as knowledge of the patient's clinical course up to that point.

Prehospital Care

The goal in caring for any trauma patient is to identify those most severely injured as early as possible and then to minimize the time from injury to definitive therapy. Unfortunately, diagnosis of shock in the field can be difficult. Blood pressure and pulse rate are crude measures of the adequacy of peripheral perfusion,[7] yet little else is available to the prehospital care provider. These individuals must make rapid decisions based on a paucity of information. Thus in most emergency medical services (EMS) systems the tendency has been to overtriage as opposed to undertriage to avoid delivering a patient to an institution not capable of providing adequate care.

Skin temperature, capillary refill, and the initial response of blood pressure and pulse rate to a fluid bolus are the primary assessment parameters available in the prehospital arena. A gauge of anatomic severity may also provide some clue as to the likelihood of blood loss. For instance, patients with multiple long-bone fractures must be presumed to have substantial blood loss and should be treated accordingly despite normal vital signs. Large scalp lacerations are notorious for producing significant hemorrhage, and patients with this type of injury must be presumed to have lost a substantial amount of blood regardless of their hemodynamic parameters. Patients with pelvic instability or a tense, distended abdomen must likewise be presumed to have bled substantially into their retroperitoneum or abdominal cavity. Physical examination of the chest provides a relatively crude indication of blood loss into the thoracic cavity. Lastly, the patient's own medical history, such as presence or absence of cardiac disease and medication use, may help determine his or her ability to withstand blood loss and respond hemodynamically. Patients taking beta blockers will not be able to use tachycardia to augment forward flow.

Several philosophies exist regarding the care of patients in the prehospital setting who are confirmed or suspected to be in shock (Table 14-3). The first is to attempt to stabilize these patients in the field. This "stay and play" philosophy is based on an assumption that time in the field can be well spent stabilizing the patient's physiologic status.[21] Correction of oxygenation or ventilatory problems can be lifesaving. The insertion of intravenous (IV) catheters for fluid resuscitation can help correct cardiovascular instability. A brief neurologic assessment can identify patients at high risk for severe brain injury, particularly those with impending herniation. Therapy can then be directed and triage possibly improved. Unfortunately, the time involved in even rapid evaluation and temporary stabilization often causes concern.

Excessive time in the field can prolong the interval from injury to definitive therapy. Proponents of the "scoop and run"

TABLE 14-3 **Field Resuscitation Strategies**

	Stay and Play	Load and Go
Time at Scene	Longer (20-30 min)	Shorter (<10 min)
Interventions	Airway stabilization Spinal stabilization IV access Fluid therapy Wound/fracture stabilization	Airway stabilization Spinal stabilization
Appropriate locale	Rural	Urban
Advantages	* Earlier fluid therapy * Earlier administration of pain control therapy * Earlier administration of effective measures for cardiac arrhythmias * Broader assessment with possible better triage	* Shorter time to definitive care
Disadvantages	* Longer time to definitive care * Potential for increased bleeding with increased fluid volume	* Delay in beginning fluid therapy * Possible increase in mistriage

Modified from Border JR, Lewis FR, Aprahamian C et al: Panel: prehospital trauma care—stabilize or scoop and run, *J Trauma* 23:708-711, 1983; and Gold CR: Prehospital advanced life support vs "scoop and run" in trauma management, *Ann Emerg Med* 16:797-801, 1987.

philosophy believe that only immediately life-threatening problems, such as airway issues, should be addressed in the field.[22] Patients should be immobilized on spine boards and external hemorrhage controlled with direct pressure. All other therapies should be attempted only en route. Prolonging field time even long enough to insert an IV catheter may negatively alter ultimate outcome.

In 1983 Smith et al reviewed the prehospital care of 52 trauma victims who underwent attempts at in-field stabilization.[23] In all cases the IV insertion time was longer than the transport time. Failure of line placement occurred 28% of the time and occurred most often in those patients most severely injured. The average IV insertion time in the field was between 10 and 12 minutes. Border et al estimated that blood loss during this time may be in excess of 1500 ml in severely injured patients.[24]

This issue was further investigated by clinicians at Los Angeles County Hospital.[25] In this study nearly 6000 trauma patients admitted via the emergency department were evaluated for field time and mode of transportation. Patients who were transported by private vehicle as opposed to the city EMS system got to the hospital statistically significantly faster. The main reason for this appeared to be the amount of time the prehospital personnel spent in the field attempting to stabilize the patient. The moderate to severely injured patients (Injury Severity Score [ISS] 15-25) arriving at the hospital without the benefit of city ambulance transport had a lower mortality than their EMS-transported counterparts. These compelling data argue strongly in favor of "scoop and run."

Some middle ground in managing trauma patients in the prehospital setting would presumably be the wisest. In dense urban areas where prehospital transport times are shorter, it is hard to imagine that spending a prolonged amount of time in the field is wise. This would be particularly true for patients with penetrating trauma, primarily penetrating torso trauma. Attempts to stabilize these patients in the field will almost certainly result in longer than necessary prehospital care. Optimal survival of these patients is a function of rapid transport and definitive control of life-threatening blood loss.

On the other hand, patients in rural areas with blunt trauma may be best served by an attempt at stabilization. An additional 10 minutes in the prehospital setting may not create an unreasonable detrimental delay in areas where long transport times are the norm. Airway control and some attempt at cardiovascular stability may be lifesaving, particularly in patients with traumatic brain injury. Each EMS system should address these issues individually. It is important to understand the skill level of prehospital care providers as well as transport time when establishing policies regarding appropriate interventions that should be carried out in the prehospital setting.

Fluid administration in the prehospital arena has evolved considerably in the past several years. Original treatment algorithms called for establishment of large-bore IV access and instillation of 2 L of crystalloid fluid as rapidly as possible, with the goal of normalizing both blood pressure and pulse rate. Early in the twentieth century, however, Cannon et al suggested that IV fluids administered in the field to patients with hypotension could be injurious.[26] He theorized that crystalloid fluid would serve only to displace hemostatic clots that may have formed on injured blood vessels as blood pressure fell. In addition, he felt that if bleeding persisted despite hypotension, administration of IV fluids would not positively influence outcome.

This thought was corroborated scientifically in 1965, when Shaftan et al investigated this theory in a canine hemorrhagic shock model.[27] They investigated various resuscitation regimens to elucidate the relative effects of pressure and volume on the hemodynamic response to crystalloid fluid resuscitation. They demonstrated that the time to hemostasis was longest and blood loss greatest in animals resuscitated to normal volume status and blood pressure. Subsequently, numerous animal models, most often a porcine aortotomy model of hemorrhagic shock, have been used to verify these findings.[28-30] All these investigations demonstrated that intraperitoneal blood loss is greatest when animals are resuscitated to normal blood pressure. The excessive amount of crystalloid fluid required to maintain normal blood pressure seems to hemodilute the available hemoglobin and increase intraperitoneal blood loss, presumably by displacing the clot that forms on top of the injured aorta at the time of hypotension. In 1994 Bickell et al randomized patients with penetrating torso trauma and hypotension in the field to receive no fluid or standard crystalloid fluid, with a target systolic blood pressure of 100 mm Hg.[31] Patients in the fluid-restricted group received fluids only at the time of anesthetic induction for surgical control of their hemorrhagic shock. In this study there was a statistically significant survival advantage to fluid restriction.

Thus it seems that moderate hypotension, although potentially detrimental, is in fact relatively well tolerated, at least for short periods. This may be better than the alternative of increased blood loss and hemodilution with crystalloid resuscitation to attain normal blood pressure. In patients with traumatic brain injury, hypotension has been shown to double mortality.[32] Thus, fluid restriction is probably not wise in these patients. Alternatively, geriatric patients with limited cardiovascular reserve may require different treatment algorithms to avoid development of acute cardiac ischemia, which almost certainly will lead to death.

The type of fluid used in the prehospital environment has likewise been called into question (Table 14-4). In most EMS systems, crystalloid fluid is the preferred volume expander. There is, however, some evidence that hypertonic saline may have the advantage of more rapid restoration of cardiovascular function with a smaller volume of fluid. As little as 4 ml/kg, if given rapidly, may have the same hemodynamic effect as several liters of crystalloid.[33] The increase in cardiac output and mean arterial pressure with hypertonic saline results from an osmotic shift of fluid from the interstitial and intracellular spaces into the intravascular space. This is mediated by rapid increases in serum osmolarity that accompany the infusion of 7.5% sodium chloride, which has a milliosmolarity of 2565. The addition of dextran prolongs this plasma expansion.[34] In several animal models of hemorrhage, hypertonic saline/dextran improved stroke volume and decreased both heart rate and systemic vascular resistance.[35,36] Enthusiasm for use of hypertonic solutions has been counterbalanced by several small studies suggesting that rebleeding and hemodynamic instability may occur after the infusion of hypertonic saline when blood loss is not

TABLE 14-4 **Fluid Therapy**

	Crystalloids	Hypertonic Saline	Hypertonic Saline/Dextran
Amount required	2 L	4 ml/kg	4 ml/kg
Osmolarity	273-308 mOsm/L	1026 mOsm/L for 3% 2565 mOsm/L for 7.5% 8008 mOsm/L for 23.4%	2400 mOsm/L for 7.5% HTS in 6% dextran 70 (will vary depending on HTS and dextran concentrations used)
Longevity	Minutes	15-30 min	3-4 hr
Advantages	* No side effects	* Faster increase in BP than with crystalloids * Requires less volume * Requires less time for infusion * May increase survival in patients with GCS ≤ 8 by decreasing intracranial pressure	* Faster increase in blood pressure than with crystalloids * Requires less volume * Requires less time for infusion * May increase survival in patients with GCS ≤ 8 by decreasing intracranial pressure
Disadvantages	* May exacerbate bleeding in large volumes * May worsen head injury in large volumes	* No increase in survival over crystalloids in the general trauma population * Potential for adverse reactions such as seizures or coagulopathies	* No increase in survival over crystalloids in the general trauma population * Potential for adverse reactions such as seizures, coagulopathies, or anaphylaxis

Modified from Mattox KL, Maningas PA, Moore EE et al: Prehospital hypertonic saline/dextran infusion for post-traumatic hypotension, *Ann Surg* 213:482-491, 1991; and Vassar MJ, Fischer RP, O'Brien PE et al: A multicenter trial for resuscitation of injured patients with 7.5% sodium chloride, *Arch Surg* 128:1003-1013, 1993.

HTS, Hypertonic saline; *BP*, blood pressure; *GCS*, Glasgow Coma Scale score.

fully controlled.[37,38] Hypertonic saline and hypertonic saline/dextran have been investigated in several randomized prospective trials in humans. Mattox et al demonstrated increases in blood pressure in a multi-institutional study on the use of hypertonic saline in the prehospital arena.[39] In the subset of patients requiring emergency life-saving surgery to control hemorrhage, survival was statistically significantly better in those who were treated with hypertonic saline compared with patients treated with dextran or crystalloid fluid. Vassar et al investigated this issue in four separate randomized trials during the early 1990s.[40-42] They were unable to demonstrate any survival advantage in the broad group of patients randomized to hypertonic saline compared with crystalloid fluid. However, in the subset of patients with severe traumatic brain injury, there appeared to be a survival advantage to using hyperosmotic resuscitation. This may have been due to a decrease in secondary brain injury from the more rapid restoration of cardiovascular function or decreases in intracranial pressure, as seen with the administration of hypertonic saline. The cerebral osmotic effects of hypertonic saline are similar to those of mannitol. In a meta-analysis Wade et al demonstrated a distinct survival advantage for patients with serious traumatic brain injury treated with hypertonic saline.[34] In a more recent study, 229 hypotensive patients with severe traumatic brain injury were randomized to receive a rapid IV infusion of either 250 ml of Ringer's lactate solution or 250 ml of 7.5% saline in addition to other resuscitation fluid provided in the prehospital setting, Cooper et al found a small trend toward greater survival in those patients who received hypertonic saline during resuscitation. However, neurologic outcome at 6 months after injury was identical to that found in the group that received only crystalloid resuscitation.[43]

There are some distinct disadvantages to the use of hypertonic saline. Although the hemodynamic effects are rapid and profound, they are relatively short lived. At some point, the intracellular hypernatremia can become problematic, and sufficient free water must be administered to repay the intracellular debt. Rapid instillation of hyperosmotic saline may be unsafe in patients with limited cardiac reserve (e.g., elderly patients), as it may precipitate heart failure. The lack of convincing randomized prospective data and the concerns about potential disadvantages of hypertonic saline have combined to limit its widespread use in the prehospital arena.

In the late 1980s, military antishock trousers (MAST) were thought to be useful in the resuscitation scheme after trauma. MAST were thought to autotransfuse volume by applying pressure to the capacitance vessels in the lower extremities. Added advantages included the potential stabilization of long-bone fractures and reduction of pelvic fractures. Data, however, have failed to demonstrate any real utility to MAST. In fact, increases in blood pressure seen with the use of MAST seem to be secondary to increases in systemic vascular resistance, and MAST do not augment cardiac preload. In a randomized trial of 911 patients, Mattox et al demonstrated no survival advantage with use of MAST.[44] Wangensteen et al reported that pneumatic external compression without concomitant intravascular volume replacement accelerated the development of lactic acidosis and decreased the survival rate in animal models.[45] In general, the widespread use of MAST has fallen out of favor, and many EMS systems have abandoned their use in the prehospital arena. However, there may be some uses for MAST. They may be useful during long transports to help support at least some blood pressure when no other mode of therapy is available. MAST can be helpful as a temporary splint in patients with extensive long-bone fractures. In addition, they can be helpful in patients with complex pelvic fractures by reducing the fracture, limiting pelvic volume, and potentially reducing blood loss. They do, however, introduce the possibility of cardiovascular effects resulting from increased intraabdominal pressure. Potential complications of MAST have prompted many trained prehospital and emergency room practitioners to use a sheet or binder wrapped around the circumference of the pelvis to achieve the same temporary stabilization without the MAST-related adverse effects (e.g., increased intrathoracic, intraabdominal pressures).

Transport Decisions

Transport decisions are as important as any other prehospital decisions. The goal of triage is to deliver each patient to the most appropriate facility as quickly as possible. Rapid transport to an emergency department or hospital that does not have the capability of providing the appropriate level of care to the patient may only jeopardize long-term outcome. All emergency departments should be able to provide immediately life-saving therapies such as establishing an airway and shock resuscitation. However, more sophisticated diagnostics and therapeutics are available in a limited number of facilities. For instance, access to a computed tomography (CT) scanner and the ready availability of a neurosurgeon may be lifesaving in a patient with operable traumatic brain injury. The ready availability of a general surgeon and an operating room likewise can be the only method of salvaging a patient who is in hemorrhagic shock from blunt or penetrating torso trauma.

In the United States, there has been an attempt to classify hospitals to rank the degree of care they may reasonably be expected to provide 24 hours a day, 365 days a year. Various agencies (e.g., local EMS systems or state governmental agencies) are responsible for this designation and verification process. Decisions regarding criteria for the various levels of trauma centers and the number of centers necessary in any given locale vary among municipalities. In some locations, any center that meets the criteria is designated. This makes the highest number of centers available but dilutes each center's experience. In other areas the issue of capacity is more important and there is a limit on the number of centers that can be designated within each geographic location. This may increase transport times slightly but concentrates experience in a smaller number of hospitals.

The American College of Surgeons (ACS) has a verification process that provides a national standard (Table 14-5).[46] To be verified as a Level I trauma center by the ACS, a hospital must have continuous coverage by an attending trauma surgeon and must provide care for at least 1200 patients each year, at least 20% of whom have an ISS greater than 15. Level I centers must also be leaders in education, prevention, and trauma research. A Level II designation allows for consultation specialties, such as orthopedics and neurosurgery, to be available on an on-call basis. Level II centers are generally not teaching or research facilities. Level III centers are equipped to deal with life-threatening injuries only on a short-term basis.

Triage of severely injured patients remains somewhat controversial. Should a badly injured patient be transported directly to a Level I trauma center, bypassing a Level II or Level III center? Alternatively, is that patient best seen at the nearest trauma center for stabilization and then transferred to a Level I trauma center if deemed necessary? Unfortunately, this debate is often fueled more by economic agendas than a real concern about the patient's welfare. The data to guide system decisions are scant. In addition, triage criteria are often vague, which has the advantage of allowing prehospital care personnel the latitude to make triage decisions in the field but also opens them to criticism should they bypass any center.

MacKenzie et al conducted a large multi-institutional trial to study the effectiveness of care provided at trauma centers versus non-trauma centers following moderate to severe injury. Mortality outcomes were compared among 5191 patients treated at any of 18 Level I trauma centers or one of 51 non-trauma centers located in 14 states. After case mix adjustment they concluded that the overall risk of death was 25% lower when injured patients received care at a Level I trauma center rather than a non-trauma center.[47]

In a study of 4364 significantly injured patients (mean ISS of 14), Sampalis et al demonstrated that patients who were transferred from the initial receiving hospital had an adjusted increase in odds of dying of 57% compared with equally injured patients taken directly to a Level I trauma center.[48] However, this study included only urban hospital transfers. Young et al demonstrated that patients with traumatic brain injury have a statistically significant increase in survival when transported directly to trauma centers in Virginia, a state that has a much more rural appearance.[49] In another study conducted in a rural setting, Rogers et al[50] found that patients transferred to a Level I trauma center from outlying hospitals had the same mortality as those admitted directly to a Level I center. This was true of even more severely injured patients. However, twice as many patients died at the scene in rural environments than in more urban environments (72% vs 40%). The authors postulated that this difference was due to delay in discovery of patients and to prolonged EMS arrival and transport times even to the regional hospitals.

The Evaluation Process

The evaluation of patients after trauma must be rapid, systematic, and organized (Table 14-6). Injuries must be identified in the order in which they are likely to produce death or serious disability. These must then be dealt with in the same order in which they are identified. It is also important to remember that injury is a tremendously dynamic process. A seemingly stable patient can rapidly become unstable, and injuries that seem minor initially can evolve into life-threatening ones in a very short time. Thus the evaluation process must be repetitive to avoid missing this progression. A primary survey is usually conducted first; it is designed to identify immediately life-threatening injury. The survey should be followed by a resuscitation period, during which patients are reevaluated and monitored. The secondary survey, a head-to-toe physical examination, follows the resuscitation phase. At the end of the secondary survey, radiographic evaluation and other diagnostic tests should be performed. The results should be compiled to determine a definitive plan of care.

Primary Survey

A primary survey is done specifically to identify and treat immediately life-threatening injury. Airway issues always assume the highest priority. In any severely injured patient, airway control must be accomplished immediately. Consideration should be given to definitive airway management in patients who present in shock and those who have significant traumatic brain injury (a Glasgow Coma Scale [GCS] score < 8), neck injuries, significant maxillofacial injury, or any other injury that potentially compromises airway integrity. Airway control in the field is generally accomplished by the orotracheal route, though nasal intubation is a viable alternative as well. Disposable end-tidal CO_2 detectors, if available, are extremely useful to confirm endotracheal tube position. However, CO_2 may be impossible to detect in profound shock due to lack of cellular respiration. Breath sounds may be difficult to interpret as well. In these cases, further attempts at airway control in the field should be abandoned and the patient should be transferred to the hospital as quickly as possible.

In the resuscitation unit, airway control is most often obtained via the orotracheal route using a rapid-sequence technique with strict in-line stabilization of the cervical spine. Once the patient has been intubated, the endotracheal tube must be properly secured. Tube position should be confirmed, documented, and periodically rechecked.

Once the patient's airway has been controlled, rapid assessment of the adequacy of oxygenation and ventilation is the next highest priority. Supplemental oxygen should be administered to all patients in order to maximize peripheral oxygen delivery. The assessment of breathing includes evaluating for the six most life-threatening injuries: tension pneumothorax, open pneumothorax, massive hemothorax, pericardial tamponade, airway obstruction, and flail chest.

Tension pneumothorax and massive hemothorax should be diagnosed and treated based on clinical assessment. Relying

TABLE 14-5 **Trauma Center Descriptors**

	Level I	Level II	Level III	Level IV
Admission requirements	1200 trauma patients per year or 240 admissions with an ISS >15 or average 35 patients per surgeon with ISS >15	Depends on geographic area served, population density, resources available, and maturity of system	No requirement; should be able to initially manage most injured patients and have transfer agreements with higher-level trauma centers; well-defined transfer plans are essential	No requirement; provide initial assessment and evaluation of injured patients but most patients require transfer to higher-level trauma centers; well-defined transfer plans are essential
Surgeon availability	Qualified surgeon must be present and participate in major resuscitations, therapeutic decisions, and operations; 24-hour in-house attending surgeon is most direct means to provide this service; a resident in PGY 4 or 5 may be approved to initiate resuscitation while awaiting the attending surgeon, whose maximal response time should not exceed 15 minutes from time of patient's arrival	Qualified surgeon must participate in major therapeutic decisions, be present for major resuscitations and operations; 24-hour in-house attending surgeon is most direct means to provide this service; a resident in PGY 4 or 5 or an emergency physician who is part of the trauma team may be approved to initiate resuscitation while awaiting the attending surgeon, whose maximal response time should not exceed 15 minutes from time of patient's arrival	A general surgeon must be promptly available; maximal response time is 30 minutes from time of patient's arrival	24-hour emergency coverage by a physician
Critical care	Must maintain a surgically directed critical care service; physician coverage available in-house 24 hours	Qualified surgeon must be involved in critical care of all seriously injured patients; physician coverage promptly available 24 hours	Qualified surgeon must be involved in critical care of all seriously injured patients	No requirement
Research center	Required	Not required	Not required	Not required
Education, prevention, and outreach	Leader in these efforts	Required	Required	Required

PGY, Postgraduate year.
The reader is referred to the current American College of Surgeons, Committee on Trauma: *Trauma Center Designation Guidelines* for a complete list of criteria.
Source: Committee on Trauma, American College of Surgeons: *Resources for Optimal Care of the Injured Patient: 2006,* Chicago, 2006, The American College of Surgeons.

TABLE 14-6 **Initial Evaluation**

Phase	Evaluation/Intervention
Primary survey	**A**irway with cervical spine precautions **B**reathing **C**irculation with control of external hemorrhage **D**isability – brief neurological assessment **E**xposure/Environment – unclothe patient but prevent hypothermia
Resuscitation	Oxygenation and ventilation Shock management; two large-bore peripheral IV lines (cutdown and central access as necessary) and warmed IV fluids Manage life threatening problems
Adjuncts to the primary survey and resuscitation	Monitoring Arterial blood gas analysis (with high index of suspicion) and respiratory rate End-tidal carbon dioxide Electrocardiogram Pulse oximetry Blood pressure Routine lab work Blood for type and crossmatch Urinary and gastric catheters X-rays and diagnostic studies Chest Pelvis C-spine DPL or FAST
Secondary survey	Head-to-toe physical assessment and history
Adjuncts to secondary survey	Computed tomography Contrast radiographs Extremity x-rays Thoracic and lumbar spine films if needed Angiography Ultrasonography

Adapted from information obtained from American College of Surgeons, Committee on Trauma. *Advanced Trauma Life Support for Doctors, Student Course Manual,* ed 7, Chicago, 2004, American College of Surgeons.
DPL, Diagnostic peritoneal lavage; *FAST,* focused assessment with sonography for trauma.

on breath sounds to make the diagnosis is unwise and could prove to be fatal. Chest decompression with tube thoracostomy is definitive therapy. However, a tension pneumothorax may be temporized by placing a 14-gauge IV catheter in the chest anteriorly through the second intercostal space. An open pneumothorax should be treated with semi-occlusive dressing immediately followed by placement of a chest tube. Flail chest is a clinical diagnosis in which a portion of the chest wall moves paradoxically from the remainder of the thoracic cage. This is caused by at least two ribs broken in at least two places. Endotracheal intubation should be considered for all patients with flail chest. However, most of the pulmonary dysfunction is from underlying pulmonary contusions and lacerations, not from the mechanical problems of the injured bony segment. Some patients can be managed without endotracheal intubation using good pain control techniques and directed pulmonary therapy. Intravenous or epidural patient-controlled analgesia (PCA) or an intrathoracic anesthetic block can be efficacious.

The physical findings often associated with the most life threatening of these conditions are depicted in Table 14-7. Unfortunately, these conditions often occur simultaneously, and the physical findings can be confusing. For instance, the patient who has exsanguinated from concomitant pulmonary hilar injury and has cardiac tamponade will not have jugular venous distention until very late, if at all, as intravascular volume loss may prohibit vascular congestion. Therefore these conditions should be treated aggressively based on clinical suspicion.

Circulation, or the adequacy of peripheral oxygen delivery, is the next highest priority. Adequate perfusion depends on oxygen delivery meeting oxygen demand. The body cannot store oxygen; therefore, an oxygen debt can be incurred rapidly. As previously noted, clinical signs often occur late in the trauma cycle, after oxygen debt is well established.

The degree of hemodynamic instability will be a function of the rapidity of ongoing blood loss and the degree or efficacy of compensation. Vasoconstriction may mask clinical signs until very late in the clinical course.[6] This is particularly true in young patients, most of whom have extremely compliant capacitance vessels. More than 50% of total circulating blood volume can be lost before patients show clinical signs.

TABLE 14-7 **Physical Findings in Thoracic Trauma Patients**

	JVD	Resonance	Breath Sounds	Tracheal Position
Cardiac tamponade	Yes	Normal	Normal	Normal
Tension pneumothorax	Yes	Hyper	Decreased	Deviated airway
Massive hemothorax	No	Hypo	Decreased	Normal

JVD, Jugular vein distention.

These patients often develop relatively sudden cardiovascular collapse. Commonly used parameters such as heart rate, blood pressure, pulse pressure, and urine output grossly underestimate the degree of blood loss. Calculation of base deficit via arterial blood gas analysis can be extremely useful in estimating blood loss and should be routine in any patient suspected of having significant blood loss.[51]

Large-bore IV access should be established and blood obtained for laboratory values. Two peripheral IV lines usually are sufficient. However, vasoconstriction may make placement of large-bore peripheral IV lines problematic or impossible in patients who are in shock. In this case central access must be obtained. Percutaneous placement of pulmonary artery catheter introducers for infusion of volume is the method most commonly used. Peripheral cutdown can take an excessive amount of time. The saphenous vein at the ankle is unlikely to be suitable for large-bore access. Saphenous cutdown in the groin risks iatrogenic injury to the femoral artery or femoral vein. Percutaneous access has been shown to be safe if done by experienced practitioners or residents with adequate supervision.[52] Flow characteristics of the fluid infused are a function of the length and diameter of the catheter. Short, wide catheters impede flow the least. Therefore long central venous pressure lines are not ideal because flow through this type of catheter will be much slower than via an introducer.

A brief neurologic assessment (D for disability) is the next highest priority. Usually patients are asked to wiggle their toes, which assesses mentation and the ability to process information. In addition, it allows early identification of complete spinal cord injuries. In patients with some degree of mental obtundation, a GCS score should be calculated (see Chapter 20). This should be compared with the neurologic assessment obtained by the prehospital care providers in the field. Focal signs on physical examination, such as a unilaterally dilated pupil or a decrease of 2 or more points in the GCS score, particularly if that decrease is in the motor component, are strong predictors of an intracranial lesion requiring evacuation.[53] This is an emergency situation that demands immediate CT examination, if the patient is hemodynamically stable, to plan operative decompression. Performing blind burr holes in the emergency department is useful only in very remote locations when patients are dying and transfer is not possible.

Any patient with a significant decrease in mental status should have airway control before leaving the emergency department. Progressive neurologic decline or evidence of transtentorial herniation not attributable to an extracranial cause suggests increased intracranial pressure that can be controlled temporarily with hyperventilation or administration of intravenous mannitol.[54] Although hyperventilation can reduce intracranial pressure (ICP), prophylactic use ($paCO_2 < 25$ mmHg) is not recommended, and this therapy should be avoided within the first 24 hours after injury when cerebral blood flow may be reduced.[54] The diuretic effect of mannitol may make patients hypovolemic in 15 to 20 minutes. These patients should be adequately hydrated before mannitol administration and may require additional intravenous fluid or blood transfusion to maintain circulating blood volume.

Complete exposure of the patient, with environmental precautions, is the next essential step in completing the primary survey. Many patients present with obvious injury, and the natural tendency is to focus on that injury. It is important to totally examine the patient to avoid missing a subtle but potentially life-threatening injury. Patients must be log rolled and their back examined, as well as the perineum and axillae. Despite the need for complete exposure, the patient must be kept warm and dry. Hypothermia depresses cardiac performance, impedes pulmonary function, and worsens any coagulopathy. Hypothermia often begins either in the field or in the emergency department. Warming fluids and autotransfusing any blood collected from the thoracic cavity can be helpful in preventing hypothermia. In addition, the ambient temperature in the resuscitation area should be kept above 70° F and patients should be covered after thorough examination.

Resuscitation

The primary survey should have identified all immediately life-threatening injuries, and those injuries should be dealt with as they are discovered. Resuscitation often occurs in concert with the primary survey because resuscitation accompanies therapy for life-threatening injuries. If the patient has been deemed stable after the primary survey, the resuscitation phase is the period in which the patient is monitored and cardiovascular stability is repeatedly reassessed. If large-bore peripheral access was not established during the primary survey, it is important to obtain at this point. Patients should be connected to a cardiac monitor and a pulse oximeter. End-tidal CO_2 monitors should be used in patients who have undergone intubation. A Foley catheter and gastric tube should be inserted if there are no contraindications.

Contraindications to nasal insertion of a gastric tube include any significant midface fracture. In patients with a cribriform plate fracture, a nasogastric tube may inadvertently be placed within the cranium. Evidence of a urethral injury is a contraindication to bladder catheterization. Physical findings, such as a high-riding prostate on rectal exam, blood at the urethral meatus, or a scrotal hematoma, are absolute contraindications to placement of a Foley catheter. In male patients with clinical evidence of a pelvic fracture, bladder catheterization can be deferred until imaging studies are completed if the patient remains stable. It may be wise to obtain a urethrogram to document the integrity of the urethra in men with complex pelvic fractures before inserting a Foley catheter, even in the absence of clinical signs.

The initial fluid bolus given is generally 2 L of isotonic crystalloid. Patients who present in shock can be stratified over several response groups. The immediate responders are those who have a complete response to the initial crystalloid fluid bolus and show no evidence of ongoing blood loss or perfusion deficits. In general, these patients have Class I or Class II shock (see Table 14-2). Transient responders are those who initially respond but ultimately show signs of ongoing blood loss or perfusion deficit. These patients generally have Class II or Class III hemorrhage or have bled once and then rebled. Fluid should be continued and a rapid search for the source of hemorrhage undertaken. Real consideration should be given to early transfusion in these patients. Patients who do not respond have life-threatening hemorrhage. The highest priority must be given to ascertaining the site of blood loss and stopping it immediately. These patients all require blood transfusion; uncrossmatched blood is the best choice.

The transition between primary survey and resuscitation into the secondary survey is an appropriate time to obtain initial radiographs. It is also important to ensure that laboratory tests have been ordered and that blood has been sent to be typed and crossmatched.

Secondary Survey

The secondary survey consists of a careful examination of the entire patient to elucidate injury and areas of potential injury. It is generally done in a head-to-toe fashion. It is important to remember to examine the pupils for reactivity and the tympanic membrane for evidence of membrane rupture and cerebral spinal fluid leak. Battle's sign—ecchymosis over the mastoid area—may be the only presenting indication of a basilar skull fracture. The midface area should be examined for swelling, tenderness, and stability. The neck should be kept immobilized until a cervical spine injury has been ruled out. However, it is possible to remove the collar carefully and examine for the presence or absence of cervical spine tenderness. The neck should also be examined for the presence of subcutaneous air, as well as ecchymoses or abrasions. The chest wall should be palpated for evidence of subcutaneous air, instability, or tenderness. The lungs and heart should be carefully auscultated. The presence of hyperresonance or dullness on percussion of the chest wall along with diminished or absent breath sounds can raise suspicion of pneumothorax or hemothorax. The abdomen should be auscultated, inspected, and palpated. The presence or absence of tenderness will help determine the need for further investigation. The pelvis should be examined gently for evidence of tenderness and stability. It is important to avoid rocking the pelvis because unstable pelvic fractures have a tendency to bleed with any motion. The patient should be log rolled and the back examined. It is necessary to carefully palpate all bony prominences over the spine and examine any tender areas of the flank. Bruising and soft tissue injury should be noted. All four extremities should be examined for pain, tenderness, ligamentous stability, and adequacy of pulses. Finally the patient should undergo a complete neurologic evaluation.

Clinical Decision Making

At this point the clinician should have identified all areas of defined and potential injury. It is now time for further diagnostics and definitive care. A priority must be assigned to each injury. Several principles apply.

Injuries should be investigated in the order in which they are likely to cause death or permanent disability. Most severely injured trauma patients require a multiplicity of diagnostic imaging, particularly radiographs and scans. The plan should maximize efficiency. Transporting patients can divert precious resources and may pose an increased risk for patients who may become unstable. When nurses transport patients for diagnostic testing, they are unable to care for other patients. Therefore it is important to realistically approximate the time needed for a diagnostic examination. An urgent CT scan of the head should not be delayed to obtain all the plain films simply for convenience.

The initial films obtained are of the lateral cervical spine, the chest, and the pelvis. These are good screening examinations to detect potentially life-threatening injuries and areas of possible blood loss. They can be obtained rapidly without transporting the patient from the resuscitation area.

Patients can lose blood internally into the chest, abdomen, pelvis, retroperitoneum, or muscle compartments or externally, outside the body. Intrathoracic injury can be diagnosed with a combination of clinical suspicion, physical examination, and a plain chest x-ray examination. Pelvic bleeding can be extremely substantial and produce life-threatening hemorrhage. Virtually every patient who has significant retroperitoneal bleeding has a pelvic fracture. This diagnosis can be made with a combination of physical examination and a pelvic x-ray examination. Muscle compartment bleeding, if significant, will be obvious on physical examination.

External blood loss can be life threatening and may occur from injuries, such as scalp lacerations, that appear innocuous at the time of initial presentation. It is difficult to quantitate blood at the scene, but the prehospital care providers will be the best gauge as to whether there was substantial external blood loss in the field. It is important to remember that even major vascular injury or significant scalp bleeding may stop, particularly if the patient develops hypotension. These injuries may rebleed once the patient's blood pressure is normalized.

Intraabdominal bleeding can be more difficult to detect. A plain film of the abdomen is not helpful and physical examination is not at all specific or sensitive. Bedside ultrasonographic examination can be helpful in determining the presence or absence of intraabdominal bleeding, particularly in a patient in shock (Figure 14-3).[55] Focused assessment with sonography for trauma (FAST) provides a rapid, noninvasive, and inexpensive means of diagnosing hemoperitoneum. During resuscitation, views of the pericardial sac, hepatorenal fossa, splenorenal fossa, and pelvis can be obtained at the bedside using portable sonography. Sequential scans can be performed easily to determine progression of blood acculmulation.[56] Diagnostic peritoneal lavage is also a rapid diagnostic test for intraabdominal hemorrhage and can be performed at the bedside, although it has largely fallen out of favor since the advent of high-resolution CT scanning and FAST. Although CT scanning is the most precise method of diagnosing abdominal blood loss, it is time consuming and usually takes the patient out of the resuscitation area. This technique should be reserved for patients who are hemodynamically stable (see Chapter 25.)

Resuscitation Fluids

The goal of fluid administration in the trauma patient is to support cardiovascular function and maintain adequate peripheral oxygen delivery. Volume increases cardiac preload, thus supporting cardiac output. The standard initial fluid is isotonic crystalloid, although colloids and hypertonic saline can also be used.[57-59] Both hypertonic saline and colloid infusion have the advantage of supporting cardiac function with a limited amount of fluid. Both rely partially on recruitment of interstitial volume to achieve this. Crystalloid fluid in adequate volume is as capable of cardiac augmentation as either of the other two choices. None of these fluids increase oxygen-carrying capacity. Overzealous administration of any resuscitative fluid can limit oxygen delivery by diluting hemoglobin levels. If hemoglobin falls dangerously low and myocardial oxygen delivery becomes insufficient, cardiovascular function may be compromised. If the heart is unable to accept a large volume load, be it colloid, crystalloid, or hypertonic saline, the heart can fail as it is pushed over the peak of its myocardial performance curve.

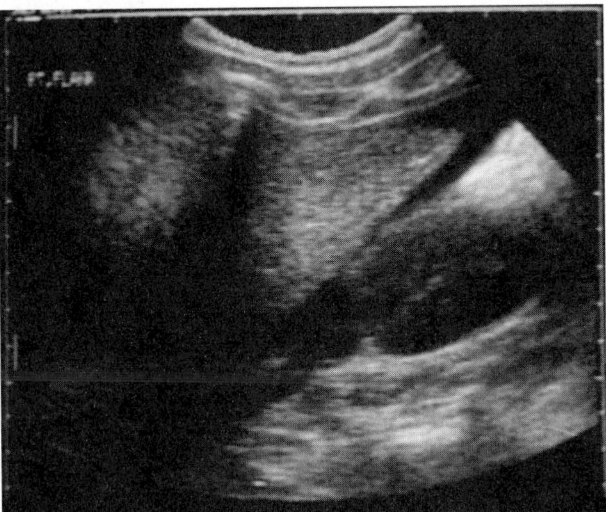

FIGURE 14-3 Focused assessment with sonography for trauma (FAST) demonstrates free intraperitoneal blood.

The only readily available fluid that increases oxygen-carrying capacity and preload is blood. Although clinicians are aware of bloodborne pathogens and transfusion reactions, equal concern must be raised regarding the consequence of delaying transfusion when blood is needed. The exact indication for transfusing blood remains controversial.[60-62] Several principles seem reasonable, however.

Patients who are hemodynamically unstable and those with evidence of persistent tissue hypoxia despite fluid resuscitation should be given blood transfusions. Cross-matched blood is preferable, but the patient's clinical condition must dictate whether delaying transfusion is prudent. Major transfusion reactions are uncommon given today's level of sophistication in blood banking. Even transfusion with type O blood is safe if necessary after major blood loss.

Some patients may have a dangerous tissue hypoxia despite relatively normal vital signs. Patients with sufficient metabolic acidosis, as indicated by arterial blood gas values, must be presumed to be in shock. Clinicians should give strong consideration to transfusing these patients, even if they are not significantly hypotensive. All patients whose metabolic acidosis persists after initial fluid resuscitation should likewise be given blood transfusions. Insertion of central monitoring devices and measurement of central venous oxygen saturation can be helpful. Patients with central venous oxygen saturations lower than 55% should be presumed to be in shock and bleeding. Consideration should be given to empiric blood transfusion.

Hematocrit, expressed in percent, is a ratio of red blood cells to circulating intravascular volume. If patients bleed acutely, they lose cells and volume equally. Thus patients who are bleeding acutely will maintain a normal hematocrit during the initial resuscitation. Hematocrit falls when patients receive exogenous fluids that dilute the red blood cells, and the kidney compensates for blood loss by retaining salt and water. Initial hematocrit should not be used as the trigger for transfusion. Serial hematocrits may be better, but the time required to obtain laboratory results makes this impractical as a minute-to-minute guide during the initial phase of care.

In addition to red blood cell transfusions, use of fresh frozen plasma (FFP) and platelets plays an important role in the care of the patient who requires massive blood transfusion. Standard blood transfusions replace only red blood cells, not coagulation factors or platelets. Coagulopathy after significant injury is common.

Thrombocytopenia is the most common disorder after massive transfusion. Although platelet counts of 20,000/mm^3 are generally sufficient to prevent spontaneous bleeding, patients in shock who are being resuscitated with large volumes of fluid and blood have much less predictable platelet function. Platelet counts must be monitored closely. In general, platelets should be given if the platelet count is less than 100,000/mm^3 or if there is clinical evidence of ongoing bleeding. Alternatively, platelets can be given empirically as part of the massive resuscitation.

The subset of trauma patients who take drugs that alter normal clotting function presents a significant challenge. Many patients take nonsteroidal anti-inflammatory drugs on a regular basis. These drugs, as well as aspirin and clopidogrel, inhibit platelet function, increasing bleeding after injury. International normalized ratio (INR) must be closely monitored in those patients who have been taking warfarin, and rapid transfusion of fresh frozen plasma may be necessary to control active blood loss, particularly in the presence of traumatic brain injury.

Like platelets, massive transfusion also rapidly depletes coagulation factors. Hepatic function may be impaired in the patient who is in shock, thus limiting the ability to rapidly mobilize additional coagulation factors. FFP can be lifesaving. It is easy to underestimate the need for plasma, and delays will certainly impede hemostasis. Prothrombin and partial thromboplastin times should be carefully monitored and normalized.

Holcomb et al recently published an observational study of the transfusion requirements of severely injured combat casualties in Iraq and Afghanistan.[63] They found that the most severely injured trauma patients presenting with the lethal triad of hypothermia, acidosis, and coagulopathy had less bleeding and a more rapid return to homeostasis when transfused with FFP as a primary resuscitation fluid in at least a 1:1 ratio with packed red blood cells. Their data, albeit anecdotal, call into question our standard crystalloid resuscitation regimen in this subset of patients.

Hypothermia

Hypothermia is a common problem in patients with serious injury and shock. Hypothermia can be classified as moderate or severe. In general, core body temperature is regulated and even relatively small changes in body temperature trigger a compensatory mechanism. This generally involves cutaneous vasoconstriction, which reduces heat loss, and shivering, which increases heat production. Unfortunately, many injured patients are subjected to environmental factors that predispose them to hypothermia. Shock, particularly if profound, is almost always accompanied by hypothermia. Patients who are injured and lie at ambient temperature on the street often become hypothermic even before they are discovered, particularly if they lie in wet clothes or are exposed to ambient temperatures significantly less than core body temperature. Decisions made by health care providers can significantly exacerbate hypothermia. Infusion of room-temperature intravenous fluids or cold blood can drop core body temperature. If patients are exposed and examined for potential injuries, care might not be taken to cover them or to warm the ambient temperature of the resuscitation area. Thus hypothermia begins in the field and can be exacerbated during resuscitation. In a series of patients requiring operation, Gregory et al demonstrated that most patients are hypothermic at the time of anesthetic induction.[64] These problems can be compounded by heat loss in the operating room from open body cavities, ongoing resuscitation, and cool irrigation fluids. In addition, anesthetic agents and narcotics suppress compensatory mechanisms.

Hypothermia affects all body systems. The extent to which each system is affected depends on the severity of the hypothermia and its duration. Initial cardiovascular response includes increases in heart rate, cardiac output, and mean arterial pressure secondary to increases in circulating catecholamines, peripheral vasoconstriction, and the resultant increase in central blood volume. Ultimately, however, cardiac output, heart rate, and blood pressure fall. There is a generalized slowing of myocardial conduction, often accompanied by T-wave inversion and increases in the QT interval. A J wave may be seen as hypothermia worsens. Both atrial and ventricular arrhythmias such as atrial fibrillation can occur. Ventricular fibrillation can be seen as temperature falls below 30° C.

Initially, hypothermia produces central stimulation of the respiratory system with an increased respiratory rate. However, as cooling progresses, respiratory depression ensues with decreased respiratory rate and tidal volume. This is often accompanied by marked increases in dead space. Epithelial mucosa may become swollen and the ability to clear secretions is depressed.

Decreased tubular enzymatic activity in the kidneys secondary to increased circulating blood volume from vasoconstriction produces a cold diuresis. This may be seen relatively early after a drop in core temperature of only 2° to 3° C.[65] This can give the false impression of an adequately resuscitated patient as vasoconstriction maintains blood pressure at normal despite a drop in cardiac output and urine output remains normal or even above normal. Oliguria and azotemia occur late. Cerebral blood flow decreases as temperature decreases and may be accompanied by impaired mentation, agitation, drowsiness, or seizure.

The diagnosis of hypothermia depends on accurate measurement of temperature. Peripheral determinations of temperature, such as oral or tympanic membrane temperature, may not accurately reflect core temperature, particularly as vasoconstriction and other cardiovascular compensatory mechanisms increase. In addition, some methods of measuring body temperature are not designed to measure temperatures below 35° C. Core body temperature can best be measured by the thermistor on a pulmonary artery catheter. In addition, thermistors have been incorporated into Foley catheters and provide continuous readout of core body temperature in the bladder. Nierman demonstrated good correlation between pulmonary artery temperature and bladder temperature as long as the bladder is not being irrigated.[66] Esophageal or rectal temperature probes may also be used to continuously measure core body temperature.

Clearly the best treatment of hypothermia is to limit heat loss and prevent it if at all possible. Treatment of mild to moderate hypothermia can be passive. This involves preventing additional heat loss and allowing the body to compensate by covering the patient with a blanket, increasing the ambient temperature, or using devices such as aluminum caps to prevent heat loss from the head. Convective air blankets can be beneficial as well.

When patients have developed severe hypothermia, active rewarming is generally wise. Heat can be exchanged across any membrane, such as the lungs, pleural cavity, or peritoneal cavity. The efficacy of rewarming is a function of the surface area across which heat can be exchanged. Thus peritoneal dialysis or irrigation of a chest tube with warmed, sterile fluid can increase body temperature. Warming inspired gases via the ventilator is another option. Intravenous fluids, including blood, should be warmed at least to body temperature. Convective warming units can be used, but they are not as efficient as the aforementioned methods. Finally, extracorporeal rewarming techniques can be used in some cases. Gentilello et al described continuous arterial venous rewarming via modification of the commercially available warmers used to warm IV fluids.[67] Impressive rates of rewarming can be achieved using this or another type of extracorporeal circuit. Cardiopulmonary bypass can also be helpful for profound hypothermia.

Hypothermia may be a marker of the severity of injury as opposed to an independent predictor of mortality. Some patients, such as those with brain injury, may actually benefit from hypothermia. Marion et al demonstrated improved survival among patients with traumatic brain injury who were randomized to sustained core body temperatures of 32° to 33° C for 24 hours.[68] Qui et al found that patients with severe traumatic brain injury cooled to 33° to 35° C for 3 to 5 days after injury had lower mortality and significantly better outcomes when compared with patients randomized to remain normothermic.[69] Pooled data from a number of studies suggest prophylactic hypothermia does not significantly reduce mortality in patients with traumatic brain injury, although it is associated with significantly better neurologic outcomes when compared with normothermic controls.[54] There also are case reports of patient survival when usually fatal injuries were repaired while the patient was in hypothermic circulatory arrest. A number of researchers have demonstrated the cerebral protective effects of deep hypothermia, up to 60 minutes in dogs, even in the face of cardiac arrest.[70,71] The potential applications in humans involve inducing a state of suspended animation accompanied by deep hypothermia to allow repair of injuries during heroic resuscitation.

Hemodynamic Monitoring

Evidence of inadequate perfusion should prompt simultaneous investigation and therapy. Patients who demonstrate inadequate resuscitation despite seemingly adequate treatment for the injuries identified may well have a missed injury. Untreated, these often are fatal. This should prompt a rapid but comprehensive search for injuries that were missed at the time of initial investigation, or that were thought to be minor but have now become more profoundly symptomatic. In addition, resuscitation efforts should be continued.

Virtually every patient who has been inadequately resuscitated is volume depleted and can benefit from increased cardiac preload. Thus a reasonable response would be to augment cardiac preload with increased intravenous fluid. Blood may be an excellent choice because it has the ability to increase cardiac output by increasing preload and to increase oxygen delivery by increasing hemoglobin. Serial measurements of serum lactate levels can be used to demonstrate the return of aerobic metabolism. Patients who undergo resuscitation efforts and then have their lactate cleared to normal can reasonably be assumed to be fully resuscitated.[72] It is important to remember that serum lactates can be misleading, especially when followed over a short period. In severely injured patients, serum lactate may be high initially and either fails to fall or actually increases after resuscitation. This represents washout as resuscitation reperfuses beds that were previously underperfused. Subsequent serum lactate measurements then begin to show normalization.

Patients who are not fully resuscitated often benefit from more sophisticated monitoring. Occult cardiovascular dysfunction is common after injury. An 80% incidence of inadequate resuscitation has been demonstrated in seriously injured patients with traumatic brain injury despite normal vital signs.[73] In addition, patients with significant penetrating torso trauma often have substantial perfusion abnormalities despite normal vital signs. In patients such as these, measurement of cardiopulmonary hemodynamics can help define the problematic cardiovascular parameters. A more sophisticated understanding of vascular resistance and preload issues allows the resuscitation to be guided more precisely.

SPECIAL CONSIDERATIONS

PEDIATRIC TRAUMA

Although the pathophysiology of shock does not differ remarkably between children and adults, the manifestation does. Pediatric patients develop system dysfunction and organ failure in a consuming manner rather than the slower, progressive organ failure seen in adults. Children normally have a higher metabolic rate than adults, and trauma and sepsis only increase their metabolic needs. This hypermetabolic state quickly depletes the limited energy stores available to a child, and anaerobic metabolism occurs earlier. Liver failure can rapidly ensue, and the hypermetabolic state cannot be sustained. Cellular energy production becomes further decreased, thus limiting oxygen supply and ultimately producing cellular death.

The most frequent cause of shock in children and adults is hypovolemia.[74] Although the circulating blood volume in a child is relatively larger than in an adult, absolute blood volume is small. Most of the total fluid volume in children is extracellular and can be lost even without extensive hemorrhage. The early symptoms of hypovolemia in children are decreased peripheral perfusion, oliguria, and tachycardia. As with adults, blood pressure is not an accurate indicator of shock in children. As cardiac output decreases, vasoconstriction increases, artificially maintaining blood pressure. Cardiac failure follows hypotension relatively quickly. Stroke volume is relatively fixed in children and thus responds to shock by increasing heart rate. Thus, to maintain adequate cardiac output in critically ill children, heart rates should be maintained within the high normal range.

Respiratory failure also occurs relatively quickly in pediatric patients. Children have little respiratory reserve because their chest wall is more compliant and their abdomen is larger, decreasing the ability to raise intrathoracic pressure. Children's thoracic musculature tires more easily than adults, predisposing them to respiratory failure.

There are also differences in the immune system in children relative to adults. Young children have few neutrophils and are not able to produce white blood cells in the face of stress as well as an older child. Complement levels do not reach adult normal ranges until the age of 3 to 6 months.[75] In addition, because immunoglobulin levels are transferred from mother to child, they wane at 4 to 5 months of age, at which point infants become extremely susceptible to viruses, *Candida* infections, and bacteria. The child does not have the ability to launch an immune response to these contagions and may develop acute organ dysfunction as a result of infection after injury.

Trauma in the Elderly

During the past 10 years geriatric trauma has become an increasingly important segment of injury care. Several principles are important to maximize functional outcome and survival of this special subset of patients. The presentation of injured geriatric patients differs from that of their younger counterparts. As with everyone, the triage and initial care of geriatric patients must be based on a stepwise evaluation of anatomy, injury, and stability. Undertriage in the field can be particularly lethal in geriatric trauma patients. Injuries are often occult. Symptoms such as confusion or pain may be ascribed to preexisting disease. Unfortunately, the margin of error that a geriatric patient will tolerate is small. In fact, Osler et al found that, when controlled for degree of injury (using the Trauma and Injury Severity Score), six times as many elderly die as younger victims.[76] Despite this, most trauma systems currently do not have specialty centers for geriatric injury or different triage protocols for the elderly. Yet these same systems often subsegment the pediatric population because of its special needs.

The care of the elderly patient in the prehospital phase should be modified. Conditions as simple as isolated fractures can be life threatening. The loss of tissue turgor and the atherosclerosis that affect virtually every elderly person may limit tamponade and increase blood loss into muscle compartments.[77] The lack of cardiovascular reserve limits the heart's ability to rapidly accept fluid volume delivered during resuscitation. Cerebral atrophy may make potentially life-threatening, traumatic brain injury relatively asymptomatic initially. Elderly patients can then become suddenly and profoundly symptomatic even hours after injury. Outcome at that point is likely to be poor, particularly if the patient has been undertriaged to a local emergency department. Paramedics should be advised to recognize that occult injuries can kill elderly patients. Intravenous fluids are best given in small boluses, such as 250-ml aliquots to avoid precipitating heart failure. Fractures should be splinted and patients transported rapidly. The suspicion of traumatic brain injury should prompt transport to a trauma center.

The physiology of aging limits the elderly patient's ability to respond to the stresses of injury. This is perhaps most important in the cardiovascular system. Cardiac output remains relatively stable as the patient ages, but the ability to augment cardiovascular performance is blunted. The same is true for heart rate, a compensatory mechanism used to maintain peripheral oxygen delivery. Autoregulation attempts to hold coronary perfusion stable over a wide range of physiologic states. This becomes particularly problematic when fixed coronary artery lesions begin to limit flow. The coronary circulation is significantly venous extracted even at rest.

Increased peripheral oxygen demands after injury can precipitate a dangerous set of circumstances. As oxygen demand increases, cardiac output must likewise increase. Blood loss limits peripheral oxygen delivery and myocardial oxygen demands increase as the heart attempts to compensate and increase cardiac output. Coronary ischemia can occur, which itself limits cardiac output. This can quickly lead to irreversible shock.

Other organ systems, such as the lungs and kidneys, behave similarly. Ventilation/perfusion mismatch can approach 15% to 20% in the elderly.[77] A drop in cardiac output may itself be sufficient to precipitate hypoxia. Nephron mass decreases as people age, and creatinine clearance follows. However, the loss of muscle mass generally means that blood urea nitrogen and creatinine levels remain normal. Even dehydrated elderly patients may produce large volumes of relatively dilute urine secondary to a loss in the reabsorptive capacity of the distal tubule. Finally, diuretic medications, which are used by many elderly people, may make the average elderly person dehydrated. Thus these patients may have significant renal impairment, even though at first glance renal function is normal.

The role of occult hypoperfusion and its impact on outcome have been recognized. Cardiovascular insufficiency is common in elderly people, even in those who appear relatively stable.[78] Early recognition of this condition is extremely important because delays in therapy can be lethal. High-risk patients include those with traumatic brain injury or multiple long-bone fractures, those who were struck by an automobile, and those who present with initial hypotension. Invasive hemodynamic monitoring can be lifesaving in these patients.[1] In a prospective study of elderly patients at high risk, Scalea et al demonstrated that half these high-risk patients were in cardiogenic shock.[78] Survival was no different when monitoring was initiated late in the patient's course of treatment. However, when the initial evaluation process was truncated, mean time to monitoring fell from 5.5 to 2.5 hours. Mortality was reduced by approximately 50% when important cardiovascular issues were identified and treated early. Thus it seems that the degree of physiologic alteration at the time of admission is not as important as early recognition and treatment.

The cause of this cardiovascular dysfunction has been thought to be pump failure secondary to a combination of chronic illness and acute cardiovascular need. However, the possibility of occult acute cardiac ischemia precipitating pump failure has been raised. This unstable angina may go unrecognized by both the patient and the physician. Chest pain may be masked by pain from other injuries. If the patient has not had angina previously, this may be dismissed as indigestion or thought to be secondary to the injury. Patients who are critically ill may be intubated and sedated and thus be unable to complain of chest pain even if it is present. If acute cardiac ischemia does occur, a different strategy is mandated. Cardiac support for the failing pump from nonischemic causes generally involves volume loading and inotropic support to maximize peripheral oxygen delivery. Acute cardiac ischemia, however, requires a strategy of myocardial protection involving beta blockade, judicious fluid administration, and nitrates. A 12-lead electrocardiogram (ECG) and a single set of cardiac enzymes may be insufficient to detect cardiac ischemia. More work is needed to determine the exact incidence of cardiac ischemia and whether a different algorithm alters outcome in these high-risk patients.

THE FUTURE OF TRAUMA RESUSCITATION

Heart rate, blood pressure, and urine output have long been recognized as inadequate parameters with which to gauge traumatic shock severity, particularly in young people.[1] In the search for a more precise yet equally obtainable method of determining impending hemodynamic instability, several researchers have successfully investigated heart rate variability as a predictor of mortality in hemorrhagic patients.[79,80] Adequate hemodynamic response to injury depends primarily on a functioning autonomic nervous system. In 1996, Winchell et al determined the R-R interval in approximately 740 ICU patients using a standard ECG tracing.[81] Heart rate variability was calculated by separating high-frequency from low-frequency bands. R-R interval oscillations of high frequency were found to correlate with parasympathetic activity. Low-frequency R-R variations represent sympathetic activity. Total power (HF/LF) estimated overall autonomic tone. They concluded that patients with low parasympathetic and high sympathetic response to injury (low HF/LF ratio) had higher associated survival rates. Conversely, a high HF/LF ratio (an indicator of parasympathetic predominance) was associated with mortality. In 1997 Winchell et al extrapolated these findings to patients with severe head injury.[82] Cooke et al explored the feasibility of applying this noninvasive technique in the prehospital setting.[80] As the field environment is notoriously noisy and requires extensive patient maneuvering, heart rate variability currently has limited application. This technology requires further refinement before it is recommended for use in the prehospital setting to assist in appropriate patient triage and to guide precise resuscitation interventions.

Another area of research involving the early recognition of compensated shock centers on the cellular hypoperfusion that occurs minutes after injury. During acute blood loss compensatory mechanisms exist to maintain oxygen perfusion to critical organs and away from noncritical organs. Chiara et al investigated splanchnic regional blood flow in a porcine model of acute hemorrhage.[83] They concluded that the gastrointestinal mucosa, perfused by the splanchnic circulation, becomes ischemic soon after bleeding begins. Gastric tonometry was developed as a method to evaluate gastric pH as an indication of gastrointestinal ischemia. However, the Miami Trauma Clinical Trials Group demonstrated that there was no advantage to using gastric tonometry as a therapeutic end point for managing shock in trauma patients.[84] Technical drawbacks also have discouraged use of this monitoring technique during trauma resuscitation.

Sublingual capnometry was developed to overcome the limitations of gastric tonometry.[85] Grundler et al[86] and Weil et al[87] demonstrated that the esophageal tissue pCO_2 mirrors the changes seen in the stomach during shock and resuscitation. In 2004, Baron et al studied the use of sublingual capnometry in patients with penetrating torso trauma.[88] They found that an $SLCO_2 > 45$ mm Hg on admission to the emergency department accurately predicted hemodynamic stability with a 90% confidence interval. More recently Baron et al demonstrated that $SLCO_2$ was comparable to base deficit and serum lactate in predicting mortality among hypotensive trauma patients.[89] Thus, the portability and accuracy of the sublingual capnometer makes it an attractive tool for use in determining the depth of shock and adequacy of resuscitation. Current technology allows sublingual capnometry data within 5 minutes. It seems likely that, within a few years, the data will be available in real time, allowing for instantaneous decision making. The most exciting future application for the sublingual capnometer is its use in the prehospital setting, where it may allow for improved triage and resuscitation schemes.

Undoubtedly the trend toward development of less invasive, easy-to-use devices that rapidly obtain repeated, and preferably continuous, accurate measures of parameters that can be used to diagnose and guide management of shock will continue. For example, there are now devices available that can be placed in line with an arterial pressure monitor to provide continuous determination of stroke volume and cardiac output as well as stroke volume variation, systolic pressure variation, and pulse pressure variation that may aid in evaluating the trauma patient's response to fluid administration.[90] Esophageal Doppler probes to evaluate cardiac output and transesophageal echocardiography probes to evaluate cardiac function and volume sufficiency are also available. A central venous catheter capable of providing continuous central venous oxygen saturation ($ScvO_2$) measurements allows insight into global tissue oxygen supply-demand balance and has already proven value as a therapeutic end point in resuscitation of sepsis.[91] Work is under way to develop monitors that may provide continuous measure of other therapeutic end points used in shock resuscitation, such as lactate. Further research is warranted to determine the effectiveness of these and other measures in guiding management of shock in trauma patients.

Likewise, technological advances have enabled devices that can provide faster, more accurate, and detailed information for diagnoses of injuries (e.g., three-dimensional thin-slice CT) and less invasive options for intervention (e.g., interventional radiology). These developments have revolutionized clinical decision making during resuscitation. Refer to the chapters on systemic injuries for further information on diagnostic and treatment strategies used for specific types of injuries.

Despite all the advances in care of the trauma patient, hemorrhage remains a leading cause of death in severely injured individuals.[92] This fact means that trauma patients may require transfusion and in some instances massive transfusion of blood products. Concerns about the safety and availability of blood have fueled an effort to look at alternative oxygen-carrying solutions.

The blood supply today is the safest it has ever been. However, the risks of hepatitis and human immunodeficiency virus (HIV) transmission via blood are real. In addition, the availability of blood for transfusion is at risk and the available allogenic blood product pool is shrinking. A shortage of 4 million units of packed red blood cells per year is projected by the year 2030.[93]

The storage of red blood cells has distinct limitations. Ideally, red blood cell storage maximizes the number of available viable red cells. The lower limit for successful transfusion is 70% red blood cell survival 24 hours after transfusion.[94] As storage time increases, red cell viability decreases as a result of a myriad of biochemical changes, such as depletion of ATP 2,3-DPG. Stored blood becomes depleted of 2,3-DPG within 3 weeks. These cells regain the ability to synthesize DPG once they are infused, but this does not occur for approximately 24 hours.[94] Animal studies have shown a significant increase in mortality and development of multiple organ failure when blood low in 2,3-DPG is transfused.[95]

Blood substitutes, now termed *oxygen therapeutic agents,* are an extremely attractive alternative. Unlike blood, hemoglobin substitutes do not require crossmatching and should carry no risk of bloodborne viral pathogens. Ideally hemoglobin-based red cell substitutes are readily available, have a long shelf life, and are not immunosuppressive. In general, they have a lower viscosity than blood, which enhances flow through smaller capillaries and potentially increases peripheral oxygen delivery.

In initial trials hemoglobin substitutes produced toxicities of great concern, particularly in the kidney. However, the methods for polymerization and tetrameric formation of free hemoglobin have vastly improved. Therefore, toxicity occurs less often and circulation times, a problem in earlier trials, have been prolonged. In addition, oxygen-loading properties have been improved.

Hemoglobin-based red cell substitutes come from various sources of hemoglobin. Human hemoglobin-based preparations are naturally occurring; however, there is limited availability of outdated units of blood, which are the sources of this hemoglobin substitute. Bovine hemoglobin-based products offer the advantages of near limitless supply and lower cost. The last option is recombinant therapy to produce synthetic hemoglobin substitutes.

The current status of various oxygen therapeutic agents is summarized in Table 14-8. Human polymerized hemoglobin (human glutaraldehyde polymerized solution) has been administered safely in Phase III trials during both elective and urgent surgery, as well as to trauma patients requiring up to 6 units of transfusion in 24 hours. Data from a recent randomized clinical trial comparing human glutaraldehyde polymerized solution with normal saline for management of hemorrhagic shock in the prehospital and emergency department settings are currently being analyzed.[96] Hemapure, a chemically stabilized bovine hemoglobin prepared in a saline solution, has been approved for human use in South Africa. A multicenter Phase III clinical trial will soon be initiated in the United States.[96]

Perfluorochemical emulsions have also been clinically evaluated as another possible alternative to human blood. Perfluorochemicals are organic liquids derived from hydrocarbons, which are able to carry large amounts of dissolved oxygen. However, they are cleared quickly from plasma and require a high partial pressure of oxygen, thus potentially limiting their clinical use. One of their greatest advantages is that the purity of perfluorocarbons can be more easily controlled. Certainly one of the potential uses for these compounds is in patients whose religion does not allow them to accept donated blood or products prepared from blood. Due to unexpected poor neurologic outcomes, the manufacturer voluntarily suspended a Phase III multicenter trial of their second-generation perfluorocarbon compound, as well as further research efforts investigating use of this drug as an oxygen therapeutic solution.[96]

It is widely recognized that acute traumatic hemorrhage begets coagulopathy, which only serves to increase the degree of hemorrhage. Resuscitation with crystalloids, colloids, or

TABLE 14-8 **Current Oxygen Therapeutic Solutions**

Company	Product	Type	Clinical Trial Status
Northfield Laboratories	PolyHeme®	Human glutaraldehyde polymerized	Awaiting results of recently completed phase 3 multicenter trials in North America in trauma patients
Biopure Corporation	Hemopure® (hemoglobin glutamer-250 [bovine])	Bovine glutaraldehyde	Approved for patient use in South Africa; awaiting initiation of phase 3 trauma trial in the United States
Hemosol, Inc.	Hemolink® (hemoglobin raffimer)	Human o-raffinose polymerized	Completed phase 3 multicenter trial in coronary bypass patients, but was not approved for clinical use in Canada; company filed bankruptcy 2005
Baxter International, Inc.	DCLHb (diaspirin cross-linked hemoglobin)	Human cross-linked hemoglobin	Terminated phase 3 trauma trial after mortality increase in experimental arm; company ended research efforts on product
Alliance Pharmaceuticals	Oxygent™ (perflubron emulsion)	Perfluorocarbon	Voluntarily suspended a phase 3 multi-center trial of transfusion avoidance in cardiac surgery in the United States

packed red blood cells dilutes the body's supply of clotting factors and increases blood pressure, which may effectively "wash out" any previously formed clots. Hemorrhage increases, shock and acidosis ensue. Efforts to quickly halt hemorrhage to reduce the need for transfusions would be an ideal management strategy.

In 2004, Dutton et al completed a study using activated factor VIIa (FVIIa) to treat the coagulopathy associated with traumatic blood loss.[97] Factor VIIa was developed to treat hemophiliacs with antibodies to factor VIII. FVIIa initiates thrombin formation by binding with exposed tissue factor. Dutton et al[97] found that FVIIa leads to an immediate reduction in coagulopathic hemorrhage, regardless of the source of coagulopathy. Although it is not a cure for surgical hemorrhage, FVIIa did allow the surgeon time to repair injuries. Additionally, Boffard et al demonstrated that factor VIIa not only did not increase the incidence of adverse events such as thromboembolism and systemic coagulation, but it was also associated with a trend toward fewer complications, such as acute respiratory distress syndrome (ARDS) and multiple organ dysfunction syndrome (MODS).[98] In a retrospective review of 285 trauma patients who received factor VIIa, Thomas et al found that 9.4% developed thromboembolic complications (e.g., cerebrovascular accident, ischemic bowel, myocardial infarction), and of these events, 33% where thought to have a high correlation with factor VIIa administration.[99] Further study is necessary, but judicious use of FVIIa in the actively hemorrhaging trauma patient shows great promise.

Despite the use of state-of-the-art diagnostics, monitoring, and management during the resuscitation of an exsanguinating trauma victim, survival is extremely low if blood loss leads to cardiac arrest. Realistically it is very difficult to transport, resuscitate, diagnose, and achieve surgical hemostasis in a patient with active hemorrhage during the "golden hour." One possible solution is to stop the clock by placing the patient in a state of suspended animation. Suspended animation is the rapid induction of hypothermia (10° to 15° C) via cardiopulmonary bypass or the induction of ice-cold saline into the aorta. This effectively preserves the brain and essential organs, allowing time for transport and resuscitative surgery. Current studies in dog models are showing survival without cerebral compromise when suspended animation is used for up to 60 minutes.[71] This holds promise for future management of severely injured trauma patients.

SUMMARY

The evaluation process and initial resuscitation of patients after significant injury is a tremendously dynamic process. It is important to identify injuries in the order in which they are likely to produce death or disability. Vital signs are imprecise, and although they can identify patients in extremis, they often underestimate the magnitude of physiologic derangement. Resuscitation schemes must be tailored to the population being treated. Some groups, such as pediatric and elderly patients, may well require specialized evaluation and resuscitation schemes.

Far and away the most important principle is for clinicians to remain suspicious. Nothing should be taken for granted; the trauma team should assume patients are severely injured with significant physiologic derangement until proven otherwise. A healthy skepticism and real clinical suspicion may prove to be the difference between survival and death.

REFERENCES

1. Abou-Khalil B, Scalea TM, Trooskin SZ et al: Hemodynamic responses to shock in young trauma patients: need for invasive monitoring, *Crit Care Med* 22(4):633-639, 1994.
2. Scalea TM, Duncan AO: Initial management of the critically ill trauma patient in extremis, *Trauma Q* 10:3-11, 1993.
3. Cottingham CA: Resuscitation of traumatic shock: a hemodynamic review, *AACN Adv Crit Care* 17(3):317-326, 2006.
4. Ozawa K: Energy metabolism. In Cowley RA, Trump BF, editors: *Pathophysiology of Shock, Anoxia and Ischemia,* Baltimore, 1982, Williams & Wilkins.
5. Hasdai D, Califf RM, Thompson TD et al: Predictors of cardiogenic shock after thrombolytic therapy for acute myocardial infarction, *J Am Coll Cardiol* 35(1):136-143, 2000.
6. American College of Surgeons, Committee on Trauma: *Advanced Trauma Life Support (ATLS Instructor's Manual),* ed 7, Chicago, 2004, The American College of Surgeons.
7. Scalea TM, Holman M, Fuortes M et al: Central venous blood oxygen saturation: an early, accurate measurement of volume during hemorrhage, *J Trauma* 28(6):725-732, 1988.
8. Scalea TM, Hartnett R, Duncan AO: Central venous oxygen saturation: a useful clinical tool in trauma patients, *J Trauma* 30(12):1539-1543, 1990.
9. Sinert RH, Baron BJ, Low RB et al: Is urine output a reliable index of blood volume in hemorrhagic shock? *Acad Emerg Med* 3:448, 1996.
10. Baron BJ, Scalea TM: Acute blood loss, *Emerg Med Clin North Am* 14(1):35-55, 1996.
11. Bania TC, Baron BJ, Almond GL et al: The hemodynamic effects of cocaine during acute controlled hemorrhage in conscious rats, *J Toxicol* 38(1):1-6, 2000.
12. Dutton RP: Shock and trauma anesthesia, *Anesth Clin North Am* 17:83-95, 1999
13. Gomersall CD, Joynt GM, Freebairn RC et al: Resuscitation of critically ill patients based on the results of gastric tonometry: a prospective, randomized, controlled trial, *Crit Care Med* 28(3):607-614, 2000.
14. Soderstrom CA, McArdle DQ, Ducher TB et al: The diagnosis of intra-abdominal injury in patients with cervical cord trauma, *J Trauma* 23(12):1061-1065, 1983.
15. Zipnick RI, Scalea TM, Trooskin SZ et al: Hemodynamic responses to penetrating spinal cord injuries, *J Trauma* 35(4):578-583, 1993.
16. Downing SE: The heart in shock. In Altura BM, Lefer AM, Schumer W, editors: *Handbook of Shock and Trauma,* New York, 1983, Raven.
17. Muller JE: Treatment of myocardial infarction. In Cowley RA, Trump BF, editors: *Pathophysiology of Shock, Anoxia, and Ischemia,* Baltimore, 1982, Williams & Wilkins.
18. Centers for Disease Control and Prevention website. Available online at http://www.webappa.cdc.gov/cgi-bin/broker.exe. Accessed April 26, 2007.
19. Rivara FP, Grossman DC, Cummings P: Injury prevention: first of two parts, *N Engl J Med* 337(8):543-548, 1997.
20. Scalea TM, Low RB: Approach to multiple trauma. In Howell JM, editor: *Emergency Medicine,* vol 2, Philadelphia, 1998, WB Saunders.
21. Reines HD, Bartlett RL, Chudy NE et al: Is advanced life support appropriate for victims of motor vehicle accidents: the South Carolina Highway Trauma Project, *J Trauma* 28(5):563-570, 1988.
22. Sampalis JS, Lavoie A, Williams JI et al: Impact of on-site care, prehospital time, and level of in-hospital care on survival in severely injured patients, *J Trauma* 34(2):252-261, 1993.
23. Smith JP, Boda BI, Hill AS et al: Prehospital stabilization of critically injured patients: a failed concept, *J Trauma* 25:65-70, 1985.
24. Border JR, Lewis RF, Aprahamian C et al: Panel: prehospital trauma care—stabilize or scoop and run, *J Trauma* 23(8):708-711, 1983.
25. Cornwell EE III, Belzberg H, Hennigan K et al: Emergency medical services (EMS) vs non-EMS transport of critically injured patients: a prospective evaluation, *Arch Surg* 135:315-319, 2000.
26. Cannon WB, Fraser J, Cowell EM: The preventive treatment of wound shock, *JAMA* 70:618-621, 1918.
27. Ryzoff RI, Shaftan GW, Herbsman H: Selective conservatism in penetrating abdominal trauma, *Surgery* 59(4):650-653, 1966.
28. Marshall HP, Capone A, Courcoulas AP et al: Effects of hemodilution on long-term survival in an uncontrolled hemorrhagic shock model in rats, *J Trauma* 43(4):673-679, 1997.
29. Bickell WH, Bruttig SP, Millnamow GA et al: The detrimental effects of intravenous crystalloid after aortotomy in swine, *Surgery* 110(3):529-536, 1991.
30. Kowalenko T, Stern S, Dronen SC et al: Improved outcome with hypotensive resuscitation of uncontrolled hemorrhagic shock in a swine model, *J Trauma* 33(3):349-362, 1992.
31. Bickell WH, Wall MJ Jr, Pepe PE et al: Immediate versus delayed fluid resuscitation for hypotensive patients with penetrating torso injuries, *N Engl J Med* 331(17):1105-1109, 1994.
32. Chesnut RM, Gautelle T, Blunt BA et al: Neurogenic hypotension in patients with severe head injuries, *J Trauma* 44(6):958-963, 1998.
33. Younes RN, Aun F, Accioly CQ et al: Hypertonic solutions in the treatment of hypovolemic shock: a prospective, randomized study in patients admitted to the emergency room, *Surgery* 111(4):380-384, 1992.
34. Wade CE, Kramer GC, Grady JJ et al: Efficacy of hypertonic 7.5% NaCl/6% dextran-70 in treating trauma: a meta-analysis of controlled clinical studies, *Surgery* 122(3):609-616, 1997.
35. Maningas PA, Volk K, DeGuzman L: Resuscitation with 7.5% NaCl/6% dextran-70 for the treatment of severe hemorrhagic shock in swine, *Crit Care Med* 15(12):1121-1126, 1987.
36. Velasco IT, Rocha-e-Silva M, Oliveira MA et al: Hypertonic and hyperoncotic resuscitation from severe hemorrhagic shock in dogs: a comparative study, *Crit Care Med* 17(3):261-264, 1989.
37. Krausz MM, Landau EH, Klin B et al: Hypertonic saline treatment of uncontrolled hemorrhagic shock at different periods from bleeding, *Arch Surg* 127(1):93-96, 1992.
38. Bickell WH, Bruttig SP, Millnamow GA et al: Use of hypertonic saline/dextran versus lactated Ringers solution as a resuscitation fluid after uncontrolled aortic hemorrhage in anesthetized swine, *Ann Emerg Med* 21(9):1077-1085, 1992.
39. Mattox KL, Maningas PA, Moore EE et al: Prehospital hypertonic saline/dextran infusion for post-traumatic hypotension: the U.S.A. multicenter trial, *Ann Surg* 213:482-491, 1991.
40. Vassar MJ, Fischer RP, O'Brien PE et al: A multicenter trial for resuscitation of injured patients with 7.5% sodium chloride: the effect of added dextran 70: the multicenter group for the

study of hypertonic saline in trauma patients, *Arch Surg* 128:1003-1013, 1993.

41. Vassar MJ, Perry CA, Holcroft JW: Prehospital resuscitation of hypotensive trauma patients with 7.5% NaCl versus 7.5% NaCl with added dextran: a controlled trial, *J Trauma* 34:622-632, 1993.
42. Vassar MJ, Perry CA, Gannaway WL et al: 7.5% sodium chloride/dextran for resuscitation of trauma patients undergoing helicopter transport, *Arch Surg* 126:1065-1072, 1991.
43. Cooper DJ, Myles PS, McDermott FT et al: Prehospital hypertonic saline resuscitation of patients with hypotension and severe traumatic brain injury: a randomized controlled trial, *JAMA* 29:1350-1357, 2004.
44. Mattox KL, Bickell W, Pepe PE et al: Prospective MAST study in 911 patients, *J Trauma* 29(8):1104-1112, 1989.
45. Wangensteen SL, Deoll JD, Ludwig RM et al: The detrimental effect of the G-suit in hemorrhagic shock, *Ann Surg* 170(2):187-192, 1969.
46. Committee on Trauma, American College of Surgeons: *Resources for Optimal Care of the Injured Patient: 2006*, Chicago, 2006, American College of Surgeons.
47. MacKenzie EJ, Rivara FP, Jurkovich GJ et al: A national evaluation of the effect of trauma-center care on mortality, *N Engl J Med* 354(4):366-378, 2006.
48. Sampalis JS, Denis R, Frechette P et al: Direct transport to tertiary trauma centers versus transfer from lower level facilities: impact on mortality and morbidity among patients with major trauma, *J Trauma* 43(2):288-295, 1997.
49. Young JS, Bassam D, Cephas GA et al: Interhospital versus direct scene transfer of major trauma patients in a rural trauma system, *Am Surg* 64(1):88-92, 1998.
50. Rogers FB, Osler TM, Shackford SR et al: Study of the outcome of patients transferred to a level I hospital after stabilization at an outlying hospital in a rural setting, *J Trauma* 46(2):328-333, 1999.
51. Mikulaschek A, Henry SM, Donovan R et al: Serum lactate is not predicted by anion gap or base excess after trauma resuscitation, *J Trauma* 40(2):218-224, 1996.
52. Scalea TM, Sinert R, Duncan AO et al: Percutaneous central access for resuscitation in trauma, *Acad Emerg Med* 1(6):525-531, 1994.
53. Gallbraith S, Teasdale G: Predicting the need for operation in the patient with an occult traumatic intracranial hematoma, *J Neurosurg* 55(1):75-81, 1981.
54. Brain Trauma Foundation, American Association of Neurological Surgeons, Congress of Neurological Surgeons, AANS/CNS Joint Section on Neurotrauma and Critical Care. Guidelines for the Management of Severe Traumatic Brain Injury, ed 3. *J Neurotrauma* 24(supplement 1), 2007.
55. Scalea TM, Rodriguez A, Chiu WC et al: Focused assessment with sonography for trauma (FAST): results from an international consensus conference, *J Trauma* 46(3):466-472, 1999.
56. American College of Surgeons, Committee on Trauma: *Advanced Trauma Life Support (ATLS Student Course Manual)*, ed 7, Chicago, 2004, The American College of Surgeons.
57. Mustafa I, Leverve XM: Metabolic and hemodynamic effects of hypertonic solutions: sodium-lactate versus sodium chloride infusion in postoperative patients, *Shock* 18(4):306-310, 2002.
58. Kaplan LJ, Philbin N, Arnaud F et al: Resuscitation from hemorrhagic shock: fluid selection and infusion strategy drives unmeasured ion genesis, *J Trauma* 61(1):90-98, 2006.
59. Moore FA, McKinley BA, Moore EE et al: Guidelines for shock resuscitation, *J Trauma* 61:82-89, 2006.
60. McIntyre L, Hebert PC, Wells G, et al: Is a restrictive transfusion strategy safe for resuscitated and critically ill trauma patients? *J Trauma* 57(3):563-568, 2004.
61. McIntyre LA, Fergusson DA, Hutchison JS et al: Effect of a liberal versus restrictive transfusion strategy on mortality in patients with moderate to severe head injury, *Neurocrit Care* 5(1):4-9, 2006.
62. Shapiro MJ, Gettinger A, Corwin HL et al: Anemia and blood transfusion in trauma patients admitted to the intensive care unit, *J Trauma* 55(2):269-273, 2003.
63. Holcomb JB, Jenkins D, Rhee P et al: Damage control resuscitation: directly addressing the early coagulopathy of trauma, *J Trauma* 62(2):307-310, 2007.
64. Gregory JS, Flancbaum L, Townsend MC et al: Incidence and timing of hypothermia in trauma patients undergoing operations, *J Trauma* 31(6):795-800, 1991.
65. Fisher DA: Cold diuresis in the newborn, *Pediatrics* 40(4):636-641, 1967.
66. Nierman DM: Core temperature measurement in the intensive care unit, *Crit Care Med* 19(6):818-823, 1991.
67. Gentilello LM, Cobean RA, Offner PJ et al: Continuous arteriovenous rewarming: rapid reversal of hypothermia in critically ill patients, *J Trauma* 32(3):316-327, 1992.
68. Marion DW, Obrist WD, Carlier PM et al: The use of moderate therapeutic hypothermia for patients with severe head injuries: a preliminary report, *J Neurosurg* 79(3):354-362, 1993.
69. Qiu WS, Liu WG, Shen H, et al: Therapeutic effect of mild hypothermia on severe traumatic brain injury, *Chin J Traumatol* 8(1):27-32, 2005.
70. Tisherman SA, Rodriguez A, Safar P: Therapeutic hypothermia in traumatology, *Surg Clin North Am* 79(6):1269-1289, 1999.
71. Nozari A, Safar P, Wu X et al: Suspended animation can allow survival without brain damage after traumatic exsanguination cardiac arrest of 60 minutes in dogs, *J Trauma* 57(6):1266-1275, 2004.
72. Abramson D, Scalea TM, Hitchcock R et al: Lactate clearance and survival following injury, *J Trauma* 35(4):581-589, 1993.
73. Scalea TM, Maltz S, Yelon J et al: Resuscitation of multiple trauma and head injury: role of crystalloid fluids and inotropes, *Crit Care Med* 22(10):1610-1615, 1994.
74. McKiernan CA, Lieberman SA: Circulatory shock in children An overview. *Pediatr Rev* 26(12):451-460, 2005.
75. Moloney-Harmon PA, Czerwinski SJ: The pediatric patient with multiple organ dysfunction syndrome. In Secor VH, editor: *Multiple Organ Dysfunction & Failure,* ed 2, St. Louis, 1996, Mosby.
76. Osler T, Hales K, Baack B et al: Trauma in the elderly, *Am J Surg* 156(6):537-543, 1988.
77. Scalea TM, Kohl L: Geriatric trauma. In Feliciano D, Moore EE, Mattox K, editors: *Trauma,* ed 3, Stamford, 1996, Appleton & Lange.
78. Scalea TM, Simon HM, Duncan AO et al: Geriatric blunt multiple trauma: improved survival with early invasive monitoring, *J Trauma* 30(2):129-136, 1990.
79. Cooke WH, Convertino VA: Heart rate variability and spontaneous baroreflex sequences: implications for autonomic monitoring, *J Trauma* 58(4):798-805, 2005.

80. Cooke WH, Salinas J, Convertino VA et al: Heart rate variability and its association with mortality in prehospital trauma patients, *J Trauma* 60(6):363-370, 2006.
81. Winchell RJ, Hoyt MD: Spectral analysis of heart rate variability in the ICU: a measure of autonomic function, *J Surg Res* 63(1):11-16, 1996.
82. Winchell RJ, Hoyt DB: Analysis of heart rate variability: a noninvasive predictor of death and poor outcome in patients with severe head injury, *J Trauma* 43(6):927-933,1997.
83. Chiara O, Pelosi P, Segala M et al: Mesenteric and renal oxygen transport during hemorrhage and reperfusion: evaluation of optimal goals for resuscitation, *J Trauma* 51(2):356-362, 2001.
84. Miami Clinical Trials Group: Splanchnic hypoperfusion-directed therapies in trauma: a prospective, randomized trial, *Am Surg* 71(3):252-260, 2005.
85. Boswell SA, Scalea TM: Sublingual capnometry: an alternative to gastric tonometry for the management of shock resuscitation, *AACN Clin Issues* 14(2):176-184, 2003.
86. Grundler W, Weil MH, Rackow EC: Arteriovenous carbon dioxide and pH gradients during cardiac arrest, *Circulation* 74(5):1071-1074, 1986.
87. Weil MH, Rackow EC, Trevino R et al: Difference in acid-base state between venous and arterial blood during cardiopulmonary resuscitation, *N Engl J Med* 315(3):153-156, 1986.
88. Baron BJ, Sinert R, Zehtabchi S et al: Diagnostic utility of sublingual PCO_2 for detecting hemorrhage in penetrating trauma patients, *J Trauma* 57(1):69-74, 2004.
89. Baron BJ, Dutton RP, Zehtabchi S et al: Sublingual capnometry for rapid determination of the severity of hemorrhagic shock, *J Trauma* 62(1):120-124, 2007.
90. Headley JM: Arterial pressure-based technologies: a new trend in cardiac output monitoring, *Crit Care Nurs Clin North Am* 18(2):179-187, 2006.
91. Rivers E, Nguyen B, Havstad S et al: Early goal-directed therapy in the treatment of severe sepsis and septic shock, *N Engl J Med* 345(19):1368-1377, 2001.
92. Sauaia A, Moore FA, Moore EE et al: Epidemiology of trauma deaths: a reassessment, *J Trauma* 38(2):185-193, 1995.
93. Scott MG, Kucik DF, Goodnough LT et al: Blood substitutes: evolution and future applications, *Clin Chem* 43(9):1724-1731, 1997.
94. Ketcham EM, Cairns CB: Hemoglobin-based oxygen carriers: development and clinical potential, *Ann Emerg Med* 33(3):326-337, 1999.
95. Harmening DM: *Modern Blood Banking and Transfusion Practices,* ed 3, Philadelphia, 1994, FA Davis.
96. Cohn SM: Advances in oxygen therapeutic agents, *Critical Connections* 6(1):8, 2007.
97. Dutton RP, McCunn M, Hyder M et al: Factor VIIa for correction of traumatic coagulopathy, *J Trauma* 57(4):709-719, 2004.
98. Boffard KD, Riou B, Warren B et al: Recombinant factor VIIa as adjunctive therapy for bleeding control in severely injured trauma patients: two parallel randomized, placebo-controlled, double-blind clinical trials, *J Trauma* 59(1):8-18, 2005.
99. Thomas GO, Dutton RP, Hemlock B et al: Thromboembolic complications associated with factor VIIa administration, *J Trauma* 62(3):564-569, 2007.

15

INFECTION AND INFECTION CONTROL

Patricia B. Casper, Manjari Joshi, Marilyn C. Algire

Rapid evacuation and transport to trauma centers and sophisticated medical technologies facilitate successful resuscitation and life support after trauma, thereby saving more lives of critically injured patients. Survivors of traumatic events experience compromise of innate host defense mechanisms, increasing their risk for infection.[1] It is a medical paradox that the invasive therapies needed to resuscitate and sustain critical trauma patients increase the risk of life-threatening infections, a predominant complication of severely traumatized patients.

Trauma patients have a predisposition to infection, owing to disruption of major protective barriers. In a recent study of 1277 trauma patients, 45.4% had nosocomial infections.[2] Of the nosocomial infections, 22% were respiratory infections (including pneumonia, sinusitis, and tracheobronchitis), 22% were intraabdominal/gastrointestinal infections, 21% were genitourinary infections, 20% were bacteremias, and 10% were wound/skin infections.[2] Nosocomial infections are a significant complication in trauma patients and are associated with prolonged length of stay, higher health care costs, and increased mortality rates.[3] These infections can also lead to the development of severe sepsis and septic shock.[2,4] In 2004, The Joint Commission recognized that nosocomial infections are a frequent safety issue for hospitalized patients and issued new patient safety goals aimed at reducing the risk of nosocomial infections.[5,6] Early diagnosis and treatment of infection are essential to improve outcome and decrease length of stay and mortality rates of trauma patients.

The purpose of this chapter is to increase the reader's knowledge about the prevention, development, and treatment of infection in trauma patients. By understanding predisposing factors, clinical findings, and effective preventive and therapeutic interventions associated with trauma-related infection, nurses can avoid, recognize, and appropriately intervene to treat this complication. Reducing infection promotes optimal patient outcomes.

HOST DEFENSE MECHANISMS

Natural host defenses against infection include external mechanisms, or the body's anatomic barriers, and internal mechanisms, consisting of humoral and cell-mediated immune responses. These protective defense mechanisms can be impeded, or in some cases completely obliterated, as a consequence of injury, invasive therapy, nutrition, or age. Disruption of mechanisms by trauma is a major risk factor for subsequent infections. Understanding the relationship between the body's defense mechanisms and the disruption caused by trauma helps the bedside nurse decrease infection risk and promote optimal patient care.

The immunosuppression seen in trauma patients affects both external and internal mechanisms. External immunosuppression is a result of a break in the integument or impairment of other protective mechanisms. Humoral and cell-mediated immunosuppression is a result of stress, malnutrition, and other factors. Unlike cancer patients, trauma patients have functioning immune systems (though they may be profoundly disrupted) and thus are able to respond to exogenous antigen invasion. Immunosuppression does not appear to be sustained in trauma patients.

EXTERNAL DEFENSE MECHANISMS

The body has innate protective mechanisms within the skin and the respiratory, gastrointestinal, and genitourinary tracts, all of which prevent the entry and proliferation of microorganisms. Pathogens can bypass the external, first-line defense when the skin or mucosal linings are broken during initial injury or later when surgery and other invasive procedures are performed. Compromised local tissue perfusion, aggressive tissue manipulation, hematoma formation, and the creation of dead space associated with injury or surgical intervention further increases risk of infection. Placement of invasive monitors, drains, vascular cannula, urinary catheters, external fixators, endotracheal tubes, or feeding tubes further compromises the external defense mechanisms.

Skin

The major mechanical barrier to invading pathogens is the skin. The skin's protective ability is enhanced by its natural acidic pH, which inhibits growth of some organisms. Also, sebum, the oily secretion of the sebaceous glands, contains long-chain fatty acids that act as a germicide. Antimicrobial peptides, which are small-molecular-weight proteins secreted by epithelial cells, are toxic to some bacteria, fungi, and viruses.[7] Normal skin flora include coagulase-positive and coagulase-negative staphylococci, streptococci, and diptheroids, which act as a potential reservoir of invading organisms.

In addition to interruption of the skin from injury or surgery, this protective barrier may be disrupted by pressure, shearing, moisture, or friction after patient admission. Pressure from maintaining a body position for a prolonged period, especially when on an unpadded surface (e.g., backboard), retraction by surgical instruments, or therapeutic devices applied to the patient (e.g., traction, braces, splint) can cause tissue ischemia. Any ischemia and subsequent necrosis of the skin provides a rich environment for bacterial growth. Excessive exposure to moisture from secretions, drainage, and incontinence can macerate skin. Friction and shearing created by movement on sheets or against restraints cause mechanical irritation that can abrade skin. Chemical irritation from degerming and defatting agents, adhesive tapes, incontinence, and excoriating exudates can also inhibit innate skin defenses.

Elderly patients have the added burden of the age-related changes that affect the skin's normal function.[8] Their skin has less oil secretion, blood flow, innervation, and subcutaneous fat,[9] which increases the incidence of skin breakdown and wound infection.[10] Similarly, obese patients are also at higher risk for skin breakdown because of impaired mobility and decreased tissue perfusion.

Nursing interventions to enhance the skin's defense mechanisms include using meticulous aseptic technique, handwashing, handling tissue gently, minimizing the use of adhesive tape, optimizing control of wound drainage with appropriate dressings, alleviating pressure areas, and using the most effective yet least irritating antiseptic solutions. The patient's risk for skin breakdown should be assessed on admission and regularly during hospitalization. Skin integrity should be evaluated each shift to detect areas with actual or potential breakdown.

Respiratory Tract

The respiratory tract has a complex system of host defense mechanisms. Mucociliated epithelium cleans and protects airway passages to prevent microbial overgrowth. Coughing, sneezing, and deep breathing provide mechanical clearing of the airways. Lung surfactant proteins appear to promote phagocytosis.[11]

Pathogens can gain access to lower airways during intubation, by inhalation, or from bloodstream infections, aspiration of gastric contents, or spread from nearby areas.[12] The major loss of defenses in trauma patients occurs with placement of an artificial airway. With this intevention, all natural defense mechanisms are circumvented, and microorganisms from the environment can be afforded unobstructed entry into the lungs. Contamination of airway circuits can allow rapid replication of pathogens that are aerosolized into the lungs. Endotracheal tubes allow pooling of oropharyngeal secretions, which contain a variety of pathogens that can pass the inflated cuff and move into distal airways.[12]

Respiratory tract defense mechanisms can be compromised with thoracic or abdominal injury or surgery, after chest tube placement, and when central nervous system (CNS) dysfunction, paralytics, sedatives, or analgesics impair ventilation and effective secretion clearance. Immobility as a result of decreased level of consciousness, neuromuscular blockade, traction and fixation devices, or spinal injury can also contribute to alveolar collapse and secretion retention. Suppression of protective cough and gag reflexes and impaired swallowing associated with traumatic brain injury increase the risk of aspiration and ineffective secretion clearance. Damage from inhalation injuries caused by heat, vaporization of toxic chemicals, and smoke can produce both temporary and permanent destruction of lung defense mechanisms.

Placement of nasal tubes can increase the risk of upper respiratory tract infections. Indwelling nasogastric and nasoendotrachael tubes can obstruct airflow to and drainage from sinuses, resulting in nosocomial sinusitis, or impede flow through the eustachian tubes, resulting in otitis media. The presence of chest tubes and retained hemothoraces are significant factors in the development of nosocomial empyema.

Elderly patients are further compromised by age-related physiologic changes. A gradual decline in many immune functions, including cell-mediated and humoral aspects of acquired immunity, contributes to an increased risk of pneumonia.[13] Decreased alveolar elasticity, reduced intercostal muscle and diaphragm tone, and diminished vital capacity hinder the elderly patient's ability to cough and expectorate sputum, increasing the risk of respiratory tract infection.[14]

Nurses can promote respiratory tract defense mechanisms by frequently repositioning unconscious and immobile patients and, in awake patients, encouraging the use of incentive spirometry, coughing, and deep breathing to facilitate removal of pulmonary secretions. Chest physiotherapy is vital to critically ill patients, especially those with new pulmonary infiltrates, fever, leukocytosis, or purulent sputum. In a study of critically ill ventilated patients, Joshi et al[15] demonstrated the benefits of vigorous chest percussion. Within 8 hours after chest physical therapy, 80% of patients had partial or complete resolution of pulmonary infiltrates. Another important maneuver that increases coughing and deep breathing to promote aveoli opening and secretion removal is getting patients moved out of bed to a chair and assisting with ambulation as soon as their condition permits. Specific interventions to prevent pneumonia are described later in the chapter.

Gastrointestinal Tract

Heavily colonized by a variety of bacteria, the gastrointestinal tract is a major reservoir of microorganisms that can cause nosocomial infection. An intact mucosal epithelium, the acidic gastric barrier, and continuous peristaltic evacuation throughout the tract constitute the external defenses in the gastrointestinal tract. Lytic enzymes in saliva, secretory antibody immunoglobulin A (IgA), lysozyme, and phagocytic cells work to destroy ingested bacteria. Normally the stomach, duodenum, and jejunum are colonized with low concentrations of mouth flora. However, the trauma patient soon loses this protection because normal gut flora is disrupted by injury, ischemia, decreased gut motility, pH changes, and fasting. Decreased visceral perfusion, seen for example in patients in shock, decreases gut barrier function and raises the potential for "translocation" of bacteria out of the gastrointestinal tract.[16]

Drug therapy may have a negative impact on gastrointestinal tract defense mechanisms. Antacids and H_2-blocking agents used to prevent or treat mucosal bleeding elevate the normal gastric pH, eliminating the acidic barrier. Gastric pH greater than 4 facilitates bacterial overgrowth.[17] Muscle relaxants, sedatives, and analgesic agents reduce gastric motility. Last, antibiotics change the composition of the normal gut flora.[18]

Genitourinary Tract

Ciliated mucosa lines the normal genitourinary tract, blocking bacterial adherence. The flushing action of the bladder evacuates microorganisms. The acidic pH and hyperosmolar composition of normal urine is bacteriostatic. Therefore, urine is normally sterile because the bladder environment is not conducive to bacterial growth.

Use of an indwelling urinary catheter in any patient breaches normal external defenses, heightening the risk of infection by creating an easy portal of entry for microorganisms. Susceptibility to infection also increases with urinary tract obstruction, renal failure, changes in the chemical composition of urine, and manipulations of the indwelling drainage system. Other factors known to increase the risk of urinary tract infections (UTIs) include increased age, obesity, and length of time an indwelling catheter has been used. Interventions to prevent UTI are addressed later in the chapter.

Internal Defense Mechanisms

This aspect of the immune system defends against infectious microbes that breach external defenses and helps eliminate foreign substances. This innate resistance is designed to limit tissue injury and prevent infection by environmental organisms.[11] The human body is designed with various physical, mechanical, and biochemical barriers that protect it from environmental substances and microbial pathogens. When the external barriers are compromised, the body's inflammatory response is activated by internal defense mechanisms (the immune system) to provide protection, prevent infection, and promote healing.[11]

Injury to vascularized tissue prompts the initiation of a characteristic inflammatory response with clinical manifestations that include redness, heat, swelling, and pain. Redness and warmth result from the increased blood flow to the affected area. Local blood vessels in the microcirculation dilate, and vascular permeability increases, allowing fluid to leak from the vessels. Leukocytes and plasma enter the tissues as the result of increased vascular permeability brought on by chemical reactions of histamine, bradykinin, leukotrienes, substance P, and prostaglandins.[19] White blood cells (WBCs) migrate from inside the blood vessels to the site of injury. These effects are visible within seconds.

The inflammatory response initiated to prevent infection includes activation of three plasma protein systems: complement, clotting, and kinin systems.[11] The complement system has a dual role in directly destroying pathogens and activating other inflammatory response systems. The clotting system uses a group of plasma proteins to form a fibrinous meshwork at the site of injury or inflammation. This meshwork prevents spread of infection by containing the microorganisms and foreign bodies. It also controls bleeding and creates a framework for tissue repair. The kinin system activates inflammatory cells and works in conjunction with the coagulation system to trap pathogens. Bradykinins, along with prostaglandins, induce pain, produce smooth muscle contraction, increase vascular permeability, and enhance leukocyte chemotaxis.[11]

Activation of these proteins recruits granulocytes and specialized cells, including neutrophils, eosinophils, basophils, and mast cells to the site of inflammation or infection. Mast cells are found in large numbers in skin and lining the gastrointestinal and respiratory tracts. They are activated and begin synthesizing inflammatory mediators (e.g., histamine, bradykinin, leukotrienes, substance P, and prostaglandins), which increase vascular permeability, activate platelets, and enhance adhesion of leukocytes to endothelial cells. These cells provide an early response to microbes even before infection. The leukocyte response is initiated within 6 to 12 hours after injury, when polymorphonucleocytes (neutrophils) infiltrate the area.[11] Their role is to ingest or phagocytize bacteria, dead cells, and cellular debris. The number of circulating neutrophils increases, usually accompanied by an increase in the ratio of immature cells (bands, metamyelocytes, myelocytes) to mature neutrophils-known as the "left shift." Neutrophils, also called polymorphonuclear cells (PMNs), are granulocyte cells that serve as the predominant phagocytes of early inflammation.[11] They are incapable of division and sensitive to acidic environments. As inflammation persists, capillary congestion at the site leads to tissue anoxia, anerobic metabolism, and decreased pH of the exudate, which is lethal to neutrophils. They have a short life span and degrade to become a component of purulent exudates (pus), which is composed of dead and dying leukocytes, blood, plasma, fibrin, cellular debris, and living and dead microorganisms.[11] It is not uncommon to have a very high WBC count (20,000-40,000 cells/mm^3) immediately after severe traumatic injury because of the inflammatory response.

Other WBC lines that are induced by "protein" messengers are monocytes and macrophages. They are similar to neutrophils in characteristics and functions, but they have a longer life span. Produced in the bone marrow as monocytes, they circulate in the bloodstream, becoming macrophages when they infiltrate the tissues.[20] Macrophages and lymphocytes may arrive at the site within 24 hours of injury but are often slow to respond, arriving 3 to 7 days later.[11] They can survive in acidic environments and therefore provide long-term defense against infectious agents. They have bactericidal activity against most microorganisms. Macrophages also stimulate other inflammatory factors and initiate the healing process.[11]

Fever/Thermoregulation as Part of the Immune Sytem

Under normal conditions, body temperature is determined by the "set point" of the hypothalamic thermoregulatory system and a delicate balance between production and loss of body heat. Heat is produced from food metabolism and body activity. Heat loss occurs by radiation, convection, and vaporization, which are regulated by peripheral blood flow to the skin, sweating, and vaporized loss from the lungs.

Fever (defined as core temperature >100.4° F [38° C])[21] results from any disturbance in the hypothalamic thermoregulatory activity that leads to an increase of the thermal set point. Fever can be an infectious or a noninfectious inflammatory response. The infectious fever response is initiated when exogenous pyrogens, such as lipopolysaccharide complexes in the cell wall of gram-negative bacteria, invade the body. Endogenous pyrogens, fever-causing cytokines, are released by neutrophils and macrophages in response to exposure to bacterial endotoxins or to antigen-antibody complexes. Endogenous pyrogens include interleukin-1 (IL-1), interleukin-6 (IL-6), tumor necrosis factor (TNF), and interferon. These pyrogens act on the preoptic nucleus of the hypothalamus to change the body's thermostat.[22] The hypothalamus and the brainstem signal increased heat production and conservation to raise the body temperature. Peripheral vascular vasoconstriction causes blood to shunt to the body's core, thereby creating a new temperature level.[22]

A febrile response may have beneficial effects by killing temperature-sensitive microbes. Fever also causes decreased levels of iron, zinc, and copper, which are needed for bacterial replication. In addition, elevated body temperature changes metabolism to lipolysis and proteolysis, thereby depriving bacteria of glucose sources. Fever can also increase neutrophil mobility, which increases their killing capability by enhancing their phagocytic capability.[22] Because of the beneficial effects of fever, antipyrogenic medications should be used judiciously. Antipyretics can negate the protective fever response and may increase the mortality rate.[21]

Fever may also be harmful by increasing the effects of endotoxins from gram-negative bacteria.[11] Also, pyrexia exacerbates ischemic neuronal damage and physiologic dysfunction after acute brain injury.[23] To avoid increasing the cerebral metabolic rate, which can increase the risk for intracranial hypertension and brain ischemia, hyperthermia is typically aggressively treated in patients with acute severe brain injury. Hypermetabolism caused by fever may not be well tolerated by trauma patients in need of nutrients for healing.

In trauma patients, many of the thermoregulatory mechanisms can be compromised by the nature of the injury. Patients sustaining massive burns or extensive soft tissue injury lose the skin's thermoregulatory functions. Spinal cord injury at the T6 level or above cuts the sympathetic nervous system off from the hypothalmic control center, causing loss of thermoregulatory capability. Patients with these injuries may have a hypothermic set point—that is, a set point below 96° F (35.5° C). Therefore, a sudden increase of temperature to 99° F (37.2° C) may be indicative of fever in these patients. Elderly patients also can have a lower thermal set point, which is attributed to the deterioration of the skin's normal function. On the other hand, activation and chronic stimulation of the inflammatory response (e.g., rheumatoid arthritis, lupus erythematosus, sarcoidosis) may cause some patients to establish a higher than normal set point. These patients appear to have a persistent fever. Patients sustaining severe brain injury resulting in compromise or injury of the hypothalamus may have irregular, widely variant temperature patterns. Fever resulting from this condition is known as central fever, which is often resistant to antipyretics.

Because fever is a manifestation of both infectious and noninfectious inflammatory responses and its presentation can be modified by many concurrent injuries, its utility for the diagnosis of infection is limited. Therefore, continuous evaluation of the patient's overall clinical condition compared with the temperature pattern trend is essential.

Acquired Immunity

When a microbe bypasses external defenses and the initial inflammatory cascade system is primed, additional mechanisms are triggered. By this adaptive or acquired immunity, the human body is able to develop powerful specific immunity against invading bacteria, viruses, and toxins. This is often thought of as the humoral or antibody response. The innate and adaptive immune systems are linked. Stimulation of the innate immune system, as described previously, initiates the adaptive immune response, which is slower acting, specific, and very long lived.[24] When challenged by substances identified by the body as "foreign," the adaptive immune system responds with lymphocytes, the WBCs that make antibodies. Foreign antigens include microbial pathogens (bacteria, fungus, virus, or parasites), noninfectious environmental agents (pollen, food, venom), and clinical mediators (drugs, vaccines, transfusions, transplants). Repeated exposure causes the adaptive immunity to "remember" the invader and increase the number of lymphocyte-produced specific antibodies.[24] When activated, lymphocytes migrate through lymphoid tissues and become either B lymphocytes, responsible for humoral immunity, or T lymphocytes, responsible for cell-mediated immunity. Although B lymphocytes make antibodies, T lymphocytes are involved in complex cell-mediated responses that provide resistance to infection.[25] The human body produces millions of T and B lymphocytes, each capable of recognizing one specific foreign antigen. B cells secrete specialized antibodies that attack antigens. For example, antibodies bind to extracellular microbes and toxins, facilitating elimination of bacteria and viruses. T cells undergo differentiation with maturation and develop into subgroups. Some stimulate leukocytes, whereas others become cytotoxic cells that directly attack and kill antigens. This immunity provides defense against intracellular viruses and bacteria that can live within phagocytes inaccessible to circulating antibodies, thereby eliminating reservoirs of infection.

The body's response to the threat of injury or infection, though usually protective, can be inadequate or excessive and uncontrolled. Understanding how tissue damage can be contained, how infection can be prevented and detected, and how best to treat injuries and promote healing enables nurses to provide optimal patient care.[11]

INFECTION

When the internal and external host defenses are overwhelmed by microorganisms, infection ensues at the site of damage or contamination. Tissue inundated by invasive infection may exceed the usual inflammatory response mechanisms that compensate for such an insult, and bacteremia ensues. In this condition, bacteria invade the bloodstream, producing a variety of symptoms, which may include fever, rigors, confusion, hypotension, tachycardia, tachypnea, and oliguria. Activation of cytokines, despite their importance in combating organisms, causes increased vascular permeability, significant loss of intravascular plasma volume into the interstitium, and cardiovascular dysfunction, which can lead to organ failure or death.

In an attempt to categorize and study the protean manifestations of the body's response to invasion, various definitions are used. Experts from a number of North American and European intensive care societies have agreed on consistent terminology and definitions for the response to insults that may trigger inflammation, namely, infection.[26] Infection is defined as the pathologic process that occurs when microorganisms invade a normally sterile body fluid, tissue, or cavitiy.[26] The definitions of systemic inflammatory response syndrome (SIRS), sepsis, severe sepsis, septic shock, and multiple organ dysfunction syndrome (MODS) are presented later in this chapter.

INFLAMMATORY RESPONSE

Inflammation is the normal response of living tissue to injury or infection.[27] This complex process mediated by the internal immune system is described earlier in this chapter (see Internal Defense Mechanisms). Inflammation is a nonspecific response[27] to tissue damage that can be caused by direct trauma or induced by a variety of mechanical, chemical, and biologic stimuli. In addition to tissue trauma, inflammation can be induced by the presence of foreign objects such as bullets, stones, sutures, catheters, and orthopedic hardware; exposure to toxic agents such as extremes of temperature, ionizing radiation, and chemicals; and the presence of biologic agents such as microorganisms, bacterial toxins, antigen-antibody complexes, and devitalized and necrotic tissue. The more extensive the tissue destruction, the greater the inflammatory response.[28] When the inflammatory response results from tissue necrosis, the progression of systemic inflammation is rapid and blood cultures often have negative results.

It is important to determine the source of the inflammation so that appropriate therapy can be initiated. It may be virtually impossible to distinguish an inflammatory response that is induced by infection from one that is not. In such cases, the diagnosis of infection must be determined by the overall trend of the patient's clinical condition. As the patient progresses through the trauma cycle, the precipitating events of inflammation resolve, cell function is restored, and fewer invasive interventions and mechanical support devices are required. Therefore, a new onset of inflammation during later phases of recovery may be more easily attributed to infection than to the systemic inflammatory response. Strategies to facilitate this diagnosis are outlined later in this chapter.

Systemic Inflammatory Response Syndrome

SIRS is a complex overall inflammatory response affecting multiple organs with or without infection. It can be precipitated by insults such as trauma, infection, pancreatitis, or surgery. It is seen in almost 70% of patients in critical care and is also common to trauma patients.[2] SIRS is a massive response of intrinsic mediators and proinflammatory cytokines indicated by the presence of at least two of the following clinical criteria: fever (temperature $\geq$38° C) or hypothermia (temperature $\leq$36° C), tachycardia ($\geq$90 beats/min), tachypnea ($\geq$20 breaths/min) or partial pressure of carbon dioxide in arterial blood (Pa_{CO_2}) $<$32 mm Hg, leukocytosis ($\geq$12,000 cells/μL) or leukopenia ($\leq$4000 cells/μL), or a left shift in the immaturation of granulocytes (bands) $>$10%.[29]

A SIRS diagnosis does not confirm presence of infection or sepsis but is associated with adverse outcomes.[2] In trauma patients, the SIRS score on admission is an independent predictor of nosocomial infection and mortality. A SIRS score $>$2 continues to be predictive of nosocomial infection through 21 days after injury.[2] SIRS scores have poor specificity, and studies are being done to explore a combination of other biomarkers (e.g., CRP, procalcitonin [PCT]) that can provide a reliable early indicator of infection.

Sepsis

In the United States, sepsis accounts for more than 210,000 deaths each year. It is the leading cause of death among critically ill patients.[30] Sepsis has been denoted as a malignant intravascular inflammation because it is uncontrolled, unregulated, and self-sustaining. Extension of the normal local inflammatory response to infection into normal tissue is termed *sepsis*, an autodestructive process.[31] Sepsis is a complex, systemic inflammatory response to infection, with or without positive blood cultures. In addition to infection, at least two of the SIRS criteria must be present to meet the definition of sepsis.[26] Sepsis is a proinflammatory response and, because it activates the coagulation system, thus altering the procoagulation-anticoagulation balance, it is also a procoagulant response. The activated coagulation system depletes plasmin and antithrombin III and activates protein C, leading to hemorrhage when anticoagulation factors are depleted. Activation of the coagulation cascade and the resultant coagulopathy produce diffuse microthrombi. As microthrombi obstruct flow through capillaries, the tissues become unable to to receive and extract oxygen. Arterial vascular tone decreases and endothelial permeability increases, causing a redistribution of intravascular fluid volume, which fosters progression to severe sepsis. Acute respiratory alkalosis, resulting from stimulation of ventilation, may be seen in early sepsis; however, as deterioration progresses to septic shock, lactic acidosis develops.[32]

Severe sepsis is defined as sepsis with organ dysfunction, hypotension, or hypoperfusion.[26,33] It is a leading cause of death in noncoronary intensive care units (ICUs).[34] In the United States, patients with severe sepsis have a mortality rate of 28% to 50%.[35] Annually, 200,000 patients in the United States die of severe sepsis.[36] With an average individual cost of care of $22,000, health care for sepsis accounted for expeditures of $16.7 billion in the United States in 2000.[34] It is anticipated that these figures will rise as the population ages, the number of immunocompromised patients increases, more antibiotic-resistant organisms emerge, the use of invasive procedures and monitoring devices expands, and the awareness of severe sepsis criteria increases.[21]

Organ dysfunction in severe sepsis results from hypotension and tissue hypoperfusion. Hypotension is defined as mean arterial blood pressure (MABP) <60 mm Hg, systolic blood pressure (SBP) <90 mm Hg, or a decrease in SBP of >40 mm Hg from baseline without other causes.[26] Hypoperfusion leads to tissue hypoxia and ischemia. Clinical signs of tissue hypoperfusion may include oliguria, lactic acidosis, or acute alterations in mental status.[26]

Septic Shock. Septic shock is sepsis accompanied by hypotension and tissue hypoperfusion, despite adequate fluid resuscitation, with other systemic abnormalities, which may include lactic acidosis, oliguria, and acute mental status changes.[26,29] Infection from a variety of bacteria, fungi, and, rarely, viruses can cause septic shock. These pathogens or exotoxins produced by bacteria interact with the host immune cells to incite a massive inflammatory response. Noncytokine and cytokine mediators (e.g., IL-1, TNF-α, IL-6) are released, activating systemic inflammation and release of mediators (e.g., thromboxane A_2, prostaglandins, and nitric oxide), which causes vasodilation and endothelial damage. Cytokines also activate the coagulation pathway, creating capillary microthrombi.[37] The inflammatory and procoagulant responses initiated by bacterial toxins result in capillary leakage, inadequate circulatory volume, circulatory collapse, and potentially profound hypotension despite adequate fluid resuscitation. This leads to impaired tissue perfusion and ischemia. As perfusion of nonvital tissues, and eventually vital organs, decreases and the body shifts to anaerobic cellular metabolism, lactate production increases, leading to metabolic acidosis. To compensate for hypoxia and acidosis, respirations become rapid and shallow. Uncorrected, this respiratory insufficiency can lead to acute respiratory failure. If the shock state is not corrected quickly, the patient's survival is jeopardized. The mortality rate from septic shock is 50% to 60%.[34]

As sepsis progresses, organ system function becomes compromised. MODS occurs when organ function is altered and homeostasis cannot be maintained without intervention. The first systems affected are usually the cardiovascular and pulmonary systems, followed by hepatic, gastrointestinal, and renal systems, and, finally, the brain.[21] As one or more organ systems fail, the mortality rate increases; with failure of three or more systems, the mortality rate reaches 70%.[38] Organ system failure is closely linked to a hypercoagulable state.

It is a paradox that progress in the management of severe medical and surgical diseases has increased the patient population now at risk for sepsis. As the population continues to age and more pathogens develop resistance to antibiotic therapy, the number of patients at risk will continue to increase. Therefore, it is extremely important that nurses be able to recognize the early, subtle signs of SIRS and sepsis and re-establish perfusion by instituting optimal supportive care and therapy.

Assessment for Sepsis/Septic Shock. Critical nursing management includes regular screening of patients for evidence of infection, SIRS critieria, and acute organ dysfunction. Nurses have a crucial role in monitioring for subtle clinical changes to recognize sepsis promptly. Signs and symptoms of specific acute infections affecting various body systems are described later in this chapter.

Vital signs, particulary changing trends in these measures, should be noted.[32] Increasing heart and respiratory rates and elevated or reduced body temperature could meet the criteria for SIRS. In early septic shock, the increase in cardiac output offsets low systemic vascular resistance; therefore, systolic blood pressure is maintained. Over time, as circulating blood volume is further depleted and compensatory mechanisms are exhausted, blood pressure will decline. Assessment of WBC count (either leukocytosis or leukopenia) and differential is also important, although leukocytosis is neither sensitive nor specific for infection. As a result of inadequate tissue perfusion, organ dysfunction affecting one or more organs can become apparent. It is important to monitor for signs of altered tissue perfusion, including altered mentation, systemic hypotension, decreased urinary output, prolonged capillary refill time, hypoxemia, respiratory compromise requiring ventilation, and respiratory alkalosis progressing to metabolic acidosis.[26] Earliest signs can include increased apprehension, confusion, and decreased sensorium (in a sedated or brain-injured patient, these findings may not be evident).[26,39] Signs of coagulation imbalance, such as decreased platelet count, abnormal coagulation studies, increased bleeding at venipuncture sites, and petechiae, may also indicate sepsis.[26,39] If two or more of the SIRS criteria are met, infection is deemed present or suspected, the patient is hypotensive or has evidence of tissue hypoperfusion, and one or more organs is dysfunctional, severe sepsis is suggested.[34]

Investigations continue in attempting to identify a biologic marker that would provide early, accurate detection of sepsis with good specificity and sensitivity. As mentioned earlier, the host response in sepsis is modulated by a cascade of pro-inflammatory cytokines or mediators (e.g., TNF, IL-1, IL-6, and interleukin-8 [IL-8]) followed by immunomodulators that down-regulate the response (e.g., anti-inflammatory mediators include interleukin-4 and interleukin-10). Markers of interest include IL-6 and IL-8, which may correlate with patient outcome. High IL-6 levels are associated with death in septic patients. However, the cytokines are not specific and are also induced by various noninfective stimuli, including surgery, viral infections, and autoimmune disorders.[40] There is great clinical interest in using these markers for predicting patients most at risk for sepsis.

Currently available markers include PCT, CRP, and the erythrocyte sedimentation rate (ESR). PCT is a propeptide produced in the thyroid gland. Usually at low systemic levels (<0.1 ng/ml), the PCT concentration rises dramatically in sepsis to more than several hundred nanograms per milliliter. PCT levels seem to reflect increasing severity of the systemic inflammatory response.[2] Another early marker is CRP, a liver-produced protein released after inflammation or tissue damage. It has both proinflammatory and anti-inflammatory actions and is frequently used to detect the presence and severity of infection or sepsis. However, multiple-trauma patients and elective surgery patients may show an increase of PCT, CRP, and other biomolecules, indicating inflammation during the early postoperative or posttraumatic period independent of the diagnosis of sepsis or infection.[41-43]

The ESR is a nonspecific blood test used to detect inflammation. Normal erythrocytes are negatively charged and repel each other. In the presence of positively charged plasma proteins, the surface charge of the erythrocytes is neutralized and they are able to aggregate. Sedimentation rate testing demonstrates the ability of the red blood cells (RBCs) to settle to the bottom of a glass tube. This rate is increased in the presence of infection, rheumatoid arthritis, lupus erythematosus, leukemia, and cancers.

Recent investigations have identified a new potential sepsis biomarker, sTREM-1. This soluble triggering receptor expressed on myeloid cells has a sensitivity of 96% and a specificity of 89% in determining the presence of infection.[44] Other biomarkers being studied for their potential prognostic ability include endotoxin (a component of gram-negative cell walls), brain natriuretic peptide (a myocardial dysfunction indicator), and endogenous protein C.[45] Much research is under way to determine the accuracy of these biomarkers in identifying and guiding the treatment of sepsis.

Management of Sepsis and Septic Shock. In 2003, critical care and infectious disease experts convened at an international conference to develop evidenced-based guidelines for the management of sepsis and to launch an initiative to encourage use of these interventions to improve patient outcomes from sepsis—the Surviving Sepsis Campaign. Key recommendations focus on the need for early syndrome recognition. New monitoring and therapy developments place great importance on the early identification and aggressive management of the septic patient. Meta-analysis of sepsis resuscitation trials showed that early interventions before organ dysfunction provide better outcomes.[45] Rivers et al[46] showed that the timeliness of treatment significantly improves the mortality rate when hemodynamic optimization is achieved within the first few hours after disease presentation. Patients with septic shock have a significantly greater risk of death when antibiotics are started more than 1 hour after initial presentation or diagnosis of septic shock.[47] These and other recommendations for managing sepsis are included in the established guidelines. The guidelines continue to evolve, and the reader is referred to the latest published recommendations for up-to-date suggestions for the management of sepsis.

The key recommendations of the evidence-based guidelines for management of sepsis and septic shock are highlighted in Box 15-1. Many instituations have developed treatment algorithms on the basis of these evidence-based recommendations. An example of an algorithm is found in Figure 15-1.

Numerous research initiatives for the treatment of septic shock are under way. New modalities for management of septic shock include investigation of the safety and efficacy of nitric oxide (NO) synthase inhibitor. NO is a highly reactive free radical found in the endothelium that maintains vascular tone.[48] NO affects blood pressure regulation and blood flow distribution. Endotoxin and cytokines released in response to infection induce NO synthase, with subsequent NO hyperproduction, which is associated with development of hypotension, decreased responsiveness to vasopressors, tissue dysoxia, and multiple organ dysfunction. Several small studies reported that NO inhibitors can restore hemodynamics and vasopressor responsiveness in patients with septic shock. Other researchers are investigating the use of the supplemental infusion of arginine vasopressin to increase MABP above 65 mm Hg.[49] Scientists are also developing novel fluids for resuscitation that will improve microcirculatory flow of hypovolemic patients. One such fluid is Ringer's ethylpyruvate, in which lactate has been replaced with pyruvate, creating a resuscitative fluid with antioxidant properties, which could reduce inflammatory cytokine production.[50]

THE MICROBIOLOGIC RESERVOIR

The presence of microorganisms in a culture does not necessarily mean that an infection is present. Positive cultures mean that an organism is growing in the culture medium.

BOX 15-1 Guideline Recommendations for Management of Sepsis and Septic Shock

- Initial resuscitation
  - Resuscitation should begin immediately upon recognition of sepsis-induced tissue hypoperfusion
  - During the first 6 hours, the desired therapeutic end points for initial resuscitation of hypoperfusion caused by sepsis include:
    - — Central venous pressure (CVP) 8 to 12 mm Hg
    - — Mean arterial pressure ≥65 mm Hg
    - — Urine output $\geq 0.5 mL/kg^{-1}/hr^{-1}$
    - — Central venous (superior vena cava) ($ScvO_2$) or mixed venous oxygen saturation (SvO_2) ≥70% or ≥65% respectively
  - During the first 6 hours of severe sepsis or septic shock resuscitation, if the $ScvO_2$ or SvO_2 does not reach 70% or 65%, respectively, once fluid administration achieves a CVP of 8 to 12 mm Hg, transfuse red blood cells to obtain a hematocrit of ≥30% and/or administer dobutamine to reach SvO_2 goal
- Diagnosis
  - Obtain appropriate cultures (e.g., urine, cerebrospinal fluid, wound, respiratory secretions, body fluids, at least 2 blood cultures [one percutaneously and one from each vascular access in place over 48 hours]) before antimicrobial therapy is begun if not associated with a significant delay in starting antibiotics
  - When possible, promptly perform diagnostic/imaging/ultrasound studies to identify infection source and causative organism
- Antibiotic therapy
  - Initiate intravenous antibiotics within 1 hour of severe sepsis or septic shock recognition
  - Consider combination antibiotic therapy with *Pseudomonas* infections
  - Consider empiric combination antibiotic therapy for neutropenic patients
  - Do not continue combination antibiotic therapy given empirically >3 to 5 days
  - Initial empiric intravenous antibiotics should have activity against likely pathogens and should penetrate in sufficient concentrations to the probable septic source
  - Duration of antibiotic therapy is typically 7 to 10 days, although longer courses may be necessary in certain patients
  - Reassess antimicrobial selection daily; optimize to narrowest effective spectrum
  - Discontinue antibiotics if noninfectious source is discovered
- Source control
  - Identify a specific site of infection as soon as possible
  - Remove potentially infected devices, drain abscess or local infection, debride necrotic tissue. If a suspected source of infection, promptly remove vascular access after new site is established
  - Choose the source control intervention least likely to cause physiologic upset
  - Once identified, perform the intervention to control the source as soon as possible (except delay surgical intervention for infected pancreatic necrosis)
- Fluid therapy
  - Resuscitate with colloids (300 to 500 mL) or crystalloids (≥1,000 mL) over 30 min. Provide additional fluid at perhaps a faster rate based on patient's condition and response (e.g., blood pressure, urine output, heart rate, CVP)
  - Reduce fluid administration when cardiac filling pressures increase without improving hemodynamics
- Vasopressors
  - Maintain mean arterial blood pressure ≥65 mm Hg
  - Norepinephrine or dopamine are first-choice vasopressor agents; vasopressin (0.03 units/min) may subsequently be administered with norepinephrine
  - Epinephrine is the first alternative in treating hypotension from septic shock that is refractory to norepinephrine or dopamine
  - Low-dose dopamine should not be used for renal protection
  - If vasoactives are needed, an arterial line should be placed as soon as possible
- Inotrope therapy
  - Dobutamine may be used to treat myocardial dysfunction evidenced by low cardiac output and high cardiac filling pressures
  - Increasing cardiac index levels to achieve a predefined elevated target is not recommended
- Steroids
  - Consider intravenous hydrocortisone (≤300 mg/day) for patients in septic shock who, despite sufficient fluid administration and vasoactives, have persistent hypotension; hydrocortisone is preferred over dexamethasone
  - Oral fludrocortisones may be added if hydrocortisone is unavailable and steroid used doesn't have mineralocorticoid activity; optional with hydrocortisone
  - ACTH stimulation testing is not recommended to determine which patients should receive steroids
  - Wean steroids once vasopressors no longer required
  - Without shock, corticosteroids not recommended for treatment of sepsis unless patient has history of steroid use
- Recombinant human activated protein C (rhAPC)*
  - Recommended for patients with sepsis-related organ dysfunction at high risk of dying (i.e., multiple organ failure, Acute Physiology and Chronic Health Evaluation II [APACHE II] score of >25) and no contraindication due to bleeding risk

*NOTE: Used in an attempt to re-establish coagulation balance. It is an analog of a native protein C that inhibits coagulation, increases fibrinolysis, and may inhibit synthesis of tumor necrosis factor. Although rhAPC may prolong partial thromboplastin time (PTT), it has minimal effect on prothrombin time (PT). Administration of rhAPC should be discontinued 2 hours before invasive surgical procedures, but it can be restarted 12 hours after the procedure. Nurses need to be aware and monitor for bleeding.

Continued

BOX 15-1 Guideline Recommendations for Management of Sepsis and Septic Shock—cont'd

- Blood product administration
  - Once tissue hypoperfusion is resolved and without extenuating circumstances (e.g., acute hemorrhage, myocardial ischemia, severe hypoxemia, cyanotic heart disease, lactic acidosis), give red blood cells if hemoglobin <7 g/dL; Target hemoglobin 7 to 9 g/dL
  - Erythropoietin is not recommended for severe sepsis-related anemia but may be used for other appropriate reasons
  - Administration of antithrombin is not recommended for treatment of septic shock or severe sepsis
  - Routine administration of fresh frozen plasma to correct coagulopathy in the absence of bleeding or a planned procedure is not recommended
  - Consider platelet transfusion for counts 5,000 to 30,000/mm^3 when there is risk of bleeding. Platelet counts of at least 50,000/mm^3 are usually required for invasive procedures. Administer platelets if counts are <5,000/mm^3
- Mechanical ventilation of sepsis-induced acute lung injury (ALI) or acute respiratory distress syndrome (ARDS)
  - In patients with ALI or ARDS, goal should be to lower tidal volumes to 6 mL/kg of predicted body weight and maintain plateau pressures ≤30 cm H_2O
  - Hypercapnia may be tolerated to lower plateau pressure and tidal volumes
  - Utilize positive end-expiratory pressure to prevent end-expiration lung collapse
  - Consider prone positioning in patients requiring high FiO_2 or plateau pressures
  - Unless contraindicated, maintain head of bed at a 30- to 45-degree elevation
  - Noninvasive mask ventilation should be considered only in a minority of select patients with mild/moderate respiratory failure
  - Utilize a weaning protocol and spontaneous breathing trials to discontinue mechanical ventilation as soon as the patient is arousable, hemodynamically stable without vasopressors, has no new serious conditions, requires low ventilatory and end-expiratory requirements, and has FiO_2 requirements that are achieveable via face mask or nasal cannula
  - Routine use of a pulmonary artery catheter is not recommended for patients with ALI or ARDS
  - Administer fluids conservatively in patients with ALI without evidence of tissue hypoperfusion
- Sedation, analgesia, and neuromuscular blockade
  - Use a sedation protocol that guides administration of intermittent or continuous sedation to achieve a goal measurable by a standard subjective sedation scale
  - Interrupt sedation administration daily to allow awaking and retitration
  - Avoid use of neuromuscular blocking agents
- Glucose control
  - Use a validated insulin protocol to maintain blood glucose below 150mg/dL
  - Use IV insulin to control hyperglycemia
  - If receiving insulin, provide a glucose source and monitor blood glucose every 1 to 2 hours until insulin infusion and glucose levels are stable, then every 4 hours
  - Interpret with caution any low glucose levels obtained by point-of-care testing
- Renal replacement
  - Consider continuous renal replacement therapies (CRRT) and intermittent hemodialysis equivalent, except in hemodynamically unstable patients when CRRT offers easier fluid balance management
- Bicarbonate therapy
  - Not recommended to reduce vasoactive use or to achieve hemodynamic stability in patients with hypoperfusion-induced lactic acidemia and pH ≥7.15
- Deep vein thrombosis (DVT) prophylaxis
  - Provide DVT prophylaxis with either low-dose unfractionated heparin (UFH) or low-molecular weight heparin (LMWH) unless contraindicated. LMWH preferred over UFH in patients at high risk
  - For patients with heparin contraindication (i.e., coagulopathy) use mechanical prophylaxis (e.g., intermittent compression devices, graduated compression stockings)
  - In very high-risk patients (i.e., severe sepsis with history of DVT, orthopedic surgery, or trauma) use combination pharmacologic and mechanical therapy
- Stress ulcer prophylaxis
  - Give H_2 blocker or proton pump inhibitor to patients with severe sepsis
- Support limitations
  - Appropriate provider/family/patient discussion about outcomes and goals of treatment should take place

SOURCES: Dellinger RP, Levy MM, Carlet JM et al: Surviving sepsis campaign: international guidelines for management of severe sepsis and septic shock: 2008, *Crit Care Med* 36(1):296-327, 2008; Bernard GR, Vincent JL, Laterre PF et al: Efficacy and safety of recombinant human activated C for severe sepsis, *N Engl J Med* 344:699-709, 2001

The reader is referred to these sources for more detail on these recommendations and for considerations with pediatric patients.

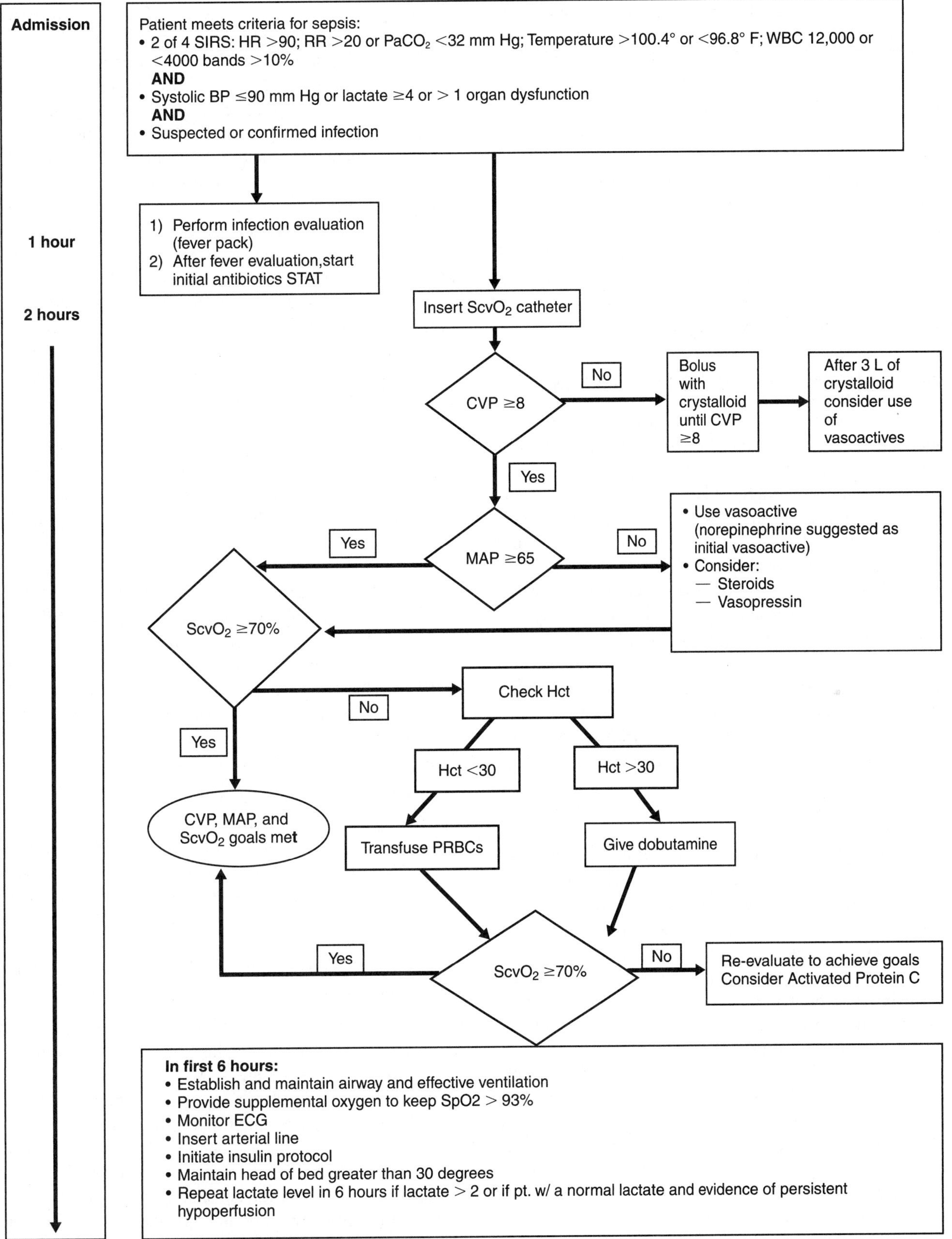

FIGURE 15-1 Treatment algorithm for initial management of sepsis on the basis of recommended sepsis guidelines. (From the R Adams Cowley Shock Trauma Center, University of Maryland Medical Center, Baltimore, MD.)

Culture results must be evaluated in relation to the clinical picture. Colonization exists when the microorganism is present without detrimental effect. Open wounds and respiratory secretions may be abundantly colonized without actual infection. However, when bacteria are cultured from areas where body fluids are normally sterile (the pleural space, the peritoneal cavity, or the CNS), this constitutes an infection. Infection occurs when the organism causes injury or damage to the tissues.

Any microorganism has the potential to cause serious or even fatal disease. The number of severe invasive infections and infections caused by drug-resistant pathogens is increasing annually. The nurse plays a pivitol role in recognizing possible infection so that appropriate diagnostics can be performed to identify the infectious source and causative organism(s) so that therapy can be initiated in a timely fashion.

SURVEILLANCE AND IDENTIFICATION OF INFECTION

Nurses must be vigilant in assessing factors that increase a patient's predisposition to infection or that indicate infection may be present. Careful assessment of all patients on admission, especially the elderly, identifies preexisting factors (e.g., advanced age, chronic obstructive pulmonary disease, alcoholism, malnutrition, diabetes, or cancer) that could increase the risk of nosocomial infection.[21,51,52] Daily monitoring of SIRS scores has been found useful in predicting infection and trauma outcome.[53] Persistent elevations in SIRS scores warrant investigation for infectious sources, enhancing early diagnosis of infection.[53] Research also supports the use of injury severity scores as an independent predictor of nosocomial bloodstream infections.[54] The combination of increased age and decreased serum albumin levels has been found to be predictive of infection and death.[55] Identifying trauma patients at increased risk for infection promotes early therapeutic intervention and decreases deaths from infectious causes.[56,57]

Evaluating trauma patients for infection can be a complex process. As a result of decreased consciousness, sedation, endotracheal intubation, or head injury, the patient's history is often unavailable. The physical examination is hampered by dressings, devices, immobility, and the use of isolation procedures. Some diagnostic tests are difficult to obtain because patient transport is too cumbersome or risky. At times, indwelling metallic implants preclude patients from imaging studies.

The classic indicators of infection—fever, tachycardia, tachypnea, and leukocytosis (SIRS)—are not specific for infections only. Table 15-1 lists various infectious and noninfectious causes of the fever/SIRS response in trauma patients at different periods of hospitalization. In general, unless a premorbid infection is present at the time of admission, very few infections occur in the first 48 hours after admission.

All through the trauma cycle, it is extremely important to distinguish infectious causes from noninfectious causes of SIRS; otherwise, an inaccurate diagnosis will be made, which will not only result in unnecessary use of antibiotics and subsequent complications but also delay the correct diagnosis and appropriate therapy. Because of all the complexities of the evaluation of infection in a critically ill trauma patient, an infectious disease team dedicated to the trauma unit could provide one of the most effective surveillance systems. An infectious disease physician can help determine difficult diagnoses in patients with atypical presentations of illnesses or clinical deterioration and institute effective treatment, thereby decreasing morbidity and mortality rates and containing the cost of care.[58] Clinical parameters such as trends in body temperature, other vital signs, oxygenation requirements, condition of the wounds, and character of drainage should be monitored closely. The presence of invasive devices and the administration of medications (antibiotics, steroids, immunosuppressives) should be noted every day. Laboratory tests such as WBC counts, hepatic/renal function studies, radiographs, and any cultures sent for analysis should be evaluated daily.

Prospective evaluation translates into early diagnosis and effective treatment of infection. Continuous surveillance includes daily evaluation of the need for various invasive devices and ensures that appropriate infection prevention measures are in place. Tracking the incidence of infection defines endemic infection rates and monitors the effectiveness of infection control practices. Additionally, close scrutiny of the cultures can result in early detection of outbreaks with resistant organisms, allowing prompt institution of appropriate infection control measures.

In our institution, when a patient has a fever of new onset (101° F [38.3° C]) or an increase in temperature by 1.8° F or 1° C above baseline, or unexplained hemodynamic instability, then a "fever protocol" is initiated by the nursing staff. This protocol includes the following laboratory tests:

- WBC count with manual differential
- Urinalysis and culture
- Two sets of aerobic and anaerobic blood cultures drawn from a venipunture unless otherwise stated
- Sputum Gram stain and cultures in ventilated patients
- Chest radiograph
- Central venous catheter (CVC) and wound cultures, if pertinent

Additionally, a sinus x-ray film may be required if patient has indwelling nasal tubes. Other studies such as computed tomography (CT) scan and magnetic resonance imaging (MRI) may be obtained. If relevant and otherwise not contraindicated, a lumbar puncture may be performed.

Because the bedside nurse often receives microbiology reports, understanding these results is important so that appropriate antibiotic therapy can be initiated promptly. Gram stain, culture, and sensitivity testing are key diagnostic tools for evaluating infection. The results of a Gram stain may be known within minutes. The Gram stain offers preliminary identification of a microorganism by its general classification (gram

TABLE 15-1 Time Sequence of Causes of Fevers or Systemic Inflammatory Response Syndrome in Critically Ill Trauma Patients*

Time from Admission	Infectious Causes	Type of Organisms	Noninfectious Causes	Comments
0 to 24 hours (early cycle)	Aspiration pneumonia (usually chemical); preexisting infection	MSSA, anaerobes, *S. pneumoniae*, streptococci, *Hemophilus* spp, enteric GNRs	SIRS response from trauma or surgery; missed injury; necrotic tissue	Noninfections causes are more common; ↑community pathogens
>1 to 3 days (early cycle)	Aspiration pneumonia; wound infection/ cellulitis	As above for lungs; wound infection: group A *Streptococcus*, *Clostridial* spp	As above; atelectasis; allergic reaction	Noninfectious causes are more common
>3 to 5 days (early cycle)	VAP; wound infection; UTI; CVC-related infection	As above for lungs and wounds; ↑nosocomial GNRs	As above; PE; DVT; drug fever; MI; spine trauma; intracranial blood; pancreatitis	Infections are becoming more common
>5 to 7 days (mid cycle)	As above	As above, MRSA	Missed injury is unlikely; rest as early cycle	Infections are very common; ↑nosocomial pathogens
>7 days (mid cycle)	As above; sinusitis; *C. difficile*; abdominal infection; meningitis (if dura is violated)	↑Resistant GNRs; MRSA; *C. difficile*; enterococci (VSE/VRE); fungus	SIRS response; rest as early/mid cycle, acalculous cholecystitis	Almost all nosocomial pathogens
2 weeks (late cycle)	As above; osteomyelitis	Off antibiotics: early pathogens On antibiotics: mid/late pathogens	As >7 days mid cycle; heterotopic ossification	Similar infections to mid cycle
After discharge (chronic)	UTI; *C. difficile*; decubitus ulcer; osteomyelitis; CVC-related infection	No devices: early pathogens Invasive devices: mid pathogens	As late cycle	Infections are dependent on devices, mobility and antibiotics

Nosocomial GNRs, *P. aeruginosa*, *Enterobacter* species, *Acinetobacter* species; *MSSA*, methicillin-susceptible *staphylococcus aureus; SIRS*, systematic inflammatory response syndrome; *VAP*, ventilator-associated pneumonia; *UTI*, urinary tract infection; *CVC*, central venous catheter; *PE*, pulmonary embolism; *MI*, myocardial infarction; *MRSA*, methicillin-resistant *S. aureus; VSE*, vancomycin-susceptible enterococci; *VRE*, vancomycin-resistant enterococci.

*All infectious and noninfectious causes of fevers/SIRS can occur at any time during hospitalization; however, these time associations are seen most frequently.

positive, gram negative, or yeast) and its shape (rod, cocci, diplococcus) (Table 15-2). Early results may identify the pathogen as small or large rods or the grouping as cocci in pairs, chains, or clusters. This gives insight into what the organism may be. Depending on the pathogen's rate of growth in culture, it may take 2 to 5 days or longer to obtain culture results that identify the specific organism. Organisms are reported as sensitive, resistant, or intermediate to specific antibiotics. Sensitivity patterns are influenced by the environmental flora in each institution.

As the patient recovers, the incidence of infections decreases. However, resistant bacteria become more prevalent and such infections require different antibiotic regimens. Infection during any phase of the trauma cycle jeopardizes the final outcome and prolongs recovery.

PRINCIPLES OF ANTIMICROBIAL THERAPY[59-61]

Several factors come into play when the appropriate antibiotic therapy for a given infection is chosen. These factors can be grouped under three categories: infecting organism (its virulence, identity, and susceptibility), host factors, and antimicrobial properties.

INFECTING ORGANISM

Microorganisms are a formidable force that are constantly adapting and developing new mechanisms of resistance. To develop an effective therapy, health care providers need to be knowledgeable about a number of facts:

- Certain bacteria possess virulence factors that lead to more severe infections. Meningococcal, group A *Streptococcus,* and clostridial infections are prime examples of severe infections caused by toxin-producing bacteria.
- In a substantial number of patients, the initial treatment of an infection is based on a reasonable statistical guess as to the most likely infecting pathogen. However, rapid identification of the pathogen is vital to optimize treatment. In many cases, a Gram stain of

TABLE 15-2 Specific Pathogens

Aerobic Bacteria

Gram-Positive

Streptococcus pneumoniae (encapsulated diplococcus)
Streptococcus viridans
Streptococcus pyogens
Streptococcus agalactiae
Enterococcus species: either α- or β-hemolytic
When resistant to vancomycin, this is a VRE.
Enterococcus faecalis normal gut flora; can access into blood
Staphylococcus aureus (cocci)
Colonizes anterior nares, skin, groin, axillae, and perineal region; easily spread on hands of health care personnel; can adhere to endothelial structures
Methicillin-sensitive *S. aureus* (MSSA) sensitive to Ancef
Methicillin-resistant *S. aureus* (MRSA); may also be termed ORSA because the organism can also be tested against oxacillin; resistant to Ancef; sensitive to vancomycin, linezolid, Synercid, Tigecycline
Staphylococcus epidermidis (cocci) coagulase negative, skin contaminant
Bacillus cereus (rod) food poisoning
Listeria transmitted to humans via animals or their feces

Gram-Negative

Escherichia coli (rod)
Klebsiella species (rod)
Klebsiella pneumoniae is most commonly isolated
Enterbacter species (rod)
Enterobacter cloacae
Enterobacter aerogenes
Proteus species (rod)
Proteus vulgaris
Proteus mirabilis
Serratia marcescens (rod)
Citrobacter (rod)
Salmonella (rod) causes typhoid fever, gastroenteritis, or sepsis; fecal-oral
Shigella (rod) causes bacterial dysentery, ulcerative colitis; fecal-oral
Neisseria species
Neisseria meningitides (diplococci) causes meningitis, petechial rash
Neisseria gonorrhoeae (cocci)
Pseudomonas species (coccobacillus)
Pseudomonas aeruginosa is one of the leading causes of GNR pneumonia
Haemophilus (coccobacillus)
Haemophilus influenzae is frequently found with chronic obstructive pulmonary disease; colonizes oropharynx
Brucella (coccobacillus) is found in contaminated milk and cheese

Anaerobic Bacteria

Gram-Positive

Actinomyces israeli (filamentous)
Clostridium botulinum (rod) causes weakness and respiratory paralysis; found in contaminated foods
Clostridium difficile (rod) causes pseudomembranous colitis, diarrhea
Clostridium perfringens (rod) causes gas gangrene, food poisoning
Clostridium tetani (rod) causes tetanus, lockjaw, spastic paralysis; spore enters puncture wound
Peptostreptococcus

Gram-Negative

Bacteroides fragilis (bacilli) causes sepsis, peritonitis, bacteremia; produces foul-smelling abscess; found in deep penetrating wounds

Acid-Fast Bacilli

Mycobacterium avium-intracellulare causes tuberculoisis-like disease
Mycobacterium leprae causes leprosy
Mycobacterium tuberculosis causes tuberculosis by droplets from cough
Nocardia asteroidies causes abscesses in heart, lung, and brain

body fluid or immunologic methods are rapid and inexpensive ways to identify the pathogen. Definitive identification is based on culture techniques.

- Antimicrobial susceptibility testing can indicate whether an organism is susceptible or resistant. Susceptibility testing is extremely important because certain organisms have acquired widespread resistance.

HOST FACTORS

A number of host factors influence antimicrobial efficacy and toxicity and the selection of antibiotic therapy:

- Age: Older adults have decreased excretion and absorption of antimicrobial agents because renal function is age dependent. Many older individuals have been previously sensitized or are taking other medications, which heightens the risk of drug interactions and hypersensitivity reactions.
- Genetic variations: The rate at which certain drugs are metabolized and acetylated in the liver is determined genetically. Asians are more rapid acetylators than are northern Europeans. As a result, the levels and hepatotoxicity of certain drugs can be very different in these populations.
- Metabolic abnormalities: Diabetics taking oral hypoglycemic agents are more prone to drug interactions. In patients with gastric achlorhydria, the absorption of certain antibiotics is altered.
- Pregnancy: All antibiotics cross the placenta to a varying degree; therefore, the fetus can be exposed to the adverse effects of a drug. Serum levels of the antibiotic can be affected by alterations in drug clearance seen in many pregnant women. Antibiotics are secreted in

breast milk and thus can produce unacceptable side effects in the infant.

- Renal and hepatic function: The kidney and liver serve as the major routes of inactivation and excretion of antibiotics. In patients with impaired renal or hepatic function, toxic levels of antibiotics can cause severe side effects.
- Site of infection: Of all the factors, the site of infection is probably the most important determinant in the choice of antimicrobial therapy. For an antibiotic to be effective, a few factors must be considered when making the appropriate selection:
    - Antibiotic concentration at the site of infection (above the minimum inhibitory concentration [MIC] of the organism); certain sites of infection (e.g., the heart, cerebrospinal fluid [CSF], bone, prostate) require specific antibiotics that can penetrate to the location.
    - Serum concentration of the drug
    - Local factors: Decreased activity of β-lactams and aminoglycosides in pus resulting from the presence of anaerobes and decreased activity of penicillins and tetracyclines in hematomas from binding to hemoglobin. Changes in pH and oxygen tension can also alter antimicrobial activity. Bacteria are present in an altered metabolic state around foreign bodies and develop novel resistance mechanisms to antibiotics. In trauma patients, the presence of devitalized tissue, foreign bodies, or surgical implants can interfere with the action of the antibiotic.
- History of allergy or adverse reaction to the drug
- Patients with a prolonged hospital stay and with a history of recent antibiotic use or health care–associated infections are more likely to harbor antibiotic-resistant organisms.

Antimicrobial Properties

Selection of antibiotic therapy for an infection is based on clearly defined antimicrobial properties:

- Penetration into the infected site
- Adequate susceptibility of the infecting pathogen
- Acceptable toxicity
- Bioavailability, especially when oral agents are used
- Local antibiograms, which demonstrate activity against the pathogens
- Less frequent dosing
- Cidal or killing activity for infections such as meningitis or endocarditis. For most other infections, static or inhibitory activity is acceptable.
- Drug interactions
- Renal or hepatic metabolism or excretion
- Ability to cause drug allergy or a significant side effect profile
- Acceptable route of administration
- Lipid solubility
- Protein binding
- Cost
- Synergy: Combinations of antibiotics are used in certain situations where a single drug may not have the same efficacy as the combination therapy. One example is the treatment of serious enterococcal infections. Penicillin acts as a static agent and by itself has a high failure rate. When given with aminoglycosides, its uptake is enhanced. As a result of this interaction, there is synergistic killing of the organism. Similarly, synergistic combination therapy may be useful in the treatment of infections with *Streptococcus viridans*, *Staphylococcus aureus*, and *Pseudomonas aeruginosa*.
- Antimicrobial combinations: Most infections can be treated with a single agent, but combination therapy is indicated for certain situations. Antimicrobial combination therapy may be needed for more broad-spectrum coverage in infected patients where polymicrobial or resistant organisms are suspected.

Inappropriate use of multiple antibiotics may have a detrimental effect. The two drugs may be antagonistic and may interfere with each other's activity. The use of multiple drugs may heighten the risk of adverse events, the cost of therapy, and the potential for emergence of resistant bacteria.

General rules for selection of effective antimicrobial therapy in trauma patients with severe infection are as follows:

- Start therapy with a broad-spectrum antibiotic, singly or in combination.
- Monitor cultures and the patient's condition.
- Observe a "3-day rule" in all patients: when the final cultures are obtained at the end of day 3, therapy should be streamlined and the most narrow-spectrum antibiotic should be used.
- When all things are equal, use the time-honored and less expensive drugs.

Antibiotoics for specific pathogens are listed in Table 15-3.

Antimicrobial Resistance

Survival of a microorganism depends on its ability to adapt to the changing environment. Microbes possess tremendous genetic variability, which helps them not only survive but also continuously adapt. Genetic variability occurs by the following mechanisms[62,63]:

- Point mutations or microevolutionary change: These mutations may occur spontaneously during replication of deoxyribonucleic acid (DNA).
- Macroevolutionary change: Large segments of the bacterial genome can be rearranged by segments of DNA called transposon or insertion sequences. The transposon units are small mobile genetic elements capable of mediating transfer of DNA within a single cell or by jumping to other cells by removing or inserting themselves into host chromosomal and plasmid DNA. Transposons are essential in the evolution of multiantibiotic-resistant organisms (MARO).

TABLE 15-3 **Choice of Antimicrobial Therapy for Selected Pathogens**

Pathogen	Recommended	Alternative	Also Effective
Gram-Positive Cocci			
S. aureus (methicillin-sensitive)	Oxacillin Nafcillin Cefazolin	Clindamycin Vancomycin	Carbapenems BL/BLI FQ Linezolid Daptomycin Tigecycline
S. aureus (methicillin-resistant)	Vancomycin	Daptomycin Linezolid TMP/SMX (some strains resistant)	Tigecycline
S. aureus (methicillin-resistant, community-acquired)	TMP/SMX or Doxycycline ±Rifampin	Vancomycin Clindamycin (if susceptible)	Daptomycin Linezolid Tigecycline
Coagulase-negative staphylococci	Vancomycin ±Rifampin	TMP/SMX ±Rifampin	Daptomycin* Linezolid* Tigecycline*
S. pyogenes (A, B, C, F, G)	Penicillin (add clindamycin for serious group A streptococcal infections; add gentamicin for group B streptococcal infections)	All β-lactams All macrolides First-/second-generation cephalosporin	Clindamycin
S. pneumoniae (penicillin-sensitive)	Penicillin	Multiple agents	—
S. pneumoniae (penicillin-resistant)	Vancomycin ±Rifampin or Gatifloxacin/Levofloxacin/Moxifloxacin	Ceftriaxone Cefotaxime	For nonmeningeal infections: Linezolid Tigecycline*
Enterococcus (penicillin-sensitive)	Penicillin or Ampicillin ±Gentamicin	Vancomycin ± Gentamicin	—
Enterococcus (penicillin-resistant)	Vancomycin ±Gentamicin	Linezolid	Daptomycin Tigecycline
Enterococcus (penicillin, vancomycin, gentamicin-resistant)	Linezolid	FQ ± Rifampin ± Doxycycline ± Chloramphenicol	Daptomycin* Tigecycline*
Gram-Negative Rods and Anaerobes			
E. coli *Klebsiella*	Third-generation cephalosporin FQ	Second-/fourth-generation cephalosporin Carbapenems TMP/SMX	BL/BLI Aminoglycosides Tigecycline Aztreonam
Enterobacter *Serratia* *Citrobacter*	FQ Carbapenems	BL/BLI Cefepime	Aminoglycosides Aztreonam TMP/SMX
Acinetobacter species	IMP/MERO or FQ + aminoglycosides	Ampicillin-Sulbactam Colistin	Polymyxin B Tigecycline*
P. aeruginosa	Piperacillin-tazobactam Ceftazidime/cefepime IMP/MERO Aminoglycosides	FQ (↑resistance) Aztreonam	Combination therapy for serious infections
H. influenzae	Second-/third-generation cephalosporin TMP/SMX Ampicillin-sulbactam	FQ Macrolides	Third-generation cephalosporin for life-threatening illnesses

TABLE 15-3 Choice of Antimicrobial Therapy for Selected Pathogens—cont'd

Pathogen	Recommended	Alternative	Also Effective
Anaerobes			
Bacteroides fragilis	Metronidazole	Clindamycin	Cefoxitin Carbapenems BL/BLI Tigecycline
C. perfringens	Penicillin + clindamycin	Erythromycin Cefoxitin BL/BLI	—
C. difficile	Metronidazole	Vancomycin	—

BL/BLI, β-lactam/β-lactamase inhibitors (ampicillin-sulbactam, piperacillin-tazobactam); *FQ,* fluoroquinolones (moxifloxacin, levofloxacin, gatifloxacin, ciprofloxacin);, *IMP,* imipenem; *MERO,* meropenem; *TMP/SMX,* trimethoprim/sulfamethoxazole.

Sources: Abramowicz M: The choice of antibacterial drugs, *Med Lett Drugs Ther* 43:69-78, 2001; Gilbert DN, Moellering RC, Eliopoulos GM, et al: *Antimicrobial therapy, the Sanford guide to antimicrobial therapy,* 35th ed, pp 47-49, Hyde Park, Vermont, 2005, Antimicrobial Therapy, Inc.

*Activity demonstrated in a few published studies; NOT Food and Drug Administration approved for this indication.

- Acquisition of foreign DNA, which is carried by plasmids, bacteriophages, and transposon/insertion sequences. Plasmids are extrachromosomal genetic elements that are common in bacteria. Plasmids existed even in the preantibiotic era, but the advent of antibiotics in the twentieth century has favored the dissemination of these mobile elements.

The organism could have inherent resistance to the drug (intrinsic resistance). A change in the genetic composition of the organism can render a previously effective drug ineffective (acquired resistance). The major mechanisms that bacteria use to develop antimicrobial resistance are outlined in Table 15-4.

Several factors unique to ICUs contribute to the proliferation and spread of MARO. The emergency nature of care

TABLE 15-4 Mechanisms of Resistance of Antimicrobial Agents

Mechanism of Resistance	Examples of Antibiotics	Type of Bacteria	Frequency of Mechanism
Enzymatic inactivation	β-lactams	GNRs Staphylococci, anaerobes	Very common Common
	Aminoglycoside-modifying enzyme	GNRs, staphylococci, enterococci	Very common
↓Permeability			
Outer membrane	Quinolones, Carbapenems*	GNRs	Common
Inner membrane	Aminoglycosides	GNRs	Not common
Antimicrobial efflux	Tetracyclines Macrolides Quinolones	GPCs/few GNRs GPCs/GNRs GNRs/GPCs	Very common Common Not common
Altered target site			
Ribosomal	Macrolides Aminoglycosides	GPCs/anaerobes Enterococci	Very common Common
Target bypass	Vancomycin	Staphylococci, enterococci	Very common
Alteration of target enzymes	β-lactams Quinolones Trimethoprim, sulfamethoxazole	Pneumococci† GNRs‡/ GPCs§ GPCs/GNRs	Very common Very common Common
Protection of target	Tetracyclines	GPCs/few GNRs/anaerobes	Common
Overproduction of target	Trimethoprim, sulfamethoxazole	GNRs/GPCs	Common

GPC, Gram-positive cocci; *GNR,* gram-negative rod.

*Loss of channels (porins) required for bacterial entry.

†Changes in penicillin-binding proteins.

‡DNA gyrase is altered; therefore, cell division of GNRs is altered.

§Topoisomerase IV is altered; therefore, cell division of gram-positive cocci is altered.

in the ICU leads to less focus on aseptic techniques and fosters transmission of MARO from health care workers to patients and also among patients. Close proximity of infected patients, use of invasive devices, prolonged length of hospital stay, and transfer of colonized patients to and from long-term care facilities also aid in the spread of MARO. Prior use of antibiotics, multiple surgical procedures, and the presence of chronic wounds in a critically ill patient are other risk factors associated with the emergence of MARO.[64,65]

Methods to prevent MARO infection/colonization are summarized below[64,65]:

- Handwashing is clearly the most important strategy.
- Place patients with MARO on isolation, which includes mandatory use of a gown and gloves for all individuals who enter the patient's room and use of dedicated medical equipment.
- Initiate education programs for health care workers, followed by reinforcement.
- On admission to the ICU, patients who have health care–associated risks for MARO need to be placed in presumptive isolation, and surveillance cultures should to be obtained.
- Any invasive devices (e.g., intravenous catheters, bladder catheters) should be used only when essential and should be removed as soon as possible. Use of aseptic technique during insertion and appropriate maintenance of the device are also important to prevent infection.
- Infection must be diagnosed and treated effectively. Culture the patient. Target empiric therapy toward the likely organism. Optimize timing, regimen, route, dose, and duration of treatment. Streamline therapy once cultures are finalized.
- Use antibiotics appropriately and wisely. Know your antibiogram, the formulary, and the patient population. Treat infection, not just the contaminants/colonizers. Use recommended guidelines and a computer-assisted antibiotic management program for appropriate antibiotic use. To discourage inappropriate antimicrobial use, some broad-spectrum antibiotics should be formulary restricted and susceptibility reporting should be limited on certain other restricted antibiotics. Cycle or rotate antibiotics; preferentially use narrow-spectrum and older antibiotics; and stop antimicrobials as soon as possible. Consult with infectious disease specialists when necessary.

Throughout the trauma cycle, nurses need to recognize risk factors for the presence and acquisition of MARO. There needs to be a targeted focus on establishing evidence-based infection control policies and procedures. Staff education on these established protocols must be performed and reinforced.

ANTIMICROBIAL PROPHYLAXIS FOR SURGERY

Forty million surgical procedures are performed annually in the United States.[66] Approximately 1 million surgical site infections complicate these procedures.[66] Patients with infections have a prolonged hospital stay, higher readmission rates, and increased mortality rates.[67]

DETERMINANTS OF SURGICAL WOUND INFECTION

The interplay of many different forces determines whether a surgical wound infection will develop.[68]

- Patient-related factors (nutrition, comorbidities, immune function)
- Procedure-related factors (foreign body, extent of trauma)
- Microbial concentration, resistance, and virulence
- Perioperative antibiotics may augment natural host immunity and definitely decrease the risk of surgical wound infections.[66]

SOURCES OF INFECTING PATHOGENS

Historically, operative procedures have been classified on the basis of anticipated bacterial contamination. The procedures are subdivided into clean, clean contaminated, contaminated, and dirty (Table 15-5). Numerous sources of bacterial contamination have been described. The most common mechanism of contamination is surgery, when the patient's endogenous flora is inoculated into the wound. Transmission from the staff and equipment has also been documented. Hands are one of the most frequent sources of

TABLE 15-5 Classification of Surgical Procedures

Class I: Clean Surgical Procedures
Definition: Nontraumatic, uninfected operative wounds in which no inflammation is encountered; there is no break in technique; and neither the respiratory, alimentary, or genitourinary tract nor the oropharyngeal cavities are entered
Expected infection rate: 1%-5%

Class II: Clean-Contaminated Surgical Procedures
Definition: Operations in which the respiratory, alimentary, or genitourinary tract is entered under controlled conditions and without unusual contamination
Expected infection rate: 8%-11%

Class III: Contaminated Surgical Procedures
Definition: Operations associated with open, fresh accidental wounds; major breaks in sterile technique or gross spillage from the gastrointestinal tract occur; or acute, nonpurulent inflammation is encountered
Expected infection rate: 15%-20%

Class IV: Dirty and Infected Procedures
Definition: Operations involving old traumatic wounds with devitalized tissue and those that involve existing clinical infections
Expected infection rate: >25%

Source: Altemeier WA, Burke JF, Pruitt BA et al: *Manual on control of infection in surgical patients,* Philadelphia, 1984, JB Lippincott.

contamination. Occasionally, hematogenous seeding from a preexisting infection can infect the wound.

Microbiology

The National Nosocomial Surveillance System[69] evaluated 17,671 wound isolates obtained from different parts of the United States over a 5-year period. *S. aureus* was the most common infecting agent associated with clean surgical procedures. It is also the most common organism infecting trauma patients. The nares were colonized with *S. aureus* in more than 50% of patients with diabetes or receiving hemodialysis, and this process was an important risk factor in the development of *S. aureus* infections. Coagulase-negative staphylococci are common isolates in surgical implant infections. Enteric gram-negative rods (GNRs) and anaerobes are associated with gastrointestinal and genitourinary surgeries.

Antimicrobial Prophylaxis

In 2004, the Surgical Infection Prevention Guideline Writers Workgroup, hosted by the Medicare National Surgical Infection Prevention Project, issued a consensus paper on antimicrobial prophylaxis for surgery. This document was endorsed by many regulating agencies and medical societies.[67] This section summarizes those guidelines and recommendations provided by the American Society of Hospital Pharmacists.[70]

Timing of Prophylaxis

To achieve the best results, the first dose of antibiotic(s) should be infused 60 minutes before surgical incision.[71] The goal is to achieve antibiotic levels in tissue and blood that exceed the MIC of the organism. In an injured patient who requires emergency surgical intervention, achieving this goal may not be possible, but in trauma centers appropriate antibiotics should be kept readily available so they can still be administered before incision.

Duration of Prophylaxis

Multiple studies have demonstrated no added benefit to antimicrobial prophylaxis after wound closure. For the majority of procedures, antibiotics should be discontinued 24 hours after surgery.[72]

Allergy to β-Lactam Drugs

Many patients give a history of allergy to the penicillin group of drugs. A true allergy or a severe reaction is rarely documented. Cephalosporins are most frequently the prophylactic agents of choice. Therefore, the potential cross-allergenicity among penicillins and cephalosporins is of clinical significance. Although each procedure must be evaluated separately, if coverage for gram-positive cocci is required, then clindamycin or vancomycin is a reasonable alternative to cephalosporins.

Premorbid History of Methicillin-Resistant *Staphylococcus aureus* or Other Resistant Bacteria

Over the past two decades, the incidence of *S. aureus* (resistant to both penicillins and cephalosporins) has been increasing across the United States. Patients are increasingly being admitted to hospitals with a history of being either colonized or infected with methicillin-resistant *S. aureus* (MRSA). In institutions with a high frequency of MRSA, vancomycin should be used for prophylaxis.[72] However, there is no consensus as to what constitutes "high," and it is not known whether substitution with vancomycin instead of a cephalosporin will lower overall rates of surgical site infection. Increased use of vancomycin has been associated with higher methicillin-sensitive *S. aureus* (MSSA) infection; therefore, there have been no changes in overall rates. Surveillance cultures should be obtained for patients at high risk of MRSA carriage.[73]

Antimicrobial Dosing

An adequate dose based on the patient's adjusted body weight should be provided. The dose should be repeated if the surgery is still in progress two half-lives after the first dose of the drug or if the patient has had significant blood loss.

Novel Methods of Antimicrobial Prophylaxis

Antibiotic-impregnated beads/cement have been used during orthopedic procedures. This form of prophylaxis is commonly used during replacement of an infected prosthetic joint or to fill the dead space in open fracture wounds. The two antibiotics that have been used extensively are vancomycin and aminoglycosides. Both are heat stable and have an appropriate spectrum of activity against anticipated pathogens. The majority of elution of the drug occurs during the first few days after placement. Although the use of this therapy is very common, published reports present conflicting views on its safety and efficacy.[74]

Side Effects of Prophylaxis

A number of side effects to prophylactic agents have been reported. The most common is allergic reaction of varying severity. Diarrhea related to *Clostridium difficile* is a rare complication. Antimicrobial use can also lead to selection of antibiotic-resistant flora. Additionally, an inappropriately long duration of prophylactic antibiotics can lead to higher costs with no added benefit and an increased incidence of nonsurgical site infections.[75]

Recommendations for Specific Sites

The authors of several reports from studies of antimicrobial prophylaxis have made specific recommendations related to specific surgical sites.[67,70] Key points to consider in selecting appropriate prophylactic antibiotic therapy are listed below:

- Expected flora requiring coverage
- Patient allergies
- Antimicrobial costs
- Penetration of antibiotic into the required site

- Type of procedure (Table 15-6)
- Knowledge of local flora and resistance patterns in the community
- Patient-related risk factors for acquisition of resistant pathogens
- Patient has features requiring a different approach to prophylaxis

During 2002 and 2003, the National Surgical Infection Prevention Collaborative, a collaboration of hospitals in the United States, sponsored by the Federal Centers for Medicare and Medicare Services, focused on three performance improvement processes to decrease surgical site infections: administration of antibiotics within 60 minutes of surgical incision, use of appropriate antibiotics, and discontinuation of antibiotics 24 hours after surgery. Other areas of performance improvement included control of glucose levels during surgery, use of supplemental oxygen during surgery and recovery intervals, and clipping rather than shaving the surgical site. These improved infection prevention practices led to a reduction in surgical site infections from 2.3% to 1.7%.[76]

STRATEGIES FOR PREVENTION OF INFECTION

GENERAL CARE CONSIDERATIONS

Health care workers need to maintain strict compliance with infection control guidelines and wash their hands frequently to reduce the incidence of infection. The Centers for Disease Control and Prevention recommend alcohol-based hand scrub use before and after each patient contact. The use of gloves can reduce bacterial contamination by 70% to 80%.[77] Prohibiting acrylic fingernail overlays and the wearing of rings by direct care providers can also reduce risk of the health care worker unknowingly carrying pathogens that can be transmitted to the patient.

Meticulous aseptic technique and proper cleaning and maintenance of equipment counteract environmental infection risks. Tape and scissors are common vehicles of cross-contamination. Tape strips placed on bedside rails may inoculate dressings with bacteria. Scissors may be vehicles for cross-contamination when they are used to remove wound dressings because the notches and grooves in the blades can become contaminated with bacteria from wound drainage, which can then be introduced into another patient's wound at a subsequent dressing change. Use of stethoscope covers and nonreusable equipment such as disposable blood pressure cuffs may also limit transmission of pathogens between patients.

ROLE OF INTENSIVE INSULIN THERAPY IN CRITICALLY ILL PATIENTS

Hyperglycemia and insulin resistance are common in critically ill patients. Traditionally, patients with hyperglycemia have been managed by maintaining a blood glucose level under 200 mg/dl. A prospective controlled study evaluated 1548 surgical ICU patients.[78] Patients were assigned to an intensive insulin therapy group with a target blood glucose level of 80 to 110 mg/dl or to a standard therapy group with a target blood glucose level of 180 to 200 mg/dl. The

TABLE 15-6 **Antimicrobial Prophylaxis by Procedure and Site***

Procedure	First-Choice Treatment	Alternative Treatment
Cardiothoracic/vascular surgery	Cefazolin or cefuroxime	Clindamycin or vancomycin
Colon surgery	Oral: neomycin + erythromycin or metronidazole Intravenous: cefoxitin or cefazolin + metronidazole	Oral: None Intravenous: Clindamycin or metronidazole + ciprofloxacin or aztreonam
Head and neck surgery (clean contaminated)	Cefazolin or clindamycin	Addition of gentamicin remains controversial
Hip or knee arthroplasty	Cefazolin or cefuroxime	Clindamycin or vancomycin
Hysterectomy	Cefoxitin or cefazolin	Clindamycin or metronidazole + gentamicin or ciprofloxacin or aztreonam
Facial fractures†	Cefazolin or clindamycin	None
Neurosurgical‡ (closed-head)	Cefazolin or nafcillin	Vancomycin
Neurosurgical (open head)	No antibiotics§	Use of antibiotics remains controversial
Orthopedic procedures (excluding joint replacements)	Cefazolin	Clindamycin or vancomycin (addition of gentamicin for grade III fractures remains controversial)

*Sources: Bratzler DW, Houck PM: Antimicrobial prophylaxis for surgery: an advisory statement from the National Surgical Infection Prevention Project, *Clin Infect Dis* 38:1706-1715, 2004; American Society of Health-System Pharmacists: ASHP therapeutic guidelines on antimicrobial prophylaxis in surgery, *Am J Health Syst Pharm* 56:1839-1888, 1999.

†Source: Chole RA, Yee J: Antibiotic prophylaxis for facial fractures: a prospective, randomized clinical trial, *Arch Otolaryngol Head Neck Surg* 113:1055-1057, 1987.

‡Source: Korinek AM, Golmard JL, Elcheick A et al: Risk factors for neurosurgical site infections after craniotomy: a critical reappraisal of antibiotics prophylaxis on 4,578 patients, *Br J Neurosurg* 19:155-162, 2005.

§Current practice at authors' institution.

following benefits were noted in the intensive insulin therapy group:

- During ICU stay, the overall mortality rate decreased to 4.6% (standard therapy group, 8.0%).
- Among patients who remained in the ICU >5 days, the mortality rate decreased to 10.6% (standard therapy group, 20.2%). The overall in-hospital mortality rate decreased by 34%. The greatest reduction in mortality rates involved deaths from multiple organ failure with a proven septic focus.
- Bloodstream infections decreased by 46%.
- The rate of acute renal failure requiring dialysis or hemofiltration was reduced by 41%.
- Requirements for blood transfusion decreased by 50%.
- The rate of critical illness neuropathy was reduced by 44%.
- The chance of requiring prolonged mechanical ventilation and intensive care was decreased.

It is proposed that the beneficial effect of glucose control during critical illness is related to improved mitochondrial function.[79]

The association of hyperglycemia and worse outcomes has been demonstrated in other patient populations as well. A study conducted by Sung et al[80] in trauma patients demonstrated that hyperglycemia at admission was associated with increased infection rates and a greater risk of death. Therefore, most critical care specialists are now advocating tight glucose control in all critically ill patients.

Early Versus Late Tracheostomy

Several studies have addressed the timing of tracheostomy in critically ill patients. The first study compared early (<48 hours) with late (14-16 days) tracheostomy in a group of patients in a medical ICU. The early group had a lower mortality rate, fewer pneumonias, fewer days in the ICU, and less requirement for mechanical ventilation.[81] A second retrospective study evaluated 185 surgical patients over a 2-year period. The investigators compared early (<7 days) versus late (>7 days) tracheostomy and reached a similar conclusion.[82] A third study in a small number of head-injured patients noted that, although early tracheostomy decreased the total days of mechanical ventilation, it did not decrease the frequency of pneumonia.[83] At our institution, unless there is a contraindication, early tracheostomy is generally recommended.

Infections Related to Disruption of the Skin

Necrotizing Soft Tissue Infections

Necrotizing soft tissue infections (NSTIs) are extensive infections of skin, subcutaneous fat, and soft tissue, extending to the fascial plane, the tissue sheath covering muscle. They characteristically are abrupt in onset and can extend, often visibly, in a matter of hours. An early symptom may be increasing unexplained pain. However, in diabetics with peripheral neuropathies, pain may be absent. Initially the skin is tender, edematous, hot, and shiny. NSTI is often difficult to distinguish from cellulitis.[84] Sloughing may occur as a result of microvascular thrombosis and destruction of subcutaneous tissue. In well-established infections, necrosis of superficial fascia and fat causes watery, foul-smelling exudates. Systemic signs, which may develop rapidly, include tachycardia, tachypnea, fever, chills, malaise, myalgia, diarrhea, anorexia, oliguria, hypotension, leukocytosis, acidosis, and altered mental status. NSTIs are characterized by fulminant tissue destruction, blood vessel thrombosis, systemic toxicity, and high rates of mortality.[85]

Type II NSTI, usually caused by group A β-hemolytic *Streptococcus* (GAS) (the "flesh-eating bacterium"), can occur in any age group, without complicated medical illness. Organisms can gain entry through a surgical wound or as a result of minor trauma, such as a broken limb or removing a cuticle, or even without any known injury. It is theorized that GAS may lie dormant in deep tissues and reactivate after trauma.[85] Within the host, the bacteria multiply rapidly, giving off toxins and enzymes that destroy soft tissue, producing gangrenous tissues. GAS avoids phagocytosis because it has the antiphagocytic properties of an M protein.[86]

Necrotizing fasciitis may progress rapidly to septic shock.[87] Any streptococcal infection with sudden onset of shock and organ failure is referred to as *streptococcal toxic shock syndrome* (STSS).[86] A complete blood cell (CBC) count with a marked left shift, elevated serum creatine kinase and creatinine levels, hyperbilirubinemia, elevated liver functions, metabolic acidosis, hypoalbuminemia, and electrolyte disturbances (e.g., hyponatremia, hypokalemia, and hypocalcemia) may be seen. Blood cultures and cultures of aspirated fluid from bullae may be done. In type II GAS, approximately 60% of patients have positive blood cultures. Cultures from deep surgical samples offer the most reliable data. Radiology studies such as a CT scan or MRI may help define whether gas is present within the tissues; this aids in differentiating GAS from gas produced by anaerobic organisms such as clostridia in patients with gas gangrene. However, imaging studies may reveal only soft tissue edema. Surgical exploration is needed to determine whether NSTI is present.[85]

Treatment is aggressive, prompt debridement and appropriate early antibiotic therapy. Initial empiric antibiotic treatment should include anaerobic coverage. Early treatment could begin with intravenous ampicillin-sulbactam with clindamycin; however, in patients who recently received an antibiotic, broader gram-negative coverage is prudent. If MRSA is suspected, treatment should include vancomycin or another agent effective against this organism. Antibiotic therapy should be optimized on the basis of specific culture and sensitivity data.

Hemodynamic monitoring and support may be needed, including aggressive fluid resuscitation and vasoactive or inotropic agents. Interventions to sustain or compensate for other organ dysfunction may also be required (e.g., mechanical ventilation, dialysis). Hyperbaric oxygen (HBO) therapy may be used as an adjunct.

Despite prompt, aggressive treatment, patients with NSTI have a high rate of mortality. The mortality rate from STSS is 30% to 34%.[88] Survivors tend to have lengthy hospitalizations, multiple operative procedures, disfigurement, prolonged rehabilitation, and residual physical limitations.

Clostridial Infections

Infections by *Clostridium* species are relatively rare; however, they are rapidly progressive and frequently fatal. *Clostridium* organisms are gram-positive, anaerobic, spore-forming pathogens that reproduce rapidly. They are widely found in soil and in the intestines of humans and domestic and feral animals.[89] *Clostridium* can also be found in operating room air, dust, and food and on clothing.[89] Contamination of open wounds is quite common. All *Clostridium* species produce potent exotoxins that foster rapid disease progression with extensive tissue damage.

Gas Gangrene

Gas gangrene, clostridial myonecrosis, is a rapidly progressing, life-threatening toxemic infection associated with skeletal muscle necrosis and systemic toxicity caused by clostridial entotoxins. It is usually induced by trauma, especially deep penetrating wounds. Eighty percent of posttrauma clostridial infections are caused by *Clostridium perfringens.*

Gas gangrene is most frequently associated with open bone fractures, crush injuries, and agricultural or industrial incidents. It is estimated that 30% to 80% of open wounds may be contaminated with *Clostridium.*[89] Wounds may become contaminated with *Clostridium* but not become infected if devitalized tissue is not present in sufficient quantity.[89] In postsurgical wounds, the incidence of clostridial infection is greatest after colon resection and biliary surgery.[89] Even a small amount of devitalized tissue will support growth of clostridial strains. The release of toxins causes massive hemolysis, platelet destruction, and capillary damage and may lead to death as a result of inhibited myocardial contractility and hypotension.

Symptoms of gas gangrene usually begin less than 24 hours after injury but may appear several days later. Initial symptoms include severe local pain with tense edema at the wound site, which undergoes a change in skin color from pale to bronze then purplish red. Bullae with a foul-smelling exudate may form. Gram stain of exudates shows gram-positive rods and an absence of PMNs because PMNs are sequestered and adhere in the vascular endothelium and released toxins lyse neutrophils.[89] Muscle necrosis is marked by distinct, advancing margins and crepitus is usually present. Systemic signs include tachycardia, fever, diaphoresis, agitation, and disorientation. In contrast to most soft tissue infections, the tissues involved in gas gangrene do not bleed because blood flow is obstructed by intravascular platelet aggregation. Bacteremia occurs in about 15% of patients. Late in the course, marked intravascular hemolysis may result in the hematocrit falling by half within hours, along with hemoglobinuria, hypotension, renal failure, and metabolic acidosis.[89]

Initiation of treatment is urgent and requires extensive surgical debridement of all necrotic tissue and prompt antibiotic treatment with large doses of penicillin. There is concern over possible resistance to penicillin.[89] Other antibiotics that are effective include chloramphenicol, metronidazole, and clindamycin. Combination treatment with penicillin and clindamycin is recommended because penicillin alone may fail because of continued toxin production. Some strains have developed resistance to clindamycin.[90] HBO treatments may be used to increase oxygen delivery to the tissues, although consensus regarding its value has not been reached.[89]

Tetanus

Clostridium tetani is a rod-shaped, spore-creating, toxin-producing, obligate anaerobe found widely in soil. The organism produces a metalloprotease, tetanospasmin, which is known as tetanus toxin. *C. tetani* can enter tissues through a simple puncture wound from a nail, splinter, or thorn; a compound fracture; or use of a contaminated intravenous needle. The organism irreversibly binds to spinal cord and brainstem receptors, where tetanospasmin blocks the disinhibition of excitatory impulse modulators from the motor cortex. The net effect is increased muscle tone, painful spasms, and autonomic instability. Symptoms include sweating, tachycardia, hypertension, profound neuromuscular rigidity, spasms of the face and the pharyngeal and laryngeal muscles (lock jaw), nuchal rigidity, and hyperextension of the paraspinous muscles (opisthotonos). *C. tetani* will not normally grow in healthy tissue. To thrive, this organism must be inoculated into areas of devitalized or ischemic tissue or where a coexistent infection or foreign body is present.[91]

Tetanus is a disease that can be prevented with immunization. Best clinical practice for any trauma patient with potentially contaminated wounds (i.e., open fractures, severe degloving, areas of abrasion, burns, deep penetrating wounds, unsterile intramuscular or cutaneous injections from substance abuse) who has not received tetanus immunization within 5 years, is to administer 0.5 ml tetanus toxoid intramuscular injection.[92,93]

Tetanus is rarely seen in the developed world; the annual number of cases in the United States averages only 43.[94] However, tetanus should be suspected in patients with risk factors and neuromuscular dysfunction. Tetanus incubation can occur from 1 to 3 days after injury or as long as several months.[91,94]

Treatment includes wound debridement to eliminate spores and necrotic tissue; aggressive antibiotic therapy with penicillin, metronidazole, or a cephalosporin if polymicrobial infection exists; human tetanus immune globulin to neutralize unbound toxin; and antispasmotics, sedatives, and neuromuscular blocking agents. Tetanus does not confer immunity after active infection. Patients with tetanus must receive active immunization with three doses of tetanus and diphtheria toxoid 2 weeks apart.

Burn Wound Infections

Burns predispose the patient to infection because of extensive loss of tissue. Systemic infection inevitably develops in patients with full-thickness burns involving more than 30% of their body surface area (BSA).[95] Patients with extensive tissue injury, invasive infections, and multisystem organ dysfunction can have mortality rates as high as 75%.[95] Large burn wound injuries substantially impair host defense mechanisms because of the loss of tissue and excessive inflammatory response. External defenses are destroyed when the innate skin barrier is compromised by the initial injury, which can extend if a partial-thickness burn converts to a full-thickness burn, resulting in progressive tissue destruction and formation of eschar. The presence of a protein-rich avascular eschar promotes bacterial growth because the eschar prevents migration of immune cells (e.g., phagocytes) and the distribution of antibiotics.

Burn injuries involving >20% of BSA incite an overwhelming SIRS response, which causes an increase in serum proinflammatory cytokine levels.[96] The sequence of events resulting in subsequent immunosuppression is related to the overwhelming inflammatory and hypermetabolic response seen in burned patients.[96-98] Evidence suggests that decreased macrophage activation and impaired neutrophil chemotaxis associated with the exaggerated inflammatory response increase susceptible burned tissue to act as a site for opportunistic invasion by endogenous and exogenous organisms.[95]

Infection is the leading cause of death in hospitalized burn patients.[95] Infection risk is decreased by rapid wound debridement, judicious use of effective topical and systemic antimicrobial agents, and early wound closure. Burn wounds and the surrounding tissue need to be evaluated frequently for signs of infection. Subtle changes in wound appearance (e.g., change in color, separation of the eschar from the wound bed), failure in wound closure, or increased drainage or hemorrhage from the wound site are reasons to explore for the presence of infection. The presence of blackened or discolored tissue may indicate a fungal infection. Fungal infections are especially prevalent in patients with more than 40% BSA burns who have received multiple doses of broad-spectrum antibiotics or who are significantly immunocompromised.[95]

Antibiotic choice for burn infection is based on the microbial flora of the patient and in the burn unit environment. Tissue biopsy with subsequent tissue culture and test for antibiotic sensitivity may be useful in determining the presence of invasive burn wound infection and identifying the pathogen so that appropriate antibiotics can be prescribed.[99,100] Progression to invasive infection generally is accompanied by physiologic changes that resemble a septic clinical presentation.

Nursing goals for burn patients include reducing the risk of infection and promoting wound healing through careful surveillance, minimizing cross-contamination by frequent handwashing, avoiding the sharing of supplies and equipment between patients, and use of appropriate barriers by visitors and staff. The basal metabolic rate is increased by 100% in patients with burns of more than 40% BSA; therefore, aggressive nutritional supplementation is important to maintain immune function.[101] Patients should be encouraged to be as active as possible, and physical therapy should be initiated early.[101] The reader is referred to Chapter 32 for additional information on burn injuries.

Wound Care Through the Trauma Cycle

The primary objectives of wound care throughout the trauma cycle are promotion of healing and the prevention and early recognition of infection. Tissue hypoxia, the presence of necrotic tissue, foreign bodies or fluid collections, acidic pH, and vascular insufficiency promote bacterial growth and increase the risk of wound infection. Pathogens that are introduced at injury or during hospitalization and allowed to remain in the wound and proliferate also increase the likelihood of wound infection.

Careful nursing assessment can detect early signs of infection. Assessment should involve analyses of trends in wound appearance, vital signs, and laboratory values (e.g., WBC count and differential). Expanded areas of inflammation, changes in the character or quantity of wound drainage, breakdown of suture or staple margins, and systemic or hemodynamic deterioration should be reported promptly. Practices that avoid introducing microorganisms into the wound are essential (e.g., good hand hygiene, appropriate use of gloves, avoiding use of uncleaned instruments between patients). Surgical wound debridment may be necessary to decrease contamination or remove foreign bodies, collections of fluid (e.g., hematoma, pus), or necrotic tissue from the wound bed. Frequent turning is essential to promote tissue perfusion and maintain skin integrity. Nurses can promote wound healing and enhance patient resistance to infection by providing adequate nutrition and ensuring sufficient oxygenation and tissue perfusion. The reader is referred to Chapter 16 for additional interventions that promote wound healing.

Infections Related to Orthopedic Injuries

One million infections related to devices placed in patients occur each year in the United States.[102] These include the more common catheter-related infections and the less frequent surgical implant–related infections. The latter are more difficult to manage because they require prolonged antimicrobial therapy and multiple surgical procedures.

Orthopedic implants include joint prostheses and fracture-fixation devices. Approximately 2,000,000 fracture-fixation devices are inserted in the United States annually. Each year, 100,000 (5%) of them become infected. It is estimated that for each infected patient, one or two extra surgical procedures are required. The combined surgical and medical cost for each infection is approximately $15,000 per patient.[102]

Open Fractures

Open fractures result from high-energy trauma and produce soft tissue and skeletal injury. Both types of injury, in turn, can cause vascular impairment and nerve damage. Open fractures communicate with the outside and therefore become contaminated with environmental microorganisms. A contamination rate of 65% has been reported.[74] The risk of infection is related to the classification of fractures, which is based on degree of soft tissue damage, wound contamination, vascular compromise, and stability of the fracture. The most widely used fracture classification system is the one described by Gustilo et al[103]:

- Type I: a small laceration (<1 cm), minimal contamination, and intact vascular status. The infection rate in this group is 0% to 2%.
- Type II: a larger laceration (>1 cm), minimal or moderate contamination, and variable soft tissue injury. The infection rate is 2% to 10%.
- Type III: high degree of contamination with severe comminuted and unstable fracture and extensive soft tissue damage involving muscle, skin, and neurovascular structures. It is subdivided into three groups:
  - IIIA: Extensive soft tissue wound but with viable soft tissue to ensure coverage of all bony surfaces
  - IIIB: Extensive soft tissue wound, massive contamination, periosteal stripping, and bone exposure requiring a flap for soft tissue coverage
  - IIIC: Open fracture with associated arterial injury that requires repair

  The infection rate is 4% in the IIIA group but up to 50% in the IIIB and IIIC groups.[103]

This is an effective classification system because it helps define the prognosis of the injury and assists in development of a treatment plan.[74,104]

Risk Factors

Multiple factors predispose patients to increased rates of early wound infections or osteomyelitis[105-108]:

- Systemic: malnutrition, renal failure, hepatic failure, diabetes, disease causing immunosuppression (e.g., human immunodeficiency virus [HIV] infection), malignancy, extremes of age, taking immunosuppressive agents, absence of appropriate antibiotic use
- Local: chronic lymphedema, small vessel disease, vasculitis, venous stasis, extensive scarring, radiation fibrosis, neuropathy, tobacco use, absence of local antibiotics, previous surgeries
- Fracture characteristics: type of fracture, as previously described, considers degree of soft tissue damage (devitalized area), size of the open wound, vascular damage, and extent of contamination; mechanism of injury; foreign material in wound
- Trauma (response to injury/wound): hypovolemia, hypoxia, presence of other acute injuries resulting in delayed orthopedic stabilization (according to priorities in resuscitation), glucose intolerance, catabolic state

Pathogenesis

Organisms are inoculated into the wound at the time of injury, or pathogens from the hospital environment (e.g., from contaminated hands and equipment) colonize open wounds associated with a fracture. Biofilms, made up of host cell adhesions, planktonic bacteria (free-floating bacteria), and bacterial glycocalyx (community of sessile bacteria surrounded by extracellular matrix), form around implanted devices and shield the bacteria from antibiotics. Infection sets in the wound or the bone.

Etiologic Agents

S. aureus remains the most common agent causing infections related to orthopedic injuries, but the incidence of enteric organisms and *P. aeruginosa* is increasing. Open injuries exposed to dirt tend to be contaminated with anaerobic flora.[104]

Diagnosis

The usefulness of initial cultures from the wound is debatable. The bacteria isolated from these cultures often do not correlate with the organisms associated with wound infection. Postdebridement wound cultures are recommended. They correlate with the flora associated with early infections. These cultures also indicate whether any unusual pathogens are present.[74]

Management of Fractures

The timing of orthopedic surgery is critical to the successful management of the fracture. Clearly, resuscitation takes priority and a wrongly timed early aggressive orthopedic intervention can worsen the initial SIRS response. On the other hand, a delay in appropriate orthopedic intervention will increase the soft tissue damage and ischemia at the fracture site and create an environment ripe for bacterial proliferation. Additionally, a delay in fracture fixation will prevent early mobilization of the patient and increase the risk of pulmonary complications, deep vein thrombosis (DVT), skin breakdown, infections, and organ failure, which will prolong the hospital stay.[105,106] An evaluation of orthopedic injuries sustained during Operation Enduring Freedom demonstrated that early and aggressive debridement of contaminated wounds in the forward-deployed area resulted in very low infection rates.[109] General principles that are useful in making management decisions include: adequately debride devitalized areas, remove or revascularize dead space, close the wound, and treat premorbid conditions.

Prevention

Orthopedic interventions must minimize the consequences of bacterial contamination and remove devitalized tissue. Acceptable measures to prevent infection related to orthopedic injuries include early fixation/stabilization, adequate debridement, irrigation of the wound, meticulous surgical techniques, and proper administration of antibiotics.

Several studies have demonstrated the benefits of damage control orthopedics and early fixation of femoral shaft fractures.[110] On the basis of these data, the American College of Surgeons' Committee on Trauma recommends that in a hemodynamically stable patient a femoral shaft fracture should be fixed within 2 to 12 hours after the onset of injury.[111] There are conflicting opinions as to which method—internal fixation (intramedullary nailing or plating) or external fixation—is superior.[112] Internal fixation translates into placement of a foreign body into the contaminated field of an open fracture and therefore encourages bacterial adhesion and infection. In certain patient groups (e.g., multiple trauma patients, patients with intra-articular fractures, those with associated vascular injury, and elderly people with open femur fractures), the benefits of stabilization outweigh the risk of infection; therefore, internal fixation is recommended. The advantages of external fixation include relative ease and speed of application, minimal soft tissue trauma, and reasonable anatomic stabilization. The disadvantages include interference with soft tissue reconstructive surgery, delayed union, need for a second definitive procedure, and possible development of pin tract infections.[74,113] If the patient is unstable, external fixation is used initially and intramedullary nailing is performed later.

The importance of meticulous surgical techniques and adequate debridement of the wound cannot be overemphasized; these practices clearly reduce the infection risk.[109] Devitalized tissue creates an environment that supports bacterial growth and therefore needs to be removed. Stabilization of the fracture aids in re-establishing the microcirculation, decreases injury to the local soft tissue from the fracture fragments, and reduces the infection risk. Irrigation of the wound is essential. However, the type of irrigating fluid, optimal volume, and method of delivery are not clearly established. Primary closure of the wound can increase the risk of infection with organisms such as *Clostridia*; therefore, it is generally not recommended. A few studies have demonstrated that primary wound closure can be done without dire consequences; however, if extensive soft tissue damage is present, wound coverage should be accomplished at a later time.[74]

The beneficial role of antibiotics in the management of open fractures is well established. For open fractures, antibiotics are considered therapeutic, not prophylactic. The type of antibiotic, of course, is based on the knowledge of wound microbiology. Therefore, gram-positive skin flora should always be covered. There are conflicting reports on the need to cover GNRs. The recommended duration of therapy is 1 to 3 days. Local administration of antibiotic-impregnated beads has been associated with decreased infection rates.[74] For more details on antibiotic use, refer to the section titled "Antimicrobial Prophylaxis for Surgery."

Throughout the trauma cycle, nurses need to be aware of the following points about orthopedic infections:

- Massively contaminated fractures have a high incidence of infection.
- Proper wound care and pin care will minimize infection rates in patients with orthopedic injuries.

Posttraumatic Osteomyelitis

Osteomyelitis is an infection-related inflammatory process that causes bone destruction. The involvement can be limited to a small portion of the bone, or several areas of the bone may be involved. The classification of osteomyelitis is summarized in Table 15-7. This chapter focuses on one type of osteomyelitis, posttraumatic contiguous osteomyelitis.

In some series, posttraumatic osteomyelitis accounts for 47% of all cases of osteomyelitis.[114] Motor vehicle crashes, sports injuries, and the use of orthopedic hardware contribute to its increased incidence. The tibia is most susceptible to infection, with an infection rate 10- to 20-fold higher than that associated with other bones.

Pathogenesis

Microorganisms are introduced at the time of trauma or from the contiguous devitalized tissue. Local and systemic risk factors for osteomyelitis after trauma are described in the section on open fractures. To understand the pathogenesis and mechanism of posttraumatic osteomyelitis, one needs to appreciate the concept of biofilms.[115,116] The complex process of biofilm formation is summarized below:

- Bacteria attach to an inert or nonviable surface.
- Bacteria colonize and grow and secrete glycocalyx. Platelets and fibrinogen are deposited onto the biofilm.
- Host immunity attempts to eradicate the bacteria. Activated WBCs produce more degradative enzymes and eventually become depleted.
- A community of sessile bacteria develops intricate mechanisms of obtaining nutrients and communicating with other colonies through special signals.[116]
- Phenotypic changes occur in the bacteria, which translate into slower growth, requirement for minimal nutrients, and development of antibiotic-resistant types.
- Biofilms can bind antibiotics and render them ineffective; the biofilm also decreases the penetration of antimicrobials into the bacteria.
- Bacterial colonies can break off and seek new locations.

TABLE 15-7 Classification of Osteomyelitis

Duration of disease	A. Acute osteomyelitis evolves over a few days B. Chronic osteomyelitis develops over months or years
Pathogenesis (Waldvogel's classification)*	A. Hematogenous Seen in children, drug abusers, elderly patients Bacteria initially seed blood and secondarily infect bone B. Vascular insufficiency† Vascular insufficiency, neuropathy, and hyperglycemia commonly occur in diabetics, resulting in increased incidence of skin, soft tissue, and bone infections C. Contiguous focus of infection Infection seen after trauma and at the base of a soft tissue infection
Anatomic/physiologic classification (Cierny-Mader staging)‡	A. Anatomic type defines the extent of the infection 1. Medullary is confined to the intramedullary bone and is usually a hematogenous process. 2. Superficial is similar to contiguous osteomyelitis and occurs at the base of a soft tissue wound. 3. Localized infection involves the medulla and the external surface but is a stable process. 4. Diffuse is a permeative and an unstable process. B. Physiologic type defines the condition of the host 1. No compromise 2. Systemic or local compromise 3. Severe compromise

*Source: Lew DP, Waldvogel FA: Osteomyelitis, *N Engl J Med* 336:999-1007, 1997.

†Source: Newman LG, Waller J, Palestro CJ et al: Unsuspected osteomyelitis in diabetic foot ulcers: diagnosis and monitoring by leukocyte scanning with indium in 111 oxyquinoline, *JAMA* 266:1246-1251, 1991.

‡Source: Ziran BH, Rao N: Infections. In Baumgaertner MR, Tornetta PT, editors: *Orthopedic knowledge update,* 3rd ed, pp 131-139, Rosemont, IL, 2005, American Academy of Orthopedic Surgeons.

The body ultimately tries to control the infection by forming an abscess or developing a sinus tract in the bone.

Clinical Features

Classic signs of inflammation such as fever, leukocytosis, and erythema of the wound occur early in the hospital course and are difficult to distinguish from normal healing. Later in the disease process, poor wound healing and nonunion of the fracture may herald the onset of osteomyelitis. Posttraumatic osteomyelitis is a continuous latent disease with periods of acute symptoms. The indolent infection presents later, with features such as intermittent drainage and periodic expulsion of pus. At times, some bacteria become metabolically active and start producing toxins and acute symptoms, such as fever, malaise, and local changes in the wound.

Microbiology

Posttraumatic osteomyelitis is often polymicrobial. The organisms are acquired from the skin flora, the environment, or hospital equipment and personnel. Staphylococci, GNRs, and anaerobes account for most of the organisms. *S. aureus* is primarily responsible for early-onset infections, and coagulase-negative staphylococci are responsible for those of late onset. Clostridial and *Bacillus* infections can result from contamination with soil, and *Aeromonas* infection can occur after exposure to fresh water. *P. aeruginosa* is seen as a nosocomially acquired pathogen in severely ill trauma patients.[117,118] MRSA may also be acquired nosocomially but is increasingly being seen in the community as well.

Diagnosis

In most cases, the infection is suspected clinically. Other modalities used to diagnosis osteomyelitis include the following:

- Cultures should be obtained from the deep infected tissue and the biopsied bone. Swabs from the sinus tracts and bone have low sensitivity.[117,118]
- An elevated CRP and ESR are nonspecific markers of inflammation. A negative CRP and ESR usually indicate a lesser likelihood of infection.
- Plain x-ray films of the bone are not positive in the early phases of infection but can show changes in 2 to 4 weeks. In the later phase, the two hallmark findings of posttraumatic osteomyelitis are nonunion of the fracture site and lucency around the hardware. It is often difficult to distinguish postoperative/trauma changes from osteomyelitis.

- MRI is highly sensitive and provides an accurate image of the bone and soft tissue; however, false-positive tests can occur. MRI cannot be performed in patients with metallic implants.[117,118] CT scan is inferior to MRI.
- Radionuclide scans have a very high sensitivity but low specificity. These tests have difficulty in distinguishing between postoperative/trauma changes and osteomyelitis.

Management

The general principles of surgical management are similar to the treatment of open fractures already described. The hallmark of surgical treatment is debridement and removal of all infected tissue. When a healed fracture becomes infected, the clinician must decide whether to treat with the implanted hardware in place or to remove the hardware. In the first scenario, infection is suppressed with antibiotics while attempting to obtain bony stability. Once stability is achieved, the implant needs to be removed. Alternatively, if the bony stability can be maintained with debridement, then aggressive debridement can be undertaken right away.

Antimicrobial therapy is prolonged (4 to 6 weeks) and requires outpatient management. Selection of antibiotics should be based on in vitro susceptibility of the organisms causing the infection. The treatment also needs to meet the specific needs of each patient.[115,117]

Desired features of antimicrobials selected to treat osteomyelitis are listed below:

- Adequate bone penetration
- Nontoxic
- Convenient to administer
- Cost-effective
- Less frequent administration/day
- Oral agent if good bioavailability; otherwise, intravenous therapy

Factors to consider when choosing an appropriate antibiotic are discussed in the section on selection of antimicrobial therapy.

Prevention

The principles for prevention of osteomyelitis are similar to those for infections of open fractures.

INFECTIONS OF THE CARDIOVASCULAR SYSTEM

BACTEREMIA

Bacteremia, or bloodstream infection (BSI), is the documentation of cultivatable bacteria in the bloodstream, which may be transient, inconsequential, or of great significance.[26,119] Nosocomial BSIs are important causes of morbidity and death, with approximately 250,000 infections occurring in the United States each year.[119] BSI in the intensive care unit is associated with an attributable mortality rate of 35% and an additional hospital cost of $40,000 per episode. A BSI may be either primary (no other source of infection) or secondary (related to another site of infection). Sixty-four percent of BSIs are primary, and the most common secondary sites of infection are intravascular catheters and urinary catheters.[120]

Significance of Positive Blood Cultures

It is important to differentiate clinically significant blood cultures from contaminants. If blood cultures are positive for organisms considered to be skin contaminants, then the following clinical criteria need to be fulfilled before the diagnosis of bactermia is established: presence of fever (>100.4° F [>38° C]), chills, or hypotension. In addition, one of two other criteria need to be met: the skin contaminant must be isolated from two blood cultures and not related to another site of infection, or there must be a single positive blood culture with an intravascular device, which requires treatment with an antimicrobial. The most common contaminants are coagulase-negative staphylococci, diphtheroids, propionibacterium, and *Bacillus*.

Microbiology

In 1999, more than 10,000 nosocomial BSIs in 49 U.S. hospitals were analyzed.[121] Sixty-four percent of the infections were caused by gram-positive organisms, 27% by gram-negative organisms, and 8% by fungi. The most common organisms were coagulase-negative staphylococci (32%), *S. aureus* (16%), and enterococci (11%).

Proper Technique for Drawing Cultures

To enhance detection of the causative organism and avoid contamination of the blood culture medium, the technique for drawing a blood culture, the timing of the collections, and the number of samples drawn are critical.[122,123] Proper technique has the following aspects:

- Prepare skin with 70% alcohol, followed by 2% chlorhexidene or as per specific institutional practice.
- Obtain cultures from a peripheral vein rather than an existing line.
- Disinfect the membrane of the blood culture bottle before inoculation.
- Obtain at least the minimum amount of blood required for each culture bottle.
- Obtain cultures from two separate sites.
- Under optimal circumstances, the cultures should be obtained within one to several hours of each other. However, cultures can be obtained from a critically ill patient within a few minutes of each other.
- Promptly transport the culures to the laboratory.

One blood sample is not sufficient: if the culture becomes positive for a skin contaminant, it is difficult to distinguish a true infection from a contaminated culture. A total of two blood culture sets is often enough. If endocarditis or an endovascular infection is suspected, then more than two cultures are required.

Throughout the trauma cycle, the nurse needs to be aware of the following information about bacteremia:

- Infections are common in the critically ill population.
- Signs and symptoms of bacteremia can vary widely from fever to full-blown septic shock.
- It is important to distinguish between colonization and true infection.
- To obtain an adequate blood sample for culture, it is vital to use the proper method.

Intravascular Catheter-Related Infections

In the United States, more than 5 million CVCs are inserted every year. CVC-related bacteremia remains one of the most common causes of nosocomial BSIs. Furthermore, CVC-related infections can result in increased hospital length of stay, higher mortality rates, and increased health care costs.

Risk Factors

The risk of infection associated with the use of a CVC depends on the following:

- Site of insertion: Femoral sites are more prone to infection than CVCs placed in the subclavian vein.
- Method of insertion: Numerous attempts to penetrate the skin and poor aseptic technique increase the risk of contamination.
- Duration of cannulation: The longer the catheter remains in place, the greater the risk of infection.
- Number of line manipulations: The greater number of line manipulations, the higher the risk of introducing infection.
- Site care: Poor site care increases infection risk.
- Underlying comorbid illnesses such as diabetes, end-stage renal disease, and low albumin levels increase risk.[124]
- Type of unit: units use intravenous devices differently, resulting in varied rates of infection.[125]

Pathogenesis

The CVC may become infected by four major sources: extraluminal colonization of the catheter from the skin, hematogenous seeding, intraluminal colonization of the hub or the lumen, and, rarely, contamination of the infusate.[126] The most common source of CVC-related infection is colonization of the external and internal portions of the intracutaneous segment of the CVC. Microorganisms usually gain access from the skin of the patient or the hands of the health care worker. The organisms form biofilms (composed of the bacterial glycocalyx and the host fibrin) over the surface of the catheter. For CVCs in place for more than 2 weeks, intraluminal/hub contamination also becomes an important source.

Microbiology

Gram-positive organisms such as the coagulase-negative staphylococci are overwhelmingly the most common infecting pathogens, followed by *S. aureus* and enterococci. Gram-negative bacilli such as *Klebsiella* species, *Enterobacter* species, *Pseudomonas* species, and *Acinetobacter* species account for 33% of CVC-related infections. Fungi are the causative agents in 20% of CVC-related infections.[126]

Diagnosis

The diagnosis of a CVC-related infection is based on the clinical presentation and the results of microbiologic studies[126,127]:

- Clinical features of an infection, such as fevers and chills, may be present. The following clinical findings may also be associated with a CVC infection: purulence at the CVC site, absence of an alternative source of infection, dysfunction of the catheter, rapid clinical improvement after removal of the catheter, and isolation of skin organisms or fungi from the blood cultures.
- More specific microbiologic studies are required to confirm the diagnosis of CVC infection.[126,127] Demonstration of positive blood cultures and documentation of a relationship between the BSI and the CVC are required to diagnose a CVC infection. Positive blood cultures without an identifiable source increase the suspicion of a CVC infection. It is vital that two sets of blood cultures are drawn from peripheral sites, not from the catheter ports (which are often contaminated). A negative blood culture obtained from a CVC has excellent negative predictive value, but positive cultures require clinical interpretation. A comparison of cultures drawn from a CVC and another simultaneously drawn from a peripheral vein can sometimes provide helpful information.[126,127]
- Once the CVC is removed, specific tests required for the diagnosis of CVC-related infection can be performed. This technique requires external cultures or the semi-quantitative cultures of the intracutaneous segment of the CVC. If the catheter tip has >15 colony-forming units (CFU) and yields the same organisms identified as causing the BSI, then the diagnosis of CVC infection is confirmed. However, this procedure does not identify the organism present in the lumen of the CVC. To identify the luminal pathogens, quantitative procedures are performed; this includes sonicating or vortexing the catheter tip. For the best yield, the catheter tip should be immersed in broth for 24 to 72 hours, followed by semi-quantitative cultures.[126,127] However, this method of attempting to identify luminal pathogens can be overly specific (providing false-positive findings) and is not routinely done.

Treatment

Several factors influence the management of CVC-related infections:

- The infecting pathogen
- The underlying medical condition of the patient
- The severity of the infection
- The anticipated duration of venous access
- The presence of alternative venous access
- Percutaneously inserted catheter versus surgically implanted catheters

The severity of illness should be assessed in a febrile patient who has a nontunneled CVC and is suspected to have a CVC-related infection. The CVC should be either removed or exchanged over a guidewire in all patients and antimicrobial therapy should be started. Blood and CVC culture results should be used to adjust antibiotic coverage and catheter management.[126] If blood cultures become positive, a previously wired line must be removed. For tunneled devices, the treatment includes removal of the catheter, appropriate antimicrobial therapy, and management of complications such as endocarditis, septic thrombophlebitis, and osteomyelitis.

Antimicrobial therapy for CVC-related infections should be instituted before the microbiology results are available. Empiric therapy is based on knowledge of the patient's flora, the most prevalent pathogens in the hospital environment, and the incidence of the most common organisms associated with CVC-related infections. Antimicrobial treatments for specific pathogens are listed in Table 15-3.

Prevention

Guidelines for the prevention of CVC-related infection were published in 2002 by members of various disciplines and endorsed by several professional organizations.[128,129] These guidelines provide evidence-based recommendations for the prevention of CVC-related infections (Table 15-8).

Throughout the trauma cycle, nurses need to be aware of the following information about cather-related infection:

- CVC-related infections are common.
- The most frequent source of CVC-related infection is colonization at the catheter site or contamination of the hub.
- Nurses can help prevent CVC-related infection by ensuring use of recommended aseptic techniques for catheter insertion and following evidence-based guidelines regarding the care of the insertion site and infusion line.

PHLEBITIS/SEPTIC THROMBOPHLEBITIS

Phlebitis (inflammation of the vein) can develop as a reaction to the catheter material or as drugs being infused into the catheter irritate the vessel or infiltrate into nearby soft tissue. Phlebitis can be either chemical or infectious (septic thrombophlebitis). The signs and symptoms of chemical or infectious phlebitis are similar: pain, tenderness, erythema, and a palpable cord over the affected site. Infectious phlebitis (septic thrombophlebitis) is suspected if the patient has a high fever and if purulent drainage can be expressed from the insertion site. CVC-related septic thrombophlebitis can present with persistent bacteremia or fungemia and metastatic infectious complications such as endocarditis and septic pulmonary emboli.[126,130]

Septic thrombophlebitis in a trauma unit is almost always associated with indwelling intravascular catheters. Gram-positive organisms are the most frequent causative agents. *S. aureus* is the most common infecting pathogen, followed by coagulase-negative staphylococci, gram-negative bacilli such as *Klebsiella* species, *Enterobacter* species, *Pseudomonas* species, anaerobes, and fungi. Eighty to ninety percent of patients with septic thrombophlebitis are also bacteremic.

Antimicrobial treatment is indicated for septic thrombophlebitis. Empiric treatment must always include coverage for *S. aureus*. When the blood and the catheter cultures become positive, the antimicrobial therapy should be tailored accordingly. The infected catheter should always be removed. Local heat and elevation may be useful. Surgical intervention is needed if there is persistent bacteremia, metastatic infection, local spread into the soft tissue, or persistent purulent discharge. Thrombolytic agents may also be used in the treatment of CVC-related thrombophlebitis.[126,131]

INFECTIVE ENDOCARDITIS

An estimated 10,000 to 20,000 new cases of infective endocarditis (IE) are diagnosed in the United States each year. Over the past 30 years, the epidemiology and etiology of IE have changed. Most of these changes relate to the types of susceptible hosts and new therapeutic modalities. The incidence of predisposing conditions such as rheumatic heart disease has declined, but new risk factors have emerged. These include intravenous drug use, prosthetic heart valves, invasive vascular procedures (e.g., angiography), intravascular devices (e.g., catheters, inferior vena caval filters), and structural heart disease.[132] More than half of all IE cases in the United States now occur in patients over the age of 60 years. This trend is probably related to two factors: (1) elderly patients are more likely to have underlying structural heart disease, and (2) elderly patients are more likely to undergo invasive procedures.[133]

Generally, in a critical care setting, endocarditis is infrequently diagnosed. When it is present, there is usually an association with indwelling devices or invasive procedures. Therefore, this section focuses on health care–related endocarditis.

Several studies have documented the increasing incidence of nosocomial and health care–associated IE. Nosocomial endocarditis is usually a complication of bacteremia induced by therapeutic modalities (pacemakers, dialysis) or vascular

TABLE 15-8 Guidelines for Prevention of Hospital-Associated Intravascular Catheter-Related Infections

Catheter	General	Catheter Insertion	Maintenance
Peripheral Venous Catheters			
Bloodstream infection risk: low	Educated HCW in insertion and maintenance practice Standardized aseptic care Dedicated "IV teams" Ensure appropriate nurse-to-patient ratios Mix all routine IV fluids in pharmacy by sterile technique Use single-dose vials for parenteral medications when possible Do not combine single-use vials for later use Do not use suspicious-appearing parenteral fluid	Hand hygiene Skin antiseptic Record time and date of insertions and dressing changes Select the catheter insertion technique and insertion site with lowest risk of complication	Hand hygiene Clean injection ports with antiseptic agent before accessing Aseptic technique during manipulation: clean gloves Replace and relocate device at least every 96 hours Replace dressing when catheter is changed and when the dressing becomes damp, loosened, or soiled Visually inspect catheter and insertion site at least daily; if unable to visualize site, remove dressing and apply new dressing Replace IV tubing no more frequently than 72-hour intervals unless clinically indicated No recommendation for hang time of intravenous fluids Complete infusion of blood within 4 hours of hanging Complete infusion of lipid-containing parenteral nutrition fluids within 24 hours of hanging the fluid Complete infusion of lipids alone within 12 hours of hanging fluid Avoid use of stopcocks and cap all ports when not in use Never reuse caps; always use a new sterile cap to close off an opening in the line
Peripheral Arterial Catheters			
Bloodstream infection risk: increased (approaching CVC risk)	As above	As above Skin antiseptic: 2% aqueous chlorhexidine gluconate lowered BSI rates compared with 10% povidone-iodine or 70% alcohol Do not use systemic antimicrobial prophylaxis before insertion	As above Promptly remove catheter if not essential Replace all catheters not inserted under aseptic technique as soon as possible but within 48 hours

devices. In some areas, it now accounts for almost 10% of all cases of IE. With this emergence of nosocomial and health care–associated endocarditis, the incidence of *S. aureus* (including MRSA) has increased, whereas the incidence of *S. viridans* has declined. Fowler et al[134] evaluated 1,779 patients with IE in 39 medical centers in 16 countries. *S. aureus* was the most common pathogen (558 patients, 31.4%) and health care–associated infection was the most common form of *S. aureus* IE (218 patients [39.1%]). Patients in the United States with IE were most likely to be hemodialysis dependent, have diabetes, have a presumed intravascular device source, be infected with MRSA, receive vancomycin, and have persistent bacteremia.[134]

If IE is suspected in a critically ill patient, the following evaluation is recommended:

- A meticulous clinical history and examination focusing on recent procedures and the presence of devices
- A leukocyte count and urinalysis for microscopic hematuria

TABLE 15-8 **Guidelines for Prevention of Hospital-Associated Intravascular Catheter-Related Infections—cont'd**

Catheter	General	Catheter Insertion	Maintenance
Central Venous Catheters			
Bloodstream infection risk: increased	As above Conduct surveillance to determine infection rates and monitor infection control lapses	As above Upper extremity site; subclavian site has lowest risk of infection in adults Choose CVC with minimal number of ports necessary Use antimicrobial/antiseptic-impregnated CVC if catheter is expected to remain >5 days and CVC infection rate is above goal Use of bedside ultrasonography for placement decreases risk of mechanical complications Maximal sterile barrier precautions: (1) cap, (2) mask, (3) sterile gown, (4) sterile gloves, (5) large sterile drape Do not routinely culture catheter tips Do not routinely replace catheters Replace CVC if purulence at site or if CVC-related infection is suspected and patient is unstable Do not use guidewire change if CVC-related infection is suspected	As above Designate one port for TPN infusion Do not use filters for infection control purposes Minimize interruptions to the CVC line and use strict sterile technique when accessing any CVC line Do not use topical antibiotics at the site of insertion Do not submerge CVC in water Change gauze dressing every 2 days and transparent dressings every 7 days on short-term catheters. Replace dressing if it becomes damp, loosened, or visibly soiled

HCW, Health care worker; *IV,* intravenous. Sources for complete recommendations: Mermel LA, Farr BM, Sherertz RJ et al: Guidelines for the management of intravascular catheter-related infections, *Clin Infect Dis* 32:1249-1272, 2001; Guidelines for the prevention of intravascular catheter-related infections, *MMWR Morbid Mortal Wkly Rep* 51:1-32, 2002.

- Three blood cultures
- An electrocardiogram and a chest radiograph
- An echocardiogram

Management of IE includes at least 4 to 6 weeks of antimicrobial therapy targeted at the causative agent and close monitoring for complications. The need for surgical intervention should be assessed at the time of diagnosis. Clear-cut guidelines have been established as to when and why a patient needs cardiac surgery.[135]

Central Nervous System Infections

Risk Factors

Major risk factors for the development of CNS infection after trauma include disruption of the dural membrane from penetrating injury, Le Forte II and III fractures, nasal and basilar skull fractures, intraventricular catheter placement, and neurosurgical procedures. Medical devices placed through the nasal passage can also increase the risk of CNS infections. Nasogastric and nasotracheal tubes should not be placed in patients with known or suspected CSF leaks. Also, nasopharyngeal suctioning should not be performed in these patients. Use of nasal tubes can significantly increase the risk of sinusitis and subsequent meningitis.[136,137]

Prophylactic Antibiotics for Prevention of Intracranial Infections

In a retrospective review of penetrating craniocerebral civilian injuries, Doherty and Rabinowitz[138] found no relationship between the use of prophylactic antibiotics and the risk of infection. Standard surgical prophylaxis after civilian gunshot wounds to the head was sufficient; however, brief antibiotic therapy in injuries involving the air sinuses may be used. No role for a prolonged antibiotic course was found. Prophylactic antibiotics after open CNS injuries specifically to reduce CNS infections are not recommended because they are costly, may not be effective, may cause adverse drug reactions, and may shift normal flora toward more antibiotic-resistant bacteria.[138] Antibiotics are not effective in treating infections associated with foreign bodies (e.g., a bullet lodged in the brain) or in devascularized or necrotic tissues. Optimal treatment consists of adequate surgical debridement, thorough irrigation, and standard surgical site antibiotic prophylaxis.

Infections Associated with Intracranial Pressure Monitoring Devices

Use of intracranial monitors is associated with the development of meningitis and ventriculitis.[139] This risk tends to be highest with placement of an intraventricular catheter. Catheters in place longer than 5 days have an increased incidence of infection.[140] Infection sources include the skin at the insertion site, the connection between the drainage tubing and the ventricular catheter, and connections and stopcocks within the drainage system.[141] CSF leakage at the insertion site also increases the risk of ventriculitis.[140]

When intraventricular catheters are used and intracranial infection is suspected, a CSF sample withdrawn from the catheter should be sent for the following studies: culture and Gram stain, CBC with differential, and protein and glucose determinations. A CSF sample is obtained whenever the patient has unexplained increasing leukocytosis or is febrile without another source or if the patient has a change in mental status without apparent cause. Results and trends of blood cell counts and glucose levels allow early detection of infection. If the CSF glucose level is low (less than two thirds of the serum value) and the WBC count is high with a predominance of polymorphonuclear leukocytes, the patient may have meningitis. Because culture results require a minimum of 72 hours before identification and antibiotic susceptibility patterns can be determined, empiric antibiotic therapy should be initiated and then adjusted when results are available.

Intraventricular catheters should be inserted by use of strict sterile technique and maintained with care. Antibiotic prophylaxis for placement of an intraventricular catheter and catheter exchange at routine intervals are not recommended as effective measures to prevent CNS infection.[142] To reduce the risk of infection, it is very important to maintain a closed system and to use meticulous sterile procedure if the drainage system must be accessed. Catheters should be removed by aseptic technique. The infectious hazards related to monitoring intracranial pressure can be reduced if, when possible, subarachnoid/subdural or parenchymal devices are used instead of the more invasive intraventricular catheters.[140]

Infections Associated with Cerebrospinal Fluid Shunts

Posttraumatic hydrocephalus can be a complication of head injury and often necessitates the use of CSF shunts. There are various types of shunts: ventriculoatrial, ventriculoperitoneal, lumbar-peritoneal, and ventriculopleural.

Complications of infection resulting from the placement of CSF shunts can lead to impaired intellectual and neurologic function and, in some cases, death.[143] These infections can include meningitis, brain abscess, wound infection, and peritonitis (in patients with peritoneal shunts). The clinical manifestations may consist of fever alone or other systemic signs of infection. Risks for CSF shunt infection are related to the operative procedure, the presence of intracerebral hemorrhage, intracranial pressure ≥20 mm Hg, irrigation of the system, and ventricular catheterization lasting more than 5 days.[143] The most common pathogens associated with CSF shunt infection are coagulase-negative staphylococci (*Staphylococcus epidermidis*), *S. aureus*, diphtheroids (*Propionibacterium acnes*), and gram-negative bacilli (*P. aeruginosa*).

Treatment of infection associated with CSF shunts depends on the site and type of infection. Brain abscess may require aspiration or surgical removal. Intracranial infection will necessitate treatment with antibiotics that penetrate the blood-brain barrier. Antibiotic therapy will likely also be necessary for infection of the insertion site or of the peritoneum. In some instances, the shunt must be removed and can be replaced after the CSF is sterile.

Meningitis

The pia, arachnoid, and dura mater constitute the meninges, the tissues that surround the brain and spinal cord. Inflammation of the meninges (i.e., meningitis) reflects infection of the arachnoid mater and the CSF in the subarachnoid space and the cerebral ventricles.[144] Meningitis is a devastating infection. Survivors are at risk for neurologic sequelae. Nosocomial meningitis is not transmissible from the patient to the health care worker, unlike community-acquired or infectious meningitis. Major risk factors for nosocomial meningitis are neurosurgery, head trauma within the previous month, placement of a neurosurgical device, and CSF leak.[144] Classic signs of meningitis—headache, nausea, vomiting, nuchal rigidity, and mental status changes—may be obscured in patients after severe brain injury or attributed to other causes. Fever and leukocytosis may be absent, intermittent, or the result of blood in the CSF. If intracranial pressure is elevated, it may be impossible to perform a lumbar puncture to obtain CSF for culture because of the risk of inducing brain herniation.

Diagnosis of meningitis is based on a CSF sample with increased WBCs in the CSF (pleocytosis) (>20/mm^3), decreased CSF glucose concentration (hypoglycorrhachia) (<40 mg/dl, <40% of serum glucose level), increased CSF protein (>10 to 500 mg/dl), and isolation of an organism. When the health care provider suspects CSF infection and the patient exhibits clinical deterioration, empiric antibiotic therapy should be initiated. Typically, the maximal dose of each antibiotic is used. If the collection of CSF is delayed, empiric therapy should be initiated promptly on the basis of the patient's age and the underlying disease/trauma status. If CSF is not obtainable, diagnosis and treatment are more difficult. Effective empiric antibiotic therapy should provide coverage against both gram-positive and gram-negative organisms. When the infecting meningeal pathogen is identified and its sensitivity pattern is known, antibiotic therapy should be optimized.

INFECTIONS OF THE RESPIRATORY TRACT

HOSPITAL-ACQUIRED PNEUMONIA

Hospital-acquired pneumonia (HAP) accounts for 25% of all ICU-related infections and is the second most common nosocomial infection in the United States.[145] It is estimated that HAP results in increased hospital stay and an excess cost of $40,000 per patient. Half the antibiotics prescribed in the ICU setting are for patients with HAP. Ninety percent of HAP cases arise in ventilated patients; mechanical ventilation results in a 6- to 20-fold increase in the incidence of HAP.[145,146]

Ventilator-associated pneumonia (VAP) occurs most frequently during the first few days of mechanical ventilation. The risk of VAP is 3% during the first 5 days of intubation, 2% during days 5 through 10, and 1% thereafter. Overall, VAP occurs in 20% of intubated patients.[145,147] The attributable mortality rate for HAP is between 33% and 50%. Increased mortality rates are associated with *P. aeruginosa* infections, *Acinetobacter* infections, bacteremia, and ineffective therapy. VAP is an independent predictor of mortality in trauma patients.[148]

Microbiology

Early onset HAP (occurring within the first 4 days of hospitalization) is typically caused by community-acquired antibiotic-sensitive pathogens, such as *Haemophilus influenzae*, *Streptococcus pneumoniae*, *S. aureus*, enteric GNRs (*Klebsiella* species, *Escherichia coli*), and anaerobes (if aspiration is documented). Late-onset HAP (after 5 days) is caused by more resistant pathogens. Gram-negative bacilli, such as *P. aeruginosa*, *Acinetobacter* species, *Klebsiella* species, and *Enterobacter* species cause 60% of HAP. During this late period, *S. aureus* (particularly MRSA) continues to be one of the major causes of HAP. In patients with head trauma, diabetes mellitus, and hospitalization in the ICU, *S. aureus* is the most frequent etiologic agent.[149] In patients with acute respiratory distress syndrome (ARDS), polymicrobial infections are more common.

Unfortunately, over the past decade, it has become apparent that certain risk factors in the community predispose patients to harbor MARO.[145] Risk factors for acquisition of MARO include the following:

- Current hospital stay of 5 or more days or hospitalization in the past 90 days
- High frequency of antibiotic resistance in the patient's community
- Receipt of antimicrobial therapy in the past 90 days
- Immunosuppressive state
- Recipient of chronic dialysis or wound care at home
- Family colonized with a multidrug-resistant pathogen

Last, patients residing in a long-term care facility are more likely to have pneumonia with pathogens similar to those responsible for late-onset HAP. In these patients, the most frequently isolated pathogens are *P. aeruginosa*, MRSA, enteric GNRs, and *S. pneumoniae*.[148]

In the immunocompetent host, the incidence of viral and *Legionella* pneumonia is low. Influenza virus, respiratory syncytial viruses, and other viruses may be seen in certain seasons. *Legionella* pneumonia has a geographic distribution and emerges if *Legionella* contaminates the hospital water supply.

Pathogenesis

The respiratory system has a formidable array of defenses against invasion by microbial pathogens. To produce HAP/VAP, the delicate balance among the host, the organism, and the environment needs to be substantially disrupted (Figure 15-2).

Diagnosis

Diagnosis of HAP and VAP is fraught with problems. Unfortunately, clinical and microbiologic criteria are oversensitive but not extremely specific.[150,151] In most cases, the clinician faces the dilemma of whether to treat the patient on clinical grounds alone or resort to invasive methods for the sake of obtaining a sputum sample to identify the specific etiologic agent. The clinical criteria used to diagnose HAP/VAP are listed below:

- Temperature >100.4° F
- Purulent sputum
- Leukocytosis or leukopenia
- A new or progressive radiographic infiltrate
- A decline in oxygenation

Although the clinical criteria raise the suspicion of HAP, they are not diagnostic of HAP. Several noninfectious conditions such as ARDS, atelectasis, heart failure, and pulmonary contusion can mimic the clinical features of HAP.[150,152] Identification of the specific organism is generally more helpful later for adjustment of antimicrobial

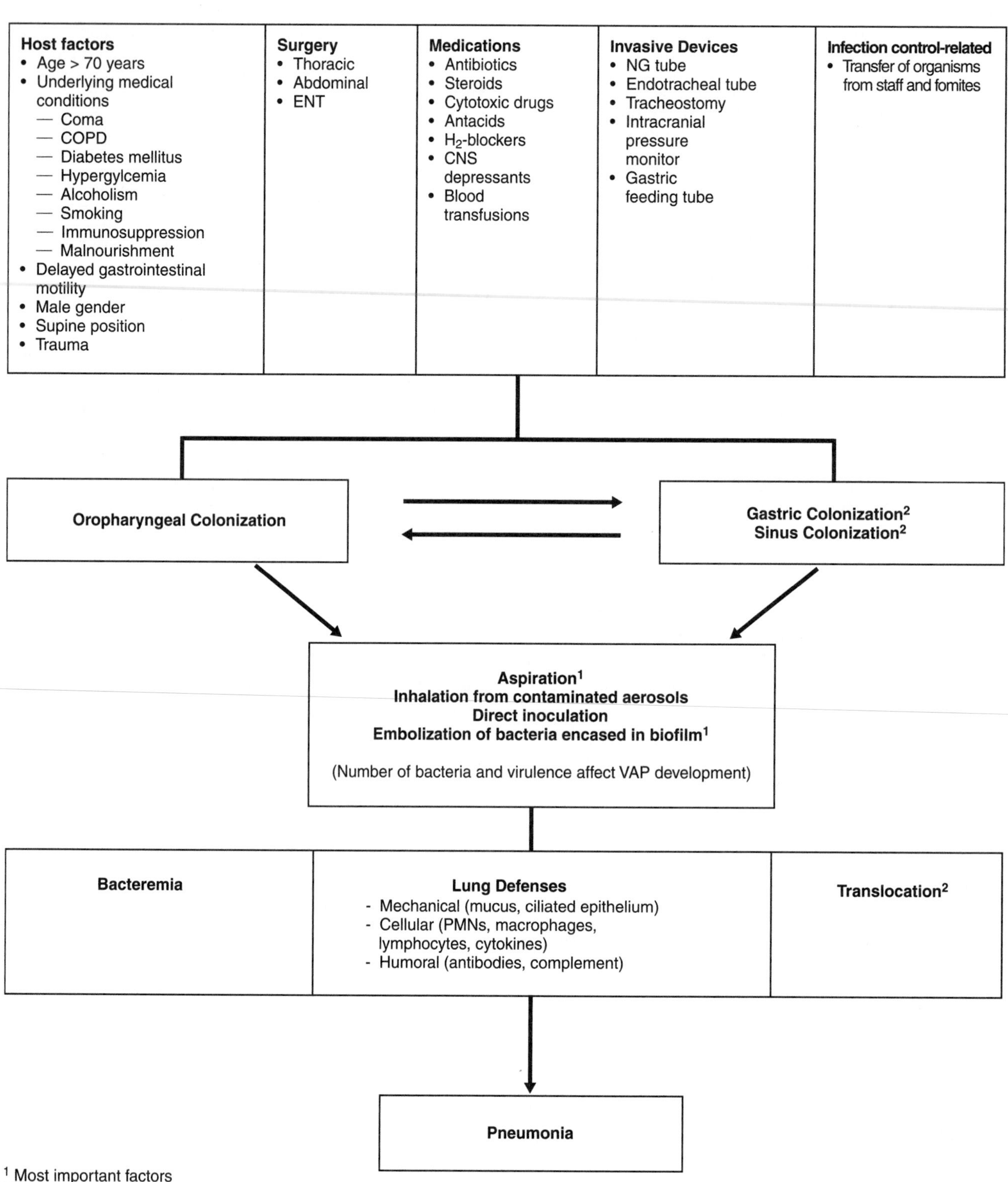

FIGURE 15-2 Pathogenesis and risk factors associated with nosocomial pneumonia. *COPD,* Chronic obstructive pulmonary disease; *ENT,* ear, nose, and throat; *CNS,* central nervous system; *NG,* nasogastric; *VAP,* ventilator-associated pneumonia; *PMN,* polymorphonuclear cells. (Adapted from Seickel JM, Joshi M: Nosocomial respiratory infections, *Ochsner Clin Rep Serious Hosp Infect* 8:1-12, 1996.)

therapy. Microbiology studies on the following fluids are recommended when the presence of HAP is suspected:

- Blood: Fewer than 10% of patients have positive cultures.
- Pleural fluid: If a large pleural effusion is present, then diagnostic thoracentesis should be performed to rule out empyema.

For lower respiratory tract Gram stain and cultures, tracheal suctioning or bronchoalveolar lavage (BAL) can be performed. The merits and disadvantages of both are discussed below.

The ideal Gram stain of the tracheal aspirate can help in the selection of empiric antimicrobial therapy and should have fewer than 10 epithelial cells and a predominance of a morphologically distinct organism. The laboratory performs semiquantitative cultures on these specimens and reports the growth as light, moderate, or heavy. However, tracheal cultures are usually contaminated with oral flora and therefore have a limited role in the diagnosis of HAP. BAL, on the other hand, is more invasive and directed at the lower airways; therefore, the sample more accurately reflects the specific pathogens causing VAP. Significant growth is considered to be $>10^4$ organisms. In some studies, microbiologic results from blind BAL techniques have shown results comparable to those from directed BAL.[153]

In summary, the diagnosis of HAP remains difficult. There is tremendous variation in the use of specific clinical and laboratory methods for the diagnosis of HAP. The use of various tests often depends on local experience and expertise. Clinical criteria, although sensitive, are nonspecific and subject to a significant percentage of error. The lower airway sampling method (BAL) appears to have more acceptable sensitivity and specificity.

Treatment

The management of patients with suspected HAP/VAP is outlined in guidelines published jointly by the American Thoracic Society (ATS) and the Infectious Diseases Society of America (IDSA).[145] The guidelines are summarized below.

In intubated patients, colonization of the respiratory tract is a universal phenomenon. For the sake of treatment, it is important to distinguish colonization of the respiratory tract from a pneumonia process. Therefore, initially, the clinical criteria and Gram stain of the sputum are used to diagnose HAP/VAP, and empiric treatment is initiated. The key features involved in the decision making involve the time of onset of HAP, disease severity, and the presence of risk factors for MARO. Additionally, the design of the empiric therapy should be based on the most likely etiologic organism, the presence of underlying disease(s), the duration of ventilation, previous use of antibiotics, and the resistance patterns in each hospital. Initial therapy, which should include intravenous antibiotics at optimal doses, should be given promptly because delay in treatment results in increased mortality rates. Combination therapy is recommended for patients likely to be infected with MARO pathogens. If the patient has a good clinical response to the empiric treatment and is not infected with *P. aeruginosa*, a shorter course of therapy (7 days) is recommended.[145,154]

At day 3, clinical features such as fever, WBC count, chest radiograph results, oxygenation, presence of purulent sputum, and organ function are assessed. Microbiologic data are also reviewed. If there is clinical improvement and cultures are positive, then antimicrobial therapy is tailored for the specific pathogen. If cultures are negative or there is no improvement, then antimicrobial therapy should be stopped or changed and another diagnosis should be considered.[145,155]

Prevention

Interventions to prevent pneumonia in the ICU are targeted at reducing microbial colonization, decreasing aspiration of pathogens into the lung, and general infection control measures.[156,157] Table 15-9 summarizes the recommendations for prevention of VAP/HAP.

Throughout the trauma cycle, nurses need to be aware of the following information about VAP/HAP:

- VAP and HAP are two of the most common nosocomial infections.
- Diagnosis of VAP/HAP is fraught with problems. An adequate sample of respiratory secretions must be obtained before treatment is initiated.
- Proper positioning, vigorous pulmonary hygiene, and oral care are vital for prevention of VAP/HAP.

Nosocomial Sinusitis

Nosocomial sinusitis is an infection that occurs in critically ill patients. Patients can have fever, leukocytosis, and occasionally purulent drainage from the nose. An extensive evaluation for other sources of fever is often negative. The prime inciting factors include mechanical ventilation, nasal and oral tubes, facial trauma, inability to mobilize the patient, and nasal packing.[158,159] Additional risk factors in the ICU have been identified as nasal colonization with enteric GNRs, sedation, and feeding through nasoenteric tubes.[160] Caplan and Hoyt[158] surveyed 2368 trauma patients over a 2-year period and reported the incidence of nosocomial sinusitis to be 1.4%. George et al[160] reviewed 366 patients hospitalized in an ICU and found the incidence of sinusitis to be 17.4 cases per 1000 patient days. A number of complications associated with nosocomial sinusitis, including direct extension to the brain, lung, and bloodstream and sepsis and even death, have been described. A few reports indicate that a search to identify and then treat maxillary sinusitis in nasotracheally intubated patients can decrease the incidence of VAP.[159] However, this concept is not universally accepted.

TABLE 15-9 **Recommendations to Decrease Risk Factors Associated with Ventilator-Associated Pneumonia***

General	Intubation and Mechanical Ventilation	Management
Staff education	Avoid intubation and reintubation	Semirecumbent position (30 to 45 degrees) is preferred to supine to prevent aspiration, unless medically contraindicated†
Hand hygiene	Noninvasive ventilation should be used when possible	Verify placement of feeding tubes
Surveillance of infections in high-risk population	Orotracheal intubation and orograstic tubes are preferable to the nasal route	Routine mouth care. Chlorhexidine oral wash may be beneficial
Assess need for endotracheal and nasogastric tube daily	Maintain endotracheal tube cuff pressure at less than 25 cm H_2O with minimal occlusive volume	Suction oral secretions as needed to avoid accumulation and aspiration
Chest physical therapy and postural drainage for patients with atelectasis and copious sputum‡	Suction secretions above the cuff before deflating	Subglottic suctioning decreases the risk of aspiration
Surveillance of infections in the high-risk patient‡	Condensation from ventilator circuits should be emptied carefully and prevented from entering the endotracheal tube or the in-line medication nebulizers	Use closed endotracheal suction system‡
	Avoid interrupting the ventilator circuit	Maintain sterile technique during suctioning and refrain from use of endotracheal saline solution lavage
	Do not routinely change ventilator circuit. Change when visibly soiled or malfunctioning	Avoid gastric overdistention‡
	Use sterile water for humidifier fluid	Intensive insulin therapy; maintain serum glucose between 80 and 110 mg/dl
	Follow protocols to improve the use of sedation and accelerate weaning to reduce duration of intubation and mechanical ventilation. Protocols for performing spontaneous breathing trials can foster timelier endotracheal extubation	Control pain that interferes with patient's ability to cough and deep breathe
		Avoid unnecessary use of antibiotics
		Ensure adequate peptic ulcer disease prophylaxis
		Early gastrostomy in patients with head injury or stroke§
		Early tracheostomy (<7 days) in surgical ICU¶
		Continuous lateral rotation therapy in a select group of patients
		Encourage mobilization of the patient as soon as possible

Sources for complete recommendations: Guidelines for the management of adults with hospital-acquired, ventilator-associated, and healthcare-associated pneumonia, American Thoracic Society documents, October 2004; Tablan OC, Anderson LJ, Besser R, Bridges C, Hajjeh R: Guidelines for preventing health-care-associated pneumonia, 2003: recommendations of CDC and the Health Care Infection Control Practices Advisory Committee, MMWR *Morbid Mortal Wkly Rep* 53:1-36, 2004.

*Sources: Safdar N, Christopher JC, Maki DG: The pathogenesis of VAP: its relevance to developing effective strategies for prevention, *Respir Care* 50:725-739, 2005; Dodek P, Keenan S, Cook D et al: Evidence-based practice guideline for the prevention of ventilator-associated pneumonia, *Ann Intern Med* 141:305-313, 2004.

†Source: Hess DR: Patient positioning and ventilator-associated pneumonia, *Respir Care* 50:892-899, 2005.

‡Authors' recommendation.

§Source: Kostadima E, Kaditis AG, Alexopoulos EI et al: Early gastrostomy reduces the rate of ventilator-associated pneumonia in stroke or head injury patients, *Eur Respir J* 26:106-111, 2005.

¶Source: Moller MG, Slaikeu JD, Bonelli P et al: Early tracheostomy versus late tracheostomy in the surgical ICU, *Am J Surg* 189:293-296, 2005.

The diagnosis is usually made with the help of specific radiographs or CT scans that demonstrate opacification or air-fluid levels in the sinus cavity. To establish whether the fluid in the sinus is infected, an antral puncture is perfomed. The specimen is submitted for Gram stain and culture.

The microbiology of nosocomial sinusitis is quite different from that of sinusitis in the community. *Staphylococcus* species, *Pseudomonas* species, and other nosocomial organisms are frequently isolated when specific cultures from patients suspected of having nosocomial sinusitis are obtained. Treatment usually consists of removing the tubes, mobilizing the patient, and instituting broad-spectrum antibiotics aimed at the offending organisms. A majority of patients respond to medical treatment within 2 to 5 days. A small number require surgical drainage.[159]

INFECTIONS OF THE INTRAABDOMINAL REGION OR CAUSED BY ALTERED INTRAABDOMINAL ORGAN FUNCTION

The gastrointestinal tract is home to a complex ecosystem of more than 400 bacterial species, predominantly anaerobic. Most of these organisms come from the oropharynx and travel through the gut. Although the flora is sparse in the stomach and upper intestine, it becomes abundant in the lower bowel.[161] Bacteria are found in the lumen and attached to the mucosa but do not normally penetrate the bowel wall. Intestinal flora can aid in prevention of infection; however, when the bowel is breached, the organisms can penetrate into the peritoneum and cause peritonitis or intraabdominal abscess.

Bacteria cultured from abdominal infections frequently include enterococci, which are part of the normal gut flora in humans and the second or third leading cause of nosocomial gastrointestinal tract infections.[161] *Pseudomonas*, an opportunistic pathogen common in soil and water and on plant surfaces and animals, exploits breaks in a host's defense. It is able to break down physical barriers with extracellular enzymes and toxins and can resist phagocytosis because it has a natural mucoid capsule.[162] This nosocomial pathogen is the fourth most common cause of gastrointestinal infection.[162]

The diagnosis of intraabdominal infections in trauma patients is complicated by a number of factors. The presence of drainage tubes, bulky dressings, and open wounds may inhibit physical assessment. Concomitant CNS injury, anesthetic agents, or analgesics may limit a patient's response to palpation. Diagnostic tests such as CT scan and MRI may be unobtainable if the patient is too critically ill to be moved and appropriately positioned.[161]

Clostridium Difficile Infection

C. difficile causes an infectious diarrhea when reduction of the normal gut flora allows overgrowth of the organism, which is an anaerobic, fast-growing, spore-forming, gram-positive bacillus that produces toxins. It is the most common cause of nosocomial diarrhea in hospitals, extended-care facilities, and rehabilitation facilities.[163] This pathogen is endogenous, found in the stool of healthy people, in soil, in various water sources (including swimming pools, beaches, rivers, seas, and tap water), and in animals (including household dogs and cats).[163] Studies have recovered spores from hospital toilets, metal bedpans, thermometers, and cultures of health care workers.[164] In one report, 59% of health care workers caring for a patient with *C. difficile* diarrhea had positive hand cultures.[163] The organism has also been recovered from stethoscopes and telephones.[164,165]

The organism proliferates when the microecology of the gut is changed by the use of stool softeners or gastrointestinal stimulants, frequent enemas, gastrointestinal surgery, or administration of antibiotics.[163] Lengthy hospital stays, interacting with infected patients, and prolonged use of nasogastric tubes are also risk factors. The loss of normal stomach acidity when the gastric pH increases after the use of proton pump inhibitors and H2-receptor antagonists facilitates colonization of the upper gastrointestinal tract and increases the risk of contracting community-acquired *C. difficile*.[166] Clinadmycin, cephalosporins, and penicillin are associated with an increased incidence of *C. difficile* infection. Symptoms can develop up to 8 weeks after antibiotic therapy.

Transmission is fecal-oral. It is estimated that 20% to 40% of hospitalized patients become colonized by health care workers.[167] The pathogen produces an inflammatory response syndrome to toxin-induced cytokines (toxins A and B), which bind to receptor sites in the colon. Toxins produced by overgrowth of *C. difficile* cause severe colon inflammation and colon cell destruction. Symptoms usually begin 4 to 9 days after initiation of antibiotic therapy and include increased WBC count, which can be >50,000, bandemia, and abdominal pain with or without diarrhea. Diarrhea is watery and foul smelling, occurring 10 to 20 times a day. Diagnosis is made with detection of *C. difficile* toxins in a cytotoxicity stool assay. This is a highly sensitive and specific test. The levels of toxin do not correlate with severity of disease. Results are reported as positive or negative and become available within 24 to 48 hours.

C. difficile infection can produce pseudomembranous colitis, toxic megacolon, sepsis, and death. In pseudomembranous colitis, plaque-like pseudomembranes become scattered in the colon. If the disease progresses to its fulminant stage, it can cause severe colon inflammation, severe lower abdominal pain, bloody diarrhea, high fever, chills, and tachycardia and can be life threatening. New strains of this pathogen exhibit increased virulence and antimicrobial resistance. Highly virulent strains produce *C. difficile*–associated disease, in which toxin levels can be as much as 23 times amounts previously seen.[166]

Treatment consists of oral administration of metronidazole or vancomycin. In patients unable to tolerate oral therapy, antibiotic therapy can be given intravenously, by nasogastric tube, or by enema. Despite appropriate antibiotic therapy, colitis may progress, necessitating colon resection.

Appropriate use of short-course antibiotics and frequent handwashing by health care workers are important in the prevention of *C. difficile* infection. *C. difficile* spores can be resistant to many disinfectants.

Acalculous Cholecystitis

Acalculous cholecystitis is distention of the gallbladder in response to cystic duct obstruction, progressing to mucosal ischemia and necrosis. Trauma patients are at risk of acute acalculous cholecystitis because of debilitation, biliary stasis, major surgery, sepsis, long-term TPN, and prolonged fasting. The mortality rate associated with acalculous cholecystitis is 10% to 50%, so early detection is important.[168] Typical symptoms include fever, nausea, vomiting, tube feed intolerance, tachycardia, and epigastric or right upper quadrant tenderness or rebound. Ten percent of patients have jaundice.[169] Many of these symptoms are masked in trauma patients, and the patient may have fever and sepsis alone.[169]

Peritonitis and Intraabdominal Abscess

Peritonitis is an inflammation of the serosal membrane lining the abdominal cavity and its organs. The peritoneal environment is normally sterile, but it can become inflamed by chemical irritants from a perforation of the stomach, bowel, or gallbladder or a liver laceration. Inflammation can also be triggered by spillage of bacteria from disruption of the gastrointestinal tract (e.g., trauma, necrotic bowel, anastomotic leakage, or enterotomy closure breakdown). When bacteria are present in this normally sterile cavity, the host defense mechanisms produce fibrinous exudates, which can sequester large amounts of bacteria in the fibrin matrix and lead to abscess formation. Bacteria frequently found in intraabdominal infections include *Bacteroides, E. coli, Klebsiella, Pseudomonas*, and *Proteus*. Patients with previous exposure to broad-spectrum antibiotics, gastric acid suppression, CVCs, hyperalimentation, diabetes, steroids, or immunosuppression are felt to be at increased risk for abdominal candidiasis. Untreated peritonitis can be fatal.[170]

Diagnostic tests include laboratory and radiologic studies. CBC results usually show leukocytosis, often with a left shift. Liver function tests may show elevations. Because genitourinary tract infection can occasionally mimic abdominal infections, a urinalysis should be done to rule out UTI. CT scans done with enteral and intravenous contrast are very useful in diagnosing intraabdominal abscesses. Aspiration of an abscess under CT guidance is a mainstay of therapy and provides specimens for culture to identify causative pathogens.[170]

Intraabdominal infections necessitate aggressive fluid resuscitation, correction of electrolyte and coagulation abnormalities, prompt initiation of systemic broad-spectrum antibiotics, and possibly antifungal therapy. Adequate drainage of abscesses either surgically or percutaneously is vital. Therapy must control the source of infection, eliminate bacterial pathogens, support organ function, and control inflammation.[170]

Persistent infection or necrosis may necessitate multiple operative procedures. Modalities that provide coverage and temporary closure of the abdomen, such as vacuum-assisted closure (VAC) dressings, can aid in management of these complicated wounds, although the open abdomen remains vulnerable to contamination with pathogens. A new advance in the treatment of intraabdominal abscesses is staged abdominal repair (STAR), in which daily surgical reexplorations are undertaken, with fascia closure over time; this approach appears to reduce mortality rates.[170,171]

Pancreatic Injury/Pancreatitis

The pancreas is rarely injured because it is protected within the retroperitoneal space. Significant blunt force is needed to injure this organ. Pancreatic injury could be indicated by a patient complaint of dull epigastric or flank pain; abdominal seat belt marks, flank ecchymosis, or penetrating injury found on examination; or retroperitonal hematoma, abdominal free fluid, or pancreatic edema on CT scan. CT scan is the safest and most reliable method of diagnosis.[171] The serum amylase level may be elevated as much as three times the upper limit; however, this test is nonspecific because other conditions can also cause this rise. Lipase is more specific than serum amylase.[172]

Pancreatitis is an inflammatory process of the pancreas associated with severe pain of rapid onset, usually in the mid epigastrium or right upper quadrant.[172] Pancreatic pain frequently radiates to the back. Systemic symptoms can include fever, vomiting, and tachycardia. Pancreatitis may progress to pancreatic necrosis, secondary infection throughout the peritoneum, shock, renal failure, or ARDS.[173] Early surgical debridement and drainage are important. The use of prophylactic antibiotics in the early stages of pancreatitis has been shown to be ineffective in preventing progression to pancreatic abscess.[174]

Infection Control Measures Through the Trauma Cycle

Gastrointestinal tract infections can occur at any part of the trauma cycle, but they are most frequent in later stages. Nurses should guard against introduction of bacteria during enteral feeding, monitor abdominal wound appearance and changes in the characteristics or quantity of wound drainage, evaluate for increased abdominal discomfort or distention, and assess for changing trends in the patient's ability to tolerate feeding. Deviations from an established baseline can signal early infection.

Spleen

The spleen is important in the immune response: it filters aging and deformed blood cells, synthesizes antibodies, and promotes phagocytosis. The spleen provides protection against bacteria because it contains macrophages that phagocytize bacteria that require opsonization. The polysaccharide sugar capsules on the bacteria enable them to evade macrophage phagocytosis. Both the invader and the phagocytizing cells are negatively charged and unable to approximate. However, by opsonization, antigens are bound by antibodies to enhance the process of phagocytosis.[175]

The spleen is a solid, highly vascularized organ that acts as a blood reservoir and can release 300 ml of blood into the circulation.[176] During trauma, splenic rupture can result in massive hemorrhage. In the past, emergency splenectomy was common; however, awareness of the spleen's role in immunity and the potential for overwhelming postsplenectomy infection have made splenic salvage by embolization or splenorrhaphy the treatment of choice.[177]

Asplenic patients are at increased risk for infection with encapsulated bacterial pathogens that normally require opsonization and phagocytosis by splenic macrophages (e.g., *Neisseria meningitis, S. pneumoniae, H. influenzae, Salmonella typhi*). These organisms can cause morbidity and death from bacteremia, meningitis, and pneumonia. Overwhelming postsplenectomy sepsis in the adult trauma patient, although rarely seen, has a high mortality rate. In a study done in the United Kingdom, Waghorn[178] found that

48% of patients with postsplenectomy sepsis died.[178] The greatest risk of infection is in the first 2 to 3 years after splenectomy, but it is a life-long risk.

Prevention of infection includes ensuring that all splenectomy patients receive the pneumococcal polysaccharide vaccine, which provides immunity for 23 of the pneumococcal capsular antigens. Investigators recommend vaccination within 72 hours after splenectomy.[179] Antibody response to the polyvalent pneumococcal vaccine in postsplenectomy trauma patients has been shown to be similar to that in healthy control patients.[179] Recommendations have also been made for giving postsplenectomy patients the meningococcal polysaccharide and *H. influenzae* type B vaccines,[180] but further clinical studies are needed to develop clinical evidence for this recommendation.

Nurses can aid in prevention of infection and optimize positive outcomes for a postsplenectomy patient by ensuring that vaccination is given. Throughout hospitalization, the patient should be monitored closely for signs of infection. Although leukocytosis is a normal sequela after splenectomy, by postoperative day 5 the persistence of WBC counts higher than 15,000/mm^3 and platelet-to-WBC ratios >20 should be considered reliable markers of infection.[181]

Patients should be educated about the signs and symptoms of infection and the necessity of prompt medical treatment if infection is suspected. They should inform their private physicians about the splenectomy so that vaccinations can be updated. Patients should be encouraged to wear medical alert bracelets and understand the risk of infection during travel. They are at increased risk for falciparum malaria, infection from animal bites, and babesiosis from tick bites.[182]

Infections of the Urinary Tract

UTIs are the most common bacterial infections in hospitalized patients. UTIs are not a reportable disease; therefore, it is difficult to assess their true incidence. According to national surveys, UTIs account for 7 million office visits, 1 million emergency department visits, and 100,000 hospitalizations per year.[183]

Risk Factors

All humans are susceptible to UTIs. The risk factors for UTIs can be divided into three categories: host susceptibility; increase in exposure to uropathogens, especially those that promote bladder colonization; and interventions involving the genitourinary tract. Risk factors that predispose patients to UTIs are listed in Table 15-10.[184]

At all ages, women have more UTIs than men. More than half of all women report having one or more UTIs in their lifetimes. The higher incidence is attributed to moister periurethral spaces and shorter distances between the urethral opening and the bladder and the anus. These factors lead to increased exposure and colonization with potential pathogens and therefore subsequent infections. Changes in vaginal flora, obstruction to urinary flow, pregnancy, and hormonal alterations set the stage for the development of UTI (Table 15-10).

An increased incidence of UTIs in the elderly is related to multiple factors, including anatomic changes (cystocele, prolapse, enlarged prostate), impaired mobility, and poor hygiene. In elderly women, changes in vaginal pH and flora also increase the incidence of UTIs.[183,184] Patients with diabetes mellitus have a twofold to fourfold increase in the incidence of UTIs because of impaired emptying of the neuropathic bladder. In addition, their uroepithelial cells may be more susceptible to bacterial binding.[183]

Certain bacteria possess characteristics that make them more efficient as uropathogens and colonizers of the gut, perineum, and urinary tract. Certain strains of *E. coli* possess adhesions on the bacterial fimbriae, which help them attach to the uroepithelial cells. Certain types of fimbriae also promote persistence of infection and prevent clearance of urinary infection. *Proteus mirabilis* also has several virulence factors. The most important is that the bacterium produces the enzyme urease, which hydrolyzes urea to ammonia. This results in the urine becoming more alkaline, which promotes UTIs and formation of struvite stones.[185]

TABLE 15-10 Risk Factors for Urinary Tract Infections

Host	Host *(continued)*
Genetic	Changes in vaginal flora
Nonsecretor status	Vaginal intercourse
ABO blood group antigens	Spermicide use
Biologic	Diaphragm use
Female sex	Antibiotic use
Older age	Menstrual cycle
Estrogen deficiency	Hormone replacement therapy
Exprosure to cold	Trauma
Diet?	Vaginal intercourse
Comorbid conditions	Condom use
Sickle cell disease	Diminished ability to empty bladder
Diabetes mellitus	Spinal cord injury
Incontinence	Neuropathy
History of UTIs	Decreased bladder tone
Congenital abnormalities	**Interventions**
HIV	Bladder catheterization
Obesity	Urogenital surgery
Urinary obstruction	Renal transplantation
Diaphragm use	**Bacterial Characteristics**
Enlarged prostate	*E. coli* with certain adhesions
Pregnancy	

Sources: Foxman B: Epidemiology of urinary tract infections: incidence, morbidity, and economic costs, *Am J Med* 113:5S-13S, 2002; Foxman B, Brown P: Epidemiology of urinary tract infections: transmission and risk factors, incidence, and costs, *Infect Dis Clin North Am* 17:227-241, 2003; Leithauser D: Urinary tract infections, *Infect Control Epidemiol* 25:1-15, 2005; Bochicchio GV, Joshi M, Shih D et al: Reclassification of urinary tract infections in critically ill trauma patients: a time-dependent analysis, *Surg Infect (Larchmt)* 4:379-385, 2003.

Classification of Urinary Tract Infections

UTIs can be classified in three ways:

- Site: bladder (cystitis) or kidney (pyelonephritis)
- Symptomatic or asymptomatic
- Uncomplicated or complicated (structural or functional abnormality, instrumentation)

A complicated UTI develops in most critically ill patients. Therefore, this section focuses on this subcategory of health care–associated UTIs, emphasizing patients who undergo urinary tract instrumentation.

Health Care–Associated Urinary Tract Infections

More than 90% of health care–associated UTIs are related to instrumentation or the presence of a urinary catheter. In patients who are catheterized, bacteriuria develops in 3% to 10% per day. Of these bacteriuric patients, 10% to 25% have a catheter-associated UTIs. On the basis of surveillance systems, the rate of catheter-associated UTIs is two to eight episodes per 1,000 catheter days. Patients with catheter-associated UTIs typically stay an additional day in the hospital, at an annual cost of $450 million.[183,186] In an acute setting, 1% to 4% of catheter-associated UTI episodes result in bacteremia, with an attributable mortality rate of 13%. Rosser et al[187] evaluated 126 septic patients in a trauma ICU and found a 15.8% incidence of urosepsis. The risk factors for urosepsis included age greater than 60 years, extended ICU stay, and prolonged urinary catheterization.

Pathogenesis

Bacteria are acquired predominantly by the extraluminal route (at the time of catheter insertion or by migration from the urethra where the catheter enters) and less often by the intraluminal route (contamination of the collection bag or failure of a closed drainage system). The surface of the catheter provides a site for microbial adherence. Bacteria generate a complex extracellular matrix that attaches to the catheter surface and forms a complex biofilm.[188] The biofilms harbor slow-growing bacteria, which can develop unique methods of antimicrobial resistance and migrate to the bladder. In the bladder, deposition of bacteria, changes in the urinary pH, and obstruction caused by formation of encrustations can further increase the incidence of catheter-associated UTI.[188] However, the duration of catheterization remains the single most important risk factor for UTI and bacteriuria. Other risk factors for catheter-associated UTI are female sex, catheter care violations, older age, presence of diabetes, and renal failure. Use of systemic antibiotic therapy has been associated with lower risk of catheter-associated UTIs; nevertheless, prophylactic antibiotic therapy has been discouraged. Antibiotic therapy can lead to higher cost, increased adverse effects, and the potential for selecting drug-resistant pathogens.[188]

Etiologic Agents

The most common pathogens implicated in catheter-associated UTIs are Enterobacteriaceae, such as *E. coli*, *Klebsiella* species, and *Enterobacter* species. GNRs and yeasts are associated with intraluminal origin, whereas the gram-positive cocci and yeasts migrate along the extraluminal surface. Infections with gram-positive cocci and susceptible GNRs occur earlier, whereas those with the resistant GNRs and yeasts occur later.[188] Monomicrobial infections occur in short-term indwelling catheters, and polymicrobial infections are associated with long-term catheters. Bochicchio et al[189] demonstrated that *P. aeruginosa*, enterococci, and yeast are also among the organisms more frequently seen in critically ill trauma patients with urinary tract infections.

Clinical Features

Patients with health care–associated UTIs can be symptomatic or asymptomatic. Symptomatic patients have lower abdominal or flank pain, nausea, vomiting, and fever. The majority of patients with long-term catheters either have nonspecific symptoms or are asymptomatic. In these circumstances, to avoid overdiagnosis and inappropriate treatment, infection needs to be clearly delineated from mere colonization.[188]

Diagnosis

The diagnosis of health care–associated UTIs is based on obtaining a proper urine specimen before administration of antibiotics. Sterile technique should be used to obtain a urine specimen from the designated port in the collection tubing or from the catheter itself. Urine should not be obtained from a collection bag. To enhance the yield, the specimen should be transported promptly to the laboratory. The tests used to make the diagnosis of the health care–associated UTIs include the following[190]:

- Urinalysis: The presence of pyuria ($>$10 neutrophils/μl) is associated with infection.
- Dipstick for leukocyte esterase and nitrites: An abnormal leukocyte esterase is associated with an inflammatory response. In some studies, leukocyte esterase has been associated with the presence of pyuria; in other studies, this test yielded false-negative and false-positive results. The presence of nitrite denotes infection with Enterobacteriaceae, which convert urinary nitrates to nitrites. However, the dipstick diagnostic tests are of limited value, and their results should be used in conjunction with evaluation for pyuria and cultures.
- Urine cultures: A positive urine culture result is $\geq 10^5$ CFUs/ml. A lower colony count can progress to significant bacteriuria in a few days. Therefore, if clinically relevant, a count lower than 10^5 CFU/ml may also be significant.
- Imaging studies: For patients with complicated UTIs, imaging studies may demonstrate renal abscesses or stones.

Management

In an uncatheterized patient, asymptomatic bacteriuria should generally not be treated with antibiotics. Asymptomatic bacteriuria should be treated only when a patient has an abnormal urinary tract or will soon undergo genitourinary instrumentation. Among patients with catheter-associated cystitis 5 to 7 days of therapy and in patients with pyelonephritis 10 to 14 days of antibiotics is sufficient.[188] Treatment of bacteriuria in patients with indwelling bladder catheters is much more controversial. Antibiotics delay the emergence of bacteriuria but do not alter the incidence of infection.

Antimicrobial therapy for health care–associated UTIs is based on the antimicrobial sensitivity patterns of the organisms in the hospital, the patient's comorbid history, severity of illness, previous antibiotic use, presence of renal failure, and history of residence in a long-term care facility. On the basis of these criteria, empiric therapy is initiated. Once the final cultures are received, the regimen should be de-escalated to the narrowest-spectrum drug[188] (see Table 15-3). Empiric antimicrobial therapy for health care–associated UTIs is summarized below:

- In a patient with symptomatic infection without suspicion of bacteremia, use fluoroquinolones, the preferred agents for the treatment of catheter-associated UTIs. However, during the past 10 years, surveillance systems have demonstrated increasing resistance patterns in *P. aeruginosa* (30%) and *E. coli* (5% to 15%). Alternative choices for these pathogens would be ceftazidime, trimethoprim-sulfamethoxazole (TMP-SMX), or aminoglycosides. TMP-SMX is an excellent choice for nonpseudomonal UTIs, but the empiric use of this drug is discouraged. On the basis of surveillance system data, the rate of *E. coli* resistance to TMP-SMX is increasing (20%).[191]
- In a patient with symptomatic infection with a suspicion of bacteremia, if enterococcal infection is suspected, use ampicillin or vancomycin (if ampicillin resistant) plus gentamicin. If GNRs are suspected, use fluoroquinolones or ceftazidime. If resistant GNRs are suspected, then use cefepime, aminoglycosides, imipenem, or piperacillin/tazobactam.

Prevention of Catheter-Associated Urinary Tract Infections

Catheter-associated UTIs carry a significant morbidity. Although the cost per episode is low, the added morbidity is enormous. Patients with UTIs possess a continual transmissible source of organisms, require antibiotic therapy, and acquire resistant organisms. Therefore, prevention of catheter-associated UTIs is an important issue.[186,188] Specific methods for preventing catheter-associated UTI are described in Table 15-11.

To decrease the incidence of UTIs, different types of urinary catheters have been recommended:

- External (condom) catheters can be used to collect urine from incontinent patients, which may permit removal of indwelling bladder catheters, thereby lowering the risk of catheter-associated UTI. On the basis of patient comfort, external catheters are preferred over indwelling catheters. However, they increase the risk of skin maceration and phimosis. Meticulous skin care is essential to prevent this process.
- Intermittent catheterization has a lower risk of catheter-associated UTI compared with the use of indwelling catheters.
- Suprapubic catheters have a lower risk of bacteriuria and higher amount of patient satisfaction than indwelling catheters placed through the urethra. They are not recommended for short-term use because the incidence of mechanical complications is higher.
- Older studies indicate that silver-coated catheters may reduce the risk of bacteriuria.[192] However, the effect of these catheters on prevention of catheter-associated UTI has not been clearly demonstated.[193] Several antimicrobial catheters have been evaluated. Minocycline/rifampin catheters may prevent bacterial migration along the surface of the catheter but offer protection against gram-positive cocci only. Nitrofurazone catheters may provide protection against GNRs during the first week of catheterization. Chlorhexidine gluconate catheters may provide improved protection against gram-positive and *P. aeruginosa* over other antimicrobial catheters.

Throughout the trauma cycle, nurses need to be aware of the following points pertaining to catheter-associated UTIs:

- Catheter-associated UTI is the most common nosocomial infection.
- It is important to distinguish between true infection and colonization of the urinary tract.
- The need for a urinary catheter must be assessed every day. The best method for preventing catheter-associated UTI is to remove the catheter.
- Nurses need to be aware of how to provide catheter care and how to properly obtain an adequate urine sample.

INFECTION CONTROL IN THE HEALTH CARE SETTING

Prevention of health care–associated infections is a priority for infection prevention and control programs. Approximately two million patients admitted to hospitals acquire infections not related to their admitting diagnoses. Health care–associated infections lead to an estimated 90,000 deaths a year and add a substantial amount of money to patient care costs ($4.5 to 5.7 billion per year).[194] The goal of an infection control program is to reduce the risk of acquisition and transmission of these infections through the following: (1) continuous assessment of infectious agents, (2) use of an epidemiologic approach for surveillance, data collection, and trend identification, (3) effective implementation of infection prevention and control processes, (4) staff education and

TABLE 15-11 Guidelines for Prevention of Catheter-Associated Urinary Tract Infections

General	Catheter Insertion	Catheter Maintenance
Educate staff, patient, and family members on care of urinary catheter When possible, use other methods of urinary drainage, such as a condom catheter, suprapubic catheter, or intermittent catheterization Limit use of urinary catheters for specific indications and discontinue use when no longer indicated	Hand hygiene Use aseptic technique and sterile equipment Choose smallest catheter Secure catheter properly to avoid movement up and down urethra Choose a sterile continuously closed system for drainage	Hand hygiene before and after manipulation of catheter or apparatus Use standard precautions when manipulating urine collection bags Daily meatal care with soap and water Avoid irrigation of indwelling catheters Urine should flow unobstructed by (1) maintaining collection bag below the level of the bladder, (2) prevent catheter from kinking Use a separate designated collection container for each patient; empty urine bag frequently The urine catheter's drainage spigot should not contact the collection container or the floor Avoid interrupting the drainage system Junction between the catheter and tubing should be disinfected before disconnection, if necessary to disconnect Disinfect sampling port before obtaining urine specimen Do not routinely change urinary catheters.

Sources: Leithauser D: Urinary tract infections, *Infect Control Epidemiol* 25:1-15, 2005; Wong E, Hooton T: *Guidelines for prevention of catheter-associated urinary tract infections,* Atlanta, 1981, Centers for Disease Control and Prevention.

collaboration with hospital leadership, and (5) collaboration with community agencies and leaders around emergency preparedness.[195] All members of the trauma team must be educated about infection control principles and guidelines and must understand their individual responsibilities in infection control to ensure consistency of patient care and compliance with infection control measures.

Occupational Exposure to Bloodborne Diseases

Occupational concerns about acquisition of an infectious disease during performance of emergency medical services (EMS) have intensified largely as a result of HIV/acquired immune deficiency syndrome (AIDS). Although needlestick injuries are the most common method of exposure to bloodborne pathogens, mucous membranes and nonintact skin can also be pathways of transmission. Health care workers in trauma settings are at increased risk because of the nature of the patient population and the need for expedited invasive procedures. Trauma centers located in urban settings serve a high-risk population, putting health care workers at higher risk for exposure to bloodborne pathogens (HIV, hepatitis B and C) than those caring for a general hospital population.[196]

Prehospital Phase

Prehospital care providers deal with unique and complex infection control issues. At the time of initial resuscitation of a patient, the presence of bloodborne pathogens is generally unknown because emergency care providers usually do not know the patient's medical history or lifestyle. In fact, this information may never be known if the patient dies or has permanent cognitive impairment as a result of the trauma.

Prehospital infection control guidelines and programs have been developed to help ensure patient and practitioner safety during delivery of EMS care. Prehospital care providers must be protected from both biologic and physical hazards. EMS procedures are often performed in inclement weather, in confined spaces, with limited supplies and equipment, and without adequate lighting or water sources. These situations underscore the importance of wearing appropriate protective attire. Heavy-duty hand protection such as leather gloves or gauntlets should be available to prevent hand injuries during extrication procedures. Hand hygiene should be performed as soon as patient care allows. Gowns are not recommended because they can be dangerous and cumbersome in rescue operations and are generally inadequate in the field. Turnout coats offer a better alternative. If a patient is discovered to be infected with a bloodborne pathogen or infectious disease, federal law stipulates that the EMS providers who treated and transported that patient must be notified.[197]

Hospital

Infection control throughout the trauma cycle is a multifactorial problem. Trauma patients can have injuries that involve every organ system, and the severity of injuries is highly varied. The infection risks and the reservoir of microorganisms are continually changing. Therefore, infection control guidelines must offer protection for both patients and staff. Recommendations for prevention and exposure resources are listed in Table 15-12.

SPECIFIC INFECTIONS

Human Immunodeficiency Virus

Exposures by percutaneous injury or contact with mucous membranes or nonintact skin place health care workers at risk for transmission of HIV and other bloodborne pathogens. The average risk of HIV infection after a needlestick or a cut with HIV-infected blood is 0.3%. The risk of infection after exposure to a mucous membrane is lower, on average 1 in 1,000.[198] Multiple factors affect the risk of transmission after an exposure. Studies have shown an increased risk for transmission in health care workers exposed to large quantities of infectious blood, in those exposed to infectious blood from terminally ill patients, and in those who have a severe injury when they are exposed.[199] Semen and vaginal secretions are considered infectious but have not been shown to be an occupational risk for health care workers. However, cerebrospinal, synovial, amniotic, pleural, peritoneal, and pericardial fluid are potentially infectious.

A vaccine is not available at this time. Focus on prevention strategies is key because of the toxicity and inconvenience of the postexposure prophylaxis (PEP) medications.[200] Recommendations for prevention can be found in Table 15-12. After certain occupational exposures, some antiretroviral drugs may reduce the chance of transmission; therefore, PEP is recommended for exposures that pose a high risk of transmission.[175] When transmission occurs, HIV-specific antibodies usually appear 6 weeks to 4 months after exposure. Rapid HIV antibody testing is now available and may reduce the time to initiation of PEP.[200]

TABLE 15-12 **Recommendations for Prevention of Bloodborne Infections in the Health Care Environment**

Prevention	Compliance with standard precautions Compliance with hand hygiene Vaccination program for hepatitis B Do not recap needles Protect broken skin Use devices with safety features Disinfect equipment Wear personal protective equipment Prehospital providers should wear heavy-duty gloves during extrication procedures.

Health care exposure	Treatment of exposure site (wash with soap and water; flush mucous membranes with water). There is no evidence that use of antiseptics for wound care or squeezing fluid from the wound reduces the risk of transmission.
	Exposure report
	  Date and time of exposure
	  Details of procedure (the type of sharp involved)
	  Details of exposure
	  Details about exposure source
	  Details about exposed person
	Immediate evaluation of exposure for potential transmission
	  Type of exposure
	  Type and amount of fluid
	  Infectious status of source
	  Susceptibility of exposed person
	Postexposure prophylaxis as indicated

Exposure management resources	National Clinicians' Postexposure Prophylaxis Hotline: 888-448-4911; http://www.ucsf.edu/hivcntr Needlestick: http://www.needlestick.mednet.ucla.edu Hepatitis Hotline: 888-443-7232; http://www.cdc.gov/hepatitis Reporting to Centers for Disease Control and Prevention: 800-893-0485 HIV Antiretroviral Pregnancy Registry: 800-258-4263; http://www.glaxowellcome.com/preg_reg/antiretroviral HIV/AIDS Treatment Information Services: http://www.hivatis.org
Facility practice recommendation	Implement a blood-borne pathogen policy Establish laboratory capacity for blood-borne exposure testing Use appropriate PEP regimens Provide exposed health care worker with access to counseling Monitor adverse effects, seroconversion, exposure management programs

Sources: Centers for Disease Control and Prevention: *Exposure to blood: what healthcare personnel need to know,* Atlanta, 2003; U.S. Department of Health and Human Services; Updated U.S. Public Health Service guidelines for the management of occupational exposure to HBV, HCV and HIV and recommendations for postexposure prophylaxis, *MMWR Morb Mortal Wkly Rep* 50:1-43, 2001.

Initially, a health care worker should be tested for HIV as soon as possible after exposure to determine baseline. After appropriate exposure assessment, a 4-week course of a combination of two or three antiretroviral drugs may be recommended for those at high risk of virus transmission.[198] When indicated, PEP treatment should be initiated as soon as possible, preferably within 2 hours. The health care worker should continue to be tested for HIV for at least 6 months after exposure, preferably at 6 weeks, 12 weeks, and 6 months.[198]

Hepatitis B

The highest seroprevalences for the hepatitis B virus (HBV) have been found among emergency department nurses, pathology staff, blood bank staff, laboratory technicians, intravenous teams, and surgical house officers.[198] The prevalence of HBV infection in the patient population influences the risk of occupational exposure. Thus, urban trauma centers are at higher risk because HBV prevalence is higher in urban settings. Percutaneous injuries are the most efficient mode of transmission; however, many health health care workers do not recall an overt percutaneous injury.[201] Among health care workers who do not recall an overt injury, HBV may have been acquired from direct or indirect blood or body fluid exposures that entered the body through a cutaneous scratches, abrasions, burns, or lesions or through mucosal surfaces. HBV can also be found in breast milk, bile, CSF, feces, nasopharyngeal washings, saliva, semen, sweat, and synovial fluid. With the exception of blood, most other body fluids contain low quantities of infectious HBV, despite the presence of hepatitis B surface antigen and thus are not considered efficient vehicles of transmission.[201]

Effectively immunized health care workers have almost no risk of infection.[198] After exposure of a health care worker who has not been vaccinated, the hepatitis B vaccine is recommended as the first step in PEP (Table 15-13). After assessment of the exposure, hepatitis B immune globulin may also be recommended. Postexposure treatment should be initiated as soon as possible, preferably within 24 hours and no later than 7 days. Postexposure treatment is very effective and there is no recommendation for routine follow-up after treatment. To determine whether a person has responded to the hepatitis B vaccine, testing should be done 1 or 2 months after the series is completed.[198]

Hepatitis C

The hepatitis C virus (HCV) causes chronic liver disease and damage, leading to cirrhosis, liver cancer, and liver transplants. Most people are chronically infected but are unaware of their disease because of the slow progression without symptoms or physical signs for two or more decades after infection.

Individuals most at risk of infection are those with large or repeated exposures to HCV-infected blood. However, the risk of HCV infection among health care workers is low.[202] The average risk of a needlestick or cut exposure to infected blood is 1.8%. The risk associated with mucous membrane exposures is unknown but is believed to be very low.[198] There is no vaccine available and no treatment after exposure that will prevent infection. Testing for HCV antibody and liver enzyme levels should be initiated as soon as possible after exposure and at 4 to 6 months after exposure. It is possible to find HCV within 1 to 2 weeks after infection.[198] Prevention activities focus on (1) education of health care workers about the prevention of exposure, (2) adoption of safety-designed medical devices, and (3) maintenance of infection control practices.[203]

Decreasing Transmission of Antibiotic-Resistant Organisms

Resistance to antimicrobial therapy is increasing in hospitals nationwide, resulting in an increase in disease severity, patient mortality rates, and health care costs. People at risk of contracting antibiotic-resistant organisms will often have a history of (1) long-term hospitalization, (2) treatment with antibiotics, (3) a weakened immune system, (4) a surgical procedure, and (5) indwelling medical devices. Through hospital surveillance, patients colonized or infected with MAROs can be treated appropriately and isolated. MAROs and infectious diseases are transmitted through various methods. The most common in a hospital setting is through the hands of health care workers (direct) and contaminated surfaces (indirect). Close compliance with hand hygiene protocols and following appropriate isolation precautions for patients with known colonization/infection or suspected colonization with MAROs (Table 15-14) decrease the risk of contamination and transmission to health care workers and patients.

Methicillin-Resistant *Staphylococcus aureus*

The genus *Staphylococcus* is widespread in nature and considered to be part of the normal flora of the skin and respiratory tract. MRSA is one of the most commonly encountered resistant organisms in hospital settings. It is resistant to several antibiotics, including methicillin, oxacillin, cephalosporins, and quinolones.[204] MRSA can cause several infections: impetigo, cellulitis, pneumonia, wound infections, surgical site infections, central line infections, urinary tract infections, and endocarditis. Known to release endotoxin toxic shock syndrome toxin-1, MRSA can cause toxic shock syndrome.[204] MRSA usually is carried or colonized in the nose, which, in an acute care setting, is frequently cultured in high-risk populations for surveillance purposes. Standard and contact precautions are indicated for patients known or suspected to carry MRSA (Table 15-14). The traditional first-line agent to treat MRSA infections is vancomycin; however, patients colonized only in the nose may be treated with mupirocin (a topical antibiotic used for skin infections) to eradicate colonization before surgery, specifically cardiac surgery.

MRSA is also found in the community. Community-associated MRSA (CA-MRSA) infections are seen with

TABLE 15-13 Vaccination Guidelines for Health Care Personnel

Vaccine	Dose Schedule/Route	Comments
HBV vaccine recombinant	Dose: three doses; first and second dose are 4 weeks apart and third dose is 5 months after second dose Route: intramuscular injection	No known adverse effects
Influenza vaccine inactivated or live attenuated	Dose: one dose annually Route: intramuscular injection or nasal spray (live attenuated)	Nasal spray is approved for healthy people between 5 and 49 years of age Nasal spray should not be given to pregnant women or persons allergic to eggs or who have had complications with live viruses
Measles vaccine* live attenuated	Dose: two doses; second dose at least 1 month later Route: subcutaneous injection	Precautions in pregnant women, immunocompromised persons, in persons with a history of reaction to gelatin, and in persons with recent receipt of immune globulin or neomycin
Mumps vaccine* live attenuated	Dose: one dose; no booster Route: subcutaneous injection	Precautions in pregnant women, immunocompromised persons, in persons with a history of reaction to gelatin, and in persons with recent receipt of neomycin
Rubella vaccine* live attenuated	Dose: one dose; no booster Route: subcutaneous injection	Precautions in pregnant women, immunocompromised persons, and in persons with a history of reaction after receipt of neomycin
Pneumococcal polysaccharide vaccine Inactivated This disease is not spread by health care workers to patients as easily as influenza and infection may not lead to clinical illness; thus at this time routine vaccination is not recommended for all health care workers	Dose: one dose; booster may be recommended; see Centers for Disease Control and Prevention recommendations Route: intramuscular injection	Recommended for individuals over 65 years old; individuals with long-term health problems; immunocompromised persons; certain Native Americans and Alaskan Natives; individuals on long-term steroids. Mild side effects have been reported in less than 1% of people vaccinated (fever, muscle aches) •No evidence of contraindication for pregnant women

Sources: Centers for Disease Control and Prevention: *Guidelines for infection control in health care personnel,* Atlanta, 1998, U.S. Department of Health and Human Services; Centers for Disease Control and Prevention: *National immunization program,* Atlanta, 1997, U.S. Department of Health and Human Services. Note: This is not an exhaustive list; please see the sources for complete recommendations.

*Health care workers with documentation of receipt or those with laboratory evidence of immunity do not require vaccine.

increased frequency in emergency departments and community clinics. CA-MRSA varies from the hospital-acquired strain genetically, in its susceptibility, and in regard to infectivity. CA-MRSA usually presents as a skin infection, such as a pimple or boil, and is commonly susceptible to clindamycin. In a study by Naima et al,[205] CA-MRSA afflicted healthy young persons and was associated with skin and soft tissue infections and toxin production. The community strain is of concern to health care workers because of its potential to become an in-hospital pathogen.

Vancomycin-Resistant Enterococci

Enterococci are bacteria present in the environment, in the gastrointestinal tract, and in the female genital tract. Enterococci are hardy microbes that tolerate a variety of environments. Vancomycin-resistant enterococci (VRE) surfaced around 1989 and the incidence of infection has increased steadily.[206] Patient populations at risk for infection and colonization include the critically ill and those with a history of intraabdominal or cardiothoracic surgery, prolonged hospital stay, a history of vancomycin therapy, and indwelling medical devices. Data suggest that resistant enterococci are transmitted to patients by the hands of health care workers and by contaminated medical devices.[207] Strict adherence to standard precautions and contact precautions is essential in the prevention of transmission among inpatients (Table 15-14). Other in-hospital control methods include active surveillance for VRE, routine screening for use of vancomycin, and establishing recommendations for treatment of infections.[208]

TABLE 15-14 **Guidelines for Isolation Precautions in Hospitals***

Type of Isolation	Description	Personal Protective Equipment/ Patient Management	Pathogens/Diseases (not an exhaustive list)
Standard precautions	Apply to all patients, regardless of diagnosis or presumed infection status, when there is possibility of exposure to body fluids (blood, body fluids, secretions, and excretions)	Hand hygiene before patient contact, after contact with body fluid or contaminated surfaces, and after gloves are worn Don gloves when touching nonintact skin, body fluids, and contaminated surfaces Change gloves between tasks or procedures and discard gloves after use, before touching clean surfaces when gloves are contaminated, and before going to another patient's room Wear a gown, mask, and eye protection during procedures and activities that may generate splashes or sprays of body fluids Respiratory Hygiene/Cough Etiquette: Educate health care workers, visitors, and patients on control measures: covering the mouth/nose with a tissue when coughing; using a surgical mask on persons coughing (when tolerated); hand hygiene after contact with respiratory secretions; and spatial separations in waiting rooms (>3 feet) for persons with respiratory infections Safe Injection Practices: Use sterile, single-use disposable needle and syringe for each injection given If possible, use single-dose vials, especially when using medication for several patients	Use for the care of all patients
Contact precautions (in addition to standard precautions)	Implemented to reduce the risk of transmission by direct or indirect contact. Apply to patients known or suspected of colonization or infection with highly contagious or resistant organisms	Hand hygiene according to standard precautions Don gloves when entering the patient's room and according to standard precautions Don a gown when entering a patient room and according to standard precautions Eye protection according to standard precautions Place patient in a private room. If not available, cohort patients Limit movement and during transport ensure that precautions are maintained If possible, avoid equipment sharing Thoroughly clean and disinfect equipment and environment	MRSA Vancomycin-resistant enterococci Resistant gram-negative organisms *C. difficile* Scabies Zoster Respiratory syncytial virus

TABLE 15-14 Guidelines for Isolation Precautions in Hospitals—cont'd

Type of Isolation	Description	Personal Protective Equipment/ Patient Management	Pathogens/Diseases (not an exhaustive list)
Droplet precautions (in addition to standard precautions)	Implemented for patients suspected or known to have microorganisms transmitted by droplet. Transmission can occur when the patient coughs, sneezes, talks, or during the performance of a procedure	Hand hygiene, gown, and gloves according to standard precautions Place in private room or cohort (consult infection control personnel if cohorting) Wear a mask for close contact with infectious patient and according to standard precautions Limit movement, and during transport, if tolerated, patient must wear a surgical mask and follow respiratory hygiene/cough etiquette. Certain microorganisms require both droplet and contact precautions: respiratory syncytial virus, adenovirus in infants and children	*H. influenzae* *N. meningitidis* Pertussis Pharyngeal diphtheria *Mycoplasma* pneumonia Mumps
Airborne precautions (in addition to standard precautions)	Implemented for patients suspected or known to have microorganisms transmitted by airborne droplet nuclei. These organisms remain suspended in the air and can disperse widely by the ventilation system	Hand hygiene, gown, and gloves according to standard precautions Patients must be placed in a private negative-pressure room with appropriate air release to the outdoors or through high-efficiency filtration before circulation into air-handling system On entry into the room, wear respiratory protection in the form of a properly fitted respirator or powered air-purifying respirator Limit movement, and during transport patient must wear a surgical mask at all times. Staff transporting patient follows standard precautions	Tuberculosis Measles Varicella (chickenpox) Disseminated zoster

Source: Siegel JD, Rhinehart E, Jackson M et al: *2007 Guidelines for isolation precautions: preventing transmission of infectious agents in healthcare settings* (2007): http://www.cdc.gov/ncidod/dhqp/pdf/isolation2007.pdf.
*For complete recommendations, please visit http://www.cdc.gov/ncidod/dhqp/pdf/isolation2007.pdf.
MRSA, Methicillin-resistant *Staphylococcus aureus; VRE,* vancomycin-resistant enterococcus; *RSV,* respiratory syncytial virus; *HCW,* health care worker.

Resistant *Acinetobacter baumannii*

Acinetobacter baumannii is an emerging pathogen in health care environments. It is widely distributed in the soil and in fresh water and can be found as normal flora in the skin and pharynx of many healthy people. *A. baumannii* can survive on surfaces for many days. Carriage on the hands of health care workers has been documented. Colonization of this bacterium is commonly found in the respiratory and digestive tracts. The risk factors for *A. baumannii* infection are similar for those associated with VRE and MRSA infections: long hospital stay, previous antibiotic use, and severe illness.[209] At the moment, the mechanism of resistance is not well understood and thus control measures are similar to those for MRSA and VRE (Table 15-14).

Decontamination, Disinfection, and Sterilization

Guidelines on these topics are confusing. The terms *decontamination*, *disinfection*, and *sterilization* are often misused or interchanged. Decontamination is a process that removes soil

TABLE 15-15 Emerging Diseases and Infectious Agents

Pathogens/Agent	General	Incubation	Presenting Infection	Preparedness*†
Avian influenza "bird flu"	Influenza caused by the avian influenza virus (H5N1). Mode of transmission is uncertain; however, additional precautions are recommended	6-10 days	Resembles influenza (fever, cough, sore throat, and muscle aches) Abnormal chest film Dyspnea Diarrhea	Place under airborne and contact precautions No vaccine available for avian flu; however, health care workers should be vaccinated with the most recent seasonal flu vaccine
Anthrax	Bacterial disease caused by *Bacillus anthracis. B. anthracis* produces spores that can remain in the soil for many years. Mode of transmission is by contact with infected animals or contaminated animal products. Person-to-person transmission is rare. Three routes of infection: skin, lungs, digestive. Respiratory form is most lethal	<2 weeks Inhalation: up to 42 days (because of spore dormancy and slow clearance from the lungs)	Cutaneous: sores that develop into ulcers with a black center Gastric: nausea, loss of appetite, bloody diarrhea, fever, and stomachache Respiratory: flu-like symptoms, cough, chest discomfort, malaise, dyspnea. Hallmark signs include hemorrhagic mediastinal lymphadenitis, hemorrhagic pleural effusion, and bacteremia	Standard precautions are recommended Contaminated dressings or linens require incineration or steam sterilization to kill spores Vaccine is available. Postexposure prophylaxis with antibiotics
Plague	Acute bacterial disease caused by *Yersinia pestis*. Most common form is bubonic plague. Transmission occurs by infected fleas; however, a bioterrorism-associated outbreak may be airborne, causing pneumonic plague. Person-to-person transmission is possible through large droplets	Bubonic plague: 2-6 days Pneumonic plague: 2-4 days	Bubonic plague: Painful, swollen regional lymph nodes Fever Pneumonic plague: Fever Cough Dyspnea Sputum with GNRs Bronchopneumonia on chest film	Standard precautions for patients with bubonic plague Place on droplet precautions for pneumonic plague May discontinue droplet after 48 hours of appropriate therapy Vaccine available but not proven to be effective for pneumonic plague Vaccination requires multiple doses given over several weeks Immunization after exposure is not recommended
SARS	Acute respiratory infection. Suspect in persons with symptoms and travel within 10 days of onset to areas of SARS transmission: China; Hong Kong; Hanoi, Vietnam; Singapore; Toronto, Canada	6 days	Fever Headache Malaise Myalgias Cough Dyspnea	Place under airborne and contact precautions Vaccine is not available

TABLE 15-15 **Emerging Diseases and Infectious Agents—cont'd**

Pathogens/Agent	General	Incubation	Presenting Infection	Preparedness*†
Smallpox	Acute viral disease caused by the variola virus. Smallpox is associated with severe morbidity. Transmission is airborne and by contact with skin lesions or secretions. Individuals become infectious at onset of rash and remain so until the scabs heal (approximately 3 weeks)	7-17 days Average: 12 days	High fever Skin lesions develop into hard pustules described as "pearls of pus." Most prominent in face and extremities, including palms and soles, surfacing at the same time, unlike varicella. Influenza-like symptoms	Place under airborne and contact precautions Vaccine is available Routine public vaccination has not been recommended

SARS, Severe acute respiratory syndrome. Sources: Pickering LK, editor: *Red Book: 2003 report of the Committee on Infectious Disease,* 26th ed, Elk Grove Village, IL, 2003, American Academy of Pediatrics; Hien TT, De Jong M, Farrar J: Avian influenza: a challenge to global health care structure, *N Engl J Med* 351:2363-2365, 2004; Centers for Disease Control and Prevention: *Key facts about avian influenza (bird flu) and avian influenza A (H5N1) virus,* Atlanta, 2006, U.S. Department of Health and Human Services.

*See hospital-specific guidelines.

†For complete recommendations, visit local health department and Centers for Disease Control and Prevention Web sites.

and disease-producing microorganisms and renders an object or the environment safe, for example, washing a surface with hot soapy water. Disinfection is a process that destroys most disease-producing microorganisms except the resistant bacterial endospores. Disinfection levels can vary from low to high. Low-level disinfection kills bacteria, fungi, and viruses. High-level disinfectants kill bacteria, tubercle bacilli, some spores, and viruses. Sterilization is a chemical or physical process that results in the total destruction of all microorganisms, including highly resistant bacterial spores. Sterilization methods used by hospitals include steam autoclaving and dry heat. Methods used to sterilize temperature-sensitive equipment include ethylene oxide gas and low-temperature sterilization technology (hydrogen peroxide plasma).[210,211]

The choice of procedure is based on the specific use of the equipment or instrument. Sterilization is required for critical items (e.g., surgical instruments, cardiac catheters, orthopedic implants, and other devices placed into normally sterile body environments). Disinfection is required for semicritical items such as those that touch or invade mucous membranes. High-level disinfection is recommended for respiratory equipment to ensure eradication of mycobacteria. All other items and surfaces that contact intact skin but not mucous membranes are considered noncritical and require cleaning, decontamination, and sanitizing (low-level disinfection).

Disinfection and sterilization procedures must be performed on precleaned surfaces because disinfectants are inactivated by the presence of organic matter. Concentrations of disinfectants and sterilants must be exact and in accordance with label instructions. Most disinfectants can be toxic, requiring personnel who use them to wear appropriate protective attire. The toxicity of products can be assessed from a material safety data sheet. In addition, it is federal law that all employees using disinfectants must be educated about and protected against associated hazards.

Chemical germicides registered with the U.S. Environmental Protection Agency as "sterilants" and cleared by the Food and Drug Administration for use on medical devices are appropriate high-level disinfectants. These agents should be used at the recommended dilutions and for the suggested contact time to decontaminate equipment/surfaces. These chemical germicides used in hospitals can quickly inactivate HIV and HBV.[212]

EMERGING PATHOGENS AND INFECTIOUS AGENTS

Emerging infectious agents and pathogens present a significant problem for health care professionals around the globe. Effective emergency preparedness programs require awareness, surveillance, and training of health care workers about such pathogens. Trauma centers in particular may have an increased burden for surveillance and containment of possible outbreaks because health care workers at these sites are likely to be among the first to encounter infected individuals. Once an outbreak is suspected, communication with local agencies is vital. Health care providers are required by law to report suspected or known cases of notifiable diseases and cases of unusual illness to the state and local health departments.[213] Health care workers play an important role in initiating the emergency response system to threats posed to the community (Table 15-15).

SUMMARY

Infection control throughout the trauma cycle is a challenge. Infection will always be a potential complication of traumatic injuries and their management. No matter the causative factor, infection can increase morbidity, prolong hospitalization, increase the cost of care, and jeopardize the patient's outcome. Therefore, every effort must be taken to prevent and minimize infection risks.

Despite all the advances in the care of trauma patients, early lessons on the importance of handwashing, meticulous aseptic technique, and careful attention to evidence-based interventions known to reduce infection risks are most important in preventing infection in this patient population. Nurses have a vital role in these infection prevention initiatives. By reducing risk of infection, recognizing onset promptly, and intervening appropriately the nurse can improve outcomes among trauma patients.

REFERENCES

1. Papia G, McLellan BA, El-Helou P et al: Infection in hospitalized trauma patients: incidence, risk factors and complications, *J Trauma* 47:923-927, 1999.
2. Hoover L, Bochicchio GV, Napolitano LM et al: Systemic inflammatory response syndrome and nosocomial infection in trauma, *J Trauma* 61:310-317, 2006.
3. Lazarus HM, Fox J, Burke JP et al: Trauma patient hospital-associated infections: risks and outcomes, *J Trauma* 59: 188-194, 2005.
4. Bochicchio GV, Joshi M, Knorr K et al: Impact of community-acquired infection on acquisition of nosocomial infection, length of stay, and mortality in adult blunt trauma patients, *J Surg Infect (Larchmt)* 3:21-28, 2002.
5. Hill CD: *Joint Commission announces 2004 national patient safety goals:* JCAHO. Accessed May 15, 2007.
6. Burke JP: Infection control: a problem for patient safety, *N Engl J Med* 3487:651-666, 2003.
7. Gantz T: Defensins: antimicrobial peptides of innate immunity, *Nat Rev* 3:710, 2003.
8. Scheinfeld N: Infections in the elderly, *Dermatol Online J* 11:8, 2005.
9. Yaar M, Gilchrest BA: Skin aging: postulated mechanisms and consequent changes in structure and function, *Clin Geriatr Med* 17:617-630, 2001.
10. Gosain A, DiPetro LA: Aging and wound healing, *World J Surg* 28:321-326, 2004.
11. Trask BC, Rote NS, Huether SE: Innate immunity: inflammation. In McCance KL, Huether SE, editors: *Pathophysiology: the biologic basis for disease in adults and children,* 5th ed, pp 175-209, St. Louis, 2005, Elsevier.
12. Mandell GL, Donowitz GR: Acute pneumonia. In Mandell GL, Bennett JE, Dolin R, editors: *Principles and practice of infectious diseases,* pp 819-841, New York, 2005, Churchill Livingstone.
13. Meyer KC: Aging, *Proc Am Thorac Soc* 2:433-439, 2005.
14. Wood KA, Ely EW: What does it mean to be critically ill and elderly? *Curr Opin Crit Care* 9:316-320, 2003.
15. Joshi M, Ciesla N, Caplan E: Diagnosis of pneumonia in critically ill patients, *Chest* 94:4S, 1988.
16. Baldwin KM, Cheek DJ, Morris SE: Shock, multiple organ dysfunction syndrome, and burns in adults. In McCance KL, Huether SE, editors: *Pathophysiology, the biologic basis for disease in adults and children,* 5th ed, p 1645, St. Louis, 2005, Elsevier.
17. Mandell LA: Hospital-acquired pneumonia, *Mediguide Infect Dis* 21:2, 2001.
18. Hayetian F, Brozovich M, Garvin R et al: Ileal perforation secondary to *Clostridium difficile* enteritis: report of 2 cases, *Arch Surg* 141:97-99, 2006.
19. Guyton AC, Hall JE: *Textbook of medical physiology,* 11th ed, Philadelphia, 2006, W. B. Saunders Elsevier.
20. Dale DC: *Nonmalignant disorders of leukocytes: monocytes and macrophage physiology:* ACP Medicine Online (2006): www.medscape.com/viewarticle/535036. Accessed June 16, 2007.
21. Balk RA, Ely EW, Goyette RE: *Sepsis handbook,* Nashville, 2001, Vanderbilt University Medical Center.
22. Huether SE, Defriez CB: Pain, temperature regulation, sleep, and sensory function. In McCance KL, Huether SE, editors: *Pathophysiology: the biologic basis for disease in adults and children,* 5th ed, pp 464-470, St. Louis, 2005, Elsevier.
23. Ghajar J: Traumatic brain injury, *Lancet* 356:923-929, 2000.
24. Trask BC, Rote NS: Adaptive immunity. In McCance KL, Huether SE, editors: *Pathophysiology: the biologic basis for disease in adults and children,* 5th ed, pp 211-248, St. Louis, 2005, Elsevier.
25. Abbas AK, Lichtman AH: General properties of immune responses. In *Cellular and molecular immunology,* 5th ed, pp 3-15, Philadelphia, 2005, Elsevier Saunders.
26. Levy MM, Fink MP, Marshall JC: 2001 SCCM/ESICM/ACCP/ATX/SIS International sepsis definitions conference, *Crit Care Med* 31:1250-1256, 2003.
27. Rankin JA, Van Soren M: Biological mediators of acute inflammation, *AACN Clin Issues* 15:3-17, 2004.
28. Baue AE, Durham R, Faist E: Systemic inflammatory syndrome (SIRS), multiple organ dysfunction syndrome (MODS), multiple organ failure: are we winning the battle? *Shock* 10:79-89, 1998.
29. Bone RC, Balk RA, Cera FB et al: American College of Chest Physicians/Society of Critical Care Medicine Consensus Conference: definitions for sepsis and organ failure and guidelines for the use of innovative therapies in sepsis, *Chest* 101:1644-1655, 1992.
30. Hotchkiss RS, Karl IE: The pathophysiology and treatment of sepsis, *N Engl J Med* 348:138-148, 2003.
31. Neviere R: *Pathophysiology of sepsis:* UpToDate ONLINE 15.2: at utdol.com. Accessed July 16, 2007.
32. Neviere R: *Sepsis and the systemic inflammatory response syndrome: definitions, epidemiology, and prognosis:* UpToDate ONLINE 15.2: www.utdol.com. Accessed July 16, 2007.
33. Russell JA: Management of sepsis, *N Engl J Med* 355:1699-1713, 2006.
34. Townsend S, Dellinger RP, Levy MM et al, editors: *Implementing the surviving sepsis campaign.* Presented at the Society of Critical Care Medicine, the European Society of Intensive Care Medicine, and the International Sepsis Forum, 2005.
35. Angus D, Wax R: Epidemiology of sepsis: an update, *Crit Care Med* 29:S109-S116, 2001.
36. Angus DC, Linde-Zwirble WT, Lidicer J et al: Epidemiology of severe sepsis in the United States: analysis of incidence, outome and associated costs of care, *Crit Care Med* 29:1303-1310, 2001.
37. Filbin MR, Stapczynski JS: *Shock, septic:* eMedicine (2006): www.emedicine.com/emerg/topic533.htm. Accessed July 20, 2007.
38. Dhainaut JF, Shorr AF, Macias WL et al: Dynamic evolution of coagulopathy in the first day of severe sepsis: relationship with mortality and organ failure, *Crit Care Med* 33:341-348, 2005.

39. Opal SM, Huber CE: *XXX Sepsis. Section 7,1-17. American College of Physicians:* www.samed.com/sam/chapters/07/0730.htm. Accessed April 29, 2001. [No longer available online.]
40. Reinhart K, Meisner M, Hartog C: Diagnosis of sepsis: novel and conventional parameters, *Adv Sepsis* 1:42-47, 2001.
41. Meisner M, Tschaikowsky K, Hutzler A et al: Postoperative plasma concentrations of procalcitonin after different types of surgery, *Intensive Care Med* 24:680-684, 1998.
42. Meisner M, Rauschmayer C, Schmidt J et al: Early increase of procalcitonin after cardiovascular surgery in patients with post-operative complications, *Intensive Care Med* 28:1094-1102, 2002.
43. Wanner GA, Keel M, Steckholzer U et al: Relationship between procalcitonin plasma levels and severity of injury, sepsis, organ failure, and mortality in injured patients, *Crit Care Med* 28:950-957, 2000.
44. Gibot S, Kolopp-Sarda MN, Béné MC et al: Plasma level of a triggering receptor expressed on myeloid cells-1: its diagnostic accuracy in patients with suspected sepsis, *Ann Intern Med* 141:9-15, 2004.
45. Rivers EP, McIntrye L, Morro DC et al: Early and innovative interventions for severe sepsis and septic shock: taking advantage of a window of opportunity, *CMAJ* 173:1054-1065, 2005.
46. Rivers E, Nguygen B, Havstad S et al: Early goal-directed therapy in the treatment of severe sepsis and septic shock, *N Engl J Med* 345:1368-1377, 2001.
47. Kumar A, Roberts D, Wood KE et al: Delays in antimicrobial therapy for sepsis, *Crit Care Med* 32:A11, 2004.
48. Bakker J, Grover R, McLuckie A et al: Administration of the nitric oxide synthase inhibitor NG-methyl-L-arginine hydrochloride (546C88) by intravenous infusion for up to 72 hours can promote the resolution of shock in patients with severe sepsis, *Crit Care Med* 32:1-12, 2004.
49. Luckner G, Dunser MV, Stadlbauer KH et al: Cutaneous vascular reactivity and flow motion response to vasopressin in advanced vasodilatory shock and severe postoperative multiple organ dysfunction syndrome, *Crit Care* 10:R40, 2006.
50. Sibbald W: *Update on current treatment modalities in shock:* www.medscape.com/viewarticle/420361. Accessed June 16, 2007.
51. Bochicchio GV, Joshi M, Knorr KM et al: Impact of nosocomial infections in trauma: does age make a difference? *J Trauma* 50:617-619, 2001.
52. Bochicchio GV, Joshi M, Bochicchio K et al: Incidence and impact of risk factors in critically ill trauma patients, *World J Surg* 30:114-118, 2006.
53. Bochicchio GV, Napolitano LM, Joshi M, et al. Persistent systemic inflammatory response syndrome is predictive of nosocomial infection in trauma, *J Trauma* 53:245-251, 2002.
54. El-Masri MM, Joshi M, Hebden J et al: Use of the injury severity score to predict nosocomial bloodstream infections among critically ill trauma patients, *AACN Clin Issues* 13:367-372, 2002.
55. Sung J, Bochicchio GV, Joshi M et al: Admission serum albumin is predictive of outcome in critically ill trauma patients, *Am Surg* 70:1099-1102, 2004.
56. Papia G, McLellan BA, El-Helou P et al: Infection in hospitalized trauma patients: incidence, risk factors and complications. *J Trauma* 47:923-927, 1999.
57. Napolitano LM, Ferrer T, McCarter R et al: Systemic inflammatory response syndrome (SIRS) score at admission independently predicts mortality and length of stay in trauma patients, *J Trauma* 49:647-652, 2000.
58. Yapar N, Erdenizmenli M, Oguz VA et al: Infectious disease consultations and antibiotic usage in a Turkish university hospital, *Int J Infect Dis* 10:61-65, 2006.
59. Moellering RC, Eliopoulos GM: Principles of anti-infective therapy. In Mandell LM, Bennett JE, Dolin R, editors: *Principles and practice of infectious diseases,* 6th ed, vol 1, pp 242-253, Philadelphia, 2005, Elsevier Churchill Livingstone.
60. Abramowicz M: The choice of antibacterial drugs, *Med Lett Drugs Ther* 43:69-78, 2001.
61. Gilbert DN, Moellering RC, Eliopoulos GM, et al: *Antimicrobial therapy, the Sanford guide to antimicrobial therapy,* 35th ed, Hyde Park, Vermont, 2005, Antimicrobial Therapy, Inc.
62. Opal SM, Medeiros AA: Molecular mechanisms of antibiotic resistance in bacteria. In Mandell LM, Bennett JE, Dolin R, editors: *Principles and practice of infectious diseases,* 6th ed, vol 1, pp 253-270, Philadelphia, 2005, Elsevier Churchill Livingstone.
63. Kaye SK, Henry SF, Abrutyn E: pathogens resistant to antimicrobial agents, *Inf Dis Clin North Am* 14:293-318, 2000.
64. Kollef HK, Fraser VJ: Antibiotic resistance in the intensive care unit, *Ann Intern Med* 134:298-314, 2001.
65. Baumgarten KK, Pankey GA: Multidrug-resistant bacterial nosocomial infections: strategies to prevent emergence, *Ochsner Clin Rep Serious Hosp Infect* 14:1-8, 2002.
66. Talbot TR, Kaiser AB: Postoperative infections and antimicrobial prophylaxis. In Mandell LM, Bennett JE, Dolin R, editors: *Principles and practice of infectious diseases,* 6th ed, vol 1, pp 3533-3545, Philadelphia, 2005, Elsevier Churchill Livingstone.
67. Bratzler DW, Houck PM: Antimicrobial prophylaxis for surgery: an advisory statement from the National Surgical Infection Prevention Project, *Clin Infect Dis* 38:1706-1715, 2004.
68. Culver DH, Horan TC, Gaynes RP et al: Surgical wound infection rates by wound class, operative procedure, and patient risk index, *Am J Med* 91:152S-157S, 1991.
69. National Nosocomial Infections Surveillance (NNIS) report, data summary from October 1986–April 1996. A report from the National Nosocomial Infections Surveillance (NNIS) system, *Am J Infect Control* 24:380-388, 1996.
70. American Society of Health-System Pharmacists: ASHP therapeutic guidelines on antimicrobial prophylaxis in surgery, *Am J Health Syst Pharm* 56:1839-1888, 1999.
71. Classen DC, Evans RS, Pestotnik SL et al: The timing of prophylactic administration of antibiotics and the risk of surgical-wound infection, *N Engl J Med* 326:281-286, 1992.
72. Mangram AJ, Horan TC, Pearson ML et al: Guideline for prevention of surgical site infection, 1999. Hospital infection control practices advisory committee, *Infect Control Hosp Epidemiol* 20:250-278, 1999.
73. Muto CA, Jernigan JA, Ostrowsky BE et al: SHEA guideline for preventing nosocomial transmission of multidrug-resistant strains of *Staphylococcus aureus* and *Enterococcus, Infect Control Hosp Epidemiol* 24:362-386, 2003.
74. Zalavras CG, Patzakis MJ: Open fractures: evaluation and management, *J Am Acad Orthop Surg* 11:212-219, 2003.
75. Namias N, Harvill S, Ball S et al: Cost and morbidity associated with antibiotic prophylaxis in the ICU, *J Am Coll Surg* 188:225-230, 1999.
76. Dellinger EP, Hausmann SM, Bratzler DW et al: Hospitals collaborate to decrease surgical site infections, *Am J Surg* 190:9-15, 2005.
77. *Hand hygiene guidelines fact sheet,* Atlanta, U.S. Department of Health and Human Services, Centers for Disease Control

and Prevention, Office of Communication (2002): www.cdc.gov. Accessed March 15, 2006.
78. Van den Berghe G, Wouters P, Weekers F et al: Intensive insulin therapy in the critically ill patients, *N Engl J Med* 345:1359-1367, 2001.
79. Vanhorebeek I, De Vos R, Mesotten D et al: Protection of hepatocyte mitochondrial ultrastructure and function by strict glucose control with insulin in critically ill patients, *Lancet* 365:53-59, 2005.
80. Sung J, Bochicchio GV, Joshi M et al: Admission hyperglycemia is predictive of outcome in critically ill trauma patients, *J Trauma* 59:80-83, 2005.
81. Rumbak MJ, Newton M, Trucale T et al: A prospective, randomized, study comparing early percutaneous dilational tracheotomy to prolonged translaryngeal intubation (delayed tracheotomy) in critically ill medical patients, *Crit Care Med* 32:1689-1694, 2004.
82. Moller MG, Slaikeu JD, Bonelli P et al: Early tracheostomy versus late tracheostomy in the surgical intensive care unit, *Am J Surg* 189:293-296, 2005.
83. Bouderka MA, Fakhir B. Bouaggad A et al: Early tracheostomy versus prolonged endotrachel intubation in severe head injury, *J Trauma* 57:251-254, 2004.
84. Stevens DL, Tanner MH, Winship J et al: Severe group A streptococcal infection associated with a toxic shock–like syndrome and scarlet fever toxin, *N Engl J Med* 321:1-7, 1989.
85. Stevens DL: *Necrotizing infections of the skin and fascia:* www.uptodate.com. Accessed February 13, 2006.
86. Bisno AL, Stevens DL: *Streptococcus pyogenes.* In Mandell GL, Bennett JE, Dolin R, editors: *Principles and practice of infectious diseases,* 6 ed, pp 2362-2379, Philadelphia, 2005, Elsevier Churchill Livingstone.
87. Lancefield RC: Current knowledge of type-specific M antigens of group A streptococci, *J Immunol* 89:307-313, 1962.
88. Wong CH, Chang HC, Pasupathy S et al: Necrotizing fasciitis: clinical presentation, microbiology and determinants of mortality, *J Bone Joint Surg Am* 85A:1454-1460, 2003.
89. Stevens DL: *Clostridial myonecrosis (gas gangrene):* www.utdol.com. Accessed February 13, 2006.
90. Wilson SE, Campbell BS: *Clostrtidium dificile*–associated disease: diagnosis and management of an increasing postoperative complication, *Serious Hosp Infect* 10:1, 1998.
91. Sexton DJ, Westerman EL: *Tetanus:* www.utdol.com. Accessed February 13, 2006.
92. Hibberd PL: Tetanus-diptheria toxoid vaccination in adults: UpToDate: www.utdol.com. Accessed July 5, 2007.
93. *R Adams Cowley shock trauma clinical manual,* R Adams Cowley Shock Trauma Center, Baltimore, Md, 2005.
94. Pascual FB, McGinley EL, Zanardi LR et al: Tetanus surveillance—United States, 1998-2000. *MMWR Surveil Summ* 52:1, 2003.
95. Schwarz K, Dulchavsky S: *Burn wound infections:* eMedicine (2005): www.emedicine.com/med/topic258.htm. Accessed July 27, 2007.
96. Ahrns KS: Trends in burn resuscitation: shifting the focus from fluids to adequate endpoint monitoring, edema control, and adjuvant therapies, *Crit Care Nurs Clin North Am* 16:75-98, 2004.
97. Church D, Elsayed S, Reid O et al: Burn wound infections, *Clin Microbiol Rev* 19:403-434, 2006.
98. Supple KG. Physiologic response to burn injury, *Crit Care Nurs Clin North Am* 16:119-126, 2004.
99. Pruitt BA, Foley FD: The use of biopsies in burn patient care, *Surgery* 3:887-897, 1997.
100. McManus AT, Kim SH, Mason AD, et al: A comparison of quanitative microbiology and histopathology in divided burn wound biopsies, *Arch Surg* 122:64-66, 1987.
101. Bauer GJ, Yurt RW: Burns. In Mandell GL, Bennett JE, Dolin R, editors: *Principles and practice of infectious diseases,* 6th ed, pp 3547-3551, Philadelphia, 2005, Elsevier Churchill Livingstone.
102. Darouiche RO: Treatment of infections associated with surgical implants, *N Engl J Med* 350:1422-1429, 2004.
103. Gustilo RB, Mendoza RM, Willams DN: Problems in the management of type III (severe) open fractures: a new classification of type III open fractures, *J Trauma* 24:742-746, 1984.
104. O'Meara PM: Management of open fractures, *Orthop Rev* 21:1177-1184, 1992.
105. Menth-Chiari WA, Norris B, Richart CM et al: Pathophysiology of the polytrauma patient. In Baumgaertner MR, Tornetta PT, editors: *Orthopedic knowledge update,* 3rd ed, pp 93-103, Rosemont, IL, 2005, American Academy of Orthopedic Surgeons.
106. Bosse MJ, Kellam JF: Orthopaedic management decisions in the multiple-trauma patient. In Browner BD, Jupiter JB, Levine AM et al, editors: *Skeletal trauma: basic science, management and reconstruction,* 3rd ed, vol 1, pp 133-146, Philadelphia, 2003, W. B. Saunders.
107. Stawicki SP, Hoff WS, Hoey BA et al: Human immunodeficiency virus infection in trauma patients: where do we stand? *J Trauma* 58:88-93, 2005.
108. Mader JT, Shirtliff ME, Calhoun JH: Staging and staging application in osteomyelitis, *Clin Infect Dis* 25:1303-1309, 1997.
109. Lin DL, Kirk KL, Murphy KP et al: Evaluation of orthopaedic injuries in Operation Enduring Freedom, *J Orthop Trauma* 18:S48-S53, 2004.
110. Bone LB, Johnson KD, Weigelt J et al: Early versus delayed stabilization of fractures, *J Bone Joint Surg Am* 71:336-339, 1989.
111. American College of Surgeons' Committee on Trauma: *Advanced trauma life support,* ed 7, Chicago, 2004, American College of Surgeons.
112. Bosse MJ, MacKenzie EJ, Riemer BL et al: Adult respiratory syndrome, pneumonia, and mortality following thoracic injury and femoral fracture treated with intramedullary nailing with reaming or with a plate: a comparative study, *J Bone Joint Surg Am* 79:799-809, 1997.
113. Scalea TM, Boswell SA, Scott JD et al: External fixation as a bridge to intramedullary nailing for patients with multiple injuries and with femur fractures: damage control orthopaedics, *J Trauma* 48:613-623, 2000.
114. Mader JT, Cripps MW, Calhoun JH: Adult post traumatic osteomyelitis of the tibia, *Clin Orthop* 360:14-21, 1999.
115. Ziran BH, Rao N: Infections. In Baumgaertner MR, Tornetta PT, editors: *Orthopedic knowledge update,* 3rd ed, pp 131-139, Rosemont, IL, 2005, American Academy of Orthopedic Surgeons.
116. Donlan RM, Costerton JW: Biofilms: survival mechanisms of clinically relevant microorganisms, *Clin Microbiol Rev* 15:167-193, 2002.
117. Lew DP, Waldvogel FA: Osteomyelitis, *Lancet* 364:369-379, 2004.
118. Gross T, Kaim AH, Regazzoni P et al: Current concepts in posttraumatic osteomyelitis: a diagnostic challenge with new imaging options, *J Trauma* 52:1210-1219, 2002.

119. American College of Chest Physicians/Society of Critical Care Medicine Consensus Conference Committee: Definitions for organ failure and guidelines for the use of innovative therapies in sepsis, *Crit Care Med* 20:864-874, 1992.
120. Wisplinghoff H, Bischoff T, Tallent SM et al: Nosocomial bloodstream infections in U.S. hospitals: analysis of 24,719 cases from a prospective nationwide surveillance study, *Clin Infect Dis* 39:309-317, 2004.
121. Edmond MB, Wallace SE, McClish DK et al: Nosocomial bloodstream infections in U.S. hospitals: a three-year analysis, *Clin Infect Dis* 29:239-244, 1999.
122. Norberg A, Christopher NC, Ramundo ML et al: Contamination rates of blood cultures obtained by dedicated phlebotomy vs intravenous catheter, *JAMA* 289:726-729, 2003.
123. Weinstein MP: Current blood culture methods and systems: clinical concepts, technology and interpretation of results, *Clin Infect Dis* 23:40-46, 1996.
124. Katneni R, Hedayati SS: Central venous catheter-related bacteremia in chronic hemodialysis patients: epidemiology and evidence-based management, *Nat Clin Pract Nephrol* 3: 256-266, 2007.
125. Jarvis WR, Edwards JR, Culver DH et al: Nosocomial infection rates in adult and pediatric intensive care units in the United States, NNISS, *Am J Med* 91:185S-191S, 1991.
126. Mermel LA, Farr BM, Sherertz RJ et al: Guidelines for the management of intravascular catheter-related infections, *Clin Infect Dis* 32:1249-1272, 2001.
127. Safdar N, Fine JP, Maki DG: Meta-analysis: methods for diagnosing intravascular catheter-related infections, *Ann Intern Med* 142:451-466, 2005.
128. Grady NP, Alexander M, Dellinger EP et al: Guidelines for the prevention of intravascular catheter-related infections, *Clin Infect Dis* 35:1281-1307, 2002.
129. McGee DC, Gould MK: Preventing complications of central venous catheterization, *N Engl J Med* 348:1123-1133, 2003.
130. Khan EA, Correa AG, Baker CJ: Suppurative thrombophlebitis in children: a ten-year experience, *Pediatr Infect Dis* 16:63-67, 1997.
131. Fry DE, Fry RV, Borzotta AP: Nosocomial blood-borne infection secondary to intravascular devices, *Am J Surg* 167:268-272, 1994.
132. Moereillion P, Que YA: Infective endocarditis, *Lancet* 363:139-149, 2004.
133. Cantrell M, Yoshikawa TT: Infective endocarditis in the aged patient, *Gerotonlogy* 30:316-326, 1984.
134. Fowler VG Jr, Miro JM, Hoen B et al: *Staphylococcus aureus* endocarditis: a consequence of medical progress, *JAMA* 293:3012-3021, 2005.
135. Fowler VG, Scheld WM, Bayer AS: Infective endocarditis. In Mandell LM, Bennett JE, Dolin R, editors: *Principles and practice of infectious diseases,* 6th ed, vol 1, pp 975-1022, Philadelphia, 2005, Elsevier Churchill Livingstone.
136. Huggins S: Reducing morbidity of acute respiratory distress syndrome in hospitalized patients: preventing nosocomial infection or aspiration, *Topics Adv Pract Nurs eJournal* 6: 2006. www.medscape.com/viewarticle/537255. Accessed July 24, 2007.
137. Sato T, Takayama T, So K, et al: Is retention of a nasogastric tube after esophagectomy a risk factor for postoperative respiratory tract infection? *J Infect Chemother* 13:109-113, 2007.
138. Doherty PF, Rabinowitz RP: Gunshot wounds to the head: the role of antibiotics, *Infect Med* 21:297-300, 2004. www.medscape.com/viewarticle/482814. Accessed July 24, 2007.
139. Barnes BJ, Wiederhold NP, Micek ST et al: *Enterobacter cloacae* ventriculitis successfully treated with cefepime and gentamicin: case report and review of the literature, *Pharmacotherapy* 23:537-542, 2003.
140. Lozier AP, Sciacca RRE, Romagnoli MF et al: Ventriculostomy-related infections: a critical review of the literature, *Neurosurgery* 51:170-182, 2002.
141. Lyle KE, Obasanjo OO, Williams MA et al: Ventriculitis complicating use of catheters in adult neurosurgical patients, *Clin Infect Dis* 32:2028-2033, 2001.
142. Brain Trauma Foundation, American Association of Neurological Surgeons, Congress of Neurological Surgeons, AANS/CNS Joint Section on Neurotrauma and Critical Care: Guidelines for the management of severe traumatic brain injury, *J Neurotrauma* 24(1 Suppl):S1-S106, 2007.
143. Pangilinan PH, Kelly BM: *Posttraumatic hydrocephalus:* www.emedicine.com/pmr/topic113.htm. Accessed July 24, 2007.
144. Mayhall CG, Archer NH, Lamb VA et al: Ventriculostomy-related infections: a prospective epidemiologic study, *N Engl J Med* 310:553-559, 1984.
145. American Thoracic Society: Guidelines for the management of adults with hospital-acquired, ventilator-associated, and healthcare-associated pneumonia, *Am J Respir Care Med* 171:388-416, 2005.
146. Rello J, Ollendorf DA, Oster G et al: Epidemiology and outcomes of ventilator-associated pneumonia in a large U.S. database, *Chest* 122:2115-2121, 2002.
147. Cook DJ, Walter SD, Cook RJ et al: Incidence of risk factors for ventilator-associated pneumonia in critically ill patients, *Ann Intern Med* 129:433-440, 1998.
148. El Solh AA, Sikka P, Ramadan F et al: Etiology of severe pneumonia in the very elderly, *Am J Respir Care Med* 163:645-651, 2001.
149. Rello J, Torres A, Ricart M, et al: Ventilator-associated pneumonia by *S. aureus:* comparison of methicillin-resistant and methicillin-sensitive episodes, *Am J Respir Care Med* 150:1545-1549, 1994.
150. Seickel JM, Joshi M: Nosocomial respiratory infections, *Ochsner Clin Rep Serious Hosp Infect* 8:1-12, 1996.
151. Markowicz P, Wolff M, Djedaini K, et al: Multicenter prospective study of ventilator-associated pneumonia during ARDS: incidence, prognosis and risk factors, *Am J Respir Crit Care Med* 161:1942-1948, 2000.
152. Cabello H, Torres A, Celiss R et al: Bacterial colonization of distal airways in healthy subjects and chronic lung diseases: a bronchoscopic study, *Eur Respir J* 10:1137-1144, 1997.
153. Torres A, EL-Ebiary M: Bronchscopic BAL in the diagnosis of ventilator-associated pneumonia, *Chest* 117:198S-202S, 2000.
154. Chastre J, Wolff M, Fagon JY et al: Comparison of 8 vs 15 days of antibiotic therapy for ventilator-associated pneumonia in adults: a randomized trial, *JAMA* 290:2588-2598, 2003.
155. Singh N, Rogers P, Atwood CW et al: Short-course empiric antibiotic therapy for patients with pulmonary infiltrates in the ICU: a proposed solution for the indiscriminate antibiotic prescription, *Am J Respir Care Med* 162:505-511, 2000.
156. Safdar N, Christopher JC, Maki DG: The pathogenesis of VAP: its relevance to developing effective strategies for prevention, *Respir Care* 50:725-739, 2005.
157. Dodek P, Keenan S, Cook D et al: Evidence-based practice guideline for the prevention of ventilator-associated pneumonia, *Ann Intern Med* 141:305-313, 2004.

158. Caplan ES, Hoyt NJ: Nosocomial sinusitis, *JAMA* 247:639-641, 1982.
159. Stein M, Caplan ES: Nosocomial sinusitis: a unique subset of sinusitis, *Curr Opin Infect Dis* 18:147-150, 2005.
160. George DL, Falk PS, Umberto MG et al: Nosocomial sinusitis in patients in the medical ICU: a prospective epidemiological study, *Clin Infect Dis* 27:463-470, 1998.
161. Gorbach SL: *Microbiology of the gastrointestinal tract:* www.gsbs.utmb.edu/microbook/ch095.htm. Accessed July 24, 2007.
162. Pier GB, Ramphal R: *Pseudomonas aeruginosa.* In Mandell GL, Bennett JE, Dolin R, editors: *Principles and practice of infectious diseases,* 6th ed, pp 2587-2609, Philadelphia, 2005, Elsevier Churchill Livingstone..
163. Schroeder MS: *Clostridium difficile*–associated diarrhea, *Am Fam Physician* 71:921-928, 2005.
164. Dallal RM, Harbrecht BG, Boujoukas AJ et al: Fulminant *Clostridium difficile:* an underappreciated and increasing cause of death and complications, *Ann Surg* 235:363-372, 2002.
165. Gerding DN, McDonald LC et al: Satellite symposium. Presented at the 43rd annual meeting of the Infectious Diseases Society of America, San Francisco, October 6-9, 2005.
166. Dial S, Delaney JA, Barkun AN et al: Use of gastric acid-suppressive agents and the risk of community-acquired *Clostridium difficile*–associated disease, *JAMA* 294:2989-2995, 2005.
167. Poutanen SM, Simor AE: *Clostridium difficile*–associated diarrhea in adults, *CMAJ* 171:51-58, 2004.
168. Shojamanesh H, Roy PK: *Acalculous cholecystitis:* www.emedicine.com/med/topic3526.htm. Accessed July 26, 2007.
169. Todar K: *Textbook of bacteriology:* www.textbookofbacteriology.net. Accessed July 27, 2007.
170. Peralta R, Genuit T, Napolitano L et al: Peritonitis and abdominal sepsis, *eMedicine* 2006. www.emedicine.com/med/topic2737.htm. Accessed July 27, 2007.
171. Sawyer RG, Barkun JS, Smith R et al: *Intra-abdominal infection: recognition and management of intra-abdominal infection:* www.medscape.com/viewarticle/525772. Accessed July 26, 2007.
172. Bjerke HS: Pancreatic trauma, *eMedicine* 2006. www.emedicine.com/med/topic2801.htm. Accessed July 27, 2007.
173. Chari St, Vege SS: *Clinical manifestations and diagnosis of acute pancreatitis:* http://www.utdol.com. Accessed March 6, 2006. [No longer available on UpToDate.]
174. Romero-Urquhart G, Phillips J: Pancreatitis, acute, *eMedicine* 2007. www.emedicine.com/radio/topic521.htm. Accessed July 27, 2007.
175. Lee CJ, Lee LH, Koizumi K: Polysaccharide vaccines for prevention of encapsulated bacterial infections, I, *Infect Med* 19:127-133, 2002.
176. McCance KL: Structure and function of the hematologic system. In McCance KL, Huether SE, editors: *Pathophysiology: the biologic basis for disease in adults and children,* 5th ed, pp 898-899, St. Louis, 2005, Elsevier.
177. Lutwick LI: Infections in asplenic patients. In Mandell GL, Bennett JE, Dolin R, editors: *Principles and practice of infectious diseases,* pp 3524-3532, New York, 2005, Churchill Livingstone.
178. Waghorn DJ: Overwhelming infection in asplenic patients: current best practice preventive measures are not being followed, *J Clin Pathol* 54:2214-2218, 2001.
179. Caplan ES, Boltansky H, Synder MJ et al: Response of traumatized splenectomized patients to immediate vaccination with polyvalent pneumococcal vaccine, *J Trauma* 23:801-805, 1983.
180. Brender E, Burke A, Glass RM: The spleen, *JAMA* 294:2660, 2005.
181. Weng J, Brown CV, Rhee P: White blood cell and platelet count can be used to differentiate between infection and the normal response after splenectomy for trauma: prospective validation, *J Trauma* 59:1076-1080, 2005.
182. Spelman D: Prevention of overwhelming sepsis in asplenic patients: could do better, *Lancet* 357:2072, 2001.
183. Foxman B: Epidemiology of urinary tract infections: incidence, morbidity, and economic costs, *Am J Med* 113:5S-13S, 2002.
184. Foxman B, Brown P: Epidemiology of urinary tract infections: transmission and risk factors, incidence, and costs, *Infect Dis Clin North Am* 17:227-241, 2003.
185. Oelschlaeger TA, Dobrindt U, Hacker J: Virulence factors of uropathogens, *Curr Opin Urol* 12:33-38, 2002.
186. Leithauser D: Urinary tract infections, *Assoc Professions Infect Control Text Infect Control Epidemiol* 25:1-15, 2005.
187. Rosser CJ, Bare RL, Meredith W: Urinary tract infections in the critically ill patient with a urinary catheter, *Am J Surg* 177:287-290, 1999.
188. Saint S, Chenoweth C: Biofilms and catheter-associated urinary tract infections, *Infect Dis Clin North Am* 17:411-432, 2003.
189. Bochicchio GV, Joshi M, Shih D et al: Reclassification of urinary tract infections in critically ill trauma patients: a time-dependent analysis, *Surg Infect (Larchmt)* 4:379-385, 2003.
190. Wilson ML, Gaido L: Laboratory diagnosis of urinary tract infections in adult patients, *Clin Infect Dis* 38:1150-1158, 2004.
191. Gupta K: Emerging antibiotic resistance in urinary tract pathogens, *Infect Dis Clin North Am* 17:243-259, 2003.
192. Liedberg H, Lundeberg T: Silver alloy coated catheters reduce catheter-associated bacteriuria, *Br J Urol* 65:379-381, 1960.
193. Srinivasan A, Karchmer T, Richards A et al: A prospective trial of a novel, silicone-based, silver-coated Foley catheter for the prevention of nosocomial urinary tract infections, *Infect Control Hosp Epidemiol* 27:38-43, 2006.
194. Mckibben L, Horan T, Tokars J et al: Guidance on public reporting of healthcare-associated infections: recommendations of the Healthcare Infection Control Practice Advisory Committee, *Am J Infect Control* 33:217-226, 2005.
195. Association for Professionals in Infection Control and Epidemiology: *Surveillance, prevention and control of infection,* 2nd ed, Washington, DC, 2005, Association for Professionals in Infection Control and Epidemiology.
196. Xeroulis G, Inaba K, Stewart TC et al: Human immunodeficiency virus, hepatitis B, hepatitis C seroprevalence in a Canadian trauma population, *J Trauma* 59:105-108, 2005.
197. Strathdee SA, O'Shaughnessy MV, Montaner JS et al: A decade of research on the natural history of HIV infection, I: markers, *Clin Invest Med* 19:111-120, 1996.
198. Centers for Disease Control and Prevention: *Exposure to blood: what healthcare personnel need to know,* Atlanta, 2003, U.S. Department of Health and Human Services.
199. Updated U.S. Public Health Service guidelines for the management of occupational exposure to HIV and recommendations for postexposure prophylaxis, *MMWR Morbid Mortal Wkly Rep* 54:1-17, 2005.

200. Mayhall CG: *Epidemiology and infection control,* 3rd ed, Philadelphia, 2004, Lippincott Williams & Wilkins.
201. Updated U.S. Public Health Service guidelines for the management of occupational exposure to HBV, HCV and HIV and recommendations for postexposure prophylaxis. *MMWR Morbid Mortal Wkly Rep* 50:1-43, 2001.
202. Centers for Disease Control and Prevention: *Guidelines for infection control in health care personnel,* Atlanta, 1998, U.S. Department of Health and Human Services.
203. Recommendations for prevention and control of hepatitis C virus infection and HCV-related chronic diseases, *MMWR Morbid Mortal Wkly Rep* 47:1-39, 1998.
204. National Institutes of Health, National Institute of Allergy and Infectious Disease: *The problem of antibiotic resistance,* Bethesda, MD, 2004, National Institutes of Health, National Institute of Allergy and Infectious Diseases.
205. Naimi TS, LeDell KH, Como-Sabetti K et al: Comparison of community- and health care–associated methicillin-resistant *Staphylococcus aureus* infection, *JAMA* 290:2976-2984, 2003.
206. Centers for Disease Control and Prevention: *Information for the public about VRE,* Atlanta, 2005, U.S. Department of Health and Human Services.
207. Huycke MM, Sahm DF, Gilmore MS et al: Multiple-drug resistant enterococci: the nature of the problem and an agenda for the future, *Emerg Infect Dis* 4:239-249, 1998.
208. Recommendations for preventing the spread of vancomycin resistance recommendations of the Hospital Infection Control Practices Advisory Committee (HICPAC), *MMWR Morbid Mortal Wkly Rep* 44:1-13, 1995.
209. El Shafie SS, Alishaq M, Leni Gracia M: Investigation of an outbreak of multidrug-resistant *Acinetobacter baumannii* in trauma intensive care unit, *J Hosp Infect* 56:101-105, 2004.
210. Centers for Disease Control and Prevention: *Sterilization or disinfection of medical devices,* Atlanta, 2002, U.S. Department of Health and Human Services.
211. Rutala WA, Weber DJ: New disinfection and sterilization methods, *Emerg Infect Dis* 7:348-353, 2001.
212. Centers for Disease Control and Prevention: *Sterilization or disinfection of patient-care equipment,* Atlanta, 2000, U.S. Department of Health and Human Services.
213. U.S. Government Accountability Office: *Emerging infectious diseases: review of state and federal disease surveillance efforts,* Washington, DC, 2004, U.S. Government Accountability Office.

16

WOUND HEALING AND SOFT TISSUE INJURIES

Mary Beth Flynn Makic, Karen A. McQuillan

The skin is the enveloping external organ of the human body and it is the first line of defense in any injury. Thus the skin is nearly always injured when trauma occurs. The extent of traumatic wounding varies from minor abrasions to large gaping wounds. Procedures and surgical interventions to treat injury also may create punctures, incisions or large openings in the skin. Injury to the skin and soft tissues predisposes the individual to secondary complications such as (1) localized and systemic infection, (2) hypoproteinemia, (3) hypothermia, and (4) sequelae related to tissue necrosis. Minimizing the risk of secondary complications and maximizing wound healing are optimal goals of all trauma patients with soft tissue injury.

Traumatic wounds differ from wounds that occur as a consequence of surgery, and this has implications for both the healing process and treatment. In contrast to the controlled nature of surgical wounds, traumatic wounds are often multiple in nature, induce extensive stress with catecholamine release, are often concomitant with shock and hypoxemia, and lead to depletion of physiologic reserves as the body responds to the traumatic insult and attempts to normalize. The likelihood of bacterial contamination at the time of injury presents the potential for wound infection and delayed healing.

All wounds, regardless of their origin, heal through the interaction of complex physiologic and biochemical responses. Tissue integrity is re-established through a highly orchestrated tissue regeneration process, which can be supported by therapeutic management that optimizes the wound bed for healing. This chapter provides a basis for understanding treatment modalities of wound healing and soft tissue injury by addressing the physical properties of the skin, the physiology of wound healing, and factors that affect healing. Selected aspects of wound assessment and management throughout the trauma cycle also are discussed.

ANATOMY OF SKIN

The skin has a surface area of 1.5 to 2 m^2 and accounts for one sixth of total body weight, making it the largest organ of the body. It is one of the fastest growing tissues of the body, evidenced by complete replacement every 4 to 6 weeks. Healthy skin is critical to survival through its prevention of dehydration, its function as a barrier to external insults such as chemicals and microorganisms, and its role in the provision of thermal regulation. Regulation of body temperature is aided by the skin through covering and insulating the body to prevent heat loss, sweating to cool the body, and cutaneous vasodilation and constriction to release or retain body heat. The skin receives about one third of the circulating blood volume and plays an important role in maintaining homeostasis. The skin also provides sensory feedback about pressure, thermoperception, touch, and pain. Finally, body image, personal self-perception, and cultural values are affected by an individual's physical appearance. Traumatic injury, specifically traumatic wounds and scarring, can influence a person's self-perception and body image.[1]

Skin is an organ with great variety: it is thin and mobile in some parts, such as the eyelids, and thick and immobile in others, such as the back and soles of the feet. It overlies other soft tissues in some areas and various bony protuberances in others (e.g., the mandible, zygoma, and malleoli). Because of this diversity, the pattern and degree of injury will vary. Injurious modalities may impart low, medium, or high amounts of energy to the soft tissue envelope, depending on the particular mechanism of injury (e.g., motor vehicle crash, animal or human bites, blunt assault, or ballistic penetrating trauma). The skin may be abraded, avulsed, amputated, lacerated, contused, punctured, crushed, or bitten.

The integumentary system is composed of the skin and its appendages: hair, nails, and sweat and sebaceous glands. The skin is divided anatomically into two major layers: the epidermis and the dermis. The epidermis is the external protective layer, and the dermis, composed largely of collagen and elastic fibers, provides strength, elasticity, and protection against mechanical shearing forces. The epidermis is the outermost layer of the skin. It is further divided into the *stratum corneum* (cornified layer), *stratum lucidum* (clear layer), *stratum granulosum* (granular layer), *stratum spinosum* (prickle cell layer), and *stratum basale* (basal layer). The stratum corneum, which makes up the most superficial skin layer, is composed of nonviable keratinized cells, desiccated cells that are shed continually. The stratum corneum is also referred to as the horny layer. The stratum lucidum, located below the stratum corneum, is the transitional layer. Cells in this layer release lipid granules into extracellular spaces before movement to the stratum corneum layer. This lipid-rich coating protects the epidermis against aqueous solutions. The stratum granulosum lies below the stratum lucidum and is known as the granular layer. The next layer is the stratum spinosum, in which cells have spinelike structures that create bridges between them.[2] Stratum basale, also called the stratum germinativum or basal layer, is the mitotically active layer. Keratinocytes divide and begin the process of differentiation in this layer. This single layer of cells runs along the dermis, creating epidermal rete ridges. These cells engage in mitotic division in response to multiple stimuli, such as growth factors and chemoattractants (e.g., cytokines). The columnar basal cells undergo continual mitosis and are the source of new cells that eventually reach the stratum corneum. The epidermis is avascular, receiving nutrients from the blood vessels in the dermis and subcutaneous tissues.[3,4]

Migrating cells—melanocytes, Merkel cells, and Langerhans' cells—are distributed uniformly throughout the basal and suprabasal layers of the epidermis.[1-4] Melanocytes are responsible for producing melanin and giving rise to skin color. Carotene, oxyhemoglobin, and circulating substances in the plasma (e.g., bilirubin) are also present in the epidermis and will influence skin color. Merkel cells make up a small part of the basal layer and are believed to participate in the sensation of touch. Langerhans' cells are macrophages that function primarily in delayed hypersensitivity reactions. They also produce interleukin-1, which aids T-cell activation[2,4,5] and thus serve an important immune function. The basement membrane zone lies below the basal keratinocytes and is a very thin layer separating the epidermis from the dermis. The basement membrane provides mechanical support for the epidermis and allows for the transport of material between the layers.

The dermis lies between the epidermis and the subcutaneous tissue. The dermis is a connective tissue composed of fibrous proteins (collagen and elastin). The junction between epidermis and dermis is undulated with upward-projecting dermal papillae and downward-projecting epidermal rete ridges. The dermis nourishes the epidermis through its rich supply of vascular and lymphatic structures. There is a superficial layer, the papillary dermis, composed of interlacing fine collagen fibers, blood vessels, nerve endings, and thermoreceptors, and a deeper reticular layer of thicker bundles of collagen that provide the skin with structural support (Figure 16-1). Fibroblasts, located in the dermis, are the major differentiating cell type that becomes active during the wound-healing process. Fibroblasts are responsible for the secretion of collagen and elastin. Sensory receptors within the papillary dermis respond to pain, cold, heat, touch, and pressure. Dermal appendages, hair follicles, and sweat glands reside within the reticular dermis and extend upward through the epidermis to serve as an important source of epidermal regeneration during wound healing.

The subcutaneous tissue lies between the lower border of the dermis and the deeper fascia and muscle tissues. Although not generally considered a true part of the skin, it is closely associated with the dermis and is an important tissue to consider in terms of wound healing. The subcutaneous tissue functions to absorb shock, insulate, store nutrients, and

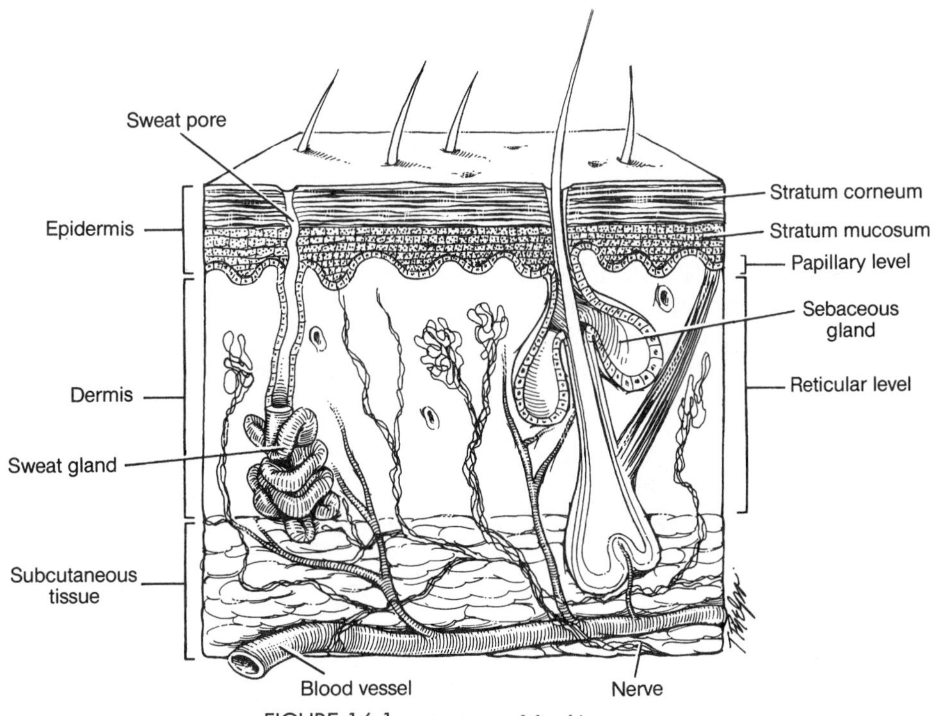

FIGURE 16-1 Anatomy of the skin.

shape the body contour. It is composed of many cells, including adipocytes, histiocytes, plasma cells, lymphocytes, and mast cells. Fat lobules of the subcutaneous tissue are surrounded by strands of collagen that contain nerves. Vascular and lymphatic networks travel from the fascia through the subcutaneous tissue and supply the dermis. There are few vascular connections between fat lobules and neighboring structures, which leaves the subcutaneous tissue vulnerable to decreased perfusion.[2-5] Altered vascular supply, or hypoperfusion of the subcutaneous tissue, has implications for wound healing. Complications of impaired healing such as infection often have their origin in subcutaneous tissue.

Traumatic injury may result in damage to any or all layers of the integument. A superficial abrasion involves the epidermal layer of the skin. Partial thickness injuries, the most common wound, involve the epidermal layer and a portion of the dermal layer. Full thickness injuries involve all epidermal and dermal skin layers and may affect subcutaneous tissue, muscle, and bone.

MUSCLE

Another soft tissue is muscle, which directly lies beneath the skin everywhere except at the bony protuberances. This chapter limits the discussion to the skeletal musculature. From a functional viewpoint, muscles accomplish motion—acting on bones across joints or acting directly on skin, as with the muscles of facial expression. Muscle has a high metabolic demand and is relatively intolerant of ischemia. Vascularity to muscle is immense, serving its higher metabolic demand. Although muscles provide important functions, some are expendable because of either redundancy in the system, whereby many muscles accomplish the same motion (e.g., gracilis and adductor magnus, which both adduct the thigh), or the vestigial nature of some muscles (e.g., palmaris longus or plantaris longus, which perform no function whatsoever in humans but are used by lower primates to cup the palm or sole).

NERVES

Nerves in the soft tissue serve two functions. The first is an afferent function, the retrieval of sensory information from the periphery to the central nervous system. These sensory nerves relay information on temperature, pain, pressure, position, and vibration from the joints and skin. The second function is efferent, signaling nerves leaving the central nervous system to execute action in the periphery. These motor nerves are directed to muscles or autonomic nerves that regulate involuntary functions such as sweating or vessel dilation.

Nerve injuries can be classified according to the Sunderland system (Table 16-1), which prognosticates the time and degree of functional recovery.[6] The extent of nerve damage is often unclear at the initial evaluation and can be surmised only by neurometric tests and serial examinations to evaluate functional progress.

PHYSIOLOGY OF WOUND HEALING

When the skin or internal organs are disrupted by trauma or surgery, a series of interdependent physiologic events occur that result in tissue repair (Figure 16-2).[7] The wound healing process is frequently described as three overlapping phases of healing—inflammation, proliferation, and remodeling. The tissue response has several major components: (1) hemostasis, (2) inflammation, (3) epithelialization, (4) angiogenesis, (5) fibroblast proliferation, (6) matrix deposition, (7) contraction, and (8) remodeling.[2-5] Through these responses, the process of wound healing is initiated, directed, and finally completed.

Wound healing occurs through primary or secondary intention or, alternately, by delayed primary closure, also called tertiary intention. In primary intention healing there is limited tissue loss, the wound is clean, and the wound edges are easily approximated with suture material or staples. In secondary intention healing, a large amount of tissue has been lost or the wound may be heavily contaminated. The wound is left open, and healing occurs through formation of granulation tissue, contraction, and re-epithelialization. In wounds with high bacteria counts, delayed primary closure is often used. The wound is cleaned and temporarily left open until the bacterial load decreases, at which point wound edges are approximated.

Tissue repair requires complex, overlapping, interdependent processes with multiple vascular, cellular, and biochemical responses. The actual time frame for healing varies depending on several factors, such as type of wound closure (e.g., primary or secondary intention) and patient factors (e.g., perfusion, nutritional status, edema, tissue oxygen

TABLE 16-1 **The Sunderland Classification System for Nerve Injuries**

Grade	Structures Injured	Name	Prognosis
I	Loss of myelin sheath	Neurapraxia	Complete recovery in days to months
II	Neural death but intact sheath	Axonotmesis	Complete return in months
III	Neural and endoneurial injury		Mild/moderate reduction in function
IV and V	Disruption of all nerve structures	Neurotmesis	Marked reduction in function

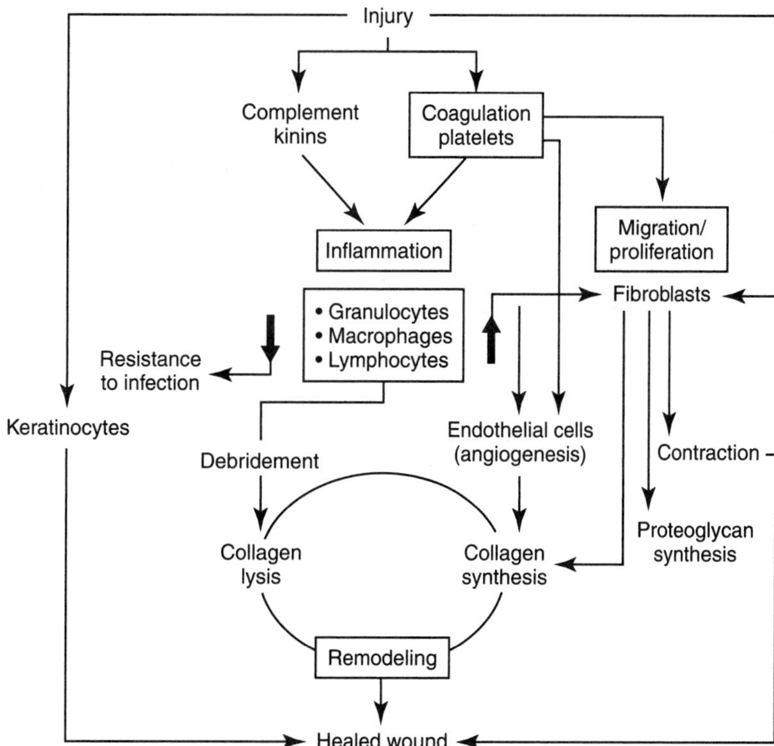

FIGURE 16-2 Schematic representation of wound healing. (From Hunt TK, Hopf HH, Hussain Z: Physiology of wound healing, *Adv Skin Wound Care* 13:6-11, 2000.)

tension, presence or absence of infection, and comorbid metabolic diseases). Generally, in acute wounds, hemostasis and the inflammatory phase begin the first day after injury. Migration and the proliferation phase begin shortly after inflammation and peak at 7 to 21 days. Remodeling and wound contraction begin about 3 weeks after injury and may continue for 6 months to a year (Figure 16-3).[8] The first days and weeks after injury are critical periods in the healing process because multiple cellular events occur.

HEMOSTASIS AND INFLAMMATION

When a wound extends through the epidermis, blood vessels are disrupted and collagen is exposed, activating the clotting cascade and initiating an inflammatory response. A clot is formed at the injured site and vascular vasospasm occurs, providing hemostasis. The clot that forms is made of platelets, collagen, thrombin, and fibronectin, and these factors release chemoattractants (e.g., cytokines) and growth factors that initiate an inflammatory response. The fibrin clot, in addition to hemostasis, provides a scaffold for the migration and proliferation of cells.[2-5,9-11] The initial response to injury and formation of a clot attract inflammatory cells (i.e., neutrophils) and several chemoattractants and growth factors, which orchestrate the inflammatory response.[9,10]

The complement system is activated with inflammation. Components of the complement system are proteins that facilitate bacterial destruction. Vasoconstriction at the wound site curtails blood flow and depletes oxygen delivery to the wounded tissues. Hypoxia after immediate wounding stimulates macrophages and initiates angiogenesis. Angiogenesis is the development of new blood vessels, a process that is essential in the proliferative phase of wound healing. Macrophages are considered vital to wound healing because they secrete essential cytokines that debride the wound, stimulate fibroblasts to produce collagen, promote angiogenesis, and stimulate keratinocytes.[2-5,11] Prolonged hypoxia impairs wound healing because it impairs the function of neutrophils and macrophages, increasing the risk of bacterial invasion.[4] Vasodilation of adjacent vessels follows vasoconstriction at the wound site, increasing perfusion and permitting plasma proteins to migrate into the wounded area with consequent edema, erythema, and pain.[4,11] Increased metabolic activity and blood flow elevates the temperature of the wound and surrounding tissue, resulting in the symptoms of erythema and warmth. Finally, fibroblasts respond to the multiple chemoattractants activated by the inflammatory process with stimulation of granulation tissue formation.

Inflammation is the body's immune system reaction to injury and is essential to normal wound healing.[4] The early physiologic responses to tissue injury accomplish hemostasis through clot formation with initiation of an inflammatory response. This vital inflammatory response begins to clear the wound of cellular debris and activates a series of cellular interactions necessary for repair of the wound.

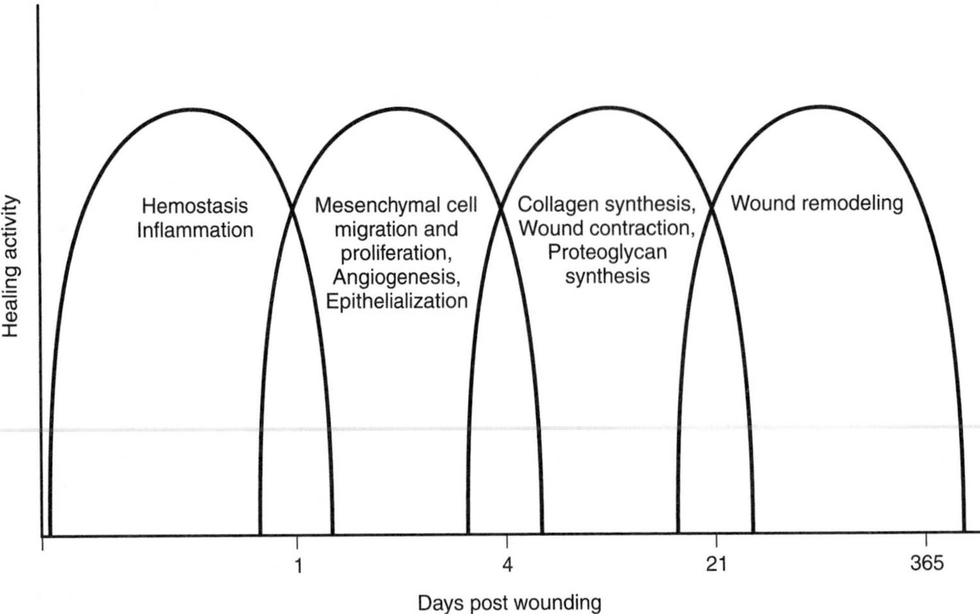

FIGURE 16-3 Phases of the healing wound. (From Lawrence WT: Physiology of the acute wound, *Clin Plast Surg* 25:321-340, 1998.)

CELL MIGRATION AND PROLIFERATION

The processes of cell migration and proliferation predominate 2 to 4 days after wounding and are mediated by chemoattractants and growth factors. This phase of healing is characterized by epithelialization, angiogenesis, and formation of collagen. The primary migratory cells are epithelial cells (keratinocytes), fibroblasts, and endothelial cells. Goals of this phase are effective resurfacing of the wound.[2-5]

The migration of epithelial cells across a wound provides protection against entry of bacteria into the wound and fluid loss. Within 24 to 48 hours of wounding, epithelial marginal basal cells enlarge, flatten, undergo mitosis, and migrate to cover the wound bed. The epidermal covering, composed of primarily keratinocytes, begins to differentiate and re-establish the protective barrier. This process is referred to as epithelialization. Cells migrate from one wound edge to an adjacent wound edge and from dermal appendages such as hair follicles. Cells move across the denuded area in a leapfrog fashion.[4,12] A moist wound environment enables the migrating cells to move across the wound surface more easily and quickly. Desiccation of wounds and eschar on the wound surface act as a deterrent to movement of epithelial cells. In wounds allowed to heal in a moist, protected environment, epithelial cells migrate on top of the wound. This is in contrast to wounds that epithelialize by cell migration under eschar that forms when a wound is allowed to become dry.

Angiogenesis occurs along with epithelialization, providing neovascularization of the wound bed. New tissue generation is dependent on nutrients supplied by the newly developed capillaries.[2] Concurrently, fibroblasts migrate to the wound site to synthesize and deposit collagen and extracellular matrix. Fibroblasts are sensitive to the partial pressure of oxygen and acidosis.[13] Local acidosis and hypoxemia initially stimulate fibroblast activity and angiogenesis; however, prolonged states of acidosis and hypoxemia will inhibit these same cells and their functions, slowing wound healing. Fibroblasts proliferate and synthesize collagen and extracellular matrix, resulting in granulation tissue covering the wound bed. New granulation tissue first appears as pale pink buds; as it fills with new blood vessels, it becomes bright, "beefy," and red.[4] This newly formed granulation tissue is very fragile.

New collagen provides strength and support to new tissues through its deposition and cross-linking in the injured area. Collagen is both synthesized and degraded in a continual process of wound repair. Over several weeks the collagen is remodeled and this process of collagen reorganization results in a stronger, tighter wound matrix. Unfortunately, the new tissue lacks the tensile strength of uninjured tissue and its strength is estimated to be no more than 80% that of healthy uninjured tissue.[5]

Wound contraction occurs during the proliferative phase of wound healing. It is the active process by which the area of a wound is decreased by contracting the extracellular matrix and wound edges. In this process new tissue is not formed; inward movement of existing tissue at the wound edge closes the area of the wound. Myofibroblasts, in granulation tissue, extend and retract pseudopods attached to collagen fibers, contracting the wound bed slowly (0.6-0.75 mm/day).[2-5,9-13] Wound contraction and remodeling will occur for approximately 6 to 24 months after injury.

REMODELING

As healing progresses, edema decreases and the numbers of fibroblasts recede. The local metabolic needs of the tissue decrease and the tissue enters into the final repair process, remodeling. This begins approximately 3 weeks after injury and continues for up to 24 months. The collagen is reorganized to increase strength of the new tissue. If there is excessive collagen synthesis, then a hypertrophic scar or keloid can result.[2-5] As the scar tissue matures, it also generally changes color and form. The early red, edematous, firm scar softens, lightens to pink, and becomes smaller. The scar tissue is strengthened through remodeling; however, the tissues only achieve approximately 80% of their original strength.

TYPES OF TRAUMATIC WOUNDS AND SOFT TISSUE INJURIES

CONTUSION

A contusion, or bruise, arises from rupture of subcutaneous blood vessels and extravasation of erythrocytes (Table 16-2). There is no break in the skin, but discoloration or ecchymosis, swelling, and pain are present at the site of contusion. A hematoma may accumulate at the site of ecchymosis.

HEMATOMA

A hematoma, resulting from rupture of a deeper and larger vein or artery, will expand in soft tissues until pressure in the area of hemorrhage exceeds the pressure within the disrupted artery or vein (see Table 16-2). Thus arterial hematomas, elaborated by arteries under greater pressure (mean arterial pressure is approximately 80-100 mm Hg) accumulate at a more rapid rate and to a larger size than do hematomas of venous origin. The size of the hematoma is also related to the capacitance of the tissues in which it forms. For instance, in the hand, where the tissues are not so distensible, the pressure will rise quickly as the skin starts to distend and tamponade the extravasation. However, in a region such as the thigh, several liters of blood may extravasate because the soft tissue envelope is more accommodating.

If a hematoma is present, fluid fluctuance, or a doughy ballotable mass, is appreciated on palpation. Postinjury edema makes distinguishing between hematoma and profound edema challenging. Focal ecchymosis overlying an area of swelling should signify a hematoma as well.

ABRASION

Abrasions suggest a friction mechanism of injury such as dragging (see Table 16-2). These injuries may be superficial (i.e., involving only the epidermis or partial thickness of the dermis) or they may be deep (i.e., violating the full thickness of the dermis). A partial-thickness abrasion demonstrates erythema and punctate bleeding and is painful. It is not unlike a partial-thickness burn. A full-thickness abrasion is white, does not bleed, and is painless because of injury to the sensory nerves as well. A partial-thickness abrasion may progress to a full-thickness loss of skin if it is not treated appropriately or if systemic resuscitation is suboptimal, resulting in tissue hypoxia and ischemia.

Traumatic abrasions are often contaminated with debris implanted into the skin, resulting in traumatic tattooing.[14] Gravel or road debris may become embedded, for instance, in a patient ejected during a motor vehicle crash. This mechanism of injury is suggested by linear streaking within the abrasion.

AVULSION

Avulsions result from stretching or tearing away of the soft tissues, creating a full-thickness loss (see Table 16-2). Unfortunately, the magnitude of an avulsion injury is often underestimated. Tissues that appear viable and salvageable on admission are frequently devitalized and unsalvageable the following day. This scenario is often repeated every 24 hours, with progressive loss of tissue. The tissue that remains behind is thus significantly compromised and declares itself viable or not over 48 to 96 hours.

LACERATION

Lacerations, compared with other soft tissue injuries, can appear to be a more elementary problem (see Table 16-2). Lacerations may be caused by trauma with a sharp object such as glass or a knife wound. The adjacent area of crush and devitalization in these mechanisms may be small, approaching surgical incisions. These linear lacerations approximate well and have an optimal chance to heal. Lacerations from a blunt mechanism of injury are associated with larger margins of contused and compromised tissues. Often visible around the laceration is a halo of erythema or ecchymosis, indicating that the absolute zone of injury is larger than that of a laceration caused by the sharp object (e.g., a knife), with a relative zone of injury quite large.

Lacerations that disrupt muscular tissues gap widely because of muscle contraction. Thus lacerations that divide muscles (e.g., across the full-thickness lip or eyelid) often give the appearance that tissue has been avulsed and is absent. By meticulously examination the functional elements, it can be ascertained that the tissues are present and can be reapproximated.

PUNCTURE WOUND

Puncture wounds carry a heightened risk of infection (see Table 16-2). Although they do not cause vast soft tissue destruction or lacerations, puncture wounds can set up an aggressive infection because they deliver bacteria or foreign inoculum deep into the body. Puncture wounds should not be closed so that any infections that may develop can be optimally treated. Animal bites are notorious causes of puncture wounds. A bite from a dog with large teeth often causes lacerations that have a lower likelihood of getting infected

TABLE 16–2 **Summary of Traumatic Wounds**

Type	*Description*	*Mechanism of Injury*	*Assessment*
Contusion/ hematoma	An injury that does not involve a break in the skin. Characterized by swelling, pain, and discoloration. The rupture of blood vessels causes extravasation of blood into the tissues, forming a hematoma	Caused by blunt trauma	Test for sensation and movement. Assess vascular involvement by measuring changes in the surface area of the bruise. Check for any underlying fractures
Crush injury	A composite injury involving two or more tissue types and graded severity of injury	Incident involving high energy exchange such as a fall of significant distance or a motor vehicle crash in which a part of the body is run over and crushed	Assess for size and anatomic location of crushed area. Check neurologic status and test for loss of function. Assess for tissue and blood loss and effect on underlying structures. Use invasive or noninvasive transcutaneous monitoring to detect increased compartment pressure (pressure exceeds diastolic arterial pressure)
Abrasion	A scraping or rubbing away of a layer or layers of the skin caused by friction with a hard object or surface. Abrasions vary in depth but are never deeper than the dermis	Often caused by motorcycle crash or any incident in which the patient is dragged or slides across a rough surface	Assess for size, depth, location, and degree of contamination. An abrasion covering a large amount of the body surface should raise concern for lost body fluids. Depth and number of exposed nerve endings affect the amount of pain felt. Location affects limitation of movement, especially if the abrasion occurs over a joint. Dirt and debris are commonly embedded
Avulsion	A tearing away of tissue, resulting in full-thickness loss. Wound edges cannot be approximated. Degloving injuries, which result from shearing types of force, are one type of avulsion	Caused when an extremity is cut by a meat slicer or saw or when an individual is thrown through the window in a motor vehicle crash	Assess for amount of lost tissue, location, loss of function, and damage to underlying structures. The amount of tissue lost determines the course of treatment (e.g., grafting vs. revision and use of a flap). A large avulsion may result in fluid loss. Disability and disfigurement particularly occur when the avulsion involves the hand or face
Amputation	An avulsion in which the affected limb is completely separated from the body	Caused when a digit or extremity is caught in a piece of equipment and is sheared off. Guillotine type of injury is caused when a digit or extremity is cleanly cut off by a power saw or similar tool	As with avulsion, assess for amount of lost tissue, location, loss of function, and damage to underlying structures. In addition, the separated part must be assessed for its viability after transport
Laceration/ incision	An open wound resulting from tearing or cutting of the skin. It is termed *superficial* if it involves only the dermis and epidermis and deep when it extends into the underlying tissues or structures	Caused by rupture of the skin when struck by a blunt force, producing a torn, jagged wound; or a sharp object such as a shard of glass can cut the soft tissue	Assess for damage to underlying structures and degree of contamination. Perform neurovascular checks to determine any sensory or motor deficits. Assess age of injury for degree of contamination and desiccation.
Puncture wound	A wound in which there is a small external opening in the skin but deep penetration of the underlying tissue	Caused by the penetration of the skin by a sharp or pointed object. A high-pressure spray gun or similar equipment produces numerous punctures	Assess for depth of penetration, degree of contamination, and any retained or injected foreign material. Appearance of surface injury may be benign. Assess for underlying tissue damage
Mammalian bites	An animal or human bite causing puncture and a crushing wound by the teeth and jaws of the mammal and resulting in a grossly contaminated injury	Caused by animal or human teeth and pressure from jaw force	Determine the source of the bite and potential for infection. Assess wound's age, depth, and size and damage to underlying tissue

Therapeutics	*Complications/*
Elevate the injured part and apply cold packs. Administer mild analgesics as required. May require up to 2-3 weeks for the hematoma to be reabsorbed	Development of compartment syndrome, in which blood and edema accumulates and increases pressure within a fascial compartment, compromising circulation and function of the affected area
Elevate and cool. Treat open portions as described above. Surgical intervention may be required for serial debridement, fasciotomy, and fracture stabilization. Measure urine myoglobin when extensive muscle damage is present	Complications include those of abrasions, avulsions, amputations, lacerations, and contusions. High risk of compartment syndrome. Amputation of crushed extremity may result
Local infiltration or topical application of anesthetic. Parenteral sedation for extensive abrasions. Meticulous cleansing by scrubbing with a saline solution– or surfactant cleanser–soaked sponge or surgical brush and copious irrigation. Do not use detergents because they produce additional pain. A needle, No. 11 surgical blade, or forceps may be required to remove embedded particles. Coat with antibiotic ointment and leave open or cover with nonadherent or occlusive dressing. Healing time varies with depth, location, and degree of contamination.	Direct sunlight may cause changes in skin pigmentation. "Traumatic tattooing," or the retention of foreign debris such as gunpowder, asphalt, and sand in the wound after healing, is characterized by a blue hue and a rough appearance
Thorough cleansing as described above. Control bleeding by direct pressure. Thorough irrigation with saline solution and early debridement of damaged tissue. Split-thickness grafting for closure when required. Complex avulsions may require use of a free flap placed with microvascular surgical techniques	Disfigurement and loss of function of the affected limb may result in changes in patient's body image and may affect vocation and avocations
Thorough cleansing as described above. Wrap amputated part in a dry, sterile dressing and place in a sterile plastic bag or container. Place wrapped part in an insulated cooler with ice. Do not freeze the amputated part. Properly managed, the part may be maintained for 6-12 hours before replantation	Infection and hypertropic scarring are the most frequent complications of amputations. Loss of viability or inability to replant the amputated part is related to mechanism of injury and warm ischemic time. Muscle in the amputated part is sensitive to ischemia and a large amount of muscle may have an adverse effect on the part's viability
Thorough cleansing and irrigation, with hemostasis by pressure and elevation. Necrotic wound edges should be excised and edges approximated and closed with suture or skin tape. Use antibiotic ointment and nonadherent or occlusive dressing. Dressing should provide some pressure to reduce swelling and hematoma formation. Splints or casts are used when immobilization is required	Sutures too tight or left in too long cause unsightly cross-hatching; sutures too loose cause wide scars. Improper approximation of the wound edges causes raised scars or tunnels that permit infection and hematoma formation. A loose dressing permits the wound to bleed and gaping to occur; a dressing applied too tight causes wound ischemia
Soak the wound and examine the tract of the penetrating object. Remove any foreign bodies and irrigate the wound. Filling the wound space may be required for adequate healing	Complications most frequently involve infection related to retained foreign material
Scrub and irrigate with povidone-iodine solution and apply cold pack. Bites more than 12 hours old should not have primary closure except in the face. Hand bites should be covered with a large bulky dressing. Plastic surgery may be required for facial bites. Antibiotic treatment is required in human and some animal bites. Tetanus and rabies prophylaxis may be needed	Infection from microorganisms in the saliva. Human bites produce both gram-negative and gram-positive infections

because the bacteria can work their way out. However, in contrast, because of their fine, needlelike teeth, cats can cause a deeper bacteria inoculum that seals over. Bacteria then flourishes and cannot egress, leading to a virulent infection.[15]

DETERMINANTS OF THE HEALING PROCESS

Physiologically, wound and soft tissue healing begins at the moment of injury and proceeds until tissue continuity is reestablished. Several local and systemic factors influence the healing process. These can be organized conceptually into a human response model that includes factors inherent in the person that increase vulnerability for impaired healing and environmental factors that present a risk for impairment of healing (Figure 16-4). Some factors may be modifiable, whereas others cannot; all are worthy of consideration to provide appropriate therapy and an environment that supports healing.

AGE

Advancing age influences healing. The elderly have slower cellular activity and multiple concurrent conditions, predisposing them to impaired healing.[16] In aging skin the epidermis thins gradually and is more easily stretched because of a decrease in elastin fibers. The dermal layer undergoes many changes with aging. There is a loss of approximately 20% in dermal thickness, which may account for the thinning appearance of elderly skin. Decreases in dermal cells, blood vessels, nerve endings, and collagen alter thermoregulation, sensation, and protective functions (e.g., moisture retention) of the skin with aging. The subcutaneous layer atrophies, decreasing the mechanical protection and insulation provided to the dermis. Additional factors such as lowered immunologic resistance, circulatory changes, and poor nutritional status seen in the elderly also contribute to altered wound healing. Older individuals frequently have more comorbidities (e.g., coronary artery disease, diabetes, pulmonary disease, etc.) that also compromise wound healing.[5] Because of these changes, aging skin is more prone to traumatic injury and generally takes longer to heal.

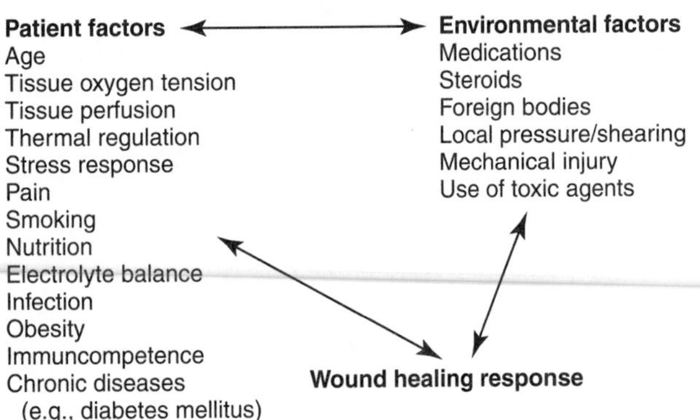

FIGURE 16-4 Human response model of factors that influence wound healing.

TISSUE OXYGEN TENSION

Oxygen is essential to meet the energy needs of biologic activity. In wounds, oxygen and perfusion play critical roles in the healing process and are related to many patient factors that influence healing. Ischemic and hypoxic tissues do not heal. An adequate supply of oxygen to the wounded area is needed for phagocytic activity of neutrophils and macrophages, angiogenesis, epithelialization, and synthesis and accumulation of collagen,[2-5,9-13] Compromised oxygen delivery to the wounded tissue will result in higher risk of infection, development of weaker collagen, and decreased tensile strength in the repaired tissues.[2,5,10,17] The rate of epithelialization is also dependent on tissue oxygen tension. Keratinocyte replication and migration requires oxygen.

Initially the disruption of the blood vasculature creates a local hypoxemic state that stimulates cytokines and growth factors to begin angiogenesis. Once angiogenesis begins, the success of new endothelial development is dependent on an adequate tissue oxygen tension.[2-5,9-13,17,18] Tissue oxygenation is essential for normal wound healing. It has increased importance when subcutaneous tissue and fascia are involved in the wounding process. Wound healing is slower in these tissues because of limited vascular supply and is further compromised in the presence of low oxygen tension.

PERFUSION

Oxygen delivery, along with the supply of neutrophils, macrophages, cytokines, growth factors, and nutrients, is closely linked to perfusion. Measurement of tissue oxygen tension provides information about blood flow to peripheral tissues. Decreases in tissue oxygen reflect insufficient blood flow, provided pulmonary status is normal. Changes in blood volume and perfusion during states of physiologic stress divert perfusion away from the skin, compromising oxygen delivery to cutaneous tissues.[17,18] Thus, tissue perfusion assessment should include evaluation of local vasoconstriction compromise at the wound as well as general perfusion (e.g., shock states).[5]

Multiple factors influence perfusion in the trauma patient. Excessive catecholamine release with traumatic injury and hypothermia induce vasoconstriction, which will compromise tissue oxygen tension. Intraoperative and vasoactive agents used to support the cardiovascular system may compromise peripheral perfusion to tissues.[2,5,10,17,18] Sepsis and systemic inflammatory response syndrome may further alter tissue perfusion and oxygenation through maldistribution of blood flow and excessive cytokine release.[9,17] Interventions to maximize perfusion to enhance wound healing should be addressed in the trauma patient's plan of care. Management should include support of cardiovascular and pulmonary systems, sometimes above normal, to preserve wound perfusion and tissue oxygenation.

Severe Anemia

Several factors can restrict tissue oxygen supply. Severe anemia is a patient element that influences tissue oxygen and, potentially, healing. Because oxygen is transported primarily by hemoglobin, there is concern that oxygen supply will be limited in patients with severe anemia. However, a number of studies indicate that anemia is not as serious a threat to healing as was once thought. Anemia in the presence of normal vascular volume and cardiac function does not impair wound healing until the hematocrit reaches a very low level (15%-18%).[13] At that point, transfusion is beneficial in terms of maintaining tissue oxygen supply.

Infection

Traumatic wounds are often contaminated with bacteria from the environment where the wound occurred. Wounds that contain more than 100,000 organisms per gram of tissue are at risk for subsequent infection. Fewer bacteria may result in wound infection in cases where local defense is compromised by necrotic tissue, dead space, or foreign bodies.

Again, tissue oxygenation is essential for the prevention and treatment of wound infection. Oxygen is used in the aerobic pathway of leukocytes for the killing of bacteria that have been introduced or that have migrated to the wound site. Oxygen is converted into free radicals that form a system of bactericidal agents. As leukocytes phagocytose bacteria, a primary oxidase in the cell membrane is activated that catalyzes an oxidation reaction, with subsequent killing of the bacteria. Recent evidence has shown that sufficient tissue oxygen levels are needed to resist infection.[10,17]

Immuncompetence of the patient will also influence the ability to resist wound infection. States of chronic stress, sepsis, and disease or drugs that compromise immunologic cells will deter the healing process but not absolutely inhibit healing.[2-5] A patient with a compromised immune system may require more meticulous wound cleansing and vigilance in the assessment for wound infection and progression of healing. The ability of the patient to mount an inflammatory response is essential to normal healing. Equally important, is that the inflammatory process proceed in an orderly fashion (i.e., initiate and cease) for wounds to heal. Wounds in which the inflammatory process is prolonged because of local or systemic factors heal more slowly and may be categorized as chronic.[13]

Smoking and Temperature

Smoking has several detrimental effects, including decreasing the amount of functional hemoglobin, causing peripheral vasoconstriction, and lowering tissue oxygenation. Smoking also increases platelet aggregation and blood viscosity and decreases collagen deposition, which negatively affect wound healing.[2-5]

Hypothermia may indirectly influence healing through the thermoregulatory responses it elicits, with subsequent vasoconstriction and lowered tissue oxygen. During and after extensive surgery, body temperature may drop below 36° C, invoking cutaneous vasoconstriction and shivering mediated through the sympathetic nervous system. Energy and oxygen consumption rise above resting levels, further increasing the need for adequate oxygen supply to tissues. In addition, leukocyte activity is also adversely affected by decreases in body temperature. It is well documented that prevention or correction of hypothermia decreases wound infection rates.[5,9,10,17]

Pain

When patients are in pain, the sympathetic nervous system is activated and catecholamines are released, increasing vasomotor tone.[5,17,19,20] The resultant vasoconstriction depresses wound tissue oxygen tension, compromising the healing process. Local perfusion to the wound cannot be ensured until patients have normal intravascular volume, are warm, are receiving no vasoconstrictive drugs, and are pain free. Cortisol is an adrenal glucocorticoid released in response to stimulation of the sympathetic nervous system. It is well documented that glucocorticoid impairs collagen synthesis.[20] However, it is not known whether physiologic levels of cortisol and adrenal glucocorticoids negatively affect the wound healing process.

Stress

Physical and psychologic stressors may impair healing. Physical stress to the edges of a wound can lead to partial or complete separation. The stress may be the result of strain, movement, or weight bearing on an injured extremity. Vomiting and abdominal distention also can disrupt chest or abdominal wounds. For this reason, adequate gastric decompression and drainage of bladder or wound cavities are important to avoid unnecessary stress on healing suture lines.

Psychologic stresses created by trauma evoke a neuroendocrine response. The sympathetic nervous system stimulation increases metabolic rate, catecholamine-induced vasoconstriction, oxygen consumption, and glucocorticoid levels. Collective responses decrease tissue oxygen tension and perfusion, negatively affecting wound healing.[17,21] Minimizing stressors may indirectly influence wound healing by reducing the stress response.[17]

Nutritional Status

Assessment and maintenance of nutritional status in trauma patients are discussed in detail in Chapter 17; however, several areas are notable for their effect on healing. Inadequate amounts of protein, fat, carbohydrates, calories, vitamins, and minerals contribute to impaired healing, problems with collagen formation, delayed development of wound tensile strength, and increased incidence of infection.[16,22,23]

Multiple trauma initiates a state of significant physiologic stress. The stress response is quite complex, encompassing inflammatory, endocrine, and central nervous system functions. The collective result is a catabolic state, frequently leading to depleted protein status and lowered serum proteins. Fewer amino acids are available for neovascularization, fibroplasia, collagen synthesis, and the formation of antibodies and leukocytes. Nutrients are needed to support the body's efforts in tissue reconstruction and the elevated metabolic demands.

Hypoalbuminemia itself is not a direct cause of poor wound healing.[23] However, hypoalbuminemia has been linked to increased morbidity and mortality rates.[17] Hypoalbuminemia is associated with a decrease in plasma oncotic pressure, tissue edema, and slowed oxygen diffusion. Albumin also serves as an important carrier for many substances, including cortisol and drugs. Adequate protein supplementation is necessary for tissue regeneration.[23]

Carbohydrates are needed in wound healing to provide glucose as the main substrate for energy production. Glucose is important as an energy source for leukocytes, cell proliferation, phagocytic activity, and fibroblast function. In the absence of glucose the body will continue the process of gluconeogenesis, further depleting protein stores and compromising wound healing. Maintaining normal glycemia is an important element in managing effective wound healing and minimizing infection.[24]

Water is a major constituent of the body and it is required for oxidation of nutrients. Water intake needs to meet metabolic needs. It needs to be sufficient to replace insensible fluid losses, gastric and fistula fluid losses, and fluid lost with diarrhea. Estimated fluid needs are generally equivalent to 1 ml of water for each calorie provided. Fluid intake should be sufficient to maintain good skin turgor and urine output. Maintaining adequate nutrition is complex in the multiple trauma patient and has a profound impact on the success of wound healing.

Electrolyte and Acid-Base Balance

Normal serum electrolytes and acid-base balance are essential for cell function. Potassium is necessary for maintaining protein anabolism for wound repair and may be lowered through loss of body fluids and in response to adrenocortical hormone release in trauma. Release of aldosterone can result in potassium loss and sodium retention, which in turn alters cellular responses. Phagocytosis is inhibited by hypernatremia and by elevated serum glucose levels. Serum pH has direct effects on cell motility. Acidosis decreases phagocytosis, thereby diminishing an essential component of the inflammatory response.

Preexisting Health Conditions

Primary vascular disease, diseases in which the immune system is compromised or depressed, states of malnutrition, and diabetes make an individual vulnerable to impaired healing.[2-5,9,13,17] Primary vascular disease compromises perfusion and interferes with the delivery of oxygen to the tissues. Immunocompetence is necessary for an appropriate inflammatory response and expression of macrophages needed for wound healing. Nutrition is essential for the anabolism required for tissue repair. Diabetes is associated with small-vessel disease, which can limit blood supply to the wound area, and hyperglycemia retards neutrophil function so that infection becomes a greater risk. Control of serum glucose levels to below 150 mg/dl is important in the prevention of wound healing complications.[24]

Principles of Wound Assessment Throughout the Trauma Cycle

Traumatic wounds result from the impact of an energy source applied against the skin and underlying structures. Initial assessment of the trauma patient is focused on the treatment of life-threatening conditions and, of necessity, precedes the exterior wound assessment and subsequent treatment. Once the patient's condition is stabilized, wound assessment is done as part of a thorough physical examination and the patient's history is obtained. Assessment information throughout all the phases of the trauma cycle provides the basis for development of the wound management plan. During this process, the patient is assessed thoroughly and is included as an active participant to the greatest extent possible. Patient involvement is generally limited only by physical condition. Many injuries that involve the skin are not life threatening, but they may have considerable psychologic impact, depending on a number of factors. For this reason, information about the patient's perception of the injury, its impact on daily living, and available support systems are included in the assessment.

Wound History

The wound history includes the details of the incident, including the time and the mechanism of injury. The age of the wound and the environment in which it occurred must be identified. It is important to estimate the time at which inoculum or bacteria was introduced into the wound. Efforts should focus on cleaning the contaminated wound before critical numbers of bacteria are reached, increasing the likelihood of local and systemic infection.[17,19,25-28] The environment of the wound includes both the location on the body and the source of the injury. The distribution of microorganisms on the body varies; in general, moist body folds harbor greater numbers than dry body areas. Information about the physical environment in which the wound occurred helps to predict the existence of foreign bodies in the wound space, such as clothing fragments and types of soil and dirt, which vary depending on the source. Similarly, an injury caused by a clean knife from the kitchen has different implications than one caused by mechanical equipment on a farm or a motorcycle crash on a city street. The organic components of soil and inorganic clay fragments have been associated with the development of wound infections, presumably because of their inhibitory effect on host defense systems.[5] Organic fractions are heavily concentrated in swamps, bogs, and marshes; clay fractions are largely located in the subsoil. Thus there is an increased risk of contamination and wound infection if injury occurs in swamps or excavation areas. Injuries that occur on farms have the potential for contamination with *Clostridium tetani;* the bacteria's natural habitat is the intestinal tract of domesticated animals, and it is consequently found in their excretions.

The patient's history also includes an assessment of concomitant disease, which may influence the course of healing, as discussed earlier. History of medication use, allergies, previous healing impairment, and tetanus immunization status are also pertinent to the wound treatment regimen.

Physical Examination

The physical examination is intended to detect sensory, motor, and vascular complications that may have resulted from the injury in addition to the physical wound. It is followed by assessment of the wound status, location, and configuration and the viability of tissue in and around the site of injury. Once this assessment is complete, initial wound treatments are planned and implemented.

Neurovascular Assessment

A comprehensive neurovascular assessment should be performed and documented before wound treatment is initiated to document the existence of complications related to the injury itself as opposed to treatment-induced complications. The components of the assessment are movement, sensation, color, temperature, presence of pulses, and edema. Comparison of the affected wounded area with its contralateral anatomic site is useful to determine disruption in neurovascular function.

The patient is tested for both sensory and motor integrity in the affected area. Both gross and fine motor functions are tested, including the flexion and extension of each joint and full range of motion of each extremity. Sensation distal to the wound can be tested grossly by discrimination between sharp and dull sensations. Systematic evaluation is based on knowledge of the major nerves serving the extremities (see Figures 16-5 and 16-6).

Perfusion and Tissue Oxygenation

The critical components of wound repair during the resuscitation phase, hemostasis, and initiation of the inflammatory process depend on perfusion and delivery of oxygen to the wounded tissues. Therefore clinical monitoring of circulation is essential. Distal and proximal pulses are

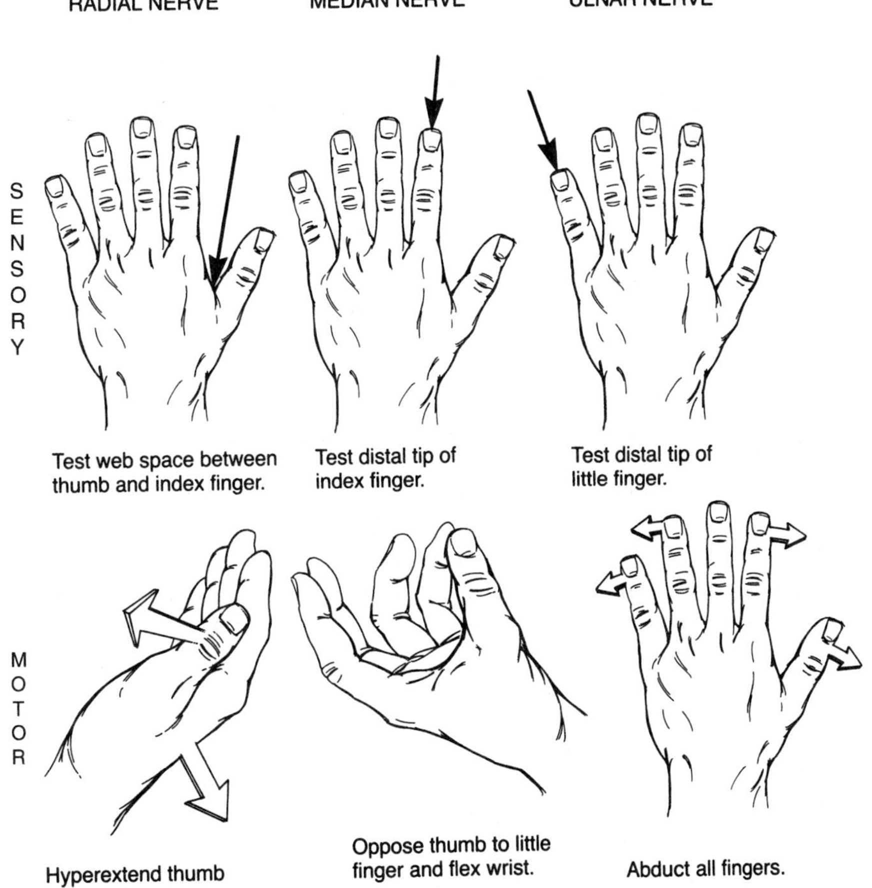

FIGURE 16-5 Upper Extremity Sensory-Motor Assessment.

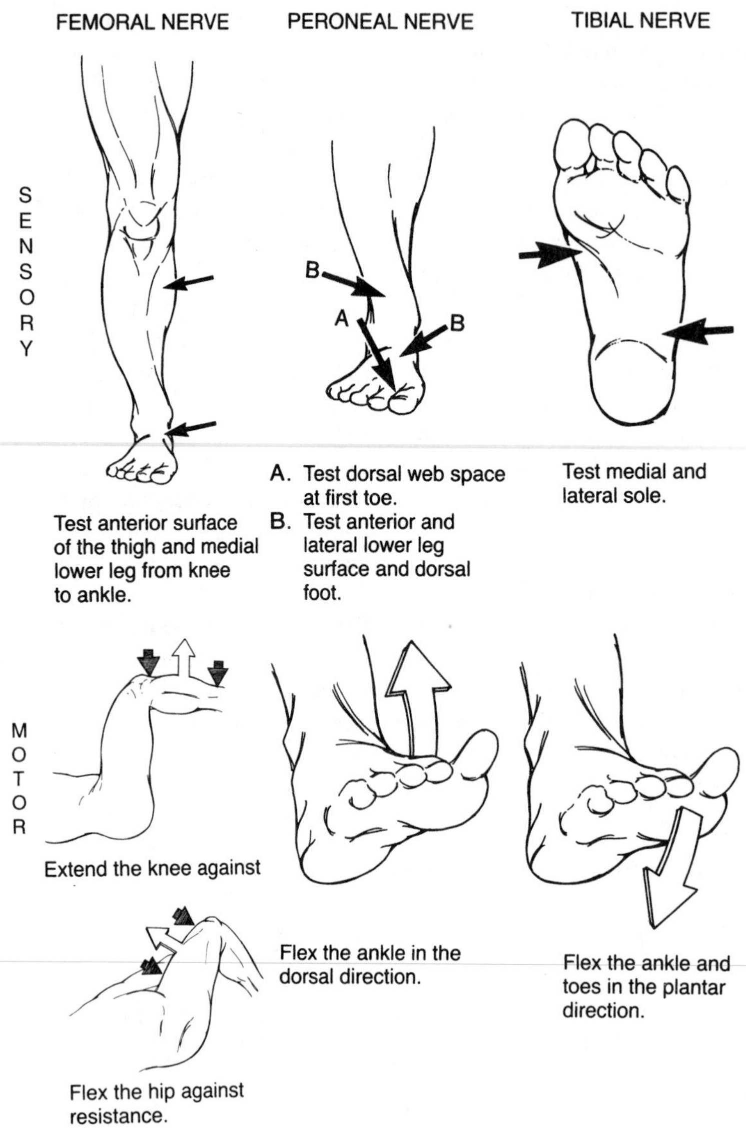

FIGURE 16-6 Lower Extremity Sensory-Motor Assessment.

assessed during the neurovascular examination to confirm the presence or absence of circulation to the affected area. Strong distal pulses provide a gross estimate of vascular supply. Pulses are palpated bilaterally and documented according to a 0 to 3+ scale, characterizing the pulse as absent (0), weak or thready (1+), normal (2+), or full or bounding (3+). Use of a Doppler ultrasound blood flow detector provides an auditory pulse when palpation is not possible. When wounds of the extremities cause tissue edema and diminished pulses, tissue pressure should be measured before the pulses are completely lost to detect the possible presence of compartment syndrome.[5] Arterial oxygenation should be assessed critically, both the saturation of hemoglobin with oxygen and the partial pressure of oxygen. As previously discussed, wound healing and prevention of infection rely on adequate tissue oxygenation.

The temperature of the wounded area is assessed by palpation with the dorsum of the hand. Wound area temperature is compared with the same region on the opposite side of the body. Temperature is significant to perfusion in the sense that cold elicits catecholamine release, which in turn decreases blood flow to the tissues.

Depth of Wound Injury

Assessment of the depth of tissue injury is necessary for the development of a plan of care. Depth of the wound bed can be described as superficial, partial thickness, deep partial thickness, or full thickness. Involvement of subcutaneous tissue, tendons, muscles, and bones is also evaluated. The extent of injury and tissue loss is considered, as is the presence of nonviable tissue. The location of the wound will also influence treatment choices (e.g., facial wounds versus lower extremity wounds).

Other Diagnostic Studies

Soft tissue damage often overlies other injuries such as fractures. For instance, periorbital ecchymosis ("black eyes" or "raccoon's eyes") is virtually pathognomonic for orbital, nasal, or basilar skull fractures. Findings of soft tissue disruption often trigger additional diagnostic studies to rule out or determine the extent of underlying injury.

Concern about the presence of an embedded foreign body may prompt additional diagnostic tests to confirm the presence, size, and location of the object. Radiographs can usually detect foreign objects that are radiopaque (e.g., metal, gravel, glass) if they are large enough to be visualized.[3,5,8] A computed tomography scan may also be useful in locating a foreign body and determining what disruption the object caused to surrounding tissues.

Wound Assessment in the Resuscitation Phase

Initially wound location and configuration are assessed. The location is considered in terms of the distribution of microflora on the skin and also the proximity of the wound to sources of contamination and the vascular supply. The effects that weight bearing and static and dynamic stress will likely have on the injured tissue also require consideration. The natural static and dynamic skin tensions that occur after wound closure influence the final appearance of the scar. Noting the extent that the wound edges are retracted and the difficulty in which the edges are reapproximated can predict the final wound appearance. Wound edges that are retracted more than 5 mm are exposed to stronger static skin tensions and heal with wider scars than do wounds with edges separated by less than 5 mm. Static tension is also influenced by wound configuration. It is sometimes not fully appreciated that jagged edged wounds, if carefully reapproximated, yield narrower scars than straight wounds because the magnitude of static tension is less per unit of wound length.[9]

Wound Assessment in the Critical Care Phase

Healing processes that typically coincide with the critical care phase include hemostasis, inflammation, fibroplasia and matrix deposition, angiogenesis, and epithelialization. Wounds that have been incised cleanly and closed will generally heal without problems; inflammation is minimal, and the distance required for new vessels to re-establish capillary networks is small. There is also relatively little need for matrix deposition and epithelial repair. These wounds present the patient with less of a metabolic burden than open wounds; however, in a compromised patient, healing may be problematic. Assessment of primary closure wounds includes observation initially for normal responses of inflammation, erythema, warmth, and induration along the suture line. Inflammation usually abates by the third to fifth day after injury, and by the seventh to ninth day a palpable healing ridge of collagen is present. The wound edges should be approximated. Impaired healing is indicated by the absence of an inflammatory response, absence of a healing ridge by the ninth day, and continued drainage along the incision, which indicates the lack of an epithelial seal.

Assessment of open wounds is vital to evaluate the progress of healing so that appropriate decisions are made regarding therapy. The location, size, and depth of open wounds need to be documented. This can be accomplished with wound tracings or by measuring the wound length, width, and depth. When the wound is measured, the patient should be in the same position each time measurements are made to control for the influence of body position on wound shape and dimensions. The wound is also assessed for tunnels (tracts) and undermining (pockets), and the location and depth of these are noted. It is important to remember that when wounds are debrided, they will likely increase in size, and this need not be interpreted as a delay in healing but as a necessity for healing to proceed.

Critical aspects of the wound, including the character of tissue in the base and sides and new epithelium on the edges and the presence of exudates, should be evaluated and documented. The characteristics of tissue, including color, moisture, and distribution, are documented. Healthy granulation tissue is deep pink to bright red and moist, with minimal amounts of exudate. Exudate, when present, varies in amount, consistency, color, and odor; these characteristics should be documented, as well as its distribution. Characteristics of exudate (purulent or serous) and amount of moisture in the wound bed may dictate different management regimens. For example, a dressing that is more absorbent may be necessary for a wound with a lot of exudate, whereas a moist wound that appears to be healing well may only require a protective dressing. Tissue that is very dark or black is necrotic and must be removed for healing to progress. True wound assessment cannot be completed in the presence of eschar.[29,30]

Growth of new epithelium is assessed on the wound edges. Its color and extent are important to note. Normally it is a light pink or pearl color. It should eventually be observable around the entire edge, extending across the wound as healing progresses. New epithelium also may be present, forming small pink islands around hair follicles.

A thorough wound assessment with documentation of the character of tissue, exudate, and epithelium is made daily or with each dressing change. Exceptions to daily assessment are made when the type of dressing dictates a less frequent changing schedule, which is the case with some of the biosynthetic dressings. In the acute-care setting, wound size should be documented weekly and with every dressing change, especially if the wound is actively debrided (e.g., sharp debridement).[31]

Wound Assessment in the Intermediate and Rehabilitation Phases

The extent to which a wound heals after trauma depends on many factors. These include the balance between metabolic demand and nutritional supply, cardiovascular and pulmonary status, and the existence of pertinent patient and environmental factors (reviewed previously). As the patient enters the intermediate and rehabilitation phases, the process of wound healing should be well established. The biologic processes of collagen synthesis, angiogenesis, and epithelial regeneration will likely continue through the intermediate phase, whereas remodeling and contraction will be the predominant processes in the rehabilitation phase. Primarily closed wounds should at this point have an epithelial seal and be gaining strength. The tensile strength of wounds cannot be observed or measured. However, the wound can be assessed for complete closure and the absence of inflammation and infection. If the wound is healing by secondary intention, the assessment strategy used in the critical-care phase remains appropriate. Generally, the wound should decrease in both size and volume as granulation tissue accrues and contractile forces operate to close the wound.

WOUND MANAGEMENT THROUGHOUT THE TRAUMA CYCLE

SYSTEMIC SUPPORT

Perfusion and Oxygenation

In the resuscitation and critical-care phases of recovery, adequate perfusion and supply of oxygen and nutrients to the wound area are crucial for optimal healing, in particular for the avoidance of infection. Systematic clinical assessment of perfusion, and in some cases oxygen tension and blood flow, as described in the section on assessment, remain appropriate evaluation strategies. Support of vascular volume is essential to ensure that needed nutrients reach the reparative cells. Clinical studies have documented that low tissue oxygen tensions are most common in the first 24 to 48 hours after surgery or injury, highlighting the necessity of maintaining tissue perfusion in the critical care period.[2,5,10,17] Treatment of hypothermia is important to consider, particularly if the patient has undergone surgery. Restoring normothermia will help prevent cutaneous vasoconstriction and may be important for resistance to infection by maintaining perfusion to injured tissues. In the presence of adequate perfusion, the use of supplemental oxygen is a rational therapeutic choice to sustain tissue oxygenation. An aggressive pulmonary hygiene plan, position changes, and, if possible, ambulation should also be considered in an effort to optimize tissue oxygenation.

In certain cases where tissue oxygen needs cannot be met through standard treatment modalities, hyperbaric treatment may be considered. Hyperbaric delivery of oxygen increases oxygen levels in soft tissues that are infected (e.g., necrotizing fasciitis) or slow to heal because of damage to the circulation. Although these tissues may be hypoperfused, at least some degree of blood supply must be present to effectively deliver oxygen to the wound site. With hyperbaric oxygenation, the cellular use of oxygen is the same as in any wound; leukocytes, fibroblasts, endothelial cells, and other cells in their reparative roles of bacterial control, collagen synthesis, and angiogenesis use oxygen.[2,5,32,33]

As healing progresses in the intermediate and rehabilitation phases of recovery, perfusion and tissue oxygen supply remain important and should continue to be supported. The emphasis and extent of treatment depend on wound status, which highlights the importance of continuing, thorough assessment of the injured site. In primarily closed wounds that are healing without complications, interventions focused on optimizing cardiopulmonary status and ensuring adequate oral intake to support nutrition and avoid dehydration are likely to be sufficient. Wounds healing by secondary intention presents greater metabolic demands. Maintenance of sufficient peripheral perfusion and oxygenation, with careful attention to volume status and in some cases supplemental oxygen, may be necessary to sustain healing.

Nutrition

Nutritional status should be assessed early in the critical-care phase and a plan for support developed. In the critical-care phase it is important to provide energy for phagocytosis and the beginning reparative processes such as angiogenesis, collagen synthesis, and matrix deposition. It is also critical to the support of wound healing that provision of nutrients be implemented quickly in the course of treatment and not be delayed. Chapter 17 presents detailed information on nutritional therapy during this phase.

Depending on the status of the wound, nutritional demands for healing will vary during subsequent trauma phases. Open wounds that continue to synthesize new tissue will naturally have greater energy requirements than wounds that simply have the edges reapproximated. For wounds demonstrating evidence of progressive healing, if the nutritional needs of the whole patient are met, it is likely that nutrition is adequate.

INFECTION CONTROL AND ANTIBIOTICS

Prevention of wound infection is best accomplished by ensuring adequate debridement of the injured tissue. Removal of devitalized tissue, fluid collections, and foreign matter eliminates a nidus for infection, thereby reducing risk. Irrigation to rinse away contaminants also reduces the bacteria load in the wound. As previously described, efforts to ensure adequate tissue perfusion and oxygen delivery, adequate nutrition, normoglycemia, and electrolyte and acid-base balance all promote wound healing and lower the likelihood of infection.

The use of antibiotics can affect the outcome of healing, but successful therapy depends largely on when they are administered. Prophylactic antibiotics are considered when the risk of infection is high or when the results of an infection would be life threatening.[5,9,10,17] However, wound infection must be treated regardless of when it occurs.

With traumatic wounds, a heavy bacterial load is most common early after the patient's injury, (i.e., prehospital and resuscitation phases of trauma care). In addition to early, aggressive cleansing of the wounds, possible use of prophylactic antibiotics may be indicated, depending on circumstances surrounding the traumatic event (e.g., farming or industrial incident) causing soft tissue injury. Tissue in which repair is well established or the wound bed has healthy granulation tissue is usually resistant to infection. Ideally this situation exists by the time the patient enters the intermediate and rehabilitation phases of recovery.

If the wound is healing by secondary intention, the presence of foul drainage, increased amount of wound exudates, a pale wound bed, failure for granulation tissue to progress, erythema at the wound edges, leukocytosis, and pain at the wound site are signs and symptoms that should be further explored for a possible wound infection. The presence of wound infection may be evaluated by clinical examination, swab culture, or tissue culture. Although swab cultures are the most frequently used method, they are easily contaminated, leading to false-positive results and may significantly underestimate bacterial counts in the wound bed.[15] Tissue cultures, although more invasive (requiring a sample of tissue), are more accurate in isolating wound bacteria.[15] As soon after a wound infection diagnosis is made, systemic antibiotics should be instituted and should be matched to the sensitivities of the infecting organism.[5,9,10,17,34] Local antibiotics may be used alone to treat a focal wound infection or may be used as an adjunct for patients already on systemic antimicrobials to obtain high concentrations in the wound without systemic side effects. However, local antibiotics have several disadvantages: cutaneous sensitization, development of bacterial resistance, inhibition of wound healing, and inactivation of the antibiotic by the wound.[17]

PROGRESSIVE PHYSICAL ACTIVITY

The effects of activity on wound healing are not well documented. In the early phases of recovery from trauma some immobilization and physical support of the wound area to avoid stress on newly injured tissues are important. Wounds, when immobilized, should be in the position of maximal function. Splinting may be required to optimize wound positioning and function. At the same time, any activity that the patient can tolerate (e.g., turning) is likely to be beneficial through indirect cardiopulmonary effects. Physical activity improves oxygenation in peripheral tissues through improvement of the ventilation to perfusion, provided that cardiac output and peripheral flow are adequate.

In the intermediate and rehabilitation phases a progressive plan for physical activity may enhance healing. Motion and mild stress applied to wounds have been associated with increased wound strength, although the mechanism is not clear.

WOUND CLOSURE AND DEBRIDEMENT

Wound Closure

Decisions about wound closure depend on the type of wound, amount of tissue loss, and extent of contamination. When tissue loss and contamination are minimal, primary closure is the likely method of choice. Factors that influence the decision regarding the type of closure material include wound location, configuration, tension that will be applied to the wound, and desired cosmetic result. Sutures are used most commonly for primary closure (Figure 16-7).[35] Sutures that lose their tensile strength within 60 days are classified as *absorbable; nonabsorbable* sutures maintain their tensile strength beyond 60 days. Techniques of suture closure for skin include percutaneous (passing through epidermal and dermal layers) and dermal. Small wounds that are not exposed to significant tension or stress can be closed with adhesive strips. Tape closure is useful for linear wounds in areas where tensions are low. If tissue loss is extensive, grafts or flaps will be required.

In some cases the wound heals by secondary intention through the processes of granulation tissue formation, contraction, and epithelial migration. However, the final scar is generally larger and the resulting deformity greater. The timing for wound closure is dependent to a large extent on the degree of contamination. Delayed primary closure, or tertiary closure, may be used with contaminated wounds. The benefits of delayed wound closure for contaminated wounds are well recognized; wound infection and dehiscence can often be avoided. The use of delayed primary closure enhances the development of a healthy granulation bed that resists infection and is prepared for subsequent grafting or closure, usually within a few days of the original injury.

Debridement

Debridement is a traditional, accepted approach for the removal of necrotic tissue (eschar) and debris from the wound. Devitalized tissue promotes bacterial growth and diminishes leukocyte function. Epithelialization cannot progress until the wound is free of eschar. Eschar may be removed by sharp, autolytic, mechanical, or chemical debridement.

The most rapid and efficient method of debridement is sharp surgical debridement.[30] Sharp debridement is the process of excising necrotic devitalized tissue from the wound bed. Healthy tissue is usually lost in the process, creating a larger wound. Sharp debridement gives the rapid result of a clean wound bed and it is the method of choice when the wound is creating a source of potentially life-threatening infection. Disadvantages include pain and creation of a larger wound.

Autolytic debridement is a process initiated by covering the eschar with a synthetic dressing (gel, hydrocolloid, or film). The body's moisture, macrophages, and cytokines are trapped over the necrotic tissue and begin to rehydrate, soften, and, finally, liquefy the hard eschar.[35] Autolytic debridement is a selective process that destroys only the

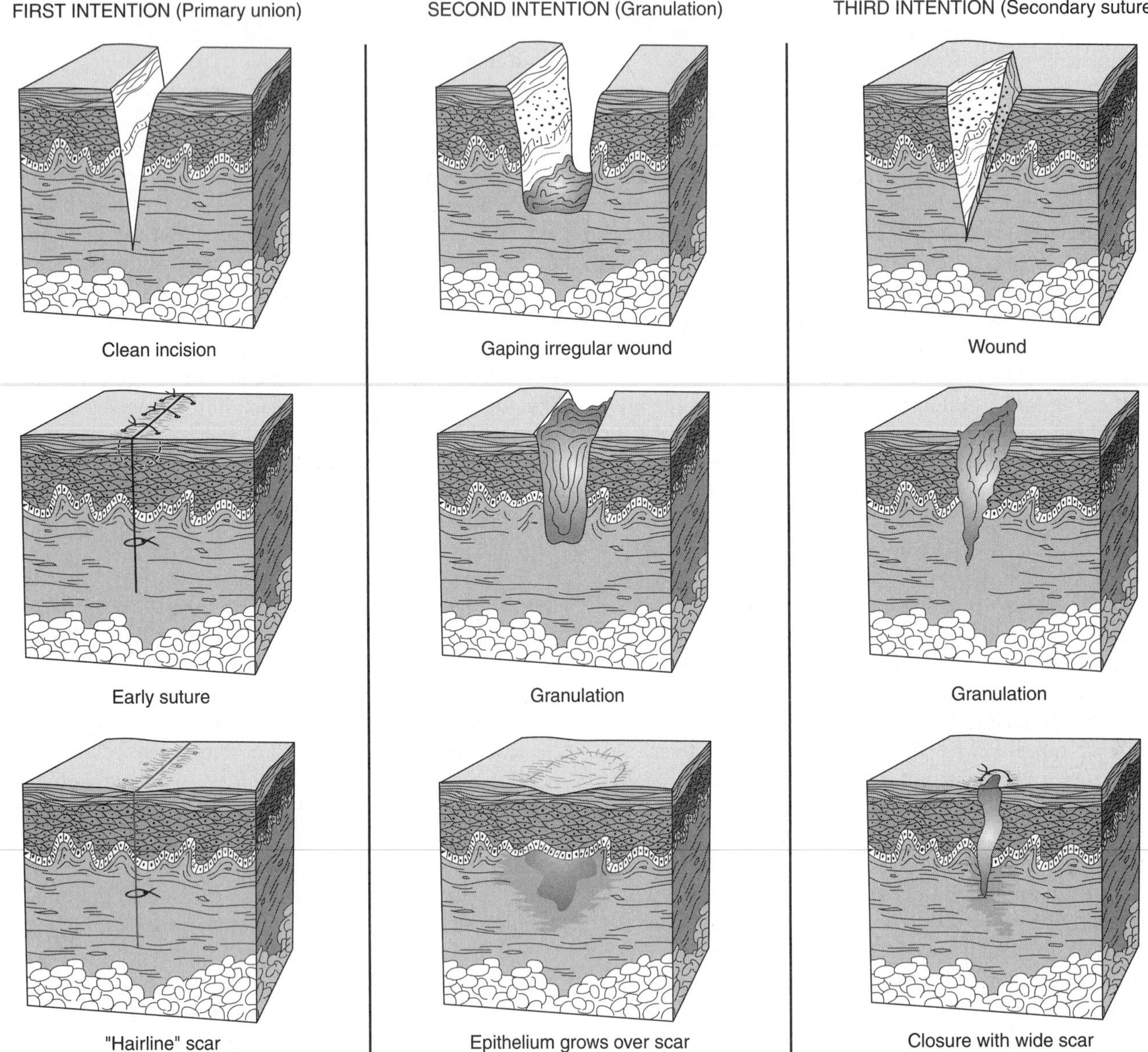

FIGURE 16-7 Wound healing by primary, secondary, and tertiary intention. (From Makic MB: Cleaning, irrigating, culturing, and dressing an open wound. In Wiegand DJ, Carlson KK, editors: *AACN procedure manual for critical care,* pp. 1103-1111, St. Louis, 2005, Elsevier.)

necrotic tissue. The process takes about 4 to 7 days, does not cause pain, and is the best option when a wound is not in need of immediate debridement.[36] Mechanical debridement is a nonselective procedure in which wet dressings are placed in the wound bed, allowed to dry, and then removed. On removal of the dry dressing, healthy granulation tissue as well as the necrotic tissue is removed. The process is very painful and damaging to viable tissues. The primary advantages of mechanical debridement include effective wound irrigation with dressing changes and familiarity of the procedure by the health care provider.[36] Disadvantages include the nonselective debridement of necrotic and healthy tissue, pain, maceration to surrounding tissue, and increased cost of supplies and nursing time associated with this method of debridement.[31,36,37] Despite the disadvantages noted, mechanical debridement with wet-to-dry gauze dressings continues to be a commonly used debridement technique.

Hydrotherapy is also considered a means of mechanical debridement. Irrigation uses mechanical force to remove debris and bacteria from the surface of wounds. Contaminants and particles are removed when irrigation pressure exceeds adhesive forces.[35,38] High-pressure irrigation, defined as 4 to 25 pounds/square inch (psi), will remove particulate matter and bacteria more effectively than will low-pressure irrigation. Low-pressure syringe irrigation, such as with a bulb syringe, removes large particles but not smaller contaminants and bacteria. An effective high-pressure system can be created with a 19-gauge plastic needle, a 35-ml syringe, and sterile normal saline solution to achieve an approximate psi of 15.[35,38,39] Concern has been raised about potential damage to tissues from high-pressure irrigation systems. The pressure needs to be sufficient to clean the wound effectively, but it should not traumatize the healing tissue. Pressure greater than 25 psi will traumatize the healing tissues and impair the wound's ability to resist infection.[39]

Chemical, or enzymatic, debridement is accomplished by applying topical debridement agents to remove devitalized tissues on the wound surface.[36] Enzymatic debridement may be used when the patient cannot tolerate sharp debridement and removal of necrotic tissue may be achieved more gradually. Debridement with enzymatic agents will be complete in 3 to 30 days, depending on the agent used.[31] Enzymatic agents are highly selective, causing debridement of only the devitalized tissue, thus promoting wound healing simultaneously.

Antiseptic Agents

Adequate and aggressive wound cleansing with use of controlled irrigation and nontoxic solutions will assist the healing process. Antiseptic agents such as povidone-iodine, sodium hypochlorite solution (Dakin's fluid), acetic acid, and hydrogen peroxide should not be used to cleanse the wound because they are toxic to fibroblasts and delay healing.[12,21-24] If an antiseptic is needed for cleaning, chlorhexidine (Hibiclens) has been shown to reduce bacterial counts and have less toxic effects on wound tissue. The use of nontoxic normal saline solution and high-pressure irrigation remains the best method for removing bacteria and particulate matter and cleansing a wound.[38,39]

Dressings: Principles and Techniques

Once the wound has been cleansed, debrided if necessary, and assessed, appropriate dressing materials must be chosen. Before the early 1960s, wounds were thought to heal more quickly and better if kept open to the environment and allowed to form a dry crust. Classic work by Winter[40] and Hinman and Maibach[41] revealed that partial thickness wounds heal twice as fast under occlusion than wounds exposed to air. Numerous studies have since supported this early work, advocating the provision of a moist wound environment to enhance and expedite the wound healing process.[12,13,42] In a dry environment epidermal cells are inhibited from migrating and resurfacing the wound because they must burrow between eschar and the underlying tissues. In a moist environment cells migrate more easily and enhance the resurfacing process. A moist environment enhances healing, but a wet environment may hinder healing by macerating healthy tissues that surround the wound. Excessive drainage and perspiration need to be considered when selecting an appropriate wound dressing so that excessive moisture in the wound bed is prevented. Infections are reduced in a moist wound environment. Wound occlusion actually reduces the risk of infection by maintaining the inflammatory cells that destroy bacteria and foreign materials in the wound bed.[12,13,42]

The dressing of choice during any phase of wound healing depends to a large extent on the characteristics of the wound, including whether it is closed primarily or left open. A myriad of wound-covering products are available, and it is probably best to make choices on the basis of some simple but important moist-wound healing principles. In general, wound treatments (dressings) should protect the wound from further injury, remove infection and necrotic tissue, support the body's tissue defenses, eliminate dead space, prevent excess exudates in the wound, and provide an optimal moist environment for healing.[31,42] Table 16-3 illustrates the basic characteristics and designs of commonly available dressings. Dressings that come in contact with a wound bed are considered primary dressings. Secondary dressings are those dressings that cover a primary dressing or secure a dressing in place. Dressings listed in Table 16-3 may be either primary or secondary dressings, depending on the application.

Wounds with excessive exudate need special consideration. Wound care should minimize periwound maceration to prevent destruction of healthy tissue because of excessive moisture. Periwound protection can be achieved by using protective barrier creams around the healthy skin. Excessive exudate can be managed with absorbent dressings (i.e., calcium alginate dressings) or more frequent dressing changes. Wound drainage systems that remove exudate and enhance angiogensis by application of negative pressure therapy may also be used with highly exudative wounds.[12,38]

Primary Closure Wounds

A primarily closed wound is most often covered with a protective dressing that may be layered if drainage is expected. A nonadherent dressing may be used as the first layer to avoid disruption of new epithelium when the dressing is removed. The next layer is absorbent to collect exudate, provide light pressure and support, and immobilize the local tissues. The top layer provides external support and protection. Coverings over primary closure wounds are usually needed for 2 to 3 days until the wound surface is sealed with epithelial cells.

Partial-Thickness Wounds

Wounds that are open will require different dressings depending on their characteristics. Partial-thickness wounds, such as dermabrasions, that mainly require epithelialization to heal and that are not heavily exudative can be covered with a product designed to provide a moist environment that supports cell migration. Several types of semiocclusive/occlusive dressings may be used to heal a partial-thickness wound. Polyurethane film dressings trap fluid next to the wound, do not adhere to the wound surface, and do not absorb fluid. Hydrocolloid and hydrogel dressings absorb moderate amounts of fluid, do not adhere to the wound, provide autolytic debridement, and can be used to cover partial-thickness wounds.

Although risk of infection is not increased with the use of occlusive dressing, caution should be used in the presence of

TABLE 16-3 **Categories of Wound Dressings**

Category of Wound Dressing	Characteristics/ Functions	Advantages	Disadvantages
Gauze	Coarse or fine mesh cotton dressing Size of pore in dressing will determine absorptive and debridement qualities of dressing	Primary dressings for wet-to-moist nonselective mechanical wound debridement May be used as a secondary absorptive layer	Nonspecific debridement Painful on removal May damage healthy granulation tissue with removal and cause minor bleeding
Nonadhesive dressings and nonadhesive impregnated gauze (e.g., Telfa, Vaseline gauze)	Nonadherent fine-mesh gauze impregnated with emollient or hydrophilic agent Does not adhere to wound May assist in creating a moist wound environment that promotes autolytic debridement	Primary dressing over a wound closed by primary intention to protect the wound and enhance healing Nonadherent Provides moisture to wound surface Reduces pain; provides comfort May require a secondary dressing to secure	Nonabsorptive May require a secondary dressing
Film dressings	Semipermeable dressings Waterproof yet permeable to oxygen and water vapor Prevent contamination of wound by exogenous bacteria Maintain moist wound environment, facilitate cellular migration, and promote autolytic debridement Minimal absorptive properties	Transparent, so wound progress can be evaluated without removal of dressing Waterproof and gas permeable Maintain moist environment Dressing may remain in place for up to 7 days Best used on superficial wounds Retention of a primary moist healing dressing	Adhesive, so they can tear healthy tissue with removal Minimally absorptive Tend to roll off wounds in high friction areas (e.g., coccyx)
Hydrocolloid dressings	Occlusive and adhesive wafer dressings Combine absorbent gel-forming agents with outer adhesive film or foam dressing Can be used on light to moderately draining wound Most react with wound exudates to form gel-like covering that protects wound bed and maintains moist wound environment Hydrocolloid powders and pastes also available for increased absorptive capacity	Waterproof Protects granulating and epitheli-zing wounds with low to moderate amounts of exudate Comfortable for easy application to body sites with curves and creases (e.g., coccyx, heel) May reduce pain at wound site Promotes autolytic debridement May be left in place for 3-5 days	Moderate to heavy exudative wounds overwhelm hydrocolloid dressings and create leakage Impermeable to oxygen; not recommended for wounds with suspected or known anaerobic infections Odor on removal of dressing may be unpleasant (from mixture of wound fluid and dressing matrix materials) Increased awareness is necessary when used around the rectum because of possible contamination More frequent dressing changes are needed with increased wound exudate
Hydrogels	Broad classes of polymer dressings that are hydrophilic and provide a moist wound environment Provide moisture to dry wounds Free flowing and can be used to fill wound spaces; easily conform to large wounds to fill cavity spaces	Effective cleansing and debride-ment of necrotic and sloughy wounds by increasing moisture contents, aiding in autolytic debridement Decrease pain at wound site Do not adhere to wound	Require a secondary dressing Caution should be used with infected wounds Minimally absorptive

TABLE 16-3 **Categories of Wound Dressings—cont'd**

Category of Wound Dressing	Characteristics/ Functions	Advantages	Disadvantages
Hydrogel sheet dressings	Most hydrogel sheets are cross-linked polymer gels in sheet form Similar properties to hydrogels; provide moisture to the wound; are minimally absorptive	Comfortable dressings that help reduce pain Aid in autolytic debridement	Minimally absorptive May require a secondary dressing to secure in place
Foam dressings	Highly absorbent dressings, generally made from hydrophilic polyurethane foam Some have adhesive backing; others require secondary dressing to secure to wound surface Foam dressings absorb large amounts of exudate, reducing maceration while promoting healing	Comfortable and easily conformable to body contures Very absorbent Can be left on wound 3-4 days, depending on amount of drainage No dressing residue in wound bed on removal Provide thermal insulation May be used under compression dressings	May dry wound if there is too little exudate May require a secondary dressing to secure in place
Alginates	Consist of calcium and are usually made from seaweed Absorb wound exudate and form moisture/vapor-permeable, gel-like covering over wound Maintain moist environment while absorbing excess exudate Highly absorbent dressing	Very useful for packing wounds with moderate to large amounts of exudate Conform to wound contours Several have good "wet strength" and can be removed in one piece	Require secondary dressing Risk of drying wound bed with low volumes of exudates Wound may need to be well irrigated with some alginates to ensure full removal of product from wound cavity
Silver-impregnated dressings	Silver ions are incorporated into dressings to provide antimicrobial activity	Provide antimicrobial activity to wound bed Available in multiple forms from creams, to nonadherent dressings, to alginates with silver	Absorptive properties are related to the dressing in which the silver has been added; may range from nonabsorptive to moderately absorptive Amount of silver is not consistent in all dressings; refer to manufacturer product information for contents of silver found in a dressing product
Antimicrobial gauze dressings	Combines absorptive properties of gauze with antimicrobial properties of polyhexamethylene biguanide	Effective in packing wounds with high amounts of exudate Effective in local treatment of wounds contaminated with *P. aeruginosa*	Frequent dressing changes necessary Nonselective debridement

gram-negative bacteria, which thrive in moist environments, and in patients who are immunosuppressed. More frequent assessment of the wound under occlusion may be necessary with contaminated wounds and immunosuppressed patients. Care also should be taken to avoid the entry of microorganisms from outside the wound through the provision of a tight wound dressing seal.

An additional apparent benefit of semiocclusive/occlusive dressings is the relief of pain associated with the wound, particularly for dermabrasions and skin graft donor sites. In addition to pain relief, there are advantages in terms of the final cosmetic result when semiocclusive dressings are used.[31] Although semiocclusive dressings may be more expensive, the cost for treatment is lowered by virtue of the decreased frequency of dressing changes. The relevance of these benefits should not be minimized. Increasing patient comfort is a significant contribution to care. Also, as mentioned previously, effective pain management enhances wound healing by limiting catecholamine response. Semiocclusive/occlusive dressings also improve scar appearance and are particularly important for wounds in highly visible areas.

Healing of Deep Partial-Thickness and Full-Thickness Wounds by Secondary Intention or Delayed Closure

Deep partial-thickness and full-thickness wounds may require more extensive dressings that offer greater absorption in addition to maintaining wound moisture. In wounds that are not necrotic or heavily exudative but have some depth, a simple wet-to-damp saline solution, fine-mesh gauze dressing will provide a moist environment for the wound bed and margins. If removal of exudate is needed, coarse gauze is recommended because fluids will move from the wound into the interstices of the gauze layers and then can be removed when the dressing is changed. Wet-to-damp or wet-to-wet dressings are removed before they dry, thus protecting fragile new capillaries from damage when dressings are allowed to dry and adhere to the wound bed.

Hydrocolloid, hydrogel, alginate, or foam dressings can be applied to deep partial-thickness and full-thickness wounds. In wounds with exudate, they are absorbent to the extent that there is moisture available. These dressings, as discussed earlier, provide a moist healing environment, conform to the wound, occupy dead space, enhance healing, and increase comfort. Absorptive properties of these dressings vary, and the amount of wound exudate should determine which dressing is selected.

Open wounds that produce large amounts of exudate can be dressed traditionally with gauze packing and multiple superficial layers to absorb fluid. Frequent changes of these dressings will manage excess drainage and remove contaminants from highly exudative wounds. Absorbent dressings are also available. They are placed into the wound cavity and covered with a secondary dressing. Again, interventions to protect the periwound tissue are necessary in the treatment of draining wounds. Wound fluid and bacteria become trapped in the spaces of the absorbent materials and are removed from the surface of the wound, reducing mediators of inflammation and infection and improving the granulation bed environment. Negative-pressure therapy or vacuum-assisted closure can be used to effectively remove excess exudate and has the added benefits of helping to reduce edema, promote angiogenesis, and enhance wound closure.[38] This therapy uses a sponge dressing placed inside the wound attached to a drainage tube and covered with an airtight outer dressing. Vacuum pressure is attached to the drainage tube to create a prescribed negative pressure (i.e., 125 mm Hg). The vacuum removes exudate from the wound to a collection container.

Grafts, Flaps, and Biologic/Biosynthetic Techniques for Wound Closure

A deep partial-thickness or full-thickness wound may require 14 to 21 days to heal on its own.[43-45] Grafting of the wound may be necessary to decrease the risk of infection, speed healing, and provide better cosmetic results. Skin grafts may be full-thickness sheet grafts or meshed partial-thickness grafts. Location of the wound, donor sites available, and cosmesis are factors used to determine the type of autograft. Skin graft "take" is a process that lasts several days. The grafted skin needs to maintain a close approximation to the wound bed for optimal adhesion of the graft. It is important that no fluid collections, such as seroma or hematoma, arise between the skin graft and the wound bed because this will impair diffusion and lead to graft loss.[38,43,44] Nursing care after a skin graft includes assessment of the external dressing, notifying the physician of a seroma or hematoma, and prevention of sheering or friction forces in the area of the skin graft. Physician orders may restrict patient movement for 12 to 24 hours to allow the graft to adhere to the wound bed for optimal "take." Chapter 32 on burn injuries provides more detailed discussion on the management of grafts for wound closure

Flaps

Wounds that cannot be closed by primary or secondary intention healing or with skin grafts may require a flap for closure. Flaps are necessary when vital structures such as nerves, blood vessels, tendons, or bones without any overlying vascular tissue are exposed. Because these vital structures need more padding than can be provided by a skin graft or they are no longer vascularized to support a skin graft (e.g., tendon without paratenon or bone without periosteum), they must be covered with tissue that brings its own vascularity—namely, a flap.

Flaps may be composed of various tissues. Skin and subcutaneous tissue flaps are called fasciocutaneous flaps. Flaps may also incorporate muscle, in which case they are termed musculocutaneous flaps. Complex composite tissues including bone, muscle, skin, and fat may also be moved as a flap. These are termed osseomusculocutaneous or osseofasciocutaneous free flaps. Flaps may be obtained from local or remote tissue. A flap from local tissue involves leaving the blood supply intact and rotating, transposing, or tunneling locally available tissue into the wound.[46] Appropriate flap selection requires attention not only to the needs of the recipient site but also to minimizing undesirable alterations at the donor site. When possible, donor sites are located in inconspicuous areas and leave little scarring to minimize undesirable appearance of the site. Preservation of function at the donor site is probably a more important consideration when selecting tissues (i.e., muscle, nerves, and blood vessels) for transfer. Preferably tissues selected for transfer should be expendable or cause minimal functional loss at the donor site.[46]

Assessment of the flap includes evaluation of color, edema, turgor, moisture, temperature, and presence of pulses. The flap should appear pink and moist with good adherence to the wound bed. There should be no excessive edema or atrophy of the flap, pulses should be palpable or audible, and drainage from the site should be unremarkable. Close monitoring of the flap is undertaken to recognize abnormal assessment findings which, if noted, should be reported immediately to the physician. Dressings over flaps are loose and nonrestrictive. Maintaining a moist wound environment; avoiding compression or manipulation; and positioning the patient to prevent obstruction of arterial or venous flow are important interventions postoperatively to promote flap viability.

Biologic/Biosynthetic Dressings

A number of dressings categorized as biologic and biosynthetic dressings have been developed in recent years and may be used on deep partial-thickness and full-thickness wounds.

Cultured epidermal autografts are created by collecting a tissue biopsy specimen from the patient and growing keratinocytes over a 3- to 4-week period in a cultured medium. The tissue is then grafted on to the patient's wound bed. Composite grafts are skin substitutes containing dermal and epidermal layers. Composite grafts are autografts grown from a dermal tissue culture and a biosynthetic biodegradable layer over 3 to 4 weeks and then grafted over the wound.[43-45] Composite grafts provide increased tensile strength. Cultured epidermal allografts use tissue such as neonatal foreskin as donor tissue for developing grafts.[43]

Biosynthetic dressings consist of synthetic materials (nylon/silicone) that may be used to close a deep partial-thickness wound. Biosynthetic dressings have a prolonged shelf life and are intended for application on to a debrided wound bed until re-epithelialization is complete. The dressing does not have adhesive materials but adheres to the wound surface by entrapment of fibrin.[5,43-45] Nonliving skin substitutes include chemically treated cadaver allografts and artificial skin.[43] Deep partial-thickness and full-thickness wounds should be closed as quickly as possible to decrease the chances of infection and optimize healing. Dressing choices will depend on patient factors (perfusion, oxygenation, nutritional status, immunocompetence) and available tissue donor sites. Chapter 32 on burn injuries provides a more detailed discussion on biologic dressings for wound closure.

ALTERATIONS IN HEALING

KELOIDS AND EXCESSIVE SCARRING

Hypertrophic scarring and keloids are two alterations in healing that may become evident in the rehabilitation phase of trauma. They are significant because of their cosmetic and symptomatic consequences for the patient. Hypertrophic scars are an overgrowth of collagenous scar tissue within the wound margins; they may regress spontaneously. A keloid is distinguished as a fibrous growth resulting from an abnormal connective tissue response, which extends beyond the wound margins and rarely regresses. The risk for keloid formation is higher in African-Americans and Asians and lowest among whites. Hypertrophic and keloid scars are managed similarly. Initial early management includes the application of compression stockings. Silicone gel contact sheeting is also recommended.[47] Eventually, revision of a scar by surgery or lasers may be attempted.

SCAR CONTRACTURE

Scar contracture is the result of contractile processes in healed scars that result in a fixed, rigid scar that causes functional or cosmetic deformity. Wound contraction begins as a beneficial process that facilitates earlier wound closure by reducing the surface area of the wound bed. Continual contraction by myofibroblasts tends to pull points of flexion together, limiting movement and causing considerable disability.[3] The most common sites involve areas of flexion, such as fingers, arms, legs, and neck. Treatment modalities include physical therapy, splinting, and surgical release with grafting. Range-of-motion exercises affect the remodeling of collagen as it is deposited within the wound. Splinting procedures impede contraction mechanically. Spilt-thickness skin grafts are less effective than full-thickness grafts, which are less effective than flaps. Control of contraction appears closely related to elements of the dermis, so grafts containing dermis provide more effective therapeutic treatment.[46]

PRESSURE ULCERS

Although pressure ulcers are not the direct result of trauma, they are associated with acute illness and surgery. Immobility is the greatest risk factor for development of a pressure ulcer. Other risk factors include frequent operations, advancing age, fecal incontinence, hypoalbuminemia, impaired circulation, use of vasoactive agents, and high injury severity scores.[48-50] The critical nature of many trauma patients, immobility, and frequent surgeries place them at risk for development of pressure ulcers.

Pressure ulcers occur in areas where pressure, shearing force, friction, and moisture have damaged the epidermis, dermis, and underlying tissue layers. They occur over a bony prominence. The smaller the area over which the pressure is distributed, the greater the potential for the development of an ulcer. Shearing forces caused by sliding adjacent surfaces produce friction and tissue damage. Excess skin moisture from perspiration and incontinence increases the risk of skin breakdown and development of a pressure ulcer. Patients who remain immobile or who have other factors that place them at risk for pressure ulcer development need to be assessed continually throughout all the phases of trauma care. Additionally, vigilant assessment is important for pressure ulcers in the following groups of high-risk patients: those with spinal cord injuries, diabetes, multiple diseases, a history of pressure ulcer, low ejection fractions, malnutrition, and incontinence; patients undergoing orthopedic surgery; those in intensive care units; and elderly patients.[51]

Guidelines for pressure ulcer prevention issued by the Agency for Health Care Policy and Research (AHCPR)[52] stress the need for assessment of risk at admission. The AHCPR recommends the Braden and Norton scales, which incorporate the following categories for assessment of skin breakdown risk: level of consciousness (sensory perception), moisture, mobility (activity), nutrition, friction, and shear. If a patient is found to be at risk, risk reduction methods should be implemented. The trauma patient population would benefit from the bedside nurse completing a thorough assessment for risk of pressure ulcers on admission and at a set frequency throughout the hospital stay. Prevention of nosocomial pressure ulcers in trauma patients can be attributed to proactive nursing interventions.

Assessment is accompanied by preventive measures to relieve pressure through frequent turning, avoiding friction and shearing forces, providing meticulous skin care, nutritional support, and patient education. The skin should be kept dry, warm, well moisturized, and protected with lubricants or protective coverings. Regular use of a mild pH-balanced skin cleanser and the use of barrier sprays and creams to repel moisture when needed are suggested. Massage over bony prominences is contraindicated.[52,53] To relieve pressure, patients require repositioning every 2 hours at a minimum if on bed rest. Static support surfaces filled with foam, water, gel, or air can be used, as well as dynamic systems such as alternating-pressure mattresses, air-fluidized systems, low air loss support systems, and viscoelastic and elastic surfaces.[54] Smaller supports such as foam cushions, wedges, pillows, or blankets can keep knees, elbows, ankles, and heels from receiving too much pressure. To avoid shearing and friction during positioning, patients should be lifted with linens or a lifting device.

The principles of assessment for open wounds apply to pressure ulcers. Location, size, and tissue and exudate characteristics are evaluated on a regular basis. A plan of treatment is established on the basis of assessment of the wound and risk factors specific to the patient. In addition to choosing an appropriate dressing, a plan of care that incorporates positioning and pressure relief is essential.

SUMMARY

Development of knowledge in the area of wound healing has advanced rapidly in recent years. An increased understanding of this complex process and the effects of various therapies on its progression has altered some traditional beliefs about wound care and healing and has provided an empiric basis for treatment. There is still much to learn. Available data emphasize the need for early assessment of the patient's status and the wound and maintaining an optimal environment for wound healing. Steps taken to provide systemic support in the early trauma phases of care contribute significantly to the healing process and can prevent a number of complications, including infection. Many therapies for wound healing have yet to be studied to discern their mechanism of action and to define the limits of their use clinically to promote and improve healing. Continued research will extend the science of wound healing and provide a rational direction for optimal assessment and treatment strategies.

REFERENCES

1. Jackson LA: Physical attractiveness: a sociocultural perspective. In Cash TF, Pruzinsky T, editors: *Body image: a handbook of theory, research, and clinical practice,* pp 13-37, New York, 2002, Guilford Press.
2. Broughton GH, Janis JE, Attinger CE: The basic science of wound healing, *Plast Reconstr Surg* 117(Suppl):12S-34S, 2006.
3. Gurtner GC: Wound healing: normal and abnormal. In Thorne CH, Beasley RW, Aston SJ, et al, editors: *Grabb and Smith's plastic surgery,* 6th ed, pp 15-22, Philadelphia, 2007, Wolters Kluwer.
4. Sussman C, Bates-Jensen B: Wound healing physiology: acute and chronic. In Sussman C, Bates-Jensen B, editors: *Wound care: a collaborative practice manual for health professionals,* 3rd ed, pp 21-51, Philadelphia, 2007, Wolters Kluwer.
5. Broughton HG, Janis JE, Attinger CE: Wound healing: an overview, *Plast Reconstr Surg* 117(Suppl):1eS-32eS, 2006.
6. Sunderland S: The anatomy and physiology of nerve injury, *Muscle Nerve* 13:771-784, 1990.
7. Hunt TK, Hopf HH, Hussain Z: Physiology of wound healing, *Adv Skin Wound Care* 13:6-11, 2000.
8. Lawrence WT: Physiology of the acute wound, *Clin Plast Surg* 25:321-340, 1998.
9. Williams DT, Harding K: Healing responses of skin and muscle in critical illness, *Crit Care Med* 31(8 Suppl):S547-S557, 2003.
10. Ueno C, Hunt TK, Hopf HW: Using physiology to improve surgical wound outcomes, *Plast Reconstr Surg* 117(Suppl): 59S-71S, 2006.
11. Stramer BM, Mori R, Martin P: The inflammation-fibrosis link? A Jekyll and Hyde role for blood cells during wound repair, *J Invest Dermatol* 127:1009-1017, 2007.
12. Okan D, Woo K, Ayello EA, et al: The role of moisture balance in wound healing, *Adv Skin Wound Care* 20:39-53, 2007.
13. Sibbald RG, Orsted HL, Coutts PM, et al: Best practice recommendations for preparing the wound bed: update 2006, *Adv Skin Wound Care* 20:390-407, 2007.
14. Troilius AM: Effective treatment of traumatic tattoos with a Q-switched Nd:YAG laser, *Lasers Surg Med* 22:103-108, 1998.
15. Bates-Jensen BM, Ovington LG: Management of exudates and infection. In Sussman C, Bates-Jensen BM, editors: *Wound care: a collaborative practice manual for health professionals,* 3rd ed, pp 215-233, Philadelphia, 2007, Wolters Kluwer.
16. Zulkowski K, Albrecht D: How nutrition and aging affect wound healing, *Nursing 2003* 33:70-71, 2003.
17. Nortcliffe SA, Buggy DJ: Implications of anesthesia for infection and wound healing, *Int Anesthesiol Clin* 41:31-64, 2003.
18. Ahrns KD: Trends in burn resuscitation, *Crit Care Nurs Clin North Am* 16:75-98, 2004.
19. Montgomery RK: Pain management in burn injury, *Crit Care Nurs Clin North Am* 16:39-51, 2001.
20. Sussman C, Bates-Jensen BM: Management of wound pain. In Sussman C, Bates-Jensen BM, editors: *Wound care: a collaborative practice manual for health professionals,* 3rd ed, pp 278-307, Philadelphia, 2007, Wolters Kluwer.
21. Habib AS: Postoperative nausea and vomiting following inpatient surgeries in a teaching hospital: a retrospective database analysis, *Curr Med Res Opin* 22:1093-1099, 2006.
22. Arnold M, Barbul A: Nutrition and wound healing, *Plast Reconstruct Surg* 117:42-58, 2006.
23. Posthauer ME: The role of nutrition in wound care, *Adv Skin Wound Care* 19:43-54, 2006.
24. Khour W, Klausner JM, Ben-Abraham R, et al: Glucose control by insulin for critical ill surgical patients, *J Trauma Inj Infect Crit Care* 57:1132-1138, 2004.
25. Attinger CE, Janis JE, Steinberg J, et al: Clinical approach to wounds: debridement and wound bed preparation, *Plast Reconstruct Surg* 117(Suppl):72S-109S, 2006.
26. Ryan TJ: Infection following soft tissue injury: its role in wound healing, *Curr Opin Infect Dis* 20:124-128, 2006.
27. Sibbald RG, Woo K, Ayello EA: Increased bacterial burden and infection: the story of NERDS and STONES, *Adv Skin Wound Care* 19:447-461, 2006.

28. Edwards R, Harding KG: Bacteria and wound healing, *Curr Opin Infect Dis* 17:91-96, 2004.
29. Grey JE, Enoch S, Harding KG: Wound assessment, *BMJ* 332:285-288, 2006.
30. Kirshen C, Woo K, Ayello EA, et al: Debridement: a vital component of wound bed preparation, *Adv Skin Wound Care* 19:506-519, 2006.
31. Sussman C: Management of the wound environment with dressings and topical agents. In Sussman C, Bates-Jensen B, editors: *Wound care: a collaborative practice manual for health professionals,* 3rd ed, pp 250-277, Philadelphia, 2007, Wolters Kluwer.
32. Broussard CL: Hyperbaric oxygenation and wound healing, *JWOCN* 30:210-216, 2003.
33. Boykin JV, Baylis C: Hyperbaric oxygen therapy mediates increased nitric oxide production associated with wound healing: a preliminary study, *Adv Skin Wound Care* 20:382-388, 2007.
34. Richards CF, Mayberry JC: Initial management of the trauma patient, *Crit Care Clin* 20:1-11, 2004.
35. Makic MB: Cleaning, irrigating, culturing, and dressing an open wound. In Wiegand DJ, Carlson KK, editors: *AACN procedure manual for critical care,* pp 1103-1111, St. Louis, 2005, Elsevier.
36. Bates-Jensen BM, Apeles NC: Management of necrotic tissue. In Sussman C, Bates-Jensen BM, editors: *Wound care: a collaborative practice manual for health professionals,* 3rd ed, pp 197-214, Philadelphia, 2007, Wolters Kluwer.
37. Mulder GD: Cost effective managed care: gel versus wet to dry for debridement, *Ostomy Wound Manage* 41:68-76, 1995.
38. Hess CL, Howard MA, Attinger CE: A review of mechanical adjuncts in wound healing: hydrotherapy, ultrasound, negative pressure therapy, hyperbaric oxygen, and electrostimulation, *Ann Plast Surg* 51:210-218, 2003.
39. Loehne HB: Pulsatile lavage with suction. In Sussman C., Bates-Jensen BM, editors: *Wound care: a collaborative practice manual for health professionals,* 3rd ed, pp 665-682, Philadelphia, 2007, Wolters Kluwer.
40. Winter GD: Formation of the scab and the rate of epithelialization of superficial wounds in the skin of the young domestic pig, *Nature* 193:293-294, 1962.
41. Hinman CD, Maibach H: Effects of air exposure and occlusion on experimental human skin wounds, *Nature* 200:377-379, 1963.
42. Fleck CA: Wound assessment parameters and dressing selection, *Adv Skin Wound Care* 19:364-370, 2006.
43. Clark RA, Ghosh K, Tonnesen MG: Tissue engineering for cutaneous wounds, *J Invest Dermatol* 127:1018-1029, 2007.
44. Collier M: The use of advanced biological and tissue-engineered wound products, *Nurs Stand* 21:68-76, 2006.
45. Woo K, Ayello EA, Sibbald RG: The edge effect: current therapeutic options to advance the wound edge, *Adv Skin Wound Care* 20:99-117, 2007.
46. Mathes SJ, Levine J: Muscle flaps and their blood supply. In Thorne CH, Beasley RW, Aston SJ, et al, editors: *Grabb and Smith's plastic surgery,* 6th ed, pp 42-51, Philadelphia, 2007, Wolters Kluwer.
47. Chen MA, Davison TM: Scar management: prevention and treatment strategies, *Curr Opin Otolaryngol Head Neck Surg* 13:242-247, 2005.
48. Ayello EA, Baranoski S: Examining the problem of pressure ulcers, *Adv Skin Wound Care* 18:192-194, 2005.
49. Fife C, Otto G, Capsuto E, et al: Incidence of pressure ulcers in a neurologic intensive care unit, *Crit Care Med* 29:283-290, 2001.
50. Keller B, Wille J, Van Ramshorst B, et al: Pressure ulcers in intensive care patients: a review of risks and prevention, *Intens Care Med* 28:1379-1388, 2002.
51. Calianno C: Assessing and preventing pressure ulcers, *Adv Skin Wound Care* 13:244-246, 2000.
52. Agency for Health Care Policy and Research: *Pressure ulcers in adults: prediction and prevention,* Rockville, MD, 1992, U.S. Department of Health and Human Services, Publication No. 92-0047.
53. Ratliff CR, Bryant DE: *Guidelines for prevention and management of pressure ulcers,* Glenview, IL, 2003, Wound, Ostomy, and Continence Nurses Society.
54. Brienza DM, Geyer MJ: Understanding support surface technologies, *Adv Skin Wound Care* 13:237-243, 2000.

17

METABOLIC AND NUTRITIONAL MANAGEMENT OF THE TRAUMA PATIENT

Catherine J. Klein, Gena Stiver Stanek

OVERVIEW OF METABOLISM AND NUTRITION IN TRAUMA

The most significant factor influencing the outcome of the trauma patient is the severity of the injury.[1] Nutrition care can either assist or complicate recovery. Clinical nutrition science is evolving as further evidence of care is tied to outcomes, incidence of complications, and the length of stay in the intensive care unit (ICU). This chapter addresses evidence-based nutrition management of trauma patients to enhance the nurse's understanding and ability to be actively involved in an important interdisciplinary aspect of trauma care.

In healthy adults, catabolism of old cells is balanced with the synthesis of vital constituents and new cell growth. Food intake replenishes body stores of carbohydrate and fat, which are oxidized for energy, and provides protein and micronutrients to maintain the integrity and function of body cells, tissues, and organs. In contrast, traumatic injury accelerates catabolic processes to remove damaged tissue. Portions of healthy tissue are broken down as well to supply nutrients to tissues undergoing repair. This heightened metabolic activity increases the rate that energy substrate is consumed and is referred to as hypermetabolism. Increased energy and nutrient demands coupled with an inability to ingest food after traumatic injury set the stage for nutrient deficiencies, which can decrease resistance to infection and hinder wound healing.

A well-planned system for interdisciplinary nutrition care is needed to optimally assist recovery of critically ill trauma patients. Feeding modalities change as the patient recovers. Therefore, this chapter addresses phase-specific nutrition assessment, feeding, and monitoring.

METABOLISM

NORMAL METABOLISM

Metabolism constitutes the cyclic physical and chemical changes that occur within cells during anabolism and catabolism. Normally there is a balance between these two processes. During anabolism nutrients from food are assimilated and tissue repair and growth occurs. In contrast, catabolism involves a series of changes by which living matter is broken down into simple and less stable substances within a cell or organism. Carbohydrate, fat, and to a lesser extent, protein are used to produce energy in the human body. These substrates are available from the digestion and absorption of food and from the breakdown of endogenous body tissue. Cellular mechanisms translate chemical energy into growth of new tissue and physical work, such as breathing. In general, energy substrate is first allocated to meet energy demand. Then, excess substrate is stored in the liver and muscle as glycogen and in adipose tissue as fat.

Carbohydrate and Energy Production

The major purpose of dietary carbohydrate is to supply glucose, which is the preferred energy currency of all cells (particularly for the brain and formed blood elements). Most dietary carbohydrate is in the form of long chains of sugar, which are clipped into smaller segments during digestion. Simple sugars are converted to glucose during absorption from the gut into the bloodstream.

Insulin and glucagon are the two principal hormones that control the blood glucose concentration. After a meal, absorption of glucose raises blood glucose levels, which triggers beta cells of the pancreas to release insulin. The presence of insulin facilitates transport of blood glucose into cells. Potentially life-threatening problems, as might occur in insulin-dependent diabetes, develop rapidly if the body is unable to control the blood glucose concentration within the normal range. Extra glucose that is not used for energy is stored in the form of glycogen in liver and muscle. The process of forming glycogen is called glycogenesis (Figure 17-1). Over time, as cells continue to take up glucose for energy, the blood glucose concentration decreases to the lower end of the normal fasting range. This stimulates alpha cells of the pancreas to secrete glucagon. Glucagon targets hepatic and muscle glycogen stores and triggers glycogenolysis, which is the process of breaking down glycogen to release glucose molecules into the bloodstream to maintain sufficient blood concentration.

The primary role of glucose is to provide an adequate, ready supply of adenosine triphosphate (ATP), the major chemical form of energy necessary for cell life. Glucose is converted to ATP in three steps: first, glucose is broken down

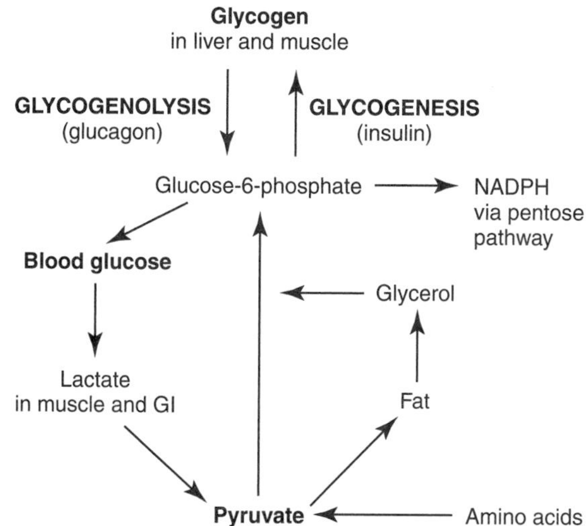

FIGURE 17-1 Glycogenesis and glycogenolysis.

to pyruvic acid during glycolysis (+2 ATP); second, pyruvic acid is converted to acetyl coenzyme A (CoA) in the cell mitochondria (+6 ATP); third, acetyl CoA is broken down in the tricarboxylic acid (TCA) cycle and hydrogens (electrons) generated from these reactions enter the electron transport chain (+24 ATP). The second and third steps in this process require oxygen consumption ($V{O_2}$) and generate carbon dioxide ($V{CO_2}$), free water, and heat. If sufficient oxygen is not available, pyruvic acid is converted to lactate and less ATP is produced. Hydrolysis of high-energy phosphate bonds in ATP supplies energy for biochemical reactions. Muscle contraction, hormone secretion, membrane transport, and synthesis of new substances are examples of functions that depend on ATP.

Lipid

Four types of body fat are especially important: (1) triglyceride molecules consisting of three fatty acids bound to a glycerol backbone, which are stored in adipose tissue and serve as a reservoir of energy; (2) phospholipids, which form plasma membranes and internal compartment membranes of all cells; (3) cholesterol, a vital structural component of cell membranes and the building material for steroid hormones (e.g., cortisol, estrogens, progesterone); and (4) the essential fatty acids, linoleic acid and α-linolenic acid (converted as needed into eicosapentaenoic acid and docosahexaenoic acid, which is important for cell membrane structure in the brain and retina).[2]

After a meal, free fatty acids (FFAs), glycerol, phospholipids, and cholesterol are absorbed through the lymph system, enter the bloodstream by the portal vein, and are taken up by the liver. The liver forms triglyceride molecules by packaging together three FFAs and a glycerol. Triglyceride and cholesterol are carried from the liver in globules of very-low-density lipoproteins (VLDL) for transport to other tissues. When VLDL reaches the capillaries, it is partially degraded by lipoprotein lipase (whose activity is stimulated by insulin), releasing FFAs. Once in the cell, FFAs are broken down through the process of β-oxidation to form molecules of acetyl CoA, which enter the TCA cycle to generate ATP. Excess FFAs are reesterified into triglyceride and stored. Under normal circumstances, triglyceride is degraded and replaced every 2 to 3 weeks. Any condition that increases energy demand also increases the release of FFAs from adipocytes. Once in the bloodstream, FFAs attach to albumin for transport to other tissues. The rate of turnover of FFAs in the plasma is rapid (every 2 to 3 minutes).

Endogenous fats are not typically lost by excretion except in the case of cholesterol, which is a component of bile and is secreted into the intestines. Although most fats can be synthesized in the body as needed, the essential fatty acids must be consumed in the diet. Essential fatty acid deficiency (EFAD) interferes with wound healing and impairs the body's resistance to infection. Signs of EFAD include hepatomegaly, elevated liver enzymes, hematuria, anemia, thrombocytopenia, scaly skin, and hair loss. The Holman index is a marker of EFAD and is calculated as the ratio of 20:3n-9 fatty acid to 20:4n-6 fatty acid. Values > 0.2 are indicative of EFAD. Safflower, sunflower, corn, and soybean oils are particularly rich sources of linoleic acid and linseed and canola oils are excellent sources of α-linolenic acid.

Protein

Proteins serve specific and vital functions: (1) protein enzymes catalyze biochemical reactions; (2) plasma proteins, such as albumin, transport nutrients through the bloodstream and protect nutrients from renal excretion (under normal conditions, intact blood proteins are too large to be filtered and excreted by the kidneys); (3) structural proteins frame cellular compartments and are particularly concentrated in muscle; and (4) peptide hormones regulate metabolism and homeostasis. There are two main classifications of biologically available protein: somatic protein (skeletal muscle proteins) and visceral protein (internal organ proteins and plasma proteins). Under normal circumstances, proteins in the liver, kidneys, and in the lining of the gastrointestinal tract turn over every 3 days, whereas proteins in skeletal muscle turn over every 18 days. Despite this turnover, the total body protein pool remains relatively constant in healthy adults because the amount of protein synthesized is generally equal to the amount of endogenous protein that is degraded and lost through secretion of digestive proteins.

Amino acids released during protein degradation are mostly conserved and reused to construct whatever proteins the body currently requires. All leftover amino acids are deaminated. The resulting amino group is converted to urea for excretion and the carbon-chain portion of the degraded amino acid is recycled into acetyl CoA for energy substrate or converted to glycerol to make triglyceride. Of the 20 common amino acids, nine are considered essential because they cannot be synthesized in the body and must be supplied in the diet. These essential amino acids are histidine, lysine, phenylalanine, threonine, tryptophan, the sulfur-containing amino acid, methionine, and the three branched-chain amino acids: isoleucine, leucine, and valine.

Protein is an integral component of most foods and is particularly concentrated in legumes, nuts, seeds, eggs, seafood, and meat. All food protein, except gelatin, contains some of each essential amino acid, but some foods are richer in certain amino acids than other foods. Food protein is digested to its constituent amino acids, which are absorbed from the gut directly into the bloodstream and are taken up by tissue. Protein intake in the United States far exceeds the minimum requirement and is usually not deficient in the diets of average persons, including vegetarians. Protein deficiency may be a problem for those who have limited access to food or have severely restricted intake for other reasons. Early biomarkers of protein deficiency in uninjured individuals include depressed concentrations of plasma prealbumin and albumin. General signs of protein deficiency include hair loss, loss of muscle mass, and edema.

Vitamins and Minerals

There are 14 essential vitamins, 12 essential minerals, and a requirement for sodium, chloride, and potassium. These nutrients play unique roles in metabolism of human life and must be consumed in the diet. An overview of the roles of essential nutrients in health and recovery is provided in Table 17-1.[3] Nutrient requirements differ among healthy individuals depending on age, body size, activity level, and other factors. The body has intricate homeostatic mechanisms to maintain adequate content of essential vitamins and minerals. For example, calcium homeostasis is regulated by hormones that control the amount absorbed by the intestine, the concentration in the bloodstream, the amount deposited and resorbed from the skeleton, and the amount excreted in urine. Figure 17-2 depicts the risks of adverse effects associated with extreme levels of intake ranging from deficient to toxic.[4]

In summary, carbohydrates, fats, and proteins are used as energy substrates. After a meal, the body stores a portion of dietary carbohydrate as glycogen to provide a ready supply of blood glucose between meals and fat serves as a vast reservoir of calories for the body to siphon in times of stress. Normal protein degradation is typically countered by a comparable rate of protein synthesis. The body uses intricate homeostatic mechanisms to absorb and retain sufficient quantities of essential vitamins and minerals. If the body is depleted of nutrients, the resulting cellular dysfunction will eventually give rise to the physical manifestations of malnutrition.[5]

METABOLIC ALTERATIONS IN STARVATION

Starvation occurs when there is a lack of food intake for several days or longer. The overriding goal of metabolism in starvation is to conserve energy while providing sufficient substrate to fuel processes that are vital for survival. Under these circumstances, the body is forced to lower its metabolic rate and increasingly uses fat and ketone bodies (from partially oxidized fat) as energy substrate to supplement the limited availability of glucose.[6]

Early Starvation

Similar to the fasted state between meals, blood glucose levels decrease in early starvation accompanied by a fall in circulating insulin levels. Alpha cells in the pancreas respond by secreting glucagon, which stimulates glycogenolysis and the release of free glucose to increase the blood concentration. However, without replenishment, tissue stores of glycogen are depleted in approximately 24 to 72 hours. To some extent, the liver and kidneys are capable of synthesizing de novo glucose from glycerol, lactate, and pyruvate and from carbon segments produced during deamination of amino acids. The process of gluconeogenesis is up-regulated by glucagon. The brain and central nervous system use about 80% of the glucose produced through gluconeogenesis. Other tissues that rely primarily on glucose for energy are red blood cells, white blood cells, bone marrow, and cells of the renal medulla. The remainder of the body, including skeletal muscle, will use both fatty acids and ketones as energy substrate. Therefore, the need for glucose is minimized and protein is spared to some extent. Catecholamine levels (e.g., epinephrine, norepinephrine) are increased during the first several days of starvation. These, along with low concentrations of glucose and insulin, trigger an accelerated release of FFA from adipose tissue and stimulate muscle catabolism for release of constituent amino acids.[7,8] The effects of early starvation are outlined in Table 17-2.

Prolonged Starvation

As starvation continues, overall body temperature and metabolic rate decrease further to conserve energy. The brain and other normally glucose-dependent tissues increasingly rely on ketone bodies for energy. As the concentration of circulating ketones increases, a mild metabolic acidosis might occur, but it is usually of little consequence unless the patient is severely stressed. Fat stores eventually become depleted, requiring that even more endogenous proteins be destroyed to meet energy demands, and eventually protein compartments (both visceral and somatic) become seriously depleted. A low concentration of blood proteins decreases the osmotic gradient along the vascular lining, causing fluid to leak into third spaces, resulting in edema, particularly in the lower extremities. A lack of protein also impairs immune competence and the body's ability to repair physical injury. Weight loss, sunken facial appearance, muscle wasting, and protruding rib bones are evident. Other signs and symptoms of nutrient depletion from prolonged starvation include anemia, fatigue, extreme weakness, decreased tolerance to cold, dizziness, muscle soreness, hair loss, skin changes, reduced coordination, ringing in the ears, apathy for matters other than food, irritability, decreased ability to concentrate, loss of sex

TABLE 17-1 **Nutrition and Implications for Wound Healing and Recovery**

Total Energy	
Primary functions	Sufficient ATP production to sustain metabolism, spare lean body mass, and promote wound healing
Indicators for assessment	Indirect calorimetry, calorie counts, body weight, BMI
Outcomes: undernutrition	Local infection, slowed wound healing, weight loss, muscle wasting (amino acids used for energy), loss of body's fat pads, increased risk of pressure ulcers at bony prominences, increased dependence on mechanical ventilation, slow progress in physical therapy
Outcomes: overnutrition	Increased body fat, increased health risk with increasing overweight
Essential Amino Acids (Protein)	
Primary functions	Protein synthesis, enzyme activity, growth of new tissue and maintenance of body cell mass, host defense, neural and muscular function, nutrient transport, oncotic pressure; synthesis of glutathione, creatine, taurine, and neurotransmitters; secretion of mucin; gluconeogenesis
Indicators for assessment	Diet records, blood albumin and prealbumin, arm muscle area, BUN, nitrogen balance
Outcomes: undernutrition	Delayed wound healing; muscle wasting; edema; dull, dry, sparse, depigmented hair; psychomotor changes; decreased resistance to local infection; weight loss
Outcomes: overnutrition	Dehydration, azotemia with possible alterations in acid-base balance
Glucose (Carbohydrate)	
Primary functions	Primary source of energy, especially for central nervous system, red blood cells, leukocytes, fibroblasts
Indicators for assessment	Blood glucose, intake records
Outcomes: undernutrition	Muscle wasting (amino acids channeled to gluconeogenesis), loss of sodium and dehydration
Outcomes: overnutrition	Decreased resistance to local infections
Fiber (carbohydrate)	
Primary functions	Gastrointestinal regularity and preservation of gut barrier as host defense
Indicators for assessment	Diet analysis, stool consistency and regularity
Outcomes: undernutrition	Constipation; strain of defecation may increase perianal wound dehiscence
Outcomes: overnutrition	Diarrhea with increased risk of stool contamination of perianal wounds
Fats	
Primary functions	Constituent of cell membrane, needed for cell growth, source of energy for resting skeletal muscle, absorption of fat-soluble vitamins in gut, synthesis of eicosanoids
Indicators for assessment	Triglyceride level, ratio of essential fatty acids in blood, intake records
Outcomes: undernutrition	Impaired wound healing, decreased resistance to infection, disruption of epidermal water barrier, hair loss, possible decreased attention and cognition
Outcomes: overnutrition	Congestion of reticuloendothelial system, increased fat deposition
Water	
Primary functions	Nutrient transport, elimination of waste, matrix for chemical reactions, dissipation of metabolic heat, cellular growth and survival
Indicators for assessment	Intake-output records: abnormal fluid loss (seeping wounds, drains, diarrhea, sweating) or retention (renal failure); blood sodium; osmolality; urine volume
Outcomes: water deficit	Decreased blood flow to skin, elevated body core temperature, headache, mental confusion, physical fatigue, renal failure
Outcomes: overhydration	Cardiovascular stress, pulmonary edema and respiratory failure
Electrolytes (Sodium, Potassium, Chloride)	
Primary functions	Regulate blood volume; needed for normal blood pressure, acid-base balance, nerve transmission, muscle contraction, and hormone secretion
Indicators for assessment	Blood electrolytes, intake records
Outcomes: undernutrition	Physical weakness, anorexia, nausea, drowsiness, irrational behavior, gastric hypomotility, cardiac arrhythmia
Outcomes: overnutrition	Edema, hypertension, cardiac arrest
Vitamin C	
Primary functions	Collagen formation; needed for the function of leukocytes and macrophages; enhances iron absorption; protects DNA, proteins, and lipids from oxidation; preserves integrity of capillary structure; hormone biosynthesis; formation of norepinephrine from dopamine
Indicators for assessment	Blood vitamin C, intake records

Continued

TABLE 17-1 Nutrition and Implications for Wound Healing and Recovery—cont'd

Outcomes: undernutrition	Collagen synthesis impaired, poor wound healing, infection, fatigue, ecchymoses and petechiae, hair follicles with a hemorrhagic halo, joint pain, swollen or bleeding gums, dry eyes and mouth
Outcomes: overnutrition	False-negative results for detection of occult blood; diarrhea, flushing, hyperuricosuria, hyperoxaluria, effects on red blood cell transfusions are still unknown, destruction of vitamin B_{12}
Vitamin B Complex (Thiamine, Riboflavin, Niacin, Pyridoxine, Folic Acid, Biotin, Pantothenic Acid, Vitamin B_{12})	
Primary functions	ATP production; protein metabolism; metabolism of therapeutic drugs; protects cell membranes and DNA from oxidation; nucleic acid synthesis and cell division for tissue growth; cell-mediated immune response; maintains integrity of hepatocytes, adrenal cortex, and nervous system; steroid synthesis and function; gluconeogenesis; neurotransmitter production
Indicators for assessment	Blood vitamin levels, erythrocyte transketolase activity, urinary excretion of metabolites, intake records
Outcomes: undernutrition	Slow growth of new tissue; fatigue, muscular weakness, and peripheral paralysis; tachycardia; respiratory distress; conjunctivitis; fissures at corners of mouth; swollen, beefy red tongue; papillary atrophy with smooth appearance; dermatitis; "burning feet" syndrome; neuropsychosis; nausea and abdominal distress; anemia
Outcomes: overnutrition	Gastric upset, flushing, ataxia, sensory neuropathy, drug-nutrient interaction of folate and phenytoin
Fat-Soluble Vitamins (A, D, E, K)	
Primary functions	Cell differentiation and proliferation; integrity of the immune system, particularly the function of T lymphocytes; vision; calcium homeostasis and bone mineralization; protects cell membranes from oxidation; synthesis of prothrombin and clotting factors II, VII, IX, X; regulation of blood clotting
Indicators for assessment	Blood vitamin levels, intake records
Outcomes: undernutrition	Impaired epithelialization, cross-linking of newly formed collagen, and poor closure of wounds; dermatitis; peripheral edema; dry, rough inflamed skin; bruising; malaise; night blindness; higher incidence of severe infections; neuromuscular degeneration; anemia; impaired blood clotting
Outcomes: overnutrition	Headache, emesis, alopecia, dryness of mucous membranes, and blurred vision; loss of muscle coordination; calcification of soft tissue; altered platelet adhesion; nutrient-nutrient interaction between vitamin E and function of vitamin K
Calcium, Phosphorus, and Magnesium	
Primary functions	Energy metabolism, protein synthesis, bone mineralization, nerve conduction, muscle contraction, blood clotting, β-oxidation of fatty acid
Indicators for assessment	Blood and urine concentrations, intake records
Outcomes: undernutrition	Weakness; tetany, tremors, spasms; cardiomyopathy; anemia; nausea and gastrointestinal distress; hypokalemia, refractive to treatment; personality changes; bone demineralization
Outcomes: overnutrition	Nausea, hypotension, bradycardia
Zinc, Iron, Selenium, Copper, Manganese	
Primary functions	Cross-linking of collagen and elastin, cell growth and repair; oxygen transport and energy production; defense against oxidative injury; formation and inactivation of hormones; biosynthesis of catecholamines; urea production
Indicators for assessment	Blood minerals, ferritin, mean cell volume, hemoglobin, transferrin saturation, erythrocyte protoporphyrin; intake records
Outcomes: undernutrition	Impaired thermoregulation, immune competence, wound healing, and growth of bone and cartilage; reduced life of erythrocytes; anemia; neutropenia; impaired taste; muscle weakness; cardiomyopathy; koilonchia (spoon-curved nails)
Outcomes: overnutrition	Constipation, gastrointestinal discomfort, reduced immune function, nutrient-nutrient interaction of zinc and copper, psychiatric disorders, fatigue

ATP, Adenosine triphosphate; *BMI,* body mass index; *BUN,* bood urea nitrogen.

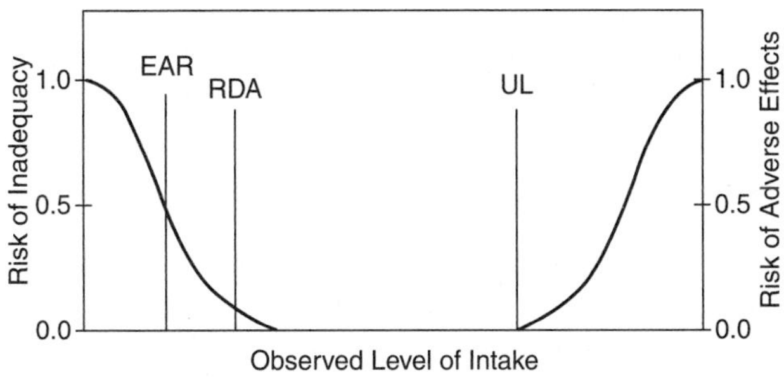

FIGURE 17-2 The risk of complications from malnutrition across the spectrum of observed levels of intake, accounting for variability in requirements and tolerance among healthy individuals. Observed intake increases from left to right. For any given nutrient, the estimated average requirement (EAR) is the intake at which 50% of individuals of the same sex and similar age group would be undernourished. The recommended dietary allowance (RDA) is a level of intake that meets the needs of nearly all (97% to 98%) individuals of the same sex and similar age group. When fed the RDA, a portion of individuals will be overfed, yet under normal health conditions, individual homeostasis will suffice to rid the body of excess nutrients. Above the tolerable upper intake level (UL), the risks of intolerance and toxic effects increase. The UL is not a level of recommended intake. (Reprinted with permission from National Academy of Sciences: *Dietary reference intakes for energy, carbohydrate, fiber, fat, fatty acids, cholesterol, protein, and amino acids (macronutrients)*, Washington, DC, 2005, courtesy of the National Academies Press, Figure 1-1, p. 23.)

drive, and altered personality.[5] Tragic circumstances demonstrate that humans will not survive much longer than 60 days without nutrient intake. Death would result sooner if the body did not have the capacity to adapt somewhat to periods when food is scarce. Death ensues when one third of the endogenous protein supply is exhausted, even if some fat stores remain available.

In summary, starvation rapidly depletes glycogen stores. Then the body is forced to catabolize endogenous proteins and fat to supply substrate for gluconeogenesis in the liver and kidneys. Body tissues that normally depend on glucose to supply energy adapt to use ketone bodies (from fat catabolism). Starvation results in severe depletion of nutrients and body mass. After a critical amount of protein is degraded and not replaced, continued starvation is fatal.

METABOLIC ALTERATIONS IN INJURY

Trauma, thermal injury, and sepsis evoke a hypermetabolic response. This increased energy demand arises from degradation of injured tissue and repair of wounds, which require synthesis of large amounts of proteins and other constituents. Thus the physiologic milieu of critical illness can result in accelerated glycogenolysis, proteolysis, lipolysis, ketogenesis, and gluconeogenesis, depleting the body's endogenous stores of protein and fat.[9] Hypermetabolism coupled with the inability to ingest food set the stage for serious nutrient deficiencies.

Ebb and Flow Phases

The acute period after traumatic injury is characterized in two phases, an "ebb" phase and a "flow" phase. The ebb phase is triggered by blood loss, hypoxia, and pain and may last up to 48 hours during which cardiac output, oxygen consumption, and body temperature decline.[10] Glycogen stores are rapidly depleted. Once the patient is adequately resuscitated and the initial insult is being managed effectively, the patient enters the flow phase, characterized by elevated cardiac output, oxygen consumption, elevated body temperature,

TABLE 17-2 **Characteristics of Starvation and Injury**

	Starvation			
Characteristic	**Early**	**Intermediate**	**Late**	**Injury**
Metabolic rate		↓	↓	↑
Body temperature	No change	↓	↓	↑
Gluconeogenesis				
From protein	↓	↓	↑	↑
From fat	↓	↑	↓	↑
Blood glucose levels	↓	↓	↓	↑
Serum insulin	↓	↓	↓	↑ or no change
Glucagon levels	↑			↑
Catecholamines	Slight ↑			↑
Cortisol levels				↑*
Blood lactate				↑
Free fatty acids	↑	↑		↑
Urine nitrogen excretion	↑	↓	↓	↑
Urine ammonia		↑		
Interleukin-1				↑
Body weight	↓	↓	↓	Varies
Muscle mass	↓	↓	↓	↓
Visceral protein		↓	↓	↓

*Might decrease with prolonged critical illness.

and hypermetabolism (see Table 17-2).[10] Many factors contribute to the intensity of the hypermetabolic response, which may last for weeks. Such factors include the patient's age, sex, previous health status, extent of the primary injury, the loss of normal barriers to infection, medical complications, and lack of nourishment. The primary drivers of the stress response are blood-borne chemical mediators, liberated directly from the site of injury (Figure 17-3).[11] In particular, interleukin-1 and tumor necrosis factor produce fever, tachycardia, and leukocytosis. These cytokines also stimulate release of growth hormone and the stress hormones (glucagon, catecholamines, and cortisol) and cause the liver to increase uptake and retention of iron and zinc.[12]

Macronutrient Substrate and Depletion

The stress hormones accelerate glucose oxidation and ATP production to provide for the high energy demands of maintaining vital physiologic functions in the flow phase. If tissues become hypoxic, which is common in critical illness, anaerobic conditions are created in the cells. Without sufficient oxygen, pyruvate (from glucose) is unable to convert to acetyl CoA and produce ATP. Under these conditions, pyruvic acid accumulates and reacts with hydrogen ions (NADH + H^+) to form lactic acid, which diffuses out of cells into extracellular fluids, resulting in elevated blood lactate concentration.[13] The heart muscle is able to take up some of the lactate and use it to produce ATP. The liver takes up another portion of the lactate for use in gluconeogenesis, which is up-regulated by cortisol and glucagon.[2] Excessive liver gluconeogenesis is the primary factor contributing to hyperglycemia in unfed trauma patients.[13]

Growth hormone, cortisol, epinephrine, and norepinephrine trigger lipolysis and release of FFAs, which supply a considerable portion of energy in critical illness. In general, blood concentration of FFAs and clearance of triglycerides are elevated in septic patients, yet some patients have less capacity to metabolize fat than others and are prone to hypertriglyceridemia.

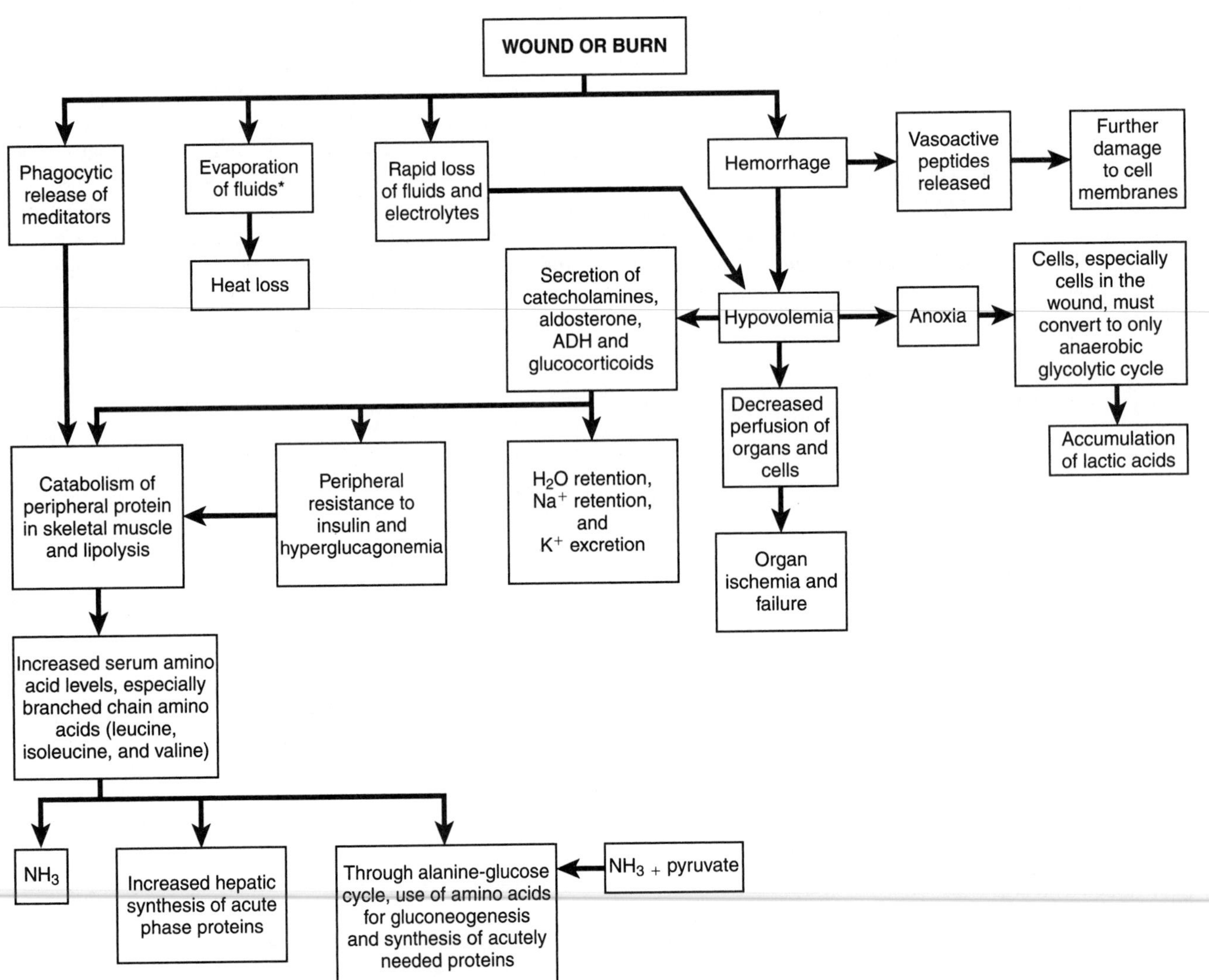

FIGURE 17-3 Physiologic and metabolic changes immediately after an injury or burn. The extent of these changes depends on the severity of the trauma. *ADH,* Antidiuretic hormone; *NH_3,* ammonia. *Occurs mainly in patients with extensive burns. (From Mahon LK, Escott-Stump S: *Krause's food nutrition and diet therapy,* 11th ed, Philadelphia, 2003, W. B. Saunders, Figure 33-1, p. 723.)

All aspects of protein metabolism are accelerated in critical illness. Although the synthesis of some proteins, such as the acute-phase proteins (e.g., C-reactive protein, ceruloplasmin) is increased, catabolism of protein is disproportionately greater than anabolism, resulting in net loss of protein (and nitrogen).[9,14,15] In particular, albumin, transferrin, and skeletal muscle proteins undergo degradation (triggered by catecholamines and glucocorticoids) at a greater rate than their synthesis. On the basis of studies of intracellular amino acid concentrations in muscle, it has been suggested that some normally nonessential amino acids may become "conditionally essential" after traumatic injury, particularly when kidney function is impaired.[16] The protein compartment in muscle suffers considerable loss in critical illness. For example, during the first week after head trauma, approximately 70% of total protein losses are derived from skeletal muscle. Alanine and glutamine comprise approximately 50% of the amino acids released from skeletal muscle,[7] which are shuttled to the liver and kidneys for degradation to produce carbon chains for gluconeogenesis. After the first week, nonmuscle proteins make up an increasing percentage of protein losses.[9] The hypercatabolic response peaks approximately 10 days after injury and then gradually decreases as medical status improves.[15] By day 21 after blunt trauma, patients have lost an average of 6.4 kg of skeletal muscle. Trauma patients may eventually exhibit wasting of arm and calf muscle. The patient's previous nutrition status, age, and the duration of the hypermetabolic flow phase will influence the total amount of lean body mass catabolized. Young, healthy, muscular patients have a relatively greater degree of protein wasting than leaner patients. It has been hypothesized that a reduction in release of growth hormone from the anterior pituitary gland may contribute to the wasting syndrome that characterizes prolonged illness, particularly in men.[12] Proteolysis cannot be substantially modified by feeding during critical illness. Hence, lean body tissue is sacrificed regardless of whether the patient is fed enough to achieve energy balance.[9,17]

In summary, extended periods of hypermetabolism can lead to depletion of nutrients and loss of substantial muscle mass, even for previously healthy patients of normal weight and those who appear overweight. These losses occur at a faster rate than depletion during total starvation without traumatic injury. Prolonged protein catabolism could result in muscular weakness, contributing to inadequate pulmonary ventilation and cardiac insufficiency. Poor nutritional status could weaken the immune system and undermine wound healing.

THE NUTRITION CARE PROCESS

Nutrition care should occur as an interdisciplinary, standardized process encompassing five main functions: (1) screen patients to identify those at nutritional risk, (2) assess the nutritional status and needs of high-risk patients, (3) diagnose nutrition problems, (4) formulate nutrition goals, plan to meet those goals, and implement interventions, and finally (5) monitor progress and evaluate outcomes. The model for care endorsed by the American Dietetic Association is presented in Figure 17-4.[18] This process is cyclic, so low-risk patients are periodically rescreened and high-risk patients are periodically reassessed. In this way, patients whose risk of malnutrition has worsened since their initial screens are identified for nutrition assessment. Periodic reassessment of high-risk patients is necessary to revise nutrition plans when the patient's status changes or if there are problems in achieving nutrition goals. Thus, the nutrition care process is designed to meet the needs of the patient throughout each phase of recovery. An added benefit from optimal nutrition care is decreased health care costs.[19]

NUTRITION SCREENING

Nutrition screening enables the hospital to consistently direct nutritional care to those patients most in need of these resources in a timely manner. Therefore, screening should identify patients who are already malnourished or who are at moderate to high risk for rapid development of malnutrition or a nutrition-related complication. Current standards of The Joint Commission (TJC) specify that all hospitalized patients must be screened for nutritional risk within 24 hours of admission by a qualified individual (Elements of performance for PC.2.1.120).[20] This time frame was endorsed by the American Society for Parenteral and Enteral Nutrition Board of Directors, who specified that results from nutrition screening should be documented.[21]

After traumatic injury, medical information is collected and documented by a succession of health care providers beginning with first responders. Family members often provide initial information about the patient's medical history, which can be refined once previous medical records are obtained. Nurses are in a strategic position to quickly identify and refer potentially at-risk patients for an in-depth nutrition assessment to determine whether special intervention is required.[22,23] Early intervention can prevent malnutrition or help correct existing deficiencies.

Screening Tools and Data Collection

Most trauma centers have created their own admission screening forms. For such tools to be effective, they should be quick, easy to use, and cost-effective. An example of a nutrition screening form that can be completed within 5 minutes is presented in Table 17-3.[23] Because screening is not meant to precisely categorize mild- or moderate-risk patients, some overestimation of risk may result to not miss identifying patients who are truly at risk.[22] Many screening tools used in clinical practice have not been validated.[24-26] Standardized examinations or tests are needed that are capable of reliably identifying all high-risk patients and minimizing the misclassification of low-risk patients.

Nutrition screening criteria include questions focusing on items that help direct the assessor to dietary or medical

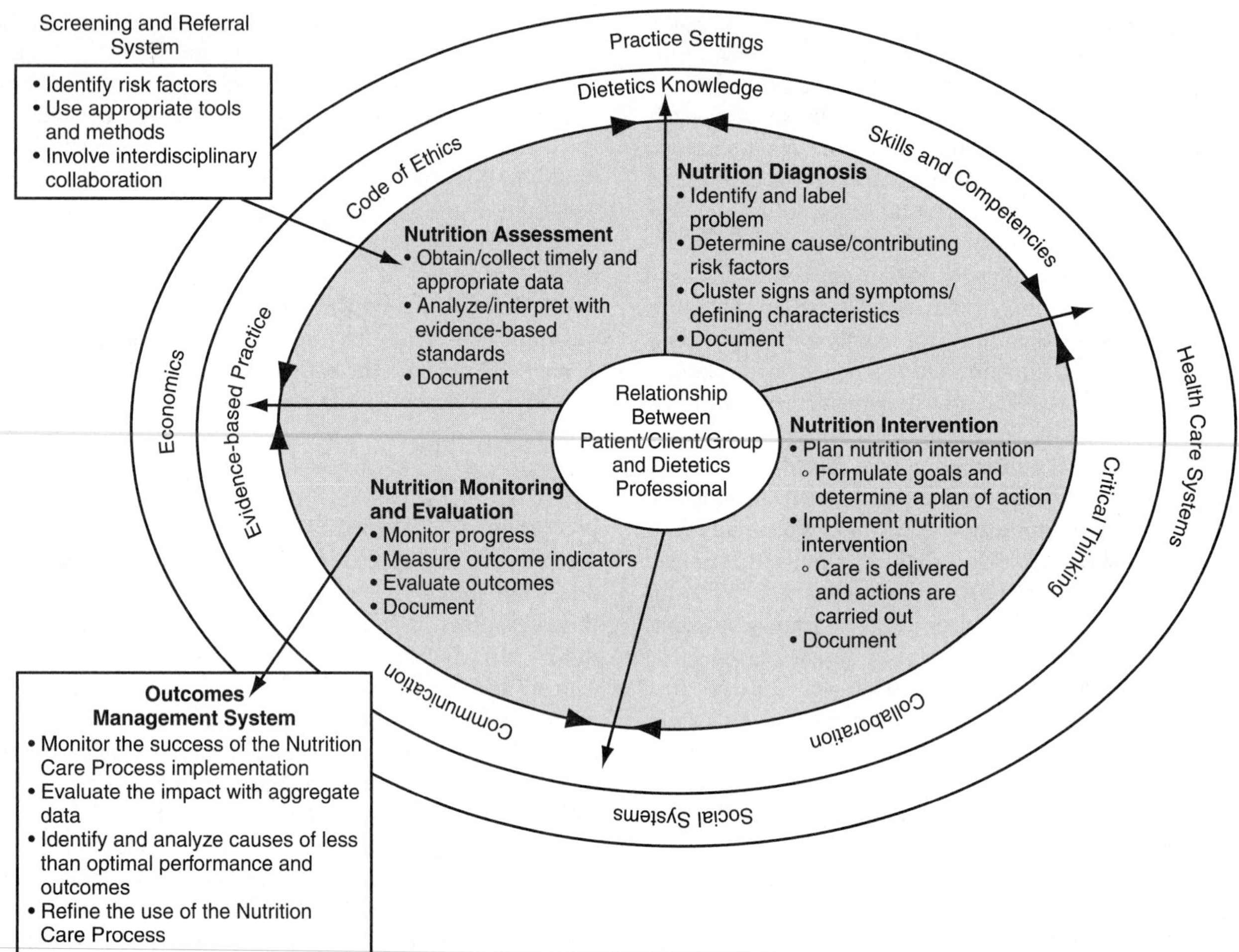

FIGURE 17-4 Nutrition care process. (Reprinted from Lacey K, Pritchett E: Nutrition care process and model: ADA adopts road map to quality care and outcomes management, *J Am Diet Assoc* 103:1061-1072, 2003, with permission from the American Dietetic Association, Figure 1, p. 1062.)

TABLE 17-3 **Example Nutrition Screening Form**

	Rating*	
Factors to Rate	**Minimal Risk**	**Potentially at Risk**
Body weight		
Unintentional change in usual body weight in last 6 months	Less than 10%	10% or more
Appearance	Relatively normal	Moderate to pronounced underweight
Food intake		
Appetite and intake	Relatively good	Poor; or physician ordered nothing by mouth; or currently receives nutrition support
Feeding	Requires little help	Only able to eat with assistance; chewing or swallowing problems
Tolerance	Good; minor gastrointestinal complaints	Regular vomiting or diarrhea, moderate to severe gastrointestinal complaints
Seriousness of illness, treatment, intervention		Admission to an ICU

*If one or more ratings of "potentially at nutrition risk," refer to nutrition specialist for comprehensive nutrition assessment. All other patients are rescreened for nutritional risk within 10 days.

imbalances that might result in nutrient deficiencies. Trauma patients with chronic illness need early identification and intervention. For example, chronic renal disease is associated with protein deficiency, which can complicate recovery. The nurse should document relevant observations such as a patient's emaciated appearance, reflecting depleted fat and muscle stores. Survey instruments are being developed for use in long-term care facilities to identify adult patients with failure-to-thrive syndrome.[27]

Assigning Level of Risk

On the basis of screening criteria, each patient is assigned a level of nutrition risk (e.g., either "minimal risk" or "potentially at risk"). The traumatic event itself is critical to assignment of risk in that the greater the magnitude of injury, the greater the risk for development of protein-calorie malnutrition. Patients who are not expected to consume food for a prolonged period because of severe traumatic brain injury, bowel resection, or other nutritionally disabling trauma are at high risk for malnutrition. Adults are considered nutritionally at risk if they have any of the following risk factors: (1) involuntary change in body weight of 10% or more within the past 6 months, a change of 5% to 10% within the past month, or having an emaciated appearance; (2) having a body weight above or below cutoff values for normal (e.g., 20% above or below ideal body weight, <19 body mass index [BMI]); (3) a restricted or required diet (e.g., diabetic diet, renal diet); (4) inadequate intake for more than the past week or orders for nutrition support; (5) the expectation that medical condition/injury will prohibit consumption of food for 5 or more days; (6) admission to an ICU; and (7) repeated episodes of nausea, vomiting, or diarrhea. Any one of these indications of nutrition risk would necessitate referral to a nutrition specialist.[1] High-risk patients are then provided with a comprehensive nutrition assessment to determine whether a special diet, supplement, or nutritional support is needed. Patients who are at minimal risk should be periodically rescreened according to hospital protocols (e.g., within 10 days, or when the nutritional or clinical status changes).[1]

Screening for Risk of Pressure Ulcers

Because pressure ulcers can develop in the first week in the ICU, it is important to screen patients for ulcer risk at admission.[28] The Braden score (i.e., Braden Scale for Predicting Pressure Sore Risk) is used to categorize the patient's risk.[29] Dietary status is a component of calculating the total Braden score and is scored as follows: 1 = eats less than one third of meals; 2 = eats about 50% of meals; 3 = eats more than 50% of meals or is on nutritional support; or 4 = eats most of every meal. This score is added to the other component scores to arrive at a total Braden score where ≤9 = very high risk; 10-12 = high risk; 13-14 = moderate risk; 15-18 = mild risk; and 19-23 = not at risk.[28] Weight status (i.e., BMI) should be assessed as well because underweight increases the risk of ulcer development and weight status is not directly measured by the Braden scoring system. A full nutritional assessment should be conducted on all patients who are substantially underweight or who have Braden scores of ≤14.[28]

Documenting the Care Process

The level of nutrition risk assigned during screening should be documented on the screening form or otherwise tracked in the referral system. Dietitians or other trained professionals who are responsible for conducting in-depth nutrition assessments of high-risk trauma patients will provide nutrition diagnostic statements of problems and will suggest plans for nutrition care.[30] Because this process is highly dependent on collaboration and integration within the health care team, timely, accurate, and relevant communication of nutrition risk, assessment, problems, goals, interventions, monitoring, and progress is vital to ensure the best opportunity to achieve favorable outcomes for the patient.[31]

Assessment

Those patients who were rated as high risk during nutrition screening should be given an in-depth nutrition assessment as soon after referral as possible (e.g., within 48 hours of admission). TJC specified that hospitals should define in writing the type of data and information gathered during nutrition assessments. The assessment should include the patient's nutritional status, appropriateness of the route and type of feeding, adequacy of intake, recognition of complications of nutrition therapy, and identification of education and discharge needs.[18]

All pertinent nutrition data are compared with reference standards for healthy individuals to determine whether the patient's status is suboptimal. In the case of reassessment, current measures are also compared with earlier measures and with nutrition goals to assess progress after intervention and over time. The assessment of nutrient requirements should be summarized in the nutrition note, particularly recommendations for protein and calorie goals and fluid, electrolyte, and micronutrient requirements that will not be met by standard oral, enteral, or parenteral feedings.

Diagnostic Statement

Key concerns that need to be addressed through intervention by the nutrition care team are stated as nutrition diagnostic problems.[18] Those most common among high-risk trauma patients often relate to a delay in feeding, underfeeding, feeding intolerance, overfeeding, electrolyte abnormalities, sudden changes in the ability to deliver nutrients through a specified route of feeding, and changes in medical status. Whenever possible, interventions are targeted at correcting the causes of high-priority problems.

Nutrition Plans, Interventions, and Monitoring

After reviewing the nutrition assessment and diagnostic statements, the patient's physician, nurse, and the nutrition support service develop a comprehensive care plan, tailored to the needs of the individual patient, designed to achieve immediate and long-term nutrition goals. Patient-specific outcome goals must be measurable and realistic. Input is obtained as needed from family members and other relevant health care personnel. Interventions are planned, targeting the highest priority problems first, to achieve nutrition goals within an anticipated time frame. An appropriate route of feeding and type of nutrition support formula, if needed, will be identified. Whenever possible, the application of nutrition interventions should be based on available evidence that is grounded in high-quality research. The American Society for Parenteral and Enteral Nutrition is an expert organization that periodically reviews and evaluates nutrition interventions for critically ill trauma patients and publishes their consensus and guideline statements.[19,31]

Periodic monitoring and reassessments are conducted to evaluate the efficacy of nutrition therapy. Daily or more frequent monitoring may be required for critically ill patients, especially those at risk for refeeding syndrome and those transitioning between total parenteral nutrition (TPN), tube feeding, or an oral diet.[21] For example, electrolyte monitoring may be monitored several times in one day, whereas calorie counts to evaluate progress in achieving energy goals might be conducted every 4 days. In stable patients, monitoring of nutrition support might occur weekly. Nutrition goals and plans may need to change over time to enhance the patient's recovery and they should address discharge planning, patient and family education about nutrition therapy, and the need for home training.

The ABCs of Assessment

A variety of techniques used to assess nutrition status are available; the most common measures are discussed briefly. The nutrition assessment of a critically ill patient cannot depend on a single parameter but should involve multiple parameters and should take into account the entire medical status of the patient.[31] Typically, the nutrition assessment is based on an evaluation of anthropometric measures (height and weight), biochemical data (composition of blood and urine), clinical data (from physical examination and medical records), dietary data (calorie counts), and measures of energy expenditure and fluid status.

Anthropometrics and Body Composition Techniques

Physical Measures

Body size and composition reflect a long-term history of energy and protein status. Anthropometric measures include all physical measures of the body, such as height, weight, weight history, triceps skinfold, and mid arm circumference (MAC). In general, anthropometric data derived from a given individual are interpreted by comparison with normal values obtained from a healthy population of the same sex and age. Weight is the most widely used measure of nutrition status because it is a general indicator of malnutrition. If past weight and height measures are not available, the clinician can measure recumbent length, calculate ideal body weight, and estimate weight on the basis of visual observation of whether the patient appears underweight, normal weight for height, or overweight. Weight relative to height is an indicator of body composition and nutrition risk compared with standards for underweight and obesity. Underweight is defined as having a BMI <18.5, whereas obesity is a BMI of 30 or greater (Table 17-4). Both extremes are associated with greater morbidity. Measures of skinfold thickness using specially designed calipers at specific locations (e.g., triceps, subscapular) are a reflection of the body's energy storage (fat). In addition, waist circumference is an indicator of the distribution of body fat. The risk for chronic disease, such as diabetes, is increased with excessive deposition of abdominal fat. MAC and arm muscle area (derived from skin fold and MAC measures) are indicators of body protein mass. Measures of triceps skinfold or MAC falling below the 15th percentile of normal are indicative of chronic undernutrition.

Technical Measures

Bioelectrical impedance analysis (BIA) is used to estimate body composition in healthy young adults but assumes that fluid and electrolyte status are stable and normal. Other methods to assess body composition, primarily used in research, include dual-energy x-ray absorptiometry scanning to determine fat and muscle mass, gamma neutron activation analysis to measure total body protein, and in vivo tritiated water and sodium bromide dilution techniques to measure body water.[32]

Anthropometrics in Critical Care

Measuring actual body weight and BIA has little value for nutrition assessment in trauma care because abnormal fluid status and body casts, braces, Hoffman apparatus, and other devices confound the measures. Hence, preinjury weight and weight/height ratios, such as BMI, provide a baseline index to estimate nutrient reserves in the trauma patient. In cases of amputation, adjustments are made to subtract the estimated weight of the missing limb to estimate the patient's weight for purposes of calculating nutrient needs. For a below-the-knee amputation, 6% of preinjury weight is subtracted, and for an above-the-knee amputation, 12% of preinjury weight is subtracted.[33] However, for calculating BMI to assess overall energy reserves, the preamputation weight is used. Typically, the early postadmission weight of the patient with multiple traumas is elevated above the preinjury weight as a consequence of fluid resuscitation. Approximately 5 L or more of resuscitation fluid might be retained by the patient by the time he or she is hemodynamically stable, which adds approximately 10 kg in weight. Body weight is then lost at a rate of approximately 0.8 kg/day until the preinjury weight is restored around day 10. Weight loss will be due to loss of fluid, muscle and some fat, depending on injury severity and the adequacy of nutrition support. Patients admitted into the ICU with

TABLE 17-4 Equations Used in Nutrition Assessment

1. BMI is used as an evaluation of weight status: BMI = kg/m^2, where weight is in kilograms and height is in meters
2. Adjusted body weight (ABW) combines ideal body weight (IBW) and metabolically active weight of overweight (estimated)
   ABW = [(Preadmission weight − IBW) × 0.25] + IBW
3. Hamwi equation for IBW
   IBW men: 106 pounds for the first 5 feet + 6 pounds for each additional inch
   IBW women: 100 pounds for the first 5 ft + 5 pounds for each additional inch
4. Percentage of usual body weight (UBW) is used as a reflection of weight change and the adequacy of energy intake
   % UBW = (Actual body weight/UBW) × 100
5. Nitrogen (N) balance is a marker of severity of the acute phase response and a rough estimate of protein need in malnourished but otherwise healthy individuals:
   N balance (g) = N intake − (N output in urine + 4), where 4 is an estimate of fecal and obligatory losses
   The amount of nitrogen in protein is calculated according to the following equation:
   $$\text{Nitrogen intake (g)} = \frac{\text{Protein (g)}}{6.25}$$
6. The Harris Benedict energy equation (HBEE) is an estimate of basal energy requirements of normal-weight adults, where weight (W) is in kilograms, height (H) is in centimeters, and age (A) is in years:
   HBEE men: 66 + (13.8 × W) + (5 × H) − (6.8 × A)
   HBEE women: 655 + (9.6 × W) + (1.8 × H) − (4.7 × A)
7. Ireton-Jones equations to estimate energy expenditure in critical illness, where age (A) is in years, weight (W) is in kilograms, sex (S) is 1 if male or 0 if female, and obesity (O), trauma (T), and burn (B) are 1 if present or 0 if not[57]:
   Spontaneously breathing patients (kcal/d): 629 − 11(A) + 25(W) − 609(O)
   Ventilated patients (kcal/d): 1784 − 11(A) + 5(W) + 244(S) + 239(T) + 804(B)
8. TEE for normal-weight, overweight, and obese adults aged 19 years and older[4]
   For men, TEE: 864 − (9.72 × Age [y]) + PA × (14.2 × Actual weight [kg]) + 503 × Height [m])
   Where the physical activity (PA) coefficient is:
   1.00 for sedentary (REE × 1.0 to 1.39)
   1.12 for low active (REE × 1.4 to 1.59)
   1.27 for active (REE × 1.6 to 1.89)
   1.54 for very active (REE × 1.9 to 2.5)
   For women, TEE: 387 − (7.31 × Age [y]) + PA × (10.9 × Actual weight [kg]) + 660.7 × Height [m])
   Where the PA coefficient is:
   1.00 for sedentary (REE × 1.0 to 1.39)
   1.16 for low active (REE × 1.4 to 1.59)
   1.27 for active (REE × 1.6 to 1.89)
   1.44 for very active (REE × 1.9 to 2.5)

preexisting severe protein depletion (extremely low muscle mass), often with low body weight, are less likely to survive.[34] Such severely malnourished patients should be provided with nutrition support without delay.

Anthropometrics in Intermediate and Rehabilitative Care

Calculating the percentage of usual preadmission body weight is helpful to assess the degree of depletion since admission (Table 17-4). Many patients recovering from critical illness are able to regain body protein in the months after release from the hospital. However, patients with spinal cord injuries continue to incur significant reductions in bone and muscle tissue during the first year after injury. Muscle paralysis and subsequent immobility contribute to changes in body composition. In long-term care, the typical body weight in the spinal cord–injured population is less than normal. It may be appropriate for the spinal cord–injured patient with paraplegia to be 10 to 15 pounds lighter than normal and those with tetraplegia to be 15 to 20 pounds lighter.[33] Body size and composition measures may be useful to monitor patients receiving long-term care on an annual basis or when body weight changes more than 5 kg. Depending on the instrument selected, BIA may be acceptable for monitoring changes of body composition for stable patients in long-term care if the equation used is validated for age, sex, and race.[35,36]

BIOCHEMICAL TESTS AND NITROGEN BALANCE

Analysis of blood, urine, and other body fluids yields data that are used to help assess the status of body protein, vitamins, minerals, and essential fatty acids and for identifying issues that can be influenced by nutrition intervention.

Biochemical Tests in Critical Care

Before feeding is initiated, routine clinical laboratory tests are reviewed by the clinician to assess the patient's potential tolerance for carbohydrate, fat, and protein. Depending on the degree of organ failure, patients may have hyperglycemia, hypertriglyceridemia, and other derangements that can limit their ability to tolerate feeding. Biochemical measures during critical illness, however, are not helpful in depicting nutrient stores in tissue. This is particularly true for blood concentrations of hepatic proteins (e.g., albumin, prealbumin) and minerals (e.g., zinc, iron), which decrease during the acute phase response to stress for reasons other than nutritional status. For example, albumin levels below 3 g/dl are common in critical illness and are correlated with increased morbidity, higher costs of care, and death because of the stress response.[37] Moreover, blood products can contain prealbumin (transthyretin). Therefore, if the patient receives massive transfusions, the prealbumin test may reflect exogenous prealbumin rather than that synthesized by the patient. Thus, neither albumin nor prealbumin are necessarily reflective of protein status or the adequacy of nutrition support in critical care.[38] Similarly, urea nitrogen loss serves as an indicator of the magnitude of injury rather than as an indicator of the amount of protein needed.

In the critical care environment, electrolytes and minerals are monitored one or more times each day and abnormalities are corrected. For example, hyponatremia can be caused by fluid overload during resuscitation or cerebral salt-wasting syndrome in patients with traumatic brain injury. Because treatment is distinctly different depending on the etiology of the disorder, electrolyte disorders such as hyponatremia are carefully managed by the physician (e.g., sodium, chloride, and fluid replacement for cerebral salt wasting).[39] In contrast, vitamin levels are not routinely measured. Critically ill adults with multiple trauma receiving specialized nutrition support commonly have hypocalcemia.[40] Numerous calculations have been used to estimate serum ionized calcium and "corrected" total calcium, such as the McLean-Hastings nomogram method. However, these estimation methods are not valid for use with trauma patients.[41] Serum ionized calcium should be directly measured to assess calcium status.

Blood Proteins and Vitamins in Intermediate and Rehabilitative Care

Once the patient has stabilized and is past the period of acute stress, monitoring trends in prealbumin concentration might reflect nutrition status and the adequacy of feeding.[15] The half-life of prealbumin is only 2 to 3 days. Hence, prealbumin concentration decreases with even short periods of underfeeding and increases rapidly with diet therapy. Corticosteroid therapy or renal failure might alter prealbumin concentration independent of nutrition status. In the absence of inflammation in the rehabilitative and long-term care setting, monitoring albumin concentrations over time is a useful indicator of protein status, but the clinician should recognize that blood albumin concentration can decline during physical stress, infection, and overhydration, even when body protein stores are ample. Because albumin has a 14- to 20-day turnover, it is not typically very sensitive to short-term changes in feeding. Yet with prolonged underfeeding of more than 2 weeks, poor protein status is associated with low serum albumin levels.

Patients whose treatment requires partial or total gastrectomy should be followed up with yearly serum vitamin B_{12} tests. Parietal cells of the stomach produce a factor that is required for vitamin B_{12} absorption. Irreversible neurologic disease from vitamin B_{12} deficiency has been documented, developing 10 years after gastric surgery.

Nitrogen Balance

Nitrogen is an integral component of amino acids in food and body protein. Nitrogen balance is positive during anabolism when the body accumulates new tissue, such as during pregnancy or during growth in children. Nitrogen balance is negative when the body loses muscle mass, such as during weight-loss diets and in critical illness.[15] For typical healthy adults, nitrogen balance is approximately zero when body weight, body composition, and dietary intake are relatively constant and intake is adequate. To obtain data for a nitrogen balance study, food records are kept for 24 hours. During this same period, all urine is collected and analyzed for urea nitrogen (urea reflects the amount of amine groups derived from body protein). Nitrogen balance is calculated by subtracting nitrogen losses (i.e., total urea nitrogen and obligatory nitrogen lost in skin, feces, drains, and menstruation) from nitrogen intake. On average, every 6.25 g of dietary protein contains 1 g of nitrogen. Hence, the amount of nitrogen in the diet is estimated by dividing the total grams of protein consumed by 6.25. Typically, a factor of 4 is used to estimate obligatory losses (Table 17-4).[4]

Nitrogen Balance in Critical Care

Many trauma patients in the ICU are highly catabolic and lose large amounts of urinary nitrogen because of metabolic stress. In general, the more severe the traumatic injury, the greater the amount of urinary nitrogen excreted. Peak nitrogen excretion typically occurs between 5 and 10 days after injury, which corresponds to the peak period of total body protein loss.[9,15] The usefulness of nitrogen balance in the clinical setting is controversial. First, calculating balance depends on small differences between two large numbers of nitrogen intake and nitrogen output, whose measure may be inaccurate.[16] Nitrogen output may be underestimated in patients with burns, diarrhea, vomiting, fistula drainage, and other abnormal nitrogen losses unless all body fluid losses are analyzed. Moreover, day-to-day measures of nitrogen balance in critically ill patients can be highly variable even when feeding remains consistent; these measures are not likely to represent the adequacy of nutrition support. Because of difficulties in accurately measuring and interpreting nitrogen balance, further research to develop new methods to better evaluate amino acid requirements after trauma must receive high priority.[16]

Nitrogen Balance in Intermediate and Rehabiliative Care

Once the patient is transferred to home or the long-term care setting and feeding regimens and intake are stable and consistent, then nitrogen balance may be indicative of the adequacy of feeding. At this point in recovery, one would expect the patient to be moving toward a neutral or more positive nitrogen balance. However, skeletal muscle protein can continue to break down at an accelerated rate during convalescence, even when stress hormones have returned to normal levels. Not all causes of continuing protein catabolism are known. Patients who have spinal cord injury may continue to lose nitrogen because of denervation and disuse of paralyzed muscles. Persistent negative nitrogen balance studies or studies that are not showing progress toward a positive balance might reflect failure of the prescribed nutrition plan, necessitating reassessment of energy and protein requirements.

Clinical Examination and Review of Systems

Clinical data are reviewed to understand how the patient's past and current medical status may affect nutritional status. Of particular importance is the type and severity of injuries and a current review of systems (e.g., neurologic, pulmonary, renal). Certain medical conditions might indicate a need to modify the route of feeding or the type of nutrients in the feeding solution. For example, maxillofacial trauma may limit the patient's ability to chew or to take any nourishment orally. A visual examination of the patient contributes to identification of nutrient deficits, excess, or fluid imbalance (Table 17-1). Also, observations of the setting and current circumstances, such as the elevation of the head of the bed, volume of output in drains, whether the patient has gastric tubes, and whether the patient is mechanically ventilated will supplement and update information obtained in the medical chart. An assessment of the patient's capacity to tolerate feeding and the likely start time for feeding should be made as soon as possible. Most multitrauma patients have disruption of several physiologic systems and have undergone extensive surgical interventions, which render the stomach useless for 48 hours or longer because of gastric ileus. Paralytic ileus is also common initially in the spinal cord–injured population because of autonomic disruption and ischemia at the time of injury.[15] Gut function is assessed by tracking the volume of nasogastric aspirate, stool output, abdominal distention, pain or tenderness, and the presence of bowel sounds.[42] Abdominal trauma requiring bowel surgeries might eliminate the upper gastrointestinal tract as a route for nutrient intake and a jejunostomy tube for feeding might be required.

Patients with severe head injuries are initially dependent on nutrition support. The risk for swallowing impairment and aspiration is increased with neurologic injury, particularly if the patient was intubated for 2 or more weeks or has a tracheostomy. The level of impairment should be assessed by a trained professional (i.e., speech pathologist). Symptoms of dysphagia that the nurse might observe include drooling, choking, coughing during or after meals, lack of gag reflex, and gurgle noises while talking.[33] A patient whose level of consciousness improves may be ready to convert from enteral to oral feedings if the gag reflex returns.

Diet and Fluid Status

Diet

During the dietary assessment, the clinician evaluates the adequacy of previous, current, and prescribed diets, including the number of days of restricted oral intake (i.e., nil per os, NPO). Food intolerance and allergies are taken into account, as are religious, cultural, ethnic, personal food preferences, any past eating disorders, and the potential for drug-nutrient interactions. Intake and output records and other food records (calorie counts and TPN prescriptions) are essential for nutrition assessment. The dietitian reviews these records and calculates the actual nutrient intake by converting food amounts into values of energy, protein, lipids, vitamins, minerals, and fluid. Hence, the nurse should record all volumes of oral, enteral, and parenteral nutrition taken in by the patient. In some cases, family members might participate in accurately recording the type of food and quantity ingested on calorie count records. This information is helpful to assess whether the patient can take in adequate nutrients on his or her own. For example, adequate calories may be consumed, but protein intake may be below ideal levels. In this case, protein supplements might be ordered to improve dietary intake. When several days of adequate oral intake are documented, enteral tube feeding may be decreased or discontinued. Often, feedings are held for therapeutic interventions. Attempting to minimize this loss of intake and ensure that the patient receives the prescribed feedings is an important nursing responsibility. Information the nurse provides regarding excessive diarrhea, vomiting, drainage, and the duration that feedings are held can assist the team in determining feeding adequacy or complications related to prescribed nutrition regimens.

Diet Assessment in Rehabilitation

During the rehabilitative phase of care, the nutrition assessment should include a patient/family interview to obtain additional information about the patient's food, cultural, and meal pattern preferences. Otherwise, nutrition interventions may fail to individualize feeding to the patient.[33] The interview also permits clarification and correction of the patient's nutritional history including weight, intake, activity level, and feeding disabilities.

Fluid Status

Water consumption and adequate body hydration is necessary for metabolism and other physiologic processes, including cognitive function and regulation of body temperature and blood pressure. The average 70-kg man has approximately 42 L of total body water, dispersed primarily in lean body mass with about 3.2 L in plasma.[43] For healthy individuals, the requirement for water depends on diet, physical activity, and environmental temperature. Most body water is lost through urination, and evaporation accounts for additional losses from lungs and skin. Increased sodium and protein intakes lead to increased obligatory water loss in urine. Drinking and eating in response to thirst and hunger sensations helps maintain water balance. Men and women typically consume 3.7 and 2.7 L per day, respectively, of total water (in food and beverages).

Plasma or serum osmolality is a widely used hematologic index of hydration status. Normal plasma osmolality is in the range of 280 to 290 mOsmol/kg. Plasma osmolality must be measured directly after a blood sample is collected and centrifuged because changes in pH, dissolved carbon dioxide, and lactic acid during cool storage can decrease and confound measures of plasma osmolality.[44] The kidneys help regulate water homeostasis by altering the concentration of urine to excrete more or less water as needed to maintain normal plasma osmolality. On average, healthy women excrete a little more than 1 L per day of urine (30 to 65 ml/h) and men, on average, excrete 1.4 L per day of urine (38 to 75 ml/h).[44] The specific gravity of urine (density as mass per volume) can be measured to assess hydration status. During dehydration, urine specimens normally range from 1.013 to 1.029 but can exceed 1.03 if the urine is especially concentrated to conserve water. Values >1.02 should be further monitored. In contrast, when the kidneys dilute urine to rid the body of excess fluid, the specific gravity of urine decreases (1.001 to 1.012).[44]

Isotope dilution techniques are the gold standard for assessing body water. However, reference tables of normal values for total body water by age and sex still need to be compiled.[44] Combined tracer dilution methods with deuterium to measure total body water and bromide to measure extracellular fluid are being used in research hospitals to assess hydration and body cell mass in pediatric patients with thermal injuries.[32] In the future, noninvasive whole body scans for total body chloride, potassium, and sodium by neutron activation analysis may be available to calculate intracellular and extracellular body water.

Fluid Status in Critical Care

In critical illness, after initial fluid resuscitation, the need for fluids continues to be increased above normal by thermal injury, hemorrhage, hyperventilation, mechanical ventilation, fever, wound drainage, neurosweats, elevated urine output, and protracted vomiting and diarrhea. Critically ill trauma patients with functioning kidneys have urine outputs of more than 0.5 ml/kg per hour (e.g., ≥35 ml/h for 70-kg man) and are often polyuric, excreting in excess of 2.5 L per day.[40] Adding another layer of complexity, the regional distribution of fluid in the body is altered in critical illness, with increased fluid volume in the thoracic region. Moreover, distribution of body water between intravascular and extravascular spaces and intracellular and extracellular spaces is often altered in critical illness. These alterations in fluid status are frequently accompanied by electrolyte abnormalities. The medical team attempts to tightly monitor and control fluid balance during the acute phase of care by calculating fluid input and losses and by tracking measures of electrolytes. Renal failure and diuretic therapy alters the renal response to fluid, and these factors should be considered when interpreting urine study tests such as specific gravity and urine osmolarity.[45] Kraft et al[46] reviewed the etiologies of fluid and electrolyte disorders in the ICU and provided guidelines for correcting such disorders. In general, overhydration seems to be more common than dehydration in the ICU.

Fluid Status in Intermediate and Rehabilitative Care

In contrast to acute care, dehydration seems to be more of an issue in intermediate and rehabilitative care. The following patients should be monitored regularly for hydration: those who have language barriers, cognitive deficits, require assistance with eating and drinking, have orders for fluid restriction or NPO, sweat excessively, are under restraint, are dependent on nutrition support, or receive medications or feedings that promote diuresis.[47] In particular, concentrated tube feedings that are high in protein can cause urea diuresis with subsequent dehydration. In general, urine osmolality near 900 or greater is an indication of dehydration. Metabolic signs of dehydration include elevated blood urea nitrogen (BUN), increased BUN/creatinine ratio, and increased blood sodium levels. Clinical signs of dehydration include oliguria, poor skin turgor, dry mouth and increased thirst, dizziness, weight loss, and an elevated heart rate (to compensate for reduced central venous pressure).[48] Dehydration is a risk factor for pressure ulcers because of reduced skin turgor and circulation,[49] it can result in constipation, and even mild dehydration of 1% to 2% of body mass can reduce alertness and cognitive function.[44] Consensus guidelines are available for assessing hydration status of patients in rehabilitative and long-term care and include strategies for maintaining adequate hydration.[47,50]

Volume overload is possible during nutrition support, infusion of intravenous fluids, or organ failure. Acute weight gain is a sensitive sign of volume excess and edema may be evident once 2 to 4 kg of fluid weight is gained.[45] Note that edema can also be caused by protein deficiency. For ambulatory patients, excess fluid can accumulate in the lower extremities, whereas fluid settles in the sacrum and buttock regions in patients who are bedridden.

ENERGY

Energy expenditure, energy requirements, and food energy all use the kilocalorie (kcal) unit. A kcal is the amount of heat required to raise the temperature of 1 g of water 1° C at a pressure of 1 standard atmosphere. The purpose of calorimetry measures is to assess the energy expenditure of the patient, which helps in setting appropriate goals for feeding.

Basal and Resting Energy

The amount of energy needed for the involuntary work of the body to sustain life is referred to as the basal metabolic rate (BMR). The BMR corresponds to caloric expenditure (heat production) in an awake, rested state and reflects functional activity of vital organs, gland secretion, cellular metabolism, and maintenance of muscle tone and body temperature. The

BMR varies between individuals depending on body surface area, body weight, age, and sex. In general, larger individuals have a greater volume of metabolically active tissue and have a higher BMR. Studies show that women who are matched with men of the same body size actually have a lower BMR because of differences in body composition. Typically, women have a smaller proportion of lean muscle mass (and more fat mass) and therefore less metabolically active tissue. At rest, women expend 0.8 to 1.0 kcal/min (1150 to 1440 kcal/d) and men expend 1.1 to 1.3 kcal/min (1580 to 1870 kcal/d).[4] For comparison, the heat released by a burning candle or a 75-watt light bulb is similar, about 1 kcal/min. In stable, mechanically ventilated patients, the energy expenditure measured at rest is not only dependent on body weight and height but is also significantly correlated with body temperature, minute ventilation, and arterial blood saturation.[51] Resting energy expenditure (REE) measures of 110% or greater than normal are indicative of hypermetabolism.

Total Energy Expenditure

Physical activity, BMR, and the thermogenic effect of food all contribute to the body's total energy expenditure (TEE). The thermogenic effect of food is the energy required for digestion and absorption of food and the stimulating effect of nutrients on metabolism but this represents only a small portion of energy. The major variable of energy expenditure in ambulatory patients is the intensity and duration of physical activity. Additional factors that can influence energy expenditure in critical illness are presented in Table 17-5.[51-54]

The method of choice for determining energy expenditure in the clinical setting is indirect calorimetry, which measures respiratory gas exchange and is closely correlated to direct calorimetry (measuring heat generated). Indirect calorimetry is based on the principle that a standard amount of oxygen is consumed for each mole of glucose oxidized in the body; that is, Vo_2 and Vco_2 are quantified and related to heat production. Indirect calorimetry is often conducted while the patient is being fed continuously. Therefore, these measurements already include the thermogenic effect of food. Indirect calorimetry is helpful to prevent overfeeding of patients who are elderly, obese, very short, severely malnourished, or diabetic. Measures should also be obtained in patients who have difficulty weaning from the ventilator, such as might be expected for patients with low cervical and upper thoracic spinal cord injuries, pulmonary contusions, rib fractures, hemopneumothoraces, and patients with pulmonary disease. For patients to be measured, the fraction of inspired oxygen should be $<60\%$ to 80% and there must not be any gas leaks in the collecting system, such as pleural leaks through chest tubes or leaks around endotracheal tubes.

The indirect calorimeter equipment is calibrated before each use by the respiratory therapist or other trained personnel. Tests begin once a steady state has been reached, meaning that average Vo_2, Vco_2, and respiratory quotient (RQ) vary $<10\%$ to 15% from minute to minute for 5 consecutive minutes. Typically, patients are measured at rest for a 15- to 30-minute stable period. This value is then extrapolated to 24 hours. Although a 30-minute measure may not reflect all energy changes that occur throughout the day, it has been shown to be reasonably reflective of the 24-hour metabolic rate. In the past, activity factors were added to the 30-minute REE for nonambulating patients to predict TEE; however, this practice was shown to be inaccurate.[55] Clinicians may prefer to extend measures of mechanically ventilated patients for a full 24-hour period to obtain an accurate TEE. Obtaining repeated 24-hour measures through indirect calorimetry is the best method available to predict energy expenditure in critically ill patients. Limited use of metabolic carts to perform indirect calorimetry is primarily related to the expense of equipment, the need for trained personnel, and

TABLE 17-5 **Clinical Factors Associated With Altered Energy Expenditure**

Clinical Factor	Increases Expenditure	Depresses Expenditure
Feeding	Glucose infusion Feeding Overfeeding	Underfeeding
Medication	Glucocorticoids	Neuromuscular blocking agents Sedation (nonspecific) Sodium pentobarbital Morphine
Activity	Dressing changes Agitation Motor activity (muscle rigidity, fine motor tremors) Shivering	Bed rest
Patient status	Traumatic injury Traumatic head injury Severe thermal injury Surgery Minute ventilation/ventilator dependence Body temperature/fever	Body temperature/external cooling (no shivering) Protein-calorie malnutrition Spinal cord motor deficit

the number of patients requiring this service.[55] Some new bedside monitors integrate indirect calorimetry with the breathing circuit during mechanical ventilation to provide continuous measures of energy expenditure.[56]

The RQ is a ratio calculated by dividing the volume of carbon dioxide produced by the volume of oxygen consumed during the same period (V_{CO_2}/V_{O_2}). This ratio varies depending on the primary substrate being consumed for cellular energy. If a normal mix of substrates (fat, carbohydrates, and amino acids) is "burned" in the cells, the RQ will be approximately 0.85.[54] When glycogen is depleted and glucose is scarce, as in prolonged fasting or underfeeding, the RQ decreases toward 0.7, reflecting a shift to oxidize more fat. An RQ <0.70 is associated with oxidation of ketones. In contrast, when the supply of carbohydrates exceeds the requirement for glucose substrate, glycogen stores are filled and cellular oxidation shifts to consume a greater percentage of carbohydrate. This produces proportionately more carbon dioxide than the amount of oxygen consumed, resulting in an RQ close to or slightly >1.00. The RQ is used to confirm that current feeding and substrate mix are yielding an RQ in the physiologic range. Extreme values outside the range of 0.67 to 1.3 may reflect methodologic error and are invalid.[55] The RQ is not reliable enough to use for minor adjustments to macronutrient composition of feeding.[55]

Energy Estimates

Numerous equations have been developed to predict energy expenditure, each with varying accuracy.[57] The Harris and Benedict energy equation (HBEE, Table 17-4) is one such multiple linear regression formula derived from measures of indirect calorimetry. The predictive value of other equations, such as the Schofield equation, is poor.[58] Weight, height, and age are included in the HBEE calculation to predict BMR. Separate regression equations are used for women and men. Compared with measures of indirect calorimetry in healthy subjects, HBEE consistently overestimates REE by 5% to 14%.[58] The HBEE has been validated for use in predicting REE in mechanically ventilated, critically ill patients when it is multiplied by an activity factor of 1.2 (i.e., HBEE × 1.2) to account for the hypermetabolism of disease.[15,59] Although trauma patients as a group are more hypermetabolic than other critically ill patients, oxygen consumption, and hence energy expenditure, can be depressed in very ill patients who have a high risk of death, resulting in REE approximately equal to normal (i.e., HBEE × 1.0). Thus, assigning ever-increasing injury factors to amplify feeding as the injury severity and the number of failed organs increases is not necessarily of benefit. In fact, erring on the side of underfeeding is preferable to overfeeding because macronutrient loads are less likely to be tolerated by the sickest patients. Moreover, it is possible for patients with significant spinal cord deficit to have caloric requirements lower than basal levels because of subnormal activity levels in affected tissue. A patient's physical activity level varies much more during the intermediate and rehabilitative phases of care than during critical care. The HBEE is usually multiplied by a factor of 1.3 for a patient who is ambulating.

The daily REE for healthy, normal-weight adults is 21 to 25 kcal/kg of body weight. On average, the daily TEE for sedentary and/or older adults is 30 kcal/kg and it is approximately 41 to 43 kcal/kg (approximately 1.75 × REE or HBEE) for healthy, active younger adults.[4] In 2005, new predictive equations to estimate energy expenditures of healthy individuals were developed by the Food and Nutrition Board on the basis of extensive data from double-labeled water studies. Age, weight, height, and activity level of the individual are the factors required to generate the TEE (Table 17-4).[4] Because of the extensive amount of data used, these equations provide the most accurate estimates available for healthy individuals of normal weight, overweight, and obese weight. Whether these equations will be incorporated into clinical practice for use with trauma patients awaits research validation and decision by consensus groups of experts.

In the past, the Fick equation was used in combination with thermodilution techniques as an estimate of energy expenditure. Substantial evidence now exists to conclude that this approach differs from indirect calorimetry measures by 350 kcal or more and that it is unreliable.[56]

Range of Motion, Quality of Life, and Psychosocial Issues

Range of Motion and Ergometry

Ergometric tests can be used to measure the patient's strength in performing physical tasks. Such measures assist in assessing skeletal muscle status and the adequacy of nutritional status. These tests are most suited to research and to long-term care settings. One example is the measure of hand grip strength. Patients are asked to grip, with the nondominant hand, a strain gauge that has a graduated scale. The best value obtained after three or four attempts is compared with age- and sex-specific reference values and the patient's past performance. Another example, the arm crank ergometry test is performed to assess upper body strength and function of paraplegic patients while the patient is sitting in a wheel chair. Other types of ergometric tests, such as treadmill tests and bicycle exercise tests, are commonly used to assess cardiopulmonary status.

Quality of Life and Psychosocial Issues

Survey tools can be used in the home and long-term care settings to assess quality of life and to document the patient's general sense of well-being in living with nutrition support. The *Short Form 36 Questionnaire*, the *Quality of Life Index*, the *Sickness Impact Profile*, and the *Nottingham Health Profile* are some of the more frequently used instruments for measuring quality of life on long-term TPN.[60] Quality-of-life measures attempt to describe aspects of physical, social, and emotional health that are relevant to the patient. These measures include: (1) subjective indications of clinical status (e.g., pain, dysphagia, nausea); (2) function (e.g., energy level, ability to participate in activities of daily living); (3) emotional health (e.g., happiness, depression, anxiety); (4) socialization and family relationships (e.g., ability to communicate); and (5) treatment satisfaction (including financial cost of treatment).[61] Psychosocial factors influencing nutrition status include family dynamics, language barriers, psychiatric disorders, finances, and patient preferences and directives with regard to intensity and invasiveness of care.

Optimal nutritional status will promote better function and quality of life during intermediate and rehabilitative care.[62] Because the technical aspects of nutrition support can interfere with routine activities at home, the health care team should consider how home management will affect the patient's quality of life and select the best options. Patients on long-term TPN report numerous psychosocial problems.[63] In particular, depression, drug dependence, sleep disturbance, frequent urination, fear of therapy-related complications, and inability to eat can negatively affect quality of life.[60] There is a need for standardized and validated survey instruments to measure quality of life for patients receiving long-term nutritional support.[64]

GOALS OF NUTRITION CARE

The overall goal for nutrition intervention during critical care is provision of nutrients and energy for metabolic support and, when possible, to protect lean body mass and function.[65] The determination of nutrition goals should be individualized on the basis of an assessment of the patient's body composition and function. Expert groups periodically evaluate the published literature to provide consensus opinions for feeding goals for trauma patients and for the nutrient content of enteral and parenteral formulations. In general, nutrient goals are set for an average daily intake level that will provide sufficient nutrients for optimal recovery and health, to include restoring body reserves and covering periods between feedings. Because some nutrients can have pharmacologic effects at megadose levels and are associated with toxicity at even higher levels, the dose and rate of delivery of nutrients is controlled through standard or prescribed nutrition support. For any nutrient, tolerance might be lower in critical illness than in health. If it is expected that the patient will not able to safely or adequately eat or drink by mouth for a period of 5 to 10 days or longer, then an alternative route for nutrition and hydration support is a priority nutrition goal.[31] Once access for nutrition support is established, nutrition support is initiated and gradually increased to the feeding goal as tolerated by the patient. The individual patient's energy and nutrient requirements are likely to fluctuate over time, depending on changes in medical and nutritional status. Thus, periodic reassessment is needed for updating nutrition goals and plans for nutrition care.

ENERGY, FLUID, AND NUTRIENT GOALS

Total Energy and Carbohydrate Goals

When selecting an energy goal, the clinician considers the patient's energy reserves (e.g., underweight, overweight), the estimate/measure of energy expenditure, the likely accuracy of that estimate, the patient's response to feeding to date, and possible future tolerance of feeding. The current goal may be to achieve energy balance (maintenance of body mass) or the goal may be to feed lower or higher than actual energy expenditure depending on medical and nutritional status. For example, slightly underfeeding may be desirable for critically ill patients who have limited tolerance for overfeeding or whose energy expenditure is estimated rather than measured.[66] Even when measures are obtained, it is not known if providing sufficient calories to achieve energy balance during critical care is ideal for recovery.[17] In contrast, feeding excess energy might be desirable in long-term care to promote weight gain in an underweight patient who is at high risk for pressure ulcers. The daily dose of carbohydrate, as a component of total energy provision, should not exceed 7 g/kg of body weight (or 5 mg/kg per minute) to minimize the risk of adverse consequences.[1,19,31]

In recent studies that include patients with moderate to severe traumatic injuries, REE is 120% to 155% above normal, averaging 1,600 to 2,650 kcal/day (approximately 22 to 35 kcal/kg).[15,52,57] Consensus groups recommend feeding trauma patients within a range of 20 to 35 kcal/kg per day.[1,19,31] When actual measures are not possible, 30 kcal/kg can be fed daily on a trial basis to adults of normal weight who are under the age of 65 years (Table 17-6). For amputees, adjusted body weight is inserted into the estimate equations (Table 17-4). Once the patient has recovered sufficiently to progress past the flow phase of hypermetabolism, metabolism shifts to favor anabolism and the level of nutrition support may need to be reassessed to provide increased energy and nutrients to promote health and continued recovery.

Muscle paralysis, extreme inactivity, and wheelchair confinement can reduce energy expenditure in patients with spinal cord injuries. Persons with injury to the upper spine, such as those with quadriplegia, are expected to have lower energy expenditures. One consensus group recommends feeding patients 20 to 22 total kcal/kg per day in the first 2 weeks after quadriplegic injury and 22 to 24 kcal/kg after paraplegic injury.[1] Studies have shown that 2 or more years after spinal cord injury men who can perform all their own activities of daily living expend approximately 27 kcal/kg per day.

TABLE 17-6 **Energy and Protein Daily Recommendations for Adults**

Phase	Total Energy Needs	Protein Needs
Critical care	20-35 kcal/kg	1.2-1.5 g/kg
Intermediate	25-30 kcal/kg	1.0-1.5 g/kg
Rehabilitation	25-40 kcal/kg	0.8-1.5 g/kg
Normal	30-40 kcal/kg	0.8 g/kg

Protein Goals

Rather than specifying requirements for individual amino acids, goals are expressed in terms of total protein. The recommended dietary allowance (RDA) for average daily protein for healthy adults is 0.8 g/kg of body weight, with 10 g per day additional needed during pregnancy. After prolonged starvation, refeeding should be initiated conservatively because the body is not accustomed to processing large quantities of nutrients. Under these conditions, refeeding with 40% to 60% of the RDA for protein is suggested and then advancing feeding as tolerated to the nutrition goal. Consensus groups suggest that protein (containing 25% to 30% essential amino acids) be administered within the range of 1.0 to 2.0 g/kg body weight per day, with 1.3 to 1.5 g/kg sufficing for most injured patients.[1,19,31] Little evidence supports an outcome benefit from feeding critically ill patients protein in excess of 1.3 to 1.5 g/kg per day, yet there is wide variation in practice.[1,67] Isotonic formulas tend to be better tolerated than elemental or peptide-based formulas, especially when feedings are initiated. Thus, whole-protein (polymeric) enteral formulas are recommended for general use.[68]

In intermediate and rehabilitative phases of care, 0.8 g/kg of protein daily may be sufficient for the unstressed adult patient with adequate organ function.[4,19,31] Research supports an average daily protein intake of approximately 120% of the RDA, or 0.96 g/day, with adequate calories to protect patients from developing pressure ulcers. Some suggest that severely underweight patients may benefit from protein intake up to 2.0 g/kg.[65]

Lipid Goals

Essential fatty acids are provided by most tube feeding formulas and parenteral lipid emulsions. Approximately 20 to 40 g of linoleic acid and 2 to 10 g of α-linolenic acid are needed each week. This translates to a minimum of 1 L per week of 10% soybean oil emulsion for intravenous use (2 × 500-ml bottles) to prevent EFAD in most adult patients who require TPN. Without essential fats, as might occur from fat-free TPN, EFAD could develop within a matter of days or weeks. The daily dose of lipids should not exceed 1.0 g/kg of body weight in unstable critically ill patients or 2.5 g/kg in more stable patients to minimize adverse consequences.[19,31] Propofol (Diprivan) is administered in a lipid solution and this fat should be counted toward the daily dose of lipid.

Vitamin and Mineral Goals

Consensus recommendations for general ranges for safe administration of nutrients in healthy adults are provided in Table 17-7.[19,31] Various solutions are available for tube feeding and the selection is determined on the basis of the nutrition assessment (Table 17-8). Most full-strength enteral formulas come with a standard mix of vitamins and minerals designed to meet nutrient requirements of adults when 1700 to 2400 ml of solution is provided daily. Hence, feeding goals tend to focus on rates of macronutrient feeding.

The vitamin and mineral content of TPN is similarly standardized but can be altered as needed. In the past, vitamin K was either not added to TPN or added once each week. On the basis of the recommendations of the U.S. Food and Drug Administration (FDA), vitamin K is now included in the multivitamin supplement added daily to TPN.[69]

Long-term alcohol consumption can result in thiamine deficiency, leading to serious brain disorders, including Wernicke-Korsakoff syndrome. Hence, trauma patients with a history of heavy alcohol consumption are often given supplemental infusions of thiamine soon after admission, but this practice varies by facility and physician. Further research is needed to determine the optimal content of vitamins and minerals in formulas for trauma patients.

Fluid Goals

The medical and fluid status of the patient will dictate the care plan for hydration. The physician may seek a negative fluid balance to reduce systemic edema for those patients who sustained large-volume resuscitation. Excess fluid might be retained in the extracellular space for several weeks after trauma and sepsis.[9] Consensus groups suggest that, in general, 30 to 40 ml/kg per day can meet the fluid requirement for adults.[19,31] However, more or less fluid administration may be indicated depending on the patient's clinical condition.

OUTCOME GOALS IN CRITICAL CARE

Outcome goals are an integral part of the plan of care and should be patient-focused, quantifiable, and realistic. Individualized goals help to prioritize the plan for care and specific time frames should be set for goal achievement. For example, if a patient in whom hyperglycemia has recently developed is receiving an infusion of dextrose solution and nutrition support (that exceeds the estimated energy requirement), a short-term goal might be "patient's blood glucose is maintained in the normal range without a requirement for insulin." After consultation with the health care team, the planned intervention might be to immediately discontinue the extra dextrose infusion. Other example patient goals, some of which might not be achieved until intermediate or long-term care, include (1) maintains a normal BMI, (2) attains a blood prealbumin concentration of 0.2 g/L (20 mg/dl) or greater, and (3) consumes/receives, on average, 90% to 100% of the estimated energy and protein needs per day. Appropriate assessment, monitoring, and interventions by the interdisciplinary team in the critical care phase will minimize complications from nutrition support and allow early goal achievement.

Avoid Overfeeding

Multiple complications can occur if energy and nutrient needs are overestimated or if patients are fed more than prescribed, which is not uncommon.[70] Health professionals need to evaluate the actual amount of calories fed compared

TABLE 17-7 **Daily Dosing Ranges for Safe Administration of Electrolytes, Vitamins, and Trace Elements in Adults***

	Enteral	Parenteral
Electrolyte Requirements		
Sodium	22 mEq (500 mg)	1-2 mEq/kg
Potassium	51 mEq (2 g)	1-2 mEq/kg
Chloride	21 mEq (750 mg)	As needed to maintain acid-base balance
Acetate	—	As needed to maintain acid-base balance
Calcium	60 mEq (1200 mg)	10-15 mEq
Magnesium	35 mEq (420 mg)	8-20 mEq
Phosphorus	23 mmol (700 mg)	20-40 mmol
Vitamin Requirements		
Thiamine	1.2 mg	6 mg† (was 3 mg*)
Riboflavin	1.3 mg	3.6 mg
Niacin	16 mg	40 mg
Folic acid	400 mcg	600 mcg† (was 400 mcg*)
Pantothenic acid	5 mg	15 mg
Vitamin B_6	1.7 mg	6 mg† (was 4 mg*)
Vitamin B_{12}	2.4 mcg	5 mcg
Biotin	30 mcg	60 mcg
Choline	550 mg	Not defined
Ascorbic acid	90 mg	200 mg† (was 100 mg*)
Vitamin A	900 mcg	1,000 mcg (3300 IU)
Vitamin D	15 mcg	5 mcg (200 IU)
Vitamin E	15 mg	10 mg (10 IU)
Vitamin K	120 mcg	150 mcg†
Trace Element Requirements		
Chromium	30 mcg	10-15 mcg
Copper	0.9 mg	0.3-0.5 mg
Fluoride	4 mg	Not defined
Iodine	150 mcg	Not defined
Iron	18 mg	Not routinely added
Manganese	2300 mcg	60-100 mcg†
Molybdenum	45 mcg	Not routinely added
Selenium	55 mcg	20-60 mcg
Zinc	11 mg	2.5-5 mg

*Nutrient prescriptions must be individualized for each patient and clinical situation.[31]
†Monitor serum manganese concentrations during long-term use.[19]

with the energy goals for the patient. Overfeeding critically ill patients is defined as the administration of energy and substrate in excess of the amount required for metabolic homeostasis. In practical terms, feeding in excess of 110% of the total energy requirement is considered overfeeding.[70] If nurses have not been trained to recognize metabolic complications of overfeeding, symptoms may be attributed inaccurately to other causes, delaying appropriate intervention. For example, excessive dextrose administration can cause metabolic changes such as hyperglycemia, fatty liver (hepatic steatosis), hypercapnia (elevated carbon dioxide), hypertriglyceridemia, and the refeeding syndrome. Patients at risk for overfeeding include very small, cachectic, or elderly patients. Also, obese patients might be overfed if their weight was overestimated or not adequately adjusted when equations based on normal-weight individuals are used. Moreover, patients receiving concentrated formulas (e.g., TPN dextrose >20%) and patients just beginning TPN or making the transition from TPN to tube feeding are at risk for overfeeding. Other patients at risk include those receiving lipids with propofol or peritoneal dialysis with dextrose in the dialysate. Patients with organ failure have reduced tolerance for certain nutrients.

GOALS IN INTERMEDIATE CARE

Chief nutritional goals during the intermediate phase of care are (1) advancing nutrition routes from parenteral to enteral tube to oral diet, (2) stabilizing muscle and visceral protein compartments, (3) maintaining immune function, and (4) patient and family education. During the intermediate phase of care, neurotrauma patients, especially spinal cord–injured patients, have increased risk for malnutrition and related conditions of pulmonary infection, pressure ulcers, and constipation.

TABLE 17-8 **Classification of Enteral Tube Feeding Formulas**

Product Class	Product Characteristics	Patient Indications
Standard	• Intact macronutrients • Mimics typical American diet	• Fully functional gastrointestinal tract
High nitrogen	• Intact macronutrients • >14% total calories from proteins	• Malnourished, catabolic, and/or obese
Elemental and semi-elemental	• Hydrolyzed macronutrients • Hyperosmolar • Low in total fat; may contain 30% of calories as fat with <50% from long-chain triglyceride	• Severe maldigestion and malabsorption
Concentrated	• Intact macronutrients • Mimics typical American diet	• Restricted fluid intake
Fiber containing	• Fiber from natural food or added soy polysaccharide	• Bowel function regulation
Specialty	• Varies depending on disease state	• Renal or hepatic failure or pulmonary compromise

Transition to Oral Feeding

Once a patient is extubated, swallowing ability and safety need to be assessed before an oral diet can be initiated. Speech pathologists test the patient's swallowing ability with foods of varying consistency, such as thin liquids, pudding, and mashed potatoes. Consistency restrictions might be recommended, which may be modified over time as the patient recovers function. Patients who have their jaws wired shut will also require meals of special consistency (blenderized/liquid). The dietitian ensures that patients with consistency restrictions are provided with adequate and appropriate meals. Patients with marginal intake because of anorexia, poor chewing ability, or other reasons can be provided with oral supplements, fortified shakes, puddings, and food bars to supply added calories, protein, vitamins and minerals. Family input may be valuable to identify special likes, dislikes, and psychologic or cultural considerations. Families can be encouraged to bring in special foods the patient may desire, and their presence during mealtime may be helpful.

To encourage appetite during the transition from tube feeding to an oral diet and to continue to meet nutrient goals, it might be necessary to use partial enteral tube feedings at night, while the patient is sleeping, and discontinue them during the day. If appetite problems persist because of fullness from continued enteral tube feedings, a trial period in which tube feedings are discontinued may help. The nasogastric tube may need to stay in place for several days until satisfactory oral intake is ensured. Another option is to tube feed a portion of the patient's requirements throughout the day, turning off feeding 2 hours before meals and reinstituting it 1 to 2 hours after a meal. Negotiating feeding schedules when appropriate may help the patient gain control over feedings and increase motivation. Tube feeding is not stopped completely until calorie counts confirm that the patient is meeting 50% to 75% of the estimated nutrient and fluid needs by oral means.[1]

Goals for Education

Often, patients are ready to begin learning more about nutrition requirements and interventions during the intermediate phase of care. The health care team determines what nutrition education is appropriate on the basis of the patient's needs, abilities, readiness, and length of stay. Traumatic illness can cause psychologic stress, anger, dependence, and depression, which can potentially alter the success of the prescribed nutrition regimen. In particular, neurologic and physical deficits may prevent independent feeding. Family members play an increasing role in nutritional interventions during this phase of care. Interdisciplinary assessment, planning, and intervention are critical to address barriers to nourishment and successful achievement of goals.

Goals for Bowel Management

Patients with spinal cord injuries, particularly neurogenic bowel dysfunction, are prone to disruption of function of the lower intestine. Lesions of the sacral spine may damage the defecation center, requiring the manual removal of stool (flaccid bowel dysfunction). Spinal cord injuries above the sacral level can eliminate the normal sensation to defecate (spastic bowel dysfunction). Therefore, regularly scheduled, well-balanced meals with plenty of fiber and fluids are important for bowel management. Patient education might include avoidance of foods causing gas (e.g., onions) and encourage foods having natural laxative effects (e.g., prune juice) and stimulate defecation (e.g., tea, coffee).

Goals for Exercise

Promoting physical activity improves muscle function and growth. Patients may be fearful of medical tubes and hardware and need to be encouraged to exercise as tolerated. Those who have been on long-term controlled mechanical ventilation need extra encouragement to increase their respiratory muscle activity. The physical therapist should assist in maintaining appropriate progress in the patient's activity level. Frequent range-of-motion exercises should be incorporated into daily activities. As activity increases, the well-nourished patient can regain protein stores and rebuild the muscle lost during critical care.

GOALS IN REHABILITATIVE CARE

Patient's who are admitted to the rehabilitation unit with severe malnutrition (i.e., BMI under 15) are more prone to pressure ulcers and delayed wound healing and are expected to have substantially longer lengths of stay than those patients with better nutritional status.[28,71] This underscores the importance of preventing severe nutrient depletion by providing adequate nutritional support throughout all phases of care. Malnourished patients will require sufficient feeding to gain weight and develop strength to mobilize and perform daily activities. A rate of weight gain of 0.5 to 2.0 kg per week is possible for severely malnourished patients during rehabilitative treatment if they can tolerate more than 2500 kcal per day.[71] The nutrition plan focuses on increasing the patient's ability to be independent and should be updated periodically to meet the individual needs. Physical and occupational therapists are actively involved in assisting the patient to achieve levels of independent functioning. Teaching the patient to understand the rationale behind proper nutrient intake is essential to help overcome disabilities.

During rehabilitation, patients adjust psychologically to their situation, although depression may still be present, boredom may exist, and patients may be eager to return home. Problems related to the experience of traumatic injury, such as loss of friends, loss of employment, and depression, can diminish self-esteem and the relationship with caregivers. Family coping skills and concerns over health insurance and financial status also affect rehabilitation. These factors affect the patient's capacity to achieve optimal nutrition status and should be addressed as appropriate to improve the patient's quality of life.

Considerations for Oral Intake

When possible, the best position to prevent aspiration while eating is to have the patient sit upright, as erect as possible, with both feet resting on the floor.[33] Independence in self-feeding is assisted with specially designed plates and utensils, such as use of a scoop plate if the patient has the strength to push food to the side of the plate. The plate is designed to allow food to fall onto the spoon.[33]

The National Pressure Ulcer Long-Term Care Study analyzed data collected from 95 long-term care facilities on 1524 residents who were at risk for pressure ulcers at the beginning of a 12-week study.[49] Oral problems with eating and weight loss were both associated with a higher risk for development of pressure ulcers. In contrast, patients who receive nutritional intervention are more likely to receive adequate calories, protein, and other nutrients to maintain their nutritional status and prevent weight loss and pressure ulcers. For example, in that study, the use of oral nutritional supplements or high-calorie (>1.5 kcal/ml) or high-protein/disease-specific formulas for ≥21 days was associated with a decreased likelihood of pressure ulcers.[49]

The clinician should ascertain reasons for poor intake, such as ill-fitting dentures, missing teeth, oral infections, or discomfort after oral procedures. Changes in the food consistency may improve intake in these situations, especially if discussed with the patient.[33] If oral intake does not improve, between-meal snacks based on the patient's preferences can supplement meals. An alternative location for mealtime may be advisable for those patients whose roommates have a persistent cough, vomiting, diarrhea, or other conditions that might interfere with the patient's appetite and oral intake.[33] Family members can be encouraged to visit at mealtime and bring a favorite food.

Goals for Discharge Education

Patients going home with physician orders for special diets or nutrition support must be educated, and further health care assistance at home may be required. A coordinated approach to home nutrition support requires appropriate selection of educational materials, training, and follow-up. Involving social workers, nurses, dietitians, pharmacists, and a home health care agency representative to prepare and educate the family may be beneficial. Most patients are anxious to go home but may be frustrated if all procedures are not mastered. Therefore, adequate time for preparation is essential.

The teaching process for transitioning to home nutrition support begins with assessing the patient and home caregiver to (1) identify learning needs, (2) determine readiness to learn, (3) establish mutual goals and objectives, and (4) choose an appropriate method/plan for teaching. Health personnel teach by demonstration, with a return demonstration by the patient to determine acquisition of skills. In addition, detailed written instruction is necessary. The nurse should document the educational process. Major problems may be prevented by keeping lines of communication open and reinforcing the need to communicate questions and concerns. Content covered for nutrition support should include all technical aspects of TPN or tube feeding, material storage, line/tube care, site care, dressing changes, infusion pump functions, nutrient delivery systems, catheter complications (infection), preparation of solutions if premixed solutions are not used, and metabolic assessment (intake and output, urine testing). Complications such as diarrhea, dehydration, and feeding tube blockage should be discussed. Patients must be taught to report symptoms such as nausea, vomiting, and abdominal distention because these may indicate feeding intolerance. In addition, the patient should report weight loss or excessive weight gain because this could indicate inadequate feeding or overfeeding. For oral diets, the dietetic specialist should educate patients and caregivers on how to select nutritious foods, plan meals, and prepare foods to address patient-specific nutrition issues. High-energy, low-quality diets can increase the risk of cardiac disease and insulin resistance among patients with spinal cord injuries. Excess weight gain should be prevented.[72] Model education that incorporates nutrition education programs is available for health promotion in the spinal cord–injured population.[73]

The Transition to Nutrition Support

The majority of critically ill patients will receive some form of nutrition support during their stay in the ICU, and a substantial proportion of patients continues to require nutrition support during the intermediate and rehabilitative phases of care.[74] Nutrition support must be prescribed before it can be administered to the patient, and an access route must be available. In-house enteral and parenteral prescription forms can assist with ordering.[19,75] Nursing procedures for nutrition support, including placement and care of lines and tubes, have been published.[76]

Timing

Fluid resuscitation and medical control of major electrolyte and acid-base disturbances should be achieved before nutrition support is initiated. Patients who are in shock and those requiring substantial amounts of fluids and inotropic agents will likely have poor perfusion of the gastrointestinal tract. Feeding increases the demand for oxygen, so feeding into a poorly perfused gut can exacerbate gastrointestinal ischemia and even lead to bowel necrosis.[1] The physician usually has some idea of how long a patient will be NPO and whether a patient will tolerate a certain feeding modality. Patients with mild injuries who were previously well nourished might be provided with 5% dextrose in water if they are expected to resume oral intake within 5 to 7 days unless free water is contraindicated. This can provide 120 to 180 g per day of dextrose (400 to 600 kcal/d), an amount that should meet the glucose requirements of the brain and formed blood elements.

The goal for initiating nutrition support is to begin as soon as the patient will likely tolerate it and within 24 to 48 hours of admission to the ICU.[68,75] Regarding enteral support for severely injured trauma patients, Jacobs et al[1] concluded that there appeared to be no outcome advantage from initiating feeding within 24 hours of admission compared with within 72 hours of admission. In practice, enteral tube feeding is typically initiated on the second day in the ICU and, for those patients who require it, TPN is typically initiated on the third day, although practice varies across facilities.[74] Patients with severe head injury should receive early rather than delayed feeding[77] and early enteral support is preferred.[1] In particular, the Brain Trauma Foundation recommends that patients with severe traumatic brain injury receive complete caloric replacement by 7 days after injury.[78]

Stress Ulcer Prophylaxis

Histamine-2 receptor antagonists are the most prevalent medication administered to NPO trauma patients and to those with postpyloric feeding tubes to decrease the risk of gastric ulcer. Proton pump inhibitors, sucralfate, and antacids are also used.[74] In the case of sucralfate, the stomach is the target site of its antiulcer effects so that the placement of a tube with a gastric port for medication delivery is important. The implementation of stress ulcer prophylaxis guidelines in trauma ICUs can decrease inappropriate use of prophylaxis (and associated charges).[79]

Route of Feeding

Several algorithms were developed by consensus groups to provide assistance in selecting an appropriate route and tube for feeding (Figure 17-5).[1,80] Ideally, an interdisciplinary nutrition support team uses an algorithm or a clinical pathway approach to guide the selection of feeding tubes and feeding route and tailors the plan of care to suit the needs of the individual patient. The type of feeding modality depends largely on the severity and type of injury and the expected recovery period. The route selected for nutrition support is that which minimizes risk to the patient.[21] Because enteral nutrition is physiologically normal, the common rule of thumb for feeding is that oral is better than tube feeding, which is preferable to parenteral nutrition. In randomized controlled trials that compared tube feeding with parenteral nutrition in hospitalized patients, the parenteral route was associated with increased infective complications and longer length of hospital stay.[77,81] Yet the difference between routes of feeding on outcome of the critically ill trauma population is less clear. When jejunal tubes are available as an option for feeding, it has been demonstrated that jejunal feeding reduces the days of TPN use.[82] Randomized controlled trials of patients with moderate to severe acute pancreatitis demonstrate that enteral feeding into the jejunum is associated with fewer infectious complications and reduced length of hospital stay than if TPN is used.[83] In practice, parenteral nutrition should only be initiated in those patients requiring nutrition support for whom enteral nutrition is not possible.[1,19] Mechanical bowel obstruction, bowel ischemia, fistulas, and anastomosis are examples of indications where TPN might be used.

Specialized Formulas

It is the responsibility of the dietitian to recommend a specific tube feeding formula on the basis of the patient's condition. Some specialized enteral formulas are commonly referred to as "immune enhancing" because they contain supplements thought to decrease infectious complications and promote healing. Although several early reports indicated that specialized formulas might reduce infection rates and length of stay, recent meta-analyses of clinical trials fail to demonstrate a reduction in risk of infectious complications, length of ICU stay, or mortality rates.[84] Well-controlled and sufficiently powered clinical trials and dosing studies of individual nutrients are needed to identify whether particular ingredients added above amounts in standard formulas might have beneficial effects on patient outcome and the dose at which effects are realized.[84,85] Hence, the use of specialized

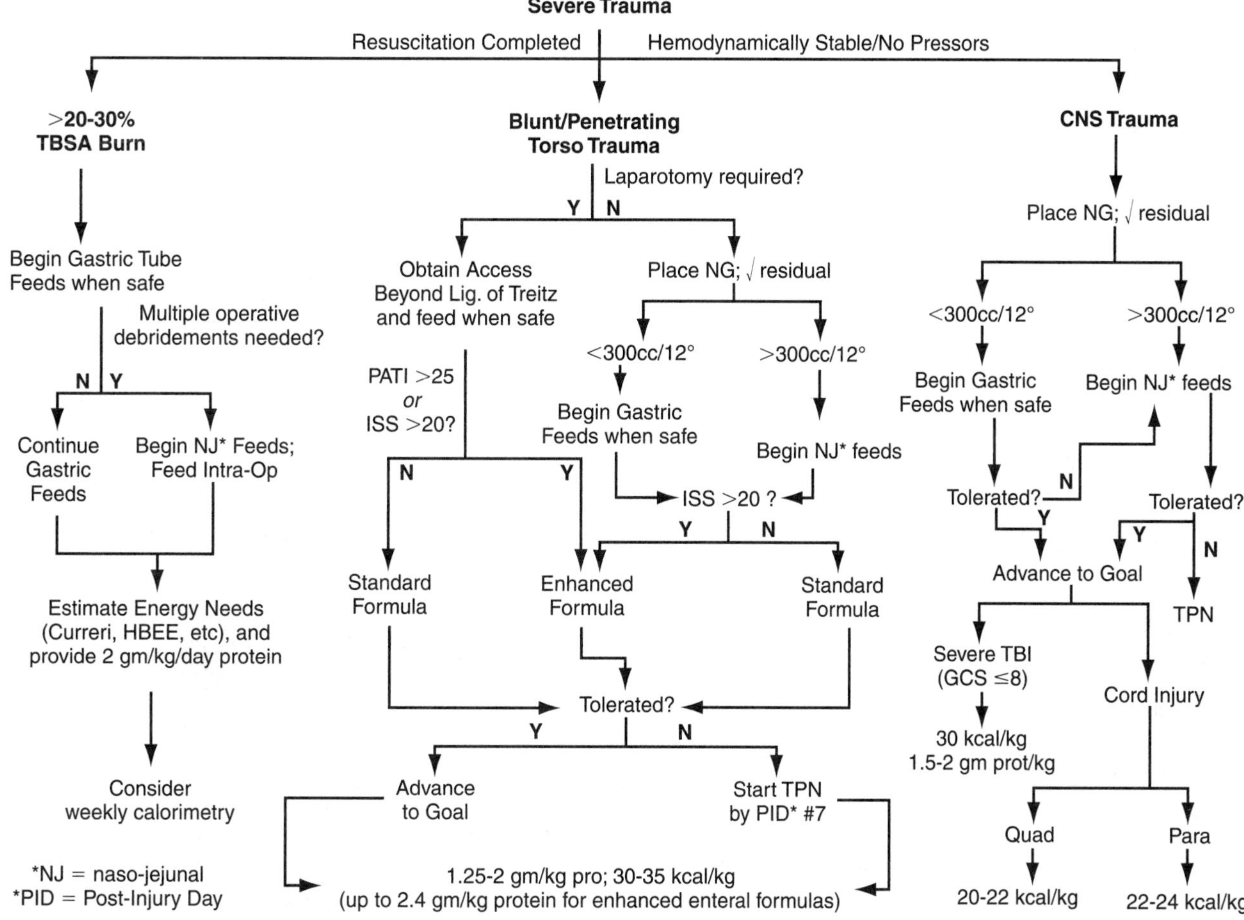

FIGURE 17-5 Summary algorithm for nutritional support of the adult trauma patient. *TBSA,* Total body surface area; *NG,* nasogastric; *PID,* post-injury day; *CNS,* central nervous system; *TBI,* traumatic brain injury; *GCS,* Glasgow coma score; *Lig,* ligament. (From Jacobs DG, Jacobs DO, Kudsk KA, et al: Practice management guidelines for nutritional support of the trauma patient, *J Trauma* 57:660-679, 2004, Fig. 1, p. 661.)

formulas and extra supplementation of individual nutrients, such as vitamin C and vitamin E, remains controversial and practice varies among hospitals.

Branched-Chain Amino Acids

Formulas enriched with essential branched-chain amino acids have been considered for patients with chronic hepatic encephalopathy who are intolerant of protein and are unresponsive to pharmacotherapy,[31] yet administration of such formulas lacks conclusive evidence of benefit for trauma patients. Further research is needed.

Arginine

The nonessential amino acid arginine enhances the synthesis of nitric oxide in endothelium. When produced in small amounts, it plays a major role as a vasodilator. However, when released in large amounts by macrophages, nitric oxide promotes autoimmune tissue damage. Another concern with arginine supplementation is that it can increase azotemia and raise the concentration of plasma ornithine (a prosclerotic agent). One clinical trial of 153 patients after myocardial infarction had to halt further recruitment of subjects because arginine supplementation was associated with increased mortality rates compared with placebo.[86] Arginine research is of interest for trauma care because, under experimental conditions, arginine increases plasma concentration of insulin-like growth factor-1, which may be beneficial if it augments hydroxyproline in wounds to promote wound healing. At this time, it is not known whether arginine-enriched diets are safe for trauma patients and whether they influence outcome.

Glutamine

The nonessential amino acid glutamine is depleted from muscle and plasma during critical illness. The largest clinical trials of enteral glutamine supplementation to date have not demonstrated a benefit for critically ill patients. One trial enrolled 85 trauma patients in addition to other critically ill patients and randomized them to a standard formula or an isonitrogenous, isocaloric formula providing a median of 19 g glutamine for 10 days.[87] Glutamine had no effect on the incidence of infection, severe sepsis, or death at 6 months. In another trial of 185 trauma and surgical patients who were fed a standard formula with or without supplemental glutamine or a specialized nutrition formula with added glutamine, no significant differences were found in morbidity or mortality rates.[88] Glutamine is not yet approved by the FDA for use in intravenous form in humans outside of investigational protocols.[89] In its free form, glutamine has limited solubility and is unstable in solution. Recently, dipeptide forms (e.g., alanyl-glutamine) demonstrated superior manufacturing potential and rapid hydrolysis to free glutamine after infusion.[90] Further studies are needed to investigate the outcome of intravenous infusion of high-dose glutamine in trauma patients, independent of effects of added protein, and to determine the mechanism of action.[91,92] Because the metabolism of glutamine can increase ammonia formation in the regulation of acid-base balance, supplemental glutamine is contraindicated in patients with renal disease or hepatic insufficiency who have decreased abilities to eliminate ammonia.[89] Glutamine supplementation might also be problematic for those with glutamine-expansion disorders such as Huntington disease and, at least initially, after focal contusions and ischemic events in the brain, particularly if there is a disruption of the blood-brain barrier.

ENTERAL SUPPORT AND MONITORING

Enteral nutrition should be initiated if the patient's gastrointestinal tract is functioning. Many trauma patients require tube feeding because altered consciousness, mechanical ventilation, or diminished gag or cough reflex puts them at risk for aspiration. Primary considerations in choosing the access route and formula include the degree of gastrointestinal function, the expected duration of nutrition therapy, aspiration risk, and the degree of organ dysfunction.[1] Nurses play key roles in enteral nutrition, inserting the feeding tubes, maintaining patency, administering formula, documenting accurate intake/output, preventing complications, and assessing the response and tolerance to feedings.[93]

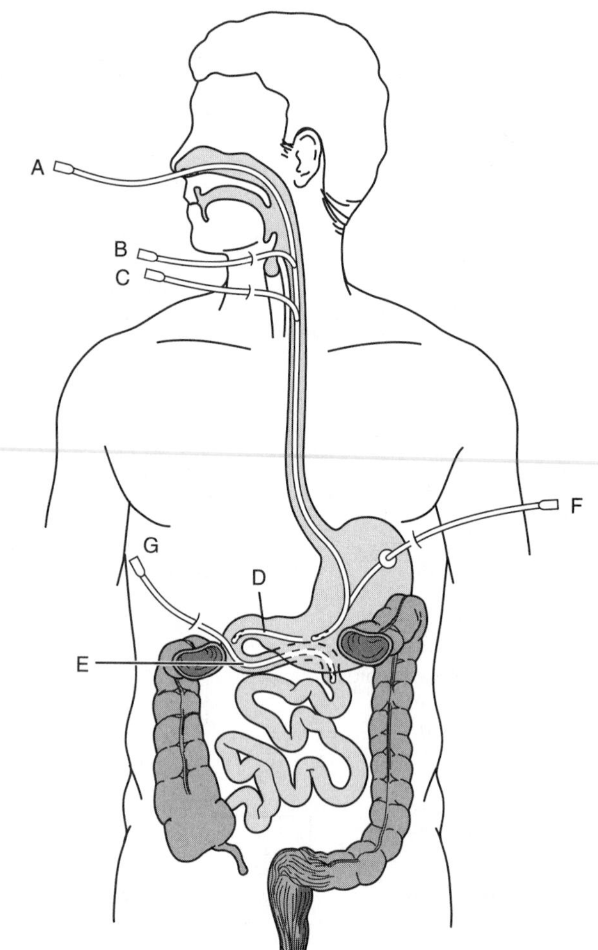

FIGURE 17-6 Tube feeding routes. *A,* Nasogastric; *B,* pharyngostomy; *C,* esophagostomy; *D,* nasoduodenal; *E,* nasojejunal; *F,* gastrostomy; *G,* jejunostomy. (From Veldee MS: Nutritional assessment, therapy, and monitoring. In Burtis CA, Ashwood ER, editors: *Tietz textbook of clinical chemistry,* 3rd ed, Philadelphia, 1999, W. B. Saunders, Figure 28-2, p. 1369.)

FEEDING TUBES

Tube Location

Nasogastric, nasoduodenal, and nasojejunal routes provide short-term (<3 to 4 weeks) access for enteral support.[80] For trauma patients needing long-term support (4 weeks or longer), gastrostomy or gastrojejunostomy routes are preferred.[80] A selection of feeding tube entrance and exit-port locations are portrayed in Figure 17-6.[94] In general, many patients with head trauma and spinal cord injuries can be fed through a nasogastric tube if the head-of-bed elevation is not medically restricted. For many patients with neurotrauma, the initial posttraumatic paralytic ileus resolves sometime during the first 72 hours after injury and then gastric feeding is well tolerated. Patients with blunt or penetrating trauma to the torso might also tolerate nasogastric feeding. The nasal route is typically contraindicated for trauma patients who have coagulopathies, basilar skull fractures, or nasal fractures. The orogastric route is usually chosen for patients with facial trauma or at risk for sinusitis if the risk of aspiration is not high. The rigid, large-bore tube that is initially placed for gastric decompression may be problematic if left in place for long-term feeding. This type of tube exerts pressure on the trachea and esophagus and over time can lead to necrosis and a tracheoesophageal fistula. A rigid tube may also prevent sufficient closure of the cardiac sphincter, permitting reflux of acidic gastric contents into the esophagus, leading to esophagitis.

Despite injury and surgery, small bowel motility and absorption may remain intact, and feeding into the jejunum should be considered even if gastric motility is impaired. Jacobs et al recommended that patients with severe head injury who do not tolerate gastric feeding be switched to postpyloric feedings, preferably beyond the ligament of Treitz (in the fourth portion of the duodenum), as tolerated.[1] Although challenging, enteral support is even feasible in some patients with abdominal compartment syndrome.[95] Patients with small bowel feeding tubes often also require a gastric tube for decompression and suction of fluids. Therefore, tubes are available that have two ports, a gastric port for suction, decompression, or medication delivery, and a separate, extended tube for simultaneous small bowel feeding. If there is lack of postpyloric access, an initial attempt at gastric feeding may be warranted to avoid delaying enteral support. However, patients at high risk for pulmonary aspiration because of prone or supine positioning, gastric retention despite prokinetic agents, or gastroesophageal reflux should receive enteral support through the jejunum.[1,80,96]

Tube Placement and Care

The method and route of tube insertion depends on the preference, training, and availability of staff. If a laparotomy is required, often a tube will be placed for feeding beyond the ligament of Treitz.[1] Otherwise, tubes for postpyloric feeding can be inserted by blind passage at the bedside or by fluoroscopic or endoscopic placement.[74,80,97] A soft, small-bore tube should be used. Small tubes (8- to 10-gauge French) made of polyurethane or silicone are less irritating to mucous tissue, especially in the nasal passage, than larger tubes. A tube that is at least 105 cm in length is required for postpyloric feedings past the ligament of Treitz. Both weighted and nonweighted tubes are used, and neither has been proven superior to the other.

Inadvertent placement of the feeding tube into the respiratory tract occurs in fewer than 5% of new tube insertions.[98] Hence, many institutions require radiographic confirmation before feeding through any blindly placed feeding tube, regardless of size.[98] The radiograph remains the gold standard to verify tube location. During and immediately after insertion, the following additional supportive methods can be considered to recognize potential problems with tube placement: marking the point at which the tube exits the patient, noting the color of the tube aspirate, noting changes in residual volumes, testing the pH of aspirate during fasting, and observing for signs of respiratory distress. The tubes should be stabilized and cleaned as needed with normal saline solution. Gastrostomy and jejunostomy tubes should be dressed daily with dry gauze and anchored. The skin surrounding the tube site should be evaluated daily for redness, swelling, warmth, skin breakdown, and drainage. Verifying tube placement and patency is a routine but essential practice and should be performed at initial placement, before medications are administered, after replacement, when proper placement is questioned, and routinely on the basis of hospital protocols. The nurse should check for the length of tube external to the body and document changes. Some advocate assessing tube patency every 2 hours[76] and tube placement at least once per shift.[99] Gastric leakage or tube displacement of more than 1 inch needs to be reported, and a radiograph should be taken if the tube is displaced.

Maintaining tube patency requires frequent tube irrigation. Water is the most effective irrigant. The ports should be flushed every 6 hours during continuous feeding, after any bolus feedings, and after residuals are assessed. If the enteral infusion is turned off for any length of time, the tube should be flushed before feeding is restarted. Obstruction of the feeding tube can result from caking of medications and residual tube feedings on the inner lumen. Furthermore, gastric acid can coagulate protein in enteral formulas at the end of the tube. The clog may be loosened by flushing the tube with warm water, alternating attempts to irrigate and aspirate in a rhythmic motion, and allowing for slight expansion of a flexible tube with a 60-ml syringe. If this approach fails, a declogging device might be used to remove the clog mechanically. The nurse should never attempt to force a clog through the tube because the tube may rupture. Prevention remains the best solution to clogged tubes.[76] Research is needed to support further development of evidence-based protocols for the nursing care of enteral feeding tubes.[76,100,101]

Aspiration Risk

Aspiration of tube feeding is potentially serious and sometimes fatal. Aspiration means that material has been inhaled into the airway below the level of the vocal cords.[102] A patient who has aspirated enteral nutrition formula can have aspiration pneumonitis or aspiration pneumonia. Signs and symptoms include cough, tachypnea, and respiratory distress.[103] Conditions that increase the risk of aspiration during nutrition support include endotracheal intubation, a head-of-bed restriction, periodic alternating supine and prone repositioning, chest physiotherapy, a malpositioned feeding tube, vomiting, and persistently high gastric residual volumes.[102] In mechanically ventilated patients, those in a prone position (face downward) have greater residual gastric volumes and more frequent episodes of vomiting in response to early nasogastric feeding than those in a supine position (lying on the back).[104]

Increasing the head-of-bed elevation to 45 degrees (or above 30 degrees if 45 degrees is not attainable), with the bend of the bed at the patient's lower back, is believed to reduce the incidence of tube feeding aspiration.[103] Maintaining the minimal occlusive volume within the endotracheal and tracheostomy cuffs of mechanically ventilated patients has also been suggested to lessen the possibility of aspiration.[103] Nurses need to be cautious to ensure that the lowest cuff pressure necessary to maintain a seal is used. This will minimize the risk for tracheal erosion. For gastric feeding, promotility agents (e.g., metoclopramide) have been used to reduce the likelihood of gastroesophageal reflux and pulmonary aspiration[105,106] yet for high-risk patients, postpyloric feedings past the ligament of Treitz with simultaneous decompression of the stomach are preferred to more proximal feeding.[107] Tube feedings should be interrupted and or gastric residuals adequately assessed when the head-of-bed is flat or lower.[99] In most cases the risk of aspiration is small relative to the benefit of feedings when appropriate nursing interventions are instituted. Tube feeding is initiated and advanced according to protocols for safety that incrementally increase the volume of formula to the target rate over several days as tolerated. Continuous feedings during critical care are thought to be associated with a reduced risk of aspiration compared with large-volume, intermittent bolus feedings.[102] Gastric residual volumes of 200 to 500 ml indicate that the patient should be monitored closely, and residual volumes >500 ml indicate the need to withhold tube feedings and reassess tolerance.[102] The use of glucose detection methods to signal aspiration events has been abandoned for lack of sensitivity and specificity. The use of blue dye in tube feeding to detect aspiration is unsafe.[103,108]

Initiation and Advancement of Enteral Support

Aspiration risk strategies should be reviewed and implemented before feeding is introduced. The patient's access device and insertion site should be visually inspected and formula label and orders should be checked.[21] Once correct tube placement is confirmed, tube feeding can be initiated. Feeding through a jejunal tube can begin as soon as the patient is hemodynamically stable, whereas gastric feeding may be delayed depending on gastric function (e.g., a single gastric residual volume >250 ml). Enteral support should not be withheld or reduced for lack of bowel sounds or diarrhea.[80]

The pump-assisted method for administering formula is strongly recommended for critically ill patients and is required for those who are continuously fed into the small bowel. Continuous feeding at a low-volume rate of delivery helps to minimize gastric complications such as nausea, cramping, and diarrhea. In addition, automated pump control of continuous feedings enables more reliable records of intake and calculation of fluid balance and energy intake. Consensus recommendations advocate initiating feeding at a low rate (e.g., 25% of the goal rate) and progressing as tolerated with caution to the goal rate by 48 to 72 hours.[102] Generally, enteral support is begun with full-strength formula at 20 to 40 ml per hour.[10] The rate is increased on the basis of physician order or hospital protocol. Typically the rate is increased by 20 to 25 ml every 4 to 8 hours as tolerated until the target rate is achieved.[80] Attempts should be made to assess residual gastric contents every 2 to 4 hours and as needed. Consensus groups strongly recommend tight glycemic control, correction of electrolyte abnormalities, and minimizing the use of narcotics for patients on enteral nutrition support.[102] It is the nurse's responsibility to ascertain whether the patient is tolerating the administration of formula and to communicate findings regarding vomiting, bowel sounds, residual volume, flatus, and amount and consistency of stools to the nutrition care team. If the patient complains of any abdominal discomfort, the abdomen becomes distended, or the patient has nausea/vomiting, the feeding should be discontinued for further evaluation. Periodic measures of abdominal girth might be useful. High aspirates are the primary reason why tube feedings are interrupted.[109] When gastric motility is a problem, a prokinetic agent (i.e., metoclopramide) can be considered.[68] If residual volumes continue to be elevated after repeated doses (e.g., four doses) of a prokinetic agent or there is repeated emesis, a jejunal feeding tube may be needed.[80]

Once the goal rate is achieved, the nurse should continue monitoring for tolerance and communicate any signs of deterioration in clinical status to the nutrition care team. Feeding may need to be temporarily discontinued or changed if the patient becomes unstable or requires ventilatory support and neuromuscular blockade.[102] Surgery or radiologic procedures may delay or reduce the amount of nutrition support the patient receives. Moreover, clogged or dislodged tubes that are not rapidly restored can also interfere with provision of adequate nutrition support. The nurse should try to minimize the amount of time that tube feedings are held for preventable or correctable reasons. Typically for trauma patients who are tube fed, enteral support is provided for approximately 8 days.[109]

Complications of Tube Feeding During Critical Illness

Several complications associated with tube feeding during critical illness can be prevented or minimized. These include constipation, tube clogging, and small bowel necrosis.

Considerations for Drug Administration

Medications should not be mixed with formulas or other medications unless they have been shown to be compatible to avoid clogging and altering absorption. In general, medication should be given separately from enteral formulas, and the tube should be flushed with water before and after medication is administered. Diluting hyperosmotic drugs with water may decrease the risk of side effects. Elixers and suspensions are a better choice for administering through a feeding tube than are syrups, a number of which are incompatible with enteral formulas. If only solid forms of medication are available, they should be crushed into a fine powder and mixed with 30 ml of water to form a slurry to prevent clogs during administration.[110] An adequate drug dosage may be difficult to achieve with soft gelatin capsules, which must be poked open, squeezed of their contents, and diluted for administration down the tube. Sustained release and enteric-coated pills should not be administered through feeding tubes. The hospital pharmacist should be consulted when questions arise about drug-nutrient compatibility. Some drugs can interact with nutrients in formula, altering absorption or metabolism. Such drug-nutrient interactions can interfere with the intended action of the drug or impair nutrition status.[111] Tube feeding may need to be delayed 30 minutes to 2 hours before and after some medications are administered.[111] For example, tube feedings are held for 2 hours before and after administration of phenytoin (Dilantin). In this case therapeutic levels of the drug need to be monitored to maintain seizure prophylaxis. The dose rate of medication may need to change when the patient is transitioned to oral feeding or TPN.

Bowel Management

Optimally, the patient should resume excreting stool on a daily basis. Adequate hydration and regular bowel care will assist in preventing constipation. The failure to pass stool after substantial amounts of tube feeding have been delivered may indicate bowel obstruction, impaction of fecal matter, or other serious problems. If these problems are ruled out, natural fiber (e.g., Metamucil), stool softeners, or fiber-containing tube feeding formula may help the gut retain moisture and give form to stool. Moreover, dietary fiber is consumed by neutral bacteria in the lower intestine that produce short-chain fatty acids that are an energy substrate for enterocytes, improving the health of the intestinal lining and supporting sodium and water absorption. Diarrhea is a common complication in critically ill patients and is not usually related to the nutrition formula.[10] When bowel irregularities occur, drug administration and infection should be considered as possible causes in addition to feeding intolerance. A thorough medical workup should be undertaken if the patient has prolonged constipation or diarrhea, and dehydration should be prevented. Nosocomial pathogens, such as *Clostridium difficile* can spread in the ICU and outbreaks often result from poor hygiene and noncompliance with standard precautions. Adult patients receiving antibiotics for several days may be susceptible to bowel infection from *C. difficile* bacteria.[112] Bacterial or viral toxins trigger the enterocytes lining the intestine to secrete fluid and electrolytes into the intestinal lumen, causing secretory diarrhea. Symptoms of *C. difficile* can include foul-smelling diarrhea, abdominal cramps, fever, persistent nausea and vomiting, and blood in the stool. Testing of stool specimens (not rectal swabs) for toxins A and B provides diagnosis. Fasting will not resolve this type of diarrhea.

Food-borne illness and diarrhea may result from microbial contamination of tube formulas from tap water, prolonged hang times, and reuse of tubing and other apparatus.[10] Commercially prepared, ready-to-use formulas that do not require the addition of water or supplements are least likely to contribute to microbial growth. Once tube feedings are contaminated, rapid growth of gram-negative bacilli can occur. For this reason it is imperative that nurses follow procedures for sanitary handling, holding, and administration of formula and manage hydration with water boluses and intravenous fluids rather than risk contamination by diluting the formula. Proper handling and cleaning of the lid before pouring the formula into the feeding bag are important. Unused portions should be covered, labeled, and refrigerated. Tube feeding formula bags should contain no more than a 4-hour supply, particularly if the formula was altered after the manufacturer's seal was opened. The maximal time a given lot of formula should hang is 8 hours.[76] Changing the feeding bag every 24 hours using clean technique and use of closed system enteral products can help minimize microbial contamination and growth.

Malabsorption of tube feeding formula can be caused by use of cold formula or a concentrated hyperosmolar solution, such as an elemental feeding formula or medication. The pharmacist can assist with determining whether drugs may have induced diarrhea. A hyperosmolar solution causes excess amounts of water to remain in the intestinal lumen, resulting in osmotic diarrhea. Conditions of maldigestion, such as lactose intolerance or dumping syndrome after gastric surgery, accelerate release of hyperosmolar stomach contents into the intestine. Osmotic diarrhea should resolve within 24 hours of stopping the concentrated feeding or medication. Depending on the etiology of the diarrhea, an antimotility medication may be indicated (rule out *C. difficile* before use of antimotility drugs).[10]

Small Bowel Ischemia and Necrosis

The risk of bowel necrosis is rare in tube-fed patients, approximately 1 in 900 (0.1%); however, its development in critically ill patients is nearly always fatal.[113] Initiating enteral feeding before the patient is completely resuscitated or feeding during hypotensive episodes may complicate bowel ischemia and contribute to the development of necrosis.[93] A majority of patients in whom bowel necrosis develops had previous small bowel resections and jejunal tubes for feeding. Early clinical signs associated with bowel necrosis resemble that of bacterial sepsis and include increased heart rate (>100 beats/min), abnormal white blood cell count (>15 10^9/L), and fever (>100.5° F) coupled with abdominal distention and the need to accelerate doses of vasopressor agents.[113] To help prevent bowel necrosis, delay tube feedings until after the patient is hemodynamically stable, carefully select routes of feeding for patients having small bowel resections, and closely monitor the response to feeding.

Intermediate and Rehabilitative Enteral Support

Many patients having paraplegia or quadriplegia from complete spinal cord transection will leave the ICU on enteral support.[109] For those patients continuing to require nutrition support, the percutaneous endoscopic gastrostomy (PEG) tube is the most common device for long-term enteral access.[114] Gastrostomies eliminate nasal irritation and the discomfort of nasotube replacement. The decision for placement of a PEG tube should include ethical considerations and always be individualized rather than the result of a general algorithm.[115] When patients require long-term respiratory support, PEG tubes are frequently inserted at the time of the tracheostomy procedure.[114] Contraindications for PEG or percutaneous endoscopic jejunostomy include serious coagulation disorders, severe ascites, peritonitis, or a clearly limited life expectancy.[115]

Guidelines are available to help maintain standards for care and to avoid aspiration, wound infection, and other complications of PEG placement and care.[115,116] Because PEG tubes exit from the stomach through an external opening, there is increased risk of infection. Antibiotic prophylaxis before placement is recommended to prevent infection.[116] Care should be given to the exit site by checking for redness, edema, exudate, and leakage of acidic stomach contents that might break down the skin barrier. Dry sterile dressings and antimicrobial ointment may be applied to protect the exit site. Patients should be fed in a semirecumbent position to help prevent aspiration. To prevent blockage, the tube should be flushed with 50 ml of water before and after every feeding or medication.[116] Assessment of fluid status continues to be an important component of nutrition care to avoid dehydration in the long-term care setting.[117] By 6 weeks after insertion of the PEG tube, the stomach should have adhered to the abdominal wall, which will help to prevent leakage of stomach contents into the peritoneum. Therefore, the initial PEG tube should not be replaced or interchanged with another model for at least 6 weeks if possible.[114]

Tube Feeding Syndrome

Overfeeding protein, especially by tube feeding without adequate water provision, can lead to azotemia (elevated BUN), hypertonic dehydration, and metabolic acidosis (i.e., tube feeding syndrome). When large amounts of protein are fed, excess amino groups are converted to urea, increasing the risk of azotemia in elderly patients and others with compromised renal function. Because high-protein diets increase the renal solute load, they cause increased urination so a patient could become dehydrated if not provided with sufficient water. Moreover, for each molecule of urea produced, one molecule of bicarbonate is spent, which could lower blood pH. Severe dehydration, with or without acidosis, can lead to mental confusion, abnormal neuromuscular activity, rapid pulse, and decreased urination.

Protein-Calorie Malnutrition

It is not uncommon for tube-fed patients to be underfed. Malnutrition can develop rapidly in patients who have continuing severe catabolic stress, low nutrient intake, and are dependent on others for feeding. Health professionals need to compare the actual amount of calories and protein fed with the nutrition goals. Factors contributing to malnutrition include impaired digestion, malabsorption, and problems with utilization once the nutrient has been absorbed. Patients with high-output fistulas are at higher risk for malnutrition.

Prolonged inadequate caloric replacement has been associated with medical complications that can alter the body's reparative processes and impair wound healing.[17] Poor nutrition status and weight loss are contributing factors to the development of pressure ulcers during this phase of care.[49] Thinning fat padding between bones and skin allows bony prominences to compress and restrict circulation to the skin, raising the risk of pressure sores.

Parenteral Support and Monitoring

Parenteral nutrition is an effective route for delivery of nutrients. It should be considered for critically ill patients if enteral feeding is not possible for 5 days or longer (Figure 17-5). Also, according to Jacobs et al,[1] TPN should be initiated by post-injury day 7 if attempts at enteral feeding were not successful, failing to achieve at least 50% of feeding goals within 1 week of injury. Many patients think they are being starved when they receive TPN; in fact, they are receiving maintenance nutrition until they can eat. Parenteral feeding modalities include peripheral (PPN) for short-term therapy and central (TPN) routes for patients who will require more than 7 days of parenteral support. PPN is typically administered as a three-in-one solution in one bag containing fat, dextrose, amino acids, electrolytes, vitamins, and minerals, whereas TPN is typically administered in two solutions: (1) a lipid-based emulsion and (2) a bag containing everything else. A complete nutrition assessment should be conducted and fluid and electrolyte abnormalities should be addressed before parenteral nutrition is initiated. Consensus recommendations for prescribing, compounding, and administering parenteral nutrition are available.[19] A delivery pump is used to avoid erratic flow rates as is a filter device to trap particulate matter.[93] Before infusing parenteral therapy, the nurse plays a critical safety role by visually inspecting the patient's access device and insertion site and checking formula orders, label, solution, and infusion rate on the pump.[21] The safety role of the nurse is of utmost importance in administering formula, maintaining accurate infusion/output records, using meticulous aseptic techniques when handling and changing the dressing for catheters, closely monitoring for infectious complications, and assessing the response and tolerance to infusions.[93]

Peripheral Parenteral Nutrition

Patients are candidates for PPN therapy if they (1) have peripheral access, (2) can tolerate approximately 3 L per day of fluid, although less may be needed for very small patients, (3) have adequate platelet counts, (4) do not have a history of hyperlipidemia, and (5) are expected to be able to transition to enteral nutrition in less than 1 week. Before initiation of PPN, routine biochemical blood tests should be assessed and monitored. PPN is less likely than TPN to cause metabolic complications of hyperglycemia, hypophosphatemia, or increased carbon dioxide production because the calorie and carbohydrate load is relatively low (1000 to 1500 kcal).[118] On the other hand, there are several disadvantages to PPN therapy. A limited amount of protein and calories can be infused into the small peripheral veins, and it requires more volume to deliver calories and protein than does TPN. Complications of phlebitis, thrombosis, and leakage of the PPN into local tissue can occur at the infusion site. Such complications can result in pain and fever. Selection of a small gauge (20 or 22), short catheter, and use of upper extremity veins exclusively reduces the risk of serious complications.

Nurses should carefully observe PPN sites to detect any infusion into subcutaneous spaces. Using other peripheral sites to infuse medications such as antibiotics is better than interrupting PPN to flush the tubing and infuse antibiotics and other medications in the PPN site. Short peripheral catheter sites are typically rotated every 72 to 96 hours to decrease the risk of infection and phlebitis.[119] Unit bags of PPN containing lipid (i.e., three-in-one solution) should not hang longer than 24 hours to decrease risk of bacterial growth and infection.[119]

A lack of consensus guidelines for PPN undoubtedly contributes to variation in its use. Further research is required to identify those trauma patients who would benefit most from PPN. In particular, research is needed to determine whether PPN through midline or midclavicular catheter placements offer any advantage over TPN given through a central line for patients requiring parenteral support for more than 1 week.

TOTAL PARENTERAL NUTRITION

Some patients who would have received TPN in the past are now better identified and provided with small bowel enteral nutrition support. Yet for others in which enteral feeding is not safe or possible, TPN is a necessary, life-saving therapy. Compared with enteral nutrition, parenteral nutrition is associated with a significant increase in the incidence of infections, particularly catheter-related bloodstream infections.[81] The nurse must monitor the patient closely for signs and symptoms of infection that may be catheter related. If the patient suddenly has an elevated temperature, blood samples for cultures and a fever workup based on clinical signs should be conducted according to hospital policy. The source of sepsis might not be related to the feeding line. If catheter-related sepsis is suspected, the line should be removed and a new catheter inserted. The length of time the catheter remains in place is the most critical factor associated with the development of infections. It is prudent to discontinue use of the site and TPN as soon as the patient no longer requires it.

Central Line and Infection Control

TPN is hyperosmolar, so it must be infused through a central line into the superior vena cava or right atrium by the subclavian route.[31] Central venous catheter (CVC)–related infections remain a serious complication of TPN.[120] In the United States, approximately 80,000 CVC-associated bloodstream infections occur in ICUs each year at a cost of $35,000 to $56,000 per infection, some of these related to TPN.[119] Coagulase-negative staphylococci and enterococci are the most frequently isolated cases of hospital-acquired bloodstream infections, but pathogen populations can change over time. Rates of colonization are lowest for catheters used solely for TPN.[121] Risk factors for infection include method and site of catheter insertion, noncompliance with aseptic techniques, use of a multiple-lumen catheter, use of the TPN line for fluids other than TPN, and length of time the catheter remains in place. Standardizing insertion techniques, proper preparation of the patient, and good surgical technique minimize the risk of catheter-related infections. Insertion site dressings should be changed when the catheter is replaced, when the dressing becomes damp, loosened, or soiled, and when inspection of the site is necessary. Nurses should have full knowledge of infection control policies related to central line insertion procedures, site preparation and care, dressing, tubing replacement, and infusion of parenteral solutions.[31] TPN lines should be used exclusively for TPN, except in a life-threatening emergency. If a multiple-lumen catheter is used, one port should be reserved for the exclusive use of TPN infusion.[119] Maintaining a closed system minimizes the chance for contamination.

Contamination from the TPN admixture bag is rare. The nurse should check TPN products for label information and expiration date and examine for turbidity, leaks, cracks, or particulate matter before infusion.[119] The TPN bottle of lipid solution is prone to bacterial growth, so it should be infused over 12 hours. If the dosing period needs to be extended because the patient had problems with tolerance or for other reasons, the Centers for Disease Control and Prevention state the infusion should be completed within 24 hours.[119] Lipid tubing should be discarded after the 12-hour infusion is completed. TPN tubing should be changed every 24 hours when lipids are administered through any portion of the line.

Admixture

In the critical care setting, TPN is prescribed and produced daily to tailor the composition of the solution to the patient's acute condition. The parenteral fluids must be admixed (compounded) in a laminar flow hood in the pharmacy using aseptic techniques.[119] Once mixed, TPN solutions are stored under refrigeration (avoiding any ice crystal formation) until 1 or 2 hours before use at room temperature. Each liter of standard TPN typically contains 4% to 6% amino acids, 15% to 20% glucose, electrolytes, trace elements, vitamins, and sometimes insulin and histamine blockers. In the past, omissions of vitamins and minerals in TPN resulted in serious disorders and even death. Overdoses of nutrients can also be dangerous. Standard TPN is formulated with nutrients in amounts that are estimated to meet health needs, with some exceptions. Physicians can order varying amounts of electrolytes from day to day to tailor the prescription as much as possible to the patient's need. Patients with diabetes or at high risk of glucose intolerance may need a low dose dextrose solution or a reduced rate of infusion.[31] Compounding problems with some minerals, such as calcium, limit the amount that can be added to TPN, and doses may not be sufficient for long-term health. Too much calcium can cause crystalline precipitates in TPN, which if infused, can occlude the pulmonary artery branches and cause severe ventilatory defects, arterial hypoxemia, and decreased oxygen saturation.[122]

Parenteral Lipid

Lipid is an energy substrate and a source of essential fatty acids. Lipid infusion protects the venous endothelium from injury related to hypertonic glucose solutions. Typically, ready-to-use lipid emulsions (e.g., 10% or 20%) are purchased in 250- or 500-ml bottles. One 500-ml bottle of 10% lipid emulsion provides 50 g of fat and 550 kcal (as much as 25% to 30% of the total calories in TPN). Fluid-restricted patients may need calorie-dense lipids (9 kcal/g) to obtain sufficient energy substrate. For example, a 500-ml bottle of a 20% lipid emulsion provides 100 g of fat and 1,000 kcal. A minimum of 100 g of lipid (two bottles of 10% or one bottle of 20%) is given each week to prevent EFAD.

If the blood triglyceride concentration is mildly elevated, a trial dose of 10% lipids can be given and serial triglyceride levels should be followed daily. There have been rare reports of fever, chills, vomiting, urticaria, chest pain, and back pain during lipid infusions. Moreover, infusing lipids too rapidly can result in palpitations, tachypnea, wheezing, cyanosis, nausea, pain at injection site, and headache. Infusing lipids over a 12-hour period appears to be well tolerated by most patients, with minimal, if any, adverse effects. Overfeeding fat can congest the reticuloendothelial system and compromise immune function. Possible consequences of lipid administration concomitant with hypertriglyceridemia include pancreatitis and altered pulmonary status.

Biochemical and Clinical Monitoring

Before TPN is initiated, serum samples should be obtained for measurement of glucose, triglyceride, bicarbonate, renal markers (e.g., creatinine, BUN), liver markers (e.g., alkaline phosphatase), phosphorus, magnesium, and other standard electrolyte levels (sodium, potassium, chloride) and any fluid or electrolyte abnormalities should be addressed. Patients who are malnourished before admission are susceptible to abnormalities from nutrition support so TPN must be provided cautiously. Patients who are at risk for the refeeding syndrome may need additional mineral supplementation. Blood glucose and serum electrolytes should continue to be monitored frequently until measurements are stable and after any change in insulin dose.[31] Intake/output, electrolyte status, results of kidney and liver function tests, serum glucose, and triglyceride levels should be evaluated on a regular basis. Such monitoring is particularly important for patients with impaired renal function or impaired cardiac function because they are prone to fluid overload. The dietitian uses the volume of TPN administered along with the TPN prescription to calculate the actual intake of energy, protein, and other nutrients.

Complications of Parenteral Nutrition

Blood Glucose Control

Hyperglycemia is a risk factor for morbidity and death. Nurses who provide good blood glucose control may decrease their patients' risk of infection, even for those who do not have preexisting diabetes. Good blood glucose control involves providing appropriate nutrition support, adequate blood tests, hypoglycemic agents when needed, timely assessments by qualified staff, and controlling use of dextrose solutions. Strict normalization of blood glucose levels to 80 to 110 mg/dl with intensive insulin therapy decreases morbidity and mortality rates for medical and surgical ICU patients compared with those whose blood glucose is permitted greater fluctuation, up to 215 mg/dl.[123,124] Accelerated weaning from mechanical ventilation and sooner discharge from the ICU is related to improvements in blood glucose control. In addition, the infusion of exogenous insulin may exert beneficial effects that reduce kidney injury.[12,17,124] The use of insulin therapy requires close monitoring because it places the patient at risk for hypoglycemia, especially if nutrition support is unexpectedly decreased or discontinued. Guidelines for insulin therapy are available.[125]

Carbohydrate Overfeeding and the Refeeding Syndrome

The risk of overfeeding trauma patients during initiation of nutrition support is greater with use of parenteral nutrition than with enteral tube feeding. Glucose feeding stimulates insulin production. Increased insulin triggers cells to rapidly take up circulating minerals, particularly phosphorus, magnesium, and potassium, depressing their concentration in the blood. The early stages of carbohydrate overfeeding are also associated with sodium and water retention, which stresses the heart. The accompanying elevations in minute ventilation, Vo_2, and Vco_2 act to increase the workload of the lungs, which may precipitate respiratory failure in the compromised host or otherwise impair the ability to wean from a ventilator. Moreover, excessive carbohydrate loading may precipitate respiratory acidosis in patients who are unable to adequately improve alveolar ventilation when compensating for increasing Vco_2. The characteristic features of the refeeding syndrome, which is precipitated by carbohydrate overfeeding, are hypophosphatemia, arterial hypotension, tachycardia, and acute respiratory failure, resulting in heart failure if not corrected.

Blood minerals (particularly phosphorus, magnesium, calcium, and potassium) should be brought to normal levels before parenteral nutrition is initiated, particularly in malnourished patients, and feeding should be advanced gradually as tolerated, with continued mineral repletion and blood glucose monitoring as needed.[31,46] Administration of an intravenous dose of thiamine to at-risk patients at least 30 minutes before parenteral nutrition is started might also be considered. Guidelines are available to assist in selection of replacement treatment.[46,126]

Chronically malnourished patients, such as those who are anorexic or addicted to alcohol, have a nutritionally depleted cardiac mass and are not prepared to deal with the circulatory demand caused by aggressive nutrition support. Moreover, many patients have pulmonary contusions, rib fractures, and hemopneumothoraces, which can limit their ability to compensate for increased Vco_2. Patients with cervical and upper thoracic spinal cord injuries are also vulnerable to effects of overfeeding because of their inability to use intercostal, abdominal, and/or diaphragm muscles to compensate for increased Vco_2. Even for less vulnerable patients, carbohydrate overfeeding causes a shift in substrate oxidation so that glucose oxidation increases and fat oxidation decreases.[53] Despite the shift toward less fat oxidation, lipolysis persists in critical illness. This surplus of endogenous fatty acid increases the risk of hypertriglyceridemia and hepatic steatosis during feeding.

Lipid Overfeeding

The parenteral administration of lipids in excess of 2 g/kg per day is associated with hypertriglyceridemia. Some drugs, such as propofol, are administered in a lipid solution and if these fat and calories are substantial, they should be counted toward the nutrition prescription to prevent overfeeding. Fat overload syndrome is a sudden onset of multiple complications leading to multiple organ dysfunction syndrome and can be fatal. Complications can occur within days of lipid overfeeding or not appear until after weeks of apparent tolerance. Platelets take up excess fat in the blood, which interferes with their clotting function. Hence, prothrombin time and partial thromboplastin time are prolonged and the patient may have bloody diarrhea, bloody urine, bleeding gums, or other bleeding. In addition to sudden and extreme hypertriglyceridemia and signs of coagulopathy, other early signs of fat overload syndrome include hypercapnia, tachycardia, hypertension, fever, elevated bilirubin, elevated liver enzymes, and decreased hemoglobin. Moreover, the reticuloendothelial cells become distended by fat, impairing immune function.

Transitional Feeding

Temporary Discontinuation and Termination

Abrupt discontinuation of TPN (as might occur if delivery of the next TPN bag is delayed or access to the central line is lost) is not recommended because it may result in acute hypoglycemia. If TPN is suddenly halted, initiating infusion of a standard dextrose solution (e.g., dextrose 5% or 10% in water) at 100 ml per hour minimizes the potential for rebound hypoglycemia until TPN can resume.

Transition to Enteral Feeding

Most trauma patients who initially need parenteral nutrition as the primary source of feeding are able to progress partially or completely to enteral feeding once their condition stabilizes and the gastrointestinal tract becomes a viable feeding route.[1] The transition should be planned in an organized fashion by the interdisciplinary team. Continuous nursing, dietary, and medical assessments are necessary to determine the earliest possible transition time.

Some reduction in the mass of the large intestine occurs during TPN; in fact, small bowel biopsy specimens from patients receiving long-term TPN have shown dramatic atrophy of the microvilli height, mass, and absorptive area. In addition, patients with preexisting malnutrition might have additional loss of absorptive surface and further depressed enzyme production, contributing to even greater malabsorptive problems, particularly of milk products (lactose). Therefore, patients who are changing from parenteral to enteral feeding need special consideration. Before a patient returns to an oral diet, a speech pathologist may need to conduct a swallowing evaluation. Disuse, general muscle weakness, endotracheal tube placement, and neurologic alterations can lead to swallowing problems, which increase the risk of aspiration.

As use of the new route for feeding increases, feeding through the previous route is gradually decreased. It may take several days for the gut to readjust to enteral feeding. This is why patients on an oral diet progress from ice chips to clear liquid, then full liquid, and finally to a regular diet as tolerated. Initially, high residuals caused by decreased peristalsis may occur when a patient is making the transition from TPN to enteral feeding. Medications that increase gastrointestinal motility may decrease problems with high residuals. Calorie counts should be initiated to determine whether intake is adequate. TPN can be partially reduced and then eliminated once enteral feedings meet >50% to 60% of the goal for energy, protein and fluids.[1]

Long-Term Total Parenteral Nutrition

Long-term home TPN (HPN) may be required for patients whose injuries resulted in short bowel syndrome or other severe malabsorption disorders. HPN can be complicated by catheter-related infections, liver disease, and metabolic bone disease. The predominant histologic finding in adults with HPN-associated liver disease is steatosis, and signs of cholestasis are usually evident as well.[127] Although it is not definitively known whether choline is a required component for optimal HPN, preliminary data suggest that de novo endogenous synthesis may be insufficient and that choline supplementation may help normalize parameters of liver health.[128] Protocols are available to guide biochemical monitoring of patients receiving HPN.[129] Bone density measurements should be performed as soon as feasible and then periodically to monitor for indications of osteoporosis.[31] Patients are periodically reassessed to delineate transient from permanent intestinal failure, which includes evaluation for surgery and intestinal transplantation.[130]

Nutritional Considerations for Special Populations

Geriatric Trauma Patients

Elderly patients (age >65 years) often have chronic disease and nutrient deficits that increase the risk of protein-calorie malnutrition after traumatic injury. Fixed income, impaired physical mobility, lack of transportation to acquire food, dental issues, loneliness, and drug-nutrient interactions are some of the circumstances that affect the nutritional status of the geriatric patient before and after hospitalization.[131] Thus, elderly patients need early identification, assessment, and intervention. Moreover, protein-calorie malnutrition at discharge is a strong independent risk factor for subsequent death within 6 years.

Energy

As people age, their lean body mass tends to decline, which results in lower BMR relative to body weight. Basal energy expenditure for healthy elderly individuals is approximately

21.5 kcal/kg per day.[4] Hence, elderly patients may be at risk for overfeeding if estimated energy expenditure is not adjusted for age and they may be less able to tolerate overfeeding than do younger patients. Repeatedly obtaining 24-hour energy expenditure measures through indirect calorimetry is the best method available to predict energy expenditure in critically ill elderly patients. When actual measures are not possible, 25 kcal/kg per day can be fed on a trial basis to normal-weight adults over the age of 65 years, in place of calculating by using the more traditional regression equations (Table 17-4).

Fluid and Protein

Monitoring hydration is especially important for elderly patients, who often have reduced thirst. A decline in renal function with advancing age leads to excess water loss because the capacity to concentrate urine may be impaired. Those who have lost the ability to concentrate urine could become dehydrated if fed a high-protein diet without sufficient water because high-protein diets cause increased urination. For this reason, protein overfeeding can lead to azotemia, hypertonic dehydration, and metabolic acidosis.

Periodic Screening in Rehabilitation

Inadequate hydration has been a persistent problem in long-term care.[132] Many elderly are diapered because of incontinence, making it difficult to assess daily urine volume.[44] Consensus guidelines are available for maintaining adequate hydration in at-risk elderly patients and for assessing hydration status.[47,50,133] On average, total fluid of 3.7 L/day for men and 2.7 L/day for women is expected to be adequate.[48]

Obese Trauma Patients

Obesity is defined as a BMI of 30 or greater (Table 17-4). Special attention must be paid to the obese patient, who is commonly mislabeled as overnourished for all nutrients. In fact, hypermetabolism of trauma combined with severe underfeeding can result in protein and micronutrient malnutrition in these patients.

Energy

The basal energy expenditure of free-living obese adults is 20 kcal/kg per day of actual body weight for men and 18.5 kcal/kg of actual body weight for women, a distinct gender difference.[4] Obtaining 24-hour energy expenditure measures repeatedly through indirect calorimetry is the best method available to predict energy expenditure in obese critically ill patients.[31] Obese patients are at risk for overfeeding if energy needs are estimated from equations, unless obese-appropriate equations are used or body weight is adjusted in normal-weight equations, because BMR is reduced relative to body weight (Table 17-4). Only 6 of 239 subjects in the study used to generate the traditional HBEE estimates were obese, so HBEE is not applicable for estimating resting expenditure unless an adjusted weight is used. Recently, TEE equations were developed for use with both normal-weight and obese adults (Table 17-4).[4]

Protein

Dietary recommendations for average adults suggest providing 25% to 30% of energy intake as protein. Hence, a similar range for obese patients might be a reasonable minimum for initiation of feeding. For the patient who is tube fed, standard formulas contain a balanced ratio of protein to energy, so that basing feeding on calculated energy goals will deliver a set amount of protein, vitamins, and minerals. More studies of the efficacy of hypocaloric protein-controlled diets are needed to determine the best formula for obese patients.

Periodic Screening in Rehabilitation

Body weight measures may be challenging to obtain for the obese patient if the patient exceeds the weight and girth range of available equipment.[134] Yet, periodic body weight measures are important and should be combined with dietary assessment and other evaluations of nutrition status. If weight is used as the only criterion of nutrition status, an obese person who has lost substantial weight from muscle tissue might be mistakenly categorized as adequately nourished.

Pediatric Trauma Patients

Many children admitted to the ICU endure substantial energy and protein deficits. Once nutrition support is initiated, fluctuations in feeding, including periods of overfeeding (>110% of actual energy expenditure), are not uncommon.[135] Fluid volume restriction, interruption of feeding for procedures, and feeding intolerance can limit the provision of nutrients. In general, tube feeding into the small bowel allows a greater amount of nutrition to be successfully delivered to critically ill children than does gastric feeding. Yet, small bowel feeding does not necessarily prevent aspiration of gastric contents.[136] In the ICU, waist circumference has been used in infants to assess tolerance to enteral feeding.

Gastrointestinal surgery is the most frequent indication for use of parenteral nutrition in infants and children. Parenteral nutrition might be infused for 11 days or longer.[137] More than one fifth of pediatric patients receiving parenteral nutrition have one or more complications.[137] Consensus guidelines are available to select relevant parameters and to establish plans for the frequency of monitoring pediatric patients, which should be tailored to the patient's clinical course.[31,138,139]

Detailed recommendations are published for both enteral infant formulas[140] and for TPN content.[19] In general, adult doses of parenteral electrolytes are used for children weighing more than 50 kg. Similarly, adult doses of parenteral multivitamins are used for children weighing more than 40 kg or who are older than 11 years of age.[19] Care should be coordinated among the health care team members to provide optimal nutrition and to minimize secondary complications.[141] A family-centered care approach is particularly important for the pediatric trauma patient.

Energy

In the case of infants and older children who are confined to bed, obtaining 24-hour energy expenditure measures repeatedly through indirect calorimetry is the best method available to predict energy expenditure. Otherwise, prediction equations will need to be used. Unfortunately, equations overestimate actual energy requirements for many ventilated, critically ill children during the early postinjury period.[142,143] The daily TEE of healthy active infants up to 6 months of age averages 71.5 kcal/kg per day with an additional 20 kcal/kg per day required for growth. From 6 months to 2 years, TEE averages 78.5 kcal/kg per day with an additional 2.5 kcal/kg per day needed for growth. On average, daily basal requirements of healthy children 3 to 8 years is 44 kcal/kg for girls and 51 kcal/kg for boys; from 9 to 13 years daily basal requirements are 33 kcal/kg for girls and 37 kcal/kg for boys; and from 14 to 18 years daily basal requirements are 25 kcal/kg for girls and 29 kcal/kg for boys.[4] Estimated energy requirements that include factors for growth for sedentary healthy children 3 through 18 years can be calculated as follows:

- Boys: 88.5 − (61.9 × Age in years) + (26.7 × Weight in kilograms) + (903 × Height in meters) + 20 to 25 kcal
- Girls: 135.3 − (30.8 × Age in years) + (10 × Weight in kilograms) + (934 × Height in meters) + 20 to 25 kcal

Fluid and Protein

On average, total fluid is expected to be adequate at 1.3 L per day for children 1 to 3 years old, 1.7 L per day for children 4 to 8 years old, 2.1 L per day for girls 9 to 13 years old, 2.3 L per day for girls 14 to 18 years old, 2.4 L per day for boys 9 to 13 years old, and 3.3 L per day for boys 14 to 18 years old.[48] Protein of 2 to 3 g/kg in daily nutrition support is likely to meet or exceed protein requirements for infants less than 1 year of age, 1 to 2 g/kg for children 1 to 10 years of age, and 0.8 to 1.5 g/kg for children 11 to 17 years of age.[4,19]

Rehabilitation

Malnutrition is a major problem in pediatric ICUs, yet the outlook is bright for children who recover as many develop good long-term nutritional status.[144] After traumatic brain injury, swallowing function and advancement to normal diets may be achieved by 12 weeks after injury in most children who initially exhibited dysphagia.[145] For those requiring long-term feeding tubes, the decision for parents is difficult and emotional. There is need for information and decision support before placing PEG tubes in children.[115] If further surgery is required, in general, clear fluids may be allowed up to 2 hours before anesthesia and light meals up to 6 hours. For infants less than 6 months of age, consensus recommendations permit breast milk or formula feeding up to 4 hours before anaesthesia.[146]

Burn Patients

Patients with second or third degree burns are at nutritional risk.[31] Early enteral feeding within 18 hours of admission is preferred to delayed feeding.[1,147] Attainment of energy and protein goals are more likely if enteral feedings are continued intraoperatively during wound debridement than if feedings are interrupted.[1] Attention to the provision of adequate nutrition is particularly important for prevention of pressure sores after thermal injuries.[148] When possible, energy requirements should be assessed by using measures of indirect calorimetry because energy expenditure fluctuates over the course of recovery and overfeeding should be avoided.[1,31,149] Substantial redistribution of fluid with tissue edema is common after thermal injury and patients have an increased requirement for fluids. Severely burned patients may also require increased intake of protein until significant wound healing is achieved (Figure 17-5).[1,31] Poor protein status has been associated with increased risk of infection, delayed healing at the skin graft donor site, and increased length of stay compared with better-nourished burn patients.[150] Enteral glutamine supplementation may offer some benefit for reduced morbidity and mortality in patients with thermal injuries, but duration and dosing compared with standard treatment need further investigation, as does the mechanism of effect.[151-153]

Imminently Terminal Patients

According to Barrocas et al,[154] the role of health care professionals is to "cure rarely, treat often, and comfort always." Nutrition support is a medical therapy that can be life saving when indicated, yet it is not without risk of complications. Because artificial nutrition and hydration are a medical therapy in the same category as ventilators and hemodialysis (which can be withheld or withdrawn under certain circumstances), nutrition support is distinct from food and water. Moreover, adult patients (or their legally authorized surrogates) have the right to accept or refuse nutrition support.[61,154] In situations in which the administration of nutrition support is of questionable benefit, but not definitively futile, a time-limited intervention might be undertaken. Under these circumstances, open communication among the health care team, patient, and family is required to convey the clear expectation of terminating the therapy when it is no longer thought to be effective.[154,155] Institutions should develop clear policies regarding the withdrawal or withholding of nutrition support and communicate these policies to patients in accordance with the patient Self-Determination Act.[61,154] Note that "do not resuscitate" orders are event specific and do not necessarily preclude the provision of nutrition support.

Interdisciplinary Strategies

Collaborative, interdisciplinary strategies are essential for a comprehensive, outcome-oriented nutrition program for the trauma population. Such strategies should include clarifying interdisciplinary role responsibilities, identifying nutrition clinical pathways, and establishing an interdisciplinary communication system. Finally, clinical quality measures should be established to determine the effectiveness of the nutrition program and to make continuing improvements. These interdisciplinary strategies must extend to rehabilitative and long-term care facilities.[156]

THE NUTRITION CARE TEAM

The nutrition care team consists of all clinicians providing nutrition care to the patient as well as formally defined nutrition support service members. Nutritionally at-risk patients should be assessed and managed by a nutrition support service or interdisciplinary team.[21]

Roles and Responsibilities

Certainly, all health care clinicians must meet performance standards of their job description. The added roles and responsibilities of the nutrition care team will vary from organization to organization. Determining roles and responsibilities for the team members is a natural part of the nutrition care pathway development process. If pathways are not used, the group can review nutrition support activities (e.g., nutrition assessment, patient care rounds, daily assessment, surveillance) to delineate specific associated tasks and assign responsibilities. This helps the team have clear expectations. Routine documentation procedures can serve to reinforce and clarify role expectations. The responsibility for overall coordination and communication of nutrition care may be shared among the disciplines, but these efforts should be reviewed periodically to identify improvements for process and patient outcome. To capitalize on collaborative expertise, clinical guidelines (clinical pathways, algorithms, and protocols) should be established by an interdisciplinary team.

Nurses are key participants in nutrition care. Major nursing responsibilities include identifying high-risk patients by screening procedures, participation in plans for care, ensuring that orders are executed correctly, and collecting samples for blood tests and nutritional measures. Moreover, reviewing laboratory data is an essential aspect of the nurse's role. Furthermore, the nurse at the bedside provides constant surveillance and feedback to the team such as communicating the patient's tolerance of tube feeding and documenting the patient's signs and symptoms. Nurses also provide patient and family education. Nurse practitioners serving on a nutrition support service can promote the use of disease-specific pathways and improve communication and collaboration between floor nurses, physicians, and others to improve the nutrition care process.[157] For nurses who are interested in specialty certification, the American Society for Parenteral and Enteral Nutrition created a credentialing program for Nutrition Support Nursing (http://www.nutritioncare.org/).

Dietitians perform nutrition assessments that include calculating energy, protein, carbohydrate, and fat requirements and actual amounts fed. Pharmacists are responsible for reviewing each parenteral nutrition prescription for dose and route of administration. Any major deviations from the previous day's prescription, including omissions, should be questioned. The potential for enteral and parenteral drug-nutrient interactions should be identified collaboratively by the nurse, pharmacist, and physician so that appropriate drug dosing can be altered. One or more trauma physicians who have a special interest in nutrition care are valued members of the interdisciplinary team. Physicians work collaboratively with the nurse, dietitian, and pharmacist to finalize nutrition support orders, review laboratory values, and write orders for additional laboratory work, indirect calorimetry, and supplemental vitamins, minerals, and electrolytes. Speech pathologists evaluate the safety of oral diets and recommend specific modifications, such as a thick liquid diet. Respiratory therapists might conduct tests of indirect calorimetry to obtain measures of energy expenditure.

Personnel Education and Training

Continuing and appropriate training sessions are needed to educate interdisciplinary team members as they are hired. All members of the nutrition care team need a sound knowledge base in metabolism and nutrition relevant to trauma care. Weaknesses in nutrition knowledge, such as lack of recognizing symptoms of overfeeding, need to be addressed so that patients are provided with appropriate and timely interventions. Attempts to solely address signs and symptoms of inappropriate feeding by adjusting ventilator settings (to correct blood gases), dialysis (to control azotemia), and insulin doses (to control hyperglycemia) may not be successful unless the nutrient prescription is also adjusted. An orientation to in-house clinical guidelines, pathways, protocols, and algorithms with a description of the various interdisciplinary role expectations should be provided to all new team members. Individual role responsibilities and collaborative activities (e.g., rounds) that are critical to successful patient outcomes should be specified and reinforced. For nursing staff, this education should include a general overview of metabolic and endocrine responses to injury, the importance of nutrition status to wound healing and recovery, instruction on administering nutrition support, and infection control principles related to nutrition. Continuing in-service education is needed to disseminate changes in the nutrition program, the latest nutrition research, and quality improvement issues or initiatives. Finally, physicians and nurses who are involved in inserting and caring for the vascular access devices should have hands-on experience and receive mentoring and supervision as part of their comprehensive nutrition support education.

Communication

Better communication between members of the health care team has contributed to improvements in patient safety related to medication administration.[158] Monitoring the patient's response to feeding is particularly challenging in the critical care setting, especially when patients undergo numerous and unpredictable changes in medical status unrelated to nutrition support. Thus, the need for communication among the clinical team is important. The process of rounding, in which all disciplines pull together to discuss and evaluate each patient individually, is instrumental to fine tune the nutrition plan of care and monitor patient response so that optimal patient outcomes can be achieved. Bedside nurses have a responsibility to speak up when they have a concern and listen carefully when others have concerns.[158] Ideally, an interdisciplinary computerized medical record with a specific nutrition screen that is integrated with laboratory data and other nutrition-related information should be created to facilitate the interdisciplinary rounding structure. Communication of nutrition care plans and future goals should be included with other care information when patients are transferred from the ICU to the acute care unit or rehabilitative facility.

Clinical Pathways and Quality Measures

Clinical pathways help articulate practice expectations along the continuum of care and generally work best for select populations. Ideally, nutrition-related care should be integrated into the overall plan of care. The pathway document serves as a mechanism for communication, an approach for documentation, and a method to evaluate processes and outcomes of care.[159,160] If specific practice interventions or outcomes do not occur in the time frame specified in the pathway, then a variance has occurred. Variances are outcomes, missed interventions, or complications that need to be reviewed and may represent opportunities to improve the care process. Complications such as hyperglycemia and diarrhea represent variances. The most common variances in nutrition support of trauma patients are due to underfeeding, overfeeding, delays in correcting electrolyte abnormalities, lack of precautions for patients at high risk of aspiration, and errors in nutrition orders. All complications cannot be prevented, yet tracking their incidence represents an opportunity for nutrition care evaluation and improvement. Any sentinel events related to the administration of nutrition support should be reported according to hospital protocol to ensure that they are properly documented. A corrective action plan can be instituted to improve the care process and reduce incidence future adverse events.[21] Consensus algorithms for delivery of parenteral and enteral nutrition are available to assist nutrition care teams in customizing plans of care for their facilities.[1,80] Developing these approaches requires intense work and keeping the team focused on patient care and clinical outcomes.

Quality Measures

The nutrition care team must determine appropriate quality measures of structure, process, and outcome. Structure indicators relate to characteristics of the staff. For example, inadequate nurse/patient ratios are associated with deficient charting of the measures of fluid balance for at-risk patients in the step-down wards, which can short change nutrition monitoring.[156] Process indicators assist in verifying that appropriate steps in the process or procedure are performed, such as timeliness, route, and adequacy of nutrition support. For example, how early were at-risk patients identified and is the nutrition care team following TJC standards? Outcome measures, such as length of stay, functional status, complications relative to overfeeding, and mortality are essential to evaluating overall clinical care.[161] Quality indicators need to be evaluated using the hospital's baseline quality data and benchmark data available in published literature. If such data are not available, a brainstorming session with all the disciplines present should be held to set priorities for data to be collected and monitored for use as an internal benchmark.

Future Research

Independent and collaborative research opportunities exist to improve the quality of nutrition care for the trauma population. The newly developed research specialty of metabolomics offers an opportunity to study metabolic profiles of biofluids and how they respond to changes in diet after traumatic injury. Through the collection of comprehensive data sets of metabolites and use of pattern recognition statistics, differences in feeding on outcomes might be elucidated.[162] Further research with preclinical animal models of traumatic injury is also encouraged to learn more about the critical effect of feeding on recovery. Subgroups of trauma patients need additional consideration. For example, elderly and obese patients have more complications when traumatically injured and head-injured patients have highly variable metabolic rates. Are there specific metabolic or nutrition interventions that might improve their prognoses? Are there differences in metabolic rate and injury response in other subgroups (e.g., men versus women) that necessitate different nutrition interventions? Previous research emphasized the need to prevent severe underfeeding. Although this is an important finding, recent studies suggest equally significant consequences related to overfeeding. Future research will distinguish between various types of fats, amino acids, and carbohydrate substrate and provide more information on vitamin and mineral needs during recovery and the special needs of subpopulations. This information is needed to better tailor nutrition care to the type and severity of injury and to individual patient characteristics, thus improving overall outcome and reducing excessive costs caused by less appropriate feeding.

Summary

This chapter provided an overview of normal metabolism and metabolic alterations after traumatic injury, most notably the hypermetabolic response. The protein compartment is substantially depleted during recovery and preservation of protein status is a primary goal of nutrition care. A multitude of factors need to be assessed in relation to the patient's medical status to administer and monitor nutrition care. An interdisciplinary team approach that involves close communication among the nurse, physician, pharmacist, dietitian, and allied health professionals is necessary to achieve nutrition goals. By providing optimal nutrition care, nurses and the rest of the health care team support wound healing, limit complications, reduce the length of hospital stay, and improve chances for long-term survival. Current practices must continue to be evaluated in relation to emerging research to provide comprehensive and appropriate nutrition care for patients recovering from traumatic injury.

REFERENCES

1. Jacobs DG, Jacobs DO, Kudsk KA et al: Practice management guidelines for nutritional support of the trauma patient, *J Trauma* 57:660-678, 2004.
2. Stipanuk MH: *Biochemical and physiological aspects of human nutrition,* Philadelphia, 2000, W. B. Saunders.
3. Posthauer ME: The role of nutrition in wound care, *Adv Skin Wound Care* 19:53-54, 2006.
4. Institute of Medicine, Food, and Nutrition Board: *Dietary reference intakes for energy, carbohydrate, fiber, fat, fatty acids, cholesterol, protein, and amino acids (macronutrients),* Washington, DC, 2005, National Academy Press.
5. Kalm LM, Semba RD: They starved so that others be better fed: remembering Ancel Keys and the Minnesota experiment, *J Nutr* 135:1347-1352, 2005.
6. Svanfeldt M, Thorell A, Brismar K et al: Effects of 3 days of "postoperative" low caloric feeding with or without bed rest on insulin sensitivity in healthy subjects, *Clin Nutr* 22:31-38, 2003.
7. Brosnan JT: Interorgan amino acid transport and its regulation, *J Nutr* 133(6 Suppl):2068S-2072S, 2003.
8. Hammarqvist F, Anderson K, Luo JL et al: Free amino acid and glutathione concentrations in muscle during short-term starvation and refeeding, *Clin Nutr* 24:236-243, 2005.
9. Plank LD, Hill GL: Similarity of changes in body composition in intensive care patients following severe sepsis or major blunt injury, *Ann N Y Acad Sci* 904:592-602, 2000.
10. Cartwright MM: The metabolic response to stress: a case of complex nutrition support management, *Crit Care Nurs Clin North Am* 16:467-487, 2004.
11. Mahan LK, Escott-Stump S, editors: *Krause's food, nutrition and diet therapy,* 11 ed, Philadelphia, 2003, W. B. Saunders.
12. Vanhorebeek I, Van den Berghe G: The neuroendocrine response to critical illness is a dynamic process, *Crit Care Clin* 22:1-15, 2006.
13. Thorell A, Rooyackers O, Myrenfors P et al: Intensive insulin treatment in critically ill trauma patients normalizes glucose by reducing endogenous glucose production, *J Clin Endocrinol Metab* 89:5382-5386, 2004.
14. Abu-Zidan FM, Plank LD, Windsor JA: Proteolysis in severe sepsis is related to oxidation of plasma protein, *Eur J Surg* 168:119-123, 2002.
15. Barco KT, Smith RA, Peerless JR et al: Energy expenditure assessment and validation after acute spinal cord injury, *Nutr Clin Pract* 17:309-313, 2002.
16. Furst P, Stehle P: What are the essential elements needed for the determination of amino acid requirements in humans? *J Nutr* 134(6 Suppl):1558S-1565S, 2004.
17. Plank LD, Hill GL: Energy balance in critical illness, *Proc Nutr Soc* 62:545-552, 2003.
18. Lacey K, Pritchett E: Nutrition care process and model: ADA adopts road map to quality care and outcomes management, *J Am Diet Assoc* 103:1061-1072, 2003.
19. Mirtallo J, Canada T, Johnson D et al: Task Force for the Revision of Safe Practices for Parenteral Nutrition: safe practices for parenteral nutrition, *JPEN* 28:S39-70, 2004.
20. The Joint Commission: *Comprehensive accreditation manual for hospitals: the official handbook, standards, rationales, elements of performance, scoring,* Oakbrook Terrace, IL, 2005, The Joint Commission.
21. Russell MK, Andrews MR, Brewer CK et al: American Society for Parenteral and Enteral Nutrition Board of Directors; Task Force on Standards for Specialized Nutrition Support for Hospitalized Adult Patients, standards for specialized nutrition support: adult hospitalized patients, *Nutr Clin Pract* 17:384-391, 2002.
22. Burden ST, Bodey S, Bradburn YJ et al: Validation of a nutrition screening tool: testing the reliability and validity, *J Hum Nutr Diet* 14:269-275, 2001.
23. de Kruif JT, Vos A: An algorithm for the clinical assessment of nutritional status in hospitalized patients, *Br J Nutr* 90:829-836, 2003.
24. Kondrup J, Allison SP, Elia M et al: Educational and Clinical Practice Committee, European Society of Parenteral and Enteral Nutrition (ESPEN): ESPEN guidelines for nutrition screening 2002, *Clin Nutr* 22:415-421, 2003.
25. Cooper N: Audit in clinical practice: evaluating use of a nutrition screening tool developed for trauma nurses, *J Hum Nutr Diet* 11:403-410, 1998.
26. Green SM, Watson R: Nutritional screening and assessment tools for use by nurses: literature review, *J Adv Nurs* 50:69-83, 2005.
27. Higgins PA, Daly BJ: Adult failure to thrive in the older rehabilitation patient, *Rehabil Nurs* 30:152-159, 2005.
28. Braden BJ, Maklebust J: Preventing pressure ulcers with the Braden Scale: an update on this easy-to-use tool that assesses a patient's risk, *Am J Nurs* 105:70-72, 2005.
29. Panel for the Predicting and Prevention of Pressure Ulcers in Adults: *Pressure ulcers in adults: prediction and prevention,* Clinical Practice Guidelines No. 3, AHCPR Publ No. 92-0047, Rockville, MD, 1992, Agency for Health Care Policy and Research, Public Health Office: http://www.ncbi.nlm.nih.gov/books/bv.fcgi?rid=hstat2.chapter.4409. Accessed December 23, 2005.
30. Fuhrman MP, Winkler M, Biesemeier C et al: The American Society for Parenteral and Enteral Nutrition (A.S.P.E.N.) standards of practice for nutrition support dietitians, *J Am Diet Assoc* 101:825-832, 2001.
31. ASPEN Board of Directors and the Clinical Guidelines Task Force: Guidelines for the use of parenteral and enteral nutrition in adult and pediatric patients, *JPEN J Parenter Enteral Nutr* 26(1 Suppl):1SA-138SA, 2002. Erratum in: *JPEN J Parenter Enteral Nutr* 26:144, 2002.
32. Prelack K, Dwyer J, Sheridan R et al: Body water in children during recovery from severe burn injury using a combined tracer dilution method, *J Burn Care Rehabil* 26:67-74, 2005.
33. Scott DD, Chase M: *Nutritional management in the rehabilitation setting* (2003): http://www.emedicine.com/pmr/topic159.htm. Accessed January 4, 2005.

34. Ravasco P, Camilo ME, Gouveia-Oliveira A et al: A critical approach to nutritional assessment in critically ill patients, *Clin Nutr* 21:73-77, 2002.
35. Buchholz AC, Bartok C, Schoeller DA: The validity of bioelectrical impedance models in clinical populations, *Nutr Clin Pract* 19:433-446, 2004.
36. Kyle UG, Bosaeus I, De Lorenzo AD et al: ESPEN: bioelectrical impedance analysis, II: utilization in clinical practice, *Clin Nutr* 23:1430-1453, 2004.
37. Brugler L, Stankovic A, Bernstein L et al: The role of visceral protein markers in protein calorie malnutrition, *Clin Chem Lab Med* 40:1360-1369, 2002.
38. Fuhrman MP, Charney P, Mueller CM: Hepatic proteins and nutrition assessment, *J Am Diet Assoc* 104:1258-1264, 2004.
39. Cole CD, Gottfried ON, Liu JK et al: Hyponatremia in the neurosurgical patient: diagnosis and management, *Neurosurg Focus* 16: Article 9, 2004.
40. Klein CJ, Moser-Veillon PB, Schweitzer A et al: Magnesium, calcium, zinc, and nitrogen loss in trauma patients during continuous renal replacement therapy, *JPEN J Parenter Enteral Nutr* 26:77-93, 2002.
41. Dickerson RN, Alexander KH, Minard G et al: Accuracy of methods to estimate ionized and "corrected" serum calcium concentrations in critically ill multiple trauma patients receiving specialized nutrition support, *JPEN J Parenter Enteral Nutr* 28:133-141, 2004.
42. Dorman BP, Hill C, McGrath M et al: Bowel management in the intensive care unit, *Intensive Crit Care Nurs* 20:320-329, 2004.
43. Sawka MN, Cheuvront SN, Carter R III: Human water needs, *Nutr Rev* 63:6:S30-S39, 2005.
44. Armstrong LE: Hydration assessment techniques, *Nutr Rev* 63:6:S40-S54, 2005.
45. Elgart HN: Assessment of fluids and electrolytes, *AACN Clin Issues* 15:607-621, 2004.
46. Kraft MD, Btaiche IF, Sacks GS et al: Treatment of electrolyte disorders in adult patients in the intensive care unit, *Am J Health Syst Pharm* 62:1663-1682, 2005.
47. American Medical Directors Association: *Dehydration and fluid maintenance,* Columbia, MD, American Medical Directors Association (2001): http://www.guidelines.gov/summary/summary.aspx?doc_id=3305&mode=menu&ss=15. Accessed January 25, 2005.
48. Institute of Medicine, Food, and Nutrition Board: *Dietary reference intakes for water, potassium, sodium, chloride, and sulfate,* Washington, DC, 2004, National Academy Press.
49. Horn SD, Bender SA, Ferguson ML et al: The National Pressure Ulcer Long-Term Care Study: pressure ulcer development in long-term care residents, *J Am Geriatr Soc* 52:359-367, 2004.
50. Mentes JC: *Hydration management,* University of Iowa Gerontological Nursing Interventions Research Center. Research Dissemination Core (2004): www.guidelines.gov. Accessed January 25, 2005.
51. Faisy C, Guerot E, Diehl JL et al: Assessment of resting energy expenditure in mechanically ventilated patients, *Am J Clin Nutr* 78:241-249, 2003.
52. McCall M, Jeejeebhoy K, Pencharz P et al: Effect of neuromuscular blockade on energy expenditure in patients with severe head injury, *JPEN J Parenter Enteral Nutr* 27:27-35, 2003.
53. Minehira K, Bettschart V, Vidal H et al: Effect of carbohydrate overfeeding on whole body and adipose tissue metabolism in humans, *Obes Res* 11:1096-1103, 2003.
54. Zauner C, Schuster BI, Schneeweiss B: Similar metabolic responses to standardized total parenteral nutrition of septic and nonseptic critically ill patients, *Am J Clin Nutr* 74:265-270, 2001.
55. Holdy KE: Monitoring energy metabolism with indirect calorimetry: instruments, interpretation, and clinical application, *Nutr Clin Pract* 19:447-454, 2004.
56. Headley JM: Indirect calorimetry: a trend toward continuous metabolic assessment, *AACN Clin Issues* 14:155-167, 2003.
57. Ireton-Jones C, Jones JD: Improved equations for predicting energy expenditure in patients: the Ireton-Jones Equations, *Nutr Clin Pract* 17:29-31, 2002.
58. Reeves MM, Capra S: Predicting energy requirements in the clinical setting: are current methods evidence based? *Nutr Rev* 61:143-151, 2003.
59. Alexander E, Susla GM, Burstein AH et al: Retrospective evaluation of commonly used equations to predict energy expenditure in mechanically ventilated, critically ill patients, *Pharmacotherapy* 24:1659-1667, 2004.
60. Winkler MF: Quality of life in adult home parenteral nutrition patients, *JPEN J Parenter Enteral Nutr* 29:162-170, 2005.
61. McMahon MM, Hurley DL, Kamath PS et al: Medical and ethical aspects of long-term enteral tube feeding, *Mayo Clin Proc* 80:1461-1476, 2005.
62. Neumann SA, Miller MD, Daniels L et al: Nutritional status and clinical outcomes of older patients in rehabilitation, *J Hum Nutr Diet* 18:129-136, 2005.
63. Persoon A, Huisman-de Waal G, Naber TA et al: Impact of long-term HPN on daily life in adults, *Clin Nutr* 24:304-313, 2005.
64. Baxter JP, Fayers PM, McKinlay AW: A review of the instruments used to assess the quality of life of adult patients with chronic intestinal failure receiving parenteral nutrition at home, *Br J Nutr* 94:633-638, 2005.
65. Hoffer LJ: Protein and energy provision in critical illness, *Am J Clin Nutr* 78:906-911, 2003.
66. Jeejeebhoy KN: Permissive underfeeding of the critically ill patient, *Nutr Clin Pract* 19:477-480, 2004.
67. Berger MM, Chiolero RL: Trauma and burns. In Rombeau JL, Rolandelli R, editors: *Clinical nutrition: parenteral nutrition,* 3rd ed, Philadelphia, 2001, W. B. Saunders.
68. Heyland DK, Dhaliwal R, Drover JW et al: Canadian Critical Care Clinical Practice Guidelines Committee: Canadian clinical practice guidelines for nutrition support in mechanically ventilated, critically ill adult patients, *JPEN J Parenter Enteral Nutr* 27:355-373, 2003.
69. Bern M: Observations on possible effects of daily vitamin K replacement, especially upon warfarin therapy, *JPEN J Parenter Enteral Nutr* 28:388-398, 2004.
70. Kan MN, Chang HH, Sheu WF et al: Estimation of energy requirements for mechanically ventilated, critically ill patients using nutritional status, *Crit Care* 7:R108-R115, 2003.
71. Denes Z: The influence of severe malnutrition on rehabilitation in patients with severe head injury, *Disabil Rehabil* 26:1163-1165, 2004.
72. Tomey KM, Chen DM, Wang X et al: Dietary intake and nutritional status of urban community-dwelling men with paraplegia, *Arch Phys Med Rehabil* 86:664-671, 2005.
73. Block P, Skeels SE, Keys CB et al: Shake-It-Up: health promotion and capacity building for people with spinal cord injuries and related neurological disabilities, *Disabil Rehabil* 27:185-190, 2005.

74. Heyland DK, Schroter-Noppe D, Drover JW et al: Nutrition support in the critical care setting: current practice in Canadian ICUs—opportunities for improvement? *JPEN J Parenter Enteral Nutr* 27:74-83, 2003.
75. Canadian Critical Care Guidelines Committee: Critical Care Connections, Inc (2005): [http://www.criticalcarenutrition.com/tableofcontents.htm. Accessed January 15, 2006.
76. Wiegand DJ, Carlson KK, editors: *AACN procedure manual for critical care,* 5th ed, St. Louis, 2005, Elsevier.
77. Yanagawa T, Bunn F, Roberts I et al: Nutritional support for head-injured patients, *Cochrane Database Syst Rev* 3: CD001530, 2002. Updated February 25, 2003.
78. Brain Trauma Foundation, American Association of Neurological Surgeons, Congress of Neurological Surgeons, AANS/CNS Joint Section on Neurotrauma and Critical Care: Guidelines for the management of severe traumatic brain injury, third edition, *J Neurotrauma* 24 (1 suppl): S1-S106, 2007.
79. Mostafa G, Sing RF, Matthews BD et al: The economic benefit of practice guidelines for stress ulcer prophylaxis, *Am Surg* 68:146-150, 2002.
80. Greenwald J, CCCCPGC: Critical Care Connections, Inc: *Routes of nutrition support guideline* (2003): http://www.criticalcarenutrition.com/pdf/trainingtools/routes%20of%20nutrition%20suport.pdf. Accessed January 14, 2006.
81. Peter JV, Moran JL, Phillips-Hughes J: A metaanalysis of treatment outcomes of early enteral versus early parenteral nutrition in hospitalized patients, *Crit Care Med* 33:213-220, 260-261, 2005.
82. Nicholas JM, Cornelius MW, Tchorz KM et al: A two institution experience with 226 endoscopically placed jejunal feeding tubes in critically ill surgical patients, *Am J Surg* 186:583-590, 2003.
83. Marik PE, Zaloga GP: Meta-analysis of parenteral nutrition versus enteral nutrition in patients with acute pancreatitis, *BMJ* 328:1407, 2004.
84. Heyland D, Dhaliwal R: Immunonutrition in the critically ill: from old approaches to new paradigms, *Intensive Care Med* 31:501-503, 2005.
85. McCowen KC, Bistrian BR: Immunonutrition: problematic or problem solving? *Am J Clin Nutr* 77:764-770, 2003.
86. Schulman SP, Becker LC, Kass DA et al: L-arginine therapy in acute myocardial infarction: the Vascular Interaction With Age in Myocardial Infarction (VINTAGE MI) randomized clinical trial, *JAMA* 295:58-64, 2006.
87. Hall JC, Dobb G, Hall J et al: A prospective randomized trial of enteral glutamine in critical illness, *Intensive Care Med* 29:1710-1716, 2003.
88. Schulman AS, Willcutts KF, Claridge JA et al: Does the addition of glutamine to enteral feeds affect patient mortality? *Crit Care Med* 33:2501-2506, 2005.
89. Buchman A: The role of glutamine: counterpoint, *Nutr Clin Pract* 18:391-396, 2003.
90. Berg A, Rooyackers O, Norberg A et al: Elimination kinetics of L-alanyl-L-glutamine in ICU patients, *Amino Acids* 29:221-228, 2005.
91. Goeters C, Wenn A, Mertes N et al: Parenteral L-alanyl-L-glutamine improves 6-month outcome in critically ill patients, *Crit Care Med* 30:2032-2037, 2002.
92. Wilmore DW: Why should a single nutrient reduce mortality? *Crit Care Med* 30:2153-2154, 2002.
93. Fox VJ, Miller J, McClung M: Nutritional support in the critically injured, *Crit Care Nurs Clin North Am* 16:559-569, 2004.
94. Veldee MS: Nutritional assessment, therapy, and monitoring. In Burtis CA, Ashwood ER, editors: *Tietz textbook of clinical chemistry,* 3rd ed, p 1369, Philadelphia, 1999, W. B. Saunders.
95. Cothren CC, Moore EE, Ciesla DJ et al: Postinjury abdominal compartment syndrome does not preclude early enteral feeding after definitive closure, *Am J Surg* 188:653-658, 2004.
96. Heyland DK, Drover JW, Dhaliwal R et al: Optimizing the benefits and minimizing the risks of enteral nutrition in the critically ill: role of small bowel feeding, *JPEN J Parenter Enteral Nutr* 26(6 Suppl):S51-S57, 2002.
97. Vanek VW: Ins and outs of enteral access, 3: long-term access—jejunostomy, *Nutr Clin Pract* 18:201-220, 2003.
98. Metheny NA, Meert KL: Monitoring feeding tube placement, *Nutr Clin Pract* 19:487-595, 2004.
99. Cottrell DB, Asturi E: Gastric intubation: assessment and intervention, *Crit Care Nurs Clin North Am* 16:489-493, 2004.
100. Williams TA, Leslie GD: A review of the nursing care of enteral feeding tubes in critically ill adults: I, *Intensive Crit Care Nurs* 20:330-343, 2004.
101. Williams TA, Leslie GD: A review of the nursing care of enteral feeding tubes in critically ill adults: II, *Intensive Crit Care Nurs* 21:5-15, 2005.
102. McClave SA, DeMeo MT, DeLegge MH et al: North American Summit on Aspiration in the Critically Ill Patient: consensus statement, *JPEN J Parenter Enteral Nutr* 26(6 Suppl):S80-S85, 2002.
103. Sanko JS: Aspiration assessment and prevention in critically ill enterally fed patients: evidence-based recommendations for practice, *Gastroenterol Nurs* 27:279-285, 2004.
104. Reignier J, Thenoz-Jost N, Fiancette M et al: Early enteral nutrition in mechanically ventilated patients in the prone position, *Crit Care Med* 32:94-99, 2004.
105. Booth CM, Heyland DK, Paterson WG: Gastrointestinal promotility drugs in the critical care setting: a systematic review of the evidence, *Crit Care Med* 30:1429-1435, 2002.
106. Metheny NA, Schallom ME, Edwards SJ: Effect of gastrointestinal motility and feeding tube site on aspiration risk in critically ill patients: a review, *Heart Lung* 33:131-145, 2004.
107. McClave SA, Snider HL: Clinical use of gastric residual volumes as a monitor for patients on enteral tube feeding, *JPEN J Parenter Enteral Nutr* 26(6 Suppl):S43-S50, 2002.
108. Maloney JP, Ryan TA: Detection of aspiration in enterally fed patients: a requiem for bedside monitors of aspiration, *JPEN J Parenter Enteral Nutr* 26(6 Suppl):S34-S42, 2002.
109. Rowan CJ, Gillanders LK, Paice RL et al: Is early enteral feeding safe in patients who have suffered spinal cord injury? *Injury* 35:238-242, 2004.
110. Sacks GS: Drug-nutrient considerations in patients receiving parenteral and enteral nutrition, *Pract Gastroenterol* July:39-48, 2004.
111. Harrington L, Gonzales C: Food and drug interactions in critically ill adults, *Crit Care Nurs Clin North Am* 16:501-508, 2004.
112. Posani T: *Clostridium difficile:* causes and interventions, *Crit Care Nurs Clin North Am* 16:547-551, 2004.
113. Gervasio JM, Ednalino R, Reynolds J et al: *Bowel necrosis associated with enteral feeding,* American Society for Parenteral and Enteral Nutrition, program syllabus, vol 2, Clinical Nutrition Week, Dallas, February 12-15, 2006.
114. Vanek VW: Ins and outs of enteral access, 2: long term access—esophagostomy and gastrostomy, *Nutr Clin Pract* 18:50-74, 2003.

115. Loser C, Aschl G, Hebuterne X et al: ESPEN guidelines on artificial enteral nutrition—percutaneous endoscopic gastrostomy (PEG), *Clin Nutr* 24:848-861, 2005.
116. Ditchburn L, Chapman W: Joint primary-secondary care design of PEG care pathways, *Nurs Times* 101:34-36, 2005.
117. Dickerson RN, Brown RO: Long-term enteral nutrition support and the risk of dehydration, *Nutr Clin Pract* 20:646-653, 2005.
118. Correia MI, Guimaraes J, de Mattos LC et al: Peripheral parenteral nutrition: an option for patients with an indication for short-term parenteral nutrition, *Nutr Hosp* 19:14-18, 2004.
119. O'Grady NP, Alexander M, Dellinger EP et al: Guidelines for the prevention of intravascular catheter-related infections, *MMWR Recomm Rep* 51:1-29, 2002. [Erratum appears in *MMWR Wkly Rep* 51:71, 2002.]
120. Wojcik J: Central venous catheters, *Adv Nurses* 27-30, 2005.
121. Dimick JB, Swoboda S, Talamini MA et al: Risk of colonization of central venous catheters: catheters for total parenteral nutrition vs other catheters, *Am J Crit Care* 12:328-335, 2003.
122. McNearney T, Bajaj C, Boyars M et al: Total parenteral nutrition associated crystalline precipitates resulting in pulmonary artery occlusions and alveolar granulomas, *Dig Dis Sci* 48:1352-1354, 2003.
123. Van den Berghe G, Wilmer A, Hermans G et al: Intensive insulin therapy in the medical ICU, *N Engl J Med* 354:449-461, 2006.
124. Van den Berghe G, Wouters P, Bouillon R et al: Outcome benefit of intensive insulin therapy in the critically ill: insulin dose versus glycemic control, *Crit Care Med* 33:359-366, 2003.
125. Roberts SR, Hamedani B: Benefits and methods of achieving strict glycemic control in the ICU, *Crit Care Nurs Clin North Am* 16:537-545, 2004.
126. Oxford Radcliffe Hospitals: *Parenteral nutrition guidelines,* version 2.7 (revised August 2005): http://static.oxfordradcliffe.net/med/gems/TPNprotocol.pdf. Accessed August 26, 2005.
127. Buchman A: Total parenteral nutrition–associated liver disease, *JPEN J Parenter Enteral Nutr* 26:S43-S48, 2002.
128. Buchman AL, Ament ME, Sohel M et al: Choline deficiency causes reversible hepatic abnormalities in patients receiving parenteral nutrition: proof of a human choline requirement: a placebo-controlled trial, *JPEN J Parenter Enteral Nutr* 25:260-268, 2001.
129. Kelly DG: Guidelines and available products for parenteral vitamins and trace elements, *JPEN J Parenter Enteral Nutr* 26(5 Suppl):S34-S36, 2002.
130. Messing B, Joly F: Guidelines for management of home parenteral support in adult chronic intestinal failure patients, *Gastroenterology* 130(2 Suppl):S43-S51, 2006.
131. Reid MB, Allard-Gould P: Malnutrition and the critically ill elderly patient, *Crit Care Nurs Clin North Am* 16:531-536, 2004.
132. Castellanos VH, Silver HJ, Gallagher-Allred C et al: Nutrition issues in the home, community, and long-term care setting, *Nutr Clin Pract* 18:21-36, 2003.
133. Hudgens J, Langkamp-Henken B: The Mini Nutritional Assessment as an assessment tool in elders in long-term care, *Nutr Clin Pract* 19:463-470, 2004.
134. Ecklund MM: Meeting the nutritional needs of the bariatric patient in acute care, *Crit Care Nurs Clin North Am* 16:495-499, 2004.
135. Hulst JM, van Goudoever JB, Zimmermann LJ et al: The effect of cumulative energy and protein deficiency on anthropometric parameters in a pediatric ICU population, *Clin Nutr* 23:1381-1389, 2004.
136. Meert KL, Daphtary KM, Metheny NA: Gastric vs small-bowel feeding in critically ill children receiving mechanical ventilation: a randomized controlled trial, *Chest* 26:872-878, 2004.
137. Moreno Villares JM, Fernandez Carrion F, Sanchez Diaz JI et al: Current use of parenteral nutrition in a pediatric hospital: comparison to the practice 8 years ago, *Nutr Hosp* 20:46-51, 2005.
138. Weckwerth JA: Monitoring enteral nutrition support tolerance in infants and children, *Nutr Clin Pract* 19:496-503, 2004.
139. Wessel J, Balint J, Crill C et al: Standards for specialized nutrition support: hospitalized pediatric patients, *Nutr Clin Pract* 20:103-116, 2005.
140. Raiten DJ, Talbot JM, Walters JH: Assessment of nutrient requirements for infant formulas, *J Nutr* 128:2059S-2294S, 1998 [erratum *J Nutr* 129:1090, 1998].
141. Kline AM: Pediatric catheter-related bloodstream infections: latest strategies to decrease risk, *AACN Clin Issues* 16:185-198, 2005.
142. Taylor RM, Cheeseman P, Preedy V et al: Can energy expenditure be predicted in critically ill children? *Pediatr Crit Care Med* 4:176-180, 2003.
143. Vazquez Martinez JL, Martinez-Romillo PD, Diez Sebastian J et al: Predicted versus measured energy expenditure by continuous, online indirect calorimetry in ventilated, critically ill children during the early postinjury period, *Pediatr Crit Care Med* 5:19-27, 2004.
144. Hulst J, Joosten K, Zimmermann L et al: Malnutrition in critically ill children: from admission to 6 months after discharge, *Clin Nutr* 23:223-232, 2004.
145. Morgan A, Ward E, Murdoch B: Clinical progression and outcome of dysphagia following paediatric traumatic brain injury: a prospective study, *Brain Inj* 18:359-376, 2004.
146. Soreide E, Eriksson LI, Hirlekar G et al: Task Force on Scandinavian Pre-operative Fasting Guidelines, Clinical Practice Committee Scandinavian Society of Anaesthesiology and Intensive Care Medicine), pre-operative fasting guidelines: an update, *Acta Anaesthesiol Scand* 49:1041-1047, 2005.
147. Lee JO, Benjamin D, Herndon DN: Nutrition support strategies for severely burned patients, *Nutr Clin Pract* 20:325-330, 2005.
148. Gordon MD, Gottschlich MM, Helvig EI et al: Review of evidenced-based practice for the prevention of pressure sores in burn patients, *J Burn Care Rehabil* 25:388-410, 2004.
149. Flynn MB. Nutritional support for the burn-injured patient, *Crit Care Nurs Clin North Am* 16:139-144, 2004.
150. Demling RH: The incidence and impact of pre-existing protein energy malnutrition on outcome in the elderly burn patient population, *J Burn Care Rehabil* 26:94-100, 2005.
151. Garrel D, Patenaude J, Nedelec B et al: Decreased mortality and infectious morbidity in adult burn patients given enteral glutamine supplements: a prospective, controlled, randomized clinical trial, *Crit Care Med* 31:2444-2449, 2003.
152. Peng X, Yan H, You Z et al: Clinical and protein metabolic efficacy of glutamine granules–supplemented enteral nutrition in severely burned patients, *Burns* 31:342-346, 2005.
153. Zhou YP, Jiang ZM, Sun YH et al: The effect of supplemental enteral glutamine on plasma levels, gut function, and outcome

in severe burns: a randomized, double-blind, controlled clinical trial, *JPEN J Parenter Enteral Nutr* 27:241-245, 2003.
154. Barrocas A, Yarbrough G, Becnel PA III et al: Ethical and legal issues in nutrition support of the geriatric patient: the can, should, and must of nutrition support, *Nutr Clin Pract* 18:37-47, 2003.
155. Carter BS, Leuthner SR: The ethics of withholding/withdrawing nutrition in the newborn, *Semin Perinatol* 27:480-487, 2003.
156. Chellel A, Fraser J, Fender V et al: Nursing observations on ward patients at risk of critical illness, *Nurs Times* 98:36-39, 2002.
157. Vazirani S, Hays RD, Shapiro MF et al: Effect of a multidisciplinary intervention on communication and collaboration among physicians and nurses, *Am J Crit Care* 14:71-77, 2005.
158. Ball M: Culture of safety, *Adv Nurses* Oct:31-32, 2005.
159. Aihara R, Schoepfel SL, Curtis AR et al: Guidelines for improving nutritional delivery in the intensive care unit, *J Healthc Qual* 24:22-29, 2002.
160. Martin CM, Doig GS, Heyland DK et al: Southwestern Ontario Critical Care Research Network: multicentre, cluster-randomized clinical trial of algorithms for critical-care enteral and parenteral therapy (ACCEPT), *CMAJ* 170:197-204, 2004.
161. Harrington L: Nutrition in critically ill adults: key processes and outcomes, *Crit Care Nurs Clin North Am* 16:459-465, 2004.
162. Gibney MJ, Walsh M, Brennan L et al: Metabolomics in human nutrition: opportunities and challenges, *Am J Clin Nutr* 82:497-503, 2005.

18

Analgesia, Sedation, and Neuromuscular Blockade in the Trauma Patient

T. Catherine Bower, Jameson P. Reuter

Introduction

Pain management in the adult trauma patient is multifactorial and complex, which presents unique challenges to nursing care. Traumatic injuries are the consequence of external forces, and subsequent delayed sequelae are multifaceted and painful. Throughout the various stages of the trauma care continuum that follows blunt or penetrating injuries, a patient may require a balanced regimen of analgesia, sedation, and possibly neuromuscular blockade (NMB). It is imperative that health care practitioners apply evidence-based practice principles to the management of an injured patient. This chapter reviews current consensus guidelines and multimodal approaches to individualize quality patient care through the phases of resuscitation to rehabilitation.

Negative Consequences of Undertreated Pain

Unabated acute pain creates negative consequences and can lead to persistent pain.[1] Physiological, psychosocial, and economic parameters can be affected throughout the trauma continuum. Table 18-1 summarizes the consequences of inadequately controlled pain. Despite high technologic advances in analgesic delivery, negative outcomes of atelectasis, hypoxemia, pneumonia, deep vein thrombosis, and ileus continue to prevent successful recovery after surgery and traumatic injury. Anxiety, fear, and depression are likely to occur if pain is persistent and goes untreated. The economic impact of undertreated pain can result in prolonged hospital stay and continued health care resource utilization on discharge.[2]

Undertreated pain has been well documented in the literature, spanning more than 30 years.[3] The term "oligoanalgesia" has evolved in the emergency medicine arena to demonstrate the practice of undermedication in patients who report pain as their chief complaint. Health care practitioners in the past were known to withhold analgesics to prevent masking of clinical findings despite the report of pain. Puntillo et al[4] reported clinically significant differences between nursing and patient pain rating scores, documenting that emergency department nurses underestimated musculoskeletal pain 95% of the time. Emergency department studies showed that 53% of patients admitted waited more than 60 minutes before analgesics were administered and those reporting a mild pain score of less than 4 (out of 10) received no analgesics.[5] Although prehospital protocols have been established for first responders to administer analgesics in the field, in one study of analgesic administration in more than 1,000 patients, only 18 (2%) were given morphine or nitrous oxide for suspected extremity fracture.[6] Young children under 6 years of age, individuals with cognitive impairment, the elderly, female patients, ethnic minorities, and those with psychiatric illness are at the greatest risk for undermedication during an emergency department admission.[7-9] At a Level I trauma center, patients at risk for oligoanalgesia were identified as those more seriously injured, as defined by a lower Revised Trauma Score, a lower Glasgow Coma Scale score, and those who were intubated.[10]

Many factors contribute to the underuse of analgesics during various points of care when a patient seeks medical attention for pain relief from injury or disease. Lack of knowledge regarding pharmacologic management appears to be a common theme among many disciplines.[11] Some care providers want to make a diagnosis before administering analgesics.[12] Lack of consistent assessment of pain is another factor that affects analgesic administration, especially when pain severity scores are not documented in the medical record. Those patients unable to communicate pain, such as the very young, the unconscious, and the elderly, usually do not receive analgesics.[7] Another barrier is the belief among emergency care physicians that a valid, informed consent needs to be obtained before administration of opioids, to prevent interfering with the patient's decision-making capability.[3,13]

Undertreatment of pain may be a risk in the critical care environment, especially when vital organ function becomes the priority. The administration of analgesics is limited during events of hemodynamic instability or in the presence of deteriorating mental status with head injury. Assessment of pain in the critically ill is limited as a result of the lack of self-report, especially if the patient is intubated and sedated.[14] Patients unable to report pain are at

TABLE 18-1 Consequences of Uncontrolled Pain: A Systems Overview

System	Response	Outcome
Neurologic	↓Mental function, ↓cognitive function	Anxiety, fear, anger, depression, confusion
Respiratory	↓Vital capacity, ↓functional residual capacity, ↓tidal volume, ↓cough effort, ↓thoracic and abdominal muscle movement, ↓alveolar ventilation, ↓oxygen saturation	Atelectasis, pneumonia, hypoxemia
Cardiovascular	↓Heart rate, ↓cardiac output, ↓peripheral vascular resistance, hypercoagulation, ↓systemic vascular resistance, hypertension, ↓coronary vascular resistance, ↓myocardial oxygen consumption	Angina, deep vein thrombosis
Gastrointestinal	↓Gastric and bowel motility	Ileus, nausea and vomiting, constipation
Genitourinary	↓Urinary output, ↓urinary sphincter tone	Urinary retention
Musculoskeletal	Impaired muscle function	Weakness, muscle spasm, fatigue
Metabolic/endocrine	Hyperglycemia, gluconeogenesis, glucose intolerance, insulin resistance, ↓ACTH, ↑cortisol, ↑ADH, ↑epinephrine, ↑norepinephrine, ↑growth hormone, ↑catecholamines, ↑renin, ↑angiotension II, ↑aldosterone	Weight loss, fever, tachycardia

ACTH, Adrenocorticotropin; *ADH,* antidiuretic hormone. Adapted from McCaffery M, Pasero C: *Pain: clinical manual,* St Louis, 1999, Mosby, p 24, Joshi GP, Ogunnaike BO: Consequences of inadequate postoperative pain relief and chronic persistent postoperative pain, *Anesthesiol Clin North Am* 23:21-36, 2005.

risk for undermedication, especially if pain behaviors such as facial expression or body movement are absent because of paralysis or because of administration of sedatives and paralytics.[15]

In 1992 the Agency for Health Care Policy and Research (AHCPR), which is now the Agency for Healthcare Research and Quality, published the first clinical practice guideline (CPG) on pain management in operative or medical procedures and trauma.[16] This publication was the springboard for the development of subsequent CPGs that address other pain syndromes and conditions. The Joint Commission (TJC) applied pain management assessment and management requirements in many practice arenas in 2001. Both these organizations have been instrumental in the formation of a standardized practice of pain assessment and delivery of quality pain management. Undertreatment of acute pain can lead to the development of chronic pain states or syndromes.[17,18]

DEFINITIONS/CLASSIFICATIONS/PHYSIOLOGIC PATHWAYS

DEFINITIONS

More than 35 years ago, McCaffery defined pain as "whatever the experiencing person says it is, existing whenever she/he says it does." This exemplifies the importance of the patient's perspective and input, which supports the individual's self-report as the most reliable indicator of pain.[16] The most widely recognized definition of pain, "an unpleasant sensory and emotional experience associated with actual or potential damage," was introduced by the International Association for the Study of Pain (IASP) in 1979.[19] It is a sensation that is strictly subjective in nature. Pain is a very complex, individualized experience with many dimensions.

Pain experienced during the various stages of the trauma continuum can be acute, intermittent or procedural, chronic (persistent), or neuropathic in nature (Table 18-2). Acute pain can be considered short in duration, as a result of direct tissue trauma. The perception of discomfort declines as tissue inflammation diminishes and healing occurs over time. Intermittent or procedural pain can be the result of routine care interventions, such as venous puncture, dressing changes, or suctioning. Turning has been recognized as one of the most painful and intermittent distressing events endured by patients in the intensive care unit (ICU).[20] Chronic pain is acquired from long-standing processes of tissue injury or unrelieved pain that results from tissue hypersensitity. Neuropathic pain can be derived from damage or dysfunction in the peripheral or central nervous system (CNS) that displays sensory symptoms and signs[21] (Table 18-3). The trauma patient can also have acute pain in addition to coexisting pain syndromes.

PAIN CLASSIFICATIONS

One way to classify pain is by inferred pathophysiologic mechanisms[22] (Table 18-3). *Nociception* refers to the body's response and processing to a noxious (or painful) stimulus along an ascending pathway. The peripheral nervous system contains free nerve endings, called nociceptors, that are responsible for pain. These receptors transmit the sensation of painful stimuli from peripheral tissues that have been injured to the cerebral cortex. Nociceptors are located in skin, joints, muscle, fascia, viscera, and the smooth muscle of the arterial walls. Two types of afferent nerve fibers or first-order neurons, A-delta and C-fibers, transmit pain through neural pathways. These fibers are located in the dorsal horn of the spinal cord (Figure 18-1). A-delta fibers are large diameter and myelinated fibers that transmit fast-moving impulses caused by thermal

TABLE 18-2 Pain Definitions

Type of Pain	Characteristics
Acute pain	Warning signal for potential of injury (protective reflex); complex, individualized experience; nociceptive in nature; usually some degree of tissue damage; hyperdynamic response related to hormone release; pain experience declines with tissue healing; may convert to chronic or neuropathic pain
Intermittent pain	Nociceptive in nature; predictable or unpredictable; pain intensity experience increases as stimulus exposure is prolonged; procedural pain (venipuncture, dressing changes, movement); "breakthrough" pain or end of dose pain from scheduled analgesic; procedural pain can induce suffering perception/anxiety
Chronic (persistent) pain	Persistent pain extending beyond a period of healing; disrupts activities of daily living and sleep; interrupts functional status; no adaptive or physiologic response; may be nociceptive or neuropathic or both; environmental and affective behaviors may exacerbate or perpetuate
Cancer pain	Malignant pain; acute and chronic components; pathology and level of pain are related
Chronic noncancer pain	Subtype of chronic pain; acute injury related or no discernible cause; prolonged, possibly life-long pain; affects daily activities, relationships, physical deconditioning; psychologic symptoms develop

Adapted from Turk DC, Okifuji A: Pain terms and taxonomies of pain. In Loeser JD et al, editors: *Bonica's management of pain,* 3rd ed, pp. 17-25, Baltimore, 2001, Lippincott Williams & Wilkins.

and mechanical stimuli. Pain sensations can be described as sharp and sudden. C-fibers are small diameter and unmyelinated fibers that transmit delayed, slow pain that has been activated by chemicals (neurotransmitters) released after cellular trauma. These neurotransmitters include histamine, serotonin, and acetylcholine. Pain descriptions verbalized by the patient include dull, diffuse, and prolonged.

Neuropathic pain arises from abnormal processing of a sensory stimulus by the peripheral nervous system or the CNS.[22] The *N*-methyl-D-aspartate (NMDA) receptor is believed to be involved in neuropathetic and chronic pain states.[23] Nerve injury can also activate changes in the CNS and result in central sensitization and "wind-up." Wind-up or hyperexcitibility occurs at the dorsal horn level as an outcome of persistent noxious stimuli.[22] Peripheral sensitization occurs related to the endogenous chemical release and inflammation that follows. Characteristics of neuropathic pain include hyperalagesia, burning, tingling, and electric-shock pain perception.

TABLE 18-3 Pain Classifications

Nociceptive Pain		**Neuropathic Pain**	
Normal process of stimuli that damages normal tissues or has the potential to do so if prolonged; usually responsive to nonopioids or opioids.		Abnormal processing of sensory input by the peripheral or central nervous system; treatment usually includes adjuvant analgesics.	
Somatic Pain	**Visceral Pain**	**Centrally Generated Pain**	**Peripherally Generated Pain**
Arises from bone, joint, muscle, skin, or connective tissue. It is usually aching or throbbing in quality and is well localized.	Arises from visceral organs, such as the gastrointestinal tract and pancreas. This may be subdivided: Tumor involvement of the organ capsule that causes aching and fairly well-localized pain. Obstruction of hollow viscus, which causes intermittent cramping and poorly localized pain.	Deafferentation pain: injury to either the peripheral or central nervous system. Examples: Phantom pain may reflect injury to the peripheral nervous system; burning pain below the level of a spinal cord lesion reflects injury to the central nervous system. Sympathetically maintained pain: associated with dysregulation of the autonomic nervous system. Examples: May include some of the pain associated with reflex sympathetic dystrophy/causalgia (complex regional pain syndrome [CRPS]: type I, type II)	Painful polyneuropathies: pain is felt along the distribution of many peripheral nerves. Examples: diabetic neuropathy, alcohol-nutritional neuropathy, and those associated with Guillain-Barré syndrome. Painful mononeuropathies: Usually associated with a known peripheral nerve injury, and pain is felt at least partly along the distribution of the damaged nerve. Examples: nerve root compression, nerve entrapment, trigeminal neuralgia

From McCaffery M, Pasero C: *Pain: clinical manual,* p. 19, St. Louis, 1999, Mosby. Reprinted with permission.

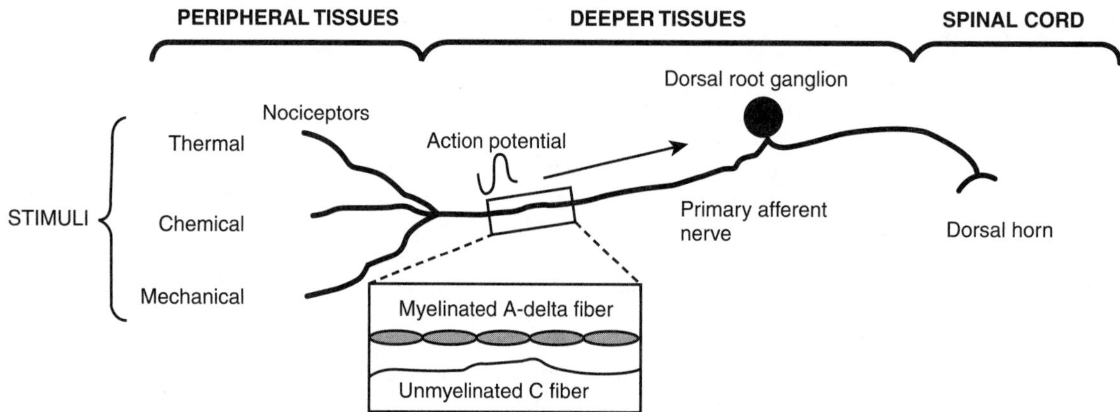

FIGURE 18-1 The physiology and processing of pain. *(Redrawn from Renn CL, Dorsey SG: The physiology and processing of pain: a review,* AACN Clin Issues *16:277-290; quiz 413-415, 2005.)*

Physiologic Pathways

There are four processes in the sensory pathway, which include transduction, transmission, perception, and modulation (Figure 18-2). Within each of these processes, analgesic therapy can be targeted to attenuate the pain experience. Transduction involves the process of converting chemical, mechanical, or thermal energy into neural impulses. In the presence of trauma or infection, chemical substances and enzymes are released from the damaged tissues, increasing the transduction of painful stimuli. Byproducts of the arachidonic acid pathway, which include prostaglandins (PG) and leukotrienes, are the major mediators of hyperanalgesia with inflammation. Histamine (H) is released from mast cells and acts directly on sensory neurons to produce itching and pain. Other sensitizing chemicals include bradykinin, serotonin (5HT), and substance P (SP). The pain stimulus causes an action potential where ion transfer occurs before impulse conduction.

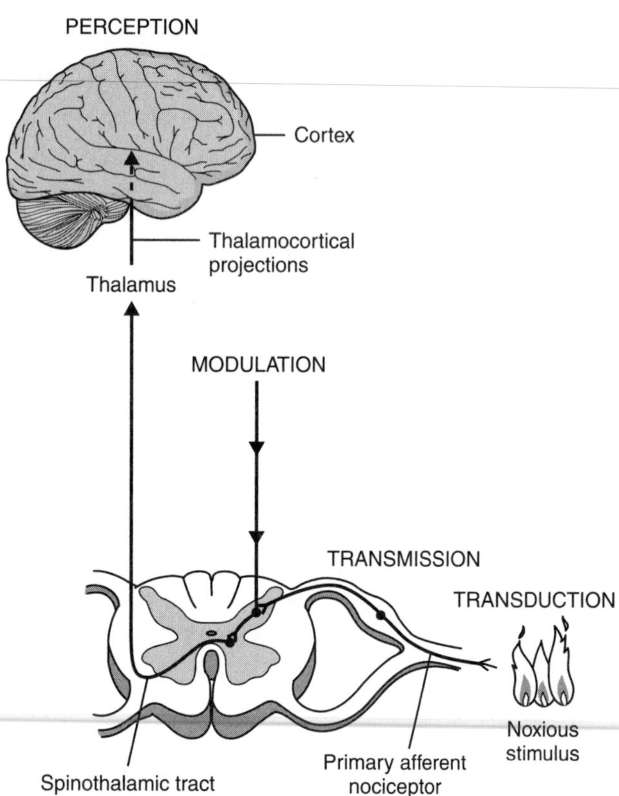

FIGURE 18-2 Four processes in sensory pathway: transduction, transmission, perception, and modulation. *(From Ferrante and VadeBoncouer, editors:* Postoperative pain management, *New York, 1993, Churchill-Livingstone.)*

The CNS has two mechanisms that are part of pain transmission: the ascending pathway through conduction and the descending pathway through modulation (Figure 18-3). Pain receptors may be stimulated by temperature extremes, mechanical injury, or chemical irritation. The ascending tracts synapse with the first-order A-delta and C-fibers located in laminae I through V of the spinal cord. Type C fibers are mainly found in lamina I and II, known as the substantia gelatinosa, and synapse with neurons in the dorsal horn. The second-order neurons, arising from the dorsal horn, travel cephalad to the thalamus.

Several pathways for afferent pain signals traverse the ascending spinal cord to the cortex. The spinothalamic pathway is regarded as the most important pathway, and it can be subdivided into the neospinothalamic (lateral spinothalamic) pathway and the paleospinothalamic (medial spinothalamic) pathway.[24] The neospinothalamic is the primary pathway for sensations of pain, temperature, and touch initiated by fast pain signals.[25] The paleospinothalamic pathway is principally for the transmission of unmyelinated type C fibers that are conductive of slow or chronic pain sensations.[26] SP is believed to be the main neurotransmitter of the paleospinothalamic pathway in the dorsal horn.[24] The spinomesencephalic pathway plays a role in the activation of descending control systems and endogenous opioid systems. It begins with the nociceptors in laminae I and V and terminates in the roof of the midbrain and the periaqueductal gray matter.[27]

Cortical understanding of the noxious stimulus occurs at the somatosensory cortex, where perception of pain is processed and individualized. The spinothalamic tract moves

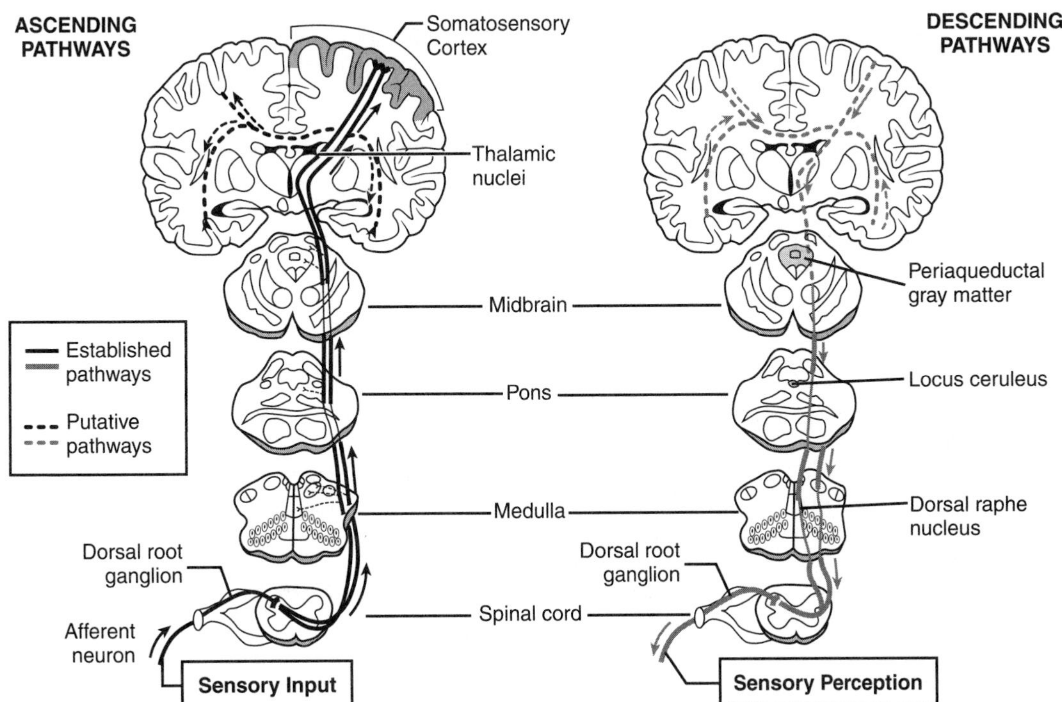

FIGURE 18-3 Normal processing of acute nociceptive pain. *(Redrawn from Hainline B: Chronic pain: physiological, diagnostic, and management considerations [review].* Psychiatr Clin North Am *28:713-735, 2005.)*

through the pons, medulla, and midbrain and terminates in the thalamus. Pain location, intensity, and emotional processing occur at this level. The reticular system is responsible for the autonomic response to pain and the emotional-affective components.[28] The somatosensory cortex localizes and characterizes pain. The limbic system is responsible for emotional processing and the behavioral reaction to pain.[22]

The descending pain pathway is the endogenous pain modulation system. Modulation involves the modification of nociceptive transmissions in the dorsal horn or spinal reflexes. Neurons originating from the brainstem descend to the dorsal horn, releasing endogenous opioids, (5HT, norepinephrine, and γ-aminobutyric acid (GABA), which inhibit the transmission of noxious stimuli and produce analgesia. Three subtypes of endogenous opioids include β-endorphin, met- and leu-enkephalins, and dynorphins.[24,29,30] Endogenous and exogenous opioids activate dorsal horn receptors mu (μ), delta (δ), and kappa (κ) to inhibit pain impulses.[22]

Pain Assessment in the Adult Trauma Patient

Pain assessment in the acutely injured is a clinician's challenge in a fast-paced environment of rapid response and resuscitation. Pain assessment must be individualized, and basic principles of a comprehensive analgesic plan can be applied using the ABC method as described by the AHCPR (Table 18-4).[31] Instituting pain protocols after the primary survey and a pain assessment may be an opportunity to facilitate analgesic administration for traumatic injuries and during pain-provoking activities.[32]

A comprehensive approach to trauma pain assessment requires the careful evaluation of key elements (Table 18-5). Although the self-report of pain is the gold standard, the unconscious, the cognitively impaired, the young and the old, the intoxicated, and those with communication or language barriers offer unique assessment challenges to the trauma team. A systematic pain assessment should include a general patient health history, pain history, a physical examination with behavioral observations, and further diagnostic investigation as needed. When the self-report cannot be articulated, other measures must be used to detect the presence of pain.

The patient history should explore the medical history, the presence of comorbities, and the mechanism of injury. With regard to previous hospitalizations, previous surgical interventions should be detailed, along with analgesic methods and agents that were effective in the past. In addition to

TABLE 18-4 **Pain Assessment and Management Mnemonic**

A	**A**sk about and **A**ssess pain regularly and systematically.
B	**B**elieve the report of pain.
C	**C**hoose the best pain control options.
D	**D**eliver pain interventions consistently and timely.
E	**E**mpower the patient and family to control the course.

Modified from Jacox A, Carr DB, Payne R et al: *Management of cancer pain,* Clinical Practice Guideline No. 9, AHCPR Pub. No. 94-0592, Rockville, 1994, Agency for Health Care Policy and Research, U.S. Department of Health and Human Services, Public Health Service.

TABLE 18-5 Pain Assessment Factors in the Critical, Intermediate, and Rehabilitative Phases of Trauma

1. Patient history
   a. Medical history/comorbidities
   b. Mechanism of injury: systems analysis/type of injury
   c. Past pain experiences and trauma; coexisting pain syndromes/functional status
   d. Past surgery
   e. Medication reconciliation (list current analgesics) and herbal supplements
   f. Medication allergies versus past opioid side effect experience
   g. Social history: use of tobacoo, alcohol, illicit drug use
   h. Cultural/religious beliefs
   i. Cognitive/memory status
   j. Emotional response to pain/hospitalization/support network
   k. Social functioning: education/employment
2. Pain assessment: self-report
   a. Provoking factors/onset: episodic; constant; triggering factors: movement/immobilization
   b. Quality/character: use patient's own words: "sharp," "dull," "ache," etc.
   c. Region/location: encourage patient to point to pain
   d. Severity/intensity: use a pain scale appropriate to patient (e.g., 0-10 scale)
   e. Timing/duration: percentage of time in pain, procedural events, time of day, sleep pattern
3. Nursing observations: behavioral assessment
   a. Vital signs: blood pressure, pulse, respiratory fluctuations with pain events
   b. Mood/affect: withdrawn, anxious, sad, fearful, tearful, worried, angry
   c. Sleep intervals
   d. Appetite
   e. Energy levels
   f. Level of consciousness/behaviors: restlessness, facial expressions, guarding, moaning, groaning, ventilator synchronization
4. Clinical workup
   a. Laboratory tests/toxicology results
   b. Radiographic studies/scans
   c. Future diagnostic follow-up/interventional studies

the patient's medical history, medication reconciliation will validate current analgesic exposure and alert the health care team to anticipate the response to analgesic treatments chosen. A pain history should include information regarding pain medication allergies or sensitivities and further investigation is warranted if previous adverse reactions are mentioned. Current use of analgesics, whether over-the-counter products or prescription analgesics and sedatives, should be validated and current frequency of administration investigated. Smoking, alcohol consumption patterns, and history of substance abuse and detoxification require further elaboration with regard to patterns of use and duration. Cultural and religious beliefs and emotional response to past pain experiences should also be explored.

A history of chronic pain syndromes, previous pain treatments, and psychosocial responses to pain and stress should be interconnected to the initial pain assessment. Patient personality and expectations concerning pain and its management must be considered. Identifying individual coping responses, pain behaviors, and cultural interpretations are important. Patient responses to painful situations can be obtained from the patient or validated by a family informant. Establishing a comfort goal[33] or acceptable pain rating should also be included during the initial pain screen if possible.

Pain assessment and history should be included with the initial nursing survey. Clarification of a pain rating system requires patient instruction and understanding. Foreign language tools are available or can easily be devised with input from an interpreter. Validation of pain rating scale education will ensure consistent use of the same rating tool throughout the trauma continuum. Behavioral presentations indicating pain may be the only aspect to rely on if the patient is unable to communicate pain because of neurologic insult or sedation.

The initial pain screen will identify patient treatment requirements and goals throughout the various stages of trauma recovery. The PQRST mnemonic is a quick and lenient method for the trauma nurse to apply the key elements of the comprehensive pain assessment for the verbal patient. The characteristics of pain expressed by the patient formulate a personal narrative. Verbalization of what **p**rovokes/**p**alliates pain, the **q**ualities of the pain, the **r**egion and **r**adiation of pain, the **s**everity and **s**trength of the pain, and length of **t**ime the pain has persisted ensures a thorough assessment.

The provoking aspects and causes of pain must be investigated thoroughly. Inquiries should include what triggers the pain (such as movement or deep breathing), specific treatments and procedures (such as wound dressing changes), and its duration: is the pain constant or episodic? Does tactile stimulation, such as pressure from orthopedic appliances or bed linens, cause discomfort? Palliative measures may include analgesic administration, elevation, realignment, and support of the injured body part.

The quality aspect of assessment uses the patient's own descriptors. Request of the patient, for example, "Tell me how your pain feels." Particular words will alert the assessor to common pain states. Acute nociceptive pain has been described as sharp, dull, or aching. Visceral pain can be characterized as cramping, twisting, or tight. Neuropathic pain has been known to produce burning, shock-like, or electric-type pain sensations. After orthopedic injury, lower extremity pain that is excruciating with passive motion may indicate early development of compartment syndrome.

Encourage the patient to point to the region of pain or use a body diagram to locate pain. Obvious injuries may not be the source of pain; for example, nasal drainage tubes can cause more distress than surgical incisions. Further explore reports of phantom limb sensation and other types of pain reported by amputees. Investigate any report of pain radiating to other areas besides that of obvious injury.

Pain rating scales offer a quick and simplified means for a patient to rate pain severity. Consistently using the same rating tool is imperative throughout the trauma continuum for assessment and documentation. Verbal rating intensity scales (Figure 18-4) aid the practitioner evaluating traumatic pain complaints. Unidimensional scales, such as the numeric scale (where 0 is no pain and 10 is the worst pain imaginable), word descriptor scales (no pain, mild, moderate, severe), or visual scales (Faces Pain Scale-R) allow the clinician to determine the patient's pain intensity within a short time frame. Many tools are available, with some using horizontal or vertical linear orientation or variations of color. The Bieri FACES-R pain rating scale can be used in patients older than 3 years of age and those with cognitive impairment (Figure 18-5). Multidimensional tools, such as the McGill Pain Questionnaire, provide in-depth pain information and effects on daily living and require a motivated patient to complete. These instruments

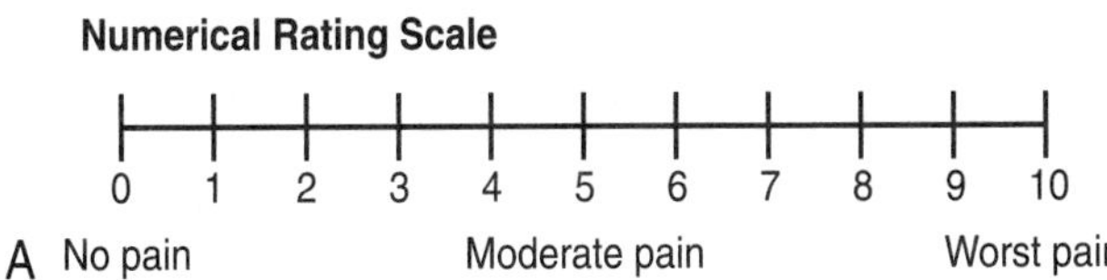

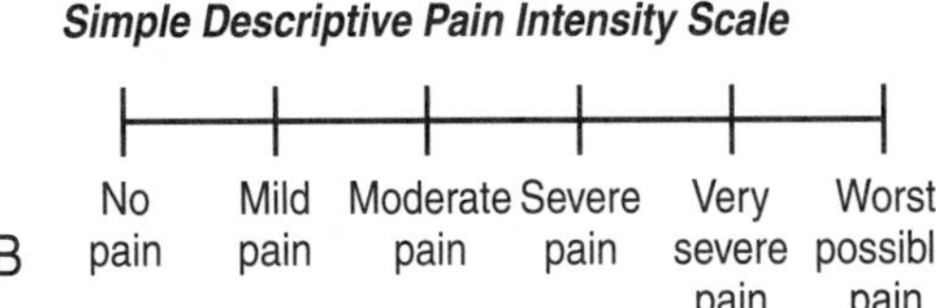

FIGURE 18-4 Verbal rating intensity scales. **A,** Numerical rating scale. (Redrawn from McCaffery M, Beebe A: *Pain: clinical manual for nursing practice,* 2nd ed, Philadelphia, 1999, Mosby.) **B,** Simple descriptive pain intensity scale. (From *Acute pain management: Operative or medical procedures and trauma,* Clinical Practice Guideline No. 1, AHCPR Pub. No 92-0032, Rockville, Md, Feb 1992, Agency for Healthcare Research and Quality, pp 116-117.)

are more helpful during the intermittent and rehabilitative phase of care when complex, persistent pain may require specialized care and follow-up.

Timing refers to when pain occurs and how long it lasts. Does it vary with activity or intensify during certain time frames? Episodic or procedure-related pain can be correlated with therapeutic activities, such as turning, endotracheal suctioning, and removal of drains from wound beds.

For the unconscious, sedated, or nonverbal patient, accurate pain assessment is difficult and results in underrated and undertreated pain.[34,35] These patients are unable to verbalize a self-report of pain. Pain in this patient population can be perceived as suffering, which presents a distinctive set of behaviors perceived by caregivers.[36] Behavioral manifestations such as restlessness, moaning, crying, or guarding the injured body part can cue the nurse to the presence of pain or discomfort. Other behaviors include teeth clenching, forehead wrinkling, restlessness, withdrawal reflexes, thrashing, rocking, kicking, and tensing muscles.[37]

Behavioral assessment tools have been frequently used in the pediatric population, with specific tools developed for certain patient age groups and diagnoses (Table 18-6). Historically, nurses relied on physiologic indicators such as increased heart rate or blood pressure, which are now considered the least sensitive indicators of pain.[38] With behavioral indicators, the nurse must assume that pain is present[15] and provide nursing interventions, such as repositioning, and offer an analgesic trial.

A behavioral tool has been validated in the critically ill, sedated, and mechanically ventilated patient population[35,39] (Table 18-7). It scores facial expression, movement of upper limbs, and ventilator compliance. Other pain-related behavioral checklists available include domains of agitation, anxiety, ventilator synchrony, facial tension, muscle tone, body movement, vocalizations, and consolability.[40-42] Adoption of a single behavior tool exclusively for the trauma patient is limited because of many variables, especially when the patient requires tracheostomy and mechanical ventilation. For the behavior scale to be valid, the patient must be able to score in all behavior categories.[15] Vocalization or expressions of pain cannot be verbalized, especially when concurrent sedation or NMB is administered. Diaphoresis and lacrimation have been observed in patients receiving NMB during painful stimulation.[43] Patients who are undergoing procedures that would be painful for others should be treated pre-emptively for pain.[34] Use of a sedation assessment tool, such as the Ramsay Sedation Rating Scale, the Richmond Agitation-Sedation Scale (RASS), or the Motor Activity Assessment Scale (MASS) is an appropriate alternative, as long as pain is assumed present with analgesics administered. Discussion of these tools occurs later in the chapter.

For the patient who is cognitively impaired, perhaps from the aging process or brain injury, the self-report of pain can be elicited through the use of standardized pain rating scales.[44,45] It is important for the nurse to determine whether the patient is able to provide a self-report and to modify the approach for assessment on the basis of the patient's cognition. Simplifying

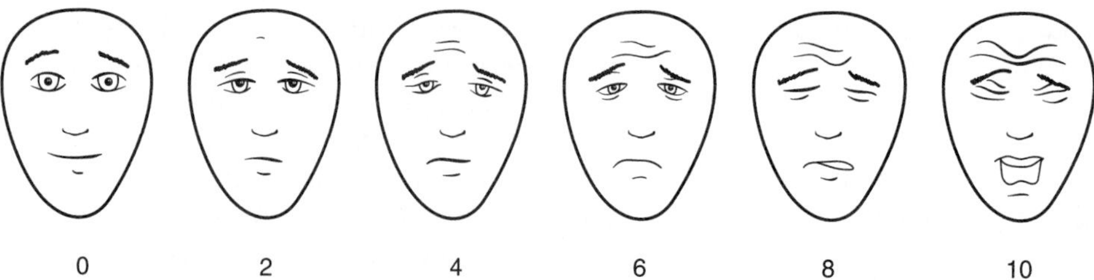

FIGURE 18-5 Bieri Faces-R Pain rating scale. When the faces pain scale is used, these instructions may be given: "These faces show how much something can hurt. This face [point to left-most face] shows no pain. The faces show more and more pain [point to each from left to right] up to this one [point to right-most face]—it shows very much pain. Point to the face that shows how much you hurt [right now]." *(From Hicks CL, Von Baeyer CL, Spafford P et al:* The Faces Scale-Revised: toward a common metric pediatric pain measurement, Pain *93:173-183, 2001. Adapted from Bieri D et al: Pain 41:139-150, 1990.)*

the descriptive anchors on the intensity scale may be required, as well as using another scale to validate the patient's response. Use of words such as mild, moderate, and severe, with explanation of their meanings on a number scale is one strategy. If the verbal descriptor scale is inclusive, validation with a visually enlarged Faces Pain Scale is an alternative.[46] Behavioral patterns can also be incorporated into the pain assessment, especially with movement. Baseline behavior and activity patterns should be documented so that changes can be further investigated.[46] Behavioral tools can also be applied for those patients unable to articulate a pain rating.[47]

Assessment of pain has been endorsed as the fifth vital sign[48] and should be adopted as a standing routine for any point-of-care documentation throughout the trauma continuum. This approach to assessment is useful in making pain assessment and treatment a priority. Frequency of assessment is directly related to its presence and severity. Current pain intensity, worst pain experienced, level of pain relief achieved, and acceptable and not acceptable pain ranges should be incorporated within the patient's plan of care. If the intensity rating is high, pain assessment should be performed more frequently, as often as every 2 hours or more as needed to address the patient's report of pain effectively. As pain is controlled and becomes less acute, the frequency of assessment can decrease. It is imperative to explore new reports of pain and the effectiveness of analgesic therapeutics, at rest and with movement.

TJC has developed standards for assessment and reassessment of pain.[49,50] Because pain should be assessed in all patients, the clinical documentation process should be institution specific and should incorporate key elements within the permanent record. Quality indicators and electronic prompts within the information system can facilitate compliance with practitioner documentation. Consistency with recording the pain rating is important. If the numeric scoring system is used, the patient rating over the range is suggested. For example, if a patient reports a pain rating of 5 on the 0 to 10 scale, nursing documentation would be "5/10." For those patients unable to verbalize a pain rating, a behavior tool can be used for documentation trends. It is imperative for clinicians to understand that a pain behavior score does not equate to a pain score rating.[15] The pain rating, along with medication recording, can track trends with effectiveness during reassessment. Reevaluation of analgesic effectiveness is recommended within

TABLE 18-6 **FLACC Scale: Pediatric Behavioral Tool**

Category	Scoring		
	0	1	2
Face	No particular expression or smile	Occasional grimace or frown, withdrawn, disinterested	Frequent to constant quivering chin, clenched jaw
Legs	Normal position or relaxed	Uneasy, restless, tense	Kicking, or legs drawn up
Activity	Lying quietly, normal position, moves easily	Squirming, shifting back and forth, tense	Arched, rigid or jerking
Cry	No cry (awake or asleep)	Moans or whimpers; occasional complaint	Crying steadily, screams or sobs, frequent complaints
Consolability	Content, relaxed	Reassured by occasional touching, hugging or being talked to, distractible	Difficult to console or comfort

Each of the five categories (F) Face; (L) Legs; (A) Activity; (C) Cry; (C) Consolability is scored from 0-2, which results in a total score between 0 and 10.
From Merkel S et al: *The FLACC: a behavioral scale for scoring postoperative pain in young children, Pediatr Nurse* 23:293-297, 1997.

TABLE 18-7 **Behavior Pain Scale***

Item	Behavior	Score
Facial expression	Relaxed	1
	Partially tightened (brow lowering)	2
	Fully tightened (eyelid closing)	3
	Grimacing	4
Upper limb movements	No movement	1
	Partially bent	2
	Fully bent with finger flexion	3
	Permanently retracted	4
Compliance with mechanical ventilator	Tolerating movement	1
	Coughing but tolerating ventilation for most of the time	2
	Fighting ventilator	3
	Unable to control ventilation	4

From Payen J-F, Bru O, Bosson J-L, et al: Assessing pain in critically ill sedated patients by using a behavioral pain scale, *Crit Care Med* 29:2258-2263, 2001.
*The Behavior Pain Scale allows the assessor to derive a score of between 3 (no pain) and 12 (highest pain score).

15 to 30 minutes of parental administration and within 1 hour of oral administration.[16]

Opioids

Effects of Opioids

Nurses routinely administer parental analgesics for the effective management of pain. Knowledge of opiate receptors and their response is essential to monitor and treat adverse effects. Opioids produce analgesia by binding to specific receptors in the peripheral and central nervous systems.

Three major classes of opioid receptors have been clinically relevant for analgesia: mu (μ), delta (δ), and kappa (κ).[51] Other receptors have been identified, including varespsilon, zeta, iota, sigma, and lambda.[52,53] Mu opioid receptors are found in the periphery after inflammation, the dorsal horn of the spinal cord, the brainstem, the thalamus, and the cortex.[54] At the cellular level, opioids decrease calcium ion entry, thus blocking SP release from the primary afferents in the dorsal horn of the spinal cord.[55] Mu-1 receptors have been linked to mediate supraspinal and spinal analgesia, whereas mu-2 receptors are responsible for respiratory depression and decreased gastrointestinal motility.[51] The delta receptors are responsible for spinal and supraspinal analgesia; kappa receptors are responsible for spinal analgesia and psychometric effects (dysphoria, sedation, miosis, respiratory depression).[52]

Opioids produce their major effects on the central nervous and gastrointestinal systems. Some of these effects are analgesia, sedation, mood changes, pupillary constriction, respiratory depression, decreased intestinal motility, nausea, and vomiting. Opioids produce a dose-dependent reduction in the responsiveness of the brainstem respiratory center, making it less responsive to increases in carbon dioxide retention. This leads to a reduction in the rate of breathing, prolonged pauses between breaths, delayed exhalation, and periodic breathing.[56] Sedation, drowsiness, and mental clouding can be potentiated when opioids are administered concurrently with antianxiety and sedative-hypnotic agents. Opioids have no significant amnestic or anxiolytic properties; therefore, coadministration of a benzodiazepine or propofol is necessary to achieve controlled levels of sedation and amnesia when patients require conscious sedation or prolonged mechanical ventilation.

Types of Opioids and Other Analgesic Agents

See Table 18-8 for a summary of opioids.

Morphine

Morphine is the most commonly used opiate agent and the standard of comparison for other analgesic agents. It has a plasma half-life range of 2 to 3 hours with a 4- to 6-hour duration of analgesia. Peak effect after a single intravenous bolus of morphine occurs within 15 to 30 minutes,[34] and the duration of clinical effects is 2 to 7 hours. Morphine is hydrophilic, a property that results in a slower onset of analgesia. When it is administered epidurally, its onset is between 30 and 60 minutes.[57] It is metabolized by the liver to water-soluble glucuronides. Morphine-3-glucuronide has no analgesic activity and is readily excreted by the kidney. Morphine-6-glucuronide (M6G) is an active metabolite that produces potent opioid effects.[58] In patients with renal impairment, M6G accumulates and can result in persistent sedation and respiratory depression after discontinuation of morphine.

Meperidine

Meperidine is less potent and has a shorter half-life than morphine. Clinically, meperidine is not recommended for more than 48 hours because of the active metabolite normeperidine, which produces neurotoxicity, clinically evidenced by anxiety, tremors, myoclonus, and generalized seizures.[34]

TABLE 18-8 **Opioid Agents and Doses***

Drug	Usual Dose: Intermittent	Usual Dose: Infusion	Advantages	Disadvantages
Morphine	1-5 mg IV every 1-2 hours	2-15 mg/hr	Inexpensive	Active metabolite Histamine release Vasodilation
Fentanyl	25-100 mcg IV every 0.5-1 hours	50-200 mcg/hr	Rapid onset No active metabolite Useful in morphine allergy Minimal cardiovasculr effect	Single-dose short duration Lipid accumulation with continued use
Meperidine	Not recommended	Not recommended	Inexpensive	Active metabolite Risk of seizures Drug interactions
Sufentanil	—	10-100 mg/hr	Short-acting	Expensive Chest wall rigidity with high dose
Alfentanil	—	250-2500 mg/hr	Short-acting	Expensive Chest wall rigidity with high dose
Remifentanil	—	Unknown	Continuation of intraoperative analgesia Very short-acting	Expensive Pain recurrence if stopped acutely Chest wall rigidity with high dose
Hydromorphone	0.15-1.5 mg IV every 1-2 hours	0.45-1.5 mg/hr	Potent Useful in morphine allergy	

IV, Intravenous.
*These are routinely used opiate agents and doses recommended in trauma patients. Patient needs may vary. Titrate to desired response.

Normeperidine is excreted in the urine and accumulates in the elderly or patients with renal insufficiency after doses of 600 mg per 24 hours.[34] Serotonin syndrome resulting from reactions with monoamine oxidase inhibitors, tricyclic antidepressants (TCAs), or selective serotonin reuptake inhibitor (SSRI) antidepressants has been implicated with concurrent use of meperidine.[59] This is an excitation syndrome characterized by hypertension, hyperpyrexia, muscle rigidity, and changes in level of consciousness.

Fentanyl

Fentanyl is a semisynthetic, lipophilic opioid, 80 to 100 times as potent as morphine.[29] By the intravenous route, it has a rapid onset of action (1-5 minutes) and a short duration of action (about 1 hour).[57] Onset of analgesia after intraspinal administration occurs in 5 to 15 minutes.[22] It is metabolized by the liver and undergoes substantial biotransformation.[60] The elimination half-life ranges from 3 to 12 hours and is affected by storage in fatty tissue, especially with prolonged administration.[61] Norfentanyl, the primary metabolite, is inactive.[62] Intermittent doses of fentanyl are used for procedures requiring conscious sedation. It can be administered as a continuous infusion for sustained effects in monitored settings. In comparison with morphine, fentanyl does not induce H release and produces minimal cardiovascular effects.[57] However, hypotension can still occur in the volume-depleted patient. Slow incremental titration is recommended because of reports of bradycardia, severe respiratory depression, and chest wall rigidity with rapid, high-dose intravenous administration.[57]

Sufentanil, Alfentanil, and Remifentanil

These fentanyl analogs have been used in trauma patients, but higher cost has limited their use. Sufentanil is approximately 10 times more potent than fentanyl.[63] It is highly lipophilic and has a faster onset and shorter duration of action than fentanyl. By the intravenous route, it has a rapid onset of action (1-3 minutes), with a peak at 8 to 15 minutes.[64] Through the epidural route, peak action is seen in 20 minutes.[65] It is metabolized by the liver and small intestines and has minimal cardiovascular effects.[66]

Alfentanil is superior to fentanyl and sufentanil and is one fourth as potent as fentanyl.[67] Its onset of action (within 2 minutes) and duration of action (10 minutes) are shorter than those of fentanyl.[67] Alfentanil offers intense analgesia and is highly useful for potentially painful procedures such as dressing changes.[68]

Remifentanil is an ultra-short-acting fentanyl congener, with a potency roughly 20 to 30 times that of alfentanil.[69] Its onset of action is 1 to 3 minutes, with a duration of 3 to 10 minutes.[70] Unlike other opioids, the liver does not metabolize remifentanil. Instead, it is rapidly hydrolyzed by plasma and tissue esterases.[71] This ultra-short-acting agent (half-life of 3 minutes) is expected to produce tolerance more rapidly; thus, its use is limited in the ICU environment.[72]

Hydromorphone

Hydromorphone is a potent, hydrophilic synthetic derivative of morphine that produces less sedation, pruritus, nausea, and vomiting than do equivalent doses of morphine. It is five to ten times more potent than morphine and can be given orally, parenterally, or neuraxially. The onset of analgesia after epidural administration is 15 to 30 minutes.[22] Hydromorphone offers minimal hemodynamic effects and no H release. It may cause a cross-reaction in morphine-allergic patients. It is the third-line agent recommended by the Society of Critical Care Medicine (SCCM) for use in hemodynamically unstable patients or patients with renal impairment because it produces no active metabolites.

Methadone

Methadone, which binds to the mu opioid receptor centrally and peripherally, also antagonizes the MNDA receptor.[73] It is known for its use with opioid dependence, but it can be used as an alternate agent for patients who have moderate to severe pain that is unresponsive to morphine. Because the half-life range is 13 to 50 hours, sedation, confusion, and respiratory depression can occur, requiring careful monitoring.[74] With repeated administration, cumulative effects are seen, and dose titration with longer intervals and lower doses may be necessary. As a result of complete incomplete cross-tolerance between morphine and methadone, equianalgesic dose calculation is complicated and requires expertise when switching to methadone.[75] Several days of administration may be required to reach a steady state that provides effective analgesia.

Oral Opioids

Oxycodone, which is available as an immediate-release and an extended-release preparation, can be used to treat moderate to severe pain. Lower doses (5 mg) in combination with nonopioids (aspirin or acetaminophen) are frequently used to treat mild to moderate pain. Planned dosing should consider the limits of acetaminophen to 4 g per day when oxycodone is administered as a combination agent. Some patients receive no analgesic benefit from this agent because of a cytochrome P450 interaction.

Codeine is structurally related to morphine and exerts its analgesic effect through demethylation to morphine. In comparison with morphine, these agents cause minimal sedation and rare respiratory depression as a result of their lower potency. These agents may cause a cross-reaction in morphine-allergic patients.

Tramadol is a centrally acting analgesic with no anti-PG activity. Analgesia is produced by inhibition of the reuptake neurotransmitters serotonin and norepinephrine.[76] Because of its mild analgesic properties, application for use may be limited in the patient with severe acute pain, with benefit in the treatment of chronic pain.[77] A major advantage is the minimal sedative and respiratory depressant effects and that it comes in parenteral formulations.[78]

Adverse Effects of Opioids

In most patients, opioid-related side effects are transient and tend to resolve with continuing treatment. Common opioid-related adverse effects include drowsiness, sedation, respiratory depression, pruritus, constipation, nausea and vomiting, and urinary retention (Table 18-9). Most opioid-related adverse effects are dose dependent, which is why it is important to initiate therapy with the lowest effective dose. CNS depression usually occurs with repeated dosing with opioids. Sedation and pruritus are typically addressed by decreasing the opioid dose rather than by treating the symptom.[22] In addition to dose reductions, other strategies to minimize opioid-related adverse effects include changing the route of administration (from parental to the oral) when possible and switching to a different opioid.[79]

Respiratory depression is the most serious adverse outcome with opioid administration. Diligent nursing assessment and monitoring of respiratory status, along with end-tidal carbon dioxide monitoring, are means of preventing negative outcomes. Patients who are unresponsive to tactile stimulation, with shallow breathing or a respiratory rate less than 8 breaths a minute and miosis can have these narcotic side effects reversed with the administration of naloxone.[22]

TABLE 18-9 **Comparison of Opioid Adverse Effects**

Drug	Analgesia	Constipation	Respiratory Depression	Sedation	Emesis
Morphine	++	++	++	++	++
Hydromorphone	++	+	++	+	+
Meperidine	++	+	++	+	nr
Fentanyl	++	nr	+	nr	+
Sufentanil	+++	nr	nr	nr	nr
Alfentanil	++	nr	nr	nr	nr
Codeine	+	+	+	+	+
Oxycodone	++	++	++	++	++

nr, Not reported. Modified from Kastrup E, editor: *Facts and comparisons*, p. 1376, St. Louis, 1999, Facts and Comparisons, 1376.

Naloxone is a competitive antagonist at the mu, kappa, and delta receptors. Careful titration of naloxone in small increments is advised if reversal is necessary. Dilution of 0.4 mg naloxone hydrochloride to a volume of 10 ml is one recommendation for 1-ml titration.[80,81] Abrupt reversal of opioid analgesia can result in withdrawal and may cause nausea, pulmonary edema, hypertension, tachycardia, and ventricular arrhythmias.[82]

Nausea and vomiting are common after opioid administration and are the direct result from stimulating the chemoreceptor trigger zone, depressing the vomiting center, and slowing gastrointestinal motility.[83] Antiemetic therapy can be supportive. Opioids slow gastric emptying time by reducing peristalsis and decreasing intestinal secretions.[84] All patients taking opioid analgesics are at risk for constipation and should be given stool softeners and laxatives to diminish this adverse effect. Increased bile duct pressure may result from opioid-induced contraction of the sphincter of Oddi.[85] Naloxone has been used to treat biliary spasm and constipation.[86,87] Opioids are known to increase smooth muscle tone, causing increased sphincter tone, which can lead to urinary retention. Closely monitoring spontaneous voiding and bladder emptying is required, along with provisions for catheterization.

Opioid rotation has been shown to be an effective strategy for managing adverse events or inadequate analgesia in patients taking opioids.[88] When opioid rotation is used, patients should be monitored closely to assess the adequacy of pain relief and the effect on opioid-related adverse events. As with any opioid regimen, subsequent dose adjustments will probably be necessary. Use of opioid rotation requires familiarity with a range of opioids and with the use of equianalgesic dose tables (Table 18-10).[89]

CLINICAL USE OF OPIOIDS

Knowledge of the various methods used to administer opioids and of how opioids are absorbed is helpful in understanding why one technique of providing analgesia may be superior to another in certain phases of the trauma cycle. The methods discussed include oral, intravenous, neuraxial, transdermal, and patient-controlled analgesia (Table 18-11).

Oral Route

The oral route usually is chosen because it is the easiest and most convenient route of administration. Absorption of orally effective opioids by the gastrointestinal tract usually is complete, but the rate of absorption varies. Onset of action usually occurs within 45 minutes, with peak drug effects 1 to 2 hours after oral administration for most immediate-release analgesics.[34] Most drugs undergo significant first-pass hepatic metabolism after absorption. First-pass hepatic metabolism is the effect seen after drugs are absorbed from the stomach and the intestine, thus passing through the liver before entering the systemic circulation. Most marketed drugs are metabolized in various ways by the cytochrome P450 (CYP450) system.[90,91] Most opioids are metabolized through the CYP3A4 or CYP2D6 pathways.[92] In the liver, the drugs are metabolized so that some of the active drug is inactivated before it is delivered to the tissue receptors. This effect explains the discrepancy between intravenous and oral doses.

The oral route is not suitable for patients with severe or acute pain because of the slower onset of action and the variability of absorption. In addition, the oral route is not useful during the early phases of the trauma cycle if patients are to receive nothing by mouth, are unable to swallow, or are hemodynamically unstable. Oral analgesics are used in the intermediate and rehabilitation phases of the trauma cycle, when the pain is less severe and the patient is able to take oral medications.

Intravenous Route

Patients in critical care areas are often given analgesics by intravenous infusion or bolus. When morphine and other opioids are given intravenously, they quickly exert an effect. Time to peak effect varies with drug lipid solubility, ranging from 1 to 5 minutes for fentanyl to 15 to 30 minutes for morphine.[34] Intravenous administration of opioids allows for more rapid access to the sites where they exert an effect (i.e., the central nervous system and the opioid receptors). The intravenous route is used during the resuscitation and critical care phases and in the post-anesthesia care unit.

Intravenous infusions of opioids provide steady blood levels and the ability to rapidly titrate relief in patients with

TABLE 18-10 Equianalgesic Doses of Commonly Used Analgesics*

Drug	Route	Equianalgesic Dose	Comments
Fentanyl (Sublimaze)	IV	100 mcg	Highly potent; monitor for chest wall rigidly
Hydromorphone (Dilaudid)	IV/IM	1.5 mg	
	PO	7.5 mg	
Methadone (Dolphine)	IV/IM	10 mg	Duration of action 4-8 hours
Meperidine	IV/IM	100 mg	Toxic metabolite normeperidine
Morphine	IV/IM	10 mg	
	PO	30 mg	
Oxycodone	PO	30 mg	Usually in combination with acetaminophen or aspirin

IV, Intravenous; *IM,* intramuscular; *PO,* oral.
*All doses are equal to 10 mg of intravenous/intramuscular morphine.

TABLE 18-11 **Analgesic Delivery**

Route of Analgesic Administration	Indication	Application to Trauma Phase	Common Agents	Disadvantages
Oral	Mild to moderate pain Scheduled dosing to maintain steady state	Critical care phase (adjunct) Intermediate Rehabilitative (postoperative)	Nonopioids Opioids (immediate release and sustained release)	Slow onset of action Metabolite association Active gastrointestinal function required
Oral transmucosal	Moderate to severe breakthrough or procedural pain	Critical care phase Intermediate Rehabilitative (postoperative)	Oral transmucosal fentanyl citrate	Requires monitoring in the opioid-naive patient
Transdermal	Moderate to severe chronic nonmalignant pain Cancer pain	Intermediate Rehabilitative	Fentanyl (Duragesic)	Not recommended for application on irriated skin Increased absortion with febrile state Takes up to 18 hours to reach steady state, thus requiring breakthrough agents
IV route	Moderate to severe pain Treatment of acute or procedural pain Rapid administration-titration Rapid effect on the CNS and opioid receptors (titration) Given as a bolus or continuous infusion	Resuscitative phase Critical care phase Operative phase Intermediate Rehabilitative	Fentanyl Morphine Hydromorphone	Requires venous access Monitoring requirements with a skilled clinician
PCA IV	Treatment of acute/postoperative pain Patient self-administers opioid by pressing a demand button Can be combined with basal infusion or demand mode Requires patient participation	Critical care phase Intermediate Rehabilitative (postoperative)	Morphine Hydromorphone Fentanyl	Requires venous access Monitoring requirements with a skilled clinician
PCEA	Analgesia to specific dermatone distribution Thoracic or lumbar area Reduce opioid requirements to enhance optimal function	Critical care phase Intermediate Rehabilitative (postoperative)	Local anesthetics: Bupivacaine/ropivacaine Opioids: Fentanyl Morphine Hydromorphone	Monitoring requirements with a skilled clinician Contraindicated in some instances
Peripheral nerve block	Analgesia to specific nerve distribution Reduce opioid requirements	Critical care phase Intermediate Rehabilitative (postoperative)	Local anesthetics: Bupivacaine/ropivacaine	Monitoring requirements with a skilled clinician Motor response assessment limited until local anesthetic recovery

IV, Intravenous; *PCA,* patient-controlled analgesia; *PCEA,* patient-controlled epidural analgesia.

acute pain that is severe and continuous. This eliminates the "peaks" and "troughs" seen with traditional intramuscular injections and provides consistent pain management. When increased analgesia is necessary, an additional opioid bolus totaling 1 hour of infusion should be administered.[34] Upward titration of the infusion rate may take up to five elimination half-lives to reach steady state.[34] Activities such as turning, chest physical therapy, or chest tube removal may require additional analgesic coverage for breakthrough pain.

Patient-Controlled Analgesia

Patient-controlled analgesia (PCA) is a technique that allows the patient to self-administer analgesics by way of the intravenous route, an epidural catheter, regionally by delivery to a specific nerve or nerve plexus or by a transdermal system in response to pain.[93] Intravenous PCA is the standard for parenteral opioid administration for pain control after many types of surgery.[94] PCA has been reported to provide consistent drug concentrations, less sedation, less opioid consumption, and potentially fewer adverse effects compared with alternative means of opioid administration.[95,96] Safety program initiatives with PCA therapy include the use of standardized solutions, protocols for pump programming and patient assessment, and education for hospital staff, the patient, and family.[93,94]

Most PCA pumps feature options of initial loading dose, demand dose, lockout interval, hour limits, and continuous infusion rate. The loading dose is clinician activated and can be used as part of the opioid titration with initiation. The demand dose (or PCA dose) is the patient-activated request by use of a demand button. To limit patient-activated dosing, a lockout interval is used to prevent overmedication between successful patient demands. Dosing limits, either in 1- or 4-hour intervals, allow programming to limit cumulative dosing. The continuous infusion (or basal infusion) is usually limited to those patients who are opioid tolerant. Risk factors for respiratory depression with intravenous PCA include advanced age greater than 70 years; basal infusion; renal, hepatic, pulmonary, or cardiac comorbidities; sleep apnea; and concurrent administration of CNS depressants.[80,97] Table 18-12 shows common PCA settings.

Transdermal Route

The transdermal route provides steady, therapeutic plasma levels without the peaks and troughs seen with intermittent dosing. The advantages of transdermal application include the avoidance of the first-pass effect, prolongation of effect, and its ability to be used when the oral route cannot be used. Fentanyl transdermal gelled reservoir and fentanyl matrix delivery systems are available for slow release in 12.5-, 25-, 50-, 75-, and 100-mcg doses.[98] The plateau of plasma fentanyl concentration is achieved during the second 12-hour period of the first patch.[99] Half-life values after the removal of the patch were between 13 and 25 hours.[100] This must be considered if opioid rotation is considered, especially by another route.

The transdermal route may be effective in the latter part of the intermediate phase and in the rehabilitation phase of the trauma cycle. Transdermal opioids have been used successfully in patients who have chronic pain from cancer, with application to other chronic pain states as well.[101] A new system involving the technology of iontophoresis for a fentanyl patient-controlled transdermal delivery system has been developed for use in the treatment of acute postoperative pain.[102,103] This novel concept requires further investigation for its application in the trauma population.

Neuraxial Opioids and Local Anesthetics

Neuraxial analgesic techniques involve the principle of interfering with pain transmission at the spinal cord level. The resulting analgesia is superior and longer lasting compared with large doses of intravenous opioids.[104] A meta-analysis compared epidural analgesic regimens with intravenous PCA and demonstrated statistically significant analgesic benefit with epidural therapy for all types of surgery.[105] The use of epidural analgesia for pain control after severe blunt chest injury and nontraumatic surgical thoracic pain has been shown to improve pulmonary function tests compared with parental opioids.[106] Epidural analgesia in the critically ill has been linked to improved patient comfort with rib fractures and chest trauma,[107,108] and is the standard for analgesia for thoracic surgery.[109,110]

The epidural space (Figure 18-6) lies within the spinal canal, which runs from the foramen magnum to the sacral hiatus. It is highly vascularized and contains fat, connective tissues, a lymphatic network, and dorsal and ventral roots of spinal nerves. Agents administered are proximal to the opioid receptors and diffuse across the dura (Figure 18-7). Morphine and hydromorphone have hydrophilic properties, with onset of analgesia between 30 and 60 minutes with neuraxial administration.[56] This creates a higher incidence of side effects

TABLE 18-12 **Guidelines for Intravenous Patient-Controlled Analgesia in Adults in Acute Pain**

Analgesic (min)	Bolus PCA Dose After Frontloading	Usual Dose Range	Usual Starting Lockout	Usual Lockout Range
Morphine (1.0 mg/ml)	1.0 mg	0.5-2.5 mg	8 min	5-10 min
Hydromorphone (0.2 mg/ml)	0.2 mg	0.05-0.4 mg	8 min	5-10 min
Fentanyl (50 mcg/ml)	10 mcg	10-50 mcg	6 min	5-8 min

Standard concentrations for most PCA machines are listed in parenthesis.
Source: American Pain Society: *Principles of analgesic use in treatment of acute pain and chronic pain,* 5th ed, p. 20, 2003, American Pain Society.

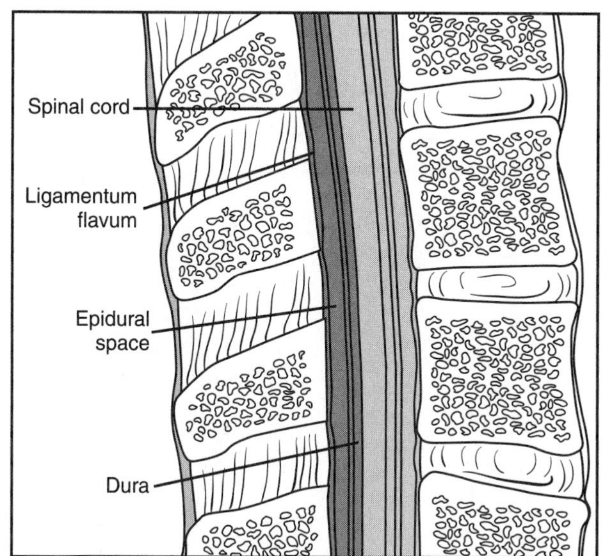

FIGURE 18-6 The epidural space and associated structures. (Weetman C, Allison W: Use of epidural analgesia in postoperative pain management, *Nurs Standard* 20: 54-64, 66, 68, 2006.)

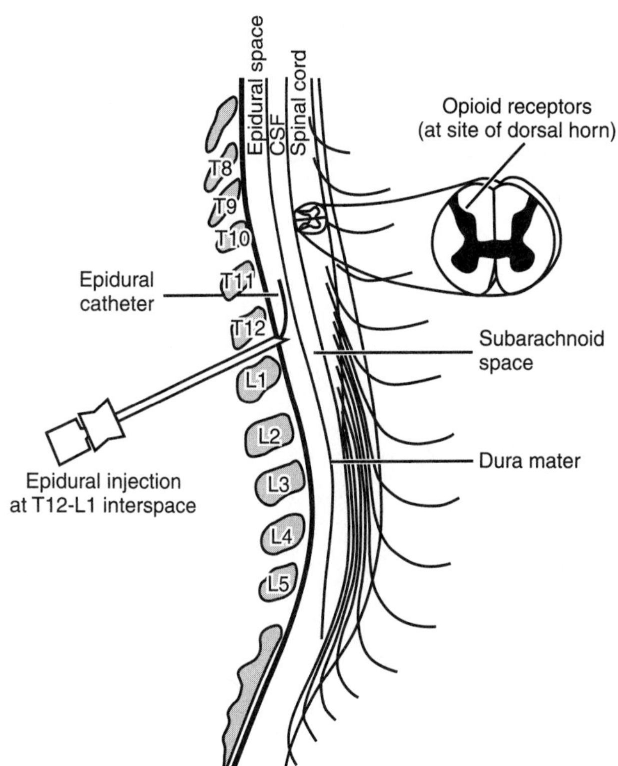

FIGURE 18-7 Agents are administered proximal to opioid receptors in the dorsal horn. Delivery of analgesics by the intraspinal routes can be accomplished by inserting an epidural needle into either the epidural space (as shown) for epidural analgesia or the subarachnoid space for intrathecal analgesia and injecting the analgesic or threading a catheter through the needle and taping it in place temporarily for bolus dosing or continuous administration. *(Redrawn from McCaffery M, Pasero CL:* Pain: clinical manual, *p. 218, ©1999, with permission from Elsevier.)*

related to cephalad spread in the cerebrospinal fluid.[111] Lipophilic opioids, such as fentanyl and sufentanil, have a shorter onset of analgesia, which is between 5 and 10 minutes,[56] and produce segmental analgesia across few dermatomes.[112] Dermatomes are cutaneous sensory bands that are 1 to 2 inches wide and that correspond to a specific nerve root (Figure 18-8). After neuraxial injection, the presence of an analgesic block is assessed through the loss of sensation and temperature discrimination along the dermatomal tracts. Temperature discrimination can be distinguished with the use of an alcohol wipe or ice bag. Emerging formulations involving liposome delivery by single injection of morphine have extended analgesic benefit without the use of an indwelling catheter.[113]

Opioids combined with diluted local anesthetics provide synergistic analgesic effect. Local anesthetics, such as ropivacaine and bupivacaine, produce analgesia through blockade of impulse conduction along nerve fibers within the spinal nerves. There is an interference with the function of sodium channels during nerve conduction, when sodium ions enter and potassium ions exit the cell. Blockade occurs first in the small C fibers to alter slow pain and then in the large A fibers for fast pain. High concentration anesthetics, such as 0.5% bupivacaine, block all types of fibers, including sympathetic, pain, sensory and motor fibers, and are used for surgical anesthesia neural blockade. Low concentrations, or dilute solutions, such as 0.1% bupivacaine, will selectively affect very fine sympathetic and pain fibers, with little effect on larger sensory fibers, responsible for touch and pressure. Large motor fibers are spared with low-concentration local anesthetics, characterizing a differential nerve block, thus facilitating mobility and ambulation.[114]

Factors that influence the onset of an epidural blockade include the site of injection and nerve root size, height and weight of the patient, positioning, and the volume, concentration, and dose of local anesthetic. Nurses caring for patients with regional analgesia require specialized training and must be able to identify potential complications. Common side effects related to epidural analgesia include hypotension related to sympathetic blockade, motor block, nausea and vomiting, pruritus, urinary retention, and respiratory depression.[115] These are more prominent with bolus dosing and hypovolemia. Nursing diligence is directed to physiologic support and monitoring. Education regarding the signs and symptoms of local anesthetic neurotoxicity and cardiotoxicity is essential. Recommendations by the American Society of Regional Anesthesia should be followed with regard to administration of anticoagulants and timing of catheter removal.[116]

Peripheral Nerve Blocks

Peripheral nerve blocks can be used in selected patients with crush injuries, fractures, and burns as part of a multimodal analgesia plan to provide analgesia with minimal side effects.[117,118] The local anesthetics used prevent or relieve pain by interrupting nerve conduction specifically aiming to block the nociceptive impulses transmitted along peripheral nerves. The action of local anesthetics prevents the transmission of nerve impulses by changing the permeability of the cell

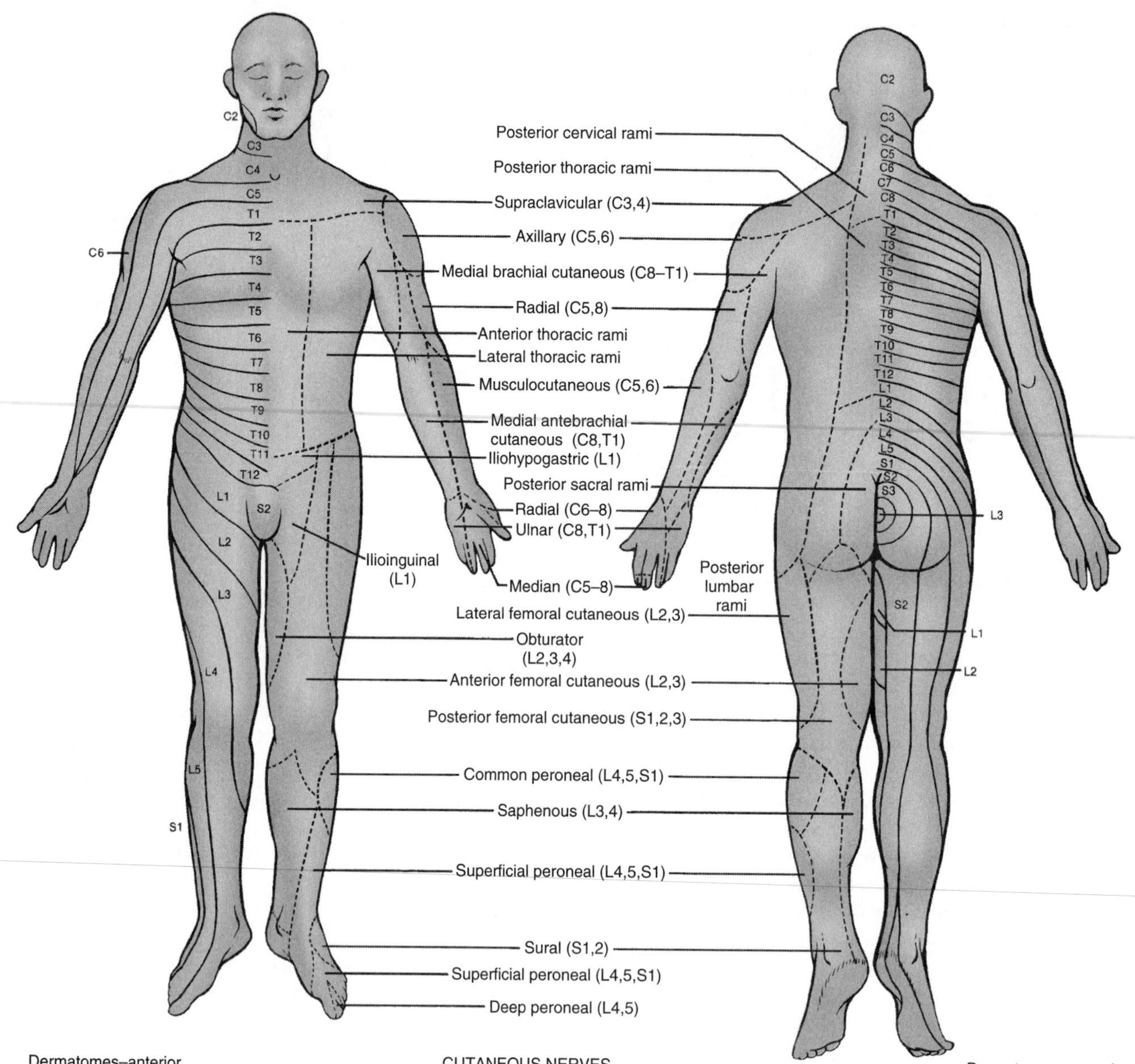

FIGURE 18-8 Dermatomes and peripheral sensory nerves. (Modified from Auerbach P: *Wilderness medicine*, 7th ed, p. 483, Philadelphia, 2007, Mosby.)

membrane to sodium.[119] Local anesthetics are classified as esters or amides and are categorized by onset and duration of action. Certain conditions may contraindicate the use of peripheral nerve blocks, such as the presence of coagulopathy, preexisting neuropathies, deviations of anatomic landmarks, and known allergies to local anesthetics.[120]

A local anesthetic is injected or delivered near and around the nerve or nerve plexus that supplies the surgical area or traumatic injury. The duration of action for each anesthetic medication depends on several factors, including concentration of the agent, the volume injected, site of injection, and absorption. The addition of a vasoconstrictor, such as epinephrine, constricts blood vessels and reduces vascular uptake, which further prolongs the duration of the anesthetic.[121,122] Clonidine acts peripherally through conduction blockade, thus increasing duration of analgesia when added to the local anesthetic.[123] For surgical procedures that are associated with mild to severe pain, the use of long-acting local anesthetics, such as bupivacaine, can provide extended postoperative analgesia. Continuous analgesia can be achieved by placing a catheter into the nerve sheath and infusing local anesthetics for several days.

Several techniques can be used to provide surgical anesthesia and analgesia for the upper and lower extremities. For upper limb injuries, regional techniques include the interscalene, supraclavicular, infraclavicular, and axillary approaches. The interscalene block provides the best analgesic coverage for the shoulder, the supraclavicular and infraclavicular blocks work best for injuries below the shoulder and above the elbow, and axillary blocks cover pain transmission in the hand and forearm.[124] Femoral nerve combined with sciatic nerve blocks may be used for the lower extremity pain control after femoral neck fractures.[115]

Nursing assessment and care is focused on intensive monitoring. After interscalene and infraclavicular approaches to the brachial plexus, there is risk for tension pneumothorax.[120] Other complications include ipsilateral phrenic nerve paralysis and Horner's syndrome.[125] General complications associated with peripheral nerve blocks include hematoma, injury or anesthetic blockade of adjacent structures, nerve damage, and systemic local anesthetic toxicity.[126]

OTHER ANALGESICS AND ADJUNCTIVE AGENTS

ACETAMINOPHEN

For the treatment of mild to moderate pain, acetaminophen is an effective nonsalicylate agent that has antipyretic qualities, without anti-inflammatory or antiplatelet effects. Acetaminophen's mechanism of action is not clearly defined. This agent can be delivered orally or rectally, at a recommended dose of 65 mg/kg per day. Hepatotoxicity may occur at doses greater than 4 g per 24 hours in adults with normal liver function.[127] The drug has a ceiling effect: once the maximum dose is reached, no additional efficacy can be expected. Caution should be taken with administration in those patients with a history of long-term alcohol consumption and liver disease. Direct comparative studies between acetaminophen (1,000 mg dose) and nonsteroidal anti-inflammatory drugs (NSAIDs) have shown acetaminophen to be equivalent in treating pain associated with orthopedic surgery and headache.[128]

NONSTERIODAL ANTI-INFLAMMATORY DRUGS

NSAIDs are antipyretic, anti-inflammatory, and analgesic agents that decrease prostaglandin production through variable inhibition of cyclo-oxygenase-1 (COX-1) and COX-2.[129] NSAID administration has a reported dose-sparing effect when administered concurrently with opioids during certain operative procedures.[130,131] Unlike opioids, these agents have an analgesic ceiling effect. Oral NSAIDs are frequently prescribed for patients with more severe pain caused by osteoarthritis.[132]

Most of the analgesic effects of NSAIDs have been attributed to COX-2 inhibition, whereas undesirable side effects are caused by the inhibition of COX-1. The disadvantage to these agents is that they carry the risk of gastrointestinal, hepatic, hematologic, cardiovascular, and renal adverse effects.[128,133] Thus, caution must be taken with administration during the trauma continuum. COX-2 inhibitor agents were developed to spare the gastrointestinal side effects of COX-1 inhibitors. This drug class has been associated with significantly greater numbers of thrombotic cardiovascular events, which has offset the gastrointestinal adverse effects caused by NSAIDs.[134] In the orthopedic patient population, NSAIDs and COX-2 inhibitors have been reported in the literature as a negative influence on bone growth.[135,136] The Food and Drug Administration (FDA) has asked manufacturers of nonprescription NSAIDs to revise their labeling to include gastrointestinal risks and cardiovascular risks to the general public.[137]

NSAID-induced renal failure can occur with the clinical presentation of hypovolemia, fluid and electrolyte imbalance, congestive heart failure, nephrotic syndrome, and kidney failure.[138] NSAIDs block the protective effects that vasodilator prostaglandins (e.g., prostaglandin D_2 and prostacyclin) present to the renal circulation by opposing the vasoconstrictor effects of angiotensin during times of stress. Peripheral edema, hypertension, and congestive heart failure may occur.[139] Patients with altered renal function should avoid NSAID administration.

α_2-AGONIST

Clonidine, which was initially introduced as an antihypertensive, is a selective partial α_2-adrenoceptor agonist, which can provide sedative, analgesic, and anxiolytic effects depending on route of administration.[140] Stimulation of the receptors in the brain and spinal cord inhibits neuronal firing, causing hypotension, bradycardia, sedation, and analgesia. The responses include decreased salivation, secretion, and bowel motility; inhibition of renin release; increased glomerular filtration; and increased secretion of sodium and water in the kidney; decreased intraocular pressure; and decreased insulin release from the pancreas.[141] Clinically, administration can occur preoperatively, intraoperatively, postoperatively, and with long-term intrathecal administration. Clonidine, in doses of 0.5 mcg/kg, enhances and prolongs the effect of local anesthetics.[142]

ANTICONVULSANTS

Gabapentin is the first-line agent recommended for the treatment of neuropathetic pain.[143] Efficacy in the reduction of postoperative pain, anxiety, and opioid requirements has also been reported with the use of this agent.[144,145] Although similar to the structure of GABA, the mechanism of action is thought to be on calcium channels, and the suppression of SP neurotransmission.[140] Dizziness and somnolence are common side effects. Doses up to 3,600 mg in a 24-hour period can be given, with dose adjustments considered with altered renal clearance.[146] Pregablin is a gabapentin analog, with a higher calcium-channel affinity and superior bioavailability.[147]

ANTIDEPRESSANTS

The use of TCAs has been shown to reduce neuropathic pain.[148] Analgesic action is the result of norepinephrine and serotonin reuptake blockade, NMDA receptor antagonism, and sodium channel blockade.[149] The TCAs provide the best analgesia compared with SSRIa and mixed serotonin-norepinephrine reuptake inhibitors but with the most side effects.[150] The TCAs (amitriptyline, nortriptyline, and imipramine) require baseline electrocardiogram evaluation because of the side effects of cardiotoxity and hypotension. These drugs are contraindicated when there is a history of glaucoma.[151] Urinary retention, constipation, and dry mouth can also occur.

N-Methyl-D-Aspartate Receptor Antagonists

Ketamine, commonly used as an induction anesthetic agent, has analgesic, sedative, amnesic, and dissociative properties. Clinical applications include acute pain management, especially in wound and burn management, procedural pain management, and as a third-line option in chronic nonmalignant pain and neuropathetic pain.[152] It noncompetitively blocks NMDA receptors in the dorsal horn of the spinal cord, which has been implicated in its mechanism to promote analgesia and reverse hyperalgesia.[117,153,154] The dissociative properties between the thalamoneocortical and limbic systems prevent the perception of visual, auditory, or painful stimuli.[155] Ketamine also inhibits the reuptake of dopamine and serotonin, which elevates circulating levels of epinephrine and norepinephrine, causing increases in heart rate, blood pressure, cardiac output, and vascular resistance.[152]

Ketamine preserves airway reflexes and maintains spontaneous ventilation with proper administration, requiring slow intravenous delivery and patient monitoring. The "emergence phenomena," in which patients experience hallucinations and nightmares, can be decreased when midazolam is administered concurrently.[156] Other side effects include excessive salivation, hypotension, and nausea and vomiting. Contraindications of administration include a history of airway instability, laryngospasm, cardiovascular disease, and increased intracranial and intraocular pressure.[157]

Topical Agents

The Lidoderm (lidocaine) patch 5% is a topical analgesic patch that has been used to relieve localized pain in postherpetic neuralgia. It may have benefits with other pain conditions, such as low back pain and osteoarthritis, and it must be applied to only intact skin.[158] Lidoderm produces an analgesic effect by the penetration of lidocaine from the patch into the epidermal and dermal layers of the skin, without loss of sensation or numbness. Capsaicin, an ingredient of hot peppers, has mixed reviews in some patients in the treatment of neuropathetic pain.[150]

Selection of Analgesic Agents

Selecting the ideal analgesic agent and mode for delivering the agent in a trauma patient can be difficult during the various phases of the trauma continuum. A thorough patient history is needed when deciding the best analgesic course. Things to consider are comorbid medical conditions, pharmacokinetic properties of the agent, potential drug interactions, adverse side effects, age, previous analgesic exposure, hemodynamic stability, and the presence of multisystem organ failure.

Comorbid conditions directly affect the choice of analgesic and sedative administration. Nonselective NSAIDs have been associated with undesired cardiorenal effects and pose risk to those patients with a history of hypertension, congestive heart failure, or kidney or liver disease.[159] Patients with significant coronary artery disease may preclude the administration of sedatives and opioids for procedural sedation and analgesia in the emergency department.[160] Patients with limited pulmonary function should have sedatives and opioids administered in a monitored setting.[161] Thoracic epidural analgesia with local anesthetics may improve coronary blood flow, which can benefit those patients with a history of myocardial ischemia.[162]

When opioid therapy is prescribed or recommended, it is important to consider the possibility of drug-drug interactions. The pharmacodynamic or pharmacokinetic profiles of many medications, including opioids, may be altered by other medications that are being taken concurrently. Oxycodone, hydrocodone, codeine, and tramadol may not be effective analgesics when given with other agents that strongly inhibit the cytochrome P4502D6 liver enzymes. Common agents with this characteristic include the SSRIs sertraline (Zoloft) (doses greater than 150 mg), paroxetine (Paxil), and fluoxetine (Prozac).[163]

Pain in the absence of disease is not a normal part of aging, yet it is experienced daily by a majority of older individuals in the United States.[164] Add trauma to the equation and the management becomes more complex in the elderly. Barriers to adequate pain management in this age group include the patient's altered level of cognition, fear of addiction, beliefs that pain is a part of aging, and the fear of side effects by the clinician.[165,166] With the use of more technology for analgesic delivery, the older individual may underuse devices such as PCA machines because of unfamiliarity and fear of overuse. Education on technology use, monitoring patient response, and minimizing distractions are important nursing strategies with advanced-age patients.

As aging occurs, metabolism and elimination of drugs is altered. Factors affected by aging include diminished renal function, decreased hepatic function, interactions of multiple drugs with the CYP 450 system, and decreased serum protein.[167] The concurrent use of herbal medications and vitamin supplements can also affect drug-drug interactions.[168]

The American Geriatric Society recommends acetaminophen as the first-line agent for treatment of mild pain.[44] The incidence of gastric irritability and the development of peptic ulcers warrant judicious administration with NSAIDs. Opioid dosages should be 25% to 50% lower than those recommended for the young, healthy patient.[34] A rule of thumb in the advanced-age population with opioids is to lower the dose and administer agents slowly. Dosing intervals should be longer, and diligent nursing assessment for sedation and confusion is imperative.

Most of the clinical pharmacology of opioids for the management of pain has been cited in the cancer literature.[169] The World Health Organization (WHO) Analgesic Ladder (Figure 18-9) was introduced to improve pain control in patients with cancer pain. However, this conceptual framework can be selectively applied to the management of acute traumatic pain because it uses a logical strategy to pain management. Step one, which provides a guide for mild pain, uses peripherally acting drugs such as aspirin, acetaminophen, or NSAIDs. With moderate pain, the second step of the ladder introduces oral opioids, such as a codeine agent combined with a nonopioid agent or adjuvant. For severe pain, the third step includes strong opioid drugs such as morphine, along with nonopioids and adjuvants to provide multimodal therapy. The synergistic effects of combining nonopioids and adjuncts are the basic principle to this paradigm.

For acute, severe traumatic and postoperative pain, a variation to the WHO analgesic ladder was introduced by the World Federation of Societies of Anaesthesiologists (Figure 18-10).[170,171] This concept shifts to address severe pain intensity first, where strong parental analgesics and regional anesthetic blocks are used as first-line therapy. As pain intensity declines, the introduction of oral opioids and nonopioids are added to the parenteral and regional techniques. As the pain decreases over time, the parenteral and neuraxil techniques are weaned and discontinued, and pain control continues with oral opioids or oral nonopioids. This model can be applied to the severely injured patient sustaining multiple traumas.

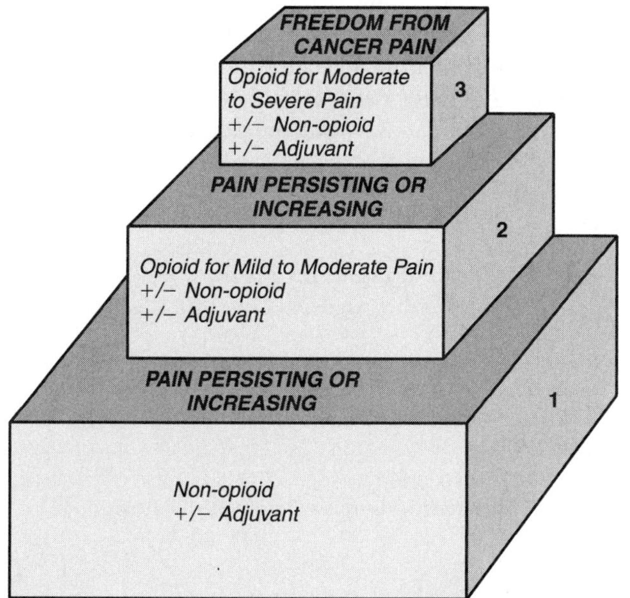

FIGURE 18-9 World Health Organization analgesic ladder. *(Redrawn with permission of World Health Organization. From* Cancer pain relief, *2nd ed, Geneva, 1996, World Health Organization.)*

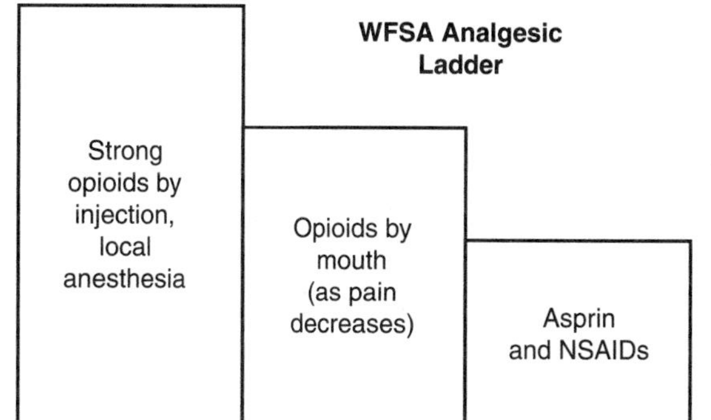

FIGURE 18-10 The World Federation of Societies of Anaesthesiologists Analgesic Ladder has been developed to treat acute pain. *(Redrawn from Charlton E: The management of postoperative pain,* Updates Anaesth Practical Proc, *7:1-7 (1997): www.nda.ox.ac.uk/wfsa/html/u07/u07_003.htm.)*

MULTIMODAL ANALGESIC TECHNIQUES

Multimodal or "balanced" analgesic techniques involving the use of smaller doses of opioids in conjunction with nonopioid analgesic agents have been the mainstay for postoperative pain treatment for several years.[130,172,173] Coadministration of agents results in additive or synergistic analgesic benefit on different areas in the pain pathway, reducing opioid requirements and diminishing adverse side effects.[52,174] Although the WHO analgesic ladder incorporates the model of selecting the simplest noninvasive approach to pain control, severe traumatic pain may require a more complex approach incorporating invasive techniques. Multimodal analgesic regimens include the use of nonopioid agents such as local anesthetics, NSAIDs, acetaminophen, and ketamine. Because of the recent controversies regarding cardiac effects of cyclo-oxygenase inhibitors (COX-2), their use in trauma pain management may be limited. Nonpharmacologic interventions, such as transcutaneous electrical nerve stimulation (TENS), has been recently suggested as a more important adjuvant therapy to pharmacologic interventions in the management of acute postoperative pain.[175]

Multimodal therapy has been used preoperatively to prevent or diminish postoperative pain. Pre-emptive analgesia has been defined as treatment that starts before surgery that prevents the establishment of central sensitization caused by incisional injury or inflammatory injuries.[176] Regional anesthesia used before elective surgical incision and continued postoperatively is helpful in diminishing postoperative pain.[177] The pre-emptive placement of thoracic epidural anesthesia has been associated with reducing the severity of acute and chronic pain after thoracotomy.[178,179]

NONPHARMACOLOGIC PAIN INTERVENTIONS

Although there is much emphasis on the administration of pharmacologic agents to control pain, nonpharmacologic methods of relieving pain and complementary therapy can be applied in the trauma setting.[180] Massage, music, and the cognitive behavioral interventions of self-guided imagery are strategies that can be used.[181] Individual innovation and refinement can be applied to the patient's unique pain experience. The patient must be willing to accept the application of these techniques. Eliciting family support can aid the nurse in the education and application of nonpharmacologic interventions and create a climate where education can take place. These techniques allow the patient to actively participate and control his or her pain.

Examples of nonpharmacologic interventions for postoperative and traumatic pain include cognitive-behavioral techniques and application of physical agents. Cognitive-behavioral techniques include relaxation, breathing techniques, guided imagery, and music distraction. Jaw relaxation, combined with slow breathing, requires only a few minutes of patient instruction and can be performed at regular intervals.[182] Breathing exercises offer both relaxation and distraction. Slow, regular breathing, particularly during potentially painful interventions, helps reduce muscular tension.[183] Imagery is the use of the imagination to alter the present situation of emotional distress or pain.[184] Guided imagery is a strategy of focused concentration where visual images of sights, sounds, music, and words are used to create feelings of empowerment and relaxation.[185] The patient must be in a mild frame to accept this form of distraction. Thinking of a pleasant situation or a place associated with happy memories is a simple approach to imagery. Specialized training or expert consultation is required for complex imagery, hypnosis, and biofeedback techniques. Nurses can teach patients how to use music to enhance the effects of analgesics, decrease pain and depression, and promote feelings of power over painful situations.[186-188]

Physical techniques include the application of moist heat or cold, massage, pressure, physical therapy, and TENS. The application of cold through compresses or packs aids in the reduction of edema and pain.[189] Cold application is usually recommended during the acute injury phase, particularly after muscle twisting and strain, except in patients with compromised vascular perfusion. Heat application increases blood flow and is usually reserved for postacute phases of injury, such as after physical therapy during the rehabilitation phase. Education in regard to application and the potential for damage to skin integrity and circulation must be provided before initiation of this therapy.

Massage can be accomplished by rubbing the affected area of discomfort. Touch is fundamental to massage therapy and allows the therapist to locate areas of muscle tension. These areas can be treated, with the clinician conveying a sense of caring using touch with the optimal amount of pressure individualized.[190] Ointments, lotion, and aromatherapy can also enhance the relaxing and sedative effects of massage and should be applied to intact skin.[191] An individualized exercise and physical activity plan are best formulated with input from the patient and physical therapist. TENS is a battery-operated device that transmits electrical impulses over a painful area. Individualized responses to TENS have been reported after postoperative incisional and chronic muscle pain.[192,193] Acupuncture and Reiki therapy are other nonpharmacologic interventions available that have been used to relieve pain in injured patients.

SEDATION

PATIENTS REQUIRING SEDATION

Anxiety, fear, and agitation are common in critically injured patients. The ICU environment and the various invasive procedures can be antagonistic and frightening. Patients in the ICU have multiple psychologic and physical stressors that are responsible for their anxiety and agitation. Because of these stresses, agitation has been found to occur in up to 71% of medical-surgical ICU patients.[194] Table 18-13 highlights some of the most common indications for sedation.

SEDATION ASSESMENT

Treating agitation is important. There are several consequences of untreated agitation, including inadvertent removal of arterial or venous catheters, self-extubation from mechanical ventilation, increased myocardial oxygen consumption, development of posttraumatic stress disorder (PTSD), and failure to participate in necessary therapeutic interventions.[195]

Most ICU patients exhibit physical signs and symptoms of agitation, but some do not. Difficulty lies in determining the source of these physical signs and symptoms and determining whether there is continuing pain or delirium adding to the agitation. Careful monitoring of physical signs and symptoms with the addition of sedatives, analgesics, or agents for delirium can give a clue to the cause. Additional things that must be considered when evaluating agitation are listed in Table 18-14. Determining a patient's sedative needs can be difficult. One clue to the sedative needs of patients can come from a detailed history and physical examination. Intubated patients may not be able to provide much information, but consultation of family members to elicit a social history may provide insight into the need for

TABLE 18-13 **Indications for Sedation in the Intensive Care Unit**

Adjuncts for the treatment of anxiety and agitation
Amnesia
Facilitate mechanical ventilation
Promote sleep
Improve patient comfort
Prevent posttraumatic distress syndrome
Facilitate NMB
ICP control

Source: Jacobi J, Fraser GL, Coursin DB et al: Clinical practice guidelines for the use of sedatives and analgesics in the critically ill adult, *Crit Care Med* 30:119-141, 2002.

TABLE 18-14 Underlying Physiologic Disturbances That Can Promote Agitation

Advanced age
Severity of illness
Liver or kidney impairment
Patient allergies/drug intolerances
Alcohol withdrawal
Substance abuse withdrawal
Hypoxemia
Hypoglycemia

Source: Jacobi J, Fraser GL, Coursin DB et al: Clinical practice guidelines for the use of sedatives and analgesics in the critically ill adult, *Crit Care Med* 30:119-141, 2002.

sedation. Multidisciplinary consultation with respiratory therapists, other nurses, physicians, pharmacists, and physical therapists can prove to be helpful.

Attention to the degree of lung injury of ICU patients is important. Reported discomforts experienced by patients during ventilatory therapy include anxiety and fear, inability to communicate because of the presence of an endotracheal tube, shortness of breath, persistent coughing, difficulty clearing secretions, and hallucinations. Patients with severe respiratory failure may require ventilation modes that are especially uncomfortable, such as inverse ratio ventilation or oscillator ventilation. As a result, these patients are typically prescribed sedation and may require pharmacologic paralysis to facilitate mechanical ventillation. Daily assessment of the patient's mechanical ventilatory mode and settings and arterial blood gas determinations can indicate whether there is a need for deeper or lighter sedation to optimize ventilation.

Sedation assessment is more difficult and less reproducible than pain assessment. The appropriate level of sedation is defined by the clinicians caring for the patient. Different practitioners caring for a patient may have different interpretations of sedation. To prevent variation, a sedation goal that is based on a standard sedation scale should be defined daily and individualized for the patient's needs.[194] Patients with mild symptoms of anxiety require low doses for comfort, whereas others may need heavy sedation to facilitate mechanical ventilation. Additionally, levels of activity may vary throughout the day, necessitating customization of sedation to provide a cooperative patient for the more awake periods and sleep at night. Recently, the American Association of Critical-Care Nurses has proposed a sedation assessment scale that incorporates the domains of consciousness, agitation, anxiety, sleep, and patient-ventilator synchrony, which will need future clinical trials to determine reliability and validity.[41]

Several sedation scales have been developed, but no one scale seems to be better than the rest.[194] Additionally, none of the scales have been shown to be better than the others regarding response to sedative dose or withdrawal. It is recommended that all sedative orders accompany some kind of sedation scale monitoring. This is important to prevent oversedation and undersedation. The numeric ratings of all the available scales are different, but they all share a common theme: they rely on responses to verbal stimuli. This can be problematic in patients who are hearing impaired, those with extensive brain injury, or those receiving pharmacologic paralysis. Current sedation scales focus on agitation and consciousness and fail to address other reasons for sedation such as anxiety, comfort, ventilator synchrony, or sleep and rest.[196]

One sedation scale that has been widely used is the Ramsay scale.[194,197] The Ramsay scale (Table 18-15) was developed to quantitate an objective end point for sedation therapy. For most patients a sedation level of 2 to 3 is considered desirable. Patients who are maintained at this level are at minimal risk for prolonged sedation upon sedation discontinuation.[194,198]

The Ramsay scale is limited by its lack of description for degrees of agitation. The Sedation-Agitation Scale (SAS)[199] developed by Riker and colleagues (Table 18-16) or the MAAS[200] may be more useful in settings that require both sedation and agitation assessment (Table 18-17). The acceptable goal of sedation on the SAS or MAAS ranges from 4 to 2. The newest and one of the most descriptive sedation scales is the RASS.[201,202] This scale, depicted in Table 18-18, has the added benefit of correlating with the administered dose of sedative and analgesic medications. It is different in that it has positive and negative variables and is more descriptive than others, such as the Ramsey, in terms of the level of sedation. An optimal score for sedation in ICU patients with the RASS is −1 to −2.

The best sedation plans allow for sedative medications to be titrated on the basis of a sedation scale. Implementing this kind of strategy relies on the nurse to make adjustments when the patient's need for sedation increases or decreases. Sedation plans of this nature need to be adaptable for changes in patient status and require that all caregivers assess the continual need for sedation and analgesia.

Monitoring the depth of sedation can be facilitated with computer analysis of electroencephalogram (EEG) patterns with bispectral (BIS) monitoring. BIS monitoring

TABLE 18-15 Ramsay Scale

Level	Description
Awake Levels	
1	Patient anxious and agitated, restless, or both
2	Patient cooperative, oriented, and tranquil
3	Patient responds to commands only
Asleep Levels, Depends on Response to a Light Glabellar Tap or Loud Auditory Stimulus	
4	Patient responds briskly
5	Patient responds sluggishly
6	Patient does not respond

Modified from Ramsay MAE, Savage TM, Simpson BRJ et al: Controlled sedation with alphaxalone/alphadolone, *BMJ* 2:656, 1974.

TABLE 18-16 **Sedation-Agitation Scale (SAS)**

Score	Description	Example
7	Immediate threat to safety	Pulling at endotracheal tube or catheters, trying to climb over bed rail, striking at staff
6	Dangerously agitated	Requiring physical restraints and frequent verbal reminding of limits, biting endotracheal tube
5	Agitated	Anxious or mildly agitated, attempting to sit up, calms down to verbal instructions
4	Calm and cooperative	Calm, arousable, follows commands
3	Oversedated	Difficult to arouse, awakens to verbal stimuli or gentle shaking but drifts off again, follows simple commands
2	Very oversedated	Awakens to physical stimuli but unable to communicate or follow commands
1	Unarousable	Does not awaken to stimuli, unable to communicate or follow commands

From Riker RR, Picard JT, Fraser GL: Prospective evaluation of the sedation-agitation scale for adult critically ill patients, *Crit Care Med* 27:1325-1329, 1999.

TABLE 18-17 **Motor Activity Assessment Scale (MAAS)**

Score	Description	Example
6	Dangerously agitated	No external stimulus is required to elicit movement and patient is uncooperative, pulling at tubes or catheters or thrashing side to side or striking at staff or trying to climb out of bed and does not calm down when asked
5	Agitated	No external stimulus required to elicit movement and attempting to sit up or move limbs out of bed and does not consistently follow commands
4	Restless and cooperative	No external stimulus required to elicit movement and patient is picking at sheets or tubes or uncovering self and follows commands
3	Calm and cooperative	No external stimulus required to elicit movement and patient is adjusting sheets or clothes purposefully and follows commands
2	Responsive to touch or name	Opens eyes or raises eyebrows or turns head toward stimulus or moves limbs when touched or name is loudly spoken
1	Responsive only to noxious stimulus	Opens eyes or raises eyebrows or turns head toward stimulus or moves limbs with noxious stimulus
0	Unresponsive	Does not move with noxious stimulus

From Devlin JW, Boleski G, Mylnarek M et al: Motor activity assessment scale: a valid and reliable scale for use with mechanically ventilated patients in an adult surgical intensive care unit, *Crit Care Med* 27:1271-1275, 1999.

TABLE 18-18 **Richmond Agitation-Sedation Scale (RASS)**

Score	Term	Description
+4	Combative	Overtly combative or violent; immediate danger to staff
+3	Very agitated	Pulls on or removes tube(s) or catheter(s) or has aggressive behavior toward staff
+2	Agitated	Frequent nonpurposeful movement or patient-ventilator dyssynchrony
+1	Restless	Anxious or apprehensive but movements not aggressive or vigorous
0	Alert and calm	
−1	Drowsy	Not fully alert, but has sustained (more than 10 seconds) awakening, with eye contact to voice
−2	Light sedation	Briefly (less than 10 seconds) awakens with eye contact to voice
−3	Moderate sedation	Any movement (but no eye contact) to voice
−4	Deep sedation	No response to voice, but any movement to physical stimulation
−5	Unarousable	No response to voice or physical stimulation

From Sessler CN, Gosnell MS, Grap MJ et al: The Richmond agitation-sedation scale: validity and reliability in adult intensive care unit patients, *Am J Respir Crit Care Med* 166:1338-1344, 2002.

TABLE 18-19 **Bispectral Index Range Guidelines**

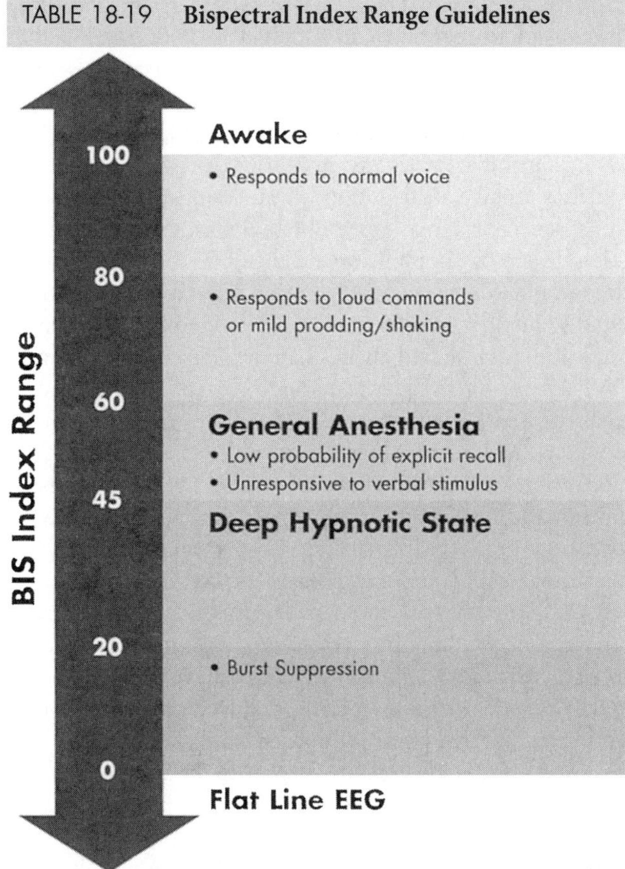

From Bispectral Index Product Brochure. BIS and the BIS logo are trademarks of Aspect Medical Systems, Inc.

provides a bispectral index parameter indicating the depth of sedation, which has been correlated to RASS scores, SAS scores, and Glascow Coma Scale scores in brain-injured patients.[203] The benefit of this type of monitoring is that it does not rely on physical response to stimuli, thus providing better sedation assessment in brain- or spinal cord–injured patients and those patients receiving neuromuscular blockade. This method of sedation monitoring can assess patients receiving intensive care, moderate sedation, and anesthesia. Table 18-19 gives a scale for the bispectral index provided by BIS monitoring.

SLEEP IN THE INTENSIVE CARE UNIT

Physiologic sleep is an organized pattern involving distinct stages and successive cycles of slow-wave sleep and rapid eye movement (REM) sleep. Critical care patients are found to have 22 to 42 arousals or wakenings per hour in the ICU on EEG.[204] The ICU environment, which may lack clocks visible to the patient and has constant noise from intravenous pumps, ventilators, and monitors, is not conducive to sleeping. Untreated anxiety and pain further contribute to sleep deprivation by causing difficulties with initiation and maintenance of sleep. This disorients a patient's normal sleep-wake cycle and results in poor quality sleep. Sleep deprivation can be exhibited as delirious behavior with auditory and visual hallucinations, paranoia, and disorientation. Sedation was thought to ensure a proper day-night cycle and prevent sleep deprivation. However, it is not known whether sedative agents such as propofol and benzodiazepines produce physiologic sleep. In fact, benzodiazepines and opioids are known to disturb the normal balance between REM and slow-wave sleep.[205] Nevertheless, it seems appropriate to administer sedatives and possibly sedative-hypnotics to prevent the disorientation attributed to undefined day-night cycles. Some of the more commonly used sedative hypnotics include chloral hydrate, temazepam, and zolpidem.

MONITORING SEDATION IN SPECIAL POPULATIONS

Sedation is always indicated in patients receiving neuromuscular blocking agents. Without sedative and anxiolytics, pharmacologic paralysis is a frightening experience. Patients would be forced to lie in bed hearing everything in the room without being able to move or respond. In the literature there are many patient accounts of the fear, or even PTSD, related to loss of muscle function and the nightmares that resulted after hospital discharge in patients not prescribed appropriate sedative and anxiolytics.[206-208] In these patients sedatives should be administered continuously or on a regular schedule to optimize their anxiolytic and amnestic effects. BIS monitoring can be performed to assess the depth of sedation in these patients.

Untreated agitation may be a symptom of physiologic conditions such as hypoxemia, sepsis, brain injury, various electrolyte abnormalities, chronic pain, and recreational drug use. When a patient becomes agitated, the clinician must identify and treat all the underlying causes so as to not sedate inappropriately. Medical conditions known to cause agitation are listed in Table 18-20. If the patient's agitation is not a result of a medical condition or its treatment, adequate pain control should be addressed while sedation is assessed.

A conscious patient can respond appropriately to a pain assessment tool, and adequate analgesic relief can be provided. An unresponsive patient will not, and a clinician may need to rely on nonspecific signs to indicate inadequate analgesia, such as restlessness, tachycardia, hyperventilation, and hypertension. Unfortunately, many times the specific cause of a patient's agitation is not established. Patients taking long-term pain medications and patients with a significant history of alcohol use can be difficult sedation cases. Both may require large sedative doses, but for different reasons. The patient with chronic pain should be supplemented with pain medication and have pain assessed before sedative doses are increased, whereas the patient undergoing alcohol withdrawal should have sedative doses escalated while being assessed for delirium tremens.

TABLE 18-20 Common Medical Causes of Agitation

Hypoxia	Sedative withdrawal syndrome
Hypercarbia	Narcotic withdrawal syndrome
Hypoglycemia	Drug intoxication
Hyperosmolar state	Digitalis toxicity
Addisonian crisis	Paradoxic effect, sedative drugs
Cerebral event	Histamine blockers
Cerebral thrombosis, embolism	Atropine, scopolamine
	Others
Subarachnoid hemorrhage	Partial drug-induced paralysis
	Antibiotic induced
Intracranial bleeding	Electrolyte disorders
Cerebral vasospasm	Hypermagnesemia
Cerebral edema	Hypophosphatemia
Inadequately treated pain	Hyponatremia
Infection	Hypercalcemia
Meningitis	Hypocalcemia
Encephalitis	Steroid psychosis
Brain abscess	Thyrotoxicosis
Sepsis syndrome	Organic brain syndrome
Delirium tremens	Mental retardation
Hepatic encephalopathy	Fear
Uremic encephalopathy	Anxiety disorders
	ICU psychosis

From Durbin CG: Sedation of the agitated critically ill patient without an artificial airway, *Crit Care Clinics* 11:915, 1995.

PHARMACOLOGIC AGENTS FOR SEDATION

Sedative, anxiolytic, and amnestic effects can be achieved with a variety of medications. Few of the commercially available sedatives provide analgesia; thus pain control must be addressed in addition to the provision of sedating agents. The drug's onset, duration, side effects, and cost dictate the choice of sedative. Sedatives can be administered "as needed," intermittently scheduled, or as a continuous infusion depending on the agent. Intermittent administration of sedatives is used to calm a patient and to induce amnesia before a procedure. Long-acting sedatives such as diazepam will provide a sustained state of sedation. However, with repetitive dosing there is a risk of drug accumulation that can prolong respiratory depression.[194] The risk of accumulation can be minimized with short-acting agents (e.g., midazolam), but these agents require either frequent administration necessitating a great deal of nursing time or use of a continuous infusion. In addition, these agents can cause sudden awakening if the infusion is disconnected or interrupted.

In 2002, the SCCM updated recommendations for sedation and analgesia in the adult critically ill patient. Their recommendations are summarized in Figure 18-11.

Benzodiazepines

Benzodiazepines are the agents most commonly used to produce sedation in trauma patients. Benzodiazepines achieve their effects by binding to and activating a high-affinity benzodiazepine receptor within the GABA receptor in the CNS. As the dose of a benzodiazepine is increased, anxiolysis progresses to sedation and sedation to hypnosis.[209] Three benzodiazepines are commonly used in the trauma setting: diazepam, midazolam, and lorazepam (Table 18-21).

Pharmacokinetics. The clinical differences observed with these benzodiazepines are primarily due to differences in potency, uptake, distribution, elimination, and the presence or absence of active metabolites. Benzodiazepines have a high degree of lipophilicity and therefore distribute quickly into the CNS to induce sedation. Because of its lower lipid solubility, lorazepam has a slower onset and longer duration of action than does midazolam or diazepam.[194] Termination of the effects of benzodiazepines is related to redistribution of the drug from the CNS to the peripheral compartments and elimination of the parent drug or metabolites from the kidney or liver. As a result of redistribution, the clinical effects of benzodiazepines have a shorter duration than the plasma terminal elimination half-life. Benzodiazepines are metabolized in the liver with renal excretion of the metabolites. Diazepam and midazolam undergo hepatic microsomal oxidation, which is influenced by age, liver disease, and some other drugs (e.g., cimetidine, phenytoin). Lorazepam, metabolized by glucuronide conjugation in the liver, is less influenced by these factors.[210]

Midazolam is short-acting agent with duration of sedative action ranging from 30 to 120 minutes.[211,212] However, a continuous infusion for more than 24 hours in critically ill patients has led to prolonged effects.[194] The longer half-life (i.e., 39 hours) in critically ill patients is the result of an increase in the volume of distribution, decreased elimination, and accumulation of the active metabolite hydroxymidazolam.[194] These parameters are difficult to predict in patients, and therefore nurses should be aware that patients receiving midazolam infusions may have a prolonged recovery.[213]

Lorazepam has peak effects that are not observed for 30 minutes and duration of 10 to 20 hours after a single bolus. This agent has the advantage of having no active metabolites. Unlike midazolam and diazepam, elderly patients or patients with significant liver disease do not appear to have prolonged sedative effects after a single bolus injection.[194]

Diazepam has slow elimination of both itself and its active metabolites, with half-lives of 20 to 50 hours for diazepam and 30 to 200 hours for metabolites.[194,213] Initially, diazepam may promptly produce sedative effects, but sedation wanes rapidly as the drug moves to other tissues. Subsequently, as tissues are saturated, the sedative effects become dependent on metabolism and the duration of action is prolonged.

Indications and Administration Methods. Midazolam is the most widely used agent for the treatment of acute agitation or sedation for short procedures, such as dressing changes and invasive procedures. A single intravenous dose of midazolam, 0.02 to 0.08 mg/kg, or diazepam, 0.03 to 0.1 mg/kg, administered 5 minutes before the procedure should provide safe and effective sedative and amnestic effects for short procedures for most patients.[194] Patients that are mechanically ventilated or who have developed tolerance to benzodiazepines may require higher doses, and those with

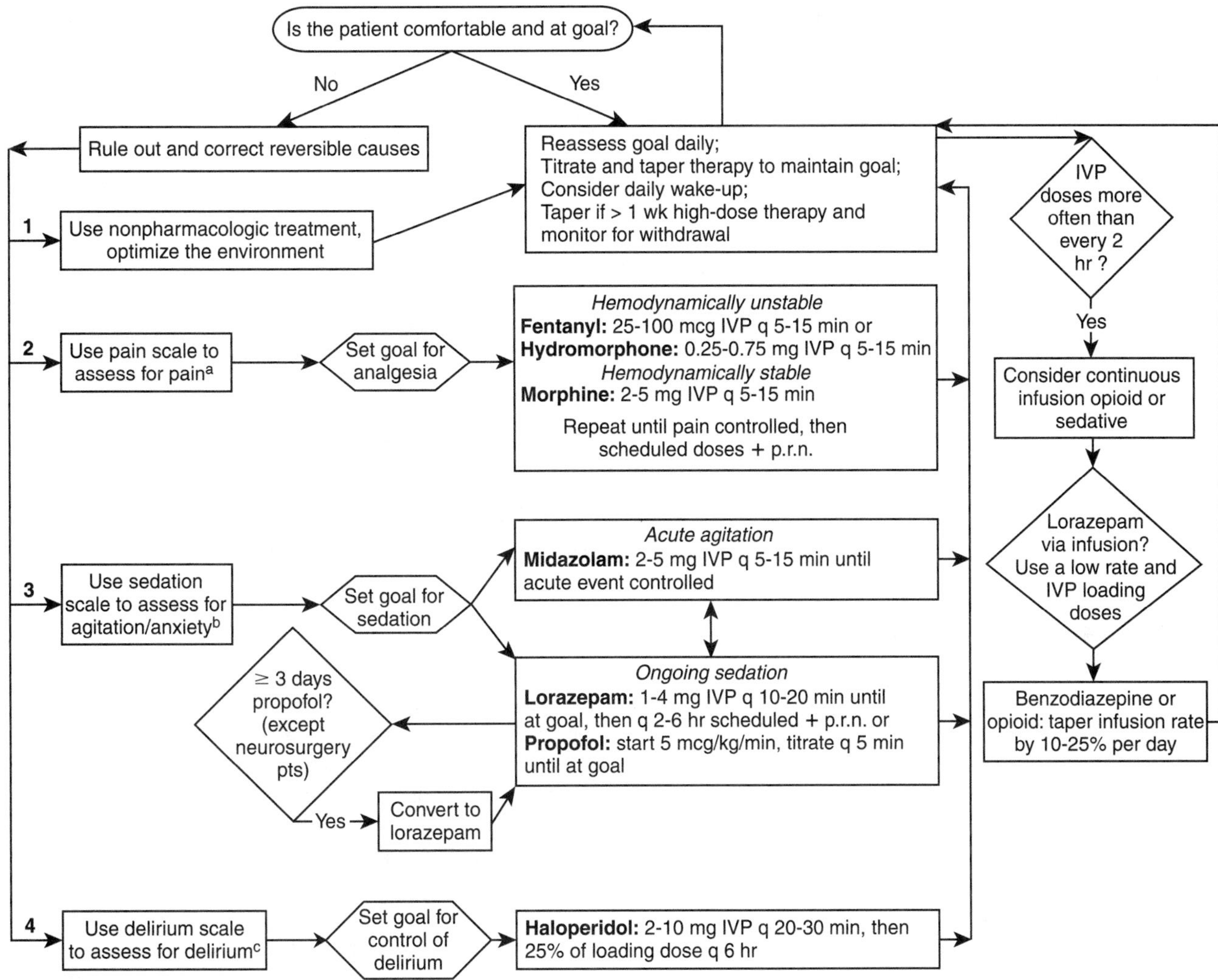

FIGURE 18-11 SCCM sedation and analgesia algorithm. (Redrawn from Jacobi J, Fraser GL, Coursin DB et al: Clinical practice guidelines for the use of sedatives and analgesics in the critically ill adult, *Crit Care Med* 30:119-141, 2002.)

advanced age or renal or hepatic damage may require less. Because of these factors, doses must be individualized.

For patients requiring prolonged sedation the SCCM guidelines stipulate that scheduled intermittent or continuous infusion dosing of agents be used.[194] Continuous infusion provides an easily titratable delivery method that most institutions use. Continuous infusions of lorazepam or propofol were selected as agents of choice. Midazolam can be administered as a continuous infusion, but several studies have demonstrated unpredictable awakening times compared with propofol as a result of the accumulation of active metabolites.[194]

Several factors must be considered when choosing between agents. Lorazepam is not as water soluble as midazolam, and precipitation is avoided by preparing infusions with a final concentration of 0.2 to 1.0 mg/ml in glass containers.[214] Second, high doses (>10 mg/hour) of lorazepam have been associated with polyethylene glycol and propylene glycol toxicity.[215-217] The toxicity is characterized by lactic acidosis, nephrotoxicity, and hyperosmolarity with hypotension.[218] Each milliliter of lorazepam contains 0.18 ml of polyethylene glycol 400 and 0.8 ml of propylene glycol. Patients receiving high doses of lorazepam, long-term infusions, and coadministration of drugs that contain propylene glycol should be monitored for these effects. Table 18-22 lists the characteristics of propylene glycol toxicity.[194,218] A list of drugs that contain propylene glycol is provided in Table 18-23.[219] Continuous infusions of lorazepam can be safely initiated at 0.01 mg/kg per hour.

Diazepam is a long-acting agent that can be useful in cases when a prolonged duration of sedation is anticipated, such as a patient with severe respiratory failure requiring intensive mechanical ventilatory support. Sedation levels must be monitored so that doses can be modified in anticipation of awakening the patient. If doses are not appropriately adjusted, the patient will have a prolonged recovery that may extend the need for mechanical ventilation and increase the length of stay.

TABLE 18-21 Commonly Used Sedatives in the Intensive Care Unit

Drug	Onset (min)	Half-Life (hr)	Advantages	Disadvantages
Diazepam	2-5	20-120	Inexpensive Rapid onset Long duration of action	Long-acting metabolites Extensive metabolism Phlebitis
Midazolam	2-5	3-11	Rapid onset	Oversedation from accumulation of active metabolite
Lorazepam	5-20	8-15	Preferred for long-term sedation No active metabolites	Slow onset Limited solubility for continuous infusion Propylene glycol toxicity
Propofol	1-2		Rapid onset Short duration of action with short-term use No pharmacokinetic changes in renal or hepatic impairment	Cost Continuous infusion only Accumulation with infusions >12 hours Changing of bottle and intravenous tubing every 12 hours Dedicated line for administration Risk of fungal infections Excessive calories (1.1 kcal/ml administered) Hypertriglyceridemia Pancreatitis "Propofol infusion syndrome"

TABLE 18-22 Characteristics of Propylene Glycol Toxicity

Metabolic acidosis with anion gap (Lactic acidosis)
- Serum sodium (mEq/L) − Serum chloride (mEq/L) + Serum bicarbonate (mEq/L)
- Elevated anion gap >12

Osmolarity gap
- (2 × Serum sodium [meq/L]) + (Blood glucose [mg/dL] /18) + (Blood urea nitrogen [mg/dL]/2.8)
- Osmolarity gap is measured osmolality − Calculated osmolarity
- Elevated osmolarity gap >10

Acute renal failure from acute tubular necrosis (elevated serum creatinine)

From Yaucher NE, Fish JT, Smith HW et al: Propylene glycol-associated renal toxicity from lorazepam infusion, *Pharmacotherapy* 23:1094-1099, 2003.

TABLE 18-23 Common Intravenous Drugs Containing Propylene Glycol

Etomidate
Diazepam
Esmolol
Lorazepam
Nitroglycerin
Pentobarbital
Phenytoin
Phenobarbital

Adapted from Yaucher NE, Fish JT, Smith HW et al: Propylene glycol-associated renal toxicity from lorazepam infusion, *Pharmacotherapy* 23:1094-1099, 2003.

A dosage of 0.03 to 0.1 mg/kg every 0.5 to 6 hours is generally administered by slow intravenous injection.[220] SCCM's practice parameters did not recommend routine use of diazepam because of the concerns for phlebitis, its long duration of action, and the accumulation of active metabolites.[194]

Enteral administration of lorazepam or diazepam is a cost-effective alternative. Caution should be exhibited when administering large doses of liquid lorazepam (i.e., 60 mg of 2 mg/ml every 6 hours) because it may lead to diarrhea from the high polyethylene glycol 400 and propylene glycol content.[194] As with any sedation plan, the dose and frequency should be evaluated daily to prevent the oversedation or undersedation that may occur when feedings are adjusted or interrupted.

Tapering. Long-term administration and high dosages of benzodiazepines are associated with tolerance and physical dependence. Unfortunately, data are limited on the development of tolerance and dependence with administration of continuous-infusion benzodiazepines in critically ill patients. The amount of time or dosage required to produce physical dependence that will predispose patients to withdrawal with abrupt discontinuation is unclear. Thus, gradual tapering of the dosage is recommended when discontinuing therapy; the SCCM guidelines recommend a taper of 10% to 25% per day.[194] One method of achieving this is through administering lorazepam or diazepam through nasogastric or feeding tubes.

Side Effects. Benzodiazepines have a low incidence of side effects. The greatest concern is respiratory and cardiovascular depression. As a class, benzodiazepines depress central respiratory drive. The effect is less profound than with opiates, but it can be additive when the agents are used together.[194] The somnolence associated with these agents can lead to a decrease in minute ventilation.

Midazolam and diazepam have few hemodynamic effects. Sedative doses have produced a slight increase in heart rate and a mild decrease in blood pressure and systemic vascular resistance.[221-223] However, in a volume-depleted state the hemodynamic effects can be more pronounced.

Flumazenil is the only benzodiazepine antagonist approved by the FDA. Flumazenil competitively inhibits benzodiazepines from binding to its receptor site, facilitating reversal of the deleterious effects associated with benzodiazepine overdose. For prolonged benzodiazepine sedation in a patient who fails to awaken after an appropriate duration after discontinuation, low doses (0.1-0.2 mg given intravenously over 1 minute) of flumazenil have been used. However, even if an improvement in the level of consciousness is noted transiently, flumazenil should not be used for reversal of long-term benzodiazepine sedation because this may induce withdrawal symptoms, elicit seizures, and increase myocardial oxygen consumption with as little as 0.5 mg of flumazenil.[194] Intravenous doses of as little as 0.15 mg of flumazenil have been associated withdrawal symptoms when administered to patients receiving continuous infusions of benzodiazepines.[194]

Propofol

Propofol is an ultra-short-acting intravenous alkylphenol amnestic agent. Sedation, anxiolysis, and some amnestic effects are produced at subanesthetic doses. Propofol is equally effective as a sedative compared with midazolam.[224] SCCM recommends using propofol as a continuous infusion for <3 days except in neurosurgery patients. In this patient population the ultra-short duration of action allows for rapid awakening for frequent neurologic examinations and it may decrease elevated intracranial pressure (ICP).[194]

Pharmacokinetics. Propofol is an ultra-short-acting sedative hypnotic with anxiolytic and amnestic properties. Like the benzodiazepines, propofol does not provide analgesic effects and produces respiratory depression. Propofol is highly lipophilic with a rapid onset and short duration of action. Sedation can be produced within 1 to 2 minutes, and recovery usually occurs within 10 to 15 minutes, allowing for easy titration, control of sedation depth, and rapid awakening. Propofol's rapid onset of action paired with the marked respiratory depression limit its use to intubated patients in most insitiutions. Bolus dosing of propofol has been described; however, many critically ill patients are not able to tolerate boluses because of the hypotension or myocardial depression that can occur.

Critically ill, elderly, and obese patients have prolonged elimination half-life and an increase in volume of distribution, so they may require dosage adjustments.[194,225] Dosing in obese patients should be based on lean body weight, and elderly patients will generally require a lower dosage.[225]

Propofol is metabolized by the liver by glucuronide and sulfate conjugation. These metabolites do not seem to elicit sedative activity, and in patients with hepatic damage or cirrhosis receiving propofol there does not seem to be a significant alteration in pharmacokinetics. This would suggest that extrahepatic clearance may be contributing to elimination.[226] Also, because there is no renal elimination of propofol, it can be used safely in patients with hepatic or renal impairment without concern for accumulation.

Indications and Administration Methods. Propofol is indicated as a sedative and amnestic agent for short-term use in mechanically ventilated patients (Table 18-24). Long-term use lends itself to neurosurgical or traumatic brain injury patients. Because of the short onset of action and duration of effect seen with short-term administration, propofol is limited to continuous infusion starting at 5 mcg/kg per minute. Doses can be titrated every 5 minutes until the patient achieves the desired sedation scale number. Propofol requires a dedicated line for administration because of the lipid emulsion. The manufacturer states that both the propofol bottle and tubing should be changed every 12 hours to prevent fungal infections.

Side Effects. Adverse effects most commonly seen with propofol include hypotension, bradycardia, phlebitis, and greenish discoloration of the urine. Hypotension seems to be dose related and more frequent after bolus doses. Care should be taken to avoid the administration of large doses or coadministration of agents (i.e., opiates) capable of hypotension.[227] Patients who are elderly, hypovolemic, or suffering from severe cardiac disease are at increased risk for development of hypotension.

Propofol is formulated in a 1% soybean oil, glycerol, and egg phosphatide emulsion. It can cross-react, resulting in anaphylaxis in patients with allergies to eggs. Also, because of the high lipophilic nature of propofol, there is an immediate redistribution out of CNS, heart, and liver on discontinuation. The terminal half-life of propofol can approach 1,900 minutes after long-term administration as a result of the slow redistribution from poorly perfused tissues.[226] Elevation of serum triglycerides or pancreatic enzymes and pancreatitis has been reported with prolonged infusions of propofol.[228] Neurosurgical patients receiving propofol for >3 days, patients receiving high doses of propofol, and those with a history of hypertriglyceridemia should have triglycerides monitored periodically. The lipid content of propofol can provide 1.1 kcal/ml infused. For short-term use this is thought to be insignificant, but in patients that are obese, receiving large doses, or receiving infusions >3 days the calories must be included in the total nutrition support prescription.

Manufacturers of propofol have placed edetic acid or sodium metabisulfate in the formulations as a preservative. A

TABLE 18-24 **Propofol Doses**

Sedation Dose	
mcg/kg/min	**mg/kg/hr**
6-53	0.4-3.2
9-131	0.5-7.9
13-37	0.8-2.2
100-150 for 3-5 min, then 25-75	6-9 for 3-5 min, then 1.5-4.5

drug holiday is recommended after 7 days in formulations with edetic acid to minimize the risk of trace element abnormalities. Products with sodium metabisulfite can cross-react in patients who have sulfite allergies. Care should be taken to identify the product administered to patients with food or drug allergies and monitor for the above adverse events.

Prolonged use (>48 hours) or high doses of propofol (>66 mcg/kg/min infusion) have resulted in "propofol infusion syndrome." Propofol infusion syndrome consists of sudden onset of bradycardia with progression to asystole, lipidemia, hepatomegaly from fatty infiltration, severe metabolic acidosis with anion gap (from lactic acidosis), and the presence of rhabdomyolysis or myoglobinuria.[229,230] This syndrome was first described in pediatric patients and in those receiving high doses (>83 mcg/kg/min).[230] Because of this, the FDA has specifically recommended against the use of high doses of propofol for adult and pediatric patients.

α_2-Agonists

Dexmedetomidine is the first in the α_2-agonist class to be developed specifically for ICU sedation. It is eight times more specific for α_2-adenoreceptors than is clonidine.[231] Clinical trials have demonstrated marked sedation with only mild reductions in minute ventilation.[231] Dexmedetomidine produces sedative and analgesic effects when administered in critically ill adults. It also produces dose-dependent declines in blood pressure and heart rate, especially when bolus doses are administered. Studies in healthy adults demonstrated a 17% decline in heart rate and a 23% decline in blood pressure.[231]

Pharmacokinetics. Dexmedetomidate has a favorable pharmacokinetic profile for ICU use. The onset of action ranges from 1 to 2 minutes and the half-life is 2 hours.[231] It is highly plasma protein bound to both albumin and α_1-glycoprotein and is extensively metabolized by the liver to methyl and glucuronides, which are eliminated by the kidneys. Patients with severe hepatic failure have significant increases in half-life and decreases in clearance.[231]

Indications and Administration Methods. Dexmedetomidine is indicated for short-term (<24 hour) infusions as a sedative agent for the critically ill. It is initiated with a bolus infusion of 1 mcg/kg administered over 10 minutes and then a maintenance infusion of 0.2 to 0.7 mcg/kg per hour. The bolus infusion can be omitted in patients where there is a concern for hypotension. Although dexmedetomidine provides sedative and analgesic effects, nearly 40% of patients receiving dexmedetomidine require additional sedative and analgesic agents for breakthrough.[231] When analgesics (e.g., narcotics) and sedatives (e.g., benzodiazepines) are used in conjunction with dexmedetomidine, the necessary dosages of these medications can usually be reduced to achieve the pain control or sedation desired.

The majority of data on dexmedetomidine is in the cardiac surgery population. The largest study to date compared (1) midazolam or propofol with (2) midazolam or propofol and dexmedetomidine.[232] Researchers found that the addition of dexmedetomidine decreased hospital length of stay by 0.6 days ($P < .0001$), decreased days on mechanical ventilation by 0.5 days ($P < .01$), decreased ICU length of stay by 3.87 days ($P < .0001$), and increased drug costs about $4,000 per patient.

Pharmacologically, dexmedetomidine may also have benefical effects similar to clonidine in patients admitted to the ICU with a history of drug or alcohol abuse. A large randomized clinical trial has not substantiated this, but case reports seem promising.[233] The utility of this agent for spinal cord injuries or traumatic brain injury is unknown.

Side Effects. Hypotension is the most commonly occuring side effect of dexmedetomidine administration. This was noted in healthy adults (28% dexmedetomidine versus 13% placebo) and was more pronounced in hemodynamically unstable critically ill patients.[234] Because of this potential complication, bolus dosing is most often omitted in the critically ill patient who may not tolerate hypotension.

Dexmedetomidine shows a lot of promise as an adjunct for sedation and analgesia in the critically ill. The potential for marked hypotension may limit its use as an adjunct to benzodiazepines and propofol and analgesics at this time. No formal trials have been conducted in the trauma population as of yet, but the theoretic advantanges in patients with hypertension, a history of substance abuse, or pain suggest that this agent may be effective.

Barbiturates

Barbiturates produce sedation by depressing excitable tissues throughout the CNS. They suppress transmission of excitatory neurotransmitters (e.g., acetylcholine) and enhance transmission of inhibitory neurotransmitters (e.g., GABA). Barbiturates are usually administered as adjuvents only when the usual agents have failed to produce the desired level of sedation. These agents are effective sedatives at low doses but have no amnestic or analgesic properties. In fact, they sometimes appear to have antianalgesic effects by lowering the pain threshold. Because agents with amnestic properties and a more favorable adverse effect profile have been developed, the routine use of barbiturates is no longer recommended.

The highly lipophilic barbiturates have a rapid onset and short duration of action. For example, thiopental typically produces a loss of consciousness within 30 seconds and recovery within 20 minutes. Barbiturates are degraded by hepatic microsomal enzymes to inactive metabolites. Tolerance to the sedative effects quickly develops, and this tolerance is conferred to most CNS depressant drugs as well.

Thiopental and pentobarbital are most often used occasionally to manage refractory intracranial hypertension in patients who do not respond to conventional therapy. However, a beneficial effect on outcomes has not been demonstrated and there is a lack of data comparing it with currently available agents.[235]

Complications associated with barbiturate administration include myocardial depression, hypotension, and respiratory depression. Patients who are elderly or who are intravascularly volume depleted are especially prone to these adverse effects.

Ketamine

Ketamine is an intravenous anesthetic agent that produces analgesia and sedation when administered in low doses.[236] It is occasionally used for repeated painful procedures such as dressing changes.[236] Ketamine causes a functional dissociation between the thalamus (which relays sensory impulses from the reticular activating system to the cerebral cortex) and the limbic cortex (which is involved with the awareness of sensation). The patient appears conscious (e.g., eyes opening, swallowing) but is unable to process or respond to sensory input. Because of its sympathomimetic properties, increases in blood pressure and heart rate are typical. However, an unexpected hypotension can occur in critically ill patients as a result of a direct myocardial depressant property.

Ketamine is used often in children younger than 10 years of age. Use in adults is limited by an emergence phenomenon characterized by hallucinations and nightmares. Pretreatment with a benzodiazepine may minimize this reaction. Ketamine is a bronchodilator and has been used to treat severe asthma exacerbations.[237] Pretreatment with atropine may diminish upper airway secretions. The place of this agent in routine ICU sedation remains to be determined.

Nonpharmacologic Therapeutic Approaches to Sedation

The stressful environment of the ICU can induce patient anxiety and fear because of a loss of independence, sensory overload, immobility, and loss of control.[238] Nonpharmacologic modalities can be used to decrease the anxiety associated with ICU care. Efforts to reduce night noise, lighting, and staff conversation promote regular sleep-wake cycles.[239] Reinstitution of patient control and family visitors can also help to relieve anxiety nonpharmacologically.[240] In addition, successful relaxation of ICU patients has been achieved with alternative therapies such as relaxation techniques, hypnosis, music therapy, breathing instruction, and massage.

ICU Delirium

ICU delirium is thought to occur in up to 20% to 80% of all ICU patients.[241] It is characterized by an acutely changing or fluctuating mental status, inattention, disorganized thinking, and an altered level of consciousness that may or may not be accompanied by agitation.[194] Delirious patients often exhibit random, purposeless movement and may harm themselves or others as a result of their agitation. Hypoactive or mixed types of delirium can occur, and these patients typically exhibit fewer physical signs and symptoms. Patients exhibiting these types of delirium can account for up to 45% of all ICU delirium patients, making the diagnosis difficult.[241] Also complicating the diagnosis is the difficulty in distinguishing patients exhibiting outward signs of untreated pain or agitation. One distinguishing feature is that delirious patients may have impaired short-term memory and may hallucinate or misinterpret stimuli.

Screening for delirium in the critically ill can be difficult. One method of screening is the Confusion Assessment Method for the ICU (Cam-ICU).[242] The Cam-ICU scale examines four criteria: (1) acute onset of mental status changes or fluctuating course, (2) inattention, (3) disorganized thinking, and (4) altered level of consciousness. Patients are diagnosed with delirium if they have both features 1 and 2 and either 3 or 4. Each of the variables has separate subpoints, which are summarized in Table 18-25.

Haloperidol

Haloperidol is considered by many clinicians to be the drug of choice for reversing the behavioral manifestations of ICU delirium. The mechanism by which haloperidol reduces delirium is not clear. Actions other than blockade of central dopamine receptors are thought to be responsible for haloperidol's calming effect in patients with delirium.[243,244] Because of the need for rapid control of acute delirium, haloperidol should be administered intravenously. Although the intravenous route is not FDA approved, there is extensive literature demonstrating its safe and effective use.[245]

For the severely agitated patient, the recommended dosage regimen uses a 2 mg intravenous dose and progressive dose doubling at intervals of no less than 15 to 20 minutes while agitation persists.[194] If the desired calming effect is not produced after several doses, the initial dose may be doubled and administered at 30-minute intervals until an adverse effect develops or a total of 400 mg has been administered. Rarely are doses of 400 mg required to treat delirium.

After the delirious patient is calmed, haloperidol should be given on a scheduled basis every 4 to 6 hours. If agitation remains controlled, the dose is tapered over several days. Intravenous infusions have been reported for patients who require frequent intravenous administration for agitation control[199,246]; however, the agent is usually administered by intermittent intravenous push.

Haloperidol should not be used as a single agent to control agitation in patients withdrawing from alcohol or benzodiazepines. Although haloperidol reduces some of the signs and symptoms associated with these withdrawal syndromes, it increases the risk of seizures by lowering the seizure threshold. Patients who cannot tolerate the hemodynamic effect of other sedatives or who are weaning from mechanical ventilation may be sedated with haloperidol alone.

Adverse effects associated with intravenous haloperidol include neurologic and cardiovascular toxicities. The neurologic toxicities are extrapyramidal effects such as akathisia and dystonia. Patients with akathisia often have the clinical symptoms of restlessness, irritability, and thought or speech disorders. Akathisia is often mistaken for continued or worsened delirium, and accurate differentiation is necessary for proper treatment. Both dystonia and akathisia respond to treatment with anticholinergic agents (e.g., diphenhydramine or benztropine). With akathisia unresponsive to anticholinergics, propranolol or amantadine may be useful.[247] The extrapyramidal effects are

TABLE 18-25 **Diagnosis of Delirium Based on the Cam-ICU**

Feature	Assessment Variables
1. Acute onset of mental status changes or fluctuating course	Is there evidence of an acute change in mental status from the baseline? Did the [abnormal] behavior fluctuate during the past 24 hours (i.e., tend to come and go or increase and decrease in severity)? Did the sedation scale (e.g., SAS or MAAS) or coma scale (GCS) fluctuate in the past 24 hours?
2. Inattention	Did the patient have difficulty focusing attention? Is there reduced ability to maintain and shift attention? How does the patient score on the Attention Screening Examination (ASE)? (i.e., Visual Component ASE tests the patient's ability to pay attention by recall of 10 pictures; auditory component ASE tests attention by having patient squeeze hands or nod whenever the letter "A" is called in a random letter sequence)
3. Disorganized thinking	If the patient is already extubated from the ventilator, determine whether the patient's thinking is disorganized or incoherent, such as rambling or irrelevant conversation, unclear or illogical flow of ideas, or unpredictable switching from subject to subject. For those still on the ventilator, can the patient answer the following four questions correctly? 1. Will a stone float on water? 2. Are there fish in the sea? 3. Does 1 pound weigh more than 2 pounds? 4. Can you use a hammer to pound a nail? Was the patient able to follow questions and commands throughout the assessment? 1. "Are you having any unclear thinking?" 2. "Hold up this many fingers." (Examiner holds two fingers in front of patient.) 3. "Now do the same thing with the other hand." (not repeating the number of fingers)
4. Altered level of consciousness (any level of consciousness other than alert [e.g., vigilant, lethargic, stupor, or coma])	Alert: normal, spontaneously fully aware of environment, interacts appropriately Vigilant: hyperalert Lethargic: drowsy but easily aroused, unaware of some elements in the environment, or not spontaneously interacting appropriately with the interviewer; becomes fully aware and appropriately interactive when prodded minimally Stupor: difficult to arouse, unaware of some or all elements in the environment, or not spontaneously interacting with the interviewer; becomes incompletely aware and inappropriately interactive when prodded strongly; can be aroused only by vigorous and repeated stimuli and as soon as the stimulus ceases, stuporous subjects lapse back into the unresponsive state Coma: unarousable, unaware of all elements in the environment, with no spontaneous interaction or awareness of the interviewer, so that the interview is impossible even with maximal prodding
Patients are diagnosed with delirium if they have both features 1 and 2 and either feature 3 or 4	

GCS, Glasgow Coma Scale. Jacobi J, Fraser GL, Coursin DB et al: Clinical practice guidelines for the use of sedatives and analgesics in the critically ill adult, *Crit Care Med* 30:119-141, 2002. Adapted from original by Ely EW, Inouye SK, Bernard GR, et al: Delirium in mechanically ventilated patients: Validity and reliability of the confusion assessment method for the intensive care unit (CAM-ICU), *JAMA* 286:2703-2710, 2001.

not dose related and are sudden in onset, and the incidence of these symptoms after intravenous use is lower than it is after oral or intramuscular administration.[248]

Cardiovascular consequences consist of the rare occurrence of QT interval prolongation or polymorphic ventricular tachycardia such as torsades de pointes.[194] The majority of these cases have occurred in patients receiving more than 50 mg per day.[199,249,250] All patients receiving intravenous haloperidol should have continuous electrocardiogram monitoring, and haloperidol should be discontinued or the dose reduced if the QT interval is prolonged by 25% or more over baseline, the interval is longer than 440 milliseconds, or polymorphic ventricular tachycardia is observed.[249] Hypotensive episodes after the administration of intravenous haloperidol are rare and almost always attributed to hypovolemia. One way to minimize cardiac and neurologic toxicities is to use lorazepam in combination with haloperidol. Combination therapy may allow lower total doses of each agent, and this combination may have a synergistic effect.

NEUROMUSCULAR BLOCKING AGENTS

Neuromuscular blocking agents (NMBAs) are used to facilitate endotracheal intubation and to help prevent laryngospasm. Once intubated, however, only a small fraction of ICU patients are treated with continuous infusion or scheduled

NMBAs. Aggressive use of analgesia and sedation is preferred initially, and NMBAs are reserved for patients who fail to meet desired ventilatory goals despite maximal sedative therapy. NMBA therapy is frequently used in an attempt to improve chest wall compliance. NMBAs can assist ventilation therapy in at least three ways: (1) reducing or eliminating spontaneous breathing, (2) preventing motor activity that can dislodge artifical airways, catheters, surgical dressings, or chest tubes, and (3) decreasing oxygen consumption by patients with severely diminished cardiopulmonary function.[251] Patients who are maximally sedated may have only minimal improvements in ventilatory mechanics and chest wall compliance with the addition of NMBAs.

NMBAs are often used during surgical procedures when complete muscle block is desirable. Examples of surgeries where NMBA may be used include abdominal or cardiothoracic, and procedures to set traumatic dislocations or fractures.[252] Postoperative NMB can be a useful adjunct to promote healing of specific surgical wounds (e.g., vascular anastomosis) by immobilizing the patient for a defined period.[252] Immobilization may prove of particular benefit when wound closure has been difficult or disruptive and loss of wound integrity would place the patient at great risk.

Apart from mechanical ventilation and postoperative indications, several situations in the ICU may justify the use of NMBAs. NMB can prevent unacceptably high oxygen consumption as a result of the profound shivering that frequently accompanies rewarming from hypothermia.[253] Furthermore, therapeutic paralysis has been used in the treatment of tetanus,[251] status epilepticus,[254] hypermetabolism resulting from burns, and uncontrolled intracranial hypertension.[254,255]

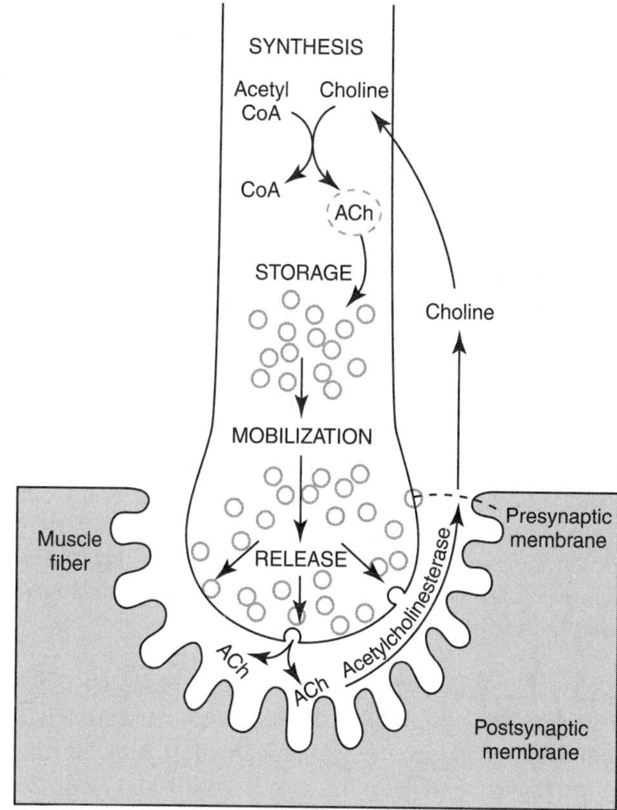

FIGURE 18-12 Neuromuscular junction. The neuromuscular junction consists of the nerve axon and muscle fiber. The neurotransmitted acetylcholine is released from axonal vesicles in response to nerve action potentials. The combination of acetylcholine with the receptor results in a depolarization of the muscle cells and contraction of the muscle fiber.

PHYSIOLOGY

The neuromuscular junction consists of the motor nerve terminal, the synaptic cleft, and the muscle's end plate, which contains nicotinic receptors (Figure 18-12). The motor nerve terminal synthesizes and stores the neurotransmitter acetylcholine. On arrival of a nerve impulse at the nerve terminal, acetylcholine is released by the nerve terminal into the synaptic cleft and binds to the nicotinic receptor, initiating the opening of a potential channel. The opening of this channel allows the influx of sodium and calcium ions and the efflux of potassium ions, thereby triggering depolarization of the motor end plate. This depolarization leads to muscle contraction. Acetylcholine can attach to or detach from the receptor. Unbound acetylcholine is metabolized by the enzyme acetylcholinesterase, thus terminating the depolarization of the end plate and the resultant contraction.

NMBAs induce paralysis of the skeletal muscle by disrupting normal neuromuscular transmission. The currently available agents structurally resemble acetylcholine and occupy the nicotinic receptors on the muscle fiber, which prevents the binding of acetylcholine to the receptors. The NMBAs are classified as depolarizing or nondepolarizing relaxants according to their effect on the motor end plate. Succinylcholine, the only depolarizing agent currently used, attaches to the receptor and depolarizes the motor end plate. The depolarizing action of succinylcholine is more sustained than that of acetylcholine, and the end plate remains refractory to the effects of acetylcholine. Transient twitching of skeletal muscle (fasciculations) is briefly produced, followed by paralysis. Nondepolarizing relaxants bind to the same receptors as acetylcholine, establishing a competitive inhibition of the attachment of acetylcholine to the receptor. In contrast to succinylcholine, nondepolarizing agents do not depolarize the end plate and cause muscle contraction.

SEQUENCE OF ONSET

When an appropriate dose of a neuromuscular blocking agent is injected intravenously, the onset of blockade is rapid. Motor weakness progresses to total flaccid paralysis. Small rapidly moving muscles such as those of the eyes are involved before those of the limbs, neck, trunk, and abdomen. Ultimately, intercostal muscles and finally the diaphragm are paralyzed and respiration ceases. Recovery of skeletal muscles usually occurs in reverse order to that of paralysis so that the diaphragm is the first to regain function. Intravenous injection of a neuromuscular blocking agent to a person who is awake initially produces difficulty in focusing and weakness in the mandibular muscles, followed by ptosis, diplopia, and dysphagia. Consciousness and sensorium remain undisturbed even in the presence of complete neuromuscular blockade.

Comparison of Agents

Neuromuscular blocking agents available for clinical use are listed in Table 18-26. These agents can be classified according to the duration of blockade they produce: short, intermediate, or long acting. Selection is based on the patient's needs and medical condition and the treatment goals. Some agents produce cardiovascular effects such as hypotension and arrhythmia. In patients with cardiovascular impairments, vecuronium, doxacurium, cisatracurium, and rocuronium may be preferred. Pancuronium has vagolytic effects that produce tachycardia and an increase in blood pressure and should be avoided in patients who cannot tolerate further increases in heart rate (coronary heart disease, valvular heart disease).[251] However, in the absence of cardiovascular disease, the increase in heart rate is well tolerated by many young patients. Hepatic and renal failure also should be considered when choosing a neuromuscular blocking agent, but they are not contraindications to agents metabolized or eliminated by these routes as long as appropriate monitoring is performed. Atracurium and cisatracurium undergo Hoffman elimination, which does not depend on hepatic or renal organ function. Because of this, these agents may be a good choice for patients with renal or hepatic failure. Pancuronium, vecuronium, rocuronium, cisatracurium, or doxacurium may be preferred for patients with asthma because they are not associated with significant histamine release. The SCCM practice guidelines recommend pancuronium as the preferred agent for most critically ill patients because it is inexpensive and the relative tachycardia and mild hypertension are seldom of clinical consequence and are presumed to be related to the dosage and rate of administration.[251]

TABLE 18-26 Currently Available Neuromuscular Blocking Agents

Drug	Onset (min)	Duration (min)
Depolarizing Agent		
Succinylcholine	0.5-1	3-6
Nondepolarizing Agents		
Short-Acting		
Mivacurium	1.5-3	15-20
Rapacuronium	1.0-1.5	15-25
Intermediate-Acting		
Atracurium	3-5	20-35
Cisatracurium	1.5-3	40-60
Rocuronium	0.5-6	20-40
Vecuronium	3-5	25-40
Long-Acting		
Doxacurium	5	100-160
Pancuronium	2-5	50-60
Metocurine	3-5	25-90
Pipecuronium	2.5-5	60-120
Tubocurarine	3-5	35-45

Bolus Dosing Versus Continuous Infusion

Neuromuscular blocking agents are usually administered as a bolus-loading dose followed by repeat bolus or continuous infusion. With short-acting or intermediate-duration drugs such as mivacurium, rocuronium, atracurium, or vecuronium, continuous infusions may be preferred.

Facilitating Endotracheal Intubation

Succinylcholine is commonly administered as an intravenous bolus of 1.5 mg/kg in adults to facilitate endotracheal intubation because its onset of 60 seconds is faster than many of the nondepolarizing relaxants. Large doses of the nondepolarizing agents mivacurium and rocuronium approach the rapid onset of succinylcholine, with muscle relaxation occurring within 2 to 2.5 minutes and 1 to 1.5 minutes, respectively.[256] However, rocuronium is very expensive, and large doses of mivacurium may cause histamine release and hypotension in patients with preexisting cardiovascular instability. Unfortunately, the side effects associated with succinylcholine may limit its usefulness for intubation in some patients.

The other nondepolarizing relaxants have an onset of about 3 to 4 minutes, limiting their use for rapid tracheal intubation. However, two techniques can speed the onset of neuromuscular blockade. The first technique involves the administration of a priming dose, one tenth of an intubating dose, several minutes before the bolus dose. Ideally, after the priming dose patients should be able to breathe spontaneously, maintain a patent airway, and avoid aspiration so that intubation can occur within 100 seconds. Some patients, however, experience weakness or respiratory distress and fear and anxiety from diplopia and dyspnea after the priming dose.

Another technique involves the administration of a dose two times the intubating dose of nondepolarizing relaxants. The large dose saturates the receptors and speeds up the onset of paralysis. The risks of this method are related to the cardiovascular effects of the relaxant, which can be avoided by using a drug with a stable cardiovascular profile such as vecuronium, doxacurium, cisatracurium, or rocuronium.[257]

Factors Affecting Paralysis

Many factors affect the degree of paralysis induced by neuromuscular blocking agents.[251] These factors may inhibit or potentiate NMB depending on the degree of blockade induced, the agent used, and individual patient characteristics. Table 18-27 lists clinical conditions and medications capable of altering the effects of these agents. Trauma patients are at risk for many of these conditions or may require many of the interacting medications, so careful monitoring is recommended.

TABLE 18-27 Factors Capable of Altering the Effects of Neuromuscular Blocking Agents

Potentiate Blockade or Decrease Drug Requirement	Antagonize Blockade or Increase Drug Requirement
Drugs	**Drugs**
Halogenated anesthetics	Phenytoin
Local anesthetics	Carbamazepine
Antibiotics	Anticholinesterase agents
Aminoglycosides	Edrophonium
Clindamycin	Neostigmine
Vancomycin	Pyridostigmine
Antiarrhythmics	Theophylline
Procainamide	Azathioprine
Quinidine	Ranitidine
Bretylium	
Calcium channel blockers	
β-Adrenergic blockers	
Cyclosporine	
Dantrolene	
Cyclophosphamide	
Lithium	
Mineralocorticoids	
Clinical Conditions	**Clinical Conditions**
Acidosis	Alkalosis
Electrolyte abnormalities	Hypercalcemia
Severe hyponatremia	Demyelinating lesions
Severe hypocalcemia	Peripheral neuropathies
Severe hypokalemia	Diabetes mellitus
Hypermagnesemia	
Neuromuscular diseases	
Myasthenia gravis	
Muscular dystrophy	
Amyotrophic lateral sclerosis	
Poliomyelitis	
Multiple sclerosis	
Eaton-Lambert syndrome	
Hypothermia	
Acute intermittent porphyria	
Renal failure	
Hepatic failure	

Nursing Assessment

Monitoring of NMB therapy by train-of-four (TOF) stimulation is widely recommended.[251] Routine monitoring by this method helps avoid excessive or insufficient use of paralytics and may prevent prolonged effects of neuromuscular blocking agents. Changing organ function and addition of medications that potentiate these drugs can foster accumulation of the agent or its active metabolites, which will be undetected without TOF monitoring. Investigators have documented that adjusting the dose of neuromuscular blocking agents by TOF monitoring versus standard clinical examination in the critically ill patient reduces drug requirements and allows a faster recovery from NMB.[251]

TOF measurement is the most common method used to monitor neuromuscular blocking agents in the ICU. Four stimuli are delivered along the path of the nerve at a frequency of 2 Hz for 2 seconds. Muscle response is measured to evaluate the number of stimuli blocked versus delivered. Electrodes should be placed over skin that is clean, dry, and hairless and replaced every 24 hours. Substantial edema or obesity may result in insufficient current being delivered to the nerve by surface electrodes. Needle electrodes (23 gauge) are available if electrocardiogram electrodes are ineffective.

The ulnar nerve at the wrist is most frequently used to evaluate neuromuscular function (Figure 18-13). Stimulation of the ulnar nerve results in the adduction of the thumb. Peripheral nerve monitoring may be performed on the facial nerve, which results in movement of the orbicularis oculi muscle (Figure 18-14). Because it is blockade of the neuromuscular junction that needs to be monitored, direct stimulation of muscle should be avoided by placing electrodes over the course of the nerve and not over the muscle itself.

In the absence of neuromuscular blocking agents, four equal muscle contractions should be observed in response to the four stimuli (4/4). In the presence of nondepolarizing agents, a progressive loss of twitch height and number of twitches represent a progressive degree of NMB. When 90% of the receptors are blocked, the muscle will only respond once (1/4). At greater than 90% blocked, no movement of the muscle may be seen (0/4). If two, three, or four twitches are observed, a block less than 90% has been quantified.

Although no prospective, controlled trials have determined the degree of NMB required to achieve optimal mechanical ventilation in patients, the recommended rate of infusion is that titrated to a minimal presence of one or two twitches (80%-90% blockade) at all times. TOF stimulation should be monitored and recorded every 8 hours, or more frequently when patient status dictates. Ablation of all four

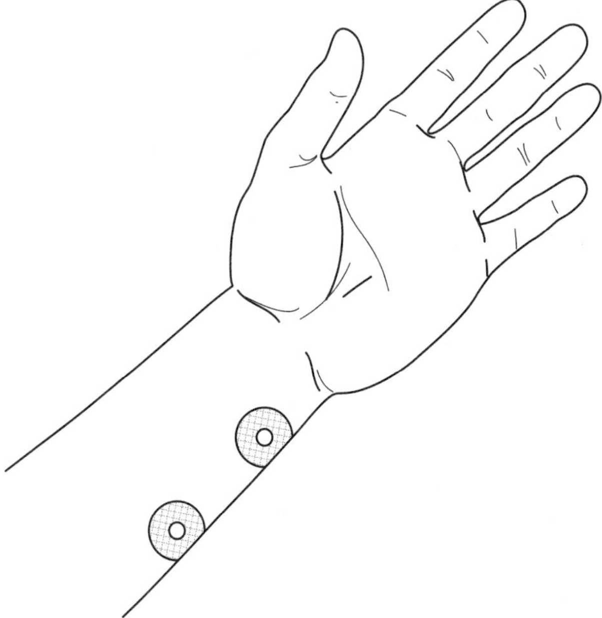

FIGURE 18-13 Ulnar nerve placement for TOF stimulation of the ulnar nerve. Electrodes are positioned in a direct line along the lateral side of the wrist. The thumb adducts to stimulation.

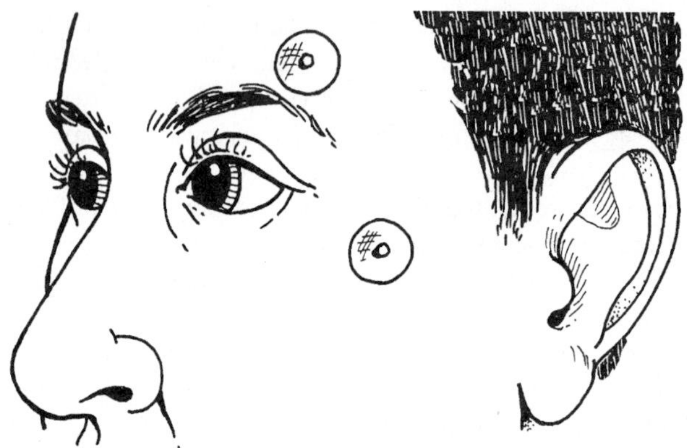

FIGURE 18-14 Facial nerve placement for TOF stimulation of the facial nerve. Electrodes are placed on either side of an imaginary line between the outer canthus of the eye and the tip of the ear. The muscles of the face will twitch when stimulated.

twitches during continuous infusion is a sign of a relative overdose of a neuromuscular blocking agent. In this situation the infusion should be discontinued until the one or two twitches return and then reinstated at a lower infusion rate.[258] If intermittent boluses are used, TOF should be repeated every 15 to 30 minutes and the next bolus not administered until at least a single twitch appears.

If TOF monitoring is not available, continuous infusion of the neuromuscular blocking agent should be stopped once a day and the time for return of some neuromuscular function noted. If this time is longer than 1 hour, the rate of infusion is empirically decreased on reinstatement of the continuous infusion. The amount of the decrease is related to the duration of prolonged NMB. For example, if a 1-hour recovery was expected but if 4 hours were required before movement, the dose may be decreased by 25% compared with 50% if 8 to 12 hours pass before movement. This prevents accumulation of the neuromuscular blocking agent. Regardless of whether TOF is used, all patients who receive infusions of these agents should have the infusions stopped once daily to assess blockade and to provide an opportunity for clinical evaluation to assess the adequacy of concomitant sedation and analgesia.

Problems With Train-of-Four Monitoring

Substantial edema and obesity are the most common factors affecting TOF monitoring. Electrode placement too far from the nerve and pressure applied to the electrodes can also affect response. Pressure decreases the electrode skin resistance and distance from the skin to the nerve, thus increasing the amount of current delivered and possibly leading to overstimulation. Use of surface electrodes and marking the location on the skin minimize variability between observers. Operator assessment of TOF is subjective and prone to misinterpretation. For example, two equal, strong thumb twitches with a faint third twitch may be interpreted as two twitches by one observer and as three twitches by another. Whether faint twitches should be included in the assessment is controversial and not addressed in the literature.

Equipment malfunction can produce a TOF error. Variability in current output has been documented at higher impedance with some peripheral nerve stimulators. Faulty connections of the stimulator to the electrodes, inadequate battery power, and improperly lubricated electrodes can contribute to erroneous TOF readings.

A major limitation to peripheral nerve stimulation is that the TOF of the ulnar nerve may not accurately reflect the depth of paralysis of the diaphragmatic and accessory respiratory muscle because of differences in sensitivities to NMB.[259,260] Some patients will have no response to TOF testing but may still demonstrate movement or response to stimulation, such as cough or gag when suctioned. Clinical assessment of patient response remains the standard when monitoring these patients, and TOF testing is performed to guide the maximal dose required. The maximal acceptable dose is determined by improvement in the parameter or condition being treated. Because of the many chances to introduce errors into TOF monitoring, the SCCM guidelines recommend that NMB be stopped at least once daily for clinical evaluation to assess the adequacy of concomitant sedation and analgesia and to determine whether continued paralysis is needed.[261]

Discontinuation and Reversal of Blockade

Most patients receiving neuromuscular blocking agents are allowed to regain neuromuscular function spontaneously. Several clinical techniques can be used to assess the adequacy of recovery: ability to open the eyes wide, to sustain protusion of the tongue, to maintain an effective handgrip, and to lift the head for 5 seconds.

In rare instances, waiting for the spontaneous recovery from nondepolarizing agents may be impractical and administration of reversing agents is necessary. Acetylcholinesterase inhibitors (ACIs) are administered to inhibit the destruction of acetylcholine by acetylcholinesterases. Acetylcholine concentration increases at the neuromuscular junction, and the binding of acetylcholine occurs more readily than the binding of the neuromuscular blocking agent to the acetylcholine receptors. Neostigmine, edrophonium, and pyridostigmine are the ACIs frequently used. These antagonists are not specific for nicotinic receptors and, when administered, result in toxic effects from the stimulation of muscarinic receptors. These toxic effects include excessive oral secretions, bronchospasm, and potentially severe bradycardia, which can lead to heart block, nodal escape rhythm, and premature ventricular contractions. Anticholinergic agents, atropine, or glycopyrrolate are concurrently administered to minimize or prevent these effects. The half-life and duration of the anticholinergic should be matched to the ACI. Atropine should be administered with edrophonium, and glycopyrrolate is best administered with neostigmine or pyridostigmine. Table 18-28 summarizes the intravenous doses of anticholinergics and ACIs.

Because succinylcholine is not metabolized by acetylcholinesterase, it diffuses away from the neuromuscular junction and is hydrolyzed in the plasma and liver by another enzyme,

TABLE 18-28 Anticholinesterase Inhibitors and Anticholinergic Doses for Reversal of Neuromuscular Blockade

Neostigmine + glycopyrrolate	Pyridostigmine + glycopyrrolate	Edrophonium + atropine
25-75 mcg/kg + 5-15 mcg/kg	100-300 mcg/kg + 5-15 mcg/kg	500-1000 mcg/kg + 10 mcg/kg

pseudocholinesterase. Fortunately, this is a rapid process in most patients because there are no reversal agents available for depolarizing blockade. In rare instances patients may have a pseudocholinesterase deficiency that results in a prolonged duration of blockade after succinylcholine administration.[262] Supportive care is provided to these patients until muscle function returns.

Adverse Effects

The undesired effects seen with neuromuscular blocking agents are generally of three different domains: (1) complications resulting from immobility, (2) adverse effects associated with individual agents, and (3) residual paralysis extending after discontinuation of the agent. The immobility produced by extended use of muscle relaxants increases the risk of pressure injury to nerves, skin pressure necrosis and ulceration, cough failure and retention of secretions, impaired ability to perform abdominal and neurologic examinations, and disuse atrophy.

Succinylcholine is associated with many adverse effects.[251] Most serious of these are hyperkalemia and rarely malignant hyperthermia syndrome. Massive muscle depolarization occurs, causing hypermetabolism and hyperkalemia. Although pretreatment or early treatment with dantrolene is effective, malignant hyperthermia syndrome can be fatal. Identifying a family or medical history of malignant hyperthermia is helpful in predicting this side effect.

Depending on the patient's autonomic nervous system, succinylcholine may increase or decrease heart rate and blood pressure. Additionally, succinylcholine commonly increases the serum potassium level 0.5 to 1 mEq/L. In rare cases serum potassium levels exceeding 5.0 mEq/L can occur. Medical conditions associated with this include upper motor neuron lesions or spinal cord injury, large burns, and massive trauma, including closed head injury. Patients become vulnerable within days of the injury and remain at risk for months. The subsequent cardiac arrest can be refractory to resuscitative efforts. Table 18-29 lists contraindications to succinylcholine.

TABLE 18-29 Contraindications to Succinylcholine Commonly Encountered in the Intensive Care Unit

Burns	Disuse atrophy
Spinal cord injury	Massive trauma
Hyperkalemia	Septic or hemorrhagic shock
Peripheral nerve injury	

Succinylcholine-induced fasciculations cause increases in intraocular and intragastric pressure. The cause of increased ICP is less understood. Increased intraocular pressure might extrude vitreous from a ruptured globe. Increased intragastric pressure may cause a patient with residual gastric contents to regurgitate and possibly aspirate. Cricoid pressure is applied when securing the airway to avoid aspiration. Whether succinylcholine should be avoided because of these increases is controversial. Uncoordinated muscle fasciculations are also thought to be responsible for the myalgias experienced by some patients.

The adverse effects associated with nondepolarizing relaxants involve the cardiovascular and respiratory system. Tubocurarine, atracurium, and mivacurium cause the release of H, which can cause hypotension and tachycardia in hypovolemic patients and wheezing in some patients.[263,264] Pancuronium has vagolytic activity that in some patients results in hypertension and tachycardia.[265,266] Vecuronium, doxacurium, pipecuronium, cisatracurium, and rocuronium have minimal cardiovascular effects.

Prolonged paralysis can lead to keratitis or corneal abrasions. Prophylactic eye care with methylcellulose eye drops, ophthalmic ointment, and possibly taping the eyelids shut can help prevent abrasions.[251]

The literature contains many reports of prolonged weakness in the ICU. Several distinct clinical syndromes of prolonged weakness have been identified. Critical illness polyneuropathy is both a sensory and motor polyneuropathy commonly observed in seriously ill, septic, and elderly patients.[267] Risk factors for the development of myopathy include coadministration of corticosteroids, high APACHE (Acute Physiology, Age, and Chronic Health Evaluation) III scores (a quantative index of disease severity), and systemic inflammatory response syndrome (a screen tool for severe sepsis).[251]

In contrast, critical illness myopathy is most likely a direct myotoxic effect from combining steroids and neuromuscular blocking agents.[267] The syndrome is characterized as a persistent moderate or severe flaccid, generalized weakness that becomes apparent after the agent is discontinued while sensory function is preserved.

Prolonged NMB occurs when neuromuscular transmission remains impaired and weakness persists after neuromuscular blocking agents are discontinued. The mechanism of prolonged weakness is thought to be caused by residual drug or active metabolites.[252,267-269] Routine TOF monitoring of the degree of NMB produced by the muscle relaxant and discontinuing the relaxant once daily to assess the patient can prevent overdose of the neuromuscular blocking agent and prolonged paralysis.[270-272]

The greatest problem associated with prolonged NMB is the delay in weaning patients from mechanical ventilation as a result of diaphragmatic or intercostal muscle weakness. No specific therapy is available, so the goal is prevention. Although TOF monitoring may prevent prolonged paralysis from neuromuscular blocking agents, there is no evidence that it prevents critical illness myopathy or polyneuropathy. Use and duration of these agents should be minimized. Most trauma patients requiring mechanical ventilation should be managed with sedatives and analgesics.

An additional problem described with neuromuscular blocking agents is the development of tachyphylaxis, or rapidly decreasing response to a drug after administration of the initial doses.[273] The SCCM recommends trying another agent if tachyphylaxis is noticed.[251,273]

Special Patient Populations

Spinal Cord Injury

Central pain may be the result of a lesion or dysfunction in the CNS, and it is correlated with sensory disturbances involving temperature and pain.[274] Spinal cord injury pain related to trauma is complex and may affect the patient's ability to participate in physical rehabilitation. Pain develops after the initial injury in approximately 60% to 70% of individuals, with about one third reporting severe pain.[275-277] Several types of pain may be experienced, which can be broadly categorized as nociceptive, neuropathic or central. These categories can be subdivided into musculoskeletal or visceral nociceptive pain, and above-level, at-level, or below-level neuropathic pain.[275] Further subdivisions incorporate specific structures involved, such as bone or muscular pain, complex regional pain syndrome, nerve root compression, or central dysesthesia syndrome.[275] Post–spinal cord injury pain can be characterized as (1) transitional zone pain, which is described as band-like pain in a dermatomal pattern at the level of injury, (2) diffuse central pain below the lesion involving posterior spinal cord tracts, and (3) pain related to delayed onset of syringomyelia involving cyst formation within the spinal cord occurring years after injury.[277]

The pathophysiologic mechanisms of central pain syndromes are still poorly understood and their treatment remains a major challenge.[278] It has long been suggested that lesions of the spinothalamic pathways, which carry pain and temperature discrimination, are involved in these pain syndromes. The recently proposed thermosensory disinhibition theory suggests that a reduced inhibition of thermal sensory afferents affecting nociceptive systems may play a major pathophysiologic role.[279] Pain and hypersensitivity that is experienced is believed to be the result of increased neuronal activity and reactivity along the somatosensory pathways and decreased inhibitory mechanisms.[274] Neuronal plasticity is a key factor that essentially alters the function of neurotransmitters, receptors, ion channels, and the structure of dorsal horn neurons.[280]

Treatment remains quite difficult, and many patients experience psychosocial and physical complaints, including anxiety, depression, insomnia, anorexia, and decreased quality of life.[281] A comprehensive management approach should include pharmacologic therapy to reduce symptoms and education and psychologic support. Patients usually describe distressing burning, shooting, and electric-type pain that is constant. Stimulus-evoked pain includes allodynia (pain evoked by a nonpainful touch) and hyperalgesia (increased pain evoked by a painful stimulus) (Table 18-30). Allodynia

TABLE 18-30 Descriptions of Chronic Pain Syndromes and Definitions of Pain Terms

Addiction: A primary, chronic neurobiologic disease that is genetically, psychosocially, and environmentally influenced. Behaviors include impaired control over drug use, compulsive use, continued use despite harm, and craving.
Allodynia: pain from a source that normally does not provoke pain.
Causalgia: a cluster of symptoms resulting from a traumatic nerve lesion (e.g., burning, allodynia, hyperpathia)
Central pain: pain resulting from a lesion or malfunction in the CNS
Dysesthesia: an unpleasant sensation
Hyperalgesia: an increased sensation after a painful stimulus
Hyperesthesia: increased sensitivity
Neuralgia: pain following the path of a nerve
Neuropathic pain: pain caused by a CNS lesion or malfunction
Paresthesia: abnormal sensation
Physical dependence: State of adaptation that includes tolerance, manifested by a drug class–specific withdrawal syndrome produced by abrupt cessation, rapid dose reduction, or administration of antagonist (American Pain Society, American Society of Addiction Medicine, American Academy of Pain Medicine)
Pseudoaddiction: Patient behaviors, such as "drug seeking," "clock watching," and use of illicit drugs that occur as a result of pain undertreatment. Behaviors resolve with effective pain management.
Tolerance: State of adaptation in which exposure to a drug induces changes that result in a diminution of one or more of the drug's effects over time (American Pain Society, American Society of Addiction Medicine, American Academy of Pain Medicine)

Modified from Merskey H, Bogduk N: *Classification of chronic pain: descriptions of chronic pain syndromes and definitions of pain terms,* ed 2, Seattle, 1994, ISAP and American Pain Society: Definitions related to the use of opioids for the treatment of pain: a consensus document from the American Academy of Pain Medicine (AAPM), the American Pain Society (APS), and the American Society of Addiction Medicine. (ASAM), 2001, American Pain Society.

can be caused by the lightest stimulation, such as skin contact with clothing or a light breeze. Expectations for pain control should be outlined initially to prevent unrealistic hopes of total pain relief.

First-line agents recommended for neuropathetic pain include antiepileptic drugs (gabapentin, pregabalin, carbamazepine, lamotrigine, oxcarbazepine, topiramate), sodium channel blockers (intravenous local anesthetics,[282] lidocaine 5% patch), analgesics (tramadol hydrochlorate, opioids), and antidepressants (amitriptyline, desipramine, nortriptyline, doxepin, imipramine).[143,148,274] Introduction of concurrent agents requires careful monitoring and dose titration related to adverse effects. Gabapentin is overall well tolerated, although dose adjustment may be indicated with renal insuffiency and the elderly.[283] Muscle spasticity can cause significant pain and can be controlled with the introduction of an antispastic agent (baclofen, tizanidine, benzodiazepines, dantrolene sodium).[277]

Amputation and Phantom Limb Pain

Phantom pain after amputation requires differentiation from phantom sensation, stump pain, and stump contractions.[284,285] A nonpainful phantom sensation is a continued perception of the missing limb. The phenomenon of telescoping is described as the gradual shortening of the sensation over time. Stump pain is the experience of localized pain near the end of the stump after amputation. Phantom pain is the distressing pain felt in the missing body part, with an incidence as high as 60% to 80%.[284] One retrospective study of traumatic amputees reported about a 25% incidence of phantom pain impeding prosthetic comfort and satisfaction.[286] Stump contractions are usually intermittent, spontaneous movements of the stump.

After an amputation, nociceptive activity is theorized to become overactive and hyperexcitable with reorganization of (1) peripheral afferent pathways, (2) the dorsal root ganglion, (3) the dorsal horn, (4) the brainstem and thalamus, (5) cortical structures, and (6) sympathetic activation.[284] Amputees have described stump pain as burning, throbbing, and squeezing pain.[287,288] Phantom pain has been described as pins and needles, throbbing, burning, shooting, tingling, and stabbing in the toes and foot after lower extremity amputation.[288,289] The nurse caring for the amputee must fully investigate all complaints of pain from the absent limb. It is not unusual for a lower leg amputee to complain of toes that are curling in an awkward position and ask for the nurse to straighten them out. Pain can also be described as intermittent and episodic.

Pharmacologic treatment for stump pain during the initial postoperative phase includes the use of traditional analgesics previously discussed. Phantom pain management requires a multimodal approach that can be directed at all levels of pain transmission and perception.[289] Sodium channel blockers, tricyclic antidepressants, MNDA antagonistic drugs, opioids, and clonidine have all been used for phantom pain control.[284] Intravenous ketamine is recommended as a third-line option for chronic, nonmalignant pain and has been cited in reducing postamputation phantom limb pain.[290,291]

The most common treatment modality for phantom pain is analgesic medication, including acetaminophen, combination acetaminophen-opioid agents, and NSAIDs.[292] Rehabilitative modalities, such as TENS application to the stump, physical therapy to prepare for prosthesis application, nerve blocks at trigger points and surgical interventions for neuroma removal can be used. Complementary methods, such as massage, acupuncture, chiropractic care, and hypnosis have also been used with some anecdotal success.[293-295]

Management in the Head-Injured Patient

After traumatic brain injury, the goal of care is to preserve neurologic function during the critical care phase. Sedative techniques are widely used to prevent secondary neurologic insult by stabilizing cerebral blood flow and metabolism during intensive monitoring. Patients receiving analgesia and sedation require frequent neurologic and hemodynamic assessment. Behavioral (increased posturing and agitation) and physiologic manifestations (increase in blood pressure and pulse) may be the only manifestations of pain.[296] The proactive treatment of pain may decrease the physiologic sequelae of the stress response after multisystem injury.

Pharmacologic pain management in acute head injury has a direct effect on the CNS, including cerebral blood flow and metabolism and ICP. Signs of neurologic deterioration must be appraised immediately. For example, decreased responsiveness, pupillary changes, motor function deterioration, cerebral hypoxia, or intracranial hypertension may indicate that cerebral metabolism is compromised and immediate intervention is indicated. Bolus dosing of fentanyl, alfentanil, and sufentanil have been linked to a significant but transient increase in ICP in patients with head trauma.[297] The use of short-acting agents should be individualized and titrated in small increments. Sedation, analgesics, and NMB can be used to treat intracranial hypertension by controlling agitation and pain and reducing oxygen demand. Appropriate monitoring of these medications is indicated. Sedation-level monitoring can be performed by clinical assessment and the BIS index monitor.[298]

With coma emergence, patient response to sedatives should be assessed and documented after each administration, including level of consciousness, respiratory rate, blood pressure, and pulse rate. Use of a sedation algorithm, with a sedation scale, is recommended to provide consistency among different practitioners. Hypotension must be avoided after head injury to prevent secondary brain injury; thus, close monitoring of hemodynamic and volume status is indicated with analgesic or sedative use. Narcotic effects are reversed by the antagonist naloxone, which may be needed for a neurologic examination.

The most frequently reported complaints of pain with coma emergence after traumatic brain injury include headache, muscloskeletal pain, spasticity, neuropathetic pain, and facial pain.[299] Persistent neck pain and occipital headaches are reported as a major source of disability after whiplash injury.[300] Pharmacologic options include acetaminophen, NSAIDs, antiepileptics, SSRIs, β-blockers, calcium-channel blockers, and steroids.[299] Intrathecal baclofen infusions for lower limb hypertonia and botulinum toxin injections for spasticity have provided positive outcomes.[301,302] Nonpharmacologic interventions, which include positioning and massage, can also be applied to promote relaxation and comfort.

NURSING CARE THROUGH THE PHASES OF TRAUMA

RESUSCITATIVE PHASE

Goals during the resuscitative phase of care include minimizing physical pain and anxiety, decreasing negative psychologic responses, and maximizing amnesia during painful procedures. Priorities of care regarding airway, ventilation, and circulation are paramount. Respiratory monitoring, continuous pulse oximetry and capnography trending, and sedation appraisal are priority nursing actions during this phase of care. Considering the mechanism of injury, patient appearance, and associated injuries can aid the nurse in identifying potential areas of pain or discomfort. Baseline neurologic assessment and presentation of deficits should be documented during the primary survey before analgesics, sedatives or paralytics are administered. Short-acting analgesics and sedatives can be titrated in incremental doses to effect if emergency intubation is required. Careful monitoring of patient response to agents delivered is important.

Providing procedural sedation and analgesia before painful procedures requires specific nursing competence and expertise. The Emergency Nurses Association and the American College of Emergency Physicians (ACEP) support the administration of medications used for procedural sedation and analgesia by credentialed emergency nurses while directly supervised.[303,304] Practice guidelines and standards of care for sedation and analgesic administration have been established by specialty organizations such as the American Society of Anesthesiologists (ASA), the American College of Critical Care Medicine, and ACEP and should be considered when developing trauma analgesic and sedation protocols for use in the emergency department setting.[305] Use of evidence-based clinical practice protocols has the potential to improve the quality of nursing knowledge in the resuscitative environment as well as improve patient care. Specific institutional policies and procedures should address education and training for the trauma team, monitoring standards, documentation, availability of anesthesiologists, and the use of a dedicated pain service.[305]

Before the administration of analgesic and sedative agents in the nonemergent situation, a thorough history and physical examination is indicated to establish any preexisting comorbid medical conditions, especially those that may affect airway condition.[306] For those administering sedatives and analgesics, expertise and advanced training in airway Mallampati classification and management is required, along with physical status classification according to the ASA.[160] Fasting guidelines should be followed before elective sedative and analgesia administration as recommended by the ASA: a 2-hour fast for clear liquids and a 6-hour fast for solids and other fluids.[307,308] Expert management of airway and resuscitation at a Level 1 trauma center should include immediate 24-hour availability of specialized anesthesiologists and nurses who provide advanced life support.[309]

Administration of analgesic agents and sedatives will greatly depend on the acuity of the patient and the need to perform pain-producing interventions. The goal of procedural analgesia is to minimize adverse psychologic responses to pain with preservation of airway. The intravenous route is the preferred method of administration during this phase of care because a more predictable response can be attained. However, the manual administration of an opiod bolus has been associated with a significant increase in ICP related to a decrease in blood pressure in severely brain-injured patients receiving mechanical ventilation.[310]

Nursing responsibilities include preparation of the patient, monitoring during the procedure, ensuring that emergency equipment availability, and demonstration of appropriate actions in the event of complications. Ensuring the readiness of resuscitative equipment and reversal agents is imperative. Standards for monitoring and documenting patient response, safety of airway, return to baseline level of consciousness, and vital signs determines the necessary level of intensive nursing care. Using standardized sedation and pain scales across the trauma continuum is recommended.

Analgesic and sedative agents should be administered before start of pain-producing procedures, such as orthopedic realignments. Verbal reassurance and explanation of procedures, along with nonpharmacologic interventions, can be used with some patients. The frequency of analgesic and sedative administration should be individualized and titrated to a desired end point. Effective analgesia and sedation is a reduction in the pain intensity rating according to a standardized pain scale without compromised ventilation or side effect presentation. A decrease in pain behaviors, such as resolution of thrashing movements, would be an indication of pain relief in the patient unable to verbalize pain. Compromised ventilation and oxygenation may be the root cause of agitation and must be corrected before administration of analgesic and sedative agents.

PERIOPERATIVE PHASE

Perioperative nursing care is directed to assessment and preparation of the patient for operative management of injuries and promoting a safe environment as the patient transitions from one phase to another on the trauma continuum. Offering education related to expected procedures, monitoring equipment, airway control, and expected disposition should be introduced once a definitive plan is established. Application of TJC's National Safety Goals[311] can provide a framework for care. Proper identification of the patient before insertion of analgesic catheters, applying a time out protocol to ascertain correct location of catheters, and accurately communicating and documenting patient information are goals specific to safe analgesic care.

Ensuring that the correct analgesic agent is correctly labeled on and off the sterile field in the perioperative and procedural area is required. The perioperative nurse has a role in maintaining aseptic technique when connecting analgesic infusions and validating the right route for delivery through line reconciliation. Protecting the patient from fall or injury during periods of sedation administration or positioning for analgesic catheter placement remains an important responsibility. Hand-off communication can be accomplished through a thorough systems report, with a review of agents administered during the operative course.

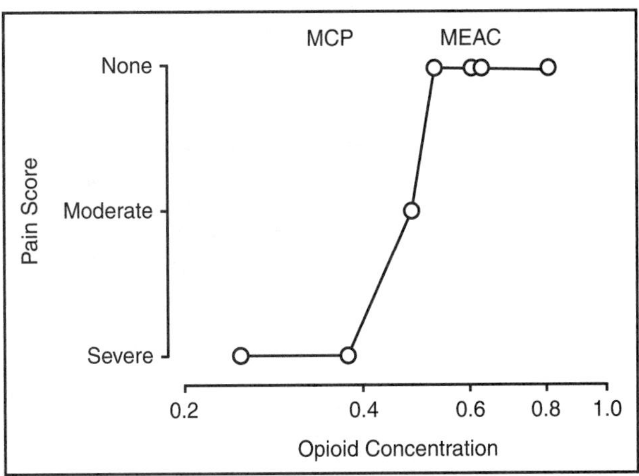

FIGURE 18-15 A theoretic representation of the steepness of the concentration/response curve for opioids is shown. The x-axis is plasma opioid concentration; the y-axis is pain rated from severe *(bottom)* to none *(top)*. *Circles* represent sequential measurements of opioid concentration and the corresponding pain values during an interval when opioid concentration is increasing. With increasing opioid concentrations, progressive increases in concentration initially produce no change in pain, then over a finite range of concentrations, pain is attenuated, and then further increases in opioid concentration produce no additional effect. MCP or "maximum concentration pain" is the maximum concentration of opioid associated with severe pain. MEAC or "minimum effective analgesic concentration" is the smallest opioid concentration at which pain is relieved. (Adapted from Austin KL, Stapleton JV, Mather LE: Relationship between blood meperidine concentrations and analgesic response: a preliminary report, Anesthesiology 53:460-466, 1980.)

Critical Care Phase

Analgesic, sedation, and neuromuscular blockade delivery during the critical care phase offer both risk and benefit to critically ill patients. Integrating critical thinking nursing skill and wireless networking is one strategy to improve medication delivery safety. Networking can accelerate best practice and process improvements with intravenous drug infusions.[312] An optimal plan of care considers several factors, including the presence of comorbid medical conditions, the hemodynamic stability of the patient, and the potential for complications. Clinical practice guidelines for the care of the patient receiving analgesia, sedation, and NMB should be integrated in the development of evidence-based critical care nursing practice and protocols.[194,313] Continuous quality programs should monitor clinical issues.[314]

An analgesic plan for the multi-injured patient should include multimodal analgesic regimens that will optimize pain control, reduce opioid requirements and potential opioid-related side effects, and enhance overall patient outcome. Analgesic techniques used in the critically ill include administration of opioids through continuous infusions, intravenous bolus dosing, and PCA or patient-controlled epidural analgesia therapies. The therapeutic window for attainment of effective analgesic effects is between a minimal effective concentration (MEC) and maximal effective concentration (MaxEC) (Figure 18-15). Pain relief within this therapeutic window involves repeatedly titrating or front-loading small doses of analgesic agents until the desired effect is achieved (Figure 18-16).[93] Insufficient analgesia and the perception of pain occur below the MEC. Side effects of agents, or toxicity, such as respiratory depression, occur above the MaxEC. Pain assessment and response to analgesic therapy must be performed regularly by use of a pain scale appropriate to the patient. Setting individualized acceptable pain goals and maintaining the therapeutic analgesic level can be accomplished with a basal infusion. "Rescue" dosing for breakthrough pain can be administered by the nurse or patient if analgesic effect decreases below MEC.

Safe practice recommendations for intravenous PCA therapy include criteria for patient selection, standardized order sets and protocols, monitoring protocols, two-clinician double-checks, patient and family education, and hospital staff education.[315,316] A selection criterion requires an awake, cooperative patient who has the ability to understand and interface with the device. This therapy gives the patient the ability to titrate his or her opioid dose to achieve an acceptable pain rating. Preemptive use of intravenous PCA is encouraged before pain-related activities and mobilization. Standardized order sets and protocols should include drug selection, dosing, lock-out intervals, precautions with concomitant analgesics, oxygen delivery recommendations, and naloxone reversal guidelines.[317]

Capnography has been successfully shown to detect hypoventilation with PCA therapy, and it can be incorporated into a monitoring protocol that identifies at-risk patients. Patients who are known retainers of carbon dioxide, have a history of congestive heart failure, are at high risk for pulmonary embolism or deep venous thrombosis, and have an oxygen saturation <92% require a higher level of monitoring.[318] Pulse oximetry monitoring can supplement the nursing assessment of respiratory rate, depth, and rhythm, and sedation assessment. The use of multimodality PCA pumps that can monitor oxygenation (pulse oximetry) and ventilation (capnography) during parenteral administration of narcotics seems a promising new direction for the future.[319] This technology can follow the patient through the trauma continuum because critical care monitoring decreases with patient status improvement to nonintensive care settings.

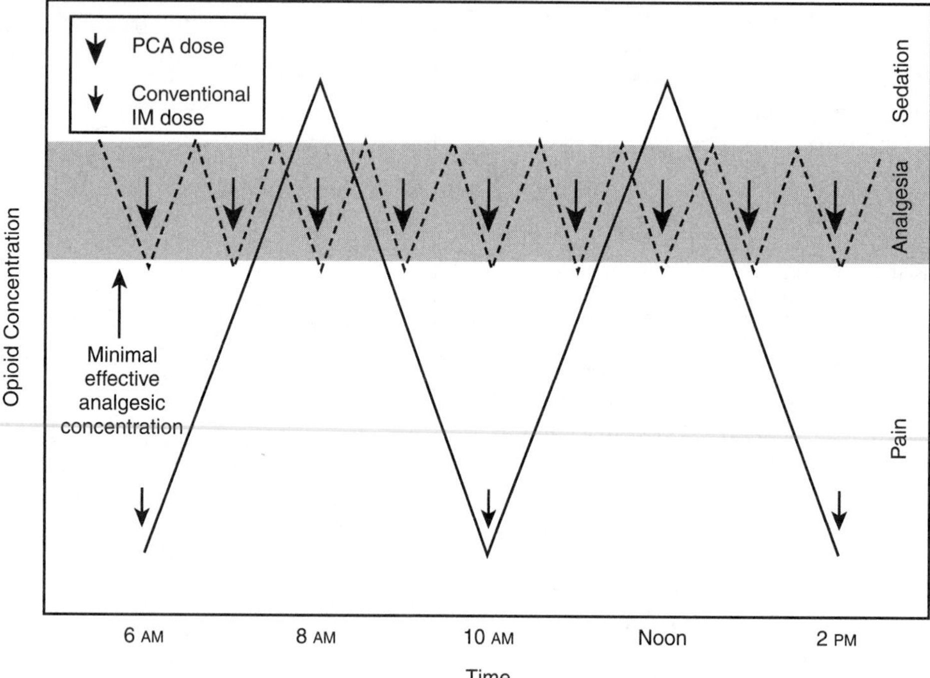

FIGURE 18-16 Pain/sedation/respiratory depression therapeutic window. Analgesia achieved with intermittent bolus administration (nurse-administered analgesia) is compared with that obtained through frequent small doses (PCA). The *shaded area* represents the target analgesic concentration. With intermittent bolus administration, there are frequent periods with concentrations more than and less than the target range. In contrast, PCA results in the opioid concentration being in the target range for a large percentage of the time. *(Adapted from Ferrante FM, Covino BG: Patient-controlled analgesia: a historical perspective. In Ferrante FM, Ostheimer GW, Covino BG, editors:* Patient-controlled analgesia, *pp 3-9, Boston, 1990, Blackwell Scientific Publications.)*

Epidural catheter placement to deliver analgesia to selected areas of painful injury includes thoracic level to be used for chest and higher abdominal discomfort and lumbar catheters to manage lower extremity pain. Regional catheters offer analgesia to a directed dermatomal region. A higher skill level is required for nurses caring for patients with epidural or regional catheters, thus necessitating institutional-specific educational programs to addresses competence within regulatory practice parameters. Elements of nursing competence include patient assessment, catheter and analgesic pump maintenance, knowledge of agents used for analgesia, treatment and prevention of side effects, and management of potential complications related to catheter technique (Table 18-31). Epidural and regional catheter technique protocols can be established to standardized infusion composition, to define duration of therapy to coincide with clinical pathways, and to outline frequency of patient assessment. Standardized pain assessment and documentation of vital signs is frequent during the initiation of therapy to establish stable analgesic levels and patient response to therapy. Unit-specific protocols can be established to address patient monitoring and treatment of analgesic gaps related to technologic difficulties of the pump, catheter problems, and breakthrough pain.[320] Loading doses through the pump, upward titration, and supplemental systemic opioid delivery for severe pain should be included in the standing order set.

Nursing priorities include monitoring patient response to analgesic therapy, preserving hemodynamic status, assessing motor strength, preserving skin integrity, and treatment of side effects. Patient education with regard to catheter technique, technology interface, and expected analgesic effects is important. Managing breakthrough pain requires a thorough dermatomal assessment, catheter integrity check, pump history interface, and evaluation of level of consciousness. Optimizing the analgesic level may require titration of the analgesic volume or drug concentration. With patient-controlled epidural analgesia therapy, orthostasis with mobilization requires treatment to support hemodymic status and protect perfusion of vital organs. Fluid replacement, reduction of the epidural infusion or concentration, or the addition of a vasoconstrictor agent are strategies to reduce the vasodilation effects of the local anesthetic.[321]

Falls precautions should be instituted on all patients until motor strength assessment is completed and deemed sufficient before mobilization.[322] Motor strength assessment is required before weight bearing with lumbar-level patient-controlled epidural analgesia. Using the modified Bromage assessment method ensures that consistent evaluation technique and reporting is used by all health care team members.[323] On a three-point scale (0-3) 0 means that there is no motor impairment and the patient is able to move joints of the hip, knee, and ankle; Bromage 1 presents the patient with an inability to raise

TABLE 18-31 **Side Effects and Complications Related to Epidural Technique**

Potential Side Effects Related to Local Anesthetics	Potential Side Effects Related to Opioids	Complications of Catheter Technique
Hypotension caused by sympathetic response	Decreased gastrointestinal motility	Catheter displacement (intrathecal migration) or dislodgement
Increased gastrointestinal motility	Nausea and vomiting	Dural puncture
Motor block resulting in leg weakness to complete loss of function	Pruritus	Epidural hematoma
Urinary retention	Urinary retention	Epidural abscess
Neurotoxicity progresses to cardiotoxicity resulting from excessive plasma levels; signs and symptoms are listed in order of severity as plasma concentration increases:	Sedation/respiratory depression	
Light-headedness		
Circumoral numbness or numbness of the tongue		
Tinnitus, visual disturbances		
Muscular twitching		
Drowsiness		
Convulsions		
Coma		
Respiratory arrest		
Cardiovascular depression		

Adapted from Weetman C, Allison W: Use of epidural analgesia in post-operative pain management, *Nurs Stand* 20:54-64, 2006.

the extended leg but able to move joints of the knee and ankle; Bromage 2 motor block has the patient unable to raise the extended leg and flex the knee but is still able to flex the ankle joint; and Bromage 3 is considered a total motor block with no movement of the knee and foot. With partial or complete motor block, downward titration of rate or concentration of infusion may be considered, and special attention should be given to skin integrity. Frequent assessment of bony prominences, with change in position, is required, especially in the heels and buttocks. Patients with isolated regional blocks need special attention to extremity position to avoid nerve compression and stretching injuries.[324]

Side effect management should be included in a standing management protocol. Pruritus, common in the facial region, is likely due to the cephalad spread of neuraxial opioids in the cerebrospinal fluid and trigeminal nucleus.[325] H is not released, so antihistamine administration is unlikely to prevent neuraxial opioid-induced pruritus.[326] Naloxone infusions at 2 mcg/kg per hour or less, ondansetron, and propofol at 30 mg per 24-hour infusion have been suggested as treatment options.[327] Nausea and vomiting can be controlled through decreasing or eliminating the opioid in the patient-controlled epidural analgesia, downward titration of the infusion, administering low-dose naloxone, and offering antiemetics.[328,329] Urinary retention, related to parasympathetic nervous system inhibition, can be treated through bladder assessment and catheterization.[330]

The SCCM practice guidelines can be applied when individualized protocols are developed for the critically ill adult requiring mechanical ventilation, analgesia, and sedation. An algorithm can be used to differentiate the need for analgesia, sedation, or anxiolytic therapy in the critically injured patient (Figure 18-11). This allows the nurse to choose interventions on the basis of the current assessment of pain and patient behavioral presentation and to provide consistency in goal setting. For patients unable to self-report pain, listing conditions and procedures that cause pain, documenting "assume pain present," and delivering pre-emptive analgesics before painful procedures, as well as delivering analgesics continuously, is suggested.[39] Fentanyl, hydromorphone, and morphine are suggested analgesic agents.[194] Patients should be closely monitored for self-extubation during periods of awakening or weaning.

Technology has been developed to enhance the assessment of sedation level, and it can be applied in the critical care environment. BIS index monitoring (Figure 18-17) has been used to measure the effects of sedatives and anesthetics on the brain.[331] Patients at risk for awareness while receiving anesthetics include those with a history of substance use or abuse, chronic pain with high-dose opioid use, and intraoperative awareness.[332] The BIS device can aid the health care team by providing EEG data that can be used in conjunction with patient presentation, clinical vital signs, and sedation scale assessment to modify sedation. The temporal sensor must be applied accurately to the patient's forehead. Muscular twitching from pain, seizures, and eye movement may alter BIS index parameters.[333]

Sedative and analgesic medications should be maximized before the institution of NMB. Long-term use of sedation, analgesia, and NMB alters physical conditioning.[334] Nursing care measures for the patient receiving NMB include frequent

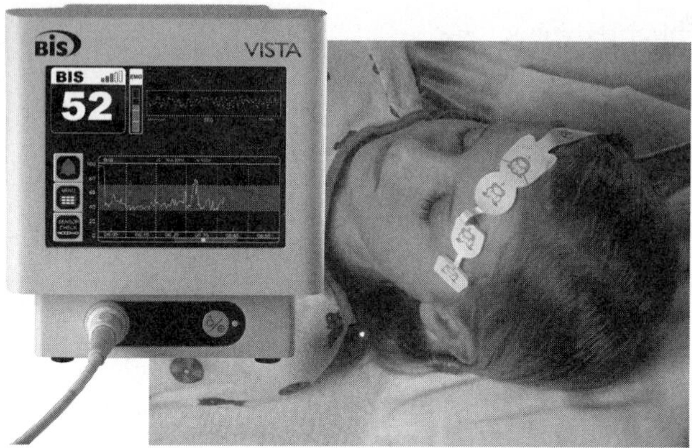

FIGURE 18-17 BIS monitor and electrode placement. *(Courtesy of Aspect Medical Systems: http://inservice.aspectmedical.com/500/200.htm. Accessed May 21, 2006.)*

position changes and turning at least every 2 hours to prevent atelectasis and pressure injuries to skin and nerves. Specialty beds can be instituted to assist in relieving pressure and to facilitate frequent repositioning. Maintaining good body alignment to promote comfort and obtaining consultation from physical and occupational therapists for positioning splints and joint support are important interventions during NMB. Muscle deconditioning occurs, and scheduled range-of-motion exercises for extremities are indicated on a regular basis. Deep vein thrombosis prophylaxis through use of extremity compression devices and anticoagulant therapy will minimize the risk of deep vein thrombosis and pulmonary embolus. The blink reflex is absent during NMB, necessitating ocular administration of polyethylene film, ointments, or drops to prevent corneal abrasions.[335] Professional staff must monitor bedside conversation, and verbal reassurances and explanations of care should occur frequently and consistently. A visual reminder for staff and family that the patient is chemically immobilized should be placed near the patient's bedside.

Environmental control of temperature, lighting, and excessive noise are nursing measures to decrease unnecessary stimulation during this phase of care. Time for rest and promotion of sleep should be provided at scheduled intervals. Liberal visiting policies offer friends and family the opportunity to provide verbal reassurances and support.

Intermediate Phase

Pain in the intermediate phase remains acute, with varying degrees of intensity, and may become episodic as a result of operative or therapeutic procedures as recovery from injury continues. When planned surgical interventions occur, patient preparation and inclusion of an analgesic plan is recommended. This allows the patient to establish acceptable levels of pain and expectations of analgesia postoperatively. Preoperative teaching offers preparation for patients to effectively communicate their pain rating and to operate PCA devices that may be used postoperatively. Repetitive procedures are causes of episodic pain, and pretreatment with short-acting opioids and nonpharmacologic strategies may be warranted. Pain may linger after the procedure, and reassessment of analgesic requirements is indicated.

Tolerance is a gradual loss in drug effect on repeated administration, requiring increasing doses to maintain analgesia. Dependence reflects a change in neuronal homeostasis that results in withdrawal symptoms on cessation of drug administration.[336] Abrupt discontinuance of the opioid can elicit withdrawal syndrome. Tapering or weaning the dose of the agent over time helps to alleviate withdrawal symptoms. There is accumulating evidence that opioid therapy might not only be associated with the development of tolerance but also with an increased sensitivity to pain, a condition referred to as opioid-induced hyperalgesia.[337] Morphine is the first-line opioid of choice for most patients with severe acute pain. Although most patients achieve adequate analgesia with morphine, some may have intolerable side effects or inadequate pain relief. Switching to an alternative opioid is becoming established clinical practice, although the evidence for the effectiveness of opioid switching does not appear to be established.[338]

As the control of pain stabilizes, with the return of gastrointestinal function parental or neuraxil analgesics can be converted to an equivalent oral route. Pharmacologic principles of equianalgesia can be applied to facilitate the transition from one route or agent to another. *Equianalgesia* refers to the dose of one agent producing the same analgesic effect as another agent or route. An equianalgesia chart or opioid conversion chart (Table 18-10) is a guide to establish doses of another agent on the basis of morphine equivalent. Patient reluctance to switch from one effective route to another may be encountered. Patient education regarding the method and agent delivery schedule may decrease anxiety related to change.

Practices of pre-emptive dosing before painful events and automatic around-the-clock dosing are recommended during the intermediate phase of care. Combined with oral analgesics, nonpharmacologic measures can be applied to promote comfort. Patient participation and interest in using alternative modalities may be suggested. Massage of painful joints, stretching and relaxation, along with the application of heat and cold, can also be therapeutic.

Rehabilitation Phase

The need for specialty services identified during the intermediate phase will determine the level of care required for rehabilitation, which may include home health care, inpatient rehabilitation, long-term care, or a skilled nursing facility.[339] Goals related to analgesia include promoting an effective plan for participation in rehabilitative therapy and achieving optimal functional status.[340] A multidisciplinary assessment and functional evaluation should be performed during this phase of care,[341,342] and functional recovery expectations need to be outlined.[343] Balancing an integrative analgesic regimen with achieving goals related to return to functional employment, reintegration to the community with positive socialization skills, and promotion of sleep and nutritional intake are important considerations when establishing a plan for effective analgesia.

Pain during the rehabilitative phase of care is usually still acute in nature, particularly from injuries requiring lengthy healing, immobilization, and repetitive reconstructive surgery. Patients with complex orthopedic injuries continue to have significant pain, and oral narcotic opioid administration should continue. The choice of agent should be individualized, and pharmacologic safety is important. For the patient requiring increasing doses of products containing acetaminophen or aspirin, a sustained-release opioid preparation may be indicated. Equianalgesic dose conversion, careful monitoring, and a tapering plan can be coordinated with a pain management team. Reassessment of pain in conjunction with healing is paramount, especially when the patient is seen in an outpatient environment. Nursing pain assessment should be detailed, and formalized pain questionnaires are useful in obtaining a comprehensive pain history after traumatic injury.

Physical therapy is an important aspect of this phase of care. Complaints of dull pain with muscle ache and spasm may occur as a result of muscle stretching and activity. Rest, elevation, massage, and the application of moist compresses are nonpharmacologic interventions that can decrease the stress and strain of exercise and activity. Adjunct medications can be offered if pain is not relieved by nonpharmacologic interventions and nonopioid analgesics. Muscle relaxants decrease muscle spasm and tension that could be the cause of pain. Major side effects from these agents include drowsiness, sedation, and gastrointestinal upset.

After complex traumatic injuries, some patients may have chronic persistent pain, which requires specialized assessment and care. Patients with posttraumatic stress symptoms have been reported to experience more physical impairment, psychologic distress, and maladaptive pain-coping strategies.[344] The International Association for the Study of Pain has classified, defined, and described chronic pain syndromes and terms. Table 18-30 offers a synopsis of terms and syndromes. A multidisciplinary approach to chronic pain management requires expertise and follow-up. Referral to a specialist in chronic pain management may be indicated.

SUMMARY

Cost-effective protocol- and pathway-driven pain and sedation management must become standard in the current climate of health care cost containment. Consistent monitoring for appropriate response and side effects related to therapies requires specialized skill and knowledge. Trauma patients often require aggressive analgesia and sedation management. Maintaining a current knowledge base of target analgesic techniques and new analgesic agents will enable the nurse to offer patients safe quality care.

REFERENCES

1. Arnstein P: Optimizing perioperative pain management, *AORN J* 76:812-818, 2002.
2. Emons MF: Persistent nonmalignant pain: implications and opportunities for managed care, *Manag Care* 12(8 suppl):2-7, 2003.
3. Rupp T, Delaney KA: Inadequate analgesia in emergency medicine, *Ann Emerg Med* 43:494-503, 2004.
4. Puntillo K, Neighbor MI, O'Neil N et al: Accuracy of emergency nurses in assessment of patients' pain, *Pain Manag Nurs* 4:171-175, 2003.
5. Silka PA, Roth MM, Moreno G et al: Pain scores improve analgesic administration patterns for trauma patients in the emergency department, *Acad Emerg Med* 11:264-271, 2004.
6. White LJ, Cooper JD, Chambers RM et al: Pre-hospital use of analgesia for suspected extremity fractures, *Prehosp Emerg Care* 4:205-208, 2000.
7. Brown JC, Klein EJ, Lewis CW et al: Emergency department analgesia for fracture pain, *Ann Emerg Med* 42:197-205, 2003.
8. Richards CF: Establishing an emergency department pain management system, *Emerg Med Clin North Am* 23:519-527, 2005.
9. Garbez R, Puntillo K: Acute musculoskeletal pain in the emergency department: a review of the literature and implications for the advanced practice nurse, *AACN Clin Issues* 16:310-319, 2005.
10. Neighbor ML, Honner S, Kohn MA: Factors affecting emergency department opioid administration to severely injured patients, *Acad Emerg Med* 11:1290-1296, 2004.
11. Pasero C: Pain in the emergency department: withholding pain medication is not justified, *Am J Nurs* 103:73-74, 2003.
12. Ritsema TS, Kelen GD, Pronovost PJ et al: The national trend in quality of emergency department pain management for long bone fractures, *Acad Emerg Med* 14:163-169, 2007.
13. Phelan C, Todd KH, Nichols R et al: Pain management issues for the emergency department and trauma patients, *Nurse Reporter* 1:25-29, 2003.
14. Stanik-Hutt JA: Pain management in the critically ill, *Crit Care Nurse* 23:99, 2003.
15. Pasero C, McCaffery M: No self-report means no pain-intensity rating: assessing pain in patients who cannot provide a report, *Am J Nurs* 105:50-53, 2005.
16. Public Health Service, Agency for Health Care Policy and Research: *Acute pain management: operative or medical procedures and trauma,* Clinical Practice Guideline No. 1, Publication No. 92:0032, Rockville, MD, 1992, U.S. Department of Health and Human Services.
17. Kehlet H, Jensen T, Woolf C: Persistent postsurgical pain: risk factors and prevention, *Lancet* 367:1618-1625, 2006.
18. Brennen TJ, Kehlet H: Preventive analgesia to reduce wound hyperalgesia and persistent postsurgical pain, *Anesthesiology* 103:681-683, 2005.
19. Merskey H, Bugduk N: *Classification of chronic pain: descriptions of chronic pain syndromes and definitions of pain terms,* 2nd ed, Seattle, WA, 1994, International Association for the Study of Pain Press: www.iasp-pain.org. Accessed July 30, 2007.
20. Pasero C, McCaffery M: Pain in the critically ill, *Am J Nurs* 102:59-60, 2002.

21. Clevlen E: From mechanisms to management: translating the neuropathic pain consensus recommendations into clinical practice, *J Am Acad Nurse Practitioners* 17(6 Suppl):4-17, 2005.
22. McCaffery M, Pasero C: *Pain: clinical manual,* 2nd ed, St. Louis, 1999, Mosby.
23. De Pinto M, Dunbar PJ, Edwards WT: Pain management, *Anesthesiol Clin North Am* 24:19-37, 2006.
24. Fink WA: The pathophysiology of acute pain, *Emerg Med Clin North Am* 23:277-284, 2005.
25. Renn C, Dorsey S: The physiology and processing of pain: a review, *AACN Clin Issues* 16:277-290, 2005.
26. Beaulieu P, Rice AS: Applied physiology of nociception. In Rowbotham DJ, Macintyre PE, editors: *Clinical management of acute pain,* pp 4-14, New York, 2003, Arnold Publishers.
27. Terman GW, Bonica JJ: Spinal mechanisms and their modulation. In Loser JD, Butler SH, Champion CR, editors: *Bonica's management of pain,* 3rd ed, pp 84-122, Philadelphia, 2001, Lippincott Williams & Wilkins.
28. Bushnell MC, Apkarian AV: Representation of pain in the brain. In McMahon SB, Koltzenburg M, editors: *Wall and Melzack's textbook of pain,* 5th ed, New York, 2005, Churchill Livingstone.
29. Gutstein HB, Akil H: Opioid analgesics. In Brunton LL, Lazo JS, Parker KL, editors: *Goodman and Gilman's the pharmacological basis of therapeutics,* 11th ed, pp 547-590, New York, 2006, McGraw-Hill.
30. Waldhoer M, Bartlett S, Whistler JL: Opioid receptors, *Annu Rev Biochem* 73:953-990, 2004.
31. Agency for Health Care Policy and Research: *Management of cancer pain,* Clinical Practice Guideline No. 9, Publication No. 94-0592, Rockville, MD, 1994, U.S. Department of Health and Human Services.
32. Seguin D: A nurse initiated pain management advanced triage protocol for ED patients with an extremity injury at a level I trauma center, *J Emerg Nurs* 30:330-335, 2004.
33. ASPAN pain and comfort clinical guideline, *J PeriAnesthesia Nurs* 18:232-236, 2003.
34. American Pain Society: *Principles of analgesic use in the treatment of acute pain and cancer pain,* 5th ed, Glenview, IL, 2003, American Pain Society.
35. Young J, Siffleet J, Nikoletti S et al: Use of Behavioural Pain Scale to assess pain in ventilated, unconscious and/or sedated patients, *Intensive Crit Care Nurs* 22:32-39, 2006.
36. Li D, Puntillo K: What is the current evidence on pain and sedation assessment in nonresponsive patients in the intensive care unit? *Crit Care Nurse* 24:68-72, 2004.
37. Kwekkeboom KL, Herr K: Assessment of pain in the critically ill, *Crit Care Nurs Clin North Am* 13:181-194, 2001.
38. Pasero C, McCaffery M: When patients can't report pain, *Am J Nurs* 100:22-23, 2003.
39. Herr K, Coyne PJ, Key T et al: Pain assessment in the nonverbal patient: position statement with clinical practice guidelines, *Pain Manage Nurs* 7:44-52, 2006.
40. Erdek M, Pronovost P: Improving assessment and treatment of pain in the critically ill, *Int J Qual Health Care* 16:59-64, 2004.
41. DeJong MM, Burns S, Campbell ML et al: Development of the American Association of Critical-Care Nurses' Sedation Assessment Scale for critically ill patients, *Am J Crit Care* 14:531-544, 2005.
42. Nygaard HA, Jarland M: The Checklist of Nonverbal Pain Indicators (CNPI): testing of reliability and validity in Norwegian nursing homes, *Age Ageing* 35:79-81, 2006.
43. Guignard B: Monitoring analgesia, *Best Pract Res Clin Anaesthesiol* 20:161-180, 2006.
44. American Geriatric Society Panel on Chronic Pain in Older Persons: The management of persistent pain in older persons: AGS panel on persistent pain in older persons, *J Am Geriatr Soc* 6:S205-S224, 2002.
45. Herr KA, Garand L: Assessment and measurement of pain in older adults, *Clin Geriatr Med* 17:457-478, 2001.
46. Herr K: Pain assessment in cognitively impaired older adults: new strategies and careful observation help pinpoint unspoken pain, *Am J Nurs* 102:65-67, 2002.
47. Abbey JA, Pillar B, De Bellis A et al: The Abbey pain scale: a 1-minute indicator for people with end-stage dementia, *Int J Palliat Nurs* 10:6-13, 2004.
48. Campbell J: Presidential address. Presented at the annual meeting of the American Pain Society. Los Angeles, CA, November 11, 1995.
49. Cohen MZ, Easley MK, Ellis C et al: Cancer pain management and the JCAHO's pain standards: an institutional challenge, *J Pain Symptom Manage* 25:519-527, 2003.
50. The Joint Commission: http://www.jointcommission.org/JCAHO. Accessed July 19, 2006.
51. Abbadie C, Pasternack G: Opioid receptors. In Quirion A, Bjorkland T, Hokfelt R, editors: *Handbook of chemical neuranatomy: peptide receptors, part ii,* pp 1-29, Amsterdam, 2003, Elsevier.
52. Hartrick CT: Multimodal postoperative pain management: clinical advances in the management of postoperative pain: symposium, *Am J Health System Pharm* 61:(1 Suppl):S4-S10, 2004.
53. Snyder SH, Pasternak GW: Historical review: opioid receptors, *Trends Pharmacol Sci* 24:198-205, 2003.
54. Terman G, Bonica JJ: Spinal mechanisms and their modulation. In Loeser JD, Butler SD et al, editors: *Bonica's management of pain,* 3rd ed, pp 73-152, Baltimore, 2001, Lippincott Williams & Wilkins.
55. Inturrisi CE: Clinical pharmacology of opioids for pain,. *Clin J Pain* 18:S3-S13, 2002.
56. Miller RD, editor: *Miller's anesthesia,* 6th ed, Philadelphia, 2005, Elsevier Churchill Livingstone.
57. Pasero C: Fentanyl for acute pain management, *J PeriAnesthesia Nurs* 20:279-284, 2005.
58. Skarke C, Langer M, Jarrar M et al: Probenecid interacts with the pharmacokinetics of morphine-6-glucuronide in humans, *Anesthesiology* 101:1394-1399, 2004.
59. 2006 Pennsylvania Patient Safety Authority: *Demerol: is it the best analgesic?* PA-PSRS Patient Safety Advisory, vol 3, No. 2 (2006): www.psa.state.pa. Accessed July 22, 2006.
60. Kurella M, Bennett WM, Chertow GM: Analgesia in patients with ESRD: a review of available evidence, *Am J Kidney Dis* 42:217-228, 2003.
61. Hanks G, Cherny N, Fallon M: Opioid analgesics. In Doyle D, Hanks G, Cherny N, editors: *Oxford textbook of palliative medicine,* 3rd ed, pp P316-P341, New York, 2004, Oxford University Press.
62. Dean M: Opioids in renal failure and dialysis patients, *J Pain Symptom Management* 28:497-504, 2004.
63. Ahonen J, Olkkola KT, Hynynen M et al: Comparison of alfentanil, fentanyl and sufentanil for total intravenous anaesthesia

with propofol in patients undergoing coronary artery bypass surgery, *Br J Anaesth* 85:533-540, 2000.

64. Howie MG, Reitz J, Reilley TE et al: Does sufentanil's shorter half-life have any clinical significance [abstract], *Anesthesiology* 59:A146, 1983.
65. Lejus C, Schwoerer D, Furic I et al: Fentanyl versus sufentanil: plasma concentrations during continuous epidural postoperative infusion in children, *Br J Anaesth* 85:615-617, 2000.
66. Sebel PS, Bovill JG: Cardiovascular effects of sufentanil anesthesia: a study in patients undergoing cardiac surgery, *Anesth Analg* 61:115-119, 1982.
67. Clotz MA, Nahata MC: Clinical uses of fentanyl, sufentanil, and alfentanil, *Clin Pharm* 10:581-593, 1991.
68. Gallagher G, Rae CP, Watson S et al: Target-controlled alfentanil analgesia for dressing change following extensive reconstructive surgery for trauma, *J Pain Symptom Manage* 21:1-2, 2001.
69. Cohen J, Royston D: Remifentanil, *Curr Opin Crit Care* 7:227-231, 2001.
70. Glass P: Remifentanil: a new opioid, *J Clin Anesthesiol* 7:558-563, 1995.
71. Westmoreland CL, Hoke JF, Sebel PS et al: Pharmacokinetics of remifentanil (GI87084B) and its major metabolite (GI90291) in patients undergoing elective inpatient surgery, *Anesthesiology* 79:893-903, 1993.
72. Glass PSA, Hardman D, Kamiyama Y et al: Preliminary pharmacokinetics and pharmacodynamics of an ultra-short-acting opioid: remifentanil (GI87084B), *Anesth Analg* 77:1031-1040, 1993.
73. Brown R, Kraus C et al: Methadone: applied pharmacology and use as adjunctive treatment in chronic pain, *Postgrad Med J* 80:654-659, 2004.
74. Inturrisi CE: Clinical pharmacology of opioids for pain, *Clin J Pain* 18:S3-S13, 2002.
75. Toombs JD, Kral LA: Methadone treatment for pain states, *Am Fam Physician* 71:1353-1358, 2005.
76. Duncharme J: Acute pain and pain control: state of the art, *Ann Emerg Med* 35:592-603, 2000.
77. Garbez R, Puntillo K: Acute musculoskeletal pain in the emergency department: a review of the literature and implications for the advanced practice nurse, *AACN Clin Issues* 16:310-319, 2005.
78. *Physician's desk reference,* 58th ed, pp 2495-2496, Montvale, NJ, 2004, Thomson PDR.
79. Dews TE, Mekhail N: Safe use of opioids in chronic noncancer pain, *Cleve Clin J Med* 71:897-904, 2004.
80. Hagle ME, Lehr VT, Brubakken K et al: Respiratory depression in adult patients with intravenous patient-controlled analgesia, *Orthop Nurs* 23:18-29, 2004.
81. Strasselels S, McNicol E, Suleman R: Postoperative pain management: a practical review, 2, *Am J Health System Pharm* 62:2019-2025, 2005.
82. Clarke SF, Dargan PI, Jones AL: Naloxone in opioid poisoning: walking the tightrope, *Emerg Med J* 22:612-616, 2005.
83. McNicol E, Horowicz-Mehler N, Fisk RA et al: Management of opioid side effects in cancer-related and chronic non-cancer pain: a systemic review, *J Pain* 4:231-256, 2003.
84. Bates JJ, Foss JF, Murphy DB: Are peripheral opioid antagonists the solution to opioid side effects? *Anesth Analg* 98:116-122, 2004.
85. Wu SD, Kong J, Wang W et al: Effect of morphine and M-cholinoceptor blocking drugs on human sphincter of Oddi during choledochofiberscopy manometry, *Hepatobiliary Pancreat Dis Int* 2:121-125, 2003.
86. Butler KC, Selden B, Pollack CV: Relief by naloxone of morphine-induced spasm of the sphincter of Oddi in a post-cholecystectomy patient, *J Emerg Med* 21:129-131, 2001.
87. Avila JG: Pharmacologic treatment of constipation in the cancer patient, *Cancer Control* 11(3 Suppl):10-18, 2004.
88. Grilo RM, Bertin P, Scotto di Fazano C et al: Opioid rotation in the treatment of joint pain: a review of 67 cases, *Joint Bone Spine* 69:491-494, 2002.
89. Ginsberg B, Sinatra RS, Adler LJ et al: Conversion to oral controlled-release oxycodone from intravenous opioid analgesic in the postoperative setting, *Pain Med* 4:31-38, 2003.
90. Flockhart DA: Cytochrome P450 drug interaction table. Indiana University School of Medicine: medicine.iupui.edu/flockhart/. Accessed August 2, 2007.
91. Ludo RA, Kern SE: The pharmacokinetics of oxycodone, *J Pain Palliat Care Pharmacother* 18:17-30, 2004.
92. Sinatra R: Opioid analgesics in primary care: challenges and new advances in the management of noncancer pain, *J Am Board Fam Med* 19:165-177, 2006.
93. Grass JA: Patient-controlled analgesia, *Anesth Analg* 101 (5 Suppl):S44-S61, 2005.
94. Weir VL: Best-practice protocols: preventing adverse drug events, *Nurs Manage* 36:24, 26, 28-30, 2005.
95. Viscusi ER, Schechter LN: Patient-controlled analgesia: finding a balance between cost and comfort, *Am J Health System Pharm* 63(1 Suppl):S1-S13, S15-S16, 2006.
96. Chang AM, Ip WY, Cheung TH: Patient-controlled analgesia versus conventional intramuscular injection: a cost effectiveness analysis, *J Adv Nurs* 46:531-541, 2004.
97. Mann C, Pouzeratte Y, Eledjam J: Postoperative patient-controlled analgesia in the elderly: risks and benefits of epidural versus intravenous administration, *Drugs Aging* 20:337-345, 2003.
98. Sathyan G, Guo C, Sivakumar K, et al: Evaluation of the bioequivalence of two transdermal fentanyl systems following single and repeated applications, *Curr Med Res Opin* 21:1961-1968, 2005.
99. Solassol I, Bressolle F, Caumette L et al: Inter- and intraindividual variabilities in pharmacokinetics of fentanyl after repeated 72-hour transdermal applications in cancer pain patients, *Therapeutic Drug Monit* 27:491-498, 2005.
100. Muijsers RB, Wagstaff AJ: Transdermal fentanyl: an updated review of its pharmacological properties and therapeutic efficacy in chronic cancer pain control, *Drugs* 61:2289-2307, 2001.
101. Langford R, McKenna F, Ratcliffe S et al: Transdermal fentanyl for improvement of pain and functioning in osteoarthritis: a randomized, placebo-controlled trial, *Arthritis Rheum* 54:1829-1837, 2006.
102. Koo PJ: Postoperative pain management with patient-controlled transdermal delivery system for fentanyl, *Am J Health Syst Pharm* 62:1171-1176, 2005.
103. Viscusi ER, Reynolds L, Tait S et al: An iontophoretic fentanyl patient-activated analgesic delivery system for postoperative pain: a double blind, placebo-controlled trial, *Anesth Analg* 102:188-194, 2006.
104. Weetman C, Allison W: Use of epidural analgesia in post-operative pain management, *Nurs Stand* 20:54-64, 2006.
105. Wu C, Cohen SR, Richman JM et al: Efficacy of postoperative patient-controlled and continuous infusion epidural analgesia

versus intravenous patient-controlled analgesia with opioids: a meta-analysis, *Anesthesiology* 103:1079-1088, 2005.

106. Eastern Association for the Surgery of Trauma: *Pain management in blunt thoracic trauma (BTT),* Winston-Salem, NC, Eastern Association for the Surgery of Trauma (2004): www.guideline.gov. Accessed August 2, 2007.
107. Holcomb JB, McMillian NR et al: Morbidity from rib fractures increases after age 45, *J Am Coll Surg* 196:549-555, 2003.
108. Karmaker MK, Ho AM: Acute pain management of patients with multiple fractured ribs, *J Trauma* 54:615-625, 2003.
109. Soto RG, Fu ES: Acute pain management for patients undergoing thoracotomy, *Ann Thorac Surg* 75:1349-1357, 2003.
110. Ochroch EA, Gottschalk A: Impact of acute pain and its management for thoracic surgical patients, *Thorac Surg Clin* 15:105-121, 2005.
111. Richman JM, Wu CL: Epidural analgesia for postoperative pain, *Anesthesiol Clin North Am* 23:125-140, 2005.
112. Pasero C: Epidural analgesia for postoperative pain, *Am J Nurs* 103:63-64, 2003.
113. Viscusi ER: Emerging techniques in the management of acute pain: epidural analgesia, *Anesth Analg* 100:S23-S29, 2005.
114. Ready LB: Acute pain: lessons learned from 25,000 patients, *Reg Anesth Pain Med* 24:499-505, 1999.
115. Schulz-Stubner S, Boezaart A, Hata S: Regional analgesia in the critically ill, *Crit Care Med* 33:1400-1407, 2005.
116. Horlocker TT, Wedel DJ, Benzon H et al: Regional anesthesia in the anticoagulated patient: defining the risks (the second ASRA Consensus Conference on Neuraxial Anesthesia and Anticoagulation), *Reg Anesth Pain Med* 28:172-197, 2003.
117. Cohen S, Christo PJ, Moroz L: Pain management in trauma patients, *Am J Phys Med Rehabil* 83:142-161, 2004.
118. Capdevila X, Pirat P, Bringuier S et al: Continuous peripheral nerve blocks in hospital wards after orthopedic surgery: a multicenter prospective analysis of the quality of postoperative analgesia and complications in 1,416 patients, *Anesthesiology* 103:1035-1045, 2005.
119. Murauski JD, Gonzalez KR: Peripheral nerve blocks for postoperative analgesia, *AORN J* 75:136-153, 2002.
120. McCamant KL: Peripheral nerve blocks: understanding the nurse's role, *J PeriAnesth Nurs* 21:16-26, 2006.
121. Sinnott CJ, Cogswell LP III, Johnson A et al: On the mechanism by which epinephrine potentiates lidocaine's peripheral nerve block, *Anesthesiology* 98:181-188, 2003.
122. Crystal CS, Blankenship RB: Local anesthetics and peripheral nerve blocks in the emergency department, *Emerg Med Clin North Am* 23:477-502, 2005.
123. Habib AS, Gan TJ: Role of analgesic adjuncts in postoperative pain management, *Anesthesiol Clin North Am* 23:85-107, 2005.
124. Morgan GE, Mikhail MS, Murray MJ: Peripheral nerve blocks. In Morgan GE, Mikhail MS, Murray MJ, editors: *Clinical anesthesiology,* 3rd ed, pp 283-308, New York, 2002, Lange Medical Books.
125. Liu S, Salinas FV: Continuous plexus and peripheral nerve blocks for postoperative analgesia, *Anesth Analg* 96:263-272, 2003.
126. Klein SM: Continuous peripheral nerve blocks: fewer excuses, *Anesthesiology* 103:921-923, 2005.
127. Kuffer EK, Dart RC, Bogdan GM et al: Effect of maximal daily doses of acetaminophen on the liver of alcoholic patients: a randomized, double-blind, placebo-controlled trial, *Arch Intern Med* 161:2247-2252, 2001.
128. Sachs CJ: Oral analgesics for acute nonspecific pain, *Am Fam Physician* 71:913-918, 2005.
129. Bell GM, Schnitzer TJ: COX-2 inhibitors and other nonsteroidal anti-inflammatory drugs in the treatment of pain in the elderly, *Clin Geriatr Med* 17:489-502, 2001.
130. Task Force on Acute Pain Management: Practice guidelines for acute pain management in the perioperative setting: an updated report by the American Society of Anesthesiologists, *Anesthesiology* 100:1573-1581, 2004.
131. Elia N, Lysakowski C, Tramer M et al: Does multimodal analgesia with acetaminophen, nonsteriodal anti-inflammatory drugs, or selective cyclooxygenase-2 inhibitors and patient-controlled analgesia morphine offer advantages over morphine alone? Meta-analyses of randomized trials, *Anesthesiology* 103:1296-1304, 2005.
132. Glass GG: Osteoarthritis, *Clin Family Pract* 7:161-179, 2005.
133. Barkin RL, Barkin SJ, Barkin DS: Perception, assessment, treatment, and management of pain in the elderly, *Clin Geriatr Med* 21:465-490, 2005.
134. Mukherjee D, Nissen SE, Topol EJ: Risk of cardiovascular events associated with selective COX-2 inhibitors, *JAMA* 286:954-959, 2001.
135. Einhorn TA: COX-2: where are we in 2003. The role of cyclooxygenase-2 in bone repair, *Arthritis Res Ther* 5:5-7, 2003.
136. Koester MC, Spindler KP: Pharmacologic agents in fracture healing, *Clin Sports Med* 25:63-73, 2006.
137. U.S. Food and Drug Administration: *Public health advisory for NSAIDs* (2004): www.fda.gov/cder/drug/advisory/nsaids.htm. Accessed August 2, 2007.
138. Whelton A: Renal aspects of treatment with conventional nonsteroidal anti-inflammatory drugs versus cyclooxygenase-2-specific inhibitors, *Am J Med* 110 (3A Suppl):33S-42S, 2001.
139. Brater DC: Effects of nonsteroidal anti-inflammatory drugs on renal function focus on cyclooxygenase-2-selective inhibition, *Am J Med* 107:65S-71S, 1999.
140. Habib AS, Gan TJ: Role of analgesic adjuncts in postoperative pain management, *Anesth Clin North Am* 23:85-107, 2005.
141. Guay DR: Adjunctive agents in the management of chronic pain, *Pharmacotherapy* 21:1070-1081, 2001.
142. Erlacher W, Schuschnig C, Koinig H et al: Clonidine as adjuvant for mepivacanie, ropivacaine and bupivacaine in axillary, perivascular brachial plexus block, *Can J Anaesth* 48:522-525, 2001.
143. Dworkin RH, Backonja M, Rowbotham MC et al: Advances in neuropathetic pain: diagnosis, mechanisms, and treatment recommendations, *Arch Neurol* 60:1524-1534, 2003.
144. Menigaux C, Adam F, Guignard B et al: Preoperative gabapentin decreases anxiety and improves early functional recovery from knee surgery, *Anesth Analg* 100:1394-1399, 2005.
145. Turan A, Karamanlioglu B, Memis D et al: The analgesic effects of gabapentin after spinal surgery, *Anesthesiology* 100:935-938, 2004.
146. Olorunto WA, Galandiuk S: Managing the spectrum of surgical pain: acute management of the chronic pain patient, *J Am Coll Surg* 202:169-175, 2006.
147. Gilron I, Flatters SJL: Gabapentin and pregabalin for the treatment of neuropathetic pain: a review of laboratory and clinical evidence, *Pain Res Manage* 11(A Suppl):16A-29A, 2006.
148. Gilron I, Watson C, Cahill CM et al: Neuropathic pain: a practical guide for the clinician, *CMAJ* 175:265-275, 2006.

149. Golembiewski J: Antidepressants: pharmacology and implications in the perioperative period, *J PeriAnesthes Nurs* 21: 285-287, 2006.
150. Finnerup NB, Otto M, McQuay HJ et al: Algorithm for neuropathic pain treatment: an evidence based proposal, *Pain* 118:289-305, 2005.
151. De Pinto M, Dumbar PJ, Edwards WT: Pain management, *Anesthesiol Clin North Am* 24:19-37, 2006.
152. Pasero C, McCaffery M: Ketamine: low doses may provide relief for some painful conditions, *Am J Nurs* 105:60-64, 2005.
153. Reves J, Glass PSA, Lubarsky DA et al: Intravenous nonopioid anesthetics. In Miller RD, editor: *Miller's anesthesia,* pp 317-378, Philadelphia, 2005, Elsevier, Churchill Livingstone.
154. Hocking G, Cousins MJ: Ketamine in chronic pain management: an evidence based review, *Anesth Analg* 97:1730-1739, 2003.
155. Bahn EL, Holt KR: Procedural sedation and analgesia: a review and new concepts, *Emerg Med Clin North Am* 23:503-517, 2005.
156. Dalens BJ, Pinard AM, Letourneau DR et al: Prevention of emergence agitation after sevoflurane anesthesia for pediatric cerebral magnetic resonance imaging by small doses of ketamine or nalbuphine administered just before discontinuing anesthesia, *Anesth Analg* 102:1056-1061, 2006.
157. Cromhout A: Ketamine: its use in the emergency department, *Emerg Med* 15:155-159, 2003.
158. Tennant FA editor: Lidoderm studied for new applications, *Practical Pain Manage* vol 3, no. 4 (2003): http://www.ppmjournal.com. Accessed August 6, 2007.
159. Whelton A: Clinical implications of nonopioid analgesia for relief of mild-to-moderate pain in patients with or at risk for cardiovascular disease, *Am J Cardiol* 97(9 Suppl):3-9, 2006.
160. Miller MA, Levy P, Patel MM: Procedural sedation and analgesia in the emergency department: what are the risks? *Emerg Med Clin North Am* 23:551-572, 2005.
161. Gruber EM, Tschernko EM: Anaesthesia and postoperative analgesia in older patients with chronic obstructive pulmonary disease, *Drugs Aging* 20:347-360, 2003.
162. Richmann JM, Wu CL: Epidural analgesia for postoperative pain, *Anesthesiol Clin North Am* 23:125-140, 2005.
163. Institute for Clinical Systems Improvement: *Assessment and management of acute pain,* Bloomington, MN, Institute for Clinical Systems Improvement (2006): www.guideline.gov/summary/summary.aspx?doc_id59009. Accessed March 22, 2006.
164. Jakobsson U, Klevsgard R, Westergren A et al: Old people in pain: a comparative study, *J Pain Symptom Manage* 26:625-636, 2003.
165. Hanks-Bell M, Halvey K, Paice JA: Pain assessment and management in aging, *Online J Issues Nurs* 93:8, 2004.
166. Polomano RC: Pain. In Cotter V, Strumpf N, editors: *Advanced practice nursing with older adults: clinical guidelines,* pp 333-360, New York, 2002, McGraw-Hill.
167. Barkin RL, Barkin SJ, Barkin DS: Perception, assessment, treatment, and management of pain in the elderly, *Clin Geriatr Med* 21:465-490, 2005.
168. Kaufman DW, Kelly JP, Rosenberg L et al: Recent patterns of medication use in the ambulatory adult population in the United States: the Slone Survey, *JAMA* 287:337-344, 2002.
169. Inturrisi CE: Clinical pharmacology of opioids in pain, *Clin J Pain* 18:S3-S13, 2002.
170. World Federation of Societies of Anaesthesiologists: 1-7, 1997.
171. Greater Philadelphia Pain Society: *Pain control in the hospital: guide to prescribing oral analgesics,* Philadelphia, 2003, Greater Philadelphia Pain Society.
172. Kehlet H, Wilmore DW: Multimodal strategies to improve surgical outcome, *Am J Surg* 183:630-641, 2002.
173. Pasero C: Epidural analgesia for postoperative pain, 2: multimodal recovery programs improve patient outcomes, *Am J Nurse* 103:43-45, 2003.
174. White PF: The changing role of non-opioid analgesic techniques in the management of postoperative pain, *Anesth Analg* 101(5 Suppl):S5-S22, 2005.
175. White PF: Electroanalgesia: does it have a place in the routine management of acute or chronic pain? *Anesth Analg* 98:1197-1198, 2004.
176. Kissin I: Preemptive analgesia: clinical concepts and commentary, *Anesthesiology* 93:1138-1143, 2000.
177. Gottschalk A, Cohen SP: Preventing and treating pain after thoracic surgery, *Anesthesiology* 104:594-600, 2006.
178. Bong CL, Samuel M, Ng JM et al: Effects of preemptive epidural analgesia on post-thoracotomy pain, *J Cardiothorac Vasc Anesth* 19:786-793, 2005.
179. Karmakar MK, Ho AM: Postthoracotomy pain syndrome, *Thorac Surg Clin* 14:345-352, 2004.
180. Dillard JN, Knapp S: Complementary and alternative pain therapy in the emergency department, *Emerg Med Clin North Am* 23:529-549, 2005.
181. Tracy S, Dufault M, Kogut S, et al: Translating best practices in nondrug postoperative pain management, *Nurs Res* 55(2 Suppl): S57-S67, 2006.
182. Good M, Stanton-Hicks M, Grass J et al: Postoperative pain relief across activities and days with jaw relaxation, music, and their combination, *J Adv Nurs* 33:208-215, 2001.
183. Friesner SA, Curry DM, Moddeman GR: Comparison of two pain-management strategies during chest tube removal: relaxation exercise with opioids and opioids alone, *Heart Lung* 35:269-276, 2006.
184. Laurion S, Fetzer SJ: The effect of two nursing interventions on the postoperative outcomes of gynecologic laparoscopic patients, *J PeriAnesthes Nurs* 18:254-261, 2003.
185. Antall GF, Kresevic D: The use of guided imagery to manage pain in an elderly orthopedic population, *Orthop Nurs* 23:335-340, 2004.
186. Dunn K: Music and the reduction of post-operative pain. *Nurs Stand* 18:33-39, 2004.
187. Siedliecki SL, Good M: Effect of music on power, pain, depression and disability, *J Adv Nurs* 54:553-562, 2006.
188. Cepeda MS, Carr DB, Lau J et al: Music for pain relief, *Cochrane Database Syst Rev* 2:CD004843, 2006.
189. French SD, Cameron M, Walker BF et al: A Cochrane review of superficial heat or cold for low back pain, *Spine* 31:998-1006, 2006.
190. Ernst E: Manual therapies for pain control: chiropractic and massage, *Clin J* Pain 20:8-12, 2004.
191. Ernst E: Massage therapy for low back pain: an update, *Alt Ther Womens Health* Sept:69-71, 2001.
192. Chiu TT, Hui-Chan CW, Chein G: A randomized clinical trial of TENS and exercise for patients with chronic neck pain, *Clin Rehabil* 19:850-860, 2005.
193. Rakel B, Frantz R: Effectiveness of transcutaneous electrical nerve stimulation on postoperative pain with movement, *J Pain* 4:455-464, 2003.

194. Jacobi J, Fraser GL, Coursin DB et al: Clinical practice guidelines for the use of sedatives and analgesics in the critically ill adult, *Crit Care Med* 30:119-141, 2002.
195. Cohen IL, Gallagher, TJ, Pohlman AS et al: Management of the agitated intensive care unit patient, *Crit Care Med* 30(1 Suppl): s97-s123, 2002.
196. Consensus conference on sedation assessment: a collaborative venture by Abbott Laboratories, American Association of Critical-Care Nurses, and Saint Thomas Health System, *Crit Care Nurse* 24:33-42, 2004.
197. Ramsay M, Savege T, Simpson B et al: Controlled sedation with alphaxolone-alphadolone, *BJM* 2:656-659, 1974.
198. Avramov MN, White PF: Methods for monitoring the level of sedation, *Crit Care Clin* 11:803-826, 1995.
199. Riker RR, Fraser GI, Cox PM: Continuous infusion of haloperidol controls agitation in critically ill patients, *Crit Care Med* 22:433-440, 1994.
200. Devlin JW, Boleski G, Mylnarek M et al: Motor activity assessment scale: a valid and reliable scale for use with mechanically ventilated patients in an adult surgical intensive care unit, *Crit Care Med* 27:1271-1275, 1999.
201. Ely EW, Truman B, Shintani A et al: Monitoring sedation status over time in ICU patients: reliability and validity of the Richmond agitation-sedation scale, *JAMA* 289:2983-2991, 2003.
202. Sessler CN, Gosnell MS, Grap MJ et al: The Richmond agitation-sedation scale: validity and reliability in adult intensive care unit patients, *Am J Respir Crit Care Med* 166:1338-1344, 2002.
203. Deogaonkar A, Gupta R, DeGeorgia M et al: Bispectral index monitoring correlates with sedation scales in brain-injured patients, *Crit Care Med* 32:2403-2406, 2004.
204. Parthasarathy S, Tobin MJ: Sleep in the intensive care unit, *Intensive Care Med* 30:197-206, 2004.
205. Peruzzi WT: Sleep in the intensive care unit, *Pharmacotherapy* 25:34S-39S, 2005.
206. Perry SW: Psychological reactions to pancuronium bromide, *Am J Psychol* 142:1390-1391, 1985.
207. Blacker RS: On awakening paralyzed during surgery: a syndrome of traumatic neurosis, *JAMA* 234:67-68, 1975.
208. Kress JP, Hall JB: Sedation in the mechanically ventilated patient, *Crit* Care *Med* 34:2541-2546, 2006.
209. Amrein R, Hetzel W, Hartmann D et al: Clinical pharmacology of flumazenil, *Eur J Anaesthesiol* 5(2 Suppl):65-68, 1988.
210. Greenblatt DJ: Clinical pharmacokinetics of oxazepam and lorazepam, *Clin Pharmacokinet* 6:89-105, 1981.
211. Reves JG, Fragen RJ, Vinil HR et al: Midazolam: pharmacology and uses, *Anesthesiology* 62:310-324, 1985.
212. Ziegler WH, Schalch E, Leishman B et al: Comparison of the effects of intravenously administered midazolam, triazolam, and their hydroxymetabolites, *Br J Clin Pharmacol* 16:63S-69S, 1983.
213. Ariano RE, Kassum DA, Aronson KJ: Comparison of sedative recovery time after midazolam vs diazepam administration, *Crit Care Med* 22:1492-1496, 1994.
214. Trissel LA: Lorazepam. In Trissel LA, editor: *Handbook on injectable drugs,* 10th ed, pp 728-734, Bethesda, MD, 1998, American Society of Health-System Pharmacists.
215. Seay RE, Graves PJ, Wilkin MK: Comment: possible toxicity from propylene glycol in lorazepam infusion [letter], *Ann Pharmacother* 31:647-648, 1997.
216. Laine GA, Hossain SMH, Solis RT et al: Polyethylene glycol nephrotoxicity secondary to prolonged high-dose intravenous lorazepam, *Ann Pharmacother* 29:1110-1114, 1995.
217. D'Ambrosio JA, Borchardt-Phelps P, Nolen JG et al: Propylene glycol-induced lactic acidosis secondary to a continuous infusion of lorazepm, *Pharmacotherapy* 13:274, 1993.
218. Wilson KC, Reardon C, Theodore AC et al: Propylene glycol toxicity: a severe iatrogenic illness in ICU patients receiving IV benzodiazepines, *Chest* 128:1674-1681, 2005.
219. Yaucher NE, Fish JT, Smith HW, et al: Propylene glycol-associated renal toxicity from lorazepam infusion, *Pharmacotherapy* 23:1094-1099, 2003.
220. Amstrong DK, Crisp CB: Pharmacoeconomic issues in sedation, analgesia, and neuromuscular blockade in critical care, *New Horiz* 2:85-93, 1994.
221. Marty J, Gauzit R, Lefevre P et al: Effects of diazepam and midazolam on baroreflex control of heart rate and on sympathetic activity in humans, *Anesth Analg* 65:113-119, 1986.
222. Samuelson PN, Reves JG, Kouchokos NT et al: Hemodynamic responses to anesthetic induction with midazolam or diazepam in patients with ischemic heart disease, *Anesth Analg* 60:802-809, 1981.
223. Samuelson PN, Lell WA, Kouchokos NT et al: Hemodynamics during diazepam induction of anesthesia for coronary artery bypass grafting, *South Med J* 73:332-334, 1980.
224. Aitkenhead AR, Pepperman ML, Willatts SM et al: Comparison of propofol and midazolam for sedation in critically ill patients, *Lancet* 2:704-709, 1989.
225. White PF: Propofol: pharmacokinetics and pharmacodynamics, *Semin Anaesth* 7:4-20, 1988.
226. Mirenda J, Broyles G: Propofol as used for sedation in the ICU, *Chest* 108:539-548, 1995.
227. Fulton B, Sorkin EM: Propofol: an overview of its pharmacology and a review of its clinical efficacy in intensive care sedation, *Drugs* 50:636-657, 1995.
228. Devlin JW, Lau AK, Tanios MA: Propofol-associated hypertriglyceridemia and pancreatitis in the intensive care unit: an analysis of frequency and risk factors, *Pharmacotherapy* 25:1348-1352, 2005.
229. Kang TM: Propofol infusion syndrome in critically ill patients, *Pharmacotherapy* 36:1453-1456, 2002.
230. Vasile B, Rasulo F, Candiani A et al: The pathophysiology of propofol infusion syndrome: a simple name for a complex syndrome, *Intensive Care Med* 29:1417-1425, 2003.
231. Bhana N, Goa KL, McClellan KJ: Dexmedetomidine, *Drugs* 59:263-268, 2000.
232. Dasta JF, Jacobi J, Sesti AM, et al: Addition of dexmedetomidine to standard sedation regimens after cardiac surgery: an outcomes analysis, *Pharmacotherapy* 26:798-805, 2006.
233. Baddigam K, Russo P, Russo J et al: Dexmedetomidine in the treatment of withdrawal syndromes in cardiothoracic surgery patients, *J Intensive Care Med* 20:118-123, 2005.
234. Dexmedetomidine (Precedex™) [package insert], 2001, Abbott Laboratories.
235. Rockoff MA, Marshall LF, Shapiro HM: High dose barbiturate therapy in humans: a clinical review of 60 patients, *Ann Neurol* 6:194-199, 1979.
236. Aitkenhead AR: Analgesia and sedation in intensive care, *Br J Anaesth* 63:196-206, 1989.
237. Park GR, Manara AR, Mendel L et al: Ketamine infusion, *Anaesthesia* 42:980-983, 1987.

238. Bryan-Brown CS, Dracup K: Alternative therapies, *Am J Crit Care* 4:416-418, 1995.
239. Meyer TJ, Eveloff SE, Bauer MS, et al: Adverse environmental conditions in the respiratory and medical ICU settings, *Chest* 105:1211-1216, 1994.
240. Krapohl GL: Visiting hours in the adult intensive care unit: using research to develop a system that works, *Dimensions Crit Care Nurs* 14:245-258, 1995.
241. Pandharipande P, Ely EW: Sedative and analgesic medications: risk factors for delirium and sleep disturbances in the critically ill, *Crit Care Clin* 22:313-327, 2006.
242. Ely EW, Margolin R, Francis J et al: Evaluation of delirium in critically ill patients: validation of the confusion assessment method for the intensive care unit (Cam-ICU), *Crit Care Med* 29:1370-1379, 2001.
243. Tesar GE, Stern TA: Rapid tranquilization of the agitated intensive care unit patient, *J Intensive Care Med* 3:195-201, 1988.
244. Baldessarini RJ, Tarazi FI: Pharmacotherapy of psychosis and mania. In Brunton LL, Lazo JS, Parker KL, editors: *Goodman and Gilman's the pharmacologic basis of therapeutics,* 11th ed, pp 461-500, New York, 2006, McGraw-Hill.
245. Cassem EH, Lake CR, Boyer WF: Psychopharmacology in the ICU. In Chernow B, editor: *The pharmacologic approach to the critically ill patient,* 3rd ed, pp 651-665, Baltimore, 1994, Williams & Wilkins.
246. Fernandez F, Holmes VF, Adams F et al: Treatment of severe, refractory agitation with a haloperidol drip, *J Clin Psychiatry* 49:239-241, 1988.
247. Marsden CD, Jenner P: The pathophysiology of extrapyramidal side-effects of neuroleptic drugs. *Psychol Med* 10:55-72, 1980.
248. Menza MA, Murray GB, Holmes VF et al: Decreased extrapyramidal symptoms with intravenous haloperidol, *J Clin Psychiatry* 48:278-280, 1987.
249. Lawrence KR, Nasraway SA: Conduction disturbances associated with the administration of butyrophenone antipsychotics in the critically ill: a review of the literature, *Pharmacotherapy* 17:531-537, 1997.
250. Zeifman CWE, Friedman B: Torsades de pointes: potential consequence of intravenous haloperidol in the intensive care unit, *Intensive Care World* 11:109-112, 1994.
251. Murray MJ, Nasaraway S, Cowen J et al: Clinical practice guidelines for sustained neuromuscular blockade in the adult critically ill patient, *Am J Health Syst Pharm* 59:179-195, 2002.
252. Fleming NW: Neuromuscular blocking drugs in the intensive care unit: indications, protocols, and complications, *Semin Anesth* 13:255-264, 1994.
253. Rodriguez J, Weissman C, Damask M et al: Physiologic requirements during rewarming: suppression of the shivering response, *Crit Care Med* 11:490-497, 1983.
254. Durbin CG: Neuromuscular blocking agents and sedative drugs, *Crit Care Clin* 7:489-506, 1991.
255. Werba A, Weinstable C, Plainer B et al: Vecuronium prevents increases in intracranial response during routine tracheobronchial suctioning in neurosurgical patients, *Anaesthetist* 40:328-331, 1991.
256. Bartkowski RR, Witkowski TA, Azad S et al: Rocuronium onset of action: a comparison with atracurium and vecuronium, *Anesth Analg* 77:574-578, 1993.
257. Lennon RL, Olson RA, Gronert GA: Atracurium or vecuronium for rapid sequence endotracheal intubation, *Anesthesiology* 64:510-513, 1986.
258. Rudis MI, Guslits BG, Zarowitz BJ: Technical and interpretive problems of peripheral nerve stimulation in monitoring neuromuscular blockade in the ICU, *Ann Pharmacother* 30:165-172, 1996.
259. Harper NJN: Neuromuscular blocking drugs: practical aspects of research in the intensive care unit, *Intensive Care Med* 19(2 Suppl):S80-S85, 1993.
260. Erickson LI: Ventilation and neuromuscular blocking drugs, *Acta Anaesthesiol Scand Suppl* 102:11-15, 1994.
261. Shapiro BA, Warren J, Egol AB et al: Practice parameters for sustained neuromuscular blockade in the adult critically ill patient: an executive summary, *Crit Care Med* 23:1601-1605, 1995.
262. Prielipp RC, Coursin DB: Applied pharmacology of common neuromuscular blocking agents in critical care, *N Horiz* 2:34-47, 1994.
263. Abel M, Book WJ, Eisenkraft JB: Adverse effects of nondepolarizing neuromuscular blocking agents, *Drug Saf* 10:420-438, 1994.
264. Coursin DB, Prielipp RC: Use of neuromuscular blocking drugs in the critically ill patient, *Crit Care Clin* 11:957-981, 1995.
265. Goldberg MF, Larijani GE, Azad SS et al: Comparison of tracheal intubating conditions and neuromuscular blocking profiles after intubating doses of mivacurium or succinylcholine in surgical outpatients, *Anesth Analg* 69:93-99, 1989.
266. Montgomery CJ, Steward DJ: A comparative evaluation of intubating doses of atracurium, d-tubocurarine, pancuronium and vecuronium in children, *Can J Anaesth* 35:36-40, 1988.
267. Gorson KC, Ropper AH: Generalized paralysis in the intensive care unit: emphasis on the complications of neuromuscular blocking agents and corticosteroids, *J Intensive Care Med* 11:219-231, 1996.
268. Op de Coul AAW, Lambregts PCLA, Koeman J et al: Neuromuscular complications in patients in Pavulon (pancuronium bromide) during artificial ventilation, *Clin Neurol Neurosurg* 87:17-22, 1985.
269. Henning RH, Houwertjes MC, Scaf AHJ et al: Prolonged paralysis after long-term high dose infusion of pancuronium in anesthetized cats, *Br J Anaesth* 71:393-397, 1993.
270. Shapiro BA, Warren J, Egol AB et al: Practice parameters for intravenous analgesia and sedation for adult patients in the intensive care unit: an executive summary, *Crit Care Med* 23:1596-1600, 1995.
271. Rudis MI, Sikora CA, Angus E et al: A prospective, randomized, controlled evaluation of peripheral nerve stimulation versus standard clinical dosing of neuromuscular blocking agents in critically ill patients, *Crit Care Med* 25:575-583, 1997.
272. Hoyt JW: Persistent paralysis in critically ill patients after the use of neuromuscular blocking agents, *N Horiz* 2:48-55, 1994.
273. Kanjo S, Barletta JF, Janisse JJ et al: Tachyphylaxis associated with continuous cisatracurium versus pancuronium therapy, *Pharmacotherapy* 22:823-830, 2002.
274. Boive J: Central pain. In McMahon S, Kolzenburg M, editors: *Wall and Melzack's textbook of pain,* 5th ed, pp 1057-1075, New York, 2006, Churchill Livingstone.
275. Siddall PJ, Yezierski RP, Loeser JD: Pain following spinal cord injury: clinical features, prevalence, and taxonomy, *IASP Newl* 3-2000, 2000.

276. Siddall PJ et al: A longitudinal study of the prevalence and characteristics of pain in the first 5 years following spinal cord injury, *Pain* 103:249-257, 2003.
277. Nicholson BD: Evaluation and treatment of central pain syndromes, *Neurology* 62(2 Suppl):S30-S36, 2004.
278. Waxman SG, Hains BC: Fire and phantoms after spinal cord injury: Na^+ channels and central pain, *Trends Neurosci* 29:207-215, 2006.
279. Ducreux D, Attal N, Parker F et al: Mechanisms of central neuropathic pain: a combined psychophysical and MRI study in syringomyelia, *Brain* 129:963-976, 2006.
280. Woolf CJ, Salter MW: Neuronal plasticity: increasing the gain on pain, *Science* 288:1765-1768, 2000.
281. Irving GA: Contemporary assessment and management of neuropathetic pain, *Neurology* 64(3 Suppl):S21-S27, 2005.
282. Finnerup NB, Biering-Sorensen F, Johannesen IL et al: Intravenous lidocaine relieves spinal cord injury pain: a randomized controlled trial, *Anesthesiology* 102:1023-1030, 2005.
283. Davies PS, Rhiner M: Shooting, burning, stabbing: case studies in neuropathic pain, *J Am Acad Nurs Pract* 17(6 Suppl):4-17, 2005.
284. Nikolajsen L, Jensen TS: Phantom limb. In McMahon S, Kolzenburg, editors: *Wall and Melzack's textbook of pain*, 5th ed, pp 961-974, New York, 2006, Churchill Livingstone.
285. Finnoff J: Differentiation and treatment of phantom sensation, phantom pain and residual-limb pain, *J Am Podiatr Med Assoc* 91:23-33, 2001.
286. Dillingham TR, Pezzin LE, MacKenzie EJ et al: Use and satisfaction with prosthetic devices among persons with trauma-related amputations: a long-term outcome study, *Am J Phys Med Rehabil* 80:563-571, 2001.
287. Borsje S, Bosmans JC, Van der Schans CP et al: Phantom pain: a sensitivity analysis, *Disabil Rehabil* 26:905-910, 2004.
288. Richardson C, Glenn S: Incidence of phantom phenomena including phantom limb pain 6 months after major limb amputation in patients with peripheral vascular disease, *Clin J Pain* 22:353-358, 2006.
289. Wilder-Smith CH, Hill LT, Laurent S: Postamputation pain and sensory changes in treatment-naïve patients: characteristics and responses to treatment with tramadol, amitriptyline, and placebo, *Anesthesiology* 103:619-628, 2005.
290. Mitchell AC: An unusual case of chronic neuropathetic pain responds to an optimum frequency of intravenous ketamine infusions, *J Pain Symptom Manage* 21:443-446, 2001.
291. Hayes C, Armstrong-Brown A, Burstal R: Perioperative intravenous ketamine infusion for the prevention of persistent post-amputation pain: a randomized, controlled trial: *Anaesth Intensive Care* 32:330-333, 2004.
292. Hanley MA, Ehde DM, Campbell KM et al: Self-reported treatments used for lower-limb phantom pain: descriptive findings, *Arch Phys Med Rehabil* 87:270-277, 2006.
293. Halbert J, Crotty M, Cameron ID: Evidence for the optimal management of acute and chronic phantom pain a systematic review, *Clin J Pain* 18:84-92, 2002.
294. Oakley DA, Whitman LG, Halligan PW: Hypnotic imagery as a treatment for phantom limb pain two case reports and a review, *Clin Rehabil* 16:368-377, 2002.
295. Leskowitz ED: Phantom limb pain treated with therapeutic touch a case report, *Arch Phys Med Rehabil* 81:522-524, 2000.
296. Ivanhoe CB, Hartman ET: Clinical caveats on medical assessment and treatment of pain after TBI, *J Head Trauma Rehabil* 19:29-39, 2004.
297. Albanèse J, Viviand X, Potie F et al: Sufentanil, fentanyl, and alfentanil in head trauma patients: a study on cerebral hemodynamics, *Crit Care Med* 27:407-411, 1999.
298. Nolan S: Traumatic brain injury: a review: *Crit Care Nurs Q* 28:188-194, 2005.
299. Cohen SP, Christo PJ, Morez L: Pain management in trauma patients, *Am J Phys Med Rehabil* 83:142-161, 2004.
300. Labi M, Brentjens M, Coad ML et al: Development of a longitudinal study of complications and functional outcomes after traumatic brain injury, *Brain Inj* 17:265-278, 2003.
301. Boviatsis EJ, Kouyialis AT, Korfias S et al: Functional outcome of intrathecal baclofen administration for severe spasticity, *Clin Neurol Neurosurg* 107:289-295, 2005.
302. Francisco GE, Boake C, Vaughn A: Botulinum toxin in upper limb spasticity after acquired brain injury: a randomized trial comparing dilution techniques, *Am J Phys Med Rehabil* 81: 355-363, 2002.
303. Emergency Nurses Association, American College of Emergency Physicians: Policy statement: delivery of agents for procedural sedation and analgesia by emergency nurses, *Ann Emerg Med* 46:368, 2005.
304. Godwin SA, Caro DA, Wolf SJ et al: Clinical policy: procedural sedation and analgesia in the emergency department. American College of Emergency Physicians Clinical Policies Subcommittee on Procedural Sedation and Analgesia, *Ann Emerg Med* 45:177-196, 2005.
305. Ashburn MA: Practice guidelines for acute pain management in the perioperative setting: an updated report by the American Society of Anesthesiologists Task Force on Acute Pain Management, *Anesthesiology* 100:1573-1581, 2004.
306. Bahn EL, Holt KR: Procedural sedation and analgesia: a review and new concepts, *Emerg Med Clin North Am* 23:503-517, 2005.
307. Nagelhout JJ: AANA journal course, update for nurse anesthetists: aspiration prophylaxis: is it time for changes in our practice? *AANA J* 71:299-303, 2003.
308. Green SM, Krauss B: Pulmonary aspiration risk during emergency department procedural sedation: an examination of the role of fasting and sedation depth, *Acad Emerg Med* 9:35-42, 2002.
309. Joint Committee on Administrative Rules, section 515.2030, Level I trauma center designation criteria: www.ilga.gov/commission/jcar/admincode. Accessed October 1, 2006.
310. Bourgoin A, Albanese J Leone M et al: Effects of sufentanil or ketamine administered in target-controlled infusion on the cerebral hemodynamics of severely brain-injured patients, *Crit Care Med* 33:1109-1113, 2005.
311. Catalano K: JCAHO's national patient safety goals 2006, *J PeriAnesth Nurs* 21:6-11, 2006.
312. Vanderveen T: *Averting highest-risk errors is first priority, II: nursing satisfaction, wireless networking, "smart" pain management, best practice improvements, and ROI: patient safety and quality healthcare*, Lionheart Publishing, Inc (2005): http://www.psqh.com/julaug05/averting.html. Accessed August 6, 2007.
313. Murray MJ, Cowan J DeBlock H et al: Clinical practice guidelines for sustained neuromuscular blockade in the adult critically ill patient, *Crit Care Med* 30:142-156, 2002.
314. Arbour R: A continuous quality improvement approach to improving clinical practice in the areas of sedation, analgesia, and neuromuscular blockade, *J Cont Educ Nurs* 34:64-71, 2003.

315. Institute for Safe Medication Practices: *More on avoiding opioid toxicity with PCA by proxy: medication safety alert!* (2002): www.ismp.org/MSAarticles/PCA.htm. Accessed August 3, 2007.
316. Weir V: Best-practice protocols: preventing adverse drug events, *Nurs Manage* 36:24-30, 2005.
317. Institute for Safe Medication Practices: *II: Safety issues with PCA: how to prevent errors: medication safety alert!* (2003): www.ismp.org/newsletters/acutecare/articles/20030724.asp. Accessed August 3, 2007.
318. Maddox RR, Williams CK, Oglesby H et al: Clinical experience with patient-controlled analgesia using continuous respiratory monitoring and a smart infusion system, *Am J Health Syst Pharm* 63:157-164, 2006.
319. Overdyk F, Maddox RR: Baseline respiratory indices variation may miscalculate respiratory depression in PCA patients, *Anesthesiology* 105:A1190, 2006.
320. Viscusi ER: Emerging techniques in the management of acute pain: epidural analgesia, *Anesth Analg* 101:S23-S29, 2005.
321. Weetman C, Allison W: Use of epidural analgesia in post-operative pain management. *Nurs Stand* 20:54-64, 2006.
322. Slowikowski RD, Flaherty SA: *Epidural analgesia for the post-operative orthopaedic pain, Orthop Nurs* 19:23-32, 2000.
323. Cherng CH, Yang CP, Wong CS: Epidural fentanyl speeds the onset of sensory and motor blocks during epidural ropivacaine anesthesia, *Anesth Analg* 101:1834-1837, 2005.
324. Murauski JD, Gonzalez KR: Peripheral nerve blocks for post-operative analgesia, *AORN J* 75:136-153, 2002.
325. Krajnik M, Zylicz Z: Understanding pruritus in systemic disease, *J Pain Symptom Manage* 21:151-168, 2001.
326. Kjellberg F, Tramer MR: Pharmacological control of opioid-induced pruritis: a quantitative review of randomized trials, *Eur J Anaesth* 18:346-357, 2001.
327. Szarvas S, Harmon D, Murphy D: Neuraxial opioid-induced pruritus: a review, *J Clin Anesth* 15:234-239, 2003.
328. Cox F: Clinical care of patients with epidural infusions, *Prof Nurse* 16:1429-1432, 2001.
329. Smith DE: Spinal opioids in the home and hospice setting, *J Pain Symptom Manage* 5:175-182, 1990.
330. Durham J: Side effects of epidurals: a summary of recent research data, *Int J Childbirth Educ* 18:11-17, 2003.
331. Luebbehusen M: Bispectral index monitoring, *RN* 68:50-54, 2005.
332. Sebel PS, Bowdle TA, Ghoneim MM et al: The incidence of awareness during anesthesia: a multicenter United States study, *Anesth Analg* 99:833-839, 2004.
333. Kelley SD: *Monitoring level of consciousness during anesthesia and sedation: a clinician's guide to the bispectral index:* www.aspectmedical.com/resources/handbook/default.mspx. Accessed August 3, 2007.
334. Puntillo K, Casella V, Reid M: Opioid and benzodiazepine tolerance and dependence: application of theory to critical care practice, *Heart Lung* 26:317-324, 1997.
335. Joyce N, Evans D: Best practice: eye care for patients in the ICU, *Am J Nurs* 106:72AA-BB, 72DD, 2006.
336. Chung S, Pohl S, Zeng J et al: Endogenous orphanin FQ/nociceptin is involved in the development of morphine tolerance, *J Pharmacol Exp Ther* 318:262-267, 2006.
337. Chu LF, Clark DJ, Angst MS: Opioid tolerance and hyperalgesia in chronic pain patients after one month of oral morphine therapy: a preliminary prospective study, *J Pain* 7:43-48, 2006.
338. Quigley C: Opioid switching to improve pain relief and drug tolerability, *Cochrane Database Syst Rev* 3:CD004847, 2004.
339. Carr DD: The case manager's role in optimizing acute rehabilitation services, *Lippincotts Case Manage* 10:190-202, 2005.
340. Doran DM, Harrison MB, Laschinger HS et al: Nursing-sensitive outcomes data collection in acute care and long-term-care, *Nurs Res* 55(2 Suppl):S75-S81, 2006.
341. Garbez RO, Chan GK, Neighbor M et al: Pain after discharge: a pilot study of factors associated with pain management and functional status, *J Emerg Nurs* 32:288-293, 2006.
342. Weiner DK, Rudy TE, Morrow L et al: The relationship between pain, neuropsychological performance, and physical function in community-dwelling older adults with chronic low back pain, *Pain Med* 7:60-70, 2006.
343. Egol KA, Tejwani NC, Walsh MG et al: Predictors of short-term functional outcome following ankle fracture surgery, *J Bone Joint Surg [Am]* 88:974-979, 2006.
344. Duckworth MP, Iezzi T: Chronic pain and posttraumatic stress symptoms in litigating motor vehicle accident victims, *Clin J Pain* 21:251-261, 2005.

19

PSYCHOSOCIAL IMPACT OF TRAUMA

Ruby J. Martinez

In the midst of an acute emergency or critical care situation such as a traumatic injury, the nurses' immediate priority is to physiologically stabilize the patient. In the fast-paced, high-stress environment of the emergency department (ED) and the intensive care unit (ICU), it may seem that there is little time for anything else and the mental health needs of the patient and their loved ones can be easily overlooked. However, taking the time to address these issues may prevent psychologic morbidity. During and often long after the acute health issues have been resolved and wounds have healed, the minds of those involved may still be suffering. The psychologic impact of the illness experience for all involved must be acknowledged and addressed.

A traumatic injury often precipitates a crisis for both the patient and family. They feel vulnerable, overwhelmed, and ill prepared to deal with the ramifications of the injury. Outcomes are uncertain and difficult decisions must be made. The patient and family find themselves in a situation over which they have little control. Psychologic consequences of traumatic injury can often lead to long-term complications such as social isolation, job loss, economic problems, and decreased pleasure in leisure activities. In addition, depression, posttraumatic stress disorder (PTSD), and other psychologic morbidity contribute to postinjury functional limitations. Long-term ramifications of trauma are significant, leaving many patients and families with long-lasting psychologic scars.[1-5]

This chapter presents a discussion on the psychologic impact of trauma on both the patient and the family. Crisis intervention theory will be used as a framework for understanding how nurses can make assessments and implement interventions to address the psychologic needs of the trauma victim and his or her family. As the patient and family move through the health care continuum from acute emergency stabilization to transitional and rehabilitation care, each nurse must develop a care plan outlining how the patient and family's mental health needs will be supported. Trauma-related mental illnesses along with the symptoms, recommended strategies, and referral recommendations will be presented. A final section will be devoted to special situations including death, traumatic grief, and care worker stress.

TRAUMA AS A CRISIS

Crisis is defined as an acute emotional upset that may interfere with the ability to cope emotionally, cognitively, or behaviorally, rendering the person unable to solve problems by usual devices.[6] The often violent and unpredictable nature of traumatic injury certainly can precipitate a situational crisis for the patient and family. Because the initial traumatic injury often precipitates other stressors and the need for continuous adaptation, crisis may occur at any point along the continuum of care. Initially, during the phases of resuscitation and critical illness, the crisis may focus on whether the individual will survive the injury. Later, during the intermediate phase, the patient and the family may experience a crisis as they attempt to adjust to physical or emotional disabilities. During the rehabilitation phase, crisis may ensue as the patient and family face the difficulties of reintegrating the injured individual into the family and the community.

Infante[7] proposes a model of crisis that provides an understanding of crisis production and the potential for growth after the event. Before being injured the individual has a level of function that allows management of his or her daily needs and provides a sense of equilibrium. The individual suddenly experiences a hazardous event, perhaps a traumatic injury, and attempts to deal with the event by using familiar coping mechanisms, which have been effective in the past. In the current situation, however, these coping mechanisms prove to be inadequate, resulting in crisis. This crisis may result in the individual functioning at a lower level than before the crisis, and prolonged crisis without appropriate intervention can be devastating to the individual. He or she may experience disruption of the family, divorce, depression, or failure to return as a productive member of society. Interventions by the trauma nurse, however, can produce more positive outcomes. A realistic goal of crisis intervention is resolution and restoration to at least the precrisis level of functioning. Resolution is possible through the acquisition of new skills and the adoption of enhanced coping mechanisms. A crisis, effectively managed, can strengthen adaptive capacity, promote growth and learning, enhance problem-solving abilities, and result in a higher level of functioning. This potential growth depends on the timing and appropriateness of interventions.

CRISIS INTERVENTION

The focus of crisis intervention is to address the immediate problem or issue that is precipitating the crisis for the patient or family. It begins with an assessment of the person's view of the situation and what resources he or she has to cope with the stressor involved. Aguilera[8] presents a model of crisis intervention that incorporates three critical factors of crisis: (1) perception of the event, (2) adequacy of situational supports, and (3) effectiveness of coping mechanisms. Balancing these critical factors determines whether an event will produce a crisis for the individuals involved (Figure 19-1). When caring for an individual experiencing a crisis, assessment of the three balancing factors will provide direction for intervention. A deficit in one or more balancing factors places the individual at risk for crisis. For example, after a traumatic spinal cord injury, Patient A may perceive the event as being completely overwhelming and one with which he can never cope. He may have functioned in isolation in the past and may feel that there is no one on whom he can call for support. In addition, he may have a history of heavy alcohol use and poor coping abilities,

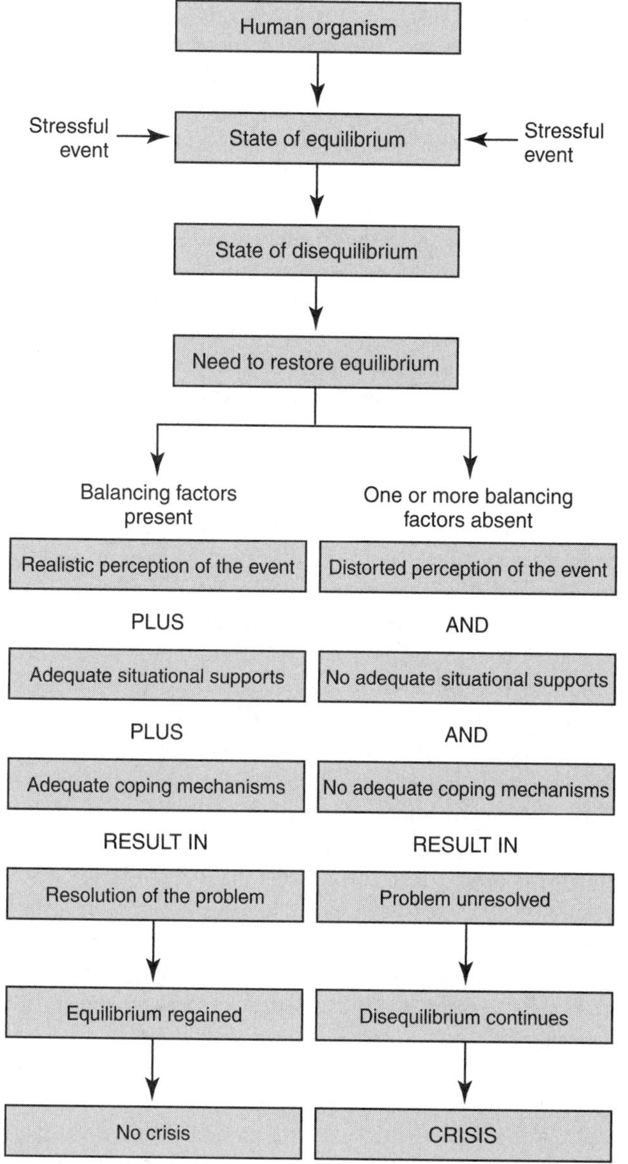

FIGURE 19-1 Paradigm: the effect of balancing factors in a stressful event. *(From Aguilera D:* Crisis intervention: theory and methodology, *p. 33, St. Louis, 1998, Mosby.)*

providing him with few effective coping mechanisms to deal with the current crisis. Patient A demonstrates deficits of all three balancing factors and is at risk for crisis development. Appropriate interventions would assist him to establish a more realistic perception of the event, use appropriate situational supports, and identify effective coping strategies. By providing support in each area of deficit, the nurse strengthens Patient A's balancing factors, reduces tension, and effectively intervenes to prevent a crisis. In contrast, Patient B has a similar spinal cord injury. This patient, however, views her injury as a challenge, one she can overcome with support from the environment. In the past Patient B has established a solid support system of friends and family on whom she can call on for help with the current event. In addition, her strong faith has assisted her to cope with past stressors and is also effective with the current stressor. Because Patient B has strengths in all three balancing factors, she is not currently crisis prone. Appropriate interventions would include support of her current resources and identification of future events that might generate a crisis.[8]

PERCEPTION

The first balancing factor is perception. Perception is defined as the subjective, individualized meaning of the stressful event and is determined by the individual's unique way of taking in, processing, and using information from the environment.[8] When confronted with an event, the individual will first perform a primary appraisal. This process allows the individual to judge whether the outcome of the event will be a threat to significant future values or goals. A secondary appraisal is then performed to determine the range of coping behaviors needed to either overcome the threat or achieve a positive outcome. If, during the appraisal stage, the stressor is perceived to be too overwhelming and not able to be handled successfully with available or typical coping mechanisms, the individual may feel forced to deny, distort, or repress the reality of the situation to cope. If, however, the appraisal process indicates that the available coping mechanisms are adequate to meet the threat, more efficient coping mechanisms may be used. If the individual distorts or denies the reality of the event, attempts to deal with the stressor will be unsuccessful, tensions will escalate, and the stress will not be reduced.[8]

The goal of intervention is to clarify the individual's perception and to focus the individual on the immediate situation. Useful questions to ask include the following:

- What does this mean to you?
- Do you understand what was just explained?
- How does it affect you right now?
- What does it mean for the future?

Intervention is directed toward determining whether the individual's perceptions are realistic or distorted. If perception is found to be realistic, support of the perception is indicated. However, if perception is distorted, it is important to use education and support to assist the individual to redefine the perception.

SITUATIONAL SUPPORTS

The second balancing factor, availability of situational supports, focuses on the evaluation of the availability of individuals in the environment who can be counted on to assist in the management of the problem. The individuals may include family members, friends, health care workers, support groups, and church or community resources. Adequate situational supports provide the individual with a source of advice, advocacy, and strength. Inadequate situational support, however, leads to feelings of isolation, loss, and vulnerability. The individual then experiences increased stress and a sense of overwhelming isolation.[8]

The goals of intervention focus on assisting the individual to identify sources of emotional, physical, social, and spiritual support that may be tapped during the crisis. To assess this balancing factor, useful questions to ask include the following:

- Are there people in your family or in your community on whom you can depend or call on for help right now? Who are they?
- Can/should they be contacted?
- Who can you most trust?
- Who is your most comfortable source of support?
- Do you have a higher power that you can call on for strength?
- With whom do you have the closest ties?

Interventions focus on connecting the individual with the most accessible and most effective sources of support and encouraging their consistent use.

COPING

The third balancing factor, availability of effective coping mechanisms, focuses on the usefulness of current coping mechanisms to deal with the stressful event. Typically individuals use a spectrum of coping mechanisms on a daily basis to handle perceived stressors. These coping mechanisms may include prayer, exercise, discussion, or crying. Others include smoking, alcohol or drug use, verbal battles, anger, swearing, or violence. When confronted with a stressor, the individual attempts to deal with it by using familiar coping mechanisms that have been effective in the past. A crisis is initiated when the individual realizes that these coping mechanisms no longer reduce the stress or provide resolution of the event. This perception of inadequate coping leads the individual to feel overwhelmed. Tension and anxiety increase, and a crisis ensues. The goal of intervention is to assist the individual to delineate methods of new or previously used coping methods to decrease anxiety and enhance coping.[8] When an individual is assessed for adequacy of coping mechanisms, it is useful to ask the following questions:

- Have you ever experienced anything like this before?
- How is this situation similar or different?
- Have you ever coped with high-anxiety situations in the past?
- What did you try? What worked? What didn't?
- What do you usually do when you feel like this?

When nurses identify use of maladaptive or self-destructive coping mechanisms such as substance abuse, violent behavior directed at self or others, or unwillingness to participate in their plan of care, psychiatric consultation may be indicated.

PREVENTION

Injuries are among the leading cause of death and disability in the world. Road traffic crashes, falls, interpersonal violence, and self-inflicted wounds are the most prevalent injury-related causes of morbidity and death.[9] Motor vehicle crashes, firearm incidents, poisonings, suffocations, falls, fires, and drownings take the lives of more than 400 Americans each day.[10] The Healthy People 2010 initiative has targeted these traumatic events as areas for intervention and prevention in the current decade. The use of safety devices such as seat belts in cars and helmets for bicyclists and increasing awareness for home safety issues including fall prevention and firearm safety were emphasized as specific interventions that would decrease the number of traumatic injuries or deaths. Characteristics of at-risk individuals and families are presented.

PERSONS AT RISK FOR TRAUMA

Age, sex, race, lifestyle, and socioeconomic factors all correlate with the likelihood of traumatic injury. For example, the young and the old are most vulnerable to fall-related injuries, men are most often the perpetrators and victims of homicide, and African-Americans are seven times more likely than whites to be murdered.[10] Injuries sustained in road traffic crashes are the leading cause of death worldwide among youth aged 15 to 44 years.[9] Choices to engage in more risky activities such as sport events or to use mind-altering substances also increase the risk for traumatic injury. For teens, sports and recreation are the most common activities associated with injury. Not surprisingly, high material wealth is positively correlated with sports injuries, whereas poverty is positively correlated with fighting injuries.[11] Low income, discrimination, and lack of education and employment are factors that are also closely associated with violent and abusive behavior.[10]

The high rate of recidivism in trauma care has prompted researchers to attempt to identify social and psychologic factors that increase the risk for traumatic injury. Poole et al[12] attempted to identify the relationship between specific psychosocial factors and the likelihood of traumatic injury.

It was discovered that individuals experiencing a traumatic injury are most likely young men who have not graduated from high school. Patients with intentional injury have a higher rate of illicit drug and alcohol use than do those with a nonintentional injury. In addition, patients experiencing intentional injury have a higher unemployment rate than those with nonintentional injury. The average intelligence score for victims of intentional injury is lower than both the national median and the scores of nonintentional trauma victims. Psychopathology is evident in the intentional trauma group, with 63% of the sample meeting diagnostic criteria for psychiatric diagnoses, including antisocial personality, depression, illicit drug abuse, and mental retardation. Results from this study indicate that, for some individuals, traumatic injury may not be a random accident but rather a result of the victim's high-risk behaviors and level of psychopathology. Social forces, such as unemployment and low education levels, may also influence the potential for traumatic injury.[12]

It is well known that alcohol use is a contributing factor in traumatic injuries. Forty percent of motor vehicle fatalities are alcohol related.[13] Ankney et al[14] analyzed the relationship among selected medical, social, and psychologic factors and alcohol-related trauma in a rural population. Their findings suggest that there are significant differences in the psychologic and social factors and medical histories of trauma victims with positive blood alcohol content (BAC) versus those with negative BAC. Patients with positive BAC were significantly more likely to be male, aged 21 to 50 years, unemployed or who had recently changed job status. In addition, this population was frequently known to the criminal justice system in that they reported a history of more arrests and criminal charges than did the BAC-negative group. The BAC-positive group also had an increased rate of inpatient mental counseling and positive drug screens. The finding that an increased number of BAC-positive patients reported having incurred a traumatic injury in the past reinforced the concept of recidivism. Several other factors approached statistical significance for the BAC-positive group: recent conflicts, interpersonal problems, or criminal sentencing; changes in financial status; and significant personal changes. The researchers conclude that trauma patients with premorbid alcohol abuse should be targeted for treatment in an effort to reduce the risk of recidivism.[14] Unfortunately, the majority of trauma patients rarely receive referral for substance abuse treatment.[15] Trauma nurses can play a key role in initiating such referrals. Trauma center administrators can set policy that requires intoxicated trauma patients to receive interventions. Research has demonstrated success in such referrals.[13]

AT RISK FAMILIES

The harsh reality of an acute health care crisis will test the strength and exploit the weaknesses of any family. For those families that have limited resources and struggle to maintain flexible and supportive interpersonal relationships among its members, the presence of a traumatic injury places them at risk for crisis. Four general functional areas are discussed in light of vulnerability to crisis: (1) levels of chronic anxiety in the family, (2) family emotional relationship structure, (3) communication process, and (4) multigenerational heritage and patterns.

Levels of Chronic Anxiety

Dysfunctional coping styles render families more vulnerable to crisis. Examples of these include very intense relationship systems: highly positive, highly negative, conflicting, or a combination. They are frequently characterized by a lesser ability to distinguish feeling process from intellectual process and are caught in a cycle of automatic emotional responses to each other, over which they perceive they have no control.[16,17] Behaviors are reactive and impulsive, with the goal of "feeling better" being paramount. Emotional responses are frequently chaotic and repetitive, reflecting a controlled, rigid, and limited repertoire of skills with which to deal with one another. In these families chronic anxiety tends to be absorbed by one family member, and that individual comes to be focused on in excess of either positive attention (i.e., "golden girl") or negative attitudes (i.e., "black sheep"). In this way the level of chronic anxiety between two family members, such as spouses, is somewhat lessened by the focus and diversion of energy onto a third person in the system. The member who is focused on in this way is the one who comes to be the most at risk for development of physical, emotional, and social problems throughout life.[17]

Emotional Relationship Structure

In times of high anxiety, dysfunctional ways of relating become even more intense. Families that tend to have a predominantly fixed and inflexible relationship structure dominated by dependence and excessive need for approval from one another will most likely react to crisis by automatic instinctual emotional forces rather than by use of intellect.[17] The concept of being enmeshed with another person implies that boundaries are diffuse and that the behavior of one family member has a direct effect on those with whom he or she is enmeshed.[18] Relationships tend to get fixed around one person underfunctioning in most of life's tasks and another reciprocally overfunctioning; there comes to be very little, if any, reciprocity within this pattern (i.e., one person always underfunctions and one always overfunctions). Members of this type of enmeshed, emotionally based family feel responsible for what another feels, whereas they do not feel much responsibility for themselves. Rather than being sensitive to another, these individuals find that they allow their behaviors to often be determined by another's desires. There is a problem distinguishing "needs" from "wants," and although family loyalty is rewarded, there may be an overall low caring index on the part of individuals for one another.

Communication Process

Crisis-prone families have few hierarchical boundaries and rules between the generations in communication and tend to be sensitive to praise or criticism for one another.[18] Communication sequences are predictable, rigid, and reactive, with low levels of conflict resolution. Confrontation of issues tends to be avoided, and many conflicting issues either are never discussed or are fought about but never resolved. Communication is closed, with little taking in of new information, and is impoverished in affect. Generalizations are frequent, and blaming is heavily used to hold someone in the family, the school, the law, the society, or the institution at fault.[17] Others are often told what to do rather than being encouraged to find their own solutions.

Multigenerational Heritage and Patterns

Often crisis-prone families are cut off from previous generations, being either geographically distant or, more frequently, emotionally disconnected.[17] Boundaries around the family are closed, with little relationship network or few social supports available to help diffuse the family's chronic anxiety. There is a strong passing down of family "myths" and expectations for behavior and feelings on the part of individuals. Most often there are multigenerational patterns of various physical, emotional, and social dysfunctions such as chronic physical illnesses, depression, violence, substance abuse, and repeated trauma.

Although an awareness of these functional areas may not prevent a future crisis or totally forestall dysfunctional family coping in light of a crisis, identification of these complex family dynamics should alert the nurse that a multidisciplinary approach to working with the at-risk family is needed. In recent years public education has played a crucial role regarding developmental family issues, parenting, adolescence, and appropriate need for counseling. More and more families are aware, as a result, of their own strengths and weaknesses and their need for appropriate direction in seeking to improve function.

In summary, adaptive coping is enhanced with low to moderate levels of anxiety, which allows the family to hear, understand, and repeat information; decreased reactivity to issues, which allows action rather than reaction and the adoption of a solution-oriented approach; high motivation and sense of personal identity distinct from an enmeshed identity with the patient; ultimate belief in one's ability to gain control over one's life again; and evidence of role flexibility and high levels of family caring and cohesion.[8,17]

RESUSCITATION PHASE

THE PATIENT

During the resuscitation phase the trauma victim feels an instantaneous, overwhelming threat to life. A study by Morse and O'Brien[19] describes a four-stage process of self-preservation experienced by trauma victims (Table 19-1). The first stage of the process begins at the time of injury, and the remaining stages continue to the point of recovery.[19]

The first stage of the self preservation model is termed *Vigilance: Becoming Engulfed.* During this stage the trauma victim initially has a significant increase in cognitive abilities. There is a heightening of senses, and survivors are able to provide extremely detailed descriptions of the incident. Time seems to slow, and the individual has difficulty with the sense of time. For example, the patient may relate that the extrication from the vehicle took hours, when in fact it took only minutes. The trauma victim often recalls the exact moment of impact of the traumatic event and immediately becomes aware of the seriousness of the injuries and that his or her life is in danger. During the prehospital phase the conscious individual becomes an active participant in his or her own care, instructing bystanders who are attempting to assist in the initial rescue. He or she will, however, relinquish control to the paramedic team if they appear to be competent.[19]

In the ED or resuscitation area, the patient may surrender the vigilant role and assume the role of detached observer. At this point, patients in the Morse and O'Brien study reported feeling calm, detached, or in a dream-like state. Although externally the individual may be demonstrating intense anxiety and panic, the internal state is described as one of detached calmness. Some revealed that they experienced an internal dialog between their objective and subjective selves. One participant in the study described her experience as follows:

> I remember lots of nurses and doctors or whatever around me. I don't remember feeling pain. I remember hearing a woman screaming for _______, who was my son who died 9 years ago. I remember wondering, "Who is that woman screaming for my son? Doesn't she know he's dead? Doesn't she know he died 9 years ago? Why is she screaming?" I could feel that it was actually me screaming and I remember thinking, it's not _______ you want. Why aren't you screaming for _______ and _______?[19]

Visual input generates fear for patients. They may have only their own damaged body to explore; the sight of tubes and machinery to which they are attached contributes to increased anxiety. If they are able to see other patients, their visual sense will be bombarded by the overwhelming mutilation of others around them. Privacy is minimal and control nonexistent. As the stage of intense vigilance ends, the individual may experience gaps in conscious awareness. These gaps may be a result of administered sedating agents or analgesics or deterioration in the patient's physical state.[19]

The intensity and degree to which the injury and resuscitation process affects the patient depend largely on the person's perception and appraisal of the situation and the level of intactness of the person's biopsychologic state. Hence, response to traumatic injury is not directly related to the severity of the injury but to the unique perception and interpretation of events and stressors and the coping strategies trauma patients are able to call forth. In effect, then, it is

TABLE 19-1 The Stages of Preserving Self

Stage I Vigilance: Becoming Engulfed	Stage II Disruption: Taking Time Out	Stage III Enduring the Self: Confronting and Regrouping	Stage IV Striving to Regain Self: Merging the Old and the New Reality
Being vigilant Experiencing clarity of thought Experiencing the expansion of time	Being in a shattered reality Experiencing memory gaps, "fog" Dreaming vividly, frequently bizarre, confused with reality	Learning to endure Living through pain and treatments Grasping the implications of the injury	Making sense Seeking information about the incident Recognizing it could be worse
Being directive, protecting the living, breathing self	Vacillating sleep/wake cycles	Trying to "bear it," learning to "take it"	
	Perceiving the world as changing and hostile	Learning to accept dependence	
Distancing subjective from objective body Observing dispassionately Becoming two-personed	Anchoring onto the significant other Trying to "keep myself together"	Latching onto the significant other Not tolerating being left alone Seeking distraction Seeking encouragement Seeking entertainment Learning physical limitations	Getting to know and trust the altered body Learning limitations Viewing life beyond self Revising/modifying life goals
Relinquishing to caregivers Surrendering Becoming calm	Recognizing reality Beginning the struggle	Doing the work of healing Living with setbacks and discouragement Keeping a score card Refusing to accept the damage	Accepting the consequences of the experience Realizing they can "hack it" Evaluating meaning Redefining self

From Morse JM, O'Brien B: Preserving self: from victim to patient, to disabled person, *J Adv Nurs* 21:888, 1995.

feasible that a minimally injured trauma patient may in fact experience and respond more intensely to stressors than a severely physiologically impaired person. The inverse also is possible: the more severely injured the patient is, the less able he or she may be to mediate the stress. It becomes clear that the nurse's assessment and understanding of the patient's perception of stressors are what guide interventions, not simply the severity of the injury.

The nursing goals during this phase are aimed at supporting patients in diminishing their anxiety level by providing them with information concerning their environment and by making the environment understandable and as safe as possible for them. By speaking calmly, empathetically, and slowly; by gently touching the patient; and by helping the patient focus his or her attention, the nurse begins a relationship with the patient that allows the patient to trust someone in a foreign and chaotic situation. Eye contact is crucial when this mode is accessible. The nurse, in fact, may have to physically hold the patient's head with her hands, look him or her in the eyes, and give short, succinct bits of information. "I'm Ann, I'm a nurse. You're in the hospital. You've been in a car crash. You've been hurt and the doctors and I are going to take care of you." Telling the patient what is going to be done before doing it allows the patient to anticipate and process what is happening. Because good communication can reduce anxiety, facilitate proper diagnoses, treatment, and outcome in trauma situations, hospitals must ensure that interpreters are available for non-English-speaking patients and their families.

The Family

During the resuscitation phase the family also experiences a state of crisis after the injury of a loved one. Fear and uncertainty regarding the severity of the patient's condition and lack of communication from the trauma team produce increased stress.[20] The stress inherent in an unfamiliar complex trauma environment and the often unstable, unpredictable nature of illness/injury can lead to enormous strain and places the family at risk for a difficult adaptation. The uncertainty of prognosis, financial concerns, role changes, disrupted daily routines, and a family's prior ability/success at managing stressful situations all affect the overall family well-being. The severity of the patient's illness/injury may be associated with a complicated, prolonged recovery, resulting in a delay in or inability in achieving an acceptable level of functional recovery. Early family contact, frequent updates and assurances (when appropriate) help foster an understanding of the situation and reduce stress. Crisis assessment and intervention is indicated with families of trauma patients.[20,21]

Assessment of the family not only involves taking into consideration the immediate needs for assistance and direction with acute crisis, but also requires an intervention framework that assists the family toward enhanced self-reliance and functional coping. The skills needed by the nurse during this acute phase incorporate a mixture of crisis intervention and beginning family system assessment as family members are struggling with the uncertainty of whether their loved one will survive or what life changes may occur if he or she does survive.

The resuscitation phase involves particularly high anxiety levels for family members, which may be exhibited in a number of ways and which are capable of being maintained for prolonged periods. Individuals may be unable to sit still; they may pace, have trouble processing verbal messages, shake, sigh deeply, or clench their fists, have difficulty breathing, not be able to complete a sentence, have flight of ideas, seem labile with mood swings, and exhibit a host of other anxious behaviors. They feel overwhelmed, powerless, out of control, frightened, and have a sense of immobilization. Even the most stable individual in the face of sufficient anxiety may behave in a bizarre fashion. One very reserved middle-aged male executive, known for his usual calm demeanor in the face of business problems, was so anxious during the first 48 hours of his son's admission to the trauma center with multiple injuries from a hit-and-run incident that he would periodically erupt from his chair in the waiting room and shout that he could not stand to hear one more announcement over the loudspeaker. His behavior frightened his family and himself because it was so out of character for him. The family was less anxious and more understanding when the nurse normalized individual responses to stress and was able to explain that the father's unusual and unexpected behavior was often encountered in such stressful situations.

Along with a high level of anxiety there may be accompanying shock, fright, disbelief, numbness, feeling of responsibility or blame, guilt, and distrust. It is important for the nurse to remember that a family's reaction to the current situation may be accentuated or blunted by previous experience with similar circumstances, and initial questioning regarding whether the family has ever experienced anything of this nature or magnitude before may provide valuable initial direction. It is very important that families be afforded the opportunity to share these initial responses because they must be dealt with for the family to move on with the crisis resolution.

Having family members present during the resuscitation phase remains controversial. Supporters believe that this is an opportunity to educate the family in a real-time/real-life situation about the medical issues confronting both their loved one and the health care team. Having the family present allows them to see and appreciate the efforts and care being provided, to understand that every reasonable effort was being attempted, and to provide them with closure to the experience. Opponents claim that having the family at bedside during resuscitation creates dangerous congestion at an already crowded bedside and that family members could become too emotional and interfere with care. The family's presence could increase caregiver stress, making them more tentative in their decisions and pressured when performing procedures. Fear of increased litigation and maintaining patient confidentiality are other often citied concerns.[22] Halm,[22] in a review of the literature, found that although families often stated a desire to be present during resuscitation efforts, whether this would have been acceptable to the patients themselves was unknown, raising significant ethical and legal issues.

In a classic study of families of trauma victims, Epperson[23] identified a six-phase recovery process that families under severe and sudden stress undergo. How individuals within the same family respond remains unique and diverse, although there does seem to be an identifiable course that is common (Figure 19-2).

Anxiety, Shock, and Fright

During periods of high anxiety, family members often need repeated clarifications and restatements of information. This information should be brief, explicit, and straightforward, and it may be more useful if it is actually written. To accurately ascertain that the family has heard what was being said, they should be asked to repeat what they understand at various points, what they have been told, and what that means to them. Even the most functional families may become dysfunctional for a time in light of enough stress, and an initial period of confusion and the need for precise reinforcement and repetition of information are normal. Often the identification of one key family member with whom the health care team communicates regarding the patient's status is useful in limiting the confusion and defusing some of the anxiety.[23]

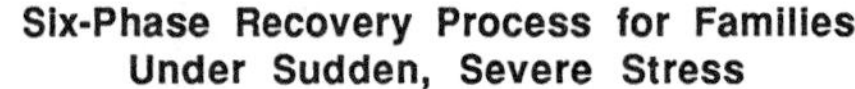

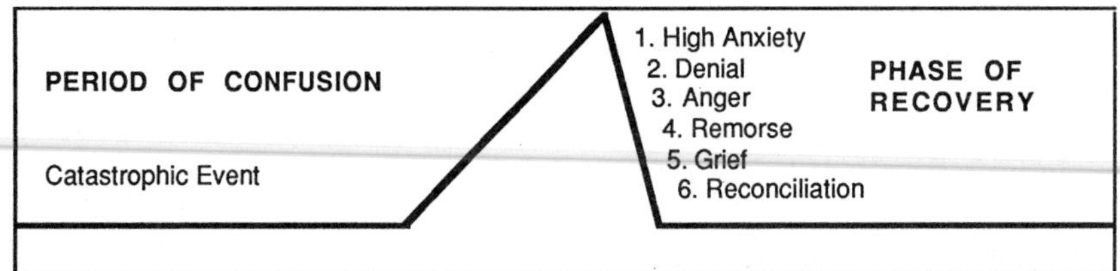

FIGURE 19-2 Six-phase recovery process for families under sudden, severe stress.
(From Epperson MM: Families in sudden crisis: process and intervention in a critical care center, *Soc Work Health Care* 2:205-273, 1977.)

Denial

Denial within the resuscitation phase serves a somewhat useful purpose for family members in that it may provide the time necessary to adapt and adjust to the actual reality of what has happened.[23] Denial, as such, buys the family "psychologic time." The nurse needs to recognize the purpose and function of denial while at the same time recognizing the family's need to deal with the reality of the present situation and still maintain hope. Statements such as, "Mrs. _____, your daughter has never been ill before and I know it must be very difficult for you to believe that she is in a coma from the car crash" are often useful. In this way the message is transmitted that the nurse is aware of the struggle between what is hoped for and what is the current reality.

If denial is prolonged and hampers the carrying out of necessary actions on the part of family members, additional interventions may have to be incorporated that are more directly unsupportive of the denial and much more directive and confrontational. In the case of one 36-year-old mother of an 11-year-old daughter who was a drowning victim and had been in a coma with no physiologic indication of functional improvement, the mother waited by the bedside every day for the child to wake up. She would say, "I just know that today Claudia's going to open her eyes and be OK." Her denial stemmed from the fact that the daughter's friend, who was with her and also had drowned and been initially unresponsive, had begun to respond and improve 3 weeks after the initial accident. Also, on the news that month was the story of a woman who had awakened after 11 years in a coma. Hence the mother's natural inclination toward denial and hope was buttressed by two cases evidencing improvement. However, given all medical indications, this was not predicted for Claudia, and her mother would make no perceptible move to investigate the possible institutional placements made available to her by the nurse and the rest of the team. A decision had to be made, and the mother had to be gently but firmly told that her daughter's case was different from the other little girl's. Clear distinctions were made in easily understandable terms as to the differences in initial signs and symptoms and the sequencing of return of function. She was shown visual pictures of the extent of brain damage and told that all indications of what was known at this time indicated that this was the state in which Claudia would remain. Hope is an important ingredient and should not be totally removed, but to break through prolonged denial that may become pathologic, a factual representation is essential, along with the notion that miracles are always possible; in this case that is what was necessary.[23] In such cases of dysfunctional denial, a team approach is recommended to ensure that a solid plan of care is constructed and a consistent message is given.

Anger, Hostility, and Distrust

Families need to be able to verbalize their anger without the health care professional personalizing it; they may be angry at the patient, at themselves, at the institutions giving care, at the physicians, at the nurses, at God, at society, and at life in general. Diffuse anger is often present and helps forestall the pain inherent in the grief that follows. Anger needs to be given expression and accepted by the nurse, while at the same time direction is given in the form of questions that help families identify the actual legitimacy of the focus of their anger. When the "real thoughts behind the anger" can be pulled out by the family, they often realize that fear, guilt, and loss of control are driving the anger. They can then put that to rest and move on with the necessary grief work before reconciliation.[23]

Remorse and Guilt

Epperson[23] refers to the remorse stage as the "if only" stage. Families struggle with sorrow and guilt over the part they played in the trauma or injury or in not preventing the possibility of it. It is important not to rationalize this phase as problem-solving questions are asked to help families reason out the thoughts, fears, and misperceptions they have. A mother's remorse and guilt over allowing her 19-year-old son to buy and ride the motorcycle on which he was struck by a truck should be listened to without judgment and without rationalization. Statements and questions such as, "19-year-olds make their own choices," "No family is without conflict," and "Is it possible for even a mom to control a 19-year-old's behavior?" may be helpful in this phase. The more verbalization the better because this will defocus the issue and work toward problem solving. However, bear in mind that wide fluctuations in mood are normal within these early phases. Many family members share the fear that they are "going crazy" because of the lability of their emotional responses during the resuscitation and critical care phases, and it is crucial for the nurse to share the "norm" in ranges of feelings experienced by most families in similar situations.[23]

Grief and Depression

Watching a family experience the necessary pain of the grief phase is especially difficult. Too often nurses intervene too rapidly to support, take care of, fix, or make better. Pain is a necessary component of grief work, and it must be allowed to run its course. To the extent that the nurse can be comfortable with staying connected to those family members who are grieving and are in great pain, the essential work for families within this phase will be augmented. This, in turn, allows the mobilization of resources and the realistic putting together of family life required for reconciliation. Table 19-2 summarizes the basic interventions for each of these initial family responses within the phases of recovery after a crisis.[24]

Throughout these phases, the art of nonjudgmental listening is essential. It is easy to allow oneself to get pulled in by emotions to giving too much support, assuming too much responsibility for others' feelings, siding, and blaming. Nontherapeutic responses, questions, and statements made by the nurse such as, "You shouldn't blame yourself," "How can you think you caused that to happen?" "Things will work out," "All things happen for a reason," "God does not give us

TABLE 19-2 **Interventions for Initial Family Responses to Crisis**

Family Responses	Interventions
Anxiety, shock, fright	Give information that is brief, concise, explicit, and concrete. Repeat and frequently reinforce information—encourage families to record important facts in writing. Ascertain comprehension by asking family to repeat to you what information they have been given. Provide for and encourage or allow ventilation of feelings, even if they are extreme. Maintain constant, nonanxious presence in the face of a highly anxious family. Inform family as to the potential range of behaviors and feelings that are within the "norm" for crisis. Maximize control within hospital environment, as possible.
Denial	Identify what purpose denial is serving for family (e.g., Is it buying them "psychologic time" for future coping and mobilization of resources?). Evaluate appropriateness of use of denial in terms of time; denial becomes inappropriate when it inhibits the family from taking necessary actions or when it is impinging on the course of treatment. Do not actively support denial but neither dash hopes for the future (e.g., "It must be very difficult for you to believe your son is nonresponsive and in a trauma unit."). If denial is prolonged and dysfunctional, more direct and specific factual representation may be essential.
Anger, hostility, distrust	Allow for ventilation of angry feelings, clarifying what thoughts, fears, and beliefs are behind the anger; let them know it's okay to be angry. Don't personalize family's expression of these strong emotions. Institute family control within the hospital environment when possible (e.g., arrange for set time[s] and set person[s] to give them information in reference to the patient and answer their questions). Remain available to families during their venting of these emotions. Ask families how they can take the energy in their anger and put it to positive use for themselves, for the patient, and for the situation.
Remorse and guilt	Do not try to "rationalize away" guilt for families. Listen, support their expression of feeling and verbalizations (e.g., "I can understand how or why you might feel that way; however, …"). Follow the "howevers" with careful, reality-oriented statements or questions (e.g., "None of us can truly control another's behavior."; "Kids make their own choices despite what parents think and want."; "How successful were you when you tried to control __________'s behavior with that before?"; "So many things have happened for which there are no absolute answers.").
Grief and depression	Acknowledge family's grief and depression. Encourage them to be precise about what it is they are grieving and depressed about; give grief and depression a context. Allow the family appropriate time for grief. Recognize that this is an essential step for future adaptation—do not try to rush the grief process. Remain sensitive to your own unfinished business and, hence, comfort/discomfort with family's grieving and depression.
Hope	Clarify with families what their hopes are, individually and with one another. Clarify with families what their worst fears are in reference to the situation. Are the hopes/fears congruent? realistic? unrealistic? Support realistic hope. Offer gentle factual information to reframe unrealistic hope (e.g., "With the information you have or the observations you have made, do you think that is still possible?"). Assist families in reframing unrealistic hope in some other fashion (e.g., "What do you think others will have learned from _______ if he doesn't make it?" "How do you think _______ would like for you to remember him/her?").

Modified from Kleeman KM: Families in crisis due to multiple trauma, *Crit Care Nurs Clin North Am* 1:23-31, 1989.

more than we can handle," and "I would agree that _______ _____ was wrong to do that!" do nothing to assist in long-term coping and may do much to alienate the nurse from the family he or she is endeavoring to support. It is not important to know the answers to many of the unanswerable questions that families pose but rather to ask the right questions so that families may begin to generate their own solutions, coping mechanisms, and resources. Questions such as "I hear what you say about ____________; how do you see that as changeable?" "What would it take for you to feel less guilty? less hostile? less ____________?" "How will your family pull together to ensure that everyone will be okay after this loss?" are examples of the types of thought-producing stimuli that facilitate the family's own problem solving and ensure the transmission of a nonjudgmental attitude on the part of the nurse.

Trauma centers must have a systematic process for accommodating and supporting large or extended families. This process must include sensitivity to cultural norms during times of crisis and illness and include discussion about how the family makes decisions and communicates information, especially during the acute phase of trauma care.

Critical Care Phase

The Patient

The critical care phase is one of great challenges to the trauma patient. Described as a time of great fear and confusion, this phase demands both physical and emotional strength. The trauma patient must deal with the pain and uncertainty of injury, separation from significant others, alteration in body image as a result of injury and treatment, inability to communicate with family and staff, impaired thinking processes, sleep deprivation, and loss of control.

During the critical care phase, the trauma victim enters stage II of the process of self-preservation as described by Morse and O'Brien[19] (see Table 19-1). Stage II, defined as *disruption: taking time out,* is described by trauma survivors as an overwhelming phase with which they had difficulty coping. The stage is often described as consisting of episodes of vivid, terrifying dreams interspersed with periods of excruciating pain. Burn patients in particular were found to experience the most terrifying and confusing of dreams. One patient describes his experience as follows: "I had a nightmare of this little kid. I was in Vietnam and I was half blown away and this kid dragged me to his mother and his mother dissected a cow and used the cow's parts and put me back together."[19]

Patients with spinal cord injuries with deficit often dream of the "old me," a dream in which the patient is intact and fully functional. On awakening, the patient is suddenly again confronted with the reality of the injury. Patients in this stage also describe intense difficulty defining reality, uncertainty as to which event is real and which is only a dream. Both sleep and wakefulness are described as being intolerable. Patients describe this period as a vicious cycle wherein they attempt to escape from the terrifying sleep state by awakening and, in contrast, escape from the pain by sleeping. The result is a state of confusion or fog in which the patient cannot determine wakefulness from sleep or sometimes life from death. During this stage, patients are most often in critical condition, receiving pain medication and sedation, both of which contribute to the confusion. The period is often recalled as one of vague, dreamlike memories or flashbacks. Patients experience altered perceptions of the environment, believing that the furnishings of their rooms are changed frequently or that they have been moved from room to room. Health providers are often viewed as hurtful, hostile, and not to be trusted. Patients report that they expected their family members to protect them from these caregivers and are hurt and confused when the family leaves at the end of the visiting session.[19]

During stage II a critical need expressed by trauma survivors is to have family members readily accessible. Patients view their family members and significant others to be essential sources of support and a safe haven in their world of pain and confusion. Often the patient is afraid to be alone and the significant other represents a sense of security, reality, and safety. The family member helps anchor the patient to reality, assists the patient to regain a sense of self and "humanness," and contributes to the healing process. Patients describe the presence of a family member as being the most important intervention during stage II.[19]

Alteration of Body Image

As the critical care phase progresses, the patient shifts from a major fear of death to increasing concerns about alterations of body function and significant losses. When it is established that life itself will not be suddenly lost, patients gradually come to terms with their altered body and with the pain that seems unceasing. At the same time, other struggles emerge; the patient must develop new ways of expressing self in relating to family, significant others, and, increasingly, the nurse.

Mutilation of the body through both trauma and subsequent treatment is stressful for the patient and the nurse. Patients recognize that their once intact body now may have holes in it, tubes that emerge from their skin, and wires and pins that hold together their flesh and bone. They must address this change by coming to terms with the reality that these apparitions are now part of self.

In a society in which youthful physical attractiveness is valued, disability, disfigurement, and scarring are likely to produce anxiety and problems with self-esteem. Sudden changes in body image, such as those brought about by unexpected traumatic injury, place the patient at risk for loss, depression, sexual problems, guilt, and grief.[25]

It is important to assist the patient with integration of this changed body image into his or her concept of self. Interventions such as facilitating open communication; conveying an empathetic, caring approach; and providing acceptance are useful. It is important to remember that each patient has a personal perception of his or her wounds. A massive abdominal wound that to the nurse is healing well may be of great worry to the patient. He or she may become anxious that the wound will not heal without great scarring or that abdominal organs will be exposed. It is important that the nurse carefully assess the patient's perceptions of his or her wounds. The patient should be asked whether he or she has any questions about the wound. His or her knowledge about the wound, its care, and the potential for healing should be assessed. The nurse should allow the patient to achieve control by answering only those questions the patient raises. This allows him or her to control the amount of potentially anxiety-producing information received at any one time. Answers to the questions should be conveyed in an accurate, factual, truthful, and reassuring manner. The provision of concrete information helps the patient become focused on reality and reduces uncertainty. The information should be communicated in easy-to-understand language.[25]

The manner in which friends, family, and staff react to the wound also greatly influences the patient's sense of self-esteem. Nonverbal body language is a powerful tool, and the health care team must be aware of its unconscious use. If the patient interprets this communication as negative, he or she will experience increased anxiety and self-doubt. In contrast, the patient will be able to begin to positively integrate the wound into his or her body image if he or she senses that the staff conveys a positive and accepting manner when caring for the wound.[25]

As a response to the mounting anxiety related to the wound and the altered body image, the patient may attempt to cope by putting into play defense mechanisms such as withdrawal, avoidance, and suppression in an attempt to maintain psychologic balance. Dressing changes and wound care are constant reminders of both the changes in the appearance of the body and the traumatic event that produced those changes. It is not unusual for the patient to respond by refusing to cooperate with dressing changes or being noncompliant with wound care. The health care team needs to be sensitive to these issues when caring for the wound, giving the patient choices such as negotiating when the wound care will occur as a strategy to increase his or her sense of control over the situation. Relief from pain is a priority for the patient during dressing changes. Pharmacologic and nonpharmacologic strategies should be instituted to manage pain. Adequate relief from anxiety must be provided. Referral to a psychiatric liaison, use of relaxation techniques, and pharmacologic methods should be explored.[25]

Impaired Verbal Communication

In the critical care phase many patients are unable to verbalize their needs because they are intubated, have facial trauma, or have tracheostomies. This compounds the problems of communication regarding the patient's psychologic needs. It is important that the nurse support patients in finding ways that they can make their needs, concerns, and feelings known. An environment that gives patients permission, creative options, and time and means to communicate at their own pace and in their own manner is crucial to effective coping.

A major component of the nursing assessment is determining the ability of patients to comprehend what is said to them. Because the patient's sensorium fluctuates in response to physiologic shifts, pain, sedation, sleep deprivation and environmental stimuli, a reliable assessment is best achieved when these factors are taken into account. Asking patients to respond to simple commands that they are physically capable of performing, such as "Raise your left arm" or "Blink your eyes twice if you understand what I'm saying," aids in determining the patients' ability to comprehend information. Once the nurse assesses that the patient comprehends what is being said, creative modes for communicating must be devised.

When patients are cognitively intact but remain intubated, it is frustrating for patients and the nurse when patients have to repeat their communications because the nurse is not able to read their lips. It is important to acknowledge that frustration and to keep trying. Questions that require short answers should be asked so as not to tire the patient. Health professionals have a tendency to speak loudly to patients who are unable to talk, forgetting that the patient's cognitive abilities are often altered and hearing may not be altered. Speaking in a normal tone, facing the patient, modifying environmental stimuli, and being patient all facilitate communication. If a patient can write or use word and picture boards, these vehicles need to be incorporated into his or her care and made known to all those interacting with the patient. Mechanisms for contacting the nurse, such as call bells or buzzers, must also be identified because the patient's sense of helplessness and level of anxiety are compounded when he or she cannot call for help. In addition, the use of therapeutic listening skills such as maintaining eye contact, sitting at eye level with the patient, and leaning forward can communicate a supportive, caring attitude to the intubated or nonverbal patient.[26]

Impaired Thinking Processes

The trauma patient's thinking processes may be radically impaired as a result of physiologic, psychosocial, and environmental factors. Hypoxia, kidney failure, electrolyte imbalances, and medications in concert with anxiety, sensory overload and deprivation, social isolation, sleep deprivation, and immobility all affect the patient's cognitive functions, resulting in disorganized thinking and behavioral patterns.

An assessment of the patient's orientation may reveal that he or she is not oriented to person, place, time, or situation. Testing of memory functioning may reveal that the patient's short-term memory and immediate recall abilities are impaired. The patient's thinking processes, as assessed through spoken or written word, may reflect an unclear and loose association of ideas, indicative of scattered thinking processes. The flow of speech may be slow, hesitant, slurred, or mumbled. The response time to questioning is often retarded. Analyzing the content of a patient's thoughts may reveal that he or she is misperceiving environmental stimuli and experiencing delusions. Repetitive themes may be present in verbalizations. Illusions or hallucinations in any of the sensory modalities may be present. The patient's affect may also be disconjugate to his or her thought content. The patient's mood may be labile: quickly cycling from crying to anger, hostility, or passive indifference.

When a patient's thought processes are impaired, his or her attention span is limited and the the patient is easily distracted by environmental stimuli. Behavior is not goal oriented and is often inappropriate. Confusion may lead the patient to pull out tubes and tear off dressings. Eye contact may be poor, and the patient may not respond as expected to touch.

When a patient has demonstrated that thinking processes are impaired, nursing goals should be directed toward providing for patient safety and helping the patient differentiate what is real from what is not. Providing patients with information that supports orientation to place, time, and situation is helpful. Consistently modifying and interpreting the environment for patients using their intact sensory modalities supports patients in differentiating real from unreal. Providing a calm, soothing environment that minimizes noise and distractions, together with frequent attempts to reorient and reassure a patient, can limit combative and disruptive behaviors. Proactively addressing these issues can minimize the need to use physical or chemical restraints that may adversely affect patient safety and worsen the confusion and agitation.[27]

Sleep Deprivation

The typical progression of sleep involves cycling through non-rapid-eye-movement (non-REM) and rapid eye movement (REM) sleep stages with a periodicity of 90 to 120 minutes. Sleep architecture is composed of three segments. Segment one involves light sleep whereas segment two involves deep sleep, often referred to as delta sleep or slow wave sleep. This is the most restorative part of sleep. Segments one and two are non-REM. The third segment is the REM stage.[28] A person passes through the stages of sleep several times, with each cycle decreasing in length until the person awakens. Trauma patients have abnormalities in sleep patterns and duration. Procedures and excessive stimulation frequently prevent extended periods of sleep, with the result that sleep deprivation can occur quickly. Medications, anxiety, fear, pain, and immobility contribute to disruption in sleep patterns. Trauma patients with sleep deprivation frequently become irritable and disoriented, displaying memory and thinking impairments.

Physical and emotional trauma disrupt the duration and quality of sleep, adversely affecting the patient's mood and healing process. Wherever possible, nonpharmacologic methods to improve sleep should be attempted. Providing appropriately timed light/daylight exposure to scheduled interventions in conjunction with a darkened, quiet comfortable sleep environment will help the patient maintain a consistent physiologic circadian sleep/wake pattern. Behavioral therapy with use of cognitive and relaxation techniques have been shown to reduce the time spent awake after sleep onset and to improve sustained sleep compared with benzodiazepines or placebo.[29]

In circumstances where pharmacotherapy is considered appropriate, the medication should be limited to the lowest effective dose to be used only intermittently and for short term (less than 2 to 3 weeks) to avoid rebound insomnia. Benzodiazapines are often used but can cause residual psychomotor slowing and daytime sedation, making the patient prone to falls. Tolerance to the hypnotic effects of benzodiazepines can develop rapidly, and addiction is always a concern.[30]

The goal of the trauma nurse is to provide an environment that not only is conducive to sleeping but also allows maximal quantity and quality of sleep. Interventions focus on minimizing interruptions when the patient is attempting to rest. This requires the nurse to structure care and treatments so that the patient has blocks of uninterrupted sleep time. Decreasing environmental noise and lighting also facilitates sleep. Relaxation techniques such as back rubs, guided imagery, and music facilitate onset of sleep. Reassuring the frightened patient that the nurse remains while the patient is sleeping diminishes anxiety and the need for constant vigilance. Many trauma patients calmly drift off to sleep in the presence of someone they trust. Taking the time to sit and do charting quietly at the bedside provides the patient with a sense of security. Because patients need between 70 and 100 minutes of uninterrupted sleep to complete one full cycle of quality sleep, a continuing chart that documents how well this is achieved is valuable. Quality sleep renews the patient both physically and psychologically and does much to enhance the healing process.[26]

Loss of Emotional Control

Because traumatic injuries are accompanied by situations and procedures that cause pain and loss of normal emotional control of behavior, the patient, in an attempt to allay anxiety, may react with loud crying, dependent behavior, use of obscenities, and questioning of the staff's ability. This may not be the person's normal repertoire of responses. The person feels extremely vulnerable to this lack of personal control because it may lead to further isolation by staff and loss of self-esteem. If the response of the staff is one of ridicule of the behavior rather than insight into the emotional needs being expressed by the behavior, anxiety and fear are increased.

As the patient moves through the critical care phase, the magnitude of the number and variety of losses experienced is startling. Throughout this cycle patients have seen losses regarding their usual communication modalities, physical functioning, interpersonal relationships, environmental issues, alterations in roles, and invasion of boundaries of the self. The threat of powerlessness is profound. Patients respond with a variety of behaviors ranging from hostility and dependence to withdrawal and lack of motivation and interest in the environment. The inability to make simple decisions or take an interest in what is happening to them reflects the deep sense of helplessness and hopelessness they are experiencing.[31]

Throughout the patient's stay in the ICU, the nurse should constantly assess and balance when and to what extent the patient can actively or passively make decisions and participate in his or her own care. A sense of personal autonomy is enhanced every time the nurse solicits the patient's views, preferences, and opinions. The more a nurse selects opportunities that allow and support the patient's decision making and control over his or her environment, personal control is enhanced. Small achievements are consistently pointed out and hope is renewed. The nurse's ability to diagnose, assess, and intervene in this phase of trauma sets the groundwork for psychologic restoration.

THE FAMILY

In our contemporary society, the concept of family has grown to encompass many different groups. Traditional heterosexual multigenerational families are now joined by blended families brought together by remarriage or death of a spouse, single-parent families, couples in committed homosexual relationships with and without children, and even, though rarely, commune-based family groups. Families usually play an important role in the care and recovery of their loved ones. They are a stabilizing force, offering hope, support, and a connection to the preinjury real life. All family members, including those considered to be nontraditional, such as gay, lesbian, or bisexual partners, must be treated with respect and afforded the opportunity to visit with and participate in the care of their significant other. Biases, real or perceived, by either clinicians or families can be disruptive and interfere with the healing process.

Pachankis and Goldfried[32] provide a discussion on key clinical considerations related to working with sexual minority populations. Although the article was written for psychotherapists, the ICU/trauma nurse can benefit from this discussion on heterocentrism, homophobia, and common biases held against people who are gay, lesbian, or bisexual. Nurses should have a grasp on these issues so that patient advocacy, a hallmark of nursing, can be ensured for all patients under his or her care. Hospital policies or practices that allow only spouses or blood relatives to visit those in the ICU will deny patients access to their loved ones at a time of severe crisis.[32]

The family faces overwhelming stresses during the critical care phase. These include the realization that their loved one is critically ill with a potentially life-threatening injury; the stresses of the critical care environment; and the disruption of family roles, routines, and plans for the future.[5] The fear of death is foremost in the minds of family members and should be acknowledged and addressed by the nursing staff. The foreign environment, frightening noises, lack of privacy, and presence of strangers further contributes to the high stress levels. Family members often judge the seriousness of the patient's condition on the basis of the number of tubes, drains, intravenous pumps, and other equipment at the bedside. Conversely, the family may interpret the removal of these items as improvement in the patient's condition.[5] Whatever the perception, the family needs validation from the nurse to facilitate effective coping during this time of high stress.

During critical illness family routines become disrupted, and key roles may have to be delegated to other members. Dreams for the future may be destroyed, producing a sense of profound loss. The need to balance household and daily routines with the demands of the hospitalization often increase anxiety for family members.[5]

Treatment goals include the establishment of a trusting relationship with both patient and family. This relationship should begin as soon as possible after the patient's admission. The family should be assessed for feelings of helplessness or loss of hope, and interventions should be put in place to strengthen coping and increase hope. Information regarding the patient's status should be provided on a continuous basis. This information must be understandable and concise, with simple terminology. It is also critical to assess the family for informational overload and provide a balance of information. Time should be set aside when possible to allow the family to participate in storytelling. This experience allows the family to discuss the impact of the injury on the patient and family system. The discussion promotes ventilation of feelings of loss, allows the family to begin the mourning process, and legitimizes the unique emotions they are experiencing.[5]

Health care providers are being challenged to provide increasingly complex care in an efficient, effective manner. As the patient population they care for grows more diverse, understanding how a patient's race, ethnicity, age, or sexual orientation can influence his or her view of health, illness, and the health care team is essential. When health care providers make the effort to respectfully inquire about cultural issues that may be important to their patients, it helps to establish a collaborative relationship based on trust, acceptance, and open communication. Culture influences behaviors and interpersonal interactions. It can have profound implications regarding issues including patient autonomy, the role of the family in decision making, end-of-life issues, and spirituality/religion. Kagawa-Singer and Blackhall,[33] in a study evaluating cross-cultural decision making regarding end-of-life care, provide insightful techniques and strategies that are applicable for negotiating all health care issues (Table 19-3). Addressing cultural differences openly, respecting individual autonomy especially when it is difficult to understand or agree with a patient's choices, and establishing a care setting that is supportive and inclusive can improve the chances that the care experience for the patient, family, and health care providers will be a positive one.

Unfortunately, the ability and willingness to effectively incorporate the family into the plan of care is not uniformly found in the critical care unit environment. A classic study by Chesla[34] revealed that some staff have difficulty balancing the need for family care with the demands of technologic care. It was found that ICU staff and policies often impede the involvement of the family. The architectural design of the ICU frequently makes it a closed environment, shutting out families. Frequently, entrance is allowed only after a phone call to the unit. Visiting hours are often restrictive and inflexible. Families are often asked to leave when the patient's condition deteriorates or when painful procedures are to be performed. Chesla[34] studied families and nursing responses in the ICU setting. Interestingly, it was found that the practice of family-centered care is most evident during birth and death, events to which the nurses are sensitive to the need for family presence. During the acute stage of illness, family-centered care

TABLE 19-3 Techniques for Negotiating Issues Influenced by Culture

Issue	Possible Consequences of Ignoring the Issue	Techniques and Strategies to Address the Issue
Responses to inequities in care	Lack of trust Increased desire for futile aggressive care at the end of life Lack of collaboration with patient and family Dissatisfaction with care by all parties involved	Address directly: "I wonder whether it's hard for you to trust a physician who is not ___ (of your same background)?" Make explicit that you and the patient and the family will work together in achieving the best care possible. Work to improve access and reduce inequities. Understand and accommodate desires for more aggressive care, and use respectful negotiation when this is contraindicated or medically futile.
Communication/language barriers	Bidirectional misunderstanding Unnecessary physical, emotional, and spiritual suffering	Take time to: Avoid medical or complex jargon Check for understanding: "So I can make sure I'm explaining this well for you, please tell me what your understanding is about your illness and the treatment we're considering." Hire bilingual, bicultural staff and train in medical translation to be bridges across cultures. Translators are preferable in person, but use AT&T language line or similar services if trained staff unavailable. Avoid use of family as translators, especially minors.
Religion and spirituality	Lack of faith in the physician Lack of adherence to the treatment regimen	"Spiritual or religious strength sustains many people in times of distress. What is important for us to know about your faith or spiritual needs?" "How can we support your needs and practices?" "Where do you find your strength to make sense of this experience?"
Truth telling	Anger, mistrust, or even removal of patient from health care system if team insists on informing the patient against the wishes of the family. Hopelessness in the patient if he or she misunderstands your reason for telling him or her directly.	Informed refusal: "Some patients want to know everything about their condition. Others prefer that the doctors mainly talk to their familes. How would you prefer to get this information?" Use a hypothetical case (e.g., "Others who have conditions similar to yours have found it helpful to consider several options for care such as nutrition, to keep them feeling as well as possible.") Be cognizant of nonverbal or indirect communication when discussing serious information.
Family involvement in decision making	Disagreement and conflict between family and medical staff when the family rather than the patient insists on making decisions	Ascertain the key members of the family and ensure that all are included in discussions as desired by the patient: "Is there anyone else that I should talk to about your condition?" Talk with whomever accompanies the patient and ask the patient about this individual's involvement in receiving information and decision making.
Hospice care	Reduced use of hospice services, leading to decreased quality of end-of-life care	Emphasize hospice as an adjunct or assistance to the family but not as a replacement: "When the family is taking care of the patient at home, hospice can help them do that."

From Kagawa-Singer M, Blackhall LJ: Negotiating cross-culture issues at the end of life: you got to go where he lives, *JAMA* 286:23, 2993-3001, 2001.

was generally less evident. Not surprisingly, some nurses described families as intrusive, meddlesome, pathologic, or a burden. The ideal family was described as compliant, passive, and uninvolved.[34]

Although the nurse's primary role in the critical care setting relates to the direct care of the patient, it remains important that family-centered care be a priority. Appropriate interventions include adequately preparing the family for entrance to the care environment, for the patient's appearance, and for the surrounding equipment. This preparation will facilitate family responses to strange and frighteningly unfamiliar sights and sounds. It is often the nurse's role modeling that is most instrumental in helping families cope with seeing a loved one. The nurse should indicate that it is okay to touch the patient ("It's okay to touch _____ and talk to her") and should model how to do that, taking family members through the experience one by one. The nurse can tell family that it is okay to show emotion in front of the patient, to be demonstrative with affection toward him or her, and in other ways "give permission" for them to be as natural as possible while helping them to feel as unafraid as possible. No matter what the appearance of the patient, it is often the actual "seeing" that is instrumental in family coping, breakdown of denial, and commencement of necessary grief work.

Families need to feel that they are being helpful to the patient. This may be accomplished by actually providing some aspect of care, by performing tasks for the patient outside the hospital setting, or even by providing valuable information to the nurse regarding the patient's previous usual functioning. This is an area where the nurse can use creativity in getting family members involved in ways most meaningful for them.

Families also need to be with or see the patient frequently. Although this is often difficult within the rigorous care schedules of a trauma unit or an ICU, family visiting is viewed as critical to the overall adaptation of family members to the crisis. As the patient's condition worsens or the family perceives that there is an increase in severity, the family's need to see the patient usually increases.[34] Visiting within a trauma unit or critical care area poses procedural difficulties for staff, but it is widely recognized and established that family members need routine and frequent access to the patient. Contact does not have to be lengthy, but it should be scheduled, predictable, and allowed. Within the uncertainties of this particular phase, one of the few things that families may count on is a visual verification of the status of their loved one. There is strong clinical evidence and substantial research to show that there are probably numerous beneficial psychophysiologic responses on the part of the patient to the presence of family.[26]

Special care should be taken to alert family members to any changes, positive or negative, in the patient's status or appearance before visits. Family members should be encouraged to communicate freely with patients even though they cannot respond. On recovery, many patients report that communication at the bedside was critical to their sense of orientation and well-being, even though they could not respond.

If family members live a great distance away, or if there are too many teenage friends of an adolescent patient to allow all to visit, innovative ways of communication and contact can be instituted. Tapes can be made by friends or family members to be played at the bedside; telephone communication can be arranged with the aid of the nurse for logistics; pictures, cards, and letters or written correspondence can all be used as effective means of communicating support and encouragement to a loved one when visiting is not possible or advisable.

Families also identify that they need support and allowance for venting of feelings. Families consistently identify their own personal needs as having low importance. Although this is important for the nurse to be aware of, families also should be apprised that they are just as much a part of the plan of care as the patient and that attention to their own personal needs can ultimately benefit the patient. Nurses should explore ways the family can care for themselves and call on resources that support family members, such as chaplain services, friends, or other relatives. Family members need to maintain adequate rest and nutrition to mobilize the energy required during the hospital course, and pointing this out in terms of their overall, long-term contribution to the patient is frequently beneficial.

Information regarding the patient's condition is also critical to the family. An overworked nursing staff, however, may perceive interruptions from family members requesting information as a burden. One strategy to meet these information needs is the distribution of pagers to family members. In this manner the family can leave the bedside, secure in the knowledge that the ICU staff can communicate with them when necessary.[35] An additional strategy is the use of structured communication programs. These programs offer focused discussion with the ICU staff within 24 hours of the patient's admission, provision of an information pamphlet describing the ICU staff and environment, and daily scheduled phone calls from the nurse caring for the patient. These strategies have been found to increase communication between the family and the ICU staff and to increase family satisfaction.[36]

Intense bonding usually occurs between family members and the nurse/health care team on the first nursing unit to which a patient is sent. This is due to the high emotional intensity and extreme interdependence that exist in the first days of the critical care phase. As patients progress, they are often transferred to a different nursing unit with strange faces, different surroundings, and divergent rules for visiting. This is an extremely difficult time for both the patient and the family, who have grown secure in the familiarity and predictability of the previous unit. It is not uncommon for families to have greatly increased levels of anxiety and even anger over the transfer, largely as a result of a lack of control and fear of the unknown once again. Special care should be taken by the primary nurse of the first nursing unit to formally introduce the patient and family to the nurse taking over on the next unit. Families should be told that an extensive report will be provided to the new team on the patient's course and that they are still available to the patient and family even though in a different capacity. Every effort should be made to inform families ahead of time of the transfer, allowing them to verbalize their feelings about the move and providing a viable explanation as to why the transfer is necessary. Adequate preparation ahead of a transfer can alleviate a multitude of adjustment problems on the part of patients and families and is well worth planned time and effort.

Many times the only other people who share in the particular horror of a traumatic injury or sudden catastrophic illness are the other families experiencing similar situations within the institution. Other families who have made it through the labile course of the critical care experience, lived through a patient transfer, and are also struggling through the aftermath of trauma that has affected their loved one can prove to be invaluable resources to one another. There is little as powerful as the support gained from others who have actually lived through a similar experience. It behooves the trauma nurse to link families whom he or she identifies as having had experiences that could be shared to benefit others. This often provides one family with the support they need and another with a sense of usefulness in providing aid and something tangibly positive and productive as an outcome of their pain.

The establishment of a trauma support group may provide the family with an opportunity to share their experiences. Led by a trained health care member, the support group brings together families at various stages of the critical care process. Information is shared among family members regarding the trauma experience. Experiences and feelings are explored. Misconceptions are clarified and reality is supported. In addition, it is a forum for the trauma family to network with other families who are currently living a similar stressful experience.[37]

Intermediate Care Phase

The Patient

As the patient's condition stabilizes and becomes less critical, he or she is confronted with reality. Wounds and injuries become more real and patients must make a decision about whether to continue to strive for survival. Patients may begin to view themselves as victims. They are now challenged by the intense work required to heal and rehabilitate. They again mourn their losses as they begin to view life as it will be after injury. Physical and psychologic challenges arise as the patient and family become fully aware of the real impact and meaning of the injuries. Morse and O'Brien call this stage *Enduring the Self: Confronting and Regrouping*[19] (see Table 19-1). Important themes during the intermediate care cycle include learning to endure the injury, learning physical limitations, latching on to significant others, doing the work of healing, and mourning losses.

During the enduring the self: confronting and regrouping stage, patients continue to experience periods of anxiety, especially when they perceive that the nurse is not available to them. Often patients are afraid of being left alone. Patients requiring increased dependence on the nurse find themselves watching the clock and fearing they have been abandoned.[19]

In the Morse and O'Brien study, patients emphasized that they counted to bring order to their days. This task allowed them to maintain a sense of control in an environment where they perceived no control. One participant states, "I would count the days. I would ask them how long I would stay in the hospital, every time they would change my bandages.... I must have driven them crazy.... I'd keep bugging the [the nurses]. How long do you figure? How long do you figure?"[19]

Participants in this study reported that they counted surgeries, dressing changes, days, hours, treatments, physical therapy sessions, and baths. Treatments that produced pain were also counted as one less to endure or a step closer to discharge. Sometimes counting was used as a mechanism to defend against having to focus on the future. The intense concentration needed to count ceiling tiles or bricks in the wall prevented them from focusing on the trauma or the difficulties that were in the future.[19]

During this stage of confronting and regrouping, patients continue to use family support as an anchor to maintain identity and begin to look to therapists and others as a source of encouragement and support. Acceptance and encouragement from the health care team takes on particular significance as patients struggle to regain independence. Patients also begin to identify with and depend on other patients.[19]

The intense therapy required during the intermediate care phase requires an enormous amount of energy expenditure by patients. Patients may view the movement toward recovery as a slow, tedious, frustrating, and exhausting process. They may find themselves on an emotional roller coaster. On one day they may be elated at a small step in the healing process; the next may find them in a deep depression because they perceive their condition to be worse, with little progress being made on the road to independence. To deal with the stresses of rehabilitation, the patients in the Morse and O'Brien study described the use of mental scorecards. Each foot walked with the prosthesis was a step closer to recovery. Each dressing change was a step closer to complete healing. These imaginary scorecards assisted the patients to begin to envision life after trauma.

As patients face the challenges of the intermediate care phase, it is important for the nurse to assist them to identify small, incremental milestones of success and to celebrate these. Encouragement of independence is essential. Independence in activities of daily living such as brushing teeth or self-feeding often help patients feel a sense of accomplishment.

During the intermediate care stage, patients may cling to the hope that a miracle will return them to their preinjury level of function. Morse and O'Brien[19] found that spinal cord–injured patients were especially prone to this type of magical thinking. One patient stated, "But I'm not going to sit down and accept the fact that I have to stay in [the wheelchair] all my life, because I might not. And I think people who accept being paralyzed defeat themselves...cause if you accept it, you shut your mind down ... to working towards getting better, or getting things back. So I was coming here with, uh, expectations of getting back ... getting as much as I could do, try to get back on my feet."[19] Maintenance of hope is critical during this stage of the healing process. Research has shown that this type of coping behavior may prompt patients to work intensely to achieve a maximal level of recovery.[19]

A major task during this phase is the task of grieving for losses incurred by self and others involved in the traumatic event. Patients who have lost family members during the traumatic event begin the task of mourning. Patients face loss of body integrity with all its attendant meanings: loss of control over their body, loss of control of the environment, and loss of control of their affective responses. Loss of function leads to loss of roles as well. Patients perceive themselves as powerless. One means of coping with these numerous losses is to become dependent on the power of others and to regress to early phases of development when the psyche could tolerate such dependence.

Patients' responses to actual or perceived losses are to mourn or grieve for them. Grieving begins the moment patients are cognitively aware that a change has occurred. The work of loss and grief is displayed affectively by patients throughout each of the phases of trauma. The most recognized expressions of loss are those identified by Kübler-Ross,[38] which includes denial, anger, bargaining, depression, acceptance and hope. Although Kübler-Ross related these stages to death and dying, they nevertheless hold true throughout the spectrum of loss. Because the expression of grief is unique for each person, it is important that the trauma nurse be cognizant of the process and recognizes each of the themes that patients are expressing. Grief work is not a systematic process consisting of stages that occur sequentially. Rather, it is a complex array of affects and cognition that patients are sorting out and attempting to make sense of to integrate the changes in their life. Through the grief process, patients are struggling to hope and find meaning in their changed life.

The patient who is grieving reflects this process in both verbalization and behavior. It is important for the nurse to obtain from either the patient or some significant other information regarding the patient's previous coping patterns when he or she experienced a significant loss. Did the patient deny the loss initially? How did the patient reflect this denial? Did his or her motor and psyche activity diminish? Was the patient verbal or nonverbal? Did he or she cry frequently? Was the patient hostile or agitated? Did he or she stop functioning in other roles, such as work? Did the patient withdraw from the people and activities in his or her environment? Did the patient's sleeping and eating patterns change? If so, how? Did the patient become dependent on others to direct his or her activities? Did the patient verbalize feelings of hopelessness? Did he or she become quiet, withdrawn, or apathetic? Was the patient preoccupied with the loss? What or who was significant in supporting the patient? What did they do or say that was helpful?[25] As the patient's history of responding to previous losses is obtained, the nurse integrates this information into workable interventions with the patient.

For patients who use denial, the nurse recognizes that their behavior serves a purpose. They are indeed buying time and preparing themselves intrapsychically to address the magnitude of the traumatic event. It is important that the nurse not strip away this defense. Reflecting verbalized content back to patients confronts their thought processes in a nonthreatening manner. For example, if a patient in traction is inappropriately attempting to get out of bed to go to the bathroom, sincerely asking him a question such as, "Do you think you would be able to walk with all that traction attached to your broken left leg?" helps the patient to focus on pieces of reality and allows the nurse to intervene with specific factual information. Simple explanations regarding the environment and procedures bring reality to the patient without forcing it on him.

Trauma patients often are hostile to and critical of staff. Anger exists because patients have lost control and are dependent on others and because what has happened to them is perceived as unfair. Because patients are virtually unable to change what has happened, by externalizing the anger to the environment they at least maintain some sense of control by finding what is at fault externally. Frequently this anger is reflected outwardly by complaining about unresponsiveness of staff to patients' needs, by questioning of staff's ability to care for patients adequately, and by constantly demanding attention from the staff. There are few, if any, answers to the question, "Why did this happen to me? It's so unfair." Blaming others initially relieves some of the patients' frustration. The astute nurse looks behind the angry verbalizations and recognizes the need they serve. The nurse must be nondefensive toward patients, recognize and acknowledge with them that they are feeling angry, and help them focus on the reasons for the anger. It is also important that nurses not be punitive in their actions or verbalizations.

Part of grief work is retreating from the environment by withdrawing invested energy from it. This internal retreat from external stimulation provides time for patients to put the pieces together. Recognizing affects of sadness and depression and verbalizing them for patients supports patients in acceptance of their loss. The nurse supports this necessary introspection by minimizing environmental input and by spending quiet time with patients. When patients are depressed, setting small achievable goals and offering choices can help the patient cope with their loss.

As the loss begins to take on perspective for the patient, he or she comes to recognize abilities that he or she does retain. Hope becomes a bigger piece of the picture at this point, and the nurse now actively presents positive aspects of his or her life situation and acknowledges independent functioning and strengths. As the patient's self-image is beginning to integrate the changes that have occurred, renewed energy is applied to the task of healing. Often at this point, the patient shifts to more independent functioning; however, the patient moves back and forth in his or her use of coping behaviors throughout the phases of trauma as he or she mourns for his or her loss.

Affective coping behaviors such as denial, regression, anger, and depression do not alter the stressors, but they alter the perception of the patient experiencing them. At this juncture in the journey to recovery is the seed of a major conflict between nurse and patient. Patients may appear less anxious because they have often transformed the stressor, such as loss of control, by becoming markedly more dependent, and they tolerate this position by regressing to a level of development when it was appropriate; the nurse, on the other hand, perceives the situation differently, perhaps without appreciation of the patient's need to feel dependent and regressive. The nurse often cannot tolerate a patient's level of dependency once there are physical signs that the patient's functioning can allow more autonomous behavior. In effect, nurse and patient may no longer be moving in the same direction. To cope with anxiety, the patient has transformed the anxiety so that it is no longer experienced. The nurse becomes more anxious as a result of a need for the patient to continue progressing in their previously mutual direction and goals. This apparent dilemma can cause an alteration in the nurse-patient relationship, as evidenced by increased conflict in their interactions. Acknowledgment of the tension by the nurse allows examination of causative factors, which in turn allows dialog and resolution. Although there are probably alterations in the patient's other relationships, the interactions that the creative, skilled nurse has with the patient can pave the way for further healing and rehabilitation.

During this stage the nurse is the dominating force that shapes the patient's experience. The nurse can tolerate the patient's dependence and regressive behavior and respond to it in such a way that hopelessness, helplessness, and powerlessness are not the patient's predominant experiences. Rather, the resourceful nurse continues to provide choices for the patient to act on. The patient's decisions in these matters of choice counteract the ever-present threat of powerlessness and helplessness. The nurse combats the patient's regressive tendencies by constantly presenting reality in terms of necessary treatments but leaves room for the patient to determine when and, as much as possible, how. The enterprising nurse constantly assesses the patient's functional level of responsibility, stepping in when the patient falters; when the patient is more active, the nurse withdraws, giving the patient freedom and legitimating these efforts to become more autonomous.

Nurses need to be extremely flexible to respond to patients' psychosocial needs. Because of pain and monotony and the constant danger of coping by regression, patients tend to be in flux. The nurse who intervenes as though patients were constantly in the same position does either too much or too little for these persons. Evaluation of patients' status is easily accomplished by assessing their capacity to problem solve. This occurs when the nurse frames the day's schedule and seeks patients' input about these events. A patient who is more regressed might simply wash her hands of the whole thing or say, "I don't care. Do what you want," or "You're going to do it anyway. Go away!" Each of these responses is a reasonably accurate reflection of the patient's willingness to act on his or her own behalf that day.

Victorson et al[4] studied whether specific coping strategies previously associated with psychologic disability were related to injury-related distress (IRD) symptoms after traumatic physical injury. With use of an ethnically diverse sample, they found that behavioral disengagement during the acute stage after trauma is related to patient reports of IRD symptoms along with use of emotional ruminating and venting. This study indicates that, although emotional rumination and venting may be a useful adaptive coping strategy initially, their protracted use can consume a patient's physical and emotional resources and inhibit the active exploration of other more constructive coping mechanisms, such as mobilizing a social network.[4] These authors report that in the acute adjustment phase after a traumatic injury persons who engage in self blame may have greater IRD symptoms. They conclude that treating hospitalized trauma patients with phase-appropriate psychosocial and educational intervention may prevent later development of depression, generalized anxiety, and PTSD.[4]

The reality of the impact of the injuries is evident as patients begin to realize how much time and work will be involved to achieve independence. Patients often experience a sense of loss of control because they are forced to depend on health care providers for everyday activities. As strength is regained, patients will begin to attempt to function as they did before the injury. Grief and loss are again experienced as patients discover the limitations of their levels of function. During this stage patients realize that the disability is permanent. On another level, however, they reject the reality of the disability and the fact that it is permanent. This notion of temporary disability is often reinforced for spinal cord–injured patients as they experience sudden spasticity and muscle contractions.

It is important to understand grief and bereavement as a normal and expected process of letting go of the past, connecting to others to build new or different relationships, and accepting one's new life with the changes brought by the loss. This painful process can appear similar to depression in that the grieving person is sad, may lose interest in pleasurable activity, and may have appetite and sleep changes. Despite this, normal grief reactions do not include thoughts of death, such as feeling that he or she would be better off dead or should have died with the deceased person or a morbid preoccupation with worthlessness.[39]

THE FAMILY

Adapting to the Injury

During the intermediate care phase the family is also confronted with the enormous physical and emotional impact of the patient's injuries. During the critical care phase the focus of the family is on the survival of the patient. The focus now shifts to the realization that the patient will indeed survive, but with associated, often devastating, disabilities and disfigurement. One relative of a severely head-injured patient stated, "For weeks we prayed he'd live. Now we know he'll live and, my God, now what do we do?"

As the crisis of the critical care phase subsides, the family may discover that its own emotional and physical resources have been depleted. Fatigue and irritability may be noted because energy runs low. It is important for the nurse to encourage the family to focus on its own restoration. The family may have to be "given permission" by the health care team to reduce visiting time to allow for refueling. Education regarding the long-term effects of chronic stress, stress management techniques, nutrition, rest, and health promotion is essential at this stage.

The intermediate care stage is the setting in which the family must become involved in the plan of care. Visiting hours should be flexible to allow the family to be present during dressing changes and therapies. Patient and family discharge education should be initiated early in this phase, not delayed until the day of discharge. During this phase it may be apparent and become a source of conflict that the patient and family are at different points in their grief work. In most cases family members are ahead of the patient because all the patient's energy has gone into fighting for life while so acutely ill. Although families may have moved through denial and resolved anger, patients may just be starting with those responses. The nurse can educate the family about the stages of grief and the fact that it is not uncommon for patients to fall behind the family in their progression through grief work. The nurse can encourage family members to be patient and tolerant, giving the patient the time necessary to progress. It is important that the nurse take an active role in supporting both the patient and the family with information regarding what the differences in responses reflect and how to understand the divergence and work with it. This is an active time in terms of education and teaching of the family by the nurse. In contrast to the empathic support and direct guidance given in the critical care cycle, the intermediate cycle necessitates a higher level intervention skill, with restructuring of family patterns, renegotiation of tasks, and more advanced application of family systems theory. Families tend to be calmer during this period but less eager for intervention and more emotionally distant from the health care team and from the patient. Once again, this is a natural progression and should not be misinterpreted. There is nothing "magic" about the time that a family has had to cope with a situation. The course of coping for families on a trauma trajectory is often erratic rather than linear, and allowances for shifts in family function should be made and accounted for on the basis of what the nurse understands regarding the need for some emotional distance and temporary emotional disengagement.

Functional Versus Dysfunctional Coping

Ambiguity and lack of resolution still remain for family members in this phase as coping demands continue to vary from day to day; however, in this phase most families who are functionally progressing have established a general system for the prolonged incorporation of the unexpected. Depending on the nurse's assessment of whether the family is functional or dysfunctional in coping at this point, consultants may be called in to deal with particular family issues of a more complex nature. Most trauma and critical care centers have highly skilled family service departments, psychiatric social workers, liaison psychiatric nurses, substance abuse counselors, and others to assist the nurse once a more complex need is identified. Also families can be directed to professional and nonprofessional support groups for additional assistance.

REHABILITATION PHASE

The rehabilitation phase is a time of active growth for the trauma patient and the family. During this phase the patient makes the transition from trauma victim to rehabilitated individual. Interventions to address continuing physical and psychologic problems become critical to a positive outcome. Chronicity becomes an issue as the family faces the great challenge of integrating the patient back into the home setting and into society.

THE PATIENT

Morse and O'Brien[19] identified the rehabilitation stage as the fourth and final stage in the trauma victim's journey to self-preservation. Stage IV is identified as *striving to regain self: merging the old and the new* (see Table 19-1). During this stage patients strive to regain the self as they perceived it to be before the traumatic injury. Goals include becoming acquainted with the new, altered body image; making sense of the trauma experience; and accepting the consequences of the traumatic event.[19]

During the rehabilitation stage, patients will attempt to clarify and piece together the details of the event leading to the injury.[19] For some patients the rehabilitation phase allows the first opportunity to compare injuries. Morse and O'Brien[19] found that participants in their study identified this as the time when they became thankful their injuries were not more severe.

Depending on the trauma suffered, many different short- or long-term physical and psychologic adaptations must be made to compensate for the injuries. Physical limitations may include sensory loss (e.g., vision, hearing, and neuropathy), inability to eat or swallow (central nervous system injury), loss of ambulation or the functional use of a limb (e.g., stroke, traumatic amputation), and sexual dysfunction (spinal cord injury), to name a few. Different strategies have been devised to accommodate these physical deficiencies and bring the patient closer to their preinjury level of functioning. Knowing how to address the psychologic needs of the trauma patient, however, is not as straightforward. Randomized prospective trials evaluating treatment strategies and outcomes for addressing the mental health needs of similar comparison groups of trauma patients are very limited.[40]

In the recovery period, elevated levels of depression, emotional distress including dysphoria, irritability, social withdrawal, rumination as the patient tries to "make sense" of what has happened to him or her, and an altered expectation of their future are all common posttrauma manifestations.

Nielson[41] evaluated the prevalence of PTSD and emotional distress in patients with recent spinal cord lesions. She found that two variables, dysphoria and decreased expectations for their future, was predictive of the development of PTSD. Thus important goals during the rehabilitation process must include treating the dysphoria and helping the patient resume prior relationships and roles. Their reintegration into the social support network of family and friends is an important aspect for minimizing the duration and impact of PTSD. Along with being an invaluable resource for the patient, the social network serves as a supportive forum for the patient to talk through the traumatic experience and its aftermath.[42]

Michaels et al[1] found that 12 months after trauma, the patient's work status, general health, and overall satisfaction with the recovery was dependent on how well his or her mental health needs had been addressed. The authors concluded that trauma centers that failed to fully treat injury-related mental illness are not fully assisting their patients to regain optimal functioning.

The Family

Leske[5] identified eight essential family outcomes after the critical care experience:

- Seeking manageable reactions to the injury
- Reframing the injury experience as a challenge
- Redefining what constitutes maximal recovery
- Maximizing family resources
- Using adaptive coping resources
- Promoting strong bonds within the family
- Maintaining family involvement in the patient's care
- Mobilizing family strengths

Achievement of these outcomes continues to be essential during the rehabilitation phase. An additional outcome during the rehabilitation phase is managing the chronicity of the injury. During this phase the family begins to better comprehend the enormous task that must be addressed to reintegrate the patient into the family. For the family of the spinal cord–injured patient, the focus becomes the development of a long-term caregiver role. A study by Weitzenkamp et al[43] demonstrated that significantly more caregiver spouses of spinal cord–injured patients experienced physical stress, emotional stress, burnout, anger, and resentment than did noncaregiving spouses. Interestingly, the caregiver, who was not disabled, reported more significant depression than did the disabled patient.[43]

Families of head-injured patients also struggle with the issue of chronicity. A study by Knight et al[44] demonstrated that caregiver burden is determined, in part, not by the severity of the head injury but by the caregiver's subjective perception of his or her ability to meet the challenges of the caregiver role. Caregivers who perceived their role as overwhelming and negative reported more physical and emotional distress than did those who viewed the role in a more positive light. In addition, families reported that the most distressing problems when caring for the head-injured family member was dealing with mood disturbances such as anxiety, lability of emotion, anger, depression, and aggression.[44] It was found that the caregivers of head-injured patients reported significant changes in family routines, financial states, social roles, and leisure activities. Perception was again an important variable. Caregivers who perceived the patient to be highly disabled reported more negative life changes than did caregivers who had a more positive appraisal of the patient's outcome. In addition, it was found that the perceived degree of social support combined with the perception of the functional deficits was a better predictor of caregiver life change than was the actual degree of head injury itself.[45]

Nursing interventions include the recognition that family involvement or lack thereof can have a powerful impact on the rehabilitation process. Assessment of family dynamics is critical, especially when family problems or conflict take precedence over the rehabilitation process. Positive communication can be achieved by inviting the family to team rounds or to the therapy sessions. Emotional support and guidance should be offered to both the patient and the family. The family should be actively involved in the development of the discharge plan.[46]

In addition, nursing care of families during the rehabilitation period must focus on providing information and networking to the family. These resources will enable the family to establish a more realistic perception of the patient's injury and rehabilitation outcomes. Preparation for discharge to home must begin early in the rehabilitation process. Too often patients are sent home to families who are ill prepared to deal with their extensive needs or intensive family education is provided on the day of discharge. Because of the stresses inherent in the discharge process, little learning is retained at that time. Families must be invited to rehabilitation therapy sessions where they are encouraged to be actively involved. Instruction regarding wound care or other procedures should be initiated early enough to allow the caregiver several practice sessions with nursing supervision available.[46]

Families of head-injured patients must establish new communication styles and relationships. Communication skills training and counseling sessions will reduce the resentment, frustration, and isolation often experienced by these caregivers.[44] Networking with other families, attending support group sessions, and contacting specialty agencies will provide a source of support to families of trauma patients.

Mental Illness Related to Trauma

People who have experienced trauma are at increased risk for depression, PTSD, and adjustment disorder. Although the trauma or rehabilitation nurse is not expected to diagnose mental illness, he or she should be able to identify symptoms that are indicative of the need for assessment and intervention from a psychiatric specialist. Major symptoms and intervention strategies are presented.

DEPRESSION

Major depression can be characterized by an almost constant depressed mood (appearing tearful or sad and feeling hopeless or empty) or loss of interest or pleasure in life lasting more than 2 weeks.[39] Other indicative symptoms include nearly daily insomnia or hypersomnia, significant weight loss or gain, psychomotor agitation or retardation (fatigue), feelings of worthlessness, excessive or inappropriate guilt (which may be delusional in nature), diminished ability to concentrate or make decisions, or recurrent thoughts of suicide and death.

According to the *Diagnostic and Statistical Manual*,[39] symptoms can develop over days to weeks, and patients frequently present with tearfulness, irritability, brooding, obsessive rumination, anxiety, excessive worry over their physical health, and complaints of pain (headache, joint, other pain). Because suicide is the most serious consequence of depression, nurses should be alert for verbalizations that indicate that patients are considering this and should be able to openly discuss and assess for suicidal ideation and to intervene as necessary. Persons with specific plans (time, place, and objects needed) are most at risk for suicidal action. Suicide risk is higher for those with psychotic features, history of prior suicide attempts, a family history of completed suicide attempts, or concurrent substance use.[39]

Treatment for depression includes pharmacologic treatment and verbal therapies. Patients need to know that antidepressants typically require 4 to 6 weeks to reach therapeutic levels and that suicidal feelings should be discussed with the health care team so that appropriate safety measures may be taken.

POSTTRAUMATIC STRESS DISORDER

PTSD is a type of anxiety disorder characterized by the development of specific symptoms after exposure to an extreme stressor where "the person experienced, witnessed, or was confronted with an event or events that involved actual or threatened death or serious injury, or a threat to the physical integrity of self or others."[39] The disorder can occur at any age and, although symptoms usually appear within the 3 months after the trauma, symptoms can be delayed for months and even years after the trauma.[35] Studies of PTSD reveal a lifetime prevalence of 8% of the adult population in the United States.[39] Spinal cord injuries and facial injuries are two types of traumas that place patients at risk for PTSD.[8,47,48]

An individual with PTSD will describe their response to the traumatic event as one of intense fear, helplessness, or horror. Victims will describe episodes of intrusion during which they experience sudden intense, vivid memories, dreams, or flashbacks of the event. These persistently recurring recollections are so real that the person may feel as if he or she is reliving the trauma. Stressful emotions such as fear, grief, and anger are common during this phase of reliving the event. In addition, exposure to internal or external cues that resemble some aspect of the traumatic event can trigger flashbacks, and intense emotional energy is needed to attempt to deal with these flashbacks.

In addition, individuals may demonstrate avoidance phenomena that relates to thoughts or feelings associated with the trauma or avoidance of activities, places, or people that arouse recollections of the trauma.[39] Relationships with family and friends often disintegrate because individuals with PTSD avoid close emotional ties, leaving them feeling detached and estranged from others. They may describe themselves as numb and emotionless, having a restricted range of affect, and a sense of a foreshortened future.[39] As this behavior continues, significant others may feel rebuffed and view victims as cold, indifferent, or preoccupied.[8]

Victims of PTSD experience a state of chronic hyperarousal and a biologic alarm reaction. Panic attacks and extreme fear may be experienced when individuals are in situations that remind them of the traumatic event. For example, a gunshot victim may feel extreme distress when hearing a car backfire. Other symptoms of hyperarousal include inability to fall or stay asleep, outbursts of anger, difficulty concentrating, hypervigilance, and an exaggerated startle response.

Holbrook et al[3] studied long-term rates of PTSD in youth aged 12 to 19 years admitted to a trauma center with an injury diagnosis. Those with severe traumatic brain injury or spinal cord injury were excluded from the study. The most common causes of injury related to motor vehicle crashes (22%), recreational incidents (13%), bike collisions (13%), intentional injury such as assaults and gunshot wounds (13%), falls (12%), and pedestrians struck (10%). They found that adolescents from lower socioeconomic families were at greater risk for PTSD. The study also focused on PTSD and injury-related factors such as perceived threat to life, mechanism of injury, sociodemographics, and postinjury behavioral problems. The rate of long-term PTSD was 27% in this sample and was associated with quality-of-life deficits throughout the follow-up period. Although more males are hurt from trauma, more females have PTSD when they are injured. This study also reported that older adolescents (ages 16 to 19 years) versus younger adolescents tend to have higher rates of PTSD. Alcohol and drug abuse, staying in school, problems with authority, social relationship problems, thoughts of suicide, and depression were also associated with PTSD. Risk factors for long-term PTSD included perceived threat to life, death of a family member at the scene of the incident, no control over the injury event, and violence-related injury.[3]

All trauma patients experiencing a traumatic event that they perceive to be stressful should be screened for PTSD. Early recognition and intervention is essential because the sooner the patient receives treatment, the better the chance for recovery. PTSD is associated with increased rates of major depressive disorder, substance abuse–related disorders, panic disorder, agoraphobia, obsessive-compulsive disorder, generalized anxiety disorder, social phobia, specific phobia, and bipolar disorder. These disorders can precede, follow, or emerge concurrently with the onset of PTSD.[39]

The goals of intervention include restoring a sense of control to the individual; diminishing the power of the traumatic event; reducing chronic hyperarousal; reducing feelings of guilt, anger, and self-blame; and restoring a sense of equilibrium for the victim.[8] Patients need to understand that their symptoms relate to a psychobiologic reaction to overwhelming stress, not to a character flaw.[49] Pharmacologic measures such as the use of serotonin reuptake inhibitors (antidepressants), tricyclic antidepressants, and monoamine oxidase inhibitors alleviate the symptoms of PTSD and improve overall functioning. Benzodiazepines are rarely, if ever, indicated and should be avoided or used judiciously in patients with PTSD.[49] Patients can also benefit from nonpharmacologic measures. These include counseling sessions by trained psychiatric professionals and involvement of the family to ensure additional support.[8]

Adjustment Disorder

An adjustment disorder occurs when an identifiable stressor such as a trauma precipitates a distress response that includes emotional or behavioral symptoms that exceed what would be expected from exposure to the stressor or that causes impairment in social or occupational (including academic) functioning.[39] Occasionally, what may initially be considered a normal reaction to a trauma may qualify as an adjustment disorder if significant adverse emotional or behavioral symptoms develop. Health impairments associated with adjustment disorders include depressed mood, anxiety, disturbance in conduct or other maladaptive reactions, and an increased risk for suicide. Symptoms typically appear within 3 months of when the stressful event occurred and typically resolve 6 months from the point when the stressor ended. In situations where the stress occurred over a prolonged period of time or had protracted repercussions, symptoms may exceed the 6-month time frame. Adjustment disorder should not be confused with bereavement, which is an expected reaction to the loss of a significant loved one.

Diagnosis of adjustment disorder requires careful consideration of patients' unique perception of and reaction to the trauma within the context of their cultures. It is important to consider the cultural aspects of a person when judging whether a reaction to a stressor is in excess of what would be expected.[39] An individual's reaction should be judged in the context of cultural norms.

It can be difficult to establish a point at which the stressor has ended for a patient because the patient may perceive the treatment for the injury (in the ED and ICU) as a continuation of the stressor. Symptoms related to their anxiety and depression can be addressed with therapy to help the patient learn new coping mechanisms and work with the associated grief and loss issues, and where appropriate, pharmacologic intervention may be initiated.

Special Situations

Death

The death of a loved one creates tremendous stresses for the person's significant others. Even in instances where the death was not necessarily unanticipated, as with patients with known poor health or advanced age, the death pronouncement is usually met with some shock and grief. Family members may respond with crying or may display feelings of guilt, anxiety, anger, and even open hostility. Denial of the event may be forcibly expressed, and the family may ask for proof of death. Some may become restless and move about aimlessly. Some will find the need to express an obsessional review of the patient's life. Others may feel profound physical distress, including nausea, chest pain, palpitations, lightheadedness, and syncope. Questions regarding the details of the death are often raised, sometimes aggressively. Information should be provided in an open, honest manner. The stress and shock associated with the death may require the information be repeated and reinforced.[50,51]

Immediate interventions include placing the family in a private area from which the body of the loved one is accessible. The pronouncement of death should be made in an empathetic manner. The term *death* should be used, rather than abstract words such as *passed away.* It is important to offer spiritual and emotional support. Consultation with clergy, a social worker, or a psychiatric nurse liaison can be beneficial. The family should always be given the option to view the body. This offer should be made in a nonjudgmental manner, allowing the family members to feel supported in their decision. The viewing should take place after the body has been washed and as much invasive monitoring equipment as possible removed. All attempts should be made to present the body in as normal a condition as possible. Disfiguring wounds should be covered with a clean dressing when possible.

Occasionally the family may decline the opportunity to spend time with the deceased loved one. It is important to give the family time to reconsider their decision to avoid future regrets. Once the family has been allowed to mobilize resources and absorb the initial shock of the situation, they may be more comfortable with a viewing. Gentle reminders that a viewing of the body is available at their request keeps the option open for them. If, however, a family ultimately refuses a viewing, the health care team should support the decision.

The amount of time spent with the loved one should be determined by the family. Some family members may wish to remain at the bedside, whereas others come and go. Chairs should be placed at the bedside for the comfort of the family. Identified clergy should be summoned as the family desires, and cultural rituals should be respected and observed when possible.

When the decision to leave is made, the family should be escorted gently from the unit. All necessary paperwork and funeral home arrangements should be completed in a quiet, comfortable area. The unit phone number and the name of a contact person should be provided to the family in the event that they have questions in the future. Sending a sympathy card to the family 2 months after the death of their loved one provides the family with a sense of comfort and caring and allows closure for the health care team.[51] Although health care workers learn to maintain a certain amount of objectivity when working with patients and families, total distancing of self is unrealistic and inconsistent with the basic values of nursing.

Traumatic Grief

The unexpected death of a loved one as a result of a motor vehicle collision, homicide, drunk driving event, or community disaster produces a profound grief event for the family. The course of bereavement is complicated by the traumatic and often violent manner of the death. Traumatic grief is defined as a complicated bereavement in which the death takes place unexpectedly, in an unfamiliar environment, often violently, allowing the family no opportunity for anticipatory grief. The surviving members feel a vicarious traumatization as a result of the death. Traumatic grief is often viewed as a combination of complicated bereavement and PTSD.[52]

The individual experiencing traumatic grief often describes an overwhelming rage, terror, and depression in response to the death of the loved one. There is an affective flooding of emotion whenever the death is remembered, often incapacitating the individual with anger, fear, and profound depression. If the individual was present during the death, as a bystander or a passenger in the vehicle, he or she may experience flashbacks of the event. Cognitively the surviving individual is preoccupied with the loss. He or she may spend inordinate amounts of time reliving the experience. Often the individual may have a morbid obsession with the loved one's thoughts and feelings at the time of the death. Regardless of whether they are accurate, these images of the loved one's physical suffering and terror and thoughts of the violent nature of the death produce significant stress for the survivor. Thoughts of real or imagined blame may be directed toward the alleged perpetrator or toward the health care team members who were not successful in saving the individual. Plans of revenge may be formed. The survivor may also have cognitive dysfunction, such as memory impairment. Physiologically the surviving individual may have a chronic state of hyperarousal in which feelings of rage and anger are intensified. The individual has an exaggerated startle response to specific cues. For example, a passenger in a motor vehicle in which the driver was killed may have feelings of acute anxiety, tachycardia, tachypnea, and hypertension when attempting future rides in motor vehicles. Behaviorally, the surviving individual may have a phobic avoidance of the stimuli related to the death. Fear exists that the traumatic event will be repeated. Family members may avoid driving on a road where a loved one was killed, taking an out-of-the way detour instead. The death event is examined to determine what could have been done to change the outcome. Often survivors feel extreme guilt over the fact that they survived the event and the loved one did not. There is real or imagined guilt over not preventing the death. Resentment toward the dead loved one is often identified as a theme after a traumatic event. The surviving individuals feel anger toward the dead loved one for not trying harder to survive and for leaving the survivors behind. Surviving individuals also report appetite disturbances, altered sleep patterns, episodes of depression, and relationship conflicts.[1,52]

In an attempt to control the intensity of the overwhelming grief, surviving individuals may feel prolonged denial after the death of the loved one. Repression of the events of the death and psychic numbing may follow, preventing survivors from effectively working through the normal grief process. Survivors may experience social isolation, overwhelming fears about the safety of self and others, and magical thinking related to keeping others safe. As a form of self-protection, survivors may use avoidance behaviors such as emotional distancing from others or the use of drugs or alcohol. On a more positive note, some survivors attempt to make sense out of the tragedy. Support groups such as Mothers Against Drunk Drivers may be joined or formed. Family members may become involved in attempting to change laws or public policies to prevent further deaths. Memorials or scholarships may be established to honor the dead individual.

Traumatic grief is further complicated by involvement with the criminal justice system. Survivors often report that they feel victimized twice: once by the actual event and again during the course of the trial. During the court process, survivors often come face to face with the alleged perpetrator. The loved ones feel a sense of loss of control and intense rage. The resolution of the grief process is interrupted as the survivors must again relive the events surrounding the death. During the course of the trial, the defendant and his or her attorney may present the deceased in a negative light. Blame for the event may be directed toward the dead loved one, producing additional pain for the survivors. Philosophic conflicts may arise if the surviving members do not believe that justice has prevailed.[53]

Individuals feeling traumatic grief must receive intervention as early as possible after the death. Immediate intervention includes guiding the survivors through the grief process. Immediate referral to a social worker or clergy is appropriate. Additionally, individuals experiencing traumatic grief may require the services of psychiatrists, psychiatric clinical nurse specialists, or grief counselors. The names and phone numbers of competent individuals in the area should be provided to survivors before they leave the hospital setting. Education regarding the issues of traumatic grief should be provided to all survivors who have experienced the unexpected, violent death of a loved one. Professional counseling focuses on crisis intervention, stabilization, and psychosocial adaptation. Assessment is made for the presence of PTSD. Substance abuse is addressed. Systematic desensitization, stress management techniques, and biofeedback are incorporated into the plan of care.

Treatment goals include allowing the survivor to ventilate, helping to identify symptoms of emotional distress, educating the individual about the normal grief process, validating the survivor's experiences, restoring control, reducing self-blame, providing support, and helping the survivor say good-bye.[54]

Care Worker Stress

Nurses enter the field with the desire to help others but without the full appreciation for what effect this type of work might have on their own well-being. The challenges of the ICU are characterized by maximum accountability, continual change of patients, changes in technology, and frequent exposure to pain, death, and sorrow.[55] Younger nurses (younger than age 30 years), those separated or divorced, and those working a full-time schedule are the most prone to burnout and emotional exhaustion.[56] Hurst and Koplin-Baucum[55] used Kobasa's concept of hardiness to analyze the responses of ICU nurses with more than 10 years of experience to determine the characteristics that allowed them to thrive in a stressful environment. Participant responses indicated that active, direct, involvement in decision making, the ability to choose among various courses of action in providing care for their patients, and the ability to view stressful events as stimulating and challenging all contributed to their sense of well-being and being cared for.[55] A collaborative effort between nurses, management, and hospital administration can foster an environment conducive to nurse retention and professional growth.

Research Indications

Although significant theories exist describing the experience of traumatic injury, little solid research is available to clearly define the psychosocial impact of the event. It is imperative that future research describe the psychologic experiences of trauma patients and families and identify the needs of these populations. Interventional studies are needed to identify the most effective interventions to assist the patient and family to overcome the crisis experience during all phases of trauma care. Studies are needed to assist in clearly identifying crisis proneness in patients and families. In addition, research targeting preventive measures will assist at-risk individuals.

Summary

A traumatic injury is a devastating event that produces both physical and psychologic injury. Both the patient and the family are affected by the injury, and significant crisis often ensues. The nurse, along with other members of the health care team, plays a significant role in assisting the patient and family to survive the crisis experience. It is clear that the psychologic impact of injury must be addressed throughout the trauma cycle. Timely application of crisis interventions assists the patient and the family as they cope with the stresses of the injury. Finally, appropriate referrals to psychiatric clinicians, clergy, spiritual advisors, social workers, and outside resources promote positive outcomes for patients and families.

References

1. Michaels AJ, Michaels CE, Smith JS et al: Outcome from injury: general health, work status, and satisfaction 12 months after trauma, *J Trauma Inj Infect Crit Care* 48:841-850, 2000.
2. Williams R, Doctor J, Patterson D et al: Health outcomes from burn survivors: a 2 year followup, *Rehabil Psychol* 48:189-194, 2003.
3. Holbrook T, Hoyt D, Coimbra R et al: Long term posttraumatic stress disorder persists long after trauma in adolescents: new data on risk factors and functional outcome, *J Trauma Inj Infect Crit Care* 58:764-771, 2005.
4. Victorson D, Farmer L, Burnett K et al: Maladaptive coping strategies and injury-related distress following traumatic physical injury, *Rehabil Psychol* 50:408-415, 2005.
5. Leske J: Treatment for family members in crisis after critical injury, *AACN Clin Issues Crit Care Nurs* 9:129-139, 1998.
6. Hoff LA: *People in crisis: clinical and public health perspectives,* 5th ed, San Fransisco, 2001, Jossey-Bass.
7. Infante MS: *Crisis theory: a framework for nursing practice,* pp 117-127, Englewood Cliffs, NJ, 1982, Prentice Hall.
8. Aguilera D: *Crisis intervention: theory and methodology,* 8th ed, pp 26-42, St. Louis, 1998, Mosby.
9. Krug EG, Sharma GK, Lozano R: The global burden of injuries, *Am J Public Health* 90:523-526, 2000.
10. U.S.Department of Health and Human Services: *Healthy people 2010: understanding and improving health,* Washington, DC, 2000,U.S. Department of Health and Human Services, Government Printing Office.
11. Pickett W, Molcho M, Simpson K et al: Cross national study of injury and social determinants in adolescents, *Inj Prev* 11:213-218, 2005.
12. Poole G, Lewis J, Devidas M et al: Risk-taking, reported injury, and perception of future injury among adolescents, *J Pediatr Psychol* 22:513-531, 1997.
13. Sommers M, Dyehouse JM, Howe SR et al: Effectiveness of brief interventions after alcohol-related vehicular injury; a randomized control study, *J Trauma* 61:523-533, 2006.
14. Ankney RN, Vizza J, Coil JA et al: Cofactors of alcohol-related trauma at a rural trauma center, *Am J Emerg Med* 15:228-231, 1997.
15. Schermer CR, Gentilello LM, Hoyt DB et al: National survey of trauma surgeons' alcohol screening and brief interventions, *J Trauma* 55:849-856, 2003.
16. Kerr ME, Bowen M: *Family evaluation: an approach based on Bowen theory,* New York, 1988, WW Norton.
17. Bowen M: *Family therapy in clinical practice,* pp 188-212, 423-450, Northvale, NJ, 1992, Jason Aronson.
18. Minuchin S: *Structural family therapy,* Cambridge, Mass, 1976, Harvard University.
19. Morse JM, O'Brien B: Preserving self: from victim to patient, to disabled person, *J Adv Nurs* 21:886-896, 1995.
20. Cross ML, Wright SW, Wrenn KD et al: Interaction between the trauma team and families: lack of timely communications, *Am J Emerg Med* 14:548-550, 1996.
21. Leske JS: Comparison of family stresses, strengths, and outcomes after trauma and surgery, *AACN Clin Issues Adv Pract Acute Crit Care* 14:33-41, 2003.

22. Halm MA: Family presence during resuscitation: a critical review of the literature, *Am J Critical Care* 14:494-511, 2005.
23. Epperson MM: Families in sudden crisis: process and intervention in a critical care center, *Soc Work Health Care* 2:265-273, 1977.
24. Kleeman KM: Families in crisis due to multiple trauma, *Crit Care Nurs Clin North Am* 1:23-31, 1989.
25. Magnan MA: Psychological considerations for patients with acute wounds, *Crit Care Nurs Clin North Am* 8:183-193, 1996.
26. Jastremski C, Harvey M: Making changes to improve the intensive care unit experience for patients and their families, *N Horiz* 6:99-109, 1998.
27. Kamel MS, Gammack JK: Insomnia in the elderly: cause, approach, and treatment, *Am J Med* 119:463-469, 2006.
28. Feinsilver SH: Sleep in the elderly: what is normal? *Clin Geriatr Med* 19:177-188, 2003.
29. Smith MT, Perlis ML, Park A et al: Comparative metaanalysis of pharmacotherapy and behavioral therapy for persistent insomnia, *Am J Psychiatry* 159:5-11, 2002.
30. Burke WJ, Folks DG, McNeilly DP: Effective use of anxiolytics in older adults, *Clin Geriatr Med* 14:47-65, 1998.
31. Schrader KA: Stress and immunity after traumatic injury: the mind-body link, *AACN Clin Issues Crit Care Nurs* 7:351-358, 1996.
32. Pachankis JE, Goldfried MR: Clinical issues in working with lesbian, gay and bisexual clients, *Psychother Theory Res Pract Training* 41:227-246, 2004.
33. Kagawa-Singer M, Blackhall LJ: Negotiating cross-culture issues at the end of life, *JAMA* 286:2993-3002, 2001.
34. Chesla C: Reconciling technologic and family care in critical care nursing, *Image J Nurse Sch* 28:199-203, 1996.
35. Olson D: Paging the family: using technology to enhance communication, *Crit Care Nurs* 17:37-41, 1997.
36. Medland J, Ferran SC: Effectiveness of a structured communication program for family members of patients in an ICU, *Am J Crit Care* 7:24-29, 1998.
37. Hsu S: Trauma support groups, *Imprint* 43:45-48, 1996.
38. Kübler-Ross E: *On death and dying,* New York, 1969, Macmillan.
39. American Psychiatric Association: *Diagnostic and statistical manual of mental disorders,* 4th ed, revised, Washington, DC, 2000, American Psychiatric Association.
40. Elliott TR, Kennedy P: Treatment of depression following spincal cord injury: and evidence based review, *Rehabil Psychol* 49:134-139, 2004.
41. Nielson MS: Post-traumatic stress disorder and emotional distess in persons with spinal cord lesions, *Spinal Cord* 41:296-302, 2003.
42. Nielson MS: Prevalence of post-traumatic stress disorder in person with spinal cord injuries: the mediating effect of social support, *Rehabil Psychol* 48:289-295, 2003.
43. Weitzenkamp DA, Gerhart MS, Charlifue SW et al: Spouses of spinal cord injury survivors: the added impact of caregiving, *Arch Phys Med Rehabil* 78:822-827, 1997.
44. Knight RG, Devereaux R, Godfrey HP: Caring for a family member with a traumatic brain injury, *Brain Inj* 12:467-481, 1998.
45. Wallace CA, Bogner J, Corrigan JD et al: Primary caregivers of persons with brain injury: life changes one year after injury, *Brain Inj* 12:483-493, 1998.
46. Rintala DH, Young ME, Spencer JC et al: Family relationships and adaptation to spinal cord injury: a qualitative study, *Rehabil Nurs* 21:67-74, 90, 1996.
47. Binks TM, Radnitz CL, Moran AI et al: Relationship between level of spinal cord injury and posttraumatic stress disorder symptoms, *Ann N Y Acad Sci* 821:430-432, 1997.
48. Bisson JI, Shepherd JP, Manish D: Psychological sequelae of facial trauma, *J Trauma* 43:496-500, 1997.
49. Yehuda R: Post-traumatic stress disorder, *N Engl J Med* 346:108-114, 2002.
50. Harrahil M: Giving bad news compassionately: a 2-hour medical school educational program, *J Emerg Nurs* 23:496-498, 1997.
51. Furukawa MM: Meeting the needs of the dying patient's family, *Crit Care Nurs* 16:51-57, 1996.
52. Spray G, McNeel J: A theoretical overview of traumatic grief. In Spray G, McNeel J, editors: *The many faces of bereavement: the nature and treatment of natural, traumatic, and stigmatized grief,* pp 55-64, New York, 1995, Brenner/Mazel.
53. Spray G, McNeel J: The process of grief following a murder. In Spray G, McNeel J, editors: *The many faces of bereavement: the nature and treatment of natural, traumatic, and stigmatized grief,* pp 65-85, New York, 1995, Brenner/Mazel.
54. Spray G, McNeel J: The treatment of traumatic grief. In Spray G, McNeel J, editors: *The many faces of bereavement: the nature and treatment of natural, traumatic, and stigmatized grief,* pp 118-135, New York, 1995, Brenner/Mazel.
55. Hurst S, Koplin-Baucum S: A pilot qualitative study relating to hardiness in ICU nurses, *Dimens Crit Care Nurs* 24:97-100, 2005.
56. Chen S. McMurray A: "Burnout" in intensive care nurses, *J Nurs Res* 9:152-164, 2001.

PART III

SINGLE SYSTEM INJURIES

20

TRAUMATIC BRAIN INJURIES

Karen A. McQuillan, Paul A. Thurman

Brain injury is the leading cause of all trauma-related deaths. It constitutes the primary cause of trauma-related death and long-term disability among young Americans.[1,2] Survivors of the initial brain insult remain at risk for various multisystem complications that can exacerbate the initial brain injury and increase mortality and morbidity. The prevention, recognition, and immediate treatment of these complications in the prehospital, resuscitation, critical care, intermediate care, and rehabilitation phases of care are of utmost importance. Recovery is often a lifelong process beset with physical, mental, emotional, and social obstacles. Brain injury and the potential long-term disabilities it creates also have a tremendous impact on the family and cost society billions of dollars each year. Because of its high incidence, mortality and morbidity, economic cost, and demand for medical resources, brain injury is a major public health problem in the United States.

This chapter provides the trauma nurse with a comprehensive review of traumatic brain injury (TBI) and its sequelae. An overview of brain injury epidemiology, mechanism of injury, and related neuroanatomy increases the nurse's knowledge about the magnitude of this disease, as well as its etiology and neurologic impact. Explanation of the various types of brain injuries and pathophysiology provides the scientific basis for interventions used to treat TBI. Strategies to monitor and assess the injured brain are reviewed so the nurse can collaborate with the other members of the health care team to properly guide and evaluate the effectiveness of treatment. Therapeutic interventions used by the multidisciplinary health care team to manage brain injury are described for each phase of trauma care. With knowledge about related anatomy and brain injury pathophysiology, assessment, and treatment, the trauma nurse can best promote optimal outcomes for patients with craniocerebral trauma.

EPIDEMIOLOGY

The precise number of TBI cases is not known; however, it is estimated that about 1.4 million Americans sustain TBI each year.[1] In 1996 the Centers for Disease Control and Prevention (CDC) was charged by Congress with developing a uniform reporting system to track the incidence, severity, causes, and outcomes of TBI (Public Law 104-166).[3] In response the CDC established guidelines for surveillance of central nervous system injury and published "Traumatic Brain Injury in the United States: Emergency Department Visits, Hospitalizations, and Deaths"[1] and "Incidence Rates of Hospitalization Related to Traumatic Brain Injury—12 States, 2002."[4] These reports are limited in that the former only provides data about patients seen in a tertiary system and the later reports data from only 12 states.

"Traumatic Brain Injury in the United States: Emergency Department Visits, Hospitalizations, and Deaths" reports that from 1995 to 2001, there were on average 1,111,000 emergency department (ED) visits for TBI, 235,000 hospitalizations, and 50,000 deaths per year. Falls are the leading cause of TBI, followed by motor vehicle crashes.[1] Of all reported TBIs, approximately 398,000 are related to falls, 280,000 to motor vehicle traffic incidents and 156,000 to assaults.[2] Each year, an estimated 80,000 to 90,000 Americans sustain permanent disability from their TBI.[2] At least 5.3 million Americans are currently living with disabilities resulting from TBI.[1]

The Traumatic Brain Injury Model Systems National Data Center, a division of the National Institute on Disability and Rehabilitation Research—United States Department of Education, established the TBI National Database.[5] Patient information for this database was contributed by 21 federally funded TBI Model Systems of Care throughout the United States. As of September 2005, the database contained information on 5756 persons age 16 and older with primarily moderate to severe TBI. More than 62% of the patients had a Glasgow Coma Scale (GCS) score ranging from 3 to 8, were intubated, or in chemical coma. According to this database the mean age of patients with TBI is 38.6; 69% are non-Hispanic Caucasian, 20% African-American, 7% Hispanic, and 2.7% Asian/Pacific Islander. Of cases admitted to the Model Systems facilities, motor vehicle crashes were the most common cause of TBI (46.9%) followed by falls (19.5%). Since 1997, 7.7% of the database sample suffered TBI from blunt assaults. More than half (63%) of the individuals were employed at the time of their injury, and by post-injury year 10, only 29% were employed. After sustaining TBI, mean length of stay for acute hospitalization was 20.0 days and 26.3 days for rehabilitation. It is important to remember that these statistics only reflect data based on a sample of patients with TBI. The true numbers of those who have sustained a TBI are not known.

The economic costs of TBI are staggering. Direct costs include initial and follow-up diagnoses, treatment, and rehabilitation. Indirect costs include societal losses secondary to restricted or lost productivity. In the United States, the estimated cost of TBI totaled an estimated $60 billion for the year 2000.[6] However the physical and psychosocial suffering endured by brain-injured persons and their families is incalculable.

CORRELATIVE NEUROANATOMY AND PHYSIOLOGY

The brain, which is part of the central nervous system, provides most of the control functions for the entire body. The brain receives and interprets sensory input and then integrates this information to determine and carry out the response to be made by the body. In general the brain maintains the quality and uniqueness of human life and behavior. The major divisions of the brain are the cerebrum, brainstem, and cerebellum (Figure 20-1), which are housed within multiple protective coverings.

COVERINGS OF THE BRAIN

Numerous protective coverings surround the brain. Outermost on top of the skull is the scalp, composed of multiple layers: skin, subcutaneous fascia, galea aponeurotica, and periosteum. The rigid, nondistendible cranium that encases the brain is made up of the sphenoid, ethmoid, frontal, and occipital bones, two parietal bones, and two temporal bones (Figure 20-2). Beneath the skull are three layers of connective tissue (the meninges) that surround the brain and the spinal cord. The meningeal layers include the outermost thick, fibrous dura mater; the fine, elastic arachnoid mater; and the innermost vascular membrane, the pia mater, which adheres to the brain's surface (Figure 20-3).

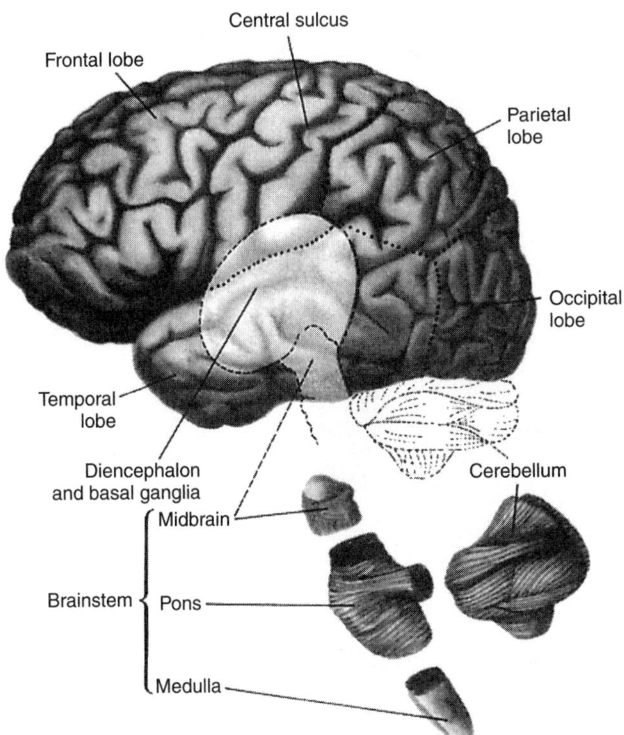

FIGURE 20-1 Major parts of the central nervous system. (From Kandel E, Schwartz J: *Principles of Neural Science,* ed 3, New York, 1991, Elsevier/North-Holland.)

CEREBRUM

The cerebrum includes the cerebral hemispheres and the diencephalon. It is capped by gray cortex (neuronal cell bodies), under which lies extensive white matter (axons). The two large cerebral hemispheres are partially separated by the great longitudinal fissure and a vertical dural fold within the fissure that creates the falx cerebri. A thick tract of white interhemispheric nerve fibers at the base of the longitudinal fissure, the corpus callosum, is the primary connective pathway between the two hemispheres.

Cerebral Hemispheres

The two cerebral hemispheres are divided into four pairs of lobes: the frontal, temporal, parietal, and occipital (Figure 20-4). Knowledge of the primary functions of the lobes (Table 20-1) and lesion location can alert the nurse to the most likely assessment findings. For example, it can be anticipated that a focal lesion in the prefrontal region may result in altered behavior, whereas a lesion in the posterior frontal region of the dominant hemisphere may result in language dysfunction. Nursing assessment and the patient plan of care should anticipate and focus on the actual or potential problems associated with lesions in specific anatomic locations.

The cerebral hemispheres are responsible for sensory and motor processes of the contralateral side of the body. Sensory information entering the spinal cord from the right side of the body crosses over to the left before reaching the cortex. Similarly, motor impulses originating from the right cerebral cortex cross over to the left before synapsing in the cord. This explains one of the fundamental principles of motor assessment; that is, structural lesions causing compression of descending motor tract fibers will almost always result in contralateral motor signs.

The basal ganglia and limbic system, which provide a number of important functions, are located deep within the cerebral hemispheres. The basal nuclei are masses of gray matter, (i.e., caudate, putamen, claustrum, amygdaloid, globus pallidus, and functionally, the substantia nigra and subthalamic nuclei), which control and regulate coordination of motor integration, voluntary movement, motion initiation, postural reflexes, and muscle tone. The basal ganglia serve as the principle center of the extrapyramidal motor system. The limbic system is composed of the limbic lobe and several other structures with which it is functionally and anatomically related, including the hippocampus, amygdala, fornix, olfactory tract, thalamus, and hypothalamus. This

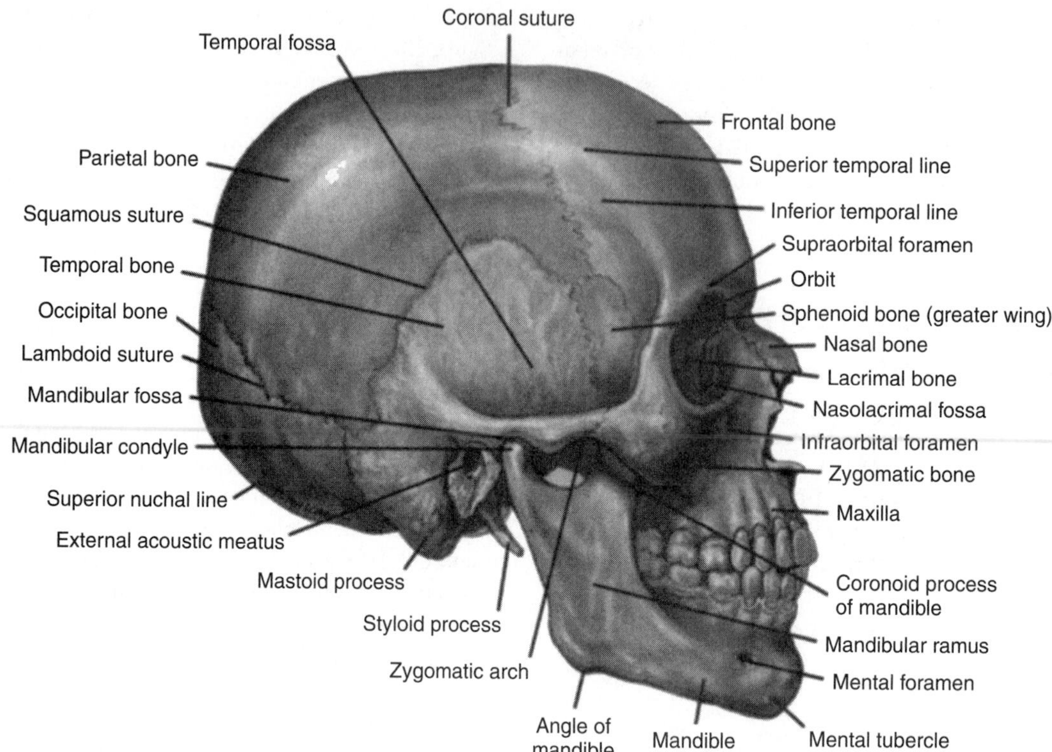

FIGURE 20-2 Right side view of the skull. (From Lindsay DT: *Functional Human Anatomy*, St. Louis, 1996, Mosby, p. 147.)

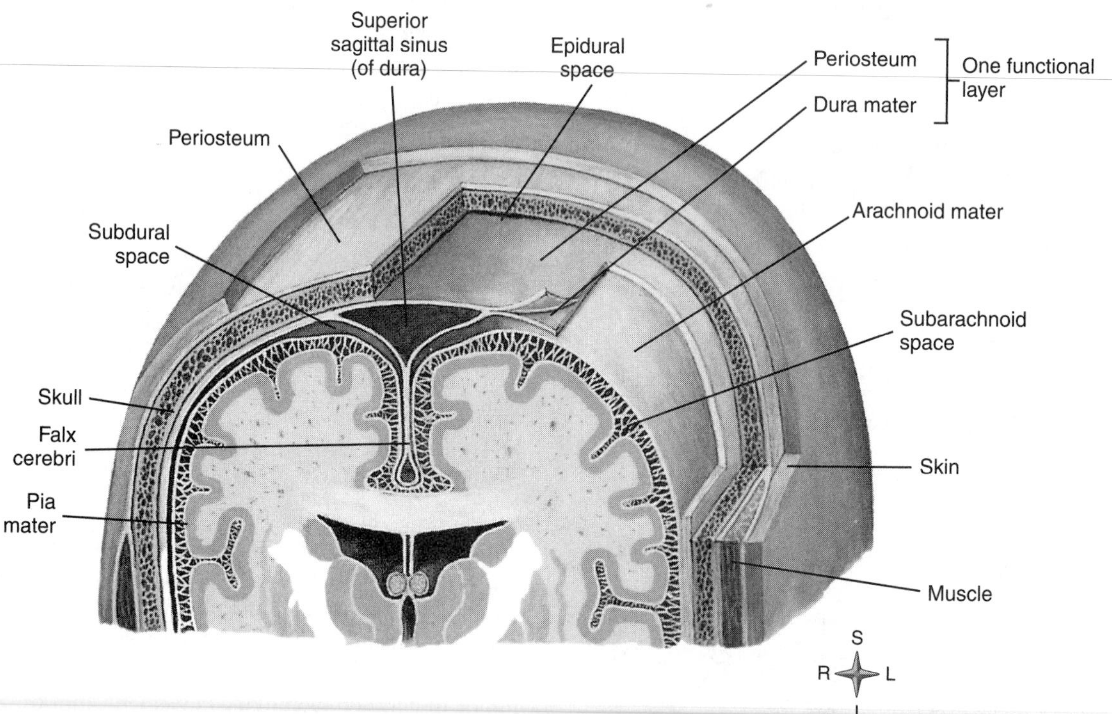

FIGURE 20-3 Coverings of the brain. *I*, Interior; *L*, left; *R*, right; *S*, superior. (From Thibodeau GA, Patton K: *Anatomy & Physiology*, ed 5, St. Louis, 2003, Mosby, p. 376.)

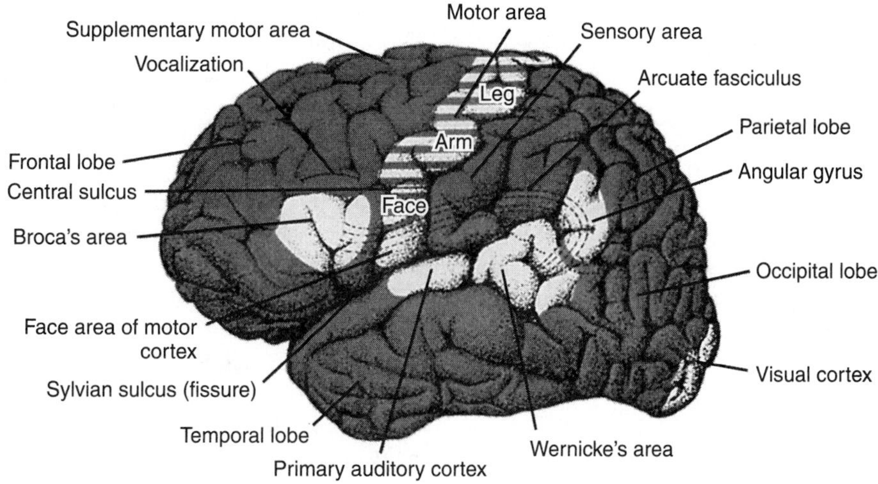

FIGURE 20-4 Lobes of the brain. (From Kandel E, Schwartz J: *Principles in Neural Science,* ed 3, New York, 1991, Elsevier/North-Holland.)

TABLE 20-1 Functional Localization in the Cerebral Cortex

Lobe	Functions

Frontal	Higher mental functions
	  Concentration
	  Abstract thinking
	  Foresight/judgment
	Behavior/tactfulness
	Inhibition
	Memory
	Personality
	Affect
	Conjugate eye movements
	Voluntary motor function (origin of the pyramidal motor system)
	Motor control of speech (dominant hemisphere*)

Temporal	Hearing Comprehend spoken language (dominant hemisphere*) Visual, olfactory and auditory perception Memory Learning/intellect Emotion
Parietal	Sensory perception of touch, pain, temperature, position, pressure, and vibration Body awareness Sensory interpretation
Occipital	Visual perception and interpretation Controls some visual and ocular movement reflexes

*Cerebral dominance: In right-handed and most left-handed people, the left cerebral hemisphere is dominant for language, mathematical, and analytic functions. The opposite nondominant hemisphere is thought to be concerned with nonverbal, geometric, spatial, visual, and musical functions.

Used with permission from McQuillan KA: The neurologic system. In Alspach GA, editor: *Core Curriculum for Critical Care Nursing,* ed 6, St. Louis, 2006, Saunders Elsevier, p. 384.

system is responsible for some aspects of learning and memory, instinctual drives (e.g., hunger, mating), and emotional behavioral responses and associated endocrine, visceral, and somatic reactions.

Diencephalon

The diencephalon is a complex of structures consisting of the hypothalamus, thalamus, epithalamus, and subthalamus. The hypothalamus, situated deep within the brain and just above the brainstem, is one of the most notable of the diencephalic structures. It is the primary regulator of autonomic function and controls numerous visceral and metabolic activities, including regulation of body temperature, blood pressure, heart rate, pupil size, shivering, sweating, gastrointestinal peristalsis, appetite, sleep-wake cycle, and water balance. Through its connection with the pituitary gland via the hypophyseal stalk, the hypothalamus directly influences pituitary hormonal activities and, in conjunction with the pituitary, mediates the body's stress/adaptation response.

Brainstem

The brainstem is a midline structure situated beneath the diencephalon. The brainstem has three sections: the midbrain is the uppermost structure, the pons lies in the middle, and the medulla is the lowest segment (see Figure 20-1). The descending medulla is contiguous with the spinal cord, which begins at the level of the foramen magnum.

The brainstem performs a variety of vital functions. It is the center of the brain that controls basic and reflexive activities, such as visual and auditory motor reflexes, wakefulness, sneezing, coughing, breathing, vasomotor activity, and heart rate regulation. It is the pathway used by sensory fibers as they ascend from the cord to the cortex. Motor tract fibers on their descent from their cerebral or brainstem origin also traverse the brainstem, and many cross over (decussate) in the medulla before exiting down the spinal cord. Many cerebellar tracts also pass through the brainstem, which allows formation of extensive connections between the cerebrum and cerebellum in this region. The reticular activating system responsible for consciousness originates in the brainstem as a dense bundle of fibers and ascends, coursing out over the cerebral cortices (Figure 20-5). The brainstem also controls many of the special senses, motor functions, and reflexes that are mediated by the cranial nerves, which arise and exit from this structure.

CEREBELLUM

The cerebellum lies within the posterior fossa behind the brainstem and beneath the cerebral hemispheres. It is separated from the cerebral hemispheres by a dural fold called the tentorium cerebelli and is attached to the three brainstem sections by three pairs of cerebellar peduncles. Cerebellar functions include control of muscle tone, coordination of muscle activity, regulation of postural reflexes, and use of feedback loops to make appropriate corrections in motor activities and to maintain equilibrium.

CEREBROVASCULATURE

The carotid and vertebral arteries deliver blood to an extensive capillary system that supplies the brain. The capillaries of the brain have a unique membranous structure that has tight junctions between the vessel wall network of endothelial cells and is surrounded by astrocyte end-feet projections. These unique capillary features, known as the blood-brain barrier, help maintain homeostasis for the neurons by limiting the transfer of substances from the intravascular space into the extracellular fluid and cerebrospinal fluid (CSF). From the capillaries, blood drains into the venous system, which differs from other veins of the body in that it lacks valves. Cerebral blood is carried by an internal and external venous system into large dural sinuses located between the dural layers, which empty into the jugular veins exiting the brain.

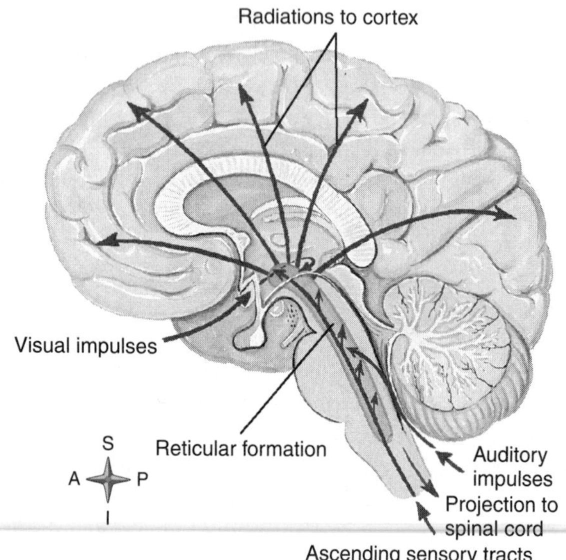

FIGURE 20-5 Reticular Activating System. Consists of centers in the brainstem reticular formation plus fibers that conduct to the centers from below and fibers that conduct from the centers to widespread areas of the cerebral cortex. Functioning of the reticular activating system is essential for consciousness. (From Thibodeau GA, Patton KT: *Anatomy & Physiology*, ed 5, St. Louis, 2003, Mosby, p. 395.)

CEREBROSPINAL FLUID

CSF supports and cushions the central nervous system. It also aids in the removal of metabolic waste products and regulates the chemical environment of the nervous system to preserve homeostasis. CSF plays an important role in intracranial dynamics and management of intracranial pressure (ICP) after severe TBI.

CSF is a clear, colorless liquid produced primarily within the choroid plexuses of the ventricles at a rate of approximately 22 to 25 ml/hr (500 ml/day). CSF contains small amounts of protein, glucose, oxygen, carbon dioxide, and potassium and relatively large amounts of sodium chloride. In adults the volume of CSF circulating through the ventricular system and subarachnoid space of the brain and spinal cord at any one time is 125 to 150 ml.

The CSF pathway (Figure 20-6) is a free-flowing system whereby CSF passes from the lateral ventricles (hollow cavities within each cerebral hemisphere) through the foramina of Monro (intraventricular foramina) into the third ventricle. From there it flows into the fourth ventricle via a small, narrow opening known as the aqueduct of Sylvius. CSF exits the fourth ventricle through the foramina of Magendie and Luschka to enter the cisterna magnum and the subarachnoid space (SAS). CSF within the subarachnoid space flows upward over the convexity of the brain and downward around the spinal cord.

Because there is continuous synthesis of CSF, it is essential that both a functional outlet system and a patent pathway be maintained to facilitate absorption and prevent fluid build-up. Arachnoid granulations or villi, outpouchings of the arachnoid membrane that herniate through the dura into the large venous sinuses, absorb most of the CSF into the venous system. These structures are pressure-dependent, one-way valves that open when CSF pressure exceeds venous pressure, allowing unidirectional flow of CSF from the subarachnoid space into venous blood.

CELLS OF THE BRAIN

The central nervous system contains two types of cells: the neuroglial, or glial cells, and the nerve cells, or neurons. Glial cells outnumber neurons by approximately 9 to 1 and are generally classified as astrocytes, oligodendroglia, microglia, or ependymal cells. Glial cells lack axons and function primarily to nourish, support, and protect the nerve cells.

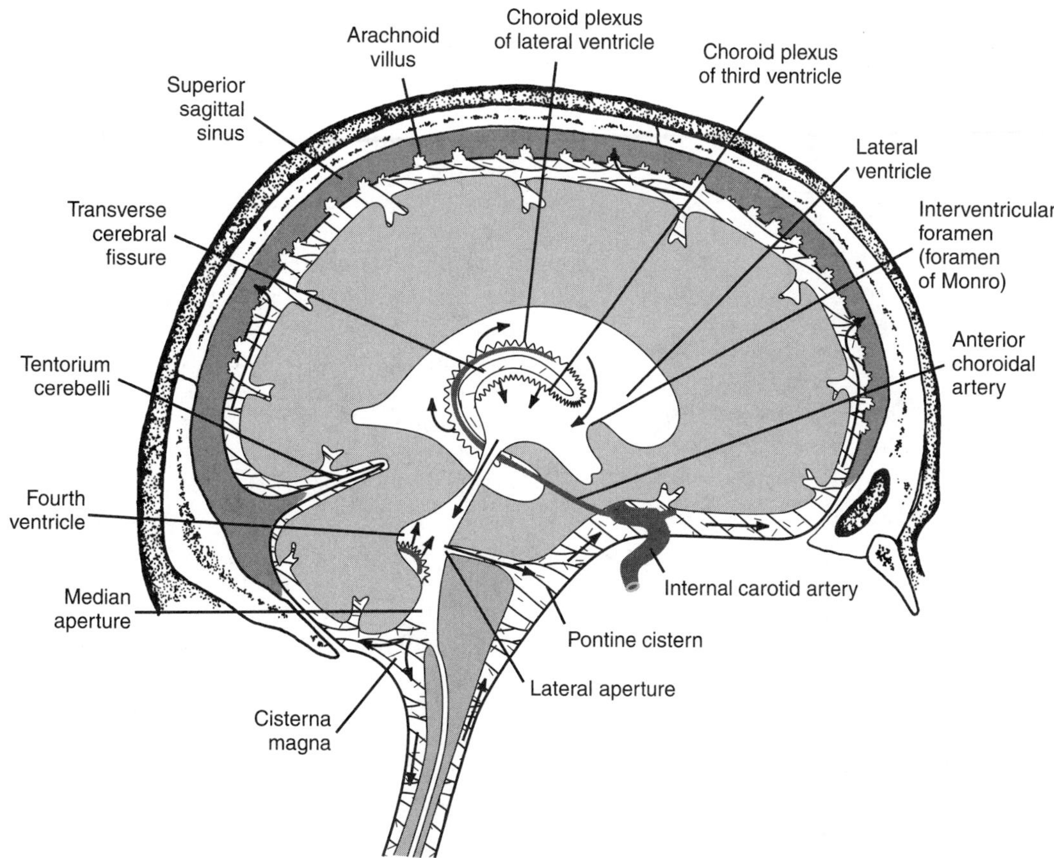

FIGURE 20-6 Path of CSF circulation. (From Nolte J: *The Human Brain: An Introduction to Its Functional Anatomy,* ed 4, St. Louis, 1999, Mosby, p. 107.)

The neuron is the functional unit of the nervous system that transmits nerve impulses. This type of cell consists of a cell body, axon, presynaptic terminals of the axon, and dendrites (Figure 20-7). Each of these cell components has a distinctive function. The cell body synthesizes and packages the products of neuronal metabolism and transports them to other regions of the cell. It exchanges nutrients, ions, and other metabolically active substances with the extracellular environment through the cell membrane. This lipoprotein membrane is crucial for depolarization of the neuron through such mechanisms as the energy-dependent sodium-potassium pump, ion-selective channels, and voltage-sensitive channels. The myelin-covered axon, a tubular extension of the cell body, is responsible for rapid nerve conduction away from the cell body. The presynaptic terminals are specialized endings at the distal portion of the axon that transmit information by chemical or electrical means to other neurons or effector cells. The specialized contact zone between the transmitting (presynaptic cell) and the receiving (postsynaptic cell) neuron is the synapse. The dendrites, unmyelinated fibers that branch extensively as they extend from the cell body, receive incoming impulses and transmit them to the cell body. The physiologic and anatomic properties of the nerve cell account for its unique ability to communicate with other cells. In general the neuron is responsible for processing, analyzing, and acting on all incoming and outgoing information, which culminates in all our behavioral responses. Neurons differ from other cells in both their communicative ability and their lack of mitotic ability. Without mitosis, neurons cannot multiply. With central nervous system maturity, the number of neurons is fixed and no new neurons are added. Injury to neurons is significant because it results in cell loss with no new cell replacement.

Cerebral Metabolism

The average brain weighs 3 pounds and accounts for 2% of an adult's body weight. Despite its relatively small size, the brain uses about 20% of the total body oxygen consumption.[7] The primary energy source for the brain is glucose, which is converted by aerobic or oxidative metabolism into a high-energy phosphate form, adenosine triphosphate (ATP). Most of the energy is used for neuronal metabolic and conductive activities. Oxygen and glucose are in continuous demand, as the brain has minimal storage capacity for either substrate. The brain's dependency on energy is so great that, without its nutrient supply, neuronal function fails within seconds of energy deprivation.

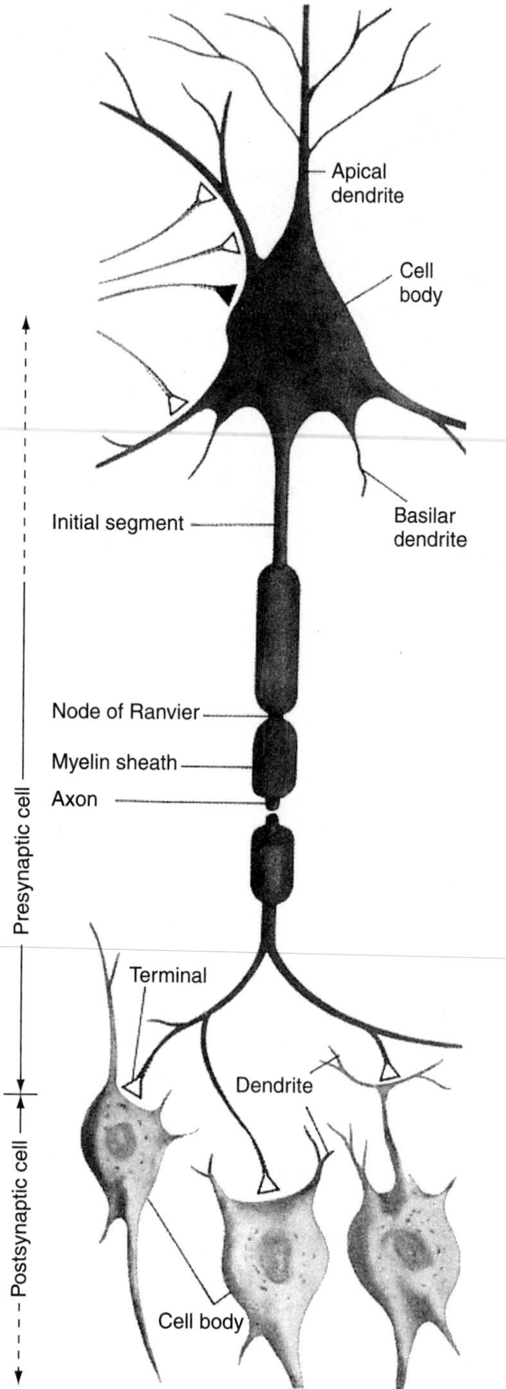

FIGURE 20-7 The neuron. (From Kandel E, Schwartz J: *Principles in Neural Science,* ed 3, New York, 1991, Elsevier/North-Holland.)

The need for oxygen and its rate of delivery depend on the degree of metabolic activity coupled with the rate of oxygen consumption. If metabolism is increased, as occurs with seizures, hyperthermia, or abnormal posturing, oxygen requirements increase. When cerebral metabolism is decreased, such as with sedation or hypothermia, oxidative requirements are reduced.

Cerebral Blood Flow

The normal brain receives an average of 750 ml of blood, or 50 ml/100 g of brain tissue, per minute. The disproportionate flow is necessitated by the brain's incessant need for oxygen and glucose delivery. Cerebral perfusion pressure and intrinsic regulatory mechanisms influence and help maintain sufficient cerebral blood flow.

Cerebral Perfusion Pressure

Cerebral perfusion pressure (CPP) is the pressure gradient that drives blood into the brain—the difference between the incoming intraarterial pressure and the outgoing intravenous pressure. Because pressure in the cerebral veins is the same as ICP, CPP can be determined by calculating the difference between the mean arterial blood pressure (MAP = 1/3 [systolic − diastolic] + diastolic) and ICP. The formula is CPP = MAP − ICP. For example, if the MAP is 90 and the ICP is 15, the CPP is 75. The normal range of cerebral perfusion in healthy adults is 50 to 150 mm Hg.

Autoregulatory Mechanisms

Pressure, or myogenic autoregulation, is the brain's ability to maintain a constant rate of blood flow over a wide range of perfusion pressures despite changes in arterial blood pressure and ICP. The cerebral arterioles or resistance vessels have an inherent self-regulatory (autoregulatory) mechanism contained within their muscular walls that allows them to change vessel diameter in response to changes in transmural pressure (Figure 20-8). As a result, an increase in arterial pressure causes vasoconstriction of the vessels, and a decrease in arterial pressure causes vasodilation. This mechanism keeps cerebral blood flow (CBF) essentially constant for a range of CPP from approximately 50 to 150 mm Hg. Intact autoregulation safeguards the brain from ischemia caused by fluctuations in arterial pressure and ICP.

Several metabolic factors also have a marked effect on cerebral blood flow, including partial pressure of arterial oxygen (Pao_2), pH, and partial pressure of arterial carbon dioxide ($PaCo_2$). A decrease in Pao_2 below 50 mm Hg causes vasodilation, which increases cerebral flow and volume.[8] Extracellular reduction in pH (cerebral acidosis) caused by hypercarbia or acid byproducts of anaerobic cellular metabolism induces vascular dilation and increases cerebral flow and volume. Carbon dioxide (Co_2) is the most potent vasoactive agent known to cerebral vessels. An increase in Co_2 causes vasodilation, increasing cerebral flow and volume. Inversely, a decrease in Co_2 constricts the cerebral vessels, decreasing cerebral flow volume. Normocapnic individuals have about a 3% alteration in CBF for every 1 mm Hg change in Co_2 between the range of 20 mm Hg and 60 mm Hg.[9]

Metabolic autoregulation causes the rate of CBF to vary depending on neuronal metabolic activity. Gray matter, which contains the metabolically active cell bodies, normally receives three to six times more flow than white matter. CBF decreases globally in coma and increases regionally with activation or

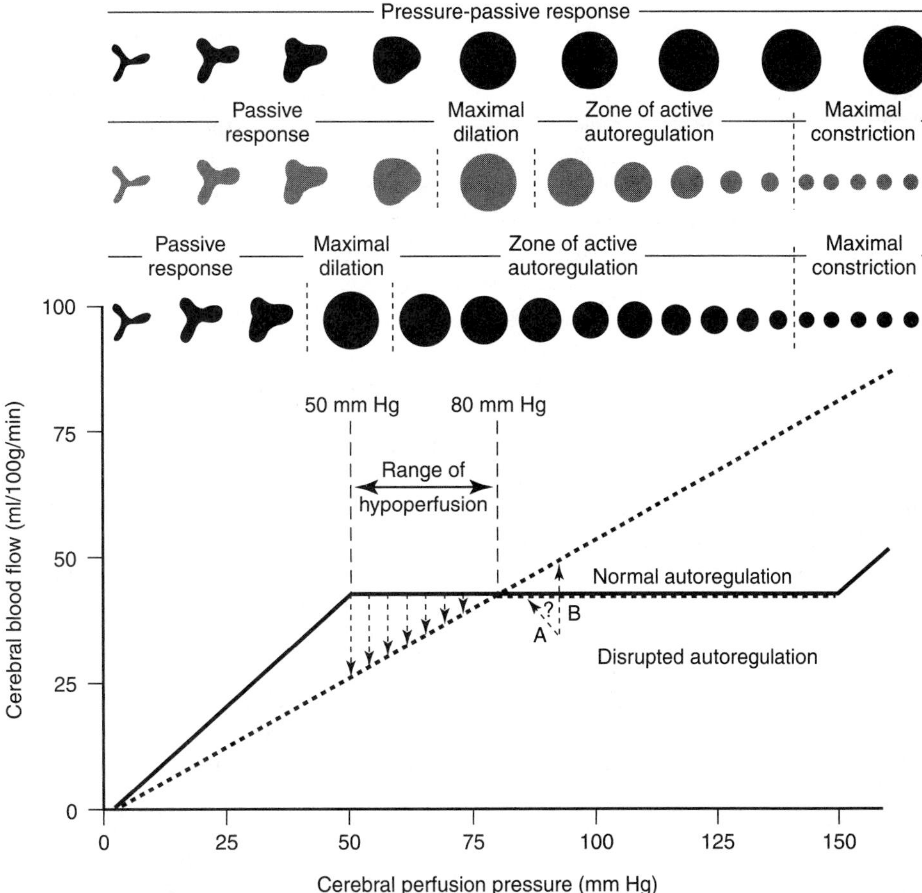

FIGURE 20-8 Normal pressure autoregulation and two possible degrees of disruption after severe traumatic brain injury. The relationship between CPP and CBF for these three states is represented by the graph. The status of the vascular system during the various stages of normal and disrupted autoregulation is represented by the *row of solid circles at the top* of the figure. The *bottom row of solid circles* represents intact autoregulation, the *middle row* corresponds to partially disrupted autoregulation (elevated lower breakpoint of active autoregulation), and the *top row* represents complete disruption of autoregulation (pressure-passive system). Cerebral blood volume (CBV) is represented by the *area of the circles.*

The ***solid line*** represents normal pressure autoregulation, with lower and upper breakpoints of active autoregulation at 50 and 150 mm Hg, respectively. Within this range, CBF is maintained at a stable value by varying the degree of vasoconstriction (zone of active autoregulation, *bottom row of circles*). A concomitant of this vasoconstriction is a progressive decrease in CBV as CPP is raised within the active range.

Disrupted pressure autoregulation is represented by the ***dashed line.*** The pressure-passive nature of complete disruption is illustrated by the straight curve ***(line B)*** where CBF is directly proportional to CPP. In a pressure-passive system, raising the CPP results in vasodilation, increased CBV, and elevated ICP throughout the range of CPP.

In the situation of partial disruption, the system is pressure-passive up to the reset breakpoint (80 mm Hg in this figure), after which pressure autoregulation occurs between 80 to 150 mm Hg ***(line A)***. The situation of cerebrovascular response and CBV changes resembles the normal situation with the exception that the transformation from pressure-passive to active occurs at a higher breakpoint.

Note that in either pathological case, there is a range of hypoperfusion between 50 and 80 mm Hg, wherein ischemia may occur despite CPP values that appear to be "within normal limits." (Courtesy Randall M. Chesnut, MD.)

specific activities (e.g., hand movement, mental processing). In coma, both cerebral metabolism and blood flow are normally depressed. Even with a blood flow reduction of as much as 40%, neuronal integrity can still be maintained as long as metabolism is equally reduced.

Neurogenic factors and mediators released from the endothelium can also affect the cerebral vasculature. Neurogenic factors work in synergy with the pressure, chemical, and metabolic factors but seem to have a less significant impact on cerebral blood flow. Multiple neurogenic systems, such as the sympathetic and parasympathetic systems, innervate cerebral arteries and may exert a vasoactive effect on these vessels. Stimuli such as shear stress and certain neurotransmitters can trigger the release of vasoactive mediators from the endothelium. Endothelin and thromboxane A_2 are examples of endothelium-derived mediators that cause vasoconstriction, whereas nitric oxide and prostacyclin dilate the cerebral vessels.

ETIOLOGY

CAUSES AND RISK FACTORS

Motor vehicle traffic incidents constitute the leading cause of TBIs that result in death or hospitalization, whereas falls are the principle cause of TBI-related ED visits.[1] Transportation-related crashes (involving motor and recreational vehicles, bicycles, and pedestrians) constitute the leading cause of TBI-related deaths and hospitalizations.[1] Of all individuals who sustained motor vehicle- or traffic-related TBI, motor vehicle occupants comprised approximately 70% of those requiring hospitalization and more than 50% of those who died.[1] Assaults cause 11% of all TBI and 13% of all TBI-related deaths.[1] Nine out of 10 people with firearm-related brain injuries die. Nearly two thirds of firearm-related brain injuries are self-inflicted.[10]

Gender, age, ethnicity, and socioeconomic status can influence the risk of TBI. Males are 1.5 times as likely to sustain a TBI as females, and the death rate from TBIs is 2.8 times higher in males than females.[1] Children ages 0 to 4 years, adolescents ages 15 to 19 and adults age 75 and older are more likely than others to sustain a TBI.[1] Young children (ages 0 to 4 years) have the highest rate of visits to emergency departments, followed by older adolescents; however, adults older than age 75 have the highest rates of hospitalization and death due to TBI.[1] Falls are the most common cause of TBI in persons younger than age 5 and those older than age 75, whereas motor vehicle crashes and assaults are the leading cause of TBI among adolescents and young adults.[1] African-Americans reportedly have the highest death rate from TBI, which is primarily due to the high rate of firearm-related deaths in this racial group.[1] Lower socioeconomic status may increase the risk of injury because of greater dependence on less safe housing and vehicles, higher likelihood of having a more physically demanding occupation, and increased exposure to personal violence.

Certain medical conditions and behavior patterns may also increase risk of TBI. Persons with medical conditions that alter level of consciousness, impair neuromuscular function, decrease visual capacity, or result in seizures are more prone to injury and therefore more likely to sustain TBI. Use of alcohol or other drugs can impair judgment, diminish reaction time, and reduce neuromuscular control, increasing the risk of TBI. Failure to use safety precautions, such as not using occupant restraint systems, refusing to wear helmets when cycling or riding a motorcycle, or exceeding the speed limit, may also increase the likelihood of sustaining TBI.

MECHANISM OF INJURY

Skull Deformation

Direct impact to the head can distort the skull's contour and injure the underlying brain tissue (Figure 20-9A). High-velocity blows to the head are most often associated with deformation injuries. Cranium indentation, fracture, or outward bowing can precipitate contusions or lacerations of the underlying brain tissue and intracranial hemorrhage.

Acceleration-Deceleration Injury

Acceleration-deceleration injuries occur when the head is thrown rapidly forward or backward, resulting in sudden alterations in movement of the skull and brain in a straight, linear path (see Figure 20-9B).[11] Acceleration injuries occur when a moving object strikes the head (e.g., a baseball bat, fist, or hammer) and the skull and the brain are set in motion. Deceleration injuries occur when a head that is in motion hits a stationary object such as a wall or windshield, causing the skull to decelerate rapidly. The semisolid brain moves slower than the solid skull; therefore, the brain collides with the cranial surface and the rough bony prominences within the skull, causing brain tissue injury. Injury caused when the brain makes contact at the site of head

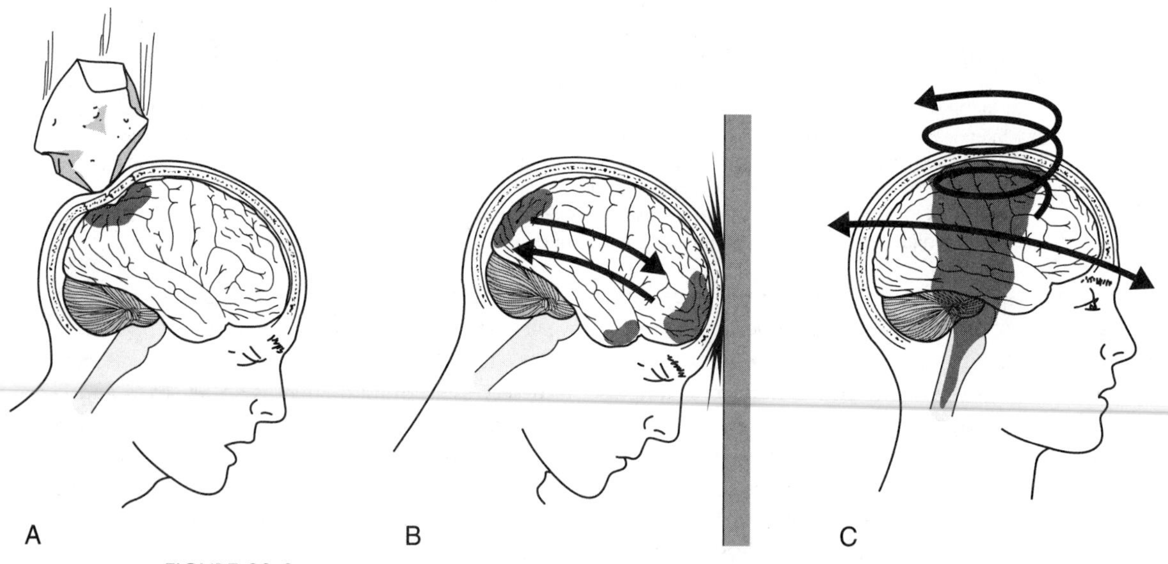

FIGURE 20-9 Mechanisms of injury. **A**, Deformation; **B**, Acceleration-deceleration; **C**, Rotation.

impact is referred to as *coup injury*. Brain injury also may occur as the brain is thrown in the direction opposite the impact, causing collision with the contralateral skull surface; this is known as *contrecoup injury*.

Rotation

Brain injury may also occur when acceleration or deceleration of the brain follows a nonlinear path, resulting in twisting or rotation of the brain within the skull (see Figure 20-9C). Rotation forces produce compressive, tensile, and shearing strains that cause distortion and injury of involved brain tissues and possible vascular disruption. Maximal stress from rotational forces is directed toward areas where tissues with different densities interface (e.g., between cerebral and fibrous tissue, between gray and white matter). The degree of injury from these rotational forces depends on the extent, rate, and direction of angular acceleration.[11,12] Motor vehicle crashes are a common cause of this type of mechanism.

Penetration

Penetrating brain injuries occur when a missile is projected, typically by a firearm, or an object is forced through the scalp and skull into the brain tissue. The penetrating object may cause brain laceration, contusion, hemorrhage, and subsequent cerebral edema and tissue necrosis. The severity of a penetrating injury depends on the size, shape, velocity, direction, and action of the foreign object that enters the brain, as well as the area of the brain involved.

A gunshot may create a single injury tract or, when a low-velocity missile is involved, it may ricochet within the cranial cavity and create multiple destructive missile tracts within the brain. A bullet projected through the skull and brain creates shock waves and a cavity that may expand to many times the bullet's diameter and then collapse, causing extensive local and remote tissue damage. High-velocity bullets that strike with much energy tend to cause greater tissue destruction from the temporary cavitation and shock waves than do low-velocity missiles, which wound primarily by direct tissue destruction.[13] Death associated with firearm-related TBI is the result of extensive structural damage and uncontrolled intracranial hypertension associated with intracranial hemorrhage and extensive cerebral edema. Patients may remain conscious immediately after gunshot wounds to the head, only to deteriorate rapidly with the onset of edema around the missile tract.

PATHOPHYSIOLOGY OF TRAUMATIC BRAIN INJURY

ASSOCIATED SCALP AND SKULL INJURIES

Scalp Injuries

Injuries to the scalp may occur in isolation or may be associated with an underlying skull fracture or brain lesion. The scalp is very prone to profuse hemorrhage as a result of its rich vascular supply and the poor ability of the scalp vessels to vasoconstrict. Blood may collect within the layers of the scalp (i.e., within the subcutaneous or subgaleal layers), or the scalp may be lacerated or avulsed, causing external hemorrhage. Subcutaneous and subgaleal hematomas generally resolve on their own without specific treatment. Direct pressure over a scalp laceration is usually sufficient to decrease bleeding until a more thorough investigation of the site can be performed to ligate any major bleeding vessels and repair the wound. Before closure, scalp wounds should be cleansed well to prevent onset of infection. If the scalp is totally avulsed, vascular reanastomosis is required to restore circulation to the segment being replaced. Skin grafts or musculocutaneous flaps may be necessary to repair areas where the scalp is missing.

Skull Fractures

Impact to the head can fracture the skull, which may or may not be accompanied by injury to the underlying brain. The presence of skull fractures has been identified as a significant predictor for injury-related abnormalities on computed tomography (CT) scan even after minor TBI.[14,15] The degree of skull injury depends on the mass, characteristics (e.g., shape), velocity, momentum, and direction of the object that impacts the head and the thickness of the skull at the point of contact.

A linear fracture is a simple break or crack in the continuity of the skull that dissects both the outer and inner tables. Linear fractures are essentially benign and require no treatment. Even though direct treatment is not required, this type of injury warrants a CT scan to rule out an underlying brain lesion. This is particularly true of linear fractures in the temporal and occipital regions, as arteries lying particularly close to the bones in these regions are susceptible to injury.

Depressed fractures are the result of the cranial bone being forced below the line of the normal skull contour. These fractures typically result from high-velocity contact sustained over a small surface area. The fragmented bone particles may be embedded into the brain tissue, resulting in cortical laceration and hemorrhage. A depressed skull fracture associated with a scalp laceration is called a *compound* or *open* fracture. These injuries are associated with an increased incidence of posttraumatic seizures and a high risk for intracranial infection.[14] Treatment of these open fractures, particularly if the fractured bone is depressed greater than the cranial thickness, usually consists of surgical debridement, evacuation of clots and bone fragments, elevation of the depressed bone, and repair of the lacerated dura as soon as possible after injury.[14] Closed depressed skull fractures may not require surgical intervention.[14]

Basilar skull fractures are located at the base of the cranium. The five bones that form the skull base are the occipital bone, the cribriform plate of the ethmoid bone, the orbital plate of the frontal bone, the sphenoid bone, and the petrous and squamous portions of the temporal bone (Figure 20-10). Basilar skull fractures are most common in the anterior and middle fossae. Fractures of the cranium base may be linear, compound, or depressed; most commonly they are linear fractures that extend downward into the base of the skull. Basilar skull fractures can be difficult to detect with routine

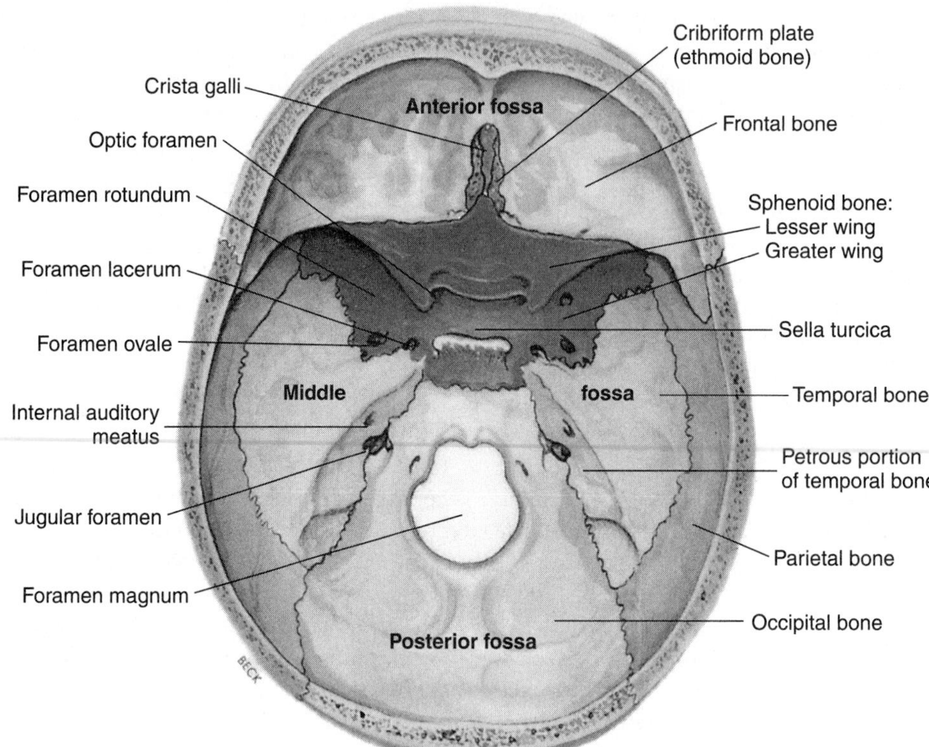

FIGURE 20-10 Base of the skull showing the cranial fossae. (From Slazinski T, Littlejohns LR: Anatomy of the nervous system. In Bader MK, Littlejohns LR, editors: *AANN core curriculum for neuroscience nursing,* ed 4, Philadelphia, 2004, W. B. Saunders, p. 32. Modified from Thibodeau GA, Patton KT: *Anatomy & physiology,* ed 5, St. Louis, 2003, Mosby.

radiographic studies. Clinical examination findings typically identify their presence. Common symptoms of an anterior fossa fracture include periorbital ecchymosis (raccoon's eyes), rhinorrhea (CSF or blood draining from the nose), and conjunctival hemorrhage without evidence of direct ocular trauma. Physical findings common in the presence of a middle fossa fracture include mastoid ecchymosis (Battle's sign), otorrhea (CSF or blood from the ears), hemotympanum, facial nerve paralysis, and hearing loss.

The presence of CSF otorrhea or rhinorrhea indicates not only that a basilar skull fracture exists, but also that the dura is lacerated, which substantially increases the risk for intracranial infection. The CSF should be permitted to drain freely by only applying a loose sterile dressing over the drainage site. Medical management typically includes observation, bed rest, head of bed elevation and precautions to prevent worsening the leak (e.g., do not blow the nose, avoid Valsalva maneuver).[16] If the CSF leak persists, a lumbar drain may be placed for a few days to divert CSF and encourage closure of the dural laceration. Although more than 80% of CSF fluid leaks stop spontaneously, those that persist after 7 to 14 days may require surgical dural repair.[16]

In addition to the possibility of intracranial infection, other potential complications associated with basilar skull fractures include cranial nerve injuries and cerebrovascular injuries. Because of their location at the base of the cranium, the cranial nerves are in jeopardy of direct injury when the basilar skull is fractured. The olfactory nerve is particularly vulnerable to fractures of the frontal bone, and the facial and auditory nerves are often injured in conjunction with temporal bone fractures. Cerebral vessels that pass through or near the base of the skull, such as the internal carotid artery, also may be injured when the cranial base is fractured, causing vessel dissection, hemorrhage, obstruction of flow, or formation of aneurysms or fistulae.

TYPE OF BRAIN INJURIES

Brain injuries can be classified as focal or diffuse. Focal brain injuries occur in a localized region, and diffuse brain injuries involve a large generalized area. Many patients with TBI, especially severe injury, have a combination of focal and diffuse injuries.[11]

Focal Brain Injuries

Focal lesions cause local brain damage at the site of injury and eventually may expand to elevate intracranial pressure and compress, shift, and damage more remote areas of the brain. Focal brain injuries are associated with lateralizing or localized signs, such as unilateral pupil dilation, hemiparesis, cranial nerve dysfunction, and speech deficit. These signs may help in localizing the site of injury. Focal injuries include cerebral contusion; epidural, subdural, and intracerebral hematomas; and subarachnoid hemorrhage.

Cerebral Contusions. Contusions are bruises of the brain tissue with associated hemorrhage and edema formation that may lead to subsequent tissue necrosis and infarction. Surrounding the contusion is a zone of edema and low cerebral blood flow that may be at high risk for ischemic insult.[17] Unlike the severely ischemic center of the contusion, the pericontusional zone or penumbra may eventually regain regional blood flow.[17]

Contusions constitute the most common type of brain injury. These lesions may occur beneath an area of skull deformation or secondary to acceleration-deceleration, rotation, or penetrating mechanisms of injury. Although contusions may occur anywhere in the brain, the most common sites are the frontal and temporal lobes.[11,17,18] Movement restrictions created by the cranial walls, dural folds, and irregular bony projections on the basilar skull surface in the frontotemporal regions explain the prevalence of brain injury in these areas. Contusions are most often multiple and frequently occur in association with other lesions.

Signs, symptoms, and severity of the injury depend on the site and extent of the contused brain. Isolated contusions generally do not produce immediate loss of consciousness. When coma is present, it is usually the result of an associated diffuse injury. Because the majority of contusions occur in the frontal and temporal lobes, patients usually present with localizing personality, memory, executive function, behavior, motor, and language deficits.[18] Progressive hemorrhage and edema formation can cause an abrupt mass effect, resulting in ICP elevation, brain compression, and, eventually, herniation.

Patients with brain contusions warrant close monitoring of their neurologic status to detect evidence of expanding mass effect and increased ICP. Special attention should be paid to patients with temporal lobe contusions, which may expand and cause brainstem compression without the warning of ICP elevation. The nurse must remain vigilant for subtle neurologic changes rather than focus solely on ICP values. Extensive contusions with mass effect require surgical evaluation as early as possible.

Epidural Hematoma. An epidural hematoma (EDH), also known as an extradural hematoma, is an accumulation of blood between the skull and dura mater (Figure 20-11). Epidural hematomas are most commonly located in the temporal region. These hematomas are often associated with a linear fracture of the thin temporal bone that lacerates the underlying middle meningeal artery, causing an accumulation of blood in the extradural space. Less frequently, the source of hemorrhage is venous (e.g., diploic veins, venous sinuses, middle meningeal vein).[19] As the hematoma accumulates, it strips the dura from the inner table of the skull and compresses the underlying brain. This local mass effect eventually causes brain herniation and can lead to death.

Signs and symptoms of EDH depend on the source and rate of blood accumulation. Clinical manifestations are usually seen within 6 hours of injury. The classic clinical presentation of a patient with an EDH is described as a period of unconsciousness believed to occur because of a concussion, followed by a lucid period of variable length, after which the level of consciousness deteriorates as the hematoma expands. The lucid interval is not pathognomonic of EDH, as it reportedly occurs in less than half of patients with epidural hematomas.[19] Other common manifestations of an expanding hematoma are pupil abnormalities (e.g., unilateral and eventual bilateral pupil dilation and decreased reactivity to light) and altered motor function (e.g., hemiparesis or hemiplegia, flexion or extension posturing).

Any EDH creating a significant mass effect requires immediate surgical evacuation and ligation of bleeding vessels. The evidenced-based *Guidelines for the Surgical Management of Traumatic Brain Injury* recommends surgical evacuation of an EDH if the size exceeds 30 cm^3 regardless of the GCS

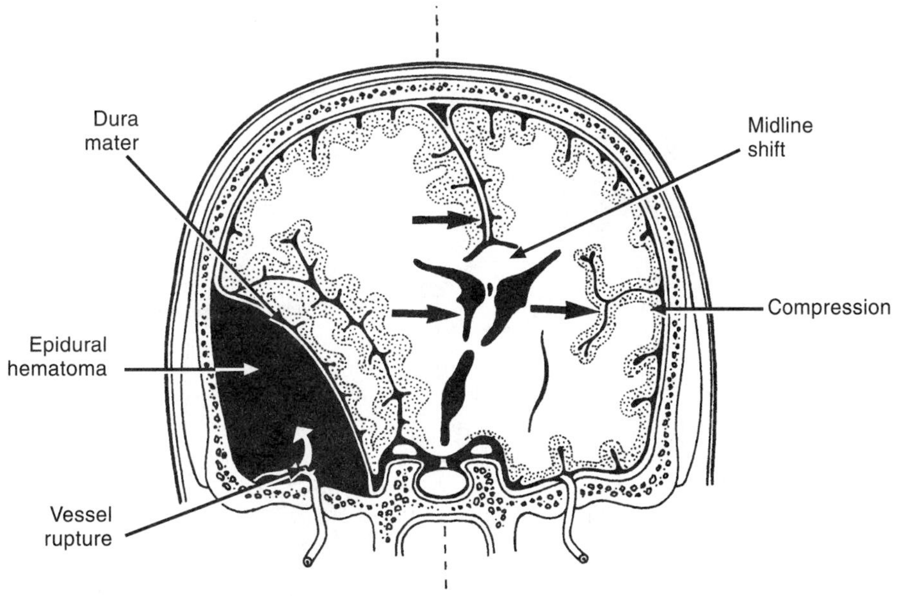

FIGURE 20-11 Epidural hematoma.

score. Nonoperative management with follow-up CT scans and close observation of neurological status can be considered if the EDH is less than 30 cm^3 with less than a 5-mm midline shift and less than 15-mm thickness in patients with a GCS score more than 8 without any focal symptomatology. In comatose patients with a GCS score of 8 or less and unequal pupil size, surgical evacuation of the EDH is strongly recommended as soon as possible.[19] If this is not possible and rapid neurological deterioration occurs, a burr hole may be placed ipsilateral to the dilated pupil or contralateral to the motor deficits to evacuate the hematoma. Although significant brain injury may result from brain compression by the hematoma, there typically is little or no underlying primary brain damage. Therefore, early diagnosis and treatment may yield a good prognosis.

Subdural Hematoma. Subdural hematoma (SDH) is a collection of blood beneath the dura mater and above the arachnoid layer of the meninges (Figure 20-12). These lesions are usually caused by rapid acceleration-deceleration mechanisms that tear veins bridging the subdural space, where they connect the brain's cortical surface to the dural sinuses. Rupture of small cortical arteries may also be the source of subdural hemorrhage, which may extend over the entire hemisphere.

SDHs may be classified as acute, subacute, or chronic, depending on the timing of symptom onset. Signs of acute SDHs become apparent within 48 hours after injury. These include indications of an expanding mass lesion, including pupil abnormalities, motor deficits, cranial nerve dysfunction, and altered level of consciousness. Patients who sustain a severe, acute SDH are usually comatose on admission, with a GCS score below 8. Other patients with acute SDH of lesser severity may be conscious or experience a lucid period prior to development of their unconscious state.

Patients with acute SDHs have one of the highest reported mortality rates of all types of TBI, averaging around 40% to 60%.[20] High mortality associated with acute SDH is believed to be associated with the large amount of primary brain damage (i.e., contusion, laceration, and vascular disruption) underlying the clot, as well as the brain compression that occurs as the lesion expands. The length of time from clinical deterioration or brain herniation to surgical intervention for SDH is significantly related to outcome.[20,21] Even with prompt surgical removal of the SDH, development of contusion, intracerebral hemorrhage or infarction of brain underlying the evacuated clot could increase mortality.

Acute SDH creating a mass effect requires rapid clot evacuation, hemorrhage control, and resection of underlying nonviable brain. *The Guidelines for the Surgical Management of Traumatic Brain Injury* recommend evacuation of a clot with a thickness greater than 10 mm or causing a midline shift of greater than 5 mm regardless of GCS score.[20] Patients with an SDH less than 10 mm thick, less than a 5 mm midline shift, and a GCS score less than 9 should undergo surgical removal of the clot if the GCS score declines by more than 2 points or the ICP is greater than 20 mm Hg, or the pupils are fixed and dilated or assymetrical.[20] Surgical evacuation of an SDH should occur as soon as possible, because data suggest those who undergo surgical SDH evacuation within 2 to 4 hours have better outcomes than those who undergo delayed operative intervention.[20] The operative procedure generally involves initial trephines or burr holes to locate the clot, followed by conversion to a craniotomy flap for optimal evacuation. A soft drain may be left in the subdural space for 24 to 48 hours. Postoperative complications may include brain swelling with subsequent increased intracranial pressure, clot reaccumulation, delayed intracerebral hemorrhage, and seizures. Small acute SDHs producing no significant mass effect may not require surgical intervention and are absorbed spontaneously.

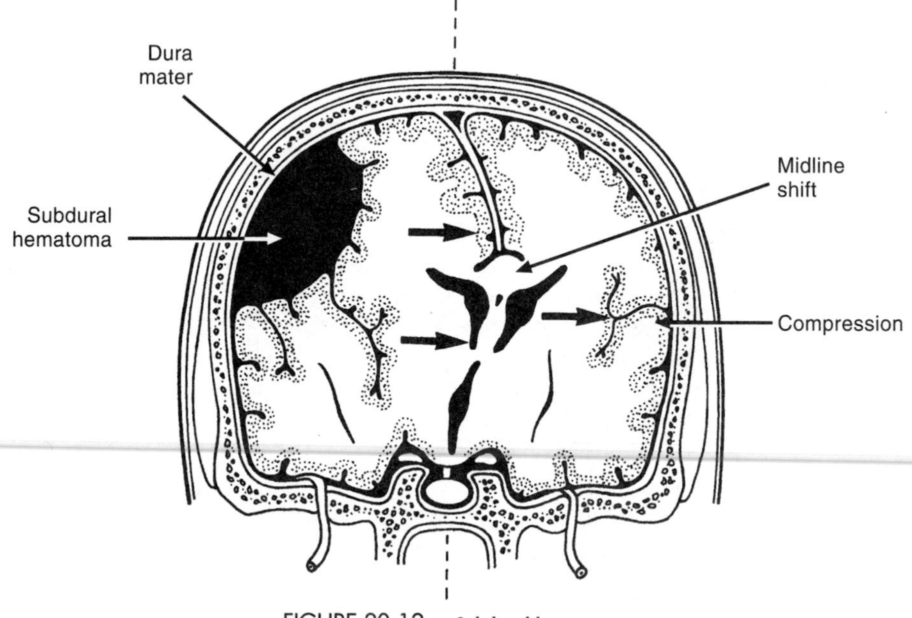

FIGURE 20-12 Subdural hematoma.

Subacute SDHs have similar but slower developing symptomatology than that seen with acute SDHs. Symptoms of a subacute SDH become apparent 2 days to 2 weeks after head injury. These symptoms tend to be more benign and the prognosis is generally better than with acute subdural hematoma. The improved prognosis is related to less severe underlying brain contusion and the decreased likelihood that the patient will deteriorate to the point of brainstem compression. Like acute SDH, subacute SDH typically requires surgical evacuation.

Chronic SDHs do not demonstrate symptoms for at least 2 weeks after relatively low impact trauma. After the traumatic event, blood slowly fills the subdural space. Over the next 2 to 4 days, that blood congeals and becomes thick and jelly-like. After about 2 weeks, the subdural clot begins to break down and becomes the consistency of thick oil. The clot then becomes more organized and encasing membranes surround the now xanthochromic fluid. Eventually the hematoma may calcify, ossify, or be absorbed. The hematoma increases in size slowly, most likely as a result of repeated small hemorrhages, causing more brain compression and eventual onset of symptoms. Signs and symptoms may include increasing headache, progressive decrease in level of consciousness, ataxia, seizures, incontinence, and eventually pupil and motor function alterations. Chronic SDHs are common among patients with brain atrophy, such as the elderly and chronic alcohol abusers. Cerebral atrophy allows a significant volume of subdural blood to accumulate, possibly resulting in considerable brain distortion, before clinical evidence of neurologic decompensation becomes apparent. Surgical evacuation of the chronic subdural hematoma usually requires craniotomy to dissect the gelatinous or calcified clot and its encasing membranes. A subdural drain may be necessary for a short time after hematoma evacuation to prevent reaccumulation of fluid.

Intracerebral Hematoma. An intracerebral hematoma (ICH) is a well-defined clot located within the brain parenchyma that, like a contusion, is typically surrounded by an area of edema and low blood flow[17] (Figure 20-13). Most likely the bleeding originates from cerebral vessels that rupture at the time of injury. Similar to contusions, most ICHs occur in the frontal and temporal lobes and, less frequently, deep within the cerebral hemispheres or in the cerebellum.[17] ICHs may be multiple and associated with other lesions, particularly contusions. When an ICH is in continuity with a SDH, it is known as a burst lobe. Evidence of an isolated ICH after head trauma should cause health care providers to consider if a hypertensive bleed may be the source of the hemorrhage.

Symptoms of ICHs are similar to those of contusions, with the course and outcome dependent on the size and location of the hematoma. Signs and symptoms may include headache, progressive deterioration in level of consciousness, motor deficits (e.g., contralateral hemiplegia), and pupil abnormalities. Dominant hemispheric lesions are frequently associated with speech deficits.

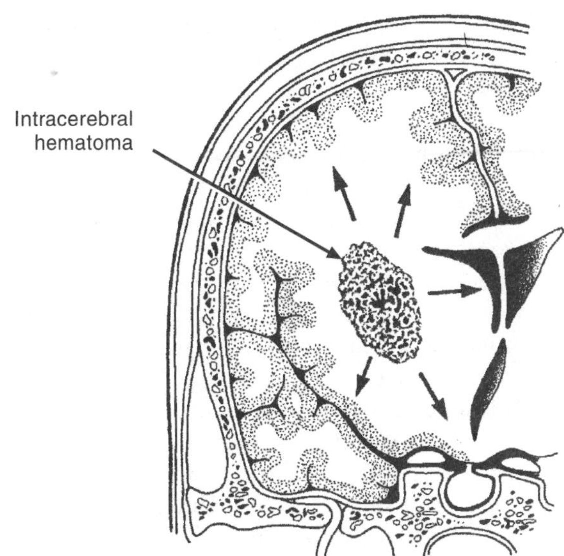

FIGURE 20-13 Intracerebral hematoma.

ICHs are complicated by aggressive focal edema and increasing mass effect, which leads to elevations in ICP and further neurologic deterioration. Deterioration can occur as late as 7 to 10 days after injury, although the majority of neurologic deterioration typically occurs in the first 48 to 72 hours.[17] The initial size of the hematoma is a predictor for subsequent lesion expansion with larger lesions demonstrating greater likelihood of enlarging than smaller ones.[17] Surgical evacuation of the ICH is not always beneficial or possible.

Subarachnoid Hemorrhage. Subarachnoid hemorrhage (SAH) is bleeding between the arachnoid and pia mater layers of the meninges. This type of hemorrhage is seen commonly in patients with severe TBI. A preexisting vascular anomaly (i.e., cerebral aneurysm) may need to be ruled out as the source of SAH. Blood from the subarachnoid space or from a coexisting ICH may extend into the ventricular system of the brain.

Signs and symptoms of SAH include decreased level of consciousness, motor deficits (e.g., hemiparesis), pupil abnormalities, and possibly evidence of meningeal irritation, such as headache, photophobia, and nuchal rigidity. Potential complications of SAH include ICP elevation, posttraumatic hydrocephalus, and cerebral vasospasm. Patients demonstrating SAH on CT scan tend to have a significantly worse outcome than those without evidence of SAH.[17] Treatment for SAH includes placement of an intraventricular catheter to drain bloody CSF and, if necessary, management of intracranial pressure.

Diffuse Brain Injury

Unlike focal injuries, diffuse injuries do not consist of damage to a single localized area of the brain; instead, damage is more widespread. Acceleration-deceleration and rotational forces, usually associated with motor vehicle crashes but sometimes falls, assaults, or other types of trauma, are the most common mechanisms that initiate the pathophysiologic process that results in diffuse injuries to the brain.[11,12] These forces create tension and compression on, and shearing of, nerve fibers, resulting in variable amounts of axonal damage. The magnitude and rate of strain and direction of the force during brain trauma determine the severity of axonal injury.[11,12] Diffuse axonal injury (DAI), also known as traumatic axonal injury, creates an injury pattern that tends to primarily affect the subcortical white matter throughout the hemispheres, especially at the gray-white matter interface, the corpus callosum, and the brainstem (Figure 20-14).[12,22-24]

Although in the case of severe TBI, a portion of axons may be disrupted physically (axonotomy) at the time of injury, more often with DAI, axons remain structurally intact but may be functionally impaired. Axons that retain structural integrity but sustain internal damage and functional disruption may recover; experimental models suggest they may suffer delayed or secondary axonotomy hours after the injury.[11] In other words, all injured axons are not transected at the time the brain is subjected to inertial forces; rather, neuronal pathology associated with DAI is a complex progressive event (described in greater detail in a later section on secondary injury).[11,18] The amount, severity, and location of axonal damage will determine the clinical severity and outcome of diffuse brain injury.[18,25] Diffuse brain injuries lie on a continuum of severity ranging from the mildest form of DAI, concussion, with little or no sustained brain dysfunction, to moderate and severe diffuse axonal injury that may produce disabling deficits or death.[11,18,22]

Patients with DAI typically progress through three phases of recovery.[18] The first phase is immediate unconsciousness, which may not occur in the mildest cases of DAI. In the next longer lasting phase, the patient regains consciousness and is confused, which is linked to anterograde amnesia.[18] In the even lengthier final phase, the patient undergoes restoration of cognitive function. Severity of DAI correlates with the duration of each phase and degree of impairment associated with the stages.[18] With mild DAI, the duration of each phase is fairly short with few if any lasting impairments, whereas the opposite is true with severe DAI.[18]

Mild Diffuse Axonal Injury: Concussion. Concussion is a transient disturbance of neurological function. Axonal shear, tension, or strain occurs, resulting in conduction impedance and transient loss of function. No anatomical evidence of brain injury is apparent on CT scan, although magnetization transfer magnetic resonance imaging (MRI), diffusion weighted MRI,[23] diffusion tensor MRI (DTI),[26] magnetic resonance spectroscopy (MRS),[27] functional MRI (fMRI), positron emission tomography (PET), and single-photon emission computed tomography (SPECT) scans,[28] though not routinely performed, are more frequently able to identify abnormalities after this type of axonal injury.[22,29] The diagnosis is based on the patient's history, clinical neurologic findings, and a CT scan that rules out other intracranial lesions.

Manifestation of a concussion may include somatic, cognitive, or psychological impairments. A temporary loss of consciousness, usually lasting only a few minutes, may or may not occur. Patients may experience retrograde amnesia (inability to recall events just preceding the injury) or posttraumatic amnesia. The duration of amnesia may predict the severity of symptoms and deficits (e.g., depression, dizziness, cognitive impairments) associated with concussion and is considered a good measure of the injury severity.[30,31] Signs and symptoms also may include headaches, confusion, dizziness, vertigo, nausea, visual disturbances, subtle personality changes, depression, difficulty in concentration, decreased

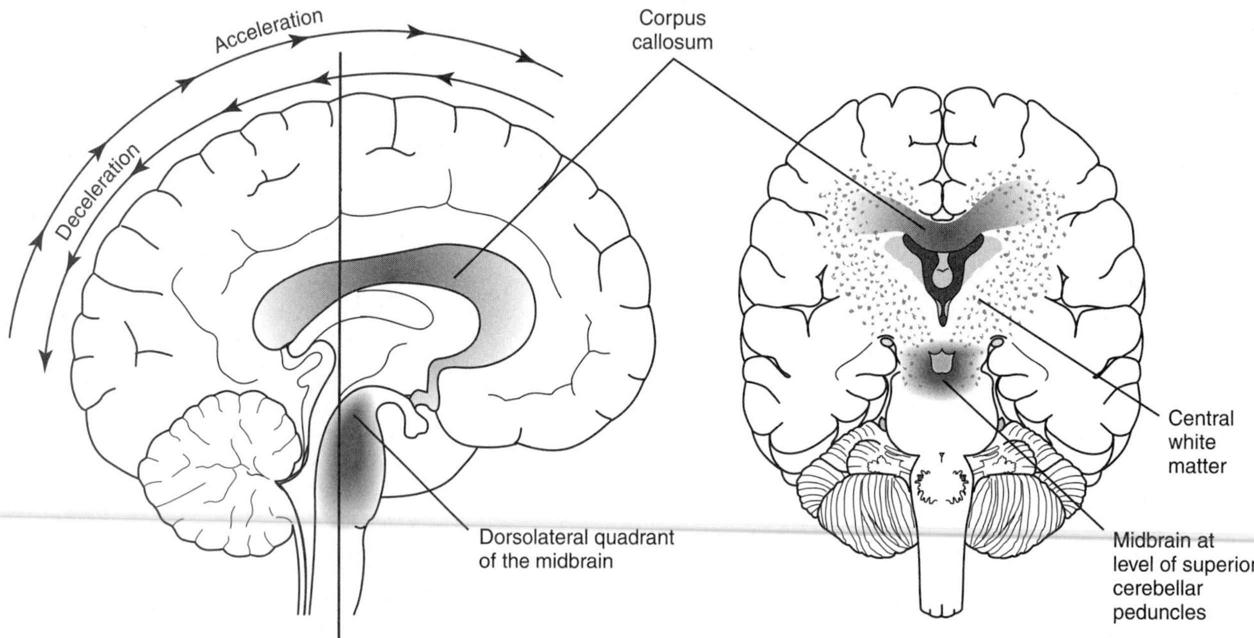

FIGURE 20-14 Diffuse axonal injury. Areas of the brain most often affected include the corpus callosum, the dorsolateral area of the upper brainstem adjacent to the superior cerebellar peduncles, and the parasagittal white matter.

information-processing speed, poor memory, behavioral disorders, emotional lability, apathy, irritability, fatigue, increased anxiety, and insomnia.[30,31] These manifestations, which can vary considerably among patients and may persist for days, weeks, or even months after the concussion, are collectively known as postconcussive syndrome (PCS). Persistence of these problems may be related to the degree of neuronal damage, emotional distress (e.g., anxiety or depression), personal set factors (i.e., older age, female gender), motivational issues, cognitive factors, or a combination of factors.[29,32]

Concussions are very common but, because of their apparently benign nature, medical attention is often not sought or there is a delay in seeking treatment for persistent symptoms. Patients who do seek medical care for an isolated concussion usually are not admitted to the hospital and receive no follow-up treatment at outpatient facilities. Patients and their families should receive information and supportive counseling on PCS, especially about the potential difficulties that may become evident after return to home, work, or school. Patients with persistent or disabling postconcussive symptoms may benefit from referral to a specialist (e.g., a neuropsychologist) for more extensive assessment and treatment. Patients should be advised to avoid activities (e.g., contact sports) that present a high risk for repeat concussion during their recovery period, because another concussion before resolution of the initial injury may cause cerebral autoregulatory dysfunction, progressive cerebral edema, neurological deterioration, and possibly death.[33] The reader is referred to expert consensus recommendations and reviews on this topic to acquire more thorough information regarding return to play recommendations for athletes who sustain a concussion.[30,34]

Moderate to Severe DAI. Tension, shearing, and compression strains created by rotational and acceleration-deceleration forces cause widespread axonal cytoskeletal and functional disruption in the cerebral hemispheres, the corpus callosum, the brainstem, and, less commonly, the cerebellum. When DAI is more severe, the duration of the recovery phases (i.e., unconsciousness, emerging consciousness, and postconfusional restoration of cognitive function) is prolonged and plagued with more significant and sometimes lasting impairments. Those with the most severe DAI may halt progression through the stages of recovery.[18]

The hallmark of moderate to severe cases of DAI is immediate and prolonged coma lasting longer than 6 hours. The prolonged coma results from severe widespread damage to conducting white matter (axons), which disrupts the brain's reticular activating system. Because diffuse axonal injury is typically microscopic, the severity of injury is not determined radiographically but by the patient's clinical characteristics and duration of coma.

In less severe cases of DAI coma may last only 6 to 24 hours. Emergence from coma may be followed by prolonged periods of restlessness or stupor and mild to moderate memory impairment. Most patients with milder DAI follow commands within 24 hours and may recover with relatively mild to moderate disabilities.

As severity of DAI increases, coma may last more than 24 hours. Confusion and long-lasting amnesia typically follow coma emergence. Most patients with moderate DAI move purposefully or withdraw from pain, but some may exhibit transient decorticate or decerebrate posturing. Mild to severe attention, behavioral, cognitive, memory, and/or executive (e.g., reasoning, speed of processing information) deficits usually persist.[25] Memory and executive dysfunction are the most common neuropsychological impairments found in patients that had CT scan or MRI findings compatible with DAI.[25]

Severe diffuse axonal injury results in extensive anatomic and functional disruption of axonal white matter fibers. Unlike less severe cases of DAI in which typically there is no visible brain injury on CT scan, in severe DAI, small tissue and vessel tears may be apparent. These tears appear as small focal lesions typically located in the hemispheric subcortical lobar white matter, corpus callosum, basal ganglia, brainstem and sometimes the cerebellum.[12,23] Involvement of the corpus callosum and dorsolateral aspect of the upper brainstem corresponds with greater severity of DAI and poorer outcome.[18] Because these lesions are small, they may be missed or difficult to appreciate on initial CT scan, and early resolution makes detection difficult in subsequent scans. MRI is more effective than CT in visualizing small lesions associated with DAI, including lesions deep in the white matter of the cerebral hemispheres.[18,22] Diffuse cerebral edema also may be seen with severe diffuse axonal injury. The extent of DAI, particularly when not severe, may be better visualized through other diagnostic technologies not typically employed in assessment of TBI as previously mentioned under the section on concussion. Extensive neuronal loss eventually results in brain shrinkage. Follow-up CT scans typically show cerebral atrophy, as evidenced by enlarged sulci and ventricular dilation.

Clinically, severe DAI is manifested by deep, prolonged coma lasting days to months. Signs of severe cerebral and brainstem dysfunction, including decorticate and decerebrate posturing, are often present on admission or develop with 24 hours of injury. Diencephalic involvement usually results in onset of tachycardia, systemic hypertension, tachypnea, hyperpyrexia, and profuse diaphoresis (hyperhidrosis) covering the face and, less frequently, the neck and upper thorax accompanied by increased muscle tone and abnormal posturing.[35] It is theorized that this syndrome, called *neurosweats, diencephalic fits, sympathetic storming, paroxysmal autonomic instability with dystonia,* or *dysautonomia,* is caused by dysfunction of the autonomic control centers (hypothalamus or thalamus) located in the diencephalic region or disruption of connections to these centers from other areas of the brain.[35] Diencephalic signs and abnormal posturing usually resolve a few weeks after injury, but may persist for months.[35]

Because of the extensive structural damage to neurons, severe DAI has a high mortality. The majority of severe DAI survivors typically have major residual disabilities that may not be evident until consciousness improves. Major sequelae of severe DAI may include cranial nerve dysfunction, sensorimotor impairments (e.g., paresis, tremors, spasticity, dyspraxia, problems with speech) and, most commonly, significant deficits in cognition and neuropsychological capability.[12] Severe DAI is the most common cause of major disability and persistent vegetative state after TBI.[36]

Primary Versus Secondary Brain Injury

Injury to neurons can be classified as primary or secondary. Primary injury to the brain tissue or brain vasculature occurs immediately on impact of mechanical force. Once primary injury occurs, the damage is done and cannot be reversed. Because there is currently no direct treatment for primary brain injury, prevention remains the only effective intervention. Not all brain injury occurs immediately at the time of initial impact. Within seconds, hours, or days after primary brain injury, a cascade of pathologic biochemical events is initiated within the injured or ischemic cells, leading to further cell death and secondary brain injury. Numerous neurologic and systemic complications after primary brain injury can also cause or exacerbate secondary brain injury.

Cellular Response to Injury

Injury, hypoxia, and ischemia are the fundamental initiators of the biochemical cascade that results in further cell death and secondary brain injury. Primary brain injury causes depolarization and halts aerobic metabolism and ATP production, quickly depleting the affected cells' energy stores, causing energy failure. When the supply of oxygen or other nutrients is inadequate to meet cellular metabolic demands, ischemia results.

Cellular ischemia or hypoxia resulting from injury causes breakdown of the energy-dependent sodium-potassium and calcium pumps, with subsequent flux of sodium, water, and calcium into the cell and potassium out of the cell.[11] Influx of sodium and water causes cellular swelling. Acidosis is produced by conversion to anaerobic metabolism, as well as ionic fluxes. Disruption of intracellular calcium homeostasis is believed to be associated with many of the pathologic mechanisms that lead to further cell death, namely by activating toxic enzymatic pathways and damaging the mitochondria, although the exact mechanisms by which calcium causes neurodegeneration remain unclear.[11,37] Calcium imbalance activates proteases (i.e., calpains) that break down cytoskeletal proteins causing cell membrane compromise and impaired structural integrity.[37] Disruption of calcium homeostasis also activates phospholipases, which hydrolyze membrane phospholipids and result in accumulation of free fatty acids (e.g., arachidonic acid). Subsequently, breakdown of arachidonic acid produces highly reactive oxygen-derived free radicals that cause further cell damage by a process known as peroxidation.[37] Metabolites (i.e., prostaglandins, leukotrienes, and thromboxanes) generated by breakdown of arachidonic acid can also foster production of free radicals.[37] Calcium also activates endonucleases that degrade DNA. Intracellular influx of calcium binds with the enzyme calmodulin, resulting in excessive nitric oxide production that, when combined with free radicals, are toxic to membrane lipids, DNA, and proteins.[37] Also, calcium can damage mitochondria, causing production of free radicals, activation of proapoptotic factors (e.g., caspases), and metabolic disruption, which leads to ATP depletion and acidosis.[37,38]

Numerous neurotransmitter system alterations, such as increased excitatory neurotransmitter release, also accompany brain cell injury and energy failure. Excitatory neurotransmitters called *excitatory amino acids* (EAA), including glutamate and aspartate, are found in high amounts around injured and ischemic brain cells.[11] Excessive activation of glutamate receptors, namely *N*-methyl-d-aspartate (NMDA) receptors, as well as non-NMDA receptors, triggers processes (e.g., opening of ion channels) that move sodium and calcium into the cell, increasing subsequent destructive processes.[37]

All these events disrupt cell structures and function. A vicious cycle is created as pathologic processes foster cellular changes that encourage further influx of extracellular ions, increased production of toxins, and eventually increased ischemia and cell death. In addition to necrosis, apoptosis, a genetically regulated, energy dependent form of cell self-destruction that normally takes place during development and natural cell turnover, has been identified as a contributor to delayed cell death after TBI.[18,37,39,40] Apoptosis is histologically unique, with distinct morphologic and biochemical features that differentiate it from necrotic cell death.[39] One hypothesized scheme of how these pathophysiologic events interact to result in loss of cell integrity and neuronal death is shown in Figure 20-15. The reader is referred to numerous reviews for a detailed description of the various processes involved in the secondary injury pathologic cascade.[11,18,39,40]

Definition of the intracellular pathological cascade initiated by injury or ischemia has prompted numerous studies investigating pharmacological agents that may target and halt these biochemical mechanisms and reduce secondary brain damage. Examples of agents that have been investigated extensively include oxygen-derived free-radical scavengers, antioxidants, excitatory amino acid antagonists, and ion-channel blockers.[41,42] Despite positive findings in numerous preliminary investigations, Phase III clinical trials have failed to identify an agent that demonstrates efficacy in the treatment of TBI. Numerous potential neuroprotective agents have been identified and several hypothetical therapeutic approaches that may reduce secondary brain injury have been suggested.[39,43] More research is needed to determine which therapy or combination of therapies is useful in improving outcomes and which targeted populations benefit from their use.

Other pathologic mechanisms that also may contribute to delayed brain injury are currently being investigated. Although inflammatory responses initiated by TBI are

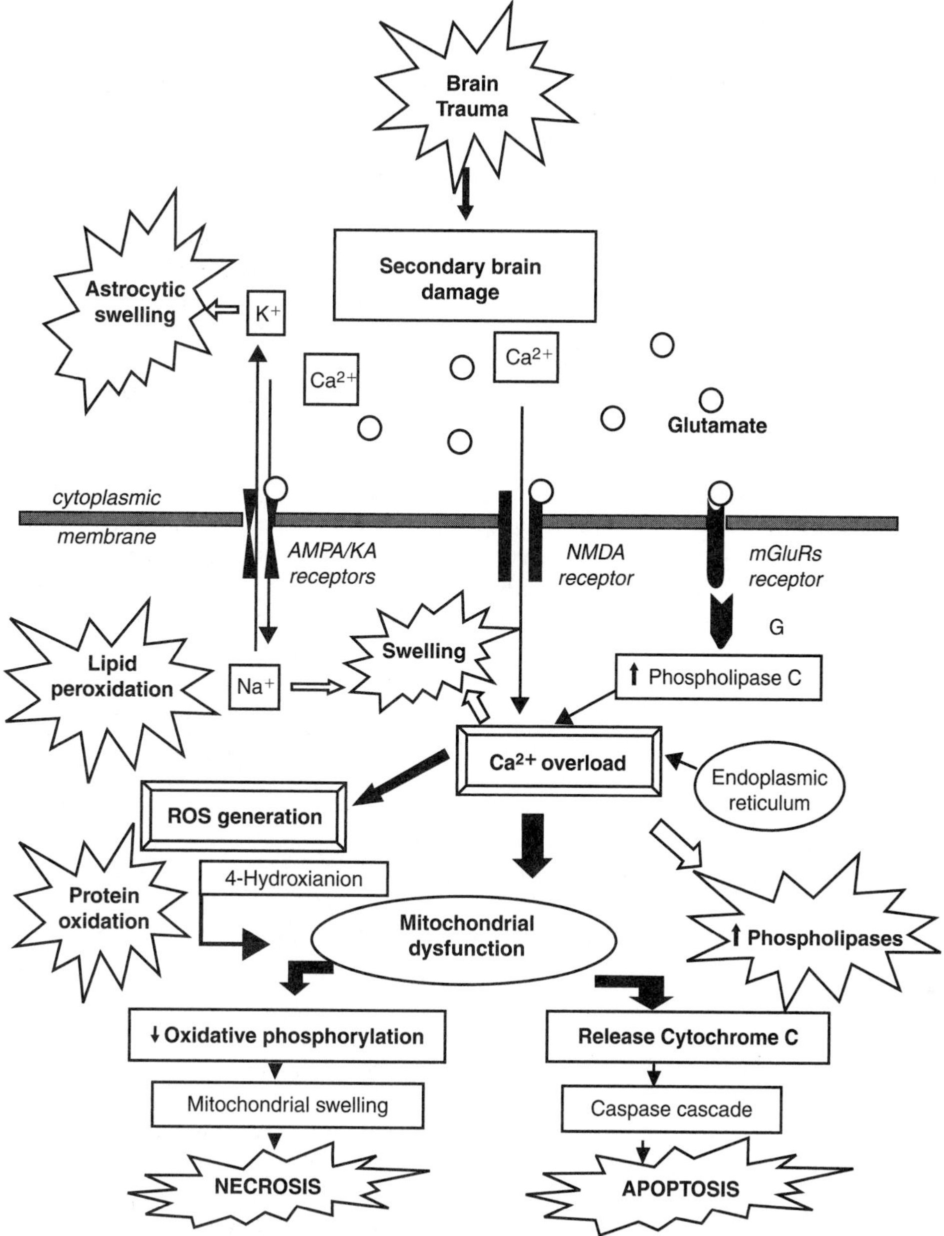

FIGURE 20-15 Selected mechanisms proposed to be involved in secondary damage after severe brain trauma. The pathways include excitotoxicity, calcium (CA^{2+}) overload, and reactive oxygen species generation. The target of these pathways is the mitochondria. (From Enriquez P, Bullock R: Molecular and cellular mechanisms in the pathophysiology of severe head injury, *Curr Pharm Des* 10:2131-2143, 2004.

believed to have some reparative functions, evidence suggests that these processes may also mediate delayed neuronal injury.[44] Inflammatory cytokines (e.g., tumor necrosis factor, interleukins) released by damaged brain cells are believed to have an important role in secondary brain injury.[37,44] Speculation that TBI may be a neurodegenerative process has been fueled by evidence that links TBI to Alzheimer's disease (AD).[45,46] TBI has been identified by some as a risk factor for AD, and β-amyloid deposits, characteristic of AD, have been identified in the brain after injury.[45] As research provides greater clarity about the various mechanisms involved in brain injury and their interactions, new opportunities to better monitor and treat TBI can be developed.

Outcome of the Injured Neuron

Once a neuron has been injured, distinct biochemical, metabolic, and morphologic changes occur throughout the cell. Depending on the severity of injury and the presence of factors that may cause or exacerbate secondary brain injury, the neuron may progress in one of two directions:

1. When injury is extensive and the damage is irreversible, progressive degeneration of the nerve cell occurs, followed by glial cell phagocytosis. The loss of relatively few neurons may be insignificant, but substantial loss results in marked cortical atrophy as brain cells literally disappear. The degree of functional disability correlates with the extent of neuronal loss.

2. When neuronal injury is less extensive, the nerve cell has the potential to restore its functional capabilities. Neurons that are functionally disrupted but have not suffered irreversible mechanical damage are particularly vulnerable to secondary insults and must be provided an environment free of these complications for recovery to occur. Restoration of function is believed to occur through neuronal rearrangement of the injured neurons themselves or of neighboring uninjured neurons.

Neuronal Repair and Regeneration. Injury to the neuron results in loss of synaptic contact or denervation. Generation of a new synapse (synaptogenesis) is essential for function to return. Structural and functional repair of the injured axons requires neuronal survival and axonal regrowth or sprouting that extends in the appropriate direction through the lesion to reinnervate the specific target neurons. Regenerating axons must also undergo remyelination and reestablish functional properties that enable impulse transmission.[47] This process is thought to play a major role in promoting recovery of function after CNS injury.[48]

Surviving neurons with the intrinsic capability for regrowth and in a supportive environment will attempt to regenerate with sprouting observed within a few days after injury.[47,48] Axonal regrowth appears to occur more readily in the immature nervous system—an observation that is reinforced by the fact that children make better recoveries than adults do after CNS injury.[47] A number of factors are believed to contribute to the limited spontaneous axonal regeneration seen in the mature central nervous system. These factors include: the neuron's intrinsic growth state; mechanical barriers (e.g., scar tissue, hematomas, infection), which may inhibit, misdirect, or block effective regrowth; lack of neurotrophic factors, proteins that direct neuronal survival and axonal regeneration; and presence of molecules that inhibit axon regeneration (e.g., three components associated with myelin have been identified as major growth inhibitors).[47,49]

Neuronal repair and axonal sprouting offer significant potential for CNS recovery and have become major foci of TBI research. Current research includes investigation of (1) neurotropic agents, such as nerve growth factor (NGF), to enhance sprouting by stimulating and guiding outgrowing neurites; (2) gene therapy to enhance neuronal survival; (3) implantation of activated macrophages to clear growth-inhibiting debris and release factors that foster regrowth; (4) reduction, neutralization, or blockade of axonal growth inhibitors; (5) transplantation or grafting of neural tissue or other growth-supportive material at the lesion site; and (6) a combination of these approaches.[47,48]

Factors that Cause or Exacerbate Secondary Brain Injury

Any systemic or neurologic complication that compromises adequate oxygen and nutrient delivery to the brain's cells, causing hypoxia or ischemia, can cause or exacerbate the pathologic cascade of events that leads to secondary brain injury. Systemic complications that cause secondary brain insult include hypotension, hypoxia, hypercapnia, hypocapnia, hyperthermia, anemia, fluid and electrolyte imbalance, acid-base alterations, systemic inflammatory disorders, hypoglycemia, and hyperglycemia.[50-53] Neurologic complications that may serve as causative factors for secondary brain injury include intracranial hypertension (any complications that may increase ICP, such as hydrocephalus, intracranial hemorrhage, cerebral edema), vasospasm, seizures, and intracranial infection.[50,54] Complications such as hyperthermia and seizures do not directly impair nutrient delivery, but they can elevate ICP and increase the brain's oxygen and nutrient requirements, making ischemia more likely. Although the healthy brain may sustain no permanent consequences with such complications, the injured brain is extremely vulnerable and can suffer irreversible damage with onset of such events.[51] Fortunately, complications that cause secondary brain injury are usually amenable to treatment.

Complications that cause secondary brain injury are not uncommon after TBI and can contribute significantly to increased mortality and morbidity. For example when systemic hypotension (systolic blood pressure <90 mm Hg) is present in the prehospital, resuscitation, or critical care phases after TBI, mortality and morbidity rises significantly.[50,51,53,55-58] In a prospective, multicenter study of 150 patients with moderate to severe TBI, those who suffered hypotension and/or hypoxia (Spo_2 $<92\%$) during prehospital transport had a longer hospital length of stay and a greater degree of disability at discharge than those without these complicating factors.[52] Occurrence of prehospital hypoxia was found to significantly increase odds of mortality following TBI.[52] Analysis of 717 patients with severe TBI from the Trauma Coma Data Bank found that early systemic hypotension (occurring between injury through resuscitation), present in approximately 35% of patients, doubled mortality and significantly increased morbidity.[59] In this same study, hypoxia (Pao_2 <60 mm Hg, apnea, or cyanosis in the field) was present in almost 46% of hospital admissions with severe TBI but had a less detrimental effect on mortality and morbidity, especially if this complication was remedied in the prehospital setting.[59] When hypotension and hypoxia coexisted, the mortality increased to 75%, suggesting a cumulative detrimental effect when more than one factor contributing to secondary brain injury is present.[59] Systemic hypotension, present in about one third of patients with severe TBI after 8 hours in an intensive care unit, tripled the rate of death or vegetative outcome.[55] A retrospective review of 81 patient records found that occurrence of hypocapnia, hypotension, acidosis, hypoxia, hyperglycemia, or hypothermia within the first 24 hours after severe TBI was associated with worse outcomes.[50] This study also demonstrated that hypotension and hypothermia were independently related to mortality.[50] In another study, the duration of hypotension, hypoxia, and pyrexia during the critical care phase were significant predictors of mortality.[56] Likewise,

Barton et al found a strong association between the depth and duration of hypotension with risk of death and functional outcome measured at 3 months after TBI.[57] Manley et al found in a prospective study of 107 patients with moderate to severe TBI that even relatively short episodes of hypotension during initial resuscitation were significantly associated with increased mortality, and repeated hypotensive events had an additive effect.[60] Hypotension, shock, hypoxia, anemia, and hyperglycemia within the first 24 hours after admission to critical care were significantly associated with progression to brain death in 59 of 404 patients with severe TBI.[51] This same study found that occurrence of shock (systolic blood pressure <90 mm Hg requiring intravascular fluids and/or vasoactives) within 24 hours of intensive care admission constituted a major independent predictor of brain death.[51] More recently, a retrospective case control study comparing 37 nonsurvivors to 37 matched survivors of TBI found that a mean arterial blood pressure <65 mm Hg in the first 4 hours after hospital admission was associated with a fourfold increase in the odds of a fatal outcome.[53]

Intracranial hypertension is another factor often associated with severe TBI that can lead to secondary brain damage and poorer patient outcomes.[54,61] One study indicated that an initial ICP reading of more than 20 mm Hg triples the risk of neurologic deterioration, resulting in higher mortality and morbidity.[61] More recently, a retrospective analysis of 429 patients with TBI demonstrated that mortality was significantly higher in those with an ICP >20 mm Hg (47%) when compared with those with an ICP below that level (17%).[54]

Ischemia may be the single most important secondary event affecting outcome after severe TBI. Even brief periods of brain ischemia can initiate mechanisms that cause cell death.[40] Brain ischemia in the acute phase following injury is associated with poor outcome.[62]

Intracranial Pressure Response

ICP, the pressure within the cranial vault, has a normal range of 0 to 15 mm Hg. Sustained pressures greater than 15 mm Hg constitute increased intracranial pressure or intracranial hypertension. The recommended threshold for treatment is 20 mm Hg.[63]

The intracranial cavity is filled with three components: brain tissue, which makes up 80% of intracranial volume; blood, 10%; and CSF, 10%. The rigid skull restricts expansion of the intracranial contents. An increase in volume of any one of the components must be offset by a reciprocal decrease in one or both of the remaining components to maintain a constant total volume. If the volume begins to exceed the normal content within the skull, the pressure starts to rise within the enclosed compartment. This is the basis of the modified Monro-Kellie hypothesis.

Intracranial volume can be increased after TBI for a number of reasons that result in added intracranial mass, blood, or CSF. Most mass or bulk is in the form of a blood clot or hematoma or, in the case of an associated infection, a suppurative process. Brain volume is also increased when there is an excess of cerebral water (cerebral edema). Cerebral edema is a sequela that often accompanies tissue damage and can occur locally around an injured site, such as a contusion, or can be diffuse throughout the brain (e.g., DAI). Cerebral edema may progress over the first 24 to 72 hours after the primary TBI and may persist much longer or, in some cases, can worsen after that time.[24,64]

The two types of cerebral edema most commonly associated with TBI are vasogenic edema and cytotoxic edema. Vasogenic edema occurs when a breakdown in the blood-brain barrier allows osmotically active proteins and electrolytes (e.g., sodium) to move out of the intravascular space into the interstitial space, which in turn attracts fluid into the extracellular space. Cytotoxic edema characterized by intracellular fluid accumulation can be caused by a number of mechanisms. When cerebral tissues are injured or deprived of adequate oxygen and glucose, energy failure followed by cellular energy depletion occurs, causing malfunction of the ATP-dependent sodium-potassium pump and accumulation of sodium and water inside the cell. Cellular energy failure precipitates lactic acidosis and increased excitatory neurotransmitter (e.g., glutamate) release, which also promote influx of ions (e.g., sodium, calcium) and water into the cells.[11,65]

An elevation in cerebral blood flow (hyperemia) may contribute to increased cerebral blood volume after TBI. Kelly et al. found that hyperemic responses associated with intracranial hypertension were most prevalent in younger patients (younger than age 35) with more severe brain injuries who may have had significant metabolic vasoreactivity and pressure autoregulation impairment.[66] Hypercarbia and hypoxemia can cause cerebral vasodilation, resulting in increased intracranial blood volume. Any obstruction of venous outflow, including simple neck flexion or rotation, also can transiently contribute to increases in cerebral blood volume.

Cerebral spinal fluid volume can be increased after TBI as a result of obstruction of CSF flow or insufficient reabsorption. Blood in the subarachnoid space after brain injury can obstruct the arachnoid villi, impairing reabsorption of CSF. This is known as communicating hydrocephalus. Accumulation of CSF may also occur from noncommunicating hydrocephalus, in which CSF flow is obstructed by cerebral edema or hematoma, for example, preventing the CSF from reaching the villi to be reabsorbed.

Mechanisms to compensate for increased intracranial volume include cerebrovascular vasoconstriction, compression of the venous system, reduced CSF production, and movement of CSF to the more dispensable spinal subarachnoid space. When these compensatory mechanisms are exhausted and intracranial volume continues to increase, a critical point is eventually reached, when the pressure within the skull starts to rise. When this occurs, even small increases in additional volume cause dramatic increases in ICP, and brain tissue is displaced.

The relationship between pressure and volume within the skull is best illustrated with an ICP/volume curve, which depicts the exponential growth of ICP in response to volume increases (Figure 20-16). The flat portion of the curve represents the compensatory phase, when vascular and CSF volume displacement buffers increased intracranial volume. During this period, intracranial homeostasis is maintained. The inflection point indicates that the displaceable volume has been exhausted, and a sharp rise in ICP is precipitated by a minimal increase in volume. The brain's inability to tolerate any increase in intracranial volume without causing a substantial rise in pressure is called *decreased compliance,* and the brain is said to be "tight" within the skull.

Cerebral Herniation

Cerebral herniation, the distortion and displacement of the brain from one intracranial compartment to another, eventually occurs if volume expansion continues within the intracranial cavity. Expanding mass lesions or hematomas are the primary causes of brain shift and herniation. The location of the lesion often determines the direction in which the brain is forcibly moved and, consequently, the type and pattern of herniation that occurs.

The majority of trauma-related mass lesions are hemispheric or supratentorial (located within the cerebral hemispheres above the tentorium). Three types of herniation are associated with supratentorial lesions: cingulate (or subfalcine), central, and uncal. All three herniation patterns can occur simultaneously as pressure gradients shift the brain laterally and eventually downward through the tentorium (Figure 20-17).

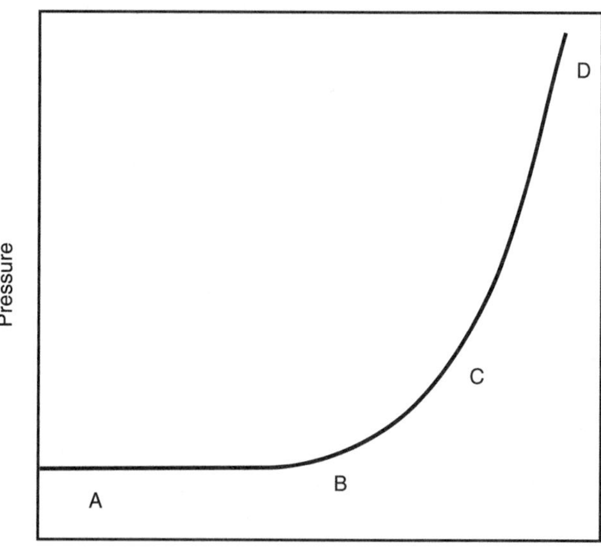

FIGURE 20-16 Pressure-volume curve. From *point A* to *point B,* ICP remains constant with addition of volume and brain compliance is high. At *point B* the brain compliance begins to change and ICP rises slightly. From *point B* to *point C,* compliance is low and ICP rises with increases in intracranial volume. From *point C* to *point D,* small increases in volume cause significant ICP elevations.

Cingulate herniation occurs when the cingulate gyrus (a convolution of brain tissue at the medial aspect of the hemispheres) is distorted beneath the falx cerebri (the dural fold that longitudinally separates the cerebral hemispheres). This type of herniation is fairly common and is caused by an expanding mass lesion in one cerebral hemisphere. Intracranial volume displaced across the midline compresses the opposite side of the brain, eventually causing more edema and ischemia. Midline shift greater than 5 mm correlates with poorer patient outcome.[67]

Central transtentorial herniation consists of downward displacement of portions of the cerebral hemispheres, diencephalon, and midbrain through the tentorium into the posterior fossa (infratentorial compartment). Clinical signs of central herniation are a reflection of compression and dysfunction of the displaced structures. These include impaired consciousness; initial contralateral hemiparesis evolving into bilateral motor dysfunction; small, equal, and reactive pupils progressing to be nonreactive and dilated; cranial nerve deficits; and vital sign alterations. Diffuse cerebral swelling, bilateral hemispheric lesions, and lesions in the midline have the greatest probability of causing central herniation.

Uncal or lateral transtentorial herniation occurs when the medial aspect of the temporal lobe (the uncus) is shifted toward the midline and then over the edge of the tentorium cerebelli. Like central herniation, uncal herniation causes life-threatening brainstem compression. Uncal herniation is most commonly associated with a unilateral hemispheric lesion, particularly epidural and subdural hematomas. Classic signs of uncal herniation include little early effect on consciousness followed by rapid deterioration, unilateral (usually ipsilateral) fixed and dilated pupils, contralateral (occasionally ipsilateral) hemiparesis or abnormal posturing, progressive dysfunction of cranial nerves III through XII, and vital sign alterations.

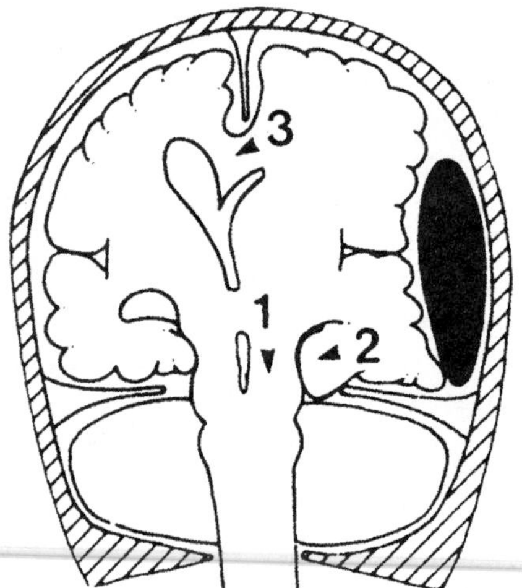

FIGURE 20-17 Brain displacement from supratentorial hematoma. *1,* Central: downward displacement of brainstem. *2,* Transtentorial: herniation of the uncus of the temporal lobe into the tentorial notch. *3,* Cingulate: herniation of cingulate gyrus below the falx. (From Jennett B, Teasdale G: *Management of Head Injuries,* Philadelphia, 1982, FA Davis.)

Infratentorial or posterior fossa mass lesions are less common with TBI. When infratentorial lesions do occur, symptoms of brainstem compression typically are evident and death is imminent. Clinical signs of infratentorial herniation include coma, motor dysfunction, abnormal eye and pupil signs, vomiting, cranial nerve dysfunction, and vital sign alterations.

CEREBROVASCULAR RESPONSE

Cerebral Perfusion Pressure and Autoregulation

Increased ICP or decreased systemic blood pressure reduces cerebral perfusion pressure. With cerebrovascular autoregulation intact, the healthy brain can maintain a constant adequate cerebral blood flow despite these pressure changes unless the normal limits of CPP are exceeded. Once outside the normal CPP range, autoregulation is impaired, CBF becomes passively dependent on the CPP, and delivery of metabolites is impaired (see Figure 20-8). Surpassing the upper CPP limit of 150 mm Hg causes passive vasodilation, which increases cerebral blood flow and fosters edema formation. When CPP falls below 50 mm Hg, cerebral blood flow is reduced. For example, if MAP is 60 mm Hg and ICP is 30 mm Hg, then CPP is only 30 mm Hg and the brain is being deprived of adequate blood flow.

After TBI, cerebral autoregulation is typically lost or impaired regionally or globally in most patients. This pathology has a variable temporal profile and occurs in patients with severe TBI, as well as those with moderate and mild brain injury.[68] Failure of the pressure autoregulatory mechanism signifies that reactivity and responsivity of the resistance vessels are lost, so changes in blood pressure and cerebral perfusion pressure cause passive changes in cerebral blood flow (see Figure 20-8). The nurse may recognize this loss of autoregulation when ICP fluctuations correlate with alterations in systemic blood pressure. When autoregulation is partially impaired, it is believed that the lower limit of CPP may reset itself so that the brain requires a higher CPP to prevent CBF compromise (see Figure 20-8). The critical threshold for CPP typically lies between 50 and 60 mm Hg, below which brain ischemia may occur.[63] Alterations in cerebral vascular autoregulation and cerebral blood flow after TBI are believed to contribute to the vulnerability of the injured brain to secondary insults.[68,69]

Cerebral Blood Flow

TBI and subsequent alterations in CPP and autoregulation have a profound effect on cerebral blood flow, which greatly influences patient outcome. A number of researchers have attempted to define a pattern of blood flow changes that occur after TBI. Cerebral blood flow studies indicate that 45% of patients with severe TBI have subnormal CBF, possibly related to reductions in cerebral metabolic rate, and 55% demonstrate a hyperemic response at some time after injury.[70] Global or localized reductions in CBF to ischemic levels (less than 18 ml/100 g brain tissue/minute) were noted in approximately one third of patients within the first 6 hours after severe brain injury.[71] Presence of regional brain ischemia within 24 hours after TBI has been demonstrated with use of oxygen-15 positron emission tomography, which confirms that blood flow was insufficient for the metabolic needs signifying true ischemia.[62] Evidence of low cerebral blood flow had a strong correlation with poor outcome.[62,71] Hyperemia may also develop early after TBI and may follow a period of brain ischemia.[72] Both hyperemia and relative ischemia have been found in the same patients, suggesting a problem with matching oxygen use to perfusion after TBI.[62] Optimal outcomes from TBI depend on prevention, early identification, and treatment of any factors that may compromise adequate CBF.

NEUROLOGIC ASSESSMENT

Once airway patency, effective ventilation, and adequate circulation have been ensured, the trauma patient's neurologic status can be assessed. Neurologic assessment after brain injury includes a comprehensive baseline evaluation followed by ongoing serial reassessment to detect changes in the patient's condition. As in all types of trauma, the assessment should include an initial injury database that provides information about the traumatic event and the probable mechanism of injury. A previous health history should be obtained from a family member or significant other as soon as possible. Neurologic assessment of the brain-injured patient also includes a clinical examination and analyses of data provided by monitoring devices and diagnostic studies.

CLINICAL NEUROLOGIC ASSESSMENT

The clinical neurologic examination is a basic yet incredibly important strategy used to assess and monitor the function of the injured brain. The nurse plays an essential role in performing a thorough baseline and serial follow-up neurologic examinations. The four major components of the examination are level of consciousness, motor and sensory function, eye and pupil signs, and vital signs.

Level of Consciousness

Level of consciousness is the most sensitive indicator of brain injury. There are two components of consciousness: arousal and cognition or awareness. Arousal is mediated by the ascending reticular activating system, which carries sensory stimuli from the environment to the cortex, activating consciousness. This system is so diffuse that injury in just about any part of the brain can disrupt or compress the reticular activating system, resulting in alteration of consciousness (see Figure 20-5). Comatose states occur when there is pressure on the dense bundle of reticular fibers that course through the brainstem or when bilateral cortical injuries affect the reticular activating system.

Arousal is assessed by determining the type of stimulus necessary to arouse the patient. The patient may be alert and responsive as soon as he or she is approached. If the patient is not alert, the assessor should begin with the least noxious stimulus (i.e., voice) to attempt to elicit a response from the patient. If that is unsuccessful, slight shaking can be attempted, then peripheral pain or nail bed pressure, and finally central pain. Central pain can be applied by sternal rub, exerting pressure to the superior aspect of the periorbital region of the eye or squeezing the trapezius muscle. Known or suspected injury to one of these specific areas would obviously contraindicate application of pressure. The assessor should document what type of stimulus was necessary to elicit a response and what the patient's response was to the stimulus (e.g., moving away from or toward the stimulus, flexing, extending, no response). Words such as *lethargic, semicomatose,* and *obtunded* are vague and should not be used to document the patient's arousal. If the patient is arousable, awareness can also be assessed. This entails evaluation of the various cerebral cortical functions, such as memory; affect; ability to perform intellectual functions (e.g., calculations); and orientation to person, place, time, and situation.

Duration and depth of coma have been identified as markers of brain injury severity. The longer the patient remains comatose, the greater likelihood of extensive severe neurologic dysfunction. Duration of coma tends to be longest in patients with severe diffuse axonal injury.

Other causes of altered level of consciousness need to be ruled out. Drug intoxication, shock, epilepsy, metabolic imbalances, infection, cerebral hypoxia, preexisting brain disease, and psychiatric disorders may alter the patient's level of consciousness. Sedatives, analgesics or paralytics administered by health care providers before or during hospitalization (e.g., during rapid sequence intubation) also can effect neurologic assessment parameters, including those used to evaluate consciousness. Even if underlying causes of altered mentation are identified, the examiner should still determine if the patient has sustained a brain injury.

Motor and Sensory Function

Motor abnormalities in brain-injured patients are primarily related to upper motor neuron dysfunction (e.g., compression of the descending pyramidal or corticospinal pathways). Corticospinal fibers normally originate in the motor strip located in the posterior aspect of the frontal lobes and descend from the cortex through the cerebral hemispheres. They are arranged in bundles as they pass through the cerebral peduncle and into the brainstem. At the level of the medulla, the fibers decussate or cross over and terminate in the opposite side of the spinal cord. The crossing over at the medullar level results in contralateral motor dysfunction when TBI affects these tracts. Occasionally motor deficit is on the same side as the lesion. This occurs when the medial temporal lobe herniates, shifting the brainstem and compressing the contralateral cerebral peduncle against the tentorium. This ipsilateral motor deficit phenomenon is known as the *Kernohan-Woltman notch phenomenon.*[73]

The first aspect of motor function to be evaluated is the patient's response to stimuli applied to assess arousal. The best possible response is that the patient consistently follows motor commands (e.g., the patient is able to hold up two fingers or protrude the tongue). It is inappropriate to evaluate ability to follow commands by asking the patient to grasp your hand, because the primitive grasp reflex, typically absent after early childhood, may return in the adult with cortical damage. Patients may be unable to follow commands but are able to localize (i.e., find offending stimuli and attempt to remove it). Localization is indicative of cortical damage. Patients in a deeper state of unconsciousness are unable to reach for stimuli and instead withdraw or pull the limb away with a normal flexor movement (Figure 20-18). This type of flexion withdraw indicates extensive cortical damage. Considerably worse motor signs are abnormal flexion (decortication), abnormal extension (decerebration), and flaccid motor responses, which are typically associated with deep coma and significant brain dysfunction. Decortication or abnormal flexion (see Figure 20-18) indicates damage to the corticospinal tracts just above the brainstem within or near the cerebral hemispheres. Extension or decerebration (see Figure 20-18) typically indicates damage to the midbrain and upper pons regions of the brainstem. These abnormal decorticate and decerebrate postures may be elicited by noxious stimuli or may occur spontaneously. Posturing may be transient or prolonged. Flaccidity with lack of a motor response after resuscitative measures is associated with lower brainstem dysfunction (death is usually imminent) or high spinal cord injury. These motor responses may be observed on one or both sides of the body. Changes in motor responsiveness may occur as the patient's condition improves or deteriorates. In general, decortication is better than decerebration, and decerebration is better than flaccidity. Deterioration in motor responsiveness indicates worsening neurologic status and warrants physician notification.

Corticospinal tract function in the conscious patient is best evaluated by assessing motor tone and strength. Muscle tone is increased in patients with upper motor neuron lesions, such as brain injuries. Increased tone and spasticity can precipitate additional complications, such as flexor extensor deformities and contractures in involved limbs.

Muscle strength is best evaluated by asking the conscious patient to pull his or her limb in opposition to the examiner (resistance measures) or by testing hand grasp. It is important to compare both sides of the patient's body to determine equality of strength. The best way to evaluate for early upper extremity motor weakness is to ask the patient to extend his or her arms outward with palms up and eyes closed and observe for "pronator drift." This response is evident when the weak or hemiparetic limb begins to pronate and drift downward, indicating the presence of motor tract compression.

If the patient is unable to follow commands, the assessor should observe the strength and equality of spontaneous movement. Awake and unconscious patients also should be evaluated for the presence of abnormal movements, such as seizures, tics, and tremors. Location and description of any

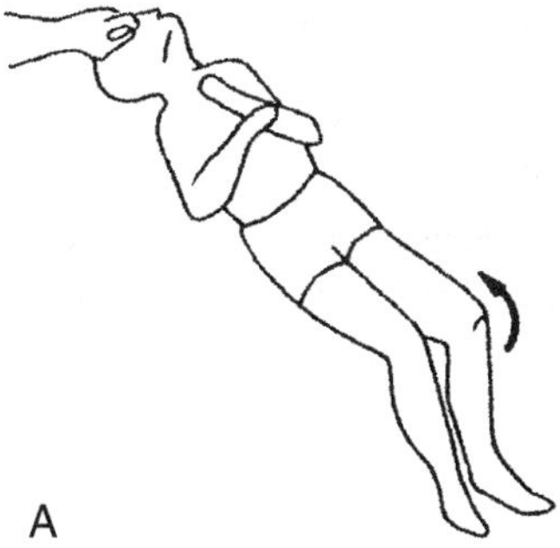

Bilateral Withdrawal (Flexion)

Arms flexed
Legs flexed
Knees come up

A

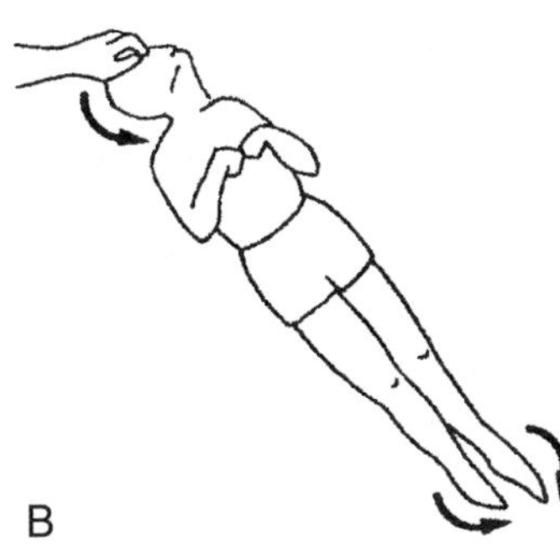

Bilateral Decortication (Abnormal Flexion)

Arms flexed
Wrists flexed
Legs extended

B

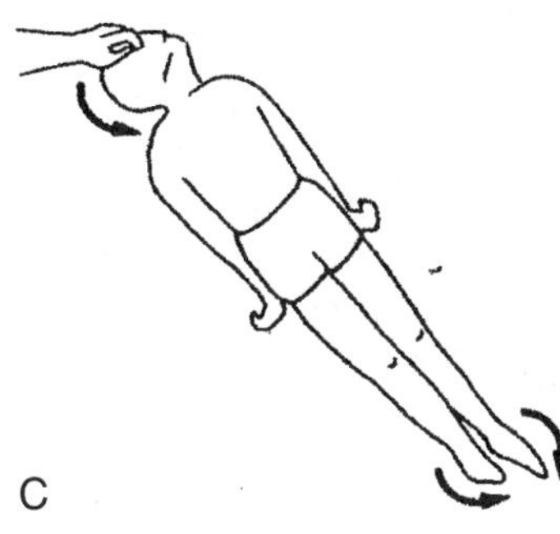

Bilateral Decerebration (Extension)

Arms extended
External rotation of wrists
Legs extended
Internal rotation of feet

C

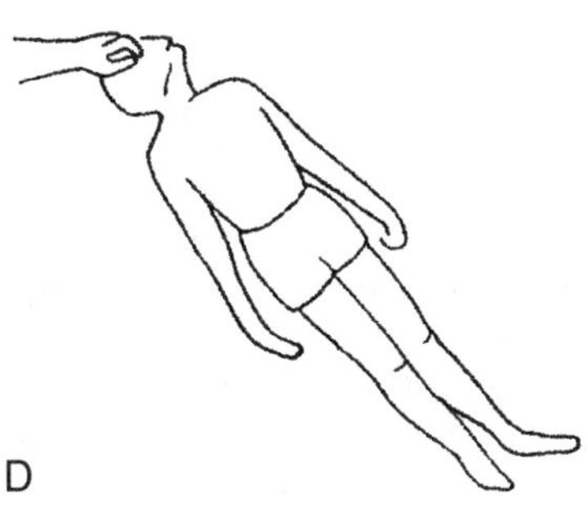

Bilateral Flaccidity

No response in any extremity to noxious stimuli
Note: Spinal cord injury must be ruled out as cause of flaccidity

D

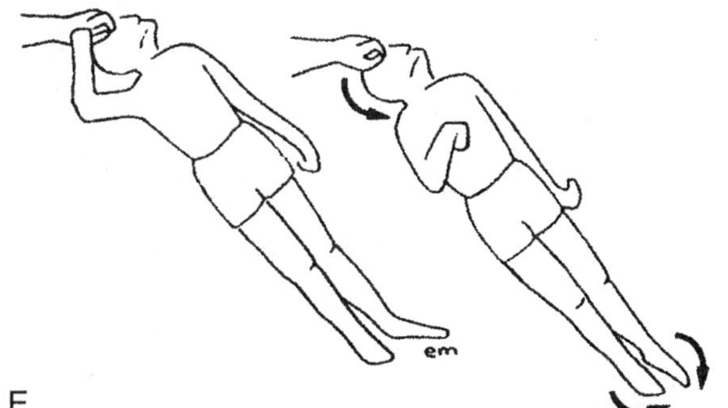

Lateralization*

Left Figure: Purposeful right side
Flaccid left side

Right Figure: Decorticate right side
Decerebrate left side

*These figures show how responses can vary from limb to limb and stress the importance of checking all extremities for motor response.

E

FIGURE 20-18 Abnormal motor responses. **A,** Bilateral withdrawal (flexion). **B,** Bilateral decorticate posturing (abnormal flexion). **C,** Bilateral decerebrate posturing (extension). **D,** Bilateral flaccidity. **E,** Lateralization. (From Marshall SB et al: *Neuroscience Critical Care,* Philadelphia, 1990, W.B. Saunders, p. 102.)

abnormal movements should be well documented and reported to the physician.

Cerebellar functions (namely, coordination and balance) can be assessed in the conscious patient. Bedridden patients can have coordination and balance evaluated by having them close their eyes and touch their finger to their nose and move the heel of one foot down the opposite shin bilaterally.

The extensor plantar reflex (Babinski's reflex) is a pathologic response that is assessed by stroking the lateral sole of the foot from the heel upward and then medially across the ball. Great toe dorsiflexion and fanning of the other toes in response to this stimulus indicates dysfunction of the corticospinal tract anywhere between the cortex and the anterior horn cell of the spinal cord. Its presence does not localize dysfunction along this tract.

The range and complexity of the sensory examination are directed by the overall clinical status of the patient. If the patient is alert and stable, complete testing of sensory function is carried out. This includes evaluation of the patient's cortical discriminatory sensation (e.g., recognition of common objects and textures by touch, discrimination between two points touched), which evaluates parietal lobe functions. The sensory examination is much more cursory if the patient is comatose or unable to communicate sensations. The practitioner makes note of the patient's response to painful or noxious stimuli applied to different areas of the body while performing various interventions (e.g., placing an intravenous catheter in an extremity).

Cranial Nerve Dysfunction

Another aspect of the clinical neurologic examination involves evaluation of the cranial nerve functions (Table 20-2). A helpful mnemonic for naming the nerves is "On Old Olympus Towering Tops, A Finn And German Viewed Some Hops," in which the first letter of each word represents the ordered sequence of nerves. Cranial nerve assessment not only gives the examiner information regarding the function of a specific nerve or nerves being tested, but also, when evaluating cranial nerves III through XII, provides vital information about general functioning of the brainstem. Cranial nerve dysfunction often provides substantive evidence of impending or actual brain herniation.

Cranial nerve injuries are not uncommon in patients with brain injury. Cranial nerve injuries can result from direct mechanical trauma; increased ICP; brain herniation; ischemia; and fractures of the face, temporal bone, or basilar skull. Documentation of cranial nerve dysfunction is an essential part of the nursing record so that deficits requiring specific nursing intervention (e.g., loss of the gag reflex, visual field deficits, or impaired hearing) receive appropriate attention and follow-up.

Eye and Pupil Signs

Pathologic eye and pupil findings can be ominous signs of neurologic deterioration, especially in the presence of concomitant motor and sensorial changes. Frequent eye and pupil checks are extremely important in nursing assessment of the brain-injured patient so that early and subtle signs of dysfunction can be recognized and reported immediately to the physician. A brief review of pupillary innervation provides a better understanding of pathologic eye signs.

Both parasympathetic and sympathetic fibers innervate the eye to control pupillary size. Parasympathetic influence provided by the oculomotor nerve (cranial nerve III) normally causes pupillary constriction, but with midbrain or third cranial nerve compression the parasympathetic innervation is blocked and the sympathetic fibers act unopposed, causing pupillary dilation (mydriasis). Inversely, if sympathetic innervation is interrupted, the parasympathetic fibers act unopposed and the result is small (miotic) pupils. There are three nuclei or points of origin for sympathetic innervation—the hypothalamus, the pons, and the cervical ganglion. A lesion at any one of these sites can result in pupillary constriction. Because the cervical ganglion is an extracranial site, miosis of intracranial origin is due to pontine or diencephalic dysfunction. Pupil constriction secondary to hypothalamic or metabolic dysfunction retains reactivity to light, whereas pontine pupils are unreactive and fixed to light.

Pupils are assessed for shape, size, equality, and reactivity to light. Pupils are normally round and regularly shaped. An early warning sign that a pupil will progress to become fixed and dilated is a change in the shape from round to oval. An oval or irregularly shaped pupil is a significant sign of impending transtentorial herniation and third cranial nerve compression. Irregularly shaped pupils also may be seen when a patient has a history of an iridectomy or has sustained ocular trauma.

Depending on the amount of light that is entering the eye, pupils can vary in diameter from 1.5 to 8 mm but generally average about 3 mm. Variation in light should be taken into consideration when assessing pupil size. Consistency in room lighting is important when performing pupil assessments that are being compared. Variation in size is generally not significant as long as both pupils are the same diameter. Pupil inequality, asymmetry, or anisocoria can have pathologic importance. A small percentage of people (11% to 16%) normally have anisocoria (inequality of the pupils), usually with a pupil size difference of less than 1 mm. Pupillary asymmetry of 1 mm or more is significant and often forewarns of subsequent progressive dilation. Unilateral pupil dilation is most commonly caused by third cranial nerve or midbrain compression but may also be due to seizures, direct orbital trauma, or optic nerve injury. Bilateral pupil dilation is seen after systemic or bilateral ophthalmic administration of mydriatics (e.g., scopolamine hydrobromide or atropine sulfate), instillation of cycloplegic agents, cerebral anoxia or ischemia, or amphetamine use. Causes of pupillary miosis include pontine or hypothalamic dysfunction, cervical ganglion lesions, instillation of ophthalmic miotic agents, and use of opiates.

Pupillary reactivity to light is mediated by the parasympathetic fibers of the oculomotor nerve, which constrict the

TABLE 20-2 **Cranial Nerves**

Cranial Nerve	Location of Cranial Nerve Nuclei	Function	Anticipated Deficits
I Olfactory	Olfactory receptor cells in the nasal mucosa	Smell	Anosmia/hyposmia
II Optic	Retina	Vision	Visual loss
		Sensory component of the light reflex	Eye with cranial nerve lesion does not have a direct light reflex; consensual light reflex is intact if cranial nerve III and midbrain connections are intact
III Oculomotor	Midbrain	Moves eyes (medially, upward and outward, upward and inward, downward and outward)	Loss of eye movements controlled by this nerve Diplopia (double vision)
		Elevation of upper eyelid	Ptosis
		Pupil constriction (parasympathetic innervation) Motor component of the light reflex	Pupil Dilated Unreactive to light
IV Trochlear	Midbrain	Moves eyes (downward and inward)	Impaired downward and inward gaze Diplopia
V Trigeminal	Pons (with branches in the midbrain and medulla)	Sensation to face, scalp, nasal and oral cavities	Absent, unequal or uncomfortable sensation when face is stimulated
		Sensory component of the corneal reflex	Absent blink/corneal reflex
		Innervate muscles for mastication	Weakness of muscles used for mastication
VI Abducens	Pons	Moves eyes (laterally outward)	Eye fails to abduct Diplopia
VII Facial	Pons (with connections in the medulla; emerges from the pontomedullary junction)	Facial muscle movement Motor component of the corneal reflex	Ipsilateral weakness of the entire side of face Loss of corneal reflex NOTE: Contralateral weakness of lower half of face indicates an upper motor neuron
		Taste, anterior two thirds of tongue	Loss of taste
		Sensation to the external auditory meatus and the auricle	Loss of skin sensation to the external auditory meatus and the auricle
		Lacrimation/salivation	Impaired/excessive salivation and lacrimation
VIII Acoustic (also known as vestibulocochlear)	Pons (with connections in the medulla; enters brainstem at the pontomedullary junction)	Vestibular: balance and coordinates head and eye movements	Dizziness; Imbalance Abnormal oculocephalic and oculovestibular reflexes
		Cochlear: hearing	Hearing loss
IX Glossopharyngeal	Medulla	Taste, posterior third of tongue	Loss of taste in posterior third of tongue
		Sensation for posterior tongue, soft palate, and pharynx	Loss of sensation in posterior tongue, soft palate, pharynx
		Pharyngeal reflex	Loss of gag reflex
		With vagus nerve participates in swallowing	Difficulty swallowing
		Sensation to carotid body and carotid sinus	Impaired blood pressure regulation
X Vagus	Medulla	Motor innervation to soft palate, pharynx, larynx Parasympathetic innervation of thoracic and abdominal viscera Conveys sensory impulses from the palate, pharynx, larynx, external auditory meatus, digestive tract, heart, and lungs	Unilateral lesion: • Ipsilateral paralysis of soft palate, pharynx, and larynx • Deviation of the uvula to the unaffected side • Impaired gag • Impaired palatal reflex • Dysphagia • Vocal cord impairment • Hoarseness Bilateral lesion: • Complete paralysis of pharynx and larynx • Vocal cord paralysis • Atonia of stomach and esophagus—vomiting • Dysphagia

Continued

TABLE 20-2 Cranial Nerves—cont'd

Cranial Nerve	Location of Cranial Nerve Nuclei	Function	Anticipated Deficits
XI Spinal Accessory (also known as accessory)	Medulla	Sternocleidomastoid and trapezius muscle movement	Inability to shrug shoulders or rotate head
XII Hypoglossal	Medulla	Motor innervation of tongue musculature	Ipsilateral tongue paralysis and atrophy Tongue deviation to side of lesion • Dysphagia • Dysarthria

pupil when light stimulates the optic nerve (cranial nerve II). When the light is shined in one eye, both pupils should constrict. Constriction of the pupil with a direct light stimulus is the direct response to light, and the constriction of the contralateral pupil is the indirect or consensual response. Both the direct and the indirect responses to light should be evaluated in both eyes. Absence of the direct response indicates either compression of the third cranial nerve or an optic nerve lesion resulting in blindness. An oculomotor nerve lesion causes loss of the direct and consensual light responses. A blind eye has no direct reaction to light, but the consensual response remains intact. Normal pupillary light response is brisk constriction of the pupils to light stimulus. Pupil size and reactivity normally decrease with age, especially in those older than age 60. The smaller the pupil, the smaller the amplitude of light reaction, so miotic pupils should be assessed carefully in a dim or darkened room to determine optimal reactivity. An early foreboding sign that a pupil will become unreactive to light is a delayed or sluggish response to light.

Pupil abnormalities can be linked to specific areas of brain dysfunction (Table 20-3). Pupil reactivity also has prognostic importance and has been identified as an independent predictor of survival.[74] Presence of at least one nonreactive pupil has been associated with less favorable outcome measured at 6 months and 1 year after TBI.[75]

Each eye is also evaluated to determine if the corneal reflex is intact. Testing this reflex entails lightly touching the cornea with a fine piece of cotton or a drop of saline and observing for a blink response. This reflex is mediated by two cranial nerves that both originate from the pons region of the brainstem: the trigeminal nerve (cranial nerve V), which provides sensation to the cornea, and the facial nerve (cranial nerve VII), which enables the eye to blink in response to the corneal stimulation. If the corneal reflex is absent, care must be taken to protect the eye from corneal abrasion or ulceration by instillation of ophthalmic lubricants, use of eye shields, or taping the eyelid closed. Prolonged contact lens use can weaken or obliterate the corneal reflex.

Other eye signs assessed as part of the clinical neurologic examination of the unconscious patient may include the oculovestibular and oculocephalic reflexes. Both these reflexes assess three cranial nerves: the oculomotor nerve (cranial nerve III), the abducens nerve (cranial nerve VI), and the acoustic nerve (cranial nerve VIII). Each of these nerves originates from a different portion of the brainstem. By evaluating these reflexes, the integrity of the three cranial

TABLE 20-3 Pupil Abnormalities Related to Specific Areas of Brain Dysfunction

Pupil Finding	Related Brain Dysfunction
Small, equal, reactive	Bilateral diencephalic damage that affects the sympathetic innervation originating from the hypothalamus; metabolic dysfunction
Nonreactive, midpositioned	Midbrain damage
Fixed and dilated	Ipsilateral oculomotor (CN III) compression or injury
Bilateral fixed and dilated	Brain anoxia and ischemia; bilateral CN III compression
Pinpoint, nonreactive	Pons damage often from hemorrhage or ischemia that interrupts the sympathetic nervous system pathways
Pupil is smaller than the other, but both reactive to light; associated with ptosis and an inability to sweat on the same side as the smaller pupil (Horner's syndrome)	Interruption of ipsilateral sympathetic innervation that can be caused by a lesion of the anterolateral cervical spinal cord or lateral medulla, damage to the hypothalamus or occlusion or dissection of the internal carotid artery

Used with permission from McQuillan KA: The neurologic system. In Alspach GA, editor: *Core Curriculum for Critical Care Nursing,* ed 6, St. Louis, 2006, Saunders Elsevier, p. 430.

nerves, as well as the brainstem, is assessed. However, the oculovestibular reflex is considered more sensitive than the oculocephalic reflex in assessing brainstem function.

After ensuring that the tympanic membrane is intact, the oculovestibular or caloric reflex can be evaluated by injecting at least 20 ml of ice water into the patient's ear while holding the patient's eyes open. During the irrigation, if the reflex is intact, the eyes should deviate first slowly toward the irrigated ear and then rapidly away from the irrigated ear. The initial deviation toward the irrigated ear is controlled by the brainstem, and the rapid movement away from the irrigated ear is controlled by the cerebral cortex. Absence of eye movement toward the irrigated ear correlates strongly with brain death or a vegetative state.

The oculocephalic (doll's eye) reflex is examined by turning an unconscious patient's head rapidly from side to side while the eyes are held open and noting if the eyes move from side to side in the opposite direction of the head movement. If the eyes move asymmetrically or if there is no eye movement, the integrity of cranial nerves III, VI, or VIII or the brainstem (from which they originate) is disrupted. *Assessment of the doll's eye reflex is contraindicated if the cervical spine has not been cleared of possible injury.*

The oculomotor nerve (cranial nerve III), the abducens nerve (cranial nerve VI), and the trochlear nerve (cranial nerve IV) enable eye movements in specific directions (see Table 20-2). Eye movements are observed to determine if the eyes move together or conjugately. In awake and cooperative patients, more detailed assessment of extraocular movements, including gaze-holding and gaze-shifting capabilities, can be assessed when time permits. Gaze deviations, which are often associated with lesions in specific areas of the brain, should be noted.

Vital Signs

Vital signs are monitored routinely in all critically ill neurotrauma patients to rapidly detect abnormalities that may cause unacceptable brain tissue hypoperfusion, hypoxemia, or hypercapnia. Abnormal respiratory patterns may have localizing value and serve as indicators of neurologic deterioration (Table 20-4). Progressively less effective patterns of respiration, characterized by slower rates and longer periods of apnea, are seen as the respiratory centers in the pons and medulla become dysfunctional. Abnormal respiratory patterns associated with brain injury may not be recognized in the patient on mechanical ventilation, and alterations in respirations may not be evident until death is imminent. Many nonneurologic factors, such as anxiety, medications, acid-base imbalance, myocardial dysfunction, shock, pulmonary injuries, hypoxia, or hypercapnia, can also influence respiration.

Brain injury can cause repolarization abnormalities (e.g., ST- and T-wave changes, prolonged QT waves, short PR intervals, Q or U waves, and myocardial infarction-like changes) and variations in heart rate and rhythm, as well as in blood pressure. Bradycardia, tachycardia, and various cardiac arrhythmias (e.g., atrial fibrillation, atrial flutter, junctional rhythm, premature ventricular contractions, ventricular tachycardia, ventricular fibrillation, and conduction blocks) may be noted after brain injury. Onset of bradycardia and increased systolic blood pressure with a widening of the pulse pressure (Cushing's response) occurs as a late sign of intracranial hypertension and brain herniation, indicating medullary compression and imminent death. Other nonneurologic causes of heart rate and blood pressure change must also be considered. Change in blood pressure and heart rate without accompanying changes in level of consciousness indicates a nonneurologic etiology (e.g., shock).

Alterations in body temperature may indicate dysfunction of the hypothalamic temperature-regulating center caused by a lesion or intracranial hypertension. Patients can have rapid alterations in body temperature, with fluctuations between hyperthermic and hypothermic states. An infectious process should be ruled out as the cause of hyperthermia.

TABLE 20-4 **Respiratory Patterns Associated with Specific Areas of Brain Dysfunction**

Breathing Pattern	Description	Location of Brain Lesions or Type of Dysfunction
Cheyne-Stokes	Regular cycles of respirations that gradually increase in depth to hyperpnea and then decrease in depth to periods of apnea	Usually bilateral lesions deep within the cerebral hemispheres, basal ganglia or diencephalon; metabolic disorders
Central neurogenic hyperventilation	Deep, rapid respirations	Midbrain, upper pons
Apneustic	Prolonged inspiration followed by a 2- to 3-second pause; occasionally may alternate with an expiratory pause	Pons
Cluster	Clusters of irregular breaths followed by an apneic period lasting a variable amount of time	Lower pons or upper medulla
Ataxic or irregular	Irregular, unpredictable pattern of shallow and deep respirations and pauses	Medulla

Used with permission from McQuillan KA. The Neurologic System. In Alspach GA. (Editor). *Core Curriculum for Critical Care Nursing,* 6th edition, St. Louis, Saunders Elsevier, 2006, p. 430.

STANDARDIZED ASSESSMENT TOOLS

Standardized assessment tools are important for quantifying the severity of injury or degree of neurologic disability. Many of these tools were created during clinical research to document consistently one or more aspects of the patient's initial condition, overall neurologic status, and response to therapy. Comparisons among groups of patients can be made using these tools. Two such tools widely used in the care of brain-injured patients are the GCS and the Rancho Levels of Cognitive Functioning: a Clinical Case Management Tool.

Glasgow Coma Scale

Brain injury severity and degree of consciousness are most commonly assessed with the internationally recognized GCS (Table 20-5).[76] Possible scores on this scale range from 3 to 15. The score is calculated by adding the values determined on three subscales: eye opening, motor response, and verbal response. The total GCS is used to classify the severity of brain injury. A score of 13 to 15 is defined as mild injury, a score of 9 to 12 is classified as moderate injury, and a score of 8 or less indicates severe head injury and coma. The lower the GCS score is, the deeper the coma and the higher the associated mortality and morbidity. This tool enables clinicians and researchers to predict more accurately brain injury outcome. Each part of the GCS may prove as important as the overall total score[77] and may be reported as E-M-V rather than the total score.

Eye Opening Assessment. Assessment of eye opening, a measure of spontaneous arousal, is most accurate within the first 5 to 7 days after brain injury. Thereafter, many patients have return of spontaneous eye opening. Crediting such a patient with reflexive eye opening erroneously increases the GCS score by 3 points despite lack of true neurologic improvement. When the patient has facial trauma and periorbital edema that inhibit voluntary eye opening, the examiner should make note of the inability to evaluate eye opening next to the total GCS score.

Motor Response Assessment. The best motor response correlates most closely with outcome and provides greater interrater reliability. A patient who exhibits two different motor responses is always given credit for the best response, although it may be evident in only one extremity. Motor responses can be ambiguous. Examiners need to be consistent in both the type of painful stimulus and limb position used to avoid influencing the patient's response.

Verbal Response Assessment. Patients with brain injuries may require endotracheal intubation, preventing the practitioner from assessing the patient's verbal response. When scoring an intubated patient, a "T" should be placed next to the total GCS score, indicating that verbal response could not be evaluated. It is controversial whether points should be awarded to the intubated patient who nods his or her head or displays other behaviors indicating that he or she would speak appropriately if able.

Considerations and Limitations of the GCS. Drug intoxication; aphasia; endotracheal intubation; periorbital swelling; and therapeutic use of sedatives, analgesics, and paralytic agents can all interfere with accurate interpretation of GCS responses. It is important therefore that the presence of these variables be noted when reporting the score. For infants and young children who are unable to produce normal adult verbal and motor responses, age-appropriate versions of the GCS must be used (see Table 29-7).

Although the GCS has been the dominant scale used internationally and has demonstrated usefulness in predicting outcome from brain injury, there have been many criticisms of its relative insensitivity to significant clinical change in the early period and to the subtleties of neurologic function in recovering patients.[78] The developers of the GCS emphasize that it cannot stand alone in evaluating overall neurologic function in the acute period but must be supplemented with evaluation of pupillary and eye movement and brainstem and cerebral function.[79] The accuracy of the GCS in predicting outcome from TBI is improved when scores are considered together with pupillary response and patient age and when broad, less-specific outcome categories are used.[77]

TABLE 20-5 Glasgow Coma Scale

Eyes	Open	Spontaneously	4
		To verbal command	3
		To pain	2
		No response	1
Best motor response	To verbal command	Obeys	6
	To painful stimulus	Localizes pain	5
		Flexion—withdrawal	4
		Flexion—abnormal (decorticate rigidity)	3
		Extension (decerebrate rigidity)	2
		No response	1
Best verbal response		Oriented and converses	5
		Disoriented and converses	4
		Inappropriate words	3
		Incomprehensible sounds	2
		No response	1
Total			3-15

From Teasdale G, Jennett B: Assessment of coma and impaired consciousness: a practical scale. *Lancet* 2:81, 1974.

Other Coma Scales

Many other scales have been proposed to replace or be used in conjunction with the GCS. Several scales incorporate indicators of brainstem function together with evaluation of consciousness and, in some cases, other aspects of neurologic function. Examples of such tools include the JFK Coma Recovery Scale–revised,[80] Reaction Level Scale (RLS85),[81] Full Outline of UnResponsiveness (FOUR) Score,[82,83] and Glasgow Coma Scale–Extended.[31,84]

Rancho Los Amigos Levels of Cognitive Functioning Scale

The Rancho Levels of Cognitive Functioning: a Clinical Case Management Tool (Rancho Tool) is a multidisciplinary tool that places the patient in one of eight categories based on observed behavioral responses to stimuli and cognitive capabilities.[85] The scale has standardized evaluation criteria for each of the levels, which range from nonresponsive to independent functioning (Table 20-6). Patient cooperation is not necessary during scoring. Several disciplines frequently use the Rancho Tool, so implications for care based on the patient's level on the scale can be coordinated among speech, occupational, and physical therapy, as well as the nursing and physician staff. This scale is also useful when educating family members about the stages of recovery typically seen after TBI. It can be used in all phases of brain injury management but is most widely used in the intermediate care and rehabilitative phases.

NEURODIAGNOSTICS AND MONITORING STRATEGIES

Alterations in results of the clinical neurologic examination typically trigger use of other neurodiagnostic and monitoring strategies. Information from these various diagnostic and monitoring strategies is used to guide therapeutic decision making and to evaluate the patient's response to treatment. Neurodiagnostics and monitoring devices are available to evaluate the brain's anatomy, pressure, function, oxygenation, biochemical environment, blood supply, metabolism, and electrical activity.

Radiographic Evaluation and Neuroimaging

Skull x-ray films have limited value in evaluating a patient with craniocerebral trauma. These films allow visualization of bony abnormalities (e.g., fractures), pneumocephalus, and metallic objects. Brain tissue and any uncalcified lesions cannot be seen on skull films.

CT scanning is the initial and primary imaging modality of choice for the patient with craniocerebral trauma. CT scanning provides anatomic localization for the majority of traumatic brain lesions. This diagnostic technique is very sensitive to the presence of intracranial hemorrhage and is superior to MRI in the diagnosis of acute hemorrhage, especially subarachnoid hemorrhage.[86] Space-occupying lesions, contusions, cerebral edema, intracranial air, and brain herniation are also identifiable. Most intracranial pathologic conditions, particularly injuries requiring surgical or medical intervention, can be diagnosed within several minutes of

TABLE 20-6 **Rancho Los Amigos Scale of Cognitive Levels and Expected Behavior**

Level	Name	Behavior
I	Unresponsive	No response to stimuli.
II	Generalized	Inconsistent, nonpurposeful, nonspecific, and reflexive reactions to stimuli.
III	Localized Response	Responsive to physical discomfort; blinks to strong light; turns toward/away from sound; inconsistently responsive to stimuli.
IV	Confused – Agitated	Alert, but disoriented and unaware of events around them; responds with bizarre and inappropriate behavior; easily distracted with impaired ability to process information.
V	Confused –Inappropriate – Nonagitated	Grossly aware of surroundings and responsive to simple commands; responses are random and nonpurposeful when lacking external structure or when task exceeds capabilities; disoriented; easily distracted requiring frequent redirection; difficulty learning new tasks but able to repeat previously learned tasks.
VI	Confused – Appropriate	Disoriented at times; responds appropriately to situations; impaired memory/attention span may make some responses incorrect; goal-directed behavior emerges; consistently follows commands; some recall of past.
VII	Automatic – Appropriate	Performs daily routine with robot-like responses in familiar environment with deterioration in unfamiliar surroundings; poor insight and judgment with impaired problem solving ability; overestimate capabilities
VIII	Purposeful – Appropriate	Responds correctly; inability to estimate abilities; easily irritable; low tolerance for stress; capable of abstract reasoning with some difficulty; Improved learning ability; minimal supervision required.
**IX*	*Purposeful – Appropriate – Self-Monitoring*	*Low frustration tolerance with need for assistance to identify and avoid problems before they occur*
**X*	*Purposeful – Appropriate – Independent*	*Able to accurately estimate abilities and adjust to task demands; may experience depression; low tolerance for frustration and irritability when stressed.*

Adapted from Hagen C, Malkmus D, Stenderup-Bowman K: *Los Amigos Research and Education,* Rancho Los Amigos Hospital, ed 3, Downey, CA, 1973. Revised by Hagen C, 1998 and www.Learningservices.com.

*A revised version of the tool includes Levels IX and X; however, the reliability and validity of the tool with these two new levels has not yet been established.

(Rancho Los Amigos National Rehabilitation Center. http://www.rancho.org/research_home.htm. Accessed August 16, 2007.)

scanning, which has been a significant factor in reducing mortality from mass lesions. Follow-up CT scans are often indicated in patients with severe or moderate brain injuries to evaluate for the evolution of pathologic brain conditions, to diagnose possible causes of any neurologic deterioration, or to determine treatment effectiveness.[87,88] Patients with neurologic deterioration after TBI benefit from a CT scan, but the indications and timing for routine follow-up CT scan in those without evidence of neurologic worsening remain unclear and require further study.[87-89] Trauma patients, who may require intravenous contrast for an abdominal CT scan, should have a head CT scan done first without contrast to avoid obscuring any intracranial pathologic conditions (e.g., an underlying contusion). Nonhemorrhagic lesions seen with diffuse axonal injury and injury in the brainstem or deep gray matter may be difficult to visualize with CT scan.[90]

MRI produces an excellent anatomic composite of the brain. The base of the brain, brainstem, basal ganglia, thalami, posterior fossa, and gray and white matter differentiation are viewed better on MRI than CT scan.[86] Compared with CT scanning, MRI is better able to detect the presence and extent of nonhemorrhagic lesions associated with diffuse axonal injury; extraaxial hematomas (i.e., subdural hematomas); and subacute or chronic intracranial hemorrhage.[86] Ischemic strokes tend to be evident sooner on MRI than on CT scan. MRI scanning may be indicated when CT findings do not explain the patient's neurologic deficits and the patient has no contraindications for the test to be performed.

Developments in MRI technology have improved the ability to detect abnormalities associated with TBI.[22,24,86] Recent improvements in MRI include fluid-attenuated inversion recovery (FLAIR), diffusion weighted imaging, diffusion tensor imaging, magnetization transfer imaging (MTI), proton magnetic resonance spectroscopy, and functional MRI. Although currently not routinely used in diagnosis of TBI, further research and continued improvements in MRI technology may make these studies more useful tools for evaluation of acute TBI in the future.[86]

Several technical disadvantages to MRI hinder its use in the unstable brain-injured patient. The magnetic field is disrupted by ferrous-containing compounds, which restricts the use of most ventilators and infusion pumps in the imaging suite. Radiofrequency waves can interfere with unshielded monitoring devices. Patients with known or suspected metallic or electronic implants are prohibited from having an MRI. Furthermore, MRI is more costly and takes longer to complete than CT.

Angiography may be indicated as an adjunct to CT when a vascular injury or disease is suspected. Angiography is essential in identifying trauma-related vascular injuries, such as vessel laceration or occlusion and aneurysms. Posttraumatic vasospasms may also be detected. Interventions to treat or repair the injured or spasmodic vessels may be performed during angiography.

Although contrast angiography is considered the gold standard for diagnosing vascular lesions, magnetic resonance angiography (MRA) and CT angiography (CTA) are other less invasive imaging modalities that may be used to visualize intracranial and extracranial vessels.[90-92] These techniques provide images of both the vessel lumen and the arterial wall while subjecting the patient to fewer potential complications than are associated with conventional angiography.[91] Multicenter trials to define better the accuracy of noninvasive diagnostics are recommended.[92]

Intracranial Pressure Monitoring

Placement of an ICP monitor provides a direct measure of pressure within the intracranial vault. Presumptive evidence of increased pressure can be obtained from clinical examination and diagnostic study, but these findings may not be apparent until after a neurologic disaster has occurred and the brain has herniated. Compressed ventricles, absent or compressed cisterns, brain shift, and vessel displacement, as demonstrated on CT, MRI, or angiography, indirectly support the diagnosis of increased ICP but do not measure the actual level of pressure.

ICP monitoring is useful in the early detection of intracranial lesions that raise intracranial pressure and may cause brain herniation. ICP serves as a guide for therapy and enables the practitioner to determine the effectiveness or response to treatment provided. Monitoring ICP is particularly helpful in patients whose clinical neurologic examination is obviated by use of excessive analgesia, paralytic agents, or anesthesia.

The *Guidelines for Management of Severe Traumatic Brain Injury* suggest that ICP monitoring is indicated for patients with a GCS score less than 9 after resuscitation and an abnormal admission CT scan.[63] Placement of an ICP monitor is also suggested in patients who have a GCS score less than 9 with a normal CT scan and in whom two or more of the following are noted on admission: (1) the patient is older than age 40; (2) the patient has unilateral or bilateral abnormal posturing; or (3) the patient's systolic blood pressure is less than 90 mm Hg.[63] Physician discretion may also determine the use of ICP monitoring. For example, a patient with a GCS score greater than 8 and at risk for brain swelling or hematoma expansion may require prolonged surgery, during which neurologic status cannot be monitored by clinical examination.

Methods of Transducing Intracranial Pressure. Four systems are currently available for transducing the pressure from the intracranial vault to the bedside monitor: the hydraulic or fluid-filled system, the fiberoptic system, the microstrain gauge system, and the air-pouch method.

Fluid-Filled or Hydraulic System. A fluid-filled or hydraulic system uses a static fluid column to transmit pressure from within the intracranial vault to an external strain-gauge transducer, which then transmits the pressure reading to a bedside monitor. This type of system is inexpensive and can be recalibrated after insertion. Inherent problems of the fluid-filled system include possible entry of air bubbles, blood clots, brain tissue, or other debris within the tubing or transducer; kinked tubing; and loose connections. These problems can dampen or distort the ICP waveform and give inaccurate measurements of ICP. Components of the system—external transducers, stop cocks, flushing devices, and pressure tubing—are prone to technical malfunction. Even when the system is functioning well, inaccurate readings can result from changes in the patient's position that cause the transducer to come out of alignment with the external anatomic reference point corresponding to the intracranial location of the fluid-filled system's distal tip at the foramen of Monro (Figure 20-6).

It is essential that the fluid-filled system be maintained optimally to reduce risk of complications and to ensure the accuracy of the ICP values. The system should be zeroed, balanced, and calibrated routinely, and the level of the transducer should be reassessed frequently to ensure that it is in alignment with a predetermined and consistently used external landmark. When the waveform becomes dampened, the system should be inspected carefully for kinks; leaks; and the presence of air, tissue, blood clots, or other debris. If there is no improvement in the waveform after the transducer is zeroed and rebalanced, the physician should be notified. The system may need to be changed or irrigated according to institution protocol. Unlike hemodynamic pressure measuring systems, a bag of flush solution should not be hung, to prevent inadvertent infusion of a large volume of fluid into the cranial vault. Interruptions to the system should be minimized, and all connections should be kept snug to avoid risk of infection.[93]

Fiberoptic Transducer-Tipped Monitoring System. Fiberoptic ICP monitoring systems use fiberoptics to transmit pressure from a transducer at the distal tip of the ICP monitoring catheter to a bedside monitor. This eliminates the need for a fluid-filled system and thus eliminates the problems inherent in a hydraulic system. Measurements are accurate and reliable compared with simultaneous standard intraventricular hydraulic system values.[94,95] One problem in this system stems from the inability to recalibrate the transducer after implantation and the possibility of drift in measured pressures over time.[63] The fiberoptics within the system are relatively fragile, but breakage can be avoided by carefully securing the cables and avoiding kinks in the catheter. Securing the cables to the patient and not the bed is important to prevent dislodging the transducer.

Miniature Strain-Gauge Transducer-Tipped System. Miniature strain-gauge transducer-tipped systems use a miniature strain-gauge pressure sensor mounted in a titanium case at the tip of a flexible nylon tube to sense ICP, which is transmitted electronically from within the cranial vault to a bedside monitor. ICP values obtained with this system have been shown to remain stable over time with negligible drift and have a good correlation with measures obtained with fluid-filled external strain-gauge transducer systems.[96] Like the fiberoptic system, this system cannot be recalibrated after insertion. It also needs to be well secured, and kinking should be avoided to prevent catheter breakage or transducer dislodgment.

Air-Pouch (Pneumatic) Pressure Sensor. This system uses a specially designed catheter with an air pouch at the tip filled with 0.1 ml of air. Intracranial pressure is transmitted through the thin wall of the pouch into the air and is converted to an electrical signal by the transducer located in the ICP monitor and connected to the catheter tip.[97] This catheter can be placed in the ventricle, brain parenchyma, subdural space, or epidural space. The sensor automatically rezeroes every hour.[97] ICP values obtained with this system in the brain parenchyma have a good correlation with measures obtained with intraventricular fluid-filled external strain-gauge transducer systems.[97,98] Because small volumes of air can be removed or added to the catheter, some models are able to provide the clinician with information about intracranial compliance.[99]

Location of ICP Monitoring Device. ICP can be monitored with a device placed in the epidural space, subdural/subarachnoid space, brain parenchyma, or intraventricular space (Figure 20-19). The advantages and disadvantages of each monitoring location are discussed next.

Epidural Monitoring. Epidural sensors are placed easily between the skull and the dura mater (see Figure 20-19). Because the dura is not penetrated, this method is considered relatively noninvasive, reducing the risk of infection and inadvertent injury to the cerebral vasculature or brain tissue. CSF cannot be drained using this system. Because the sensor may not achieve perfect placement within the plane of the dura and it must detect pressure transmitted across the inelastic dura, the measurements obtained may be less accurate and reliable than intraventricular devices.[63,93] Epidural placement for ICP monitoring is the least desirable

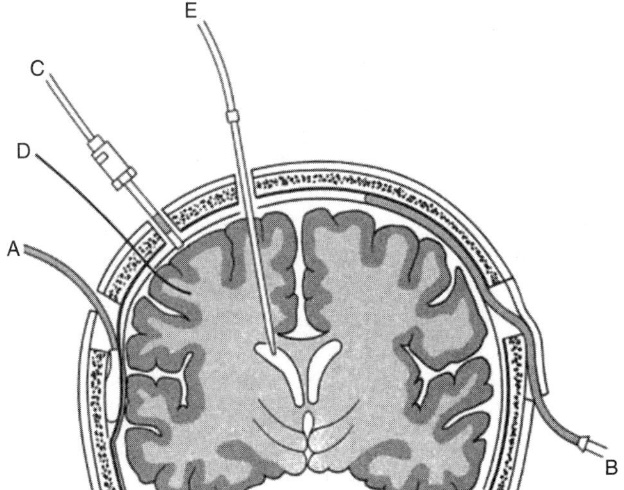

FIGURE 20-19 Coronal section of brain showing potential sites for placement of ICP monitoring devices. **A,** Epidural. **B,** Subdural. **C,** Subarachnoid. **D,** Intraparenchymal. **E,** Intraventricular. (From McNair ND: Intracranial pressure monitoring. In Clochesy JM, Breu C, Cardin S et al, editors: *Critical Care Nursing,* ed 2, Philadelphia, 1996, W.B. Saunders, p. 296.)

means of monitoring ICP when considering accuracy, stability, and ability to drain CSF.[63]

Subdural/Subarachnoid Monitoring. Fiberoptic, fluid-filled strain-gauge, miniature strain-gauge, or air pouch systems can be used to monitor ICP in the subarachnoid or subdural space (see Figure 20-19). The fluid-filled system requires a hollow bolt or screw to be inserted via a twist drill through a hole in the skull and dura into the subarachnoid or subdural space. Fiberoptic and miniature strain-gauge systems can be placed with or without a bolt. Advantages of a subdural/subarachnoid monitoring system include the relative ease of insertion, even in the presence of small compressed ventricles; the lack of brain penetration; and the reduced risk of infection compared with intraventricular monitoring. Disadvantages include possible hemorrhage or hematoma at the insertion site, risk of intracranial infection, and inability to withdraw CSF. CSF leakage from the insertion site is a possible complication with subarachnoid placement. Like epidural sensors, devices placed in these locations tend to be less accurate than monitors placed in the brain parenchyma or ventricle.[63] The skull must be intact for insertion and stabilization of a bolt. Protruding bolts may be inadvertently dislodged.

Intraparenchymal Monitoring. Fiberoptic, miniature strain-gauge, or air pouch systems can be inserted into the brain tissue to monitor intracranial pressure (see Figure 20-19). Intraparenchymal insertion is quick and easy, even when the ventricles are small and compressed. There is little brain penetration, and the readings in this location tend to be accurate and yield a good waveform. Parenchymal transducer-tipped monitoring devices are considered second only to intraventricular monitoring techniques based on their accuracy, stability, and CSF drainage capability.[63] Intracranial infection and the possibility of hemorrhage or hematoma on insertion are potential complications associated with placement of ICP monitors into the brain tissue. CSF cannot be withdrawn with systems placed into the brain parenchyma.

Intraventricular Monitoring. Monitoring intraventricular pressure involves inserting a catheter through the scalp, skull, meninges, and brain tissue into the anterior horn of a lateral ventricle (see Figure 20-19). The ventricular method is used for both diagnostic and therapeutic purposes. It is considered the most accurate and reliable of all ICP monitoring techniques and serves as the reference standard.[63] Intraventricular catheter (IVC) placement also permits CSF removal for analysis, to evaluate brain compliance, or to reduce intracranial volume and decrease ICP.

A fluid-filled, fiberoptic, miniature strain-gauge or pneumatic transducer system can be used to transmit the ICP from the intraventricular location. When a fluid-filled system is used, the transducer is leveled at a designated external anatomic landmark corresponding to the location of the foramen of Monro (Figure 20-6), where the IVC tip is situated. Suggested landmarks include the tragus of the ear, 1 cm posterior to the outer canthus of the eye, the external auditory canal, and halfway between the outer canthus and tragus. Consistent use of the same landmark for leveling the transducer is most important.

CSF may be drained continuously or intermittently through the IVC. A continuous drainage system is open at all times to facilitate the automatic egress of CSF when ICP exceeds a predetermined level. The air-fluid interface of the CSF drip chamber is leveled a prescribed number of centimeters above the designated external landmark for the foramen of Monro. It is recommended that CSF drainage be briefly stopped to obtain an ICP measure, because pressure shunted through the outflow portal may cause artificially low readings. The intermittent method of drainage is essentially a closed system that is opened periodically for drainage when the ICP rises to a specific level. The physician determines the ICP value that prompts drainage, as well as how much CSF should be drained or for how long the drainage should be continued. The nurse should monitor the amount and character of CSF drainage and notify the physician if there is a change in character of the drainage, a sudden increase in drainage, or a lack of CSF drainage.

Several disadvantages are associated with monitoring ICP in the intraventricular space. Insertion can be difficult, particularly when there is ventricular compression or shift. Each repeated attempt to pass the IVC through brain tissue increases the risk of brain or cerebrovascular injury. Excess drainage of CSF may cause ventricular collapse. This complication can be avoided by properly securing and positioning the CSF bag and draining the CSF only as prescribed. Intraventricular ICP monitoring has the highest risk of intracranial infection.[93,100] Routine exchange of IVCs at regular intervals and antibiotic prophylaxis for catheter placement are not recommended to decrease infection.[63] Nurses should ensure that the intraventricular drainage system remains closed, with all portals of entry covered, and that only strict aseptic technique is used if any interruption to the system is necessary.

Extracranial Monitoring. Research is underway to develop a noninvasive system capable of determining ICP or monitoring ICP waveforms. A number of these investigational initiatives use ultrasound technology.[101-103] This type of monitoring system would virtually eliminate any substantial risks associated with the more invasive techniques used to monitor ICP and associated waveforms. The success of such a device could expand the use of ICP monitoring to the prehospital setting and outside the critical care environment.

Quantitative measures of pupillary function obtained using a hand-held pupillometer may help detect the presence of intracranial hypertension in patients with TBI.[104] Taylor et al found that in 13 patients with ICP >20 mm Hg for 15 minutes and midline shift exceeding 3 mm, there was a reduction in ipsilateral pupil constriction velocity. In five patients with diffuse brain swelling, constriction velocities decreased when ICP was >30 mm Hg.[104] Trends indicating a decline in constriction velocity and the percent of pupil reduction are seen in brain-injured patients with intracranial hypertension.[105] There are many medications, environmental factors (light), and clinical conditions that can affect the pupillary measures.[106] Prospective clinical trials are needed to determine the significance of data provided by the pupillometer.

Interpretation of ICP Data. ICP monitoring provides a digital ICP measure. Various interventions and activities (e.g., suctioning, repositioning) may cause transient elevations in ICP. A sustained ICP elevation that reaches or exceeds 20 mm Hg typically indicates the need for therapeutic intervention.[63]

Several limitations should be considered when interpreting ICP. Pressure gradients may exist within different intracranial compartments, which may cause higher ICP in unmonitored compartments to go unnoticed. For example, ICP gradients between the supratentorial and infratentorial compartments and transient interhemispheric pressure gradients have been found in some patients after TBI.[107,108] Neurologic deterioration and CPP insufficiency can occur in the presence of normal ICP. It is essential that nurses not focus solely on the ICP but also consider the neurologic examination, neuroimaging findings, and other monitored parameters when evaluating the patient's condition.

Waveforms displayed during ICP monitoring also require close evaluation. ICP waves originate from cerebrovascular pulsations and correlate with each cardiac systole and diastole. The upward sweep of the wave reflects cardiac systole followed by the diastolic slope and dicrotic notch (Figure 20-20). Natural fluctuations in the ICP pulse wave are caused by small amounts of blood added to the intracranial volume with each systolic ejection. This natural volume stress causes the ICP to increase about 2 mm Hg with each cardiac cycle. Slow oscillation of the entire waveform by a few millimeters of mercury may also be noted, and these fluctuations correlate with the changes in intrathoracic pressure that occur during respiration.

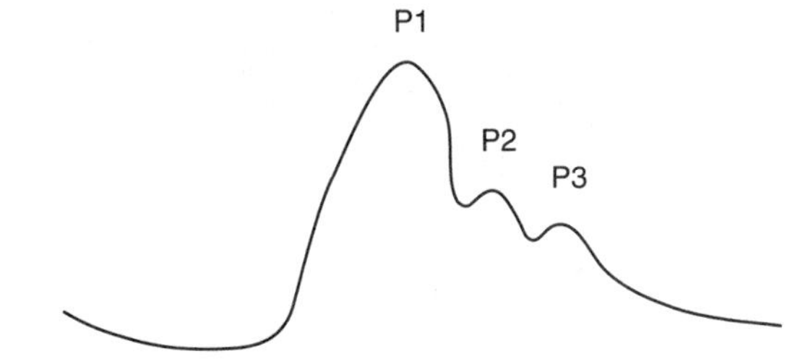

FIGURE 20-20 Components of the intracranial pressure wave.

Each individual ICP wave usually has three peaks. First is P1, the percussion wave, which has fairly consistent amplitude and is believed to originate from pulsations of the choroid plexus and intracranial arteries. P2, the tidal wave, usually has a lower but more variable amplitude. P3, the dicrotic wave, has the lowest amplitude and usually tapers back to baseline.[93]

As the ICP rises, so do the amplitudes of the various waveform components. P2 wave elevations typically exceed the P1 and P3 wave elevations, causing a more rounded appearance of the pressure waveform as the brain's blood volume increases and compliance decreases (Figure 20-21). P2 waves are thought to be a reflection of the brain's compensatory capacity or compliance. When the P2 wave amplitude is elevated (P1:P2 ratio is ≥0.8), the brain's compliance is believed to be reduced, indicating that the brain's ability to compensate for added volume is exhausted.[93] This finding should provide warning that the patient may have significant and persistent ICP elevations in response to stimuli (e.g., suctioning, repositioning), although this is not always the case and these ICP responses may occur without presence of P2 elevation.[93] Advanced ICP waveform analysis (i.e., spectral analysis) techniques require further investigation as a means of dynamically assessing brain compliance and cerebral autoregulation, which could prove helpful in managing patients with TBI.[109]

A dampened ICP waveform configuration usually indicates problems with the monitoring system, although it is often seen when a portion of the cranium has been removed (i.e., after decompressive craniectomy). When the waveform is dampened, every attempt should be made to troubleshoot the system and, if possible, alleviate any problem. If the problem cannot be resolved and an acceptable waveform regained, the physician should be notified. Never assume that the readings are accurate when the waveform is dampened.

In addition to the shape of each waveform, there are three patterns of collected waves or ICP trends: C waves, B waves, and A (plateau) waves. C waves are rapid (4 to 8 minutes), rhythmic, and small in amplitude and correspond to changes in blood pressure (Figure 20-22). No clinical significance has been ascribed to C waves.

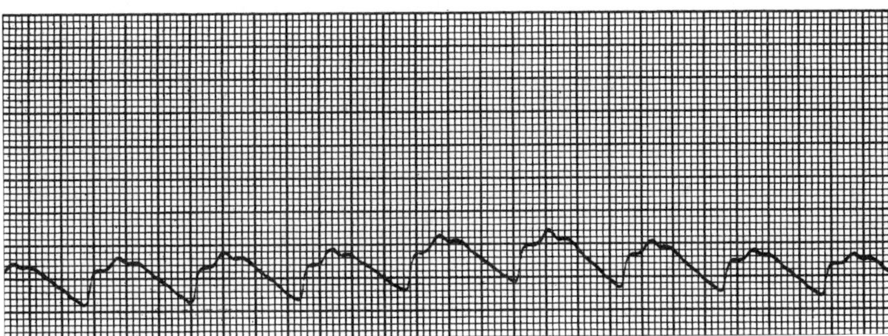

FIGURE 20-21 Intracranial pressure waveforms demonstrate elevation of the P_2 wave component.

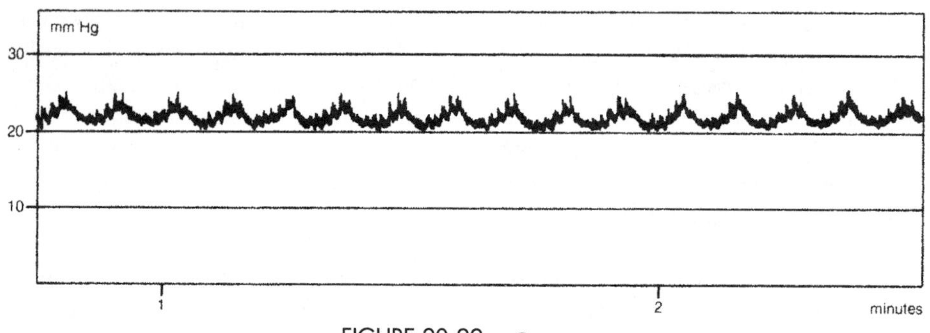

FIGURE 20-22 C waves.

B waves are characterized by sharp, rhythmic elevations of variable amplitude. These elevations occur at 30-second to 2-minute intervals and may reach levels of 20 to 50 mm Hg (Figure 20-23). Elevations typically occur from a normal or slightly elevated baseline and are only a few seconds in duration. B waves may precede the more pathologic plateau or A waves, indicating decreasing intracranial compliance.[93]

A, or plateau, waves are characterized by sustained elevations in ICP as high as 50 to 100 mm Hg, generally lasting 5 to 20 minutes. These elevations, which typically arise from an elevated baseline, can happen at varying intervals and are precipitated by physiologic alterations or occur spontaneously (Figure 20-24). During these elevations, CPP is compromised, possibly causing cerebral ischemia and neurologic deterioration. The presence of A waves demands immediate intervention to control ICP.

Intracranial Compliance. There are two established methods for estimating intracranial compliance: the pressure volume index (PVI) and the volume-pressure response. Both are determined by adding small volumes of saline or removing small volumes of CSF from the intracranial space. Due to risk for infection, potential inaccuracies, and difficulties in performing the intermittent measures, these invasive methods of estimating compliance are not routinely used.[110] Noninvasive methods that allow serial measurements of compliance have been investigated, but good data acquisition is still not possible.[111,112] A technique to continuously monitor intracranial compliance has been developed, but clinical use remains limited.[110,113]

Patient observation may provide a rough approximation of brain compliance. Brain-injured patients who show substantial or sustained ICP elevations in response to changes in head

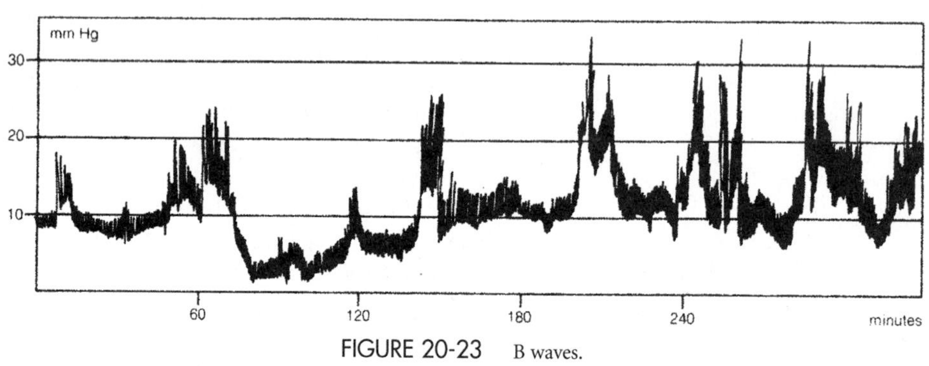

FIGURE 20-23 B waves.

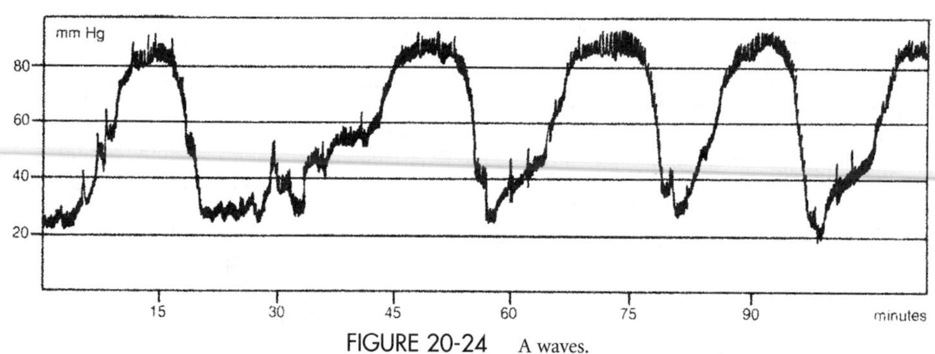

FIGURE 20-24 A waves.

position, turning, suctioning, or noxious stimulation should be suspected of having decreased compliance and should be treated accordingly. As previously described, the patient's ICP waveform can also demonstrate specific morphologic changes that indicate poor intracranial compliance.

Cerebral Blood Flow.

CBF disturbances leading to cerebral ischemia are a significant pathophysiological cause of disability or death following brain injury.[40,62,114] Unfortunately, there is no clinical symptom associated with reduced CBF until it decreases to a level that is unacceptably close to the threshold of permanent neuronal damage. Multiple techniques exist that enable practitioners to evaluate CBF directly or indirectly, although no one technique is perfect and without limitations or disadvantages.

Cerebral Perfusion Pressure. Currently the most frequently used indirect index of global cerebral perfusion is cerebral perfusion pressure. CPP is easily monitored and calculated at the bedside by subtracting the ICP from the mean arterial blood pressure. Kirkness et al found that when compared to patients randomized to have CPP displayed on a less visible traditional monitor screen, those who had a prominent, real-time, continuous display of CPP, particularly those with more severe initial TBI, had significantly better odds of survival and condition at discharge.[115] A more obvious display of active CPP may foster more timely intervention to remedy values that exceed acceptable parameters, which may contribute to poorer patient outcomes.[115,116] Although normal CPP is considered to be 50 to 150 mm Hg, after TBI it is desirable to aim for a CPP value between 50 and 70 mm Hg.[63]

CPP is not a specific or sensitive measure of CBF. CPP values may be within normal limits, even though blood flow to the brain is inadequate. This measure also does not consider regional distribution of brain perfusion.

Clinicians have questioned if therapy for the patient with severe TBI should be targeted toward minimizing ICP or maximizing CPP and CBF. Robertson et al[117] compared a CBF-targeted protocol for TBI management, in which CPP was maintained higher than 70 mm Hg and $PaCo_2$ was kept at approximately 35 torr, with an ICP-targeted protocol, in which CPP was maintained at more than 50 mm Hg and the $PaCo_2$ was kept between 25 and 30 torr. Treatment was provided for ICP greater than 20 mm Hg and jugular venous oxygen saturation (Sjo_2) less than 50% for patients randomized to either treatment group. Results showed that the risk of brain ischemia more than doubled with the use of the ICP-targeted protocol, and secondary ischemic insults could be prevented with the CBF-managed protocol. However, there was no difference in neurologic outcome. A fivefold increase in the frequency of acute respiratory distress syndrome (ARDS) was found in patients treated with the CBF-targeted protocol. Therefore, although ischemic insults were reduced substantially with the CBF-targeted protocol, the adverse effects of ARDS may offset these beneficial effects.[117] For this reason, the most recent edition of the *Guidelines for Management of Severe Traumatic Brain Injury* recommends avoiding aggressive volume loading and pressor use to maintain the CPP above 70 mm Hg.[63] Low CPP also has been associated with poorer outcomes.[61,116,118] Therefore, the *Guidelines for Management of Severe Traumatic Brain Injury* suggest avoiding a CPP less than 50 mm Hg.[63] Other studies demonstrate that ICP above 20 mm Hg can worsen outcomes in patients with TBI.[61,54] Desirable therapeutic endpoints for the patient with severe TBI should include maintaining the ICP at less than 20 mm Hg and targeting a CPP value between 50 and 70 mm Hg.[63] Other parameters, such as measures of CBF, oxygenation, or metabolism, may serve as useful guides in selecting and achieving the optimal CPP for a specific patient.[63]

Intermittent Measures of Cerebral Blood Flow: Perfusion Computed Tomography Scan. Perfusion CT provides rapid quantitative and qualitative assessment of regional cerebral perfusion, including measures of CBF, cerebral blood volume (CBV), and mean transit time ([MTT]: average time it takes for the blood to pass from the middle cerebral artery to the venous sinus).[119] This technique involves acquisition of multiple sequential CT images during or just after intravenous administration of iodinated contrast material. These CT images are analyzed with specialized software to provide maps describing the perfusion parameter values.[119,120] Wintermark et al[121] demonstrated that perfusion CT provides insight into regional perfusion alterations associated with brain injury, cerebral edema, and intracranial hypertension and is more sensitive than conventional noncontrast head CT in detecting cerebral contusions. Perfusion CT done upon admission in patients with severe TBI may provide prognostic information with respect to functional outcome.[121] When continuous CPP measures are considered together with perfusion CT results, it may allow clinicians to evaluate patients' cerebral autoregulation, which can guide interpretation of CPP measurements and ultimately therapy.[120] More recent research supports use of perfusion CT to provide direct and quantitative evaluation of cerebral autoregulation in patients with severe TBI and evidence of cerebral edema.[122]

Continuous Bedside Monitoring of Cortical Blood Flow. Regional cerebral cortical blood flow can be monitored continuously using thermal diffusion flowmetry or laser Doppler flowmetry techniques. Thermal diffusion flowmetry uses a thermal diffusion sensor placed directly on the brain cortex, away from large blood vessels. Microprobes that can be placed into the brain parenchyma have also been investigated and results are promising.[123,124] Temperature differences between two plates on the sensor can be detected, providing an inverse measure proportional to CBF.[124,125] Laser Doppler flowmetry uses a low-power laser light positioned on the cortical surface or in the brain parenchyma to provide a measure of regional CBF.[125] Continuous measure of CBF can be used to detect regional ischemia, monitor autoregulation, and serve as an additional guide for treatment of TBI.

Continuous regional cerebral cortical blood flow monitoring devices evaluate blood flow in a small focal area and do not provide information about perfusion in other areas of the brain. Both devices are invasive and, therefore, carry the risk of intracranial infection and CSF leakage. Loss of probe contact with the cerebral cortex or contact with large surface vessels causes data to be unreliable. Artifacts caused by probe movement and change in hematocrit can also alter laser Doppler flowmetry measurements.[125]

Functional Neuroimaging. Functional neuroimaging studies, including PET and SPECT, provide measures of regional cerebral blood flow and metabolic activity and thus furnish information about the functional status of brain tissue.[22,86] PET uses positron-emitting radionuclide tracers and a scanner to obtain data which are used to calculate global and regional cerebral blood flow and provide quantitative measures of other physiologic functions, such as regional variations in cerebral oxygen utilization and glucose metabolism. PET scanning affords quantitative cross-sectional or three-dimensional images depicting cerebral blood flow and metabolism.[22] Single-photon emission CT uses commercially available radionuclide tracers and a rotating gamma camera to measure and provide cross-sectional and three-dimensional images of regional cerebral blood flow distribution.[22] Because metabolism is directly linked to regional blood flow, this method provides an indirect measure of brain metabolism.[22] Although PET and SPECT scans and functional MRI are not used in routine management of acute TBI, these studies may detect areas of brain ischemia, metabolic abnormality, and cerebral dysfunction not identified on CT scan or MRI.[22,86,126,127] Findings may have some significance in determining prognosis and guiding long-term therapy after TBI.[86]

fMRI creates images of blood flow in the brain using magnetic properties of hemoglobin. Patients are scanned while performing cognitive tasks. Blood flow increases in areas of the brain where there is increased regional neuronal activity, allowing abnormal brain function to be detected.[22] fMRI may be a more sensitive indicator of brain injury than cognitive testing after concussion.[128]

Functional neuroimaging studies provide only a snapshot of cerebral blood flow, metabolism, or functional activity. Patients require transport to the scanner used for the imaging study, and the patient's head must remain immobilized during the test. Despite these limitations and disadvantages, the ability of functional neuroimaging studies to provide helpful information about the physiologic status of the injured brain is likely to expand their use in the future.

Transcranial Doppler Ultrasonography. Transcranial Doppler (TCD) ultrasonography uses a low-frequency pulsed ultrasonic signal that penetrates thin areas of the cranium to measure the velocity and direction of blood flow in major intracranial arteries. A TCD study cannot quantify blood flow to the brain, but its measures are affected by CBF. Flow velocity is proportional to CBF, as long as the vessel diameter and angle of insonation remain constant.[124] If CBF remains constant, the flow velocity is inversely proportional to the cross-sectional area of the vessel being examined.[129] The pulsatility index, describing variability in maximal systolic and diastolic flow velocities, can be calculated to provide an indirect measure of the resistance in distal vessels.[130]

This noninvasive, portable technique can be performed repeatedly or continuously (with a Doppler probe secured to the patient's temporal scalp) to detect posttraumatic cerebral hemodynamic changes and complications (e.g., vasospasm, hyperemia, cerebral blood flow reduction, and circulatory arrest). TCD studies also can be used to evaluate the status of cerebral metabolic and vasomotor autoregulation and to confirm clinically diagnosed brain death.[129,131] This assessment strategy may also be valuable in detecting emboli or identifying vascular anomalies that may be premorbid or occurred as a result of cerebrovascular injury. Despite its benefits, the measures are technician sensitive and the study is difficult to perform on uncooperative patients who do not remain still. Factors that influence CBF (e.g., $PaCO_2$, hematocrit) must be considered when interpreting TCD findings.

Cerebral Oxygenation Measures

Jugular Venous Oxygen Saturation and Arteriojugular Oxygen Content Difference. SjO_2 is a measure of the hemoglobin's oxygen saturation level as the venous blood exits the brain. SjO_2 reflects the relative balance between cerebral oxygen consumption and cerebral oxygen delivery, as long as hemoglobin levels, oxygen saturation of hemoglobin in the arterial blood (SaO_2), and the oxyhemoglobin dissociation curve remain constant.[132] Whereas CBF is normally coupled with the metabolic demand of the brain, following TBI this coupled relationship is often lost.[133] Monitoring SjO_2 allows for assessment of the global cerebral oxygen supply (flow) and demand (metabolism) balance.[134]

SjO_2 is monitored via a catheter placed into an internal jugular vein, with the catheter tip threaded retrograde to the jugular bulb, where the jugular vein curves before descending from the cranial vault. A lateral skull film typically is performed after insertion to confirm placement of the catheter tip in the jugular bulb. Intermittent jugular venous blood samples can be obtained from the catheter and sent to the lab for SjO_2 determination, or a fiberoptic oximetric catheter may be inserted into the jugular bulb to measure SjO_2 continuously.

SjO_2 values may be affected by factors that alter cerebral oxygen delivery or the cerebral metabolic rate of oxygen. When cerebral oxygen delivery is insufficient to meet the brain's metabolic need for oxygen, cerebral hypoxia and ischemia occur and SjO_2 declines. Factors that reduce the oxygen supply to the brain include systemic hypoxemia, anemia, and reduced cerebral perfusion caused by intracranial hypertension, hypotension, hypovolemia, hypocapnea, or cerebral vasoconstriction.[134] Factors that increase the cerebral metabolic rate of oxygen include seizures, pain, agitation, and hyperthermia. SjO_2 desaturations, particularly if the episodes are multiple or prolonged, are associated with poorer outcome after TBI.[134-138] If cerebral oxygen delivery exceeds the metabolic demand for oxygen in the brain, the Sjo_2 rises. Sjo_2 becomes elevated when there is an increased supply of oxygen to the brain, as seen with hyperemic or hyperoxia states, or when there is a decreased demand for oxygen utilization in the brain, as seen with sedation, hypothermia, anesthesia, or large areas of cerebral infarction.[133] Elevations in Sjo_2 caused by reduction in the cerebral oxygen metabolism rate have been associated with poor outcomes.[132]

With knowledge of the Sao_2 and Sjo_2, the cerebral extraction of oxygen (CEo_2) can be calculated (Table 20-7). A low CEo_2 indicates that the brain's supply of oxygen is greater than its demand for oxygen. A high CEo_2 indicates that the supply of oxygen is less than the demand.

Arteriojugular venous oxygen content difference ($Avjdo_2$) is calculated by subtracting the content of jugular venous oxygen from the content of arterial oxygen (see Table 20-7). $Avjdo_2$ provides an indication of the overall balance between oxygen consumption and CBF. Elevations in $Avjdo_2$ occur when the CBF and oxygen delivery are inadequate for the brain's demand for oxygen. When the $Avjdo_2$ is reduced, CBF and oxygen delivery are excessive for the brain's demand for oxygen. If the cerebral metabolic rate is constant, then relative changes in CBF can be reflected and are inversely proportional to changes in $Avjdo_2$.[124]

Direct and derived measures obtained by Sjo_2 monitoring can be helpful in the clinical setting, where practitioners are striving to ensure adequate supply of oxygen to meet the brain's metabolic demand in an effort to reduce brain ischemia and secondary injury. Cruz compared the outcomes of patients with severe TBI and intracranial hypertension whose therapy was guided by CPP only with the outcomes of similar patients whose therapy was guided by CPP and CEo_2. The use of both CPP and CEo_2 as therapeutic guides yielded better outcomes, as measured by the Glasgow Outcome Scale (GOS).[139] Sjo_2 monitoring parameters may assist the clinician in selecting the most appropriate interventions for ICP management and help define the patient's most desirable CPP (refer to the management section).

There are a number of disadvantages and limitations of Sjo_2 monitoring. Potential complications of this monitoring technique include infection, vascular injury, and vascular thrombosis. Nurses need to be proficient at maintaining, regularly calibrating, and troubleshooting the oximetric monitoring system. Artifacts are common with oximetric Sjo_2 monitoring. Catheter malposition or breakage, or formation of a fibrin clot on the tip of the catheter may make the readings inaccurate. If the catheter becomes malpositioned or blood is aspirated too quickly from the jugular line, extracranial blood contamination can artificially elevate Sjo_2.[124] Using this monitoring strategy, relatively small focal areas of ischemia may go undetected, and Sjo_2 may not decline until significant cerebral ischemia has occurred.[124]

Partial Pressure of Brain Tissue Oxygen. Continuous partial pressure of brain tissue oxygen ($Pbro_2$) can be measured after introduction of an electrode into the brain parenchyma. While always placed in the brain's white matter, there is lack of consensus, and it is the physician's preference as to where the probe is placed with respect to the injury (i.e., in the penumbra near the injured site or in the relatively uninjured hemisphere).[105] This monitoring technique is a safe and reliable method for continuous measure of regional brain oxygen tension.[140-142] Although some researchers cite the $Pbro_2$ threshold for cerebral ischemia as less than

TABLE 20-7 **Sjo_2, CEo_2, and $AvjDO_2$ Normal Values and Calculations for Derived Parameters**

Parameter	Source	Normal Values
Jugular venous oxygen saturation ($Sjvo_2$)	Directly measured	55% to 75% <50% is the recommended threshold for treatment in the *Guidelines for Management of Severe Traumatic Brain Injury,* 2007
Cerebral extraction of oxygen (CEo_2)	Calculated $Sao_2 - Sjo_2$	24% to 40% <24% oxygen supply greater than demand >40% oxygen supply insufficient for demand
Arteriojugular venous difference of oxygen ($AvjDO_2$)= $CMRo_2$/CBF	Calculated $Cao_2 - Cjvo_2$ $Cao_2 = (Sao_2 \times 1.34 \times Hb) + (Pao_2 \times .0031)$ $Cjvo_2 = (Sjo_2 \times 1.34 \times Hb) + (Pjvo_2 \times .0031)$ OR $(Sao_2 - Sjo_2) \times 1.34 \times Hb + \mathit{(Pao_2 \times Pjvo_2) \times 0.0031}$ (Sometimes the relatively small contribution of dissolved oxygen in italics is ignored to simplify calculation and value is expressed in vol %)	4.5 to 8.5 ml/dl <4.5 ml/dl oxygen supply greater than demand >8.5 ml/dl oxygen supply insufficient for demand

Sao_2, Oxygen saturation of hemoglobin in the arterial blood; *Pao_2,* Partial pressure of oxygen in arterial blood; *Hb,* Hemoglobin; *$CMRo_2$;* Cerebral metabolic rate of oxygen; *CBF,* Cerebral blood flow; *Sjo_2,* Jugular venous oxygen saturation; *$Pjvo_2$,* Partial pressure of oxygen in jugular venous blood; *Cao_2,* Arterial oxygen content; *$Cjvo_2$,* Jugular venous oxygen content.

Note: Normal values and calculations reported in the literature vary.

20 mm Hg, most report the critical value to be less than 10 to 15 mm Hg.[141,143-145] The current recommendation made in the *Guidelines for Management of Severe Traumatic Brain Injury* as an option for care is to use a Pbro$_2$ <15 mm Hg as the threshold for treatment.[63] Brain Po$_2$ is a predictor of outcome, with the duration and depth of brain tissue hypoxia related to unfavorable patient outcome and death.[141,143,144] Stiefel et al compared 28 patients who where treated with ICP (maintained at <20 mm Hg) and Pbro$_2$ (maintained at >25 mm Hg) used as therapeutic endpoints with 25 historical controls who only had ICP monitoring and found that when brain tissue Po$_2$-directed care was used, mortality decreased from 44% to 25%.[145]

Biochemical Monitoring of the Injured Brain

Brain injury and ischemia produce numerous biochemical byproducts, which can be measured in the brain tissue, cerebral spinal fluid, or blood. Examples of substrates that are elevated in response to brain tissue damage include neuron-specific enolase, glial fibrillary acidic protein, cleaved tau protein, myelin-basic protein, brain natriuretic peptide, and S-100.[146,147] Measurement of these substrates in the serum or CSF may provide information about the extent or severity of TBI, detect ongoing secondary brain injury, determine need for follow-up diagnostic studies, and help predict the patient's outcome.[146] When a retrograde jugular venous catheter is in place, the arteriovenous difference in the levels of certain metabolites, such as glucose and lactate, can be measured to detect cerebral ischemia or metabolic dysfunction.[148] Some researchers have identified variables unrelated to brain injury that may confound interpretation of these measures and have questioned the reliability of some markers in predicting brain injury or ischemia.[149-151] Additional studies are necessary to determine how these biomarkers can best guide therapy and predict outcome from TBI.[146]

The biochemical milieu of the brain tissue can be monitored directly at frequent intervals by use of cerebral microdialysis. Substances from local extracellular fluid diffuse across a semipermeable membrane into perfusate that flows continuously through a microdialysis probe inserted into brain tissue. Dialysate coming from the probe is sampled at regular intervals and analyzed to determine its chemical composition, which reflects that of the extracellular fluid in the brain. Although this technology is capable of collecting any molecule able to cross the semipermeable membrane, the metabolites typically assessed in patients with TBI are glucose, lactate, pyruvate, lactate:pyruvate ratio, glycerol, and glutamate.[152,153] Monitoring the neurochemical composition of the brain may provide insight into the pathophysiological mechanisms of secondary TBI (e.g., hypoxia, ischemia, excitotoxicity, cell membrane degradation, substrate availability), the nature and magnitude of cerebral damage, the response to therapy, and the prognosis of the patient.[152,153] Currently, cerebral microdialysis is not used extensively in clinical settings. A few centers have the capability or resources required, but developments in this monitoring technique and better understanding of how the data may guide treatment may expand its future clinical application.

MRS utilizes MRI technology to offer a noninvasive approach for measuring neurochemicals, such as *N*-acetylaspartate, lactate, lipid, choline, myo-inositol, creatine, phosphocreatine, and glutamate, in the brain. This technology can detect altered metabolite concentrations caused by brain injury, hypoxia and ischemia.[154] MRS may be useful in identifying metabolite alterations associated with brain injury not visible on conventional CT scan or MRI.[154-156] Findings from MRS may also assist in predicting patient outcome after TBI.[154,156] MRS does have technical limitations that prohibit its use with certain patients, including those with metallic implants and those who cannot remain still during the test.

Electrophysiologic Monitoring

Electroencephalogram. Using scalp electrodes, an EEG measures the spontaneous electrical activity of the superficial layers of the cerebral cortex. EEG findings are influenced by cerebral metabolism and brain ischemia or hypoxia, but they can also be affected by electrical, biologic, environmental, and movement artifacts, as well as drug therapy administered to the patient. After TBI an EEG may be used to detect electrical abnormalities associated with insufficient cerebral perfusion, cortical dysfunction, or seizure activity.[157,158] The degree of cerebral suppression achieved with induction of a drug-induced (e.g., barbiturate) coma for the management of intracranial hypertension or status epilepticus may also be determined using electroencephalographic monitoring. EEG may be used to confirm clinically diagnosed brain death.

A quantitative processed or computerized EEG, often used for continuous bedside EEG monitoring, uses a computer that manipulates and compresses data so that it can be displayed in a fashion that is easier to interpret by the bedside practitioner.[158] This technique allows evaluation of trend data and may enhance abnormalities difficult to visualize on a raw EEG, but it may miss short-lived events. In addition, results can be affected by numerous physiologic and technical variables.[158] Nurses caring for a patient on a continuous EEG monitor should be knowledgeable about the normal and abnormal EEG patterns and understand what action should be taken if abnormalities become apparent.

Bispectral Index Monitoring. Bispectral index monitoring (BIS) uses a four-lead sensor and monitor to obtain a statistically derived parameter of the EEG that is expressed as a score between 0 (no brain activity) and 100 (fully awake).[159,160] Currently this tool is used in critical care and intraoperative settings to guide and evaluate sedation and anesthetic administration. In critically ill patients with nontrauma-related brain injury, a statistically significant correlation between the BIS scores and standard sedation scale scores was found.[159] In a small study of 12 patients receiving high-dose barbiturates for high ICP, the BIS score was found to correlate well with the suppression ratio, suggesting this method of monitoring may prove helpful in evaluating the effectiveness of this therapy.[161] BIS values measured after sedation was withdrawn for at least 24 hours were shown to be significantly different between patients who regained consciousness after TBI and those who did not.[162] BIS scores measured in the emergency department prior to administration of sedation were found to be predictive of brain injury and neurologic outcome at discharge. There are some concerns about the reliability and validity of BIS monitoring in brain injured patients.[159] Potential artifact from outside interference and physiologic factors can affect BIS monitoring.

Sensory Evoked Potentials. Sensory evoked potentials (SEP) are small electrical responses generated along a sensory pathway in response to direct stimulation. Functional integrity of the visual, somatosensory, and auditory brainstem pathways can be assessed by evaluating the evoked potentials generated as each of these pathways is stimulated. SEPs are quantified by measuring the amplitude, latency from stimulation to response, and conduction time of the waveform generated by computer analysis of numerous evoked potentials.[163,164] Auditory brainstem evoked potentials, activated by tones and clicking sounds, and somatosensory evoked potentials, activated by peripheral nerve (e.g., median nerve) stimulation, are most commonly evaluated after severe TBI.[164] These studies can be performed at the bedside by a skilled technician, and results are relatively immune to the effects of sedatives. SEPs, particularly somatosensory evoked potentials, correlate well with patient outcome after severe TBI, and therefore may be considered when predicting patient prognosis.[163,165,166]

MANAGEMENT

PRIMARY PREVENTION

Because there is no treatment currently available to treat primary brain injury effectively, prevention of TBI is of utmost importance. Improvements in roadway safety measures, such as lowering speed limits, and installing red-light cameras,[167] speed enforcement detection devices,[168] area-wide traffic calming schemes,[169] roadside barriers, and traffic signage, contribute to reductions in motor vehicle crashes. Better motor vehicle safety features (e.g., improved ability to absorb impact, occupant restraint systems, and air bags)[170,171] and use of approved helmet protection[172,173] assist in decreasing the number and severity of injuries. These safety initiatives, as well as legislative and educational efforts to increase the use of seat belts, child safety seats and helmets, and to decrease the incidence of driving while intoxicated, have likely combined to reduce motor vehicle-related TBI deaths. Despite the decline in deaths caused by transportation-related TBI, the increase in falls-related TBI deaths, primarily among the elderly, indicates a need to focus strategies on curbing this problem.[174] Continued efforts to reduce violence-related trauma is another area where prevention initiatives may foster a reduction in brain injury deaths and disability. Development of new, more effective, targeted strategies to prevent TBI and continuation of initiatives with proven success require ongoing, standardized surveillance of TBI incidence, risk factors, causes, and outcomes. Refer to Chapter 6 on injury prevention for more information on this topic.

GOALS OF CARE

There are three goals that nurses, together with the rest of the multidisciplinary health care team, strive to achieve when caring for a patient who has sustained TBI. First is to restore or maintain brain function, which focuses interventions on preventing secondary brain injury. The second goal is to prevent, recognize, and treat potential neurologic and systemic complications, which may increase mortality and morbidity and can exacerbate secondary brain injury. Third is to maintain and enhance the brain-injured patient's cognitive, psychosocial, and emotional processes. Achievement of these goals fosters optimal patient outcomes.

ESTABLISHED GUIDELINES AND RECOMMENDATIONS FOR CARE

In response to study results demonstrating considerable variations in treatment among institutions,[175] the Brain Trauma Foundation, the American Association of Neurological Surgeons, and the Joint Section on Neurotrauma and Critical Care formed a panel of experts to compile evidenced-based guidelines for management of severe TBI. *The Guidelines for the Management of Severe Traumatic Brain Injury* was first published in 1995 and updated in 2000 and again in 2007.[63] In addition to these guidelines, others focusing on unique aspects of TBI management have been developed.[176-181] Adoption of evidenced-based guideline recommendations into practice has proven successful in improving outcome from TBI.[182-184]

RESUSCITATION PHASE

Priorities during resuscitation of the patient with severe TBI are the same as those used with any trauma patient—that is, ensuring adequate airway, breathing, and circulation. Accomplishing these priorities is essential to prevent numerous factors that can cause secondary brain injury, such as hypoxia, hypotension, ischemia, and hypercapnia. Once these initial priorities are accomplished, efforts can be directed toward neurologic assessment and continued treatment of the TBI.

Injury Database

As with any trauma, an injury database is obtained from the prehospital care providers. The database includes all possible information about the onset and cause of injury, as well as significant events surrounding the traumatic event. It is important to document the patient's baseline neurologic status while in the field and changes that occur during transport to the hospital. Intervention provided by prehospital care providers and the patient's responses to these efforts should be noted.

Airway Patency

Airway obstruction causing inadequate ventilation can transform a potentially mild brain injury into a severe brain injury as a result of hypoxia and hypercapnia. TBI sequelae put the patient at risk for airway obstruction. When level of consciousness decreases, the patient's upper airway relaxes and the tongue can prolapse back, obstructing the airway. Cough, swallow, and gag reflexes may be diminished or absent after TBI, which leaves the airway unprotected and puts the patient at increased risk for aspiration and secretion retention. Vomiting at or near the time of injury is common and increases the likelihood of aspiration. Possible associated maxillofacial injuries may also heighten predisposition for airway obstruction.

When airway patency is impaired, interventions to alleviate the problem take precedence and are instituted immediately. Because 4% to 8% of patients with TBI also have spinal cord injury, great care must be taken to maintain cervical alignment during any attempt to reestablish airway patency.[185,186] The chin-lift or jaw-thrust maneuver may be all that is needed to open the airway. The oropharynx should be suctioned to clear secretions and foreign debris.

Care must be taken when using devices that assist in maintaining airway patency. Oral airways are used to prevent the tongue from falling back and occluding the airway, but they may stimulate coughing and gagging, thereby exacerbating intracranial hypertension. Nasopharyngeal airways are contraindicated in patients with suspected basilar skull fractures, because intracranial intubation may result. If protective airway reflexes are depressed or the patient's decreased level of consciousness impairs airway control, tracheal intubation is required.

Patients with an initial GCS score of 8 or less generally require immediate endotracheal intubation. Intubation is usually performed in the prehospital phase by a trained provider or during the inhospital resuscitation phase using an endotracheal tube, preferably via the orotracheal route, while maintaining inline manual cervical immobilization. The reported impact of prehospital intubation on outcome has varied with some researchers suggesting intubation in the field may worsen outcomes while others have demonstrated this practice is beneficial for patients with TBI.[187-190] Ideally, a prospective randomized trial that controls for oxygenation and carbon dioxide levels is needed to better define which patients with TBI benefit from prehospital intubation. Cricothyroidotomy or tracheostomy may be necessary to establish an airway if an endotracheal tube cannot be placed. Sedative or paralytic agents are frequently required to facilitate intubation. Short-acting or easily reversible agents are preferable. If possible, a rapid neurologic assessment should be performed before administration of these pharmacologic agents.

Once a patent airway is established, measures to maintain a clear airway must be initiated. Endotracheal suctioning is provided as needed. Bronchoscopy may be used to clear secretions, vomitus, blood, teeth, and other debris from the airway. Gastric decompression using an orogastric tube in addition to early intubation reduces the risk of aspiration.

Supplemental Oxygen

Supplemental oxygen should be administered to ensure adequate cerebral oxygen supply. The initial fraction of inspired oxygen (Fio_2) delivered to patients with severe TBI is usually 100%. Once an arterial blood gas reading can be obtained, the Fio_2 can be adjusted to maintain the Pao_2 well above 60 mm Hg,[63] preferably >70 mm Hg, and some advocate around 90 to 100 mm Hg.[160] Pulse oximetry can be used to titrate oxygen administration to maintain a desired oxygen saturation well above 90%,[63] preferably >94%,[191] and, again, some advocate at 100%.[160] Administration of 100% oxygen before and after intermittent tracheal suctioning or intubation is important to prevent hypoxemia during these interventions.

A number of researchers have explored the use of hyperoxia to improve cerebral oxygen delivery and aerobic metabolism.[192-194] In patients with TBI, although cerebral oxygenation parameters increased and lactate levels fell during short-term administration of 100% Fio_2, brain oxygen metabolism did not improve.[192-194] These findings, together with lack of clarity around the amount and duration of oxygen administration that causes toxicity, and concerns about adverse effects of excessive oxygen use, particularly for prolonged periods, suggest that unnecessary administration of 100% oxygen is not indicated for routine use in management of patients with acute TBI.

Adequate Ventilation

Central nervous system injuries frequently result in abnormal and ineffective breathing patterns. Not only CNS dysfunction, but also drugs with respiratory depressant effects and chest injuries can impair ventilation. Impaired ventilation leads to hypoxia and hypercapnia, which can potentiate intracranial hypertension and exacerbate secondary brain injury. Therefore, prevention or immediate resolution of insufficient ventilation is a priority in brain injury management.

Nurses should assess the patient's respiratory status, paying particular attention to the respiratory rate and rhythm, chest excursion, breath sounds, and gas exchange effectiveness. Use of devices such as pulse oximetry and end-tidal Co_2 monitoring to continuously evaluate oxygenation and carbon dioxide levels or evaluating serial blood gases is essential in guiding oxygen and ventilatory therapy in the resuscitation phase. Once an airway is established, if ventilation is still deemed inadequate, the patient should be given assistance. Initially an Ambu bag can be used for manual ventilation. Mechanical ventilation may be required until the patient is able to breathe sufficiently without assistance. Carbon dioxide levels should be normalized and, in patients with severe TBI, should be maintained in the low normal range (around 35 to 38 mm Hg).[191] Hyperventilation of the patient should be avoided for 24 hours after injury and is only indicated if needed as a temporizing measure to decrease intracranial hypertension.[63]

Adequate Systemic and Cerebral Perfusion

Once airway patency and adequate ventilation have been established, the priority becomes circulatory stabilization. Circulatory instability resulting in hypotension rarely occurs secondary to brain injury itself, unless there has been prolonged medullary compression and brain death is imminent. Hemorrhagic shock as a result of blood loss from extracranial injury is the primary cause of systemic hypotension and consequent cerebral hypoperfusion during brain injury resuscitation. Hypotension (systolic blood pressure $<$90 mm Hg), present in approximately 35% of brain-injured patients from the time of injury through resuscitation, is predictive of a poorer outcome and should be corrected immediately.[50,51,53,55,57-59]

Intravascular volume must be restored and cardiac pump function must be optimized to restore circulatory stability. External and internal hemorrhage must be identified and controlled. Isotonic crystalloids, sometimes colloids, and, when appropriate, blood products should be infused to achieve a euvolemic state. Hypotonic solutions, such as D_5W, should be avoided because they reduce the osmolarity of the intravascular volume, which encourages fluid leakage out of the intravascular space, thereby exacerbating cerebral edema. Multiple animal and human studies have demonstrated positive effects when hypertonic saline, sometimes combined with dextran-containing solutions, are used during resuscitation of patients with TBI.[195-198] The use of hypertonic solutions to achieve cardiovascular stability is associated with a need for smaller fluid volumes and has fewer complications (e.g., cerebral edema and intracranial hypertension). Despite these findings, a double-blind, randomized, controlled trial comparing the effect of 250 ml administration of 7.5% hypertonic saline versus lactated Ringer's solution, in addition to other resuscitation fluids administered to hypotensive patients with severe TBI in the prehospital setting, failed to demonstrate any difference in the mortality or neurological outcome between the two groups.[199] The role of hypertonic saline solution for resuscitation of patients with TBI remains unclear.

The patient's hemodynamic status (e.g., heart rate, blood pressure, central venous pressure) and clinical findings indicating sufficiency of tissue perfusion (e.g., capillary refill time, urine output, acid-base balance, lactate levels) should guide the volume of fluid provided during resuscitation. Care should be taken to avoid fluid overload, which may exacerbate cerebral edema. If the patient's hypotension is unresponsive to fluid therapy, other causes, such as spinal shock, must be ruled out. Once adequate intravascular volume replacement has been ensured, consideration should be given to administration of inotropic and vasoactive agents in order to support blood pressure. Refer to Chapter 14 for additional information on the management of traumatic shock.

Baseline and Ongoing Clinical Examination

It is imperative for a baseline neurological assessment to be obtained as soon as possible and that the patient be monitored closely to determine if brain function deteriorates or improves over time. If cerebral hypoperfusion and hypoxia are contributing to the patient's altered mentation, sensorium should improve as oxygenation and perfusion deficits are corrected. Responses to various therapeutic interventions should be noted. Alterations in mental status caused by drug use generally resolve as the drugs are metabolized. If there is a high suspicion that the patient took an excessive amount of narcotic before injury, naloxone (Narcan) may be administered during resuscitation to reverse the narcotic effects. Metabolic disorders, such as hypoglycemia, hyperglycemia, and electrolyte imbalances, should be corrected promptly.

A CT scan of the brain is obtained as soon as possible for patients who present with an altered level of consciousness. If an operable lesion is confirmed, the patient should be prepared immediately for surgery. Delay in surgical intervention to remove an acute subdural hematoma can escalate patient mortality and morbidity.[21]

Analgesia, Sedation, and Control of Agitation

Pain and agitation must be controlled to decrease cerebral metabolic requirements, reduce ICP, facilitate effective ventilation, provide patient comfort and safety, and allow diagnostic and therapeutic procedures. Severe pain is most likely caused by extracranial sources, because the brain tissue itself lacks pain receptors. Agitation frequently accompanies TBI; however, other causes for agitation, such as hypoxia or electrolyte imbalance, must be ruled out before attributing the altered mental status solely to craniocerebral trauma.

Sedatives and analgesics should be administered judiciously to brain-injured patients, because their use can blunt clinical indications of neurologic deterioration. Management of pain and agitation is based on individual patient assessment. Before administration of sedatives or analgesia, a complete baseline neurologic examination and pain assessment should be completed. Precise anatomic areas of pain or tenderness should be identified when possible.

If the patient is awake and complains of mild discomfort, the first drug of choice for pain relief should be a non-CNS depressant (i.e., a mild analgesic, such as acetaminophen [Tylenol]). When other agents are necessary to control pain, the smallest possible dosages of short-acting or easily reversible analgesic agents are preferred. Morphine is one preferred agent for pain management because it is easily reversed with naloxone, has a minimal effect on cardiac output, and does not interfere with pupillary dilation if oculomotor nerve compression occurs. Fentanyl (Sublimaze) and sufentanil (Sufenta), rapid-acting synthetic opioids with a short half-life, are also reversible with naloxone, providing another option in the selection of analgesic agents that may be used after TBI. Caution is encouraged when using the synthetic opioids because reductions in mean arterial blood pressure and elevations in ICP have been reported with these agents.[63,200]

Short-acting agents, such as propofol (Diprivan), midazolam (Versed), or thiopental may be used to control agitation in the mechanically ventilated patient. In a randomized, controlled trial comparing administration of propofol with low-dose morphine versus just morphine, despite having more poor prognostic indicators, those in the propofol arm of the study required less intense ICP therapy and had long-term outcome measures similar to those in the morphine-only arm.[201] The *Guidelines for Management of Severe Traumatic Brain Injury* recommends propofol as an option for care to control ICP, but not to improve outcomes.[63] Midazolam has the advantage that its effects can be reversed with Flumazenil. No one analgesic or sedative agent has been proven most effective for all patients with TBI.

Extreme caution should be exercised when administering sedation or analgesia to patients with mild or moderate head injury who lack ventilatory support or ICP monitoring capabilities. The threat of respiratory depression inherent in the use of these agents contradicts rapid or high-dose intravenous administration in the spontaneously breathing patient. Large doses or rapid administration of analgesia or sedation also may lower blood pressure to unacceptable levels. Blood pressure response to administration of these medications should be noted, and care should be taken not to use excessive doses that may threaten hypotension.

Nursing interventions to reduce pain and agitation should complement pharmacologic agents used for these purposes. The nurse should attempt to calm, reassure, and comfort the patient. Physical restraint may become necessary to protect the patient from harm and should be applied according to institution protocol, if needed.

Patient and Family Psychologic Support

During resuscitation, emphasis is placed on treating and maintaining the patient's physical being, but the psychologic, emotional, and spiritual welfare of the patient and family must not be overlooked. Even the patient who is confused or partially responsive may be aware of the environment and treatment events. The nurse, as well as other trauma team members, should take the time to explain procedures in simple terms, offer emotional support, and reorient the patient frequently.

The patient's family is typically in crisis and requires support and information. Repeated simple and clear explanations of the patient's condition and progress must be provided at timely intervals. Family coping mechanisms and support systems should be evaluated and mobilized whenever possible.

Critical Care Phase

Nursing care in the critical care phase continues to focus on preventing or minimizing secondary brain injury to optimize functional recovery. Avoidance of factors known to exacerbate secondary brain injury (e.g., hypoxemia, hypercapnia, systemic hypotension, and intracranial hypertension) continues to be the key physiological priority. The critical care nurse is responsible for collaborating with the other trauma team members to prevent, recognize, and treat both intracerebral and systemic complications of TBI. Complications may arise in response to brain injury, nonneurologic injury, or treatment. Early aggressive intervention directed toward prevention and treatment of secondary complications reduces mortality and morbidity.[50-62]

Meticulous monitoring is essential to detect clinical changes and guide treatment. Ongoing comprehensive physical examination remains an essential aspect of assessment. In addition to physical examination findings, data from neuroimaging tests, ICP monitoring, cerebral blood flow and metabolic measures, cerebral oxygenation assessment, cerebral microdialysis, biomarker studies, CSF analysis, and electrophysiologic evaluation may be used in the critical care environment to guide therapy. Parameters that assess the function of other body systems (e.g., respiratory gases, hemodynamic measures, body temperature, fluid and electrolyte balance, coagulation factors) are also evaluated to direct care requirements for the brain-injured patient. Rather than simply directing care at optimizing any one of these variables, numerous therapeutic end points need to be considered in tandem when making clinical decisions. In an effort to ease decision making, a number of organizations have developed treatment algorithms or critical thinking pathways that direct the care provider to the most appropriate treatment option while considering numerous endpoints.

Initial Interventions to Prevent Factors that Cause Secondary Brain Injury

Initial interventions for patients with moderate and severe TBI are aimed at ensuring adequate respiratory gas exchange, optimal intravascular volume and hemodynamic function, sufficient oxygen carrying capacity, desired electrolyte and osmolarity levels, proper positioning, normothermia, and complication prevention. All seek to prevent factors that cause secondary brain injury and thereby optimize patient outcome. If factors that precipitate secondary brain injury occur, then interventions intended to quickly remedy these detrimental findings must be used.

Adequate Respiratory Gas Exchange. It remains essential that hypoxia and hypercapnia be prevented and treated aggressively during the critical care phase. Maintenance of adequate respiratory gas exchange during this phase can be challenging because of the onset of respiratory complications, which are common after TBI. Maintaining airway patency and adequate ventilation are all important to ensure adequate respiratory gas exchange. Effectiveness of respiratory gas exchange should be evaluated frequently, and preferably continuously, by monitoring oxygenation (i.e., pulse oximetry, Pao_2) and carbon dioxide levels (i.e., end-tidal Co_2, $PaCo_2$). The goals remain to keep Pao_2 >70 mm Hg, Spo_2 >94%, and $PaCo_2$ around 35 to 38 mm Hg.[191]

Airway patency is maintained by providing appropriate care for any artificial airway device in place (e.g., endotracheal tube or tracheostomy), using aspiration precautions, and performing vigorous pulmonary hygiene. The spontaneously breathing patient with a natural airway needs to be monitored carefully for any evidence of airway insufficiency. All necessary equipment for emergency intubation should be kept in close proximity. The patient who is beginning to localize to stimuli but is not yet ready for removal of the artificial airway may require soft protective restraints or hand mittens to prevent self-extubation.

Most patients with significant brain injury require mechanical ventilation to promote adequate respiratory gas exchange. Interventions aimed at minimizing ventilator-induced lung injury, such as using higher positive end-expiratory pressure (PEEP) and smaller tidal volumes, may not be well tolerated by patients with severe TBI.[202] Although mechanical ventilation techniques that increase intrathoracic pressure (e.g., high levels of PEEP) may be necessary to prevent end-expiratory alveolar collapse, support adequate oxygenation, and prevent hypercapnia, the elevated pressure within the thorax can impede cerebral venous outflow, causing ICP elevations and impair venous return, thereby reducing mean arterial blood pressure, all of which may compromise CPP.[202] Despite controversy about the use of high PEEP in patients with TBI, research suggests that its use is safe in brain-injured patients with acute lung injury, especially when the level does not exceed that of ICP, significant alveolar recruitment is appreciated, or the patient has low respiratory system compliance.[202-204] Maneuvers that drive up peak airway pressures as high as 60 cm H_2O in an effort to recruit collapsed alveoli were found to minimally improve oxygenation while causing deterioration in parameters reflecting cerebral hemodynamics.[205] Another lung-protective intervention, use of smaller tidal volumes, may prompt hypercapnia, thereby increasing CBF and ICP.[202] Practitioners must continuously monitor the effects of various mechanical ventilation settings on intracranial parameters (e.g., ICP, CPP, CBF, brain oxygenation) and balance the use of lung protective methods of ventilation with those that are more likely to optimize measured neurological variables. A number of modes of mechanical ventilation can be used to ventilate the patient with TBI effectively. Investigation continues into determining ventilation strategies that minimize lung injury while optimizing intracranial parameters. Small case series involving patients with brain injury have demonstrated initial success with high-frequency percussive ventilation,[206] high-frequency oscillatory ventilation,[207] and pumpless extracorporeal lung assist.[208]

Aggressive respiratory care, including suctioning and, when possible, chest physiotherapy (CPT), is important for removal of pulmonary secretions and prevention of atelectasis, which can compromise respiratory gas exchange. These respiratory care interventions are all known to have a potentially detrimental effect on the patient's cerebrovascular status, specifically by elevating ICP and possibly compromising CPP.[209,210] Therefore, neurologic status, including ICP, CPP, and, when possible, cerebral blood flow or oxygenation parameters, should be monitored closely while performing these activities. If monitored neurologic parameters exceed acceptable limits, pulmonary care measures should be discontinued and then reinstituted when cerebrovascular variables are brought under control. Maintaining good head and neck alignment and premedicating the patient with a prescribed sedative before performing these interventions may enhance tolerance of these activities.[209]

Suctioning is performed through the established airway as necessary. Nasopharyngeal suctioning should be avoided until the possibility of a basilar skull fracture has been ruled out. Nursing research findings provide the basis for establishing evidence-based endotracheal suctioning protocols that minimize cerebrovascular compromise during this procedure (Table 20-8).[209,211-213] Studies have demonstrated that although suctioning increases ICP, CPP values can remain sufficient.[211,213] Using measures of Sjo_2, MAP, and middle cerebral artery velocity, Kerr et al[213] demonstrated that cerebral oxygen delivery was maintained and cerebral oxygenation was preserved during endotracheal suctioning.

Fluid and Electrolyte Balance. Fluids should be administered with the goal of achieving and maintaining normovolemia. The practice of keeping the patient dehydrated in an effort to reduce brain swelling has largely been abandoned because severe dehydration compromises blood pressure, cardiac output, and renal function and increases the risk for cerebral vasospasms. Maintaining adequate intravascular volume is important to enhance perfusion to the injured brain. The patient's clinical assessment and hemodynamic parameters should continue to guide the volume of fluid administered. Patients with TBI may have multiple

TABLE 20-8 Research-Based Recommendations for Suctioning Patients With Traumatic Brain Injury

- Pass the suction catheter for no longer than 10 seconds.
- Limit the number of suction catheter passes, preferably to no more than two passes per suctioning episode.
- Hyperoxygenate the patient before and after each passage of the suction catheter (e.g., deliver four ventilator breaths at 135% of patient's tidal volume on 100% Fio_2 at a rate of four breaths in 20 seconds).
- Minimize airway stimulation (i.e., stabilize endotracheal tube, avoid passing the suction catheter all the way to the carina).

avenues of fluid loss that need to be accounted for, such as hemorrhage and fluid loss from associated injuries and surgical interventions, third-spaced fluid, and diuresis from diabetes insipidus or aggressive diuretic use.

Generally, isotonic crystalloids (e.g., normal saline, plasmalyte-A) are administered to patients with TBI and hypotonic solutions (e.g., D_5W) are avoided unless severe hypernatremia dictates judicious use. Generally, fluids administered are selected with the goal of achieving a high normal or slightly elevated serum sodium and osmolality so that volume does not easily leak out of the intravascular space exacerbating cerebral edema.[191] Colloids also may be used for fluid replacement. If the patient is anemic or coagulopathic, blood products serve as excellent replacement fluids. Inherent risks associated with blood administration (e.g., infection, transfusion-related acute lung injury, transfusion reaction, immunosuppression) should be considered prior to transfusion. Many support maintaining a hematocrit of 30% in patients with severe TBI, although there is currently no evidence that this transfusion threshold improves outcomes in this patient population and therefore there is little empiric data to support this practice.[191,214,215] Blood transfusion to attain a higher hematocrit may be considered in patients with severe TBI if CPP or blood pressure is unstable or cerebral oxygenation parameters ($Pbro_2$, Sjo_2) suggest a need to improve cerebral oxygen delivery.[191,216]

Positioning. Adhering to evidence-based recommendations for positioning of patients with TBI may reduce ICP or prevent intracranial hypertension. Patient position can affect ICP, CPP, and other cerebrovascular parameters. Changing the patient's position may elevate the ICP and possibly compromise CPP.[217,218] To minimize adverse effects associated with repositioning, rapid unexpected turning, head and neck malalignment, neck compression, and sharp hip flexion should be avoided.[217-219] The patient should be turned slowly (after being informed of the pending change) while cardiovascular, respiratory, and cerebrovascular parameters are monitored. It is important to maintain head and neck alignment. Head rotation and neck flexion, extension, or compression can inhibit cerebral venous outflow, increasing cerebral vascular volume and elevating ICP.[218,220,221] Head and neck alignment can be maintained with bilateral rolled towels, small sandbags, or other immobilization devices.

As the head of the bed is elevated, ICP typically decreases, and as the head of the bed is lowered, ICP tends to rise.[217,222-224] This ICP response is believed to occur because the head-up position facilitates cerebral venous outflow and movement of CSF out of the brain into the spinal subarachnoid space.[225] The opposite effect is usually seen with systemic blood pressure, which decreases as the head of the bed is raised and increases as the head of the bed is lowered. Although ICP may be lower with the head of the bed elevated, CPP and CBF may be reduced.[224] In most studies comparing a 0-degree versus 30-degree head-of-bed elevation on various cerebral, hemodynamic, and oxygenation parameters, ICP was lower and CPP was improved or unchanged when the head of the bed was at 30 degrees; brain tissue oxygenation parameters demonstrated no significant change.[222,224,226,227] Studies comparing the cerebral vascular responses with various head-of-bed positions have suggested that a 30-degree head-of-bed elevation tends to be optimal for a majority of patients with TBI, although there are many individualized responses to head-of-bed position.[222-224,227] Optimal head-of-bed position should be selected based on the patient's individualized response, considering which position best minimizes ICP and optimizes CPP, CBF, and cerebral oxygenation.

Prone positioning is a well-established means of improving oxygenation in patients with ARDS, which may occur following severe TBI.[228] Thelandersson et al studied the effects of a 3-hour proning period in 12 patients (six with TBI) with poor brain compliance. One patient exceeded acceptable ICP and CPP thresholds and was moved back to a supine position. Of the 11 who where proned, ICP, CPP, and mean arterial blood pressure did not change substantially, but Pao_2 and Sao_2 improved significantly.[228] Likewise, Nekludov et al. demonstrated in 12 patients with intracranial and pulmonary pathology (five with severe TBI) that proning improved oxygenation (Pao_2) and increased ICP, but found that CPP improved due to MABP elevations.[229] Results from these small studies suggest that prone positioning may benefit the oxygenation status of a number of patients with TBI as long as hemodynamic and intracranial parameters closely monitored throughout the therapy indicate the patient is tolerating the intervention.

Patients with lung pathology causing poor respiratory gas exchange and hypoxia that are intolerant of proning or chest physiotherapy due to refractory ICP elevations present a dilemma. At the R Adams Cowley Shock Trauma Center in Baltimore, Maryland patients with these findings have been secured to a tilt table and placed in a standing position to effectively improve oxygenation and ventilation. By standing the patient, the intraabdominal contents that may impinge on the thorax when the patient is sitting upright are allowed to drop down, which presumably reduces intrathoracic pressure and improves ventilation capability, subsequently lowering ICP. Additionally, shifting the position of the lungs and heart may promote better ventilation perfusion matching to enhance oxygenation. A case series describing the technique and effectiveness of standing the patient with severe TBI is being prepared for publication.

Normalize Body Temperature. Hyperthermia is prevalent in patients after severe TBI.[230,231] Temperature elevations may be caused by dysfunction of the hypothalamic temperature-regulating mechanism; cerebral inflammation and release of endogenous pyrogens stimulated by brain injury or the presence of intraparenchymal, subarachnoid, or intraventricular blood; seizure activity; or onset of an extracranial complication (e.g., infection, atelectasis, thromboembolism, drug or blood reaction).[232,233] The presence of fever has been identified as a factor that exacerbates secondary brain injury and can worsen outcomes from TBI.[56,230,234]

Nurses should monitor the patient's body temperature closely, recognizing that brain temperature is often reported to be higher than temperatures measured in the pulmonary artery, esophagus, rectum or bladder.[235] Once hyperthermia is identified, measures to reduce body temperature should be promptly implemented. An extracranial source of fever should always be ruled out and, if present, needs to be appropriately treated. Interventions used to lower body temperature include administration of an antipyretic, cool baths, ice packs, or external water- or air-filled cooling devices; and, in the last few years, placement of an intravascular thermoregulation device.[236,237] Rapid cooling of the patient or prolonged use of hypothermia blankets may precipitate shivering, which also elevates ICP. Shivering can be avoided by slowly reducing body temperature, discontinuing hypothermia use when the body temperature reaches approximately 100° F, and, in severe cases, administering sedatives such as meperidine (Demerol) or chlorpromazine (Thorazine). Strategies to reduce body temperature sometimes lack effectiveness and some may be contraindicated for certain patients.[232] More investigation is necessary to better define evidence-based best practices for fever management in patients with severe TBI.[231,237]

Specific Nursing Interventions. Nurses must remain extremely cognizant of which interventions, activities, or stimuli reduce monitored ICP, CPP, brain oxygenation, CBF, and metabolite levels and which cause elevations. There is wide variation in patient response to interpersonal, auditory, and tactile stimuli, and such responses should be considered when planning and implementing care aimed at optimizing these parameters. Additional studies evaluating the effects of various stimuli and specific nursing interventions on cerebral oxygenation, blood flow, and metabolite levels are needed.

Evidence of decreased intracranial compliance (e.g., baseline ICP elevations or P2 ICP wave amplitude that exceeds the P1 wave) is also important to recognize.[93] In patients with decreased intracranial compliance, activities, such as respiratory care procedures, and changes in head and body position that normally cause transient ICP elevations may provoke prolonged increases that may compromise cerebral perfusion. Effects of such activities should be anticipated, and nursing interventions to attenuate the ICP elevation should be initiated. It may be useful to medicate the patient with a prescribed sedative or analgesic before implementing interventions. Proper body positioning, rest periods, and removal of any unnecessary noxious stimuli are other important nursing interventions that may foster the patient's ability to tolerate a procedure.

Measures to Control Intracranial Hypertension

When ICP exceeds 20 mm Hg or the prescribed therapeutic threshold, a reevaluation should occur to ensure that all initial interventions aimed at preventing ICP elevation are in place and optimized (e.g., patient properly positioned, normothermic with adequate respiratory gas exchange, and desired fluid and electrolyte balance). If despite use of all initial prevention strategies the ICP remains above an acceptable level, a number of interventions can be used to reduce ICP. Intracranial hypertension that persists despite initial interventions should prompt the provider to determine if a repeat CT scan of the head is indicated to assess for a new, perhaps operable, intracranial lesion. Consideration is then given to use of therapies aimed at reducing ICP.

Removal of Intracranial Volume

Surgical Intervention for Removal of a Space-Occupying Lesion. Surgical intervention may be necessary to reduce intracranial hypertension by removing mass lesions or necrotic brain tissue from within the cranial vault. The evacuation of mass lesions is often a life-saving measure, with speed of treatment being crucial. A study of comatose patients with acute SDH demonstrated that those undergoing surgical evacuation within 4 hours of injury had a mortality of 30%, compared with a 90% mortality in those with surgical intervention after 4 hours.[21]

Cerebral Spinal Fluid Drainage. Reduction of CSF volume effectively but temporarily reduces ICP. Use of an intraventricular catheter allows measurement of ICP and continuous or intermittent CSF drainage. In patients with posttraumatic hydrocephalus, long-term CSF drainage via the intraventricular catheter may be necessary until a ventricular shunt can be placed.

Sedation, Analgesia, and Control of Agitation. As in the resuscitation cycle, pain and agitation must be adequately controlled in the brain-injured patient by the appropriate use of sedation and analgesia. Sound judgment is required in managing sedation and analgesia. The inability to report pain should not result in withholding analgesia particularly when the patient has injuries or is undergoing procedures known to be painful.[238] The nurse is encouraged to use a valid and reliable assessment tool designed to screen for pain in the unresponsive patient (e.g., Behavioral Pain Scale).[239] When there is no other option, the practitioner can consider patient behaviors (e.g., facial expressions, vocalizations, movements) and, although they lack specificity and may be transient, physiologic signs (e.g., heart rate, blood pressure) to screen for pain or to evaluate pain relief interventions.[240] The patient's neurologic and cerebral vascular status should be monitored closely to recognize the need for sedation when acute intracranial hypertension arises. Recognition of the need to withhold sedation when the patient must be evaluated clinically is equally important. Care must be taken to prevent systemic hypotension associated with sedation or analgesia administration. Nurses should continually evaluate the effectiveness of prescribed sedatives and analgesics and work in collaboration with the physician to find a drug and dosages that best meet the patient's needs. Small, frequent dosages of short-acting or easily reversible agents are typically preferred.

Propofol is recommended as an option for care to control ICP, but not to improve mortality or outcome in 6 months.[63] Although propofol (Diprivan) has the benefits of having a very rapid onset, short duration, and a depressant effect on cerebral metabolism and oxygen consumption, there are concerns, particularly with high-dose or long-term use, that life-threatening propofol infusion syndrome may occur.[63,241] Elevations in creatine phosphokinase (CPK), metabolic acidosis, myocardial failure, cardiac dysrhythmias, myoglobinuria, renal failure, hyperkalemia, and lipemia are common findings with propofol infusion syndrome and, if noticed, should prompt notification of the physician to discontinue the infusion.[63,241]

Therapeutic Hyperventilation. Therapeutic hyperventilation decreases $PaCo_2$, which causes cerebral vasoconstriction and a decline in CBF, subsequently reducing ICP.[7,242] When cerebral reactivity to Co_2 is intact, the effectiveness of therapeutic hyperventilation is typically apparent within 2 to 3 minutes. Eventually the cerebral vasculature adapts to prolonged periods of hyperventilation as the CSF bicarbonate level and pH return to baseline.[242] CBF returns to prehyperventilation levels despite continued Co_2 reduction, typically within 24 hours of initiating this therapy.[242] An abrupt end to therapeutic hyperventilation, especially when used for prolonged periods, can cause vasodilation of the cerebral vessels beyond the baseline diameter, thereby elevating cerebral blood flow and increasing intracranial pressure.[242]

There is concern that the vasoconstriction and marked reduction in CBF induced by therapeutic hyperventilation may actually worsen cerebral ischemia in the injured brain. A prospective, controlled, randomized clinical trial conducted by Muizelaar et al.[243] demonstrated that patients with a GCS motor score of 4 or 5 receiving prophylactic hyperventilation ($PaCo_2$ of 24 to 28 mm Hg) had a worse outcome at 3 and 6 months than patients who had their $PaCo_2$ maintained between 30 and 35 mm Hg.[243] Numerous studies have demonstrated that therapeutic hyperventilation can reduce CBF or cerebral oxygenation parameters (i.e., Sjo_2, $Avjdo_2$, $Pbro_2$) to levels at or below ischemic thresholds and may cause deleterious alterations in mediators of secondary brain injury measured by cerebral microdialysis.[7,135,143,244,245]

Based on a review of current research findings, the *Guidelines for Management of Severe Traumatic Brain Injury* do not recommend use of prophylactic hyperventilation ($PaCo_2 \leq 25$ mm Hg).[63] Lowering the $PaCo_2$ to less than 35 mm Hg should be avoided during the first 24 hours after severe TBI, when cerebral blood flow is often dangerously low and use of hyperventilation may carry an increased risk of causing cerebral ischemia.[63] Therapeutic hyperventilation may be necessary as a temporizing measure to decrease intracranial hypertension.[63] Initially, the goal of hyperventilation is to maintain the $PaCo_2$ between 30 and 35 mm Hg.[191] When hyperventilation is used, it is recommended that measures of cerebral oxygenation (i.e., Sjo_2, $Pbro_2$) be obtained to monitor cerebral oxygen delivery[63] and guide appropriate use of hyperventilation. When discontinuing hyperventilation, the $PaCo_2$ should be normalized gradually to avoid a rebound increase of cerebral blood flow and ICP.

Hyperosmolar Therapy

Osmotic Diuretics. Mannitol is widely accepted as the osmotic diuretic of choice to control intracranial hypertension. Mannitol's exact mechanism of beneficial action remains controversial. Initially, mannitol is believed to cause an immediate plasma expansion that increases CBF and oxygen delivery and reduces ICP.[246,247] By sequestering fluid into the intravascular space and increasing intravascular volume, mannitol causes hemodilution, reduced blood viscosity, and decreased red blood cell adhesiveness, which serves to improve CBF and oxygen delivery.[246-248] A transient elevation in intravascular blood volume, and possibly the systolic blood pressure, together with ICP reduction, can improve CPP.[246,248] Improved oxygen delivery triggers cerebral vasoconstriction, reducing CBF and ICP.[198] From 15 to 30 minutes after administration, mannitol creates an osmotic gradient between the blood and brain and draws fluid out of the brain, across the semipermeable blood-brain barrier, and into the intravascular space, subsequently reducing overall brain fluid volume and ICP.[63,248] Mannitol may also exert a beneficial effect by scavenging oxygen free radicals, which are known to be cytotoxic and exacerbate secondary brain injury.[249] Mannitol is typically administered to control intracranial hypertension, but it also may be indicated for a volume-resuscitated patient whose ICP is not being monitored but who has clinical evidence of transtentorial herniation or progressive neurologic decline that lacks an extracranial cause.[63] The effective dosage of mannitol generally ranges from 0.25 to 1 g/kg body weight.[63] Higher doses of mannitol may be preferable in specific subsets of patients with TBI. When high-dose mannitol (an additional dose of 0.6 to 0.7 g/kg if pupils were not widened or 1.2 to 1.4 g/kg if pupils were wide) in addition to a conventional dose (0.6 to 0.7 g/kg) of mannitol was administered prior to surgery for evacuation of an acute subdural hematoma, patients had a lower mortality and more favorable outcomes at 6 months when compared with patients who only received a conventional dose.[250] Likewise Cruz et al found that when patients with signs of impending brain death (dilated pupils; GCS score = 3) received high-dose mannitol (about 1.4 g/kg) in the resuscitation phase, they had significantly better outcomes at 6 months compared with similar patients who received only a conventional dose (0.7 g/kg) of mannitol.[251] Sufficient evidence is lacking to recommend a superior method of mannitol administration in adult patients with severe TBI; it may be given as a bolus or continuous infusion.[63,252] It is preferable to administer mannitol through a central line, because extravasation of the drug can cause skin sloughing. Mannitol may also precipitate and therefore should be administered through a filtered needle or an in-line 5 micron filter.

There is concern that mannitol may get on the wrong side of the blood-brain barrier when administered to a patient with brain injury. If this occurs, fluid could be pulled into instead of out of the brain, causing a rebound ICP elevation.[248,253,254] Prolonged circulation of mannitol (which occurs with repeated doses or continuous infusion of the drug) may exacerbate this problem.[253,254] Despite these concerns, mannitol continues to be a mainstay in the care of patients with severe TBI because of its effectiveness in reducing intracranial pressure.

Osmotic diuretic use has multiple implications for nursing practice. The nurse should be vigilant in assessing for potential complications associated with mannitol use, including systemic hypotension and renal failure. These adverse effects are more likely if the patient is not adequately hydrated prior to mannitol administration.[198] Risk of renal failure is also increased when the patient has a serum osmolality >320 mOsm/L[191,255] or a history of a premorbid disease state (e.g., hypertension, diabetes) that causes chronic renal insults.[256] The nurse must frequently monitor the patient's fluid, electrolyte, and hemodynamic status while diuretics are in use. A bladder catheter should be in place to best monitor urine output. Fluids must be administered as necessary to replace intravascular volume lost by diuresis so that the patient's overall volume status and systemic blood pressure are not compromised.

Hypertonic Saline Solutions. Hypertonic saline solutions are emerging as an alternative to mannitol for controlling intracranial hypertension. These solutions have an osmotic effect, pulling fluid from the brain's interstitial spaces into the intravascular space, reducing brain water volume where the blood-brain barrier is intact and effectively reducing ICP.[198,257,258] Hypertonic saline solutions also dehydrate the endothelial cells of the cerebrovasculature, thereby increasing vessel diameter and reducing intracellular fluid of erythrocytes to improve red blood cell deformability, which together with augmentation of intravascular volume can improve CBF and oxygen delivery.[259,260] These solutions may also provide benefit by modifying the inflammatory response associated with injury (e.g., decreases leukocyte adhesion).[261,262] Administration of hypertonic saline solutions may be particularly useful for patients in whom intravascular volume depletion (caused by osmotic diuretics) is undesirable.

Numerous researchers have explored the efficacy of bolus doses or continuous infusion of hypertonic saline (3% to 23.4%) for the treatment of intracranial hypertension after TBI.[63,198,257,263] The most efficacious method of administration and concentration of hypertonic saline remains unclear.[63,263] Whereas the desired serum osmolarity with mannitol use is generally <320 mOsm/L, with hypertonic saline the aim in managing patients who have persistent intracranial hypertension may be to have serum osmolarity 320 to 340 mOsm/L (some advocate for an upper limit of 360 mOsm/L) and serum sodium higher than 150 mEq/L (some advocate for an upper limit of 160 mEq/L).[191,263] A number of studies suggest that hypertonic saline may be more effective than mannitol in decreasing intracranial hypertension.[264-266] Studies done in pediatric patients with TBI have provided enough evidence for the *Guidelines for the Acute Management of Severe Traumatic Brain Injury in Infants, Children, and Adolescents* to make a Level III recommendation (unestablished degree of certainty) that a continuous infusion of 3% saline or a bolus dose of mannitol should be given to keep the ICP <20 mm Hg and the osmolarity within a desired range.[179] Although hypertonic saline solutions are addressed in the most recent *Guidelines for Management of Severe Traumatic Brain Injury,* there are no recommendations provided regarding use of these agents.[63] Despite preliminary evidence that supports use of hypertonic saline solutions to reduce ICP, additional controlled clinical trials are needed.

Potential complications associated with administration of hypertonic saline solutions include electrolyte imbalance, phlebitis, coagulopathies, volume overload, congestive heart failure, hyperosmolarity, acid-base imbalance, seizures, osmotic myelinolysis, renal failure, rebound cerebral edema, and subdural hematoma formation.[63] To reduce the risk of central pontine myelinolysis, which is most likely to occur in patients with chronic hyponatremia, the presence of hyponatremia should be ruled out before administration of hypertonic saline.[63] Metabolic acidosis can be prevented by supplementing the hypertonic saline with acetate.[198,257] In an effort to avoid rebound edema, continuous hypertonic infusions should be tapered off rather than abruptly discontinued.[257,263] Like with mannitol use, the nurse must monitor the patient closely for evidence of adverse effects from hypertonic saline solutions and promptly intervene if complications are identified.

Paralytic Agents. Paralytic agents may be used to eliminate posturing and other movement (e.g., shivering associated with hypothermia) that can elevate ICP or interfere with therapeutic interventions. Paralytics also prevent reflexive motor responses to tracheal stimulation (i.e., coughing) that can elevate ICP. Neuromuscular blockade can facilitate rapid sequence intubation and may be used to control the patient on mechanical ventilation. Early routine use of neuromuscular blocking agents is generally not indicated and has not been shown to improve overall patient outcomes.[267] Hsiang et al found that early routine long-term use of neuromuscular blocking agents increased rates of pneumonia and sepsis and intensive care unit length of stay.[267] Therefore, neuromuscular blockade is generally reserved for patients requiring escalation in treatment intensity for intracranial hypertension. When necessary, it is recommended that a short-acting neuromuscular blocking agent be used and, if ineffective in lowering ICP, the paralytic should be discontinued.[191]

Paralytic agents obliterate most of the neurologic examination, making the clinician dependent on pupillary activity, results of neuroimaging studies, and intracranial monitoring devices to evaluate the patient's neurologic status. Paralytic agents can also mask the motor movement associated with seizures. An unexplained elevation in ICP, heart rate, or blood pressure in the paralyzed patient may indicate an underlying seizure. The patient requires mechanical ventilation while receiving paralytic agents, and there is always a concern about prolonged weakness after discontinuation of neuromuscular blocking agents. Nurses should ensure that adequate sedation is provided, because paralytics do not block the patient's perception of painful stimuli.

Steroids. Glucocorticoids (e.g., dexamethasone or methylprednisolone) were introduced into brain injury treatment with the hope that they would reduce cerebral edema and thus ICP. However, randomized, controlled trials have failed to substantiate the benefit of steroids in the management of TBI. An extensive review of randomized, controlled trials exploring corticosteroid use in acute TBI patients suggests that steroids should not be routinely used in this patient population.[268] Likewise, the *Guidelines for Management of Severe Traumatic Brain Injuries*, provides a Level I recommendation (i.e., good quality randomized, controlled trials support the recommendation) that administration of steroids is not recommended for reducing ICP or improving outcomes in patients with TBI. In patients with moderate or severe TBI, use of high-dose methylprednisolone was found to increase mortality and is contraindicated in this patient population.[63]

Adjunct Therapies. A number of therapies are reserved for treatment of ICP elevations refractory to previously described initial interventions or are only used in addition to primary treatment options. Unfortunately, although these interventions may effectively control ICP, they put the patient at risk for other life-threatening complications that may be instigated by the therapy itself. The multidisciplinary team must carefully evaluate the patient's condition and weigh the risks and benefits of each of these therapies to determine appropriate use of these therapeutic options. If the initial adjunct therapy used proves ineffective, another may be considered for use in addition to or instead of the one initially tried.

High-Dose Barbiturate Therapy. High-dose barbiturates have been used in the management of severe TBI to reduce elevated ICP and protect the brain against hypoxia and ischemia. This therapy is believed to decrease ICP by suppressing neuronal activity and reducing the cerebral metabolic rate, which subsequently decreases CBF and intracranial volume.[63,269] Barbiturates may also have a direct cerebral hemodynamic effect that is beneficial in decreasing ICP.[269] This pharmacological intervention is also thought to inhibit certain intracellular pathological events that play a role in secondary brain injury (e.g., scavenges free radicals, inhibits lipid peroxidation by free radicals, stabilizes plasma and lysosomal membranes, reduces release of excitotoxic amino acids).[269]

Barbiturates can reduce intracranial hypertension that is otherwise refractory to other interventions.[63,269-272] A case series by Rea et al[271] and a randomized, controlled trial by Eisenberg et al[272] demonstrated that mortality is substantially less among patients with refractory intracranial hypertension that can be controlled with barbiturate therapy than among those whose elevated ICP is unresponsive to barbiturates. Clinical research does not support the prophylactic use of barbiturates in management of severe TBI.[63,273]

High-dose barbiturate therapy may be considered in the hemodynamically stable patient who has refractory intracranial hypertension.[63] Pentobarbital, a short-acting barbiturate, is usually the drug of choice. An initial loading dose of the barbiturate (e.g., 10 mg/kg over 30 minutes and then 5 mg/kg every hour for 3 hours) is typically prescribed, followed by a maintenance dose (e.g., 1 mg/kg/hr).[63,272] The maintenance dose and additional loading doses are titrated to reach a desired therapeutic endpoint, which is ICP control while maintaining a blood pressure that preserves sufficient CPP. A reliable method of monitoring barbiturate effectiveness is continuous EEG.[63] Burst suppression on EEG indicates neuronal suppression with near-maximal cerebral metabolism and CBF reductions.[63] Serum barbiturate levels may be measured routinely, but there is a poor correlation between serum drug levels, drug effectiveness, and onset of complications.[63]

High-dose barbiturate therapy is plagued with potential adverse effects. Most undesirable, barbiturates may cause myocardial depression and hypotension, which can precipitate detrimental reductions in cerebral perfusion pressure and eventually CBF, ultimately worsening patient outcome. Continual assessment of hemodynamic parameters (e.g., arterial blood pressure, central venous pressure, cardiac output) permits early recognition and prompt treatment of hypotension or myocardial depression. Vasoactive and inotropic agents (e.g., dobutamine [Dobutrex], norepinephrine [Levophed], phenylephrine [Neo-Synephrine]) are frequently necessary to support the hemodynamic state of the patient receiving barbiturates. High-dose barbiturates also obscure the results of the neurologic examination. Motor function, eye opening, and verbal response cannot be assessed reliably, and most brainstem and motor reflexes are suppressed. The pupillary dilation response to brainstem compression typically remains intact; therefore, pupil size should continue to be assessed. Suppression of most motor and sensory reflexes, including the corneal and protective airway reflexes, means that the patient is completely dependent on nursing care to protect the eyes, skin, and airway. High-dose barbiturates also induce respiratory depression, making the patient ventilator dependent. Meticulous pulmonary care must be provided. Gastrointestinal tract motility is also typically depressed by barbiturate use, which may limit use of enteral alimentation.[274] High-dose barbiturate administration may also cause immunosuppression and increased risk of infection,[275] necessitating close surveillance. Hypothermia, reversible leukopenia, and cardiovascular complications induced by high-dose barbiturates may mask early recognizable signs of infection, including fever, leukocytosis, and a hyperdynamic state.

Decompressive Craniectomy. In patients who have refractory ICP elevations with malignant brain swelling, consideration may be given to performing a unilateral or bilateral decompressive craniectomy. This surgical procedure entails removing a portion of the cranium (e.g., from the frontoparietotemporal or bifrontal region), and sometimes expanding the underlying dura mater lining (i.e., expansive duraplasty using a graft), to decompress the edematous brain and reduce ICP.[276-278] The only randomized, controlled trial evaluating the effectiveness of decompressive craniectomy was done with 27 children who received either standard therapy to manage severe TBI or standard therapy plus a decompressive craniectomy.[279] Those children who had a decompressive craniectomy were more likely to have lower ICP and fewer bouts of intracranial hypertension after the procedure, as well as better outcomes (i.e., less functional impairment, better quality of life).[279] In adults, a number of cohorts with historical controls and case series report that decompressive craniectomy can effectively reduce refractory intracranial hypertension, increase brain tissue oxygenation, and improve cerebral blood flow velocity and cerebral perfusion.[276-278,280-282] Some studies have reported better than expected functional outcomes in patients who had decompressive craniectomy when compared with other control cohorts.[276,277] Randomized, controlled trials are needed to better define the efficacy, appropriate patient selection, optimal timing, and role for this intervention in management of TBI.[278] Two such trials are currently underway.

Complications associated with decompressive craniectomy may include hydrocephalus, subdural or subgaleal hygromas, hemorrhagic swelling on the same side as the operative site, infection, delayed incision healing, resorption of the autograph, and possible injury to the unprotected brain.[277,278] After intracranial monitoring and drainage devices have been removed and cranial swelling has gone down, the patient should be fitted for a protective helmet to protect the brain where the cranium was been removed. Eventually, the portion of the skull that was removed or a synthetic implant can be used to close the cranial defect.

Minimize Intraabdominal Pressure. Elevations in intraabdominal pressure can be translated to the intrathoracic cavity, whereby cerebral venous outflow is inhibited, increasing ICP. Gastric and bladder distension can contribute to intraabdominal pressure and can be relieved by placement of drainage tubes that are typically inserted during the resuscitation phase. Elevation of pressure in the abdominal cavity may result from high intrathoracic pressures transmitted to the abdominal cavity or development of visceral and retroperitoneal edema associated with increased fluid administration to maintain sufficient CPP, as well as the injury-induced inflammatory response.[283,284] In a retrospective review of 17 patients with intraabdominal pressure of 21 to 35 mm Hg but without clinical evidence of abdominal compartment syndrome, decompressive laparotomy reduced intraabdominal pressure and decreased refractory ICP elevations by at least 10 mm Hg. Those with only transient ICP reductions died, whereas those with sustained ICP reductions lived, although there is no mention of functional outcomes of the survivors.[283] Authors of this research recommend routine measurement of intraabdominal pressure in patients with uncontrolled ICP so that high intraabdominal pressure can be identified and surgical decompression can be considered.[283] Additional research is needed to define the efficacy and indications for decompressive laparotomy in management of patients with TBI.

Hypothermia. Mild to moderate hypothermia is thought to exert a neuroprotective effect on the injured brain by a number of mechanisms, including reducing the cerebral metabolic rate to decrease CBF and ICP; inhibiting the inflammatory response; limiting blood-brain barrier damage; decreasing edema formation; and suppressing release of excitatory amino acids and production of free radicals.[285-287] Multiple clinical studies suggest a trend toward improved outcomes and demonstrate ICP is reduced when patients with TBI were treated with mild to moderate hypothermia.[286,288-291] Despite these findings, a large, multicenter, randomized, controlled clinical trial failed to demonstrate any improvement in the outcomes of patients with severe TBI who were treated for 48 hours with induced hypothermia to 33° C within 8 hours of injury.[292] To date, five meta-analyses on this subject have been published, all of which suggest that there is insufficient evidence to recommend routine use of hypothermia as a standard of care for patients with TBI.[63,293-296] The most recent meta-analysis published in the *Guidelines for Management of Severe Traumatic Brain Injury* specifically included studies that evaluated prophylactic hypothermia and found this intervention was not associated with consistent and statistically significant reductions in mortality when compared with normothermic controls.[63] Level III recommendations (unestablished degree of clinical certainty) based on preliminary findings from the analysis suggest hypothermia may have a greater chance of reducing mortality when target temperatures are sustained for over 48 hours. When compared to normothermic controls, patients managed with prophylactic hypothermia had significantly higher GOS scores.[63] Additional randomized, controlled trials are needed to better determine the efficacy of hypothermia in managing patients with TBI, as well as to define the optimal temperature management protocol, including the best temperature reduction strategies, timing for induction, target temperature, duration of treatment and method for rewarming.

Despite the fact that evidence does not consistently support a beneficial effect of hypothermia on mortality and morbidity, multiple institutions use prophylactic hypothermia at the time of admission[63] or as an adjunct therapy to manage refractory intracranial hypertension in patients with TBI. If used, nurses must remain cognizant of the potential complications associated with hypothermia, including infection, coagulopathy, hemorrhage, cardiac arrhythmias, fluid and electrolyte imbalance, skin breakdown, and shivering.[297] During hypothermia, the nurse must carefully assess for onset of potential complications; closely monitor patient's temperature to ensure the desired endpoint is achieved; and provide prescribed sedation, analgesia, and neuromuscular blocking agents.

Measures to Promote Adequate Cerebral Oxygenation

Measures of brain tissue PaO_2 or Sjo_2 provide another therapeutic endpoint that can help direct clinical decision-making for patients with severe TBI. Specifically, these parameters can direct a number of interventions aimed at optimizing cerebral oxygen delivery sufficient to meet the metabolic demands of the brain and may assist in decision making about ICP and CPP management. Measures of cerebral oxygenation are particularly helpful in guiding appropriate use of therapeutic hyperventilation and in defining the optimal CPP.

Prior to using Sjo_2 or Sjo_2-derived values in clinical decision making, the practitioner should always validate the measurement is accurate, as artifacts and erroneous readings are fairly common with this monitoring technique. When measures indicate that oxygen supply is excessive for the demand, as noted by an elevation in Sjo_2 or a reduction in CEo_2 or $Avjdo_2$, consideration must be given to why the cerebral oxygen demand is low or why the cerebral supply of oxygen is excessive. Treatment of excessive systemic blood pressure may be warranted in this situation if hyperemia is present. If the patient is hyperemic and not already hypocapnic, increasing ventilation to reduce Co_2 might be considered to treat intracranial hypertension, as long as cerebral oxygen or blood flow parameters do not near ischemic thresholds. When the oxygen supply is insufficient for the demand, as evidenced by a reduction in Sjo_2 or an elevation in the CEo_2 or $Avjdo_2$, consider why the demand for oxygen is excessive or why the supply is inadequate. It is important to ensure adequate systemic blood pressure, hemoglobin level, and oxygenation. Increasing Co_2 as tolerated and raising CPP also may effectively improve oxygen delivery. In this situation, intracranial pressure may be best managed by drainage of CSF, administration of mannitol or hypertonic saline, and providing sedation and analgesia.[105] Factors increasing cerebral metabolic demand, such as seizures and fever, should also be treated and alleviated.

When $Pbro_2$ values fall below the accepted threshold, interventions aimed at improving oxygen delivery to the brain should be initiated. This includes efforts to reduce intracranial hypertension and optimize CPP. Cerebral perfusion pressure augmentation can increase $Pbro_2$[298,299] and $Pbro_2$ monitoring can help determine the optimal CPP and aid in CPP management.[63] $Pbro_2$ monitoring is recommended as an option for care when using therapeutic hyperventilation to reduce ICP so that practitioners are alerted if the therapy is causing insufficient cerebral oxygen delivery.[63] Interventions to increase $Pbro_2$ are also aimed at optimizing cardiovascular function (e.g., ensure adequate intravascular volume, myocardial function and hemoglobin), oxygenation (e.g., provide supplemental oxygen), and respiratory status (e.g., provide pulmonary hygiene, patent airway, sufficient ventilation). Administration of supplemental oxygen was found to correlate with $Pbro_2$ elevations[298] and, in most patients, red blood cell transfusion increased $Pbro_2$.[216] Factors known to increase oxygen utilization (e.g., fever, seizures) also require prompt treatment to improve $Pbro_2$ (Table 20-9).

Measures to Promote Adequate Systemic Blood Pressure

It is essential that the patient's systemic blood pressure be sufficient. Care should be taken to avoid a systolic blood pressure below 90 mm Hg and maintain a MAP sufficient to provide the desired CPP.[63] Adequate intravascular volume should be maintained. Once adequate intravascular volume is ensured, vasoactive and inotropic medications may be needed to maintain blood pressure. Acute adrenal insufficiency, found to be present in approximately 50% of patients with moderate or severe TBI, can contribute to lower blood pressure and greater vasopressor use.[300] When brain-injured patients require vasopressors, cortisol levels should be assessed, especially when using propofol or high-dose pentobarbital, which have a strong association with low cortisol levels.[300] In patients with low cortisol levels stress-dose glucocorticoids may provide therapeutic benefit in managing hypotension. The nurse should remain cautious when administering drugs that may cause systemic hypotension, such as diuretics and sedatives. Blood pressure should be monitored frequently during administration of such agents in order to rapidly detect and treat any subsequent hypotensive episode.

TABLE 20-9 **Management Guidelines for $Pbro_2$**

$Pbro_2$ <15 mm Hg	
ICP >20 mm Hg	**ICP < 20 mm Hg**
Increase fio_2 by 20% for 5 to 15 minutes	Increase fio_2 by 20% for 5 to 15 minutes
Ensure patent airway (suction if necessary)	Evaluate and optimize hemodynamics and respiratory status to promote oxygen transport
Follow CPP management protocol to reduce ICP	Ensure patent airway (suction if necessary)
If $Pbro_2$ unresponsive, try increasing CPP	Ensure ventilator settings are set to optimize respiratory gas exchange
	Ensure euvolemia
	Consider RBCs for Hct <33%
	Optimize cardiac output
	Ensure Normothermia

R Adams Cowley Shock Trauma Center, University of Maryland Medical Center, Baltimore, Maryland
RBCs, Red blood cells.

Management of excessive hypertension is controversial. Systemic blood pressure should be maintained to ensure adequate cerebral perfusion, but excessive hypertension may cause cerebral venous engorgement, subsequent ICP elevations, and exacerbation of cerebral edema.[301] Such patients may benefit from normalization of the systemic blood pressure. Patients with cerebral ischemia (i.e., vasospasm or cerebral infarct) may benefit from a higher than normal blood pressure to enhance cerebral perfusion. The health care team must be extremely cautious when deciding to treat systemic hypertension, remembering that elevations in blood pressure occur as a compensatory response to brainstem compression. When the brain-injured patient presents with hypertension, particularly if other symptoms of brainstem compression are evident, ICP must be controlled first and CPP evaluated before considering antihypertensive therapy.

Extreme caution should be used when administering antihypertensives to prevent systemic hypotension. The patient's cerebrovascular and cardiovascular response to the antihypertensive agent should be monitored closely. Short-acting antihypertensives with a favorable safety profile and reliable response to dose relationship (e.g., labetalol) are often preferred when initiating treatment.[301]

Recognizing, Preventing, and Treating Potential Complications

Neurologic Complications. Cerebral edema, delayed intracerebral hemorrhage, reaccumulation of an evacuated hematoma, and posttraumatic hydrocephalus are possible sequelae of TBI that directly increase intracranial volume, eventually increasing ICP, and possibly causing secondary brain injury. Symptoms of these complications become evident as ICP rises and brain compression occurs. Other potential complications originating in the brain that can lead to secondary brain injury are cerebral vasospasms, seizures, and intracranial infections.

Posttraumatic Vasospasm. Cerebral vasospasms can occur after TBI, reducing blood flow and potentially causing ischemia to the region of the brain perfused by the artery in spasm. The reported incidence of posttraumatic vasospasms varies among numerous studies, but in a large investigation of 299 patients with mild to severe TBI, 36% to 37% of subjects were found to have evidence of vasospasm.[302] Occurrence of posttraumatic vasospasms is related to the presence of SAH, although vasospasms have been noted in brain-injured patients without evidence of blood in the subarachnoid space.[302,303] Posttraumatic vasospasms may become evident as soon as 2 days after brain injury and can persist for many days, although in many patients resolve within 5 days.[302] Neurologic deterioration caused by vasospasm can go unrecognized in the comatose patient and therefore clinical evidence of the immediate effects of vasospasm may go undetected.[302]

Management of vasospasm is aimed at ensuring adequate brain tissue perfusion and, if possible, relieving the vessel narrowing. Nimodipine, a calcium channel blocker, has been used in an attempt to prevent and treat posttraumatic vasospasms. A systematic review done in 2003[304] determined calcium channel blockers were beneficial for patients with traumatic subarachnoid hemorrhage, although these findings were refuted in a more recent review done on a larger sample of subjects that found the incidence of mortality and of poor outcomes was essentially the same between patients treated with nimodipine and those given a placebo.[305] Angioplasty or administration of "triple H" therapy (hypervolemia, hemodilution, and hypertension) may be considered for treatment of severe refractory vasospasms, keeping in mind the potential complications related to these therapies.[302,306] Further clinical research is needed to determine the efficacy of these or other treatments for posttraumatic vasospasm.

Seizures. Traumatic brain injury can trigger the onset of seizures, which may occur early (i.e., within 7 days of trauma) or late (i.e., more than 7 days after injury). Numerous factors have been identified that increase the risk of a patient with TBI for developing posttraumatic seizures. These risk factors include penetrating brain injury, intracranial hematoma (particularly subdural hematoma that requires surgical evacuation or intracerebral hematoma that necessitates surgical intervention), cortical contusion, depressed skull fracture (especially if not surgically elevated), parietal lesion on CT scan, prolonged inability to follow commands ($\geq$ a week), GCS score $<$10, at least one nonreactive pupil, and presence of early seizures (even seizures in the first 24 hours after injury).[63,307,308]

Seizures increase the cerebral metabolic rate, which may cause ischemia and intracranial hypertension, especially in the acute phase after TBI, when the brain is vulnerable to secondary insult and may have poor compliance. Hemodynamic instability, changes in oxygen delivery, and excessive neurotransmitter release associated with seizures may also have adverse effects on the patient with TBI.[63] Seizure activity may also result in patient injury or adverse psychosocial or emotional sequelae.[63]

Although it is desirable to prevent posttraumatic seizures, the anticonvulsants used to prevent or treat seizures may have numerous adverse side effects. After evaluating the evidence describing the efficacy of anticonvulsants administered to prevent posttraumatic seizures. *The Guidelines for Management of Severe Traumatic Brain Injury* provide Level II recommendations (moderate degree of clinical certainty), stating that although prophylactic use of anticonvulsants may be effective in preventing early seizures, phenytoin and valproate have not proven to be beneficial for prevention of late posttraumatic seizures.[63] Therefore, it is recommended that prophylactic anticonvulsants be administered for the first week to patients at high risk for seizure activity, but not be routinely administered after 7 days in an effort to prevent late seizures.[63] Routine use of valproate to prevent early posttraumatic seizures is not recommended, because it has no benefit over short-term phenytoin administration and may be associated with a higher mortality rate.[309] Haltiner et al[310] demonstrated that administration of phenytoin for the first week after TBI to prevent posttraumatic early seizures can be done without significant increase in drug-related side effects. Currently there is no evidence that preventing early seizures improves outcome by reducing death or neurologic disability after TBI.[63]

Patients with a preinjury history of seizures should have their anticonvulsant therapy continued during and after hospitalization for brain injury. Seizure precautions should be instituted in all brain-injured patients. These precautions generally include keeping an airway, suction, and anticonvulsants readily available, siderails padded and upright, and the environment free of sharp or hazardous items. In the event of a seizure, the nurse should observe and document its onset, characteristics, and duration. Maintenance of a patent airway remains the first treatment priority. Any objects in the patient's physical proximity should be removed to prevent injury, but no attempt should be made to restrain the patient. Prescribed anticonvulsants should be administered to halt the seizure activity, followed by a loading and maintenance dose of the antiepileptic agent desired for long-term seizure treatment. The nurse caring for the patient receiving anticonvulsants should monitor for adverse drug effects and ensure therapeutic drug levels are maintained.

Intracranial Infection. Meningitis and brain abscesses are examples of intracranial infections that may occur after TBI. Severe TBI is associated with changes in immunologic function, which can increase risk of infectious complications.[311,312] Administration of high-dose barbiturates to treat intracranial hypertension also can cause immunosuppression and lower white blood cell counts.[275] Patients with open head injuries are at greater risk for intracranial infection than patients with closed injuries. Intracranial surgical procedures and placement of invasive intracranial monitoring devices also predispose the patient to CNS infection.

Every effort should be made to prevent, recognize, and appropriately treat intracranial infections to minimize adverse effects on patient outcome. Strict aseptic technique is imperative when manipulating intracranial monitoring devices. The nurse should monitor the patient closely for evidence of infection, including continued assessment of body temperature and white blood cell count trends. Intracranial pressure elevations, focal neurologic deficits, and development of brain shift, which is usually visible on CT scan or MRI, are signs of a brain abscess. Bacterial meningitis is a more diffuse process characterized by signs and symptoms of systemic infection, meningeal irritation (e.g., nuchal rigidity, photophobia) and deteriorating neurologic status.

When an intracranial infection is confirmed or suspected, appropriate antibiotics should be administered. Antibiotics are selected based on the sensitivity pattern of the cultured organism and the ability of the agent to penetrate the blood-brain barrier. If drainage of an abscess is required, the patient and family should be prepared for upcoming surgery. Penetrating brain injuries (e.g., missile injuries) generally require immediate debridement of the wound, closure of CSF leaks, and administration of prophylactic antibiotics potentially to reduce the risk of intracranial infection.[178] A retrospective review of 59 patients with penetrating TBI found no relationship between risk of infection and use of prophylactic antibiotics.[313] The authors of this study suggest that in civilians with gunshot wounds to the brain, although a brief course of antibiotics may be indicated for those with injuries that involve the air sinuses, standard surgical prophylaxis without a prolonged antibiotic course is otherwise sufficient to prevent central nervous system infection.[313] Prophylactic antibiotic therapy for open brain injuries, including those associated with pneumocephalus or basilar skull fractures and dural tears that result in CSF leakage, remains controversial. Some practitioners feel that the adverse effects of the intracranial infection warrant prophylactic use of antibiotics; however, many others concerned about the onset of antibiotic-resistant infection, and drug side effects suggest that no antibiotics should be given, unless appropriate for standard surgical prophylaxis, until infection is evident.

Pulmonary Complications. Respiratory complications are prevalent after moderate and severe brain injury. Brain-injured patients with a decreased level of consciousness frequently have suppressed protective airway reflexes, with consequent increased susceptibility to secretion retention and aspiration. A decreased level of consciousness in concert with immobility and potentially abnormal respiratory patterns can lead to atelectasis and secretion retention. Endotracheal intubation is often necessary in the patient with severe TBI, causing bypass of the protective upper respiratory tract. Prolonged immobility and venous stasis pose a threat of pulmonary emboli. Severe head injury, often associated with intracranial hypertension, may trigger the onset of neurogenic pulmonary edema. Although the exact etiology of neurogenic pulmonary edema remains poorly defined, it is hypothesized that neurologic injury, possibly associated with disturbance of the hypothalamus and medulla, triggers a massive sympathetic discharge, causing severe pulmonary and systemic vasoconstriction and increased pulmonary hydrostatic pressure.[314] This, together with an inflammatory-mediated increase in pulmonary capillary permeability, leads to pulmonary edema and is frequently associated with myocardial dysfunction.[314] Direct or indirect pulmonary injury can trigger onset of acute respiratory distress syndrome, a cascade of pathologic inflammatory/immune reactions that leads to acute lung injury and respiratory failure.[315] Associated thoracic trauma may also impair pulmonary function.

Pulmonary complications can increase mortality and morbidity.[315] All respiratory complications increase the likelihood of detrimental hypoxia and hypercarbia and risk subsequent secondary brain injury. Aggressive pulmonary hygiene, aspiration precautions, and appropriate ventilator management help to reduce the incidence of these complications. When compared with prolonged endotracheal intubation, early placement of a tracheostomy (day 5 to 6 after injury[316] or <7 days[317]) in patients with severe TBI has not been shown to reduce mortality or incidence of pneumonia, but it may reduce ventilator days[316] or ICU length of stay.[317]

Therefore the *Guidelines* provide a Level II recommendation (moderate degree of clinical certainty) that early tracheostomy should be performed.[63] A Level III recommendation (clinical certainty is not established) states that early extubation of patients who satisfy respiratory criteria and have sufficient cough and gag reflexes can be performed without increasing risk for pneumonia.[63] Close monitoring of respiratory status and respiratory gas exchange is imperative to detect the onset of these complications. Once recognized, appropriate therapy should be instituted to resolve the complications immediately.

Fluid and Electrolyte Imbalance. A number of conditions leading to fluid and electrolyte imbalance may exist after TBI. Diuretics and hyperosmolar agents used in the treatment of increased ICP may create alterations in fluid and electrolyte balance. The metabolic response to stress and injury can result in the release of adrenocorticotropic hormone (ACTH) and aldosterone, resulting in sodium and water retention and hypothalamic release of antidiuretic hormone (ADH), which also causes water retention. Brain injury can cause fluid and electrolyte imbalance directly by increasing or decreasing ADH output by the hypothalamus-neurohypophyseal system or by triggering excessive sodium and water loss. Nurses must closely monitor the brain-injured patient's urine and serum electrolytes and osmolarity, fluid intake and output, and hemodynamic parameters to readily detect fluid and electrolyte imbalance so intervention to reestablish equilibrium can be quickly initiated.

Neurogenic Diabetes Insipidus (DI). Brain injury that affects the hypothalamic/posterior pituitary system may cause partial or complete cessation of ADH production or secretion, resulting in neurogenic DI.[318] Insufficient ADH decreases water reabsorption by the renal tubules, causing an increased loss of free water and hypotonic urine output. This loss of free water leaves behind a concentrated intravascular volume with increased serum osmolarity and sodium levels. Diabetes insipidus is typically recognized in the clinical setting when large volumes (≥200 ml/hr for 2 consecutive hours) of diluted urine output are noted. Treatment entails providing fluid and ADH replacement as needed (Table 20-10). Administering intravascular fluid volume is particularly important in patients with an altered level of consciousness, who are unable to self-regulate fluid intake, and therefore are at risk for dehydration.[318]

Syndrome of Inappropriate ADH. Syndrome of inappropriate ADH (SIADH) is a complication of CNS trauma that disrupts the hypothalamic-neurohypophyseal system, resulting in abnormal excretion of ADH. Abnormally elevated levels of ADH occur despite lack of a hypovolemic or hyperosmolar state that would normally trigger ADH release. This inappropriate increase in ADH secretion causes continuous reabsorption of water from the renal tubules,

TABLE 20-10 **Clinical Manifestations and Treatment of Neurogenic DI, Syndrome of Inappropriate ADH, and Cerebral Salt Wasting**

Parameter	Diabetes Insipidus	Syndrome of Inappropriate ADH	Cerebral Salt Wasting
Urine specific gravity	Low	Elevated	Elevated
Urine osmolality	Low	Increased	Increased
Urine sodium	Low in relation to serum	Elevated	Elevated
Serum osmolality	Elevated	Decreased	Decreased
Serum sodium	Elevated	Decreased	Decreased
Clinical manifestations	Hypovolemia, dehydration Intensive thirst (if mechanism is not impaired) Large volumes of poorly concentrated urine Aqueous pitressin administration causes urine osmolality increase of 9% or more	Euvolemic or hypervolemic Usually low urine output, low BUN Muscle cramps, weight gain without edema, lethargy, confusion, personality change, irritability, sluggish deep tendon reflexes, anorexia, nausea/vomiting, diarrhea, abdominal cramps, fatigue, headache, restlessness Severe signs—coma, seizures, death	Hypovolemia, dehydration Normal or increased BUN High urine output Net sodium loss
Treatment	Administer fluid to replace intravascular volume loss, urine output and insensible losses Administer exogenous ADH: • Aqueous Pitressin—commonly used in critical care phase • Pitressin tannate in oil • 1-Deamino-8-D-arginine vasopressin (dDAVP, desmopressin) • Nasal lysine vasopressin	Fluid restriction For severe symptoms: • Give hypertonic saline solution • Diurese with furosemide (Lasix) • Give demeclocycline (Declomycin) to produce renal resistance to ADH • Administer an arginine vasopressin (AVP) receptor antagonist (e.g., conivaptan hydrochloride [Vaprisol]) to cause free water diuresis	Replete salt and fluid volume Administer fludrocortisone acetate to increase renal tubule sodium reabsorption

BUN, Blood urea nitrogen; *ADH,* Antidiuretic hormone.

resulting in serum hypotonicity and hyponatremia without evidence of dehydration or peripheral edema.[319,320] High urine sodium levels and urine osmolality greater than the serum osmolarity are also noted.[319] As hyponatremia worsens, other symptoms become evident, such as neurologic deterioration, nausea, vomiting, and muscle weakness (see Table 20-10).[319] The ultimate consequence of SIADH is water intoxication with cerebral edema.[320]

Treatment depends on the severity of SIADH and typically starts with strict fluid restriction (as little as 800 ml/day). Furosemide may be used to diurese the patient and, in severe cases, hypertonic saline solutions (usually 3% sodium chloride) may be administered judiciously. Demeclocycline hydrochloride (Declomycin) may be used to produce renal resistance to ADH.[320] An arginine vasopressin (AVP) receptor antagonist (e.g., conivaptan hydrochloride [Vaprisol]) may be administered to prompt excretion of free water while sparing removal of electrolytes.[320,321]

Cerebral Salt Wasting. Brain injury may also trigger cerebral salt wasting (CSW), which causes primary sodium loss and subsequent reduction in extracellular fluid and intravascular volume. The exact etiology for this abnormal sodium loss is unknown, although it is postulated that increased circulating natriuretic peptides (perhaps the one produced in the brain) and/or reduced sympathetic input to the kidneys may play a role in this process.[322] Like SIADH, cerebral salt wasting results in hyponatremia and serum hyposmolarity, but, unlike SIADH, there is a decrease in extracellular fluid volume and a negative salt balance (see Table 20-10).[319] Normal or high blood urea nitrogen levels, excessive loss of sodium in the urine, and evidence of fluid volume deficit are noted with CSW. Treatment of CSW entails replacing fluid, as well as sodium.[319]

Coagulopathy. Severe TBI with massive brain tissue damage can activate coagulation systems, causing an increase in clotting and consumption of clotting factors, which results in coagulopathy and excessive bleeding.[323] Abnormality in coagulation parameters has been correlated with worse outcomes from TBI.[323-325] Coagulopathy can increase the risk of hematoma expansion or delayed intracranial hemorrhage.[325-327] It can also be cause for delay in necessary neurosurgical procedures. Nurses should monitor coagulation values to detect coagulopathy. Once recognized, treatment with appropriate blood products, such as fresh frozen plasma, platelets, and other sources of clotting factors, should be instituted as appropriate. Administration of even small doses (as low as 10 to 15 mcg/kg) of recombinant factor VII (FVIIa), a potent prothrombotic agent, may be considered to rapidly correct coagulation abnormalities associated with brain injury or prior use of prescription anticoagulants (e.g., warfarin, clopidogrel).[328-330] Currently, there is a lack of prospective data to establish the potential benefits of FVIIa use in patients with traumatic intraparenchymal hemorrhage or to define the risk of thromboembolism with use of this drug in patients with TBI, so careful consideration is warranted before selecting this therapy.[329]

Gastrointestinal Mucosal Erosion. Patients with severe TBI are at increased risk for erosion of the gastrointestinal mucosa. The pathogenesis of this gastrointestinal process as it relates to intracranial injury is still unclear. Posttraumatic stress and autonomic nervous system disruption associated with brain injury are thought to be two potential causes of mucosal erosion. Inadequate or delayed resuscitation can also contribute to mucosal ischemia and subsequent erosion. Venkatesh et al.[331] demonstrated that significant gastric intramucosal acidosis occurred in 9 of the 10 patients studied who had isolated, severe TBI. Proton pump inhibitors, mucosal protective agents (sucralfate), H2 antagonists, and antacids are usually routinely administered to prevent gastrointestinal erosion and possible bleeding.

Protein-Calorie Malnutrition. Severe TBI triggers a metabolic response characterized by hypermetabolism and hypercatabolism.[63,332] The metabolic expenditure of comatose patients with isolated brain injury is increased to an average of 140% of expected with variations of 120% to 250% of that expected.[63] In another systematic review of metabolism in patients with moderate to severe TBI, metabolism in sedated patients was 96% to 132% of expected, whereas it ranged from 105% to 160% in nonsedated patients.[332] Nitrogen excretion is increased with the daily nitrogen balance ranging from −3 to −16 g N each day.[332] This hypermetabolic and hypercatabolic state persists in most patients for the first 2 weeks after injury, after which there are little data to demonstrate metabolic trends.[332] Elevated catabolic hormone and cytokine levels and increased muscle tone associated with brain injury are believed to contribute to this hypermetabolic response.[63,333] This metabolic response to TBI can quickly lead to protein-calorie malnutrition, which increases the likelihood of multisystem organ dysfunction, impaired wound healing, and increased incidence of complications (e.g., skin breakdown, infection).[333,334]

Nutritional assessment and management are multidisciplinary, involving the nutritionist, physician, and nurse. Consultation with a registered dietitian is helpful for determining the patient's individualized nutritional requirements. The *Guidelines for Management of Severe Traumatic Brain Injury* provides a Level II recommendation (moderate degree of clinical certainty) that nutrition should be provided to patients to reach full caloric replacement by 7 days after TBI.[63] To attain full caloric replacement in 7 days, it is suggested that enteral or parenteral formulas containing at least 15% of their calories as proteins should be started within 72 hours and gradually increased over 2 to 3 days.[63] Evidence suggests trends toward lower mortality and morbidity when feedings are started early.[332,335] Although there are multiple advantages in using enteral nutrition, upper gastrointestinal intolerance, common in the first 2 weeks after injury, may prohibit use of gastric feedings.[332] A jejunal route for enteral feedings may be preferred, since gastric intolerance is avoided and risks of parenteral nutrition are absent.[63] Data are lacking to define clearly which location is best for feeding tube placement.[63,332] Nurses should remain cognizant of how well the patient is tolerating feedings. Hyperglycemia and hypoglycemia should be avoided to prevent a potential adverse effect on the patient's outcome.[50,51,63] See Chapter 17 for a complete review of the metabolic and nutritional management of the trauma patient.

Complications Related to Immobility. Motor deficits caused by brain injury, as well as therapy used to manage this disease (e.g., sedatives and paralytic agents), render the patients immobile, making them prone to a plethora of complications. Meticulous skin care and regular turning aid in the prevention of skin breakdown. Minimizing time on unpadded bed surfaces, adequately padding and relieving pressure on bony prominences, and avoiding placement of hypothermia blankets beneath the patient are other nursing measures that aid in preserving skin integrity. The incidence of deep vein thrombosis (DVT) may be reduced by (1) use of lower extremity pneumatic compression devices or graduated compression stockings until the patient can ambulate, together with (2) initiation of prophylactic low-dose unfractionated heparin or low-molecular-weight heparin therapy. Administration of anticoagulants for DVT prophylaxis poses the increased risk for intracranial or systemic bleeding.[63] For patients with severe TBI, data are lacking as to the preferred anticoagulant, dosage, or timing for pharmacologic DVT prophylaxis.[63] Frequent passive range-of-motion exercises are needed to reduce venous stasis and prevent contractures. Once a patient is stable and approval has been obtained from the neurosurgeon, consideration should be given to getting the patient out of bed and properly supported in a bedside chair for a limited time to help prevent complications related to immobility. Serial lower extremity casting and upper extremity splints may be used in the critical care setting to prevent or treat spasticity-induced contractures. Early initiation of physical therapy and occupational therapy in the critical care phase can be vitally important for prevention of many complications associated with immobility.

Cognitive Rehabilitation

Once the patient has been stabilized and ICP is well controlled, cognitive retraining can begin during the critical care phase. The nurse should work collaboratively with speech, physical, and occupational therapists to evaluate the patient's level of functioning and then plan appropriate therapies. In the critical care phase, a patient with severe TBI is often unresponsive to stimuli, nonpurposeful, and demonstrates an inconsistent generalized response or an inconsistent localized purposeful response to stimuli. These behaviors are synonymous with the descriptors in the first three levels of the Rancho Tool. The goal for a patient with this low level of function is to elicit behavioral responses to external stimuli and to evoke higher level motor responses (i.e., purposeful arm or leg movement). Cognitive retraining proceeds by providing meaningful stimuli to the five senses. Sensory stimulation and all components of brain rehabilitation are based on the theory that repetition and consistency of stimuli strengthen recessive or alternative pathways through which function may be regained. Sensory stimulation therapy is designed to arouse only one sense at a time for a brief period to minimize confusion and sensory overload.[336] Most stimulation occurs naturally during routine nursing interventions. For example, tactile stimulation can be provided when performing hygiene measures. Soft, smooth speech patterns during reorientation or explanation of needed procedures, as well as intermittent music or television, provide auditory stimuli. Taste can be stimulated during mouth care with the use of flavored mouth swabs or by touching the tongue with a popsicle. Placing substances with pleasant odors near the patient provides olfactory stimulus. Family photos and familiar items can be shown to the patient to provide visual input. The nurse should identify particular and preferably familiar stimuli that best elicit a response. Each period of stimulation should be preceded by a rest period.[336]

The family should be included in the cognitive retraining program. Their ability to provide familiarity for the patient is invaluable. If family members are unable to visit, they can be encouraged to make audio tapes and supply personal items that have pleasant associations for the patient.

Care of the Family

Crisis intervention that began in the resuscitation phase should continue in the critical care phase of care. Family members must be taught how to interact with a patient who is unresponsive or may respond inappropriately. The nurse should demonstrate how to speak and provide tactile stimulation to the patient. The patient's physiologic response to family interaction should be noted.

Intermediate Care and Rehabilitation Phases

Numerous complications can continue to plague the brain-injured patient throughout the intermediate care and rehabilitation phases of care. Interventions aimed at prevention, recognition, and treatment of potential complications remain important. Therapy aimed at optimizing cognitive function and resolving psychologic and emotional disturbances associated with brain injury is also important during these phases.

Maintaining Airway Patency

Maintaining a patent airway remains a priority during the intermediate care and rehabilitation phases. The patient's airway can be partially or completely obstructed by improper positioning, collection of secretions in the respiratory tract, or aspiration. The patient should be positioned so that the upper airway is completely open. A side-lying or upright position with good head and neck alignment is advisable. Aggressive pulmonary hygiene, including postural drainage and chest physiotherapy, should be continued as necessary to prevent atelectasis and possible retention of secretions. Aspiration precautions initiated during the critical care phase, when enteral tube feedings were likely started, should be continued in the intermediate care and rehabilitation phases. Before beginning feedings by mouth, a swallowing evaluation should be performed to determine if swallowing dysfunction exists, which would increase the risk of aspiration.

Hypopituitarism

The hypothalamic-pituitary system, encased within the sella turcica and perfused by a delicate vascular supply, is at high risk for injury. Direct traumatic force, compromised blood supply perhaps associated with cerebral and pituitary edema, or basilar skull fracture can damage the system.[337] The effects of posterior pituitary injury are well known as the syndromes associated with imbalance of ADH, described previously under Fluid and Electrolyte Imbalance. Until recently, anterior pituitary deficiency was thought to be relatively rare, yet it is estimated that its occurrence in patients with TBI may be as high as 40% to 50%.[338] Anterior pituitary deficiency may involve one or more of the hormones it secretes (i.e., thyroid stimulating hormone [TSH], growth hormone [GH], ACTH, follicle stimulating hormone [FSH], lutenizing hormone [LH], prolactin), most commonly, gonadotropin (i.e., LH, FSH) and growth hormone.[339] Hypopituitarism can occur after any TBI, regardless of severity. Signs and symptoms are determined by the hormone(s) that is deficient (Table 20-11). Hypopituitarism and the hormonal deficiencies that result may adversely affect recovery from TBI; therefore, its identification and treatment are imperative.[337] The reader is referred to the consensus statement developed by international experts in endocrinology for guidelines on screening for hypopituitarism following TBI.[340]

Preventing and Treating Complications Related to Immobility

Prevention and treatment of complications related to immobility, including pulmonary complications, venous thrombosis, skin breakdown, loss of joint mobility, and bowel and bladder complications, continue to be a high priority during the intermediate and rehabilitation phases of care. Occupational and physical therapists continue to play a pivotal role in prevention of immobility-related complications during these phases of hospitalization. Realistic goals to increase patient mobility should be set by the multidisciplinary health care team, taking into account the patient's tolerance of increased movement and any limitations cited by the neurosurgeon. Getting a patient out of bed at least twice a day as tolerated is helpful in preventing complications of immobility. Active and passive range-of-motion exercises remain important, and strengthening exercises can be started once the patient is actively involved in his or her therapy.

Spasticity. Spasticity, a complication of an upper motor neuron injury, is the sustained increase in involuntary muscle tone that occurs in response to muscle stretch. When subjected to passive range of motion, resistance increases in a velocity-dependent fashion.[341] Early and more aggressive onset of spasticity tends to be seen with severe TBI and in those with autonomic dysfunction.[342]

Spasticity has some potential benefits and adverse effects. Favorable aspects of spasticity include the ability to help prevent deep vein thrombosis and osteoporosis, aid in retention of muscle mass, enable reflexive bowel and bladder emptying, and assist in maintenance of posture and mobility.[341] Spasticity can also increase patient disability by reducing range of motion, decreasing the patient's functional capabilities, increasing energy requirements, interfering with positioning and sleep, and causing contractures and pain.[341]

Thorough serial assessments of joint range of motion and tone should be carried out in the acute and post-acute settings. Based on assessment findings, the multidisciplinary health care team should initiate management of spasticity in the acute care setting with the primary goal of maintaining range of motion.[342] Clear goals and treatment option selections should be based on the individual patient's spasticity assessment findings and clinical condition. Noxious stimuli (e.g., bowel impaction, urinary tract infection, decubitus ulcer) that may trigger hypertonicity should be avoided. Passive stretching of the involved muscles helps modulate spasticity and can reduce risk of contractures.[341,342] Long-duration stretching can be facilitated by application of serial casts or splints.[341] Other physical modalities used to treat spasticity include cold and heat application, cryotherapy, proper positioning, functional electrical stimulation, ultrasound and short wave diathermy, and biofeedback.[341,342] Decisions about pharmacologic intervention should consider the potential side effects of the drugs and the patient's course of neurologic dysfunction, distribution and severity of spasticity, and presence of other medical problems (e.g., hepatic dysfunction, infection).[341] Drugs that have treatment of spasticity as their primary indication include dantrolene sodium (Dantrium), baclofen (Lioresal), and tizanidine (Zanaflex). Dantrolene sodium (Dantrium) is typically the initial drug of choice, because it has a peripheral site of action and has less sedative effect.[341,342] Other drugs that may

TABLE 20-11 **Signs and Symptoms Associated With Anterior Pituitary Hormone Deficiencies**

Signs and Symptoms	Hormones Deficient
Weakness, fatigue, exercise intolerance	ACTH, GH, LH, FSH, TSH
Increased body fat, decreased muscle mass	GH, LH, FSH
Loss of libido, erectile dysfunction	LH, FSH
Weight gain	TSH
Weight loss	ACTH
Ischemic heart disease, shortened lifespan	GH

Adapted from Urban RJ, Harris P, Masel B: Anterior hypopituitarism following traumatic brain injury, *Brain Injury* 19(5):349-358, 2005.

ACTH, Adrenocorticotropic hormone; *FSH,* Follicle stimulating hormone; *GH,* Growth hormone; *LH,* Lutenizing hormone; *TSH,* Thyroid stimulating hormone.

occasionally be used to reduce cerebral spasticity include diazepam (Valium), gabapentin (Neurontin), tiagabine (Gabitril), and clonidine (Catapres).[341,342] Intrathecal baclofen can treat global tone effectively while causing fewer potential adverse CNS effects.[343] Chemical denervation using phenol or botulinum toxin has also been used to control focal spasticity.[341]

Heterotopic Ossification. Heterotopic ossification (HO) is the deposition of bone in tendons, ligaments, or muscles adjacent to joints. These ectopic bone formations can potentially cause complete ankylosis and decreased mobility of the joint, functional impairment, pain, increased spasticity, and neurovascular entrapment.[344] The etiology of HO after brain injury remains unclear. HO is most commonly seen in the hips, elbows, knees, and shoulders, but can be seen in other joints as well and may affect multiple joints in one patient.[344] Symptoms of HO include extremity or joint swelling with redness and possibly a low-grade fever. Plain x-ray films may be negative in the early inflammatory phase, but eventually can confirm presence of ectopic osseous formations.[344] HO also may be apparent on bone scan. Alkaline phosphate levels may also be increased.[345] Nonsteroidal antiinflammatory drugs (e.g., indomethacin) may be given as a prophylactic measure for patients at high risk for HO or after HO formation to help reduce pain and decrease inflammation.[343,345,346] Low-dose radiation may be provided to help prevent ectopic bone deposition.[346] Etidronate disodium (Didronel) has been used to prevent or decrease the severity of HO, although a systematic review on use of this therapy reported that there were insufficient data to recommend use of this drug or any other for the treatment of HO.[347] Surgical resection of the bone deposit may be indicated in severe cases.[343]

Management of Bowel and Bladder Function

Patients in a vegetative state may have persistent bowel and bladder incontinence. Female patients with urinary incontinence may require an indwelling catheter, intermittent catheterization, an external urine collection bag, or incontinence briefs, whereas male patients can generally be managed using an external condom device for collection of urine. Prevention of urinary tract infection is critical.

Constipation is common in the immobilized patient. A bowel regimen should be initiated once the patient tolerates enteral feedings, and the patient should be checked regularly for bowel impaction. Bowel retraining, typically initiated in the intermediate phase, can be done even when the patient is comatose. The goal is to establish an effective bowel evacuation pattern.

Cognitive Rehabilitation

Some patients who have suffered severe brain injury may continue to have very low levels of cognitive function consistent with Rancho Tool scores of I, II, or III. These patients are typically referred to long-term care facilities or to coma stimulation programs, where attempts are made to illicit a response to environmental stimuli, as described in the critical care phase.[336] Other patients have less cognitive impairment or may demonstrate improvement in their cognitive status, giving them a higher level of cognitive function.

A patient who is confused and agitated, or confused and inappropriate (Levels IV and V, respectively, on the Rancho Tool), should have stimulation and informational input drastically reduced. Patients exhibiting these behaviors have impaired ability to process information, and they rapidly reach a point of sensory overload. Short-term memory is also severely impaired, so patients are unable to ground themselves with information about people, places, or events. Bizarre behavior, such as screaming outbursts, aggression, disinhibition, delusions, hallucinations, or incoherent verbalizations may be evident. Patients have a limited attention span and may confabulate or perseverate. Confusion can contribute to difficulty in managing the patient and present safety concerns for the patient and staff.[348]

The nurse must provide a structured environment with controlled stimulation, order, repetition, and consistency to optimize the patient's cognitive processing. A break in routine can increase the patient's confusion or rebellious behavior. This can often be avoided by preparing the patient for change as far in advance as possible and providing frequent reinforcement. Choices must be restricted so that the patient's confusion is not increased. A strict schedule of therapies and activities should be established, accompanied by intermittent rest periods.

These patients have difficulty deciphering stimuli; when bombarded with sensory input, their behavior can become erratic and confused. Stimuli should not be excessive. Music and television may be productive for short periods but may become overwhelming if used excessively. Visitors should be limited to one or two persons, and conversation should involve only one person at a time. A calm, quiet atmosphere supports information processing.

Stimuli should be meaningful, and repetition should be encouraged. When patients need to relearn previous skills, it is most productive to use meaningful objects (e.g., use a cup to teach grasping and grasp release). Patients should be given only one-step commands if that is all they are capable of handling. If more steps are given, confusion results and patients are unable to carry out any of the commands. Simple mnemonics, visual imagery, and association and organizational strategies are helpful to cue patients with memory deficits. Patient teaching should be simple and concrete with positive reinforcement. Considerable time and patience are typically required to assist the patient in achieving the goal of functioning independently.

Disruptive and at times aggressive behavior is common.[349] The nurse needs to be cognizant of the potential for self-injury and injury to others. This type of behavior can be handled by use of distracting tactics, capitalizing on the patient's short-term attention span and impaired processing skills.

It is common for patients to go through a period of agitation during recovery from brain injury.[349,350] Agitation can disturb patient care, impede active patient participation in therapy and interfere with rehabilitation efforts.[349-351] Persistent agitation is associated with an increased length of stay in rehabilitation and less functional independence upon patient discharge.[350] Agitated patients are usually confused and have severe short-term memory impairment.[351] Every effort should be made to rule out other physiologic causes for agitation, such as hypoxia, sleep disturbances, seizures, fluid and electrolyte imbalance, or pain. Unnecessary noxious stimuli should be removed and avoided if possible. Psychomotor activities such as ambulation are encouraged to help decrease agitation. A quiet environment, a room with padding to prevent injury, and reassuring one-to-one supervision may be necessary during periods of extreme agitation.

When nonpharmacologic intervention proves unsuccessful in controlling agitation, pharmacologic agents may be considered.[349] The goal is to control agitation while minimizing adverse side effects of the drug used.[349] Various pharmacologic agents have been used in attempts to control agitation, including certain beta blockers, benzodiazepines, hormonal agents, neuroleptics/antipsychotics, neuroleptic butyrophenones, atypical antipsychotics, antidepressants, psychostimulants, antiparkinsonian agents, and anticonvulsants.[349,352] Despite a plethora of research evaluating the effects of medications on agitation in patients with TBI, there is limited ability to draw definitive conclusions about the efficacy of different drugs.[349,352] Therefore, consensus is lacking among practitioners about the ideal agent for managing agitation.[353]

Patients at Rancho Tool Level VI are confused but appropriate and able to accomplish tasks with supervision. Information processing has improved, although memory deficit persists and instructions may need to be repeated. A daily routine should be established and followed closely. Patients may be given more responsibility for their own activities of daily living and toileting. Feedback should be provided to reinforce appropriate behavior. Behavior modification programs can be used to control uninhibited, disruptive behavior. Cognitive remediation is based on assessment of deficits and strengths, remedial cueing interventions, and the patient's ability to respond to the interventions.

At a Level VII on the Rancho Tool, the patient's behavior is automatic and appropriate, with minimal to no confusion, but there may still be some difficulty with socialization, emotions, and returning to work. Structure should be reduced and self-care responsibilities should be increased for the patient at this level of cognitive functioning. The patient may still require information to be repeated and needs to be reminded of possible dangers associated with specific activities. It is essential to give the patient positive and constructive feedback. The patient may also require continued follow-up to deal with the emotional difficulties that may persist after TBI.

At a Rancho Tool Level VIII, the patient will be purposeful and appropriate, totally oriented with good recall, but problem solving and reasoning difficulties may continue to be challenging. The patient is typically able to compensate for these persistent difficulties (e.g., with the use of cue cards to compensate for short-term memory impairment). Involvement in a support group may prove beneficial for the patient.

Management of Psychologic and Emotional Disturbances

Emotional and psychologic disturbances associated with brain injury can increase the patient's disability and inhibit optimal recovery. Depression, mood changes, anxiety, personality disorders, substance abuse, and acute stress disorder are a few of the psychologic and emotional disturbances described after brain injury.[354,355] Depression is particularly common after brain injury and can impede achievement of optimal functional outcomes.[355-357] Involvement of specific regions of the brain and several psychosocial factors have been correlated with depression after brain injury.[356,357] The physical and psychologic sequelae of brain injury can confound the diagnosis and assessment of depression. Accurate assessment, diagnosis, and treatment of depression are essential. Antidepressants are often used to manage depression in these patients.[354] Cognitive-behavioral therapy, psychotherapy, and support groups may also be helpful for the patient.[354]

FAMILY AND RESOURCES

Trauma affects both the patient and the family, the latter usually being unprepared for the sudden onset of brain injury and the long-term rehabilitation it may require. Shock, disbelief, denial, grief, and anger are common initial feelings described by families of patients with a TBI. Caregivers of patients with TBI have said that the patient's neurobehavioral and emotional disturbances, rather than the physical disabilities, have the most significant impact on the family members' quality of life.[358] Family members often develop relationship strains, social isolation, substance abuse problems, and financial burden related to caring for the patient and lack of employment. Depression has been reported among caregivers of patients with TBI.[359]

It is extremely important to provide care and support for the family as well as the patient. Long-term monitoring of caregivers' emotional status is important to identify onset of depression or increased anxiety. The nurse should establish daily communication with the family and assist in identifying other resources that will enable the family to cope more effectively with the catastrophic event. It is important to provide families with information about the patients' quality of life after TBI. The correct information needs to be provided to the family at the right time for the message to have the most beneficial effect. Families have reported receiving limited information regarding diagnosis, prognosis, navigating the health care system, and what happens "after," which produces feelings of frustration and mistrust.[360,361] The nurse is poised to intervene. Information about behavioral and emotional changes that may be caused by TBI should be provided to enhance the family's ability to cope with these disabilities. Support and counseling to enhance coping skills are extremely important. It is important to offer frequent reassurance for their positive coping skills and to try to decrease feelings of guilt. The need for respite care should be emphasized to decrease the fatigue and emotional distress often felt when caring for the patient with TBI. In addition, support groups or individual therapy may be necessary for some family members.

Families should be made aware of all brain injury support services within the hospital, in the community, and across the nation. Sources of referral within the acute care setting may include social services, nursing psychiatric specialties, pastoral care, neuropsychologic consultations, and an in-house brain injury support group. Community and national support referrals include local brain injury support groups, the Brain Injury Association, and the state chapter of the Brain Injury Association. The family should be informed of possible benefits and sources of financial assistance at the state and federal levels for patients with TBI.

Community Reintegration

Complex emotional, psychosocial, behavioral, cognitive, and physical disabilities may persist for years after a TBI. Disposition of patients after brain injury depends on the extent of the neurologic disability. The majority of mildly brain-injured patients without obvious neurologic deficiencies are discharged home with follow-up instructions. Although superficially these patients may have normal neurologic function, after return to work or school, difficulty concentrating, poor memory, fatigue, and other types of symptoms associated with mild TBI may become evident and quite disabling. With resumption of the patient's previous lifestyle, the chronic nature of deficits and the limiting effects of disabilities become apparent. Distress is increased and patients tire easily, are overwhelmed, and may withdraw, resulting in family conflict.

Patients with obvious deficits may be discharged with plans for continued outpatient rehabilitation or to independent living programs or community reentry programs. Patients in a vegetative state or too severely disabled to actively participate in a structured rehabilitation program are typically discharged to extended care facilities or to facilities that have special coma management programs. Other specialized brain-injury programs are also available to meet the needs of brain-injured patients. In addition to acute rehabilitation and coma management programs, other options include behavioral programs, transitional living, independent living, community reentry, home-based services, and prevocational, vocational, and sheltered work training.[362]

Outcome from Traumatic Brain Injury

Improved survival after TBI is important but means little without concomitant improvement in quality of life. Epidemiologic and treatment studies done during the past decade have focused on defining more carefully outcomes of both acute and chronic care beyond merely survival.

Disability results from motor, sensory, cognitive, and behavioral deficits. Many motor and mild sensory deficits improve over time. Some patients have complete functional recovery, and the majority of those with permanent deficits generally learn to compensate or adapt to their loss. Cognitive and personality deficits, however, tend to persist even after focal deficits have resolved; they are the major cause of chronic disability after head injury. Even though a brain injury is classified as mild or moderate, with few measurable deficits, the disability resulting from a combination of cognitive, motor, and sensory dysfunction may be extremely troublesome and a source of great anxiety to the individual and the family.

Short-term memory impairment is the most persistent of all deficits. In patients with severe disability, it may not return to any functional extent. This presents a major problem in recovery because new information cannot be retained sufficiently for relearning to take place.

For research studies describing natural recovery or comparing modes of treatment, outcome is generally assessed 6 months after injury, because maximum recovery occurs in about 90% of patients during this period.[363] This is not to say that no further recovery continues, but the rate is much slower in the years after injury. It appears that physical deficits improve more quickly than cognitive ones, with the latter showing slow improvement over the years. There is growing evidence that formalized rehabilitation programs improve vocational and social function beyond that expected from spontaneous recovery alone.[364] Consequently, outcome may be reasonably assessed as early as 6 months and as long as 3 to 5 years after injury.[363]

Measures of Outcome

The formal measurement of outcome has become much more extensive in recent years as survival has increased, and there has been more emphasis on outcomes indicating quality of survival. The most commonly used outcome measure is the GOS. The original GOS has five categories (Table 20-12).[365] A more recent 8-point refinement, called the Extended Glasgow Outcome Scale (GOSE), includes two gradations within each of three categories of functional survival.[366,367] Its structured interview format[367] provides good reproducibility of classification among observers. The Disability Rating Scale (DRS), Functional Independence Measure (FIM), and Community Integration Questionnaire (CIQ) are other measures of outcome often used in studies of treatment of and recovery from TBI.[363]

Predictors of Outcome

Although some patients with a poor prognosis do well and others who should conceivably do well make poor recoveries, the outcome of most people with severe head injuries in

TABLE 20-12 **Characteristics Defining Each Category of the Glasgow Outcome Scale**

Categories	Characteristics
Good recovery (GR)	• Able to participate in normal social activities and return to work • Some restrictions in extent of social and leisure participation, or infrequent personality changes that interfere with return to normal life place person in lower GR category
Moderate disability (MD)	• Inability to work in previous capacity • Restriction on previous social and leisure activities • Frequent or constant posttraumatic personality changes • The lower range of MD is characterized by inability to work or ability to work only in a sheltered workshop or noncompetitive job, inability to participate in prior social and leisure activities
Severe disability (SD)	• Implies consciousness, but dependence on others for at least some of daily needs • Needs assistance in home for some activities of daily living, cannot shop without assistance, cannot travel locally without assistance • If person also needs someone to be around home most of the time, he or she qualifies for the lower SD category on GOSE
Vegetative state (VS)	• Have sleep and awake periods, but with no evidence of sentient responsiveness
Death (D)	

terms of survival and good versus poor recovery can be fairly well predicted from injury and clinical data. In a study utilizing the International Mission for Prognosis And Clinical Trial (IMPACT) database with 9205 patients whom sustained severe or moderate TBI, age, GCS motor score, pupil response, CT characteristics, glucose level, and occurrence of hypotension or hypoxia were found to be important prognostic factors.[368] Using the IMPACT database, the 3-month GCS score was the strongest independent predictor of long-term outcome, with prolonged hypotension, DAI, and fixed or dilated pupils also identified as independent predictors for poor outcome.[74] Considerable progress has been made in assessing a range of outcomes from TBI. These include both survival and the quality of recovery.

SUMMARY

Nurses in each phase of trauma care play a pivotal role in ensuring that the patient with TBI achieves optimal outcomes. Equipped with knowledge about TBI pathophysiology, assessment interpretation, and current evidence-based recommendations for treatment, the nurse is able to work collaboratively with the multidisciplinary team to plan and implement the most appropriate care. New developments in defining TBI pathophysiology and innovations in assessment and monitoring techniques for the injured brain open opportunities for nursing research to define the care that will best enable optimal outcomes to be achieved.

REFERENCES

1. Langlois JA, Rutland-Brown W, Thomas KE: *Traumatic Brain Injury in the United States: Emergency Department Visits, Hospitalizations, and Deaths,* Atlanta, 2006, Centers for Disease Control and Prevention, National Center for Injury Prevention and Control.
2. Centers for Disease Control and Prevention (CDC), National Center for Injury Prevention and Control: *Report to Congress on Mild Traumatic Brain Injury in the United States: Steps to Prevent a Serious Public Health Problem,* Atlanta, 2003, Centers for Disease Control and Prevention.
3. Langlois JA, Marr A, Mitchko J et al: Tracking the silent epidemic and educating the public: CDC's Traumatic Brain Injury—associated activities under the TBI Act of 1996 and the Children's Health Act of 2000, *J Head Trauma Rehabil* 20(3):196-204, 2005.
4. CDC: Incidence rates of hospitalization related to traumatic brain injury —2 states, 2002, *MMWR* 55(08):201-204, 2006.
5. TBI National Database Center: TBI national database update, *Traumatic Brain Injury Facts and Figures* 12(1):8-10, 2006.
6. Finkelstein E, Corso P, Miller T et al: *The Incidence and Economic Burden of Injuries in the United States,* New York, 2006, Oxford University Press.
7. Stocchetti N, Maas AIR, Chieregato A et al: Hyperventilation in head injury, *Chest* 127:1812-1827, 2005.
8. Kety SS, Schmidt CF: The effects of altered arterial tensions of carbon dioxide and oxygen on cerebral blood flow and cerebral oxygen consumption of normal young men. *J Clin Invest* 27:484-492, 1948.
9. Obrist WD, Marion DW: Xenon techniques for CBF measurements in clinical head injury. In Narayan RK, Wilberger JE Jr, Povlishock JT, editors: *Neurotrauma,* New York, 1997, McGraw-Hill.
10. Centers for Disease Control and Prevention (CDC), National Center for Injury Prevention and Control: *Traumatic brain injury in the United States—A Report to Congress.* Atlanta, 1999, Centers for Disease Control and Prevention.
11. Gaetz M: The neurophysiology of brain injury, *Clin Neurophysiol* 115:4-8, 2004.
12. Smith DH, Meaney DF, Shull WH: Diffuse axonal injury in head trauma, *J Head Trauma Rehabil* 18:507-516, 2003.
13. Blissett P: Care of the critically ill patient with penetrating head injury, *Crit Care Nurs Clin N Am* 18:321-332, 2006.
14. Bullock MR, Chestnut R, Ghajar J et al: Surgical management of depressed cranial fractures, *Neurosurgery* 58(3 supp):s2-56-s2-60, 2006.

15. Saboori M, Ahmadi J, Farajzadegan: Indications for brain CT scan in patients with minor head injury. *Clin Neurol Neurosurg* 109:399-405, 2007.
16. Bell RB, Dierks EJ, Homer L et al: Management of cerebrospinal fluid leak associated with craniomaxillofacial trauma, *J Oral Maxillofac Surg* 62:676-684, 2004.
17. Chang EF, Meeker M, Holland MC et al: Acute traumatic intraparenchymal hemorrhage: risk factors for progression in the early post-injury period, *Neurosurgery* 58:647-656, 2006.
18. Povlishock JT, Katz DI: Update of neuropathology and neurological recovery after traumatic brain injury, *J Head Trauma Rehabil* 20:76-94, 2005.
19. Bullock M, Chestnut R, Ghajar J et al: Surgical management of acute epidural hematomas, *Neurosurgery* 58(3 supp.):s2-7-s2-15, 2006.
20. Bullock M, Chestnut R, Ghajar J et al: Surgical management of acute subdural hematomas, *Neurosurgery* 58(3 supp.):s2-16-s2-24, 2006.
21. Seelig JM, Becker DP, Miller JD et al: Traumatic acute subdural hematoma: major mortality reduction in comatose patients treated within four hours, *N Engl J Med* 304(25):1511-1518, 1981.
22. Bazarian J, Blyth B, Cimpello L: Bench to bedside: evidence for brain injury after concussion—looking beyond the computed tomography scan, *Acad Emerg Med* 13(2):199-214, 2006.
23. Zheng WB, Liu GR, Wu RH: Prediction of recovery from a post-traumatic coma state by diffusion-weighted imaging (DWI) in patients with diffuse axonal injury, *Neuroradiology* 49:271-279, 2007.
24. Parizel PM, Van Goethem JW, Ozsariak O et al: New development in the neuroradiological diagnosis of craniocerebral trauma, *Eur Radiol* 15:569-581, 2005.
25. Scheid R, Walther K, Guthke T et al: Cognitive sequelae of diffuse axonal injury, *Arch Neurol* 63:418-424, 2006.
26. Huisman TAGM, Schwamm LH, Schaefer PW et al: Diffusion tensor imaging as potential biomarker of white matter injury in diffuse axonal injury, *AJNR Am J Neuroradiol* 25:370-376, 2004.
27. Holshouser BA, Tong KA, Ashwal S: Proton MR spectroscopic imaging depicts diffuse axonal injury in children with traumatic brain injury, *AJNR Am J Neuroradiol* 26:1276-1285, 2005.
28. Kinuya K, Kakuda K, Nobata K et al: Role of brain perfusion single-photon emission tomography in traumatic head injury, *Nucl Med Commun* 25:333-337, 2004.
29. Lewine JD, Davis JT, Bigler ED et al: Objective documentation of traumatic brain injury subsequent to mild head trauma: multimodal brain imaging with MEG, SPECT, and MRI, *J Head Trauma Rehabil* 22(3):141-155, 2007.
30. Lovell M, Collins M, Bradley J: Return to play following sports-related concussion, *Clin Sports Med* 23:421-441, 2004.
31. Drake AI, McDonald EC, Magnus NE et al: Utility of Glasgow Coma Scale-Extended in symptom prediction following mild traumatic brain injury, *Brain Injury* 20(5):469-475, 2006.
32. Ryan LM, Warden DL: Post concussion syndrome, *Int Rev Psychiatry* 15:310-316, 2003.
33. Cantu R: Recurrent athletic head injury: risks and when to retire, *Clin Sports Med* 22:593-603, 2003.
34. McCrory P, Johnston K, Meeuwisse W et al: Summary and agreement statement of the 2nd International Conference on Concussion in Sport, Prague 2004, *Br J Sports Med* 39:196-204, 2005.
35. Blackman J, Patrick P, Buck M et al: Paroxysmal autonomic instability with dystonia after brain injury, *Arch Neurol* 61:321-328, 2004.
36. Graham DI, Adams JH, Murray LS et al: Neuropathology of the vegetative state after head injury, *Neuropsychol Rehabil* 15(3/4):198-213, 2005.
37. Weber J: Calcium homeostasis following traumatic neuronal injury, *Curr Neurovasc Res* 1:151-171, 2004.
38. Chang DTW, Reynolds IJ: Mitochondrial trafficking and morphology in healthy and injured persons, *Prog Neurobiol* 80:241-268, 2006.
39. Zhang X, Chen Y, Jenkins LW et al: Bench-to-bedside review: apoptosis/programmed cell death triggered by traumatic brain injury, *Critical Care* 9:66-75, 2005.
40. Enriquez P, Bullock R: Molecular and cellular mechanisms in the pathophysiology of severe head injury, *Curr Pharm Des* 10:2131-2143, 2004.
41. Narayan RK, Michel ME, Ansell B et al: Clinical trials in head injury, *J Neurotrauma* 19(5):503-557, 2002.
42. Maas AI, Marmarou A, Murray GD et al: Clinical trials in traumatic brain injury: current problems and future solutions, *Acta Neurochir Suppl* 89:113-118, 2004.
43. Levi MS, Brimble MA: A review of neuroprotective agents, *Curr Med Chem* 11:2383-2397, 2004.
44. Lucas S-M, Rothwell NJ, Gibson RM: The role of inflammation in CNS injury and disease, *Br J Pharmacol* 147:S232-S240, 2006.
45. Olsson A, Csajbok L, Ost M et al: Marked increase of B-amyloid$_{(1-42)}$ and amyloid precursor protein in ventricular cerebrospinal fluid after severe traumatic brain injury, *J Neurol* 251:870-876, 2004.
46. Szczygielski J, Mautes A, Steudel WI et al: Traumatic brain injury: cause or risk of Alzheimer's disease? A review of experimental studies. *J Neural Transm* 112:1547-1564, 2005.
47. Selzer ME: Promotion of axonal regeneration in the injured CNS, *Lancet Neurol* 2:157-166, 2003.
48. Wieloch T, Nikolich K: Mechanisms of neural plasticity following brain injury, *Curr Opin Neurobiol* 16:258-264, 2006.
49. Domeniconi M, Filbin MT: Overcoming inhibitors in myelin to promote axonal regeneration, *J Neurol Sci* 233:43-47, 2005.
50. Jeremitsky E, Omert L, Dunham CM et al: Harbingers of poor outcome the day after severe brain injury: hyperthermia, hypoxia, and hypoperfusion, *J Trauma* 54:312-319, 2003.
51. Sanchez-Olmedo JI, Flores-Cordero JM, Rincon-Ferrari MD et al: Brain death after severe traumatic brain injury: the role of systemic secondary brain results, *Transplant Proc* 37: 1990-1992, 2005.
52. Chi JH, Knudson MM, Vassar MJ et al: Prehospital hypoxia affects outcome in patients with traumatic brain injury: a prospective multicenter study, *J Trauma* 61:1134-1141, 2006.
53. Henzler D, Cooper DJ, Tremayne AB et al: Early modifiable factors associated with fatal outcome in patients with severe traumatic brain injury: a case control study, *Crit Care Med* 35:1027-1031, 2007.
54. Balestreri M, Czosnyka M, Hutchinson P et al: Impact of intracranial pressure and cerebral perfusion pressure on severe disability and mortality after head injury, *Neurocrit Care* 4: 8-13, 2006.
55. Chesnut RM, Marshall SB, Piek J et al: Early and late systemic hypotension as a frequent and fundamental source of cerebral ischemia following severe brain injury in the traumatic coma data bank, *Acta Neurochir (Suppl)* 59:121-125, 1993.

56. Jones PA, Andrews PJ, Midgley S et al: Measuring the burden of secondary insults in head-injured patients during intensive care, *J Neurosurg Anesthesiol* 6:4-14, 1994.
57. Barton CW, Hemphill JC, Morabito D et al: A novel method of evaluating the impact of secondary brain insults on functional outcomes in traumatic brain-injured patients, *Acad Emerg Med* 12:1-6, 2005.
58. McHugh GA, Engel DC, Butcher I et al: Prognostic value of secondary insults in traumatic brain injury: results from the IMPACT study, *J Neurotrauma* 24:287-293, 2007.
59. Chesnut RM, Marshall LF, Klauber MR et al: The role of secondary brain injury in determining outcome from severe head injury, *J Trauma* 34:216-222, 1993.
60. Manley G, Knudson MM, Morabito D et al: Hypotension, hypoxia, and head injury: frequency, duration, and consequences, *Arch Surg* 136:1118-1123, 2001.
61. Juul N, Morris GF, Marshall SB et al: Intracranial hypertension and cerebral perfusion pressure: influence on neurological deterioration and outcome in severe head injury, *J Neurosurg* 92:1-6, 2000.
62. Coles JP: Regional ischemia after head injury, *Curr Opin Crit Care* 10:120-125, 2004.
63. Brain Trauma Foundation, American Association of Neurological Surgeons, Congress of Neurological Surgeons, AANS/CNS Joint Section on Neurotrauma and Critical Care: *Guidelines for the Management of Severe Traumatic Brain Injury,* ed 3, *J Neurotrauma* 24(suppl 1):S1-S106, 2007.
64. Katayama Y, Kawamata T: Edema fluid accumulation within necrotic brain tissue as a cause of the mass effect of cerebral contusion in head trauma patients, *Acta Neurochir Suppl* 86:323-327, 2003.
65. Unterberg EW, Stover J, Kress B et al: Edema and brain trauma, *Neuroscience* 129:1021-1029, 2004.
66. Kelly DF, Kordestani RK, Martin NA et al: Hyperemia following traumatic brain injury: relationship to intracranial hypertension and outcome, *J Neurosurg* 85:762-771, 1996.
67. Maas AI, Steyerberg EW, Butcher I et al: Prognostic value of computerized tomography scan characteristics in traumatic brain injury: results from the IMPACT study, *J Neurotrauma* 24:303-314, 2007.
68. Werner C, Engelhard K: Pathophysiology of traumatic brain injury, *Br J Anaesth* 99:4-9, 2007.
69. Jaeger M, Schuhmann MU, Soehle M et al: Continuous assessment of cerebrovascular autoregulation after traumatic brain injury using brain tissue oxygen pressure reactivity, *Crit Care Med* 34:1783-1788, 2006.
70. Obrist WD, Langfitt TW, Jaggi JL et al: Cerebral blood flow and metabolism in comatose patients with acute head injury. Relationship to intracranial hypertension, *J Neurosurg* 61:241-253, 1984.
71. Bouma GJ, Muizelaar JP, Stringer WA et al: Ultra-early evaluation of regional cerebral blood flow in severely head-injured patients using xenon-enhanced computerized tomography, *J Neurosurg* 77:160-168, 1992.
72. Kelly DF, Martin NA, Kordestani R et al: Cerebral blood flow as a predictor of outcome following traumatic brain injury, *J Neurosurg* 86:633-641, 1997.
73. Binder DK, Lyon R, Manley GT: Transcranial motor evoked potential recording in a case of Kernohan's notch syndrome: case report, *Neurosurgery* 54:999-1002, 2005.
74. King JT Jr, Carlier PJ, Marion DW: Early Glasgow Outcome Scale scores predict long-term functional outcome in patients with severe traumatic brain injury, *J Neurotrauma* 22(9): 947-954, 2007.
75. Marmarou A, Lu J, Butcher I et al: Prognostic value of the Glasgow Coma Scale and pupil reactivity in traumatic brain injury assessed pre-hospital and on enrollment: an IMPACT analysis, *J Neurotrauma* 24:270-280, 2007.
76. Teasdale G, Jennett B: Glasgow coma scale, *Lancet* 2:81-84, 1974.
77. McNett M: A review of the predictive ability of Glasgow Coma Scale scores in head-injured patients, *J Neurosci Nurs* 39: 68-75, 2007.
78. Segatore M, Way C: The Glasgow coma scale: time for change, *Heart Lung* 21:548-557, 1992.
79. Teasdale G, Murray G, Parker L et al: Adding up the Glasgow coma score, *Acta Neurochir* 28:13-16, 1979.
80. Giacino JT, Kalmar K, Whyte J: The JFK Coma Recovery Scale—Revised: measurement characteristics and diagnostic utility, *Arch Phys Med Rehabil* 85:2020-2029, 2004.
81. Walther SM, Jonasson U, Gill H: Comparison of the Glasgow Coma Scale and the Reaction Level Scale for assessment of cerebral responsiveness in the critically ill, *Intensive Care Med* 29:933-938, 2003.
82. Wijkicks EFM, Bamlet WR, Maramattom BV et al: Validation of a new coma scale: the FOUR score, *Ann Neurol* 58:585-593, 2005
83. Wolf C, Wijdicks E, Bamlet W et al: Further validation of the FOUR score coma scale by intensive care nurses, *Mayo Clin Proc* 82(4):435-438, 2007.
84. Nell V, Yates DW, Kruger J et al: An extended Glasgow Coma Scale (GCS-E) with enhanced sensitivity to mild brain injury, *Arch Phys Med Rehabil* 81:614-617, 2000.
85. Hagen C, Malkmus D, Stenderup-Bowman K: *Los Amigos Research and Education, Rancho Los Amigos Hospital,* ed 3, Downey, CA, 1973, Revised by Hagen C, 1998.
86. Lee B, Newberg A: Neuroimaging in traumatic brain imaging, *NeuroRx* 2:372-383, 2005.
87. Brown CVR, Weng J, Oh D et al: Does routine serial computed tomography of the head influence management of TBI? A prospective evaluation, *J Trauma* 57(5):939-943, 2004.
88. Wang MC, Linnau KF, Tirschwell DL et al: Utility of repeat head computed tomography after blunt head trauma: a systematic review, *J Trauma* 61:226-233, 2006.
89. Sifri ZC, Homnick AT, Vaynman A et al: A prospective evaluation of the value of repeat cranial computed tomography in patients with minimal head injury and an intracranial bleed, *J Trauma* 61:862-867, 2006.
90. Provenzale J: CT and MR imaging of acute cranial trauma, *Emerg Radiol* 2007. Available on-line at http://www.springerlink.com.proxy-hs.researchport.umd.edu/content/9141h04266220w6h/. Accessed August 16, 2007.
91. Goldsher D, Shreiber R, Shik V et al: Role of multisection CT angiography in the evaluation of vertebrobasilar vasospasm in patients with subarachnoid hemorrhage, *AJNR* 25:1493-1498, 2004.
92. Biffl WL, Eggin T, Benedetto B et al: Sixteen-slice computed tomographic angiography is a reliable noninvasive screening test for clinically significant blunt cerebrovascular injuries, *J Trauma* 60:745-752, 2006.

93. Fields L, Blackshear C, Mortimer D et al: *Guide to the Care of the Patient with Intracranial Pressure Monitoring,* Glenview, IL, 2005, AANN American Association of Neuroscience Nurses.
94. Gambardella G, d'Avella D, Tomasello F: Monitoring of brain tissue pressure with a fiberoptic device, *Neurosurgery* 31(5): 918-922, 1992.
95. Chambers IR, Kane PJ, Choksey MS et al: An evaluation of the Camino ventricular bolt system in clinical practice, *Neurosurgery* 33(5):866-868, 1993.
96. Koskinen L-O, Olivecrona M: Clinical experience with the intraparenchymal intracranial pressure monitoring Codman MicroSensor system, *Neurosurgery* 56(4):693-698; 2005.
97. Lang J-M, Beck J, Zimmermann M et al: Clinical evaluation of intraparenchymal Spiegelberg pressure sensor, *Neurosurgery* 52:1455-1459, 2003.
98. Chambers KR, Siddique MD, Banister K et al: Clinical comparison of the Spiegelberg parenchymal transducer and ventricular fluid pressure, *J Neurol Neurosurg Psychiatry* 71: 383-385, 2001.
99. Yau YH, Piper IR, Clutton RE et al: Experimental evaluation of the Spiegelberg intracranial pressure and intracranial compliance monitor. Technical note, *J Neurosurg*ery 93(6): 1072-1077, 2000.
100. Lozier AP, Sciacca RR, Romagnoli MF: Ventriculostomy-related infections: a critical review of the literature, *Neurosurgery* 51:170-182, 2002.
101. Schmidt B, Czosnyka M, Raabe A et al: Adaptive noninvasive assessment of intracranial pressure and cerebral autoregulation, *Stroke* 34:84-89, 2003.
102. Fountas KN, Sitkauskas A, Feltes CH et al: Is non-invasive monitoring of intracranial pressure waveform analysis possible? Preliminary results of a comparative study of non-invasive vs. invasive intracranial slow-wave waveform analysis monitoring in patients with traumatic brain injury, *Med Sci Monit* 11(2):CR58-63, 2005.
103. Ueno T, Macias BR, Yost WT et al: Noninvasive assessment of intracranial pressure waveforms by using pulsed phase lock loop technology: technical note, *J Neurosurg* 103:361-367, 2005.
104. Taylor WR, Chem JW, Meltzer H et al: Quantitative pupillometry, a new technology: normative data and preliminary observations in patients with acute head injury. Technical note, *J Neurosurg* 98(1):205-213, 2003.
105. Bader MK: Gizmos and gadgets for the neuroscience intensive care unit, *J Neurosci Nurs* 38:248-260, 2006.
106. Fountas K, Kapsalaki EZ, Machinis TG et al: Clinical implications of quantitative infrared pupillometry in neurosurgical patients, *Neurocrit Care* 5(1):55-60, 2006.
107. Sahuquillo J, Poca M-A, Arribas M et al: Interhemispheric supratentorial intracranial pressure gradients in head-injured patients: are they clinically important? *J Neurosurg* 90:16-26, 1999.
108. Slavin KV, Misra M: Infratentorial intracranial pressure monitoring in neurosurgical intensive care unit, *Neurol Res* 25(8):880-884, 2003.
109. Balestreri M, Czosnyka M, Steiner A et al: Intracranial hypertension: what additional information can be derived from ICP waveform after head injury? *Acta Neurochir* 146:131-141, 2004.
110. Kiening KL, Schoening WN, Stover JF et al: Continuous monitoring of intracranial compliance after severe head injury: relation to data quality, intracranial pressure and brain tissue PO_2, *Br J Neurosurg* 17:311-318, 2003.
111. Lang EW, Paulat K, Witte C et al: Noninvasive intracranial compliance monitoring. Technical note and clinical results, *J Neurosurg* 98(1):214-218, 2003.
112. Mase M, Miyati T, Yamada K et al: Non-invasive measurement of intracranial compliance using cine MRI in normal pressure hydrocephalus, *Acta Neurchir Suppl* 95:303-306, 2005.
113. Yau YH, Piper IR, Contant C et al: Assessment of different data representations and averaging methods on the Spiegelberg compliance device, *Acta Neurochir Suppl* 95:289-292, 2005.
114. Mazzeo AT, Kunene NK, Choi S et al: Quantitation of ischemic events after severe traumatic brain injury in humans: a simple scoring system, *J Neurosurg Anesthesiol* 18:170-178, 2006.
115. Kirkness CJ, Burr RL, Cain KC et al: Effect of continuous display of cerebral perfusion pressure on outcomes in patients with traumatic brain injury, *Am J Crit Care* 13:600-609, 2006.
116. Kirkness CJ, Burr RL, Cain KC et al: Relationship of cerebral perfusion pressure levels to outcome in traumatic brain injury, *Acta Neurochir* Suppl 95:13-16, 2005.
117. Robertson CS, Valadka AB, Hannay J et al: Prevention of secondary ischemic insults after severe head injury, *Crit Care Med* 27:2086-2095, 1999.
118. Andrews PJ, Sleeman DH, Statham PF et al: Predicting recovery in patients suffering from traumatic brain injury by using admission variables and physiological data: a comparison between decision tree analysis and logistic regression. *J Neurosurg* 97(2):326-336, 2002.
119. Hoeffner EG, Case I, Jain R et al: Cerebral perfusion CT: technique and clinical applications, *Radiology* 231:632-644, 2004.
120. Wintermark M, Chiolero R, Van Melle G et al: Relationship between brain perfusion computed tomography variables and cerebral perfusion pressure in severe head trauma patients, *Crit Care Med* 32:1579-1587, 2004.
121. Wintermark M, Van Melle G, Schnyder P et al: Admission perfusion CT: prognostic value in patients with severe head trauma, *Radiology* 232:211-220, 2004.
122. Wintermark M, Chiolero R, Van Melle G et al: Cerebral vascular autoregulation assessed by perfusion-CT in severe head trauma patients, *J Neuroradiol* 33:27-37, 2006.
123. Vajkochy P, Horn P, Thome C et al: Regional cerebral blood flow monitoring in the diagnosis of delayed ischemia following aneurismal subarachnoid hemorrhage. *J Neurosurg* 98:1227-1234, 2003.
124. Steiner LA, Andrews PJD: Monitoring the injured brain: ICP and CBF, *Br J Anaesth* 97:26-38, 2006.
125. Bhatia A, Gupta AK: Neuromonitoring in the intensive care unit. 1. Intracranial pressure and cerebral blood flow monitoring, *Intensive Care Med* 33:1263-1271, 2007.
126. Kinuya K, Kakuda K, Nobata K et al: Role of brain perfusion single-photon emission tomography in traumatic head injury, *Nucl Med Commun* 25:333-337, 2004.
127. Belanger HG, Vanderploeg RD, Curtiss G et al: Recent neuroimaging techniques in mild traumatic brain injury, *J Neuropsychiatry Clin Neurosci* 19:5-20, 2007.
128. Jantzen K, Anderson B, Steinberg F et al: A prospective functional MR imaging study of mild traumatic brain injury in college football players, *Am J Neuroradiology* 25:738-745, 2004.

129. Saqqur M, Zygun D, Demchuk A: Role of transcranial Doppler in neurocritical care, *Crit Care Med* 35(5 suppl): S216-S223, 2007.
130. Bellner J, Romner B, Reinstrup P et al: Transcranial Doppler sonography. Pulsatility index reflects intracranial pressure, *Surg Neurol* 62:45-51, 2004.
131. Sloan MA, Alexandrov AV, Tegelere CH et al: Assessment: transcranial Doppler ultrasonography, *Neurology* 62: 1468-1481, 2004.
132. Cormio M, Valadka AB, Robertson CS: Elevated jugular venous oxygen saturation after severe head injury, *J Neurosurg* 90:9-15, 1999.
133. White H, Baker A: Continuous jugular venous oximetry in the neurointensive care unit—a brief review, *Can J Anesth* 49: 623-629, 2002.
134. Perez A, Minces PG, Schnitzler EJ et al: Jugular venous oxygen saturation or arteriovenous difference of lactate content and outcome in children with severe traumatic brain injury, *Pediatr Crit Care* 4:33-38, 2003.
135. Sheinberg M, Kanter MJ, Robertson CS et al: Continuous monitoring of jugular venous oxygen saturation in head-injured patients, *J Neurosurg* 76:212-217, 1992.
136. Gopinath SP, Robertson CS, Contant CF et al: Jugular venous desaturation and outcome after head injury, *J Neurol Neurosurg Psychiatry* 57:717-723, 1994.
137. Robertson C: Desaturation episodes after severe head injury: influence on outcome, *Acta Neurochir (Suppl)* 59:98-101, 1993.
138. Fandino J, Stocker R, Prokop S et al: Cerebral oxygenation and systemic trauma related factors determining neurological outcome after brain injury, *J Clin Neurosci* 7:226-233, 2000.
139. Cruz J: The first decade of continuous monitoring of jugular bulb oxyhemoglobin saturation: management strategies and clinical outcome, *Crit Care Med* 26:344-351, 1998.
140. Dings J, Meixensberger J, Roosen K: Brain tissue Po_2 monitoring: catheter stability and complications, *Neurol Res* 19: 241-245, 1997.
141. Van der Brink WA, van Santbrink H, Steyerberg EW et al: Brain oxygen tension in severe head injury, *Neurosurgery* 46:868-878, 2000.
142. Gracias VH, Guillamondegui OD, Stiefel MF et al: Cerebral cortical oxygenation: a pilot study, *J Trauma* 56:469-474, 2004.
143. Bardt TF, Unterberg AW, Hartl R et al: Monitoring of brain tissue Po_2 in traumatic brain injury: effect of cerebral hypoxia on outcome, *Acta Neurochir (Suppl)* 71:153-156, 1998.
144. Valadka AB, Gopinath SP, Contant CF et al: Relationship of brain tissue Po_2 to outcome after severe head injury, *Crit Care Med* 26:1576-1581, 1998.
145. Stiefel MF, Spiotta A, Gracias CH et al: Reduced mortality rate in patients with severe traumatic brain injury treated with brain tissue oxygen monitoring, *J Neurosurg* 103:805-811, 2005.
146. Berger RP: The use of serum biomarkers to predict outcome after traumatic brain injury in adults and children, *J Head Trauma Rehabil* 21:315-333, 2006.
147. Sviri GE, Soustiel JF, Zaaroor M: Alteration in brain natriuretic peptide (BNP) plasma concentration following severe traumatic brain injury, *Acta Neurochir* 148:529-533, 2006.
148. Artru F, Dailler F, Burel E et al: Assessment of jugular blood oxygen and lactate indices for detection of cerebral ischemia and prognosis, *J Neurosurg Anesthesiol* 16:226-231, 2004.
149. Poca M, Sahuquillo J, Vilata A et al: Lack of utility of arteriojugular venous differences of lactate as a reliable indicator of brain anaerobic metabolism in traumatic brain injury, *J Neurosurg* 106(4):530-537, 2007.
150. Pelinka LE, Hertz H, Mauritz W et al: Nonspecific increase of systemic neuron-specific enolase after trauma: clinical and experimental findings, *Shock* 24:119-123, 2005.
151. Routsi C, Stamataki E, Nanas S et al: Increased level of serum S100B protein in critically ill patients without brain injury, *Shock* 26:20-24, 2006.
152. Ungerstedt U, Rostami E: Microdialysis in neurointensive care, *Curr Pharm Des* 10:2145-2152, 2004.
153. Tisdall MM, Smith M: Cerebral microdialysis: research technique or clinical tool, *Br J Anaesth* 97:18-25, 2006.
154. Cihangiroglu M, Ramsey RG, Dohrmann GJ: Brain injury: analysis of imaging modalities, *Neurol Res* 24:7-18, 2002.
155. Shutter L, Tong KA, Lee A et al: Prognostic role of proton magnetic resonance spectroscopy in acute traumatic brain injury, *J Head Trauma Rehabil* 21:334-349, 2006.
156. Govindaraju V, Gauger GE, Manley GT et al: Volumetric proton spectroscopic imaging of mild traumatic brain injury, *AJNR* 25:730-737, 2004.
157. Hirsch LJ: Continuous EEG monitoring in the intensive care unit: an overview, *J Clin Neurophysiol* 21:332-340, 2004.
158. Nuwer MR, Hovda DA, Schrader LM et al: Routine and quantitative EEG in mild traumatic brain injury, *Clin Neurophysiol* 116:2001-2025, 2006.
159. Deogaonkar A, Gupta R, DeGeorgia M et al: Bispectral index monitoring correlates with sedation scales in brain-injured patients, *Crit Care Med* 32:2403-2406, 2004.
160. Bader MK, Arbour R, Palmer S: Refractory increased intracranial pressure in severe traumatic brain injury, *AACN Clin Issues* 16:526-541, 2005.
161. Riker RR, Fraser GL, Wilkins ML: Comparing the bispectral index and suppression ratio with burst suppression of the electroencephalogram during pentobarbital infusions in adult intensive care patients, *Pharmacotherapy* 23:1087-1093, 2003.
162. Fabregas N, Gambus PL, Valero R et al: Can bispectral index monitoring predict recovery of consciousness in patients with severe brain injury, *Anesthesiology* 101:43-51, 2004.
163. Fischer C, Luaute J, Adeleine P et al: Predictive value of sensory and cognitive evoked potentials for awakening from coma, *Neurology* 63:669-673, 2004.
164. Lew HL, Poole JH, Castraneda A et al: Prognostic value of evoked and event-related potentials in moderate to severe brain injury, *J Head Trauma Rehabil* 21:350-360, 2006.
165. Amantini A, Grippo A, Fossi S et al: Prediction of 'awakening' and outcome in prolonged acute coma from severe traumatic brain injury: evidence for validity of short latency SEPs, *Clin Neurophysiol* 116:229-235, 2005.
166. Fischer C, Luaute J: Evoked potentials for the prediction of vegetative state in the acute stage of coma, *Neuropsychol Rehabil* 15:372-380, 2005.
167. Aeron-Thomas AS, Hess S: Red-light cameras for the prevention of road traffic crashes, *Cochrane Database Syst Rev* Apr 18(2):CD003862, 2005.
168. Wilson C, Willis WC, Hendrikz JK et al: Speed enforcement detection devices for preventing road traffic injuries, *Cochrane Database Syst Rev* Apr 19(2):CD004607, 2006.

169. Bunn F, Collier T, Frost C et al: Area-wide traffic calming for preventing traffic related injuries, *Cochrane Database Syst Rev* (1):CD003110, 2003.
170. Nirula R, Kaufman R, Tencer A: Traumatic brain injury and automotive design: making motor vehicles safer, *J Trauma* 55:844-848, 2003.
171. Bazarian JJ, Fisher SG, Flesher W et al: Lateral automobile impacts and the risk of traumatic brain injury, *Ann Emerg Med* 44:142-152, 2004.
172. Liu B, Ivers R, Norton R et al: Helmets for preventing injury in motorcycle riders, *Cochrane Database Syst Rev* (2):CD004333, 2004.
173. Ouellet JV, Kasantikut V: Motorcycle helmet effect on a per-crash basis in Thailand and the United States, *Traffic Inj Prev* 7(1):49-54, 2006.
174. Adekoya N, Thurman DJ, White DD et al: Surveillance for traumatic brain injury United States, 1989—1998, *MMWR* 51(SS10):1-16, 2002.
175. Ghajar J, Hariri R, Narayan RK et al: Survey of critical care management of comatose, head-injured patients in the United States, *Crit Care Med* 23:560-567, 1995.
176. Brain Trauma Foundation Writing Team: Guidelines for Prehospital Management of Traumatic Brain Injury, 2nd edition, *Prehospital Emergency Care* 12(Suppl),1-53, 2007.
177. Cushman JG, Agarwal N, Fabian TC et al: Practice management guidelines for the management of mild traumatic brain injury: The EAST practice management guidelines work group, *J Trauma* 51(5):1016-1026, 2001.
178. Aarabi B, Alden TD, Chesnut RM et al: Management and prognosis of penetrating brain injury, *J Trauma* 51(Suppl), S81-S86, 2001.
179. Adelson PD, Bratton SL, Carney NA et al: Guidelines for the acute medical management of severe traumatic brain injury in infants, children, and adolescents, *Crit Care Med* 31(6 Suppl), S407-S491, 2003.
180. Knuth T, Letarte PB, Ling G et al: *Guidelines for the Field Management of Combat-Related Head Trauma,* New York, 2005, Brain Trauma Foundation.
181. Bullock MR, Chesnut R, Ghajar J et al: Guidelines for the surgical management of traumatic brain injury, *Neurosurgery* 58(3 Suppl):S16-S24, 2006.
182. Palmer S, Bader MK, Qureshi A et al: The impact on outcomes in a community hospital setting of using the AANS Traumatic Brain Injury Guidelines, *J Trauma* 50:657-664, 2001.
183. Fakhry SM, Trask AL, Waller MA et al: Management of brain-injured patients by an evidence-based medicine protocol improves outcomes and decreases hospital charges, *J Trauma* 56:492-500, 2004.
184. Watts DD, Hanfling D, Waller MA et al: An evaluation of the use of guidelines in prehospital management of brain injury, *Prehosp Emerg Care* 8(3):254-261, 2004.
185. Holly LT, Kelly DF, Counelis GJ et al: Cervical spine trauma associated with moderate and severe head injury: incidence, risk factors, and injury characteristics, *J Neurosurg* 96(3 Suppl): 285-291, 2002.
186. Piatt JH Jr: Detected and overlooked cervical spine injury in comatose victims of trauma: report from the Pennsylvania Trauma Outcomes Study, *J Neurosurg Spine* 5(3):210-216, 2006.
187. Winchell RJ, Hoyt DB: Endotracheal intubation in the field improves survival in patients with severe head injury, *Arch Surg* 132(6):592-597, 1997.
188. Bochicchio G, Ilahi O, Joshi M et al: Endotracheal intubation in the field does not improve outcome in trauma patients who present without an acutely lethal traumatic brain injury, *J Trauma* 54:307-311, 2003.
189. Poste JC, Davis DP, Ochs M et al: Air medical transport of severely head-injured patients undergoing paramedic rapid sequence intubation, *Aid Med J* 23(4):36-40, 2004.
190. Davis DP, Peay J, Sise MJ et al: The impact of prehospital endotracheal intubation on outcome in moderate to severe traumatic brain injury, *J Trauma* 58(5):933-939, 2005.
191. Chesnut RM: Care of central nervous system injuries, *Surg Clin N Am* 87:119-156, 2007.
192. Magnoni S, Ghisoni L, Locatelli M et al: Lack of improvement in cerebral metabolism after hyperoxia in severe head injury: a microdialysis study, *J Neurosurg* 98(5):952-958, 2003.
193. Alves OL, Daugherty WP, Rios M: Arterial hyperoxia in severe head injury: a useful or harmful option, *Curr Pharm Des* 10:2163-2176, 2004.
194. Diringer MN, Aiyagari V, Zazulia AR et al: Effect of hyperoxia on cerebral metabolic rate for oxygen measured using positron emission tomography in patients with acute severe head injury, *J Neurosurg* 106(4):526-529, 2007.
195. Vassar MJ, Perry CA, Gannaway WL et al: 7.5% Sodium chloride/dextran for resuscitation of trauma patients undergoing helicopter transport, *Arch Surg* 126(9):1065-1072, 1991.
196. Vassar MJ, Fischer RP, O'Brien PE et al: A multicenter trial for resuscitation of injured patients with 7.5% sodium chloride. The effect of added dextran 70. The Multicenter Group for the Study of Hypertonic Saline in Trauma Patients, *Arch Surg* 128:1003-1011, 1993.
197. Wade CE, Grady JJ, Kramer GC et al: Individual patient cohort analysis of the efficacy of hypertonic saline/dextran in patients with traumatic brain injury and hypotension, *J Trauma* 42(5):S61-S65, 1997.
198. White H, Cook D, Venkatesh B: The use of hypertonic saline for treating intracranial hypertension after traumatic brain injury, *Anesth Analg* 102:1836-1846, 2006.
199. Cooper DJ, Myles PS, McDermott FT et al: Prehospital hypertonic saline resuscitation of patients with hypotension and severe traumatic brain injury. A randomized controlled trial, *JAMA* 291:1350-1357, 2004.
200. Sperry RJ, Bailey PL, Reichman MV et al: Fentanyl and sufentanil increase intracranial pressure in head trauma patients, *Anesthesiology* 77:416-420, 1992.
201. Kelly DF, Goodale DB, Williams J et al: Propofol in the treatment of moderate and severe head injury: a randomized, prospective double-blinded pilot trial, *J Neurosurg* 90: 1042-1052, 1999.
202. Lowe GJ, Ferguson ND: Lung-protective ventilation in neurosurgical patients, *Curr Opin Crit Care* 12:3-7, 2006.
203. Caricato A, Conti G, Corte FD et al: Effects of PEEP on the intracranial system of patients with head injury and subarachnoid hemorrhage: the role of respiratory system compliance, *J Trauma* 58:571-576, 2005.
204. Mascia L, Grasso S, Fiore T et al: Cerebro-pulmonary interactions during the application of low levels of positive end-expiratory pressure, *Intensive Care Med* 31:373-379, 2005.
205. Bein T, Kuhr LP, Bele S et al: Lung recruitment maneuver in patients with cerebral injury: effects on intracranial pressure and cerebral metabolism, *Intensive Care Med* 28:554-558, 2002.

206. Salim A, Miller K, Dangleben D et al: High-frequency percussive ventilation: an alternative mode of ventilation for head-injured patients with adult respiratory distress syndrome, *J Trauma* 57:542-546, 2004.
207. David M, Karmrodt J, Weiler N et al: High-frequency oscillatory ventilation in adults with traumatic brain injury and acute respiratory distress syndrome, *Acta Anaesthesiol Scand* 49:209-214, 2005.
208. Bein R, Scherer MN, Philipp A et al: Pumpless extracorporeal lung assist (pECLA) in patients with acute respiratory distress syndrome and severe brain injury, *J Trauma* 58:1294-1297, 2005.
209. Gemma M, Tommasino C, Cerri M et al: Intracranial effects of endotracheal suctioning in the acute phase of head injury, *J Neurosurg Anesthesiol* 14:50-54, 2002.
210. Leone M, Albanese J, Viviand X et al: The effects of remifentanil on endotracheal suctioning-induced increases in intracranial pressure in head-injured patients, *Anesth Analg* 99: 1193-1198, 2004.
211. Kerr ME, Rudy EB, Brucia J et al: Head-injured adults: recommendations for endotracheal suctioning, *J Neurosci Nurs* 25:86-91, 1993.
212. Brucia J, Rudy E: The effect of suction catheter insertion and tracheal stimulation in adults with severe brain injury, *Heart Lung* 25:295-303, 1996.
213. Kerr ME, Weber BB, Sereika SM et al: Effect of endotracheal suctioning on cerebral oxygenation in traumatic brain-injured patients, *Crit Care Med* 27:2776-2781, 1999.
214. Carlson AP, Schermer CR, Lu SW: Retrospective evaluation of anemia and transfusion in traumatic brain injury, *J Trauma* 61:567-571, 2006.
215. McIntyre LA, Fergusson DA, Hutchison JS et al: Effect of a liberal versus restrictive transfusion strategy on mortality in patients with moderate to severe head injury, *Neurocrit Care* 5:4-9, 2006.
216. Smith MJ, Stiefel MF, Magge S et al: Packed red blood cell transfusion increases local cerebral oxygenation, *Crit Care Med* 33:1104-1108, 2005.
217. Parsons LC, Wilson MM: Cerebrovascular status on severe closed head injured patients following passive position changes, *Nurs Res* 33:68-75, 1984.
218. Sullivan J: Positioning of patients with severe traumatic brain injury: research-based practice, *J Neurosci Nurs* 32:204-209, 2000.
219. Mitchell PH, Ozuna J: Moving the patient in bed: effects on intracranial pressure, *Nurs Res* 30:212-218, 1981.
220. Williams A, Coyne SM: Effects of neck position on intracranial pressure, *Am J Crit Care* 2:68-71, 1993.
221. Lipe HP, Mitchell PH: Positioning the patient with intracranial hypertension: how turning and head rotation affect the internal jugular vein, *Heart Lung* 9:1031-1037, 1980.
222. Winkelman C: Effect of backrest position on intracranial and cerebral perfusion pressures in traumatically brain-injured adults, *Am J Crit Care* 9:373-380, 2000.
223. Fan J-Y: Effect of backrest position on intracranial pressure and cerebral perfusion pressure in individuals with brain injury: A systematic review, *J Neurosci Nurs* 36:278-288, 2004.
224. Ng I, Lim B, Wong HB: Effects of head posture on cerebral hemodynamics: its influences on intracranial pressure, cerebral perfusion pressure, and cerebral oxygenation, *Neurosurgery* 54:593-598, 2004.
225. Rosner MJ, Coley IB: Cerebral perfusion pressure, intracranial pressure, and head elevation, *J Neurosurg* 65:636-641, 1986.
226. Meixensberger J, Baunach S, Amschler J et al: Influence of body position on tissue-Po_2 cerebral perfusion pressure and intracranial pressure in patients with acute brain injury, *Neurol Res* 19:249-253, 1997.
227. Feldman Z, Kanter MJ, Robertson CS et al: Effect on head elevation on intracranial pressure, cerebral perfusion pressure, and cerebral blood flow in head-injured patients, *J Neurosurg* 76:207-211, 1992.
228. Thelandersson A, Cider A, Nellgård B: Prone position in mechanically ventilated patients with reduced intracranial compliance, *Acta Anaesthesiol Scand* 50:937-941, 2006.
229. Nekludov M, Bellander B-M, Mure M: Oxygenation and cerebral perfusion pressure improved in the prone position, *Acta Anaethesiol Scand* 50:932-936, 2006.
230. Geffroy A, Bronchard R, Merckx P et al: Severe traumatic head injury in adults: which patients are at risk of early hyperthermia? *Intensive Care Med* 30:785-790, 2004.
231. Thompson HJ, Kirkness CJ, Mitchell PH: Intensive care unit management of fever following traumatic brain injury, *Intensive Crit Care Nurs* 23:91-96, 2007.
232. Thompson HJ, Tkacs NC, Saatman KE et al: Hyperthermia following traumatic brain injury: a critical evaluation, *Neurobiol Dis* 12:163-173, 2003.
233. Diringer MN, for the Neurocritical Care Fever Reduction Trial Group: Treatment of fever in the neurologic intensive care unit with a catheter-based heat exchange system, *Crit Care Med* 32:559-564, 2004.
234. Jiang JY, Gao GY, Li WP et al: Early indicators of prognosis in 846 cases of severe traumatic brain injury, *J Neurotrauma* 19:869-874, 2002.
235. Mcilvoy L: Comparison of brain temperature to core temperature: a review of the literature, *J Neurosci Nurs* 36:23-31, 2004.
236. Aiyagari V, Diringer MN: Fever control and its impact on outcomes: what is the evidence? *J Neurolog Sci* 261:39-46, 2007.
237. Thompson HJ, Kirkness CH, Mitchell PH: Fever management practices of neuroscience nurses, part II: nurse, patient, and barriers, *J Neurosci Nurs* 39:196-201, 2007.
238. Herr K, Coyne PJ, Key T et al: Pain assessment in the nonverbal patient: position statement with clinical practice recommendations, *Pain Manag Nurs* 7:44-52, 2006.
239. Young J, Siffleet J, Nikoletti S et al: Use of a Behavioural Pain Scale to assess pain in ventilated, unconscious and/or sedated patients, *Intensive Crit Care Nurs* 22:32-39, 2006.
240. Belden JM: Pain section of the neurologic system. In Alspach JG, editor: *Core Curriculum for Critical Care Nursing*, St. Louis, 2006, Saunders Elsevier.
241. Rosen DJ, Nicoara A, Koshy N et al: Too much of a good thing? Tracing the history of the propofol infusion syndrome, *J Trauma* 63:443-447, 2007.
242. Muizelaar JP, van der Poel HG: Cerebral vasoconstriction is not maintained with prolonged hyperventilation. In Hoff JT, Betz AI, editors: *Intracranial Pressure*, ed 7, Berlin, 1989, Springer-Verlag.
243. Muizelaar JP, Marmarou A, Ward JD et al: Adverse effects of prolonged hyperventilation in patients with severe head injury: a randomized clinical trial, *J Neurosurg* 75:731-739, 1991.

244. Marion DW, Puccio A, Wisniewski SR et al: Effect of hyperventilation on extracellular concentrations of glutamate, lactate, pyruvate, and local cerebral blood flow in patients with severe traumatic brain injury, *Crit Care Med* 30:2619-2625, 2002.
245. Soustiel JF, Mahamid E, Chistyakov A et al: Comparison of moderate hyperventilation and mannitol for control of intracranial pressure control in patients with severe traumatic brain injury—a study of cerebral blood flow and metabolism, *Acta Neurochir* 148:845-851, 2006.
246. Kirkpatrick PJ, Smielewski P, Piechnik S et al: Early effects of mannitol in patients with head injuries assessed using bedside multimodality monitoring, *Neurosurgery* 39:714-721, 1996.
247. Schrot RJ, Muizelaar JP: Mannitol in acute traumatic brain injury, *Lancet* 359:1633-1634, 2002.
248. Sakowitz OW, Stover JF, Sarrafzadeh AS et al: Effects of mannitol bolus administration on intracranial pressure, cerebral extracellular metabolites, and tissue oxygenation in severely head-injured patients, *J Trauma* 62:292-298, 2007.
249. Luvisotto TL, Auer RN, Sutherland GR: The effect of mannitol on experimental cerebral ischemia, revisited, *Neurosurgery* 38:131-139, 1996.
250. Cruz J, Minoja G, Okuchi K: Improving clinical outcomes from acute subdural hematomas with the emergency preoperative administration of high doses of mannitol: a randomized trial, *Neurosurgery* 49:864-871, 2001.
251. Cruz J, Minoja G, Okuchi K et al: Successful use of the new high-dose mannitol treatment in patients with Glasgow Coma Scale scores of 3 and bilateral abnormal pupillary widening: a randomized trial, *J Neurosurg* 100:376-383, 2004.
252. Schierhout G, Roberts I: Mannitol for acute traumatic brain injury, *Cochrane Database Syst Rev* (2):CD001049, 2000.
253. Kaufmann AM, Cardoso ER: Aggravation of vasogenic cerebral edema by multiple-dose mannitol, *J Neurosurg* 77: 584-589, 1992.
254. Wakai A, Roberts I, Schierhout G: Mannitol for acute traumatic brain injury, *Cochrane Database Syst Rev* Jan 24(1): CD001049, 2007.
255. Becker DP, Vries JK: The alleviation of increased intracranial pressure by the chronic administration of osmotic agents. In Brock M, Dietz H, editors: *Intracranial Pressure*, Berlin, 1972, Springer.
256. Gondim Fde A, Aiyagari V, Shackleford A et al: Osmolality not predictive of mannitol-induced acute renal insufficiency, *J Neurosurg* 103:444-447, 2005.
257. Ogden AT, Mayer SA, Connolly ES Jr et al: Hyperosmolar agents in neurosurgical practice: the evolving role of hypertonic saline, *Neurosurgery* 57:207-215, 2005.
258. Lescot T, Degos V, Zouaoui A et al: Opposed effects of hypertonic saline on contusions and noncontused brain tissue in patients with severe traumatic brain injury, *Crit Care Med* 34:3029-3033, 2006.
259. Shackford SR, Zhuang J, Schmoker J: Intravenous fluid tonicity: effect on intracranial pressure, cerebral blood flow, and cerebral oxygen delivery in focal brain injury, *J Neurosurg* 76:91-98, 1992.
260. Kreimeier U, Messmer K: Small-volume resuscitation: from experimental evidence to clinical routine. Advantages and disadvantages of hypertonic solutions, *Acta Anaesthesiol Scand* 46:625-638, 2002.
261. Hartl R, Medary MB, Ruge M et al: Hypertonic/hyperoncotic saline attenuates microcirculatory disturbances after traumatic brain injury, *J Trauma 42(5 Suppl)*:S41-S47, 1997.
262. Hashiguchi N, Lum L, Romeril E et al: Hypertonic saline resuscitation: efficacy may require treatment in severely injured patients, *J Trauma* 62:299-306, 2007.
263. Ziai WC, Young TJK, Bhardwaj A: Hypertonic saline: first-line therapy for cerebral edema? *J Neurol Sci* 261:157-166, 2007.
264. Vialet R, Albanese J, Thomachot L et al: Isovolume hypertonic solutes (sodium chloride or mannitol) in the treatment of refractory posttraumatic intracranial hypertension: 2 mL/kg 7.5% saline is more effective than 2 mL/kg 20% mannitol, *Crit Care Med* 31:1683-1687, 2003.
265. Battison C, Hons BA, Andrews JD et al: Randomized, controlled trial on the effect of a 20% mannitol solution and a 7.5% saline/6% dextran solution on increased intracranial pressure after brain injury, *Crit Care Med* 33:196-202, 2005.
266. Ware ML, Nemani VM, Meeker M et al: Effects of 23.4% sodium chloride solution in reducing intracranial pressure in patients with traumatic brain injury: a preliminary study, *Neurosurgery* 57:727-736, 2005.
267. Hsiang JK, Chesnut RM, Crisp CB et al: Early, routine paralysis for intracranial pressure control in severe head injury: is it necessary? *Crit Care Med* 22:1471-1476, 1994.
268. Alderson P, Roberts I: Corticosteroids for acute traumatic brain injury, *Cochrane Database Syst Rev* Jan 25(1):CD000196, 2005.
269. Goodman JC, Valadka AB, Gopinath SP et al: Lactate and excitatory amino acids measured by microdialysis are decreased by pentobarbital coma in head-injured patients, *J Neurotrauma* 13:549-556, 1996.
270. Thorat JD, Wang EC, Lee KK et al: Barbiturate therapy for patients with refractory intracranial hypertension following severe traumatic brain injury: its effects on tissue oxygenation, brain temperature and autoregulation, *J Clin Neurosci* November 2007. Epub ahead of print.
271. Rea GL, Rockswold GL: Barbiturate therapy in uncontrolled intracranial hypertension, *Neurosurgery* 12:401-404, 1983.
272. Eisenberg HM, Frankowski RF, Contant CF et al: High-dose barbiturate control of elevated intracranial pressure in patients with severe head injury, *J Neurosurg* 69:15-23, 1988.
273. Ward JD, Becker DP, Miller JD et al: Failure of prophylactic barbiturate coma in the treatment of severe head injury, *J Neurosurg* 62:383-388, 1985.
274. Bochicchio GV, Bochicchio K, Nehman S et al: Tolerance and efficacy of enteral nutrition in traumatic brain-injured patients induced into barbiturate coma, *JPEN J Parenter Enteral Nutr* 30:503-506, 2006.
275. Humar M, Pischke SE, Loop T et al: Barbiturates directly inhibit the calmodulin/calcineurin complex: a novel mechanism of inhibition of nuclear factor of activated T cells, *Mol Pharmacol* 65:350-361, 2004.
276. Polin RS, Shaffrey ME, Bogaev CA et al: Decompressive bifrontal craniectomy in the treatment of severe refractory posttraumatic cerebral edema, *Neurosurgery* 41:84-94, 1997.
277. Aarabi R, Hesdorffer DC, Ahn ES et al: Outcome following decompressive craniectomy for malignant swelling due to severe head injury, *J Neurosurg* 104:469-479, 2006.
278. Timofeev I, Hutchinson PJ: Outcome after surgical decompression of severe traumatic brain injury, *Injury* 37: 1125-1132, 2006.

279. Taylor A, Butt W, Rosenfeld J et al: A randomized trial of very early decompressive craniectomy in children with traumatic brain injury and sustained intracranial hypertension, *Child's Nerv Syst* 17:154-162, 2001.
280. Stiefel MF, Heuer GG, Smith MJ et al: Cerebral oxygenation following decompressive hemicraniectomy for the treatment of refractory intracranial hypertension, *J Neurosurg* 101: 241-247, 2004.
281. Bor-Seng-Shu E, Hirsch R, Teixeira MJ et al: Cerebral hemodynamic changes gauged by transcranial Doppler ultrasonography in patients with posttraumatic brain swelling treated by surgical decompression, *J Neurosurg* 104:93-100, 2006.
282. Heppner P, Ellagala DB, Durieux M et al: Contrast ultrasonographic assessment of cerebral perfusion in patients undergoing decompressive craniectomy for traumatic brain injury, *J Neurosurg* 104(5):738-745, 2006.
283. Joseph DK, Dutton RP, Aarabi B et al: Decompressive laparotomy to treat intractable intracranial hypertension after traumatic brain injury, *J Trauma* 57:687-695, 2004.
284. Scalea TM, Bochicchio GV, Habashi N et al: Increased intra-abdominal, intrathoracic, and intracranial pressure after severe brain injury: multiple compartment syndrome. *J Trauma* 62:647-656, 2007.
285. Mori K, Maeda M, Miyazaki M et al: Effects of mild and moderate hypothermia on cerebral metabolism and glutamate in an experimental head injury, *Acta Neurochir (Suppl)* 71: 222-224, 1998.
286. Tokutomi T, Morimoto K, Miyagi T et al: Optimal temperature for the management of severe traumatic brain injury: effect of hypothermia on intracranial pressure, systemic and intracranial hemodynamics, and metabolism, *Neurosurgery* 52:102-112, 2003.
287. Sahuquillo J, Vilalta A: Cooling the injured brain: how does moderate hypothermia influence the pathophysiology of traumatic brain injury, *Curr Pharm Des* 13:2310-2322, 2007.
288. Clifton GL, Barrodale AS, Plenger B et al: A phase II study of moderate hypothermia in severe brain injury, *J Neurotrauma* 10:263-271, 1993.
289. Shiozaki T, Sugimoto H, Taneda M et al: Effect of mild hypothermia on uncontrollable intracranial hypertension after severe head injury, *J Neurosurg* 79:363-368, 1993.
290. Marion DW, Penrod LE, Kelsey SF et al: Treatment of traumatic brain injury with moderate hypothermia, *N Engl J Med* 336:540-545, 1997.
291. Jiang J, Yu M, Zhu C: Effect of long-term mild hypothermia therapy in patients with severe traumatic brain injury: 1-year follow-up review of 87 cases, *J Neurosurg* 93:718-719, 2000.
292. Clifton GL, Miller ER, Choi SC et al: Lack of effect of induction of hypothermia after acute brain injury, *N Engl J Med* 344:556-563, 2001.
293. Harris OA, Colford JM, Good MC et al: The role of hypothermia in the management of severe brain injury, *Arch Neurol* 59:1077-1083, 2002.
294. McIntyre LA, Fergusson DA, Hebert PC et al: Prolonged therapeutic hypothermia after traumatic brain injury in adults, *JAMA* 289:2992-2999, 2003.
295. Henderson WR, Dhingra VK, Chittock DR et al: Hypothermia in the management of traumatic brain injury, *Intensive Care Med* 29:1637-1644, 2003.
296. Alderson P, Gadkary C, Signorini DF: Therapeutic hypothermia for head injury, *Cochrane Database Syst Rev* Oct 18(4): CD001048, 2004.
297. Adelson PD, Ragheb J, Kacey P et al: Phase II clinical trial of moderate hypothermia after severe traumatic brain injury in children, *Neurosurgery* 56:740-754, 2005.
298. Reinert M, Barth A, Rothen HU et al: Effects of cerebral perfusion pressure and increased fraction of inspired oxygen on brain tissue oxygen, lactate and glucose in patients with severe head injury, *Acta Neurochir* 145:341-350, 2003.
299. Johnston AJ, Steiner LA, Coles JP et al: Effect of cerebral perfusion pressure augmentation on regional oxygenation and metabolism after head injury, *Crit Care Med* 33:189-195, 2005.
300. Cohan P, Wang C, McArthur DL et al: Acute secondary adrenal insufficiency after traumatic brain injury: a prospective study, *Crit Care Med* 33:2358-2366, 2005.
301. Rose JC, Mayer SA: Optimizing blood pressure in neurological emergencies, *Neurocrit Care* 1:287-299, 2004.
302. Oertel M, Boscardin WJ, Obrist WD et al: Posttraumatic vasospasm: the epidemiology, severity, and time course of an underestimated phenomenon: a prospective study performed in 299 patients, *J Neurosurg* 103:812-824, 2005.
303. Taneda M, Kataoka K, Akai F et al: Traumatic subarachnoid hemorrhage as a predictable indicator of delayed ischemic symptoms, *J Neurosug* 84:762-768, 1996.
304. Langham J, Goldfrad C, Teasdale G et al: Calcium channel blockers for acute traumatic brain injury, *Cochrane Database Syst Rev* (4):CD000565, 2003.
305. Vergouwen MDI, Vermeulen M, Roos YBWEM: Effect of nimodipine on outcome in patients with traumatic subarachnoid haemorrhage: a systematic review, *Lancet Neurol* 5: 1029-1032, 2006.
306. Diringer MN, Axelrod Y: Hemodynamic manipulation in the neuro-intensive care unit: cerebral perfusion pressure therapy in head injury and hemodynamic augmentation for cerebral vasospasm, *Curr Opin Crit Care* 13:156-162, 2007.
307. Temkin NR: Risk factors for posttraumatic seizures in adults, *Epilepsia* 44:18-20, 2003.
308. Englander J, Bushnik T, Duong TT et al: Analyzing risk factors for late posttraumatic seizures: a prospective, multicenter investigation, *Arch Phys Med Rehabil* 84:365-373, 2003.
309. Temkin NR, Dikmen SS, Anderson GD et al: Valproate therapy for prevention of posttraumatic seizures: a randomized trial, *J Neurosurg* 91:593-600, 1999.
310. Haltiner AM, Newell DW, Temkin NR et al: Side effects and mortality associated with use of phenytoin for early posttraumatic seizure prophylaxis, *J Neurosurg* 91:588-592, 1999.
311. Quattrocchi KB, Frank EH, Miller CH et al: Severe head injury: effect upon cellular immune function, *Neurol Res* 13: 13-20, 1991.
312. Smrcka M, Mrlian A, Karisson-Valik J et al: The effect of head injury upon the immune system, *Bratisl Lek Listy* 108: 144-148, 2007.
313. Doherty PF, Rabinowitz RP: Gunshot wounds to the head: The role of antibiotics, *Infect Med* 21:297-300, 2004.
314. Baumann A, Audibert G, McDonnell J et al: Neurogenic pulmonary edema, *Acta Anaesthesiol Scand* 51:447-455, 2007.
315. Holland MC, Mackersie RC, Morabito D et al: The development of acute lung injury is associated with worse neurologic outcome in patients with severe traumatic brain injury, *J Trauma* 55:106-111, 2003.
316. Bouderka MA, Fakhir B, Bouaggad A et al: Early tracheostomy versus prolonged endotracheal intubation in severe head injury, *J Trauma* 57:251-254, 2004.

317. Ahmed N, Kuo YH: Early versus late tracheostomy in patients with severe traumatic head injury, *Surg Infect (Larchmt)* 8:343-347, 2007.
318. Agha A, Thornton E, O'Kelly P et al: Posterior pituitary dysfunction after traumatic brain injury, *J Clin Endocrinol Metab* 89:5987-5992, 2004.
319. Tisdall M, Crocker M, Watkiss J et al: Disturbances of sodium in critically ill adult neurologic patients, *J Neurosurg Anesthesiol* 18:57-63, 2006.
320. Diringer MN, Zazulia AR: Hyponatremia in neurologic patients: consequences and approaches to treatment, *Neurologist* 12:117-126, 2006.
321. Verbalis JG: AVP receptor antagonists as aquaretics: review and assessment of clinical data, *Cleve Clin J Med* 73:524-533, 2006.
322. Rabinstein AA, Wijdicks EFM: Hyponatremia in critically ill neurological patients, *Neurologist* 9:290-300, 2003.
323. Carrick MM, Tyroch AH, Youens CA et al: Subsequent development of thrombocytopenia and coagulopathy in moderate and severe head injury: support for serial laboratory examination, *J Trauma* 58:725-730, 2005.
324. May AK, Young JS, Butler K et al: Coagulopathy in severe closed head injury: is empiric therapy warranted? *Am Surg* 63:233-236, 1997.
325. Engstrom M, Romner B, Schalen et al: Thrombocytopenia predicts progressive hemorrhage after head trauma, *J Neurotrauma* 22:291-296, 2005.
326. Stein SC, Young GS, Talucci RC et al: Delayed brain injury after head trauma: significance of coagulopathy, *Neurosurgery* 30:160-165, 1992.
327. Yadav YR, Basoor A, Jain G et al: Expanding traumatic intracerebral contusion/hematoma, *Neurology India* 54:377-381, 2006.
328. Roitberg B, Emechebe-Kennedy O, Amin-Hanjani S et al: Human recombinant factor VII for emergency reversal of coagulopathy in neurosurgical patients: a retrospective comparative study, *Neurosurgery* 57:832-836, 2005.
329. Dutton RP, Stein DM: The use of factor VIIa in haemorrhagic shock and intracerebral bleeding, *Injury* 37:1172-1177, 2006.
330. Yusim Y, Perel A, Berkenstadt H et al: The use of recombinant factor VIIa (NovoSeven) for treatment of active or impending bleeding in brain injury: broadening the indications, *J Clin Anesth* 18:545-551, 2006.
331. Venkatesh B, Townsend S, Boots RJ: Does splanchnic ischemia occur in isolated neurotrauma? A prospective observational study, *Crit Care Med* 27:1175-1180, 1999.
332. Krakau K, Omne-Ponten M, Karlsson T et al: Metabolism and nutrition in patients with moderate and severe traumatic brain injury: a systematic review, *Brain Injury* 20(4):345-367, 2006.
333. Wilson RF, Tyburski JG: Metabolic responses and nutritional therapy in patients with severe head injuries, *J Head Trauma Rehabil* 13:11-27, 1998.
334. Denes Z: The influence of severe malnutrition on rehabilitation in patients with severe head injury, *Disabil Rehabil* 26:1163-1165, 2004.
335. Perel P, Yanagawa T, Bunn F et al: Nutritional support for head-injured patients, *Cochrane Database Syst Rev* Oct 18(4): CD001530, 2006.
336. Gerber CS: Understanding and managing coma stimulation. Are we doing everything we can? *Crit Care Nurs Q* 28(2): 94-108, 2005.
337. Urban RJ, Harris P, Masel B: Anterior hypopituitarism following traumatic brain injury, *Brain Injury* 19(5):349-358, 2005.
338. Agha A, Rogers B, Sherlock M et al: Anterior pituitary dysfunction in survivors of traumatic brain injury, *J Clin Metab* 89:4929-4936, 2004.
339. Bondanelli M, Ambrosio MR, Zatelli MC et al: Hypopituitarism after traumatic brain injury, *Eur J Endrocrinol* 152: 679-691, 2005.
340. Ghigo E, Masel B, Aimaretti G et al: Consensus guidelines on screening for hypopituitarism following traumatic brain injury, *Brain Injury* 19(9):711-724, 2005.
341. Saulino M, Jacobs BW: The pharmacological management of spasticity, *J Neurosci Nurs* 38(6):456-459, 2006.
342. Zafonte R, Elovic EP, Lombard L: Acute care management of post-TBI spasticity, *J Head Trauma Rehabil* 19(2):89-100, 2004.
343. Gordon WA, Zafonte R, Cicerone K et al: Traumatic brain injury rehabilitation: state of the science, *Am J Phys Med Rehabil* 85(4):343-382, 2006.
344. Hendricks HT, van Ginneken BC, Heeren AJ et al: Brain injury severity and autonomic dysregulation accurately predict heterotopic ossification in patients with traumatic brain injury, *Clin Rehabil* 21:545-553, 2007.
345. Chan K-T: Heterotopic ossification in traumatic brain injury, *Am J Phys Med Rehabil* 84(2):145-146, 2005.
346. Balboni TA, Gobezie R, Mamon HJ: Heterotopic ossification: pathophysiology, clinical features, and the role of radiotherapy for prophylaxis, *Int J Radiat Oncol Biol Phys* 65(5): 1289-1299, 2006.
347. Haran M, Bhuta T, Lee B: Pharmacological interventions for treating acute heterotopic ossification, *Cochrane Database Syst Rev* Oct 18(4):CD003321, 2004.
348. Sherer M, Nakase-Thompson R, Yablon SA et al: Multidimensional assessment of acute confusion after traumatic brain injury, *Arch Phys Med Rehabil* 86:896-904, 2005.
349. Levy M, Berson A, Cook T et al: Treatment of agitation following traumatic brain injury: a review of the literature, *NeuroRehabil* 20:279-306, 2005.
350. Nott MT, Chapparo C, Baguley IJ: Agitation following traumatic brain injury: an Australian sample, *Brain Injury* 20(11):1175-1182, 2006.
351. Lequerica AH, Rapport LJ, Loeher K et al: Agitation in acquired brain injury: impact on acute rehabilitation therapies, *J Head Trauma Rehabil* 22(3):177-183, 2007.
352. Fleminger S, Greenwood RJ, Oliver DL: Pharmacological management for agitation and aggression in people with acquired brain injury, *Cochrane Database Syst Rev* Oct 18(4): CD003299, 2006.
353. Francisco GE, Walker WC, Zasler ND et al: Pharmacological management of neurobehavioral sequelae of traumatic brain injury: a survey of current physiatric practice, *Brain Injury* 21(10):1007-1014, 2007.
354. Alderfer BS, Arciniegas DB, Silver JM: Treatment of depression following traumatic brain injury, *J Head Trauma Rehabil* 20(6):544-562, 2005.
355. Ashman TA, Gordon WA, Cantor JB et al: Neurobehavioral consequences of traumatic brain injury, *Mt Sinai J Med* 73:999-1005, 2006.
356. Dikmen SS, Bombardier CH, Machamer JE et al: Natural history of depression in traumatic brain injury, *Arch Phys Med Rehabil* 85:1457-1464, 2004.

357. Jorge RE, Robinson RG, Moser et al: Major depression following traumatic brain injury, *Arch Gen Psychiatry* 61:42-50, 2004.
358. Wells R, Dywan J, Dumas J: Life satisfaction and distress in family caregivers as related to specific behavioural changes after traumatic brain injury, *Brain Injury* 19(13):1105-1115, 2005.
359. Rivera P, Elliott TR, Berry JW et al: Predictors of caregiver depression among community-residing families living with traumatic brain injury, *NeuroRehabilitation* 22:3-8, 2007.
360. Lefebvre H, Levert M: Breaking the news of traumatic brain injury and incapacities, *Brain Injury* 20(7):711-718, 2006.
361. Duff D: Family impact and influence following severe traumatic brain injury, *Axon* 27(2):9-23, 2006.
362. Khan F, Baguley IJ, Cameron ID: Rehabilitation after traumatic brain injury, *Med J Aust* 178:290-295, 2003.
363. Van Baalen B, Odding E, Maas AI et al: Traumatic brain injury: classification of initial severity and determination of functional outcome, *Disabil Rehabil* 25(1):9-18, 2003.
364. Sorbo A: Outcome after severe brain damage: what makes the difference? *Brain Injury* 19(7):493-503, 2005.
365. Jennett B, Bond MR: Assessment of outcome after severe brain damage, *Lancet* 1:480, 1975.
366. Teasdale GM, Pettigrew LE, Wilson JT et al: Analyzing outcome of treatment of severe head injury: a review and update on advancing the use of the Glasgow Outcome Scale, *J Neurotrauma* 15:587-597, 1998.
367. Wilson JT, Pettigrew LE, Teasdale GM: Structured interviews for the Glasgow Outcome Scale and the extended Glasgow Outcome Scale: guidelines for their use, *J Neurotrauma* 15:573-585, 1998.
368. Murray G et al: Multivariable prognostic analysis in traumatic brain injury: results from the IMPACT study, *J Neurotrauma* 24(2):329-337, 2007.

21

Maxillofacial Trauma

Suzanne Frey Sherwood, Karen A. McQuillan

Introduction

The treatment of maxillofacial trauma is one of the oldest healing arts. In Hippocrates' time, skin grafts were used for facial reconstruction. The nineteenth and twentieth centuries saw major research-and-development breakthroughs in the diagnosis and treatment of facial trauma.[1] Effective management of maxillofacial injuries remains complex and challenges virtually every member of the multidisciplinary health care team. Management of these injuries requires a profound appreciation of the functional components of the orbit, nose, and oral cavity, as well as of the subtle interrelationships between skeletal and soft tissue components that define the individual's physical identity. The patient with facial injuries in conjunction with multisystem injuries requires integrated and coordinated assessment and management by multiple health care team members.

This chapter provides a review of maxillofacial anatomy then describes how to perform an assessment to detect maxillofacial injuries based on anatomical considerations. Specific types of maxillofacial injuries and current recommended treatment for these injuries are explained. Priorities of care and appropriate nursing interventions are described for each phase of the trauma cycle.

Etiology and Mechanism of Injury

Despite mandatory seatbelt laws, lower speed limits, and airbag systems, the incidence of facial injuries remains high following motor vehicle crashes due to the fact that the face is exposed and vulnerable to forces associated with rapid deceleration.[2,3] The magnitude of maxillofacial injury is directly proportionate to the velocity at impact when the face makes contact with an object. In low and mid-velocity mechanisms of injury, such as assaults, athletic incidences, falls, and low-speed motor vehicle crashes, the source of injury is usually a single-vector force and the injuries are minor, limited to soft tissue contusions, abrasions, and lacerations. However, as the velocity of single-vector injuries increases, there is greater dissipation of energy along with increased soft tissue disruption, and the underlying bone structures begin to fracture along predictable fault lines, as described by Le Fort[4] (Figures 21-1 and 21-2).

In high-speed crashes with unrestrained occupants, injury forces become exaggerated and often multivectored, resulting in even greater soft tissue disruption, bone comminution, and a loss of distinguishable Le Fort fracture patterns. In these extreme injuries, the facial structures expand outward, away from the vital orbital and intracranial structures, resulting in a distorted spherical shape.

Less common facial injuries are penetrating wounds that may result from shootings or avulsions caused by high-speed motorcycle crashes. These represent a unique subset of injuries that do not follow Le Fort's pattern of fractures and have a high potential for tissue devascularization and progressive necrosis. Patients with these injuries frequently require multiple surgeries during the early phase of hospitalization to debride necrotic tissues, followed by bone and soft tissue reconstruction performed before infection and wound contracture develop.[5,6]

Assessment of Maxillofacial Injuries With Correlative Facial Anatomy

Comprehensive management evolves from an initial, thorough clinical examination, which then directs further diagnostic studies and culminates with development of a multidisciplinary plan of care for the patient. Maxillofacial injuries can be horrific; however, these injuries must not distract the trauma team from first stabilizing the patient's airway, breathing, and circulation. Only then will the health care provider complete a thorough maxillofacial evaluation as well as a comprehensive assessment of other body systems to rule out associated injuries.[7,8] Comprehensive maxillofacial evaluation starts with a thorough assessment of soft tissue injury followed by examination of the underlying bony elements and evaluation of possible functional disruption. Knowledge of the anatomic location and function of maxillofacial structures provides rationale for strategies used to assess facial injuries and allows appropriate interpretation of assessment findings.

A generalized inspection for contusions, abrasions, and disruptive lacerations provides cues to direct a more thorough assessment of the underlying bony skeleton and functional elements. The ear canal, nose, oral cavity, and pharynx should be thoroughly assessed to identify any occult lacerations. An intraoral examination should account for all teeth and consider the possibility that a tooth is displaced into the alveolar bone (intrusion) or dislodged into the respiratory tract.[9] A seemingly simple abrasion and laceration of the lateral cheek

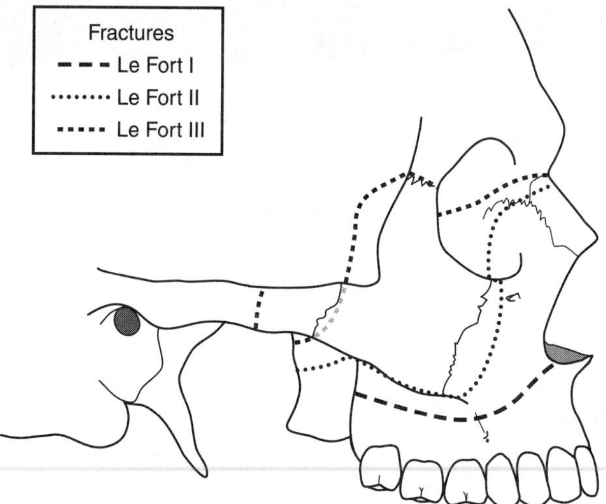

FIGURE 21-1 Le Fort lines of fracture. (From Cohen SR: Craniofacial trauma. In Ruberg RL, Smith DJ [eds]: *A Core Curriculum Plastic Surgery,* St. Louis, 1994, Mosby-Yearbook, p. 323.)

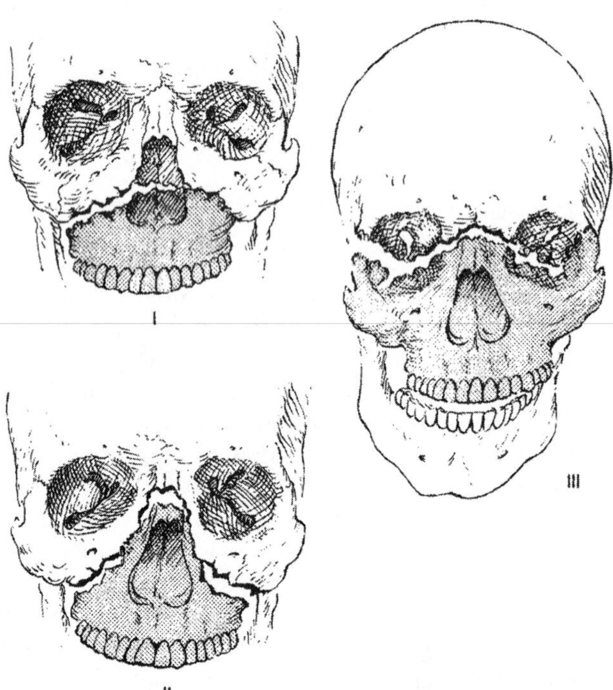

FIGURE 21-2 Le Fort classification of maxillary fractures. (From Schultz RC: Maxillofacial injuries. In Barrett BM [ed]: *Patient Care in Plastic Surgery,* ed 2, St. Louis, 1996, Mosby-Yearbook, p. 319.)

from a low-impact injury may have penetrated deep to injure the parotid gland and its duct, or may have injured the facial nerve, affecting facial animation[10] (Figure 21-3). A spectacle hematoma of the orbit is indicative of an anterior cranial base fracture with bleeding into the intracoronal fat compartment of the orbit and mandates a thorough and serial assessment of both ocular and neurological function.

Facial bones are relatively thin and arranged to allow deformation and displacement away from the associated functional elements of the orbit, airway, and brain. Surrounding each of the craniofacial functional units are dense bony struts organized in a system of vertical, transverse, and horizontal buttresses (Figure 21-4). These buttresses determine the three-dimensional structure of the face and act as energy-absorbing shields around the vital craniofacial structures.

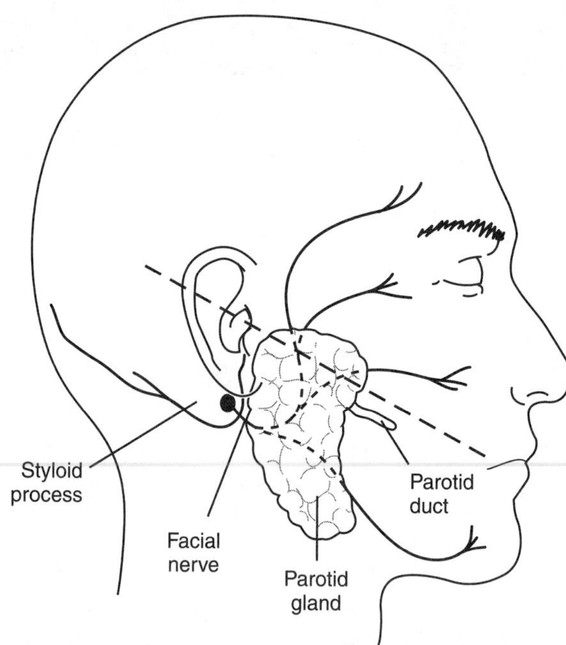

FIGURE 21-3 Lateral cheek injury and topical landmarks for localizing the parotid gland and duct and the facial nerve.

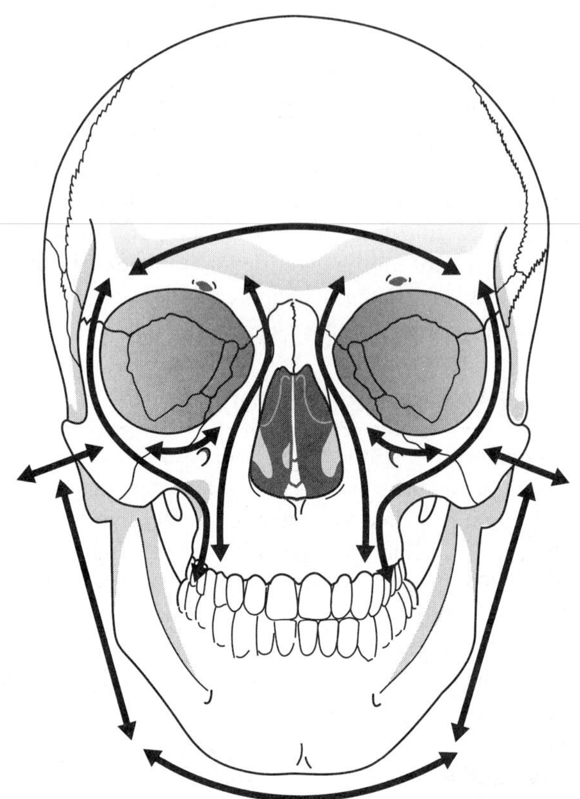

FIGURE 21-4 Craniofacial buttresses. (*Arrows* indicate buttresses.)

When the transmitted energy exceeds the absorptive capacity of these buttresses, facial fractures occur. As Le Fort described in the early 1900s, this excess force results in predictable fractures at the junction of one buttress system with another.[4]

Skeletal structures should be inspected for symmetry, irregularity of bone continuity, and functional imbalance. Palpation should also be performed to identify the abnormal presence of crepitus, tenderness, or bony irregularity. Clinical evaluation techniques are shown in Figure 21-5.

The health care provider should anticipate and recognize the functional disturbances associated with each type of facial fracture. Disturbances of vision, smell, nasal breathing, facial sensation, and the perception of bite relationship are the key dysfunctional findings, which can lead to the diagnosis of specific facial fractures. Maxillofacial clinical assessment, like any other assessment, is an orderly system-related evaluation of structures and their associated function.

Functionally, the face is most easily divided into thirds (Figure 21-6).[11] The upper third of the face includes the lower portion of the frontal bone, supraorbital ridge, nasal glabellar region, and frontal sinus. In this region, the frontal sinus, being an air cell with thin surrounding bone, is most vulnerable to injury and is referred to as a "crumple zone."[12] Fractures typically pass through its anatomic boundary. As a result, most patients present with epistaxis, absent or abnormal smell, and possible cerebral spinal fluid (CSF) drainage from the nose (rhinorrhea). If the fracture communicates more laterally through the supraorbital ridge, the patient may have decreased sensation in the upper face/forehead region, resulting from disruption of the trigeminal nerve branch (V1) innervating this area[10] (Figure 21-7). If the supraorbital ridge is depressed, this fragment may impinge on the orbit, causing inferior displacement (vertical dystopia) and double vision (diplopia). A severe fracture of the orbital roof may communicate posteriorly with the superior orbital fissure (fissure between the greater and lesser sphenoid wings through which branches of cranial nerves III, IV, V, and VI traverse to the orbit), producing an associated superior orbital fissure syndrome (SOFS). Patients with this syndrome present with absent V1 sensation, pupillary fixation and dilation, loss of extraocular eye muscle movement, a down-and-out positioning of the eye, and upper eyelid ptosis (drooping).[13,14] Finally, patients with injuries of this region often have associated injuries of the intracranial vault and an abnormal neurological assessment. Any abnormal neurological assessment mandates a complete neurosurgery consultation.

The middle facial third (midface) includes the orbits, maxillary sinuses, nose, zygoma bones, and basal bone of the

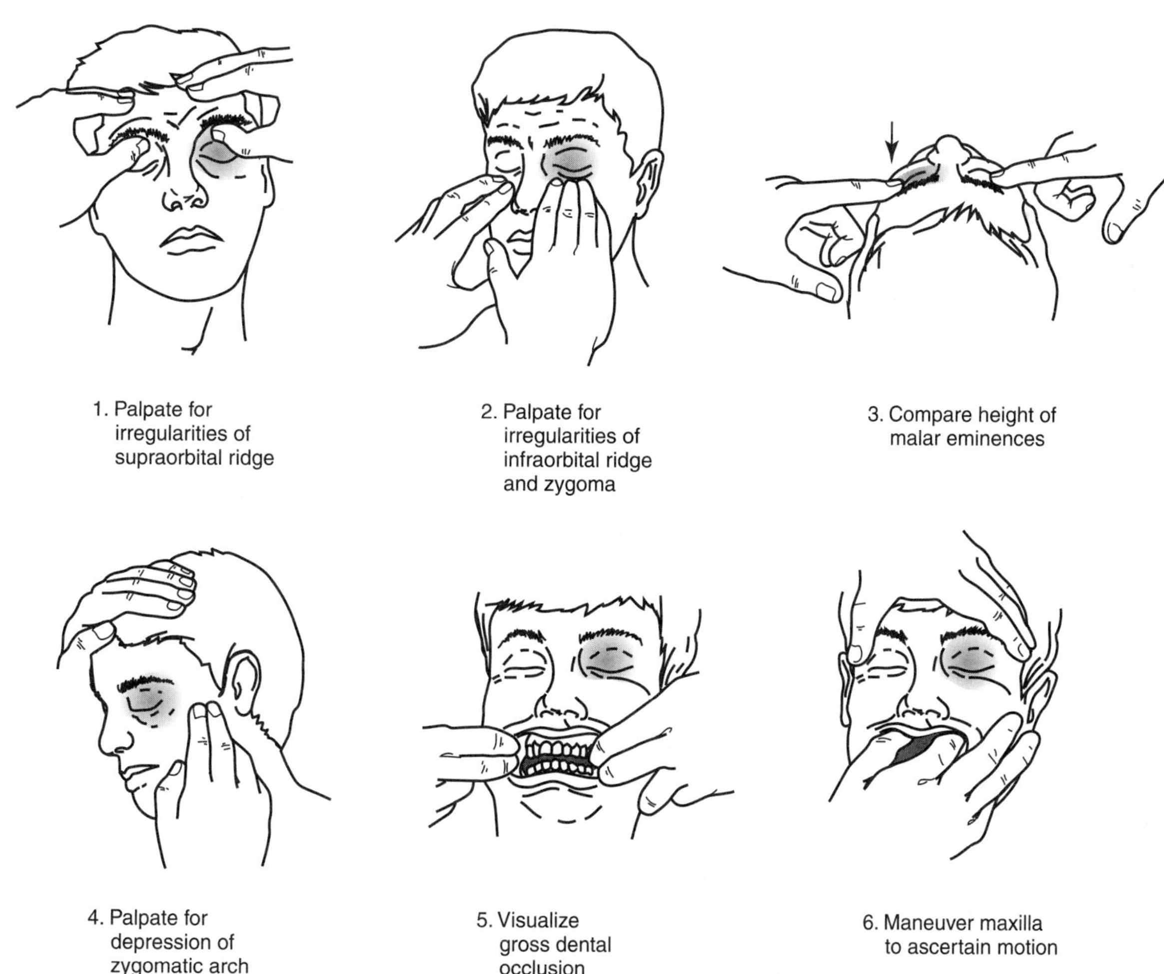

FIGURE 21-5 Techniques for palpating facial injuries.

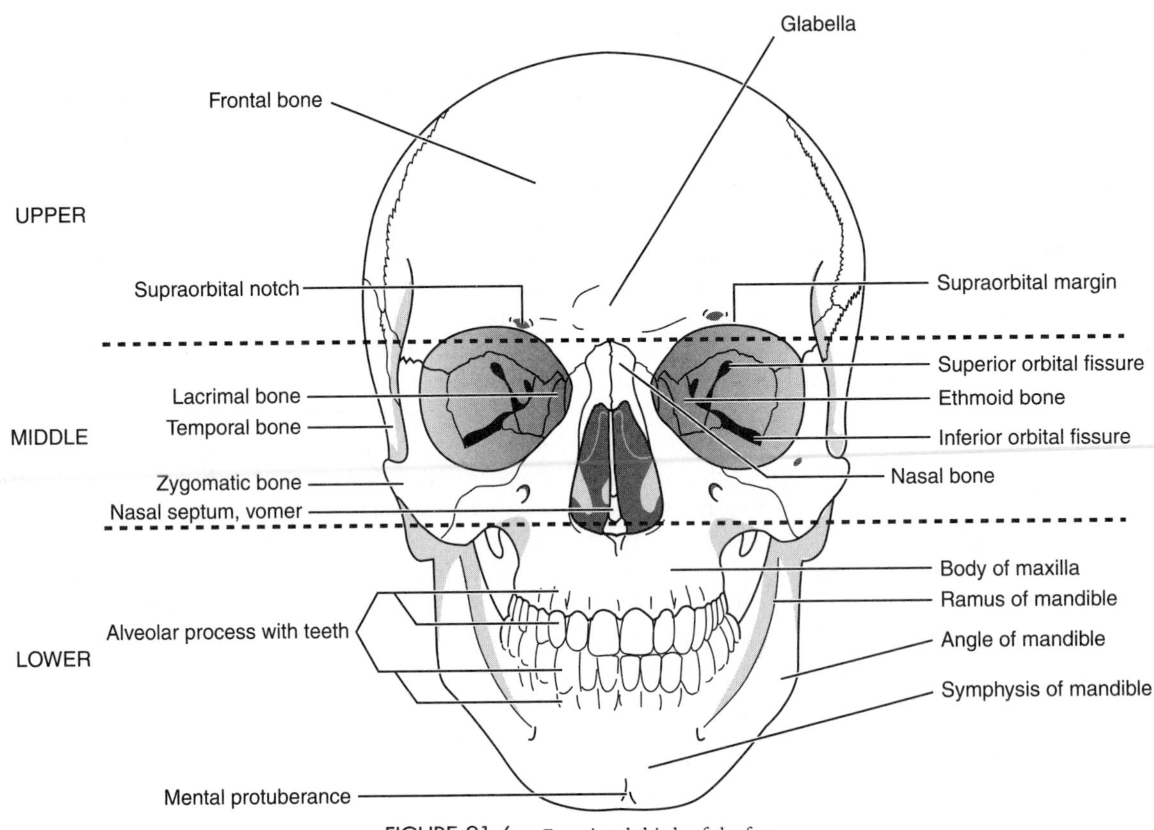

FIGURE 21-6 Functional thirds of the face.

maxilla. In this region, from a functional standpoint, fractures involve the orbit, nose, or both. The nasal bones are the most prominent structures of the midface, and therefore are the facial bones most commonly fractured. They constitute the third most commonly fractured bones in the body. Clinically, a nasal fracture presents with contour deformity and deviation, epistaxis, subcutaneous emphysema, airway obstruction, and absent or abnormal smell. In all instances, the nasal septum should be examined to rule out the presence of a nasal septal hematoma. A nasal septal hematoma must be evacuated to prevent avascular necrosis of the nasal septum and subsequent saddle-nose deformity (nasal bridge is significantly depressed) or septal perforation.[15] Sense of smell provided by the olfactory nerve (cranial nerve I) is evaluated simply by determining if the patient can smell an alcohol wipe held approximately 8 inches from the nares.

In his classic paper, Le Fort described three basic patterns of midface maxillary fractures, each of which has unique clinical findings[4] (Figures 21-1 and 21-2). A Le Fort I fracture is the transverse disarticulation of the maxillary dentoalveolar process from the remaining basal bone of the maxilla and midface. Clinically, this fracture presents with mobility of the maxillary dentition, but stability of the nose, orbit, and midface. A Le Fort II fracture is a pyramidal fracture involving the entire maxilla and nasal complex. Clinically, this fracture presents with unified mobility of the maxillary teeth along with the nose, but stability of the orbit and remaining midface. A Le Fort III fracture is a complete craniofacial-midface disassociation. Here there is unified mobility of the maxillary dentition, nose, and orbits. Other subtle clinical findings with a fracture of midface structures include an alteration of the horizontal orbital plane resulting from downward displacement of the zygoma or contour deformity of the malar eminence and nasal bony pyramid.

Most remaining midfacial fractures communicate through the orbit; therefore, a complete ocular assessment is mandatory. The eyes are assessed for obvious signs of trauma, such as conjunctival hemorrhage or ruptured globe. Vision and visual acuity should be evaluated. Movement of the eyes through the fields of gaze evaluates the ability of the extraocular muscles to move the eyes freely and the integrity of cranial nerves III, IV, and VI, which innervate the extraocular muscles. The patient should be observed closely for conjugate gaze in the horizontal, vertical, and sagittal eye positions. Impaired eye movement may result from edema restricting ocular movement; hemorrhage; direct injury to cranial nerves III, IV, or VI; contusion of the extraocular muscles, or an orbital fracture that causes extraocular muscle entrapment. Diplopia may result from dysconjugate gaze.[16]

All patients with facial fractures, in particular those with periorbital ecchymosis, should have frequent assessment of the pupillary response to light. Assessment of the pupillary light reflex evaluates cranial nerve II (optic nerve), which enables the patient to perceive incoming light stimuli, and cranial nerve III (oculomotor nerve), which causes the pupil to constrict in response to the light stimulus. The Marcus-Gunn

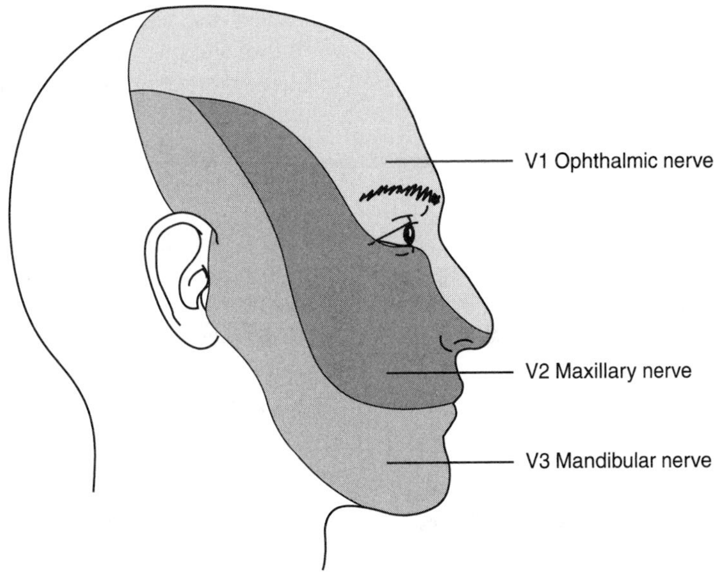

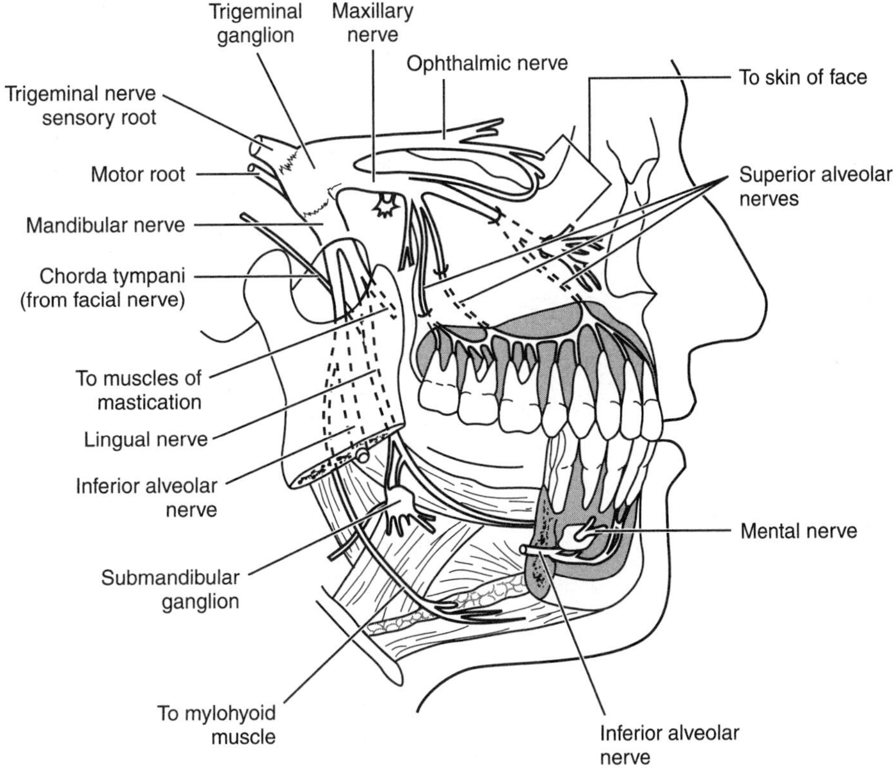

FIGURE 21-7 Trigeminal nerve (cranial nerve V) and its branches. V1 gives sensation from the upper eyelid to the apex of the scalp; V2 supplies the lower eyelid, cheek, upper lip, and lateral nose; V3 innervates the chin and lower lip.

pupil test (swinging light test) should be performed on all patients[17](Figure 21-8). When the healthy eye is illuminated with a bright light, the pupils constrict bilaterally; however, when the light is moved quickly to the diseased eye, the pupil dilates. This test can be performed even in the unconscious patient and is the single most sensitive test for injury of the visual track between the retina and optic chiasm.[17] An ophthalmology consult is indicated whenever ocular injury is suspected by evidence of diplopia, restricted eye movement, altered forehead (V1) or cheek (V2) sensation, hyphema (anterior chamber ocular hemorrhage), ptosis, or periocular fractures.[17,18] In a retrospective case review Cook found that of 365 patients with orbital fractures examined by an ophthalmologist, 22% also had ocular injuries and 24% of these

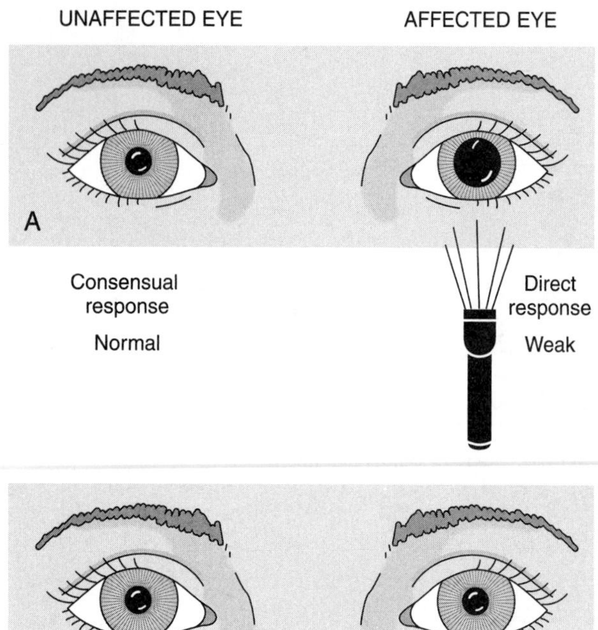

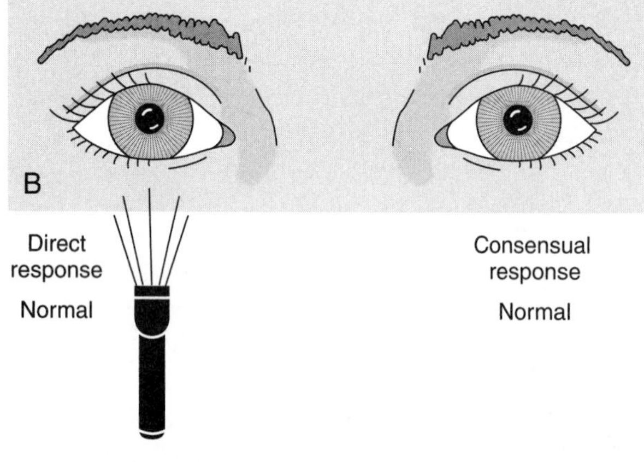

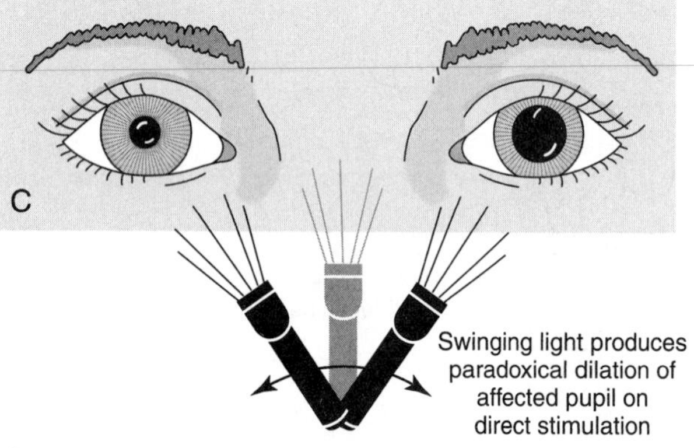

FIGURE 21-8 The Marcus Gunn (swinging light) test. Conduct test in a dark room with the patient fixing their eyes on a distant object. **A,** Shining the light in the affected eye produces minimal, weak, or no constriction of that pupil. **B,** Shining a light in the unaffected eye produces normal direct and consensual pupil constriction. **C,** When the light is moved quickly from the unaffected eye to the affected eye, a paradoxical dilatation, rather than constriction, of the affected pupil occurs, indicating a positive test.

patients required immediate interventions to prevent further ocular damage.[18] Any abnormality in the visual assessment should be regarded as emergent and warrants an immediate ophthalmology consult.[16]

The lower third of the face includes the maxillary and mandibular teeth-bearing bone and the basal bone of the mandible. The posterior/superior aspect of the mandible includes the temporomandibular joint and its associated condyle and meniscus. The position of the mandible and its functional relationship with the maxilla are directed by the muscles of mastication as they function through the temporomandibular joint. Therefore, a functional assessment of the lower facial structures involves an evaluation of the muscles of mastication and their movement of the mandible through the temporomandibular joint. The patient should be asked to open and close the mandible and move it in all directions. Any fracture of the mandible or maxilla will upset the balance of this musculoskeletal system and manifest with muscular pain, splinting, and an altered bite (malocclusion). An altered bite is often subtle and perceived only by the patient; nonetheless, any objective or subjective irregularity of the bite is always abnormal and should alert the practitioner that the maxilla, mandible, or both have been fractured.[19]

Other subtle clinical findings associated with facial fractures in any of the three facial regions include altered facial sensation and/or motor function. Facial sensation should be assessed over the areas of distribution for each of the three branches of the trigeminal nerve (cranial nerve V) (Figure 21-7). The ophthalmic or V1 division innervates the upper face; the maxillary or V2 division innervates the midface; and the mandibular or V3 division provides sensation to the lower face. Abnormal sensation in any one of these regions may indicate an associated fracture coursing through the cranial nerve skeletal foramen. In addition to supraorbital ridge fractures, which can alter V1 sensation, orbital floor, zygoma, and Le Fort II fractures typically are associated with altered V2 sensation, and a mandible fracture may manifest with diminished V3 sensation.

Any abnormality of facial animation indicates injury to the facial nerve (cranial nerve VII), which innervates the muscles of facial expression and conveys taste for the anterior two thirds of the tongue (Figure 21-9). Facial movement can be assessed by having the patient puff out his or her cheeks, smile, show the teeth, frown, raise the eyebrows, and tightly close the eyes. In the absence of a direct laceration to one of the branches of the facial nerve, a thorough neurologic evaluation should be performed to further evaluate for possible traumatic brain injury.[7] If only the lower portion of the face is paretic and the upper face is spared, an upper motor neuron lesion involving the central nervous system should be suspected. If the entire half of the face is paretic, a peripheral nerve injury involving the facial nerve is indicated.[19] When the injury is believed to be proximal to the mastoid foramen, a neurosurgery consult should be obtained in conjunction with a temporal bone and intracranial computed tomography (CT) scan. Even in the comatose patient, the motor function of the facial nerve and the sensory function of the trigeminal nerve can be assessed by testing the corneal reflex. Normally, light touch with a wisp of cotton on the cornea stimulates the trigeminal nerve, which triggers the facial nerve to cause the eye to blink.

Comprehensive assessment then directs specific radiological examination. A detailed discussion of the indications

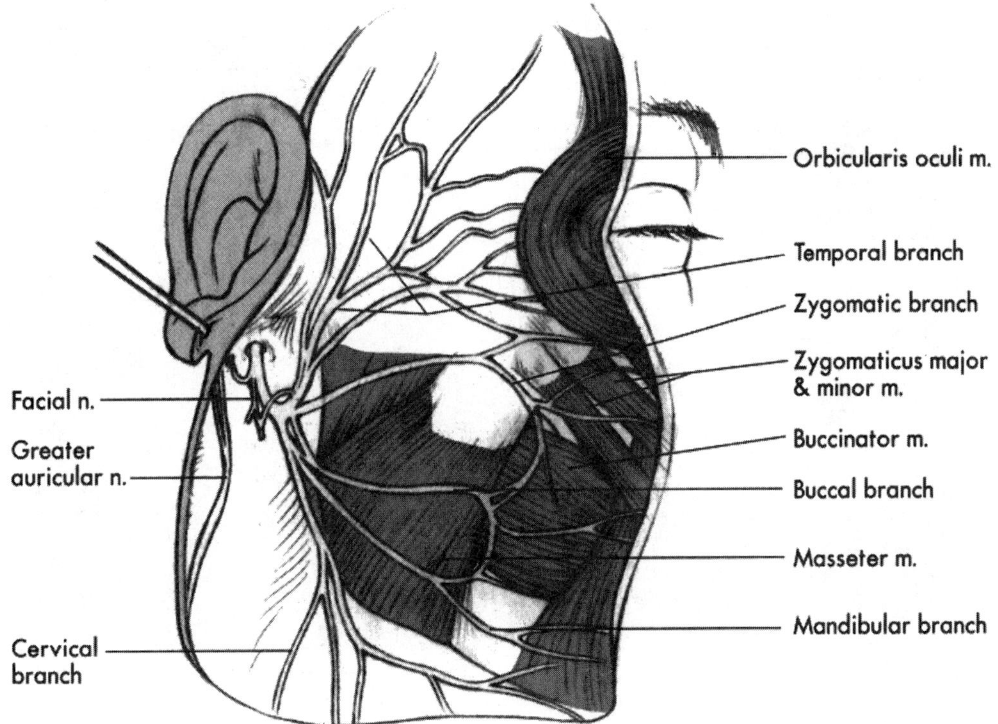

FIGURE 21-9 Facial nerve (cranial nerve VII) and it's branches. The temporal, zygomatic, buccal, mandibular, and cervical branches of the facial nerve emerge from superior to inferior along the anterior border of the parotid gland. (From Mathers LH, Chase RA, Dolph J et al: *Clinical Anatomy Principles,* St. Louis, 1996, Mosby, p. 180.)

for specific radiographs is beyond this review, but in general, the most effective method for a quick and thorough radiographic assessment of the maxillofacial structures is axial and coronal CT. The advantages of CT assessment over plain radiographs is the ability to evaluate more accurately the complexity of maxillofacial fractures, their comminuted parts, and the relationship of the fractures with the surrounding soft tissue[12] (Figure 21-10). In the absence of obtaining true coronal CT scans, a reconstructed version can be substituted.

Twelve percent of trauma patients requiring head CTs have some type of facial fracture.[20,21] Soft tissue injuries of the face can act as markers to aid clinicians in deciding if a diagnostic study should be performed to assess for facial injuries. Holmgren and Dierks propose that the acronym LIPS-N (*L*ip laceration, *I*ntraoral laceration, *P*eriorbital contusion, *S*ubconjunctival hemorrhage, and *N*asal laceration) be used during physical examination of trauma patients to indicate assessment findings that should prompt the practitioner to obtain a CT scan of the face in addition to a brain CT scan.[21]

Before formalizing the diagnosis and management plan, added information can be obtained from dental impressions, old dental records, and comparison of the clinical presentation to preinjury facial photographs. Management of complex facial injuries frequently requires nursing coordination between the patient, family, and multiple medical teams (ophthalmology, neurosurgery, orthopedic surgery, critical care, and plastic surgery). This coordination includes communication and patient advocacy; therefore, it becomes crucial for the nursing staff to be up to date with all diagnoses, individual team plans, and expectations of the patient and family.

SPECIFIC TYPES OF MAXILLOFACIAL INJURIES

SOFT TISSUE WOUNDS

All open facial soft tissue wounds have the potential for contamination; therefore, the patient's tetanus immunization status should be verified. If a patient has not been immunized, it is recommended that 250 units of tetanus immune globulin (Hyper-Tet) be administered and, with a different syringe at a different intramuscular injection site, 0.5 ml of tetanus toxoid be given. Two additional tetanus toxoid boosters should be given at 1 and 12 months after the initial dose to complete the immunization. In general, tetanus toxoid is given to individuals who have been immunized previously to ensure sufficient immunization.[22,23]

Contusions, abrasions, and lacerations are usually not life threatening, and the timing of their treatment depends on the patient's status and the ability to establish a surgically clean wound. Tissue that is obviously contaminated and crushed is susceptible to infection and should be excised, followed by delayed primary closure or primary repair with serial reexamination ("second-look procedure"). Multiple second-look procedures may be required every 24 to 36 hours for further debridement of progressive necrosis. This latter

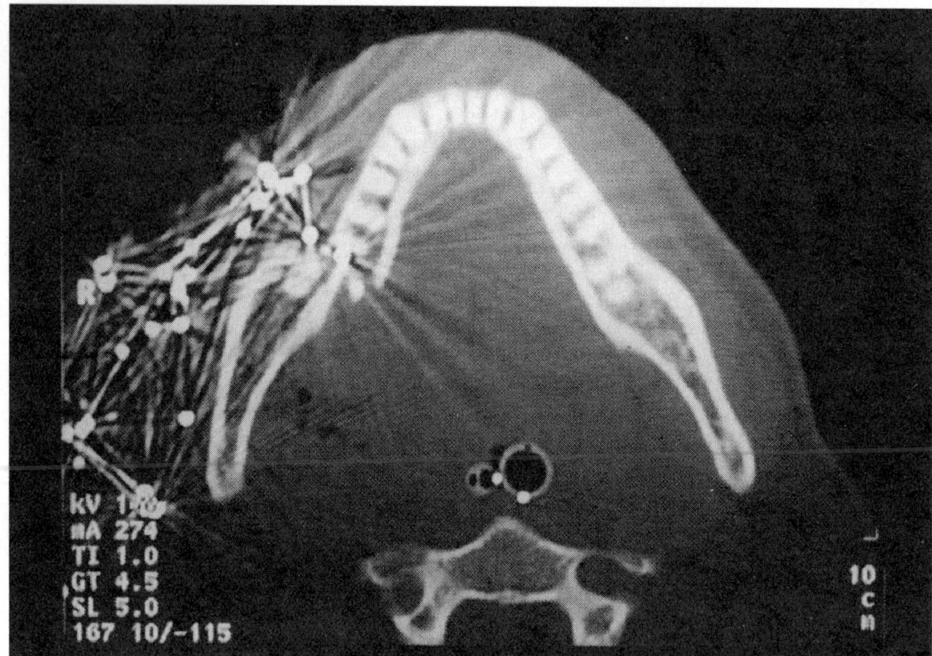

FIGURE 21-10 Computed tomography scan of facial shotgun injury demonstrating the complexity of a mandible fracture as it relates to the surrounding soft tissue envelope. (From Robertson BC, Manson PN: High-energy ballistic and avulsive injuries: a management protocol for the next millennium, *Surg Clin North Am* 6:1489-1502, 1999, p. 1493, Figure 3, **C**).

form of soft tissue management is most common for facial gunshot wounds and massive avulsive injuries.[24]

Rapid-absorbing gut suture, octylcyanoacrylate Dermabond, or nylon suture may be used for closure of facial lacerations. A comparison study of these three materials for the treatment of facial lacerations failed to show any clinically significant differences in the patient's cosmetic outcomes at 9 and 12 months.[25] Rapid-absorbing gut-suture or octylcyanoacrylate Dermabond may be preferred to eliminate follow-up visits solely for suture removal.

All wounds should be examined carefully for the presence of foreign material. The presence of foreign material increases the likelihood of infection. Meticulous hemostasis will reduce the potential for hematoma formation (a perfect medium for bacterial growth) and hence reduce the potential for infection. The use of drains may be indicated in lacerations of the parotid gland or in extensive injuries in which fluid may accumulate and produce a dead space, which fosters bacterial colonization and potentiates infection.[19]

Special attention should be devoted to the care of abrasions. Even though these injuries may be superficial, their mismanagement can lead to severe disfigurement. Entrapment of dirt, grease, or other foreign material beneath healed skin will lead to permanent tattooing, a situation extremely difficult to manage secondarily. These wounds should be cleansed aggressively with a brush while the patient is under appropriate anesthesia.

More complex soft tissue injury may require skin grafts or local or remote tissue flaps. The reader is referred to Chapter 16 for more in-depth discussion about soft tissue injury.

Nasal Fractures

The nose is a triangular pyramid with both cartilaginous and bony structural support. High-velocity injuries will create more anterior/posterior displacement and comminution. Low-velocity fractures typically cause a disjunction of the nasal cartilaginous vault from the nasal bony pyramid. In these cases, the patient has an inverted V deformity of the nasal dorsum.

Stranc and Robertson classified nasal fractures according to their anteroposterior displacement and lateral deviation (Figure 21-11).[26] In this classification, a plane 1 nasal fracture involves only the end of the nasal bony pyramid, and there is little deformity. This type of nasal fracture usually can be managed with internal reduction and nasal packing. A plane 2 nasal fracture is more extensive, involving the base of the nasal bony pyramid and nasal septum. Typically, patients with this type of injury present with a flattened nasal dorsum, obstruction of the nasal passage, and absence of smell. Treatment may require, in addition to internal reduction, some degree of external splinting and bone grafting. A plane 3 nasal fracture is in reality a nasoethmoidal-orbital fracture. This type of fracture commonly requires wide clinical exposure, bone graft reconstruction, and internal fixation techniques.

Zygoma and Orbital Fractures

The zygoma is a major buttress of the midface, and its eminence gives prominence to the cheek. Additionally, it forms the lateral portion of the orbit. The zygoma is the second most frequently fractured bone in the craniofacial skeleton.[4,7]

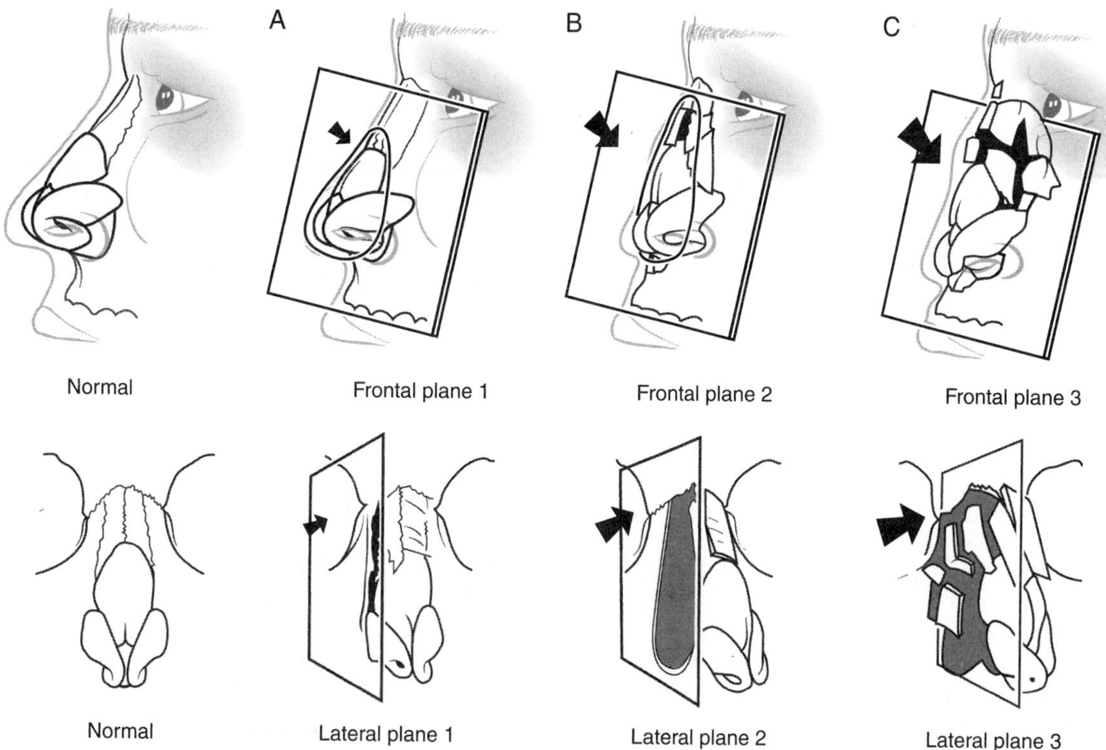

FIGURE 21-11 Stranc classification of displacement following a nasal fracture. Displacement is analyzed in terms of (1) lateral deviation and (2) anteroposterior displacement (frontal impact nasal fracture). Frontal impact nasal fractures are characterized by degrees of displacement: **A,** Plane 1 frontal impact nasal fracture. The end of the nasal bones and the septum are injured. **B,** Plane 2 frontal impact nasal fracture. The injury is more extensive, involving the proximal portion of the nasal bones and the frontal process of the maxilla at the piriform aperture. **C,** Plane 3 frontal impact nasal fracture involving one or both frontal processes of the maxilla extending up to the frontal bone. This is, in reality, a nasoethmoido-orbital fracture because it involves the lower two thirds of the medial orbital rim. (Redrawn from Stranc MF, Robertson GA: A classification of injuries of the nasal skeleton, *Ann Plast Surg* 2:468-474, 1979.)

Almost all fractures of the zygoma involve the orbital floor and the V2 division of the trigeminal nerve. Clinically, patients with this type of injury often have an abnormal ocular examination with periorbital ecchymosis, double vision (diplopia), and ocular proptosis secondary to edema. With extreme comminuted fractures, there may be acute enophthalmos (ocular recession within the orbit) secondary to severe loss of skeletal support. The eyes should be assessed for restriction of extraocular eye muscle movement. If there is restriction in any visual field, one must assume there is bony entrapment of the muscle requiring decompression as soon as possible.[27] Additional findings specific for zygomatic fractures are depression of the malar eminence and zygomatic arch (see Figure 21-5) and downward displacement of the lateral canthus. In most instances, the zygoma is depressed and displaced downward; hence, the lateral canthus of the eye follows with the lateral orbital rim (Figure 21-12). Occasionally, the zygomatic arch can be displaced inward and impinge upon the mandibular coronoid process, thereby creating a mechanical block to mandibular opening (Figure 21-13).

Surgical management of zygomatic and orbital floor fractures is directed by the presence of functional ocular impairment (e.g., reduced eye movement caused by entrapment of extraocular muscle, diplopia, enophthalmos), depressed zygoma with deformity, altered V2 sensation, and impingement on maxillary and mandibular musculoskeletal

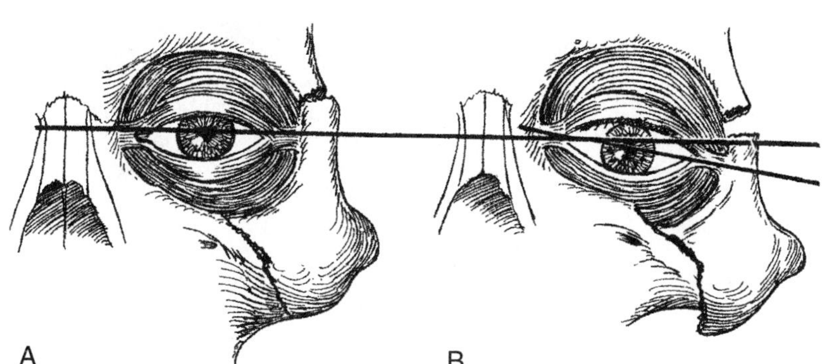

FIGURE 21-12 When the frontal process of the zygoma is depressed downward, the lateral canthal mechanism and the canthus of the eye follow. **A,** Normal position of the lateral canthus and a fracture without displacement. **B,** Downward displacement of the globe and lateral canthus as a result of frontozygomatic separation and downward displacement of the zygoma and the floor of the orbit. (Redrawn from Manson PN: Facial injuries. In McCarthy JG, editor: *Plastic Surgery,* vol 2: The Face: Part 1, Philadelphia, 1990, W.B. Saunders, p. 995.)

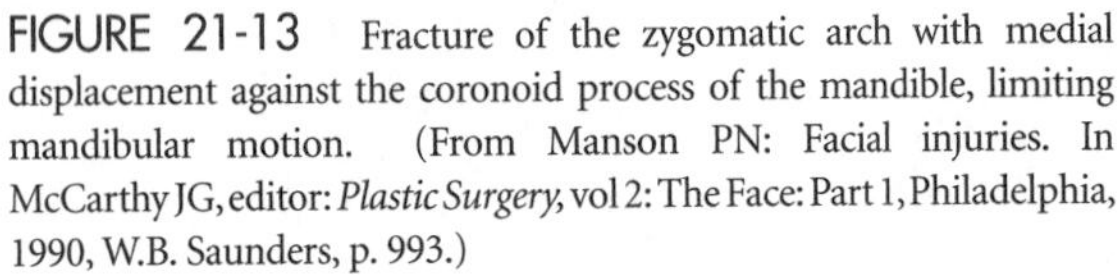

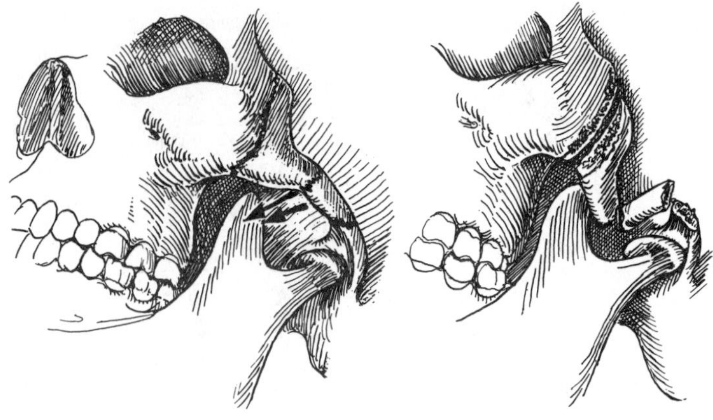

FIGURE 21-13 Fracture of the zygomatic arch with medial displacement against the coronoid process of the mandible, limiting mandibular motion. (From Manson PN: Facial injuries. In McCarthy JG, editor: *Plastic Surgery*, vol 2: The Face: Part 1, Philadelphia, 1990, W.B. Saunders, p. 993.)

function. The primary goal of treating the orbital floor component is to decompress any entrapped ocular tissue and simultaneously restore proper orbital volume to minimize the potential for secondary diplopia and enophthalmos.[28] With respect to the zygoma itself, the goal is to anatomically reposition the zygoma for proper facial midface projection and width dimension (Figure 21-14). For accurate anatomic reduction and stabilization of the quadrangular zygoma bone, three points of fixation typically are required: the frontozygomatic buttress, infraorbital rim, and zygomaticomaxillary buttress (Figure 21-15). Access to these buttresses can be obtained through a lower eyelid incision and an intraoral maxillary buccal sulcus incision. Severe high-velocity comminuted zygomatic fractures may also require a posterior approach to reconstruct the zygomatic arch.[29] The orbital floor component is explored and reconstructed through the eyelid incision using an alloplastic implant.[27]

MAXILLARY AND MANDIBULAR FRACTURES

Fractures involving the maxilla or mandible are managed functionally to restore the preinjury habitual bite relationship. The bite relationship acts as a template for accurate anatomic reduction of fractures involving the basal bone of the maxilla and mandible. By establishing this relationship, the surgeon can determine the proper facial height, width, and projection (see Figure 21-14).

In most instances, the preinjury bite relationship can be recognized and established by the wear facets on the teeth. However, in injured patients whose teeth or segments of bone are missing, it may be difficult to determine the normal occlusion relationship. In these instances, old photographs, dental records, and dental models are extremely helpful.

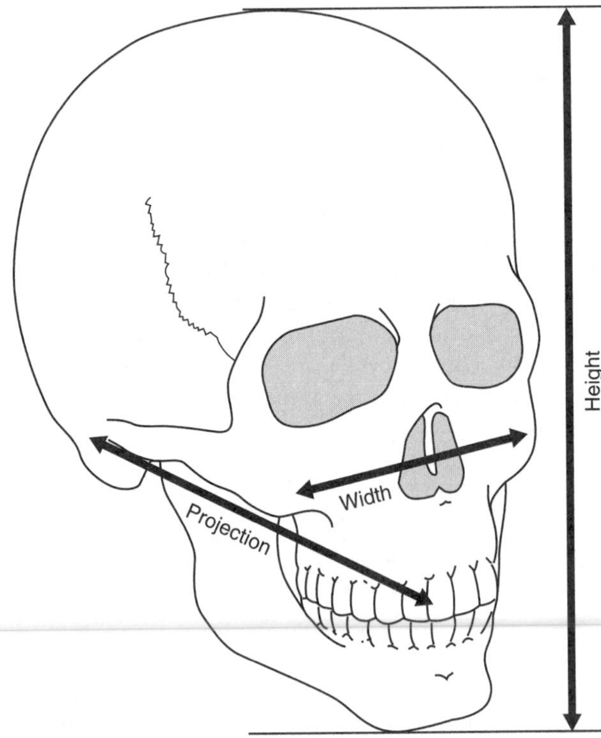

FIGURE 21-14 The goal in midface fracture repair is to reestablish normal facial width, height, and projection.

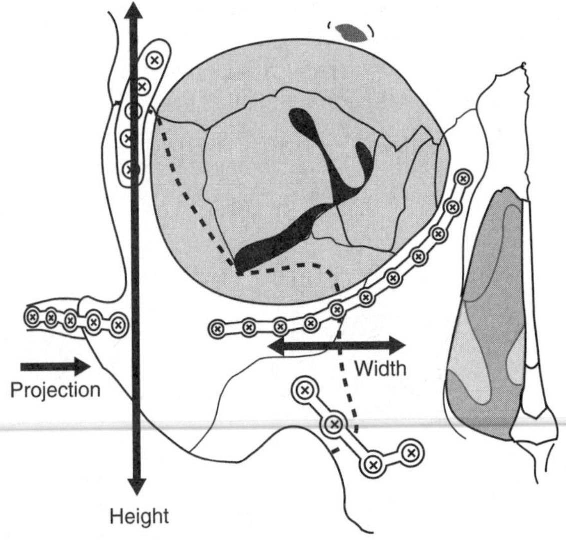

FIGURE 21-15 Technique of open reduction and internal fixation of a zygoma fracture.

The starting point for stabilizing any maxillary or mandibular fracture is placing the patient into maxillary and mandibular fixation. This is most easily accomplished by securing dentoalveolar arch bars to the dentition and wiring the jaws closed. Following this, the basal bone fractures of the maxilla and mandible are exposed, reduced anatomically, and stabilized with rigid titanium plates and screws.[11,30] Preservation of bone allows for placement of dental implants and decreases risk of bone grafts.[31]

TOOTH FRACTURES

Essentially there are four types of tooth fractures (Figure 21-16). A type I fracture involves only the insensate tooth enamel, and here the patient will complain of the sharp fractured edges but not experience significant discomfort. A type II fracture involves the tooth dentin, which contains nerve extensions from the tooth pulp. Patients with this type of fracture have moderate discomfort to hot and cold liquids but generally are comfortable at rest. A type III fracture involves exposed pulp and patients have significant pain at rest. A type IV fracture is through the root and presents as well with pain at rest. Most type II and III fractures require urgent dental attention for relief of discomfort and tooth salvage versus extraction.

MANAGEMENT

Interdisciplinary communication of assessment findings and anticipated treatment needs enable the health care team to develop a coordinated comprehensive plan for managing the patient with maxillofacial injury in each phase of the trauma cycle. Management of complex facial injuries demands an appreciation of facial anatomy and an orderly management scheme that will allow anatomic reconstruction of the facial skeletal structures, followed by redraping of the overlying soft tissue elements. Only with a consistent comprehensive approach can the harmonious balance of facial function and restoration of the patient's characteristic identity be achieved. An effective multidisciplinary plan of care considers treatment of the patient's actual injuries, interventions to avoid potential detrimental complications, and the psychological and emotional aspects of facial injury.

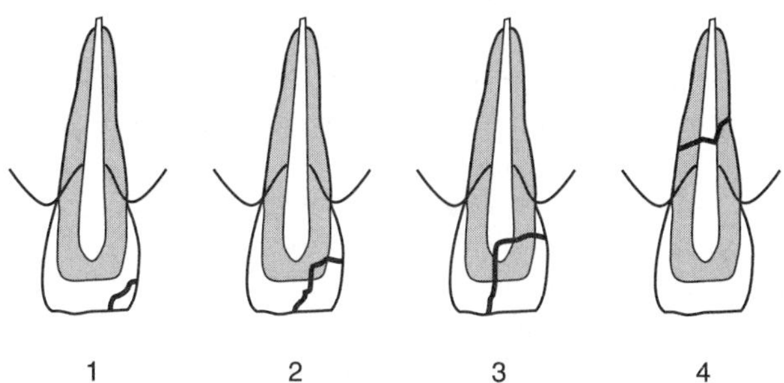

FIGURE 21-16 Types of tooth fractures. 1, Enamel injuries. 2, Dentin injuries. 3, Pulp injuries. 4, Root injuries.

RESUSCITATION PHASE

Priorities of care during the resuscitation phase are the same for all trauma patients and include the need to establish a patent airway and provide adequate ventilation and sufficient circulation.[32] Maxillofacial injuries can cause life-threatening airway obstruction, impaired ventilation, and/or hemorrhage, mandating immediate attention and nondefinitive treatment.[12] Generally, unless maxillofacial injuries pose a threat to the airway, breathing, or circulation, management falls into an urgent category and definitive treatment is not performed until all other actual or potential life-threatening injuries have been addressed.[32] In addition to managing potentially lethal injuries, interventions that recognize and treat neurologic dysfunction and those that manage pain and anxiety should be included in the resuscitation phase plan of care for patients with maxillofacial injuries.

Maintain a Patent Airway and Ensure Adequate Ventilation

In the patient with maxillofacial injury, the airway can be obstructed and ventilation compromised as a result of pharyngeal swelling or occlusion of the pharynx by the tongue. Secretions, blood, vomit, unsupported soft tissue, displaced bone, dislodged dental appliances, avulsed teeth, and tooth fragments can also obstruct the airway. Initial attempts to establish a patent airway include use of the chin-lift or jaw-thrust maneuver and suction of secretions and foreign debris from the airway. Airway obstruction due to tongue edema or loss of mandibular skeletal support may be managed by pulling the tongue forward and, if necessary, securing the tongue with sutures to prevent prolapse back over the airway. Care must be taken to maintain head and neck alignment throughout maneuvers to establish an airway until any possible cervical spine injury has been definitely ruled out.[12] If initial attempts fail to establish and maintain a patent airway, early endotracheal intubation is indicated. An oral rather than a nasal route for emergent placement of endotracheal or gastric tubes is preferred to avoid additional midfacial injury and inadvertent insertion of the tube into the brain through possible coexisting cranial base fractures.[33] A cricothyroidotomy or tracheostomy may be preferred in the presence of severe facial injuries when the patient has multiple mandible or maxillary fractures or massive soft tissue damage.

Care is also taken to ensure the airway remains patent and aspiration is prevented, as these complications are associated with high morbidity and mortality.[12] The patient is at risk for aspiration due to secretions, debris, and blood from the traumatized nasopharynx and oropharynx. Patients with multiple fractures of the mandible that involve the floor of the mouth or with profuse nasal hemorrhage are at particularly high risk for aspiration. Nursing interventions that may help prevent aspiration include suctioning the mouth and oropharynx frequently and positioning the patient on his or her side (unless otherwise contraindicated) to promote the removal of blood and secretions from the oral cavity. Placement of an orogastric tube to decompress the stomach also helps prevent aspiration. Risk of aspiration is decreased in the intubated patient by ensuring that the endotracheal or tracheostomy tube cuff remains inflated adequately. Symptoms indicating that aspiration has occurred include audible rales or rhonchi upon chest auscultation, decreased blood oxygen saturation (Spo_2) and partial pressure of oxygen (Pao_2), reduced lung compliance, and eventually infiltrates visible on chest radiographs. Aggressive pulmonary hygiene, namely endotracheal suctioning, is indicated if aspiration is suspected. Bronchoscopy may be needed to remove aspirated blood or foreign debris (e.g., a tooth) from the patient's airway.[12]

Once a patent airway is established, ensuring adequate ventilation becomes a priority. Nurses should assess the quality and effort of spontaneous respiration, symmetry of chest wall movement, and breath sounds. Noninvasive measures of Spo_2 and end tidal carbon dioxide levels provide an indication about whether respiratory gas exchange is sufficient. Inadequate ventilation may occur secondary to aspiration, associated injuries, or administration of medications that suppress respiration during resuscitation. Insufficient spontaneous ventilation is treated initially by manually ventilating the patient, followed eventually by mechanical ventilation. Supplemental oxygen is generally provided to foster adequate oxygenation.

Control Hemorrhage and Ensure Adequate Intravascular Volume

Hemorrhage is the next immediate concern. Extensive hemorrhage and significant blood loss can result from injury to one or more of the multiple facial arteries[34] (Figure 21-17). Application of direct pressure on the site of vessel injury is the primary method of hemorrhage control.[12] Circumferential pressure bandages can also be used. If these measures fail to control the bleeding and the source of blood loss is visible, clamping and ligation or repair of the vessel may be indicated.[35] Nurses should monitor dressings closely for blood saturation and keep the physician apprised of the estimated blood loss. Surgical hemostats, clamps, and suture material should be readily available. Hemorrhage caused by facial fractures such as those involving the mandible, maxilla, nose, zygoma, frontal sinus, or nasoethmoid may be controlled by reduction of the fracture.[35,36]

The health care provider must try to obtain the patient's past medical history to determine if factors that increase the likelihood of profuse bleeding are present. Patients with liver disease or blood disorders, or receiving anticoagulant therapy are at increased risk of uncontrolled hemorrhage.[12,15] Astute assessment of coagulation profiles is imperative so that coagulapathy can be readily recognized and corrected.

Profuse epistaxis (nasal bleeding) can occur with any facial fracture that communicates with the nose (e.g., nasal fracture[s], maxillary fracture[s], cranial base fracture[s], sinus fracture[s]).[15] Actively bleeding vessels in the nasal region can be compressed by inserting a 30-ml balloon or petroleum gauze into each nares. Nasal packing is removed by the physician under controlled conditions within 24 to 48 hours. Packing that remains in place for longer than 2 days becomes a source of infection and may cause compression necrosis of the mucous membranes. Early maxillary fracture surgical reduction and fixation (IMF) may be necessary to control profuse nasopharyngeal bleeding. Transvascular embolization of bleeding vessels performed during angiography may be effective in halting intractable oronasal hemorrhage when other conventional treatments have failed.[37]

Patients presenting with severe facial trauma, such as Le Fort and naso-orbital injuries, are at risk for vessel injury. Research done at the R Adams Cowley Shock Trauma Center compared the accuracy of computed tomography angiography (CTA) with more invasive angiography for diagnosis of blunt cervical arterial injury. Researchers demonstrated that CTA, which is quicker and less invasive than traditionally used studies, is an accurate diagnostic tool for blunt cerebrovascular injury.[38]

Restoration of intravascular fluid volume is achieved by intravenous administration of crystalloids, colloids, and, when appropriate, blood products. The patient's hemodynamic status, including measures such as blood pressure, heart rate and central venous pressure, and assessment parameters that indicate sufficiency of tissue perfusion (e.g., urine output, and serial lactate levels) dictate the necessary volume of fluid replacement. Serial assessment of hemoglobin, hematocrit, and coagulation factors will determine the need for blood product administration and alert the practitioner to further bleeding. Other sources of blood loss besides hemorrhage from maxillofacial injury also need to be ruled out and controlled if identified.

Recognize and Treat Neurologic Dysfunction

Brain injury may accompany maxillofacial trauma.[39] Penetrating objects causing maxillofacial injuries (e.g., bullets, knife blade) as well as maxillofacial fractures themselves can extend into the cranial vault and injure the brain. Acceleration-deceleration forces that result in maxillofacial injury can set the semisolid brain into motion within the rigid skull, possibly causing the brain to be injured as it comes into contact with the skull surface or by causing stretching, tension, and shearing of involved neurologic tissue. Brain and cervical spine injuries should always be suspected until ruled out. See Chapter 20 for more specific information on traumatic brain injuries.

Frequent neurologic assessments are warranted throughout the resuscitation phase. Any changes or abnormal findings should be reported immediately to the physician. Neurosurgical consultation is recommended to evaluate completely any suspected central nervous system injury. Radiographic studies to evaluate the cervical spine and CT scan of the head should be included in the patient's initial workup if alterations in level of consciousness, motor function, sensation, or eye and pupil function are evident during patient assessment.[39]

Intracranial injury with a dural tear and CSF leak should be suspected in any patient with severe nasal, frontal sinus,

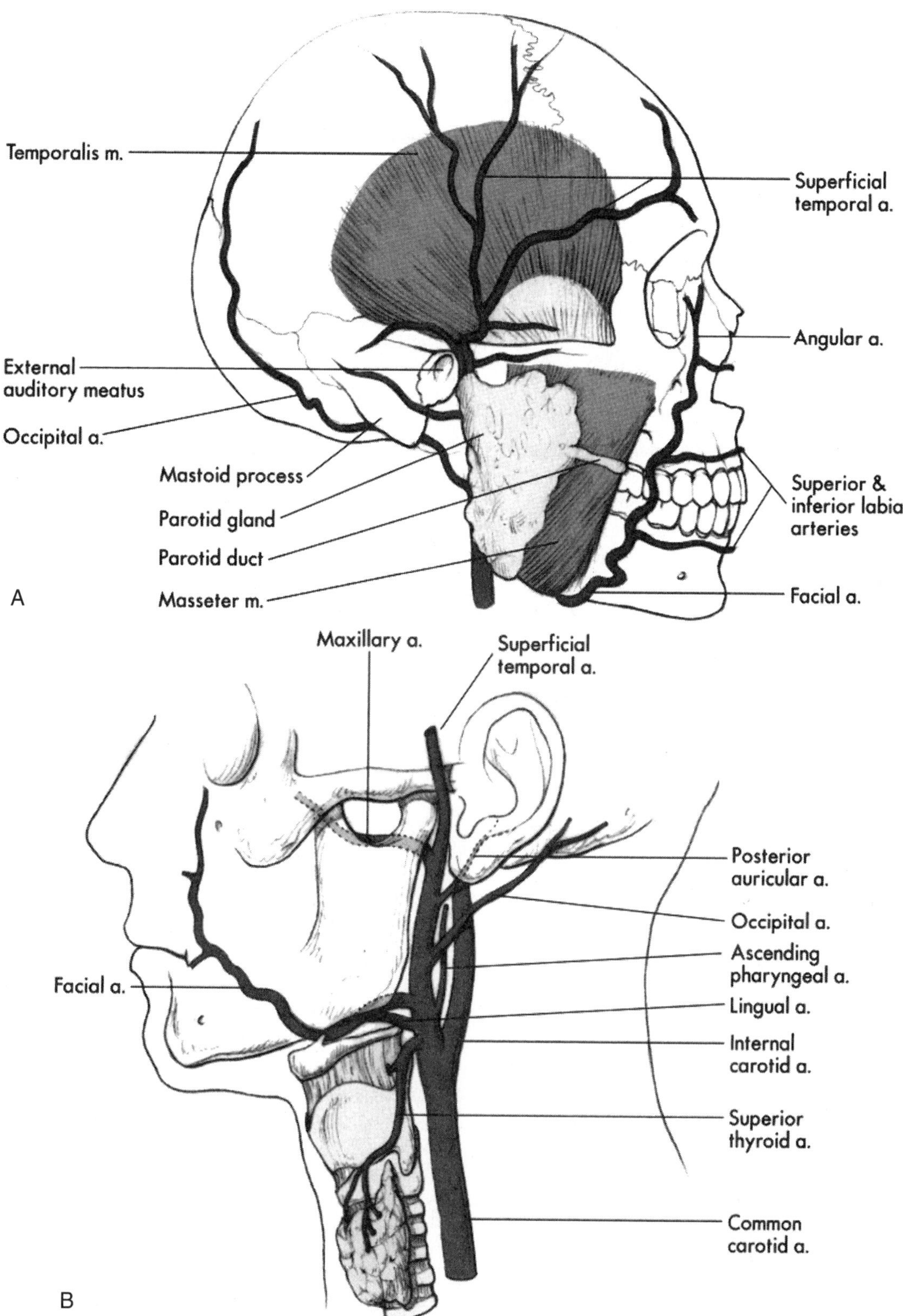

FIGURE 21-17 Vascular supply of the face. **A,** Branches of the external carotid artery. **B,** Further branches of the external carotid and the carotid bifurcation. (From Mathers LH, Chase RA, Dolph J, et al: *Clinical Anatomy Principles,* St. Louis, 1996, Mosby, p. 182.)

nasoethmoid, or Le Fort III fractures. CSF rhinorrhea is often difficult to detect when there is blood in the nares. A nasal drip pad (i.e., a folded gauze pad) should be placed loosely under the nares to collect drainage so that its amount and character can be evaluated. When drainage contains CSF, a yellowish "halo ring" typically appears around a stain of blood on the drip pad and the draining fluid will test positive for glucose (blood also contains glucose and will cause a positive test result). Although posttraumatic CSF leaks generally will heal in time without invasive actions, there are leaks that become problematic and require placement of a CSF drain or surgical intervention.[40]

Manage Pain and Anxiety

Maxillofacial injuries and associated injuries may cause substantial patient discomfort. Prescribed analgesia should be administered to achieve an acceptable level of pain control. If possible, a nonverbal mechanism should be developed with the patient unable to verbally communicate pain and pain relief (e.g., holding up 1 to 10 fingers to indicate level of pain severity). A neurologic examination should be obtained and documented before providing analgesia; preferably, short-acting or easily reversible agents (e.g., morphine, Fentanyl) are used to allow ongoing neurologic evaluation.

Nurses should orient patients to their surroundings and offer appropriate reassurance to help allay anxiety. Clear, concise explanations regarding procedures and reinforcement of physician explanations regarding diagnosis and the treatment plan should also be provided. Nurses should be aware of their own actions and behaviors (i.e., facial expressions, eye contact, and voice) while caring for the patient, taking care not to convey alarm or disgust, which can heighten the patient's anxiety.[41] Medications to reduce or alleviate anxiety may be necessary and their effect on the neurological examination should be considered before administration.

Operative Phase

During the past 100 years, three hallmark developments led to our current surgical management of facial injuries. In the early 1900s, Le Fort conducted research on the effect of injury on the craniofacial skeleton.[4] He demonstrated that the craniofacial skeleton will fracture predictably along the weak fault lines that lie between the supporting buttresses, which surround and protect the delicate functional elements of the face. Le Fort then classified three basic fracture patterns as described earlier in this chapter.

During the next 60 years, management of facial injuries focused on reducing and controlling the position of these structural buttresses via indirect techniques. Small incisions were used to identify the line of fracture, and the buttresses were stabilized with interosseous wires and external fixators. In the hands of a master surgeon, the outcome of these techniques was oftentimes exceptional; however, all too often these indirect techniques led to incomplete reduction of skeletal buttresses and distortion of the functional elements as well as facial appearance. In the late 1970s, with the advent of CT, injury patterns and the interrelationship of the soft tissue and underlying bony construct became more fully understood. Injuries were no longer diagnosed as isolated Le Fort fractures but, in addition, were classified as to the level of energy required to produce the specific pattern of injury.[42] This led to the realization that wide exposure and direct visualization of the fractured components were required for accurate anatomic reduction of the craniofacial buttresses. Perfection of diagnostic techniques, adaptation of cosmetic surgical exposure, development of biocompatible materials for rigid stabilization of buttresses, and improved understanding of bone physiology and bone healing have led to the current standards for management of facial skeletal injuries.[43]

The concept of accurate anatomic reduction and stabilization of the craniofacial buttresses can be applied to all levels of fracture patterns. Even when treating a high-velocity fracture with severe bone comminution and soft tissue disruption, adherence to this principle will allow accurate facial reconstruction. This same basic principle also can be extrapolated to low-velocity facial gunshot wounds. However, in high-velocity facial gunshot wounds and facial avulsive injuries, there is the potential for soft tissue and bone devascularization, which does not necessarily manifest at the time of initial presentation. Typically, a progressive soft tissue and bone necrosis evolves over several days.[5,6] At the R Adams Cowley Shock Trauma Center between 1977 and 1993, a high potential for complications after immediate reconstruction of missing bony components using nonvascularized bone graft was observed. A review demonstrated a failure to recognize the evolution of this necrosis phenomenon, specifically oral mucosal lining necrosis. As a result, today a rapid sequential protocol that is used calls for immediate anatomic stabilization of the bony and soft tissue elements, followed by serial take-back procedures for "second-look" debridements of necrotic tissue, and definitive vascularized bone and soft tissue reconstruction (occasionally with free tissue transfer [free flap]) during the primary phase of wound healing.[44] This provides complete vascularized soft tissue reconstruction of all missing tissue prior to the secondary phase of wound contracture, when profound soft tissue distortion can occur. With this modified technique, all craniofacial buttresses are anatomically restored within the primary phase of wound healing, and these buttresses are surrounded with stable vascularized tissue. This results in less secondary wound contraction impinging on the functional elements and less distortion of the surrounding soft tissues. Secondary soft tissue rearrangement using adjacent aesthetic units of the face for an optimal final surgical outcome is then allowed[44] (Figure 21-18).

Facial reconstruction procedures, whether simple or complex, may take several hours. Intraoperative nursing care is directed toward the anesthetized patient but must also include support of the family or significant others awaiting information about their loved one. One family spokesperson

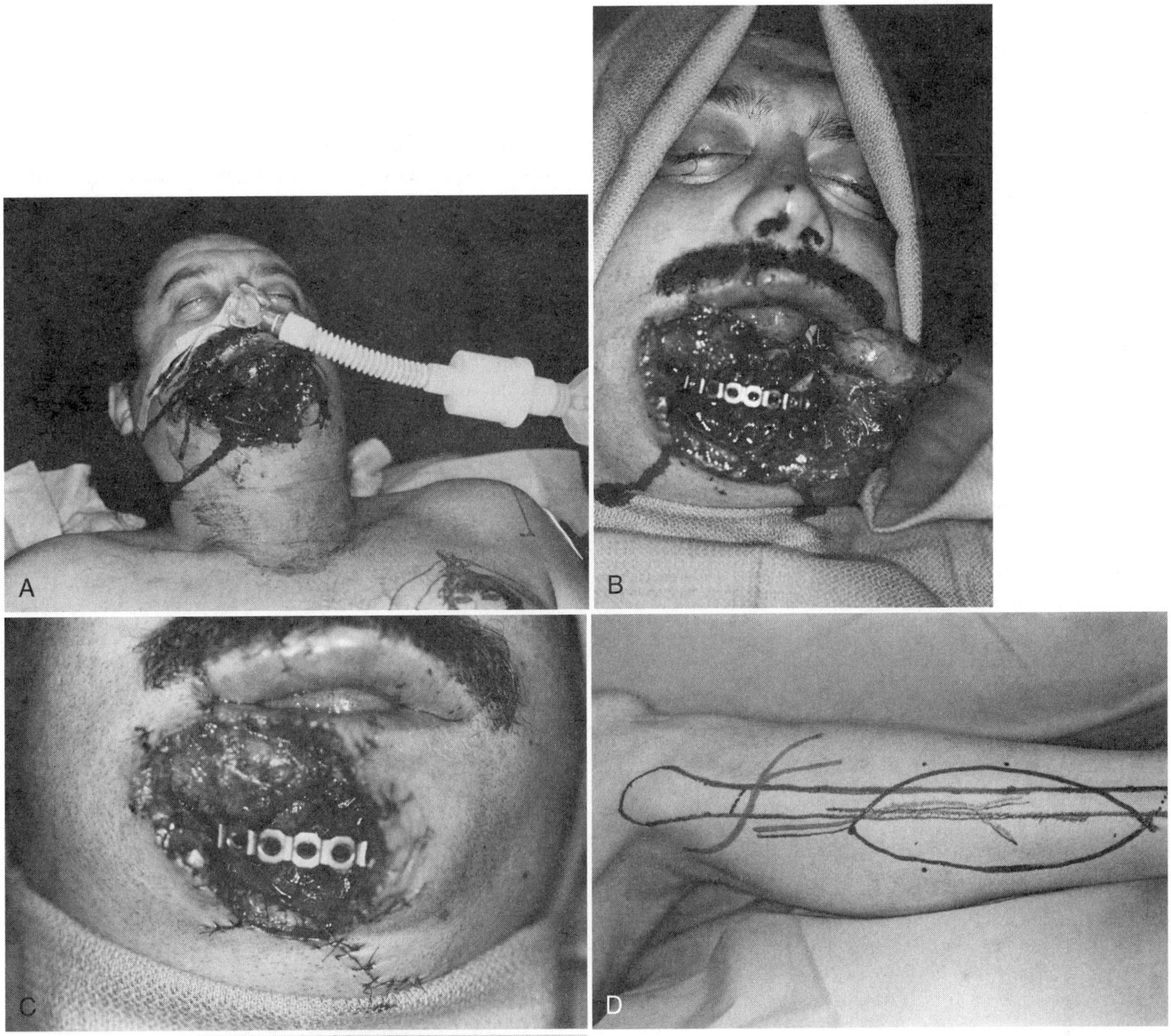

A

B

C

D

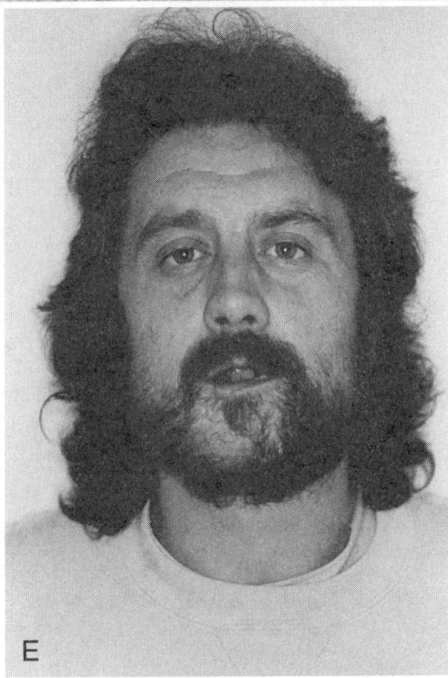

FIGURE 21-18 **A,** Initial appearance of facial gunshot wound. **B,** After initial debridement, bone stabilization, and closure of oral mucosal lining. **C,** Hospital day 5, status-post serial "second-look" debridement and now ready for free microvascular reconstruction. **D,** Site of microvascular fibula osteocutaneous flap. **E,** Six months after completed reconstruction. (From Robertson BC, Manson PN: High-energy ballistic and avulsive injuries: a management protocol for the next millennium, *Surg Clin North Am* 6:1489-1502, 1999.)

should be identified who will receive brief updates about the progress of the patient's surgery, estimated time remaining, and planned disposition of the patient postoperatively. The operating surgeon should provide specific information about the operative procedure, complications, patient diagnosis, and future treatment plan. Family members should be directed to write down questions regarding these topics and address them with the surgeon following the surgery.

Critical Care/Intermediate Care Phases

Postoperatively, the patient with maxillofacial injury may require critical care or intermediate care management, depending on the severity of injury, threat to airway, breathing or circulation, associated injuries, and medical history. Airway patency, adequate ventilation, and circulation remain the most important care priorities during these phases. Complications such as inadequate oxygenation, tissue hypoperfusion, infection, and inadequate nutrition can compromise wound and fracture healing and must be avoided. For more specific information on wound healing, the reader is referred to Chapter 16. Attention to potential neurologic compromise, pain and anxiety control, and psychological well-being must also be included in the plan of care.

Ensure Adequate Respiratory Function

Airway patency and adequate ventilation are threatened by a number of factors following maxillofacial fracture repair or soft tissue reconstruction. Upper airway edema caused by trauma, operative manipulation, or prolonged intubation can cause airway occlusion necessitating endotracheal intubation or a tracheostomy until the edema subsides (Figure 21-19). Ineffective clearance of intraoral and pulmonary secretions also can cause airway obstruction. Prolonged time under anesthesia for lengthy facial repair increases the likelihood of atelectasis formation, which compromises respiratory gas exchange. Trauma patients may also present with thoracic trauma or a past medical history significant for smoking, chronic obstructive pulmonary disease, or other pulmonary pathology, which increases likelihood of respiratory failure. A proactive approach concerning these patients allows for the best opportunity to prevent respiratory complications and promote recovery.

Indications for early tracheostomy in patients with maxillofacial injuries include complex fractures involving the nose, maxilla, and mandible and fractures associated with significant loss of mandibular or maxillary skeletal support of the surrounding soft tissue. In the latter group, the unsupported soft tissues will collapse into the airway (Figure 21-20). Patients with associated severe brain injury or pulmonary injury for whom prolonged intubation is likely are also candidates for early tracheostomy.[12]

Every effort should be made to maintain an established airway by using measures to avoid premature artificial airway removal, continuing with aggressive pulmonary hygiene, and taking precautions against aspiration. Patient positioning should ensure that unnecessary tension on an artificial airway is avoided so that the tube is not inadvertently dislodged and further airway irritation and edema formation does not occur. The patient should be kept calm through frequent verbal reassurance and appropriate use of sedation and anxiolytics. Premature self-extubation or inadvertent airway dislodgment can be life threatening for the patient with maxillofacial injury, as reintubation may be difficult or impossible because of massive upper airway edema.[19] Appropriate use of physical and chemical restraints should

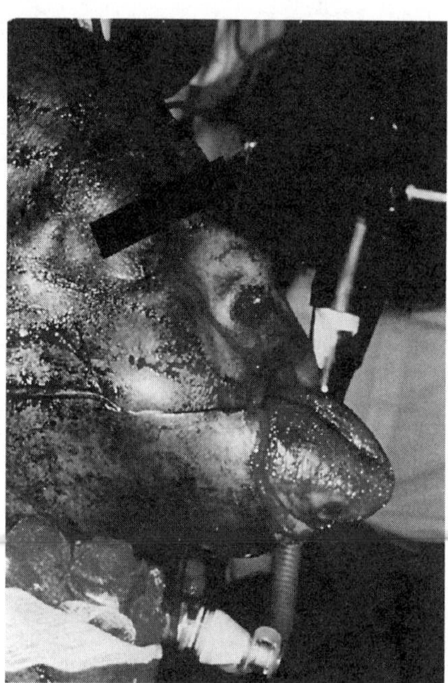

FIGURE 21-19 Postoperative edema of the face and tongue.

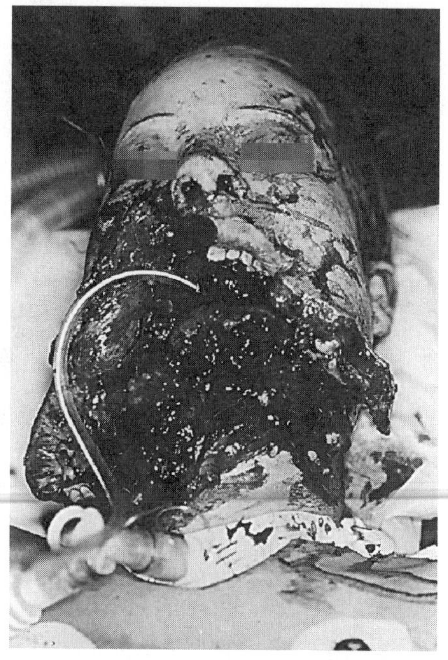

FIGURE 21-20 Unsupported soft tissue collapse.

be considered to prevent this from occurring. Patients with intermaxillary fixation should have wire cutters at the bedside or some other device that allows rapid release of the fixation in the event of an airway emergency.[19]

Aggressive pulmonary hygiene, including suctioning and chest physiotherapy (CPT), remains important to remove secretions and maintain airway patency. Sometimes the extent of the injury or type of maxillofacial reconstruction prohibits head-down positioning for postural drainage in the early period just after injury or surgical intervention. Nurses should speak with the surgeon who performed the facial repair to determine what type of patient positioning is permitted. Nonintubated patients should be encouraged to use the incentive spirometer at frequent intervals. Interventions initiated in the resuscitation phase to avoid aspiration, including ensuring tracheal cuff inflation, frequent removal of intraoral secretions, positioning the patient to enhance outflow of oral drainage, and gastric decompression, remain relevant throughout the critical care and intermediate care phases.

Adequate Hydration

Adequate intravascular volume must be maintained to ensure sufficient perfusion to the site of tissue injury and repair. After a prolonged surgical intervention for maxillofacial repair, the nurse should carefully evaluate the patient's fluid balance and hemodynamic status to determine if hydration is adequate. The physician should be notified immediately if the patient appears dehydrated or hemodynamically unstable, so that the problem can be quickly remedied.

Ongoing Neurologic Assessment

It is imperative that the nurse compares the patient's postoperative neurologic assessment with the baseline assessment obtained preoperatively. Serial neurologic assessments, including examination of consciousness, motor function, sensation, eye and pupil reflexes, and other cranial nerve functions, should be performed thereafter to detect possible deterioration. A complete neurologic assessment provides a systematic evaluation of the craniofacial structure functions. Any deterioration in the patient's neurologic function should be reported immediately to the physician.

During the critical care phase, barriers to assessment of certain neurologic parameters may exist for patients with maxillofacial injuries. Assessment of the patient's orientation, speech, and cognitive abilities is difficult if the patient is intubated. Asking simple yes or no questions that allow the patient to nod or signal the answer is one strategy that can be used to elicit this information. Periorbital edema or suturing the eyelids closed make the eyes inaccessible for evaluation. In the cooperative patient able to acknowledge simple questions, assessment of light perception by shining a light directly over the closed or covered eye is recommended every 2 to 4 hours for the first 24 hours after zygoma and orbit repair.

Nasal drainage should continue to be monitored for the presence of CSF. The nasal drip pad should be checked frequently to determine the amount, consistency, color, and odor of drainage. Any change in these characteristics should be reported immediately to the physician.[40]

Pain Management

Pain generally persists postoperatively and requires prescribed analgesics for control. Dressing changes or wound irrigations may increase pain intensity, increasing the need for analgesia and possibly sedation just before these procedures. Application of ice packs to the face for the first 24 hours after surgical intervention may help reduce facial swelling and discomfort. The reader is referred to Chapter 18 for more specific information on pain and sedation management.

Wound Care

Skin integrity is likely altered in the patient with maxillofacial injury from traumatic lacerations, degloving, abrasions, and/or surgical incisions. Suture lines and facial abrasions should be cleansed at the prescribed frequency using the method requested by the surgeon. If prescribed, a thin layer of antibiotic ointment (e.g., bacitracin) is applied over the cleaned incision or wound site. A pH-corrected ointment for ophthalmic use is applied to incisions in the periorbital region.[45] Operative incisions are often left open to air once any significant drainage from the site has ceased. Skin flaps or grafts will require unique specialized care, which is described in Chapter 16.

The operating surgeon should provide specific instructions about oral care required for the patient with intraoral lacerations or incisions. Dental hygiene is essential even when intraoral devices such as arch bars or elastics are in place. Generally, a prescribed oral rinse (e.g., chlorhexidine gluconate [Peridex]) is used to irrigate the mouth at regular intervals or as a mouthwash solution for patients with intraoral infections. Patients may continue to use warm saline as an oral rinse. Oral lavage is usually done at least four to six times a day until serosanginous secretions subside (which can be a minimum of 2 to 3 days). A large syringe with a flexible peripheral intravenous catheter sheath attached can be used to inject the rinse solution into spaces that are difficult to reach within the mouth. As the oral cavity is irrigated, a suction catheter is used to remove the rinse and secretions. Patients with a decreased level of consciousness will need to be positioned on their side to prevent aspiration during the lavage. A toothbrush or commercial toothpaste should not be used until approved by the physician. Orthodontic wax may be applied over metal arch bars to prevent irritation to the oral mucosa but should be removed daily to allow thorough cleansing of the mouth.

Nutrition

Adequate hydration and nutrition are essential to allow fractures and soft tissue to heal and to reduce the risk of infection. Wound healing depends on the intake of adequate protein, carbohydrate, and fat, as well as sufficient vitamins and minerals.[46] Consultation with a registered dietitian is helpful for determining the patient's individualized nutritional requirements. The reader is referred to Chapter 17 for a complete review of metabolic and nutritional management of the trauma patient.

If enteral feeding is contraindicated for any reason, total parenteral nutrition should be considered. A patient with intermaxillary fixation or with some other restriction to mastication may require an orogastric or intestinal feeding tube to deliver commercially prepared tube feedings. The head of the bed should be elevated at least 30 degrees (unless contraindicated) while the patient is receiving enteral feedings to promote gastric emptying and discourage reflux, thereby reducing risk of aspiration. The nurse should remain vigilant for symptoms that indicate intolerance to the enteral feedings (i.e., nausea, vomiting, diarrhea, excessive gastric residual, abdominal distention). Suction apparatus should be kept readily available to assist with removal of any vomitus, and patients should be positioned on their side to reduce risk of aspiration if vomiting occurs. Wire cutters must be readily accessible for patients with intermaxillary fixation, so that the fixation can be released if vomiting occurs and the emesis cannot be removed with suction and positioning.[19] The physician should be notified immediately if fixation is released; the patient in this situation should not be left unattended.

Once oral feedings are permitted—usually following evaluation of swallowing capability by speech therapy—the prescribed diet is initiated. Generally, clear liquids are introduced, with advancement to full and pureed liquids and foods as tolerated by the patient. A pureed or soft diet can be continued until mastication becomes more comfortable for the patient. Care should be taken to ensure that food fibers from blended foods are removed to avoid the particles becoming trapped between dentition or between fixation devices. A dietitian can assist in finding attractive and creative ways to enhance necessary caloric intake.[47]

Potential for Infection

Maxillofacial injuries, with or without penetrating wounds, are usually considered contaminated, as the fractures pass through the paranasal sinuses and communicate with teeth and the oral cavity. Despite this hostile environment, the actual incidence of infection is remarkably low unless there has been incomplete debridement of devascularized tissue and foreign material, incomplete evacuation of hematoma, failure to obliterate dead space, incomplete establishment of oral lining closure, or obstruction of glandular ducts. The incidence of infection is highest in penetrating gunshot wounds and high-speed avulsive injuries that involve the mandible. In these instances, the potential for progressive soft tissue and bone necrosis over the first several days is high; therefore, serial "second-look" operative washout and debridement procedures are advised until the wound becomes stable (see Figure 21-18, A-C). At this point, all missing tissue, including the lining, bone, and overlying skin envelope, should be reconstructed with vascularized tissue[5,44] (see Figure 21-18, D-E).

Antibiotics are usually administered during the perioperative period. Ongoing prophylactic antibiotic coverage may be considered for patients with an open brain injury (i.e., CSF leak or pneumocephalus), fractures opening into the mouth, fractures communicating with the teeth or adjacent to tooth roots, lacerations into the oral cavity, animal bites, sinus fractures, or orbital emphysema. A great deal of controversy surrounds the indiscriminate use of antibiotic prophylaxis, as it may place the patient at risk for infections caused by antibiotic-resistant organisms. More important than antibiotics is timely intervention to decontaminate the maxillofacial wound. When a clean wound cannot be established, prophylactic antibiotics are usually indicated and should be administered as prescribed. Antibiotics provided for prophylaxis are typically discontinued after 2 to 3 days.[12]

Early signs of infection unique to maxillofacial injuries include disproportionate edema and pain in the region of the parotid and submandibular glands, a persistent foul breath odor despite good oral hygiene, persistent serous or seropurulent drainage from incision lines, rapidly spreading erythema, and increasing discomfort when moving the eyes or tongue. Early detection of infection is critical because the causative organisms are usually anaerobic and spread rapidly through the head and neck tissue planes. As with any infection, early evacuation of the source, along with operative debridement of devascularized tissue and initiation of appropriate antibiotics based on organism sensitivity, is required. The surgeon must reinspect and ensure adequate drainage of the paranasal sinuses and parotid and submandibular glands, reevaluate the fracture sites that communicate through tooth sockets, remove teeth that have become mobile, and ensure a watertight closure of the oral mucosal lining.

Facial fractures, including sinus fractures, often increase the risk of sinusitis. Stein and Caplan's brief review of risk factors for nosocomial infections found that patients with facial trauma had a high risk of developing nosocomial sinusitis.[48] To prevent this infectious process, long-term placement of nasal packing and nasal gastric or endotracheal tubes should be avoided. The nasal cavity should be cleansed daily with normal saline nose drops to prevent obstruction of the paranasal sinuses and ensure a patent nasal airway. Decongestants may also be prescribed to help maintain the nasal airway and clear the sinuses, but administration of these agents should be limited to 3 to 5 days. Presence of fever, halitosis, and purulent nasal drainage should alert the practitioner to the possibility of a sinus infection. Sinusitis can be verified with radiographs demonstrating opacification of the sinuses. Needle aspiration or surgical drainage is indicated to drain the infected sinuses, and appropriate antibiotics should be initiated.[48] Follow-up sinus x-ray films may be indicated in 2 to 3 weeks to determine if sinus opacification has resolved.

Le Fort II and Le Fort III fractures as well as naso-orbital-ethmoidal and frontobasilar fractures frequently communicate with the anterior cranial base through the cribriform plate and are associated with dural lacerations and CSF leakage (CSF rhinorrhea).[49] Generally, anatomic reduction and stabilization of these fractures will allow the dural injury to seal within 24 to 36 hours. If the CSF leak does not stop spontaneously, surgical intervention to repair the dura may be necessary. Measures should be taken to avoid retrograde migration of bacteria into the cranial vault, and thus decrease the risk of meningitis. Nasal packing, nasal intubation with gastric or endotracheal tubes, and blowing of the nose should be avoided.[50] Currently there are no evidence-based guidelines that clarify what discharge instructions should be given to the patient concerning when they may or may not blow their nose or travel by plane after treatment for fractures of the zygomatic complex.[50] More research is required concerning these educational issues. Patients with these injuries should also be examined frequently for changes in their neurologic status, which may indicate intracranial infection.[40] If meningitis is confirmed or highly suspected, the patient is treated with an antibiotic that crosses the blood–brain barrier and is effective in treating the known or likely infectious organism(s).

Eye Care

When injuries occur in or near the orbital region, special attention should be given to care of the eye. Prescribed ophthalmic drops or ointment should be applied to the eye(s) at regular intervals to maintain lubrication and prevent corneal abrasions. Eyelids may also be sutured by the surgeon or taped closed to protect the eyes. Use of ophthalmic lubricant and special protective interventions for the eye are particularly important if eyelid closure is impaired, eyelid injuries are present, the corneal reflex is absent, or natural tear formation is insufficient. The reader is referred to Chapter 22 for more information on ocular injuries.

Early double vision following management of periorbital fractures is common but should gradually improve as edema resolves.[16,18] Ocular function should be compared with the findings from the preoperative baseline evaluation. Any variance should be brought to the attention of the physician. If there is a change in light perception or pupillary response, optic nerve compression from a retrobulbar hematoma or displaced bone fragment must be suspected and an emergency ophthalmology consult obtained.[51]

Altered Body Image

Any type of facial trauma threatens the concept of self. Each patient's reaction to sudden disfigurement is different, whether the injury involves a small laceration or massive tissue loss. Human interaction usually occurs face to face, and if the appearance of the face is altered, the interaction process also changes. Altered body image caused by maxillofacial injury can have a profound impact on the patient's self-esteem, interpersonal interactions, and role performance. Individuals with such alterations in body image often respond with anger, grieving, or depression.[52]

Encouraging the patient to express feelings about the injury and communicating to the patient with a caring, empathetic approach are strategies that may be helpful. Alternative modes of communication need to be established with the patient who is unable to verbalize (e.g., an intubated patient). Nurses must remain conscientious about their nonverbal communication, which should focus on maintaining eye contact and relaying an accepting and positive attitude when caring for the wound. Reinforcing positive qualities can also help enhance self-worth. Referral to a psychiatric liaison or crisis counselor may assist the patient in coping with the injury and altered body image. The reader is referred to Chapter 19 for more information on the psychosocial impact of trauma and appropriate nursing interventions.

Altered body image caused by facial wounds may prompt the patient to cope by use of denial, withdrawal, repression, suppression, or regression. Patients may turn to substance abuse to deal with their traumatic injuries.[53] The reader is referred to Chapter 33 for more information on caring for the trauma patient with a substance abuse problem. The patient may refuse wound care or prefer to isolate himself or herself from interactions with others. Adequate pain and anxiety relief should always be provided when caring for the wound site. Discussion about possible negative reactions to the facial disfigurement should be encouraged. The patient should not be forced into unwanted social interaction, but a supportive significant other may prove helpful in decreasing anxiety and apprehension about the wound and socialization.

Reintegration Into the Community

Although the hospital course for patients with maxillofacial trauma will vary depending on the type and severity of injuries they sustained, the final desired outcome for all patients is reintegration into society. After discharge from the hospital, most patients with maxillofacial injury need continued care for the physical as well as psychological aspects of their injury. A great deal of clear and comprehensible patient and family education and adequate home health care resources are required for successful reintegration of the patient back into society.[54]

Patient/Family Education

A clear plan of care and realistic outlook for the patient's facial restoration need to be communicated to the patient and family by the physician. Anticipated follow-up surgeries and expected outcomes of reconstruction should be explained to the patient and family by the surgeon. The nurse should reinforce this information. Offering false reassurances and reinforcing unrealistic hopes for a new facial appearance are strongly discouraged.

Wound care should be explained and demonstrated to the patient and family, and then a return demonstration by the individual who will be performing the care at home should be observed. Instruction and demonstration of suture line care may be best done with the patient in front of a mirror. Patients should be instructed to wash their hands frequently, to keep their hair clean and styled away from the operative incision, and to avoid air pollutants (e.g., cigarette smoke and excessive dust). Patients should be advised to avoid direct hand contact with wound sites. Education should also be provided on symptoms of potential localized, systemic, or intracranial infections and actions to take if such symptoms are recognized.[55]

Direct exposure of incisions or wounds to sunlight or ultraviolet rays should also be avoided to prevent the wound from becoming deeper in color. Patients should be taught that if sunlight exposure is anticipated, strong sunscreen or sun block should be applied over and around the facial scar. Incisions will appear red and elevated for about 6 months after repair.

Intraoral irrigations and rinses after meals are usually continued after hospitalization and must be stressed as part of discharge instructions. The patient should be taught when and if a bristled toothbrush or toothpaste can be used. A water-jet appliance can be recommended for removal of retained food residue in hard-to-reach areas of the mouth. Appropriate use of orthodontic wax is reviewed if relevant for the patient.

Patients requiring a long-term tracheostomy need education about care and safety measures concerning the artificial airway device. Patients and their families should be instructed on airway clearance techniques and tracheostomy site care. Emergency care to be taken if the airway becomes occluded or dislodged should be described and demonstrated thoroughly.

After surgical intervention for mandibular fractures, particularly condylar and subcondylar fractures, an exercise regimen may be prescribed to enhance mandibular range of motion. The surgeon determines the timing for introduction of these exercises. The patient should be encouraged to perform these exercises in front of a mirror to allow observation of progress. Other measures that may be used to increase mandibular motion include heat application and muscle relaxants.[56]

Patients and families should be informed that psychological adjustment and adaptation to facial injury might take several weeks or months. Posttraumatic stress disorder may develop in individuals who suffer facial trauma. Patients and families should be aware that reactions to such injury might include altered mood patterns, depression, increased anxiety, and nightmares or flashbacks about the injury event. Follow-up counseling or therapy is an option that the patient should consider if these or other psychological symptoms become evident and problematic.

Other late complications of maxillofacial injuries include issues related to musculoskeletal scar formation and scar contracture, persistent double vision, enophthalmos, glandular obstruction, fracture nonunion or malunion, devitalization of teeth, and malocclusion. These late complications are generally not present at the time of release from the primary acute care hospital; however, the physician, nurse, and therapist need to review symptoms of these potential problems with the patient and family at the time of discharge.[57] Scars and scar contracture can cause unacceptable alterations in appearance and function, and thus require intervention. Techniques used to treat scars and scar contracture are described in Chapter 16.

Persistent double vision from eye muscle injury may continue after edema subsides, in 6 to 8 weeks.[18] This may require treatment by an ophthalmologist with prisms or ocular muscle surgery, or both, to readjust functional movement of the eye. Post-injury enophthalmos may occur secondary to malreduction of orbital fractures with increased orbital volume, reduced ocular volume secondary to intraocular fat atrophy, retroocular scar retraction, or some combination thereof. Post-injury enophthalmos is generally corrected by surgically releasing the scar tissue or correcting the volume of the orbit by reconstructing the involved malpositioned orbital walls.[17] In general, this late form of enophthalmos takes several months to reach its final position, and correction is usually deferred until scar maturation has occurred at 6 to 12 months.

Periodically, parotid and submandibular glandular dysfunction does not manifest during the primary phase of hospitalization. Patients with this condition will complain of persistent glandular swelling and marked pain when eating. Glandular function is checked by evaluating for clear salivary flow from the parotid duct (located on the buccal mucosa opposite the maxillary second molar) and the mandibular duct (located on the floor of the mouth just behind the mandibular central incisors). If there is no flow, or if pain and a cloudy discharge are present, further investigation for glandular dysfunction is indicated. A sialogram (x-ray of the salivary ducts and related glandular structures), CT scan, or both may be warranted.

The primary focus of follow-up evaluation during the convalescent phase of recovery from maxillofacial fractures is to determine fracture union and to maintain a stable, balanced, functional occlusion. Occasionally, fracture nonunion or malunion (bony malalignment) may occur. In these cases, patients may manifest with persistent pain at the fracture site, mobility, and, if the maxilla or mandible is involved, malocclusion. Further surgery may be required to restore the proper bite relationship and to realign the bony components. A bone graft may be needed to ensure bone union.[56]

Home Health Care Resources

Home health care may be needed if facial reconstruction is extensive, complex dressing changes are required, intravenous medications must be continued, or a tracheostomy will remain in place. A home health care nurse may be needed to supervise initial wound or tracheostomy care after discharge from the hospital. Adequate supplies and resources should be arranged for the patient prior to discharge.

A number of trauma patients are unable to obtain home health care services or supplies due to their inability to pay, location, or by choice. In a prospective case-controlled study, Lento and colleagues found that indigent patients with facial trauma continued to experience significant psychological distress for up to 12 months after injury. Patients with orofacial injury tend to report more current and lifetime mental health and social service needs than patients with similar sociodemographics undergoing elective-surgery.[57] The astute trauma nurse must recognize the patient's psychosocial needs and advocate for sufficient resources to best meet those needs following discharge.

Cosmetics

A patient may be interested in using cosmetics to conceal prominent facial scars. A plastic surgeon should be consulted to verify the types of makeup that should be used during scar healing and maturation. Referral to a cosmetologist with experience in scar coverage and concealment may also be offered to the patient. The cosmetologist can educate the patient on techniques to achieve symmetry of color and contour between scarred areas and natural pigmentation. Through use of color and outline, scars and other defects can be made to appear less prominent.

SUMMARY

In the future, we look forward to adapting more biocompatible materials that are resorbable for use in facial repair and engineering specific tissue structures for improved tissue reconstruction without the morbidity currently associated with autogenous tissue transfer. Composite tissue allotransplantation (CTA) has become a reality. The end of 2005 saw the world's first partial face transplant occur in Europe amid ethical controversy. In the past, what used to be science fiction medicine is today's reality. Since *full* facial transplants are certainly in the near future, we embark on the slippery slope of balancing the risk to patients and their quality of life issues.

Work with automobile manufacturers will hopefully enable development of improved protective devices that could further reduce the incidence of facial injuries. Research to define nursing therapeutics that best promote wound and fracture healing, relieve pain, and deal effectively with the psychological effects of facial trauma will continue to be important for improving care to patients with maxillofacial injuries. Laski et al suggest that patients suffering facial trauma are at risk for recurrent facial injury. This is especially seen with those patients living in urban settings. There is a window of opportunity for the nurse, while caring for these patients, to provide education, emotional support, and reinforcement of prevention strategies to help change behavior patterns, thereby avoiding reinjury.[58]

With a comprehensive approach to managing complex facial injuries, one can achieve harmonious balance of facial function and restoration of the patient's individual characteristic identity. Nursing plays a critical role in providing the physical and psychological care necessary for patients with maxillofacial trauma. Knowledge of facial anatomy and assessment strategies to recognize maxillofacial injury prepares the nurse to anticipate and deliver the care required for specific types of maxillofacial trauma. Together with the rest of the multidisciplinary health care team, the nurse who is knowledgeable about maxillofacial injuries is able to plan and implement care in each phase of the trauma cycle to optimize outcomes for patients with these injuries.

REFERENCES

1. Edelstein L: *Ancient Medicine,* Baltimore, Md., 1994, Johns Hopkins Press.
2. Cox D, Vincent DG, MacLennan PA et al: Effect of restraint systems on maxillofacial injury in frontal motor vehicle collisions, *J Oral Maxillofac Surg* 62:571-575, 2004.
3. Brookes C, Wang S, McWilliams J: Maxillofacial injuries in North America vehicle crashes, *Eur J Emerg Med* 10(1):30-40, 2003.
4. Le Fort R: Etude experimentale sur les fractures de la machoire superieure, *Rev Chir Paris* 23:208, 360, 479, 1901.
5. Robertson BC, Manson PN: High-energy ballistic and avulsive injuries: a management protocol for the next millennium, *Surg Clin North Am* 6:1489-1502, 1999.
6. Vayvada H, Menderes A, Yilmaz M et al: Management of close-range, high-energy shotgun and rifle wounds to the face, *J Craniofac Surg* 16(5):794-804, 2005.
7. March K: Neurologic and facial trauma. In Cohen SS, editors: *Trauma Nursing Secrets.* Philadelphia, 2003, Hanley & Belfus, Inc.
8. Hohlrieder M, Hinterhoelzl J, Ulmer H et al: Traumatic intracranial hemorrhages in facial fracture patients: review of 2,195 patients, *Intensive Care Med* 29(7):1095-1100, 2003.
9. Calasans-Maia JA, Calasans-Maia MD, da Matta EN et al: Orthodontic movement in traumatically intruded teeth: a case report, *Dent Traumatol* 19(5):292-295, 2003.
10. Fogaca WC, Fereirra MC, Dellon AL: Infraorbital nerve injury associated with zygoma fractures: documentation with neurosensory testing, *Plast Reconstr Surg* 113(3):834-838, 2004.
11. Kelly KJ, Manson PN, Vander Kolk CA et al: Sequencing LeFort fracture treatment (Organization of treatment for a panfacial fracture), *J Craniofac Surg* 1:168-178, 1990.
12. Perry M, Dancy A, Mireskandari K et al: Emergency care in facial trauma—a maxillofacial and ophthalmic perspective, *Injury* 36:875-896, 2005.
13. McAvoy CE, Lacey B, Page AB: Traumatic superior orbital fissure syndrome, *Eye* 18(8):844-855, 2004.
14. Giaoui L, Lockhart R, Lafitte F et al: Traumatic superior orbital fissure syndrome: report of 4 cases and review of literature. *J Fr Ophthalmol* 24(3):295-302, 2001.
15. Mondin V, Rinaldo A, Ferlito A: Management of nasal bone fractures, *Am J Otolaryngol* 26:181-185, 2005.
16. Dancy A, Perry M, Silva DC: Blindness after blunt facial trauma: are there any clinical clues to early recognition? *J Trauma* 58(2):328-335, 2005.
17. Jabaley ME, Lerman M, Sanders HJ: Ocular injuries in orbital fractures. A review of 119 cases, *Plast Reconstr Surg* 56:410-418, 1975.
18. Cook T: Ocular and periocular injuries from orbital fractures, *J Am Coll Surg* 195(6):831-834, 2002.
19. Silegy T, Scheer P: Management of traumatic facial injuries, *J Calif Dent Assoc* 32(10):839-843, 2004.

20. Holmgren EP, Dierks EJ, Homer LD et al: Facial computed tomography use in trauma patients who require a head computed tomogram, *J Oral Maxillofac Surg* 62:913-918, 2004.
21. Holmgren EP, Dierks EJ, Assael LA: Facial soft-tissue injuries as an aid to ordering combination head and face computed tomography in trauma patients, *J Oral Maxillofac Surg* 63(5):651-654, 2005.
22. Graham JR, Scott TM: Notes on the treatment of tetanus, *N Engl J Med* 235:846-852, 1946.
23. University of Maryland Medical Center: *Tetanus Immune Globulin (Human): Drug Information,* Lexi-Comp, Inc., 1978-2006.
24. Futran ND, Farwell DG, Smith RB et al: Definitive management of severe facial trauma utilizing free tissue transfer, *Otolaryngol Head Neck Surg* 132(1):75-85, 2005.
25. Holger JS, Wandersee SC, Hale DB: Cosmetic outcomes of facial lacerations repaired with tissue-adhesive, absorbable, and nonabsorbable sutures, *A J Emerg Med* 22(4):254-257, 2004.
26. Stranc MF, Robertson GA: A classification of injuries of the nasal skeleton, *Ann Plast Surg* 2:468-474, 1979.
27. Czerwinski M, Martin M, Chen L: Quantitative topographical evaluation of the orbitozygomatic complex, *J Am Plast Surg* 115(7):1858-1862, 2005.
28. Exadaktylos AK, Sclabas GM, Smolka K et al: The value of computed tomographic scanning in the diagnosis and management of orbital fractures associated with head trauma: a prospective, consecutive study at a level I trauma center, *J Trauma* 58(2):336-341, 2005.
29. Shere JL, Boole JR, Holtel MR et al: An analysis of 3599 midfacial and 1141 orbital blowout fracture among 4426 United States Army soldiers, 1980-2000, *Otolaryngol Head Neck Surg* 130(2):164-170, 2004.
30. Manson PN, Hoopes JE, Su CT: Structural pillars of the facial skeleton: an approach to the management of Le Fort fractures, *Plast Reconstr Surg* 66:54-61, 1980.
31. Andrew JL, Gear MD, Apasova E et al: Treatment modalities for mandibular angle fractures, *J Oral Maxillofac Surg* 63(5):655-663, 2005.
32. American College of Surgeons, Committee on Trauma: *Advanced Trauma Life Support Doctors Student Course Manual,* ed 6, Chicago, 2004, American College of Surgeons.
33. Ferreras J, Junquera LM, Garcia L: Intracranial placement of a nasogastric tube after severe craniofacial trauma, *Oral Surg Med Path Radiol Endodont* 90(5):564-566, 2000.
34. Shenaq SM, Dinh T: Maxillofacial and scalp injury in neurotrauma. In Narayan RK, Wilberger JE, Povlishock JT, editors: *Neurotrauma,* New York, 1996, McGraw-Hill.
35. Sody AN, Nash M, Niv A et al: Control of massive bleeding from facial gunshot wound with a compact elastic adhesive compression dressing, *Am J Emerg Med* 22(7):586-588, 2004.
36. Yang WG, Tsai TR, Hung CC et al: Life-threatening bleeding in a facial fracture, *Ann Plast Surg* 46(2):159-162, 2001.
37. Bynoe RP, Kerwin AJ, Parker HH et al: Maxillofacial injuries and life-threatening hemorrhage: treatment with transcatheter arterial embolization, *J Trauma* 55(1):74-79, 2003.
38. Sliker C, Shanmuganathan K, Mirvis S: Diagnosis of blunt cerebrovascular injuries with 16-MDCT: accuracy of whole-body MDCT compared with neck MDCT angiography, *AJR* 190: 790-799, 2008.
39. Martin RC, Spain DA, Richardson JD: Do facial fractures protect the brain or are they a marker for severe head injury? *Am Surg* 68(5):477-481, 2002.
40. Bell RB, Dierks EJ, Homer L et al: Management of cerebral spinal leak associated with craniomaxillofacial trauma, *J Oral Maxillofac Surg* 62(6):676-684, 2004.
41. Furness PJ: Exploring supportive care needs and experiences of facial surgery patients, *Br J Nurs* 14(12):641-645, 2005.
42. Linnau KF, Stanley RB, Hallam DK et al: Imaging of high-energy midfacial trauma: what the surgeon needs to know, *Eur J Radiol* 48(1):17-32, 2003.
43. Saigal K, Winokur RS, Finden S et al: Use of three-dimensional computerized tomography reconstruction in complex facial trauma, *Facial Plast Surg* 21(3):214-220, 2005.
44. Robertson BC, Manson PN: The importance of serial debridement and "second look" procedures in high-energy ballistic and avulsive facial injuries, *Operative Techniques Plast Reconstr Surg* 5:236-245,1998.
45. Smith SC: Ocular injuries. In McQuillan KA, Hartsock RL, Von Rueden KT et al, editors: *Trauma Nursing: From Resuscitation through Rehabilitation,* ed 3, Philadelphia, 2002, W.B. Saunders.
46. Thompson C, Fuhrman MP: Nutrients and wound healing: still searching for the magic bullet, *Nutr Clin Pract* 20(3):331-347, 2005.
47. Slone DS: Nutritional support of the critically ill and injured patient, *Crit Care Clin* 20(1):135-157, 2004.
48. Stein M, Caplan ES: Nosocomial sinusitis: a unique subset of sinusitis, *Curr Opin Infect Dis* 18(2):147-150, 2005.
49. Bagheri SC, Holmgren E, Kademani D et al: Comparison of the severity of bilateral LeFort injuries in isolated midface trauma, *J Oral Maxillofac Surg* 63(8):1123-1129, 2005.
50. Mahmood S, Keith D, Lello GE: When can patients blow their nose and fly after treatment for fractures of zygomatic complex: the need for consensus, *Injury* 34:908-911, 2003.
51. Bater MC, Ramchandani PL, Brennan PA: Post-traumatic eye observations, *Br J Oral Maxillofac Surg* 43(5):410-416, 2005.
52. Levine E, Degutis L, Pruzinsky T et al: Quality of life and facial trauma: psychological and body image effects, *Ann Plast Surg* 54(5):502-510, 2005.
53. Zatzick DF, Jurkovich GJ, Gentilello L et al: Posttraumatic stress, problem drinking, and functional outcomes after injury, *Arch of Surg* 137(2):200-205, 2002.
54. Girotto JA, MacKenzie E, Fowler C et al: Long-term physical impairment and functional outcomes after complex facial fractures, *Plast Reconstr Surg* 108(2):312-327, 2001.
55. Sen P, Ross N, Rogers S: Recovering maxillofacial trauma patients: the hidden problems, *J Wound Care* 10(3):53-57, 2001.
56. Yun PY, Kim YK: The role of facial trauma as a possible etiologic factor in temporomandibular joint disease, *J Oral Maxillofac Surg* 63:1576-1583, 2005.
57. Lento J, Glynn S, Shetty V et al: Psychologic functioning and needs of indigent patients with facial injury: a prospective controlled study, *J Oral Maxillofac Surg* 62:925-932, 2004.
58. Laski R, Ziccardi VB, Broder HL: Facial trauma: a recurrent disease? The potential role of disease prevention, *J Oral Maxillofac Surg* 62:685-688, 2004.

22

OCULAR INJURIES

Martha A. Conlon

Ocular injury is the leading cause of monocular blindness in the United States and is second only to cataracts as the most common cause of visual impairment.[1] Trauma is the most frequent reason for eye-related visits to hospital emergency departments. Most eye injuries are minor and result in no permanent visual damage. For severe injuries, a substantial proportion of patients experience poor visual outcomes.[2]

Society bears a burden from ocular injury. The direct costs are linked to health-related issues, and the indirect costs are related to days lost at work. These costs are experienced over a period of many years as most trauma victims are young. The emotional costs continue over many years as well and cannot be quantified in dollar amounts.

As of 2004 the majority of eye injuries (37.8%) occurred in the home. Blunt objects (32.3%) account for the most common source of injury. Fifty-six percent of eye injuries occur in people younger than age 30, and males outpace females by a 4:1 ratio for eye trauma. The leading cause of bilateral eye injury remains motor vehicle crash. Construction injuries account for the majority of occupational-related injuries. Baseball and softball (34.6%) are two of the most common causes of sports-related eye injuries.[3] Falls account for the majority of injuries in the elderly (Table 22-1).

The immediate goals of eye injury management are:

- Protection of intact visual structures
- Prevention of further ocular damage
- Accurate assessment of the injury and appropriate triage or referral of the patient
- Timely initiation of the best possible care by qualified medical personnel

In meeting these goals, health care providers help those with eye injuries achieve optimal functional outcomes and maximum cosmetic results.

The United States Eye Injury Registry (USEIR) is a federation of 40 individual states and the U.S. Military Eye Injury Registry that collects and documents data about serious eye injuries in a standardized fashion. The injuries entered into the database are judged by the reporting ophthalmologist as to the likelihood that permanent structural or functional damage to the eye or orbit will result. Participation in USEIR is voluntary, so actual eye trauma statistics are higher than reported by this federation.

The Ocular Trauma Classification (OTS) Group developed a standardized system for classifying mechanical eye injuries based on the Birmingham Eye Trauma Terminology (BETT). BETT makes descriptions of eye trauma consistent and accurate by providing a clear framework for defining each type of injury[4] (Table 22-2). OTS categorizes both open globe and closed globe injuries by four parameters: type of injury, grade or visual acuity, pupil function, and zone of the injury.[5] Under the open-globe classification for injury type, penetrating injuries are limited to those that only have an entry site, whereas perforating injuries have entry and exit sites and rupture indicates the cause of injury is due to blunt compression of the globe.[6]

To minimize the incidence of permanent vision loss associated with ocular trauma, it is important that those caring for patients with such injuries understand ocular anatomy and function, examination techniques, and recommended therapy. This chapter explains the anatomy and physiology of the eye, prevention of ocular injuries, ocular examination, and management of a variety of traumatic eye injuries. Nursing care provided to the patient with ocular injury in each phase of the trauma cycle has a tremendous impact on the patient's recovery.

ANATOMY AND PHYSIOLOGY

During embryonic development, the ocular and periocular tissues are derived from surface ectoderm, neuroectoderm, and mesoderm. The optic nerve, retina, and portions of the iris and ciliary body are all neuroectodermal structures, as are all components of the central nervous system. These structures, when damaged, are unable to regenerate and require a continuous supply of nutrients and oxygen. If the supply is compromised for even minutes, cells will sustain permanent damage. Injury to neuroectodermal structures, particularly the optic nerve and retina, is primarily responsible for permanent visual loss in cases of trauma.

The conjunctiva, lens, corneal epithelium, and eyelid skin all are derived from surface ectoderm. Cells of these tissues are able to regenerate and repair themselves after injury and can survive a relatively long time without a constant supply of blood and oxygen.

Mesodermal structures include the bony orbit, extraocular muscles, sclera, corneal stroma, ocular and periocular connective tissue, blood vessels, and internal eyelid structures. These tissues are able to regenerate to varying degrees after damage.

TABLE 22-1 United States Eye Injury Registry: Selected Data 1982 to 2004

Age*

	Percentage	Male:Female Ratio
0-9 years	12%	2.4:1
10-19 years	23.2%	4.5:1
20-29 years	20.8%	5.2:1
30-39 years	18%	5.5:1
40-49 years	11.6%	5.3:1
50-59 years	6.2%	5.1:1
60-69 years	3.8%	3.8:1
≥ 70 years	4.5%	1:1
	100% (TOTAL)	4:1 (MEAN)

Race

Caucasian	51.2%
Black	18%
Hispanic	3.5%
Asian	0.6%
Native American	1%
Unknown	25.3%
Other	0.4%

Intention

Assault	14.7%
Self-inflicted	0.8%
Unintentional	64.5%
Unknown	19.9%

When Injured

Summer	21.7%
Winter	27.1%
Spring	29.8%
Fall	21.4%

Eye Protection

None	66.3%
Regular	2.9%
Safety	1.5%
Sunglasses	0.3%

Sports Injuries

Baseball	23.6%
Fishing	17.6%
Softball	11%
Basketball	10.4%
Soccer	5.2%
Racquetball	5.4%
Football	4.8%
Golf	5.3%
Other	16.6%

Place of Injury

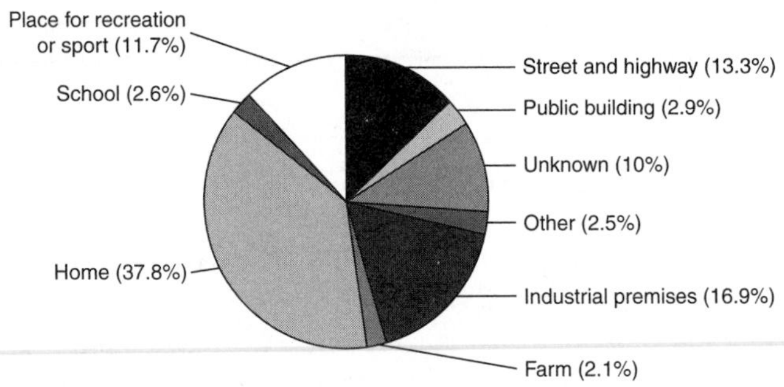

Source of Injury

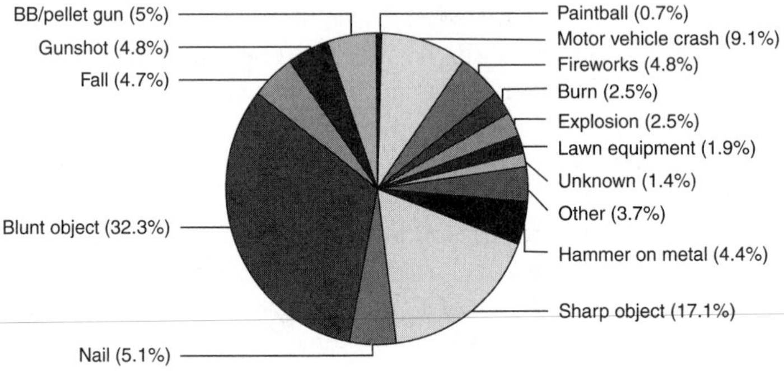

Bystanders: 19.14% (M:F: 2.9:1). Reported alcohol use when injured: 10%.
Bilateral injuries: 5%; leading source of bilateral injury: motor vehicle crash.
Open globe injuries: 43.5%.
Injured eye: OD, 48.3%; OS, 50.3%; unknown, 1.3%.
Work-related injuries: 15.29%; leading reported occupation: construction; leading reported injury source: sharp object.

This analysis reflects USEIR's database December 2004 (N = 13,061) and contains reports of serious eye injuries from Alabama, Arkansas, California, Connecticut, Florida, Georgia, Hawaii, Idaho, Illinois, Indiana, Iowa, Kansas, Kentucky, Louisiana, Maine, Maryland, Massachusetts, Michigan, Minnesota, Missouri, Montana, Nebraska, New Jersey, New Mexico, North Carolina, North Dakota, Ohio, Oregon, Pennsylvania, Rhode Island, South Carolina, South Dakota, Tennessee, Texas, Utah, U.S. Military, Virginia, Washington, and Wisconsin.

Data provided by the United States Eye Injury Registry, through funding by the Helen Keller Foundation, Birmingham, Alabama, USA.

*Range: 1-118 years; mean: 29.09 years; median: 27 years; 56% were <30 years old.

TABLE 22-2 Ocular Trauma Classification System

Open-Globe Injury Classification

Type

A. Rupture
B. Penetrating
C. Intraocular foreign body
D. Perforating
E. Mixed

Grade

Visual acuity*:
1. 20/40 or greater
2. 20/50-20/100
3. 19/100-5/200
4. 4/200-light perception
5. No light perception†

Pupil

Positive: Relative afferent pupillary defect present in affected eye
Negative: Relative afferent pupillary defect absent in affected eye

Zone

I. Isolated to cornea (including corneoscleral limbus)
II. Corneoscleral limbus to a point 5 mm posterior into the sclera
III. Posterior to the anterior 5 mm of sclera

Closed-Globe Injury Classification

Type

A. Contusion
B. Lamellar laceration
C. Superficial foreign body
D. Mixed

Grade

Visual acuity*:
1. 20/40 or greater
2. 20/50-20/100
3. 19/100-5/200
4. 4/200-light perception
5. No light perception†

Pupil

Positive: Relative afferent pupillary defect present in affected eye
Negative: Relative afferent pupillary defect absent in affected eye

Zone‡

I. External (limited to bulbar conjunctiva, sclera, and cornea)
II. Anterior segment (involving structures internal to the cornea and including the posterior lens capsule; pars plicata but not pars plana)
III. Posterior segment (all internal structures posterior to the posterior lens capsule)

Kuhn F, Pieramici D, editors: *Ocular Trauma Principles and Practice,* New York, 2002, Thieme.
*Measured at distance (20 ft, 6 m) using Snellen chart or Rosenbaum near card with pinhole when appropriate.
†Confirmed with bright light source and fellow eye well occluded.
‡Requires B-scan ultrasonography when media opacity precludes assessment of more posterior structures.

Intraocular Structures

The eye and its adnexal structures are as complex anatomically and functionally as they are in embryonic development. Light rays enter the eye through the cornea, pupil, and lens and fall on the diaphanous retina (Figure 22-1), which activates the retinal photoreceptor elements, the rods, and cones. Rods are responsible for night vision and function best in dim lighting. Cones (there are three types: red, blue, and green) are responsible for color and detailed vision; they function best in bright light. Cones predominate in the macula. The macula is the only site capable of 20/20 vision. Through complex synaptic interconnections among a variety of cell types, the rods and cones transmit the light messages they receive to the 1 million retinal ganglion cells, whose axons are gathered together at the optic disc and form the optic nerve. The optic disc (Figure 22-2) measures 1.5 mm in diameter and contains a central depression, or cup, which averages one third the disc diameter. As the axons leave the globe, they travel for approximately 1 mm through the sclera. They are then covered by dura and arachnoid while extending 25 to 30 mm through the orbit, 4 to 9 mm through the optic canal, and 10 mm intracranially before forming the optic chiasm and finally terminating deep in the brain substance.

Anterior to the retina is the vitreous, a gelatinous substance that constitutes two thirds of the volume of the eye. External to the retina is the choroid, a layer of vascular channels. Surrounding the choroid is the sclera, a tough connective tissue layer that protects the internal ocular structures and acts as the structural skeleton for the globe.

The lens lies anterior to the vitreous. This structure is approximately 9 mm in diameter and 4 mm thick. It is suspended just behind the iris by fibers that connect it to the wedge-shaped ciliary body, which consists of muscular, vascular, and epithelial elements. The ciliary body is responsible for producing aqueous humor and for changing the shape of the lens, which becomes more biconvex for near vision and flattens for distance vision. The iris is an anterior extension of the ciliary body. This flat structure lies just anterior to the lens and contains a central round aperture, the pupil. Contraction of the iris sphincter muscle, innervated by the parasympathetic nervous system, redúces pupil diameter; contraction of the iris dilator fibers, innervated by the sympathetic nervous system, enlarges the size of the pupil. These actions control the amount of light entering the eye.

In front of the iris lies the anterior chamber, which contains the aqueous fluid produced by the ciliary body. Aqueous humor is continuously produced by the ciliary body. It moves forward through the posterior chamber and pupil into the anterior chamber, where it drains out via the trabecular meshwork and Schlemm's canal. These structures are located in the angle created by the junction of the iris, cornea, and sclera. The sclera blends into the cornea, an avascular, crystal-clear, convex disc-like structure. It is

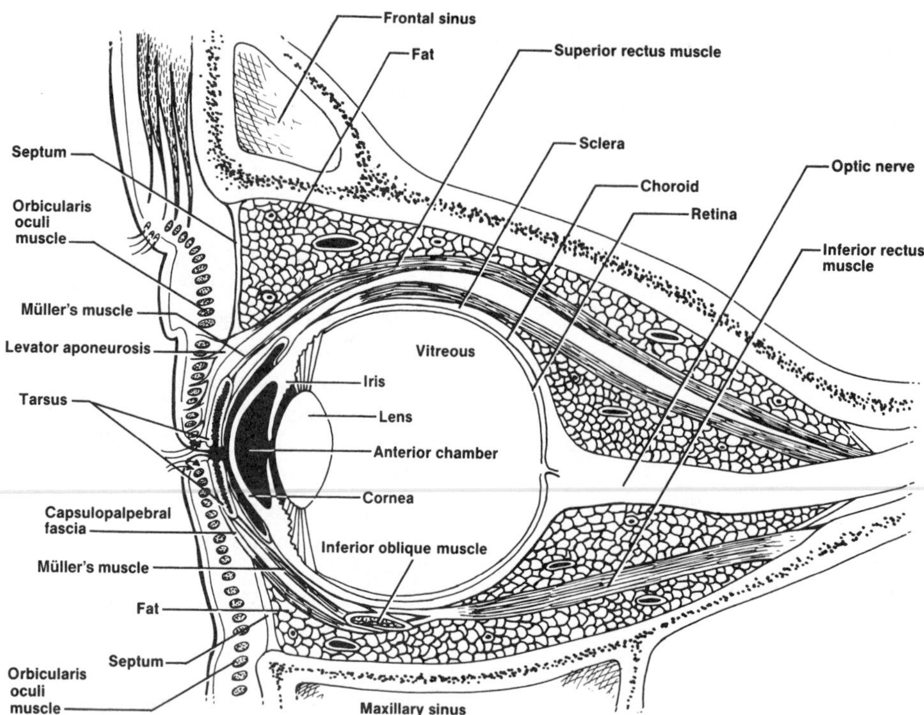

FIGURE 22-1 Ocular and periocular anatomy, including vascular supply and innervation of ocular structures.

covered by a layer of epithelium five to six cells thick, which can regenerate in 24 to 48 hours when scratched or abraded. The cornea becomes continuous with the epithelium of the conjunctiva, the mucous membrane that lines the posterior surface of the eyelids and the anterior portion of the sclera. Overlying the cornea and conjunctiva is the tear film, which is composed of lacrimal, mucinous, and lipid gland secretions. These secretions are produced by the lacrimal and accessory lacrimal glands, conjunctiva goblet cells, and meibomian glands. An adequate tear film evenly distributed across the cornea and an intact corneal epithelium are essential factors for achieving clear vision.

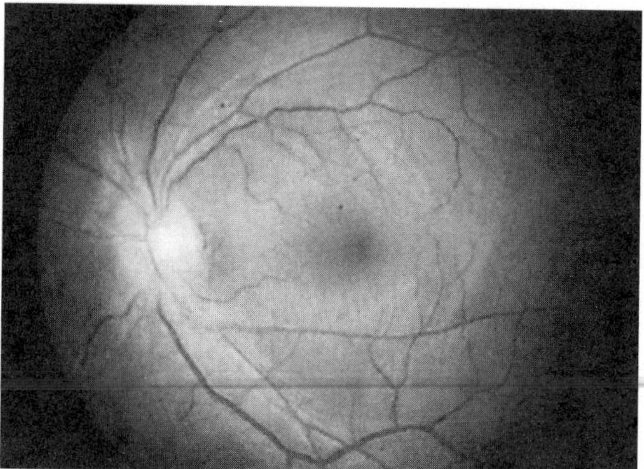

FIGURE 22-2 Normal ocular fundus with optic disc, retina, macula, and vessels.

Periocular and Orbital Structures

The eyelids cover and protect the globe. They also distribute the tear film across the cornea and aid in the removal of excess tears and tear film debris. The eyelids can be divided into five layers. Most posterior is the conjunctiva. Anterior to this in the upper lid is Müller's muscle, a structure that is partially responsible for eyelid elevation. Müller's muscle is attached to the tarsus, a dense, fibrous connective tissue structure containing the meibomian glands, that provides structural support for the upper and lower eyelids. Anterior to Müller's muscle and the tarsus is the levator muscle complex in the upper eyelid. The capsulopalpebral fascia is an analogous structure in the lower eyelid that attaches to the inferior border of the tarsus. The third cranial nerve innervates the levator muscle, which is responsible for elevating the eyelid. For this reason, ptosis (droop) (Figure 22-3) may be present with third nerve paresis. Because parasympathetic fibers to the iris sphincter muscle also travel in the third nerve, a dilated (mydriatic) pupil may be associated with third nerve paresis. Anterior to the levator muscle complex is the orbicularis muscle, a structure innervated by the seventh cranial nerve. When this nerve is paretic, as in Bell's palsy (Figure 22-4), the eyelids cannot close, resulting in tear film evaporation and corneal epithelial damage. Corneal ulceration can occur if this is not treated promptly. Skin is the final structure covering the eyelid. A component of the eyelid that cannot be overlooked is the orbital septum, which is a continuation of the periosteum covering the bony orbit. This structure extends from the orbital rim and attaches to the levator muscle complex in the upper lid and the

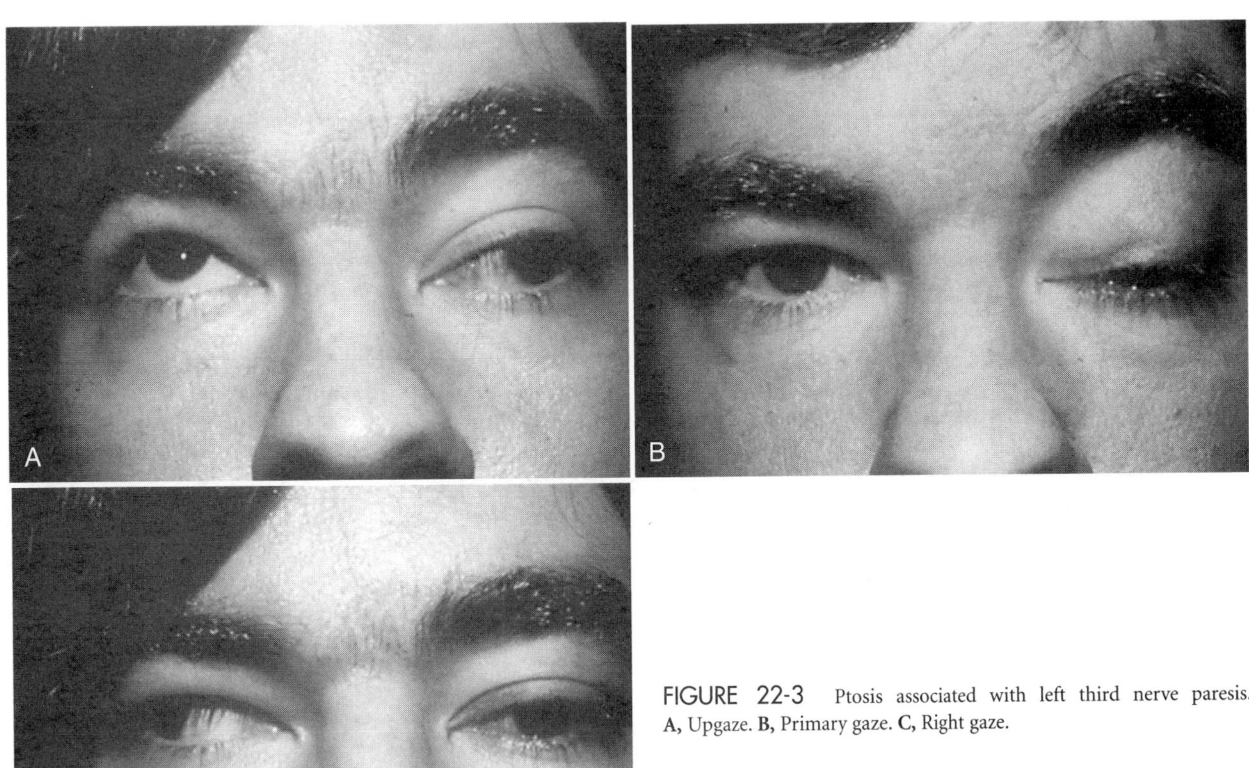

FIGURE 22-3 Ptosis associated with left third nerve paresis. **A,** Upgaze. **B,** Primary gaze. **C,** Right gaze.

capsulopalpebral fascia in the lower lid. The orbital septum represents the boundary between the orbital and periorbital structures. Violation of this protective barrier exposes the orbital contents to external forces, specifically infectious agents. Infection can involve the entire orbit, causing subsequent visual loss and possible intracranial spread, resulting in meningitis and abscess formation.

The globe lies within the bony orbit, which consists of the maxillary, lacrimal, ethmoid, greater and lesser sphenoid, frontal, palatine, and zygomatic bones. These bones are joined to form a quadrilateral pyramid with its apex located posteriorly. The anterior opening of the adult orbit measures approximately 35 mm in height and 40 mm in width. The orbit is 40 to 45 mm deep. Superior to the orbit

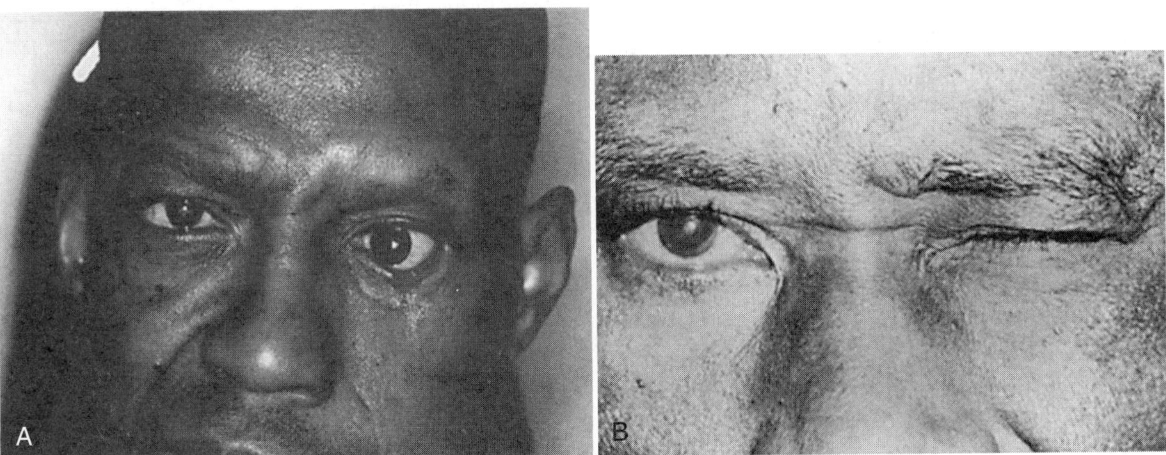

FIGURE 22-4 **A,** Left-sided Bell's palsy causing facial paralysis and lower eyelid sag. **B,** Right-sided Bell's palsy causing inability to close right eye.

are the frontal sinus anteriorly and the anterior cranial fossa posteriorly. Medial to the orbit are the ethmoid and sphenoid sinuses and the nasal cavity. Inferiorly is the maxillary sinus. Laterally are the temporalis fossa anteriorly and the middle cranial fossa, temporal fossa, and pterygopalatine fossa posteriorly. Posterior to the orbital apex are the clinoid processes, pituitary gland, cavernous sinus, carotid arteries, middle cranial fossa, and optic chiasm. Because the globe and orbit are close to many important nonocular structures, severe ocular injury is often seen in conjunction with serious nonocular injury.

In addition to many other structures, the orbit contains the extraocular muscles that are responsible for coordinated eye movements. Disruption of the third, fourth, or sixth cranial nerves that innervate the extraocular muscles may result in various abnormal alignments of the eyes.

Tear secretions exit through the lacrimal drainage system (Figure 22-5). Any damage to this system may result in epiphora (excessive tearing) and infection. Puncta (orifices leading to the lacrimal drainage system) are present in the medial aspect of the upper and lower eyelids. These lead to the canaliculi, which connect to the lacrimal sac. This latter structure lies within the lacrimal sac fossa and posterior to the medial canthal tendon. Tear secretions flow from the lacrimal sac into the bony nasolacrimal duct within the maxillary bone before entering the nose.

The arterial supply to the globe and orbit is derived almost entirely from the ophthalmic artery and its branches. This vessel is the first branch from the internal carotid artery after it enters the cranial cavity. This important factor explains the tendency for emboli flowing through the internal carotid artery to enter the ophthalmic artery, resulting in visual symptoms and deficits. The facial and maxillary arteries, which are branches of the external carotid artery, provide additional blood supply to the lower eyelid, medial canthus, and inferior orbit. The venous drainage of the eye and orbit occurs via the inferior and superior ophthalmic veins to the cavernous sinus. This is an important route for the intracranial spread of infection. There are no lymphatics within the orbit. However, the eyelids have a rich lymphatic system draining into the preauricular and submaxillary nodes.

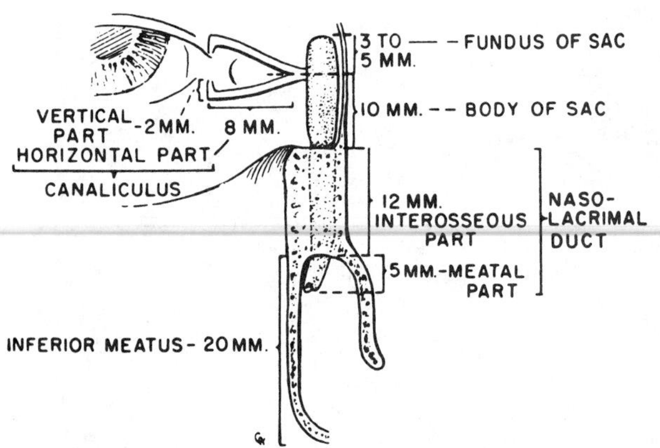

FIGURE 22-5 Lacrimal drainage system.

Sensory innervation to the ocular structures is provided by the fifth cranial (trigeminal) nerve. The ophthalmic division of this nerve supplies the forehead, upper eyelid, nose, and cornea. The maxillary division of the fifth cranial nerve supplies the lower eyelid, cheek, medial aspect of the nose, upper lip, gums, and lateral forehead. Portions of this nerve travel beneath the orbital floor. This explains the loss of sensation involving the cheek, lips, and gums after inferior orbital rim and floor fractures.

PREVENTION

The majority of eye injuries are preventable if existing protective devices, such as seat belts, safety helmets, and protective eyewear, are used. Seat belts have reduced the incidence of eye injuries from 65% to 47%.[5] Airbags have been identified as culprits of ocular injury, although it is often not possible to determine if airbag deployment coexists with or actually is the cause of eye injury. In many cases airbags can serve to protect the eyes. Without airbags the possibility exists that injury may be more serious or even fatal.[5,7]

Eye protection devices are available for specific work and recreational activities. Neither regular glasses nor contact lenses alone provide adequate protection for environments involving projectile objects, chemicals, particulate matter, intense heat or radiation energy. Polycarbonate lenses in polyamide frames with a posterior retention rim are the most effective in preventing eye injury. Solid wrap-around frames should be used (rather than hinged frames) because they better withstand lateral blows.[8] Certain athletic guards without lenses do not provide adequate protection. A high incidence of eye injuries in ice hockey players led to the mandated use of face visors in youth hockey, and, a subsequent reduction in the incidence of injuries.[6] Standards for protective eyewear for specific sports have been defined by the American Society for Testing Materials and the Canadian Standards Association.

A variety of ocular safety protectors are available for occupational uses. The United States Department of Labor Occupational Safety and Health Administration (OSHA) sets and enforces standards to improve workplace safety and health, which includes recommended protective eyewear for specific occupations. Information about occupation-specific OSHA recommended protective eyewear can be accessed on-line at www.osha.gov. In the industrial setting eye protection devices must meet the standards of American National Standards Institute (ANSI) Z87 Standard Practice for Occupational and Educational Eye and Face Protection. In addition to goggles, a face shield offers best protection for specific occupations, such as those involving radiation and light (welding) or flying particles (grinding).

Despite many educational campaigns and legislative efforts, the compliance with protective gear is low. For example, welders and grinders often lift up the face shield to inspect work or to perform touch-up grinding. A majority of injuries occur in the home, where regulations regarding protective eyewear are not enforced. It is important for educational campaigns to emphasize use of appropriate properly maintained eye protection while working in industry or the home and for consumer products to contain information regarding the need for eye protection on the labeling.

TRAUMA MANAGEMENT

When managing a trauma patient, it is essential to set priorities for the treatment of injuries. Establishing an airway, breathing, and circulation are the first management priorities during resuscitation. Examining, diagnosing, and treating ocular trauma may need to be delayed until emergency and life-threatening injuries are treated and the patient has been adequately stabilized to allow further evaluation.

Trauma patients may not be capable of assisting in an examination. Administration of paralytic agents; heavy sedation or anesthesia; intubation (which compromises communication); confusion, disorientation, or combativeness secondary to a brain injury; hypoxia; or hemodynamic instability are some of the variables inhibiting assistance by a patient. Physical examination in such instances may be limited or incomplete. Repeated examinations may be required before complete knowledge of any ocular pathology is possible.

In some areas, centers that specialize in the care of complex ocular injuries have been established and referral to such a center may be made once other life-threatening injuries are ruled out. Initial assessment and classification of patients presenting to the ophthalmic emergency room, known as ocular triage, is performed to determine the priority of treatment. An ocular triage exam consists of obtaining (1) vital signs, (2) a brief description of the injury, and (3) information about known allergies and level of pain. During triage health care professionals should initiate immediate therapy when required, for example, irrigating the eye in the setting of a chemical injury, or immobilizing or protecting an object protruding from the globe to prevent further trauma. Once the ocular triage is complete, the patient should receive an ocular screening exam, which consists of obtaining a pertinent ocular history and external examination of the eye including the periorbital area.[9]

ASSESSMENT

An ocular trauma assessment begins with an ocular history. The ocular history provides information that can help in diagnosis, initial management, and prognosis of eye injury. Patient-reported symptoms of vision loss or blurred vision that does not improve with blinking, double vision, sectorial visual loss, or ocular pain are important findings and require immediate referral to an ophthalmologist. The mechanism, time and location of injury and course of events, symptoms, and any therapeutic interventions provided must be determined. It is important to ascertain whether eye injury, ocular disease (e.g., glaucoma, macular degeneration), systemic disease that may impair sight (e.g., diabetes, hypertension), or visual impairment was present before the traumatic event. The history should also include medications the patient is taking and specifically whether the patient has received or is currently receiving any ocular therapy (i.e., medication or surgical intervention).[9] When the patient cannot provide an accurate history, it may be necessary to obtain an ocular history from other sources, when available, such as family, friends, or the patient's personal ophthalmologist.

A few instruments are needed to examine the patient with ocular trauma. A Snellen chart, near-vision card and pinhole occluder are useful to assess visual acuity. A penlight with a cobalt blue filter, tonometer, Hertel exophthalmometer, and ophthalmoscope will help in other parts of the examination. A slit-lamp biomicroscope, will aid in the examination of the conjunctiva, cornea, anterior chamber, iris, lens and anterior vitreous cavity. Topical anesthetic agents such as Proparacaine will help in examining patients who are unable to open their eye due to a corneal abrasion. A lid retractor (Figure 22-6) may be required for evaluating infants or patients with corneal injury. Sodium fluorescein test strips are needed to evaluate the extent of the corneal epithelial loss. These are used with a cobalt blue filter covering a penlight. Short acting dilating drops such as 2.5 percent phenylephrine or 1 percent tropicamide (Table 22-3), both of which have a dilatation action lasting 3 to 6 hours, are essential for adequate examination of the ocular fundus. These agents must be used with great caution with any patients with known or suspected intracranial trauma.

Visual Acuity

An essential aspect of the ocular examination is determination of visual acuity—the most crucial prognostic indicator following trauma. This assessment is preferably performed with the patient wearing his or her corrective eyeglasses. If a patient does not have spectacle correction or if there is a question concerning the adequacy of a corrective lens, a pinhole occluder may be used to measure visual acuity within one or two lines of the patient's expected best corrected vision. The pinhole occluder is an eye shield with small perforated holes that allows light rays to reach the retina without the interference of optical problems. Visual acuity should be measured in each eye separately, with the opposite eye covered but not compressed.

The most common eye chart utilized for evaluating visual acuity is the Snellen chart. The Snellen chart displays lines of block letters of diminishing size, each defined according to the distance at which the line of letters can be read by a person with normal visual acuity. Visual acuity measured using the Snellen chart is expressed by a numerator, indicating the distance the patient is from the chart during testing (20 feet), and a denominator which is the smallest line of the print the patient can read at that testing distance.[10] If a standardized distance or near visual acuity chart is not available, a newspaper or some other printed material can be substituted. Visual acuity can then be recorded as the size of print (e.g., newspaper

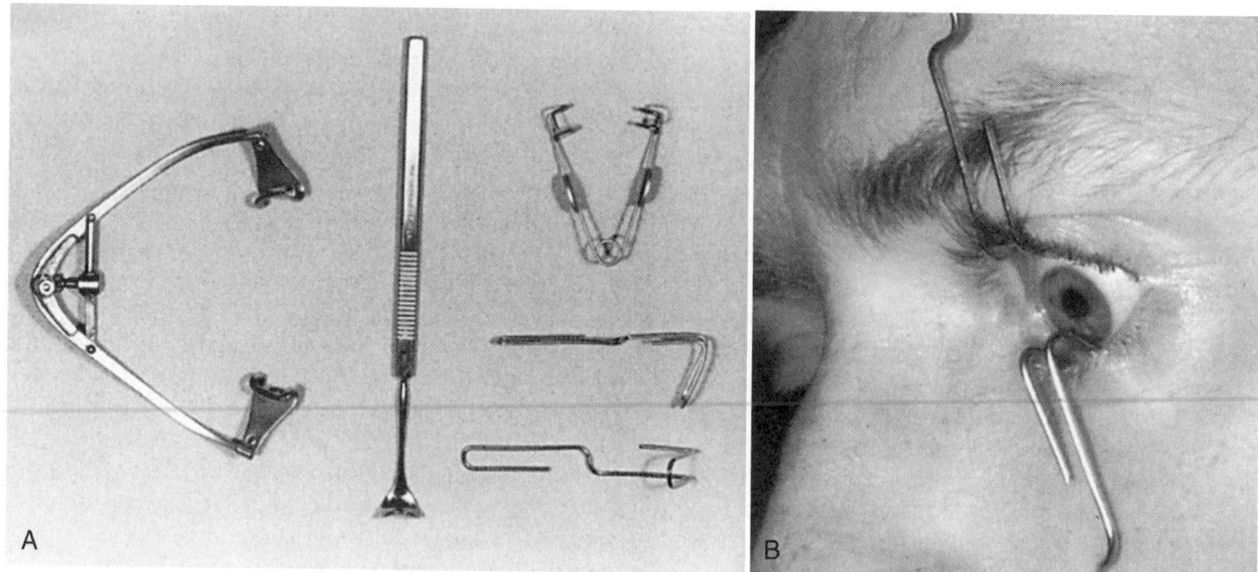

FIGURE 22-6 **A,** Eyelid retractors. **B,** Paper clip retractors.

headline, print at the top of an order sheet) the patient sees at a specified distance, usually 14 inches. For children or patients who are illiterate, a picture chart can be used.

In situations of very poor visual acuity or where determination of reading vision is not possible, vision may be evaluated by determining the patient's ability to count fingers or ascertain the direction of hand movements at a specific distance. Record the longest distance at which the patient is able to count fingers and if the patient can correctly identify hand movements performed at 1 foot away. A positive response is charted as hand movement. If the patient performs inadequately on the visual acuity tests, the ability to perceive a bright light shined directly in the eye must be ascertained. If the patient is able to see the light, chart as light perception and if no light perception is present, record as no light perception.

For children between the ages of 6 months and 2 years, vision is assessed using the fix-and-follow method. Using this method, first observe the patient with both eyes open; then, with one eye occluded at a time, determine whether the patient stares or fixates on a stationary object (e.g., face, light) and pursues or follows a moving target at arm's length.[10] If the patient is unable to appropriately fixate and follow, the response is documented as abnormal.

Pupils

Examination of the pupils helps determine the integrity of the anterior visual pathways. First, in dim light with the patient's gaze fixed on a distance object, measure the size and assess the shape of each pupil. Second, the pupil's reaction to light stimulus is tested. The pupillary light reflex evaluates the optic nerve, which must be intact to perceive the light, and the oculomotor nerve integrity, which allows the pupil to constrict. To evaluate this reflex, the patient is asked to look at a distant object while the examiner shines the light into one eye, moving the light from the side onto the eye while observing the speed and amount of pupillary constriction that occurs. Constriction of the pupil should occur within 1 second after presentation of the light stimulus. This is repeated for the other eye to evaluate each pupil's response to direct light stimulus. Next, one eye is examined while shining the light onto the opposite eye. Pupillary constriction should occur in the observed eye while shining a light in the opposite eye. This is called the consensual response. Normally the pupils are linked together in response to light stimulus, each constricting an equal amount to the stimulus. If both oculomotor nerves and one optic nerve are intact and the opposite optic nerve is damaged, the pupils both constrict equally when a light stimulus is presented to the intact side. When the light is presented to the damaged optic nerve, the stimulus will not be perceived, and the pupils will not constrict. The accommodation response is tested by having the patient look at an object at about 20 inches distance and then observing pupillary constriction as the object is moved toward the eyes. The patient's pupils should be similar in size, round, and equally reactive to light and accommodation (PERRLA).

Last, the response to the "swinging flashlight" test is observed. In a dimly lit room with the patient fixating on a distant object, light is shined on one eye for 3 seconds and is then quickly moved in a swinging motion across the bridge of the nose into the opposite eye while pupil response is noted. In patients without visual pathway disturbances and normal iris function, the eye will not constrict or dilate to the swinging light. This is because direct and consensual responses are equal in the normal patient. The examiner swings a light back and forth over the bridge of the nose from one pupil to the other. If the eye paradoxically dilates when exposed to the light source, the eye has a relative afferent pupillary defect and is sometimes known as a Marcus Gunn pupil. In trauma patients, if the optic nerve is damaged, the pupil on that side will

TABLE 22-3 Eye Medications Used For Treatment of Ocular Injuries

Ophthalmic medications may be used as:

1. Diagnostic agents
2. Treatment agents for ocular conditions
3. Adjuncts to surgical interventions

Administration considerations:

1. If administrating more than 1 eye drop wait 2 to 5 minutes between drops.
2. Digital punctal occlusion: place your finger over the patient's lacrimal sac and apply light pressure for 1 minute or more (or instruct patient to do this if able). This is indicated when (1) systemic absorption of medication may prove harmful to the patient, (2) prolonged corneal-drug contact is desired, or (3) tasting or feeling ocular medication in the nasopharyngeal mucosa is distressing to the patient.
3. Administer eye drops before ointment.
4. Instruct patient that ointment may obscure vision.

Medication	Classification	Action	Dose	Nursing Considerations
Acetazolamide (Diamox)	Carbonic anhydrase inhibitor	Reduces IOP	• 250-1000 mg orally, divided 1-4 times daily • 250-1000 mg IV divided 1-4 times daily	1. May cause nausea, vomiting (may require administration of antiemetic) and dizziness 2. Contains sulfa
Acetazolamide (Diamox sequels)	Carbonic anhydrase inhibitor	Reduces IOP	• 500 mg tablet, sustained release, every 12 hours	1. Refer to nursing considerations for acetazolamide
Atropine	Mydriatic-cycloplegic	Dilates pupil	• 1 drop of 1% solution up to 3 times a day	1. Digital punctal occlusion indicated 2. Not recommended for long term use 3. Do not use with intracranial injury without permission of neurosurgery
Cyclopentolate	Mydriatic-cycloplegic	Dilates pupil	• Diagnostic aid: 1-2 drops of 0.5%, 1% or 2% followed by another drop in 5 minutes if necessary • 1-2 drops of 0.5%-2% solution	1. Contraindicated with narrow angle glaucoma 2. Digital punctal occlusion indicated, especially with small infants
Homatropine	Mydriatic-cycloplegic	Dilates pupil	• 1-2 drops of 2% or 5% solution	1. May cause burning sensation 2. Digital punctal occlusion indicated 3. Do not use with intracranial injury without permission of neurosurgery
Mannitol	Osmotic diuretic	Reduces IOP	• 0.25-2 g/kg IV infused over 30-60 minutes as a 15%-20% solution • Max dose 6 g/kg in a 24-hour period	1. Check sodium and potassium before infusion Patient may require electrolyte replacement 2. Requires the use of a filter for infusion 3. Only compatible with normal saline—recommend dedicated IV line 4. Easily forms crystals; handle with care 5. Ensure adequate hydration before administration
Phenylephrine hydrochloride	Mydriatic-cycloplegic	Dilates pupil	• 1 drop of a 2.5% solution and may repeat in 1 hour if necessary	1. Medication may cause increase in blood pressure and pulse. Do not administer if diastolic blood pressure is >95 mm Hg 2. Do not administer to children <2 years of age 3. Digital punctual occlusion indicated 4. May cause burning sensation 5. Do not use with intracranial injury without permission of neurosurgery
Prednisolone acetate	Anti-inflammatory	Reduces inflammation	• 1-2 drops 2-4 times a day	1. Should not be used if viral or fungal infection(s) suspected 2. May raise IOP 3. Steroid taper indicated to discontinue drug
Timolol	Antiglaucoma β-adrenergic blocker	Reduces IOP	• 1 drop of a 0.25%-0.5% twice daily and may increase to 1 drop of 0.5% solution if unsatisfactory clinical response	1. Digital punctal occlusion indicated 2. Ophthalmic use may produce additional systemic effects in patients receiving oral β-blockers

paradoxically dilate. In some cases of severe retinal damage or intraocular hemorrhage, there can be some afferent pupil defect, although not always.

Unequal or nonreactive pupils can be seen in many different conditions besides ocular trauma, including brain lesions affecting the midbrain, optic nerve or oculomotor nerve, acute glaucoma, interruption of the pupillary sympathetic innervation, and previous eye surgery. Approximately 20% to 25% of people naturally have unequal pupil size, but this variation normally does not exceed 1 mm. Trauma patients with pupil abnormalities should be seen by a neurosurgeon to rule out brain injury. If pupil abnormalities are noted in a patient with an otherwise normal neurologic exam and trauma to the eye, ocular injury is a suspected cause for pupil dysfunction and an ophthalmologist should be consulted.

Ocular Motility

Examination of ocular motility screens for abnormal eye movements and ocular malalignment. Instruct the patient to follow your finger or a penlight, which is moved from straight ahead to the far right and left and then up and down. The eyes should move an equal amount at the same speed in each gaze direction. There are nine cardinal gaze positions: straight ahead, directly up, up and to the right, directly lateral, lateral and down, directly down, down and laterally left, directly left, and up and to the left. However, in most clinical situations, measuring straight ahead, directly up, left, right, and down provides enough information to assess for the presence of a deviation. In an unconscious patient with an uninjured cervical spine, the "doll's eye" maneuver, or oculocephalic reflex, can be tested to evaluate ocular motility. Rapid, passive side-to-side head turning is performed; the normal response is movement of the eyes in the direction opposite the head movement. Forced duction testing (Figure 22-7) may be indicated to rule out muscle entrapment if an orbital floor fracture is suspected. This involves anesthetizing the eye with topical anesthesia, grasping the limbal conjunctiva and sclera with toothed forceps, and rotating the globe up and down and right and left to test the muscles that control ocular motility while noting any restriction to free movement of the globe. This test is contraindicated in cases of open globe injury. Common causes of abnormal ocular movements include orbital edema or hemorrhage; extraocular muscle entrapment; and damage to cranial nerves III, IV, or VI.

Orbit

Patients with orbital trauma should undergo an examination to ascertain whether the nervous system is intact. Injuries to the orbit may be associated with severe neurological injuries, which can be life threatening and take precedence over the orbital trauma.[5] As part of the ophthalmic assessment, it is important to assess the periorbital and orbital structures and the relationship of the globe to these structures. Evaluating the position of the globe within the orbit and comparing the ocular structures of both eyes are important to diagnose such conditions as orbital fractures, the presence of foreign bodies, retrobulbar hemorrhage, and orbital cellulitis or abscess. The presence or absence of enophthalmos or exophthalmos can be detected during physical exam. Normally, a comparison of the two globes by Hertel exophthalmometry (Figure 22-8) shows less than a 2-mm difference between opposite sides in the distance from the lateral orbital rim to the corneal apex. The normal measurement for this distance is approximately 17 to 20 mm. Exophthalmos, when the difference is 2 mm or greater and the globe is pushed out of the orbit, may be found with orbital edema, a retained foreign body, retrobulbar hemorrhage, orbital abscess or cellulitis, dysthyroid ophthalmopathy, or an orbital tumor. When the globe is sunken into the orbit (enophthalmos), orbital fractures must be considered (Figure 22-9). If a straight edge is held horizontally to bisect the pupil, the center of each pupil should be on the same horizontal plane. When one eye is lower than the other, an orbital floor fracture may be

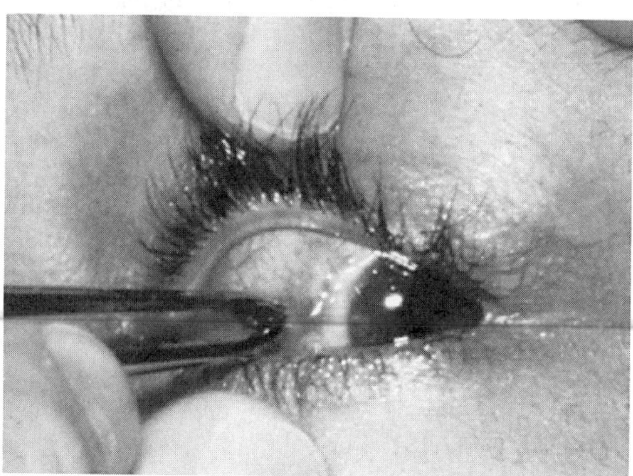

FIGURE 22-7 Forced duction.

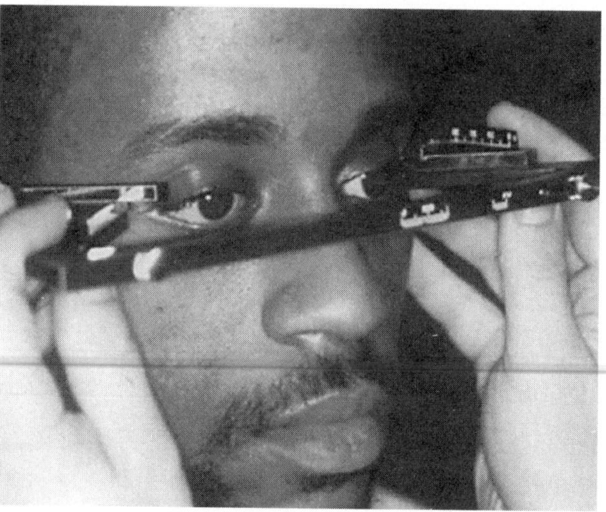

FIGURE 22-8 Hertel exophthalmometry.

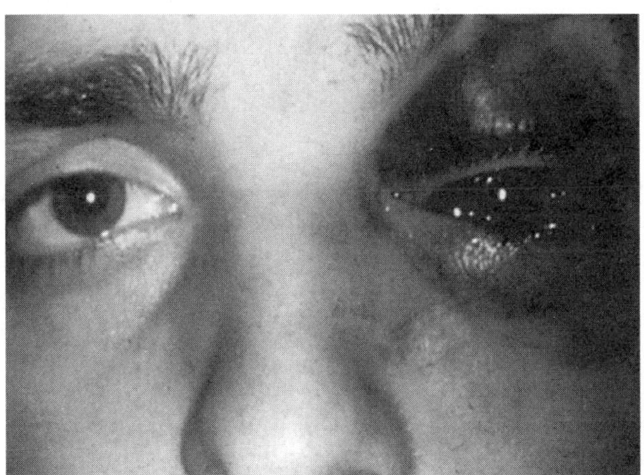

FIGURE 22-9 Acute orbital fracture with periorbital edema, ecchymosis, and hypoophthalmos. *(From American Academy of Ophthalmology: The Athlete's Eye, San Francisco, 1984, The Academy.)*

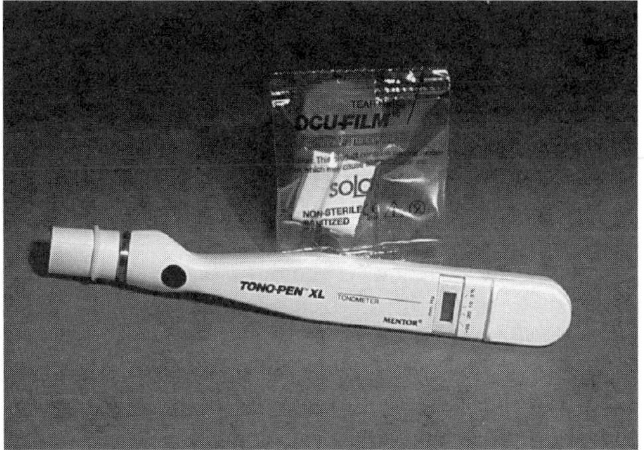

FIGURE 22-10 Tono-pen. *(Courtesy University of Iowa Health Care, Department of Ophthalmology & Visual Sciences, Iowa City, Iowa.)*

present (see Figure 22-8). The horizontal distance from the medial canthus to the middle of the nasal bones is approximately 16 mm. When this is widened or when there is inequality between opposite sides, telecanthus (a wider than normal distance between the eyes) associated with a midfacial fracture may be present. Upon palpation the orbital rim should be smooth, without any breaks or irregularities that might indicate an orbital rim fracture. Crepitus of the eyelids is another sign of an orbital bone fracture. Periorbital edema and ecchymosis commonly accompany many types of orbital, head and facial trauma and, while not specific, indicate the possibility of ocular injury. When there is the possibility of orbital fracture, retrobulbar hemorrhage, or orbital infection or foreign bodies, an ophthalmologist should be consulted to evaluate the patient.

Intraocular Pressure

Measurement of intraocular pressure (IOP) is another important aspect of the examination following ocular trauma. It is important to recognize that this should not be performed when there is any question concerning the integrity of the globe. Any pressure on the perforated globe could result in expulsion of intraocular contents and permanent loss in vision. To measure intraocular pressure, a topical anesthetic drop is instilled in the patient's eye and the patient is asked to look straight ahead. A tonometer pen (Figure 22-10) is an electronic device commonly used to measure IOP. The tip of the Tono-Pen is lightly touched to the cornea. This is repeated three times and an average is derived from the three readings. The accuracy diminishes as the pressure moves farther outside the normal range.[10] Application tonometry is another method used to measure IOP. A tonometer, found on most slit lamps, is placed on the central portion of the cornea. When performing an IOP measurement, it is important not to put any pressure on the globe while holding open the eyelids. Normal IOP is 8 to 21 mm Hg.

The IOP may rise acutely when the eye is contused, especially when blood (hyphema) or inflammatory cells are present in the anterior chamber. Persistently high IOP (greater than 30 mm Hg) may indicate presence of an outflow obstruction, acute angle closure glaucoma or retrobulbar hemorrhage. Urgent treatment (surgical or pharmacologic intervention) is needed in this case to lower elevated pressure and prevent permanent vision loss. Low IOP (less than 8 mm Hg) may indicate the patient has a perforated globe, retinal detachment, or severe intraocular trauma. These conditions require immediate evaluation and treatment by an ophthalmologist.

Eyelids and Lacrimal System

The eyelids and the canaliculus of the lacrimal system are frequently injured when ocular trauma occurs. Medial eyelid lacerations often involve the canalicular system. Direct damage to the levator muscle or Müller's muscle may result in ptosis (Figure 22-11). Ptosis may also be seen with enophthalmos associated with an orbital fracture and often accompanies periorbital edema and ecchymosis. Inability to close

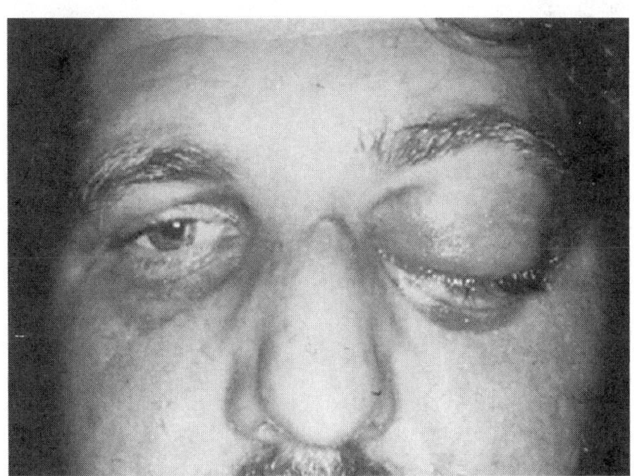

FIGURE 22-11 Traumatic ptosis.

the eyelids adequately is a more serious problem that may be indicative of damage to the seventh cranial nerve. It can also be associated with scarring after repair of an eyelid laceration. Disruption of the eyelid margin may impair the tear pump. Inability to close the eye, inadequate blinking, poor corneal wetting, or misdirected lashes may cause corneal ulceration and require immediate referral to an ophthalmologist to prevent visual loss.

Eyelid injuries require a thorough ocular evaluation to eliminate the possibility of damage to the canalicular system or severe injury to the globe (Figure 22-12). Repair of these tissues is rarely emergent. When lacerations involve the eyelid margin or canalicular system or when they are deep or complicated, repair by an experienced ophthalmologist is essential to prevent permanent functional and cosmetic deficits.

Conjunctiva

Examination of the conjunctiva, tear film, cornea, anterior chamber, iris, lens, and anterior vitreous cavity is best performed with a slit-lamp biomicroscope. However, an initial exam may be performed with a penlight or flashlight. The upper lid must be everted to assess the conjunctival surface thoroughly for foreign bodies that may be embedded in the folds of the conjunctiva. To accomplish this maneuver, the examiner grasps the upper eyelashes, and rotates the lid over a cotton-tipped applicator away from the globe. It is also important to examine the anterior conjunctiva for injection, lacerations, chemosis (edema of the conjunctiva) or hemorrhage. Presence of these findings is indicative of a ruptured globe. If a conjunctival laceration is identified, it is necessary to investigate further for a scleral laceration or subconjunctival foreign body. In addition, conjunctival injection is often present after trauma that causes ocular inflammation and in cases of infectious and noninfectious conjunctivitis, corneal abrasions, and acute glaucoma. Perilimbal (the area where cornea and sclera blend together) dilated blood vessels often associated with proptosis can be a manifestation of a post-traumatic intracranial arteriovenous fistula.

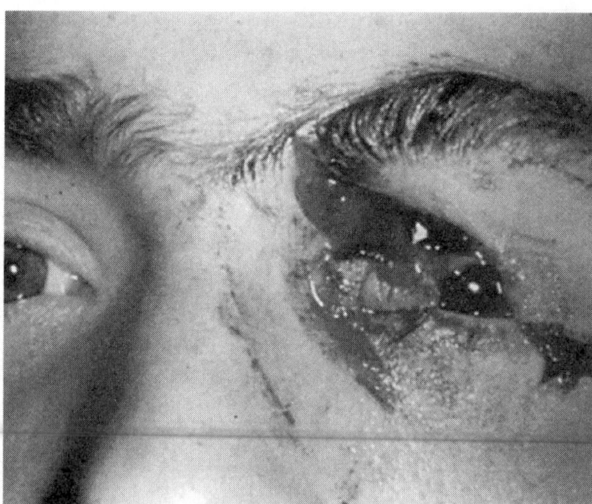

FIGURE 22-12 Severe eyelid laceration with associated penetrating trauma to globe. *(From American Academy of Ophthalmology: Eye Trauma and Emergencies, San Francisco, 1985, The Academy.)*

Cornea

Normally the cornea is clear with a bright smooth surface. Examination of the cornea can be performed using the naked eye and a penlight but is best done with a slit-lamp biomicroscope. Corneal lacerations, foreign bodies, abrasions, and irregularities may be identified. Corneal examination can be facilitated by instillation of a stain, such as sodium fluorescein, which discolors areas denuded of epithelium but not healthy tissue. With use of a cobalt blue filter over a penlight to enhance fluorescein detection, corneal defects are seen as green patches on the surface that do not move after the patient blinks. A cloudy cornea may indicate acute glaucoma, edema from trauma, a foreign body in the anterior chamber, or an infectious process.

Anterior Chamber

On penlight examination the anterior chamber should be clear and deep, with the iris well separated from the posterior corneal surface. Shallowing of the anterior chamber can be demonstrated by shining the beam from a penlight across the chamber from the temporal side of the globe. The beam should highlight the entire chamber without impediment. When the chamber is shallowed, the beam will fall on the iris, creating shadows, and will not illuminate the chamber. Areas of localized shallowing or irregularities should be noted because they can indicate underlying problems, such as choroid detachment or hemorrhage, foreign bodies in or behind the iris, or rupture of the posterior sclera with vitreous loss. Acute angle closure glaucoma is a consideration in such cases, especially if there is an associated rise in intraocular pressure; clouding of the cornea; complaints of visual loss, halos around objects, eye pain or nausea; or vomiting. When blood (hyphema) (Figure 22-13) or white cells (hypopyon) are present, serious ocular injury, inflammation, or infection has occurred and immediate attention by an ophthalmologist is required.

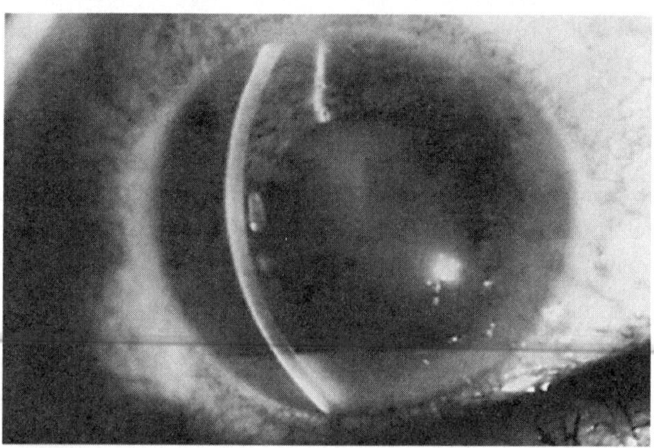

FIGURE 22-13 Hyphema involving 15% of the inferior anterior chamber.

Iris

In cases of ocular trauma, examination of the iris may reveal tears and holes. Iris injuries may cause pupil irregularities (Figure 22-14), hyphema (as a result of damage to iris blood vessels) (see Figure 22-13), or chronic glaucoma (from damage to the trabecular meshwork and aqueous drainage system). Sometimes small foreign bodies may be embedded on the iris surface or may bounce off the iris and fall to the anterior chamber. Damage to the iris is a common manifestation of severe open and closed globe injuries. In these situations immediate evaluation by an ophthalmologist is needed.

Lens

The normal lens is a crystalline structure. Opacification of the lens and cataract formation may occur after ocular trauma. The lens should be examined for clarity, position, stability, anteroposterior diameter (i.e., swelling), and capsule integrity. Examination of the lens is best performed using the slit-lamp biomicroscope. If severe inflammation is associated with ocular injury, adhesions (posterior synechiae) between the iris and the lens may develop. This may lead to an elevation of intraocular pressure and subsequent optic nerve damage. When a force of sufficient intensity is delivered to the globe, the lens can be torn away from the ciliary body and may float free in the vitreous. If the lens dislocates into the anterior chamber, acute glaucoma may develop owing to a blockage of aqueous outflow. In many situations, the cataractous lens can be removed and replaced with an intraocular lens (IOL) as a secondary procedure weeks to months after the globe repair.

Fundus

The fundus examination is the final aspect of the ocular evaluation. Normally the vitreous is a clear structure that allows an unimpeded view of the retina. Hemorrhage (Figure 22-15, A) within the vitreous occasionally occurs in association with intracranial hemorrhage. It also may occur when a retinal vessel is torn and may indicate damage from a penetrating foreign body or a retinal detachment. The normal retina is thin, relatively clear, and colorless. The orange color imparted to it on fundus examination is caused by the underlying retinal pigment epithelium and vascular choroid. Retinal edema (Berlin's edema, commotio retinae) is common after blunt ocular trauma. In such cases the retina appears milky white. Swelling around the macula can cause the fovea to look red (a pseudo-cherry-red spot). Although this condition usually subsides spontaneously, resulting in a return of vision, some patients with macular involvement (Figure 22-16) suffer permanent loss of the central visual field. Traumatic hemorrhage (Figure 22-15, B) can occur on, within, or beneath the retina or choroid when the retinal or choroidal vessels are damaged. These may be associated with retinal tears and holes, retinal detachment, and choroidal layer ruptures. Hard exudates also may be associated with retinal trauma. After retinal trauma, proliferation of glial tissue may cause neovascular fronds (abnormal new blood vessels) to develop, which cause retinal detachment or hemorrhage. Choroidal layer ruptures are another posttraumatic cause of visual loss and fibrovascular proliferation. All these pathologic processes can cause severe, and in many cases permanent, visual loss.

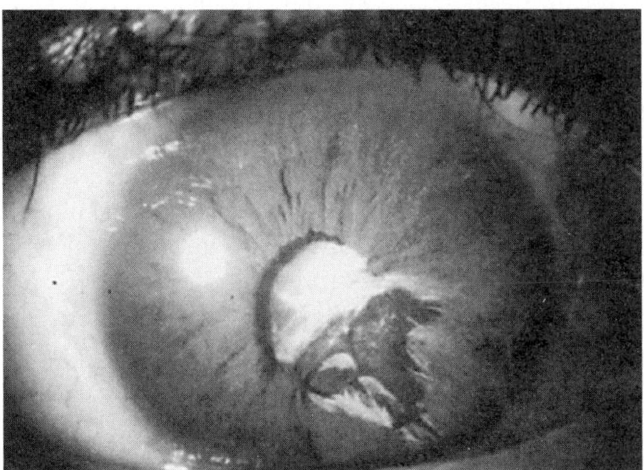

FIGURE 22-14 Traumatic pupillary irregularities with posterior synechiae and cataract formation.

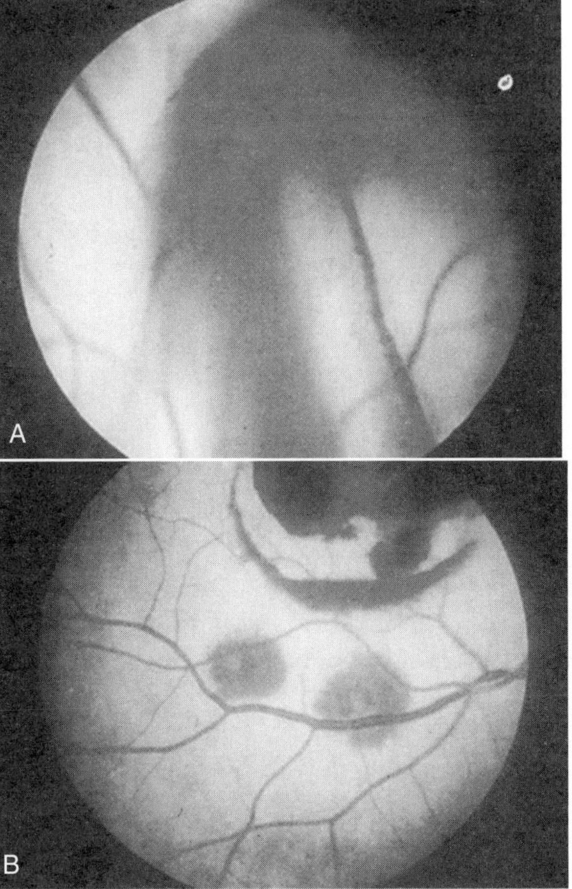

FIGURE 22-15 **A,** Vitreous hemorrhage. **B,** Traumatic intraretinal and periretinal hemorrhages.

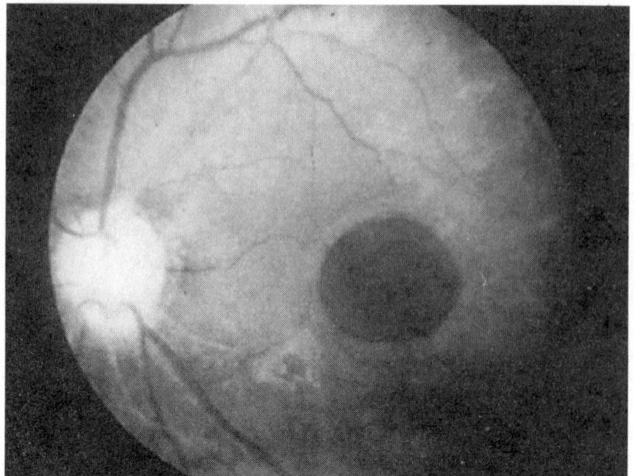

FIGURE 22-16 Macular hole.

Optic Nerve

The optic nerve normally appears somewhat yellow, with defined margins. Its central cup constitutes approximately one third of the substance and has a single branching central retinal artery and vein. Blurring of the disc margin caused by edema of the nerve fibers is seen with increased intracranial pressure or pressure on the optic nerve (Figure 22-17). Atrophy of the optic nerve after contusion or transsection injuries results in a loss of disk substance and a whitening of the nerve head. The disc will not become pale until 2 to 3 weeks after injury to the nerve.

Diagnostic Studies

In addition to the ophthalmic examination, other diagnostic modalities are available to aid in the evaluation of the eye and its adnexal structures after trauma. An imaging study is recommended to rule out pathology that may need immediate attention. Computed tomography (CT) (Figure 22-18) is the most commonly used imaging study to evaluate the injured eye. The sensitivity and specificity of CT in the detection of open globe injury are 73% and 95%, respectively.[11] Advantages of CT include that it is readily available in most

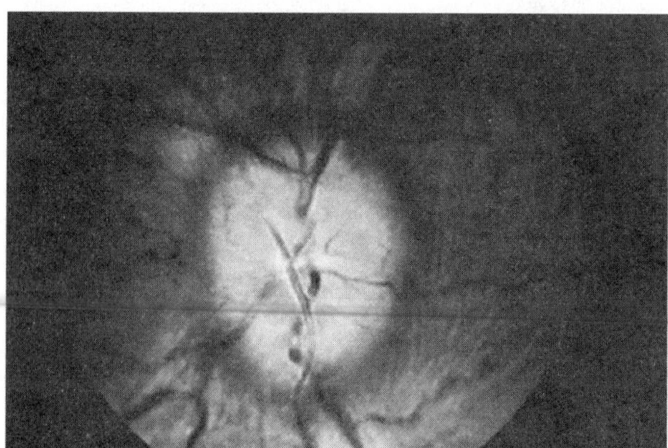

FIGURE 22-17 Edema of the optic nerve head (disc edema).

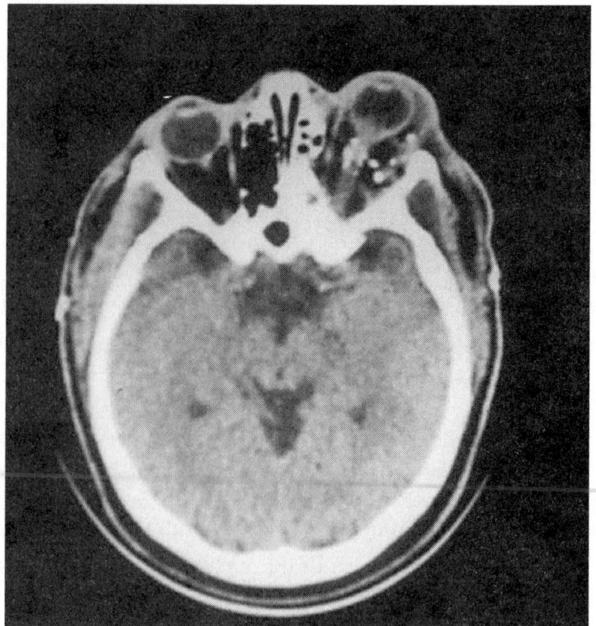

FIGURE 22-18 CT scan of bullet fragments in orbit and around optic nerve.

hospitals, direct contact with the eye is not required, and it is less expensive and has fewer limitations than magnetic resonance imaging (MRI). Computerized tomography is an ideal imaging study to rule out orbital floor fracture, and it is more sensitive than ultrasound in detecting the presence of an intraocular foreign body (IOFB).[5] A CT scan ideally should include both axial and coronal sections. Coronal views aid in visualization of the orbital roof, orbital floor, inferior and superior rectus muscles, and any IOFB. Echography (ultrasound) can be used to aid in the evaluation of the orbit, internal ocular structures and detection of IOFBs. Orbital and intraocular ultrasonography can detect retinal and choroidal detachment, posterior vitreous separation, vitreous hemorrhage and opacities, retinal tears, choroidal and scleral ruptures, and IOFBs. Ultrasound provides real time images of the eye and orbit, and serial ultrasounds allow the physician to follow the progression of a condition. It can be performed at the bedside or in the operating room and is advantageous when the patient cannot be moved. Because ultrasound requires direct contact with the eyelid, it should not be used when the eye is at high risk for expulsion of intraocular contacts or the patient is agitated. Formal visual field examination with Goldman or Humphrey perimetry is useful for delineating damage to the optic nerve, chiasm, or tract. This provides additional localizing information about intracranial pathology.

Prehospital Management

Prehospital management of eye trauma is very limited. The most important aspect is the protection of an injured eye, which is achieved by shielding it (Figure 22-19). To protect

A 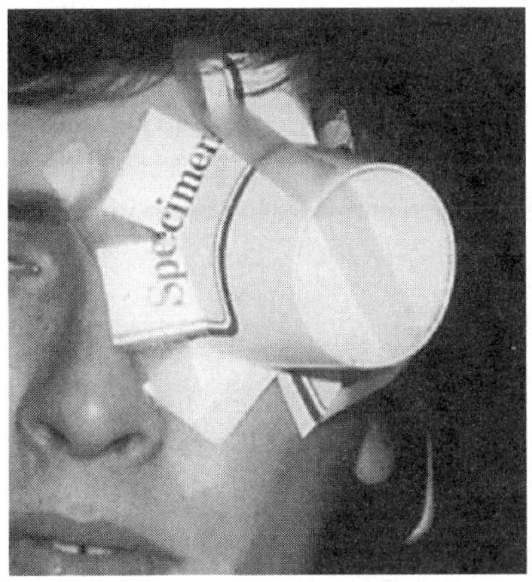

B 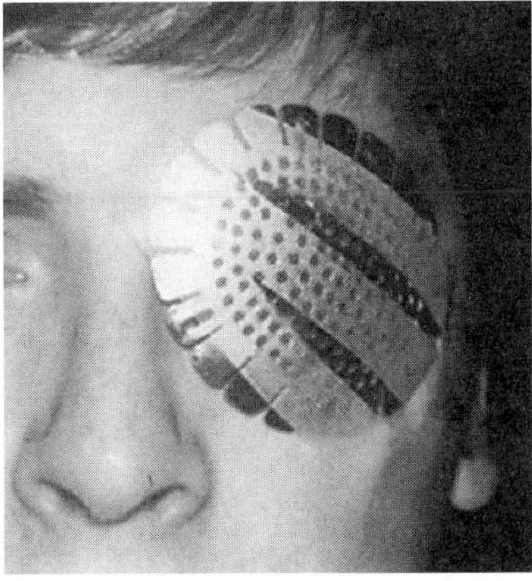

FIGURE 22-19 **A,** Cup shield. **B,** Metal shield.

the globe, a pressure dressing and vigorous cleansing or palpation of the area should be avoided. Any increased pressure on an open eye may result in loss of the intraocular contents (Figure 22-20). If active bleeding from the eye is noted, a loose gauze dressing may be applied. Ocular medicine should not be given in the prehospital phase except in cases of chemical injury, when immediate irrigation must be performed, or with severe facial burns, when the eyes must be lubricated vigorously with artificial tear ointments. The patient should be instructed to lie still and, unless contraindicated, the head should be elevated 30 degrees. To alleviate fears and decrease anxiety, all interventions must be explained to the patient.

Introduction of a chemical substance to the eye constitutes an emergency in which every second counts. Eye irrigation should start immediately in the field and continue until the patient reaches the hospital. It is ideal to irrigate with a normal saline solution or water. A loose moist saline dressing can be applied to the eyes if continuous irrigation is not possible.

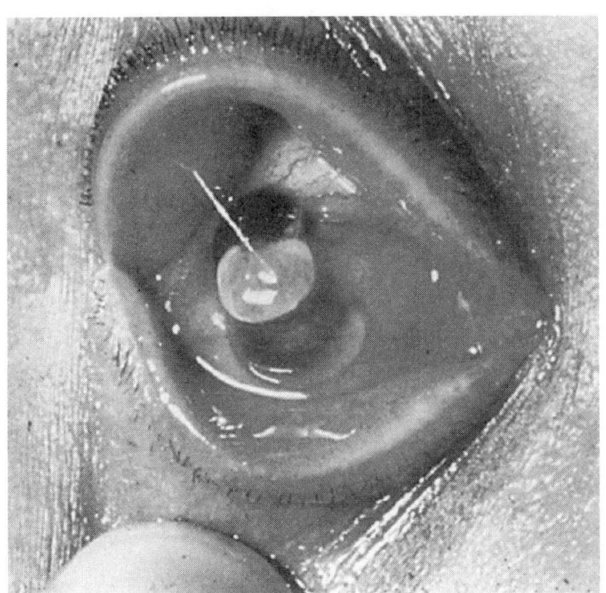

FIGURE 22-20 Extrusion of lens through corneal laceration.

Resuscitation

When ocular trauma occurs in conjunction with other injuries, treatment of life-threatening injuries is the first priority. Sight-threatening injuries can be addressed once the patient is stabilized. When any ocular injury is suspected, Ophthalmology should be consulted as soon as possible and, when possible, an ocular history should be obtained.

During resuscitation, a shield should be placed over the injured eye to provide protection. If there is any suspicion of an injury to the globe, eyelids, ocular adnexa or orbit, the facial structures should not be manipulated in any way. In addition to the eye shield, it may be necessary to immobilize the head. Analgesics and sedatives may be needed to relieve pain and anxiety and foster immobility. Periorbital lacerations must not be sutured and orbital fractures must not be palpated until perforating ocular injuries are repaired. Generally, bleeding from eyelid lacerations and orbital trauma is minimal and will stop spontaneously. Pressure should never be placed on the eyelids, eyeball or periorbital structures to stop bleeding if there is any suspicion that the globe is not intact. Any increased pressure on an open eye may result in loss of the intraocular contents and irreparable damage to the eye.

Access to a variety of items is necessary for the successful treatment of ocular injuries before ophthalmologic consultation. At least 2 L of normal saline are needed for irrigation of chemical injuries. Acetazolamide (Diamox), an osmotic diuretic such as mannitol, and β-adrenergic blocking ophthalmic solutions such as timolol maleate 0.5% or levobunolol 0.5% are needed to reduce ocular pressure associated with glaucoma. Short-acting mydriatic/cycloplegic eye drops, such as tropicamide 1% or cyclopentolate hydrochloride 1% should be on hand to dilate the pupil. Antibiotic eye drops such as ofloxacin 3%, moxifloxacin, erythromycin, or tobramycin may be necessary to treat superficial ocular infections. An antibiotic ointment, such as erythromycin or tobramycin, is needed to treat corneal abrasions. A topical cycloplegic, such as homatropine 5% and corticosteroid (prednisolone acetate 1%) are the mainstays of treatment for ocular inflammation (see Table 22-3). Artificial tears and ointments are helpful for managing patients with inadequate blinking or poor eyelid closure. If ocular medications are necessary for long-term use, the therapy should be managed by an ophthalmologist. Eye shields and tape are needed to provide a protective ocular covering.

Anesthetic ointments should never be used in the treatment of ocular trauma because their prolonged effect may result in inadvertent corneal damage. For a similar reason, anesthetic eye drops should not be used on a long-term basis. Ocular ointments should be avoided when a fundus exam is needed (they obscure visualization of the fundus) or when penetrating trauma is present (they may enter the globe). Application of artificial tear ointment may be necessary to protect the cornea in cases of eyelid avulsion or thermal injury. Corticosteroid eye drops should never be used if infection with the herpes virus or fungus is a possibility, as suppression of the body's normal defenses against these infections can occur. Atropine eye drops are not for routine use. Atropine's mydriatic effect is long lasting and can cause chemical and allergic reactions.

Acute management of ocular injuries also requires extensive emotional support. If there is any visual impairment (secondary to either patching or injury), the patient must be assured that the injury is being assessed thoroughly and treated appropriately. Explanation of what has happened and what is being done for the patient is essential to help alleviate fears of the unknown.

Management of Specific Ocular Injuries

Chemical Injury

Chemical injuries to the eyes can occur in any setting: home (e.g., ammonia found in cleaning agents), schools (e.g., chemicals from chemistry laboratories), and the work place (e.g., industrial toxins). Alkaline agents readily penetrate the eye, causing damage to the corneal stroma, endothelium, iris, lens and ciliary body. Alkali burns can cause a rise in intraocular pressure. Because of the penetrating nature of alkali substances, ocular damage continues to occur after the initial injury. Acid substances, in contrast, tend to remain confined to the ocular surface, causing formation of a precipitated necrotic barrier that tends to limit further penetration.

All chemical injuries to the eye must be considered an emergency. Immediate irrigation of the eye with water should begin in the field and continue while transporting the patient to a health care facility. The longer the time between injury and irrigation, the worse the prognosis. Once the name or type of the chemical involved is identified, information about the substance can be obtained from a Materials Data Sheet or a phone call to the local Poison Control Hotline. In the emergency center irrigation of the eye should be continued using sterile isotonic saline until the pH of the tear film in the cul-de-sac is 7.0. The lids must be held apart so that the injured eye can be irrigated copiously. Standard urethral irrigation tubing or an intravenous infusion set for irrigation, eyelid retractors to hold the eyelids apart, and topical anesthetic drops to reduce the blepharospasm caused by corneal damage will all greatly help in carrying out adequate ocular lavage (Figure 22-21). Any foreign bodies should be irrigated away from the eye and eyelids need to be everted to ensure removal of any particulate matter clinging to the conjunctiva. A cotton-tipped applicator may be used to remove any particulate matter (e.g., cement) from the fornices.

After irrigation, necrotic tissue may need to be debrided from the eye. Pharmacologic treatment includes administration of cycloplegic eye drops to reduce pain from ciliary spasm. Increases in intraocular pressure frequently accompany serious alkali injuries; therefore evaluation of intraocular pressure is important. If the pressure is elevated, it should be treated with antiglaucoma agents (e.g., acetazolamide, mannitol, and topical β-adrenergic blocking ophthalmic solutions [e.g., timolol maleate]) to reduce intraocular pressure. To decrease inflammation, topical steroid drops are prescribed for the first 2 weeks after injury. Beyond 2 weeks, steroids may inhibit reepithelialization and cause corneal melting and perforation to occur. Ascorbate (vitamin C) and citrate drops are useful in moderately severe alkali burns but only minimally effective for preventing corneal melting in patients with severe burns or persistent corneal epithelial defects.[8] Ophthalmic lubricants are applied to protect the cornea. Topical antibiotics may be considered for prophylaxis against infection. Administration of analgesics to achieve pain control is another important aspect of therapy.

Hyphema

Hyphema (see Figure 22-13), or blood in the anterior chamber, can occur as a result of blunt or perforating ocular trauma. A microhyphema is a condition in which red blood cells are suspended in the aqueous fluid. When a hyphema is present, the globe may be perforated and, therefore, should be protected with a shield. An ophthalmologist should be consulted for further management. Assessment should include examination of the globe for perforation, evaluation of visual acuity and

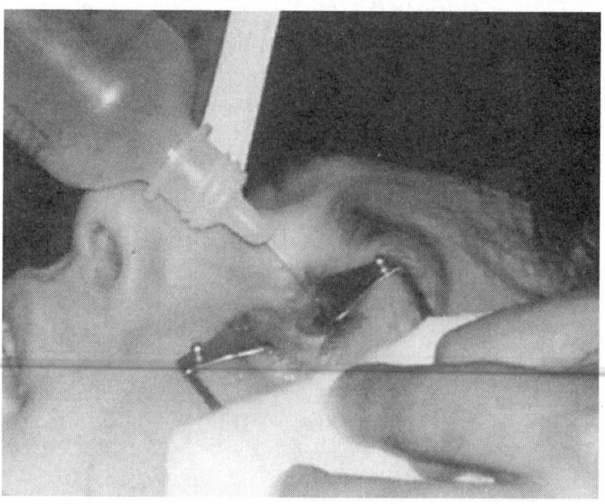

FIGURE 22-21 Ocular lavage.

measurement of intraocular pressure using caution to avoid causing rebleed. Generally, all patients with hyphema need to be examined daily to monitor intraocular pressure and measure the percentage of the anterior chamber that is layered with blood. Topical steroid drops are prescribed to reduce inflammation and promote patient comfort. If the globe is intact, cycloplegic eye drops (e.g., atropine 1%) (see Table 22-3) are prescribed to dilate the pupil and relax the ciliary body.

Red blood cells in the anterior chamber are broken down and washed from the eye through the same channels (trabecular network and canal of Schlemm) that normally route aqueous humor. Cells or cell remnants can clog the trabecular meshwork, causing significant aqueous outflow obstruction and a rise in IOP. IOP readings elevated greater than 20 mm Hg require close monitoring and aggressive treatment. Ophthalmic drops for treatment of glaucoma may be used to reduce IOP. These antiglaucoma eye drops work by causing the pupil to constrict, thereby stretching and opening the trabecular drainage canal, or by reducing the production of aqueous humor. The medications are prescribed until reabsorption of the hyphema occurs. In cases of elevated IOP that are unresponsive to antiglaucoma medication, paracentesis or anterior chamber washout of the hyphema may be performed to evacuate blood and lower the pressure

All African American patients should be screened for sickle cell trait. This hereditary condition causes normal erythrocytes to become deformed and rigid with a slightly decreased oxygen concentration. These sickled cells, when present in the anterior chamber, clog the trabecular meshwork and impede outflow of aqueous humor. As the IOP rises, further hypoxia develops, causing further sickling of the red blood cells and significant aqueous outflow obstruction.[12] Because certain drugs (e.g., carbonic anhydrase inhibitors such as dorzolamide [Trusopt] and acetazolamide [Diamox]) can potentiate sickling, pharmacologic therapy must be carefully monitored by an ophthalmologist. Central retinal artery occlusion can occur with only modest elevations of intraocular pressure in a patient with sickle trait.

Rebleeding is the most common complication of a traumatic hyphema. Incidence of rebleed is highest 2 to 5 days after the injury, when the initial clot begins to retract and lyse, causing the injured vessels to bleed again. Those at highest risk for rebleeding are those with a 50% hyphema (blood fills 50% of the anterior chamber), African Americans and those who initially have high intraocular pressure and poor vision.[13] Rebleeding increases the risk of corneal blood staining, glaucoma and vision loss. Patients must be instructed to remain on bed rest with the head of the bed elevated 30 degrees and to avoid use of anticoagulants, so that the possibility of rebleed is reduced and the red blood cells will settle to the bottom of the anterior chamber.

Penetrating and Perforating Injuries

Penetrating and perforating injuries of the ocular structures are a major cause of vision loss from trauma. Such injuries may occur in isolation or in combination with injuries to surrounding facial structures or other body systems. Failure to treat penetrating and perforating injuries aggressively will almost always result in vision loss. A patient with an open globe (ruptured globe) injury will present with a full-thickness defect in the eye wall, internal eye structures may be expelled, and signs of infection (endophthalmitis) may be present within the globe. An open globe can occur as a result of a penetrating object, a rupture of the eyeball, a through-and-through perforation, or a combination of the latter.

When it is suspected that an injured patient has an open globe, the affected eye should be protected with an eye shield or paper cup. The protective device should be placed before any manipulation of the patient takes place. This prevents any pressure on the globe or periocular structures, which can result in the extrusion of ocular contents causing severe and irreparable damage. Treatment of all non–life-threatening injuries of the face and head should be deferred until an ophthalmologist can evaluate the extent of the ocular injuries. Operative repair of penetrating or perforating ocular trauma must be performed by an ophthalmologist with use of specialized equipment and often involves multiple staged surgeries. Radiographic studies, laboratory tests, and administration of antibiotics and tetanus toxoid (if applicable) should be carried out prior to surgery. In cases where there is a high suspicion of a retained metallic foreign body, emergent surgery is indicated.

Orbital Fractures

An orbital blowout fracture is very common after a blunt injury to the orbit. In many cases the object striking the orbit has a larger diameter than the width of the orbit. With the blow, a pressure wave is generated, which travels across the orbit and eyeball. The unique configuration of the orbit predisposes the medial wall and floor of the orbit to fracture.[14]

Patients with an orbital floor fracture may present with diplopia due to edema, hemorrhage or perimuscular tissue dislocation into the fracture (Figure 22-22). This must be differentiated from trapdoor entrapment of the inferior rectus muscle. In children younger than age 18, there is an increased likelihood of trapdoor entrapment. There may be mild swelling or bruising (the "white-eyed blowout") but

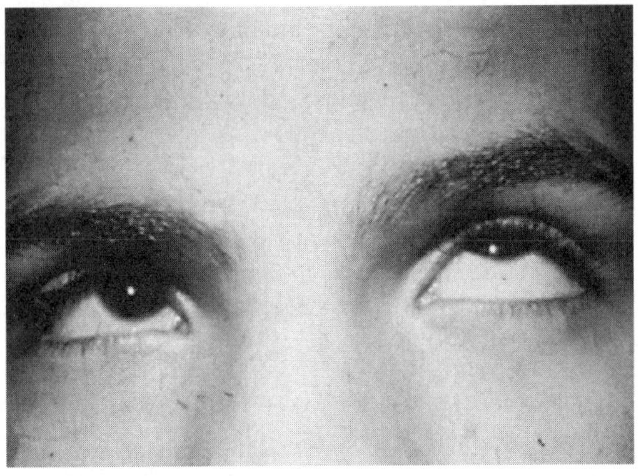

FIGURE 22-22 Orbital fracture with decreased upward mobility.

severe limitation of elevation of the eye. In this case, nausea and vomiting often are present. Forced duction testing (see Figure 22-7) demonstrates restricted eye movement with muscle entrapment. Presence of ophthalmoplegia may be caused by swelling, muscle entrapment, or associated nerve injury. In cases of orbital floor fracture, hypoesthesia may be present in the region innervated by the infraorbital nerve (i.e., upper gums, part of nose and upper lip, inferior eyelid and conjunctiva). Measuring the distance with Hertel exophthalmometry from the lateral orbital rim to the corneal apex may reveal a shorter distance on the involved side, or an increase if there is considerable swelling. Crepitus may be present upon palpation, which may indicate the presence of intraorbital air. Other signs and symptoms may include periorbital swelling, ecchymosis, proptosis, chemosis, subconjunctival hemorrhage, and palpable defects of the bony orbital rim. Orbital CT scans provide the best images of the relationship between the bone and the soft tissue. Both direct and coronal views should be obtained.

Orbital fractures can be associated with optic nerve trauma and globe perforation. Therefore, initial ocular assessment begins with a general examination to determine whether the patient's nervous system and globe are intact. These associated injuries must be managed as described elsewhere in this chapter. As previously mentioned, if the globe is perforated, there should be no manipulation of the orbital bones or eyelids.

The decision for surgical repair is based on evidence of muscle entrapment, enophthalmos, and hypoglobus (downward displacement of the globe) and massive disruption to the orbital floor. Surgery is recommended as soon as it can reasonably be scheduled (within a few days). Two exceptions for this recommended timing of surgery are a small fracture with mild diplopia and no CT evidence of entrapped tissues, and the trapdoor fracture. A waiting time of up to 2 weeks can be allowed to see if diplopia resolves in the case of the small fracture with no evidence of entrapment. If possible, urgent surgery, within 24 hours, is indicated in the case of the trapdoor fracture in a child. Ongoing crushing of the trapped inferior rectus muscle dictates the urgent approach. Complications of orbital floor fracture repair include permanent loss of vision, persistent enophthalmos and diplopia, scarring, eyelid retraction, and implant extrusion. Some patients may forgo surgical repair.

Nose blowing and sneezing should be avoided, as this may lead to intraorbital subcutaneous air, which can cause proptosis, pressure on the globe and optic nerve, with possible loss of vision. Oral steroids are prescribed and ice applied to reduce swelling. Nasal decongestants are administered on the involved side. The use of oral antibiotics is controversial but should be considered if there is a history of sinus disease. Administration of analgesics to relieve pain is also needed.

Optic Nerve Injuries

Severe penetrating orbital injury can result in optic nerve damage and sudden visual loss. Trauma to the optic nerve can also occur in association with blunt orbital trauma and orbital fractures. Loss of vision can be caused by transsection or avulsion of the optic nerve, optic nerve sheath hemorrhage, pressure on the optic nerve from bone fragments or orbital hemorrhage, direct contusion of the nerve, or disruption of the blood supply to the nerve and globe. Often such injuries are irreversible. However, every effort must be made to try to restore vision. Evaluation of such injuries should include a visual acuity assessment, if possible, and examination of the pupils for an afferent defect. Thin-cut CT or MRI scans of the optic nerve and canal are important for evaluating the extent of optic nerve injury. Surgical intervention, such as unroofing the optic canal or opening the optic nerve sheath, may be required in those cases in which there is nerve sheath hemorrhage or edema or fracture of the optic canal. In the past, intravenous high-dose steroids were recommended for managing optic nerve injuries to reduce inflammation and prevent further injury secondary to the inflammatory response. There is now controversy as to whether the high-dose steroid regimen applies to the treatment of optic nerve injury. Goldenberg-Cohen et al, concluded in a retrospective review of traumatic neuropathy among pediatric patients that medical evidence did not support one particular approach to treatment.[15] Ophthalmologists expert in the management of traumatic optic neuropathy are no longer using high-dose steroids.

Corneal Injuries and Foreign Bodies

Corneal foreign bodies may be associated with minor or major trauma (Figure 22-23). Corneal abrasions cause pain, photophobia, and tearing. Anesthetic drops and fluorescein staining facilitate corneal examination. Fluorescein stains the exposed basement membrane of the epithelial defect and can highlight leakage from penetrating wounds. It is imperative to ensure that foreign material is not inside the eye. Fluorescein staining, a penlight, and slit-lamp examination will aid in detection of intraocular foreign matter.

The cornea epithelium represents the first line of protection for the eye, and treatment efforts should be directed at achieving epithelial coverage. A tight eye-pressure patch should be avoided because it may inhibit oxygen supply to the epithelium. Patching increases corneal temperature, facilitating the growth of microorganisms. Placement of a bandage soft contact lens can provide protection without interfering with the oxygen supply to the cornea. The use of personal contact lenses should be avoided during the healing phase. Treatment with concurrent use of antibiotics and cycloplegics (cyclopentolate) (see Table 22-3) may result in faster healing than patching. Patients should never be prescribed a topical anesthetic. Extended use of topical anesthetics results in corneal hyposensitivity and significantly interferes with corneal immunity.[5] A topical lubricant is recommended and will aid in patient comfort.

Foreign bodies must be removed from the eye. Superficial foreign bodies can be removed with a cotton-tipped applicator or a sharp instrument, such as a 30-gauge needle attached to a tuberculin syringe. The material should be

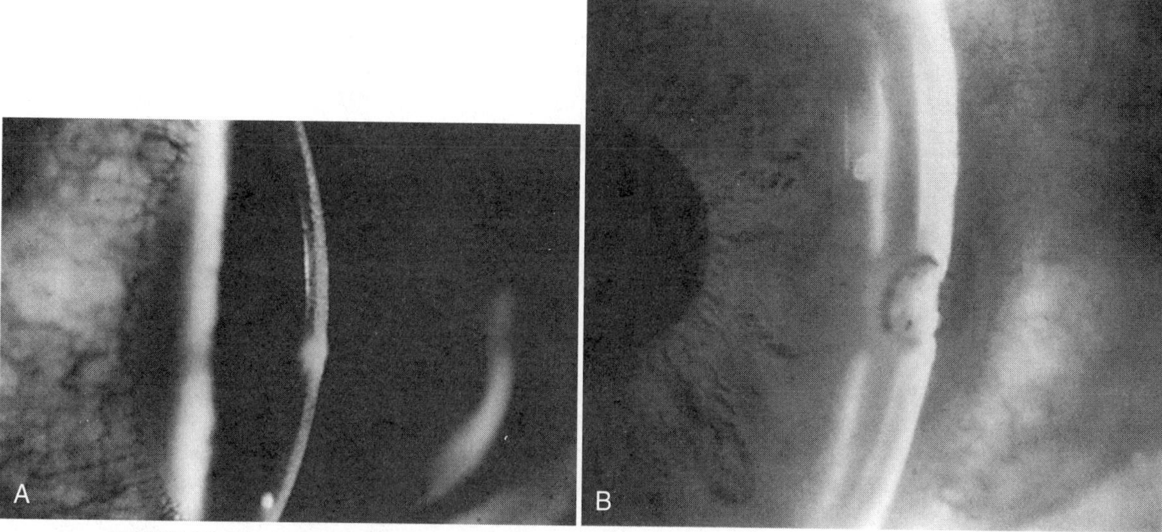

FIGURE 22-23 **A,** Foreign body (rose thorn) embedded in cornea. **B,** Rust ring after removal of foreign body.

removed gently to avoid further damage. The eyelids need to be everted, and any clinging particulate matter must be removed. Metallic rings surrounding copper or iron fragments (seen with welding) can be removed with a battery operated drill that has a burr tip. Topical anesthesia is needed when removing foreign bodies from the eye. If the matter is deeply imbedded, an ophthalmologist should be consulted for surgical removal.

Contact lenses are another type of foreign body often requiring removal. When contacts are worn for extended periods, corneal abrasions can occur. Even in the absence of ocular trauma, the eyes should be examined for the presence of a contact lens. After trauma, the lenses may become dislodged from the cornea and migrate to the superior or inferior ocular cul-de-sacs. A bulb contact lens remover (Figure 22-24) uses suction to lift hard contact lenses from the cornea or sclera. Soft contact lenses can be removed by finger manipulation or by irrigating the eye with normal saline allowing the lens to "float off" the globe. Once removed, contact lenses should be stored in a container with the appropriate storage solution.

Subconjunctival Hemorrhage

Subconjunctival hemorrhage and chemosis frequently occur after trauma. Although these may herald serious intraocular and orbital trauma, they often occur as isolated signs. In the absence of more severe trauma, the management involves waiting and watching. The hemorrhage is usually reabsorbed in 2 to 3 weeks. Reassuring the patient is important and artificial tears may alleviate any surface discomfort. If a ruptured globe is possible, a referral to an ophthalmologist is indicated.

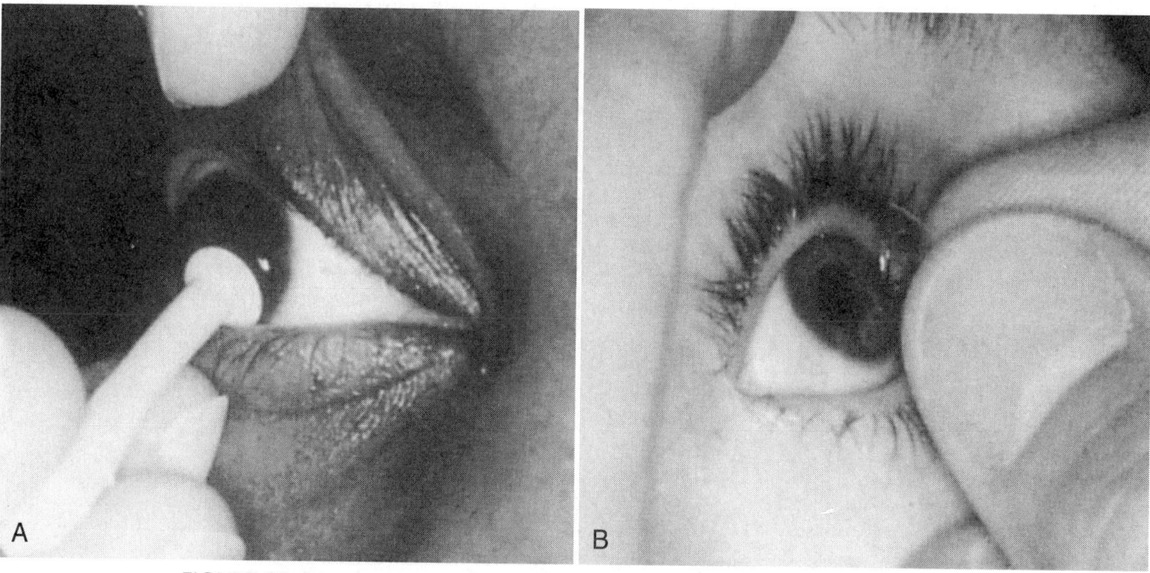

FIGURE 22-24 **A,** Bulb contact remover for hard contact. **B,** Removal of soft contact lens.

OPERATIVE CARE

Timely surgical repair of ocular injuries is almost always required. A conservative wait and see approach can lead to irreversible damage. Unlike other systems, the function of the eye depends on the exact maintenance of anatomical relationships between its structures, including the eyelids, cornea, anterior chamber, lens, retina, extraocular muscles and nerves.

If there is question of a penetrating ocular injury, the globe should be explored and repaired under general anesthesia. Every attempt should be made to salvage or repair any lacerated globe. Primary enucleation is very rare. When necessary, enucleation is a secondary surgery and should only be performed if the eye remains without light perception despite reconstructive efforts.

CRITICAL CARE/INTERMEDIATE CARE

Patients in the critical care and intermediate care phases of trauma continue to require physical, psychological, and emotional support. Reactions to ocular injury and its sequelae will be individual and support efforts should be tailored to each patient's unique needs. It is essential to monitor the patient for signs and symptoms of infection, further vision loss, pain, hemorrhage or other complications. Adverse changes should be reported promptly so that therapy can be instituted and further vision loss prevented.

Pain Management

Pain management is an important aspect of care for the patient with ocular injury. A pain assessment should be completed on a routine basis. Frequently there is minimal or moderate pain after ocular trauma or surgery to the eye, but pain medications may be helpful. For patients with moderate to severe levels of pain, patient-controlled analgesia may be indicated. Ice packs are helpful to decrease swelling and control pain, especially following orbit and eyelid surgery. Keeping the head elevated at 30 degrees may aid in patient comfort.[16] Unrelieved or increasing pain should be considered an indication for further ophthalmological evaluation.

Surgical Site/Wound Management

Patients who have had ocular surgery are at risk for disruption of the surgical site as a result of elevated intraocular pressure and inadvertent blunt trauma to the operative site. To protect the eye, a metal or plastic eye shield must be applied to the affected eye postoperatively.

Increased intraocular pressure may result from hemorrhage or edema after surgery. Nursing measures must focus on the prevention of increased pressure and assessment for early detection. Activities that should be avoided are coughing, gagging, lying flat or in the Trendelenburg position, straining for bowel movements, bending at the waist, and lifting objects greater than 10 pounds. Chest physiotherapy may be contraindicated. Patients should receive instruction to stoop to retrieve items, use a stool softener, increase fluid and fiber in the diet, and avoid all strenuous athletic activities.

Wound care should be performed as prescribed. The injury or surgical site should be assessed frequently for healing progression and signs of infection. Purulent discharge, erythema, increased tenderness, pain and inflammation at the wound or surgical site are symptoms of possible wound infection and should be reported to the physician.

Potential for Iritis

Iritis, an inflammatory reaction that involves the iris and ciliary body, frequently occurs 2 to 3 days after blunt trauma. Patients present with significant photophobia, a red sclera, tearing, and blurred vision. A complete eye exam is indicated to rule out serious ocular injury. Administration of cycloplegic agents (e.g., homatropine 5%) and corticosteroid drops will alleviate symptoms. Symptoms generally resolve in 7 to 10 days.

Potential for Cellulitis

Preseptal or periorbital cellulitis (Figure 22-25, A) is an infection of periocular tissues. Preseptal cellulitis involves the soft tissues anterior to the orbital septum, a connective-tissue curtain that separates the eyelid structures from the orbit. Blunt or penetrating trauma can be responsible for the

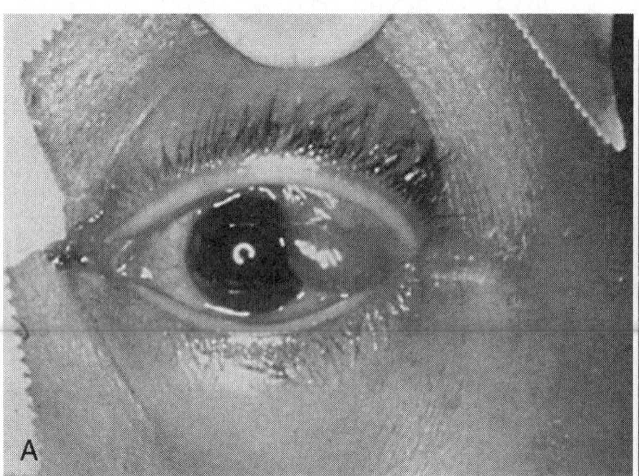

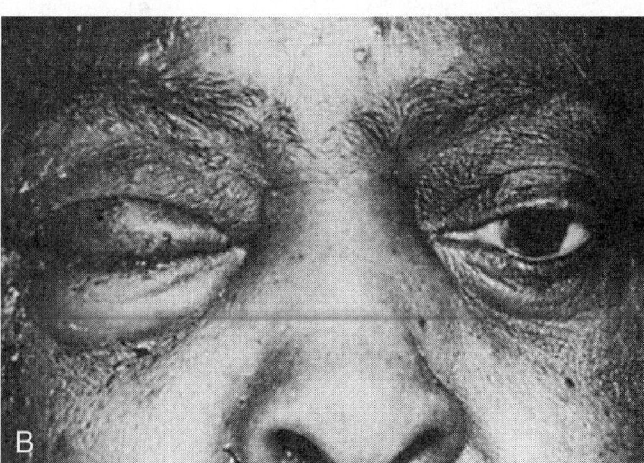

FIGURE 22-25 **A,** Periorbital cellulitis. **B,** Orbital cellulitis.

introduction of bacteria into the preseptal tissues through the breaks in the periorbital skin. The most common causative organisms are *Streptococci pyogenes* and *Staphylococci aureus.* Fungal infection is unusual but can occur if there was organic material involved in the injury. Patients with preseptal cellulitis will present with an eyelid that is erythematous, warm, tender and swollen. The swelling usually extends over the nasal bridge to the opposite side of the face and may be so severe that elevation of the eyelid is not possible. Purulent drainage may accompany these symptoms. Vision, pupillary reflexes, and extraocular movements are normal. A low-grade fever and elevated white blood cell count may be present. The workup includes obtaining a complete blood count and a culture of material from any open wound. A CT scan of the orbit and sinuses is performed. In cases of mild to moderate preseptal cellulitis, oral broad-spectrum antibiotics may be prescribed and started after the culture is obtained. In severe cases of periseptal cellulitis, or when the patient is unable to take medications orally, intravenous antibiotics may be required. Incision and drainage of any suppurative areas, such as abscesses that may have formed, is indicated.

Orbital cellulitis occurs posterior to the orbital septum[10] (Figure 22-25, B). Penetrating ocular trauma or eye surgery may cause this severe infectious process, or more frequently, it may occur secondary to a sinus or oral infection. Orbital cellulitis is a serious disease associated with severe ocular, intracranial, and systemic morbidity, which may include loss of vision from optic nerve damage, glaucoma, corneal damage or retinal injury, brain abscess, cavernous sinus thrombosis, and sepsis. Patients commonly present with fever and leukocytosis. Proptosis, restricted ocular motility, pain on eye movement, conjunctival hyperemia and chemosis, sluggish pupillary reflex, visual loss, and increased intraocular pressure may be present. An orbital or subperiosteal abscess may form. Workup is similar to preseptal cellulitis. It is essential to obtain a CT scan to determine the extent of orbital, sinus, and intracranial involvement. Patients are treated with intravenous antibiotics. Surgical drainage of an abscess or sinus may be indicated acutely or may be delayed 1 to 3 days to allow the effect of antibiotics. It is important to involve the aid of an otolaryngologist and ophthalmologist to manage orbital cellulitis.

Cavernous sinus thrombosis may result from orbital cellulitis or may occur independently. Patients with cavernous sinus thrombosis appear severely ill and have a fever, nausea, vomiting, headache, and an altered level of consciousness in addition to signs of orbital cellulitis. Orbital pain is absent and cranial nerves III, IV, and VI are impaired as a result of their compression within the cavernous sinus.

Potential for Corneal Erosion

Corneal erosion can be caused by abnormal eyelid position, poorly fitted contact lenses, contact lens over-wear, abnormalities of the eyelid margin, misdirected eyelashes, inadequate tear film, inability to close the eyelids or infrequent blinking. Trauma-related facial nerve damage that impairs eyelid closure is frequently associated with corneal abnormalities. Decreased corneal sensation from damage to the fifth cranial nerve can result in a weak or absent corneal reflex and inadequate surfacing of the pericorneal tear film resulting in injury to the cornea. During the 6 to 12 months after injury, traumatic ptosis, eyelid closure, and blinking may improve spontaneously. In the interim, vigorous use of artificial tears and ointments is essential to protect the cornea. These may be administered as frequently as every hour. If the patient does not respond to artificial tears, an extended-wear bandage contact lens may be applied. The lens should stay in place 24 hours a day and be changed every 2 weeks. If drops and ointments are inadequate to prevent continued exposure keratopathy (corneal noninflammatory dystrophy), it may be necessary to tape the eyelids shut, perform a tarsorrhaphy (temporary or permanent closure of part of or the entire eyelid) or inject botulinum toxin to maintain eyelid closure. Surgical correction of eyelid abnormalities may be required in some cases. It is essential that patients with corneal pathology caused by exposure be managed vigorously to prevent ocular discomfort, blepharospasm, permanent scarring, corneal ulcers, and corneal perforation.

Potential for Sympathetic Ophthalmia

Sympathetic ophthalmia is an inflammation in the uninjured eye after the other has been damaged by a penetrating injury.[8] It is the major indication for enucleation of a globe that had been previously injured and then repaired. Sympathetic ophthalmia is a rare condition characterized by a severe, bilateral, granulomatous inflammation of the uveal tract (uveitis), which includes the iris, ciliary body, and choroid. It may manifest as soon as 5 days after injury or years later. If untreated, the inflammatory response may result in loss of vision in the uninjured eye. The incidence of sympathetic ophthalmia has declined sharply with new advances in surgery. When sympathetic ophthalmia occurs, aggressive treatment using systemic and topical steroids is initiated. This treatment is often successful. If the traumatized eye is blind, enucleation of that eye (the inciting eye) may be helpful in the management of sympathetic ophthalmia.

Patient and Family Education

Patient and family teaching during the critical care and intermediate care phases should include information regarding the injury, the symptoms the patient may expect, and therapeutic interventions. Education regarding patching, ocular medication, pain, wound care, and restrictions on mobility and activities are especially important. Patients undergoing surgical intervention for ocular repair should also receive information about the procedure and their anticipated preoperative and postoperative management. Patients may have activity restrictions and are often discharged to home the same day or within 1 to 2 days after surgical repair of isolated traumatic ocular injuries. Potential complications and their symptomatology should be explained carefully to the patient and family.

Coping Assistance

Although any injury-related disability is stressful and undesirable, visual loss is considered by many to be one of the most devastating outcomes from trauma. According to Gallup polls, in America, blindness is one of the most feared of all disabilities, ranking fourth after acquired immunodeficiency syndrome (AIDS), cancer, and Alzheimer's disease as "the worst disease or ailment."[17] Society relies on sight for everyday activities, and an unexpected loss can have a detrimental effect on our physical, social, and emotional well-being.

If vision is lost, the patient is faced with learning new ways to receive and process information. This will impact activities of daily living and social interactions. The financial situation of the patient and the family also may be adversely affected, especially if the patient is the primary wage earner in the household.

Emotional aspects of shock, denial, anger, and depression that accompany the grieving process after a death are also associated with a loss of vision (see Chapter 19 for Psychosocial Impact of Trauma). Psychological and emotional support from health care providers, family, and friends is essential to help the visually impaired person cope with their loss. The impact of blindness may require professional counseling to adjust to this unfamiliar situation.

When the full impact of visual loss is realized by the patient and family, time and support must be allowed for grieving. Expressions of pity and being overly solicitous are counterproductive to allowing visually impaired persons to adapt to sight loss. The patient should be encouraged to express their own feelings and concerns in an accepting atmosphere. Efforts should be made to assist patients with resources to aid in transitions. It must be acknowledged that the patient's self image will be affected. A father and husband may no longer be the provider for the family; a mother may no longer be able to care for her children without assistance. The patient may no longer be able to engage in certain activities without assistance.

Nurses should frequently orient the patient to time, place, and unfamiliar environments (including noises and smells); this will alleviate fears of the unknown. Before initiating an intervention, it must be described to the patient. Each person entering the patient's immediate environment should introduce himself or herself. The patient with unilateral visual impairment should be approached from the sighted side.

Normally size, dimension, color, shape, and density of objects are all processed visually. With vision loss, this ability is lost. Patients must rely on other senses to process this information. This relearning takes time and requires sensitivity and, most of all, patience from care providers. The patient should be allowed to touch and smell objects, including objects that may be used in their care. The color of objects should be described to patients. Each time a health care team member interacts with the patient, they should describe themselves (e.g., eye color, hair, height) if the patient desires. The patient should be allowed to feel the face of the health care team member if it is helpful. Environmental stimulation is provided through conversation, radio, television, audio tapes, or a computer.

Whether the visual loss is permanent or temporary, the absence of sight is frightening and devastating. Visual loss combined with the presence of other systemic injuries, the circumstances of the trauma event, pain, and potential morbidity contribute to anxiety and fear, compounding the feelings of complete powerlessness felt by the patient. Health care workers can reduce fear by touch. A gentle touch conveys many messages to a frightened patient, including care, concern, and a willingness to help. It is reassuring and comforting to a patient to be able to identify a voice and gentle touch together. Anxiety, fear, and apprehension can be diminished, making the experience less terrifying for the patient and the recovery process easier. Understanding the patient's fears, concerns, and anxieties is imperative to enable the nurse to individualize the care given to each patient.

It is important to promote the patient's sense of independence, which may be difficult to do in the acute phase of hospitalization. Within the limitations imposed by other injuries and the patient's general condition, the patient should be encouraged to assist with tasks, even things as simple as hand washing, so that a sense of accomplishment and self-control is fostered. Occupational therapists can help a patient learn new ways to perform activities of daily living (ADL). The patient also may be taught how to perform simple tasks related to ocular therapy and management, such as the instillation of ocular medication or patching an eye. When possible, the patient should be offered choices about how and when care should be delivered.

A health care team composed of clergy, nurses, physicians, psychiatrists, psychologists, and social workers can be extremely helpful in assisting the patient and family as they adapt. Including a child-life specialist can be helpful in reducing a child's fears. Referral to rehabilitative services (e.g., occupational therapy, physical therapy, vocational rehabilitation, and community agencies providing services for the visually impaired) should be initiated. Interventions that assist the patient in coping with the visual impairment remain important throughout hospitalization and must continue after discharge.

Safety Risk Management

The environment must be safe, organized, and consistent for the person who is visually impaired and cannot see impending dangers. The environment must be free of sharp-edged furniture and equipment; items easily tripped over (e.g., scatter rugs); objects that can be easily broken and cause injury; and objects that are hanging from the ceiling or protruding from the walls. The nurse should educate the patient on the contents and layout of the room. A patient with limited vision may not have the ability to judge distance in feet. Therefore, it is helpful to instruct the patient how many steps it will take to travel from one point to another. Consistency in the placement of items in the room (e.g., phone on left side of bed, tissues on right) is helpful to facilitate the patient's independence. When preparing the patient to eat a meal, it is helpful to explain the food items on the plate as numbers on a clock. Commonly used items can be identified by touch. An easy to recognize texture (e.g., a gauze pad, wrinkled paper) can be placed on an item to make the object easier to identify. To foster a sense of security, a call bell or other means of attracting assistance should be kept in a specific location easily accessible to the patient.

REHABILITATION AND COMMUNITY INTEGRATION

Rehabilitation efforts begin soon after the injury occurs during the resuscitation and critical care phases. Some visually impaired patients may be discharged directly to home and some may require admission to a rehabilitation facility. Programs and services vary by geographic location and access to programs may be insurance dependent. Each patient's needs require individualized evaluation for safe discharge planning. Careful planning and communication between the health care team, patient, and family are essential.

The primary goal of rehabilitation is to prepare the visually impaired person for a life of independence within the limitation of his or her disability. The patient must be encouraged and motivated to attain maximal potential independent functioning. Promotion of self-esteem, personal value, and self-confidence, and learning to master living in a sightless world are essential for maximal recovery. Learning Braille, independent household management, and new modes of ambulating with a visual impairment (possibly using a seeing-eye dog or cane) are examples of priorities during this phase. Whenever possible, the patient should be encouraged to make use of adaptive equipment and techniques to enable resumption of activities.

Returning the patient to a more normal appearance also promotes self-esteem and may ease community integration. Medications to reduce eye redness, cosmetics to cover scarring, or surgery to correct strabismus or eyelid deformity may be indicated. A prosthetic eye to replace an enucleated globe can improve body image. All these measures help alleviate the patient's stress when interacting with other individuals in the community.

Rarely does a patient sustain bilateral vision loss after ocular trauma; usually monocular loss occurs. The patient's view of the world can be very different if vision is only present in one eye, especially the dominant eye. For example, depth perception may be affected. As a result, instruction on head and body movements that enable the patient to see from different

TABLE 22-4 **Resource Organizations for the Visually Impaired**

American Foundation for the Blind	11 Penn Plaza, Suite 300 New York, NY 10001 (800) 232-5463	www.afb.org
American Council of the Blind	1155 15th St. NW, Suite 1004 Washington, DC 20005 (202) 467-5081 or (800) 424-8666	www.acb.org
American Printing House for the Blind	1839 Frankfort Ave Louisville, KY 40206 (502) 895-2485	www.aph.org
Association for the Education and Rehabilitation of the Blind and Visually Impaired	1703 N. Beuregard St., Suite 440 Alexandria, VA 22311 (703) 671-4500	www.aerbvi.org
National Association for the Visually Handicapped	22 West 21st Street New York, NY 10010 (212) 889-3141	www.navh.org
Prevent Blindness America	211 West Wacker Dr., Suite 1700 Chicago, Ill 60606 (800) 331-2020	www.preventblindness.org
American Academy of Ophthalmology	655 Beach Street San Francisco, CA 94119 (415) 561-8500	www.aao.org
American Society of Ophthalmic Registered Nurses (ASORN)	P.O. Box 193030 San Francisco, CA 94119 (415) 561-8513	www.asorn.org
Social Security Administration	6401 Security Boulevard Baltimore, MD 21235-0001 (800) 772-1213	www.ssa.gov
U.S. Department of Health and Human Services	200 Independence Avenue SW Washington, DC 20201 (877) 696-6775	www.hhs.gov
State Department of Rehabilitation Services	Contact information varies by state	

viewpoints is crucial. The patient may benefit from an evaluation from a low vision specialist. This specialist can help the patient maximize use of their remaining eyesight.

Rehabilitation is carried out closely in conjunction with community integration. Community integration must be planned and initiated well before the patient is ready to go home, either from the hospital or rehabilitation facility. Appropriate housing and home care for the patient must be arranged. Supplies, equipment, and medications required for wound or injury management must be procured for the patient. Some patients may benefit from a visiting nurse to assess their progress and some may need the temporary assistance of a meal delivery program. The nurse needs to use fully the community resources for optimal patient care at home. The patient, family, and all involved health care providers should have a thorough understanding of the care required, including medications, wound management, activity restrictions, necessary safety precautions, signs and symptoms of complications, physician follow-up appointments, and actions to take in an emergency.

Patients and families need to be educated about state and federal tax relief, Social Security and Medicare benefits, travel discounts, and vocational rehabilitation. Health care providers who care for patients with ocular injuries should be knowledgeable about community agencies and services available to the visually impaired. A list of national and community organizations for the visually disabled should be provided to the patient (Table 22-4). Introductions to other patients with visual loss who have adapted to their disability and are functioning as productive members of society may help. Social workers can be of great help by providing financial, vocational, and social resources for the patient.

SUMMARY

Familiarity with ocular anatomy and function form the basis for evaluating and managing ocular trauma. Appropriate interpretation of ocular assessment findings allows recognition of eye injuries and their possible complications. The prevention of permanent damage from trauma depends on the use of appropriate management techniques. More importantly, ocular trauma may be avoided if proper safety measures are taken in the workplace, at home, and during recreational activities. If permanent visual disability occurs despite appropriate protective measures and trauma management, a variety of individuals and groups are available to aid in the patient's adjustment to a severe disability and reintegration into society.

REFERENCES

1. Leonard R. *Statistics on Vision Impairment: A Resource Manual, 2000,* New York, 2000, Lighthouse International.
2. McGwin G Jr, Owsley C: Incidence of emergency department-treated eye injury in the United States, *Arch Ophthalmol* 123:662-666, 2005.
3. United States Eye Injury Registry (USEIR). Available at http://www.useironline.org. Accessed January 14, 2006.
4. Kuhn F, Morris R, Witherspoon C: Birmingham Eye Trauma Terminology (BETT): terminology and classification of mechanical eye injuries, *Ophthalmol Clin North Am* 15:139-143, 2002.
5. Kuhn F, Pieramici D, editor: *Ocular Trauma Principles and Practice,* New York, 2002, Thieme.
6. Koo L, Kapadia M, Singh RP et al: Gender differences in etiology and outcomes of open globe injuries, *J Trauma* 59(1):175-178, 2005.
7. Pearlman JA, Au Eong KG, Kuhn F et al: Airbags and eye injuries: epidemiology, spectrum of injury, and analysis of risk factors, *Surv Ophthalmol* 46(3):234-242, 2001.
8. Riodan-Eva P, Whitcher J, editor: *Vaughan & Asbury's General Ophthalmology,* New York, 2004, Lange Medical Books/McGraw-Hill.
9. Conlon M, Navarro V, Lai J et al: EMTALA: The ophthalmic nurse as qualified medical personnel, *Insight* 29(3), 2004.
10. Trobe J, editor: *The Physicians Guide To Eye Care,* San Francisco, 2001, The Foundation of the American Academy of Ophthalmology.
11. Joseph DP, Pieramici DJ, Beauchamp NJ: Computed tomography (CT) in the diagnosis and prognosis of open globe injuries, *Ophthalmology* 107:1899-1906, 2000.
12. Sankar P, Chen T, Grosskreutz et al: *Traumatic hyphema, Int Ophthalmol Clin* 42(3):57-68, 2002.
13. Girkin C, McGwin G, Morris R et al: Glaucoma following penetrating ocular trauma: a cohort study of the United States Eye Injury Registry, *Am J Ophthalmol* 139:100-105, 2005.
14. Long J, Tann T, Orbital trauma ophthalmology, *Ophthalmol Clin North Am* 15:249-253, 2002.
15. Goldenberg-Cohen N, Miller N, Repka M: Traumatic optic neuropathy in children and adolescents, *JAAPOS* 8(1):20-27, 2004.
16. Mason G: Ocular trauma. In Goldblum K, editor: *Core Curriculum for Ophthalmic Nursing,* Dubuque, Ia, 2002, Kendall Hunt.
17. Morris R, Fletcher D, Scott S: Counseling and rehabilitation, *Ophthalmol Clin North Am* 15:167-170, 2002.

23

SPINAL CORD INJURIES

Tammy A. Russo-McCourt

Spinal cord injury (SCI) was first described in the literature in 2500 BC by Egyptian surgeons as "an ailment not to be treated."[1] This sentiment was echoed for the next several thousand years. It was not until the early 1900s when Dr. Alfred Reginald Allen developed an experimental SCI model that permitted reproducible injury that "modern-day" understanding of spinal cord injury was elicited. This model allowed Allen to study the outcomes that resulted when the spinal cord was subjected to varying forces. These experiments led to his hypothesis that traumatic SCI created two types of injury: (1) direct injury to the axons at the time of impact (primary SCI) and (2) a response of the affected nervous tissues to the initial injury that occurs over time and causes delayed cellular damage (secondary SCI). Research has consistently supported the concept of primary and secondary injury. The potential to interrupt this secondary response and prevent worsening outcome prompted early, aggressive treatment of SCI.[2,3]

A combination of many events in the late 1960s and early 1970s led the way in changing the approach to management of acute spinal injury. New technologies, such as the intraoperative microscope and neuroradiologic diagnostics, and the development of modern intensive care units have all contributed to survivability.[2] Introduction of the military model for triaging and rapid transport of trauma victims and the understanding of the multisystem effects of SCI enabled many more paralyzed individuals to survive their injury. This demonstrated both the ability to successfully treat such injuries and highlighted the need for appropriate SCI rehabilitation. The pioneering work of Sir Ludwig Guttmann identified the need to provide comprehensive multidisciplinary care from the onset of SCI through rehabilitation so that individuals can return as productive members of society. Guttmann's holistic approach serves as the model for modern-day SCI care.

Publication of the *Guidelines for the Management of Acute Cervical Spine and Spinal Cord Injuries* (2002) by the American Association of Neurological Surgeons/Congress of Neurological Surgeons joint section on Disorders of the Spine and Peripheral Nerves with the collaboration of the Joint Section on Trauma provides evidence-based recommendations for care of the patient with SCI. These *Guidelines* are the result of an extensive review and analysis of the existing literature; whereas the evidence is frequently controversial wherever convincing studies (e.g., well-designed randomized controlled trials) exist, practice standards are suggested. When the research provides moderate clinical certainty about an intervention (i.e., based on nonrandomized cohort studies, case-control studies, and randomized controlled trials with design flaws), the recommendations are termed *practice guidelines.* Whenever the consensus statements are based only on case series, expert opinion or randomized controlled trials with flaws that cause doubt about the study's conclusions, the recommendations about care are referred to as practice options. It is important to stress that while most areas lacked the necessary scientific evidence to support standard-of-care or guideline statements, the document offers practitioners a framework for evidentiary appraisal to assist in the development of clinical protocols and practices.

SCI, with its multisystem sequelae, creates a ripple effect in every facet of the patient's life, the family's life, and society at large. Enormous burdens are placed on resources to provide the necessary care for the paralyzed person; until recently, very little support existed. The United States Veterans Administration and the National Institute on Disability and Rehabilitation Research have made significant contributions in this area.

The primary goal of this chapter is to provide a thorough description of SCI and its effects. A brief review of neuroanatomy facilitates greater understanding of the mechanisms of injury and the multisystem impact of the injury. Assessment and management of SCI will be presented in a "cycle of trauma" format to highlight the importance of interventions within each phase of trauma care on patient outcomes.

EPIDEMIOLOGY

It is estimated that there are approximately 40 new cases of SCI per million U.S. citizens each year; this translates to 11,000 new cases per year.[3-6] Researchers estimate that an additional 4800 victims of SCI die before reaching the hospital.[3] It is currently estimated that between 250,000 and 400,000 individuals in the United States are living today with SCI or dysfunction.[4-6] This broad range reflects the difficulty in capturing accurate data caused by the complexity of ICD-9 codes and lack of discharge coding and reporting.[4] Recent funding within several states may support improved data collection.

While the incidence of SCI is relatively low, it is considered a high-cost disability. Depending upon age at the time of injury, average lifetime direct cost is estimated at $1.6 to $2.8 million for high tetraplegics (C1-4), $1 to $1.6 million for low tetraplegics (C5-8), and $450,000 to $1 million for paraplegics.[5] A conservative estimate of the economic burden of SCI in the United States is $7.13 billion per year.[6,7] This includes the cost of newly injured persons, acute and rehabilitation care, home environment adaptation, and care for chronic issues such as pressure sores, which alone cost on average $1.2 billion yearly.[8] This does not reflect indirect costs, such as loss of wages, fringe benefits, and productivity, which represent an additional $2.6 billion dollars annually.[6,7]

In 1973, the National Spinal Cord Injury Database was established at the University of Alabama at Birmingham. This registry captures approximately 13% of new SCI cases per year.[4] Because this group is representative of the SCI population at large, it has contributed significantly to our ability to compile incidence, prevalence, and demographic information on SCI. Since 2000, the average age at the time of SCI has risen to 37.6, up from 28.7 in the 1970s.[4,8] This trend reflects the median age increase in the population at large since the 1970s. Males continue to sustain SCIs more often than females by about a 4-to-1 margin, and the primary etiology remains motor vehicle crashes. Demographics are showing shifts in several areas: (1) an increase in the proportion of those injured who are older than age 60, again matching a rise in the median age of the general population; (2) a rise in the proportion of injuries among African-Americans (increasing from 13% in the 1970s to 22% since 2000) and Hispanics (increasing from 6% in the 1970s to 12.6% since 2000), paralleling the increase of these racial and ethnic groups in the composition of the population at large; (3) a rise in the incidence of falls, especially as age increases; and (4) more SCIs due to violent events, particularly in young African-American males.[4,8,9]

In years past, the average life expectancy of a person sustaining an SCI was less than 1 year. With the improvements made in prehospital, critical, and long-term care, life expectancies for persons with SCI that survive the first year are continuing to increase.[8,9] Because patients are living longer, more of them will receive Medicare and disability income. We can expect a continued increase in the annual expenditure for SCI-related health care.[7] There also has been a shift in the leading causes of death for patients with SCIs. Historically, the leading cause of death was renal failure, although with significant advances in urologic management, this etiology has declined. The most common causes of death have become pneumonia, heart disease (54% were sudden, unexplained heart attacks), and septicemia, most frequently related to pressure ulcers, urinary tract infections, or pneumonias.[4,9,10] Recent prospective mortality studies have disputed the long-held belief that level and extent of SCI, age at injury, and calendar year of injury are directly related to mortality.[10] Interestingly, comorbidities affecting mortality rates are the same as those without SCI: heart disease, diabetes, pulmonary function abnormalities, and cigarette smoking.[10,11] It is crucial that care during the cycle of trauma be focused on limiting complications to achieve maximum recovery and sustain optimal health.

PREVENTION

There are three general strategies to prevent injuries: persuasion, legal requirements, and provision of automatic protection. Persuasion is the most difficult strategy to apply effectively. The Think First Foundation (www.ThinkFirst.org), developed and supported by the American Association of Neurologic Surgeons and the Congress of Neurological Surgeons, is one group that assists communities in providing programs to educate children and adolescents about prevention of brain and spinal injuries. Also, changes in laws creating safer vehicles and more effective restraint systems and enforcement of these laws can help protect the public. Mandatory safety equipment for high-impact sports, particularly improved helmets and neck rolls, can help prevent SCI. Aggressive campaigns, such as those sponsored by Mothers Against Drunk Drivers (MADD), provide media attention and public education regarding the dangers of high-risk behaviors and promote social reform, which can be effective in reducing SCIs. The number one cause of SCI in persons age 65 and older is falls.[4,5,11,12] Statistically, one third of persons older than age 65 will sustain a fall resulting in a significant injury. Of this group, two thirds will sustain a second fall within the same year.[12] Fall prevention programs for the elderly should start with risk assessment of both the person and the living environment. The Centers for Disease Control and Prevention (CDC) and the National Center for Injury Prevention have published the *U.S. Fall Prevention Programs for Seniors* that provides a listing of available comprehensive programs in addition to the Senior Fall Prevention Tool Kit. Raising public awareness, providing education, using passive protective mechanisms, and enacting social and legal reform can be effective prevention methods.

BASIC SPINAL ANATOMY

Gross spinal anatomy can be divided into three categories: (1) the vertebral bony column, intervertebral disks, ligaments, and muscles; (2) the spinal cord and associated nerves and membranes; and (3) the spinal cord vasculature.

THE BONY STRUCTURES

The spinal, or vertebral, column consists of 33 vertebrae (Figure 23-1) separated and cushioned by fibrocartilaginous pads called *intervertebral disks*. The vertebrae and disks are joined by ligaments.

The majority of the vertebrae have similar anatomic features. Each vertebra can be divided into two sections: an anterior body, the segment that faces toward the front of a person, and the posterior arch (Figure 23-2). The opening created between the body and the arch is the spinal canal (vertebral foramen), where the spinal cord, its coverings, and blood vessels pass. The arch is a series of fused bony parts. Starting at the midpoint is the spinous process. These are the points that can be seen or felt protruding along the midline of the back. Moving laterally in either direction are more

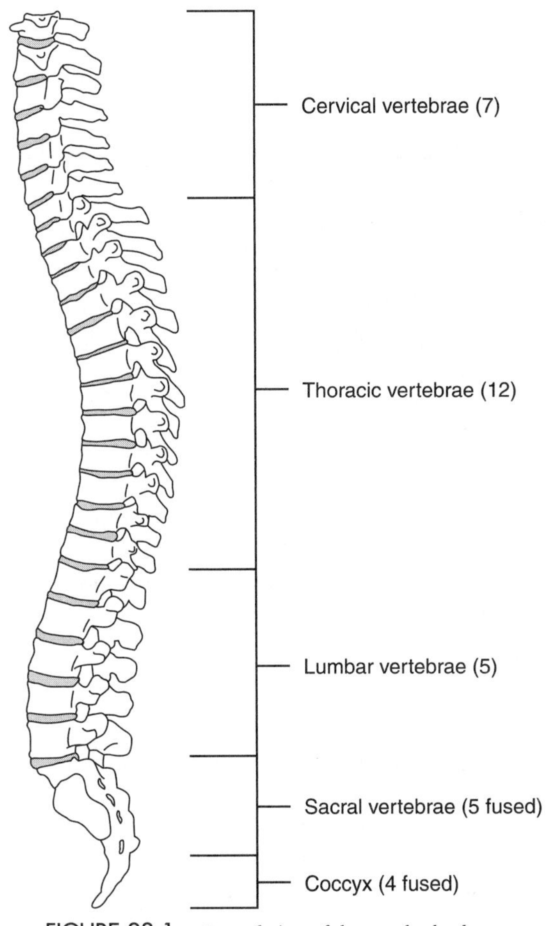

FIGURE 23-1 Lateral view of the vertebral column.

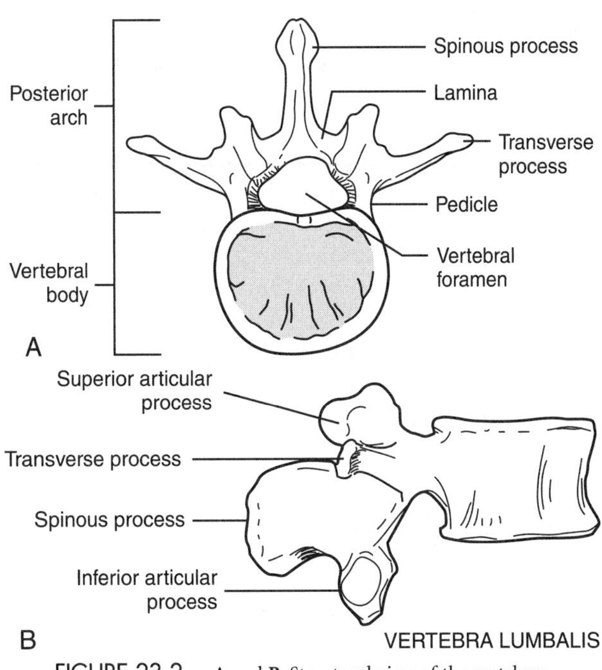

FIGURE 23-2 **A** and **B**, Structural view of the vertebrae.

distinct bony prominences called the *transverse processes* with superior and inferior articular processes or facets. These are joined to the spinous process by the lamina. The transverse processes are connected to the vertebral body by the pedicles. When the vertebrae are aligned in a column, the inferior articular processes, which project downward, meet the upward protruding superior articular processes of the vertebrae directly below. Between these processes and the bodies and disks an opening exists—the intervertebral foramen, through which peripheral nerves pass.

Of special interest are the first cervical (C1) (atlas) and second cervical (C2) (axis) vertebrae (Figure 23-3). The first cervical vertebra is called the atlas because it literally supports the "globe" of the head. By articulating with the skull, C1 provides 50% of the normal motion of the neck, mainly flexion and extension. It is an unusual vertebra in that it lacks a vertebral body. The odontoid, a bony projection jutting upward from the C2 vertebral body, protrudes through the anterior arch of C1. The odontoid process forms the pivot on which the atlas and skull rotate (hence the term *axis*). The sacrum and coccyx are also unique because the vertebral bodies of these areas are fused together.

The intervertebral disks, made up of an inner gelatinous material (nucleus pulposus) surrounded by cartilaginous

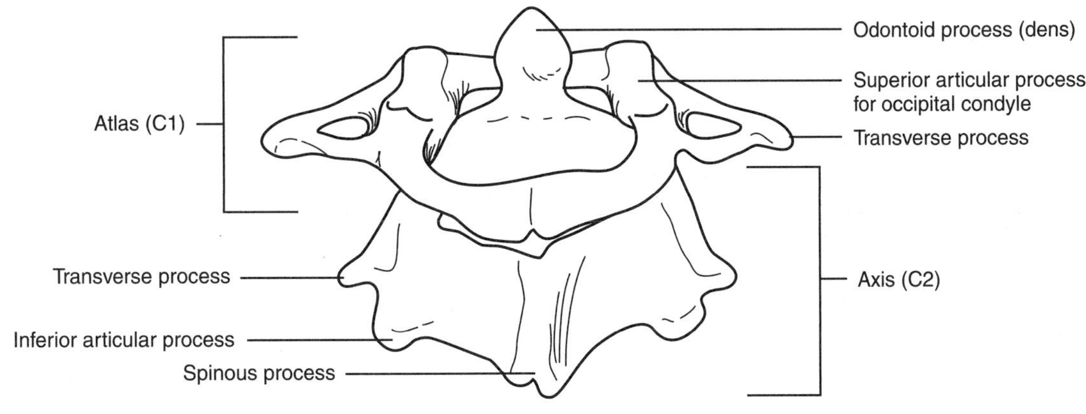

FIGURE 23-3 Articulated view of the C1-2 structure.

fibers (annulus fibrosus), confer a degree of flexibility to the spine. They act as shock absorbers by temporarily flattening and bulging from between the vertebrae when they are compressed. The vertebrae and disks are held in alignment by ligaments (Figure 23-4). The ligaments prevent extreme flexion and extension of the spine. The anterior and posterior longitudinal ligaments join the bodies of adjacent vertebrae. whereas the strong ligamenta flava join the lamina. The ligamentum nuchae extends from the skull through the spinous process of the seventh cervical vertebra. Below this level, supraspinal ligaments join the spinous processes. Adjacent spinous processes are joined from their roots to their ends by interspinal ligaments.

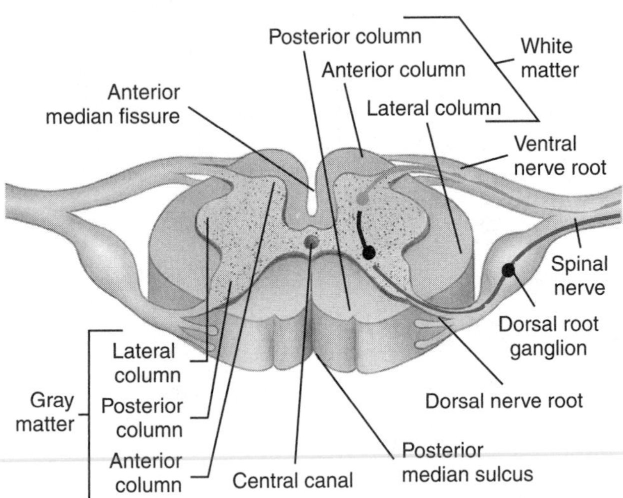

FIGURE 23-5 Transverse section of spinal cord. (From Ozuna JM: Nursing assessment nervous system. In Lewis SM, Heitkemper MM, Dirksen SR, editors: *Medical Surgical Nursing Assessment and Management of Clinical Problems*, ed 6, St. Louis, 2004, Mosby.)

THE SPINAL CORD

The spinal cord, composed of gray matter and ascending and descending nerve tracts, is covered by meninges and housed inside the vertebral column. The spinal cord, essentially an extension of the medulla oblongata, begins at the foramen magnum and terminates between the first and second lumbar vertebrae. This conical termination point is called the *conus medullaris.*

Spinal nerve roots exit from the cord at each intervertebral foramen. There are a total of 31 pairs of spinal nerves: 8 cervical, 12 thoracic, 5 lumbar, 5 sacral, and 1 coccygeal. Each spinal nerve has a dorsal (posterior) root and a ventral (anterior) root (Figure 23-5). The dorsal root consists of sensory or afferent fibers, which carry impulses from the body to the cord. The dorsal root contains a spinal ganglion, which is located outside the cord but within the intervertebral foramen. The ganglion contains the cell bodies of the sensory neurons. The ventral root consists of the motor, or efferent, fibers. The cell bodies of the motor neurons are located within the ventral horn (anterior gray matter column) of the cord. These fibers carry the impulses from the cord to the appropriate effector site.

The spinal cord is surrounded by three meninges: the dura mater, the arachnoid, and the pia mater. The meninges are continuations of the meninges covering the brain. Above the pia mater is the subarachnoid space. The subarachnoid space is filled with cerebrospinal fluid (CSF), as is the central canal that pierces the central gray matter of the cord. The central canal is continuous with the fourth ventricle. The spinal cord is tethered to the meninges via the dentate (or denticulate) ligaments.

GRAY AND WHITE MATTER

The substance of the spinal cord is divided into two types: gray matter and white matter.

The gray (unmyelinated) matter is centrally located in an H or butterfly-shaped pattern. It is composed of cell bodies and their axons and dendrites. It can be divided into three areas, columns, or horns: the anterior, the intermediolateral,

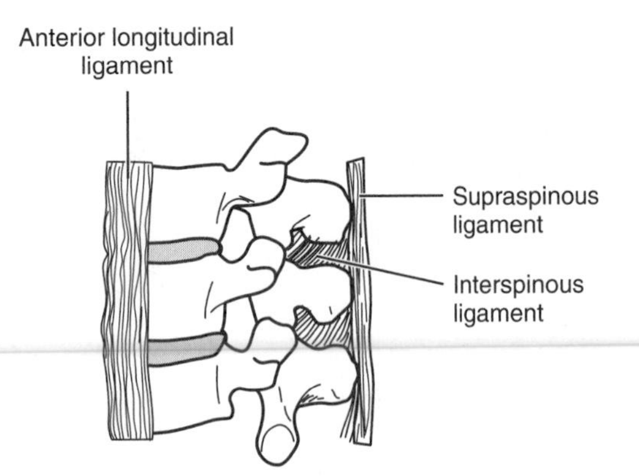

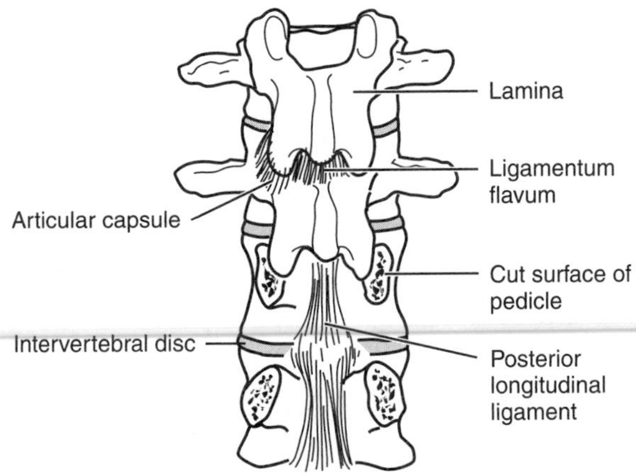

FIGURE 23-4 The chief ligaments of the vertebral column. (From Jenkins DB: *Hollinshead's Functional Anatomy of the Limbs and Back*, ed 7, Philadelphia, 1998, W.B. Saunders.)

and the posterior. The anterior horn provides the motor component of the spinal nerves, often referred to as the final common pathway. The intermediolateral horn contains cell bodies, which give rise to the preganglionic sympathetic fibers of T1-L2 and the preganglionic parasympathetic fibers of the sacral segments of the cord. The posterior horn contains axons from peripheral sensory neurons. These may terminate there or ascend or descend in the white matter.

The white (myelinated) matter surrounds the gray matter of the cord and is divided into large fiber bundles called *columns* or *funiculi*. There are three columns: the posterior, the lateral, and the anterior. Each column contains ascending sensory tracts and descending motor tracts (Figure 23-6).

The major ascending tracts include the posterior (dorsal) columns, the spinocerebellar tracts, and the spinothalamic tracts. The posterior column mediates proprioception, vibration, two-point discrimination, deep pressure, and touch.[13] These columns ascend on the ipsilateral side of the spinal cord, where they enter and decussate in the medulla and become the internal arcuate fibers of the medial lemniscus; these fibers ascend through the thalamus to the cerebral cortex.[14] There are many well-identified ascending tracts of the lateral column. The most significant of these are the spinocerebellar tracts and the spinothalamic tracts. The spinocerebellar tracts carry information on position sense and body movement (unconscious proprioception) necessary for coordination of body movement from the extremities and trunk to the cerebellum. The spinothalamic tracts carry information from the periphery to the thalamus. The anterior spinothalamic tracts transmit light touch and pressure impulses, whereas the lateral spinothalamic tract mediates most pain and temperature sensations. The spinothalamic tracts decussate almost at the level of entrance into the spinal cord and ascend in the contralateral anterolateral system to the thalamus. The anterior column tracts are primarily involved with motor function, posture reflexes, light touch, and pressure.

The major descending pathways are the corticospinal, reticulospinal, vestibulospinal, rubrospinal, and tectospinal tracts. The largest and the one of greatest clinical concerns is the lateral corticospinal, or pyramidal, tract. Fibers originate in the motor cortex, and the majority cross to the opposite side in the medulla and descend the spinal cord as the lateral corticospinal tract delivering voluntary motor function. Fibers of the lateral corticospinal tract are arranged in the spinal cord, with the motor fibers controlling the lower extremities located peripherally, and the fibers controlling the upper extremities located medially.

The descending tracts or motor pathways can be divided into two categories: upper motor neurons (UMNs) and lower motor neurons (LMNs). UMNs originate and terminate within the central nervous system (CNS) and include all neurons or nerve cells, which modulate the motor output of the anterior

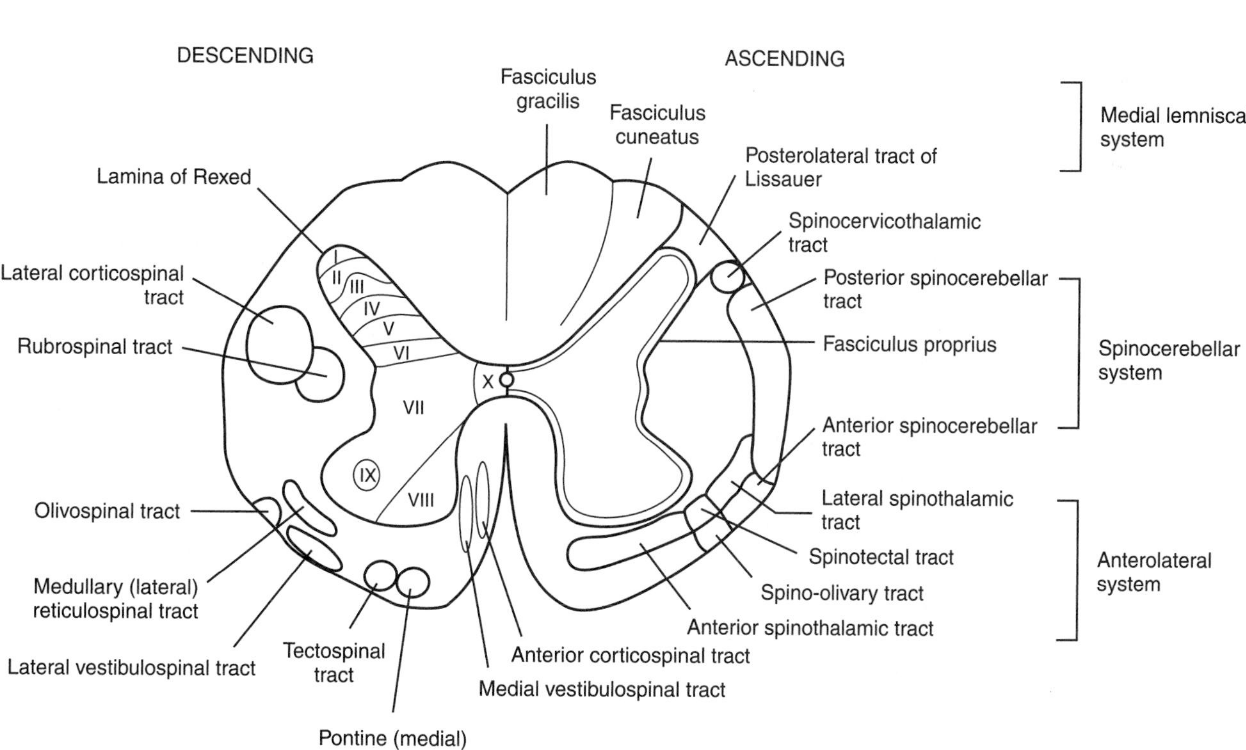

FIGURE 23-6 Cross-section of spinal cord detailing major descending (motor) and ascending (sensory) tracts.

horn cell of the spinal cord. The motor modulators that constitute the majority of the UMNs include the cerebral cortex, cerebellum, basal ganglia, red nuclei, vestibular nuclei, and reticular formation. Any lesion or trauma that disrupts these areas and their modulation of the LMNs will create an upper motor neuron deficit. This deficit is characterized by paralysis, hypertonicity in affected muscle groups, and hyperreflexia.

The LMNs constitute the anterior horn cells and their efferent motor neurons—the final common pathway. They originate in the CNS and terminate at the neuromuscular junction. All nerves that influence the final common pathway are UMNs. Destruction of the LMNs results in loss of muscle tone, muscle atrophy, hyporeflexia (absent reflexes), muscle flaccidity, and fasciculations.

In summary, the primary motor tracts are located in the anterior and anterolateral portion of the spinal cord, and the primary sensory tracts are located in the posterior and posterolateral section of the cord (see Figure 23-6). This generalization helps provide an understanding of incomplete spinal cord syndromes.

Spinal Blood Supply

Branches from the terminal portion of the vertebral artery unite at the level of the foramen magnum to form the anterior spinal artery (Figure 23-7). The artery descends down the median ventral aspect of the spinal cord, supplying blood to its anterior two thirds. The remaining blood supply is provided by the two posterior spinal arteries, which descend down the posterolateral aspect of the spinal cord from their vertebral artery source. As these three vessels descend the cord, they receive additional perfusion from branches of the cervical, intercostal, lumbar, and sacral arteries. The large artery of Adamkiewicz, which arises from the aorta, enters the cord at the second lumbar ventral root level to supply blood to most of the lower third of the spinal cord.[13]

Venous drainage of the spinal cord consists of two main systems: the intrinsic system and the extrinsic system. The intrinsic, or intradural system, closely follows the arterial system to drain blood from the spinal cord emptying into the venous plexus surrounding the cord (venous vasa corona). The extrinsic, or extradural, system forms a series of plexus from the craniooccipital junction to the sacral region. All venous drainage ultimately ends up in the vena cava.[14]

The Autonomic Nervous System

The autonomic nervous system (ANS) controls and regulates the functioning of the involuntary muscles and glands of the major body systems. It is regulated by the hypothalamus, which is located at the crossroads of the ascending

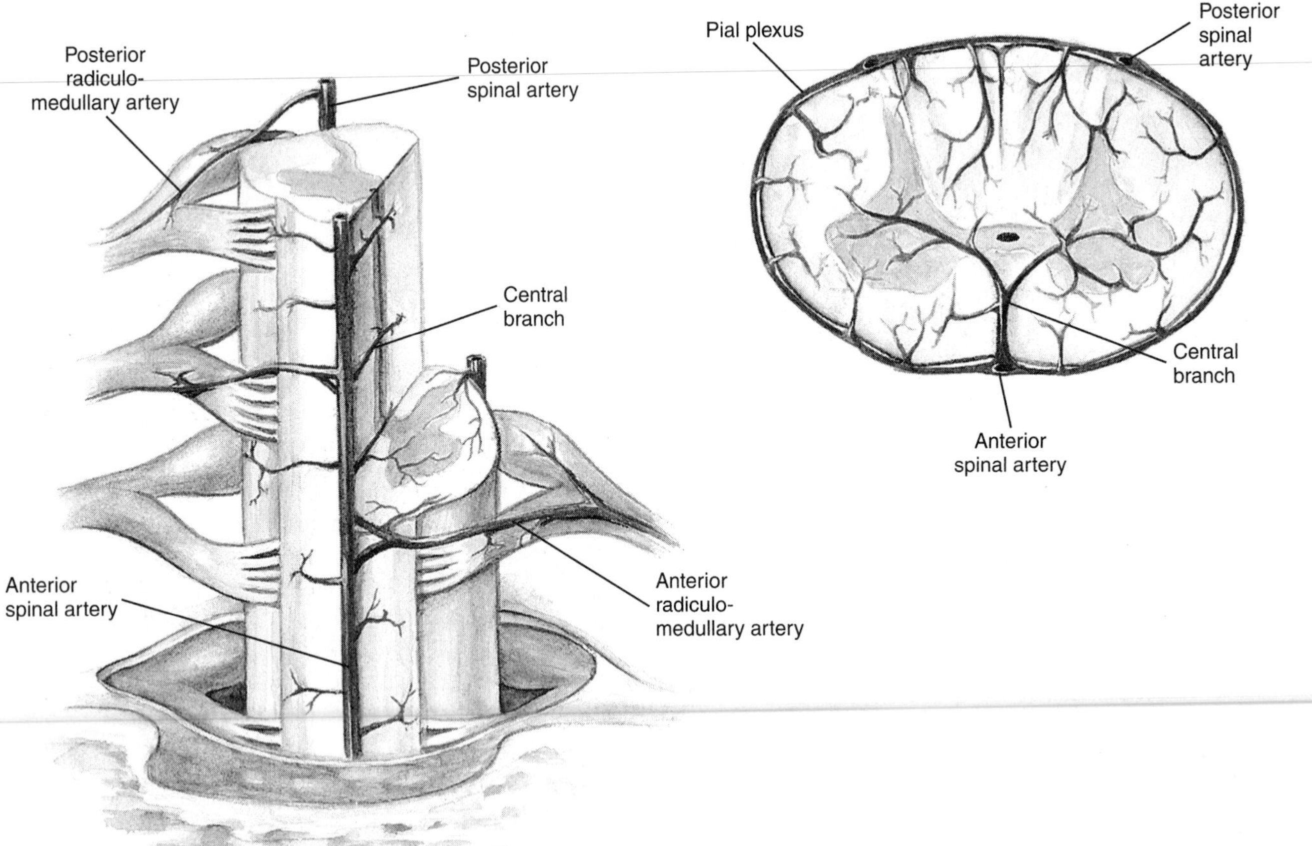

FIGURE 23-7 Arterial circulation of the cord. **A,** Cross-sectional views.

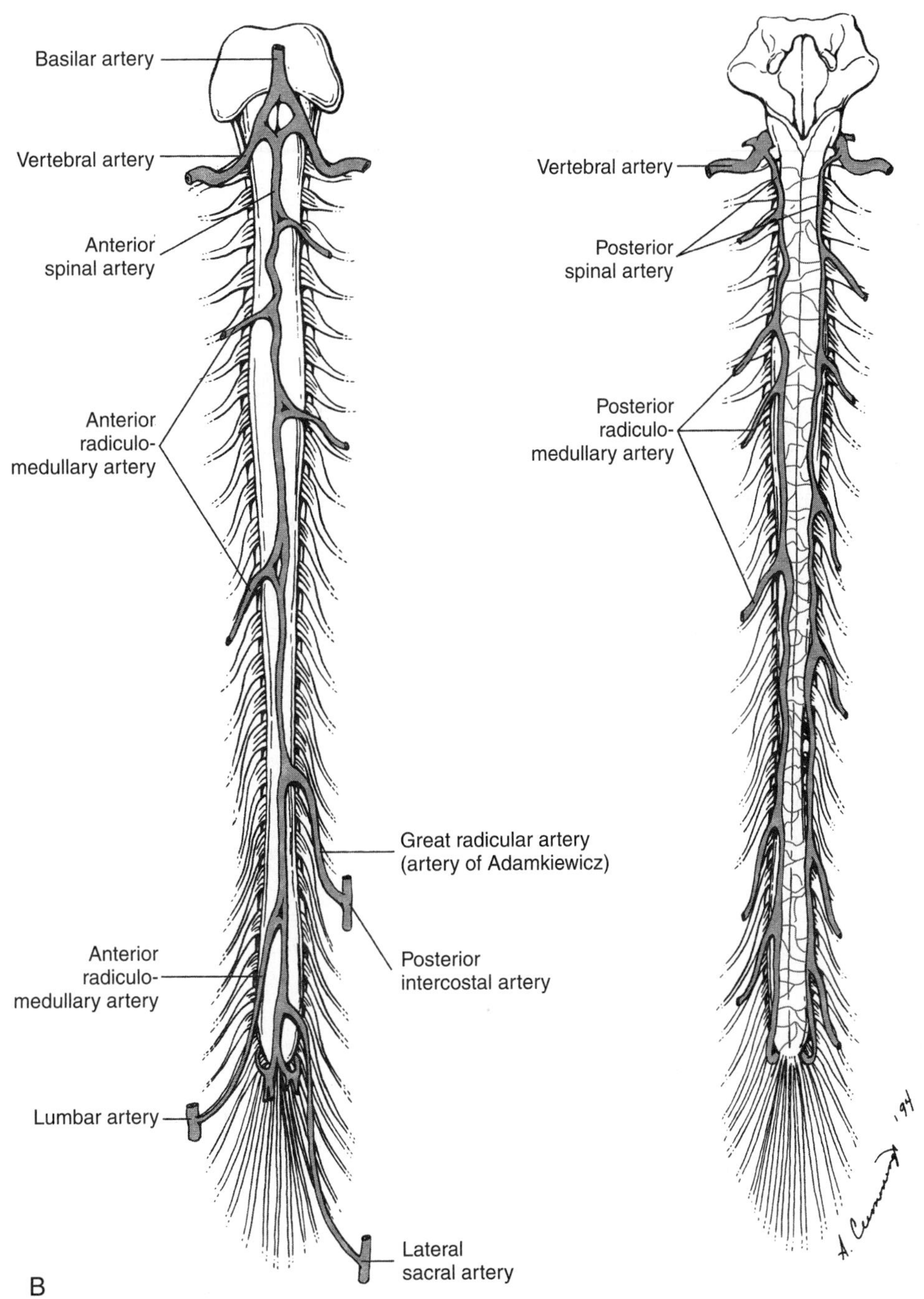

FIGURE 23-7, cont'd **B,** Anterior and posterior views. (From Darby SA. General anatomy of the spinal cord. In Cramer GD, Darby SA, editors: *Basic and Clinical Anatomy of the Spine, Spinal Cord and ANS,* ed 2, St. Louis, 2005, Elsevier Mosby.)

and descending spinal tracts in the diencephalon. The ANS is divided into two antagonistic branches: the sympathetic branch (SNS) and the parasympathetic branch (PNS).

The SNS controls functions commonly referred to as the "fight or flight" response. It exits the spine in the thoracolumbar area and prepares the body to respond to stressful situations. The parasympathetic branch is responsible for energy conservation and system relaxation. The parasympathetic system, including the third, seventh, ninth, and tenth cranial nerves, exits the spine at the cervicosacral level. This information is important in understanding the systemic consequences of a spinal cord injury (Figure 23-8 and Table 23-1).

Mechanism of Injury

The primary mechanisms that result in spinal injury are hyperflexion, hyperextension, axial loading (vertical compression), rotation, and penetrating trauma (Figure 23-9). Many injuries involve an exaggerated movement in one direction (e.g., hyperflexion), but usually there is a degree of accompanying injury on the opposite side (e.g., extension)

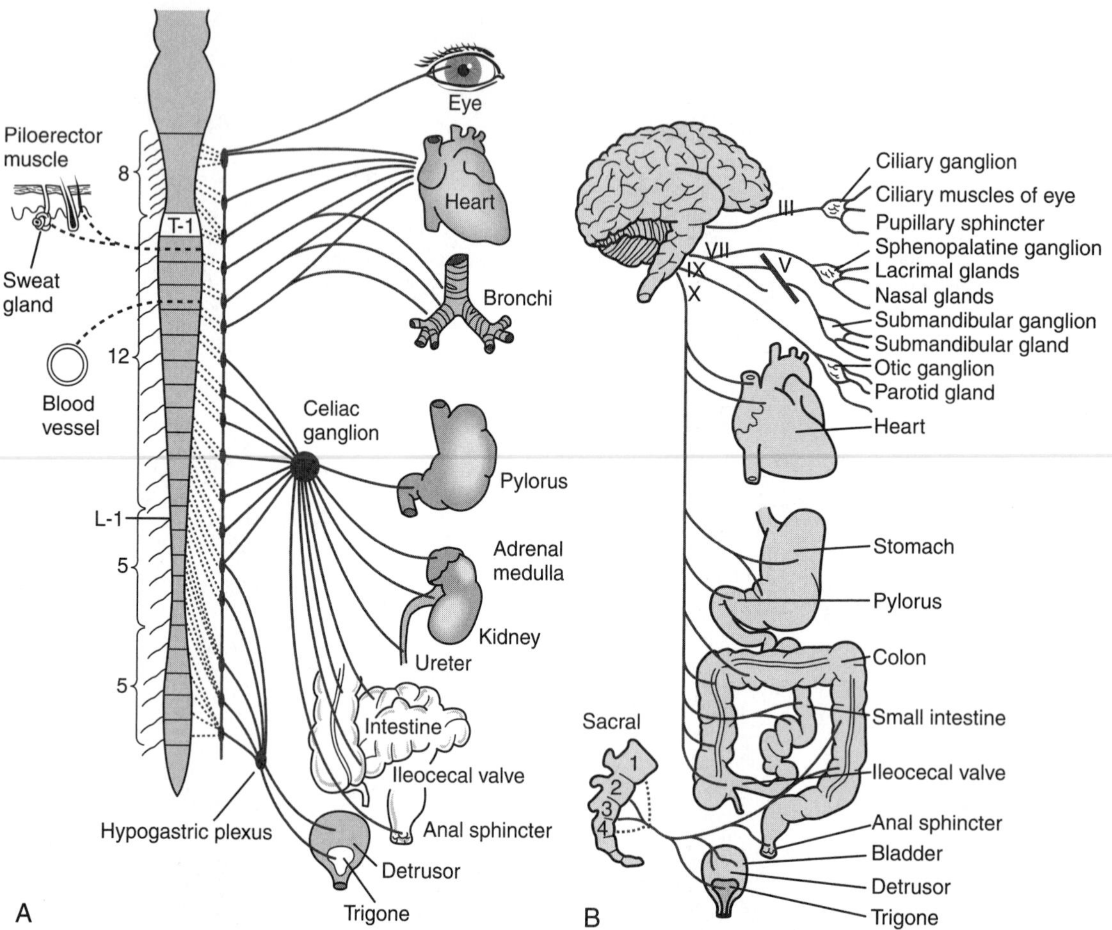

FIGURE 23-8 **A,** Sympathetic nervous system. **B,** Parasympathetic nervous system. Solid lines represent preganglionic fibers, and dashed lines represent postganglionic fibers. (From Guyton AC, Hall JE: *Textbook of Medical Physiology,* ed 10, Philadelphia, 2000, Saunders.)

as the articulated spine responds to the extreme motion. Forces that cause injury may impact the spinal column simultaneously or in succession.[15] Severity of injury is directly related to the magnitude of the force(s); in other words, the greater the force, the greater the injury.[16]

HYPERFLEXION

Hyperflexion injury occurs when a portion of the spine receives a force, direct or indirect, exerted toward the anterior surface of the vertebral body, causing flexion beyond the normal range of motion. This is often associated with head-on collisions. On impact, the driver's head continues forward, and with sufficient speed and force, the weight of the head forces the chin to the chest, causing a hyperflexion injury. In hyperflexion injuries the most flexible levels of the spine absorb this energy and act as fulcrums. This extreme force and stretch can cause an anterior vertebral compression (wedge) fracture and possible intervertebral disk herniation.[16] Posterior ligaments are stretched and may tear, allowing the vertebrae to sublux. Subluxation of the vertebral column disrupts the continuity of the spinal canal, stretching and impinging on the spinal cord and altering spinal cord blood flow. Disk matter can also extrude into the spinal canal toward the cord.

HYPEREXTENSION

Hyperextension injury results when there is extreme extension of the spinal column, such as in a fall, when the chin strikes an immovable object, or in a rear-end collision. Whiplash is a mild form of this mechanism. Once again the extreme force is absorbed by the flexible points of the spine, producing a stretch or tear of the anterior longitudinal ligaments, possible fracture, and subluxation of the vertebrae and rupture of the disks. If the integrity of the spinal canal is compromised, the spinal cord may be damaged. Injury also occurs when the hyperextended spinal cord is stretched excessively so that it is compressed by the ligamentum flavum, causing cord contusion and ischemia.[13,17] Persons with preexisting conditions, such as degenerative cervical stenosis, are at greater risk for developing SCI as the result of hyperextension because of the presence of osteophytes and narrowing of the spinal canal.[17]

TABLE 23-1 **Autonomic Nervous System: Effects on Various Effector Sites**

Effector Organ	Sympathetic Influence	Parasympathetic Influence
Eye		
Pupil	Dilation (mydriasis)	Constriction (miosis)
Glands		
Lacrimal	Decreased	Increased
Nasal	Decreased	Increased
Salivary	Decreased	Increased
Sweat	Increased	None
Heart	Increased rate Increased conduction velocity Increased contractility	Decreased rate Decreased contractility
Blood vessels		
Coronary	Vasodilation	Minimal dilation
Skeletal	Vasodilation	None
Abdominal viscera	Vasoconstriction	None
Cutaneous	Vasoconstriction	None
Blood pressure	Increased	Decreased
Lungs	Bronchodilation	Bronchoconstriction
Gastrointestinal		
Motility	Decreased peristalsis	Increased peristalsis
Sphincter	Increased tone	Relaxation
Secretions	Inhibition	Stimulation
Bladder	Decreased detrusor tone	Increased detrusor tone
Sex organs	Ejaculation	Erection
Skin		
Pilomotor muscles	Excited (contraction)	None

Modified from Guyton AC, Hall JE: *Textbook of Medical Physiology*, ed 9, Philadelphia, 1996, W.B. Saunders.

Axial Loading

Axial loading, also referred to as vertical compression, occurs when sufficient force is exerted vertically through the spinal column. The vertebral bodies and intervertebral disks attempt to absorb the energy and literally burst. This is known as a compression or burst fracture. Bone fragments and disk matter are sent in all directions, including into the spinal canal.[13] The imploding bone can tear and compress the spinal cord, which it surrounds. Additional "buckling" of the cervical spine involving a combination of flexion and extension at various vertebral levels may also occur.[18] Injury from this mechanism often occurs with shallow diving or head-first tackling and generally results in significant SCI.

Rotational Injuries

Rotational injuries are the result of twisting the spine. Lateral flexion of the cervical spine is accompanied by axial rotation. Rotational forces may stretch and rupture the posterior ligaments, dislocate the facets, and may cause compression fracture of the bony structure.[15,16] This injury may occur as a result of a side impact motor vehicle crash, particularly when occupants are unrestrained, or when force is exerted to the side of the head or jaw, such as a "hook" blow in boxing.

Penetrating Injuries

Penetrating injuries may be classified as low velocity or high velocity. Stabbings or shootings with low-caliber handguns that actually pierce or transect the spinal cord cause low-velocity wounds. They rarely disrupt spinal column integrity and therefore are typically considered "stable" injuries. Foreign objects, such as a bullet from a high-caliber gun or shrapnel from an explosion that enters the body at great force, cause high-velocity injuries. Bony injury may or may not be present. However, the concussive forces alone are sufficient to cause spinal cord damage.

Spinal Column Injuries

Soft Tissue Injuries

Injuries can affect the soft tissues that surround and support the spine, including the muscles, disks, and ligaments. Under an extreme load, the central nucleus can burst through the surrounding cartilaginous fibers, the annulus fibrosus, producing a herniated disk. Disk injury can compress and injure the spinal cord or nerve roots. Disruption of spinal ligaments can threaten vertebral column stability, allowing vertebrae to dislocate and injure the underlying spinal cord. *Whiplash* is a common term used to describe a hyperextension injury

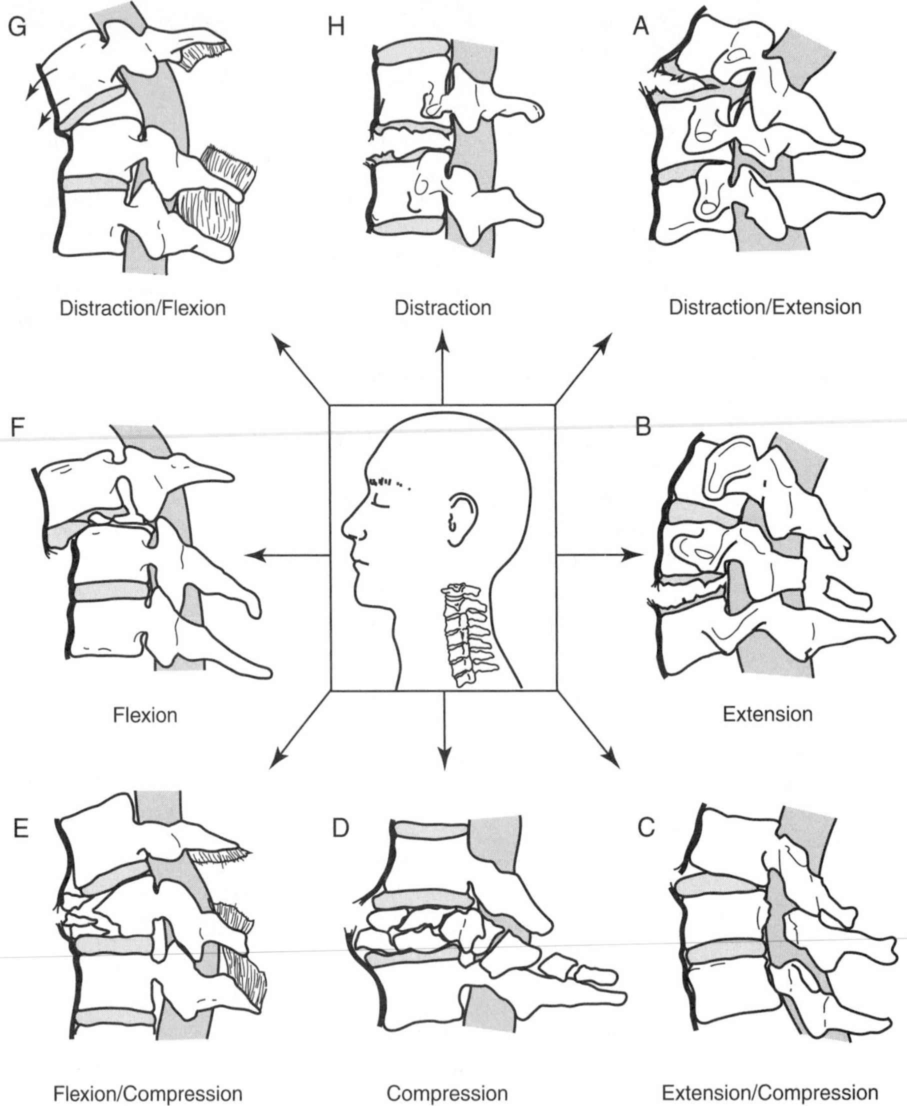

FIGURE 23-9 **Mechanisms of injury and resulting cervical pathology.** Subaxial cervical spine injuries involving C3 through C7 commonly follow a pattern. These injury patterns were developed at the University of Maryland Shock Trauma Center and incorporate the work of Allen and Ferguson. **A,** Extension injuries in the midcervical spine can cause disruption of the anterior longitudinal ligament with some posterior displacement of the superior or cephalad vertebrae on the more caudal vertebrae. **B,** When there is more forced extension, there may be fracture of the spinous process and even the lamina. This is different from the clay-shoveler's fracture, which occurs at the C7 spinous process and is thought to be an avulsion injury. **C,** A forced extension injury in which some form of fracture occurs through the facet region like an incomplete spondylolysis, which is seen in a lumbar spine. Injuries represented in **A, B,** and **C** can occur in the elderly with preexisting cervical spondylolytic stenosis. **D,** With further compression injuries, the patient typically suffers a burst fracture. **E,** A combination of flexion and compression. The vertebral body will fracture anteriorly, and there may be posterior disruption of the interspinous ligaments. Without significant canal compromise, a neurologic deficit may be absent. (Modified from Clark CR, editor: *The Cervical Spine,* ed 3, Philadelphia, 1998, Lippincott-Raven.)

of the neck that causes stress and strain injury to neck ligaments and muscles.[13] Symptoms, including headache, stiff neck, neck and shoulder pain, muscle spasm, and limitation of movement, are thought to be caused by the stretching, microhemorrhage, and edema incurred by the neck muscles.[13] The results of physical examination are usually normal except for the above symptoms, and radiologic findings are negative. Palliative treatment measures generally include mild analgesics, nonsteroidal antiinflammatory drugs (NSAIDs), heat therapy, muscle relaxants, and exercise regimens.[13,19,20] Cervical collars, although controversial, may be used.[13,19,21,22]

VERTEBRAL INJURIES

An easy method for understanding injuries to the vertebrae is to classify them by fracture type and location within the vertebral column. Fractures can occur in any part of the vertebrae. The fracture site and type are generally a result of the traumatic mechanism and forces sustained by the vertebral column.

Simple Fracture

A simple fracture is a singular break that usually occurs to the spinous or transverse process, pedicles, or facets of the vertebral arch. They may or may not be stable fractures and usually do not produce neurologic compromise. Simple fractures are usually managed conservatively; however, if over time the fracture dislocates, surgical intervention may be needed.

Wedge Fracture

Wedge (compression) fracture occurs when the anterior portion of the vertebral body becomes compressed by the force exerted on it by adjacent vertebrae.[16,17] If the posterior elements remain intact, the fracture is stable. The spinal cord may or may not be spared. It is most often associated with axial loading and hyperflexion injury.[13,15-17]

Burst Fracture

Burst fracture results from vertical forces directed onto the spinal column that shatter the vertebral body and are frequently associated with intervertebral disk rupture. Bone fragments and disk material may be driven into the spinal canal, producing serious spinal cord compromise.[13] Management is based on characteristics and stability of the fracture and presence or absence of neurologic deficit. Patients without deficit may be conservatively managed with bracing or casting.[17,23-25]

Teardrop Fracture

Teardrop fracture, usually associated with a compression-flexion force, occurs when a small fragment of bone from the anterior edge of the vertebra breaks off.[16,17] The vertebral body may be dislocated posteriorly into the spinal cord. In addition, interspinous separation (distraction) posteriorly and fractures of the lamina and spinous processes may occur.[16] Surgical intervention is required to remove the fragment and stabilize the spine.

Dislocation

Dislocation injury, a result of distractive-flexion force, occurs when one vertebrae subluxates over another, often resulting in unilateral or bilateral facet dislocation. The injury is staged based on the degree of vertebral involvement (fracture and displacement) and ligamentous disruption.[16,17] Accompanying ligamentous injury ranges from stretch or strain to complete rupture of the stabilizing ligature. Management is dependent upon severity of fracture and degree of displacement.[17]

Fracture-Dislocation

Fracture-dislocation is a term used to convey the presence of a vertebral break in combination with displacement of the vertebral body. It is associated with ligamentous injury, possible disk herniation, and usually involves spinal cord injury. Fracture-dislocation injury results from shearing force in combination with another injury mechanism, such as axial rotation or flexion.[16,17] This complex and unstable injury usually requires surgical fixation for stabilization.

High Cervical Fracture

The unique properties of the C1 and C2 vertebrae necessitate that separate attention be focused on injury to this area. The majority of head and neck movement is derived from the atlantoaxial relationship to the occiput. The wide range of motion in this area makes it highly susceptible to injury secondary to excessive rotation. Several unique patterns of injury and fracture have been identified.

Atlantooccipital dislocation (AOD) results when the occiput is avulsed from the atlas. Injury to the spinal cord and brainstem occur, causing this injury to be fatal in most cases. In addition to bony disruption and neural damage, impingement of the vertebral artery may occur. Surviving patients may have variable motor and sensory deficits, cranial nerve defects, and cardiopulmonary instability. Management of these injuries is directed toward immediate stabilization and reduction of the spine.[26,27] Early fusion and application of a halo apparatus are recommended.[26,27]

A Jefferson fracture is the result of vertical compression of the atlas ring. As the vertebra absorbs the force, it is split, or burst, into several parts. The fractures permit widening of the vertebral foramen, and therefore the spinal cord usually remains undamaged. However, any movement of the head can displace a fragment and sever the cord, which often results in death. Literature generally supports conservative management with a rigid stabilization, such as a halo apparatus, for up to 12 weeks, if the transverse ligament is intact.[28,29] Patients with ligamentous rupture may require surgical intervention with subsequent rigid stabilization.[28,29]

An odontoid or dens fracture of the C2 vertebrae is a rather common traumatic cervical injury.[29-31] It usually results from multiple extreme forces, including compression, extension, rotation, and flexion.[30,31] These fractures can be classified according to location of the dens fracture (Figure 23-10). The majority of these fractures are not associated with neurologic deficit. Odontoid fractures are best visualized radiographically with lateral or open-mouth views of the cervical spine. Management is dictated by the type of fracture and degree of dens displacement.[30] External cervical immobilization may be used initially to manage type I, II, or III fractures; however, surgical fixation should be considered if a type II or III fracture is comminuted, significantly displaced, or alignment cannot be obtained and maintained with cervical immobilization.[29,30] Persons older than age 50 with type II injuries should be

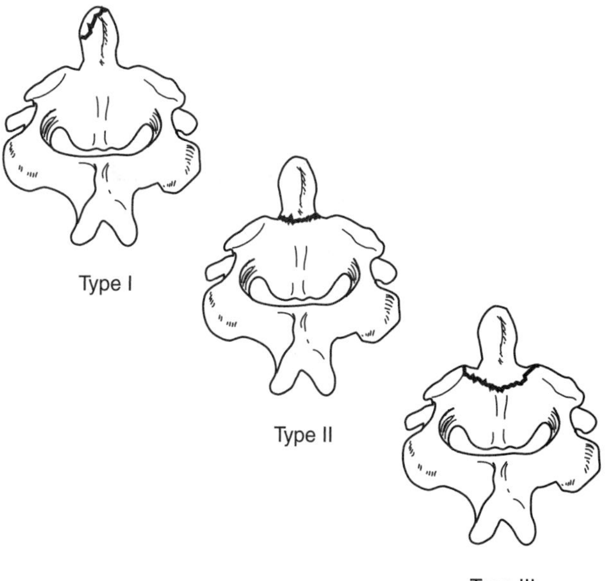

FIGURE 23-10 **Anderson and D'Alonzo classification of odontoid fractures.** Type I: fracture results from avulsion of the alar ligament. Type II: fractures are through the base of the odontoid separating it from the vertebral body. Type III: fractures occur through the C2 body.

considered for a combination of surgical and external stabilization.[30]

Traumatic spondylolisthesis of the axis, commonly referred to as hangman's fracture, is characterized by fractures through the neural arch and pedicles of the axis (C2) with possible displacement of C2 on C3. Given the large vertebral foramen of the high cervical spine and because the anterior and posterior elements generally separate, the majority of these fractures are without neurologic impingement. Treatment will vary depending on the severity of vertebral angulation, distraction, and facet dislocation.[30] Many fractures can be treated conservatively with external immobilization.[30,31]

SPINAL CORD INJURIES

Injury to the spinal cord results from direct or indirect insult. When direct insult occurs, such as when a missile or bone fragment impacts the cord, the physical severing of neural elements is clear. However, in many SCIs the damage results from the normal physiologic response to the concussive forces or impaired perfusion.

The concept of primary and secondary injuries, first proposed more than 80 years ago, has emerged as an explanation for the phenomenon of delayed neural injury.[32-34] A primary injury is the mechanical disruption that occurs to the spinal cord substance at the time of injury, whereas the progressive pathologic responses that occur subsequently over hours to days are known as secondary injury.[13,32-35] A number of factors, such as hypoxia and hypoperfusion, are known to trigger or exacerbate secondary SCI and worsen outcome. Although there is little that can be done to change the circumstances of the initial trauma, the outcome of the secondary injury may be amenable to therapeutic intervention. The intrinsic responses occurring during SCI have been well documented.[32-35] Understanding the cascade of events that ultimately lead to cellular death (necrosis) and the initiation of apoptosis is key to understanding the use of investigational agents to interrupt the sequence of biochemical interactions and improve neurologic outcomes (Figure 23-11).

Classification by Type of Injury

Types of SCI include concussion, contusion, laceration, transection, hemorrhage, and vascular disruption. A concussion of the spinal cord causes a temporary loss of function lasting no more than 24 to 48 hours. It produces a transient dysfunction of the spinal cord from jarring forces. A contusion of the spinal cord is actual bruising of the neural substance. It includes the intrinsic responses to bleeding, including edema, compression, ischemia, and possibly infarction. The severity of this injury depends on its size, location, and the physiologic response to the bleeding. A laceration is an actual tear in the cord, which results in permanent injury. Surrounding contusion and the normal physiologic response to injury accompany a tear. A transection is a complete severing of the neural elements. Complete transection results in the spinal cord being physically separated into two distinct pieces; this is a rare finding. However, in functional terms, a complete transection is frequently the result of significant injury. Hemorrhage into

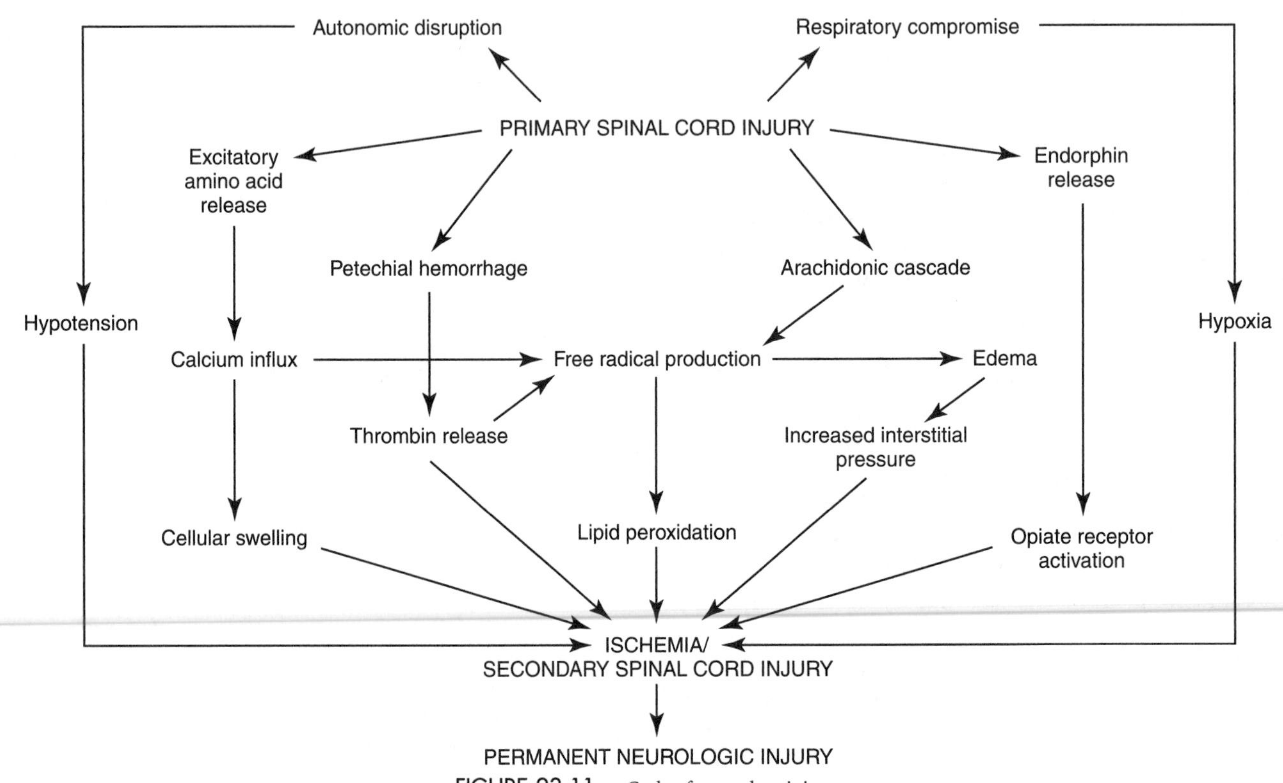

FIGURE 23-11 Cycle of secondary injury.

or around the spinal cord can compress the neural substance and initiate the intrinsic cascade. This may produce ischemia and neurologic deficits. Vascular disruption to the spinal cord causes a loss of blood flow to the neural substance and results in ischemic changes. The duration of ischemia is directly related to the neurologic outcome.[32-34]

Classification by Function

SCI can be classified as either complete or incomplete, according to functional outcome. In complete SCI, there is loss of all voluntary muscle control and sensation at and below the level of the lesion. Per the American Spinal Injury Association (ASIA), a complete SCI is defined as a loss of all voluntary muscle control and sensation in the sacral segments (S4-5); this definition simplifies classification of patients with asymmetric presentation or zones of partial preservation. Clinical implications depend on the level of injury. Injuries to the cervical spine, especially at and above C4, are typically the most life threatening secondary to the potential loss of diaphragmatic innervation and respiratory failure (Figure 23-12). Several functional outcome scales exist; the ASIA impairment scale, which uses an alphabetical system of A (complete) through E (normal), and the Functional Independence Measure (FIM), which assigns numeric value to specific functional tasks, are two of the most commonly used. Functional outcomes are covered in greater detail in the rehabilitation phase.

Classification by Spinal Cord Injury Clinical Syndrome

Incomplete spinal cord injuries are distinguished by partial preservation of neurologic function below the level of the lesion. Incomplete injuries can be grouped into several recognizable syndromes.

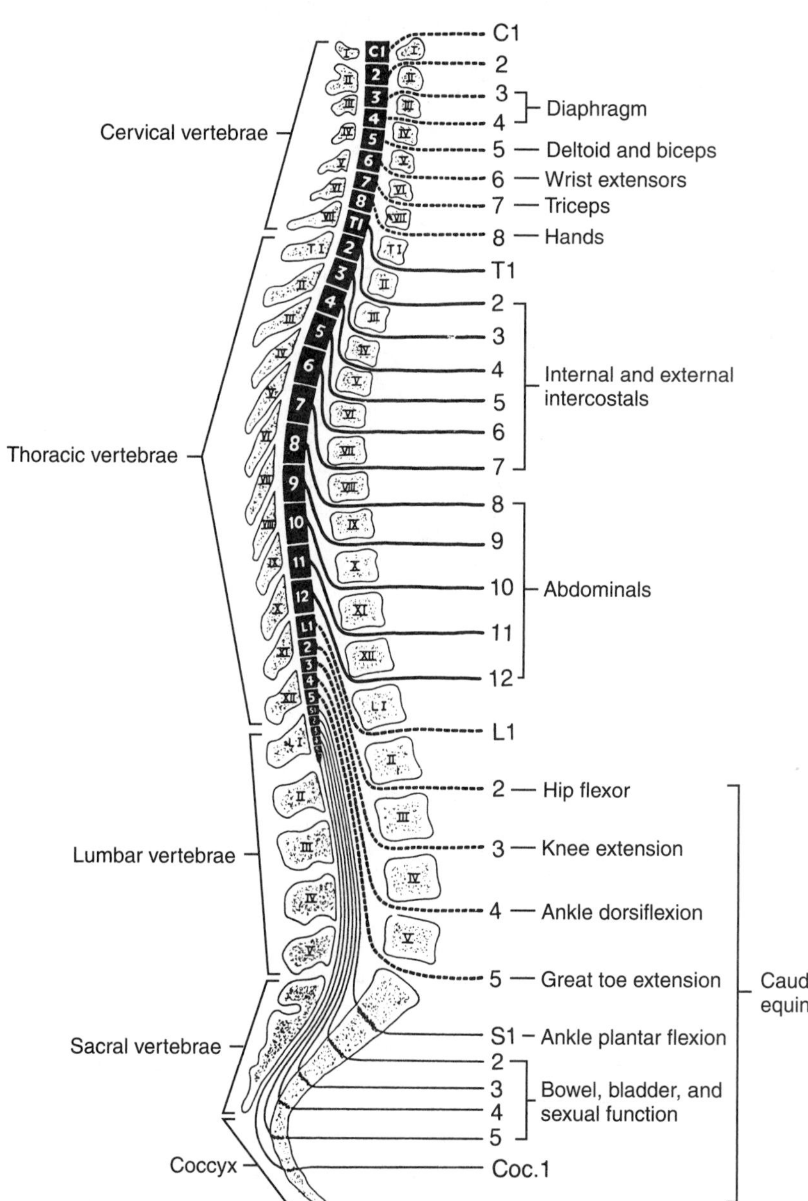

FIGURE 23-12 Spinal nerves emerging from the spinal cord through the intervertebral foramina and muscle movements that evaluate specific levels of spinal nerve function.

Anterior Cord Syndrome. Anterior cord syndrome is usually associated with flexion-dislocation injuries and may be associated with acute disk herniation.[13] An injury to the anterior part of the spinal cord or interruption of blood supplied by the anterior spinal artery results in ischemia to the anterior gray horn and the anterolateral columns of the white matter. There is usually complete motor loss accompanied by a loss of pain, temperature, and touch sensation at and below the level of the lesion. Light touch, proprioception, and vibration senses are preserved.[13,35] (Figure 23-13, *A*).

Central Cord Syndrome. The cardinal feature of central cord syndrome is a disproportionate loss of upper extremity motor function, especially fine motor movement, compared with the lower extremities. This usually occurs as the result of a hyperextension injury often seen in elderly persons who have experienced degenerative changes of the cervical spine (a natural result of aging).[13,35-40] Recent studies suggest that mechanical compression and selective injury to the lateral white matter columns that control the upper extremities may be the underlying pathogenesis for this syndrome.[36] Anatomically, the corticospinal tracts are arranged in such a way that the sacral fibers are most peripheral and the cervical fibers are most central. Thus, when contusion occurs, there is a decrease or loss of upper extremity motor function and a preservation of limb lower function (Figure 23-13, *B*). Bladder dysfunction and varied degrees of sensory loss may accompany this syndrome.[35-40] Similar to acute central cord syndrome is cruciate paralysis, in which an injury to descending corticospinal tracts as they decussate at the cervicomedullary junction results in weakness of upper extremities and relatively intact lower extremity function.[40,41] Radiologic studies including plain films, computed tomographic (CT) scans, and magnetic resonance imaging (MRI) aid in differentiating these disorders.[40,41]

Brown-Séquard Syndrome. Brown-Séquard syndrome results from a unilateral cord lesion. Ipsilateral motor deficit and loss of light touch, proprioception, and vibration sensations occur at and below the level of the lesion. There is, however, preservation of pain and temperature sensation on the same side as the SCI. On the opposite side, below the level of injury, there is nearly complete loss of pain and temperature sensations with preserved posterior column and motor function. This injury classically is caused by penetrating trauma that partially severs the spinal cord but may also result from nonpenetrating mechanisms, such as disk herniation, hyperextension injury, or unilateral articular process fracture-dislocation.[13,35] Partial Brown-Séquard syndrome can occur (Figure 23-13, *C*).

Posterior Cord Syndrome. Posterior cord syndrome is an extremely rare finding.[13,35] It is associated with hyperextension injury. In its purest form only the posterior column sensory functions are lost while motor function and pain and temperature sensation remain intact. Patients with this syndrome generally have excellent functional recovery.

Conus Medullaris Lesions. The conus medullaris is the distal portion of the spinal cord; it is the site of transition from the central nervous system to the peripheral nervous system. The termination point can be somewhat variable, but in most adults, the lumbar cord segments are anatomically located opposite the T12 vertebral body.[42] The majority of the sacral cord segments are opposite the L1 vertebral body. Over a lifetime, the vertebral levels that are in alignment with the lumbar and sacral nerve roots may become more caudal due to natural age-related changes of the bony spine.[42] Injuries at the T11-12 and T12-L1 levels are relatively common because of the great degree of mechanical flexibility that exists at these vertebral junctions. As a result, injuries to

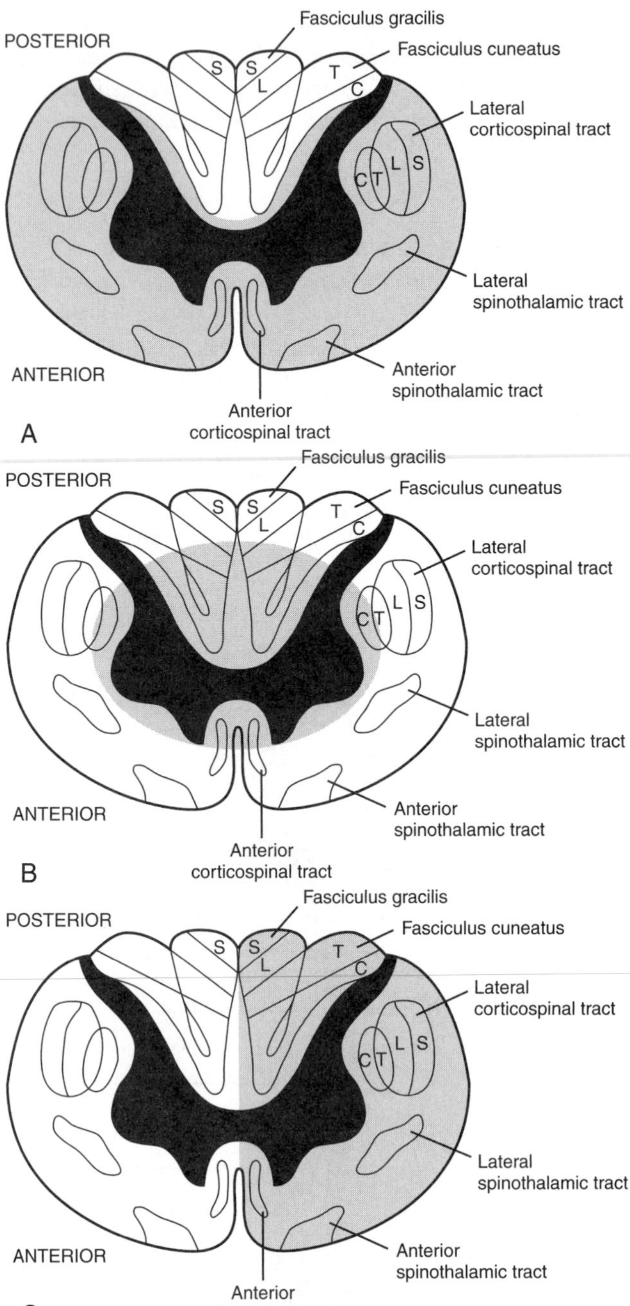

FIGURE 23-13 **Cross-sectional representation of the spinal cord syndromes. A,** Anterior cord syndrome. **B,** Central cord syndrome. **C,** Brown-Séquard syndrome. (From Browner BD, Levine AM, Jupiter JB et al, editors: *Skeletal Trauma: Fractures, Dislocations, Ligamentous Injuries,* ed 2, vol 1, Philadelphia, 1992, W.B. Saunders.)

the conus medullaris are frequent.[42] These injuries usually produce a combination of UMN and LMN deficits, including flaccid paralysis and muscle atrophy; in the chronic phase, spasticity and hyperreflexia may occur. The sensory involvement can be variable. In severe cases bowel and bladder deficits can be significant.

Cauda Equina Lesions. Cauda equina lesions involve injuries to the spinal nerve roots, usually resulting from direct fracture-dislocation trauma; disk herniation may or may not be present. The cauda equina is composed of LMNs, which originate from the spinal cord around the L1-2 disk space.[42,43] Injuries at or below this level involve the cauda equina nerve roots, although spinal origins of some roots may be affected by injuries one to two levels above L1-2. Nerve roots can be involved unilaterally or bilaterally. Saddle anesthesia; bowel, bladder, and sexual dysfunction; and progressive lower extremity weakness may be present.[42-44]

Prehospital Phase

Resuscitation of the patient with a spinal cord injury begins in the prehospital setting. The initial treatment priorities for the patient suspected of having SCI are the same as with all injured patients: (1) prevention of further injury to the patient and emergency personnel through rapid assessment of the scene and the patient; (2) initial spinal stabilization with an extrication collar; (3) extrication of the patient if necessary; (4) full systems assessment with emphasis on evaluation and interventions to ensure airway patency, ventilation, and circulation; (5) further stabilization of the spine and splinting of other fractures; and (6) transport to the nearest appropriate facility.

Examination at the scene provides rescue workers with important clues about the mechanism and pattern of suspected injury. A thorough assessment of the patient may be hampered by physical limitations, but a brief initial assessment of airway patency, ability to breathe, pulse, and level of consciousness, and a brief gross motor examination help determine how extrication should proceed. Simply because a patient appears neurologically intact does not mean a spinal injury does not exist. Any patient who has received a force to the head is at risk for SCI.[29,45-47]

Once the patient has been moved to a secure area, a detailed systems assessment is performed with strict attention given first to airway patency, effectiveness of breathing, and adequacy of circulation. Evidence of airway compromise, ineffective respiration, or inadequate circulation is remedied immediately to prevent hypoxia, hypercapnia, or hypoperfusion, which can precipitate systemic complications and exacerbate secondary SCI.[13,29,45,46] A brief assessment of the patient's neurologic status, including sensory and motor function, can then follow. When there is suspicion of SCI based on assessment findings or mechanism of injury, or if the patient is unable to cooperate with the examination due to other distracting injuries or altered level of consciousness, he is properly immobilized on a backboard with a hard cervical collar, head blocks, and forehead and chin straps or taping (Figure 23-14)[29,45-47] Recent investigations of selective prehospital cervical spine clearance suggest that an evidence-based cervical spine clearance protocol, coupled with prehospital medical provider training, may safely and successfully reduce the unnecessary implementation of full spinal immobilization for many patients with a mechanism of injury sufficient to produce cervical injury.[48-51] Finally, other body systems can be evaluated carefully for evidence of injury. Once the patient is assessed and initial spinal stabilization applied, the patient is closely monitored and rapidly transported to the nearest appropriate hospital.

Resuscitation Phase

While the patient is en route to the hospital and during admission into the acute care setting, information about the mechanism of injury, patient condition, treatment rendered, and patient response to interventions is obtained from prehospital care providers. On arrival at the hospital, a physical systems assessment is performed with attention again focusing on the airway, breathing, and circulation. Caution is used to avoid disruption of spinal alignment, which could further injure the spinal cord.

Assessment of the Spine and Neurologic Function

Once airway patency, effective ventilation, and adequate circulation are ensured, assessment shifts to evaluation of the patient's spine and neurologic function. The patient's clothing is carefully removed and he is inspected for evidence of injury. He should be log-rolled and the spinal

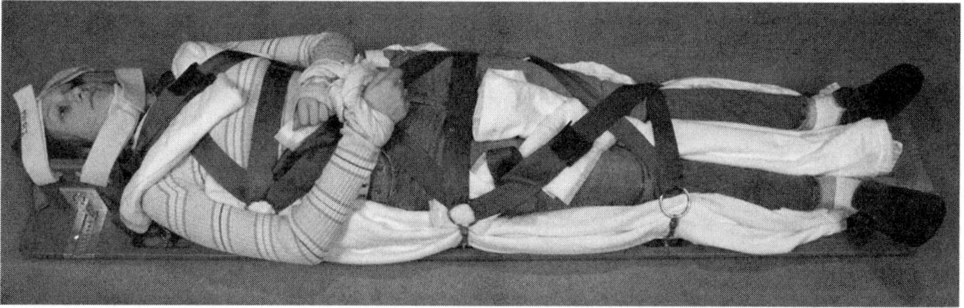

FIGURE 23-14 **Spinal immobilization.** Combined use of long board, head blocks, and a cervical hard collar for transport. (Photo provided by the Maryland Institute for Emergency Medical Services Systems.)

MUSCLE GRADING

0 total paralysis

1 palpable or visible contraction

2 active movement, full range of motion, gravity eliminated

3 active movement, full range of motion, against gravity

4 active movement, full range of motion, against gravity, and provides some resistance

5 active movement, full range of motion, against gravity, and provides normal resistance

5* muscle able to exert, in examiner's judgement, sufficient resistance to be considered normal if identifiable inhibiting factors were not present

NT not testable. Patient unable to reliably exert effort or muscle unavailable for testing due to factors such as immobilization, pain on effort, or contracture.

ASIA IMPAIRMENT SCALE

☐ **A = Complete:** No motor or sensory function is preserved in the sacral segments S4-S5.

☐ **B = Incomplete:** Sensory but not motor function is preserved below the neurologic level and includes the sacral segments S4-S5.

☐ **C = Incomplete:** Motor function is preserved below the neurologic level, and more than half of key muscles below the neurologic level have a muscle grade less than 3.

☐ **D = Incomplete:** Motor function is preserved below the neurologic level, and at least half of key muscles below the neurologic level have a muscle grade of 3 or more.

☐ **E = Normal:** Motor and sensory function are normal.

CLINICAL SYNDROMES (OPTIONAL)

☐ Central Cord
☐ Brown-Séquard
☐ Anterior Cord
☐ Conus Medullaris
☐ Cauda Equina

STEPS IN CLASSIFICATION

The following order is recommended in determining the classification of individuals with SCI.

1. Determine sensory levels for right and left sides.
2. Determine motor levels for right and left sides.
Note: in regions where there is no myotome to test, the motor level is presumed to be the same as the sensory level.
3. Determine the single neurologic level.
This is the lowest segment where motor and sensory function is normal on both sides, and is the most cephalad of the sensory and motor levels determined in steps 1 and 2.
4. Determine whether the injury is Complete or Incomplete (sacral sparing).
If voluntary anal contraction = **No** *AND all S4-5 sensory scores =* **0** *AND any anal sensation =* **No**, *then injury is COMPLETE. Otherwise injury is incomplete.*
5. Determine ASIA Impairment Scale (AIS) Grade:

Is injury Complete? If **YES**, AIS=A Record ZPP
(For ZPP record lowest dermatome or myotome on each side with some (non-zero score) preservation)

NO ↓

Is injury motor incomplete? If **NO**, AIS=B
(Yes=voluntary anal contraction OR motor function more than three levels below the motor level on a given side)

YES ↓

Are at least half of the key muscles below the (single) neurologic level graded 3 or better?

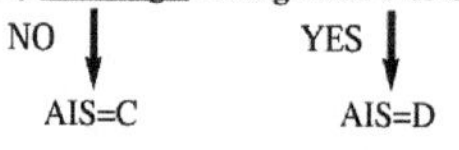

AIS=C AIS=D

If sensation and motor function is normal in all segments, AIS=E
Note: AIS E is used in follow-up testing when an individual with a documented SCI has recovered normal function. If at initial testing no deficits are found, the individual is neurologically intact; the ASIA Impairment Scale does not apply.

A

FIGURE 23-15 American Spinal Injury Association (ASIA)/International Spinal Cord Society (ISCOS) Standard Neurological Classification of Injury Worksheet. **A,** Definitions of muscle grading and ASIA impairment scale, and instructions for use of the ASIA classification tool.

column inspected for penetrating wounds, contusion, bulging, or obvious deformity, and palpated for tenderness and malalignment.[13,35,29,45,46]

A formal evaluation of neurologic function is performed. This examination includes assessment of motor, sensory, and reflex function. In the unconscious or uncooperative patient, observation of movement and response to noxious sensory stimuli are the only means of ascertaining spinal cord function on physical examination. A more thorough evaluation of motor and sensory function is done if the patient is able to follow commands reliably and can communicate sensory perceptions. It is important to assess both neurologic and functional abilities.[13,35,45,46,52,53] It is also recommended to use assessment scales that are widely accepted and have demonstrated strong interrater reliability, such as the ASIA motor and sensory scores and impairment scale and the FIM.[29,35,46,53] A comprehensive motor and sensory assessment evaluates three spinal tracts: the lateral corticospinal, lateral spinothalamic, and dorsal columns. The lateral corticospinal (motor) tract is evaluated by having the patient move all major muscle groups on both sides of the body, beginning with the deltoids and moving caudally. The strength of each movement should be graded using a 5-point scale (5 is normal and 1 is trace movement) (Figure 23-15, *A*). Assessment of proprioception, the ability to determine body position in space, evaluates dorsal column function. Proprioception is assessed by having the patient communicate if a limb or digit is being moved up or down. The lateral spinothalamic tract is evaluated by using a sterile needle to gently apply sharp stimuli and a blunt edge (head of a safety pin) to apply dull stimuli to determine if the patient can distinguish between the two in each sensory dermatome (Figure 23-15, B). Frequent examination with the use of a consistent grading system and documentation provides practitioners with an ability to monitor and communicate improvement or deterioration of function.

Reflex function is evaluated to determine sensory or motor sparing and to approximate the level of SCI. Specific nerve roots innervate each reflex. The major deep tendon reflexes (DTR) assessed are the biceps (C5–6), brachioradialis (C5–6), triceps (C7–8), quadriceps (knee jerk) (L3–4), and Achilles (S1–2). The following superficial or cutaneous reflexes should also be assessed: abdominal, cremasteric, bulbocavernosus, and superficial anal (Table 23-2). Rectal tone is evaluated to determine if sacral sparing is present. Priapism, a reflexive penile erection, may be noted initially in male patients with complete SCI.

Neurologic deficits and vital sign alterations caused by SCI can mask other systemic injuries. Intrathoracic,

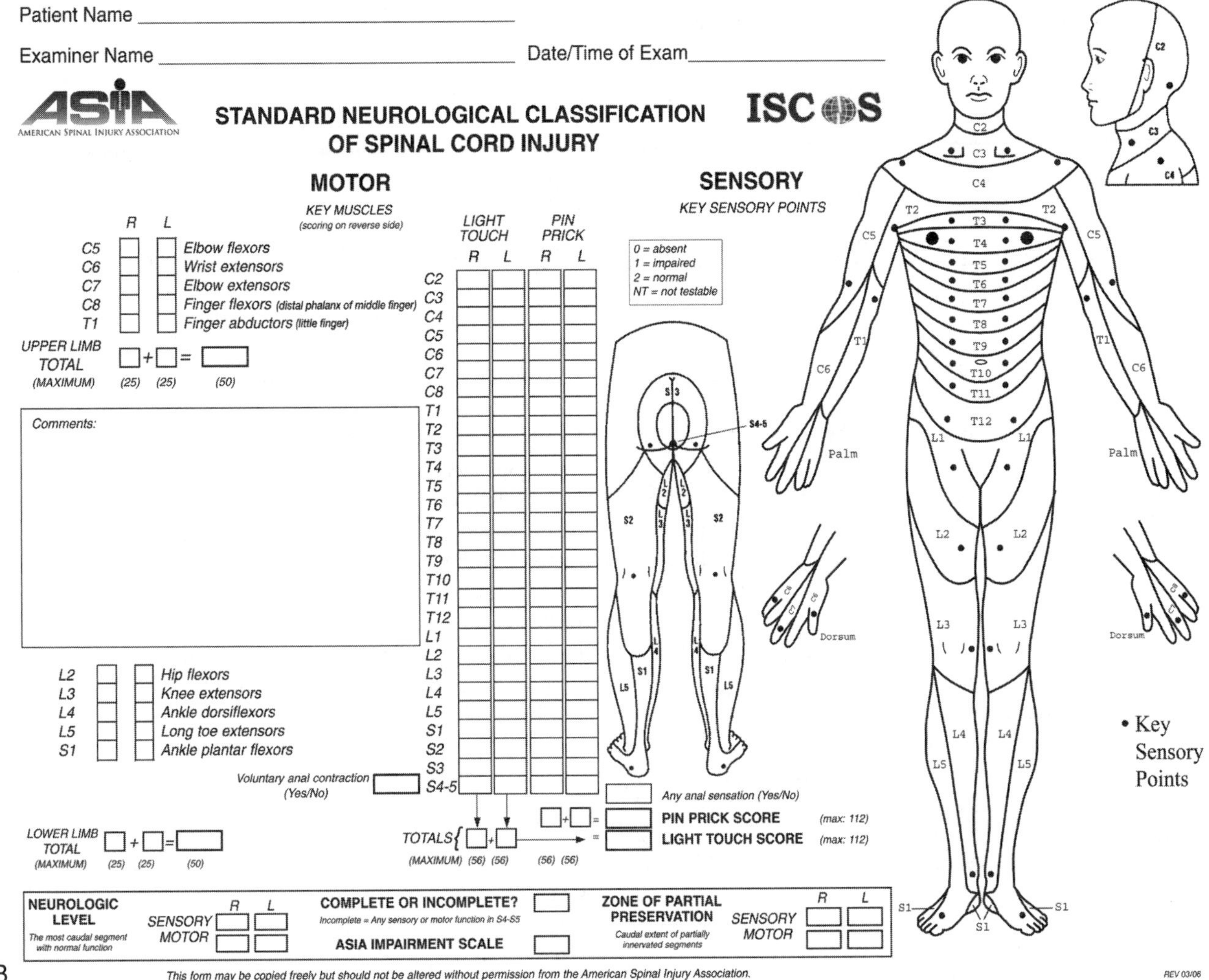

Patient Name ______________________

Examiner Name ______________________ Date/Time of Exam ______________________

ASIA
AMERICAN SPINAL INJURY ASSOCIATION

STANDARD NEUROLOGICAL CLASSIFICATION OF SPINAL CORD INJURY

ISCoS

MOTOR

KEY MUSCLES (scoring on reverse side)

	R	L	
C5	☐	☐	Elbow flexors
C6	☐	☐	Wrist extensors
C7	☐	☐	Elbow extensors
C8	☐	☐	Finger flexors (distal phalanx of middle finger)
T1	☐	☐	Finger abductors (little finger)

UPPER LIMB TOTAL ☐ + ☐ = ☐
(MAXIMUM) (25) (25) (50)

Comments:

	R	L	
L2	☐	☐	Hip flexors
L3	☐	☐	Knee extensors
L4	☐	☐	Ankle dorsiflexors
L5	☐	☐	Long toe extensors
S1	☐	☐	Ankle plantar flexors

Voluntary anal contraction (Yes/No) ☐

LOWER LIMB TOTAL ☐ + ☐ = ☐
(MAXIMUM) (25) (25) (50)

SENSORY

KEY SENSORY POINTS

	LIGHT TOUCH R	LIGHT TOUCH L	PIN PRICK R	PIN PRICK L
C2				
C3				
C4				
C5				
C6				
C7				
C8				
T1				
T2				
T3				
T4				
T5				
T6				
T7				
T8				
T9				
T10				
T11				
T12				
L1				
L2				
L3				
L4				
L5				
S1				
S2				
S3				
S4-5				

0 = absent
1 = impaired
2 = normal
NT = not testable

☐ Any anal sensation (Yes/No)

TOTALS ☐ + ☐ → ☐ LIGHT TOUCH SCORE (max: 112)
☐ + ☐ = ☐ PIN PRICK SCORE (max: 112)
(MAXIMUM) (56) (56) (56) (56)

NEUROLOGIC LEVEL		R	L
The most caudal segment with normal function	SENSORY	☐	☐
	MOTOR	☐	☐

COMPLETE OR INCOMPLETE? ☐
Incomplete = Any sensory or motor function in S4-S5

ASIA IMPAIRMENT SCALE ☐

ZONE OF PARTIAL PRESERVATION		R	L
Caudal extent of partially innervated segments	SENSORY	☐	☐
	MOTOR	☐	☐

REV 03/06

B

FIGURE 23-15 cont'd **B,** Assessment worksheet with sensory dermatomes, sensory and motor documentation by level, and neurologic summary, including ASIA impairment grade and zone of partial preservation. Available for downloading at http://asia-spinalinjury.org/publications/2006_Classif_worksheet.pdf

intraabdominal, and skeletal injuries may be present without the typical clinical findings of muscle rigidity or patient-reported pain. A thorough evaluation, including physical assessment, x-ray examination, CT scan, and other necessary diagnostic studies, should be performed as soon as possible to rule out associated injuries.[29,46,52] Hypotension and bradycardia associated with high SCI may mask signs of hemorrhagic shock. All potential sites of hemorrhage should be investigated.

DIAGNOSTICS

Radiographic assessment of the cervical spine is unnecessary in neurologically intact patients (i.e., Glasgow Coma Scale score of 15) who are unimpaired from drug or alcohol use, have a low suspicion or risk of injury, do not have an associated distracting injury or pain, and do not have neck pain or tenderness (including palpation and range-of-motion). For this population, clinical clearance is adequate to rule out injury.[54-56] In the symptomatic trauma patient or those at moderate to high risk for cervical injury, the standard of care is to obtain a three-view (anteroposterior, lateral, and odontoid) cervical spine series.[56-58] These pictures provide information about fractures and vertebral alignment. X-ray films can be obtained quickly at the patient's bedside, eliminating the need to transport the patient with suspected spinal injury. There are technical limitations with these films; therefore, they are rarely used alone to determine the extent of injury. The most common cause of missed injury is the failure to adequately visualize the region of injury.[57,58] Suboptimal films, including a failure to visualize from the occiput to T1, or suspicious areas should be supplemented with CT. AP and lateral films are considered the gold standard to evaluate the thoracic and lumbar spine.[59-64]

Reformatted CT, performed in sagittal, coronal, and axial planes, provides a close look at bony structures and disk integrity. Fractures are easily visualized, indicating high sensitivity and positive predictive value. The newer spiral CT

TABLE 23-2 **Cutaneous Reflexes, Level of Spinal Cord Innervation, and Method for Assessment**

Reflex	Spinal Nerve Innervation	Stimulus	Response
Abdominal	T8 - T12	Stroke upper and lower abdomen	Abdominal wall contracts, causing umbilicus to move toward the stimulus
Cremasteric	L1, L2	Stroke inner thigh	Testicular and scrotal elevation
Bulbocavernous	S3, S4	Squeeze the glans penis or clitoris	Anal sphincter contracts
Perianal	S3 - S5	Stroke perianal skin	Contraction of the anus

Adapted from McIlvoy L, Meyer K, McQuillan KA: Traumatic spine injuries. In Bader MK, Littlejohns L, editors: *AANN Core Curriculum for Neuroscience Nursing,* ed 4, St. Louis, 2004, Saunders.

scan allows rapid imaging and reconstruction into multiple planes and, given certain injury patterns and the degree of vertebral displacement, can infer ligamentous and cord injury.[59-64] CT can be particularly sensitive in detecting missed bony injuries of the midthoracic through lumbar spine associated with blunt trauma.[60-65] These thoracolumbar vertebral injuries can be difficult to detect on the two-view thoracic and lumbar plain film series. A growing body of evidence from studies comparing plain view radiographs to spiral CT in the detection of spinal injury suggests that in symptomatic patients, patients at significant risk for injury, or obtunded patients, spiral CT is superior to plain x-rays for the detection of spinal injury; and recommends that CT replace routine spine views as the initial screening test in this population.[60-70]

Ligamentous or soft tissue injuries cannot necessarily be excluded with the three-view cervical series and CT combination.[56,58] Dynamic flexion-extension radiographic views may be used to rule out ligamentous injury of the cervical spine in awake or obtunded patients.[56,58] These views require the awake patient to flex and extend his head and neck at least 30 degrees in each direction. When the patient is obtunded, using physician-directed dynamic fluoroscopy, the head and neck are manipulated at least 30 degrees in each direction. If adequate range of motion is achieved, information about maintenance of cervical alignment is obtained. Care must be taken by the physician during this procedure because dynamic fluoroscopy has not proven the ability to visualize ligaments or disks; it demonstrates alignment and intervertebral space changes during motion, which can infer ligamentous injury. Patients with herniated disks or stenosis are at potential risk for neurologic injury during manipulation. Recent studies assert that with the advent of CT scans with three-dimensional reconstruction and MRI, ligamentous and soft tissue injuries can be better visualized with less risk to the patient, particularly obtunded patients.[71-75]

MRI provides clear, distinct images in multiple planes without the use of radiation. This study is particularly valuable in evaluating the soft tissues of the spinal column, namely the disks, ligaments, and, most importantly, the spinal cord.[56,71] Changes in signal intensity provide the ability to see cord contusion, hemorrhage, or transection. Studies demonstrate that MRI is not particularly sensitive in detecting fractures and therefore, should not be performed in isolation.[58,59,71] Magnetic resonance angiography (MRA) enables physicians to visualize any vascular impingement or disruption, such as possible vertebral artery occlusion associated with cervical SCI.[76] The limitations of this technology are many. Because of the magnetic fields, many pumps and ventilators cannot be used in the scanning room. Any patient with metallic implants may not be able to enter the MRI field. Other disadvantages of MRI include high cost, long study time, relative inaccessibility, need for patient transport, and the inability to monitor the patient adequately within the bore of the magnet.[71] Most patients require a mild sedative to assist with overcoming the confines and noise of the scanner; any movement creates distortion of the images. If MRI is not available and vascular injury is suspected, CT angiography or conventional angiography may be performed.[58] Once a definitive diagnosis has been made, a plan for stabilization and management can be formulated.

Somatosensory evoked potential (SSEP) can be used to assess and monitor the integrity of the somatosensory pathway from the site of peripheral nerve stimulation to the cerebral cortex. Most often the ulnar or median nerve and the posterior tibial nerve are selected for stimulation, and cortical and subcortical responses are monitored via noninvasive scalp electrodes. SSEP is often used for intraoperative physiologic monitoring of the spinal cord, providing "real-time" information for surgeons regarding impending neurologic damage. Baseline studies are obtained preoperatively, and monitoring continues throughout the perioperative event. Sustained reductions in values alert the surgical team to possible mechanical or ischemic injury within the spinal cord, providing an opportunity to evaluate the patient immediately and, when possible, to take corrective action to reverse processes that may lead to permanent neurologic deficit.[77,78] SSEP monitoring is limited in that SSEPs only evaluate ascending sensory tracts, predominantly located in the dorsal columns.[77,78] To enhance cord monitoring, transcranial motor evoked potentials (TcMEPs) can be added. Transcranial electrical stimulation of the motor cortex monitors the anterior motor pathways.[77,78] Leads are placed on the scalp and over a muscle group in the hand, shin, and foot, bilaterally. In patients with significant preexisting deficits, the deltoids or biceps can also be used. In a manner similar to the SSEP, an impulse is delivered via the scalp leads and measured at the distal extremity leads. When used in conjunction with SSEPs, TcMEPs extend physiologic monitoring to provide information about evolving motor tract injury.[77,78]

SYSTEMS MANAGEMENT

Patients with acute SCI, especially cervical injury, require intensive monitoring and aggressive care to manage the complex systemic consequences. Optimally, these patients should be admitted to tertiary centers that specialize in care of SCIs. While no definitive evidence supports this as a standard of care, at minimum, these patients should be placed in an acute monitored setting with specific attention given to cardiac, hemodynamic, and respiratory function.[79]

Respiratory Insufficiency

If the patient is unable to maintain the airway or adequately ventilate, there is an increased risk of secondary hypoxic injury, particularly to the damaged cord. The jaw-thrust maneuver should be used in attempting to establish an airway in the unconscious patient with a potential cervical spine injury. When possible, patients unable to maintain their airway or ventilate adequately are intubated emergently. Every effort is made to avoid neck movement, especially hyperextension or flexion, during intubation. Manual in-line traction is applied to minimize neck motion.[29,45,46,52,80] Prevertebral swelling combined with less than optimal oroglottal alignment and impaired visualization can make intubation technically difficult in this population[80]; fiberoptic devices offer enhanced visualization and may facilitate successful intubation.[29,52,80]

When a spinal cord injury occurs at the high thoracic or cervical level, there can be paralysis of the intercostal muscles or diaphragm, which may lead to respiratory failure. The patient should be monitored for rate, depth, and pattern of breathing (use of accessory muscles or paradoxical breathing), strength and effectiveness of cough, and the ability to adequately oxygenate and ventilate. A chest film should be obtained to assess for underlying thoracic trauma, such as rib fractures, hemothorax, pneumothorax, or pulmonary contusion, as well as aspiration or atelectasis.[52,81,82] The chest film also evaluates diaphragm position. Intermittent arterial blood gases (ABGs) and continuous pulse oximetry and, when possible, end-tidal carbon dioxide should be monitored. In addition to these studies, vital capacity and tidal volume can be assessed. In most patients with a vital capacity less than 1 L (approximately 10 to 15 ml/kg), respiratory fatigue and failure can be anticipated.[29,52,81,82] Patients with declining or poor respiratory parameters are candidates for respiratory support. The use of mechanical ventilation, whether invasive or noninvasive, should be implemented to prevent hypoxia and further spinal cord insult.[52,79,81,82] Patients with complete injuries at C4 and above require invasive mechanical ventilation; most of these patients will remain ventilator-dependent for life.[82]

Spinal Shock

Spinal shock occurs when there is a loss of continuous tonic impulses from the brain, causing a transient suppression of reflexes below the SCI. Spinal shock is manifested as follows: (1) flaccid paralysis, (2) absence of cutaneous/proprioceptive sensation, (3) loss of autonomic function, and (4) deep suppression or cessation of all reflex activity below the site of injury. The degree of severity often is associated with the level of injury. Onset of spinal shock typically occurs at or near the time of injury, but there is a lack of consensus regarding duration.[83] If duration criteria are based upon the return of deep tendon reflexes, spinal shock generally lasts a few days to weeks.[83,84] If the resolution is based upon the return of any reflex, then spinal shock lasts no longer than a few hours, because hyporeflexive cutaneous responses (e.g., bulbocavernous, superficial anal, and cremasteric reflexes) may return within several hours of injury. A newer model of spinal shock proposed by Ditunno et al.[83] defines this phenomenon as a continuum or series of evolving phases, beginning with the loss or deep depression of reflexes and ending with the return of deep tendon reflexes and development of spasticity (hyperreflexia) below the level of injury (Table 23-3). Based upon this model, it can take up to a year for spinal shock to fully resolve.[83]

Neurogenic Shock

Neurogenic shock is the inadequate tissue perfusion that results from the cardiovascular events triggered by SCI at or above the T6 level. Studies suggest that cardiovascular dysfunction results from SCI that affects the posterior aspect of the dorsolateral funiculus (white matter) where the descending vasomotor tracts pass.[85] These sympathoexcitatory neurons provide input to the sympathetic preganglionic neurons located within the gray matter (intermediolateral column) of the thoracolumbar segments (T1-L2).[86,87] In the acute phase of shock, this abrupt loss of sympathetic innervation caused by a high thoracic or cervical SCI produces loss of vasomotor reflexes. Loss of vascular tone causes vasodilation, decreased systemic vascular resistance, and lowered blood pressure. Hypotension and decreased venous return lower cardiac output and reduce tissue perfusion.

Neurogenic shock must be appropriately treated to prevent hypoperfusion of the injured spinal cord, which can exacerbate secondary SCI. Increased intravenous fluid administration, the first-line therapy, rarely results in the necessary rise in central venous pressure and may lead to hypervolemia, pulmonary edema, and increased swelling of the injured spinal cord.[52] Blood pressure is managed with crystalloid administration and, once intravascular volume has been optimized, vasoactive agents (e.g., phenylephrine, dopamine) or inotropes (e.g., dobutamine) are introduced.[29,35,52,85-87] Care must be taken to avoid overcorrection of blood pressure, which could result in hyperemia, increased swelling of adjacent spinal tissues, and a greater reduction of blood flow to the area of injury.[52] Placement of a

TABLE 23-3 Ditunno's Phases of Spinal Shock

Phase*	Initiation/Duration	Presentation
Phase I	Day 0-1	Absence of DTRs Flaccid paralysis Appearance of DPR Autonomic dysfunction May see early return of cutaneous reflexes: BC, SA, and CM
Phase II	Day 1-3	Increasing strength of cutaneous reflexes May see some early return of DTRs in children and elderly
Phase III	Day 4-1 month	Return of DTRs Loss of DPR in most patients Improved autonomic function—decreased vagal mediation of profound bradyarrhythmias and hypotension Appearance of autonomic dysreflexia
Phase IV	Month 1-Year 1	Cutaneous reflexes, DTRs, and BS become hyperresponsive Detrusor sphincter reflex returns Continued stabilization of autonomic function, heart rate, and hypotension

*Should be viewed as a continuum with areas of overlap rather than phases in isolation.
CM, cremasteric reflex; *BC,* bulbocavernous reflex; *BS,* Babinski sign; *DPR,* delayed plantar response; *DTR,* deep tendon reflex; *SA,* superficial anal reflex
Adapted from Ditunno JF, Little JW, Burns AS: Spinal shock revisited: a four-phase model, *Spinal Cord* 42:383-395, 2004.

central venous catheter or a pulmonary artery catheter is desirable to gain information about intravascular volume and facilitate administration of vasoactive or inotropic agents. After an extensive review of the literature, the *Guideline* authors concluded that there was insufficient evidence to support development of a standard of care for the management of blood pressure after acute spinal cord injury. However, the group recommended two options for care: (1) systolic blood pressure below 90 mm Hg should be avoided, and (2) maintain a mean arterial pressure of 85 to 90 mm Hg for the first 7 days after injury to provide adequate blood flow to the injured spinal cord and ensure end-organ perfusion.[88] As with any other injured organ, autoregulatory function of the spinal cord may become impaired and perfusion of the cord may become dependent upon mean arterial pressure.[52] A noninvasive blood pressure monitor or an arterial line should be used to provide continuous information on the patient's response to therapy.

Bradycardia, seen with high thoracic or cervical lesions, results from the inhibition of the sympathetic cardiac accelerator fibers and unopposed parasympathetic vagal outflow.[52,86,87] This bradycardia may not be harmful to the patient, because cardiac output is maintained through increased stroke volume secondary to decreased systemic vascular resistance (SVR). When the heart rate declines below a level sufficient to maintain adequate tissue perfusion, the patient becomes symptomatic. The patient's heart rate and rhythm should be monitored continuously. The use of alpha agents to restore vascular tone facilitates the maintenance of venous return and may provide some support for the heart rate.[29,35,52,85-87] In cases of symptomatic bradycardia, administration of a positive chronotropic drug, such as atropine, may be needed.[29,35,52] In spinal cord injuries below T4, tachycardia may develop.

Temperature Regulation

Poikilothermia, a condition in which body temperature varies with the environment around it, occurs after SCI because of a disruption between the sympathetic nervous system and its control center in the hypothalamus. The lack of sympathetic function produces vasodilation, which promotes loss of body heat and inactivates the sweat glands that cool the body. Muscle paralysis eliminates shivering or muscle contractions to generate heat. Many patients arrive at the hospital with hypothermia. This may further depress heart rate and cardiac function. Frequent or continuous monitoring of the patient's body temperature is advised. Gentle warming with a hyperthermia blanket and warmed intravenous fluids will help restore core body temperature. Care must be taken to prevent overwarming.

Urinary Retention

The abrupt disruption of the spinal cord and the onset of spinal shock renders the bladder atonic. Acute urinary retention develops. Placement of an indwelling catheter permits drainage of the bladder and monitoring of urinary output.[29,35,52] Intermittent catheterization is generally not performed at this time because of the high urinary output that results from volume resuscitation.

Skin Integrity

Patients with suspected SCIs are transported on a rigid backboard to support the spinal elements. While conferring the desired immobility of the spine, it also produces pressure to multiple points along the spine, most specifically the sacral area.[47,48,89] Extrication collars, designed to be an inexpensive, easily applied means for cervical immobilization, also present significant risk to skin integrity.[47,89] The constant pressure coupled with the hypotensive state after injury reduces blood flow to the tissues, putting the patient at high risk for skin breakdown. Most SCI patients are insensate and unable to perceive pain and pressure below the level of SCI. Significant pressure sores can delay surgery if they develop in the area of surgical approach or if they become infected. It is prudent to remove the patient from the backboard and, if long-term collar use is anticipated, transition to a well-fitted and padded cervical collar as soon as possible.

Pain and Anxiety

Fear may be the greatest problem for the conscious patient. Frequent verbal and physical contact with the patient to provide information and offer reassurance can reduce feelings of anxiety, fear, and helplessness. He or she should be touched in areas where sensation remains. Patient-family contact should occur as soon as feasible. Cautious use of sedation is advised to prevent impairment of the sensorimotor examination, reduction of blood pressure, and depression of respiratory drive. Anxiety also heightens the pain experience.

Spinal cord–injured patients may experience bony pain from fractures, muscle and soft tissue pain, or neurogenic pain. Appropriate pain management should be implemented with the same precautions as for sedation. The use of short-acting, reversible medications is generally recommended in the emergent phase of care.

Pharmacologic Intervention to Reduce Secondary SCI and Optimize Outcome

Medical management of a patient with spinal cord injury is aimed at limiting secondary SCI by reducing and stabilizing the bony injury and maintaining tissue perfusion and oxygenation. Much of the treatment to optimize perfusion and oxygenation is focused on the support of other body systems. Despite much research, few drugs have demonstrated effectiveness in limiting secondary injury and improving outcomes of SCI patients. The current modalities can be loosely divided into several categories based upon their primary mechanism or site of action. Although these classifications are simplistic, most potential therapeutic strategies initiate a complex interaction that results in a combination of effects at the cellular level to attenuate spinal cord injury.

Neuroprotection

Steroids. Although the exact mechanism of action is unclear, glucocorticoids such as methylprednisolone have multiple theoretical effects derived from their ability to attenuate the inflammatory response and provide an antioxidant effect. Benefits may include suppression of vasogenic edema, enhancement of spinal cord blood flow, stabilization of lysosomal membranes, alteration of electrolyte concentrations in injured tissue, and inhibition of lipid peroxidation and cell membrane destruction.[7,32,33,52,90-94] Use of corticosteroids for SCI gained significant momentum in 1990, when Bracken et al published the results of the National Acute Spinal Cord Injury Studies (NASCIS) II trial supporting the use of methylprednisolone sodium succinate (MPSS) in acute non-penetrating SCI.[90-92] The NASCIS II trial was a multiinstitutional, randomized, double-blind study in which patients were randomized into one of three treatment arms—methylprednisolone, naloxone, or control—within 12 hours of injury. The authors concluded that the group receiving MPSS demonstrated improved neurologic outcomes at 6 weeks and at 6 months after injury if administered *within 8 hours of injury*.[92] A later clinical trial (NASCIS III) investigating the use of methylprednisolone concluded that patients initiated on the steroid protocol within 3 hours of injury should receive 24 hours of therapy, whereas patients initiated on therapy 3 to 8 hours after injury should receive steroids for 48 hours. Patients who received the 48-hour treatment were more likely to improve one full neurologic grade (ASIA) at 6 weeks and at 6 months. The authors also observed that these same patients experienced more severe sepsis and pneumonia than patients who receive methylprednisolone for only 24 hours.[93] (Table 23-4 describes guidelines for this protocol.)

The conclusions of the NASCIS II and III studies are highly controversial.[90,91,94-97] Criticism has focused upon several key points: results reporting, lack of standardization of medical management, and functional outcomes measurement.[90,94] Subsequent studies have been undertaken to address some

TABLE 23-4 Guidelines for Methylprednisolone Treatment

Loading dose: $\dfrac{\text{30 mg/kg} \times \text{(pt weight in kg)}}{\text{(mg/ml on drip concentration)}} = \text{Total bolus dosage (ml)}$

Set infusion pump to deliver total bolus in 15 minutes. Then proceed with maintenance infusion.

Maintenance dose: $\dfrac{\text{5.4 mg/kg} \times \text{(pt weight in kg)}}{\text{(mg/ml based on drip concentration)}} = \text{Maintenance dosage per hour (ml)*}$

Set infusion pump to deliver hourly maintenance dose for 23 to 47 hours.†

Note: Reconstitute methylprednisolone in sterile water to a concentration of 50 mg/ml.

*If drug infusion is inadvertently stopped, new flow rates are calculated so that the remaining drug can be administered within the time remaining for the originally planned infusion schedule.

†Treatment started within 3 hours of injury delivers a total of 24 hours of therapy; treatment started within 3 to 8 hours after injury delivers a total of 48 hours of therapy.

of these issues and although the results "suggest" neurologic benefit when MPSS is given within 8 hours of injury,[98,99] they have failed to convincingly prove that MPSS improves outcomes.[94,97] As a result, the *Guidelines* do not recommend the use of steroids as a standard of care, but offer its use as "an option that should only be undertaken with the knowledge that the evidence suggesting harmful side effects is more consistent than any suggestion of clinical benefit."[94]

Preventing Apoptosis. Apoptosis or programmed cell death is the result of a complex interaction of biochemical events, a subcycle within the cycle of secondary injury. Reduced blood flow resulting from injury and shock can lead to anaerobic cellular metabolism and a rise in local glutamate concentration, which results in a subsequent dysfunction of the normal cellular ionic gating mechanisms (NMDA receptors).[32-34,90,100] This facilitates an influx of calcium. A bifurcated pathologic pathway ensues; one direction culminates in cellular necrosis, the other in apoptosis. Rising intracellular calcium activates calpains mediating apoptosis. Calpains, calcium-activated proteases, play a role in the breakdown of the cytoskeleton.[7,32-34,90,100] This loss of cellular structure is an early event in the apoptotic process. Caspases, proteases activated by proteolysis, mediate apoptosis by cleaving other proteins. When apoptosis is initiated and a cell dies, it influences surrounding cells, extending the area of secondary injury.[7,32-34,90,100] As apoptotic bodies are released, macrophages infiltrate the area to phagocytize the debris. This leads to further cavitation of the spinal cord beyond the initial area of necrosis.[32-34,90,100]

A number of pharmacologic agents that may halt apoptosis are under investigation. Medications that can inhibit glutamate-induced processes, such as the NMDA receptor antagonist, dizocilpine (MK 801, Merck), or gangliosides (see below) may prove helpful.[32,33,90] As calcium is implicated in the activation of calpains, it has been postulated that reducing the transcellular flux of calcium into the cells might interrupt early proapoptotic events. Nimodipine, a calcium channel blocker, has been investigated; however, clinical trials have failed to demonstrate any benefit in neurologic outcomes.[90]

Miscellaneous Neuroprotective Agents

Other pharmacologic agents targeting various points in the cycle of secondary injury/ischemia have also been investigated. These agents include 21-aminosteroids, or lazaroid, and opiate antagonists. Antioxidants, such as tirilazad, scavenge lipid peroxyl and superoxide radicals and inhibit lipid peroxidation.[32,90] Opiate antagonists, such as naloxone, theoretically prevent the release of endorphins and improve microcirculation of the injured cord.[32,52,90] So far, neither agent has demonstrated benefit in treatment of SCI. Ionic channel antagonists that prevent transcellular shift of electrolytes may also be neuroprotective. Sodium channel blockade, which may prevent intracellular movement of sodium and subsequently water, is currently under laboratory investigation. In animal models, tetrodotoxin (TTX), administered into the spinal cord via microinjections, has demonstrated neuroprotection of white matter and improved functional outcomes.[32,90] Riluzole (Rilutek, Sanofi-Aventis, Bridgewater, N.J., USA), approved by the Food and Drug Administration (FDA) for the treatment of amyotrophic lateral sclerosis (ALS), has demonstrated similar benefits in animal SCI models.[90,91] Some newer agents have generated interest based upon their beneficial effects in animal model studies. Recombinant human erythropoietin (rhEPO) has demonstrated multiple potentially beneficial properties in the setting of spinal and brain injury, including antiinflammatory, antioxidant, and antiapoptotic.[90,101] Minocycline, a synthetic derivative of the drug tetracycline, has been shown to inhibit glutamate excitotoxicity and caspase activity (antiapoptotic), reduce inducible nitric oxide synthase (antioxidant capacity), and attenuate activation of microglia.[34,90,102,103] Because these drugs have current FDA approval for use in humans for other disease states, the safety profiles are well established and may facilitate the implementation of Phase I clinical trials.

Neural Regeneration

Gangliosides. Research also has been focused on attempting to identify pharmacologic agents that promote neurologic regeneration. GM-1 ganglioside, or Sygen (Fidia Pharmaceutical Corporation, Washington, D.C.), which may prevent apoptosis and augment and promote neural outgrowth, plasticity, and synaptic transmission, has demonstrated the ability to enhance recovery of white matter tracts to the lower extremities.[104] This finding suggests that the agent improved the function of axons traversing the injury site but had no effect on the gray matter at the level of injury.[32,52,90,94,104] Building upon the success of a small ganglioside trial,[105] The Sygen Study Group initiated a large Phase II multicenter double-blind trial. The primary efficacy criterion was the proportion of patients with marked recovery at week 26. Geisler et al concluded that although "the time course of recovery suggests earlier attainment of marked recovery in the Sygen-treated patients, regardless of their baseline severity," the multicenter trial failed to demonstrate any improved patient outcomes at 26 weeks with Sygen use.[104] Therefore, GM1-ganglioside can only be recommended as an option in the care of acute spinal cord injury without demonstrated clinical benefit.[94] A secondary finding was yielded from the study data. All patients in the study received MPSS per the NASCIS III protocol; however, none of the patients in the control/placebo arm demonstrated the same motor improvements as those in the original NASCIS III trial.[94,104] This finding brought forth further questions about the validity of the NASCIS II and III conclusions.

Cell Transplantation. SCI results in death of neural tissue, leaving a "gap" in the spinal cord. A large body of research has focused on the efficacy of transplanting various types of cells into the site of SCI to bridge the area unable to transmit nerve impulses. Research is currently focused on Schwann cells, olfactory ensheathing cells (OEC), stem cells, and astrocyte transplantation. Embryonic tissue or a synthetic combination of hydrogel and cells has been used to create a bridge that aids axonal elongation across the spinal lesion. While modest results have been achieved, research has demonstrated the potential of these therapies. The outcomes also reinforce that because SCI involves a cascade of events that damage the neural elements, therapeutic intervention will also require a combination of strategies to effect repair.

Miscellaneous. In addition to gangliosides, other experimental interventions have been studied regarding neural regeneration. Historically, it has been held that injured CNS tissue did not possess the ability to regenerate. It now appears that many therapeutic interventions can promote crucial aspects of outgrowth, guidance, target recognition, and synaptic stabilization in the laboratory setting. Recently, results of the Phase I trial were published demonstrating the safety of the Procord.[106] Procord (Proneuron Biotechnologies, Delaware USA / Proneuron Biotechnologies Cell Center, Ness-Ziona, Israel) is a protocol that involves injecting incubated autologous macrophages into the area of SCI.[106] Because of CNS-specific structures (e.g., blood-brain barrier), the immune system has limited access and function within the spinal cord. It has been suggested that macrophages injected into the injury site phagocytically clear myelin debris and secrete growth factors that promote a more positive environment for axonal regrowth.[32,34,106] In simple terms, it is postulated that neural deterioration is decreased and regeneration is promoted through immunomodulation of the spinal cord. Based upon the Phase I results, a Phase II multicentered trial has been initiated.[106]

Animal laboratory studies have demonstrated the ability of applied voltage currents to stimulate and direct axon growth. A Phase I trial using the Oscillating Field Stimulator (OFS) is currently under way.[107] Within 18 days of injury, three electrodes are placed one level above the level of SCI and three are placed one level below to intermittently provide the oscillating field stimulation. Based upon the results of the initial participants; permission has been granted to expand enrollment to include an additional 10 participants. Whether these trials demonstrate unequivocal outcomes remains to be seen. At minimum, they demonstrate that neural regrowth is a realistic goal for the future.

Spinal Column Alignment and Stabilization

A plan for spinal realignment, decompression, and stabilization is established as soon as possible once the diagnostic evaluation of the spinal column and cord is complete. Surgical or nonsurgical interventions may be required. The choice of surgical intervention versus conservative nonoperative management is controversial and is determined in part by physician preference.[29,108-112] Most physicians base their treatment decision on the mechanism of injury, the neurologic status, the structural dysfunction of the spine, and the patient's medical history and current condition.

The "hard" neck collar is usually maintained on patients throughout resuscitation and until a cervical spine injury is ruled out or stabilized in another way. In patients with an unstable cervical spine injury, cervical traction may be applied to assist in immobilizing the spine, realigning the vertebrae, and relieving spinal cord compression.[29,108-111] This can be accomplished with application of tongs or a halo ring; today, most apparatuses are fabricated with MRI-compatible materials to facilitate care. Initial weight for cervical injuries below C2 is 3 pounds per vertebral level (e.g., C5 = 3 pounds × 5 for 15 pounds).[108] Subsequent weight is added gently and steadily, in 5- to 10-pounds increments, to the in-line traction.[29,46] To prevent overdistraction or worsening of alignment, sequential neurologic examinations and radiologic evaluation should be performed after each traction manipulation. Radiologic evaluation may be performed either by lateral radiography after each manipulation or with the use of the C-arm fluoroscope. Once reduction and alignment are achieved, the weights are reduced to the minimal amount necessary to maintain alignment and stability. A wedge turning frame (Figure 23-16) or kinetic bed (Figure 23-17) may be used to permit pressure relief and prevent pulmonary complications while maintaining cervical traction and spinal immobility. Care must be taken to maintain cervical traction by keeping the weights hanging freely and the traction rope knot away from the traction pulley. If necessary, the patient can be pulled down in bed by several people but can never be pulled up because traction would be lost.

For stabilizing injuries below the cervical level, various types of braces can be used. Until the brace is applied, the patient is typically maintained on bed rest with the head of the bed flat. If the patient cannot be log-rolled, a specialty bed, such as a wedge turning frame or a kinetic bed, should be considered for mobilization.

Patients can be transported while maintaining spinal alignment by using the scoop or breakaway stretcher. This device separates into two halves that can be slid beneath the patient being log-rolled side to side. The two sides connect

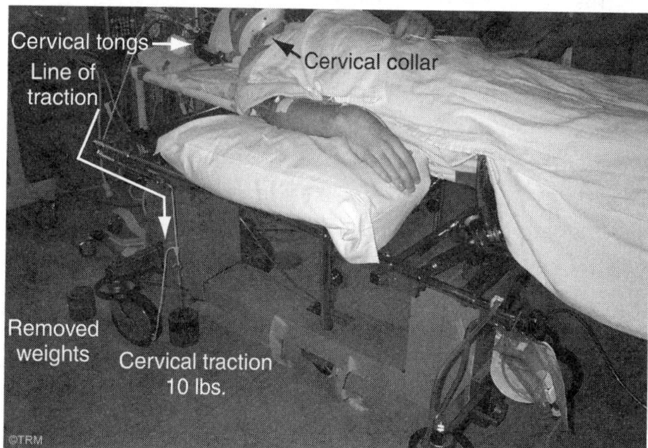

FIGURE 23-16 **The Stryker wedge turning frame.** Patient on the Stryker wedge turning frame with cervical traction. Note weights have been decreased to minimum amount necessary to maintain reduction and alignment.

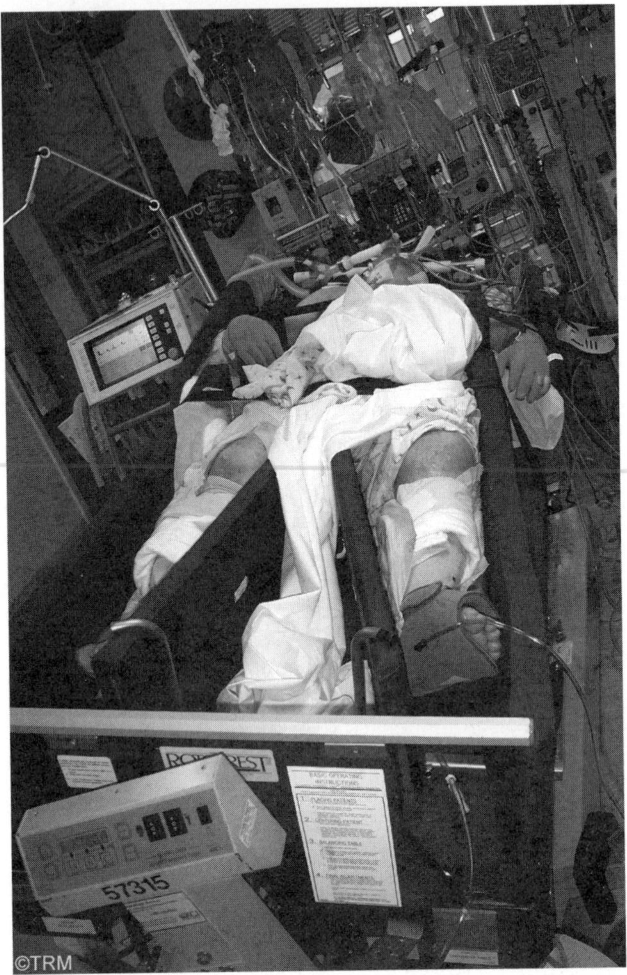

FIGURE 23-17 **The Rotorest kinetic therapy bed.** Use of Rotorest bed to maintain spinal precautions while providing some mobility to reduce the complications associated with prolonged bed rest in the enforced supine position. The degree and pattern of lateral rotation is set by the clinician.

at the head and feet to form a complete lifting device. Patients in cervical traction can be transported by having the physician maintain manual traction while log-rolling the patient onto an in-line traction board and connecting him or her to the traction weights or a traction wheel.

The timing of surgical intervention is controversial.[29,109-112] When it is not possible to reduce the spine with traction, further intervention is required to realign the spinal column and decompress the spinal cord, thereby promoting blood flow to the injured area. There is a window of opportunity to safely surgically reduce a patient within the first 72 hours after injury. After this period, the window closes because the spinal cord is extremely refractory to any manipulation because of edema and circulatory changes. The window opens again after 7 days. Early intervention, historically defined as within the first 72 hours, might improve neurologic recovery, facilitate early mobilization to reduce complication rates, decrease hospitalization time, and lower overall costs.[109-112] More recent literature has redefined early surgery as within 24 hours.[112] Advocates of delayed surgery argue that early operative intervention may increase the risk of neurologic deterioration or cause cardiopulmonary instability that compromises recovery. They also point out that early fixation failed to demonstrate improved overall outcomes in initial trials and may be prohibited by the lack of necessary resources at the admitting hospital.[29,109-112] In 2004, McKinley et al published the results of a large multicenter review that demonstrated no significant difference in neurologic outcomes based on timing of surgery; however, complications, length of stay, and hospitals costs were higher for patients who had delayed surgery.[109] A clear candidate for emergent surgical intervention is the patient with neurologic deterioration who displays evidence of spinal cord compression from bone or disk fragments, vertebral malalignment, or hematoma.[108-112]

The Operative Phase

The goals of surgical intervention are to decompress the spinal cord, align and stabilize the bony column, and promote early mobilization. This may be accomplished through the removal of bone fragments, hematoma, or extruded disk; vertebral realignment; and spinal fusion. Placement of a bone graft to maintain disk spacing, in conjunction with the use of instrumentation such as plates, screws, wires, cables, or rods, may be necessary to maintain alignment and stability until the vertebral column fuses. External orthotic devices such as a collar, halo vest, or thoracolumbar jacket may be used as adjunctive treatment to promote spinal immobilization until vertebral fusion is complete.

Care of the spinal cord–injured patient in the operative phase is the same as for any patient. Strict attention is given to respiratory, hemodynamic, body temperature, and neurologic responses. Adequate respiratory gas exchange and blood pressure must be ensured throughout the operative phase. Hemoglobin and hematocrit levels should be monitored during and after surgery. This is especially true for patients undergoing thoracic and lumbar procedures that are likely to involve large volumes of blood loss. Succinylcholine is avoided as part of balanced anesthesia in SCI patients because it may cause dangerous elevations in serum potassium levels. Postoperative sensorimotor evaluations and follow-up x-ray films are performed to detect any changes from the preoperative assessment findings.

The Critical Care Phase

Patients diagnosed with acute SCI, particularly those with cervical or high thoracic injury that require frequent respiratory and hemodynamic monitoring and intervention, are typically transferred to the intensive care unit following initial resuscitation. The patient with acute SCI should be approached as a multitrauma patient, because injury to the central nervous system affects all body systems. The goal of care is to prevent further secondary injury and neurologic deterioration. Prevention, prompt recognition, and appropriate treatment of systemic complications reduce the risk of secondary SCI and help optimize patient outcomes. These goals are best met with the use of a multidisciplinary team approach that includes physicians; nurses; respiratory, physical, occupational, and speech therapists; nutritionists; pharmacists; and social workers.

RESPIRATORY IMPLICATIONS

Injuries to the cervical or thoracic spinal cord may affect innervation to muscles used for respiration (Table 23-5). In normal respiration the inspiratory phase is an active process in which the diaphragm contracts and descends, increasing the vertical diameter of the thoracic cavity. The external intercostals elevate the ribs, causing an increase in the lateral and anteroposterior diameter. These events produce a negative pressure gradient, drawing air into the lungs. Expiration is usually passive unless a defensive process such as a cough or sneeze is required. During forced expiration the abdominal muscles contract, driving the diaphragm upward and causing the internal intercostals to contract. In a spinal cord-injured patient, paralysis of these muscles dramatically alters the mechanics of respiration, reducing inspiratory and/or expiratory flow.[52,82,113-115] SCI at or above the C4 level typically causes loss of all spontaneous respirations. With injury at the C5, C6, C7, or C8 level, the diaphragm remains functional, but there is complete loss of intercostal muscle function. In able-bodied individuals, the diaphragm generates approximately 65% of vital capacity (VC).[113] However, in acute tetraplegia at the C5 through C8 levels, VC is reduced to 20% to 50% of the predicted value.[82,113,114,116] Variable intercostal muscle dysfunction accompanies SCI at the T1 to T11 levels. If the intercostals are dysfunctional after SCI, chest wall mobility is impaired and a paradoxical breathing pattern is apparent. Lack of abdominal muscle function alters the position of the diaphragm because of the loss of viscera support. Loss of abdominal tone allows the diaphragm to sag, reducing diaphragmatic excursion and decreasing the patient's inspiratory capacity. Also, loss of abdominal muscle innervation, seen with SCI above T7, eliminates function of the major "defense" muscles needed for coughing or sneezing. Forced exhalation and cough are reduced dramatically. Once spinal shock has resolved, spasticity develops in the abdominal and thoracic muscles. This increased tone helps stabilize respiratory mechanics, although forced expiration and cough remain weakened.[52,82,113-115]

Compounding the loss of muscle function are the unopposed effects of the PNS upon the pulmonary system. The PNS innervates the M3 muscarinic receptors located in the lungs, producing vasoconstriction, bronchoconstriction, and increased mucus production. Reductions in ventilatory volumes coupled with the increased work of breathing predispose the SCI patient to significant pulmonary complications. These complications—atelectasis, pneumonia, and respiratory failure—remain the leading causes of mortality and morbidity after acute SCI.[4,52,113,114,117] Promoting optimal respiratory function and preventing pulmonary complications are primary goals for the patient with acute SCI.

Complications

The acutely injured individual is at risk for many pulmonary complications. At the time of injury the patient is at risk for aspiration and subsequent pneumonia. Placement of an

TABLE 23-5 **Innervation, Action, and Function of Respiratory Muscles**

Muscles	Innervation	Action	Function in Respiration
Accessory muscles			
Sternocleidomastoid	Cranial nerve XI, C1-C2	Draws sternum upward	These accessory muscles elevate and stabilize the chest wall to assist with inspiration and deep breathing
Trapezius	Cranial nerve XI, C3-C4	Elevates the rib cage	
Scalene	C4-C8	Lifts the sternum and first two ribs	
Clavicular portion of the pectoralis major	C5-T1	When the humerus and shoulders are fixed, can elevate the upper rib cage	
Diaphragm	Phrenic nerve arising from the C3-C5 levels	Contracts and descends, lengthening the thoracic cavity and expanding the lungs	Enables inspiration and deep breathing; the ability of this muscle to create a deep breath is the initial step in generating an effective cough
External intercostal muscles	T1-T11 levels	Lift the chest wall outward for lung expansion	Aid in inspiration and deep breathing
Internal intercostal muscles	T1-T11 levels	Pull the ribs downward and inward	Enable forced expiration and coughing
Abdominal muscles	T7-T12 levels	Depress the lower ribs and force the diaphragm upward	Aid forced expiration and coughing

(From McIlvoy L, Meyer K, McQuillan KA: Traumatic spine injuries. In Bader MK and Littlejohns L, Editors: *AANN Core Curriculum for Neuroscience Nursing*, ed 4, St. Louis, 2004, Saunders.)

artificial airway, hypersecretion, and secretion retention further increase risk for pneumonia. The use of steroid therapy to reduce spinal edema can worsen the resulting pneumonia. Swelling of injured paraspinal soft tissues may threaten airway patency. Pulmonary edema from excessive fluid infusion is always a threat during resuscitation. The presence of neurogenic shock, pneumonia, or aspiration may trigger the onset of acute respiratory distress syndrome (ARDS). Alterations in respiratory mechanics and immobility put SCI patients at high risk for the development of significant atelectasis. Immobility and decreased venous return also put them at risk of a deep venous thrombosis (DVT) and pulmonary embolism (PE). The critical care nurse must make pulmonary management a top priority to prevent life-threatening complications that can impair respiratory gas exchange and exacerbate secondary SCI. Respiratory complications also can delay surgery for spinal fixation, prolonging immobilization and increasing the length of hospitalization.[109]

Patients should be monitored vigilantly by paying strict attention to respiratory rate and pattern, work of breathing, evidence of fatigue, respiratory gas exchange, and breath sounds.[52,113,114] The use of accessory muscles is commonplace. Patients with cervical and high thoracic injuries exhibit a paradoxical breathing pattern as a result of the loss of intercostal muscle function. On inspiration, accessory muscles (see Table 23-5) expand the upper part of the rib cage anteriorly, decreasing pleural pressure and pulling the diaphragm upward. This results in a drop in intraabdominal pressure, an outward movement of the abdominal wall, and a passive collapse of the paralyzed muscles of the lower rib cage. On expiration, the intercostals passively reexpand as the diaphragm resumes resting position.[82,113,114] Resting respiratory rates and work of breathing tend to be higher in patients with SCI. By definition most SCIs result in a restrictive lung disorder.[82,113-115] Serial pulmonary function tests, which may include measures of vital capacity, tidal volume, maximum inspiratory force (pressure), and maximum expiratory force (pressure), that demonstrate worsening trends provide evidence of respiratory muscle fatigue or an ascending spinal cord lesion. In the patient with a natural airway, VC can be measured through incentive spirometry. If the VC is less than 1000 ml, mechanical ventilation may be necessary.[52,81] Pulse oximetry and routine assessment of ABGs should be performed to monitor Pao_2 and Pco_2. The addition of end-tidal Co_2 monitoring is recommended. Patients with cervical and high thoracic injuries are prone to develop mild hypercarbia. Auscultation of all lung fields can detect secretion retention and early signs of atelectasis, pneumonia, or consolidation. Routine chest films can provide additional evidence of pathologic pulmonary conditions.

If the work of breathing becomes laborious and the patient demonstrates fatigue, intubation and mechanical ventilation may be required. Patients with cervical or high thoracic SCI have diminished respiratory reserve. Expending a large amount of energy to breathe means that a great deal of energy also is required to clear secretions. If the energy for breathing cannot be redirected for use in respiratory defense, secretion retention and further increased work of breathing occurs, exhausting the patient and necessitating use of mechanical ventilation. The use of positive end-expiratory pressure (PEEP) has been recommended to increase peak inspiratory volume and lower expiratory flow rates, thus preserving "open lung" units.[118-120] Noninvasive positive- pressure ventilation has been successfully used as an alternative to intubation; it has been demonstrated to be an effective means of assisting the SCI patient in recruiting alveoli, reducing the work of breathing, and improving oxygen saturation.[81,113,114,120-124] Promoting *effective* spontaneous breathing, whether invasive or noninvasive ventilation is used, aids maintenance of open posterior lung segments, which are prone to collapse secondary to decreased tidal volumes and supine positioning that is enforced until the spine is stabilized. Spontaneous breathing offers the additional benefits of improved venous return and cardiac output.[125,126]

If the patient requires invasive mechanical ventilation, ensure use of a ventilator strategy that provides adequate tidal volumes to prevent or resolve atelectasis. Initial tidal volumes of 15 ml/kg based upon ideal body weight should be considered, with efforts made to keep peak airway pressures less than 40 cm H_2O to reduce the risk of barotrauma.[52,81,113,114] Generally, in acute spinal cord injury, the lung tissue is healthy and tolerates larger volumes and hyperinflation, which appears to aid surfactant production.[81,113,114] In tetraplegia, it is also recommended that the ventilator be set to avoid patient triggering.[81,113] Most often, injuries are not equal; in other words, one side of the body is stronger (or weaker) than the other side. This includes the diaphragm. By avoiding patient triggering, the clinician reduces the risk of preferential ventilation caused by the stronger side drawing volume from the weaker side. If unequal ventilation is allowed, persistent atelectasis may occur on the weaker side that is receiving smaller lung volumes. As atelectasis or pneumonia resolves, tidal volumes are slowly reduced to wean the patient. If the patient develops an acute lung injury, such as ARDS, an appropriate ARDS protocol for mechanical ventilation should be used to prevent potential barotrauma.[81]

Aggressive pulmonary hygiene is essential to prevent and treat pulmonary complications.[52,81,113,114,119-124] Studies using a spinal cord–injured population have demonstrated that postural drainage and percussion are effective methods to clear secretions, resolve atelectasis, and increase oxygenation.[52,81,113,114,119-124] Additional measures to enhance mobilization of secretions include intrapulmonary percussive ventilation (IPV), insufflation (with breath stacking)/exsufflation, intermittent positive-pressure breathing (IPPB) and glossopharyngeal breathing.[81,113,119-124] Combining high tidal volumes and inspiratory flows and PEEP increases collateral ventilation, which may increase the gas pressure behind secretions, aiding clearance.[119,120]

Endotracheal suctioning can effectively remove secretions from intubated patients. Mucolytics (guaifenesin and acetylcysteine) may thin secretions, aiding clearance. Bronchoscopy may be necessary to remove retained secretions and open atelectatic airways when routine suctioning, postural drainage, and chest physiotherapy (CPT) prove to be insufficient.[81,113,114] Patients with a weak cough and who have a natural airway or are intubated but stable enough to participate in pulmonary hygiene should use an assistive cough technique. The patient is instructed to take three breaths; on the expiratory phase of the third breath, the nurse places the heel of the hand halfway between the patient's umbilicus and xiphoid process and thrusts in and upward while the patient coughs. Performed correctly, this can be an effective means of clearing secreions.[81,113,114,119,120,125] Many patients can be instructed to perform this procedure on themselves. Increasing mobility reduces the patient's risk for posterior pooling of secretions and the development of lower lobe atelectasis and pneumonia. Whenever possible, patients should be repositioned at least once every 2 hours. Use of a Stryker or wedge turning frame (see Figure 23-16) or kinetic therapy bed (see Figure 23-17) provides greater mobility for the patient in cervical traction or with lower spine instability.

Bronchoconstriction resulting from the unopposed parasympathetic innervation may add an obstructive component to a restrictive lung disorder. Inhaled bronchodilators may be used to reduce bronchoconstriction and hyperreactivity of airways after injury.[52,81,113,114] The use of ipratropium should be limited to the acute phase of management because the anticholinergic effects may lead to decreased surfactant production and thickened secretions over time.[81,113] Beta agonists (albuterol or salmeterol) appear to offset some of the effects of the unopposed parasympathetic stimulation. They produce bronchodilation, increase heart rate, and may enhance surfactant production.[81,113] Use of methylxanthines to aid activation of latent diaphragmatic motor pathways remains controversial. Some studies suggest that the administration of theophylline (or IV aminophylline) improves diaphragmatic performance and aids weaning in the acute phase.[126,127] Other medications, such as leukotriene inhibitors (montelukast), to reduce airway inflammation and volume trapping may also aid weaning.[81,113]

When a person with SCI sits in an upright position, the weakened or paralyzed abdominal muscles permit the abdominal contents to relax forward, pulling the diaphragm downward and reducing excursion. Use of an abdominal binder to support the viscera can assist the patient's breathing by bringing the diaphragm into a better resting position (i.e., elevates position and promotes diaphragmatic curvature).[81,82,113,18,120] By starting inspiration with the diaphragm in a higher position, or with a lower lung volume, a more volume efficient respiratory effort results. Proper placement of the binder is important to prevent impingement of chest movement. The binder should be placed below the costal margin and extend over the iliac crests bilaterally (Figure 23-18). The lower portion of the binder should be tighter than the section running along the floating ribs.

Many patients with cervical spine injuries require mechanical ventilation. Patients with complete injuries at C3 and higher will likely remain ventilator dependent. Other patients may require prolonged mechanical ventilation until respiratory muscles can be strengthened and pulmonary complications resolve. Early tracheostomy is desirable for these patients to reduce anatomical dead space, decrease the discomfort of prolonged intubation, lower the risk of tracheal stenosis, facilitate communication, promote weaning, and shorten intensive care unit length of stay.[128,129] A weaning strategy should be devised by the multidisciplinary team caring for the patient to promote strengthening of the respiratory muscles and provide time for psychological separation from the ventilator.[81,113] Many different methods of weaning have been used, most of which are based on a work-rest principle.[81,113] Studies suggest that progressive ventilator-free breathing (PVFB), where the patient is placed on humidified oxygen for increasing periods to slowly build endurance, is more successful than synchronized intermittent mechanical ventilation (SIMV) or pressure support weaning.[81,113] Weaning can be a long process, often extending into the intermediate cycle of care.

Cardiovascular Implications

Hypotension

Decreased systemic blood pressure caused by loss of sympathetic outflow typically remains problematic in the critical care phase. Continued use of vasopressor agents such as dopamine or phenylephrine hydrochloride (Neo-Synephrine) produces vasoconstriction of the vessels, improving venous return and augmenting blood pressure. The American Association of Neurological Surgeons (AANS) guidelines recommend avoiding a systolic blood pressure below 90 mm Hg

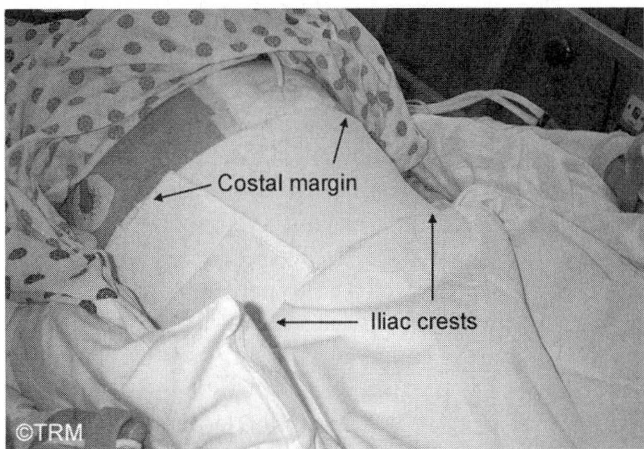

FIGURE 23-18 **Abdominal binder placement.** Proper placement of abdominal binder. Binder should be trimmed, if necessary, to sit along floating ribs (costal margin) extending down to the iliac crests. Improper placement can lead to restriction of rib cage and increased risk of atelectasis.

and maintaining a mean blood pressure of 85 to 90 mm Hg for 7 days to ensure adequate perfusion of the spinal cord and other body organs.[88,130,131] If not placed during resuscitation, invasive hemodynamic monitoring lines may be inserted during the critical care phase to assist with ongoing assessment and treatment of neurogenic shock. A central venous pressure (CVP) or pulmonary artery catheter can help guide vasoactive administration and fluid replacement. Placement of an arterial line provides constant blood pressure assessment to guide titration of vasopressors and an ability to easily access serum for laboratory analysis.

As with any critically injured patient, maintenance of cardiovascular function to ensure adequate tissue perfusion is of utmost importance. Close monitoring of the patient's hemodynamic parameters provides information helpful in guiding management decisions. Ensuring adequate filling pressures, heart rate and rhythm, blood pressure, and cardiac output promotes optimal end-organ perfusion. Administration of an inotropic agent, such as dobutamine, may be appropriate to optimize cardiac output. Monitoring intake, output, and laboratory values to ensure fluid and electrolyte balance assists in the maintenance of proper intravascular volume and cardiac function.

Venous pooling and dependent edema are other consequences of altered vascular tone. Application of pneumatic compression devices promotes venous return and reduces the risk of deep vein thrombosis. Introduction of prophylactic heparin or low-molecular-weight (LMW) heparin is appropriate once risk of any hemorrhage has been ruled out.

Bradycardia

Bradycardia resulting from sympathetic blockade can also persist into the critical care phase. The intact PNS innervates the M2 muscarinic receptors located in the heart, which slow the heart rate, decrease contractile forces of the atrial cardiac muscle, and reduce conduction velocity through the atrioventricular (AV) node.[132] The contractile force of the ventricular cardiac muscle is unaffected by the PNS. In addition to bradycardia, other arrhythmias may occur after disruption of the SNS, such as junctional escape beats, atrioventricular blocks, and premature atrial or ventricular complexes.[132] It is important to remain cognizant of the effects of hypothermia and hypoxia on heart rate and rhythm. Also, use of high tidal volumes (15 ml/kg) in mechanical ventilation is associated with a reflex cardiac depression that may worsen existing bradycardia.[133,134] For patients with symptomatic bradycardia, atropine should be given as needed. If repetitive dosing is required, clinicians need to bear in mind the impact of anticholinergic medications on secretions and gastric motility. In profound cases, temporary pacing may be necessary. Case reports offer some support for the use of various inotropic agents, chronotropic medications, and aminophylline for temporary heart rate support.[52,135-137] Generally, even the most serious cases of bradycardia resolve within 6 weeks of injury, and permanent cardiac pacing is rarely required.[52,135,137]

Vasovagal Response

In addition to baseline bradycardia, many patients experience a vasovagal response. The unopposed parasympathetic flow causes cardiac arrest. This response can be stimulated by a number of patient or nursing actions, including sudden position changes, coughing, gagging, and suctioning. Strategies to reduce the occurrence of this response are to change the patient's position slowly and to induce hyperoxygenation before suctioning. Symptomatic events can be treated by administration of atropine or, in some cases, use of a temporary pacer.

Hyponatremia

Patients with acute SCI are at risk to develop hyponatremia within the first week of injury.[52,138,139] This tends to occur more often in complete versus incomplete injuries.[138] Several mechanisms may contribute to the development of hyponatremia, including inappropriate secretion of antidiuretic hormone (ADH) and a disruption in normal sodium excretion.[52,139] ADH is released in response to increased osmolality (osmo receptors) and decreased effective circulating volume (baroreceptors). As a result, water is retained. Water retention leads to dilution of sodium and plasma water expansion. Volume expansion leads to increased atrial stretching and the release of atrial natriuretic peptide, which in turn leads to a reduction in aldosterone release. In response to the reduction in aldosterone, the distal renal tubules increase urinary sodium excretion. This worsens the hyponatremia. As the serum osmolality continues to drop, an overriding of the ADH effect occurs and excess water is excreted, leading to polyuria. In some cases, an osmostat resetting occurs and chronic hyponatremia develops.[139]

Patients are managed with 0.9% NaCl or balanced electrolyte solutions and close monitoring of serum and urinary electrolytes. Strict monitoring of intake and output should be implemented. Care must be taken to avoid misinterpretation and subsequent mismanagement of the polyuria. Invasive volume monitoring may aid in actual volume status interpretation to avoid overly aggressive fluid replacement, which may result in a worsening hyponatremia.

Deep Venous Thrombosis

Any immobilized patient is at risk for DVT formation. The SCI population is at high risk as a result of venous pooling, decreased venous return, hypercoagulability from injury-induced stimulation of thrombogenic factors, and possible presence of a vessel injury.[140,141] The greatest risk to the patient appears to be within the first 2 weeks after injury.[140-142] Clinical features of DVT, such as extremity swelling, pain, or mottling when dependent, can be obscured by the normal physical response to spinal injury. For many patients the first sign of DVT is a pulmonary embolus.[142] The nurse should remain vigilant for signs of increased lower extremity girth, redness or warmth, and elevation of body temperature, which may indicate presence of DVT. Diagnosis can be made with contrast venography, duplex ultrasonography, or impedance plethysmography of the lower extremities.

Prevention is the key to DVT management. The current guidelines for prophylaxis include prophylactic anticoagulation with adjusted-dose heparin or LMW heparin.[140-142] Anticoagulation should be initiated as soon as the physician deems the patient is not at high risk for bleeding from spinal cord or other injury. Mechanical devices such as graduated compression stockings or intermittent pneumatic compression devices may be of benefit when used with anticoagulants or when anticoagulants are contraindicated.[140-143] Because studies demonstrate a low incidence of thromboembolic event after 6 to 12 weeks, it is recommended that DVT prophylaxis be discontinued 3 months after injury unless the patient remains at high risk.[140,141] Patients with clinical contraindications for anticoagulation (e.g., high risk for exacerbation of bleeding within the injury site or intraoperatively) or use of mechanical devices or those who have failed prophylaxis should have an inferior vena cava (IVC) filter placed.[140,141,143] Some studies advocate prophylactic placement of IVC filters in SCI,[144] whereas others suggest that this may be an unnecessary procedure for the majority of patients, especially over time.[145] Retrievable vena caval filters are now available for short-term use, which may address one concern.[146,147] Heightening staff awareness and implementation of a DVT prophylaxis protocol appears to positively affect rates of occurrence. Range-of-motion exercises, early mobilization, and adequate hydration may help reduce the risk of DVT formation. If DVT is detected, full anticoagulation is initiated unless contraindicated. Patients and their families should receive education on the signs, symptoms, risk factors, and prevention of DVT.

Gastrointestinal Implications

The gastrointestinal system is disrupted by loss of sympathetic nervous system innervation, resulting in autonomic nervous system imbalance. Initially, most patients experience a loss of intestinal motility (adynamic ileus). Acute abdominal distention resulting from the paralytic ileus can further inhibit respiratory function and may harbor a large volume of third-spaced fluid, which increases risk for aspiration. This condition rarely lasts longer than 2 to 5 days. A gastric tube should be placed for decompression, and displaced intravascular volume should be replaced as necessary.

Gastritis, esophagitis (gastroesophageal reflux), and gastrointestinal mucosal erosion with associated hemorrhage can occur secondary to stress; transient reduction or loss of sympathetic innervation (unopposed vagal outflow) that leads to increased gastrin secretion and a reduction in gastric pH; steroid administration; and relative intestinal ischemia.[52,148,149] Patients should receive routine peptic ulcer disease prophylaxis with histamine blockers, antacids, or proton pump inhibitors. A gastric tube should be placed for stomach decompression, and gastric aspirate may be monitored for presence of occult blood or abnormal pH. Hemoglobin, hematocrit, blood urea nitrogen (BUN), and creatinine also should be monitored.

Pancreatic dysfunction can occur in the patient with SCI due to increased stimulation of the sphincter of Oddi, thickening of pancreatic secretions, and alterations in organ perfusion.[148,149] Serum amylase levels should be monitored, especially with the start of low-dose enteral feedings. If the amylase concentration rises as feedings are increased, the patient's oral intake should be restricted (NPO) and hyperalimentation provided until serum amylase levels return to normal.

Superior mesenteric artery syndrome is a relatively infrequent complication of acute SCI occurring more often in tetraplegia.[148] Because of alterations in the vascular tone to the viscera, the distal part of the duodenum is compressed by the superior mesenteric artery against the aorta.[148,149] Symptoms may include persistent epigastric pain (possibly referred to a shoulder) and a feeling of postprandial fullness followed by nausea and vomiting. Other conditions, such as delayed gastric emptying or ileus, may mimic this condition. Diagnosis is made with contrasted radiographic studies, such as upper GI series or abdominal CT scan.[148] Most patients respond to conservative treatment, including low-dose enteral feedings with frequent right lateral positioning or NPO status with intravenous fluids or parenteral nutrition. This syndrome frequently resolves as spinal shock begins to subside.[149]

Every effort should be made to meet the nutritional requirements of the patient with appropriate parenteral or enteral nutrition. Initiation of early enteral feeding is important to maintain GI integrity and provide nutritional support. Early enteral feeding also may help reduce septic complications, decrease the hypermetabolic response to critical injury, improve wound healing, and maintain intestinal immunologic defenses.[150-153] Patients with cervical spine injuries may experience a delay in gastric emptying.[148,149] Placement of a transpyloric tube is recommended to facilitate enteral feeding if gastric intolerance occurs. Before initiating oral feedings for a patient with a high SCI, a swallowing evaluation is often recommended.

Constipation can occur as a result of reduced GI motility, narcotic and sedative use, and immobility. Occasionally this may create a bowel obstruction. Routine rectal examination should include assessment of anal sphincter tone and presence of retained stool or impaction.[148,149,154] Evaluation of anocutaneous and bulbocavernosus reflexes determines if the patient has UMN or LMN bowel dysfunction. A bowel program, including stool softeners and stimulant cathartic suppositories (e.g., bisacodyl [Dulcolax]) should be implemented as soon as possible to assist with regular bowel emptying.[148,149,154]

Stabilization Devices

Spinal orthoses are used to protect the injured unstable spine by controlling the position and limiting the mobility of the spine or segment of the spine. Spinal motion can be loosely categorized as flexion-extension, lateral bending, or rotation and is quantified by degrees. Different orthoses restrict spinal motions in different ways and to varying degrees.[155] A brace is chosen according to location of injury, desired function, and specific treatment goals.[155] Braces are categorized by the spinal segments involved. These categories are cervical orthoses (CO), head cervical orthoses (HCO), cervical thoracic orthoses (CTO), thoracolumbosacral orthoses (TLSO), lumbosacral orthoses (LSO), and cervical thoracolumbosacral orthoses (CTLSO). Construct (rigid, semirigid, or flexible) and indication (corrective or supportive) can further stratify these categories (Figure 23-19).

Skin breakdown, loss of spinal alignment, pain, weakening of immobilized muscles, soft tissue contractures, restriction of pulmonary excursion, and increased lower extremity venous pressure, which can produce varicosities and dependent edema, are all potential complications of spinal orthoses. Proper brace fit and meticulous skin care beneath the brace are essential to maintain skin integrity. Two people are required to perform skin care. The patient is placed flat while the anterior portion of the brace is removed. The patient should be instructed to avoid movement while the brace is open. Skin is cleansed with soap and water and dried thoroughly. A light dusting of powder or cornstarch is applied. Lotion, which creates a moisture layer, is avoided. The skin is inspected for redness or breakdown. To perform back care, the anterior shell is reapplied, the patient is log rolled, and care is performed with one person stabilizing the patient and the anterior shell. Patients and their families must be educated on the proper application and fit of a brace, cleaning the brace, skin care, proper body mechanics, and appropriate exercises for reducing the deconditioning effects of the brace.

Care of the patient in a halo vest (Figure 23-20) demands special focus. The halo vest is opened at the thoracic belts only, one side at a time. Skin beneath the vest should be well cleaned and dried while the thoracic straps are open. Replacement pads or sheepskins are available, which can be rolled into and out of the vest for washing. A wrench should be kept secured to the chest plate of the vest for emergency vest removal. The skeletal traction pin insertion sites should be regularly cleansed and monitored closely for symptoms of infection. Grabbing or pulling on the support rods to position the patient or to adjust the brace fit must be avoided.

PAIN

Pain is also an issue in the acute phase of injury, and for many patients it remains a chronic issue. Individuals may experience bony pain associated with fracture or use of skeletal

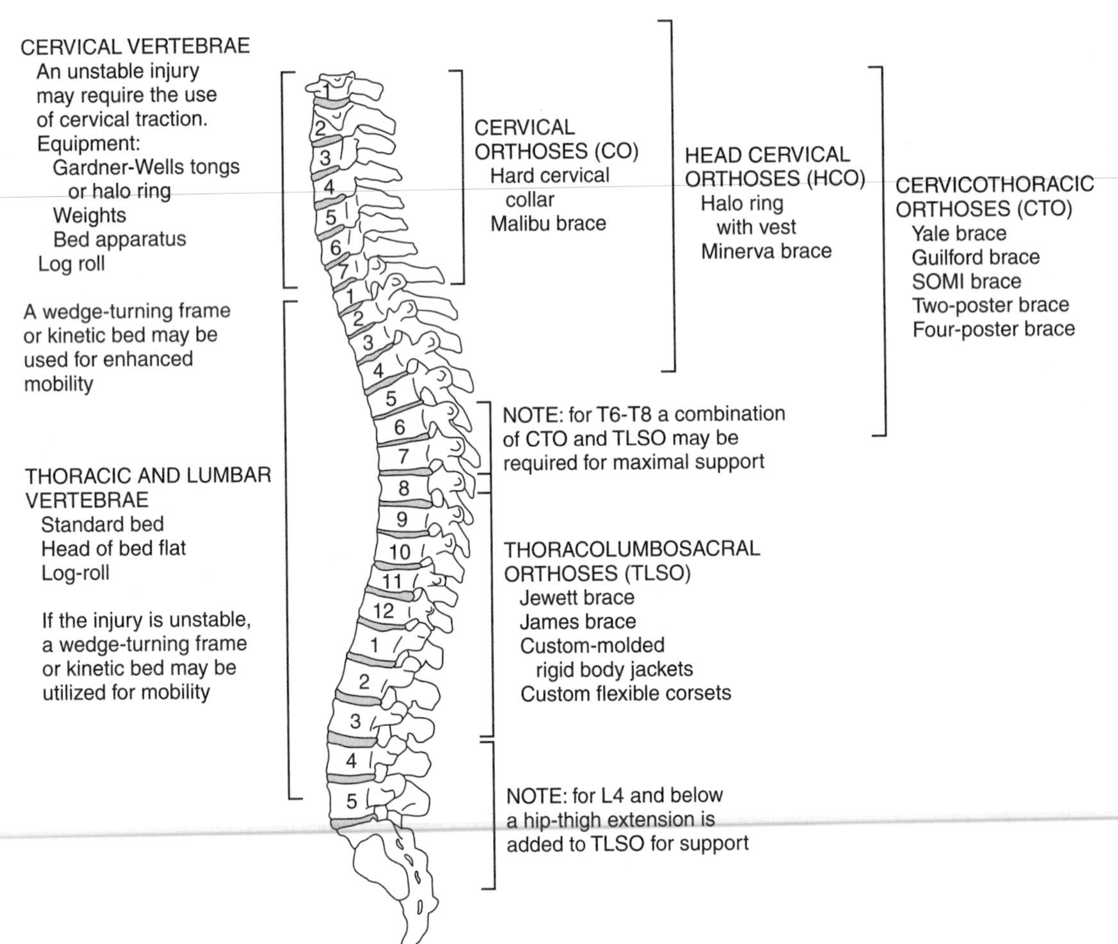

FIGURE 23-19 Spinal immobilization devices. *SOMI,* Sterno-occipital-mandibular immobilizer.

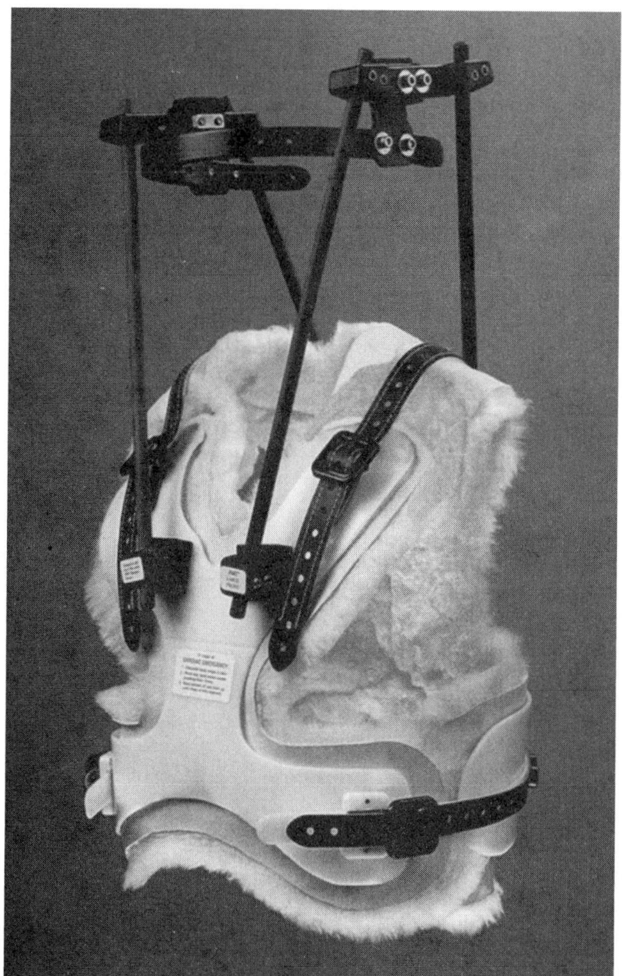

FIGURE 23-20 Halo vest. (Courtesy PMT Corporation, Chanhassen, Minn.)

traction, soft tissue and muscular pain associated with acute injury, and neurogenic pain associated with CNS trauma. Associated injuries involving areas where sensation is intact also contribute to the pain experienced by the patient. The nurse must assess carefully the patient's pain and collaborate with the physician to determine the appropriate pharmacologic intervention. If available, consultation with a pain management service to assess and coordinate pain control facilitates care.

Psychosocial Implications

Acute SCI is devastating and overwhelming for the patient and the family. Because of the sudden nature of the injury, there is no time for the patient to prepare for the event. Fear and anxiety are the primary emotions seen in the critical phase of care. Interventions should be aimed at providing reassurance and assisting patients to reassert control over their situation and environment. Initially, many patients are too ill to comprehend the long-term consequences of their injury; they exist in a state of denial, functioning only in the present. Immediate gratification of needs is desired. Early implementation of a daily schedule that includes the patient's preferences assists in providing a sense of control. Development of a stable team of care providers can help to establish trust. A means of communication should be established as soon as possible so that the patient can relay needs and ventilate feelings. This can be accomplished with a blink board, a picture board, an artificial larynx, a Passy-Muir valve (one-way, "no-leak" tracheostomy speech valve [Passy-Muir, Inc./Irvine, CA]), or other strategies. Specialized call bells should be available for the patient to use to summon the nurse. If no other alert mechanism is established, the patient may resort to "clicking" (moving the tongue and mouth to create a clicking sound) to draw the attention of caregivers. Nurses must set limits on the patient to prevent excessive clicking. The nurse should reach an agreement with the patient on when clicking is appropriate. It is imperative that when a patient uses the call bell or clicks, someone responds. This develops trust in the caregivers and decreases the patient's fears and anxiety, which ultimately reduces the frequency of calling or clicking.

It is not unreasonable to use pharmacologic interventions in the initial stages of injury to calm the patient and prevent panic attacks. Excessive anxiety resulting in flailing can cause patients to unintentionally disrupt their spinal alignment. Hyperventilation caused by anxiety can hamper the patient's pulmonary status.

It is also important to regulate the patient's sleep cycle. Sleep deprivation is a constant threat in the critical care environment. Measures should be taken to maintain a day-night cycle for patients and to allow for rapid eye movement (REM) sleep. Sleep deprivation can make the patient's pain management more difficult and reduce the patient's ability to cope with the stress caused by the injury.

Families also must be involved with the patients' care from the beginning. Patient and family education about SCI begins on admission and continues through rehabilitation. It is often necessary to share information repeatedly for the patient and family to assimilate it. Health care providers should also assist the patient and family in identifying and using support systems and appropriate coping mechanisms.

Intermediate Care and Rehabilitation Phases

After definitive spinal treatment has been rendered and body systems are stabilized, the patient enters the intermediate and rehabilitation phases of care. During this time the patient is at risk for late complications of SCI related to alterations in body functions caused by interruption of sympathetic and sacral parasympathetic outflow and immobility. The goals of intermediate and rehabilitation care are to prevent complications, enhance physical strength, relearn activities of daily living (ADLs) (Table 23-6), and regain emotional stability. When these goals are met, the outcome potential of the patient with an SCI is optimized, and return to the "outside" world is more likely to be successful.

TABLE 23-6 **Functional Goals for Spinal Cord–Injured Patients**

Level	Muscle Function	Functional Goals
C3-4	Neck control Scapular elevators	Manipulate electric wheelchair with mouth stick Dependent to limited self-feedings with ball bearing feeders Dependent transfers Dependent to assisted turn in bed with arm slings; independent pressure relief in chair with adaptive equipment Dependent bathing, grooming, and dressing Dependent bowel and bladder
C5	Fair to good shoulder control Good elbow flexion	Propel wheelchair with handrim projections Self-feeding with adaptive equipment Dependent transfer; independent pressure relief with equipment Dependent bathing Assisted grooming and dressing Dependent bowel and bladder
C6	Good shoulder control Wrist extension Supinators	Transfer from wheelchair to bed and car with or without minimal assistance Self-feeding with adaptive equipment Bowel care: assist getting to and from commode chair Bladder care: some assistance to dependent depending on strategy Assisted bathing for lower body Dressing: independent upper body, assisted lower body Driving with adapted van
C7	Weak shoulder depression Weak elbow extension Some hand function	Independent in transfer to bed, car, and toilet Independent grooming Some assistance with lower body bathing and dressing Wheelchair without handrim projections Self-feeding with no assistance devices Bowel and bladder care: independent to some assistance Driving car with hand controls or adapted van
C8-T4	Good to normal upper extremity muscle function	Wheelchair to floor and return Wheelchair up and down curb Wheelchair to tub and return
T5-L2	Partial to good trunk stability	Total wheelchair independence Limited ambulation with bilateral long leg braces and crutches
L3-L4	All trunk-pelvic stabilizers intact Hip flexors Adductors Quadriceps	Ambulation with short leg braces with or without crutches, depending on level
L5	Hip extensors, abductors, knee flexors, ankle control	No equipment needs if plantar flexion is enough for push off at end of stance

Modified from Boston University School of Nursing.

Patient goals are achieved best through a multidisciplinary team approach. The care team evaluates patients to determine the best means to achieve these goals. The SCI patient is often evaluated using the ASIA standards to determine level and completeness of injury, which assists in setting realistic functional goals (see Table 23-6). The FIM instrument (Uniform Data System for Medical Rehabilitation, a division of UB Foundation Activities, Inc., Amherst, NY), a widely used functional assessment measure, is useful in evaluating the patient's functional outcome (Table 23-7).

RESPIRATORY IMPLICATIONS

SCIs that involve paralysis of the respiratory muscles have significant impact on patients across their lifetime. In the first year after SCI and thereafter, respiratory complications, particularly pneumonia, remain one of the leading causes of rehospitalization and death, especially with tetraplegia.[4,156] Over time, the chest wall becomes more rigid, resulting in decreased lung and chest wall compliance.[114,157] Weakened or paralyzed respiratory muscles recruit the use and development of accessory muscles. Individuals with tetraplegia or high thoracic paraplegia use the spared neck muscles to aid in chest lift and expansion. It has been noted that these patients increase neck size over time.[158] Studies of pulmonary function in spinal cord–injured patients have demonstrated a reduction in vital capacity of up to 50% and loss of total lung capacity to approximately 30% of normal.[113,118,157] Autonomic dysfunction can result in both chronic bronchial hypersecretion and reactive airway disease. Weakened expiratory force and reduced ability to cough, coupled with a decrease in airway size, can lead to secretion accumulation and retention and the development of pneumonia. Long-term inhaled beta agonists

TABLE 23-7 **Functional Independence Measure Scale**

Independent	
7	Complete independence. The activity is typically performed safely, without modification, assistive devices or aids, and within reasonable time.
6	Modified independence. The activity requires an assistive device, more than reasonable time, or is not performed safely.
Modified Dependence	
5	Supervision or setup. No physical assistance is needed, but cuing, coaxing, or setup is required.
4	Minimal contact assistance. Subject requires no more than touching and expends 75% or more of the effort required in the activity.
3	Moderate assistance. Subject requires more than touching and expends 50% to 75% of the effort required in the activity.
Dependent	
2	Maximal assistance. Subject expends 25% to 50% of the effort required in the activity.
1	Total assistance. Subject expends 0% to 25% of the effort required in the activity.

The Functional Independence Measure (FIM) instrument focuses on six areas of function: self-care, sphincter control, mobility, locomotion, communication, and social cognition. The FIM rating (summed across all items) estimates the cost of disability in terms of safety issues and of dependence on others and on technical devices. FIM is a trademark of Uniform Data System for Medical Rehabilitation, a division of UB Foundation Activities, Inc.

may alleviate some of the symptoms associated with bronchoconstriction and improve feelings of breathlessness.[159,160] Home use of manual or mechanical cough techniques or noninvasive positive-pressure ventilation may reduce microatelectasis and ward off respiratory failure. Abdominal binders, which may be helpful during the acute phase of injury, become less effective once the chest wall becomes fixed. In the chronic phase, abdominal binders have been shown to increase vital capacity; however, they also have the undesirable effect of reducing functional residual capacity (FRC).[157] The loss of FRC may result in increased airway closure and atelectasis.[118]

Sleep disorders and sleep apnea occur in a large number of SCI patients. Routine care (e.g., turning, bladder management), chronic pain and depression, and muscle spasms can lead to fragmented sleep.[161-164] Disruption in melatonin levels may further contribute to sleep disturbance.[161,165] The suprachiasmatic nuclei, located in the anterior hypothalamus, is thought to control melatonin secretion via an efferent pathway that routes through the spinal cord via the superior cervical ganglion to the pineal gland.[161,165] Patients with cervical injury have a disruption of the pathway resulting in a reduction of basal melatonin and a loss of cyclic secretion. Melatonin may be involved in regulation of circadian rhythms and therefore sleep-wake patterns. Sleep apnea in SCI has been attributed to increased neck size and reduced airway diameter associated with impaired respiratory mechanics, as well as use of antispasmodic medications, particularly baclofen and benzodiazepines.[161-164] SCI patients should be routinely screened and tested for the development of sleep apnea. Treatment may include nighttime continuous positive airway pressure (CPAP)—positive-pressure stents open the upper airway and aids respiratory effort—and possibly medications.

CARDIOVASCULAR IMPLICATIONS

Autonomic Dysreflexia

After spinal shock resolves, patients sustaining an SCI at the T6 level or above are at risk for autonomic dysreflexia (AD); this syndrome occurs in 50% to 90% of tetraplegics and high paraplegics.[166] AD is an uncontrolled, massive sympathetic reflex response to a stimulus below the level of the lesion (Figure 23-21). Common stimuli precipitating AD include a full bladder, distended bowel, or skin irritation (e.g., pressure sore).[86,87,166-169] The irritant stimulates the sympathetic nervous system below the injury, resulting in severe vasoconstriction below the level of the SCI lesion. Pallor, chills, goose bumps, and cool skin are evident below the injury level. Blood volume is shunted into the nonconstricted vessels above the lesion, causing hypertension. Baroreceptors in the carotid arteries and aortic arch respond to the hypertension by sending a message to the higher vasomotor centers in the brain. These centers send messages to the heart, causing reflexive slowing, and to the blood vessels, resulting in vasodilation. Unfortunately, these messages cannot go beyond the level of the lesion; thus, vasodilation occurs only above the level of injury, producing facial flushing, nasal congestion, and a pounding headache. If left untreated, hypertension can lead to myocardial infarction, retina detachment, seizures, and cerebrovascular accident.[167,168] This syndrome is potentially life-threatening to the SCI patient.[167-169]

Nursing interventions should be aimed at recognition of the early signs and preventing stimuli that might trigger the onset of AD.[169] Baseline blood pressure in midthoracic to cervical spinal cord–injured patients tends to be lower than in the population at large (systolic 90 to 110 mm Hg), therefore, a systolic blood pressure of 140 mm Hg may indicate early AD.[169] If AD does occur, the first step in care is

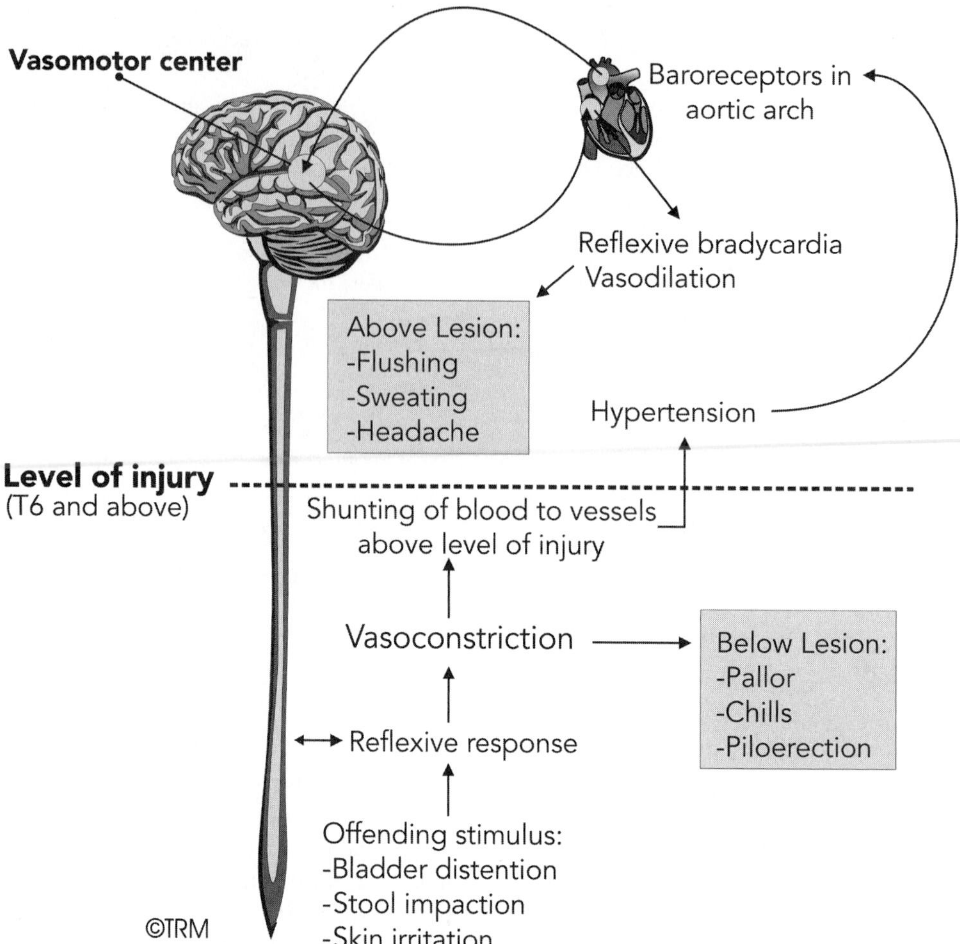

FIGURE 23-21 **Pathophysiology of autonomic dysreflexia.** A noxious stimulus initiates a reflexive response below the level of injury, which results in significant vasoconstriction. This shunts blood from the periphery to the large vessels and increases venous return to the heart. Baroreceptors in the aortic arch receive the sudden increase in pressure, then transmit information to the vasomotor center, which in turn sends messages back to the heart and other organs, resulting in a slowing of the heart rate and vasodilation. The message cannot travel below the level of injury and the result is one group of symptoms above the lesion and another constellation of symptoms below the lesion.

to sit the patient upright to induce orthostatic hypotension.[86,87,166-169] The patient's blood pressure should be monitored at least every 5 minutes during the crisis. The next step is to identify and remove the offensive stimulus. The bladder should be palpated for distention and immediate catheterization, using an anesthetic lubricant, performed.[169] If a catheter is in place, any obstruction of urine outflow should be alleviated immediately. Next, a digital rectal examination should be performed, using an anesthetic ointment, to assess for impaction. If the abdomen is distended and no impaction is noted in the rectum, a laxative should be administered. Clothing should be loosened and any adaptive splints removed. If these measures fail to resolve the problem, hypertensive management should be initiated.[86,87,166-169] Alpha-adrenergic blockers, such as terazosin, have been particularly useful in bladder-mediated AD, while reserpine and clonidine or intrathecal hexamethonium have successfully prevented symptoms in patients who experience recurrent AD in the absence of acute predisposing factors.[168] Although AD is likely to be most severe in the first 6 to 12 months after SCI, it remains a lifelong potential complication. Patients and families must be educated about the symptoms and treatment of AD.

Orthostatic Hypotension

Patients with SCI above T7 are particularly vulnerable to orthostatic hypotension. This complication results from the loss of vasoconstriction and paralysis of lower extremity muscle groups, which produce pooling of blood in the viscera and dependent extremities.[83,167,170] This leads to a reduced venous return, cardiac output, and blood pressure. Additional factors, including an impaired baroreflex and early hyponatremia, also predispose patients to the development of orthostasis.[83,170] Symptoms include a decrease in blood pressure, possibly an increased heart rate, and generalized signs of cerebral hypoperfusion—dizziness or lightheadedness, blurred vision, and even loss of consciousness—when the patient assumes an upright position.[167,170] In an emergent situation, the patient should be placed supine with their head flat and legs elevated. Treatment of orthostasis is generally successful with conservative, nonpharmacologic measures. Gradual elevation of the head of the bed, application of an abdominal binder, compression of the lower extremities with antiembolism stockings or Ace wraps when out of bed, and maintenance of hydration are interventions that can reduce postural hypotension.[86,87,167,170,171] If these measures fail, administration of salt tablets to promote volume expansion may be helpful. In severe cases, administration of a mineralocorticoid, such as fludrocortisone (Florinef), to promote salt and water retention may be effective.[86,87,170,171] The use of sympathomimetics, such as pseudoephedrine, ephedrine, or midodrine, may elevate blood pressure and reduce postural hypotension.[86,87,170-173] Recent studies demonstrated that using functional electrical stimulation to the lower extremities effectively increased blood pressure, so this therapy may be useful in treating orthostatic hypotension.[170,174,175]

Gastrointestinal Implications

Altered bowel elimination is an issue for most spinal cord–injured individuals throughout the course of their lives. Studies focusing on bowel dysfunction and life satisfaction demonstrate that this area causes most SCI persons a high degree of distress, which can lead to poor social reintegration and isolation.[149,154,176-178] The level of injury dictates the type of alteration in bowel elimination the patient experiences.

Defecation results from an intricate interplay of the intrinsic (enteric nervous system) system and extrinsic (CNS, SNS, PNS, and somatic nervous system) system.[149,154,178] The extrinsic system functions as a modulator. Reflexes in the colon, rectum, and internal and external anal sphincters send and receive impulses via intact loops that involve the pelvic nerves, pelvic and hypogastric plexi, sacral roots, and the pudendal nerve (see Figure 23-8). Sympathetic outflow to the ascending colon arises from thoracic nerve roots (T6-12); sympathetic innervation to the remaining colon through the rectum arises from the lumbar roots (L1-3). SNS effects include decreased intestinal motility and increased sphincter tone. Parasympathetic innervation involves the vagus nerve (cranial nerve X), sacral roots (S2-4), and the pudendal nerve. PNS effects include increased intestinal motility and propulsion and sphincter relaxation.

Injuries above the level of the conus medullaris (L1-2) are associated with spastic paralysis and an inability to feel the urge to defecate, although the reflex activity for defecation remains intact (reflexive bowel). With an injury to the sacral cord segments in the conus medullaris or cauda equina, the reflex center for defecation is destroyed, and there is a loss of anal tone (areflexive bowel). Fecal retention and oozing of stool through the flaccid anal sphincter are associated with this type of lower motor neuron injury.

Constipation and impaction are common complications for patients with SCI. Constipation and fecal impaction also are linked to abdominal distention, pain, and in high thoracic or cervical injuries, the precipitation of autonomic dysreflexia.[148,149,154] It is important to initiate bowel training as soon as possible. The first step in developing a bowel routine is to differentiate between a reflexive and an areflexive bowel.[154] Although the goals and global components of the bowel programs are similar, a few subtle differences exist. Consistency is the cornerstone to any successful program. A high-fiber diet, adequate fluid intake, exercise, effective positioning, set scheduling, and a combination of medications (stool softeners, stimulant cathartic suppositories, and small-volume enemas) all aid in bowel evacuation.[148,149,154,176,177] Harsh laxatives are avoided to prevent unpredictable time of defecation and diarrhea leading to incontinence.

Mechanical methods are also used to assist with bowel emptying. Digital stimulation is helpful to initiate defecation in patients with cervical or thoracic injury. Proper technique is important to avoid increased spasticity of the anal sphincter.[148,149,154,176] Digital stimulation is delivered by donning a clean glove and applying water-based lubricant. A gentle rotation of the finger around the sphincter is performed until relaxation of the external anal sphincter is felt and usually flatus is passed. Digital stimulation is performed every 5 to 10 minutes until evacuation is completed or the internal anal sphincter contracts. In patients with an areflexive bowel, manual stool evacuation is performed. This technique is performed similarly to stimulation. One or two fingers are gently inserted into the rectum and stool is broken up. Using a "hooking" motion, the stool is removed until the rectal vault is empty. For each method to be most successful, it is important to achieve the proper stool consistency. In managing patients with a reflexive bowel, stool consistency should be kept soft, but not loose, whereas in patients with an areflexive bowel, stool should be kept firm to aid manual removal.[148,149,154] Patients with lower thoracic injury frequently use a Valsalva maneuver to initiate defecation. It is crucial to empty the bladder before engaging in this maneuver to minimize the occurrence of vesico-ureteral reflux of urine. This maneuver should also be avoided if the patient has a history of cardiac disease, hypertension, or significant hemorrhoids.[154] If patients with a cervical or thoracic injury experience impaction, they are at significant risk for autonomic dysreflexia. An anesthetic lubricant should be used to reduce initiation of dysreflexia if manual disimpaction is needed.

Lifelong bowel-associated issues include chronic constipation, incontinence, hemorrhoids, and skin irritation/breakdown. For patients who fail to respond to conventional bowel programs, more aggressive measures can be considered, which include more aggressive use of medications or surgical diversion (i.e., colostomy or ileostomy).[148,149,154,176,177] Another possible intervention is implantation of the Vocare (NeuroControl Corp., Cleveland, OH, USA), a neurostimulator that is connected via subcutaneous wires to the sacral nerves. Although this system was primarily developed to improve bladder care, in a multicenter trial, it was demonstrated to be a safe and useful adjunct to bowel management.[179]

Education of the patient and the caregiver is essential.[148,149,154] A successful bowel program must meet the physiologic and lifestyle needs of the patient while remaining within the abilities of the caregiver. Socioeconomic factors directly affect home care due to the availability of resources. Cost of medication, durable adaptive equipment, and adaptability/accessibility of the home all impact long-term outcomes.[154]

Gallbladder disease is another complication that has an increased incidence after SCI. The most frequent cause of emergency abdominal surgery in spinal cord-injured persons is cholecystitis or cholelithiasis.[148] It is postulated that the causes may be abnormal gallbladder motility, abnormal enterohepatic circulation, and altered intestinal motility, which lead to abnormal biliary secretion.[148,180] Classic clinical signs of gallbladder disease, such as a rigid abdomen, tenderness, and peritoneal rebound, are often absent in patients with midthoracic and higher spinal cord lesions, leading to a delayed diagnosis. Referred shoulder tip pain, anorexia, nausea, vomiting, increased spasticity, and autonomic dysreflexia are the most important indications of gallbladder disease in patients with high SCI.[148,180]

Genitourinary Implications

Voiding results from a series of events that culminate in the reflexive micturition. Normal micturition involves coordination between the bladder, the internal and external sphincters, micturition control centers in the brain, and the autonomic nervous system (see Figure 23-8). Sympathetic innervation to the bladder, carried by the hypogastric nerves, whose cell bodies lie in the T11-12 cord segments, produces relaxation of the bladder body and narrowing of the bladder neck. Parasympathetic nervous system innervation occurs via the pelvic nerves, which enter and exit the spine at the S2-4 spinal segments. The PNS facilitates bladder emptying through contraction of the detrusor muscle and relaxation of the internal sphincter. The external sphincter is innervated by the somatic nervous system via the pudendal nerves, whose cell bodies arise from the sacral cord segments (S2-4). Stimulation of the pudendal nerves produces tightening of the external sphincter. This permits bladder filling and inhibition of urination.[181-184]

Stretch receptors in the urethra and bladder walls are stimulated when the bladder is full. Afferent fibers conduct signals via the pelvic nerves to the sacral area of the spinal cord, and an efferent response is sent back via the parasympathetic nervous system to the bladder. This causes contractions of the detrusor muscles of the bladder and concomitant relaxation of the internal sphincter. The pelvic musculature begins to relax, the abdominal muscles and diaphragm contract as the glottis closes to increase intraabdominal pressure, and urine flows into the urethra. The external sphincter reflexively relaxes once urine is released by the internal sphincter and voiding begins. When voiding is complete, reflexive and voluntary closure of the sphincters occurs and the bladder relaxes.[181-184]

The bladder and lower urinary tract are rendered flaccid and areflexive by the state of spinal shock, which results in urine retention. Once spinal shock resolves, SCI above the level of the conus causes uninhibited, involuntary contraction of the detrusor muscle, resulting in spontaneous voiding, which can occur at abnormally low bladder volumes (reflexive neurogenic bladder). If the SCI occurs in the area of the sacral plexus (i.e., conus medullaris or cauda equina injury), the bladder and sphincter are denervated and urinary retention with overflow voiding occurs (areflexic neurogenic bladder).

Initial bladder management during spinal shock requires an indwelling catheter. After the critical phase, when systems have stabilized and spinal shock is resolving, the patient is ready for implementation of a bladder management program. There is no panacea for urinary management in the SCI population. Major considerations should include gender, functional level of injury, age, body habitus, motivation, and lifestyle. Intermittent catheterization, associated with fewer complications than indwelling catheterization, is generally the best method for long-term management if a large bladder capacity can be obtained, with minimal leakage, low intravesicular pressure, and without precipitation of AD.[185-191] To begin bladder training, the patient is placed on a 2000 to 2400 ml/day fluid restriction in an attempt to limit the volume of urine produced to approximately 400 ml every 4 to 6 hours.[185] This volume should be adequate to maintain hydration and bladder flushing while preventing repetitive distention, which can damage the bladder wall and upper genitourinary tract.[185-190] Patients and caregivers are taught to perform regular palpation of the suprapubic area to assess for bladder fullness. Portable ultrasonic bladder scan devices can be used to perform volume-guided intermittent catheterizations as opposed to time-guided catheterization.[189,190] Prolonged intermittent catheterization may increase the risk of developing urethral strictures.[191] Generous lubrication, gentle insertion, and the use of hydrophilic catheters may reduce strictural development.[191] In male patients with reflexive voiding, an external condom catheter can be used. As spontaneous reflexive voiding develops, it is important to perform intermittent catheterizations to assess postvoid residuals.[186] Urodynamic studies also help to assess intravesical pressures. If postvoid residual bladder volumes exceed 75 to 100 ml or intravesical pressures are high (greater than 40 to 50 cm H_2O), intermittent catheterizations should continue.[185] Suprapubic tapping can be used to elicit reflexive voiding.[187] Reflexive voiding is often considered an inadequate means of management for females because there is a lack of appropriate external urine collection appliances. If an indwelling catheter is selected for long-term drainage, a suprapubic catheter is placed to avoid the complications associated with transurethral placement. Suprapubic catheters are associated with infection, leakage, and recurrent bladder stones.[185-187,190] Patients with a suprapubic catheter are encouraged to increase their fluid intake to up to 4 L/day to maintain bladder flushing. Many surgical procedures have been developed to assist patients in obtaining continence. Continent conduits, augmentation cystoplasty, and sphincter prostheses are options that are being used.[185,186,191,192]

A long-term complication associated with a reflexive bladder is detrusor sphincter dyssynergia (DSD). DSD is the result of a loss of coordination between the bladder and the external sphincter. As the bladder reflexively contracts in response to fullness, the external sphincter also contracts, prohibiting release of urine. DSD is associated with elevated voiding pressures, which can cause vesicoureteral reflux and hydronephrosis. Annual urodynamic evaluation should be performed to monitor for high bladder pressures and sequelae. Studies suggest that during the transition from indwelling to spontaneous voiding, bladder dynamics continue to change as spinal shock continues to resolve.[185-188] Because spinal shock may take up to a year to fully resolve, frequent titration of medication and monitoring of bladder response is necessary. Pharmaceutical management may include the use of α_1-adrenergic blockers (e.g., prazosin, terazosin) to reduce bladder outlet resistance, antispasmodic agents (e.g., dantrolene, baclofen) to reduce external sphincter spasticity, anticholinergic agents (e.g., propantheline bromide), and botulin A injection to relax the detrusor muscle and lower bladder pressures.[181,185,186] Historically, oxybutynin (Ditropan) was used to balance bladder function. Recent studies have shown this drug to be ineffective, and it may even aggravate the dyssynergia by facilitating neurotransmission to the sphincter.[185,192] Sympathomimetics, used for orthostatic hypotension, close the bladder neck and adversely affect voiding pressures. Surgical intervention for external sphincter spasticity (i.e., sphincterotomy) is usually delayed for at least a year to evaluate for spontaneous recovery of bladder contraction and external sphincter coordination and is used only when conservative treatment fails.[185,192] External sphincterotomy converts the high-pressure bladder to a low-pressure bladder with leakage. If bladder neck function is maintained, leakage may be reduced. Although this intervention affects lifestyle, it is performed to preserve the upper genitourinary tract and promote overall health. Sphincterotomy is not always successful; 15% to 40% of patients require repeat sphincterotomy in addition to pharmacologic intervention.[193]

Conus and cauda equina injuries result in the bladder being insensate and hypocontractile or noncontractile (areflexic). Patients may void by using Valsalva's maneuver or manual bladder compression (Credé's maneuver). Caution must be used when performing a Credé's maneuver; suprapubic compression increases bladder pressure and causes a compression of the urethra creating a functional obstruction. This may worsen existing high bladder outlet resistance and lead to insufficient emptying. Because of the high pressures that may be created during the Credé and Valsalva maneuvers, consensus guidelines recommend that use of these interventions be discouraged unless urodynamic testing is performed that documents acceptable bladder pressures.[185,187]

Loss of reflexive muscle tone can produce urinary incontinence. External urine collection devices, such as condom catheters for males or incontinence pads for women, can be used. Attention to maintenance of skin integrity is important with the use of these products. Condom catheters must be changed at least once a day to prevent a buildup of bacteria and promote airflow to the penile tissues.[187] Intermittent catheterizations are usually reserved for patients with elevated postvoid residuals.[185-187] Female patients present unique problems. They frequently experience breakdown of perineal tissue from incontinence, and intermittent catheterization can be technically difficult. Many women are managed with indwelling catheters. Surgical procedures, such as the continent conduit, provide women with more options for urinary management.

Functional electrostimulation (FES) has been used in an effort to use spared muscles and neuronal pathways to influence continence and voiding. Perhaps the most successful of these devices is the Finetech-Brindley Bladder system, Vocare (NDI Medical, Cleveland, OH, USA). In patients with intact parasympathetic preganglionic neurons and detrusor contractility, electrodes are surgically implanted on the sacral roots and connected via leads to a subcutaneous receiver-transmitter.[179,188] With use of radiotransmission, pulsating electrical stimulation is delivered and bladder pressure is raised. Upon cessation of electrical stimulation, the detrusor sphincter relaxes faster than the bladder, allowing for the opening of the sphincter while bladder pressure is briefly maintained. Periodic application of the radiotransmission allows for the patient to control voiding.

A sacral posterior rhizotomy (surgical severing of nerve elements) may be performed to render the bladder and sphincter areflexic. This will also result in a loss of any spared perineal sensation. Post procedure, patients are continent, have increased bladder capacity, lower post void residuals, and a reduction in urinary tract infections (UTIs). Patients also report the additional benefit of enhanced bowel control and defecation and, in males, stimulator-associated erections.[179,194] Because a rhizotomy is an irreversible procedure, careful consideration is required prior to performing this intervention.[188]

Urinary Tract Infection

UTIs are the most common complication for SCI patients in the first year after injury, and issues related to the genitourinary system are the most common reason for rehospitalization.[4,156]

Every effort should be made to prevent UTIs by removing indwelling bladder catheters as soon as possible and ensuring complete bladder emptying. Patients must be educated about the signs and symptoms of an acute UTI, which may include fever; spontaneous voiding between catheterizations; autonomic dysreflexia; hematuria; pyuria; cloudy, foul-smelling urine; and vague abdominal discomfort. It is important to recognize that patients with neurogenic bladder dysfunction usually present with persistent bacteriuria. Bacteriuria in the absence of clinical symptoms represents colonization. To reduce the risks of suprainfection and antibiotic-resistant bacteria, antibiotic treatment is typically not indicated in the asymptomatic patient.[191,195,196] UTI implies microbial invasion of any tissues of the urinary tract. UTIs are treated with appropriate antibiotics and increased fluids. Repetitive infections may indicate other urologic problems, such as renal calculi or improper lower urinary tract management. Further evaluation through renal ultrasound and urodynamic studies is recommended if other urologic problems are suspected.[181] Recent investigations studying the impact of lowering the urine pH and the use of cranberry extracts upon bacterial adhesion to the bladder wall concluded that neither strategy altered the rate of bacteriuria in patients using intermittent catheterization.[197]

Urinary Tract Calculi

The presence of urine bacteria and sediment, long-term indwelling catheters, urinary stasis, and chronic calcium loss that occurs after SCI predispose patients to the formation of urinary tract calculi.[187,198] Calculi should be suspected in the presence of persistent UTI, hematuria, or unexplained AD. A definitive diagnosis is reached through diagnostic studies (e.g., kidney/ureter/bladder [KUB] x-ray films, intravenous pyelogram [IVP], or cystogram) or with passage of a stone. Treatment modalities are based on the size and location of the stone. Patients prone to develop stones should modify their diet and increase their fluid intake to dilute and flush the urinary tract.

Skin Implications

Immobility, loss of sensation, incontinence of stool and urine, spasticity, use of adaptive splints and braces, edema, hypotension, and poor nutrition are factors that contribute to the development of skin breakdown in patients with SCI.[199,200] A pressure sore can delay surgery, prolong immobilization, increase hospital stay, and increase the risk of AD. The incidence of pressure ulcer formation during the acute and rehabilitation phases is 33% to 34%, second only to pneumonia.[5] It is the most frequent secondary medical complication in all post-injury years.[156] The most common sites for pressure sore development are the sacrum, ischium, elbows, heels, trochanteric areas, and occiput (especially when cervical collars are worn).[5,199,200] The best treatment for pressure sores is prevention.[199] Use of a pressure-relieving mattress in conjunction with log-rolling every 2 hours during bed rest will help reduce skin breakdown risk. Ensuring proper fit of braces or splints and providing good skin care beneath these devices help preserve skin integrity. The nurse should routinely inspect bony prominences and skin under splints and braces. Nutritional support to maintain healthy tissues is essential. Once the patient can be mobilized, it is imperative that the right chair (i.e., a high-back wheelchair) be used with a pressure-relieving cushion. While the patient is in the chair, weight-shifting or pressure release maneuvers should be performed every 20 minutes by the patient or caregiver. Pressure release maneuvers consist of tilting the wheelchair back for 5 minutes, leaning sideways, and lifting the hip for a few minutes or performing a pushup on the arms of the wheelchair. Patients and family members should be instructed how to perform these maneuvers.

Once a pressure sore occurs, treatment is based on its location, size, and depth.[199] The stage and measurement of the wound should be assessed routinely and documented. Consulting wound care specialists, such as wound, ostomy, and incontinence nurses, assist in developing an optimal program of wound and skin care. Frequent inspection, pressure relief, cleansing, debridement, and protection of the wound should continue during healing. If the wound has significant depth (stage III or IV), surgical intervention may be required.[199] In cases that require significant surgical intervention, the patient requires full pressure relief in the area involved. A fluid therapy bed can provide this relief if the physician determines that the patient's spinal stability can tolerate the lack of support offered by this type of bed. If this option is used, nurses must be vigilant in performing range-of-motion exercises to prevent contractures. The nurse must recognize the emotional impact of prolonged immobilization and hospitalization. Various therapies and family members should be involved in assisting the patient to attain some rehabilitation goals while waiting for skin breakdown to heal.

Musculoskeletal Implications

SCI has significant ramifications for the musculoskeletal system. Depending on the type and level of injury to the spinal cord, flaccidity, paresis, or spasticity may result. In severe injury, as spinal shock resolves, reflexes return and spasticity develops below the level of injury. A loss of muscle innervation leads to a shortening of muscle fibers, imbalance of opposing muscle group strength, and immobility of joints, predisposing the patient to the development of contractures. Also complicating matters is the potential development of heterotopic ossification and a loss of bone density over time.

Spasticity

The pathophysiology of spasticity is not clearly understood. It involves a complex interaction of the descending UMN pathways and heightened stretch reflex propagation coupled with decreased inhibition.[84,201,202] Equally elusive has been an adequate definition that encompasses the various expressions and complexities of this syndrome.[84,201-203] Decq, in 2003, proposed a modified definition of spasticity that sought to unify all the potential causes and resulting symptoms.[204] He defined spasticity as a symptom of UMN dysfunction characterized by an exaggeration of the stretch reflex secondary to hyperexcitability of spinal reflexes. Over time, increased spinal reflex excitability can be attributed to intrinsic changes in the cord. Spasticity is a sequela of UMN (cord) injury, and its onset indicates the resolution of spinal shock.

Two distinct patterns of muscle spasm often occur: flexor patterning and extensor patterning. In flexor patterning the major limb flexors contract, drawing the limb toward the body. In extensor pattern, the extensor muscles contract, resulting in rigid extension of the limbs. The pattern of spasm a patient experiences may be related to the stimulus received and the position of the limb at the time of stimulation. The patterns may also alternate.

Spasticity can have positive and negative effects. Increased muscle tone can reduce venous pooling, stabilize the thoracic and abdominal musculature used in respiration, promote or maintain muscle bulk, and assist patients in dressing and stand-pivot transfers.[202,203] Detrimental effects of spasticity have been linked to chronic pain syndrome, sleep disturbance and fatigue, joint contracture, heterotopic ossification, and skin breakdown.[202,203] Assessing resistance to passive motion of an affected extremity evaluates spasticity. The Modified Ashworth Scale is one of several methods that have been developed to quantify spasticity in terms of degree of tone and frequency of event (Table 23-8). Most important to the evaluation of spasticity is the patient's perception of its impact on quality of life.

The goals of spasticity management are to decrease muscle tone that interferes with function, retain joint range of motion, and relieve associated pain—in short, to strike a balance between the beneficial aspects and detrimental effects of muscle spasms.[201-203] These goals are best achieved with a multidisciplinary approach. Treatment of spasticity usually begins with range-of-motion exercises, positioning techniques, weight-bearing exercises, and orthoses or splinting.[201-203] If these conservative interventions fail to provide adequate relief, pharmacologic agents can be introduced. The major inhibitory neurotransmitter in the spinal cord is believed to be gamma-aminobutyric acid (GABA). Baclofen, one of the few drugs FDA approved for the treatment of spasticity related to CNS disorder, is considered by many to be the drug of first choice in the management of spasticity associated with SCI.[201-203] By binding with $GABA_B$ receptors, baclofen exerts an inhibitory effect on the monosynaptic and polysynaptic reflexes. Benzodiazepines, such as diazepam, bind presynaptically with the $GABA_A$ receptors enhancing chloride-mediated reduction in the postsynaptic action potential. $Alpha_2$-adrenergic agonists, such as clonidine and tizanidine, bind to $alpha_2$ receptors on the interneurons in the dorsal horn of the spinal cord to inhibit postsynaptic neurotransmission.[201-203,205] $Alpha_2$-adrenergic agonists have demonstrated their potential to reduce spasticity, especially when used in conjunction with baclofen. Dantrolene, which acts at the peripheral effector site (muscle tissue), reduces muscle contraction by increasing calcium binding with the sarcoplasmic reticulum; decreased release of calcium results in an inhibition of calcium-mediated excitation-contraction coupling.[201-203,205] Intrathecal delivery of antispasmodic medications via implantable pump has revolutionized the management of severe SCI spasticity. This route maximizes CSF concentrations of antispasmodics, reducing the required dosage and side effects. Injection therapy using botulism toxin or phenol has demonstrated results for regional, or *focal,* control of spasticity.[201-203,205] In severe cases that fail to respond to conservative physical and pharmacologic intervention, surgical interventions are considered. Surgical interventions tend to be drastic measures that involve severing of neural elements to prevent spasm. Given the direction of neural regeneration research, surgery should be used only for the most desperate cases.

TABLE 23-8 **Modified Ashworth Scale**

Grade	Description
0	No increase in tone
1	Slight increase in tone, giving a "catch" and release or minimal resistance at the end of the range-of-motion (ROM) when the affected part is moved in flexion or extension
1+	Slight increase in tone, giving a "catch" followed by minimal resistance throughout the remaining ROM
2	More marked increase in tone, but limb easily flexed
3	Considerable increase in tone, passive movement difficult
4	Limb rigid in flexion or extension

Modified from Bohannon RW, Smith MB: Interrater reliability of a Modified Ashworth Scale of Muscle Spasticity, *Phys Ther* 67(2):206-20a7, 1987.

Contractures

Joint contractures can occur within 1 week of injury. Imbalance of muscle innervation that occurs with paralysis causes certain muscle groups to become stronger than their opposing muscle group. This produces a shortening of the stronger, contracted muscle fibers. Additional risk factors for the development of joint contractures include high level of spine injury, presence of a pressure ulcer, concomitant head injury, spasticity, heterotopic ossification (HO), and extremity fracture.[206,207] Contractures can lead to a loss of function and functional independence, increased pain, difficulty in positioning, and skin breakdown.[206,207] It is easier to prevent contractures than to treat them. Aggressive range-of-motion exercises assist in preservation of joint movement. Antispasmodic medications to reduce tone may facilitate maintenance of joint range. Early introduction of physical and occupational therapy in conjunction with patient and family education on range-of-motion exercises, positioning, and the use of splints can combat the development of contractures. [206,207] Serial casting with weekly removal for skin assessment and further limb mobility may help reverse a contracting joint. Caution must be taken to avoid forcing joint range of motion so that bone fracture does not occur.

Heterotopic Ossification

HO is the deposition of ectopic bone within connective tissue. The cause of this complication is unclear but appears to involve a combination of humoral (osteoblast stimulating factors), neuroimmunologic (autonomic dysregulation), and local factors (tissue injury with inflammatory response).[208,209] HO usually occurs within the first 6 months after injury; it develops below the level of SCI—the most common site being the anterior aspect of the hips.[208-210] The incidence is higher in patients with neurologically complete injuries, especially those with spasticity. The classic clinical presentation of HO includes swelling, warmth, redness, possibly pain, and reduced range of motion of the affected area, and fever.[208-210] Differential diagnosis is made by bone scan. Treatment of HO in the early phases consists of aggressive range-of-motion exercises and mobilization of the patient. Treatment to reduce spasticity may be of value. Pharmacologic management consists of etidronate disodium (Didronel) to reduce ectopic bone formation.[208-210] Etidronate disodium is contraindicated in patients with actively healing fractures because it prevents ossification of the fractured bone. NSAIDs may help alleviate inflammation and pain.[208-210] In extreme cases surgical intervention to restore joint mobility may be required once the area of ectopic bone formation has matured.[208-211] Maximum maturation can take up to 2 years.

Bone Loss

Loss of bone density after injury is a common occurrence for spinal cord–injured patients. Demineralization occurs in bones below the level of injury. The exact mechanism for the development of osteoporosis is multifactorial, including disuse, neural injury, and hormonal factors.[212,213] Rapid bone loss occurs within the first 4 to 6 months of injury.[212,214] Parathyroid hormone levels are lower in the first year after injury, resulting from injury-related parathyroid gland suppression.[213,214] Within days of initial injury, an increase in bone resorption, increased renal excretion of calcium and a reduction in intestinal absorption are noted, leading to a significant reduction is calcium stores.[213,214] A rise in the rate of osteoclast production is noted within the first months after injury. Symptoms may include pain after range-of-motion exercises and stress fractures.[213,214] Fractures are reported in up to 34% of patients after SCI.[213,214] Diagnosis is made via serum blood tests, including calcium, phosphorus, alkaline phosphatase, 1,25-dihydroxyvitamin D and calcitonin, and urinary calcium and hydroxyproline. Bone density may be measured via dual-energy x-ray absorptiometry (DEXA) scan or quantitative computed tomography (QCT) scan. Treatment may include weight-bearing exercises with a standing frame, harness, or bike; use of various forms of FES; smoking cessation; limiting caffeine intake; and pharmacologic management.[212-214] Medications prescribed may include biphosphates such as pamidronate (Aredia) or alendronate (Fosamax) and parathyroid hormone (teriparatide [Forteo]) supplementation.

Improving Mobility

Loss of upper extremity function is a severe problem for tetraplegic patients because it threatens their ability to be independent. Orthoses and surgical reconstruction play an important role in the rehabilitation of the upper extremity. Techniques in FES are offering many patients restoration of function.

The goals of surgical reconstruction are to restore active elbow extension and single handgrip.[215,216] This is accomplished by muscle tendon transfer. Selection for surgical reconstruction is dependent on existing motor and sensory function. Surgical intervention is usually not performed for at least 1 year after injury. This provides adequate time for neurologic recovery to plateau, for spasticity of the extremity to become static, and for the patient to progress in adjustment to the psychological ramifications of injury.[215,216]

FES is the electrical stimulation of a muscle to provide a specific movement or function. The muscles can be stimulated by surface electrodes placed on the skin or by surgically implanted electrodes. Prerequisites for successful use of FES include control of spasticity, adequate seated balance, nearly full range of motion of the affected extremity, and an intact LMN.[216,217] FES systems can be used to facilitate upright positioning, augment walking, and allow finger movement. Surface systems can be difficult to apply and remove, cumbersome for the patient to wear, and cosmetically unattractive. Surgically implantable systems may be superior for long-term use.[216,217]

Sexual Function

Spinal cord–injured patients have the same sexual desires as any other person. The goal of sexual rehabilitation for the patient with SCI is the same as any other rehabilitative goal—to assess residual capacity and attempt to maximize posttraumatic potential. Perhaps the greatest obstacle to achieving this goal lies in the myths that society has created surrounding sex and sexual fulfillment. Phrases such as "able-bodied" or "less of a man or woman" embody the attitude that permeates society, equating physical capabilities with the ability to attain sexual satisfaction. Sexual intimacy has become synonymous with the physical act of intercourse. With the overwhelming changes in body image and self-concept, coupled with the fear of rejection, it is not surprising for patients with SCI to experience an initial reduction in libido.[218-220] Sexual counseling to explore attitudes, history, experience, and options should be offered early in rehabilitation. Sexual experimentation is necessary to discover new ways for the individual to please and be pleasured.[218,219]

The normal physiologic response centers that control sexual behavior and the conscious experience of pleasure are located in the brain. These higher centers integrate afferent input from the genitals; skin; auditory, visual, and gustatory centers; and psychogenic or fantasy information. In people with SCI, there is a break in afferent information from below the level of injury to the brain; however, sensory input from above the injury remains intact. The physical act of intercourse remains possible for most individuals. Female patients, though they lack innervation of the pelvic floor muscles, maintain reflex lubrication and congestion. For men, the ability to have and maintain an erection and to ejaculate is a significant issue. In a manner similar to bowel and bladder innervation, the sympathetic nervous system (hypogastric and lumbar sympathetic chain), PNS (sacral nerves), and somatic nervous system (pudendal nerve) are all involved in these processes.[220,221]

Erection is a function of the PNS. In men with intact sacral reflexes (SCI at T10 and higher), obtaining an erection is possible; however, the duration tends to be short-lived and of insufficient rigidity for penetration.[218,220-224] Erectile dysfunction can be managed with technical aids (rings or vacuum pumps) or pharmacologic agents. Pharmacologic agents may include intracavernous injection of vasoactive agents (phentolamine, papaverine, and alprostadil) to vasodilate penile vessels and cause an erection, or oral phosphodiesterase inhibitors (sildenafil [Viagra], tadalafil [Cialis], or vardenafil [Levitra]) to promote ability to achieve and maintain an erection.[218,220-224] Penile implants, while available, have largely been abandoned in this population due to the success of pharmacologic interventions.[218]

Ejaculation, a function of the sympathetic nervous system, is an issue when fertility is considered. Most spinal cord–injured men will not experience reflex ejaculation. Several methods for artificial ejaculation, or sperm retrieval, are available: masturbation, vibroejaculation, electroejaculation, and surgical intervention. Vibroejaculation has a high success rate for patients with injuries at T10 and higher, whereas patients with injuries below this level generally require electroejaculation.[218,220-224] Caution must be used to prevent eliciting AD when stimulating the genitals. Spinal cord–injured men tend to have poor sperm quality; serial ejaculation may improve sperm motility.[218,223,224] In vitro fertilization has been a very successful method for spinal cord–injured men to father a child.[218]

For women, fertility is generally not an issue and conception is possible.[218,219,225,226] Pregnancy and delivery may be complicated by increases in blood pressure, inability to sense contractions, and possible precipitation of AD during labor.[218-220,225,226] Close monitoring and good prenatal care and planning help prevent these complications.

Chronic Pain and Depression

Chronic pain is a significant issue for SCI patients. Studies investigating the prevalence of chronic pain in patients with SCI have found rates between 47% and 96%.[227-230] It appears to interfere less frequently with work and daily living over time.[227-229] Chronic pain limits patients' ability to perform ADLs, which diminishes quality of life and increases depression. In 2000, the Spinal Cord Injury Pain Task Force of the International Association of the Study of Pain proposed a taxonomy of pain to aid classification and treatment.[230-232] Pain can be separated into two categories: nociceptive and neuropathic. Nociceptive pain is caused by noxious stimulation of somatic or visceral receptors in normally innervated body parts. Although it is often related to traumatic injury (vertebral fractures, muscle spasms, inflammation), usually nociceptive pain is not related to the sustained sensory or motor deficit.[227,232] Neurogenic pain is related to injury of the nerve tissue in the central or peripheral nervous system; it may occur at, above, and below the level of injury.[227,232] Siddall and Middleton have proposed and advocated the development and use of algorithms, or a multitiered approach, to managing pain.[232] Using the underlying pathology to differentiate the type of pain and using type- and source-specific interventions can lead to optimal management. A combination of drugs and non-medication strategies is usually used.

In patients with SCI, there is a high incidence of shoulder pain.[227,228,230,232-234] This chronic shoulder pain is exacerbated by excessive use in ADLs and wheelchair locomotion. Range-of-motion exercises, shoulder strengthening exercises, massage, local application of heat or cold, and the use of muscle relaxants and analgesics (e.g., opioids, NSAIDS) generally help to manage this pain.[227,232,233] Electrical stimulation (transcutaneous electrical nerve stimulator [TENS] and FES) may be effective in reducing nociceptive pain.[227,232] In cervical injuries, neck pain is a frequent complaint, particularly during the early phases of rehabilitation. Neck pain is commonly attributed to spine instability, surgical intervention, inflammatory response, and neurovascular compression. Cariga et al recently noted the incidence of neck pain and orthostatic hypotension in SCI subjects, especially new cases, and hypothesized that the two events were connected rather than simply coexisting.[234] Further study demonstrated a strong association between the two events, leading to the conclusion that the neck pain resulted from ischemia. The neck and surrounding muscles are largely supplied by vessels located above the heart. When upright, gravitational forces combined with loss of vascular tone favor a reduction of flow to these areas. Most subjects report a reduction or resolution of neck pain with recumbency or head-forward positioning, such as that used for pressure relief.[234]

Neurogenic pain can be more difficult to treat. Rarely can a specific cause be pinpointed, other than the trauma to nerve tissue. Anticonvulsants such as gabapentin (Neurontin), carbamazepine (Tegretol), and antidepressant/tricyclic compounds such as amitriptyline have been used with varying success.[227,232] Recently, pregabalin has gained FDA approval for use with neuropathic pain. A more potent derivative of gabapentin, pregabalin, is capable of providing a similar effect with fewer dose-related side effects. A recent study by Siddall et al concluded that pregabalin was effective in relieving central neuropathic pain and in improving sleep and anxiety in patients with SCI.[235] In extreme cases implantable intrathecal pumps with narcotic infusion have been used. Destructive surgical procedures to control chronic pain after SCI have been largely abandoned.

The perception of pain and its severity is influenced by many factors, particularly depression and adjustment disorders.[227,232,236,237] In cases in which depression is a precipitating factor, counseling or cognitive behavior therapy can be valuable.[227,232] Pain causes psychological distress, leading to poor community reintegration and quality of life.[236] Because the ultimate goal in rehabilitation after SCI is reintegration into the community with a high perceived quality of life, breaking the pain-depression cycle becomes paramount. Studies demonstrate that patients who achieved the greatest life satisfaction were those who were able to participate in a variety of activities to the fullest of their abilities, whereas those who achieved poor social and community reintegration reported greater pain and lower life satisfaction.[237,238] Pain also reduces the ability to cope with severe impairment, producing even greater emotional distress and depression.

Given the life-altering nature of SCI, individuals are at risk of developing feelings of powerlessness. This despondency can easily develop into clinical depression. The Consortium for Spinal Cord Medicine has developed clinical practice guidelines to assist primary providers in screening and treating this disorder.[237] Routine screening done by the physician interviewing the patient and family focuses on identifying the general risk factors; specific risk factors; and biologic (sleep disturbance, anorexia, fatigue), social (living arrangements, finances, activities), and psychological (coping style, self-blame, posttraumatic stress) risk factors.[237] Once this information is compiled and depression is suspected, the patient should be referred to an appropriate mental health provider. A comprehensive treatment plan that delineates the responsibility of the primary care provider and mental health provider should be developed and articulated. This plan should provide patient and family education and counseling, appropriate pharmacologic intervention, and development of a supportive environment and social system.[237] The treatment plan should be evaluated with a focus on revitalizing the patient and restoring him or her to an optimal level of well-being and functioning. It is also important to monitor the coping ability of the family. Often family members also are the primary caretakers and are just as vulnerable to feelings of inadequacy and helplessness.

Neurologic Implications

Posttraumatic Syringomyelia

Posttraumatic syringomyelia (PTS) is a relatively late-occurring complication of SCI. A syrinx, a fluid-filled cavity within the spinal cord, may develop within a few months to decades after SCI.[239,240] It has been detected clinically in 0.3% to 3.4% of patients and, on MRI, in up to 22% of patients.[239-241] This complication is seen more often in paraplegics than in tetraplegics.[239-241] The etiology of PTS development is not well understood. Common to all theories of pathogenesis is the loss of spinal cord substance and subsequent formation of a cystic cavity within the parenchyma of the spinal cord. The most common symptom of PTS is pain, usually described as a dull ache that increases with straining, coughing, or sneezing.[239,241] Additional symptoms include ascending sensory loss, motor weakness, and changes in spasticity.[239,240] Autonomic symptoms, such as increased sweating and hypertension, may also occur. The earliest clinical sign is loss of deep tendon reflexes.[239-241] Definitive diagnosis is made through clinical examination and MRI.

Management of PTS is as controversial as the theories surrounding its development. The advent of MRI technology has increased the accuracy of imaging, permitting surgeons to detect cavitation within the cord, measure size and length, monitor progression over time, and monitor surgical decompression.[239,240] The goal of surgical intervention is to reduce pain and prevent further neurologic deterioration. Surgical intervention to drain the cavity has had unreliable success rates and exposes patients to the risk of further neurologic insult.[239,240]

Decompression techniques include laminectomy with subarachnoid space reconstruction, primary drainage, and use of shunts. In most patients surgery decreases pain and reduces motor deficit, but there is little effect on sensory deficits or spasticity.[240] There are patients who continue to deteriorate despite surgical intervention. PTS remains a threat to all SCI patients. It is important to consider the presence of PTS whenever intractable upper extremity, shoulder, or scapular pain is a presenting symptom. Early diagnosis may minimize the potentially devastating neurologic losses caused by PTS.

Summary

Although the incidence of SCI is relatively small, the effects on the individual, the family, and society are staggering. Although prevention of SCI is a daunting task, preventing just one case per year can be a tremendous cost savings, especially over time. For many years it appeared that an injured spinal cord could not be repaired or regenerated.

However, exciting progress has been made in neural regeneration and pharmacologic intervention that may interrupt the cycle of secondary injury. The burgeoning field of biomedical technology is creating many options to assist patients in becoming more independent in their daily lives. SCI is a fertile area for nursing research. The nurse is challenged in providing care, preventing complications, and facilitating the patient's reintegration into society. Social reform and legislation to protect the rights of handicapped individuals and provide accessibility have improved the quality of life for the individual with SCI. As our body of knowledge on the care of patients with acute SCI grows, our ability to limit complications and enhance outcomes improves.

REFERENCES

1. Bearsted JH: *The Edwin Smith Surgical Papyrus,* Chicago, 1930, University of Chicago.
2. Lifshutz J, Colohan: A brief history of therapy for traumatic spinal cord injury, *NeurosugFocus* 2004;16(1):Article 5. Available online at http://www.aans.org/education/journal/neurosurgical/jan04/16-1-5.pdf. Retrieved February 11, 2006.
3. Sekhon L, Fehlings MG: Epidemiology, demographics, and pathophysiology of acute spinal cord injury, *Spine* 2001;26(245): S2-S12.
4. National Spinal Cord Injury Statistical Center: *Annual Statistical Report for the Model Spinal Cord Injury Care Systems 2005,* University of Alabama at Birmingham, July 2005. Available online at http://images.main.uab.edu/spinalcord/pdffiles/facts05.pdf. Accessed January 27, 2006,
5. National Spinal Cord Injury Statistical Center: *Spinal Cord Injury Facts and Figures at a Glance,* University of Alabama at Birmingham, June 2006. Available online at http://images.main.uab.edu/spinalcord/pdffiles/Facts06.pdf. Accessed October 26, 2006.
6. Berkowitz M: The costs of spinal cord injury. In Lin VW, editor-in-chief: *Spinal Cord Medicine: Principles and Practice*, New York, 2003, Demos Medical Publishing Inc.
7. Liverman CT, Altevogt BM, Joy JE et al, editors: *Spinal Cord Injury: Progress, Promise, and Priorities*, Washington, DC, 2005, National Academies Press.
8. Centers for Disease Control and Prevention, National Center for Injury Prevention and Control: *Spinal Cord Injury Fact Sheet.* Available online at http://www.cdc.gov/ncipc/factsheets/scifacts.htm. Accessed February 11, 2006.
9. Jackson AB, Dijkers M, DeVivo MJ et al: A demographic profile of new traumatic spinal cord injuries: change and stability over 30 years, *Arch Phys Med Rehabil* 85:1740-1748, 2004.
10. Garshick E, Kelley A, Cohen SA et al: A prospective assessment of mortality in chronic spinal cord injury, *Spinal Cord* 43: 408-416, 2005.
11. Centers for Disease Control and Prevention, National Center for Injury Prevention and Control: *Web-based Injury Statistics Query and Reporting System* (WISQARS) (2005) (online database). Available online at http://www.cdc.gov/ncipc/wisqars/. Accessed February 11, 2006.
12. Centers for Disease Control and Prevention, National Center for Injury Prevention and Control: *Falls Among Older Adults: Summary of Research Findings,* (2004). Available online at http://www.cdc.gov/ncipc/pub-res/toolkit/SummaryOfFalls.htm. Accessed February 11, 2006.
13. Hickey JV: *The Clinical Practice of Neurological and Neurosurgical Nursing,* ed 5, Philadelphia, 2003, Lippincott Williams and Wilkins.
14. Slazinski T, Littlejohns LR: Anatomy of the nervous system. In Bader MK, Littlejohns LR, editors: *AANN Core Curriculum for Neuroscience Nursing*, ed 4, St. Louis, 2004, WB Saunders.
15. Iencean SM: Classification of spinal injuries based on the essential traumatic spinal mechanisms, *Spinal Cord* 41:385-396, 2003.
16. Savas PE: Biomechanics of the injured spine. In Vaccaro AR, editor: *Fractures of the Cervical, Thoracic, and Lumbar Spine,* New York, 2003, Marcel Dekker, Inc.
17. Kwon BK, Vaccaro AR, Grauer JN et al: Subaxial cervical spine trauma. *J Am Acad Orthop Surg* 14(2):78-89, 2006.
18. Nightingale RW, McElhaney JH, Richardson WJ et al: Experimental impact injury to the cervical spine: relating motion of the head and the mechanism of injury, *J Bone Joint Surg Am* 78(3):412-421, 1996.
19. Douglass AB, Bope ET: Evaluation and treatment of posterior neck pain in family practice, *J Am Family Practice* 17(Suppl): S13-S22, 2004.
20. Peloso P, Gross A, Haines T et al: Cervical Overview Group: Medicinal and injection therapies for mechanical neck disorders, *Cochrane Database Syst Rev* 18(2)CD000319, 2005.
21. Crawford JR, Khan RJ, Varley GW: Early management and outcome following soft tissue injuries of the neck: a randomized, controlled trial, *Injury* 35(9):891-895, 2004.
22. Dehner C, Hartwig E, Strobel P et al: Comparison of the relative benefits of 2 versus 10 days of soft collar cervical immobilization after acute whiplash injury, *Arch Phys Med Rehabil* 87(11):1423-1427, 2006.
23. Tropiano P, Huang RC, Louis CA et al: Functional and radiographic outcome of thoracolumbar and lumbar burst fractures managed by closed orthopaedic reduction and casting, *Spine* 28(21):249-265, 2003.
24. Butler JS, Walsh A, O'Byrne J: Functional outcome of burst fractures of the first lumbar vertebra managed surgically and conservatively, *Int Orthop* 29(1):51-54, 2005.
25. Yi L, Jingping B, Gele J et al: Operative versus non-operative treatment for thoracolumbar burst fractures without neurological deficit, *Cochrane Database Syst Rev*18(4):CD005079, 2006.
26. Milam RA, Silber JS, Vaccaro AR: Traumatic injuries of the occipital-cervical junction. In Vaccaro AR, editor: *Fractures of the Cervical, Thoracic, and Lumbar Spine*, New York, 2003, Markel Dekker, Inc.
27. Hadley MN, Walters BC, Grabb PA et al: Diagnosis and management of traumatic atlanto-occipital dislocation injuries, *Neurosurgery* 50(3):S105-S113, 2002.
28. Hadley MN, Walters BC, Grabb PA et al: Guidelines for the management of acute cervical spine and spinal cord injuries: isolated fractures of the atlas in adults, *Neurosurgery* 50(3): S120-S124, 2002.
29. Campagnolo DI, Heary RF: Acute medical and surgical management of spinal cord injury. In Kirshblum S, Campagnolo DI, DeLisa JA: *Spinal Cord Medicine*, Philadelphia, 2002, Lippincott Williams & Williams.

30. Hadley MN, Walters BC, Grabb PA et al: Guidelines for the management of acute cervical spine and spinal cord injuries: isolated fractures of the axis in adults, *Neurosurgery* 50(3): S125-S139, 2002.
31. German JW, Hart BL, Benzel EC: Nonoperative management of vertical C2 body fractures, *Neurosurgery* 56(3):516-520, 2005.
32. Hulsebosch CE: Recent advances in pathophysiology and treatment of spinal cord injury, *Adv Physiol Educ* 26:238-255, 2002.
33. Hausmann ON: Post-traumatic inflammation following spinal cord injury, *Spinal Cord* 41:369-378, 2003.
34. Ramer LM, Ramer MS, Steeves JD: Setting the stage for functional repair of spinal cord injures: a cast of thousands, *Spinal Cord* 43:134-161, 2005.
35. McIlvoy L, Meyer K, McQuillan KA: Traumatic spine injuries. In Bader MH, Littlejohns LR, editors: *AANN Core Curriculum for Neuroscience Nursing*, ed 4, St. Louis, 2004, WB Saunders.
36. Harrop JS, Sharan A, Ratliff J: Central cord injury: pathophysiology, management, and outcomes, *Spine J* 6(6 Suppl):S198-S206, 2006.
37. Hadley MN, Walters BC, Grabb PA et al: Guidelines for the management of acute cervical spine and spinal cord injuries: management of acute central cervical spinal cord injuries, *Neurosurgery* 50(3):S166-S172, 2002
38. Tow AM P-E, Kong KH: Central cord syndrome: functional outcome after rehabilitation, *Spinal Cord* 16:156-160, 1998.
39. Aito S, D'Andrea M, Werhagen L et al: Neurological and functional outcome in traumatic central cord syndrome. *Spinal Cord* 45(4):292-297, 2007.
40. Levi AD, Tator CH, Bunge RP: Clinical syndromes associated with disproportionate weakness of the upper versus lower extremities after cervical spinal cord injury, *Neurosurgery* 38(1): 179-185, 1996.
41. Hatzakis MJ Jr, Bryce N, Marino R: Cruciate paralysis, hypothesis for injury and recovery, *Spinal Cord* 38(2):120-125, 2000.
42. Harrop JS, Hunt GE, Vaccaro AR: Conus medullaris and cauda equine syndrome as a result of traumatic injuries: management principles, *Neurosurg Focus* 16(6):e4, 2004. Available online at http://www.aans.org/education/journal/neurosurgical/june04/16-6-4.pdf. Accessed February 2, 2006.
43. Strayer A: Lumbar spine: common pathology and interventions, *J Neurosci Nurs* 37(4):181-193, 2005.
44. Thongtrangan I, Hoang L, Park J et al: Cauda equina syndrome in patients with low lumbar fractures. Neurosurg Focus 16(6): e6, 1004. Available online at http://www.aans.org/education/journal/neurosurgical/june04/16-6-6.pdf. Accessed February 2, 2006.
45. Whetstone W: Prehospital management of spinal cord injured patients. In Lin VE, editor: *Spinal Cord Medicine: Principles and Practice*, New York, 2003, Demos Medical Publishing Inc.
46. Capen DA, Leppek E: Emergency management of spine trauma. In Vaccaro AR, editor: *Fractures of the Cervical, Thoracic, and Lumbar Spine*, New York, 2003, Markel Dekker, Inc.
47. Hadley MN, Walters BC, Grabb PA et al: Guidelines for the management of acute cervical spine and spinal injuries: cervical spine immobilization before admission to the hospital, *Neurosurgery* 50(3):S7-S17, 2002.
48. Domeier RM, Swor RA, Evans RW et al: Multicenter prospective validation of prehospital clinical spinal clearance criteria, *J Trauma* 53(4):744-750, 2002.
49. Domeier RM, Frederiksen SM, Welch K: Prospective performance assessment of an out-of-hospital protocol for selective spine immobilization using clinical spine clearance criteria, *Ann Emerg Med* 46(2):123-131, 2005.
50. Muhr MD, Seabrook DL, Wittwer LK: Paramedic use of a spinal injury clearance algorithm reduces spinal immobilization in the out-of-hospital setting. *Prehosp Emerg Care* 3(1):1-6, 1999.
51. Burton JH, Cunn MG, Harmon NR et al: A statewide, prehospital emergency medical service selective patient spine immobilization protocol, *J Trauma* 61(1):161-167, 2006.
52. Barboi C, Peruzzi WT: Acute medical management of spinal cord injury. In Lin VW, editor in chief: *Spinal Cord Medicine: Principles and Practice*, New York, 2003, Demos Medical Publishing Inc.
53. Hadley MN, Walters BC, Grabb PA et al: Guidelines for the management of acute cervical spine and spinal injuries: clinical assessment after acute cervical spinal cord injury, *Neurosurgery* 50(3): S21-S29, 2002.
54. Hoffman JR, Mower WR, Wolfson AB et al, for the National Emergency X-Radiography Utilization Study Group: Validity of a set of clinical criteria to rule out injury to the cervical spine in patients with blunt trauma, *N Engl J Med* 343(2):94-99, 2000.
55. Hadley MN, Walters BC, Grabb PA et al: Guidelines for the management of acute cervical spine and spinal injuries: radiographic assessment of the cervical spine in asymptomatic trauma patients, *Neurosurgery* 50(3):S30-S35, 2002.
56. Marion D, Domeier F, Dunham CM et al (Cervical Spine Clearance Committee): Determination of cervical spine stability in trauma patients. Eastern Association for Surgery in Trauma (EAST) Clinical Practice Guideline revised 2000. Available online at http://www.east.org/tpg/chap3u.pdf. Accessed November 24, 2006.
57. Stiell IG, Wells GA, Vandernheen K et al: The Canadian c-spine rule for radiography in alert and stable trauma patients, *JAMA* 286(15):1841-1848, 2001.
58. Hadley MN, Walters BC, Grabb PA et al: Guidelines for the management of acute cervical spine and spinal injuries: radiographic spinal assessment in symptomatic trauma patients, *Neurosurgery* 50(3): S36-S43, 2002.
59. Holmes JF, Mirvis SE, Panacek EA et al: Variability in computed tomography and magnetic resonance imaging in patients with cervical spine injuries, *J Trauma* 53(3):524-530, 2002.
60. *Practice Management Guidelines for the Screening of Thoracolumbar Spine Fracture.* Eastern Association for the Surgery of Trauma: Practice Management Guideline Committee, revised 2006. Available online at http://www.east.org/tpg/TLSpine.pdf. Accessed 11/24/2006.
61. Rhee PM, Bridgeman A, Acosta JA et al: Lumbar fractures in adult blunt trauma: axial and single-slice helical abdominal and pelvic computed tomographic scans versus portable plain films, *J Trauma* 53(4):663-667, 2002.
62. Sheridan R, Peralta R, Rhea J et al: Reformatted visceral protocol helical computed tomographic scanning allows conventional radiographs of the thoracic and lumbar spine to be eliminated in the evaluation of blunt trauma patients, *J Trauma* 55(4):665-669, 2003.
63. Berry GE, Adams S, Harris MB et al: Are plain radiographs of the spine necessary during the evaluation after blunt trauma? Accuracy of screening torso computed tomography in thoracic/lumbar spine fracture diagnosis, *J Trauma* 59(6): 1410-1413, 2005.

64. Hauser CJ, Visvikis G, Hinrichs C et al: Prospective validation of computed tomography screening of the thoracolumbar spine in trauma, *J Trauma* 55(2):228-234, 2003.
65. Brown CV, Antevil JL, Sise MJ et al: Spiral computed tomography for the diagnosis of cervical, thoracic and lumbar spine fractures: its time has come, *J Trauma* 58(5):890-895, 2005.
66. Antevil J, Sise MJ, Sack DI et al: Spiral computed tomography for the initial evaluation of spine trauma: a new standard of care? *J Trauma* 61(2):382-387, 2006.
67. Griffen MM, Frykberg ER, Kerwin AJ et al: Radiographic clearance of blunt cervical spine injury: plain radiograph or computed tomography scan? *J Trauma* 55(2):222-226, 2003.
68. Sanchez B, Waxman K, Jones T et al: Cervical spine clearance in blunt trauma: evaluation of a computed tomography-based protocol, *J Trauma* 59(1):179-183, 2005.
69. Gale SC, Gracias VI, Reilly PM et al: The inefficiency of plain radiography to evaluate the cervical spine after blunt trauma, *J Trauma* 59(5):1121-1125, 2005.
70. Holmes JF, Akkinepalli R: Computed tomography versus plain radiography to screen for cervical spine injury: a meta-analysis, *J Trauma* 8(5):902-905, 2005.
71. Sliker CE, Mirvis ST, Shanmuganathan K: Assessing cervical spine stability in obtunded patients: review of medical literature. *Radiology* 234(3):733-739, 2005.
72. Padayachee L, Cooper DJ, Irons S et al: Cervical spine clearance in unconscious traumatic brain injury patients: dynamic flexion-extension fluoroscopy versus computed tomography with three-dimensional reconstruction. *J Trauma* 60(2):341-345, 2006.
73. Davis JW, Kaups K, Cunningham MA et al: Routine evaluation of the cervical spine in head-injured patients with dynamic fluoroscopy: a reappraisal, *J Trauma* 50(6):1044-1047, 2001.
74. Bolinger B, Shartz M, Marion D: Bedside fluoroscopic flexion and extension cervical spine radiographs for clearance of the cervical spine in comatose trauma patients, *J Trauma* 56(1): 132-136, 2004.
75. Pollack CV Jr, Hendey GW, Martin DR et al: NEXUS Group: Use of flexion-extension radiographs of the cervical spine in blunt trauma, *Ann Emerg Med* 38(1):8-11, 2001.
76. Ren X, Wang W, Zhang X et al: The comparative study of magnetic resonance angiography diagnosis and pathology of blunt vertebral artery injury, *Spine* 31(18):2124-2129, 2006.
77. Costa P, Bruno A, Bonzanino et al: Somatosensory- and motor evoked potential monitoring during spine and spinal cord surgery. *Spinal Cord* 45(1):86-91, 2007. Epub May 2, 2006. Retrieved 12/1/2006.
78. Hilibrand AS, Schwartz DM, Sethuraman V et al: Comparison of transcranial electric motor and somatosensory evoked potential monitoring during cervical spine surgery, *J Bone Joint Surg Am* 86-A(6):1248-1253, 2004.
79. Hadley MN, Walters BC, Grabb PA et al: Guidelines for the management of acute cervical spine and spinal injuries: management of acute spinal cord injuries in an intensive care unit or other monitored setting, *Neurosurgery* 50(3):S51-S57, 2002.
80. Crosby ET: Airway management in adults after cervical spine trauma, *Anesthesiology* 104(6):1293-1318, 2006. Available online at http://www.anesthesiology.org/pt/re/anes/pdfhandler.00000542-200606000-00026.pdf;jsessionid5FztRrckRjmg38HCKyVKvh2r9JpyL4wKjhNhBQG2fSLJk9BPxNTwJ!2030273863!-949856145!8091!-1. Accessed December 01, 2006.
81. Consortium for Spinal Cord Medicine: *Respiratory Management Following Spinal Cord Injury: a Clinical Practice Guideline for Healthcare Professionals*, Washington, D.C., 2005, Paralyzed Veterans of America.
82. Brown R, DiMarco AF, Hoit JD et al: Respiratory dysfunction and management in spinal cord injury, *Respir Care* 51(8): 853-868, 2006.
83. Ditunno JF, Little JW, Burns AS: Spinal shock revisited: a four-phase model, *Spinal Cord* 42:383-395, 2004.
84. Hiersemenzel LP, Curt A, Dietz V: From spinal shock to spasticity: neuronal adaptations to a spinal cord injury, *Neurology* 54; 1574-1582, 2000.
85. Krassioukov AL: Which pathways must be spared in the injured human spinal cord to retain cardiovascular control? *Prog Brain Res* 152:39-47, 2006.
86. Krassioukov A, Claydon VE: The clinical problems in cardiovascular control following spinal cord injury: an overview, *Prog Brain Res* 152:223-229, 2006.
87. Teasell RW, Arnold JMO, Krassioukov A et al: Cardiovascular consequences of loss of supraspinal control of the sympathetic nervous system after spinal cord injury, *Arch Phys Med Rehabil* 81(04):506-516, 2000.
88. Hadley MN, Walters BC, Grabb PA et al: Guideline for the management of acute cervical spine and spinal injuries: blood pressure management after acute cervical spinal cord injury, *Neurosurgery* 50(3):S58-S62, 2002.
89. Vickery D: The use of the spinal board after the pre-hospital phase of trauma management. *Emerg Med J* 18:51-54, 2001. Available online at http://emj.bmj.com/cgi/content/full/18/1/51. Accessed October 26, 2006.
90. Kwon BK, Tetslaff W, Grauer JN et al: Pathophysiology and pharmacologic treatment of acute spinal cord injury. *Spine J* 4:451-464, 2004.
91. Schwartz G, Fehlings MG: Secondary injury mechanisms of spinal cord trauma: a novel therapeutic approach for the management of secondary pathophysiology with the sodium channel blocker riluzole, *Prog Brain Res* 137:177-190, 2002.
92. Bracken D, Shepard M, Collins W et al: A randomized controlled trial of methylprednisolone or naloxone in the treatment of acute spinal cord injury, *N Engl J Med* 322(20):1405-1411, 1990.
93. Bracken MB, Shepard MJ, Holford TR et al: Administration of methylprednisolone for 24 or 48 hours or tirilazad mesylate for 48 hours in the treatment of acute spinal cord injury. Results of the third national acute spinal cord injury randomized controlled trial. National acute spinal cord injury study, *JAMA* 277(20):1597-1604, 1997.
94. Hadley MN, Walters BC, Grabb PA et al: Guideline for the management of acute cervical spine and spinal injuries: pharmacological therapy after acute cervical cord injury, *Neurosurgery* 50(3):S63-S72, 2002.
95. Quian R, Guo X, Levi AD et al: High-dose methylprednisolone may cause myopathy in acute spinal cord injured patients, *Spinal Cord* 43:199-203, 2005.
96. del Rosario Molano M, Broton JG et al: Complications associated with the prophylactic use of methylprednisolone during surgical stabilization after spinal cord injury, *J Neurosurg (Spine 3)* 96: 267-272, 2002.
97. Short DJ, El Masry WS, Jones PW: High dose methylprednisolone in the management of acute spinal cord injury: a systemic review from a clinical perspective, *Spinal Cord* 38:273-286, 2000.
98. Bracken MB: Pharmacological interventions for acute spinal cord injury, *Cochrane Database Syst Rev* 1:1-32, 2001.

99. Bracken MB, Holford TR: Neurological and functional status 1 year after acute spinal cord injury: estimates of functional recovery in National Acute Spinal Cord Injury Study II from results modeled in National Acute Spinal Cord Injury Study III, *J Neurosurg Spine (3)*96:259-266, 2002.
100. Emery E, Aldana P, Bunge MB et al: Apoptosis after traumatic human spinal cord injury, *Neurosurg Focus* 6(1), 1999. Article 7. Available online at http://www.aans.org/education/journal/neurosurgical/jan99/6-1-7.asp. Retrieved February 8, 2006.
101. Gorio A, Madaschi L, DiStefano B et al: Methylprednisolone neutralizes the beneficial effects of erythropoietin in experimental spinal injury, *PNAS* 102(45):16379-16384, 2005. Available online at http://www.pnas.org/cgi/reprint/102/45/16379. Retrieved November 23, 2006.
102. Wells JEA, Hurlbert RJ, Fehlings MG et al: Neuroprotection by minocycline facilitates significant recovery from spinal cord injury in mice, *Brain* 126(7):1628-1637, 2003.
103. Teng YD, Choi H, Onario RC et al: Minocycline inhibits contusion-triggered mitochondrial cytochrome c release and mitigates functional deficits after spinal cord injury, *PNAS* 101(9):3071-3076, 2004. Available online at http://www.pnas.org/cgi/reprint/101/9/3071. Retrieved November23, 2006.
104. Geisler FH, Coleman WP, Grieco G et al: The Sygen acute multicenter acute spinal cord injury study, *Spine* 245:S87-S98, 2001.
105. Geisler FH, Dorsey FC, Coleman WP: Recovery of motor function after spinal cord injury—a randomized, placebo-controlled trial with GM-1 ganglioside, *N Engl J Med* 324(26):1829-1838, 1991.
106. Knoller N, Auerbach G, Fulga V et al: Clinical experience using incubated autologous macrophages as a treatment for complete spinal cord injury: phase I study results, *J Neurosurg Spine* (3)173-181, 2005.
107. Shapiro S, Borgens R, Pascuzzi R et al: Oscillating field stimulation for complete spinal cord injury in humans: a phase I trial, *J Neurosurg Spine* (2)3-10, 2005.
108. Hadley MN, Walters BC, Grabb PA et al: Guidelines for the management of acute cervical spine and spinal injuries: initial closed reduction of fracture-dislocation injuries, *Neurosurgery* 50(3):S44-S50, 2002.
109. McKinley W, Meade MA, Kirshblum S et al: Outcomes of early surgical management versus late or no surgical intervention after acute spinal cord injury, *Arch Phys Med Rehabil* 85:1818-1825, 2004.
110. Fehlings M, Tator CH: An evidence-based review of decompressive surgery in acute spinal cord injury: rationale, indications, and timing based on experimental and clinical studies, *J Neurosurg* 91(1 suppl):1-11, 1999.
111. Tator CH, Fehlings MG, Thorpe K et al: Current use and timing of spinal surgery for management of acute spinal cord injury in North America: results of a retrospective multicenter study, *J Neurosurg* 91(1 suppl):12-18, 1999.
112. La Rosa G, Conti A, Cardai S et al: Does early decompression improve neurological outcome of spinal cord injured patients? Appraisal of the literature using a meta-analysis approach, *Spinal Cord* 42(9):503-512, 2004.
113. Peterson PW, Kirshblum S: Pulmonary management of spinal cord injury. In Kirshblum S, Campagnolo DI, DeLisa JA, editors: *Spinal Cord Medicine,* Philadelphia, 2002, Lippincott Williams & Williams.
114. Sassoon CS, Baydur A: Respiratory dysfunction in spinal cord disorders. In Lin VW, editor in chief: *Spinal Cord Medicine: Principles and Practice,* New York, 2003, Demos Medical Publishing Inc.
115. Laghi F, Tobin MJ: Disorders of the respiratory muscles, *Am J Respir Crit Care Med* 168:10–48, 2003.
116. Ledsome JR, Sharp JM: Pulmonary function in acute cervical cord injury, *Am Rev Respir Dis* 124(1):41-44, 1981.
117. Aito S: Complications during the acute phase of traumatic spinal cord lesions, *Spinal Cord* 41:629-635, 2003.
118. Bodin P, Olsen MF, Bake B: Effects of abdominal binding on breathing patterns during breathing exercises in person with tetraplegia, *Spinal Cord* 43:117-122, 2005 .
119. Hess DR: The evidence for secretion clearance techniques, *Respir Care* 46:1276-1293, 2001.
120. McCool DF, Rosen MJ: Nonpharmacologic airway clearance therapies: ACCP evidence-based practice guidelines, *Chest* 129:250-259, 2006.
121. Miske LJ, Hickey EM, Kolb SM et al: Use of the mechanical in-Exsufflator in pediatric patients with neuromuscular disease and impaired cough, *Chest* 125:1406-1412, 2004.
122. Tzeng AJ, Bach JR: Prevention of pulmonary morbidity for patients with neuromuscular disease, *Chest* 118:1390-1396, 2000.
123. Bach JR: Continuous noninvasive ventilation for patients with neuromuscular disease and spinal cord injury, *Semin Respir Crit Care Med* 23(3):283-292, 2002.
124. Tromans AM, Mecci M, Barrett FH et al: The use of the BiPAP biphasic positive airway pressure system in acute spinal cord injury, *Spinal Cord* 36(7):481-484, 1998.
125. Bach JR, Miske LJ, Panitch HB: Don't forget the abdominal thrust, *Chest* 126: 1388-1390, 2004. Editorial.
126. Nantwi KD, Basura CI, Goshgarian HG: Effects of long-term theophylline exposure on recovery of respiratory function and expression of adenosine A1 mRNA in cervical spinal cord hemisected adult rats, *Exp Neurol* 182(1): 232-239, 2003.
127. Bascom AT, Lattin CD, Aboussouan LS et al: Effect of acute aminophylline administration on diaphragm function in high cervical tetraplegia: a case report, *Chest* 127:658-661, 2005.
128. O'Keefe T, Goldman RK, Mayberry JC et al: Tracheostomy after anterior cervical spine fixation, *J Trauma* 57(4):855-860, 2004.
129. Harrop JS, Sharan AD, Scheid EH et al: Tracheostomy placement in patients with complete cervical spinal cord injuries: American Spinal Injury Association Grade A, *J Neurosurg Spine (1)*100:20-23, 2004
130. Levi L, Wolf A, Belzberg H: Hemodynamic parameters in patients with acute cervical cord trauma: description, intervention, and prediction of outcome. *Neurosurgery* 33:1007-1017, 1993.
131. Vale FL, Burns J, Jackson AB et al: Combined medical and surgical treatment after acute spinal cord injury: results of a prospective pilot study to assess the merits of aggressive medical resuscitation and blood pressure management, *J Neurosurg* 87:239-246, 1997.
132. Collins HL, Rodenbaugh DW, DiCarol SE: Spinal cord injury alters cardiac electrophysiology and increases the susceptibility to ventricular arrhythmias. In Weaver LC, Polosa C, editors: *Progress in Brain Research* 152:275-288, 2006.

133. Pinsky M: Cardiovascular issues in respiratory care, *Chest* 128(5 Suppl 2):592S-597S, 2005.
134. Frisbie JH: Breathing and the support of blood pressure after spinal cord injury, *Spinal Cord* 43:406-407, 2005.
135. Sabharwal S: Cardiovascular dysfunction in spinal cord disorders. In Lin VW, editor in chief, *Spinal Cord Medicine: Principles and Practice*, New York, 2003, Demos Medical Publishing Inc.
136. Panoori VR, Leesar MA: Use of aminophylline in the treatment of severe symptomatic bradycardia resistant to atropine, *Cardiol Rev* 12(2):65-68, 2004.
137. Bilello JF, Davis JW, Cunningham MA et al: Cervical spinal cord injury and the need for cardiovascular intervention, *Arch Surg* 138(10):1127-1129, 2003.
138. Peruzzi WT, Shapiro BA, Meyer PR Jr et al: Hyponatremia in acute spinal cord injury, *Crit Care Med* 22;252-258, 1994.
139. Kahn T: Reset osmostat and salt and water retention in the course of severe hyponatremia, *Medicine* 82(3):170-176, 2003.
140. Consortium for Spinal Cord Medicine: *Prevention of Thromboembolism in Spinal Cord Injury,* ed 2: Washington, DC, 1999, Paralyzed Veterans of America.
141. Hadley MN, Walters BC, Grabb PA et al: Guideline for the management of acute cervical spine and spinal injuries: deep vein thrombosis and thromboembolism in patients with cervical spinal cord injuries, *Neurosurgery* 50(3):S73-S80, 2002.
142. Geerts WH, Pineo GF, Heit JA et al: Prevention of venous thromboembolism. The Seventh ACCP Conference on Antithrombotic and Thrombolytic Therapy. *Chest* 126:338-400, 2004. Available online at http://www.chestjournal.org/cgi/content/full/126/3_suppl/338S. Accessed November 1, 2006.
143. Velmahos GC, Kern J, Chan LS et al: Prevention of venous thromboembolism after injury: an evidence-based report—part II: analysis of risk factors and evaluation of the role of vena caval filters, *J Trauma* 49(1):140-144, 2000.
144. Wilson JT, Rogers FB, Wald SL et al: Prophylactic vena cava filter insertion in patients with traumatic spinal cord injury: preliminary results, *Neurosurgery* 34(2):234-239, 1994.
145. Maxwell RA, Chavarria-Aguilar M, Cockerham WT et al: Routine prophylactic vena cava filtration is not indicated after acute spinal cord injury, *J Trauma* 52(5):902-906, 2002.
146. Hoff WS, Hoey BA, Wainwright GA et al: Early experience with retrievable inferior vena cava filters in high-risk trauma patients, *J Am Coll Sur* 199(6):869-874, 2004.
147. Rosenthal D, Wellons ED, Lai KM et al: Retrievable inferior vena cava filters: early clinical experience, *J Cardiovasc Surg* (Torino) 46(2):163-169, 2005.
148. Stiens SA, Fajardo NR, Korsten MA: The gastrointestinal system after spinal cord injury. In Lin VW, editor in chief: *Spinal Cord Medicine: Principles and Practice*, New York, 2003, Demos Medical Publishing Inc.
149. Chung EAL, Emmanuel AV: Gastrointestinal symptoms related to autonomic dysfunction following spinal cord injury *Prog Brain Res* 152:317-333, 2006.
150. Hadley MN, Walters BC, Grabb PA et al: Guideline for the management of acute cervical spine and spinal injuries: nutritional support after spinal cord injury, *Neurosurgery* 50(3): S81-S84, 2002.
151. Rown CJ, Gillanders Lk, Paice RL et al: Is early enteral feeding safe in patients who have suffered spinal cord injury? *Injury* 35(3):238-242, 2004.
152. Romito RA: Early administration of enteral nutrients in critically ill patients, *AACN Clin Issues* 6(2):242-225, 1995.
153. Moore FA, Moore EE, Haenel JB: Clinical benefits of early post-injury enteral feeding, *Clin Intensive Care* 6(1):21-27, 1995.
154. Consortium for Spinal Cord Medicine: *Neurogenic Bowel Management in Adults with Spinal Cord Injury,* Washington, DC, 1998, Paralyzed Veterans of America.
155. Ayyappa E, Down K: Spinal orthosis. In Lin VW, editor in chief: *Spinal Cord Medicine: Principles and Practice*, New York, 2003, Demos Medical Publishing Inc.
156. Cardenas DD, Hoffman JM, Kirshblum S et al: Etiology and incidence of rehospitalization after traumatic spinal cord injury, *Arch Phys Med Rehabil* 85:1757-1763, 2004.
157. Baydur A, Adkins RH, Milic-Emili J: Lung mechanics in individuals with spinal cord injury: effects of injury level and posture, *J Appl Physiol* 90:405-411, 2001.
158. Frisbie JH: Breathing pattern in tetraplegic patients, *Spinal Cord* 40:424-425, 2002. Letter to the editor.
159. DeLuca RV, Brimm DR, Lesser M et al: Effects of a β2-agonist on airway hyperreactivity in subjects with cervical spinal cord injury, *Chest* 115(6):1533-1538, 1999.
160. Schilero GJ, Grimm DR, Bauman WA et al: Assessment of airway caliber and bronchodilator responsiveness in subjects with spinal cord injury, *Chest* 127:149-155, 2005.
161. Epstein LJ, Brown R: Sleep disorders in spinal cord injury. In Lin VW, editor in chief: *Spinal Cord Medicine: Principles and Practice*, New York, 2002, Demos Medical Publishing Inc.
162. Kelfbeck B, Sternhag M, Weinberg C et al: Obstructive sleep apneas in relation to severity of cervical spinal injury, *Spinal Cord* 36:621-628, 1998.
163. Burns SP, Rad MY, Bryant S et al: Long-term treatment of sleep apneas in persons with spinal cord injury, *Am J Phys Med Rehabil* 84(8):620-626, 2005.
164. Berlowitz DJ, Brown DJ et al: A longitudinal evaluation of sleep and breathing in the first year after cervical spinal cord injury, *Arch Phys Med Rehabil* 86(6):1193-1196, 2005.
165. Zeitzer JM, Ayas NT, Shea SA et al: Absence of detectable melatonin and preservation of cortisol and thyrotropin rhythms in tetraplegia, *J Clin Endocrinol Metab* 55(6): 2189-2196, 2000. Available online at http://jcem.endojournals.org/cgi/reprint/85/6/2189.pdf. Accessed February 11, 2006.
166. Weaver LC, Marsh DR, Gris D et al: Autonomic dysreflexia after spinal cord injury: central mechanisms and strategies for prevention, *Prog Brain Res* 152:245-264, 2006.
167. Mathias CJ: Orthostatic hypotension and paroxysmal hypertension in humans with high spinal cord injury, *Prog Brain Res* 152:231-244, 2006.
168. Vaidanathan S, Soni BM, Sett P et al: Pathophysiology of autonomic dysreflexia: long-term treatment with terazosin in adult and paediatric spinal cord injury patients manifesting recurrent dysreflexic episodes, *Spinal Cord* 36(11):761-770, 1998.
169. Consortium for Spinal Cord Medicine: *Acute Management of Autonomic Dysreflexia: Adults with Spinal Cord Injury Presenting to Health Care Facilities*, ed 2, Washington, DC, 2001, Paralyzed Veterans of America.
170. Claydon VE, Steeves JD, Krassioukov A: Orthostatic hypotension following spinal cord injury: understanding clinical pathophysiology, *Spinal Cord* 44:341-351, 2006.

171. Groomes TE, Huang CT: Orthostatic hypotension after spinal cord injury: treatment with fludrocortisone and ergotamine, *Arch Phys Med Rehabil* 1(72):56-58, 1991.
172. Mukand Karlin L, Barrs K, Luldin P: Midodrine for management of orthostatic hypotension in patients with spinal cord injury: a case report, *Arch Phys Med Rehabil* 82(5):694-696, 2001.
173. Barber DB, Rogers SJ, Fredrickson MD et al: Midodrine HCl and the treatment of orthostatic hypotension in tetraplegia: two cases and a review of the literature, *Spinal Cord* 38(2): 109-111, 2000.
174. Sampson EE, Burnham RS, Andrews BJ: Functional electrical stimulation effect on orthostatic hypotension after spinal cord injury, *Arch Phys Med Rehabil* 2(81):139-143, 2000.
175. Chao CY, Cheing GL: The effects of lower extremity functional electrical stimulation on the orthostatic responses of people with tetraplegia, *Arch Phys Med Rehabil* 86(7): 1427-1433, 2005.
176. Lynch AC, Antony A, Dobbs BR et al: Bowel dysfunction following spinal cord injury, *Spinal Cord* 39:193-203, 2001.
177. Lynch AC, Frizelle FA: Colorectal motility and defecation after spinal cord injury in humans, *Prog Brain Res* 152:335-343, 2006.
178. Brading AF, Famalingam T: Mechanisms controlling normal defecation and the potential effects of spinal cord injury, *Prog Brain Res* 152:345-358, 2006.
179. Creasey GH, Brill JH, Korsten M et al: An implantable neuroprosthesis for restoring bladder and bowel control to patients with spinal cord injuries: a multicenter trial, *Arch Phys Med Rehabil* 82:1512-1519, 2001.
180. Rotter KP, Larrain CG: Gallstones in spinal cord injury (SCI): a late medical complication? *Spinal Cord* 41:105-108, 2003.
181. Potter, PJ: Disordered control of the urinary bladder after human spinal cord injury: what are the problems? *Prog Brain Research* 152:51-57, 2006.
182. de Groat WC, Yoshimura N: Mechanisms underlying the recovery of lower urinary tract function following spinal cord injury, *Prog Brain Res* 152:58-84, 2006.
183. Wrathall JR, Emch GS: Effect of injury severity on lower urinary tract function after experimental spinal cord injury, *Prog Brain Res* 152:117-134, 2006.
184. Craggs MD: Pelvic somato-visceral reflexes after spinal cord injury: measures of functional loss and partial preservation, *Prog Brain Res* 152:205-219, 2006.
185. Stöhrer M, Castro-Diaz D, Chartier-Kastler et al: Guidelines on neurogenic lower urinary tract dysfunction, *Prog Urol* 17(3):703-755, 2007.
186. Vaidyanathan S, Soni BM, Sett P et al: Flawed trial of micturition in cervical spinal cord injury patients: guidelines for trial of voiding in men with tetraplegia, *Spinal Cord* 41:667-672, 2003.
187. Wyndaele JJ, Madersbacher H, Kovindha A: Conservative treatment of the neuropathic bladder in spinal cord injured patients, *Spinal Cord* 39:294-300, 2001.
188. Gaunt RA, Prodhazka A: Control of urinary bladder function with devices: successes and failures, *Prog Brain Res* 152: 163-194, 2006.
189. Wyndaele JJ: Intermittent catheterization: which is the optimal technique? *Spinal Cord* 40:432-437, 2002.
190. Polliack T, Bluvshtein V, Philo O et al: Clinical and economic consequences of volume- or time-dependent intermittent catheterization in patients with spinal cord lesions and neuropathic bladder, *Spinal Cord* 43:615-619, 2005.
191. Wyndaele JJ: Complications of intermittent catheterization: their prevention and treatment, *Spinal Cord* 40:536-541, 2002.
192. Chartier-Kastler EJ, Mozer P, Denys P et al: Neurogenic bladder management and cutaneous non-continent ileal conduit, *Spinal Cord* 40:443-448, 2002.
193. Reynard JM, Vass J, Mamas M: Sphincterotomy and the treatment of detrusor-sphincter dyssynergia: current status, future prospects, *Spinal Cord* 41:1-11, 2003.
194. Creasy GH, Dahlber JE: Economic consequences of an implanted neuroprosthesis for bladder and bowel management, *Arch Phys Med Rehabil* 82:1520-1525, 2001.
195. National Institute for Disability Rehabilitation Research Consensus Statement: The prevention and management of urinary tract infections among people with spinal cord injuries, *J Am Paraplegia Soc* 15:194, 1992.
196. Penders J, Huylenbroeck AAY, Everaert K et al: Urinary infections in patients with spinal cord injury, *Spinal Cord* 41: 549-552, 2003.
197. Schlager TA, Ashe K, Hendley JO: Effect of a phosphate supplement on urine pH in patients with neurogenic bladder receiving intermittent catheterization, *Spinal Cord* 43: 187-189, 2005.
198. Chen Y, DeVivo MJ, Stover SL et al: Recurrent kidney stone: a 25 year follow-up study in persons with spinal cord injury, *Urology* 60(2):228-232, 2002.
199. Consortium for Spinal Cord Medicine: Pressure ulcer prevention and treatment following spinal cord injury: a clinical practice guideline for healthcare professionals, Washington, DC, 2000, Paralyzed Veterans of America.
200. Garber SL, Rintala DH: Pressure ulcers in veterans with spinal cord injury: a retrospective study, *J Rehabil Res Dev* 40(5): 433-442, 2003.
201. Priebe MM, Goetz LL, Wuermser LA: Spasticity following spinal cord injury. In Kirshblum S, Campagnolo DI, DeLisa JA, editors: *Spinal Cord Medicine*, Philadelphia, 2002, Lippincott Williams & Williams.
202. Nance PW: Management of spasticity. In Lin VW, editor: *Spinal Cord Medicine: Principles and Practice*, New York, 2003, Demos Medical Publishing Inc.
203. Adams MM, Hicks AL: Spasticity after spinal cord injury, *Spinal Cord* 43:577-586, 2005.
204. Decq P: Pathophysiology of spasticity. *Neurochirugie* 49: 163-183, 2003.
205. Gracies JM, Elovic E, John McGuire J et al: Traditional pharmacological treatments for spasticity part II: general and regional treatments, *Muscle Nerve* 20(Suppl 6):S1-S29, 1997.
206. Dalyan M, Sherman A, Cardenas DD: Factors associated with contractures in acute spinal cord injury, *Spinal Cord* 36: 405-408, 1998.
207. Harvey LA, Herbert RD: Muscle stretching for treatment and prevention of contracture in people with spinal cord injury, *Spinal Cord* 40:1-9, 2002.
208. van Kuijk AA, Beurts ACH, van Kuppevelt HJM: Neurogenic heterotopic ossification in spinal cord injury, *Spinal Cord* 40:313-326, 2002.
209. Banovac K, Banovac F: Heterotopic ossification. In Kirshblum S, Campagnolo DI, DeLisa JA, editors: *Spinal Cord Medicine*, Philadelphia, 2002, Lippincott Williams & Williams.
210. Freebourn TM, Barber DB, Able AC: The treatment of immature heterotopic ossification in spinal cord injury with

combination surgery, radiation therapy and NSAID, *Spinal Cord* 37:50-53, 1999.

211. Garland DE: Resection of heterotopic ossification in patients with spinal cord injuries, *Arch Phys Med Rehabil* 242:169-176, 1987.
212. Weiss DR: Osteoporosis and spinal cord injury. In Yadav RR, Talavera F, Foye PM et al, editors: Available online at http://www.emedicine.com/pmr/topic96.htm. Updated December 7, 2006. Accessed December 11, 2006.
213. Jiang SD, Dai LY, Jiang LS: Osteoporosis after spinal cord injury, *Osteoporosis Int* 17(2):180-192, 2006.
214. No author. Osteoporosis and spinal cord injury, *Research Review* March 5(1), 2003. Available online at http://www.spinalcord.uab.edu. Accessed December 11, 2006.
215. Freehafer A: Tendon transfers in tetraplegic patients: the Cleveland experience, *Spinal Cord* 36:315-319, 1998.
216. Hentz VR, McAdams TR: Functional restoration of the upper extremity in tetraplegia. In Lin VW, editor in chief: *Spinal Cord Medicine: Principles and Practice,* New York, 2003, Demos Medical Publishing Inc.
217. Gorman PH: Functional electrical stimulation. In Lin VW, editor in chief: *Spinal Cord Medicine: Principles and Practice,* New York, 2003, Demos Medical Publishing Inc.
218. DeForge D, Blackmer J, Moher D et al: *Sexuality and Reproductive Health Following Spinal Cord Injury. Evidence Report/Technology Assessment No. 109 AHRQ.* Publication Rockville, MD, 2004, Agency for Healthcare Research and Quality. Available online at http://www.ahrq.gov/downloads/pub/evidence/pdf/sexlspine/sexlspine.pdf. Accessed February 11, 2006.
219. Klebine P, Lindsay L, Rivera P: *Sexuality for Women with Spinal Cord Injury.* University of Alabama at Birmingham, April 2004, Spinal Cord Injury Infosheet 21. Available online at http://images.main.uab.edu/spinalcord/pdffiles/21Women.pdf. Accessed February 11, 2006.
220. Elliott SL: Problems of sexual function after spinal cord injury, *Prog Brain Res* 152:387-400, 2006.
221. Hubscher CH: Ascending spinal pathways from sexual organs: effects of chronic spinal lesions, *Prog Brain Res* 152:401-414, 2006.
222. Johnson RL: Descending pathways modulating the spinal circuitry for ejaculation: effects of chronic spinal cord injury, *Prog Brain Res* 152:415-426, 2006.
223. Brown DJ, Hill ST, Baker HWG: Male fertility and sexual function after spinal cord injury, *Prog Brain Res* 152:427-440, 2006.
224. Sipski ML, Arenas A: Female sexual function after spinal cord injury, *Prog Brain Res* 152:441-448, 2006.
225. Atterbury JL, Groome LJ: Pregnancy in women with spinal cord injuries, *Nurs Clin North Am* 33(4):603-613, 1998.
226. Klebine P, Lindsey L, Jackson AB et al: *Pregnancy for Women with Spinal Cord Injury.* University of Alabama at Birmingham, March 2003, Spinal Cord Injury Infosheet 14. Available online at http://images.main.uab.edu/spinalcord/pdffiles/14-2003.pdf. Accessed February 11, 2006.
227. Bockenek WL, Stewart PJB: Pain in patients with spinal cord injury. In Kirshblum S, Campagnolo DI, DeLisa JA: *Spinal Cord Medicine,* Philadelphia, 2002, Lippincott Williams & Williams.
228. Salisbury SK, Choy NL, Nitz J: Shoulder pain, range of motion and functional motor skills after acute tetraplegia, *Arch Phys Med Rehabil* 84:1480-1485, 2003.
229. Cardenas DD, Bryce TN, Shem K et al: Gender and minority differences in the pain experience of people with spinal cord injury, *Arch Phys Med Rehabil* 85:1774-1781, 2004.
230. Siddall PJ, McClelland JM, Rutkowski SB et al: A longitudinal study of the prevalence and characteristics of pain in the first 5 years following spinal cord injury, *Pain* 103(3):249-257, 2003.
231. Siddall FJ, Yezierski RP, Loeser JD: Pain following spinal cord injury: clinical features, prevalence, and taxonomy, *Int Assoc Study Pain Newslett* 3:3-7, 2000.
232. Siddall PJ, Middleton JW: A proposed algorithm for the management of pain following spinal cord injury, *Spinal Cord* 44:67-77, 2006.
233. Consortium for Spinal Cord Medicine: Preservation of Upper Limb Function Following Spinal Cord Injury: A Clinical Practice Guideline for Health-Care Professionals, Washington, DC, 2005, Paralyzed Veterans of America.
234. Cariga P, Ahmed S, Mathias CJ et al: The prevalence and association of neck (coat-hanger) pain and orthostatic (postural) hypotension in human spinal cord injury, *Spinal Cord* 40:77-82, 2002.
235. Siddall PJ, Cousins MJ, Otte A et al: Pregabalin in central neuropathic pain associated with spinal cord injury: a placebo-controlled trial, *Neurology* 67(10):1792-1800, 2006.
236. Donnelly C, Eng JJ: Pain following spinal cord injury: the impact on community reintegration, *Spinal Cord* 43:278-282, 2005.
237. Consortium for Spinal Cord Medicine: *Depression Following Spinal Cord Injury: Clinical Practice Guidelines for Primary Care Physicians,* Washington, DC, 1997, Paralyzed Veterans Administration.
238. Schonherr MC, Groothoff JW, Mulder BA et al: Participation and satisfaction after spinal cord injury: results of a vocational and leisure outcome study, *Spinal Cord* 43:241-248, 2005.
239. Little JW: Syringomyelia. In Lin VW, editor: *Spinal Cord Medicine: Principles and Practice,* New York, 2003, Demos Medical Publishing Inc.
240. Perrouin B, Lenne-Aurier K, Robert R et al: Post-traumatic syringomyelia and post-traumatic spinal canal stenosis: a direct relationship: a review of 75 patients with a spinal cord injury, *Spinal Cord* 36:137-143, 1998.
241. Nielson OA, Biering-Sorenson F, Botel F et al: Post-traumatic syringomyelia, *Spinal Cord* 37: 680-684, 1999.

24

THORACIC TRAUMA

P. Milo Frawley

INTRODUCTION

Thoracic injuries account for much of the immediate life-threatening trauma encountered in the field or in the hospital setting. These injuries usually require rapid and skilled responses and considerable clinical judgment by nurses. Chest injuries and their effects on the patient are the subject of this chapter. The purpose is to educate the nurse about the most common injuries sustained in the thoracic region and about complications of these injuries throughout the phases of trauma care. This chapter describes specific injuries of the heart, lungs, lower airways, major vascular structures, and bony thorax itself and explains physiologic alterations associated with trauma that may affect the respiratory system.

The discussion of each injury includes a description of the injury's symptoms, pathophysiology, diagnosis, and management, but the patient's pain and fear of death and treatment must be considered with every injury. Each intervention begins with the nurse explaining procedures, treating pain and fear, and supporting the patient and family through medical and nursing therapies. These statements are not written over and over again but they are implied with each injury and complication. There is time to assist in treating the pneumothorax *and* to change the patient's uncomfortable position *and* to explain what having a chest tube will be like. Each of these three therapeutic actions is done in the priority order indicated by an assessment of the individual patient.

EPIDEMIOLOGY OF THORACIC INJURIES

A commonly cited statistic suggests that thoracic injuries are responsible for approximately 20% percent of all trauma-related deaths.[1] This citation, however, is not only dated but relied heavily on inference and extrapolation and not use of rigorous scientific methods for data collection. But, as the authors acknowledged, "Few statistics are available in the United States on chest trauma itself."[1] Today, published statistics on thoracic trauma remain sparse. For the 10-year period from 1996-2005, the trauma registry at the R Adams Cowley Shock Trauma Center (STC) in Baltimore, Maryland, indicates that approximately 5750 patients per annum arrived in the trauma resuscitation unit.[2] On average, 28% of admissions were classified as having an injury to the thorax. Of those patients admitted with a thoracic injury, 54% may be classified as a serious thoracic injury. With the use of the Abbreviated Injury Scale,[3] "serious thoracic injury" may be defined as a score of >2 (on a scale of 1 to 6, where 1 is considered minor and 6 virtually nonsurvivable). Patients who die and have a serious thoracic injury (as defined above), although potentially other serious injuries may be present, make up 56% of all deaths of all admissions to the STC.[2]

The epidemic of societal violence has changed the patterns of chest injuries that dominated previous decades. A significant number of violent interactions involving shootings or stabbings result in penetrating chest trauma.[4] Likewise, growth in the elderly segment of the population has an impact on the changing pattern of thoracic injury. Today, patients older than 65 years of age seen at the STC have a 30% chance of having thoracic trauma (mild, moderate, or severe).[2]

Sophisticated prehospital care and expeditious transportation to a definitive trauma care site have improved the detection, treatment, and outcome of injuries that were previously found only on postmortem examinations. Advancements in the management of thoracic trauma have occurred primarily because military campaigns, motor vehicle crashes, and societal violence have prompted clinicians to modify their practice, thereby improving response times, diagnosing more quickly, and initiating treatment earlier. Research, practice, and technology have progressed simultaneously. Type, severity, and number of various thoracic injuries will continue to evolve as long as clinicians, manufacturers, and lawmakers remain responsive to data collected by members of the health care community. Motor vehicle design modification, such as automated driver and passenger restraint systems; new laws to include zero blood alcohol tolerance for young drivers and previous offenders; and clinical interventions previously reserved for the hospital being executed in the field or ambulance are all changes that have been made with the hope of improving outcomes from trauma.

THORACIC ASSESSMENT IN TRAUMA

The assessment of patients with thoracic injury is based, as is any type of trauma examination, on a series of diagnostic clues obtained from directed data collection. Initially the data are used to form a diagnostic set known as the *index of suspicion.* In other words, given the specific details of the incident and the initial, rapid assessment, a list of injuries most likely to be present is identified.[5]

HEALTH HISTORY

In addition to the injury history, the personal health history gives insight into the individual's unique response to shock and thoracic injury. Whether the historian is the patient or a family member, the nurse attempts to determine the patient's previous respiratory, cardiac, and vascular status. Previous cardiopulmonary problems are uncovered through the usual review-of-systems approach and selective and directed questioning. The injured person is frequently young and has an unremarkable cardiopulmonary or vascular history. Nevertheless, questions should be asked specifically about the presence of persistent upper or lower respiratory infections, asthma, or chronic sinus problems; smoking, alcohol, and drug abuse history should also be investigated. Any of these problems may affect the patient's tolerance of nasal or oral endotracheal tubes or the response to mechanical ventilation. It is particularly important to ask whether there have been any previous trauma incidents or injuries.

Although it is not always possible, every endeavor is made to extract a recent health history from the patient. Chief complaints, which frequently include chest pain and difficulty with breathing, should be noted. Some patients may clearly describe or point to a specific location of pain. If a history cannot be elicited from the patient because of altered level of consciousness, intubation, or distracting injuries, emergency medical personnel and, less commonly, non-health care witnesses such as friends, bystanders, or police may be consulted for ascertaining key information. This includes information about the mechanism of injury (e.g., motor vehicle crash; size and type of weapon; number of times weapon was used; height of fall), extrication time, and fatalities at the scene. Further information to obtain about the patient includes length of time from moment of trauma to arrival in the resuscitation area, treatment administered by prehospital providers (e.g., amount of resuscitation fluid given), and patient response to interventions (e.g., trends in vital signs).

THORACIC ANATOMY

Correlation of underlying anatomy and surface landmarks is imperative in the trauma examination. The examiner must be able to identify key structures in the true thorax, the cervicothoracic inlet, and the boundaries of the thoracoabdominal cavity. Key structures include the trachea, carotid arteries, carina, lung fields, diaphragm, cardiac borders, aorta subclavian arteries, and pulmonary artery (Table 24-1). External landmarks and knowledge of the relationship with internal structures assist in identifying injuries (Figures 24-1 through 24-5).

TABLE 24-1 Thoracic Surface Anatomy

Structure	Landmarks
Aorta	
Root	Angle of Louis, midsternal line
Arch	First rib, sternal border
Pulmonary artery	Within and below aortic arch
Subclavian artery	First rib, clavicle
Cardiac borders	
Apex	Fifth left ICS, midclavicular line
Base	Second left ICS, substernal
Carina	Angle of Louis
Diaphragm	Right dome superior to left
Full inspiration	Tenth-eleventh rib posteriorly, sixth-eighth rib anteriorly
Full expiration	Tenth thoracic vertebra posteriorly, fourth-fifth rib anteriorly

ICS, Intercostal space.

PHYSICAL EXAMINATION

Primary Survey

The primary survey identifies life-threatening conditions. Management of any threat to life begins immediately, before progressing to the rest of the primary survey. Traumatic injuries to the chest can kill swiftly. On arrival the patient's airway is assessed, predominantly for obstruction. Noisy breathing or stridor indicates obstructed breathing and must be corrected or the natural airway bypassed with placement of an artificial airway. Independent of identified chest trauma, a Glasgow Coma Scale score of 8 or less is often seen as an indication for intubation for airway protection. Similarly, loss of gag, cough, or ability to protect the airway will warrant intubation. With the patient's chest completely exposed, the respiratory pattern is assessed, including the rate, depth, and chest movement, namely, noting equality of movement and possible presence of paradoxic motion of the chest wall (flail segment). Adequate ventilation must be established. Cyanosis is often a late finding in the trauma patient; thus, the absence of cyanosis does not necessarily equate to the absence of hypoxemia.

Ensuring adequate circulation is the next priority. Although blood pressure (BP) and pulse are noted, neither is a definitive sign of shock. The heart rate may be elevated in the trauma patient as a result of pain and anxiety, even in the absence of significant injury. Conversely, patients prescribed β-blockers may have a relatively slower heart rate than expected. Low BP is a late marker of shock[6] and not recommended as a sole indicator of poor tissue perfusion.[4,6] This is particularly true in young patients who have the ability to vasoconstrict and maintain a relatively normal BP despite significant intravascular volume loss. Warm extremities, brisk capillary refill time, normal mentation, and adequate urine output indicate an intact cardiovascular system providing adequate tissue perfusion. The neck veins are assessed for distention. Although jugular venous distention (JVD) may accompany injuries such as tension pneumothorax and cardiac tamponade, these conditions may be present even in the absence of JVD, which may not be evident because of hypovolemia.

During the initial survey, the presence or suspected presence of a pneumothorax or hemothorax is treated with a thoracostomy tube. A tension pneumothorax, considered a

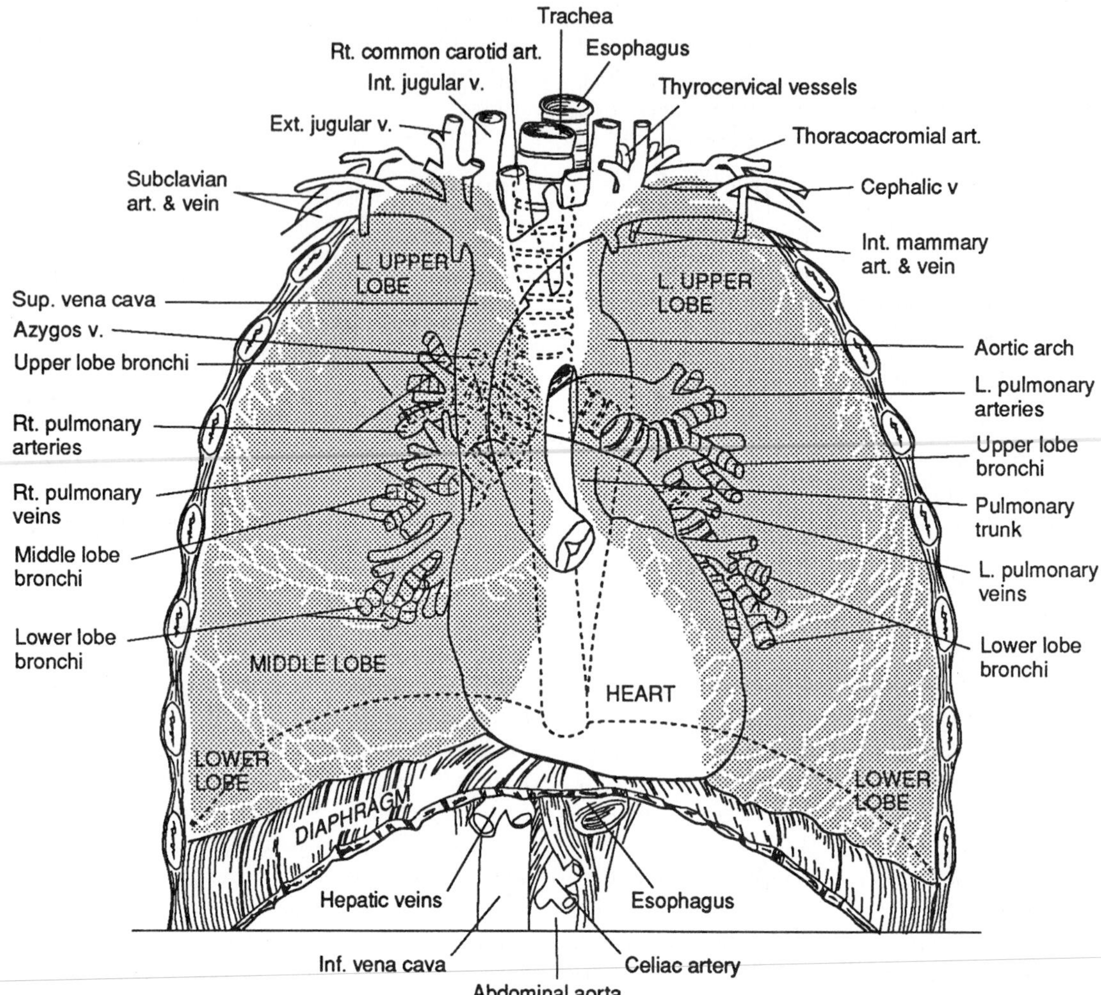

FIGURE 24-1 Anatomy of the thorax and its contents. (From Shires GT: *Care of the trauma patient,* New York, 1985, McGraw-Hill.)

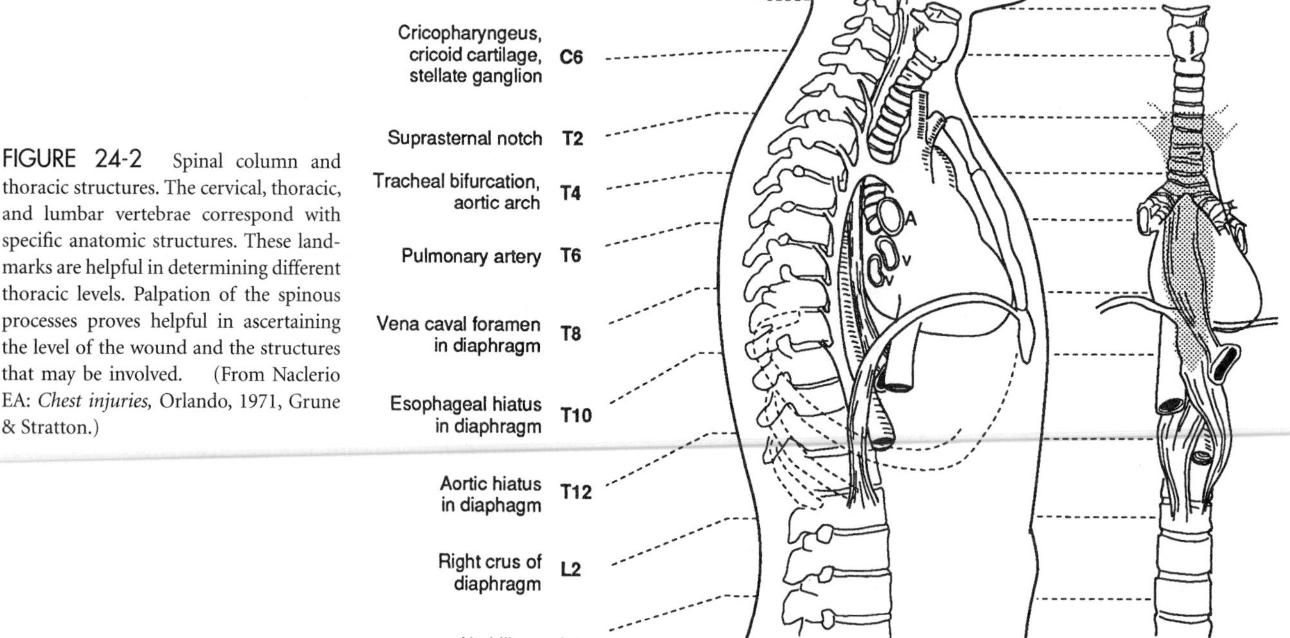

FIGURE 24-2 Spinal column and thoracic structures. The cervical, thoracic, and lumbar vertebrae correspond with specific anatomic structures. These landmarks are helpful in determining different thoracic levels. Palpation of the spinous processes proves helpful in ascertaining the level of the wound and the structures that may be involved. (From Naclerio EA: *Chest injuries,* Orlando, 1971, Grune & Stratton.)

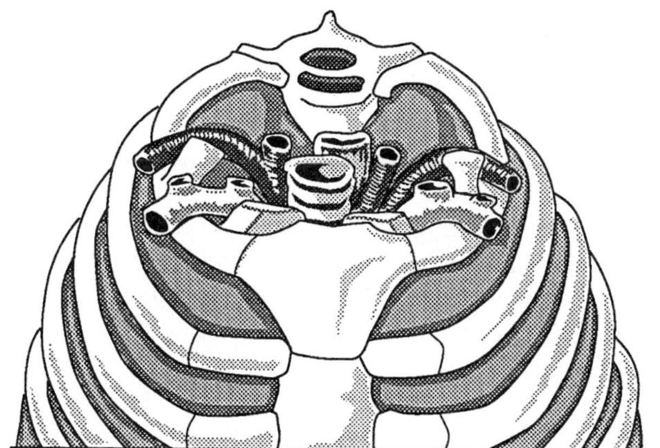

FIGURE 24-3 Cervicothoracic region. The root of the neck is actually the cervicothoracic region, which forms a boundary between the neck and the thorax. It is occupied by a number of vital structures that enter or leave the thoracic cavity. As shown, the apex of the lung rises above the level of the anterior part of the first rib. The subclavian artery lateral to the subclavian vein is separated from the lung by the membranous cervical diaphragm and the pleura. (From Naclerio EA: *Chest injuries,* Orlando, 1971, Grune & Stratton.)

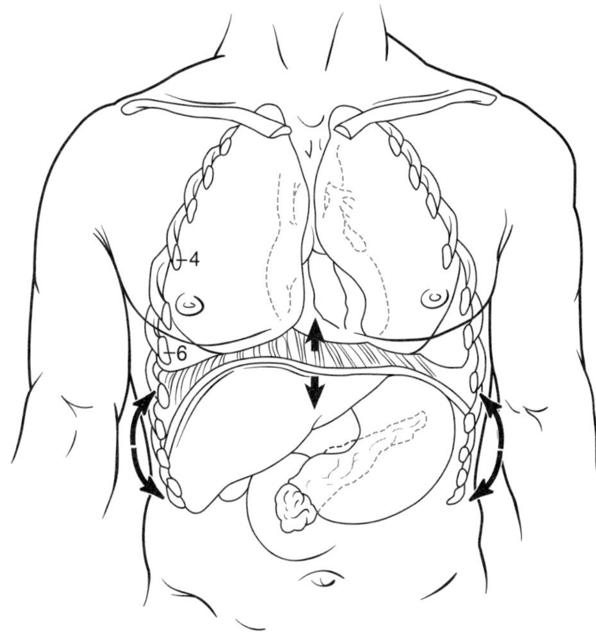

FIGURE 24-5 The thoracoabdominal region in thoracic assessment. *Arrows* indicate the variation in diaphragm and lung position during respiration.

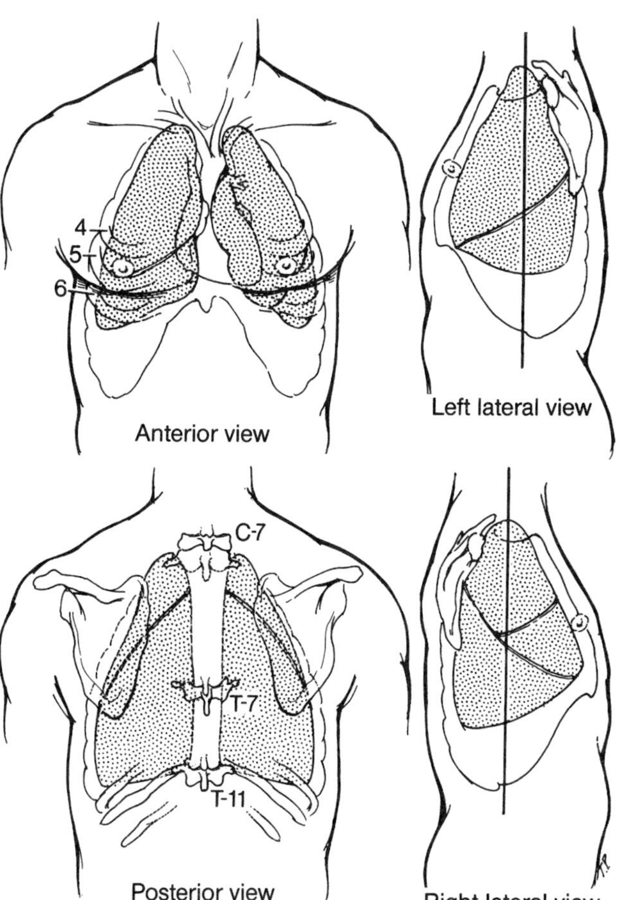

FIGURE 24-4 Correlation of surface to underlying thoracic anatomy. *Anterior view,* Note the relationship of the heart, great vessels, and lungs to bony thorax. *Posterior and right lateral views,* Major and minor interlobar fissures. *Left lateral view,* Note single interlobar fissure.

serious and often life-threatening form of pneumothorax, requires immediate decompression, which may be initially achieved by inserting a large-bore needle (e.g., 14-gauge) into the second intercostal space over the rib margin in the midclavicular line of the affected side. The tension pneumothorax is thus converted to a pneumothorax, and treatment with a thoracostomy tube may be pursued.

Finally, the patient's axillas are assessed and the patient is turned and the back inspected, and the number and location of penetrating wounds or blunt injuries are noted. To turn the patient who had sustained blunt trauma requires "log-rolling," although this technique is not always an imperative in penetrating injuries. Clinical judgment is the best guide as to whether log-rolling is indicated in the latter group.[7]

Secondary and Detailed Examinations

With the primary survey completed (which takes seconds to minutes) and with initiation of laboratory and radiographic studies (e.g., chest radiograph [CXR], arterial blood gas [ABG], electrocardiograph [ECG]), a second more detailed, although nonetheless time-efficient, physical examination must be performed. Inspection, palpation, auscultation, and percussion are used. Any deviation from normal is noted and any identified emergency condition is treated promptly.

Inspection. The chest wall is again visually inspected for bilateral equal expansion and for any discoloration, penetrating wounds, or other abnormalities. Abnormalities may include simple abrasions, contusions, flail segments, or sucking chest wounds. The number and location of wounds are documented. The location of wounds may be a guide in determining the path of a missile or weapon, although assumptions of trajectory may be wrong. Inspection of the posterior chest, back, and axilla is included in the assessment.

Palpation. Placement of both hands on the two hemithoraces permits assessment of the symmetry of chest wall motion. Furthermore, crepitance may be palpated. Crepitance is the crackling sound or the popping, grinding sensation felt with broken bones or air in the soft tissue. The clinician needs to differentiate between the finer crepitance of subcutaneous emphysema and the more coarse crepitations felt with movement of broken ribs or the sternum. Pain may also be a significant finding at this time.

Auscultation. The trauma resuscitation arena presents unique problems with auscultation. Often ambient noise is loud enough to limit auscultation to detecting only the very basic absence or presence of breath sounds. The absence of breath sounds will frequently warrant an intervention. Under such circumstances interventions will override further tests, which may cause delays in the setting of life-threatening conditions. The presence of breath sounds does not guarantee an absence of injury. Particularly in the early phase, a small pneumothorax may be readily seen on CXR or chest computed tomography (CT) but cause no appreciable difference in air entry or effect on breath sounds. Heart sounds may not be well differentiated in the trauma resuscitation area and, subsequently, are rarely helpful.

Percussion. For reasons outlined in the section on auscultation, thoracic percussion may be similarly limited in its usefulness in the trauma resuscitation arena. When it is performed and a normally tympanic area sounds blatantly dull, urgent treatment is often more appropriate than delaying management to complete a diagnostic test. This is especially true in an unstable patient.

Finally, the thoracoabdominal area is examined carefully for evidence of trauma. This is of particular concern in patients with penetrating injuries that may have had an upward trajectory with possible diaphragmatic tears and involvement of the pleural space.

PHYSIOLOGIC APPROACH

Clinical monitoring of BP, cardiac rate and rhythm, respirations, urine output, and ABGs is considered a standard part of patient management after thoracic injury. However, it is recognized that BP is frequently unaffected until a 30% loss in blood volume has been sustained.[4] Although invasive monitoring of central venous pressure may be helpful in evaluating intravascular volume, it is not routinely initiated during early fluid replacement and management of significant thoracic injuries. The time required to insert a central venous catheter cannot be afforded during initial moments of resuscitation; therefore, large-bore (14-gauge) peripheral intravenous catheters are preferable for volume repletion. If the patient has limited intravenous access, a central venous line can be placed.

Definitive management in the operative and critical care phases requires a practical yet comprehensive approach to systemic cardiopulmonary monitoring. The nurse must be familiar with an extensive array of cardiopulmonary variables and accompanying monitoring technology to be able to assess patients with thoracic trauma. The patient-ventilator system is monitored as a unit and is an important source of data about the patient's pulmonary status.

Arterial and pulmonary artery catheters provide information useful for assessing patients with extensive injuries and related complications. These hemodynamic parameters can also aid in determining the effect of therapies such as inotropes, fluids, and positive end-expiratory pressure (PEEP). When indicated, mixed venous oxygen tension and saturation monitoring may be helpful tools in determining circulatory sufficiency and global tissue oxygen consumption. In particular, geriatric patients, including the apparently clinically stable group, with multiple fractures, head injury, acidosis, initial systolic BP <150 mm Hg, or who were pedestrians struck by a motor vehicle may benefit from early invasive monitoring coupled with judicious use of vasoactive drugs.[8,9] Table 24-2 is a summary of physiologic parameters that may be obtained to monitor the patient with thoracic trauma.

NONINVASIVE MONITORING

The oxygenation status of the patient can be assessed by using noninvasive monitoring with pulse oximeters and transcutaneous, conjunctival, or tissue oxygen tension monitors. Oximetry is the determination of the oxygen-hemoglobin saturation of the blood and may be measured with an appropriate sensor that detects the pulsatile blood flow through some translucent part of the body (e.g., fingers, ear lobes, nasal septum, forehead). Pulse oximetry (Spo_2) is well accepted as a convenient, portable, noninvasive, and cost-effective indicator of arterial oxygen saturation (Sao_2). Pulse oximetry estimates the fractional hemoglobin saturation by determining the maximal light absorbance of the different hemoglobin species. Practical application of this technology aids both the detection of hypoxemia (Sao_2 <90%) and hyperoxemia (Sao_2 >98% in the presence of supplemental oxygen), allowing for appropriate titration of inspired oxygen concentration and other mechanical ventilator settings. Spo_2 measures are up to 4% higher than Sao_2 when at 90%, assuming that the only hemoglobin species present are reduced hemoglobin and oxyhemoglobin. The accuracy of Spo_2 measures may be reduced in the presence of movement, significant amounts of carboxyhemoglobin or methemoglobin, dark skin pigmentation, hypothermia, and hypovolemia, although advancements in technology continue to negate the impact of these variables. Anemia, once considered to affect accuracy, may have only a minor impact on the precision of measurements with the pulse oximeter.[10] Because pulse oximetry depends on pulse transmission, intense peripheral vasoconstriction may also be associated with lost or inaccurate readings. Generally, when the Sao_2 is greater than 90%, the accuracy of the Spo_2 increases substantially. An Spo_2 of less than 92% serves as a trigger to consider additional tests to confirm the oxygenation status of the patient.[10,11]

Noninvasive assessment of carbon dioxide (CO_2) is complex, especially in critically ill patients with significant ventilation-perfusion (V/Q) abnormalities, increased physiologic

TABLE 24-2 **Common Cardiopulmonary Parameters in Thoracic Assessment**

Variable	Abbreviation	Measurements or Calculation	Normal Range Low	Normal Range High	Units
Heart rate	HR	Direct measurement	60*	100	beats/min
Mean arterial pressure	MAP	(SBP − DBP)/3 + DBP	65	95	mm Hg
Central venous pressure	CVP	Central venous catheter	2	8	mm Hg
Pulmonary artery wedge pressure	PAWP	Pulmonary artery catheter	8	12	mm Hg
Mean pulmonary artery pressure	$\overline{PA}$	(PAS − PAD)/3 + PAD	15	20	mm Hg
Body surface area	BSA	[Ht (cm) + Wt (kg) − 60]/100	1.6 (female adults)	1.9 (male adults)	m^2
Cardiac output	CO	HR × SV	4	8	L/min
Cardiac index	CI	CO/BSA	2.5	4.0	L/min/m^2
Stroke volume index	SVI	CI/HR × 1000 (or SV/BSA)	35	65	ml/beat/m^2
Left ventricular stroke work index	LVSWI	SVI × (MAP − PAWP) × 0.0136	35	85	g-m/m^2
Right ventricular stroke work index	RVSWI	SVI × ($\overline{PA}$− CVP) × 0.0136	7	12	g-m/m^2
Systemic vascular resistance	SVR	80 × (MAP − CVP)/CO	800	1,200	dynes-s-cm^{-5}
Systemic vascular resistance index	SVRI	80 × (MAP − CVP)/CI	1,360	2,390	dynes-s-cm^{-5}/m^2
Pulmonary vascular resistance	PVR	80 × ($\overline{PA}$ − PAWP)/CO	20	250	dynes-sec-cm^{-5}
Arterial blood gases	ABGs				
Partial pressure of oxygen in arterial blood	Pao_2	Direct	80†	100	mm Hg
Partial pressure of carbon dioxide in arterial blood	$Paco_2$	Direct	35	45	mm Hg
pH	pH	Direct	7.35	7.45	
Bicarbonate	HCO_3	Calculated	22	26	mEq/L
Arterial oxygen saturation	Sao_2	Direct or calculated (technology-dependent)	96	100	%
Base excess	BE	Calculated	−2	2	
Mixed venous blood gases	MVBGs				
Partial pressure of oxygen in venous blood	PvO_2	Direct	35	40	mm Hg
Partial pressure of carbon dioxide in venous blood	$Pvco_2$	Direct	41	51	mm Hg
pH	pH	Direct	7.31	7.41	
Bicarbonate	HCO_3	Calculated	22	26	mEq/L
Venous oxygen saturation	Svo_2	Direct or calculated (technology-dependent)	60	80	%
Base excess	BE	Calculated	−2	2	
Arterial oxygen content	CaO_2	SaO_2 × (1.39 × Hb) + 0.003 × Pao_2	19	20	ml oxygen/100 ml whole blood
Mixed venous oxygen content	Cvo_2	Svo_2 × (1.39 × Hb) + 0.003 × Pvo_2	15	16	ml oxygen/100 ml whole blood
Oxygen delivery index	Dao_2I	Cao_2 × CI × 10	500	650	ml/min/m^2
Oxygen consumption index	Vo_2I	(Ca − Vo_2) × CI × 10	120	170	ml/min/m^2
Respiratory rate	RR	Direct measurement	12	20	breaths/min
Tidal volume	V_T	Spirometry	200 Varies with height and sex	500	ml
Vital capacity	VC	Spirometry	65	75	ml/kg
Inspiratory force	IF	Direct measurement	−100	−75	cm H_2O
Static compliance	Cst	V_T / (Plateau pressure − PEEP)	70	100	ml/cm H_2O
Dynamic compliance	Cdyn	V_T/(Peak inspiratory pressure − PEEP)	50	80	ml/cm H_2O

*Lower in the older and the fit. †80-1 for every year over 60, up to 80 years.

SBP, Systolic blood pressure; *DBP,* diastolic blood pressure; *PAS,* pulmonary artery systolic pressure; *PAD,* pulmonary artery diastolic pressure; *mm Hg,* millimeters of mercury; *m^2,* square meter; *SV,* stroke volume; *L/min,* liters per minute; *L/min/m^2,* liters per min per square meter; *ml/beat/m^2,* milliters per beat per square meter; *g-m/m^2,* gram-meters per square meter; *dyne,* where in physics the *dyne* is a unit of force and dyne can be defined as the force required to accelerate a mass of 1 g at a rate of 1 cm per second squared; *dynes-sec-cm^{-5}/m^2,* dynes second centimeter to the power of 5 per square meter; *mEq/L,* milliequivalents per liter.

dead space, and hemodynamic instability. When these confounding factors are stable, changes in end-tidal CO_2 ($ETCO_2$) can be assumed to reflect changes in alveolar ventilation and arterial CO_2 tension ($Paco_2$). $ETCO_2$ monitoring by mass spectrometry or an infrared analyzer correlates reasonably well with $Paco_2$ and is used in a variety of environments, including prehospital, emergency department (ED), and operating, recovery, and critical care areas.[12] In relatively healthy patients, the relationship between $Paco_2$ and $ETCO_2$ is close (less than 5 mm Hg difference), with the exhaled CO_2 ($ETCO_2$) commonly lower than the $Paco_2$. For example, a $Paco_2$ of 40 mm Hg might correlate with an $ETCO_2$ of 36 mm Hg.[12] As with other forms of monitoring, analysis of a trend over time rather than an individual value is most useful because there may be considerable breath-to-breath variability. Currently, there is some interest in the use of $ETCO_2$ to identify patients requiring more aggressive resuscitation during emergency trauma surgery[13] and as a predictor of death in patients undergoing emergency trauma surgery.[14]

Sublingual capnometry may be destined to play a role as a noninvasive indicator of the depth of shock and adequacy of resuscitation. Sublingual capnometers consist of three components: a disposable CO_2 sensor (placed under the tongue, equilibrates with the corresponding CO_2 level in the superficial mucosa), a fiberoptic cable, and, a blood gas analyzer. Within 5 minutes of connecting the components, a sublingual CO_2 measurement is attained. Such values may be useful as end points of resuscitation.[15]

INTEGRATING OTHER DIAGNOSTIC DATA

Other diagnostic data used to complete a total thoracic trauma assessment include laboratory, radiographic, ultrasonographic, and magnetic resonance imaging (MRI) data. Essential laboratory data include ABGs with base deficit measurement, complete blood cell count, including hematocrit and hemoglobin, clotting studies, serum electrolytes, osmolality, and lactate. A recent sputum or transtracheal aspirate culture may also be indicated. A drug and alcohol screen may also prove useful.

Thoracic evaluation commonly includes a CXR to visualize any significant bony, vascular, or pulmonary injuries (Figure 24-6, *A* and *B*). The appropriate angle of the film (supine, upright, or lateral) is used for best exposure of specific structures yet must consider any restrictions in positioning the patient. Often, as a result of hemodynamic instability or other suspected injuries (e.g., spinal column fracture), the CXR is a portable, supine, anteroposterior (AP) view. For penetrating injuries, a radiopaque marker is placed at suspected entrance and exit sites.[16]

One of the most valuable assessment tools in thoracic trauma is a clear, high-quality upright CXR. The patient should face the radiograph beam at a 110-degree angle to avoid unnecessary distortion of underlying structures on the CXR. A true upright film allows better visualization of vascular injuries within the chest and some estimation of the amount of blood or fluid in the chest cavity. Cardiac and aortic borders are also less distorted. Before an upright film is obtained, spine injury must be ruled out.

Digital total-body radiographic scanning (StatScan) may aid in the diagnosis of thoracic injury. StatScan is a comprehensive diagnostic total body x-ray examination that can be completed in less than 5 minutes and at a greatly reduced overall radiation dose to medical staff and patients. Initial images are available in less than 10 seconds. The quality of the x-ray film is reasonable although generally limited to one view (AP). StatScan plays a role in quickly and simultaneously identifying abnormalities of the thorax and the rest of the body[17] (Figure 24-7).

Overall, the use of plain radiographs is decreasing in the acute trauma setting in part because of the increased use of CT scanning. The CT scan is more sensitive in detecting hemothorax, pneumothorax, and pulmonary contusion than is the CXR.[18] Evaluation of underlying lung, cardiac, and mediastinal structures is also enhanced by the use of CT scans. However, a simple and rapid assessment of blunt trauma patients with CXR and abdominal ultrasonography may alert the clinician to significant injury.[19] Aortography remains the standard for evaluating aortic branch vessel injury,[20,21] although a contrast-enhanced CT may have a sensitivity and negative predictive value equivalent to that of aortography for assessment of just the aorta.[22,23] An abnormality of a branching vessel would be an indication to proceed with aortography. Assessment of penetrating trauma may also undergo a decline in use of angiography and other invasive tests as the role of contrast-enhanced CT is expanded.[24] As CT technology advances, the potential applications are increasing.[25]

Three-dimensional (3-D) images of the thorax can be obtained after multidetector row CT scanning. Certain structures may be deleted on the radiograph to allow better visualization of other structures. 3-D imaging plays a role in clarifying complex vascular and nonvascular anatomy. Further technical developments will help solidify the role of two- and three-dimensional reconstructions in the management of thoracic trauma[26] (Figure 24-8).

Ultrasonography of the thorax is a relatively new diagnostic tool. Although the surgeon-performed focused assessment by sonography for trauma (FAST) examination has become a standard part of the abdominal assessment for hemorrhage, ultrasonography of the thorax awaits mainstream acceptance and use. The exception, however, is sonography for rapid diagnosis of traumatic pericardial fluid collections.[27] Recently, use of sonography for the diagnosis of pneumothorax has gained more interest.[28,29] Although posttraumatic occult pneumothoraces may be more likely to be identified by ultrasonography than by a plain CXR,[30] the accuracy of ultrasonography continues to be limited by the expertise of the user.

The use of MRI in the acutely ill patient with thoracic trauma is limited by the incompatibility of many metallic implants and life support devices with the magnetic field. Coupled with limited visualization and the potential for

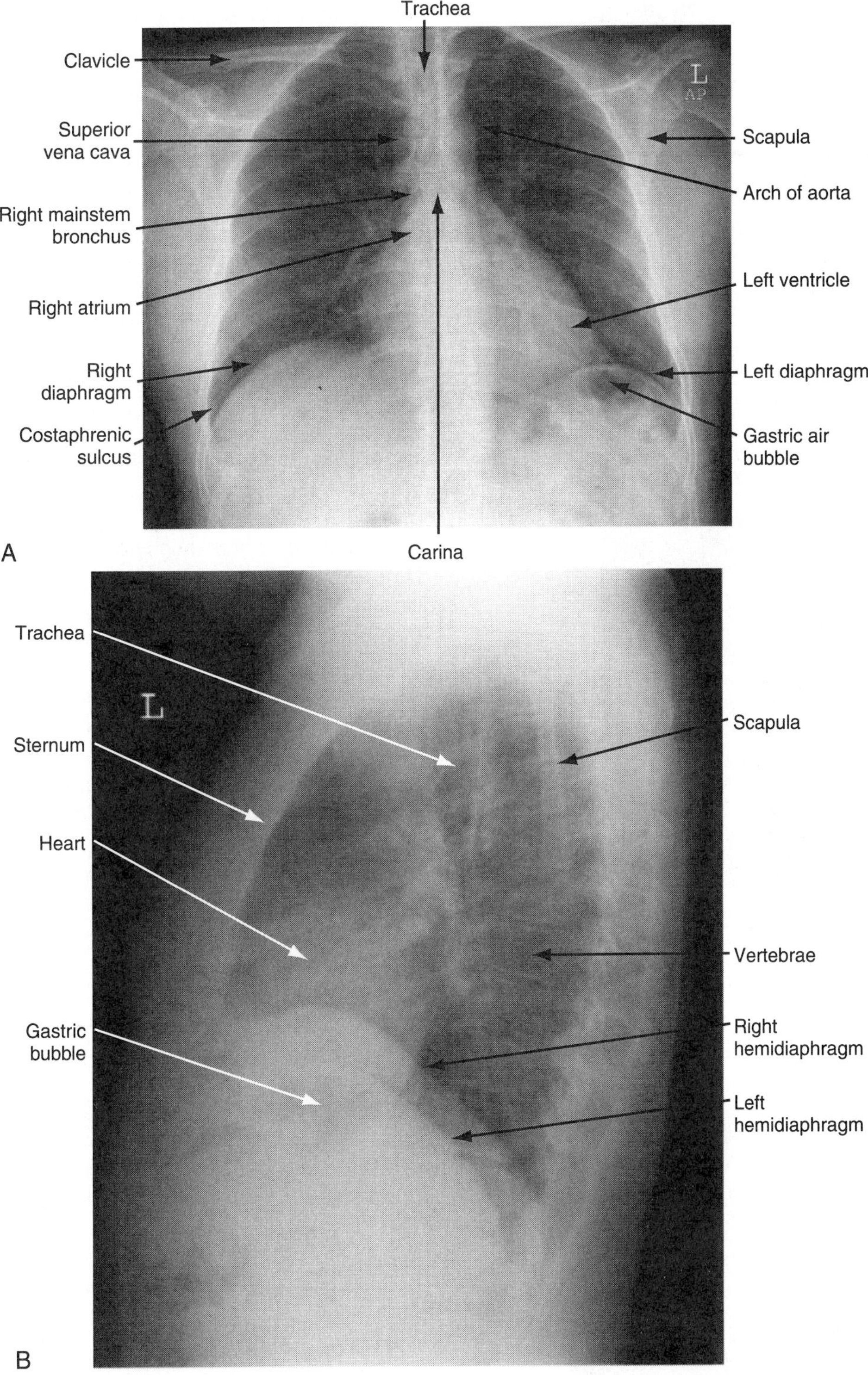

FIGURE 24-6 Normal AP (**a**) and lateral (**b**) films of the chest.

rapid hemodynamic deterioration while the patient is in the scanner, MRI is typically not a desirable diagnostic strategy for this group of patients. The use of MRI may be considered an adjunct diagnostic tool in appropriately selected patients, although it will probably have an increasing role as MRI-compatible physiologic support and monitoring devices become increasingly available.[25]

Reassessment and Early Thoracotomy

Repeated thoracic assessment is the key to determining missed or progressive injuries. Injury to the thorax requiring intervention may be broadly split into three categories: those requiring observation, tube thoracostomy (chest tube), and formal thoracotomy. The majority (85%) of thoracic trauma cases requiring intervention are managed with tube

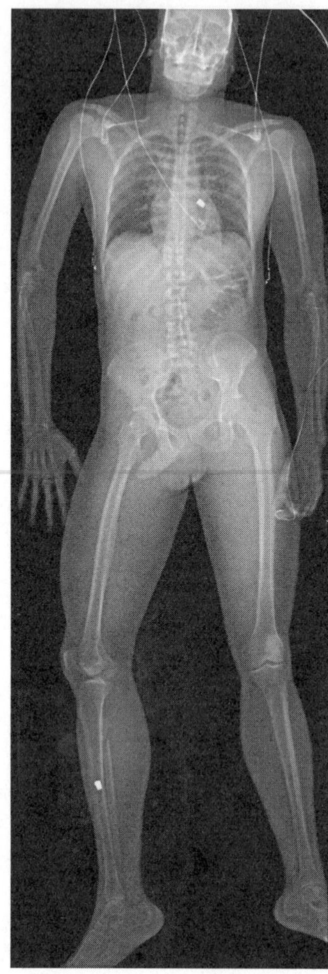

FIGURE 24-7 Image produced by the StatScan total body radiograph machine. The total body radiograph of this young man identified two bullets. One is in the region of the left chest, and the other is in the right lower extremity associated with a fractured fibula.

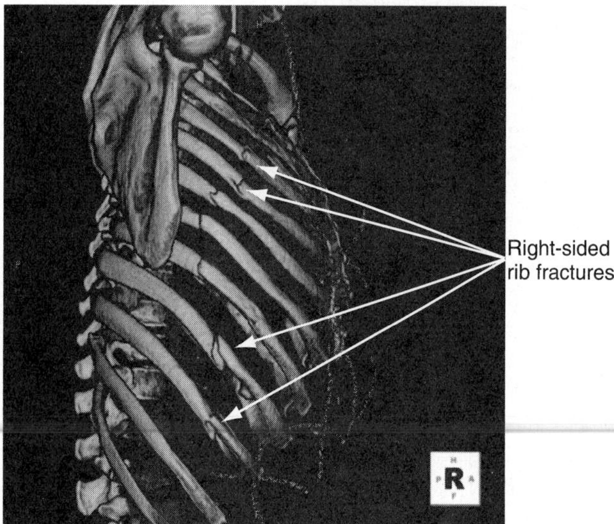

FIGURE 24-8 3-D view of right-sided rib fractures. Multiple rib fractures are identified on the right lateral view of a 3-D image.

thoracostomy (chest tube), pain control, pulmonary toilet, and observation.[31]

Should the patient's condition deteriorate or result in cardiac arrest, immediate exploratory thoracotomy may be performed. Indications for the procedure have been the subject of considerable controversy. Resuscitative ED thoracotomy may be indicated for the following:

1. Penetrating thoracic trauma with a systolic BP <40 mm Hg or prehospital signs of life
2. Penetrating nonthoracic trauma, noncranial trauma with a systolic BP <40 mm Hg and signs of life in the resuscitation area
3. Cardiac arrest after blunt chest or abdominal trauma after arrival in the ED with an obtainable BP[16]

Successful outcomes after ED thoracotomy are often related to reversible conditions such as cardiac tamponade, controllable intrathoracic bleeding, elimination of massive air embolism, or bronchopleural fistula. Thoracotomy also permits open cardiac massage and access to the descending aorta to facilitate temporary clamping to redistribute limited blood flow to the myocardium and brain while stifling any subdiaphragmatic bleeding.[32] Historically, patients were more likely to survive an ED thoracotomy if they had sustained a penetrating injury (5% to 8% survival) than a blunt trauma (<2%) or were in extremis after extrathoracic injuries (<1%).[33] Recently, a small European study suggested that patients with blunt trunk trauma and cardiac arrest after hemorrhagic shock may benefit from ED thoracotomy and open massage with a similar probability of survival as shown for patients with penetrating injury. However, the success of the intervention was contingent on early thoracotomy after closed chest resuscitation of less than 20 minutes by trained professionals. On average, the survivors of open chest cardiac massage had undergone 13 minutes of closed chest cardiopulmonary resuscitation before the thoracotomy.[34]

Thoracoscopy may be useful in limited emergency situations. This procedure may be used on stable patients with penetrating chest injuries, for diagnostic evaluation, or to control bleeding and remove blood clots.[35]

INJURIES

AIRWAY OBSTRUCTION

Airway assessment and management is the first imperative in the care of any trauma patient. Airway obstruction occurs frequently in trauma patients from primary injury to the airway (e.g., injuries to the pharynx, larynx, trachea) or as the result of some other injury. The source of an obstruction and the therapeutic approach are slightly different in the patient with a natural airway versus one with an artificial airway already in place. However, the principles of basic and advanced life support are fundamental in management of all obstructions.

The Patient With a Natural Airway

The most common sources of obstruction are the tongue and foreign bodies such as teeth, blood clots, and bone fragments. The unconscious patient in shock or one with central nervous system, maxillofacial, or neck injuries is at particularly high risk. Loss of protective airway reflexes including the cough and gag also increase risk of aspiration and loss of airway patency.

Assessment begins with rapid determination of airway patency by evaluating whether there is air passage through the upper respiratory tract into and out of the lungs. This evaluation is followed by observation of the rate and pattern of ventilation. Air movement through the airway, if any, may be noisy, indicating presence of a partial obstruction. Respiratory distress may or may not be immediately evident. Continuous pulse oximetry monitoring can detect reductions in the oxygen saturation of hemoglobin, and ABGs are measured as the most certain method of assessing oxygenation and ventilation.

Airway obstruction must be corrected immediately or the natural airway bypassed. Initially the airway is opened by a chin-lift or jaw-thrust maneuver, and the oropharynx is cleared by suction. Any obvious foreign material is removed manually. Each step is performed with great care to maintain immobility of the cervical spine until injury to the spine has been ruled out. Initial manual airway maneuvers may be inadequate or only temporary solutions; therefore, more definitive airway control is often required.

The simplest adjuncts are placement of an oral or nasal airway. Both are generally for short-term use and have restricted use in patients with facial trauma such as nasal fractures, cribriform plate fractures, or oropharyngeal injury. The oropharyngeal (or Guedel) airway is reserved for the unconscious/unresponsive patient because this device may otherwise cause gagging and vomiting. The nasopharyngeal airway (or Trumpet) may be tolerated better by the patient with a higher level of consciousness. However, this device is contraindicated with basilar skull fractures and cribriform plate defects for fear of penetration into the cranial cavity.

When positioning does not relieve the obstruction, endotracheal intubation is the management technique of choice for most types of trauma. Alternatives to conventional intubation include use of the Laryngeal Mask Airway (LMA) (Laryngeal Mask Company) or the esophageal Combitube (Sheridian Catheter, Argyle, NY). These devices are blindly inserted into the pharynx and on inflation of their seal allow for ventilation of the lungs. The Combitube is relatively easy to insert, even after only brief training. The LMA has a less well defined role in the trauma population and is generally not tolerated if the gag reflex is present.[36]

In general, oral endotracheal intubation with rapid-sequence induction using a short-acting sedative and paralytic agent is the gold standard for securing an airway. This may be done safely after cervical spine injury has been ruled out or even in cases of unknown cervical spine status provided the neck does not require aggressive manipulation to visualize the vocal cords. Cricoid pressure is applied routinely during the procedure. The rationale is that the trauma patient is likely to have a full stomach and is therefore at risk for aspiration of gastric contents. Cricoid pressure is maintained until the tube is inserted, cuff inflated, and bilateral chest sounds auscultated.

Although oral-tracheal intubation constitutes the preferred airway management, there are several caveats. If the patient is unstable but breathing and the urgency of airway management does not allow preliminary cervical spine clearance, blind nasotracheal intubation may be attempted. Conversely, an oral-tracheal route is used if the patient is apneic and the cervical spine is immobilized manually in a neutral position. Last, fiberoptic laryngoscopy and bronchoscopy may be useful to facilitate difficult intubations in stable patients, particularly in those individuals with maxillofacial or cervical spine trauma and in patients with short necks.[37] Scopes may be less practical in the emergency or urgent situation.

If the patient cannot be intubated successfully, emergency cricothyroidotomy is recommended. In the event a surgical airway is required, a cricothyroidotomy is preferred over a tracheostomy. Comparatively, a cricothyroidotomy is less bloody, quicker, and considered easier to perform.[37] There are two cricothyroidotomy procedures currently in use. The first is a surgical technique in which a transverse incision is made through the skin and the cricothyroid membrane, located below the thyroid prominence of the neck. Usually, a No. 6 endotracheal tube is inserted into the exposed airway (Figure 24-9). A second approach, needle cricothyroidotomy or percutaneous transtracheal ventilation, is initiated by insertion of a 14-gauge needle into the trachea at the cricothyroid membrane below the level of obstruction. Pressurized oxygen is insufflated intermittently through the needle into the trachea. The limitation of the needle cricothyroidotomy is that ventilation is usually impaired despite sufficient oxygenation. The choice of method depends on the injury, available equipment, and capability of the resuscitating health professional.

The choice of appropriate airway requires consideration not only of available equipment and personnel but also factors specific to the patient, the injury, and short- and long-term management plans. For example, early intubation may be indicated not only for airway management but also for intraoperative or critical care management of patients with thoracic injuries. Table 24-3 summarizes the advantages of different artificial airways, their restrictions, and their potential complications.

The Patient With an Artificial Airway

In trauma patients with an artificial airway in place (routinely an endotracheal or tracheostomy tube), obstructions or partial obstructions may occur, usually in an insidious and subtle fashion. Obstruction may be caused by thick or dried secretions or blood clots within the lumen of the airway or malposition of the airway. Assessment of airway patency and effectiveness requires continuous evaluation. Signs of airway obstruction include increasing level of agitation, rising airway

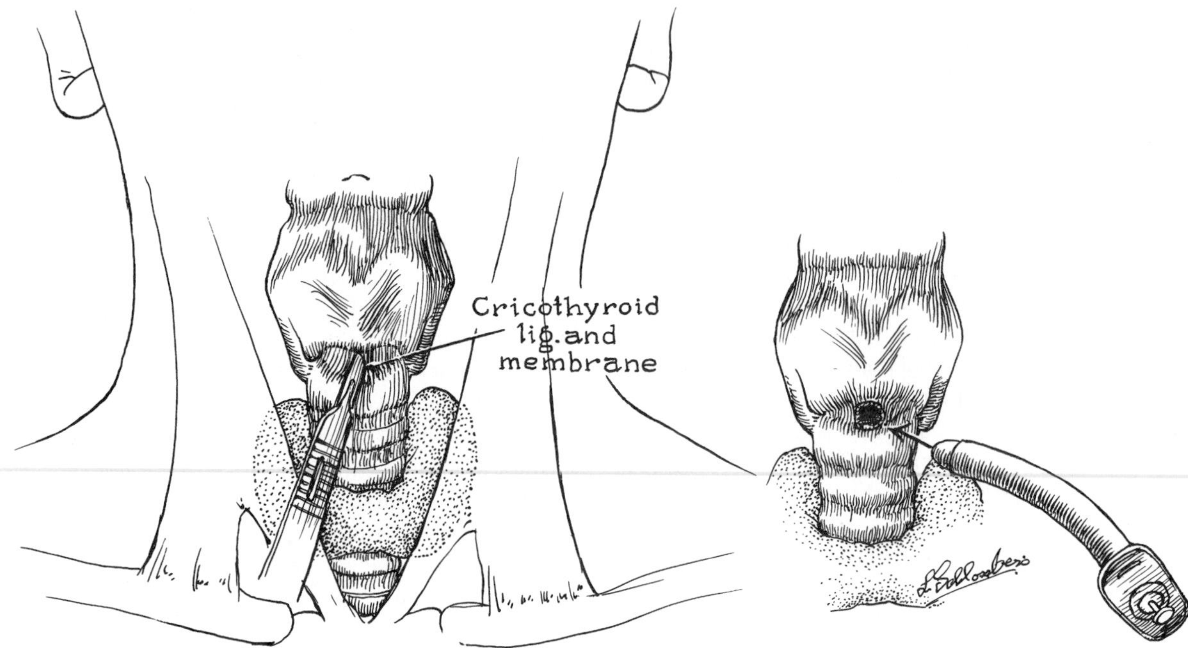

FIGURE 24-9 Cricothyroidotomy technique. (From Zuidema GD, Rutherford RB, Ballinger WF: *Management of trauma,* 4th ed, Philadelphia, 1985, W. B. Saunders.)

pressures during mechanical ventilation (peak inspiratory pressure, not plateau pressure), difficulty in advancement of a suction catheter, and decreased Spo_2 or increased $ETCO_2$. Frequent evacuation of bloody clots or mucus plugs may precede the occlusion of the airway. Humidification is a front-line measure to prevent secretions from drying in the artificial airway and causing obstruction. Inhalation of aerosolized agents aimed at loosening secretions (e.g., a mucolytic agent such as Mucomyst [acetylcysteine solution]) may also be prescribed. Ensuring that any artificial airway is well secured and supported during repositioning of the patient helps maintain appropriate placement of the device.

The optimal timing of converting an artificial airway from endotracheal to tracheostomy is controversial. Historically, a patient requiring an artificial airway for less than 10 days was managed with an endotracheal tube, and if artificial ventilation was still required after 21 days, a tracheostomy was recommended.[38] More recently, advantages to earlier tracheostomy have been suggested.[39,40] Advantages include shorter duration of ventilation, shorter intensive care unit (ICU) stay, less damage to the mouth and larynx, and facilitation of communication.

General nursing management begins by documentation of airway type and size, patient tolerance, any complications, duration of intubation, and date of tracheostomy. The patient-specific plan of care is based on such factors as a history of any airway problems, difficulty in intubation, and patient behavior, such as attempts at self-extubation or bronchospasm during suctioning. An identical spare tracheostomy tube, and second with an internal diameter 1 mm smaller than the original, and a manual resuscitator bag with face mask should be located at the bedside for rapid management of obstruction or lost airway. Emergency intubation kits that contain all the necessary equipment for rapid intubation and airway management should be strategically located on the unit. Airway hygiene is implemented on the basis of assessment findings. Tracheostomy care is patient specific depending on the newness of the stoma, the type of secretions or peritracheal drainage, and signs of infection. Commonly, the tracheostomy site is cleaned with saline solution and a gauze dressing is placed around the site at least once a shift and as required. A record is maintained of all tube changes, tube size, and any difficulties encountered in tube placement. The need for long-term airway management is apparent in the intermediate care setting, if not before. An alternative mode of communication (e.g., writing, use of a letter or picture board) must be established for the patient unable to verbally express himself or herself because of placement of an artificial airway. A speech-language pathology consultation may be helpful in determining an alternative means of communication. Insertion of a fenestrated or "talking" tracheostomy will help the patient regain the ability to verbally communicate. As soon as the patient and family indicate readiness, a teaching plan is begun that covers long-term and home management of secretions and tracheostomy care. Excellent reviews of nursing care of the patient with an artificial airway are available.[41,42]

TRACHEOBRONCHIAL TRAUMA

Description

The tracheobronchial tree may be injured by either blunt or penetrating trauma at any level. Most commonly, injury involves the mainstem bronchi within close proximity to the carina in blunt trauma and the cervical trachea in penetrating trauma (Figure 24-10). Injuries may be complete or

TABLE 24-3 **Airway Adjuncts in Trauma**

Oropharyngeal Airway	
Indications	Unconscious patients without gag reflex; short-term use
Advantages	Holds tongue away from posterior pharynx
Restrictions	Oropharyngeal injuries
Complications	Intraoral injury; induction of vomiting and aspiration; increased obstruction if positioned incorrectly by pushing the tongue back into pharynx
Nasopharyngeal Airway	
Indications	Semicomatose or arousable patients with decreased control of upper airway; prevention of tissue trauma during frequent nasotracheal suctioning
Advantages	Better tolerated in awake patients than oral airway; easily secured
Restrictions	Maxillofacial trauma such as nasal, nasoethmoid fractures
Complications	Nasopharyngeal injury; nasal bleeding
Esophageal Obturator Airway, Combitube, Pharynotracheal Lumen Airway, Laryngeal Mask Airway	
Indications	When unable to successfully place endotracheal tube
Advantages	Can be positioned quickly without direct visualization, with minimal manipulation of cervical spine
Restrictions	Cannot be used in awake or semiconscious patients
Complications	Induction of vomiting and aspiration; esophageal tears; postpharyngeal bleeding; unrecognized incorrect placement
Endotracheal Tube	
Indications	Preferred method of airway control
Advantages	Stable airway; provides protection from aspiration; permits mechanical ventilation to be used; decreases gastric distention associated with bag-mask ventilation
Restrictions	Used with caution in presence of laryngotracheal injuries (glottis, subglottis, and upper trachea)
Complications	Esophageal intubation leading to hypoxia; right mainstem bronchus intubation; induction of vomiting and aspiration; vocal cord injury; pharyngeal injury; tracheal lacerations; conversion of cervical spine injury without neurologic deficit to injury with deficit; dislodged tube
Cricothyroidotomy	
Indications	When intubation does not relieve obstruction or trachea cannot be intubated
Advantages	More rapid, greater ease of accessibility, and lower incidence of bleeding than tracheostomy
Restrictions	Children younger than 12 years old; laryngeal injury or inflammation
Complications	Subglottic stenosis; vocal cord injury; aspiration; hemorrhage; tracheal or esophageal laceration; mediastinal emphysema; dislodged tube
Standard Tracheostomy	
Indications	When intubution does not relieve obstruction or in significant laryngeal or tracheal trauma; used for prolonged ventilatory support
Advantages	Bypasses upper airway and glottis; stable airway with low resistance to air flow; easily suctioned
Restrictions	Limited use as an emergency procedure because of time requirements and potential for bleeding
Complications	Early or delayed hemorrhage; aspiration; mediastinal emphysema with or without pneumothorax; tracheoesophageal fistula; tracheal stenosis; tracheomalacia; tracheoarterial fistula; dislodged tube

incomplete, and total separation of the tracheobronchial tree can occur. However, continuity of the airway may be maintained by the fascia surrounding the trachea and bronchi. Lower airway injuries are of interest to nurses in all phases of trauma care because discovery of injury may occur dramatically during intubation and mechanical ventilation or may occur surprisingly late in the patient's posttrauma course. Tracheobronchial tears may also be caused by penetrating injury, frequently in association with esophageal, carotid artery, or jugular vein trauma.

Resuscitation/Critical Care Assessment

Tracheobronchial injuries are a rare, although often fatal injury, with many patients dying at the scene. In those who survive to reach the hospital, the index of suspicion for tracheobronchial injury is heightened by a history of violent trauma, particularly in patients with fractures of the upper five ribs. The rupture may be immediately symptomatic as evidenced by dyspnea, subcutaneous emphysema, or tension pneumothorax.[27] Hoarseness, stridor, and pneumomediastinum may also be present. A tear may be suspected in the patient with mediastinal and subcutaneous emphysema accompanied by a persistent pneumothorax that resists reexpansion. More commonly the rupture develops in two stages. The patient shows almost no symptoms until 3 or 4 days after admission, when pneumothorax or subcutaneous emphysema develops. Should the patient already have chest tubes in place, a persistent pleural air leak is evident, possibly with continued extravasation of air into tissues. Early persistent atelectasis may appear as a result of occlusion of the bronchus with blood and secretions. Bloody secretions are evident on coughing or during suctioning

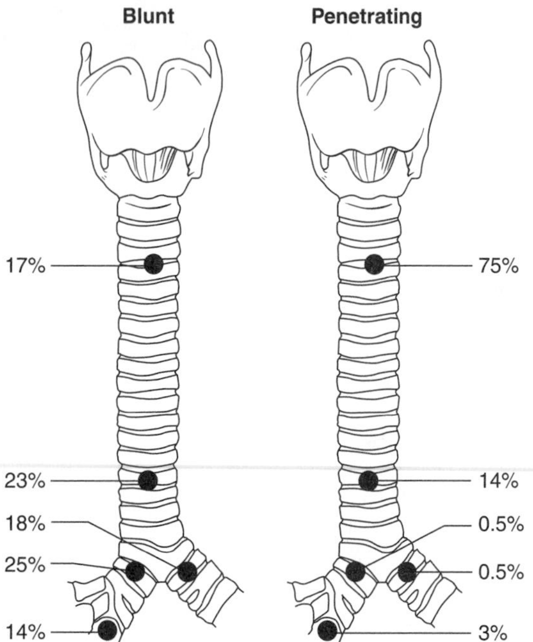

FIGURE 24-10 Tracheobronchial ruptures: general localizations based on literature review. Series included are only those that are not dedicated to a specific location. Three percent of blunt injuries occurred in major bronchi not otherwise localized. Seven percent of penetrating injuries occurred in major bronchi not otherwise localized. $N = 325$ blunt, 190 penetrating. (From Riley RD, Miller PR, Meredith JW: Injury to the esophagus, trachea, and bronchus. In Moore EE, Feliciano DV, Mattox KL, editors: *Trauma*, 5th ed, pp 539-552, New York, 2004, McGraw-Hill.)

as pleural fluid is drawn back through the damaged airway. These clinical findings require good communication and correlation of nursing and medical observations to make the diagnosis of tracheobronchial trauma. Diagnosis, early or late, is made based on clinical history and the presenting signs and symptoms. CT scanning may suggest injury (presence of mediastinal air), although diagnostic bronchoscopy is still required. Bronchoscopy allows for precise determination of site, nature, and extent of the tracheobronchial defect.[43] Presence or even suspicion of the presence of a tracheobronchial injury requires immediate surgical consultation.

Management

Initial management is dependent on the severity of the symptoms described above. A stable patient capable of maintaining the airway and ventilation does not require an immediate artificial airway. Close observation continues as the diagnostic workup proceeds. The patient with significant hemoptysis and airway obstruction must have an airway secured either by insertion of an endotracheal tube or by tracheostomy. Either procedure carries great risk, including further damage to the defect and creation of a false passage. Urgent tracheostomy performed in the operating room may be the safer option.[43] A double-lumen endotracheal tube permits the use of independent lung ventilation, thereby facilitating ventilation of the lung with an injured main bronchus with either lower ventilating pressure or straight continuous positive airway pressure (CPAP). If present, pneumothorax, tension pneumothorax, or pneumomediastinum are treated by tube thoracostomy and evacuation of pleural air by suction. The rate and amount of air evacuated by the chest tube are monitored, as is the adequacy of air intake into the lungs. Large air leaks may require a second thoracostomy tube. Immediate thoracotomy is indicated in the presence of massive air leak that prevents adequate ventilation or oxygenation.

More commonly the initial tube thoracostomy is followed by definitive diagnostic bronchoscopy and plans for injury repair. If the tear is large and irregular or is a complete rupture, early surgical repair is accomplished by a cervical or thoracic approach. A small tear may be treated conservatively solely through airway management.

Nonoperative management may be considered and implemented in patients with defects that involve less than one third of the circumference of the tracheobronchial tree. Conservative management may result in accumulation of excess granulation tissue that causes airway narrowing. If significant, this may require future long-term surgical intervention.[43]

Specific Nursing Management

The nurse must know the location of the tear and repair status to create an appropriate plan of care. If an artificial airway has been placed, the airway must be secured carefully and protected from dislodgment or inadvertent repositioning. If surgical repair has been completed, airway protection remains critical while the suture line heals. Careful suctioning technique and neck positioning to avoid increased suture tension protect the area of surgical repair.

An additional management focus is monitoring the quantity of any air leak and evaluating the effect it has on ventilation and oxygenation. Pleural drainage is inspected regularly for sudden air evacuation and increases in a known leak. Thoracic examination is repeated to appreciate changes in subcutaneous air and the development of pneumomediastinum or pneumothorax. Nursing care is directed toward avoiding sudden rises in the patient's airway pressure, which may delay healing of the injury.

Bronchial injury may be accompanied by lung injury with tears in surrounding small blood vessels, allowing air to enter the pulmonary venous circulation. Monitoring for signs of air embolism is important, particularly before repair or in the patient who is managed conservatively without repair. Sudden cardiovascular deterioration after endotracheal intubation without signs of bleeding may be indicative of air embolism. Focal neurologic signs in the non–head-injured patient are also significant. Placing the patient in Trendelenburg's position is presumably optimal to trap air in the apex of the left ventricle. Aggressive treatment includes thoracotomy to clamp the pulmonary hilum and access the left ventricle so that a cardiocentesis can be performed to aspirate air bubbles.[43] Hyperbaric oxygen therapy may also be used.

Intermediate Care Assessment and Management

Tracheobronchial tears are often diagnosed late in the assessment for occult or missed injury. Patient assessment should focus on identification of posttraumatic complications such as bronchial stenosis. The initial tracheobronchial tear results in a stenosed airway obstructed by granulation tissue and prone to repeated inflammation and infection. Delayed atelectasis appears as granulation tissue obstructs the bronchus. Resection of the area of stricture and reanastomosis may be required to prevent repeated infections and excess scar tissue formation below the level of the stenosis. Laser ablation of stenotic lesions and endobronchial stents are also used.[44]

Nursing management is directed toward chest physiotherapy for the affected lung areas to facilitate secretion clearance and maintain airway patency. The patient's vital capacity, chest film, and secretions are monitored. Assistance in coughing is a priority because the injury frequently leaves a residual decrease in bronchial sensitivity resulting in diminished stimuli to initiate a cough.[44]

Tracheal injury or, less commonly, tracheostomy may result in tracheal stenosis, which is made apparent by a hoarse, unproductive cough; wheezing; and periodic dyspnea on exertion. Occasionally assessment may reveal signs of tracheomalacia, which is a softened tracheal wall. This is the outcome of damage and loss of tracheal cartilage from tissue ischemia, necrosis, infection, and long exposure to an overinflated cuff. The patient's trachea expands and collapses during respiration (truncated loop sign). Repairs of both types of complications are achieved by surgical resection and anastomosis or stent placement.

Posttraumatic Tracheal Fistula

Description and Etiology

Tracheoarterial fistula (TAF) (including tracheoinnominate fistula) and tracheoesophageal fistula (TEF) may result from blunt injury. More commonly it is a form of endotracheal or tracheostomy tube trauma. TAF occurs when a fistula forms between the trachea and an artery, usually the innominate artery (also known as the brachiocephalic artery). TEF is a fistula between the trachea and the esophagus. Tube trauma can be a sequela of a difficult intubation or tracheostomy.[44] During these procedures a retropharyngeal or tracheal wall nick or tear can occur. The area becomes infected with upper airway secretions, erodes, and becomes a fistula. TAF[45] and TEF[46] are rare but often fatal complications after tracheostomy or intubation.

Tracheoarterial Fistula

The vessel involved may be the innominate, right carotid, or a lower thyroid artery that has been exposed to pressure from an overinflated cuff or a poorly positioned airway (e.g., a tracheostomy). As the tracheal wall erodes, the vessel is perforated and suddenly bleeds into the airway. The patient may die immediately from hemorrhage through the tracheostomy. Occasionally, sentinel bleeding may appear as hemoptysis. A patient with an artificial airway and hemoptysis warrants notification to a physician and immediate further investigation. Figure 24-11 shows how poor tube positioning and cuff overinflation may cause a hemorrhage. The incidence of TAF in patients with a short- or long-term tracheostomy is similar at 0.7% and is almost always fatal if not recognized and surgically corrected.[47]

Prevention. Physiologic cuff pressure should be maintained at less than a mean mucosal capillary pressure of 20 to 25 mm Hg. Different commercially available tracheostomy and endotracheal tubes all exert varying tracheal wall pressures, including the soft, large-volume cuffs and foam cuffs, which are autoregulated by an air valve. Proper inflation of the cuff according to product recommendations is useful; however, the actual cuff pressure must be measured. Measurement is made by a purpose-designed cuff pressure manometer or, if necessary, by a simple stopcock and manometer apparatus. If there is reason to believe that the patient is at higher risk for TAF, a shorter or longer tube of appropriate diameter may be inserted to relieve the immediate pressure at the site of tracheal erosion. A pulsating tracheostomy tube is evidence of such risk but does not confirm fistulization. Any patient at high risk can be examined by tracheoscopy for evidence of fistula formation.[48]

Immediate Management of the Fistula. An attempt is made by immediate maximal cuff inflation to stem the bleeding. If cuff overinflation fails, the tracheostomy tube is removed, and a translaryngeal tube is inserted. The cuff is again inflated at the level of the fistula to control the bleeding, or the tube may be positioned to allow direct finger pressure for control. The finger is inserted along the anterior trachea and compresses the blood vessel against the sternum. The patient is ventilated and prepared for immediate transport to the operating room. If transport is not possible, the surgical equipment necessary for artery ligation is readied in the patient's room. Suction must be immediately at hand.[45]

Definitive Management. Should the patient survive the initial hemorrhage and artery ligation, ventilation is provided by a long transtracheal tube with the cuff positioned below the necrotic area. Delayed repair of the trachea and arterial reconstruction is accomplished once the risk of infection is lessened. The repair includes resection and anastomosis or grafting if necessary. Every effort should be made to wean the patient from the ventilator and remove the tracheostomy tube as soon as possible.

Tracheoesophageal Fistula

A TEF also can be life threatening, although not as rapidly as a vascular fistula. It is not an emergency, yet it threatens life through respiratory insufficiency and infection. The injury is a pressure necrosis of the trachea and the anterior esophageal wall, most commonly from cuff-related tracheal injury. Nasogastric or orogastric tubes may also cause erosion from the esophagus through to the trachea. Rarely is it a primary

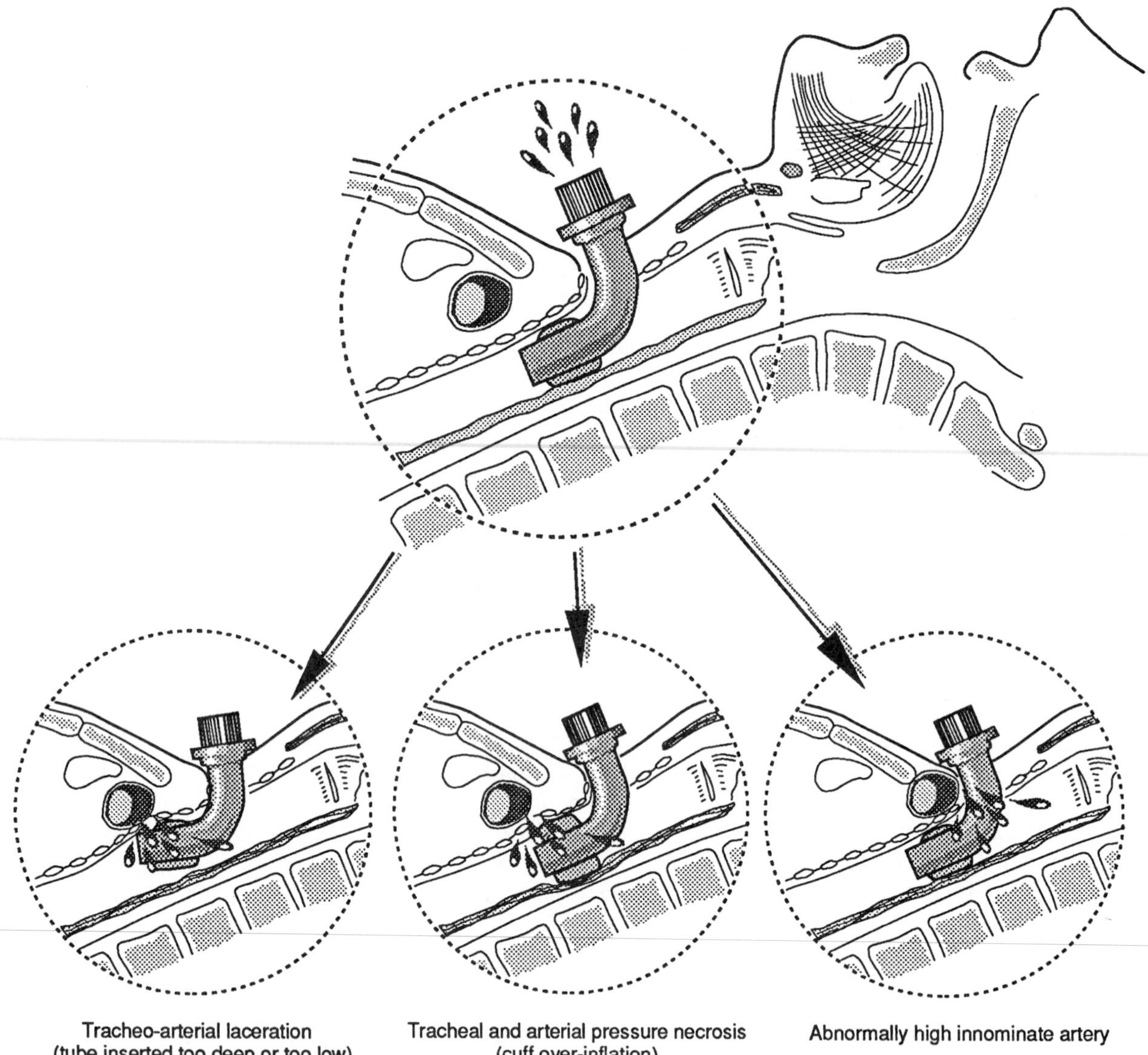

FIGURE 24-11 Tracheoarterial fistula in patients with tracheostomy. (From Besson A, Saegesser F: *Color atlas of chest trauma and associated injuries,* vol II, Oradell, NJ, 1983, Medical Economics, p 48.)

injury from blunt trauma. Figure 24-12 shows how fistulas occur from tube placement and cuff inflation.

Prevention. The techniques described for prevention of vascular fistulas are also appropriate in this case. The most likely pressure site is between the airway cuff and the nasogastric or orogastric tube. Frequent evaluation of the need for and use of these tubes is a primary preventive action. Each tube is viewed as a risk factor and should be eliminated as soon as possible. For example, a gastrostomy tube can be placed for long-term gastric decompression or feeding so that the nasogastric or orogastric tube can be removed. The risk of a fistula continues into the rehabilitative phase for the trauma patient who requires long-term tracheostomy.

Assessment. Most symptoms are usually identified by the nurse. The patient coughs on swallowing, or pulmonary secretions appear contaminated by gastric contents. The usual amount of tracheal secretions increases and constant gastric distention may be evident. The appearance of swallowed methylene blue dye in tracheal aspirate is a classic bedside test. Patients on mechanical ventilation may have a loss of tidal volume. Visualization of the fistula is accomplished by esophagoscopy or bronchoscopy. Contrast studies are associated with a high risk of aspiration and are not recommended.

Management. On a confirmed diagnosis of a TEF, the first course of action is to minimize tracheobronchial soilage by placing the cuff of the artificial airway distal to the fistula. Gastric content reflux is negated by placement of a gastrostomy tube, and nutrition is facilitated by a jejunostomy tube (preferred) or total parenteral nutrition. Spontaneous closure of the TEF is rare; thus, surgical correction is normally required. Ideally, the operation is performed after the patient is weaned from positive-pressure ventilation. An artificial airway with a large-volume, low-pressure cuff is used if positive

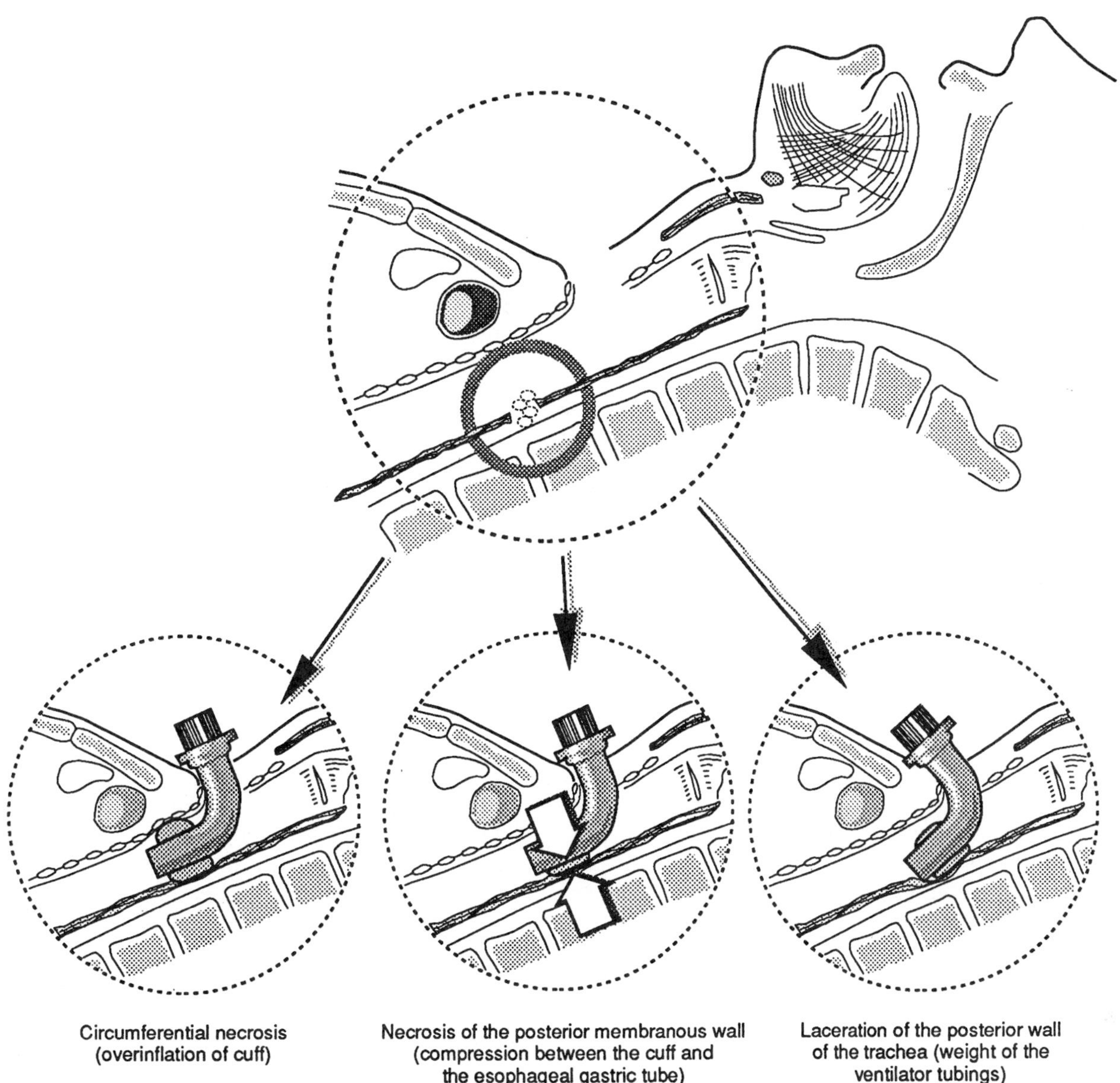

FIGURE 24-12 Tracheoesophageal fistula in patients with tracheostomy. (From Besson A, Seagesser F: *Color atlas of chest trauma and associated injuries,* vol II, Oradell, NJ, 1983, Medical Economics, p 51.)

pressure is necessary. If possible, the airway cuff is positioned away from the site of erosion within the trachea.[46]

BONY THORAX FRACTURES

Description and Fracture Sites

The triad of pain, ineffective ventilation, and secretion retention is observed consistently in patients with rib fractures, sternal fractures, or flail chest. It is from this perspective that the patient with thoracic cage fractures presents the greatest demand for creative and effective nursing care. The first two ribs are generally protected by the surrounding muscles, clavicle, scapula, and humerus. Fractures of these ribs signal high-impact trauma and are often accompanied by injury to the lungs, trachea, aortic arch, great vessels, or vertebral column. Ribs 3 through 9 are most commonly fractured in blunt trauma and are frequently associated with underlying lung injury, including pulmonary contusion and pneumothorax. The lower ribs (9 through 12) have an association with lung injury or abdominal injuries (e.g. spleen, liver, or kidney lacerations). Sternal fractures are also associated with considerable blunt trauma and may result in cardiac contusion or great vessel injury.[49] A system for classifying rib fractures may be found in Table 24-4.

Flail Chest

Flail chest is an injury of the bony thorax involving two or more contiguous ribs in two or more places.[27] Some authors state the criterion of three or more ribs.[7] Multiple rib fractures may have an associated sternal fracture. Alternatively, bilaterally fractured costochondral cartilages may present with an anterior flail segment or "flail sternum."[7] No matter

TABLE 24-4 Classification of Rib Fractures

Injury	Major Manifestations, Related Injuries, and Common Complications
Fractures of one rib	
Simple	Pain aggravated by deep breathing, coughing Localized tenderness Roentgenograms may or may not demonstrate fracture
Complicated	Pneumothorax, hemothorax Pulmonary infection or atelectasis
Multiple rib fractures	
With stable chest wall	Severe chest wall pain Underlying lung contusion or contusion of opposite lung Decreased cough and accumulation of secretions Acute gastric dilation Hemothorax, pneumomediastinum, and pneumothorax
With instability of chest wall	Generally involves fracture of each rib in two sites Panel of chest wall moves independently of thoracic cage (paradoxical respiration) Severely impaired cough and airway clearance Contusion of underlying lung Hemothorax and pneumothorax
Fractures of first rib	Usually associated with fractures of clavicle and upper ribs May involve neurovascular structures of neck Intrathoracic injuries
Fractures of lower ribs (seventh to twelfth)	Injuries to liver and spleen Acute gastric dilation

From Guenter CA, Welch MH: *Pulmonary medicine,* 2nd ed, Philadelphia, 1982, J. B. Lippincott.

the location, the continuity of the thorax is disrupted and the bony thorax no longer moves evenly and in unison. The injured parts of the bony thorax do not respond to the action of the respiratory muscles but move according to changes in intrapleural pressure. The flail segment moves paradoxically, and *paradoxical chest wall motion* may be noted during spontaneous breathing. Clinically, this appears as a "caving in" of the flail segment on inspiration followed by a "bulging out" on exhalation.[50] Gas flow within the lungs may or may not move paradoxically, but it is significantly diminished. The bellows effect of the chest is lost, intrapleural pressure is less negative than normal, and ventilation is compromised. The decreased gas flow and increased respiratory dead space are evident in lowered tidal volume, increased respiratory effort, and varying degrees of hypoxemia.

Resuscitation Assessment. The best assessment is simply to carefully observe the patient's breathing and chest wall movement. With flail chest in the spontaneously breathing patient, respirations are rapid and labored, and the chest wall moves in an asymmetric and uncoordinated manner. These findings may not be seen while the patient is on full ventilatory support. Crepitus may be palpated over bony fragments. The degree of initial hypoxemia depends on the associated pulmonary parenchymal injury (contusion) and restricted chest wall movement (from pain). The flail segment, although dramatic in appearance and an imposition on the work of breathing, does not independently cause hypoxemia. The initial chest film or chest CT scan identifies the general extent of the flail segment and additional thoracic injuries.[27] Later, without appropriate and adequate treatment, atelectasis and retention of secretions ensue.

It is difficult to characterize a specific profile for patients with flail chest because the injury is so often accompanied by either a pneumothorax or some degree of pulmonary contusion. Both conditions are discussed in detail later in this chapter. It is essential to associate flailing thoracic injuries with a high probability of underlying parenchymal damage. Serial blood gases, continuous pulse oximetry monitoring, and continuous observation of the patient's chest excursion and respiratory effort are initiated, particularly in the patient who is not immediately intubated and mechanically ventilated. Flail chest and associated injuries also frequently produce upper and lower airway obstruction from aspiration of blood, mucus, or vomit.

Initial Management. The mainstays of managing flail segment and thoracic wall fractures during both the prehospital and initial intrahospital period are the administration of analgesia, judicious use of crystalloids, and appropriate ventilatory support.[27] On stabilization, the focus becomes pain control, chest physiotherapy, and mobilization.[51] Initially, intravenous (IV) analgesia is used; however, in those patients with more than three rib fractures, epidural anesthesia/analgesia (e.g., bupivacaine/fentanyl) has been shown to be superior to IV patient-controlled analgesia (PCA) (e.g., morphine). Limitations to the use of epidural analgesia include the presence of spinal column fractures, high rib fractures (1 through 3), spinal cord injury, and traumatic brain injury.[51-53] The major advantage of epidural analgesia is its apparent effectiveness without sedation. Disadvantages include technical difficulties with initiation, hypotension, and infection. Other effective, although less commonly used, forms of pain relief include intercostal nerve block, intrapleural anesthesia, and thoracic paravertebral block. Each form of analgesia comes with advantages and disadvantages. Pulmonary contusion is almost always an associated injury with flail segment; thus, care of the flail is, in part, guided by the principles of pulmonary contusion treatment. Because the injured lung is sensitive to both underresuscitation and overresuscitation, the fluid management goal is euvolemia.[27] Humidified oxygen through a natural airway may be all that is necessary at the outset, although intubation and positive-pressure ventilation may be needed under circumstances of hypoxemia, hypercarbia, intolerable pain, or airway issues.

Various forms of surgical stabilization have been investigated.[54,55] Internal fixation may improve patient outcomes and avoid the complications associated with prolonged ventilatory support. Further research will help determine the role of internal fixation of fractured ribs and flail segments.

Ventilatory Therapy. There are several ways to support ventilation in patients with significant flail chest. Spontaneous breathing holds advantages[56,57] over conventional modes of ventilation and may be the optimal choice if the blunt chest trauma is the sole injury and analgesia is adequate. Alternatively, a combination of thoracic epidural and noninvasive ventilation (NIV) may be sufficient for those patients able to maintain their own airways who are neurologically intact and cooperative. NIV with CPAP maintains the advantages of spontaneous breathing while giving assistance to the patient to increase the functional residual capacity (FRC).[58] However, in practice, patients receiving this regimen require more attention and care, and staff generally require higher levels of expertise. Finally, some patients will need an artificial airway and positive-pressure ventilation to facilitate other aspects of their treatment or because their pulmonary status warrants it. Again, spontaneous breathing may be considered by selecting modes or means that permit spontaneous breathing (e.g., airway pressure release ventilation, CPAP).

Specific patients who benefit from mechanical ventilation include nonambulatory or disoriented patients, those with significant lung conditions, and those with poor chest excursion as a result of fatigue and other injuries. Disadvantages of mechanical ventilation include increased risk of volutrauma, pulmonary contamination, and a potentially longer need for therapy.

Critical Care Assessment and Management. In addition to factors previously discussed, the choice of therapy may depend on available equipment and nursing expertise. Intubation and ventilator therapy may not occur until admission to the critical care unit. The patient with significant flail segment and underlying lung contusion frequently has a lengthy stay in the ICU, sometimes requiring weeks of ventilator support. Appropriate equipment and effective nursing management must be available throughout the period. As stated earlier, the common triad with flail chest is ineffective ventilation, accumulation of secretions, and chest pain. Specific nursing care includes management of the patient-ventilator unit, pulmonary care, and pain control. The most important goal is to open the injured lung and to maintain alveolar recruitment.

Managing the Patient-Ventilator Unit. Most ICUs strive to minimize the number of different models of ventilators in use. This serves several practical purposes, including that staff becomes familiar with consistent alarm sounds and proficient with quick machine assessment, data extraction, and problem resolution. These advantages are true for all disciplines (nursing, medicine, respiratory therapists, and biomedical engineers). Mechanically ventilated patients must be monitored closely by pulse oximetry, blood gases, and pulmonary function assessment, including plateau pressure, mean airway pressure, tidal volume, and a measure of the work of breathing to determine the effectiveness of therapy.

Before the introduction of mainstream positive-pressure ventilation in the 1950s, flail chest was treated with some form of external splinting (sandbags or adhesive straps), operative fixation (rib plates), or an external traction device (weights and pulleys attached to the fractured ribs). In the 1950s, treatment was modified to include "internal pneumatic stabilization" with positive-pressure ventilation.[59] In treating this injury, many clinicians considered only the flail segment of ribs with the paradoxic wall motion and failed to recognize the pulmonary contusion beneath. Trinkle et al[60] in their landmark article redirected attention away from mechanical ventilation and normalization of the flail segment and focused treatment on the pulmonary contusion beneath the flail. Their retrospective review compared the outcomes of 30 patients with flail chest who received either conventional treatment with intubation and mechanical ventilation versus the experimental group with avoidance of mechanical ventilation combined with use of fluid restriction, diuretics, steroids, albumin, pulmonary hygiene, and intercostal nerve blocks. Their findings resulted in a recommendation *not* to routinely use mechanical ventilation for treatment of flail segment but rather to focus treatment on the pulmonary contusion lying beneath. Subsequently, tracheostomy and prolonged ventilation were often avoided. This method resulted in a lower ICU length of stay, decreased mortality rates, and reduced complication rates.

Current literature supports the practice of spontaneous breathing in patients with blunt chest wall trauma, although "selective" intubation and positive-pressure ventilation remain indicated at times.[61,62] Core elements in treatment of a flail chest include preventing or reversing hypoxemia; maintaining a euvolemic intravascular state, avoiding both overhydration (particularly with crystalloids) and underresuscitation; and controlling pain primarily with an intercostal or epidural nerve block.[27] The future direction of flail segment and rib fracture management will most likely continue to include facilitation of spontaneous breathing either with simple administration of oxygen, noninvasive ventilation support, or by an artificial airway with modes of mechanical ventilation that permit spontaneous breathing.

Repeated clinical examinations and periodic chest films reveal trends in respiratory complications, such as effusions or atelectasis, and progress toward chest wall stability. Chest wall rigidity is apparent at approximately 3 weeks, and a full 6 weeks are usually required before the fractures are consolidated. Significant pain may continue for weeks to months. In one study, patients with one or two rib fractures and no other extrathoracic injuries were unable to return to work or usual activity for an average of 50 days.[63]

Pulmonary Care. As ventilation becomes stabilized, pulmonary care to clear the airways and lung fields begins. Aggressive chest physiotherapy consisting of postural drainage, percussion, and vibration coupled with suctioning and early mobilization are used at varying intervals, depending on the patient's pulmonary status and tolerance. The quality and quantity of secretions are monitored for infection. A plan for patient position change is based on observation of which position provides greatest chest wall stability (such as lying on the flail segment) and best ventilation/oxygenation. These treatments are discussed in more detail in the section on critical care therapeutics.[62]

Pain Control. Pain control is critically important and may be the primary problem for patients with bony thorax fractures. A variety of useful treatments have been reported for thoracic pain; they include intercostal nerve blocks, intrapleural administration of narcotics, and PCA, both IV and epidural (EPCA). These methods are supported by research as safe and effective modalities for pain control.[53,64] Continuous infusion of IV narcotics, which can be titrated by the nurse on the basis of the patient's respiratory status, level of consciousness, and level of pain, also constitutes a well-accepted method of pain control, especially with patients not candidates for epidural or IV PCA. Research now supports the use of epidural over IV PCA for optimal pain relief and better outcomes for patients with thoracic injuries.[51] However, not all patients will be candidates for EPCA.[65] Regardless of the method or route of administration, the appropriate dosages for analgesics are established individually for each patient on the the basis of the nurse's continual assessment of pain relief, pulmonary status, and level of consciousness. Nonpharmacologically, the application of a transcutaneous electrical nerve stimulator (TENS) may relieve the pain associated with thoracic injuries. Relaxation, distraction, acupuncture, and guided imagery are also part of the nonpharmacologic armamentarium to help control the pain resulting from thoracic trauma.[66]

Intermediate/Rehabilitation Care Assessment and Management

In this phase of trauma care, new complications of bony thorax fractures may become evident. The normal healing of the fractures may be altered, and deformities may be noticeable to the patient and family. Some deformities, from flail chest in particular, are permanent, unattractive, and difficult for the individual to accept. Others may create ventilatory impairment, leading to long-term disability and changes in lifestyle. Attempts at surgical reconstruction may dominate the patient's recovery experience.

The plan of care for the patient focuses on assessment to recognize emerging complications and disability, previously described pulmonary care to prevent retention of secretions and infection, and relief of chest pain. The goal of pulmonary care is to achieve spontaneous ventilation and weaning from oxygen therapy. Chest physiotherapy and incentive spirometry are continued to clear problem areas in the lungs and to improve respiratory mechanics such as thoracic muscle strength. The patient continues to feel chest pain to some degree: some individuals endure intractable intercostal pain or neuralgia. Often, the specific cause of the pain is not known but may result from traumatic neuromas, where intercostal nerves become trapped in scarred tissue. Chest pain may be managed primarily pharmacologically. However, other methods must be initiated if they are not already in progress because pain relief is frequently a lengthy and complex problem with response more likely from synergistic therapies. TENS, massage, and positioning are only a few of the possible alternatives for relieving pain.[67]

Complications of Fracture Healing

Rib fractures usually heal within 6 weeks. Occasionally, malunion or a failure to consolidate fractures, even an entire flail segment, does occur. Inspection and palpation, as previously described, will identify the unstable chest segment and this can be confirmed radiographically. Internal fixation may be achieved by various surgical procedures, including the use of struts or insertion of a metal plate.[54,55]

Abnormal healing also can result in excessive or hypertrophic callus formation, which may be gradually reabsorbed or may require surgical excision. The callus rubs on surrounding tissue and muscle, creating considerable pain and possibly restricting chest wall movement. An abnormal union of adjacent ribs, intercostal synostosis, may occur during the months after injury. Clinical and radiographic examinations can identify abnormal healing.[68]

Posttraumatic Respiratory Disability

Observation and interview help to identify dyspnea, shortness of breath, and a feeling of chest tightness. Blood gas analysis and chest film findings are frequently unchanged. The long-term sequelae of significant bony thorax trauma are unclear, and published case reports are few. The current nursing approach includes tracking the patient's unique problems, instituting measures that provide comfort, ensuring appropriate physical therapy referrals, and providing a great deal of psychological support.[67]

Rib Fractures and the Elderly

The elderly (>65 years of age) warrant special consideration regarding trauma and in particular rib fractures. The trauma-related mortality rate is nearly twice as high in elderly patients with rib fractures as in younger patients with similar injuries.

Furthermore, the mortality rate rises in a steplike fashion with increasing numbers of rib fractures.[69,70] Epidural use may come with a slightly higher complication rate in the elderly than in the young, although these risks are outweighed by the benefits and decreased mortality rate.[71] Admission and observation is often warranted in the elderly for simple rib fractures, whereas it may not be necessary in the young.

PULMONARY CONTUSION

Mechanism and Pathophysiology

Essentially a compression/decompression injury, lung contusion occurs as the chest wall hits an object such as a steering wheel or is acted on by an outside force such as an explosion. The force against the chest wall is transmitted to the lung, rupturing tissue, small airways, alveoli, and blood vessels. The pressure wave abates, and the chest wall springs back, pulling the lung with it and causing additional injury. It is a bruising process possibly accompanied by a pulmonary tear or laceration. This injury occurs most often in young people because the chest wall is more flexible than in older individuals. Although an older person might sustain multiple rib fractures and fewer lung contusions, a young person might sustain more contusions and fewer fractures. Individuals with thin chests sustain greater contusions because there is less protection provided by muscle and adipose tissue.[72,73]

Contusions may be mild and go unnoticed in the treatment of associated injuries such as flail chest or hemopneumothorax. However, unilateral or bilateral contusion can be severe, even life threatening, and can seriously interfere with gas exchange. The contusion process is hemorrhagic and is accompanied by interstitial and alveolar edema as a response to injury. Hemorrhage and edema occur within the area of contusion and gradually involve surrounding tissue in general inflammation. Damaged or closed alveolar-capillary units produce ventilation and perfusion abnormalities and shunt. If no further lung injury occurs, the areas of infiltrate begin to clear and healing occurs. The natural course of a pulmonary contusion may demonstrate a progressive worsening over a period of the first few days.

Resolution of contusions may be detected as early as 48 to 72 hours after trauma, although many days may be required in the presence of a significant injury.[25] Alternatively, the injured area may continue to evolve as secretion retention, decreased regional lung compliance, and the presence of intra-alveolar blood and edema fluid creates an environment prime for infection. Blunt trauma that produces significant lung contusion is frequently associated with pulmonary hematoma or laceration. Severe lacerations that bleed into the pleural space or airway may require thoracotomy and pulmonary resection.

Resuscitation Assessment

During initial resuscitation, respiratory distress may be evident. Accompanying rib or sternal fractures are common but not universal. If the contusion is clinically significant, the partial arterial oxygen tension (Pao_2) is frequently less than 60 mm Hg on room air and hemoptysis is not an uncommon finding. Lung infiltrates may be seen on the admission chest film, although their appearance may not be evident until 6 or even 48 hours after trauma.[74] The CXR is relatively insensitive to contusions unless they are fairly extensive or contain large or multiple lacerations. Radiographs can show improvement as a decrease in lung opacification assuming the injury is bad enough to be recognized in the first place. CT scan is much more sensitive than CXR at demonstrating and quantifying pulmonary contusion.[25,74]

Critical Care Assessment

Predicting the outcomes of patients with pulmonary contusions is difficult at best. In the first 24 hours the patient may show progressive clinical and radiographic changes that correlate with underlying alveolar capillary injury. Patchy infiltrates persist on subsequent chest films. Bloody sputum, either fresh blood or old blood and clots in the mature contusion, may continue to be evident during suctioning or with coughing. Local areas of wheezing are a common finding. Patients with significant contusions show progressive evidence of stiff, wet lungs and increased work of breathing. Measured pulmonary compliance falls. Plateau pressure increases (in volume targeted modes) with a fall in pulmonary compliance. The degree of deterioration in Pao_2 and pH is usually a function of the severity of lung injury and failure to recognize the extent of the contusion and to institute early ventilatory support and pulmonary hygiene. The presence of associated injuries or development of complications that cause a systemic inflammatory response (e.g., shock) produce secondary changes within the lung. Posttraumatic respiratory distress syndrome may be superimposed on the evolving lung contusion. Methods of predicting the likelihood of acute respiratory distress syndrome (ARDS) development as a complication of pulmonary contusion have been proposed.[74] The release of mediators and the inflammatory cascade as a result of pulmonary contusion is also recognized. Pharmacologic treatment, such as with indomethacin, may eventually play a routine role in the management of patients with pulmonary contusion.[75]

Critical Care Management

Management of pulmonary contusion is almost entirely supportive.[7,72,73] Goals during this phase of care are to achieve adequate pain relief, ensure adequate respiratory gas exchange, and maintain euvolemia. Steroids are not considered helpful, nor are prophylactic antibiotics, and use of either is probably counterproductive.

Treatment of hypoxemia may require a range of therapy. Support of spontaneous ventilation with supplemental oxygen may be adequate for some patients. Underlying pulmonary disease, associated injuries, or massive contusion may necessitate ventilatory support in a defined subset of patients. Selection of ventilation mode will be based on available technology and clinician skills. Ideally, modes capable of facilitating spontaneous breathing would be considered first. Noninvasive ventilation may serve to help maintain functional residual capacity, provide a means of oxygenation, and decrease work of breathing, all the while allowing the patient to spontaneously breathe. Intubation with positive-pressure ventilatory techniques that can maintain airway pressure over time to facilitate lung recruitment while limiting derecruitment may be useful in patients with severe chest trauma.[76] As the physiologic effects of the contusion resolve, ventilatory support is gradually weaned.

Neuromuscular blockade (NMB), once a primary adjunct to mechanical ventilation in the acutely ill, is now recommended only "as a last resort" in mechanically ventilated septic patients.[77] The limited evidence available regarding the assumed benefits of NMB (facilitate ventilation, manage increased intracranial pressure [ICP], treat muscle spasms, and decrease oxygen consumption) are generally weak and the sequelae of postparalytic tetraparesis are well known.[78] NMB is contraindicated if a goal of spontaneous breathing is sought. During the first few days after trauma, pulmonary care to mobilize and clear bloody secretions is required in every patient as the contusion resolves. This is particularly important in management of significant lung contusions. Early institution of chest physiotherapy, postural drainage, and mobilization assists in avoiding pulmonary complications. The treatment should be specific to the lung segment involved. Within 48 to 72 hours the bloody mucus often becomes thinner and darkens, eventually clearing to normal appearance. If symptoms of infection become evident, sputum cultures and chest films may be pursued. Facilitation of chest physiotherapy, postural drainage, and ambulation is normally contingent on adequate pain relief. The nurse plays a paramount role in finding the balance between adequate analgesia and limited sedation, including the most appropriate drug, dose, and delivery method (e.g. epidural versus oral versus IV).

In all cases, gas exchange is observed over time by continuous pulse oximetry monitoring, capnography, periodic blood gas analysis, and calculating parameters such as V/Q ratio or shunt (Qs/Qt), Pao_2/fractional concentration of oxygen in inspired gas (Fio_2) ratio, and lung compliance. Repeated physical examination is essential to determine the effectiveness of therapy and progress of the lung condition.

Although trauma patients in shock may require large volumes of fluid, this practice may worsen a pulmonary contusion. In the absence of shock or hypotension, IV administration of crystalloid must be controlled with a goal of maintaining euvolemia. Both underhydration and overhydration may adversely affect pulmonary function.[27,79] Animal studies suggest that a hypertonic solution (7.5% sodium chloride) does not appear superior to isotonic solution in reducing the magnitude of lung injury after pulmonary contusion.[80] Colloid solutions have also been investigated in the treatment of pulmonary contusion without significant conclusions.[81] Volume administration is guided by using clinical indicators of tissue perfusion (e.g., urine output, mentation, lactate level) and invasive hemodynamic parameters as therapeutic end points. Pulmonary artery catheters (PACs) may hold no benefit (as measured by survival) over central venous catheters for guiding clinicians in optimal fluid therapy, although catheter-related complications (predominantly arrhythmias) are twice as likely to occur with PACs.[82] The ideal volume and type of resuscitation fluid warrants further study.[80]

Intermediate Care/Rehabilitation Management

In this phase, the focus of nursing management continues to be pulmonary hygiene and restoration of respiratory reserve. Weeks after injury a traumatic cyst may develop, which establishes a further concern for pulmonary infectious sequelae. The literature is essentially devoid of long-term studies on the effect of pulmonary contusion on overall health, although there is the suggestion that patients with pulmonary contusion may have fibrotic changes in the contused lung.

Pleural Space Injuries

Under healthy conditions, a serous membrane adheres to the lungs and then folds over itself and adheres firmly to the inner wall of the rib cage. The membrane attached to the lung is the visceral pleura, and the membrane attached to the rib cage is the parietal pleura. Between the two pleura is about 10 to 20 ml of lubricating fluid (pleural fluid) that facilitates the pleura gliding over itself during ventilatory movement. The two pleura are in constant contact and only a "potential space" exists between them. The pressure within the pleural space is subatmospheric (negative) and ranges from about 4 mm Hg to -10 mm Hg. A disruption of the pleural space will result in an alteration of pulmonary mechanics. With the lung's natural tendency to recoil no longer counteracted by the outward forces of the chest wall, the lung will tend to collapse. The left and right pleural spaces and the mediastinum are three separate compartments and their pleural spaces do not communicate. Therefore, injuries to the right pleura do not directly affect the mediastinal or left pleural space.[83]

Pleural space injuries are caused by both blunt and penetrating mechanisms. The injury may be a laceration or perforation of a thoracic structure, usually a lung or blood vessel. Blood and/or air collects between the pleural layers, and the normal negative intrathoracic pressure is lost. All or part of the lung on the affected side collapses because of its unopposed elasticity. The result may be a pneumothorax (intrapleural air collection), hemothorax (intrapleural blood collection), or, a common finding in trauma, emopneumothorax (mix of both blood and air within the pleural space). If intrapleural air or blood continues to increase within the constraints of the closed intrathoracic cavity, internal structures are compressed and displaced as tension builds. The result is a tension pneumothorax or hemothorax. Pleural space injuries may be unilateral or bilateral.

Assessment of Pleural Space Injury

Examination for any type of pleural space injury follows the thoracic assessment procedure described earlier. Several classic assessment findings are seen with significant pleural space injuries. Some degree of respiratory difficulty or dyspnea is evident. Because the primary problem is altered ventilation, there is evidence of poor gas exchange. Frequently, diminished or absent breath sounds are evident on the affected side or sides, particularly with a collapsed lung or when blood loss into the thoracic cavity is significant (generally >350 ml). There is a loss of normal resonance on percussion of the affected side. Dullness is audible in the presence of a hemothorax, and there is hyperresonance when significant pneumothorax is present.[7]

Early analysis of arterial blood gas is useful only in the context of the patient's clinical examination. The patient who is breathing rapidly because of shock and pain may have relatively normal initial blood gas levels. Alternatively, there may be hypercarbia and hypoxemia, which are often associated with ventilatory failure.

Chest film findings assist in determining injuries and must be obtained as rapidly as possible. A pneumothorax appears on the CXR as a visceral pleural line without distal lung markings (Figure 24-13, *A* and *B*). In the supine patient, the pneumothorax may be seen more readily as an enlargement of the costophrenic angle (deep sulcus sign)[84] (Figure 24-14). The erect CXR classically reveals the visceral pleural line apically or laterally. Hemothorax in the supine trauma patient appears as an opacification or haziness covering the affected lung as blood fills the posterior, dependent pleural space. In the erect patient, a meniscus sign (fluid line) with obliteration of the costophrenic and cardiophrenic angles occurs as the blood fills these spaces.[25] Approximately 200 to 300 ml of blood is required in the pleural space before a hemothorax is evident on the CXR.[7] However, in patients with acute thoracic trauma plain CXR for pneumothoraces and hemothoraces is becoming a screening tool because thoracic CT scan sensitivity exceeds that of the CXR and accessibility of scanners is increasing.[85] A growing area of interest is the use of hand-held ultrasonography in the resuscitation area for the diagnosis of pneumothorax[86] and hemothorax.[87]

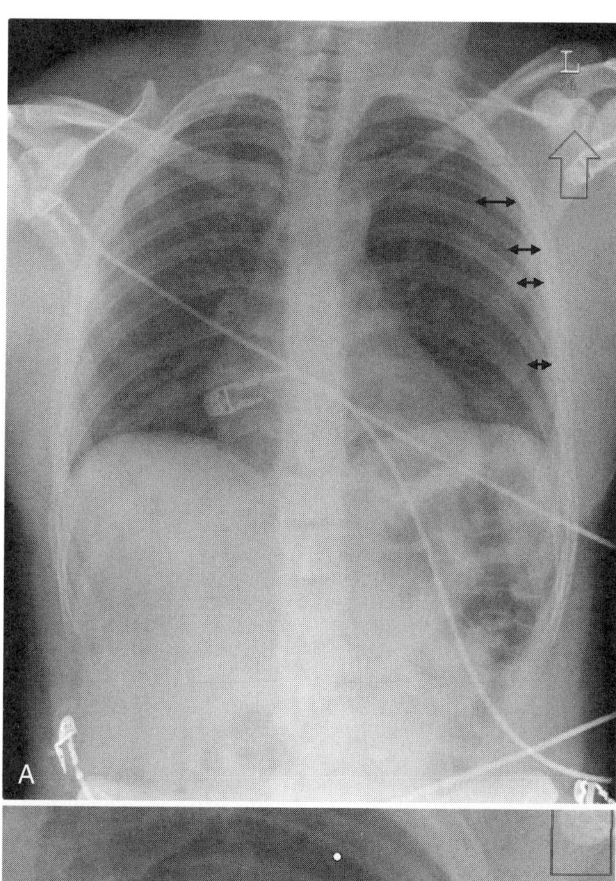

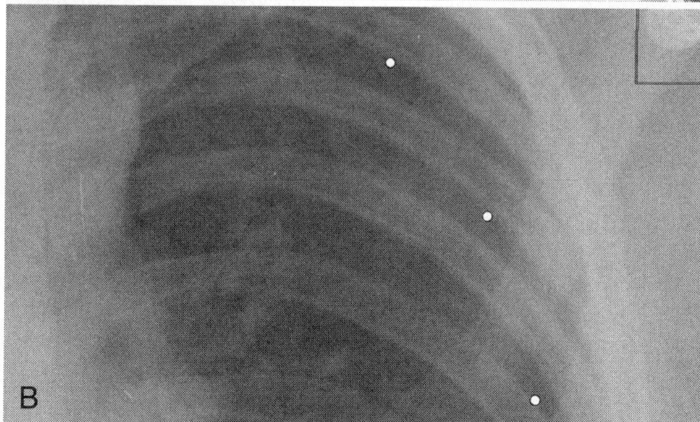

FIGURE 24-13 Pneumothorax. A large left pneumothorax extends from left lung base to apical region; however, a pneumothorax may be difficult to appreciate on CXR, particularly for the untrained eye. In this example (**A**) there is an absence of lung markings along the outer edge of the left lung (indicated by the *black arrows*). The visceral pleural line may be better visualized in the enlarged section of the left lung radiograph (**B**). By joining the white dots an imaginary curved line may be formed approximating the visceral pleural edge. To the right of the visceral pleural edge is the pneumothorax and to the left is aerated lung.

Closed Pneumothorax or Hemothorax

A simple closed pneumothorax is usually the result of a lung laceration caused by a fractured rib or penetrating wound (Figure 24-15). In more complex injuries a diaphragmatic tear allows the abdominal contents to protrude into the chest cavity. In many instances the intrapleural air leak is self-limiting in that the progressive collapse and decreasing ventilation of the affected lung seal the leak. In other cases, depending on the size and location of the injury, the lung may collapse completely.

Common sources of bleeding in hemothorax include internal mammary arteries and intercostal arteries and accompanying veins (Figure 24-16). Penetrating wounds may involve major pulmonary vessels, lung, any of the mediastinal structures, or the diaphragm. The lung is a low-pressure vascular system capable of tamponading sources of bleeding; thus, re-expansion of the lung and apposition of the parietal and visceral pleura is core to the treatment of simple hemothorax. To this end, chest tube placement and deep breathing

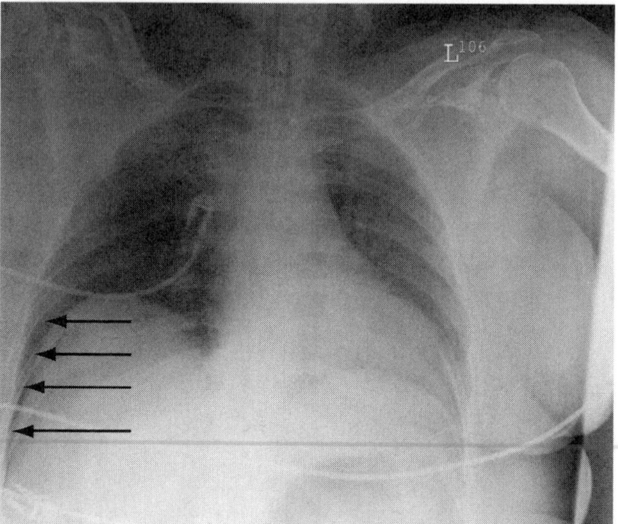

FIGURE 24-14 Deep sulcus sign of pneumothorax. CXR revealing a deep sulcus sign in the right costophrenic region.

are common treatments. Infrequently, thoracotomy may be required.[7]

Resuscitation Management. Appropriate airway, ventilatory, and oxygen therapy begins the management process. Occult pneumothoraces resulting from blunt trauma may not require chest tube placement; however, careful pulmonary assessment is paramount to recognize respiratory status deterioration, which may occur if the pneumothorax enlarges.[88,89] Up to 85% of the time small hemothoraces measuring <1.5 cm on CT scan may not require drainage.[90] A larger pneumothorax or a hemothorax requires the correct placement of a chest tube for the purposes of lung re-expansion and drainage of air, blood, and clots from the pleural space. Inadequate drainage creates short- and long-term complications, including intrapleural infections and adhesions. Insertion of a chest tube also reduces the risk of tension pneumothorax, which may develop as air fills the chest cavity (described in detail later). Explanations of the injury and treatment are offered to the patient in a manner most appropriate for his or her emotional state and level of consciousness. The patient's pain must be recognized, repeatedly measured, and appropriately treated.

A large-bore chest tube (36F-40F) is inserted, usually in the fourth or fifth intercostal space at the midaxillary line, to drain both air and blood. Alternatively, but less optimal in traumatic injuries, a tube may be placed in the second intercostal space at the midclavicular line to drain a simple pneumothorax. As soon as the tube is connected to the underwater seal system and suction drainage, the effects of the treatment are assessed by clinical examination and chest x-ray examination. Intrapleural bleeding is frequently self-limited, and blood loss is replaced as needed determined by the patient's overall status. Small to moderate air leaks will

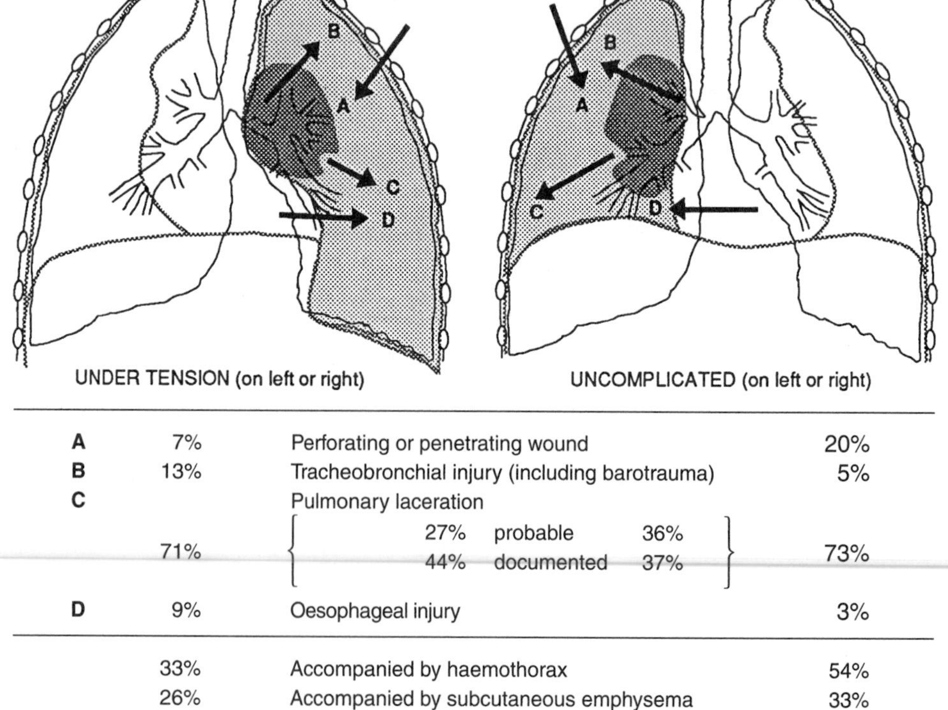

	Under tension		Uncomplicated
A	7%	Perforating or penetrating wound	20%
B	13%	Tracheobronchial injury (including barotrauma)	5%
C		Pulmonary laceration	
	71%	27% probable 36% 44% documented 37%	73%
D	9%	Oesophageal injury	3%
	33%	Accompanied by haemothorax	54%
	26%	Accompanied by subcutaneous emphysema	33%

FIGURE 24-15 Origins of pneumothorax. Uncomplicated pneumothorax and tension pneumothorax are compared with respect to the source of air causing the pneumothorax. (From Besson A, Seagesser F: *Color atlas of chest trauma and associated injuries,* vol II, Oradell, NJ, 1983, Medical Economics, p 233.)

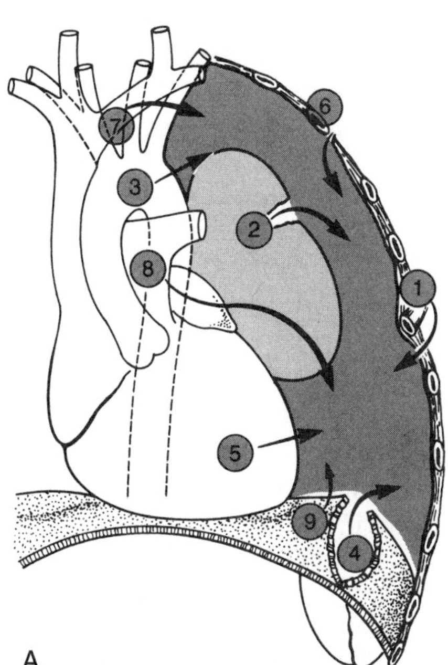

Source of bleeding in left hemothorax (moderate or massive)

1.	Rib fracture	36%
2.	Pulmonary parenchyma	35%
3.	Aortic isthmus	15%
4.	Spleen	5%
5.	Heart chamber	5%
6.	Intercostal or internal mammary artery	5%
7.	Supraaortic vessel	3%
8.	Major pulmonary vessel	2%
9.	Diaphragm	0%

There are several sources of bleeding in 6 percent of cases.

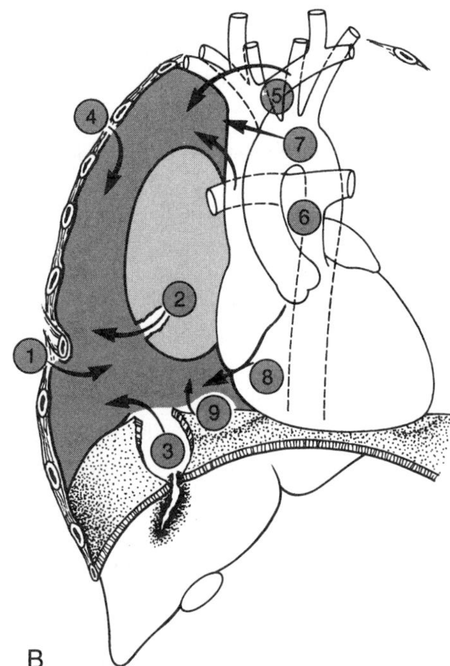

Source of bleeding in right hemothorax (moderate or massive)

1.	Rib fracture	51%
2.	Pulmonary parenchyma	27%
3.	Liver	10%
4.	Intercostal or internal mammary artery	5%
5.	Supraaortic vessel	4%
6.	Pulmonary vessel	3%
7.	Aortic isthmus	1%
8.	Heart chamber	1%
9.	Diaphragm	0%

There are several sources of bleeding in 2 percent of cases.

FIGURE 24-16 Sources of bleeding in hemothorax. (From Besson A, Seagesser F: *Color atlas of chest trauma and associated injuries,* vol I, Oradell, NJ, 1983, Medical Economics, p 280.)

usually seal over in the first few hours to days after trauma. Occasionally a major air leak persists, requiring more negative pressure in the suction drainage system or placement of an additional chest tube. Bronchoscopy and thoracotomy may be required to determine whether major bronchial injury is responsible for the continued air leak and to facilitate definitive treatment.

Critical Care/Intermediate Care Management. Patients with an isolated simple pneumothorax or a small hemothorax will not necessarily require critical care intervention. However, these injuries may be one of several thoracic or multitrauma injuries and are frequently associated with more life-threatening injuries. The use of a high concentration of inspired oxygen has been advocated as a treatment modality for nontension spontaneous pneumothoraces[91] and with experimental small pneumothoraces (<20%)[92] for some years. Research suggests that oxygen therapy may accelerate the resolution of pneumothorax by increasing the nitrogen gradient between the pneumothorax and the pleural capillaries. The denitrogenation of arterial and thus capillary blood increases the gradient for nitrogen absorption through pleural capillaries. The ideal inspired oxygen concentration and means to deliver the oxygen rich gas is controversial. Studies on rabbits suggest that a 60% oxygen concentration may be appropriate, although lower concentrations may also be effective.[92] Administration of approximately 35% to 40% oxygen by nasal cannula comes with the advantages of being more comfortable than a face mask; allows the patient to speak, drink, and eat more readily without interrupting oxygen delivery; and provides easy access to the mouth for pulmonary exercises (e.g., incentive spirometry). Further research is needed to determine the appropriateness of oxygen therapy and the best inspired oxygen concentration for a patient with traumatic pneumothorax.

Monitoring the Injury and Drainage. The nurse must regularly evaluate the functioning of the chest tube system and the progress of the injury. Repeated physical assessment and follow-up chest films determine whether the lung has re-expanded and ventilation has returned to the patient's baseline. Blood loss through or around the chest tube is measured and evaluated to determine progression of bleeding. Exploratory thoracotomy may be indicated if there is a 1500-ml blood loss within the first 24 hours[93] or drainage of 200 ml/hr or greater over 2 to 4 hours coupled with a deteriorating or poor physiologic status of the patient.[27] Trends in the patient's tidal volume and air evacuation through the chest tube system are monitored for significant air leaks and loss of ventilatory volume. Nursing management of pleural drainage is discussed in more detail later in this chapter.

Massive Hemothorax

Massive hemothorax is defined as blood loss of 1500 ml or more within the thorax. This constitutes a life-threatening situation. Frequently there are severe associated thoracic injuries, and the source of bleeding is a large blood vessel or mediastinal structure. Because the chest cavity is large enough to contain most of the patient's circulating blood volume, the bleeding slows only when the pressure within the pleural cavity is equal to or greater than the pressure within the damaged vessel. Shock associated with an absence of breath sounds or dullness to percussion over the suspected hemithorax is considered an essential finding for massive hemothorax (tension hemothorax). Distended neck veins are rare because blood loss into the thorax is substantial causing intravascular volume depletion.[27]

Resuscitation Assessment and Management. The patient may arrive in cardiopulmonary arrest and in need of immediate thoracotomy to control bleeding. The immediate clinical picture includes signs of hypovolemic shock, dyspnea, tachypnea, and cyanosis. Shock is the predominant finding before or concomitantly with impaired ventilation. Ventilation problems are caused by lung compression and collapse, and signs of mediastinal shift with cardiac compression may also be present. The initial CXR identifies the extent of the massive hemothorax, which appears as a primarily opaque chest cavity (Figure 24-17).

Hemorrhagic shock is managed by immediate insertion of a large-bore IV line and administration of resuscitation fluids. Controversy exists over the end points of resuscitation and the ideal resuscitation fluid. Although this debate continues, the use of crystalloids over colloids has gained popularity[94] along with *permissive hypotension.*[95,96] Large amounts of fluid resuscitation in patients with uncontrolled bleeding may actually worsen outcome. A core management principle of hemorrhagic shock is to find the source of bleeding and stop it. To that end, urgent thoracotomy may be necessary, but only if performed by a qualified surgeon with appropriate training and experience.[27] A delay in thoracotomy and initial insertion of a chest tube may provide an avenue for exsanguination by eliminating any tamponade effect from a closed chest injury. The practice of clamping a chest tube in the presence of large bloody output to possibly create an internal compressive effect is not supported. Clamping of chest tubes during massive hemothorax may result in tension hemothorax, further compromising patient status.

Autotransfusion of Shed Blood. Autotransfusion of shed blood is useful in the management of intrathoracic sources of bleeding. The reinfusion of blood drained from the chest may be accomplished by using one of a variety of techniques and commercially available autotransfusion devices. Basically, the

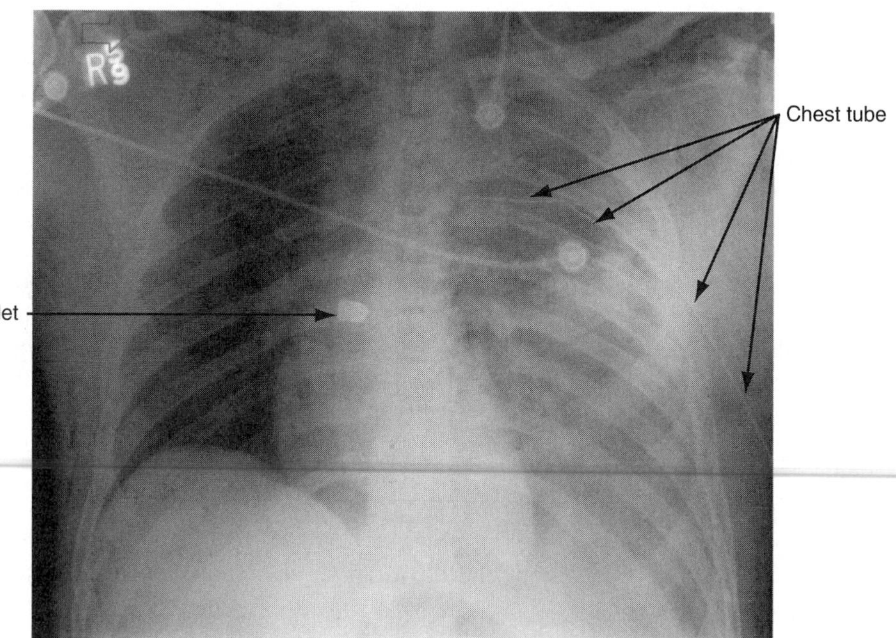

FIGURE 24-17 Hemothorax. Radiograph of a young man in profound shock from a gunshot wound to the chest. Note the bullet, which transverses the left hemithorax and is lodged in the right chest. Also, increased density over the left hemithorax represents layering of blood. Hemothorax and shock were treated by chest tube drainage and fluid administration. The patient was transported to the operating room but died there as a result of continuing hemorrhage. In massive hemothorax, exsanguination may occur after chest tube insertion.

blood is aspirated through sterile tubing, collected in a sterile reservoir, filtered, and returned to the patient intravenously. The retrieval bag may contain citrate phosphate dextrose, other types of anticoagulants, or no anticoagulant.[97]

The increasing use of autotransfusion during the resuscitation, operative, and critical care phases of care attests to the numerous advantages of autologous blood administration. These include the following:

1. The blood is readily available and particularly useful in the patient with massive hemorrhage that exhausts or severely taxes the bank blood availability.
2. Autologous blood requires no cross-matching and should be free of pyrogens, avoiding allergic and febrile reactions.
3. Autotransfusion avoids the risk of hepatitis, acquired immune deficiency syndrome, or exposure to homologous antigens.
4. Platelet counts and 2,3-diphosphoglycerate (essential for normal oxygen delivery to tissues) levels are reported to be near normal in blood that is autotransfused soon after removal. No warming is required.
5. Autologous blood may be acceptable to patients, such as Jehovah's Witnesses, who would normally refuse bank blood.
6. Cost savings generally are appreciated, depending on institutional pricing of equipment, operation, and packaging.

Specific contraindications to autotransfusion include known malignancy, inadequate renal or hepatic function, wounds more than 3 hours old, and significant contamination caused by bowel, stomach, or esophageal disruption. Clinical judgment is required as to the acceptable degree of contamination and the risk of septic complications.

Precautions and implications for nursing management center on the risk of coagulopathy, microembolism, and infection. The drained blood undergoes some hemolysis, leading to a reduced hematocrit and increased urine hemoglobin levels. Autologous blood from serosal cavities such as the thorax lacks fibrinogen, contains elevated levels of fibrin split products, and has prolonged prothrombin and partial thromboplastin times. Infusion of microembolism is of concern because of hemolytic cell debris or platelet aggregation. Filters are used during the collection of autologous blood and a 40-μm filter is used as part of the blood administration protocol to reduce the risk of emboli infusion. Air embolism is also a concern, especially when the shed blood is reinfused with a surrounding pressure bag. Extraordinary care must be used to expel all the air within the reservoir bag before application of the pressure bag.[97]

In view of these concerns, the patient who is or who has recently been autotransfused should have coagulation profiles monitored, including complete blood cell count and urine hemoglobin. Platelets and fresh-frozen plasma are given if clotting factors need to be replaced. If an anticoagulant accompanied the autotransfused blood, the same concerns are present as for banked blood. The serum calcium level is measured to assess the chelating effect of citrate on calcium. If contaminated shed blood is reinfused, the patient is monitored for symptoms of emerging sepsis.

Tension Pneumothorax

Immediate recognition of tension pneumothorax, a life-threatening condition, is required of nurses who manage patients in any phase of trauma care. The presence of hemodynamic compromise with an expanding intrapleural space air mass distinguishes a tension pneumothorax from a simple pneumothorax. Tension pneumothorax may be the immediate result of primary traumatic injury, a delayed complication of an occult injury such as bronchial tear, or the undesirable result of necessary therapies such as central line placement. Air (and possibly blood) that has entered the pleural space is trapped without exit, creating a one-way-valve closed system. One or more internal thoracic structures (most notably the trachea, lung, heart, and great vessels) are progressively compressed and fail to function adequately. The compression/failure mechanism may affect one or both sides of the chest cavity simply because pressure is transmitted through the chest as a whole. In addition to failure in ventilation, cardiovascular compromise is also noted. Mostly the superior vena cava and inferior vena cava compression, and cardiac constriction, are what eventually reduces preload, thereby decreasing cardiac output and blood pressure, eventually causing death. Assessment and treatment deal with problems in ventilation and cardiovascular performance.

Initial Assessment. Classic signs of tension pneumothorax may be obscured by hemorrhagic shock and other injuries or treatments until the patient is severely compromised. Under these circumstances the initial assessment begins by identifying the high-risk patient, such as one with an inadequately resolved pneumothorax, bronchial tear, lung contusion, or pulmonary cyst. Knowing the mechanism of the trauma may also help identify patients likely to have a pneumothorax. Positive-pressure ventilation, particularly in the presence of a simple pneumothorax, may be associated with development of a tension pneumothorax. The injury may not be discovered until the patient has a rapid and steep fall in oxygenation and displays signs of shock.[27]

The patient should be examined carefully and rapidly for clues to the reason for failure in ventilation or cardiac output. Chest wall movement is observed for asymmetry, and the chest wall is percussed for the characteristic hypertympanic note of trapped air. Tracheal shift is a classic finding but may be difficult to determine in the intubated patient. Unless the patient is hypovolemic, neck veins may be distended, reflecting increased intrathoracic pressure. Breath sounds are compared from one side to the other and are diminished. Pulse oximetry measures decline and blood gases, if available, show a sudden drop in Pao_2. Finally, cardiac output is reduced, with evidence of decrease in blood pressure, tachycardia, or a general shock state that is unexplained by other injuries. Figure 24-18 shows chest radiograph findings seen with tension pneumothorax.

Immediate Management. Once tension pneumothorax is recognized, treatment begins immediately, even before radiologic confirmation.[27] Supplemental oxygen is provided, and then the chest must be decompressed by release of the trapped air. Initial decompression can be accomplished by needle thoracentesis. A 14-gauge catheter-over-needle is inserted into the pleural space at the second intercostal space in the midclavicular line. The needle is introduced over the superior edge of the rib to minimize likelihood of damage to intercostal vascular structures. On release of air, the needle is withdrawn and the sheath advanced. The sheath may be advanced all the way to the hub and then secured in place with tape. The pleural space equilibrates with atmospheric pressure, and the tension pneumothorax is converted temporarily to an open pneumothorax. The next phase of treatment occurs as one or more chest tubes are inserted, both to re-expand the lung (or both lungs in bilateral tension pneumothoraces) and as prophylaxis for any repeated episodes. Third, the cause of the injury must be explored and managed appropriately. A CXR, ABGs, hemodynamic measurements, and clinical examination are repeated to reassess the patient's posttreatment state.

Open Pneumothorax

Penetrating chest trauma or impalement that opens the pleural space to the atmosphere creates an open pneumothorax, or sucking chest wound. A number of factors have been proposed to explain the ventilatory difficulty presented by open pneumothorax. If the size of the chest wall defect is approximately two thirds the tracheal diameter, air will preferentially enter the chest wall during ventilation. This "false airway" allows intrathoracic and atmospheric pressures to equalize, losing the essential pressure gradient required for normal ventilation.[98] Loss of normal intrathoracic negative pressure reduces venous return and cardiac performance, which is aggravated by mediastinal shift and compression of the vena cava and heart.

Resuscitation Assessment and Management. First, the open wound must be located. Careful inspection of the entire thorax, including the patient's back, should be performed to

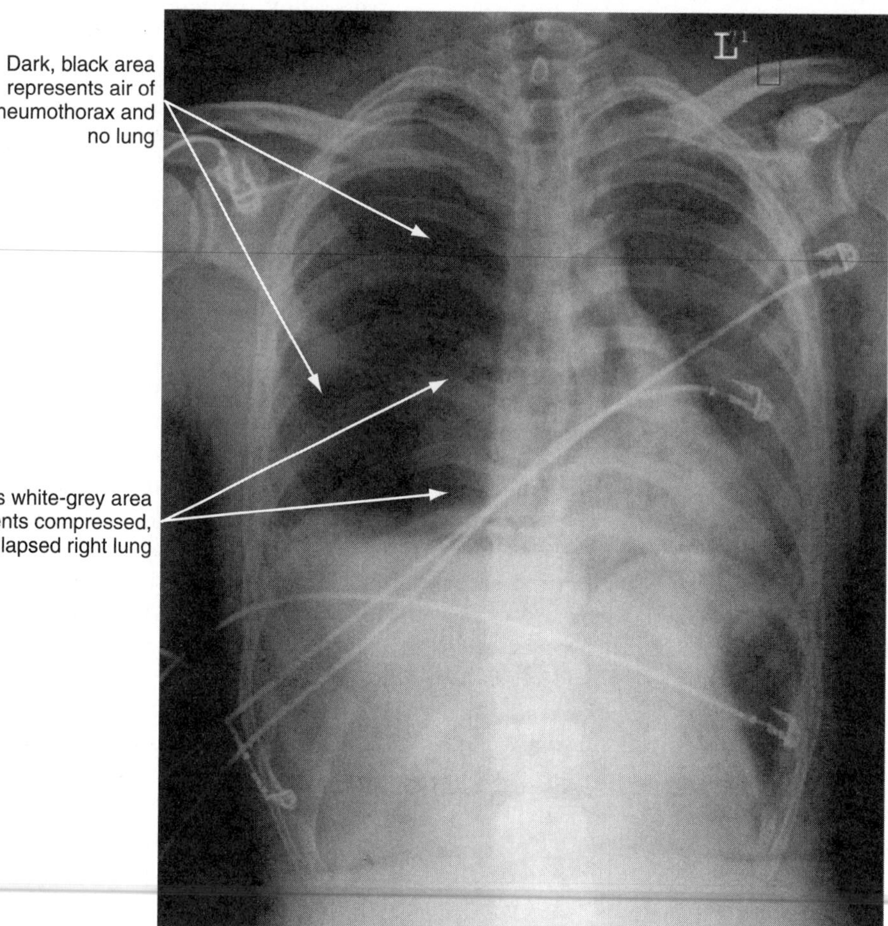

FIGURE 24-18 Tension pneumothorax. A knife wound to the lung resulting in a tension pneumothorax. Pressure builds in the hemithorax, impeding venous return, shifting the mediastinum and heart, and depressing the diaphragm. The great vessels become twisted and distorted. This decreases cardiac input and, subsequently, cardiac output, leading to shock with cyanosis, dyspnea, and possible neck vein distension. Insertion of a venting needle or chest tube may be lifesaving.

reveal the injury. Once the wound has been found, the sucking action is readily apparent. Frequently there are gas bubbles at the wound site, and a popping sound may be audible. Not all penetrating chest wounds create an open pneumothorax; some are superficial although menacing in appearance. Conversely, a small and unassuming wound may be responsible for the pneumothorax and other threatening injuries.

The management objectives are to restore ventilation and to debride and close the wound. Ventilation is, as always, the priority. Extensive open wounds, such as from a close-range shotgun blast, will require intubation and mechanical ventilation. The false airway must be sealed and re-expansion of the lung facilitated. A sterile semiocclusive dressing is applied immediately over the entire wound, the effects of which are reassessed repeatedly. An old but still useful method is three-sided taping of dressing materials to the chest wall. This creates a flutter-valve effect as the dressing is sucked down to the chest wall on inspiration yet allows air to escape on expiration. Should the occlusive dressing seal off the wound without a means of escape for the trapped air, tension pneumothorax is possible. Therefore, the effect of the dressing on ventilation is observed over time, particularly while waiting for placement of chest tube. After the dressing is applied, a chest tube is inserted at another site to treat the pneumothorax. The treatment effect is monitored without removing the dressing by noting changes in breath sounds, alterations in respiratory gas exchange, and signs of increased intrathoracic pressure (e.g., elevated plateau pressure in volume-targeted mode or decreased delivered volume in pressure-targeted mode.)

After ventilation has been managed adequately, the wound requires cleansing and debridement. The need for definitive surgical exploration and closure depends on the wound and on the presence of additional injuries requiring higher priority.

Acute Respiratory Distress Syndrome

ARDS is a form of noncardiogenic pulmonary edema with refractory hypoxemia. The mortality rate from ARDS is estimated between 35% and 65%, although review authors note a rate of <50% since the mid-1990s.[99-101] Patients with ARDS most often die of sepsis and multisystem organ dysfunction and not solely from respiratory failure.[102] Put another way, patients do not generally die from ARDS, but rather with ARDS.

Terminology used to describe posttraumatic respiratory distress can be confusing. In older literature the term "shock" lung was used and references to "traumatic respiratory insufficiency," "wet" lung, and "adult respiratory distress syndrome," which has been renamed *acute* respiratory distress syndrome (ARDS), can be encountered.[103] ARDS was originally described in 1967[104] as a cluster of clinical features with apparent similarities in pathophysiology.

Establishing a simple, uniform definition of ARDS is imperative to facilitate accurate estimates of the incidence and outcomes of ARDS. Quantifying the incidence and outcomes enables scientific study of ARDS and allows clinicians to enroll patients in clinical studies. Although a consensus conference definition for ARDS was developed in 1994,[103] a truly workable definition that is practical and reproducible both clinically and in research continues to evolve.[105,106] ARDS may be considered at the most severe end of the acute lung injury (ALI) continuum. ALI was redefined at the same time as ARDS in 1994, differentiating between mild and severe forms of the same disease. Mild ALI is reported to have a mortality rate half that of ARDS.[107] The four criteria for ARDS are as follows:

- Acute in onset
- Oxygenation: a partial pressure of arterial oxygen to fractional inspired oxygen concentration ratio (P/F ratio or Pao_2/Fio_2) <200 (regardless of PEEP)
- Bilateral pulmonary infiltrates on chest radiograph
- Pulmonary artery wedge pressure <18 mm Hg or no clinical evidence of left atrial hypertension

ALI has similar defining characteristics, with the only difference noted in the P/F ratio:

- Acute in onset
- Oxygenation: a P/F ratio <300 (regardless of PEEP)
- Bilateral pulmonary infiltrates on chest radiograph
- Pulmonary artery wedge pressure <18 mm per Hg or no clinical evidence of left atrial hypertension

An easy mnemonic using the acronym *ARDS* to recall the defining characteristics of ARDS is listed below[108].

1. **A**cute onset
2. **R**atio of Pao_2 to Fio_2 is <200 (regardless of PEEP) and <300 for ALI
3. **D**iffuse, bilateral pulmonary infiltrates on CXR
4. **S**wan-Ganz pulmonary artery pressure is <18 mm Hg or no clinical evidence of left atrial hypertension

Description and Risk Factors

ARDS is not a primary disease. It is a syndrome that is secondary to an insult or combination of injuries. Major risk factors or conditions associated with the development of ARDS in trauma patients include shock of any type (septic, hemorrhagic, cardiogenic, neurogenic, or anaphylactic), multisystem trauma with extensive tissue destruction, pulmonary contusion, multiple orthopedic injuries (particularly long bone or pelvic fractures), massive transfusions, thoracic trauma, bacterial pneumonia, sepsis, near drowning, gastric aspiration, and major head injuries.[109] There is a higher incidence of the syndrome in those patients with multiple risk factors than in those with a single risk factor.[109,110] ARDS is a sequela of hemorrhagic shock and hypotension and can develop in hypovolemic patients with other insults or predisposing problems. It has become apparent over the years that hypotensive shock per se is not the sole cause or mechanism of the syndrome. Numerous traumatic and biochemical insults produce apparently similar responses in the lung and a characteristic clinical picture. Sepsis, usually from a nonpulmonary source, is a key factor leading to ARDS. These varied insults initiate a common lung response that may be clinically evident 2 to 48 hours after injury. The major problem is respiratory insufficiency, evidenced by hypoxemia, noncardiogenic pulmonary edema, pulmonary hypertension, and intrapulmonary shunting.[109,110]

Pathophysiology

Whatever the precipitating insult(s), the central pathophysiologic component of ARDS is damage to the alveolar-capillary interface, affecting both the endothelium and epithelium. The degree of alveolar-capillary disruption varies. Studies that performed CT scans on patients with ARDS demonstrate considerable regional variability of the disease within the lung fields; normal areas are adjacent to areas of severely injured tissue.[111] Early stages of the syndrome's pathophysiologic features are explained by this primary loss of microvascular and alveolar membrane integrity, resulting in noncardiac pulmonary edema, hypoxemia, pulmonary hypertension, V/Q mismatching, and decreased pulmonary compliance. Progressive alveolitis and fibrosis occurs in later stages of ARDS, accompanied by respiratory infection and pneumonia.[112]

ARDS has often been described as "high-permeability" pulmonary edema; however, the characteristic edema is due in part to increased capillary permeability and in part to increased hydrostatic pressure resulting from pulmonary hypertension. The effect within the lung includes formation of interstitial and then alveolar edema, abnormal surfactant action, and nonuniform collapse of functional lung units. The amount of lung edema may not necessarily correlate well with the clinical findings, particularly with the severity of the early oxygenation deficit.[104] The apparent lack of correlation is related to the ability of the pulmonary lymphatics to compensate for increases in microvessel permeability. It is also related to the concept that edema, although a hallmark of ARDS, is also a consequence of lung injury.

Resuscitation Assessment

Clinical evidence of the syndrome is not typically apparent during the initial resuscitation period. It is important to assess and document the risk of posttraumatic respiratory insufficiency for each patient.

It remains unclear whether the type and volume of resuscitation fluids are implicated in causing the pulmonary edema seen with posttraumatic ARDS. With the goal of determining optimum fluid volume administration, the ARDSNet consortium (described below) completed a prospective, randomized, multicenter trial of "fluid conservative" versus "fluid liberal" management of ALI and ARDS.[113] The authors concluded that, although mortality rates did not appear affected by conservative versus liberal fluid administration, the conservative strategy improved lung function and shortened the duration of mechanical ventilation and intensive care without increasing nonpulmonary organ failures. Elsewhere, interest in transfusion-related acute lung injury has focused attention on the impact of blood transfusion and lung injury. This syndrome, highlighted by bilateral pulmonary edema, dyspnea, hypoxemia, fever, and hypotension in the presence of normal cardiac function, has been underrecognized and underreported, mostly because the symptoms can be confused with other transfusion-related events (e.g., anaphylaxis, circulatory overload).[114,115] The debate over use of crystalloid versus colloid as a resuscitation fluid remains unresolved,[116] although crystalloids are currently recommended by some authors.[94] In the future, principles of fluid resuscitation may include oxygen-carrying blood substitutes, low volume replacement, and selection of different fluids for different clinical situations (e.g., one solution for a geriatric patient with a head injury and another fluid for a teenager with a head injury).[117] Similarly, fluid administration may be specifically selected for the patient with a thorax injury and significant potential for development of acute lung injury.

Critical Care Assessment

Patients who are at risk for ARDS after major trauma are observed closely for signs of respiratory difficulty. Four clinical phases of respiratory dysfunction are defined on the basis of clinical findings and pathophysiologic changes: impending insufficiency, clinical insufficiency, severe failure, and resolution.[112]

Impending Insufficiency. The physical examination may be essentially normal. There is no evidence of excessive lung water on auscultation, and secretions are minimal or explained by other injuries. However, the patient is dyspneic, although the Pao_2 is relatively normal. ABGs also reveal decreased $Paco_2$ and respiratory alkalosis, either as a new finding or as a continuation of the tachypnea observed during initial resuscitation. Changes in the CXR that are characteristic of ARDS are rarely evident. Lung pathology is poorly defined in this early phase, except that neutrophil sequestration and some degree of interstitial edema are apparent. Knowledge of the patient's risk factors and these early assessment findings form the basis for providing supportive oxygen therapy and pulmonary care.

Clinical Insufficiency. Within the first 24 hours there are both clinical and pathologic signs of acute lung inflammation. Oxygenation is markedly decreased in relation to the delivered concentration. The patient is dyspneic and in respiratory distress. Increases in physiologic dead space and pulmonary vascular resistance are measurable. Patchy lung infiltrates are evident on the CXR, particularly in dependent areas. With appropriate ventilatory management and control of the underlying etiology, the ARDS process may resolve at this point.

Some patients continue to have progressive respiratory failure over the next 2 to 3 days and require progressive escalation of ventilatory and hemodynamic support. Physiologic dead space continues to increase, and the shunt fraction is high. The patient requires a high concentration of inspired oxygen despite PEEP. Characteristic bilateral infiltrates are recognizable on the chest radiograph. The lungs are heavy and wet, with continued white blood cell infiltration, alveolar edema, and microvascular congestion. Many individuals are in a hyperdynamic state with elevated cardiac index, regional perfusion shifts, and peripheral defects in oxygen use.[112] The hyperdynamic state may be caused by the same processes (e.g., trauma, sepsis) that originally produced the respiratory dysfunction.

Severe Failure. Frequently irreversible, pathologic respiratory conditions include fibrosis, atelectasis, and recurrent pneumonia. Hypoxemia is refractory to continued increases in delivered oxygen. Despite ventilator adjustments, impaired gas exchange and a progressive decrease in lung compliance are accompanied by impaired peripheral oxygen extraction and acidosis.

Typically the patient dies within 2 weeks of the onset of the syndrome, not because of hypoxemia or complications of respiratory support but because of an inability to eliminate the underlying disease or infectious process. This etiologic process can eventually cause multiple organ failure, which is associated with a high mortality rate.[104,110]

Resolution. Some patients do not progress to the severe failure stage. If complications such as infection are contained and the functional lung tissue is supported appropriately over time, the alveolar-capillary injury heals and clinical abnormalities abate. Although many people who survive ARDS make a full recovery, some survivors have lasting damage to their lungs.

Critical Care Management

Despite early identification of patients at high risk for ARDS and knowledge of the progressive disease pattern, preventive measures are few. However, actions within the clinician's domain include measures to prevent complications that can initiate ARDS, such as aspiration pneumonia, pulmonary emboli, and infection.[118] The primary treatment for ARDS is currently supportive. Although many studies have been undertaken and more are under way to test various treatments, no single, uniform method for intervention has emerged as the standard. Therapies may be broadly classified as either nonventilatory or ventilatory strategies.

Nonventilatory Treatment Strategies for Acute Respiratory Distress Syndrome. Pulmonary surfactant (a contraction or "surface active agent") reduces surface tension of alveoli, increasing compliance and allowing the lung to inflate more easily. Type II alveolar cells synthesize and recycle surfactant; however, in the presence of ALI/ARDS, surfactant production is decreased, modified, or unable to keep up with need. Surfactant may be administered to patients by intratracheal delivery, direct bronchoscopic instillation, or aerosolization in ventilator gas. Although successful use of surfactant in animal models and in human neonatal respiratory distress syndrome strongly suggests that surfactant replacement may play a role in ARDS treatment, currently this therapy is only considered to be experimental.[119]

Fluid management is a challenging aspect of ARDS treatment because many patients will have the cardiovascular dysfunction often associated with systemic inflammation. Some authors support keeping the intravascular volume as low as possible while maintaining adequate hemodynamics,[119] whereas others argue that the risk of fluid restriction to hemodynamics and end-organ function cannot be justified by the limited potential advantage of reducing lung edema.[118] A higher positive fluid balance in the first 96 hours of ICU admission has been linked to an increased mortality rate compared with similar patients with a lower positive fluid balance.[120] Euvolemia may be the best goal.

Nitric oxide (NO) is produced in the lung, causing pulmonary vasodilation. The gas may also be administered artificially with a goal of minimizing V/Q mismatch. Although many patients with ARDS/ALI show an improvement of more than 20% in Pao_2 when inhaled NO is used, overall NO is not associated with an improved mortality outcome in this patient population compared with control groups.[119] There may be a role for use of NO with severe refractory hypoxemia, particularly in combination with other strategies.[119]

Prostaglandin E_1 (PGE_1) has two properties of potential benefit to ARDS patients: pulmonary vasodilation and anti-inflammatory effects on neutrophils/macrophages. Although it is effective in improving Pao_2, most studies have found no difference in time to extubation or death when PGE_1 was used.[121]

Prostacyclin (prostaglandin I_2, PGI_2) is an endothelium-derived prostaglandin that acts as a bronchodilator, vasodilator, platelet aggregation inhibitor, and membrane stabilizer. It may also increase surfactant secretion. Studies have suggested an improvement in oxygenation with inhaled PGI_2 in patients with ARDS originating from an extrapulmonary source. PGI_2 remains under investigation and, as yet, no improvement in the mortality rate has been proven despite improved oxygenation seen in ARDS subsets.[121]

Use of NMB agents is controversial in the management of ALI/ARDS. Historically, paralytic agents were used for hypoxemic ventilated patients to improve oxygen consumption/delivery balance and to reduce barotrauma.[122] Over the years, scientific studies have scrutinized these beliefs and generally failed to support their use. The clinical significance of balancing oxygen consumption and delivery in the patient with ARDS has not been proved.[121] Furthermore, harmonizing the patient and the ventilator to minimize the risk of barotrauma has been accomplished with sedatives and advances in ventilator technology. Complications of NMB agent use are well reported,[77,78] and the benefits of spontaneous breathing during mechanical ventilation are also documented.[57,123] NMB use is recommended only when all other means of treatment have been tried without success.[78]

Prone positioning, like other promising therapies for ARDS, results in an improvement in oxygenation but has not demonstrated an improvement in patient survival.[124] Placing a patient with ARDS in the prone position increases oxygenation in 60% to 70% of patients.[118] This simple therapy requires only motivated clinicians and a watchful eye and is best implemented early in respiratory failure (Figure 24-19). Complications include facial edema and skin breakdown,

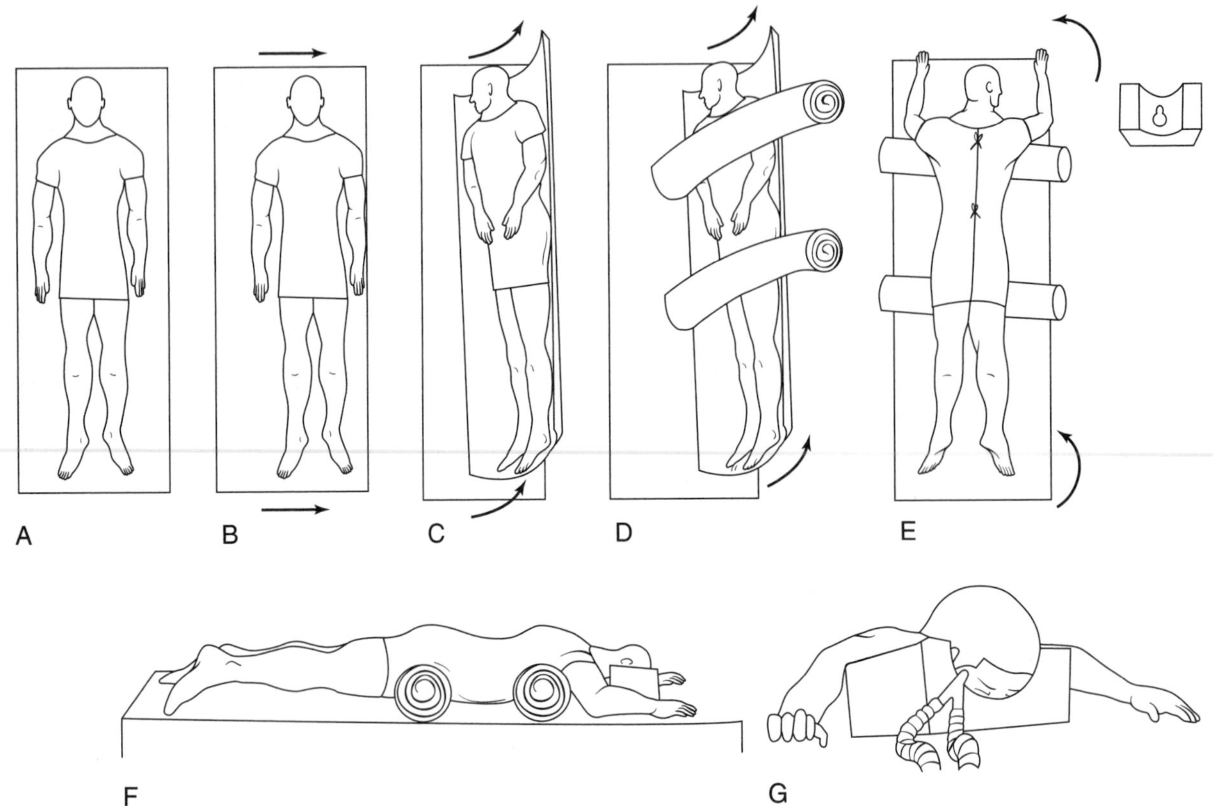

FIGURE 24-19 Prone positioning on one bed. Steps **A** through **G** depicts the turning of a patient from the supine to the prone position. (From Balas MC: Prone positioning of patients with acute respiratory distress syndrome: applying research to practice, *Crit Care Nurse* 20:24-36, 2000.)

whereas inadvertent tube or catheter removal is no more common in prone patients than in those not prone.[125] If contraindications preclude a patient from being turned to the prone position, kinetic therapy may be used to continuously rotate the patient side to side. Kinetic therapy is associated with a reduction in pneumonia and lobar atelectasis, although optimal turning frequency, angle, and duration are unknown.[126] Excellent nursing reviews are available on these topics.[126,127,128]

Steroids, more specifically glucocorticoids (i.e., corticosteroids), have been investigated in the treatment of late ARDS (>7 days after diagnosis). Glucocorticoids are believed to provide potential benefit by decreasing fibrotic lung disease and inhibiting multiple inflammatory cytokines.[121] One small study (n = 24) demonstrated that a subset of ARDS patients who received methylprednisolone (a corticosteroid) had an improved Pao_2/Fio_2 ratio and a lower mortality rate (none died in the steroid group) compared with a placebo group.[129] Many clinicians were not convinced to use corticosteroids for ARDS on the basis of this study.[121] More recently, a multicenter randomized controlled trial of methylprednisolone in patients with persistent ARDS did not support the use of steroids in ARDS.[130] Furthermore, there was an increased risk of death when steroid use commenced more than 2 weeks after the onset of ARDS.

Extracorporeal life support (ECLS) involves draining blood from the venous circulation into an external extracorporeal circuit, where it is oxygenated and carbon dioxide is removed before it is reinfused back to the patient. ECLS in adults has been used to support patients with severe reversible cardiopulmonary disease including ARDS. The technology is complex and reserved for select environments. Much of the supportive published literature for patients with ARDS is limited to either retrospective, uncontrolled prospective, or anecdotal reports.[121] ECLS, including extracorporeal membrane oxygenation and extracorporeal carbon dioxide removal, is currently considered last-resort support for adult ARDS patients and is limited to institutions capable of managing the practice. ECLS is yet another area in the treatment of ARDS ripe for large prospective studies.

Partial liquid ventilation combines mechanical ventilation with the intrapulmonary instillation of perfluorocarbon (PFC) liquid at a volume sufficient to equal FRC. PFC liquid readily dissolves oxygen and is nontoxic and minimally absorbed. Maintaining liquid in the lung supports alveoli, thus preventing collapse.[131,132] However, because inadequately powered or structured studies have been conducted, results remain inconclusive and high-quality randomized trials are still needed.[133]

Nutritional guidelines for ICU patients[134] and trauma patients[135] have been reported. Standard principles are applied when feeding the ARDS patient, with route and rate of nutrition influenced by the patient's condition, tolerance, and calculated need. Principles for providing nutrition include avoiding overfeeding, which results in increased CO_2 production and thus increased work of breathing to clear CO_2 and using the enteral route whenever possible to preserve gut integrity and reduce infectious complications,. Before specific recommendations on immunomodulatory nutritional supplementation for patients with ALI/ARDS are available, large multicenter trials are required.[136]

Ventilatory Treatment Strategies for Acute Respiratory Distress Syndrome. Probably the most stimulating and controversial ventilatory study to come out in recent years is one that compared a controlled ventilatory strategy using a tidal volume (V_T) of 12 ml/kg (on the basis of predicted body weight [PBW]) with a lung protective strategy using a V_T of 6 ml/kg PBW.[137] This multicentered randomized controlled trial performed by the ARDSNet (Acute Respiratory Distress Syndrome Network) group concluded that mechanical ventilation with a lower tidal volume (6 ml/kg) decreased the mortality rate and increased the number of days without ventilator use. Discussion on this study and several other studies conducted by the ARDSNet consortium are readily available in print and electronic form.[138-142] Although many clinicians have not adopted the practice of using low tidal volume and higher PEEP ventilation,[143,144] many other clinicians have, and most are at least aware of this research and give consideration to limiting plateau pressure to help reduce the incidence of ventilator-induced lung injury (VILI). Some authors suggest that the tidal volume used is less important than the limit applied to the plateau pressure. Generally, the recommended plateau pressure is less than 32 cm H_2O with a range of 30 to 35 cm H_2O.[145]

The goal of opening the lung (recruitment) and keeping it open (preventing derecruitment) may be achieved with varying success by use of a host of strategies. One possible method is to use the low tidal volume and higher PEEP technique, although this practice may be more adept at preventing derecruitment than actually recruiting collapsed alveoli. However, other modes, such as airway pressure release ventilation and high-frequency ventilation (discussed later) maintain a constant or near-constant airway pressure to facilitate lung recruitment and help prevent derecruitment, making them worthy of serious consideration in patients with ARDS/ALI.

An acceptable ABG for the patient with severe ALI may not be the same as a "textbook normal" ABG. Permissive hypercapnia (PHC) may be incorporated into the treatment strategy. PHC is when ventilation is intentionally limited (i.e., limiting tidal volume or plateau pressure) to protect the lung from VILI with the understanding that $Paco_2$ levels will climb, albeit in a controlled fashion.[146] PHC is not the same as caring for a hypercarbic patient on conventional ventilator settings who is not responding to mechanical ventilation in a manner desired or intended. The Pao_2 may be maintained around 60 to 80 mm Hg, which will generally provide an Sao_2 of >90%. Some authors consider a Pao_2 >80 mm Hg important to maintain a safety buffer in the event of a "sudden deterioration of oxygen saturation."[118] Conversely, the higher the Pao_2 is artificially maintained with an elevated mean airway pressure or inspired oxygen concentration, the less likely the bedside clinician will be to detect early pulmonary deterioration by oximetric measures. Vigilant bedside nursing is essential to the success of this practice. A discussion on ventilatory support and strategies is provided later.

Future of Acute Respiratory Distress Syndrome Treatment. The mortality rate for ARDS has decreased slightly in the last 10 years, although much remains to be done to improve outcomes. Future treatment will likely be developed in several areas. Improvements in the management of multiorgan failure and sepsis, greater understanding of specific pulmonary pathologic processes, and increased understanding and exploration of treatments other than conventional ventilation hold the greatest promise. Better defining the patient population with ARDS being evaluated to determine treatment effectiveness is essential to identifying appropriate therapeutic interventions. For example, one treatment option may be ineffective in a geriatric patient with comorbidities and late-stage ARDS from a pulmonary source, whereas the same treatment may prove successful in an otherwise healthy teenager with early ARDS from a nonpulmonary cause.

Intermediate/Rehabilitation Care

Published reports of respiratory abnormalities in patients recovering from ARDS differ in the patterns and severity of dysfunction. These differences may be partially explained by the variability in ARDS etiology, in the patient's health history, and in the length of time over which patients were studied. Measurable aberrations in vital capacity and FRC, respiratory mechanics, and arterial oxygenation, particularly during exercise, have been described in patients recovering from ARDS. Long-term (12-month) survivors of ARDS may expect considerable respiratory symptoms and a decreased general health-related quality of life.[147] It is not clear how long this impairment will last, nor is it clear if the physical impairment is directly related to the course of ARDS or caused by another aspect of the patient's critical illness.[148] ARDS does not appear to have an impact on the mortality rate after discharge compared with deaths of equally ill patients with trauma or sepsis.[149]

Nursing management is directed toward weaning the patient from ventilatory support and protecting the patient from further respiratory complications, particularly retained secretions and infection. Weaning from mechanical ventilation may begin at varying points in the patient's recovery course. In general, weaning is initiated once the patient has stable hemodynamic status and when respiratory drive and muscle strength are sufficient for spontaneous ventilation. Generally, withdrawal of support is unsuccessful if there is a persistent septic focus or major organ insufficiency. Most patients are successfully weaned. Weaning strategies are discussed later.

Once the patient no longer requires ventilatory support, blood gases and pulmonary function are evaluated as needed.

The patient is observed for dyspnea and shortness of breath both at rest and during exercise, and the plan of care is modified accordingly. The survivor of posttraumatic ARDS needs considerable support and information to understand the recovery process and any limitations in respiratory function and exercise tolerance.

Cardiac Tamponade

Description

The pericardium of the heart, similar to the pleura of the lung, is actually two layers. Between the visceral pericardium (inner layer) and the parietal pericardium (outer layer) is pericardial fluid. The pericardial sac normally holds approximately 25 ml of fluid that cushions and protects the heart and enables the two layers to glide over each other with minimal friction during each heart beat.[150] Usually addition of small amounts (50-100 ml) of blood or air into the sac produces only a small rise in intrapericardial pressure. Continued bleeding increases this pressure sharply and produces the symptoms of obstructive shock.[151] Cardiac output falls as the increased intrapericardial pressure interferes with venous return into the right atrium or prevents ventricular filling, thus impairing cardiac output. A decline in cardiac performance is directly related to the speed at which the pericardial sac accumulates blood and fluid and how well it can accommodate for this increase in volume. Initially a change in pericardial sac volume results in little change in pressure, although eventually very small increases in volume will result in significant elevations in pericardial sac pressure.[152] This characteristic is important because injury recognition and treatment may not occur immediately on the patient's admission to the ED or critical care unit. Both a symptom and an injury, cardiac tamponade is life threatening and requires immediate treatment. Injury to the pericardium or heart may result from a penetrating wound or, less commonly, from blunt anterior chest wall trauma (Figures 24-20 and 24-21).

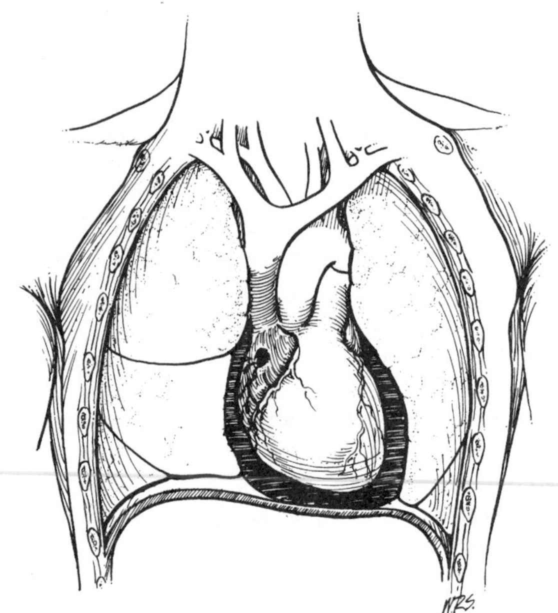

FIGURE 24-20 Cardiac tamponade resulting from a knife wound. The heart becomes compressed by blood, and cardiac output decreases, resulting in shock. Removal of blood by pericardiocentesis can restore cardiac output and allow time for definitive repair. (From Weiner SL, Barrett J: *Trauma management for civilian and military physicians,* Philadelphia, 1986, W. B. Saunders.)

Resuscitation Assessment and Management

Diagnosis can be difficult because some of the classic symptoms may be obscured by hypovolemic shock. Index of suspicion is used in discovery of the injury. The patient with an inappropriately low cardiac performance in relation to his or her injuries should make practitioners suspicious of possible cardiac tamponade. Evidence of precordial trauma, such as a wound along the lateral sternal border from the second to seventh intercostal space or a history that indicates the possibility of myocardial injury, also suggests the need to rule out cardiac tamponade. Commonly the patient has midthoracic pain and dyspnea.

"Classic symptoms" include the presence of Beck's triad: systemic hypotension, muffled heart tones, and elevated venous pressure reflected in neck vein distention. However, the latter may not be evident in the injured patient who is already volume depleted and hypotensive. Furthermore, distant or muffled heart tones are difficult to assess in noisy

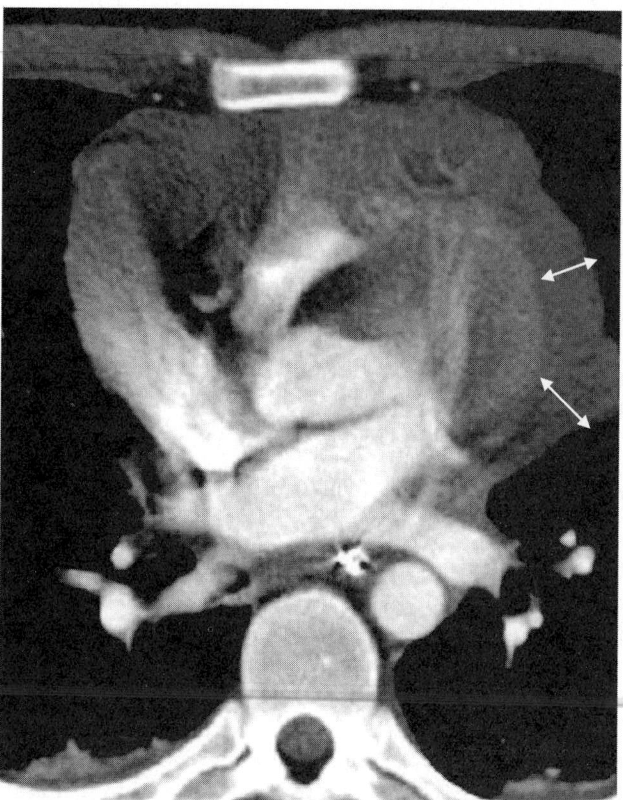

FIGURE 24-21 CT scan cross-section of the heart, with *white arrows* indicating blood in the pericardial space.

patient care areas. Pulsus paradoxus (paradoxical pulse) is an exaggeration in the normal variation in pulse volume with inspiration. This may be seen as a dip in the arterial pressure waveform during inspiration or felt as a weaker radial pulse during inspiration. Pulsus paradoxus, a swing of more than the normal 10 to 15 mm Hg in arterial pressure during inspiration, is significant but difficult to measure reliably unless an arterial line is in place. Assessment findings indicative of possible cardiac tamponade include elevated central venous pressure, narrowed pulse pressure, a precipitously falling cardiac output, a gray deathlike appearance, extreme anxiety, inability to lay supine, and tachycardia. FAST plays an important role in the rapid diagnostic examination of the patient with potential cardiac tamponade. In one study, the FAST accurately diagnosed 100% of cases of hemopericardium and there were no false-negative results.[153] The test is considered both accurate and rapid.[154]

Diagnosis and immediate treatment may occur simultaneously by performance of a pericardiocentesis or a pericardial tap (Figure 24-22). One method of pericardiocentesis is as follows. A long (6-inch), 16- to 18-gauge over-the-needle catheter attached to a stopcock is inserted 1 to 2 cm inferior to the left of the xiphochondral junction at a 15-degree angle to the skin, aimed toward the tip of the left scapula. The fluid present in the sac is aspirated, usually with immediate improvement in cardiac performance, and as much unclotted blood as possible is withdrawn. Because the pericardium is self-sealing, the tamponade may recur. Therefore the catheter is left in place and secured for possible repeated aspiration.[49]

Pericardiocentesis may be falsely negative, often because the needle becomes obstructed with tissue or clots during the procedure. When it is correctly performed, the pericardial fluid is aspirated without cardiac puncture. One indication that the heart has been entered is rapid clotting of aspirated blood. Pericardial blood should not clot because it is defibrinated by cardiac motion within the pericardium.

Ultimately, the underlying cause of the cardiac tamponade must be determined, and surgery (i.e., thoracotomy or sternotomy) may be required to identify and repair the source of bleeding. The choice of management by pericardiocentesis alone or by thoracotomy is an area of historical debate among resuscitating physicians. Generally, definitive treatment of cardiac tamponade is surgical and pericardial tap is temporizing if surgery is not available. Factors that influence management include the mechanism of injury (ice pick wound versus gunshot wound), hemodynamic status, and the response to pericardiocentesis. The resuscitation nurse needs to be aware of these factors, monitor the patient's response to pericardiocentesis, and make preparations for rapid surgery should it be required.

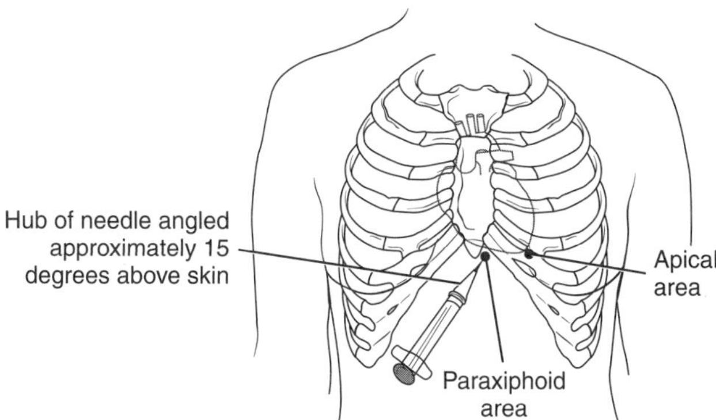

FIGURE 24-22 Technique of paraxiphoid pericardiocentesis for diagnosis and temporary treatment of cardiac tamponade. In the paraxiphoid approach, the needle should be aimed toward the left shoulder. (From Spodick DH: Acute cardiac tamponade, *N Engl J Med* 349:684-690, 2003.)

Intermediate/Rehabilitation Care

Longer-term treatment options will depend on short-term interventions. A catheter may be left in situ after pericardiocentesis, allowing for drainage and intermittent reaspiration. The plastic catheter may be sutured or taped in place. Cardiac tamponade requiring thoracotomy or sternotomy will be managed in the standard postoperative fashion. Particularly important are deep breathing exercises, management of chest tubes, and hemodynamic monitoring.

Myocardial Contusion

Description

Clinicians still debate the most accurate means to diagnose myocardial (or cardiac) contusion. Therefore, defining myocardial contusion lacks similar agreement. Characteristics of myocardial contusion include myocardial cellular injury consistent with muscle necrosis and hemorrhage infiltrate, both of which may result in arrhythmia and ventricular dysfunction.[155] The right ventricle, an anterior structure, is affected more commonly than the left ventricle.[156] Technically, diagnosis requires a direct visual inspection of the injured myocardium revealing intramyocardial hemorrhage, edema, and necrosis of myocardial muscle cells; however, the opportunity to directly inspect the heart is rarely present. Other blunt cardiac injuries include cardiac wall rupture, valvular disruption, and coronary artery dissection.

Injury Recognition During Resuscitation

The index of suspicion for myocardial contusion is high in the patient with external chest wall contusions, severe anterior blunt trauma, and fractures of the sternum and ribs. Meaningful tests in the diagnosis of myocardial contusion remain elusive. A 12-lead ECG may be useful, particularly in severe cases where ventricular dysfunction and malignant arrhythmia are more likely.[157] Abnormal ECG findings may include rhythm disturbances, localized ST-T wave changes, and atrioventricular or intraventricular conduction abnormalities. Serum cardiac troponin I has become part of the gold standard for diagnosis of myocardial infarction. This practice has been controversially extrapolated in trauma to include diagnosis of myocardial contusion. Some authors report that troponin I can be used independently in diagnosing myocardial injury.[158] Others believe it is the combination of ECG with troponin I findings that is effective in ruling in or ruling out cardiac contusion.[159] However, the current recommendation from the American College of Surgeons Committee on Trauma is that cardiac troponins "have no role in the evaluation and management of the patient with a myocardial contusion."[27]

Critical Care Assessment

Postresuscitative assessment and management is also somewhat controversial. The patient is surveyed continuously for symptomatic arrhythmias, specifically ventricular irritability and conduction defects. Two-dimensional echocardiography and multigated angiography (MUGA) may be useful in determining abnormalities in ventricular wall movement and ejection fraction. In practice, MUGA scanning and radionuclide imaging has largely given way to echocardiography (transthoracic or transesophageal).[158] Transesophageal echocardiography, although less widely available than transthoracic echocardiography, is more reliable and considered safe when performed by a skilled operator.[157] Serial monitoring of cardiac isoenzymes is supported by some authors but not by current Advanced Trauma Life Support (ATLS) guidelines.

Critical Care Management

The patient with a nonclinically significant contusion chiefly requires observation. Nearly all life-threatening ventricular arrhythmias and acute cardiac failure occur within the first 24 hours after trauma.[26,158] Therefore, hospitalization for an isolated myocardial contusion is typically brief if no complications occur. Myocardial oxygenation is maintained through appropriate ventilatory support. Continuous ECG and hemodynamic monitoring is needed to detect and manage arrhythmias. Standard antiarrhythmic agents are administered if ECG changes become clinically significant. IV fluid administration is guided by hemodynamic parameters. Low stroke volume and ejection fraction are treated pharmacologically with inotropic agents such as dobutamine. Changes in cardiovascular data are correlated with the effect of drugs, fluids, and any additional treatments the patient receives. Analgesia is important for the treatment of chest discomfort or soreness.

Nurses are caring for the equivalent of a cardiac patient in the busy environment of a surgical intensive care unit or general medical-surgical floor. This implies that nursing care should be targeted toward eliminating unnecessary stressors and preventing needless myocardial work or increases in oxygen consumption until the injury has healed. However, few nursing-centric studies have been done that help to direct the nursing care of these patients or that compare patient outcomes with those of patients with primary cardiac disease.

Intermediate/Rehabilitation Care

Late complications of cardiac contusion include ventricular aneurysm, chronic dilated cardiac dysfunction, development of structural cardiac lesions, constrictive pericarditis, and ventricular arrhythmias originating from myocardial scar tissue or aneurysm.[158] Generally, these complications are rare, and the long-term outcome and prognosis in patients with myocardial contusion is favorable.[158,160] Most issues may be managed on an outpatient basis and better addressed by a cardiologist or cardiac surgeon.

Aortic and Other Great Vessel Disruption

The great vessels of the thorax, aside from the aorta and its three arterial branches (brachiocephalic, left common carotid, left subclavian), include the pulmonary arteries and veins and the superior and intrathoracic inferior vena cava.[161] The brachiocephalic (innominate) and azygos veins are not classified as thoracic great vessels, but because of their size and high flow they are prone to generate a high-volume blood loss when traumatized. Injury to thoracic vessels occurs after both blunt and penetrating trauma. Most commonly, however, cardiovascular injuries are due to penetrating trauma.[162]

Penetrating Trauma

Generally, penetrating thoracic trauma is managed without thoracotomy, the majority of patients (approximately 85%) requiring only chest tube placement and conservative management (analgesia, pulmonary toilet, observation). Patients who do require thoracotomy have a great vessel injury approximately 25% of the time.[163] Sequelae of vascular injuries associated with penetrating trauma include exsanguination, tamponade, hemothorax, air and fragment embolism, and arteriovenous fistula and pseudoaneurysm formation. A penetrating wound should not be probed in an attempt to determine depth or trajectory because any of the above sequelae may develop.

Blunt Trauma

Leading causes of blunt thoracic trauma include motor vehicle crashes and falls from a height. Commonly, the mechanism involves severe deceleration or a high-speed impact from the front or the side. The majority of patients with blunt aortic injuries who survive to reach the hospital sustain an injury in the isthmus of the aorta between the left subclavian artery and the ligamentum arteriosum. The next most common is injury to the innominate artery. Injuries to the ascending aorta invariably result in early death, and injuries to the descending aorta are uncommon[163] (Figure 24-23).

Subsequent to thoracic trauma, an aneurysm may form. A true aneurysm is a localized dilation of the vessel wall that involves all three layers (intima, media, and adventitia) and is *not* associated with trauma. Pseudoaneurysms (false aneurysm) and saccular (dissecting) aneurysms are associated with trauma. A pseudoaneurysm results from a break in the vessel wall through all three layers, although the bleeding is contained by the blood clot and the surrounding structures. A traumatic dissecting aneurysm results from an outpouching of the adventitia layer after damage to the two innermost layers[164] (Figure 24-24). Either type of trauma-related aneurysm prolongs the survival of the patient compared with aortic rupture but may clearly have a time-limited effect.

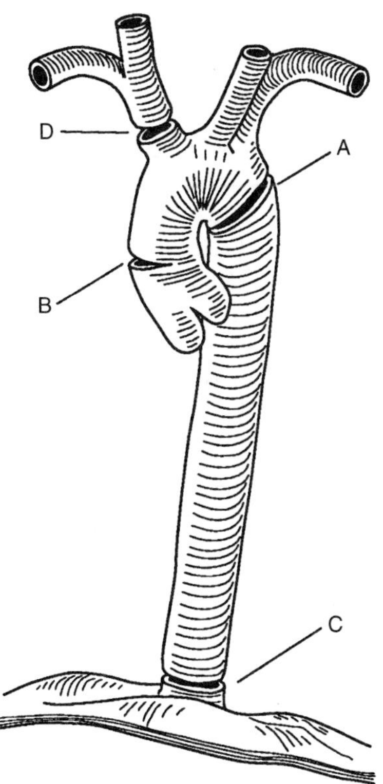

FIGURE 24-23 Sites of aortic rupture in order of frequency. *A,* Distal to left subclavian artery at the level of the ligamentum arteriosum. *B,* Ascending aorta. *C,* Lower thoracic aorta above diaphragm. *D,* Avulsion of innominate artery from aortic arch. (From Frey C: *Initial management of the trauma patient,* Philadelphia, 1976, Lea & Febiger.)

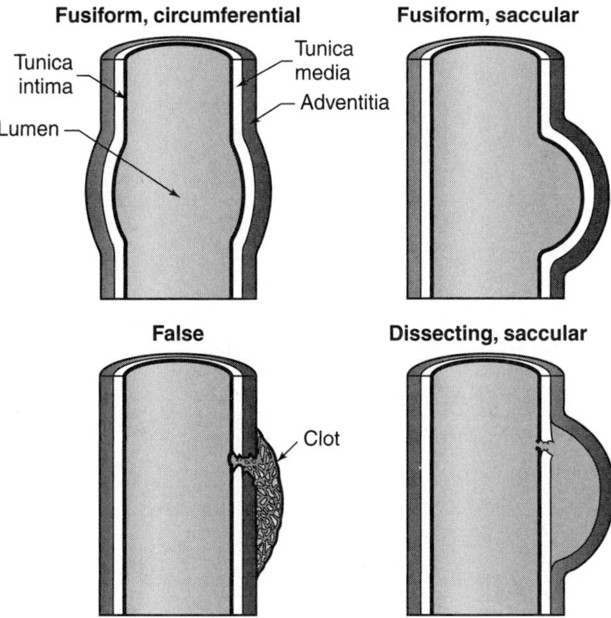

FIGURE 24-24 Longitudinal sections showing types of aneurysms. The fusiform circumferential and fusiform saccular are true aneurysms, caused by weakening of the vessel wall. False (pseudoaneurysm) and dissecting saccular aneurysms involve a break in the vessel wall, usually caused by trauma. (From Brashers VL: Alterations of cardiovascular function. In McCance KL, Huether SE, editors: *Pathophysiology: the biologic basis for disease in adults and children,* 5th ed, pp 1081-1146, St Louis, 2006, Elsevier Mosby.)

Resuscitation Assessment

The mechanism of injury, as well as associated injuries, raises the suspicion of aortic disruption. Penetrating mediastinal injuries, falls from >10 feet, pedestrians struck by motor vehicles, and unrestrained drivers or ejected passengers are mechanisms that heighten the index of suspicion.[165] Somewhat disconcerting for such a significant injury is that patients may have minimal to no complaints for the thoracic injury and may focus complaints on another injury in an unrelated body area (e.g., ankle). However, symptoms may include chest pain, back pain, dyspnea, hoarseness, dysphagia, and cough. Clinical findings may include hypotension, upper extremity hypertension, external evidence of major chest trauma, palpable thoracic fractures, systolic murmur, and acute aortic coarctation syndrome (narrowing of the lumen of the aorta).[165,166] Coarctation syndrome's classic triad of symptoms includes upper extremity hypertension, a systolic murmur (often best heard posteriorly), and delayed femoral pulses.

The initial chest film is done with the patient in the supine position for reasons related to spine immobilization and hemodynamic instability. A widened mediastinum or obscured aortic knob is highly suggestive of innominate artery injury or aortic disruption and demands further evaluation. CXR is a useful but not a definitive means of identifying aortic disruption; liberal use of angiography is recommended.[27] For penetrating trauma, a radiopaque marker should be placed to identify entrance and exit sites.[166]

Unless the patient is deteriorating rapidly, the definitive diagnosis is made by aortography, a retrograde dye study performed through the femoral artery, which allows visualization of the aneurysm or hematoma. On determination of the injury location, planning the appropriate surgical approach may take place. Although this study is essential for identifying the site or sites of the life-threatening rupture, there is risk of aneurysm rupture during transport to the angiography suite or during the procedure. The risk of rupture is greatest on catheter insertion and dye injection. Other limitations of angiography include that it is expensive, invasive, time consuming, not always immediately available, and requires the removal of the patient from the direct clinical care area for extended periods.[25]

More data have emerged regarding the accuracy of the dynamic helical and multislice computed chest tomogram for diagnosis of aortic disruption, which carries less risk and is less invasive than aortography.[25,167] In recent years, CT was introduced as part of blunt thoracic assessment to rule out great vessel injury in patients likely to have a negative aortography. After administration of contrast, the CT is performed and may identify the presence or absence of mediastinal hemorrhage and aortic injury.[25] Although CT scanning is an effective screening modality for blunt thoracic aortic injury with a high negative predictive value, there are limitations (e.g., interobserver variability, wide range for positive predictive value) to its use in comparison to angiography.[168] As technology and technique continue to improve, the role of contrast-enhanced CT scanning will likely continue to expand. Some authors suggest that patients with a positive CT proceed directly to the operating room and that angiography be reserved for scenarios involving mediastinal fluid or hematoma around the aorta and great vessels but without evidence of aortic injury.[169] An algorithm for diagnosing potential aortic injury has been suggested by Mirvis[25] (Figure 24-25).

Transesophageal echocardiography (TEE) is another method used for investigation of aortic injury. Direct sonography is capable of identifying injuries such as dissection, intimal flap, wall hematoma, aneurysm, and aortic obstruction. However, certain "blind spots" exist where not all aspects of the aorta may be visualized. Furthermore, operator expertise and availability may be limited; thus TEE at this time is limited to a screening tool for special circumstances.[25,166]

Resuscitation Management

Initial resuscitation includes establishing an appropriate airway (frequently endotracheal intubation), securing large-bore IV access, and treating other immediately life-threatening injuries. Other injuries may be treated in the operating room or be assigned a lower priority than the disrupted aorta. Should delay in repair occur (e.g., awaiting transport to a trauma center), the resuscitation nurse must keep the patient as sedate and comfortable as possible. Traumatic aortic injuries hold histopathologic similarities to nontraumatic aortic disruptions. Therefore, guiding principles for management of nontraumatic cases may be borrowed for treatment of the traumatic aorta disruptions; these principles include permissive hypovolemia and minimizing the change in left ventricular pressure (dP/dT). β-Blockade (e.g., propranolol, labetalol) for aggressive blood pressure control (i.e., systolic 80 to 90 mm Hg or slightly higher in patients with premorbid hypertension) and heart rate control (i.e., 60 to 80 beats/min) is suggested as an important aspect of early care,[170,171] although prospective studies in this area are lacking.[167] An indwelling arterial catheter is essential for continuously monitoring blood pressures. Blood is typed and cross-matched and 10 units of packed red blood cells are made available. Rupture will normally require surgical intervention and repair.

Operative Management

The operative approach and procedure is determined by the site or sites of rupture and the choice of the surgical team. Basically, repair may be performed either by the "clamp and sew" technique or the "distal aortic shunt." The latter technique may have several variations including a proximal

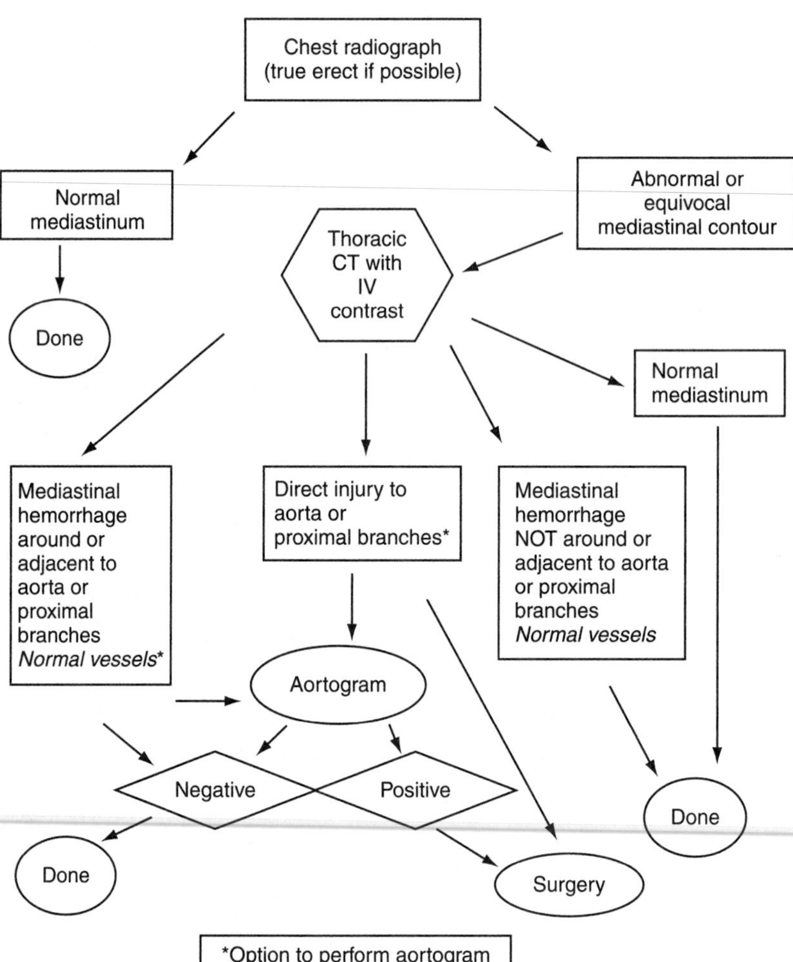

FIGURE 24-25 Algorithm for diagnosing potential aortic injury. (From Mirvis SE: Diagnostic imaging of thoracic trauma. In Mirvis SE, Shanmuganathan K, editors: *Imaging in trauma and critical care,* 2nd ed, pp 297-367, Philadelphia, 2003, Elsevier.)

shunt location of either the left atrium, left ventricle, or the ascending aorta and either a heparin or heparinless bypass. Anticoagulation presents difficulties in the multiply injured patient. A shunt bypass technique allows perfusion of the descending aorta while resection and repair are completed (Figure 24-26). If a Dacron polyester graft is inserted with anastomosis to the vessel edges, flow through the grafted vessel is observed, the shunt is removed, and insertion sites are closed with patch grafts. Chest tubes are placed for drainage, and the chest is closed.[169]

An alternative and faster approach is a cross-clamp repair without shunt. The aorta is clamped proximally and distally to the tear, the rupture site is resected, and the graft is inserted as previously described. Simple lacerations may be repaired by lateral aortorrhaphy. Cross-clamp time must be as short as possible, generally less than 30 minutes, because flow to the distal aorta is occluded. The concept of a "safe" cross-clamp time is difficult to define because of individual variation in tolerance. Long cross-clamp times are associated with markedly increased postoperative complications resulting from poor perfusion of the spinal cord, kidneys, and mesentery. All repair techniques described entail the risk of perfusion-related complications.[169]

Certain injuries may be amenable to endovascular stenting, particularly in the patient unlikely to tolerate operative repair. Advantages include a less invasive procedure avoiding many of the complications of surgery. However, until research demonstrates an advantage in stenting over other current surgical options, stenting must be considered "an experimental option best suited for patients who are too unstable to undergo operation."[166]

Critical Care Assessment and Management

Individuals who survive the operative period may die within the first week after injury. Often this is related to multisystem trauma and failure, which is often associated with this group of patients. Repair of the thoracic aorta requires postoperative monitoring and management similar to that for any patient recovering from major chest surgery. Systematic assessment for residual injury effects and complications of tissue hypoperfusion is a primary concern for these patients. Any organ below the level of aortic tear may be damaged during the period of hypoperfusion. This period extends from the time of injury until re-establishment of adequate blood transport through the vessel. It is important for the nurse to determine the hypoperfusion time, particularly the length of cross-clamp time, to predict postoperative problems. The patient's age, previous cardiovascular status, preexisting diabetes or pulmonary or renal disease, and accompanying injuries are factors that influence the incidence of postoperative problems.[172]

Postoperative respiratory complications include atelectasis, ARDS, pneumonia, and mechanical ventilator dependence. Any mechanism sufficient to cause disruption of the aorta is likely to result in pulmonary contusion or thoracic bone fractures. Modes of ventilation capable of facilitating

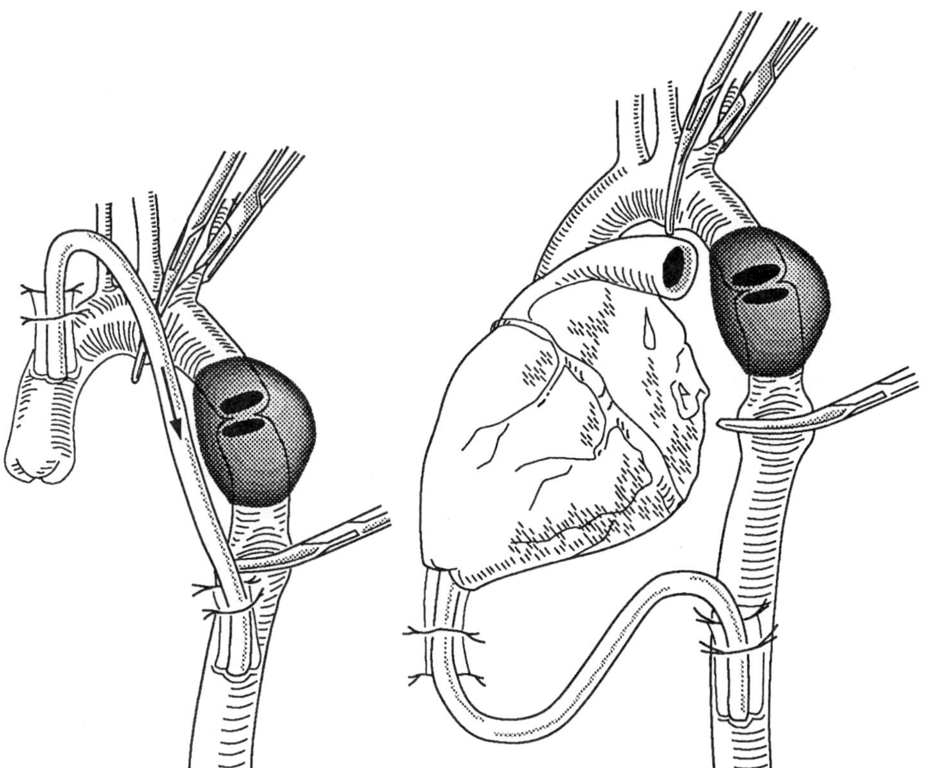

FIGURE 24-26 Shunt bypass technique in aortic repair. (From Blaisdell FW, Trunkey DD: *Cervicothoracic trauma,* New York, 1986, Thieme Medical.)

recruitment and preventing derecruitment are a first-line consideration (described later). Administration of analgesia may be by an epidural, IV, and later, an enteral route. With adequate and appropriate analgesia, patient mobility is increased to include frequent turning and getting out of bed (once cleared by the surgeon).

Hypertension and hypotension are both potentially harmful, so blood pressure must be maintained within strict parameters. Patients with aortic isthmus repairs frequently remain hypertensive postoperatively. Continuous hemodynamic monitoring is essential to track systemic and pulmonary pressures. After clear postoperative parameters for acceptable systolic, diastolic, and mean blood pressure have been established with the surgeon, antihypertensive agents are titrated to those parameters. The nurse correlates the effect of the drugs not only with mean arterial pressure but also with tissue perfusion. Dosages are balanced carefully to protect the integrity of the fresh graft and the tissue needs of the brain, spinal cord, kidneys, and other organs.

Postoperative bleeding is often associated with coagulopathy related to hypothermia, acidosis, and massive blood transfusion. The nurse must monitor laboratory values and blood loss from chest tubes and other organs potentially damaged by the trauma (e.g., spleen and liver). Appropriate blood products are administered as prescribed. Further diagnostic testing may be appropriate if bleeding continues.

Evidence of paraplegia caused by interruption of spinal cord blood supply may have been apparent during the initial resuscitation. More often, critical care assessment reveals the effect of spinal cord hypoperfusion. Lower extremity weakness or paralysis, loss of reflexes, or sensory dysfunction may be evident. Spinal cord perfusion can be compromised by preoperative hypotension or a lengthy cross-clamp time. In a review of nine studies (177 patients) of left heart bypass, postoperative paraplegia was noted in 1.1% of cases.[170] Simple cross-clamping results in a higher incidence of paraplegia because of a higher occurrence of suboptimal spinal cord perfusion intraoperatively. The use of antihypertensive drugs (as described previously) can lower the mean arterial blood pressure at a level incompatible with spinal cord perfusion. Once the paraplegia has been identified, every effort is made to maximize possible recovery of function.

Bowel is at risk for ischemia and infarction if mesenteric arterial perfusion is compromised. Older patients with primary vascular disease are particularly at risk. The nurse assesses for delayed return of bowel sounds, fever, abdominal pain, and distention. Surgical removal of dead or diseased bowel segments is required for definitive management. Hypoperfusion of the kidneys may result in poor renal function or outright failure.

Graft leaks are possible because there is little permanent bonding of the graft to the aorta. Chest tube drainage is monitored carefully for signs of rebleeding because delayed leakage is possible. Intermittent leakage and fever of unknown origin are of particular concern because these are sentinel events of graft infection. Prophylactic antibiotics and rigorous precautions are used to prevent bacteremia, which could seed the graft site. Long-term graft complications are uncommon.

Intermediate/Rehabilitation Phase Concerns

The patient's specific plan of care will depend on the resulting disabilities. For example, if postinjury paraplegia persists, spinal cord injury care and rehabilitation protocols are implemented. Frequently these patients are able to regain some lower extremity function with the help of exercise and physical therapy. Postoperative hypertension also may be encountered in the long-term survivor of a ruptured aorta. It can persist for months after aortic repair and is treated with standard antihypertensive agents if necessary.

There are also a number of general considerations for the patient during the intermediate and rehabilitative stages. Surveillance for graft leaks and infection continues throughout this part of trauma recovery. Intermittent small leaks may occur at the graft-vessel anastomosis, resulting in chronic aneurysm formation that is dangerous because of the risk of delayed hemorrhage into the pleural cavity or pericardium. Additionally, thrombus formation within the aneurysm presents a risk of embolism. Continuing assessment includes systematic inspection of all wounds, old chest tube sites, and incisions. Body temperature and white blood cell count are monitored for signs of infection and sepsis. The degree of continued chest pain is individual and is related to any associated thoracic injuries. Pulmonary care is directed toward the goal of preventing retained secretions and atelectasis. The patient and family become part of an instructional plan regarding the vascular prosthesis, the risk of infection, concern for long-term aneurysm formation, and the need for long-term follow-up care.

NURSING THERAPEUTICS FOR THE PATIENT WITH THORACIC TRAUMA

The previous description of thoracic injury management includes actions specific to a given injury and its complications. The following sections are intended to provide greater detail concerning therapies common for all patients with thoracic trauma.

THE PATIENT-VENTILATOR UNIT

Many patients with significant chest trauma require mechanical ventilation during their hospital stay and, less commonly, into the rehabilitation phase. The rationale for initiating some form of mechanical ventilation may be either as a life-saving measure to ensure oxygenation and adequate ventilation or as a supportive therapy, as with posttraumatic ARDS. It is useful to keep the goals for ventilatory therapy in mind: to improve oxygenation, correct hypoventilation and acidosis, and ease work of breathing. Although the decision to commit the trauma patient to any given form of ventilatory therapy is based on individual history, type of injury, and injury complications, some general criteria for initiating mechanical ventilation may be applied.

Open communication among the nurse, physician, and respiratory therapist is essential in determining which specific equipment and therapies are to be used. Communication is particularly important when a relatively complicated technique such as independent lung ventilation or some form of high-frequency ventilation is in progress. Whatever the type of ventilator or mode chosen, the nurse monitors not only the patient's responses to therapy but also the functional status of the patient-ventilator unit. Disconnections or leaks within the breathing circuit may or may not be obvious, and detailed assessment must be included as part of continuous monitoring. Checking to see whether alarms are functional at all times is one of the simplest and most essential nursing actions. The bedside nurse and respiratory therapist are the most likely persons to note high resistance or obstruction in the endotracheal tube, increased resistance in the inspiratory and expiratory circuits, or improper function of the exhalation valve. Changes in equipment or ventilator technique are explained to the patient, who may panic at sudden changes in airflow or work of breathing.

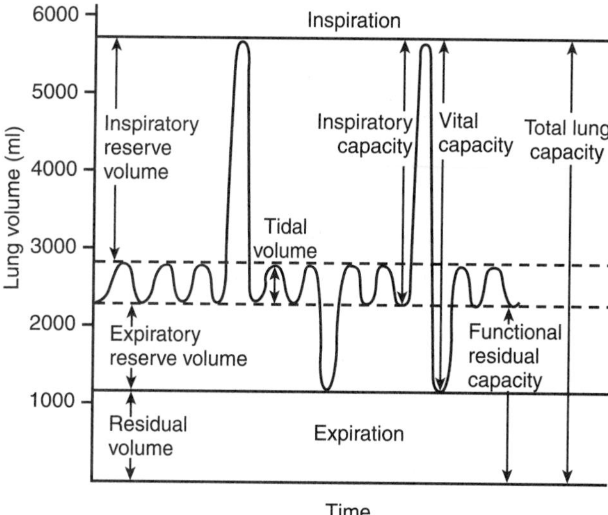

FIGURE 24-27 The spirometer curve. This diagram represents ventilatory excursions during normal breathing and during maximal inspiration and maximal expiration. Work of breathing is low when occurring on top of normal FRC, but work of breathing increases as FRC depletes. (From Guyton AC, Hall JE: Circulatory shock and physiology of its treatment. In *Textbook of medical physiology,* 11th ed, pp 471-482, Philadelphia, 2006, Elsevier Saunders.)

Mechanical Ventilation

Nurses caring for trauma patients requiring ventilatory support need a solid knowledge base in the principles of mechanical ventilation. Because mechanical ventilation uses evolving technology and current practice lacks unanimity, the challenges for the bedside clinician are significant. The modern era of positive-pressure ventilation began in the mid-1950s with the introduction of mechanical ventilators capable of delivering a fixed tidal volume for a fixed number of breaths. This mode, called volume control or controlled mechanical ventilation (CMV), has been superseded by other modes and is not used today.

Assist control volume (often called assist control or AC) developed from a need to allow the patient to "request" more breaths than the fixed set rate selected by the clinician. The practitioner may set a minimum number of guaranteed breaths, say 12 breaths per minute, and the total number delivered each minute may be 12 or greater. Responding to the patient's need for more breaths proved advantageous in many circumstances, including situations involving pain, anxiety, metabolic acidosis, impaired carbon dioxide clearance, and increased activity (e.g., turning in bed).

During the 1960s, the clinical application of PEEP developed.[173] With the initiation of PEEP, airway pressure is prevented from returning to 0 cm H_2O at the end of expiration. The concept of PEEP relates directly to CPAP. Both adjuncts act by increasing FRC (Figure 24-27) and preventing derecruitment.[174] The addition of PEEP or CPAP will keep more gas in the lung at the end of expiration than if these features are not used, thereby increasing end-expiratory lung volume (EELV). Beyond the added advantage of derecruitment prevention, an increase in EELV also results in gas exchange being maintained in more alveoli throughout the entire ventilatory cycle, thus lowering the need for increased FiO_2. The toxic effects of oxygen are well established,[175] and pursuing means to facilitate safely lowering inspired oxygen concentration is a worthy goal. Neither CPAP nor PEEP is considered a mode of ventilation because true modes of ventilation must incorporate a machine-driven dynamic change in ventilating pressure. The term "PEEP" is reserved for association with positive-pressure breathing modes, whereas the term "CPAP" is reserved for spontaneous breathing (no machine-supported breaths), but both PEEP and CPAP perform the same function of raising the baseline airway pressure above 0 (technically atmospheric pressure).

Derecruitment is the collapsing of previously gas-containing alveoli, whereas recruitment is the opening of previously gasless alveoli. The healthy lung does not require recruitment because derecruitment is not present. However, certain states can lead to derecruitment and the thoracic trauma patient is susceptible to many of these conditions.

Assist control was the first major step in ventilatory modifications that allowed patients to interact with ventilators. The primary advantage of AC is that it allows patients to initiate more breaths than the set rate; however, ironically, this was also the major disadvantage. Weaning patients from AC proved difficult. In practice, if the set rate was 15 breaths per minute and the tidal volume set at 500 ml and the patient triggered another 5 breaths, the total minute ventilation was around 10 L/min (15×500 ml $+ 5 \times 500$ ml $= 10$ L/min). If the set rate was decreased to 10 breaths/min, invariably the patient now triggered an extra 10 breaths; thus the breaths delivered by the machine (500 ml) remained at a total of 20 per minute (set breaths + patient-triggered breaths). Therefore, the minute ventilation also remained at 10 L/min with the patient still receiving significant mechanical support to achieve the total minute ventilation, whereas only exerting minimal effort to initiate a breath. Although the set rate was decreasing, weaning was not occurring. Ultimately, like in CMV, the patient was simply disconnected from the ventilator and made to breathe unsupported through the artificial airway. Humidified oxygen was normally delivered by a circuit. This configuration is known as "T-piece breathing."

A weaning alternative to the all-or-none principle of AC and CMV was suggested in the early 1970s. The new mode was named intermittent mandatory ventilation (IMV) and offered the benefits of a guaranteed clinician-selected minimal rate with the ability to incorporate spontaneous breathing from the patient.[176,177] In the late 1970s, synchronization occurred between the delivery of the mandatory breaths and the patient's spontaneous efforts with the introduction of computer technology in the ventilator. Thus, synchronized intermittent mandatory ventilation (SIMV) was created. Despite early ridicule,[178] IMV/SIMV has clearly stood the test of time.

Historically, SIMV, like AC and IMV, in adults was a volume-targeted mode (i.e., the clinician selected a tidal volume for the ventilator to target or deliver). Today, SIMV may be either volume targeted or pressure targeted. Pressure-targeted modes raise the ventilating pressure to a preset clinician-determined pressure level. Converse to the volume-targeted modes, which guarantee delivery of a minimum tidal volume with variable airway pressure, the pressure-targeted modes guarantee a fixed ventilating pressure with variable tidal volumes.

Factors affecting the variable tidal volume of pressure-targeted modes include the amount of set pressure, lung compliance, airway resistance, and patient effort. Lesser tidal volumes may be anticipated with lower set pressures, lower pulmonary compliance, higher airway resistance, and minimal to no patient effort. In practice, the tidal volume generated with pressure targeted modes will be an "average" of these four factors.

In the twenty-first century, ventilators are capable of delivering any number of modes of ventilation. The selection of a pressure-targeted versus volume-targeted mode is dependent on several factors, including disease process, model of ventilator, standard hospital practice, and attending physician preference. Historically, in general, adult patients were managed with volume-targeted modes. The concept is simple: a guaranteed tidal volume is delivered (once believed to be a good thing). For patients with minimal pulmonary disease, volume-targeted modes play a major role in their support and are well suited. However, for patients with more complex disease processes, a more complex mode may be very appropriate. Pressure-targeted modes require slightly more sophistication but may offer the skilled clinician a better option in a wide variety of circumstances.

In adults, the most commonly used pressure targeted mode is pressure-support ventilation (PSV). Introduced in the early 1980s initially as a means to help overcome increased work of breathing imposed by less-responsive inspiratory valves and airway resistance associated with breathing through an artificial airway, PSV was developed as an enhancement to CPAP.[179] Eventually, PSV found its niche as a maintenance mode for nonsevere respiratory failure and as a weaning mode.

PSV holds some unique characteristics. Every PSV breath must be patient triggered (i.e., there is no set rate). If the patient fails to trigger a breath, apnea ensues. Furthermore, the length of time of the inspiratory period cannot be preset by the clinician as can be done in other modes. With PSV, the inspiratory period is influenced by several variables, including the set pressure, the flow-cycle termination set point, patient effort, pulmonary compliance, and airway resistance. As lung function worsens and the inspiratory period shortens, PSV becomes less attractive as a primary mode of ventilation. Finally, PSV may be combined with other modes to convert spontaneous breaths to pressure-supported breaths. For example, SIMV (volume-targeted) and PSV may be combined to form a single mode resulting in a combination of volume-targeted and pressure-targeted breaths.

Pressure control (PC) and PC assist are the pressure-targeted equivalents of CMV and AC, respectively. In practice, like CMV, PC is not generally used. PC assist is more often seen in moderate to severe cases of respiratory failure, where a strategy of maintaining pressure over time is a useful means of alveolar recruitment. Prolonging the inspiratory phase of PC will result in an inversing of the normal inspiratory to expiratory ratio (1:3). PC with an inversed inspiratory/expiratory (I/E) ratio of 1:1, 2:1, 3:1, or 4:1 is known as pressure control inverse ratio ventilation (PC-IRV). Although PC-IRV may improve oxygenation and CO_2 removal in patients with poor gas exchange from acute respiratory issues, the technique often requires the use of heavy sedation and, at times, NMB. "Historical" PC-IRV is becoming superseded by PC-IRV on newer ventilator models that allow for unrestricted spontaneous breathing throughout the prolonged inspiratory period, thus possibly negating, or at least reducing, the need for NMB and heavy sedation.

In 1987, a new pressure-targeted mode, called airway pressure release ventilation (APRV), was described.[180,181] APRV is a simple concept—CPAP with release. Airway pressure is no longer held continuously but is dropped periodically (or released) for a very brief time to a lower level. APRV capitalizes on recruitment by maintaining pressure over time and allowing spontaneous breathing, which promotes alveolar recruitment and contributes to CO_2 removal. The brief releases further assist the patient with CO_2 removal. APRV holds an added advantage of being applicable through all phases of ventilatory support from acute respiratory failure through maintenance support periods to the weaning phase. Eventually, the patient is converted from APRV (CPAP with release) to straight CPAP (no release).[182,183]

High-frequency ventilation (HFV) modes adopt a strategy similar to that of APRV. By maintaining a constant mean airway pressure, recruitment is facilitated and derecruitment minimized or negated. HFV is an umbrella term for different types of high-frequency ventilation to include high-frequency positive-pressure ventilation (HFPPV), high-frequency jet ventilation (HFJV), and high-frequency oscillation ventilation (HFOV).[184] Recently, published literature holds most interest in HFOV for the adult patient with severe respiratory failure. HFOV uses small tidal volumes (approx. 1 to 3 ml/kg) at frequencies of up to 2400 breaths/min. Conceptually HFV is significantly different to conventional mechanical ventilation and requires a purpose-built machine to deliver the mode. Consequently, many clinicians do not use HFV and in those units that use it periodically, the comfort factor for many staff may be low. Despite this, encouraging data exists for HFOV. Well-designed trials comparing HFOV with APRV are needed.

In the 1990s, "dual-targeting" was used either as an individual mode (e.g., pressure-regulated volume control [PRVC] [Maquet]) or as an adjunct to volume-targeted modes (e.g., autoflow added to assist control [Draeger Medical]). Dual-targeting combines features of both volume-target and pressure-target modes. The primary target of each breath remains a clinician-set tidal volume; however, through a series of calculations performed by the ventilator on every breath, to include delivered volume and pulmonary compliance, the ventilator adjusts inspiratory gas flow to guarantee the volume but at the lowest possible ventilating pressure. The airway pressure waveform changes shape from a volume-targeted breath to appear similar to a pressure-targeted breath. Clinicians, realizing the advantages of pressure-targeted ventilation, but not comfortable with "letting go" of volume targeting, find dual-targeting an attractive alternative. (Figure 24-28, *A* through *M,* provides the airway pressure wave forms associated with each mode of ventilation.)

Keeping current with technologic advancements in the care of the mechanically ventilated patient is one of the greatest challenges for the bedside clinician. Attractive attributes, some of which are currently available, that are likely to

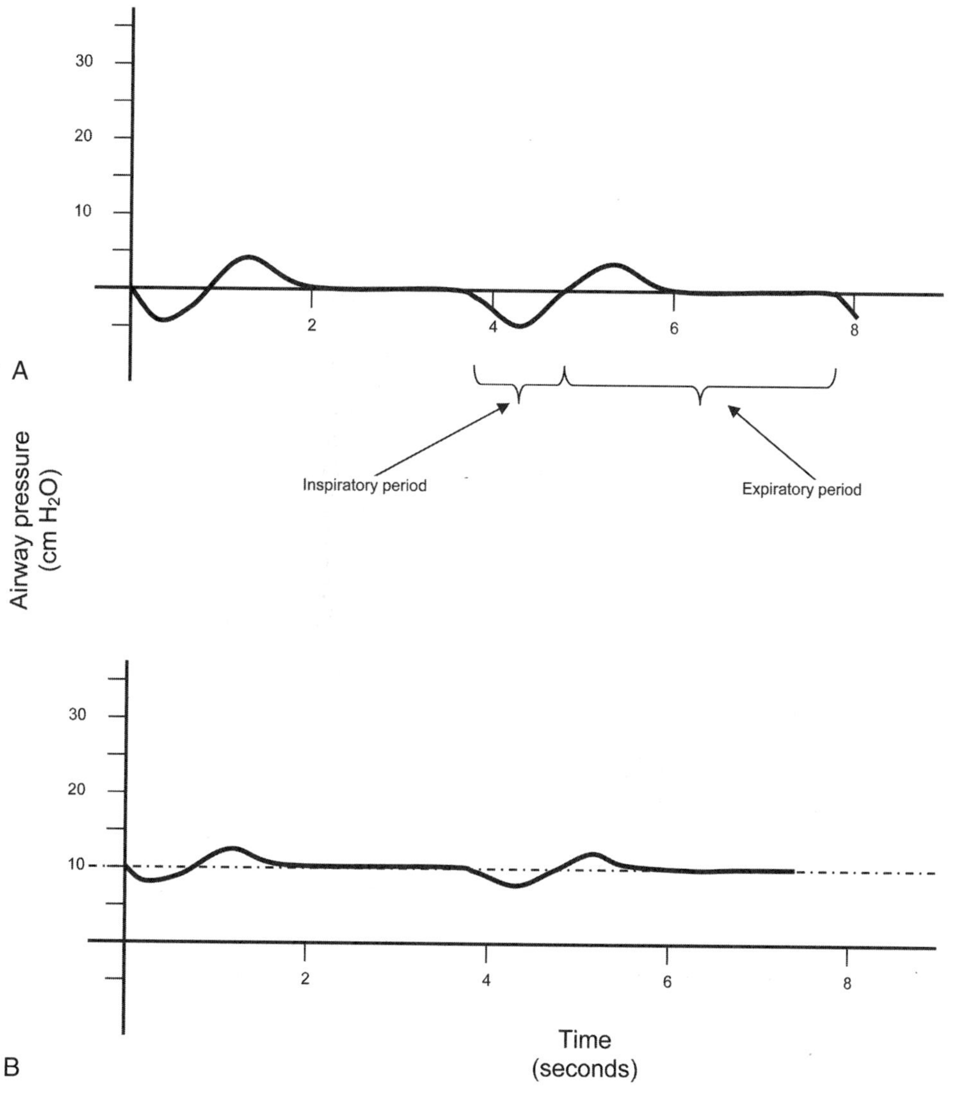

FIGURE 24-28 Airway pressure waveforms. **A,** Spontaneous breathing. This airway pressure graphic represents the change in airway pressure during normal spontaneous breathing. At the commencement of inspiration, airway pressure becomes negative relative to atmospheric pressure. At end inspiration the pressure throughout the airways down to the alveoli has returned to 0. Expiration results in a transient positive airway pressure, a return to 0, and finally a static period of no pressure change. In adults, approximately 1 second is spent in inspiration and 3 seconds in expiration, giving a normal I:E ratio of 1:3 on average. **B,** CPAP set at 10 cm H_2O. CPAP is associated with only spontaneous breathing and no positive-pressure breaths are delivered. The airway pressure graphic is very similar to spontaneous breathing, although the lows and highs may not be as noticeable in CPAP.

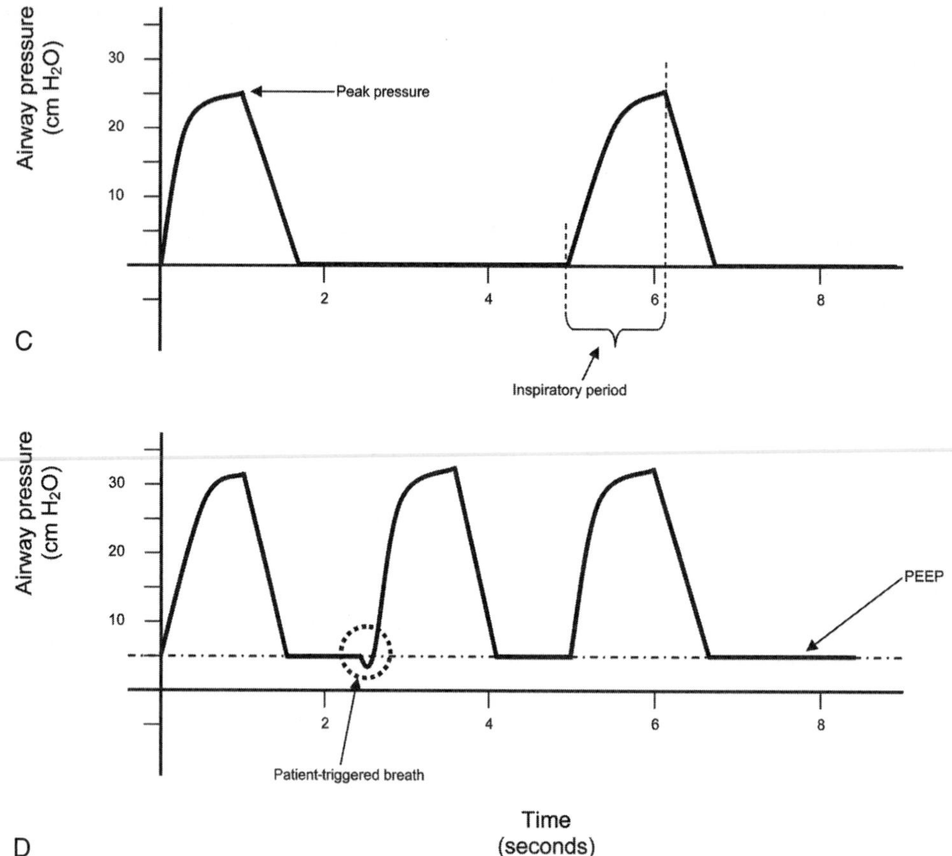

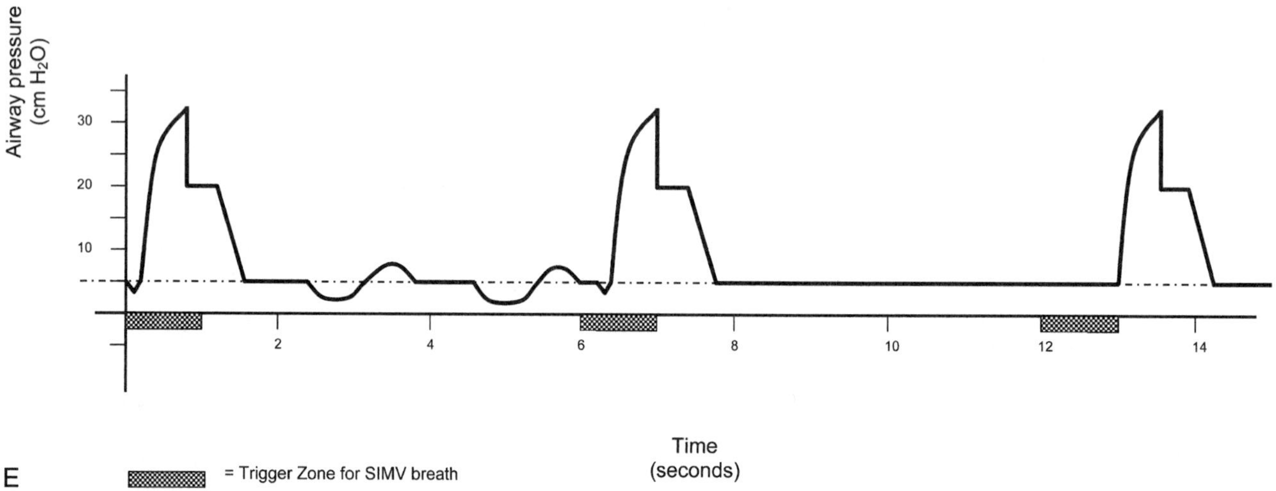

FIGURE 24-28, cont'd **C,** Volume control (or controlled mechanical ventilation). In this example, the ventilatory rate is set at 12 breaths/min, thereby delivering one breath every 5 seconds. The inspiratory period is set at 1 second and the delivered volume generated a peak pressure of 25 cm H_2O on both breaths. In volume-targeted modes, ventilating pressure may vary from breath to breath depending on compliance and resistance. Inspiratory effort between mandatory breaths does not result in gas flow from the ventilator and no breathing is permitted. **D,** Assist-control volume is similar to the outdated volume control; however, in assist control, inspiratory effort between mandatory breaths results in a machine-delivered, identical volume-targeted breath. Thus, the patient receives a minimum number of breaths (the set rate) and may "request" more breaths above the set rate. In this example, the set rate is 12 breaths/min (mandatory breath every 5 seconds) and an extra breath has been "triggered" by patient effort. Also, the clinician has selected 5 cm H_2O PEEP. **E,** SIMV with a set rate of 10 breaths per minute (one SIMV breath approximately every 6 seconds), a PEEP of 5 cm H_2O, and an inspiratory pause added during the machine-delivered breaths. During the inspiratory pause period, the inspiratory and expiratory gas flow is held, pressures within the lung equilibrate, and a plateau pressure is formed. On opening of the expiratory valve, airway pressures return to the PEEP level.

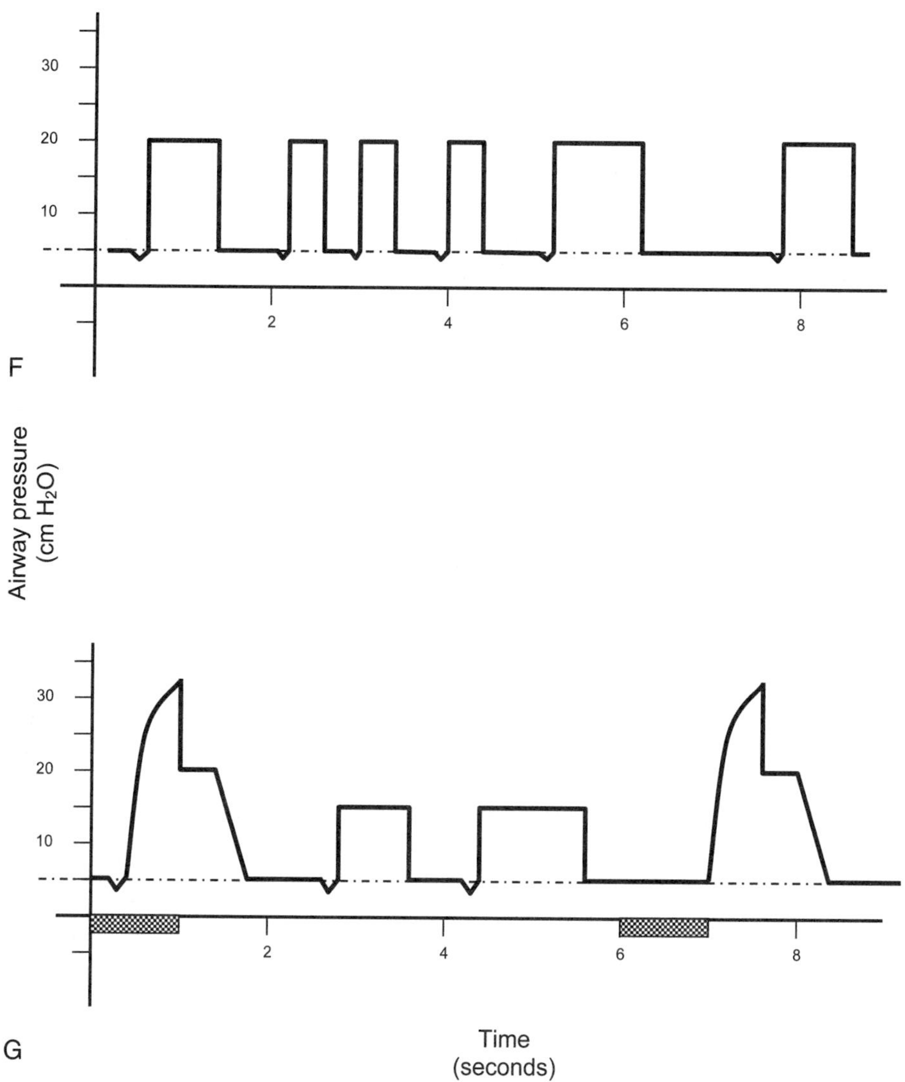

FIGURE 24-28, cont'd **F,** Pressure support ventilation with 15 cm H_2O of pressure support and 5 cm H_2O of PEEP. Note every breath is patient triggered, limited by the set pressure, and the clinician cannot set a fixed inspiratory period. The inspiratory period will vary with compliance, resistance, and patient effort, making this a less useful mode for sicker patients with varying compliance, resistance, and inspiratory effort. Pressure-targeted modes have a block-shaped waveform, unlike the shark fin–shaped waveform of conventional volume-targeted modes. **G,** SIMV (volume) with pressure support ventilation of 10 cm H_2O above PEEP. Spontaneous breaths are replaced with pressure supported breaths.

be incorporated into future modes of mechanical ventilation may include the following:

- Facilitation of spontaneous breathing. Spontaneous breathing (negative-pressure ventilation) holds several advantages over mechanically delivered breaths (positive-pressure ventilation). In the supine patient, spontaneous breathing preferentially draws gas into the dorsal lung units, helping to open derecruited alveoli and improve gas exchange. Pulmonary circulation is primarily gravity dependent; thus, patients in the supine position have the best blood flow in the posterior (lower or dependent) regions of the lung.[185] Therefore, the supine, spontaneously breathing patient has good V/Q matching.[186] Spontaneous breathing requires the muscular diaphragm to maintain tone, consequently blunting the effect of the abdominal contents wanting to push cephalad and cause compression atelectasis of dorsal alveoli. Conversely, a breath delivered by positive-pressure tends to follow the path of least resistance (i.e., toward the area of highest compliance). Gas preferentially fills alveoli in the ventral chest and may cause overdistention. The dorsal alveoli have lower compliance in the supine position and thus are less likely to fill. A V/Q mismatch occurs as ventral ventilation is *not* ideally matched with dorsal perfusion. Early model ventilators and modes did not permit spontaneous breathing. Notable exceptions included SIMV (without pressure support) and APRV. More recently, some ventilator companies incorporated a spontaneous breathing option into the inspiratory period of the machine breath. Such an option depends on an intelligent microprocessor system combined with highly sophisticated valves, flow, and pressure sensors.
- Tube compensation. The work of breathing increases as airway resistance increases. In the intubated patient, the artificial airway constitutes a major constriction within the airway. If the patient is actively inspiring, for example in APRV or CPAP, there is added work of breathing associated with resistance of the artificial airway. Tube compensation aims to negate the imposed inspiratory work of breathing by raising ventilating pressure at the proximal end of the

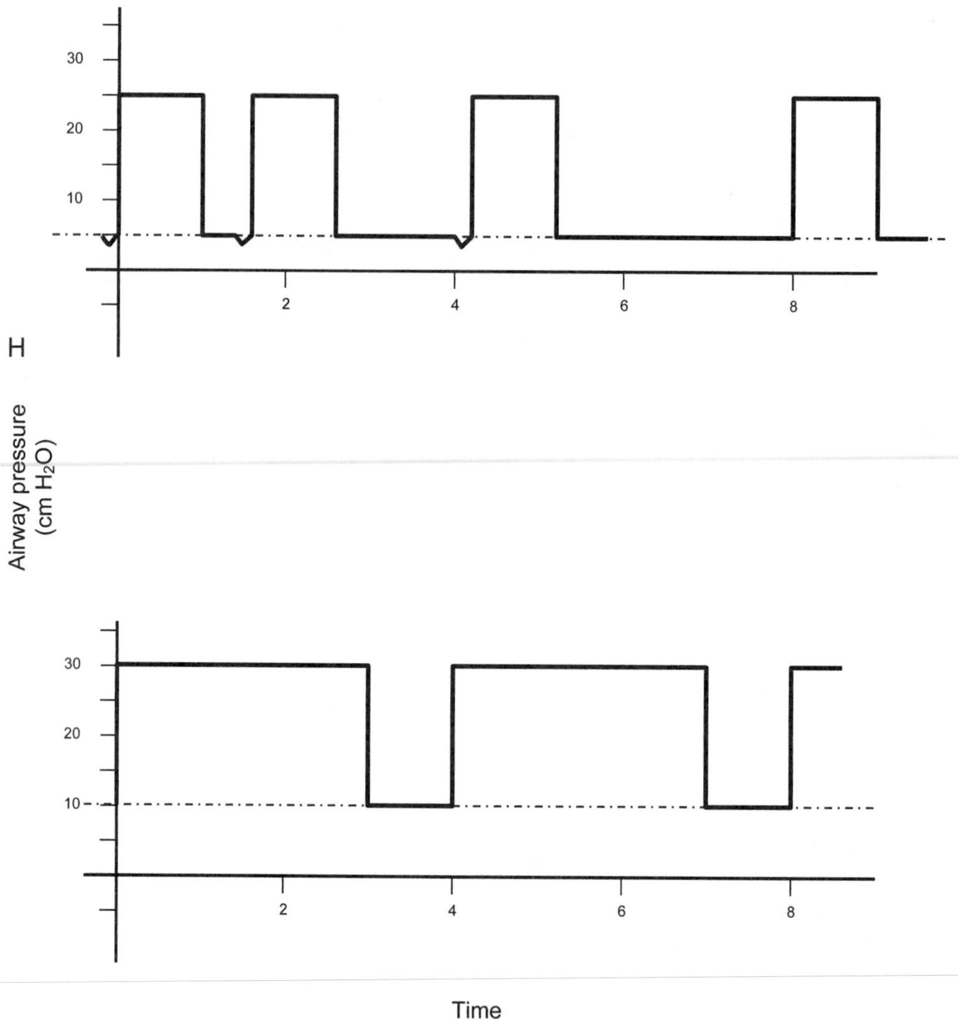

FIGURE 24-28, cont'd **H,** Assist control pressure with a rate of 15 breaths/min (i.e., a mandatory breath approximately every 4 seconds) and a pressure 20 cm H_2O above PEEP. Similar to assist control volume, the patient may trigger extra breaths if the patient initiates inspiratory effort. The inspiratory period is fixed. **I,** Pressure control inverse ratio ventilation. Pressure is set at 20 cm H_2O above PEEP (set at 10 cm H_2O). Inspiratory time has been increased to 3 seconds and expiratory period limited to 1 second, resulting in an I:E ratio of 3:1. The longer inspiratory period proves useful in the recruitment of collapsed alveoli.

artificial airway to equal the drop at the distal end. The patient's resistive work of breathing is reduced, and the patient no longer feels as if he or she is breathing through an artificial airway. Furthermore, in expiration, a momentary reduction of the end-expiratory pressure also helps lower expiratory work of breathing.

- Automation including incorporation of weaning protocols. The first steps toward automation of mechanical ventilation has already occurred. PRVC, autoflow, and tube compensation all use complex algorithms requiring measurement of variables, calculations, and modification of the breath by the ventilator. With certain features, these calculations and responses occur more than 100 times per second. In the future, ventilators will be fed information from the bedside clinician (e.g., patient history, predicted body weight, diagnosis), and therapeutic goals (e.g., target Spo_2 and $ETCO_2$, maximum minute ventilation, maximum mean airway pressure). The ventilator will commence ventilation and automatically modify settings in response to the patient's condition and measured variables. Weaning will be included.
- Abandonment of conventional volume-targeted modes. For the first three decades after the mainstream introduction of modern positive-pressure ventilation, adults were treated primarily with volume-targeted modes (CMV, AC, IMV, SIMV). These modes used fixed (or constant) gas flow. The problem with fixed gas flow is it often does not meet the patient's inspiratory demand at the beginning of the breath and exceeds demand at the end. This is because our natural inspiratory gas flow is not fixed. At rest, we inspire with a sinusoidal-shaped gas flow pattern, resulting in gas flow in an unfixed manner. Gas flow accelerates to a high point in the middle of the breath and decelerates for the second half of inspiration.[187] In a demand state, this curve may skew slightly to the left. Pressure-targeted modes use a decelerating gas flow pattern, which more closely approximates patient demand. Dual-targeting (described earlier) also uses a decelerating gas flow and has become an attractive

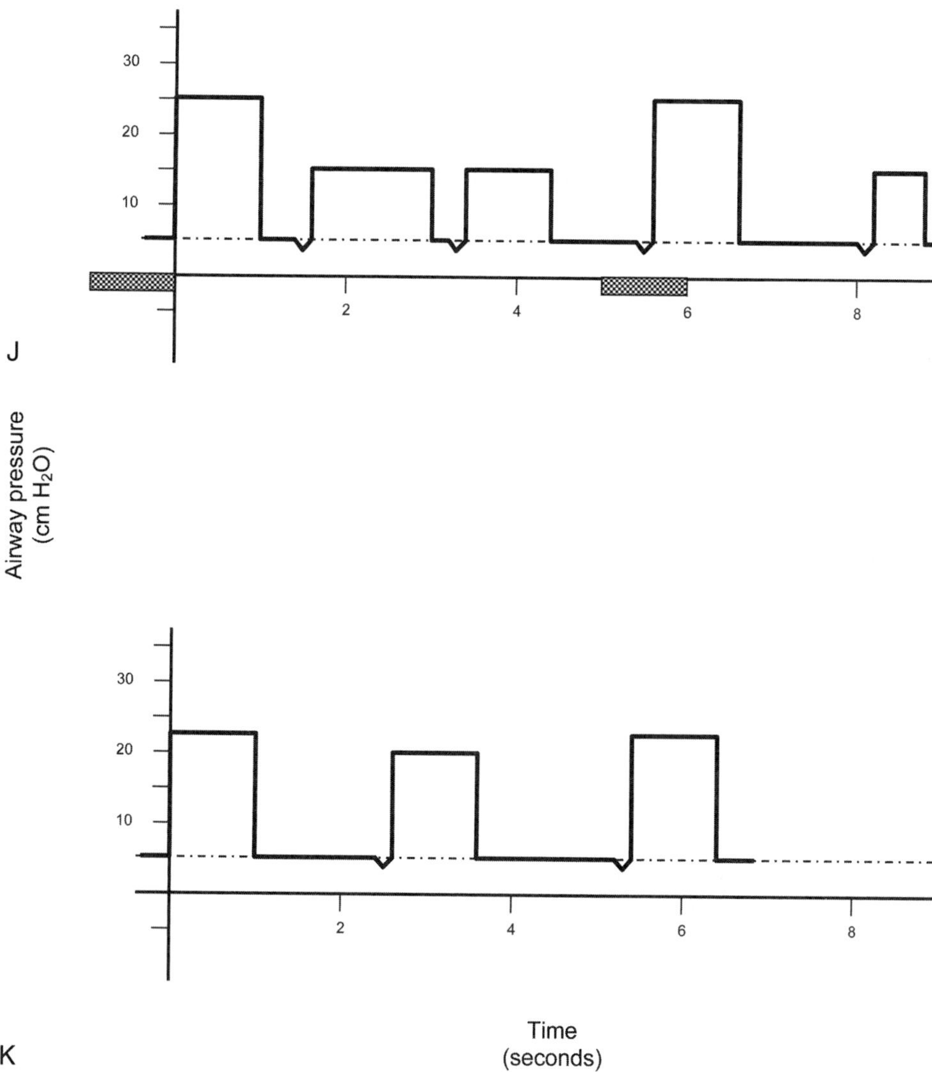

FIGURE 24-28, cont'd **J,** SIMV (pressure) with pressure support ventilation. In this example, the SIMV breaths are set at 20 cm H_2O and the pressure support breaths at 10 cm H_2O above PEEP. Spontaneous breaths are replaced with pressure-supported breaths. The inspiratory period is fixed for the SIMV breaths but variable for the PSV breaths. In practice, this mode is identical to SIMV (volume) with PSV, other than the fact that the SIMV breaths are now pressure targeted, not volume targeted. **K,** Assist control (volume) with a "dual-targeting" option activated. Note the classic "shark fin"–shaped waveform of a volume-targeted breath now takes on the appearance of the block-shaped waveform more consistent with pressure-targeting modes. However, unlike conventional pressure-targeted modes, dual-targeting may result in variable pressure levels while striving to maintain a constant delivered volume.

alternative to conventional volume-targeted modes. The popularity of conventional volume-targeted modes (which use constant gas flow) will probably decline significantly over the next decade and, eventually, be abandoned altogether.

- Noninvasive ventilation (NIV). NIV is the delivery of positive-pressure breaths or CPAP, by either a purpose-built machine or a conventional ventilator, to a patient wearing a mask device permitting access to the airway but without intubation. NIV may be applied by a device covering the nose, the nose and mouth, the entire face, or encompassing the head. NIV may decrease resource utilization and avoid complications associated with conventional invasive ventilation.[188] Studies have shown that the initial response (first few hours) to NIV is a strong predictor of success. Careful patient selection and well-designed protocols are major determinants in the successful implementation of NIV.[189] Patients with acute exacerbations of chronic obstructive pulmonary disease (COPD or COAD) appear particularly well suited and responsive to NIV. The best patients are cooperative, able to protect the airway, and otherwise medically stable.[190] The role for NIV in the patient with acute thoracic trauma is as yet undetermined, although it holds promise.[191]

Miscellaneous Concepts

Independent Lung Ventilation

In instances where the condition involves one lung exclusively or predominantly, the option exists to ventilate each lung independently. Patients with bronchopleural fistula with massive air leak may not respond well to conventional mechanical ventilation and PEEP.[192] Posttraumatic surgical repair or resection of lung may result in a need for ILV.[193] Severe asymmetric lung contusion is also a common indication.[194] In the absence of ILV, flow delivered by the ventilator will preferentially go to the more compliant lung, particularly when there are large differences in compliance between lungs. The healthy lung may be at risk of hyperinflation and volutrauma/barotrauma, whereas the diseased lung receives inadequate ventilation. Further complicating the matter,

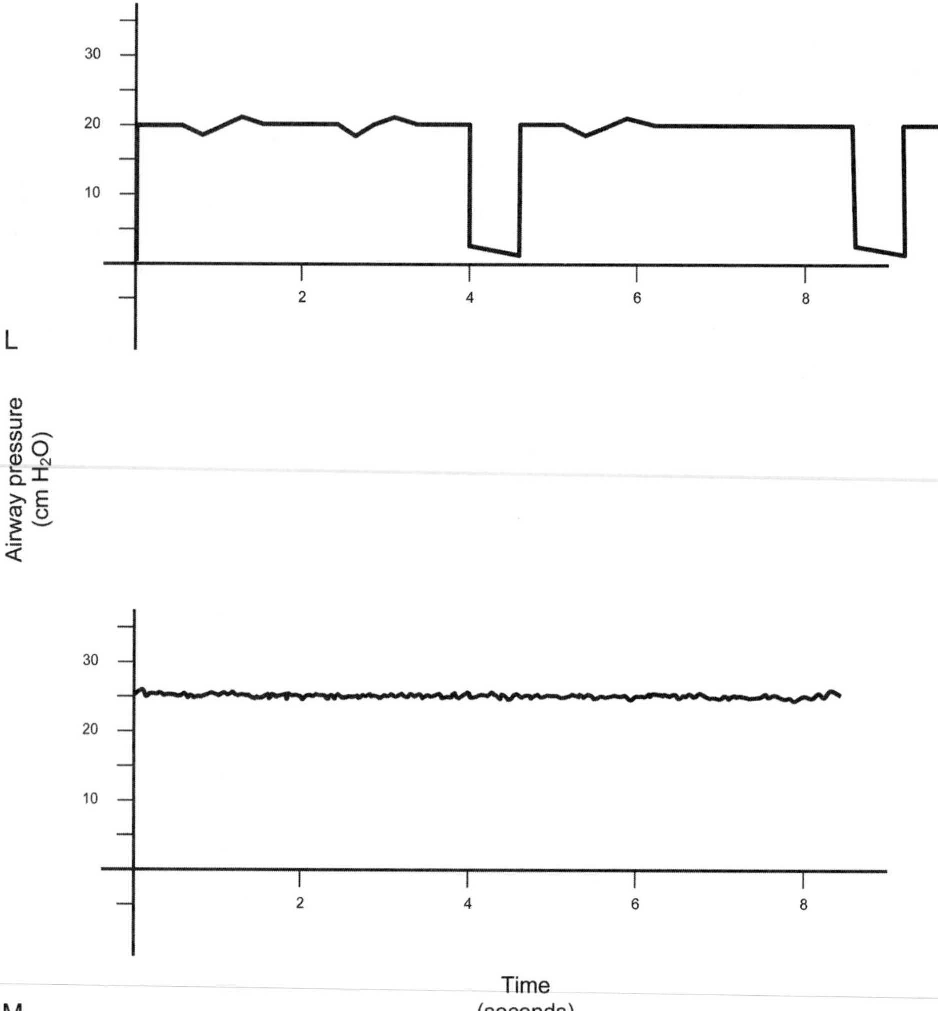

FIGURE 24-28, cont'd **L,** APRV. In this example, P High is set at 20 cm H_2O, P Low at 0 cm H_2O, T High at 4.0 seconds, and T Low at 0.6 seconds. The patient is breathing spontaneously at the upper pressure level (P High). APRV capitalizes on recruitment by maintaining pressure over time and allowing spontaneous breathing. **M,** High-frequency ventilation. Ideally, the constant airway pressure selected allows sufficient lung inflation to optimize gas exchange while protecting the already injured lung from alveolar overdistention or underdistention, and avoiding hemodynamic impediment. NMB or deep sedation are often required; thus spontaneous breathing, and its benefits, are negated.

pulmonary blood flow may be diverted from the overdistended healthty lung to the diseased lung, resulting in additional V/Q mismatch.[194] Under such circumstances, intubation of each bronchus with a double-lumen tube and ILV provides an alternative ventilatory therapy (Figure 24-29).

The endotracheal tubes may be connected to an array of systems[192]:

1. CPAP set at two different levels
2. Differential ventilation and PEEP applied with a single ventilator and a flow divider
3. Two synchronized ventilators connected by a computer cable
4. Two unsynchronized ventilators acting independently
5. Combination of different modes (e.g., APRV to right lung, PSV and PEEP to left lung)

Ventilating pressure is targeted to 26 cm H_2O or less,[194] with the diseased lung expected to receive less volume for an equipressure setting. ILV may be used with volume- or pressure-targeted modes including HFO[195] and APRV. Recruitment maneuvers may be directed preferentially to one lung.

Nursing management can be unusually demanding, depending on the complexity of ventilator setup and the cardiopulmonary stability of the patient. Blood gases, ventilatory parameters (including end-tidal CO_2 monitoring), and hemodynamic status are closely observed. Air leak through the chest tubes is monitored. The patient may have large amounts of pulmonary or bloody secretions, requiring careful airway hygiene and suctioning. It is rarely necessary or beneficial to remove the patient from the ventilator system for suctioning or changing body position, although it is useful to have two manual resuscitation bags and spare double-lumen endotracheal tubes at the bedside for machine failure or inadvertent tube dislodgment. Pharmacologic paralysis is generally required, accompanied by sedatives and analgesia. Family members need explanation of the therapy before entering the patient care area because it may appear complex and frightening.

Ventilator-Induced Lung Injury

Although critical to survival and clearly lifesaving in many circumstances, mechanical ventilation, ironically, has the potential to cause significant harm. VILI results from use of

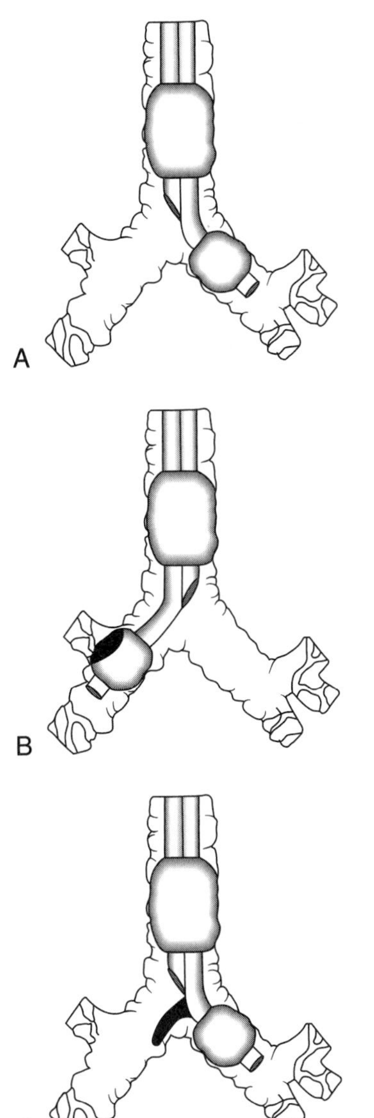

FIGURE 24-29 Distal end of endotracheal tubes used for independent lung ventilation. Design of the *(A)* left- and *(B)* right-sided Robertshaw and the *(C)* Carlens double-lumen endotracheal tubes showing relative placement of the two cuffs in the airways for each design and the carinal hook characteristic of the Carlens tube. (From Thomas AR, Bryce TL: Ventilation in the patient with unilateral lung disease, *Crit Care Clin* 14:743-773, 1998.)

mechanical ventilation and appears as both macroscopic and microscopic lung injury, similar to the diffuse alveolar damage observed in ARDS.[196] There are four basic mechanisms of VILI:

1. Volutrauma
2. Barotrauma
3. Atelectrauma
4. Biotrauma

Volutrauma results from alveolar overdistention resulting from high lung volume with or without high pressure. Barotrauma has been attributed to high ventilating pressure measured by the plateau pressure, not the peak inspiratory pressure (Figures 24-30 and 24-31). Atelectrauma occurs from the repetitive opening and closing of alveoli (recruitment/derecruitment phenomenon). Biotrauma is inflammatory in nature and associated with injury to alveoli resulting from cytokine release, most likely related to volutrauma and atelectrauma.[197,198] VILI may be prevented, or at least reduced, by ventilating patients with methods that facilitate alveolar stability. Modes of ventilation that limit airway pressure (<35 cm H_2O)[199] and regional hyperinflation, minimize derecruitment, and maintain pressure over time to facilitate recruitment serve to prevent or limit VILI.

Ventilator Dependence

The trauma patient may be difficult to wean from ventilatory support for many of the same reasons present in any group of critically ill individuals. Previous respiratory disease complicates the recovery from injury and can be anticipated from the patient's health history. Psychophysiologic factors have a profound effect on weaning success.[200,201] Ventilator dependence can arise from direct thoracic injury, or it can be a function of central nervous system injury, ARDS, other pulmonary complications (e.g., pneumonia, atelectasis, aspiration) or the enormous metabolic demand of sepsis or healing.

Ventilator Weaning. Weaning is defined as the process of gradually or abruptly withdrawing ventilatory support. Abrupt withdrawal may be successful in many patients if resolution of the underlying cause of the respiratory failure has occurred.[202] Successful weaning from mechanical ventilation culminates in removal of the artificial airway in the orally or nasally intubated patient or permanent use of the tracheostomy collar in the patient with a tracheostomy tube not ready for decannulation.

Appropriateness to wean the trauma patient is based on evaluation of the patient to include several parameters:

1. Cause for need of mechanical ventilation is resolved or significantly improved
2. Absence of high-grade fever
3. Stable cardiovascular status
4. Correction of metabolic or electrolyte disorders
5. Nutritional deficits and needs addressed
6. Pain and sedation requirements met and tapering
7. Satisfactory generic weaning parameters (see Table 24-5)

The four most commonly used and researched methods of weaning are (1) T-piece, (2) CPAP, (3) PSV, and (4) SIMV, each having its own advantages and disadvantages.[203] Weaning protocols developed by multidisciplinary protocol development teams are considered an important tool in reducing ventilator weaning time and thus complications of intubation and ventilation.[204,205] Although development of protocols tailored to an institution's needs may be time consuming[206] and breaches of protocol may occur,[207] they nonetheless are very important in facilitating weaning.[204,208] Protocol-directed weaning may be more effective if implemented as part of a quality improvement process, which may improve understanding and adherence.[209]

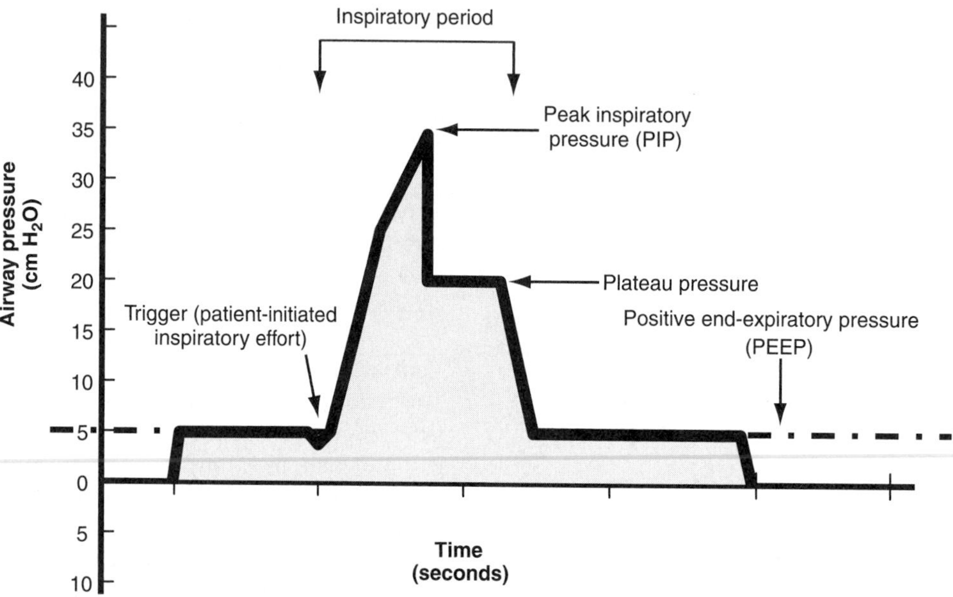

FIGURE 24-30 Airway pressure waveform of a typical volume-targeted breath. In this example, a PEEP of 5 cm H_2O and an inspiratory pause is added. An inspiratory pause involves a brief "breath-hold" at the peak of inspiration. During this time, airway pressures equilibrate and a plateau pressure is reached. Plateau pressure reflects mean alveolar pressure and is a useful determinant of lung compliance in volume-targeted modes (i.e., higher plateau pressure, lower compliance).

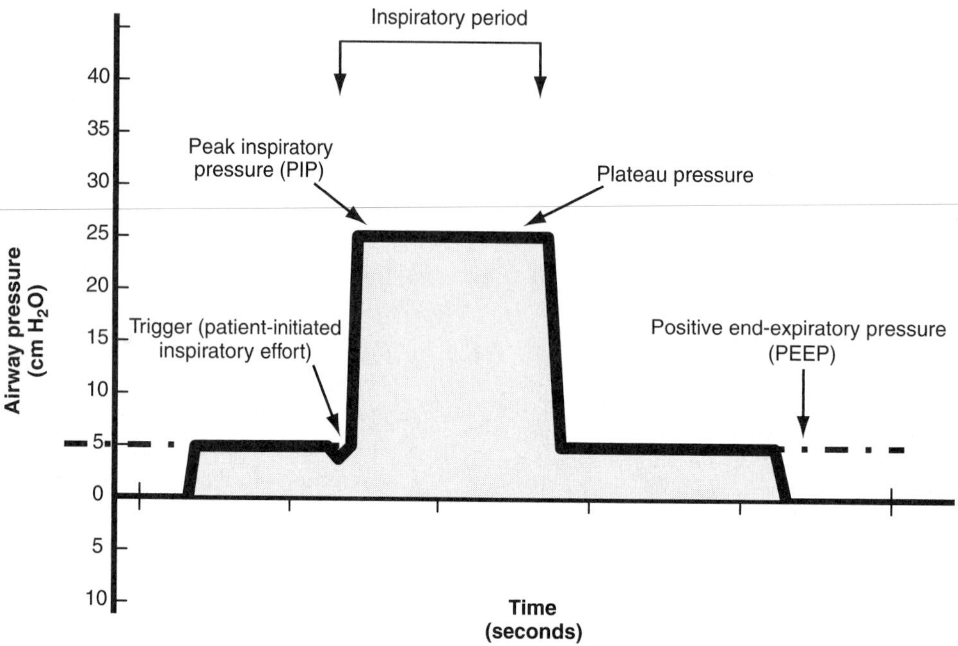

FIGURE 24-31 Airway pressure waveform of a typical pressure-targeted breath. In this example, a PEEP of 5 cm H_2O and a set pressure 20 cm H_2O above PEEP are used. Generally, the peak pressure and plateau pressure are the same in pressure-targeted modes of ventilation. Because the ventilating pressure is set by the clinician, this is no longer an indicator of compliance. However, volume will vary with compliance (i.e., lower delivered volume, lower compliance). High resistance will also lower delivered volume in pressure-targeted modes.

Spontaneous breathing trials should be conducted every 24 hours. During this trial the patient meeting established criteria is placed on minimal ventilator support to evaluate the patient's spontaneous breathing capability. If the patient performs well and is without any respiratory compromise during the 2-hour trial, consideration is given to appropriateness for extubation.[204]

The rapid shallow breathing index (RSBI)[210] is a measure of ventilatory frequency to tidal volume (f/V_T) and has been described as "the most accurate predictor of failure or success in weaning patients from mechanical ventilation." The test is achieved by counting the number of breaths in a minute and averaging the tidal volumes (measured in liters) for the same period. For example,

TABLE 24-5 Common Criteria for Assessing the Likelihood of Successful Ventilator Weaning

Parameter	Goal Value
Rapid shallow breathing index (RSBI) (unassisted breaths and minimal supplemental oxygen)	<100
Pao_2/Fio_2 ratio	>250
Minute ventilation	< 10 L/min
Unassisted breathing rate	< 30 breaths/min
Maximal inspiratory pressure	< −20 cm H_2O
Vital capacity	> 10 ml/kg
Maximal voluntary ventilation	2 × minute ventilation

20 breaths at average of 0.4 L give an RSBI of 50 (20 ÷ 0.4 = 50). Generally, a RSBI value of less than 100 breaths/min/L is predictive of successful weaning (defined as no requirement for mechanical ventilation for a period of >24/hours ± extubation).[210,211] Of note, the RSBI value of less than 100 was based on data that did not include pressure support, PEEP, or supplemented oxygen. Clinicians assessing patients with added PSV, PEEP, CPAP, or supplemental oxygen must factor this in when considering the merits of an RSBI assessment.[212]

Pulmonary Therapeutics

Procedures that effectively clear the airways at all anatomic levels and remove retained secretions are the foundation of thoracic injury management. Pulmonary care is frequently a difficult and time-consuming process in trauma patients. However, chest physiotherapy, suctioning, and injury-specific positioning are essential components of care. Inflating the lungs and keeping them inflated must remain paramount in the nurse's mind.

Physical Therapy

Postural drainage, percussion, and vibration are used to mobilize intrapulmonary secretions, accompanied by suctioning or coughing to clear the larger airways. Effective postural drainage, such as positioning the patient so that the affected segmental bronchus is uppermost, assists movement of secretions from the lung by gravity and requires knowledge of lung anatomy and which lung segments are abnormal. Percussion (rhythmic clapping with a cupped hand) is performed directly on the chest wall throughout the respiratory cycle. Vibration intermittently compresses the involved area during expiration. Percussion may be performed carefully and gently over fractures or painful areas, complemented with analgesia.[213]

Each selected component, its frequency, and the length of a therapeutic session are planned in relation to the patient's injuries and specific respiratory abnormalities. The frequency of treatment, often every 4 hours in critically ill patients, is evaluated every 12 to 24 hours on the basis of desired end points such as the appearance of the daily CXR, trends in total lung compliance, stability of blood gases, clinical examination, and patient tolerance. Patients with copious secretions or high-risk injuries, such as flail chest with significant lung contusion, may require more frequent or longer treatments. The length of treatment is determined by clinical parameters such as improved breath sounds and changes in airway pressures and lung volumes. The amount of sputum or suctioning aspirate is rarely an indicator of the therapy's effectiveness and does not serve as the sole criterion for ending a therapy session. The duration of a treatment also may be determined by adverse effects on intracranial pressure (ICP) or hemodynamic stability.[214]

Chest physiotherapy may be performed by the nurse, physical therapist, or respiratory therapist. Frequently, positioning for therapy requires an assistant to avoid inadvertent extubation, disconnection of IV or arterial lines, and physical trauma to the patient. The use of prone, head-down, or lateral positions during chest physiotherapy may be responsible for both adverse effects and benefits. Optimal positioning often requires more substantial turning than typically used for basic position changes (e.g., at least three fourths prone for drainage of posterior segments). Therapy sessions may often be coordinated with other necessary care such as linen changes.[213] When agitated patients are treated, plans for appropriate positioning and use of restraints need to be in place. The therapy session is coordinated with the patient's analgesia and sedation. In cooperation with the physical therapist or respiratory therapist, the nurse's role includes planning the treatment schedule and evaluating both desirable and undesirable effects during and after treatment.

Although the goals of physical therapy in the thoracic trauma patient are consistent with the overall treatment plan for improvement and recovery, in general, research has failed to demonstrate an overwhelming advantage to chest physical therapy in preventing postoperative pulmonary complications in broad groups of acute patients compared with other measures (e.g., incentive spirometer, CPAP).[215-217] Although no clear advantage to chest physical therapy over other means of lung expansion has been demonstrated, these techniques are superior to no intervention in the prevention of postoperative complications.[215] Studies in trauma patients are sadly lacking, and large randomized trials with clinically relevant end points and reasonable follow-up periods are needed.

Suctioning

Optimal methods of endotracheal suctioning have been the subject of nursing research and clinical review.[218] The practice of instilling isotonic saline solution into the endotracheal tube to aid in the removal of thick secretions has consistently been associated with adverse effects and no rigorously research-based benefit.[218-220] Despite overwhelming evidence disputing the practice of saline solution instillation, the dogma continues in many ICUs, with respiratory therapists twice as likely as nurses to support the practice.[218] Adverse effects associated with saline solution instillation include hypoxemia, dislodgment of bacteria, and dyspnea, although these results are not consistently reported.[221] Rather than using unproven and harmful techniques to respond to tenacious secretions, the bedside nurse should focus on prevention. Ensuring adequate patient hydration, using appropriate devices to provide sufficient airway heat and humidity, and periodically administering prescribed mucolytic agents are all means the bedside nurse may use to prevent and treat thick secretions.

Risks associated with suctioning include hypoxemia, aspiration, atelectasis, mucosal damage, hypertension, and serious arrhythmias. Use of closed suction catheter systems, preoxygenation before and after each catheter passage, limiting suction pressure to 80 to 120 mm Hg, limiting suction time to 10 seconds, limiting suction to no more than three consecutive catheter passages, and not disconnecting the patient from the ventilator are recognized means of limiting adverse events.[222] Suctioning in the multiply injured individual has not been well studied, particularly in patients with preexisting lung disease or significant physiologic instability. The need for suctioning and the technique used is best determined by the patient's injuries, clinical presentation, and assessment findings.[221]

Positioning

Another form of pulmonary therapy is therapeutic positioning, the use of specific body positions to maximize oxygenation and ventilation despite lung abnormalities. Turning the patient has long been accepted as treatment for the complications of immobility, and the effect of position on gas exchange must be considered in clinical management. The usefulness of positioning techniques is based on the effect of gravity on the lung fields, specifically on gravity-dependent V/Q matching in particular respiratory segments. By recognizing that perfusion is greatest in the dependent lung or dependent portions of the lung,[223] it is possible to position the patient so that specific lung areas receive a greater or lesser proportion of blood flow. Position is manipulated so that the healthy portion of the lung is dependent and therefore receives the greatest perfusion. In a similar way, lung areas that are compromised by injury and poor ventilation are positioned uppermost, thus receiving a gravity-dependent reduction in blood flow. The result is increased blood flow to areas of best ventilation, decreased flow to poorly ventilated areas, and overall improved V/Q matching.

The prone position is an important therapy for trauma patients who have had pulmonary collapse of the commonly affected dorsal lung units. Clinical trials have demonstrated an improvement in oxygenation in 70% to 80% of prone patients with early ARDS.[124] Despite improved oxygenation, this has not translated into improved survival.[125] The reasons for this are complex, and further studies in more select groups of patients with rigorous standards are warranted before discounting the practice of proning. The improvement seen with use of the prone position may be attributed to redistribution of ventilation (recruitment of previously collapsed dorsal regions) and more uniform distribution of perfusion[124] (Figure 24-32). The improvement may persist even when patients are returned to the supine position. A Stryker frame, two hospital beds, a single hospital bed, a proning device, or a kinetic therapy turning bed may be used to facilitate positioning the patient into the prone position.[127] The presence of skeletal traction or lower extremity external fixators does not necessarily preclude prone positioning. Modification to technique may be required and skilled handling is important, but the prone position may still often be used.

Thoracic assessment and knowledge of the most recent CXR or chest CT scan results are used to select best patient positions, which may include sitting, prone, and, most commonly, lateral decubitus. Benefits of the new position may be noted to include increased secretion production and clearance, increased chest excursion, decreased airway pressure, and improved Spo_2 and $ETCO_2$. The effect of body position may be evaluated after 30 minutes to determine changes in respiratory gases, hemodynamic parameters, and subsequent oxygen transport to tissues. In all cases body alignment, support of head and neck, and comfort are evaluated. Part of the positioning protocol is planning for

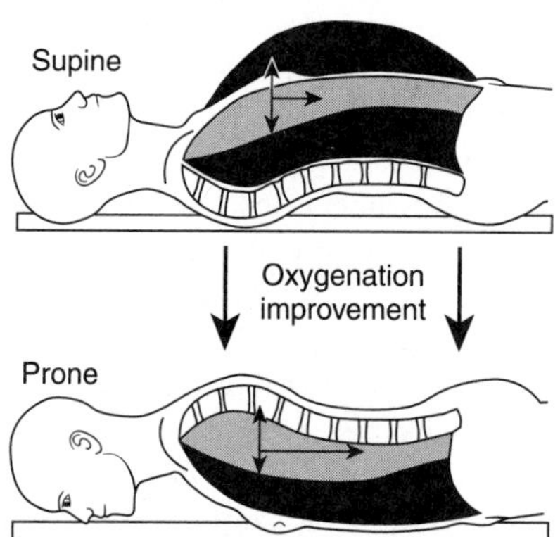

FIGURE 24-32 The effect of prone positioning on ventilation distribution. In the supine position, the distribution of positive-pressure ventilation is preferentially distributed to the ventral regions. When the patient is prone, the stiffness of the ventral chest wall help favors the distribution of ventilation to the dorsal regions, facilitating reinflation. (From Gattinoni L, Pelosi P, Brazzi L et al: Acute respiratory distress syndrome. In Albert RK, Spiro SG, Jett JR, editors: *Clinical respiratory medicine,* 2nd ed, pp 743-758, St. Louis, 2004, Mosby.)

pain relief and removing secretions mobilized by turning. The frequency of position change is determined by the results of this continual evaluation. Multitrauma patients with severe mobility limitations may be well suited for kinetic therapy (systematic mechanical rotation of patients with 40-degree turns), particularly in an attempt to reduce pulmonary complications.[126]

Role of Bronchoscopy

Fiberoptic bronchoscopy provides a means for pulmonary hygiene, foreign body removal, direct airway inspection, and diagnostic sputum or tissue sampling. Chest physiotherapy and vigorous cough are essential for the removal of central airway secretions and treatment for atelectasis. Bronchoscopy may be considered a support in this cause, not a replacement, and its role is limited to specific situations. Risks include hypercarbia, hypoxemia, pneumothorax, and cardiac arrhythmias. A paucity of scientific data exist on bronchoscopy in the thoracic trauma patient population requiring pulmonary hygiene.[224] Institutional bias probably plays a role in the acceptance and use of bronchoscopy.

Ventilator-Associated Pneumonia

Historically, pneumonia was classed as either community acquired or hospital acquired, although recently a new category, health care–associated pneumonia, has been described.[225] Hospital acquired is further categorized to include ventilator-associated pneumonia (VAP) if the pneumonia arose after the patient had been receiving at least 24 to 48 hours of mechanical ventilation.[226,227] VAP in the trauma patient is a continuing concern, imposing increased risk of death, hospital days, and hospital costs.[227] The nurse plays a crucial role in limiting the occurrence of VAP through several measures. American Association of Critical Care Nurses' guidelines for prevention of VAP include keeping the head of the bed elevated 30 degrees or higher unless medically contraindicated; use of endotracheal tubes with continuous suction above the cuff; and not routinely changing ventilator circuits.[228] Mouth care is of particular importance in reducing VAP risk, although oral care may take a lower priority among interventions performed by ICU nurses or it may be performed in an ineffective manner.[229,230] Ventilator weaning directed by a weaning protocol and implemented by the bedside nurse has also been shown to decrease VAP.[205]

Pleural Space Drainage

Most thoracic injuries are treated by the insertion of one or more chest tubes, often under emergency conditions. Although the management of pleural space drainage systems is common to all types of critical care nursing, there are some special concerns for the thoracic trauma patient. Management of pleural space drainage described here remains pertinent to intermediate and acute care settings.

Mechanics of the Chest Drain Bottle

Most drainage bottles today are of the "all-in-one" design.[231] These single units contain separate compartments that historically represented separate bottles. Initially, a single bottle was used to facilitate drainage. To ensure that air was not sucked back into the pleural space during inspiration, the end of the drainage tube was placed beneath water. In doing so, the water acted as a one-way valve allowing air to escape (bubble out) but not be sucked back in. Using just 2 cm of water to cover the end of the drainage tube provided an adequate "underwater seal" without imposing an excessive resistor to allowing air out of the pleural space. This concept was known as the single-bottle model (Figure 24-33, *A*).

The mechanics of the above system became distorted because not only air drained out, but also fluid (blood, pleural fluid). Subsequently, the underwater seal level of 2 cm increased and removal of contents from the pleural space, particularly air, was no longer guaranteed. Resolution to this issue was achieved by adding a second bottle before the first. The new bottle acted only as a collection device for draining fluid. Once again, air was prevented from returning up the circuit by an underwater seal configuration in the original bottle. This concept was known as the double-bottle model (Figure 24-33, *B*).

In the presence of a large leak, a concern rises that the above system is not sufficient in keeping up with the removal of air. Removal of air may be enhanced by adding well-controlled suction to the drainage device, which in turn, communicates with the pleural space. To accomplish this, a third bottle was added with a relay connection to the two previous bottles. The third bottle was connected to a suction source generally set between 80 and 120 mm Hg. The design of the third bottle included a straw with one end open to atmospheric pressure (outside the bottle) and the other end beneath 20 cm of water. Thus, physics ensured that, as long as any bubbling occurred through the straw, the maximum amount of negative pressure transmitted through the entire system, including the pleural space, would be limited to −20 cm H_2O. This concept was known as the triple-bottle model (Figure 24-33, *C*).

Glass bottles have long been replaced with a multichamber, disposable plastic device capable of performing the same function but in one handy unit[231](Figure 24-33, *D*). Incorporated in many single-unit devices is a graded leak indicator allowing the clinician to quantify the severity of an air leak. Also, in some units, the chamber filled with 20 cm of water has been replaced with a mechanical suction regulator that performs the same function. These units are sometimes referred to as "dry suction units."

Insertion

The chest tube chosen for trauma management is large bore, such as 36F to 40F, so as to evacuate a mixture of air, blood, and tissue fragments. Commonly, the axillary approach through the "triangle of safety" is selected. The triangle of safety is bordered by the midaxillary line posteriorly, the

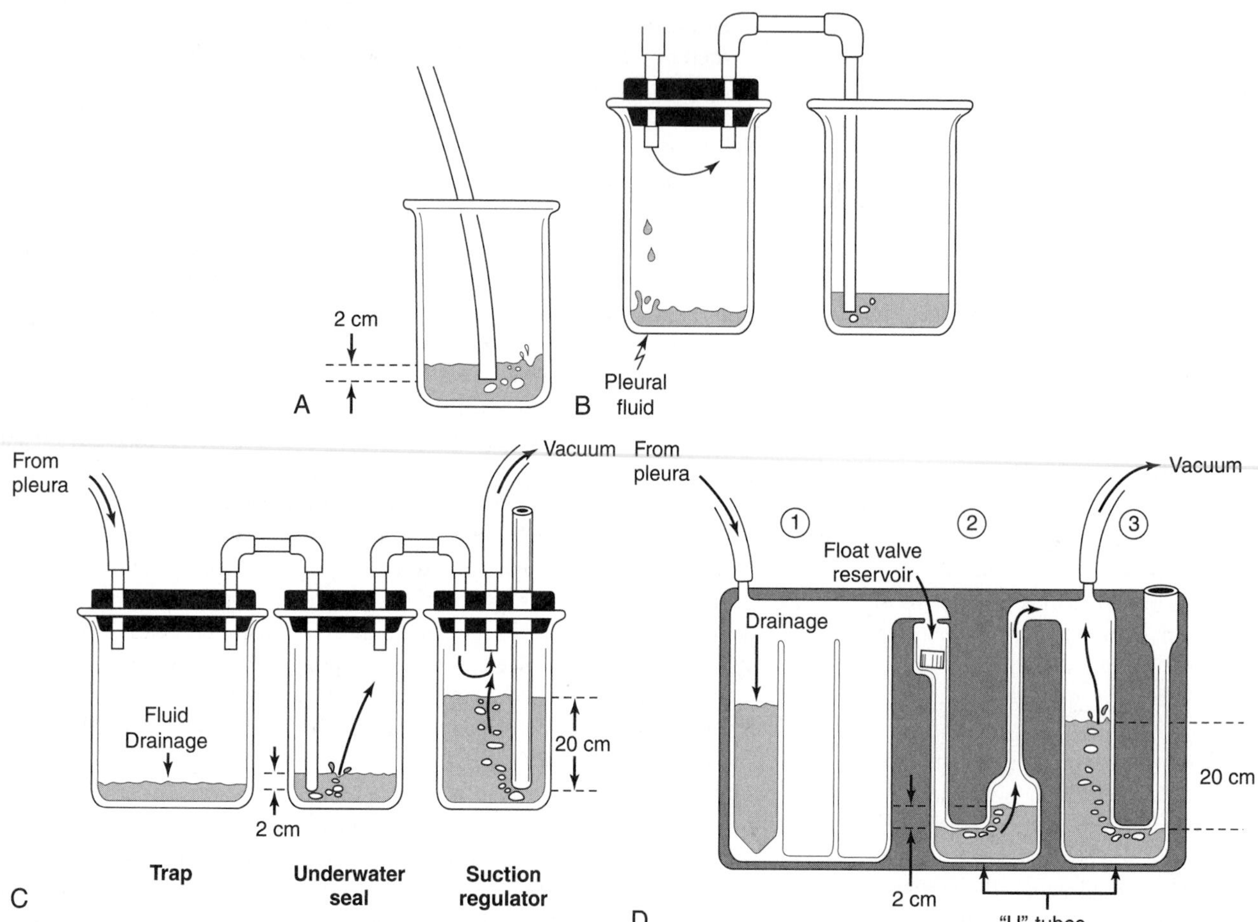

FIGURE 24-33 **A,** Single-bottle model of chest tube drainage. By placing the end of a tube under a small amount of water (2 cm), a simple one-way valve is established and air will bubble out but prevents air from re-entering the thoracic cavity. **B,** Double-bottle model of chest tube drainage. By placing a second (sealed) bottle before the first, the new bottle acts as a collection chamber while the original bottle continues to perform as a simple one-way valve. **C,** Triple-bottle model of chest tube drainage. With the addition of a third bottle, all containers sealed, and the addition of a suction regulator device, 20 cm H_2O of suction may now be consistently applied to the pleural space. **D,** Single unit combining the triple-bottle model. Many companies produce similar variations of the triple-bottle model in one self-contained disposable unit. (From Fishman NH: *Thoracic drainage: a manual of procedures,* Chicago, 1983, Year Book Medical.)

level of the nipple inferiorly, and the lateral border of the pectoralis major anteriorly. Typically, the insertion point is made anterior to the axillary line and in the fourth, fifth, or sixth intercostal space. No longer is a rigid trocar to penetrate the parietal pleura recommended because it may cause complications and is generally unnecessary. Directing a chest tube within the pleural space is challenging and a practice with questionable benefit. Intuitively, it would seem best to direct the tube apically for drainage of air or posterobasally for drainage of blood or fluid. In practice, a drain in any position within a "virgin pleural cavity" re-expands a lung by restoring negative pressure, thus expelling pleural contents. In the presence of intrapleural adhesions, directing the catheter may have potential benefit. Complications of chest tube insertion include perforation of the lung, trauma to the intercostal neurovascular bundle, re-expansion pulmonary edema, and infection.[232]

Thoracostomy Tube Care

Principles of thoracostomy tube care include the following:

- Tubing should not become occluded by excessive twisting, patient positioning, or bed rails.
- Loops of drainage tubing are not permitted to form because these may collect fluid, consequently inhibiting drainage of air.
- Every connection is taped or secured with chest tube bands.
- The drainage bottle should be kept below the level of the chest to prevent siphoning of contents back into the pleural space.
- Clamps are not used to close off the chest tube drainage (there may be rare exceptions to this rule as directed by a senior physician). Clamping a chest tube with an air leak will lead to a tension pneumothorax.

Clamping is not necessary for moving the patient as long as drainage bottles are kept beneath the level of the chest.

- Discontinuation of suction includes removal of suction tubing from the drainage bottle; otherwise, a closed system may develop, creating a potentially hazardous situation in the presence of a developing pneumothorax.
- Chest tubes may be milked to drain fluid and compressed to break up debris and clots but not stripped. Stripping increases local negative suction pressure in the area of the drainage holes of the chest tube and may damage lung and pleural parenchyma.
- Suction through the chest drain and associated tubing is normally maintained at −20 cm H_2O. The suction must be adequate to facilitate drainage of air and blood but not high enough to entrap tissue or delay healing of the injury. Occasionally the suction level is inadequate to properly evacuate air and help seal an existing air leak. Greater suction may be provided. The effectiveness of the new level of suction is evaluated clinically and radiographically. Conversely, low suction levels may be required in selected patients managed with controlled mechanical ventilation to avoid increasing the gradient between positive airway pressure and negative intrapleural suction. An increased gradient may delay healing, create additional air leak, and potentiate a bronchopleural fistula.

Examination of Air Leak

Observance for leaks occurs with each assessment. The spontaneously breathing patient (without assistance from a ventilator) may only have a minor leak represented by bubbling during a forced cough (raises intrathoracic pressure, thus forcing air out). A more serious leak would be present during a normal expiratory phase, whereas continuous bubbling is consistent with the most significant leak. In the patient receiving positive-pressure ventilation, these findings are reversed (i.e., a leak will be seen most readily during *inspiration* when pressure within the thorax increases). Patients receiving PEEP are more likely to have a continuous leak than those not receiving PEEP because pressure within the thorax, on average, is more positive.

A method of classifying a leak has been described by Cerfolio et al[233] (Robert David Cerfolio classification system) and may be modified depending on the chest tube drainage device. Basically, a leak is defined first by its appearance as either continuous (occurring during inspiration and expiration), inspiratory, expiratory, or forced expiratory. These four choices are listed in order of decreasing severity in the spontaneously breathing patient. Next, the leak is labeled by its size, as measured by a grading device within the chest tube drain unit, with a grade of 1 being the least. The specific design of the grading device may vary from manufacturer to manufacturer, although the concept is common (Figure 24-34). By use of this system, a "continuous 3" may be quantified against a "forced expiratory 2."[233]

Assessment for leak must also exclude an external source of leak. Both visual inspection and CXR will determine whether a drain side port is lying outside the pleural space and probably beyond the skin. A port outside the pleura, and not sealed with fat, muscle, or dressing, may facilitate the entrainment of air and produce bubbling in the chest tube. Furthermore, a correctly positioned chest tube, that the clinician pinches shut near the insertion point, may still yield bubbling if there is a break or crack in the tubing, its connections, or the drainage device.

Thoracostomy Tube Site Care

A pleural space injury may become infected by a break in the drainage system or by inadequate dressing techniques. Several therapeutic nursing measures can minimize this risk or prevent infection. As always, careful handwashing and skillful and careful assistance during insertion or removal of the drainage system are essential. Even under emergency conditions, the skin must be disinfected before chest tube insertion. Surveillance for aseptic technique is required on the part of all individuals during insertion, repositioning, or removal of the chest tube. All parts of the drainage system that connect to the pleural space must be sterile. Collection containers are replaced when contaminated. It is important to date the drainage system and to document when it was initiated or changed. Many patients have large amounts of drainage and require several changes of the collection system.

The chest tube is sutured in place, dressed, and carefully secured to the chest wall. The objective is to avoid slippage of the tube back and forth, which increases local injury and the possibility of infection. The dressing procedure is sterile, requiring a small sterile field, mask, and gloves. It can be done economically and quickly without compromising sterile technique.[234] The final dressing is closed to the environment by tape and changed when soiled, every 2 to 3 days, or when ordered.[235] It is useful to establish a standard for routine changing and to systematically document the date of dressing change, the appearance of the site, and the drainage apparent on the dressing. The use of prophylactic antibiotics to reduce the incidence of empyema associated with chest tube thoracostomy in the trauma patient is not supported,

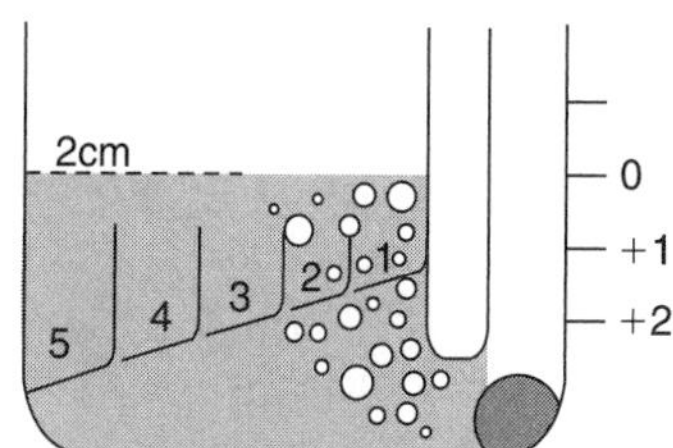

FIGURE 24-34 Graded leak indicator.

although their use may lead to a reduction in the incidence of pneumonia.[236] Further studies are needed.

Removal of the Tube

Generally, suction is maintained until air leaks resolve. In the nontrauma patient population, placing chest tubes to water seal appears superior to wall suction for stopping air leaks after pulmonary resection in patients with small leaks.[237,238] This practice warrants further study in the trauma patient population, although large leaks will require suction to prevent development of symptomatic pneumothorax. If no leak is present, a chest tube may often be placed to water seal. After a period of time, commonly between 6 and 24 hours, the chest tube on water seal with no air leak may be removed.[239,240] Drainage output of less than 200 ml per day is recommended before discontinuation of the chest tube.[232,241] Because tube thoracostomy is relatively common in trauma centers, timely safe removal of chest tubes holds significant financial and length of stay implications.

Removal of a chest tube at either end-inspiration or end-expiration is associated with equal risk for pneumothorax development.[241] Proponents of removing a chest tube at end-expiration argue that the pressure difference between atmospheric and intrapleural pressure is minimized; thus, the risk of inadvertent air flow into the pleural space during chest tube removal is also minimized. Chest tube removal at end-inspiration holds the advantage of having the lung maximally expanded and the parietal and visceral pleura most closely opposed.[241] An essential safety component of chest tube removal is to *not* have changing pleural pressure during the removal phase. This is best achieved by holding the patient's breath at maximal inspiration.[232] The tendency of patients who feel pain with the removal process is to gasp (i.e., take a short, sharp, sudden breath in). If the lungs are maximally expanded and in a breath-hold position, no further air can be drawn in and pleural pressure does not change. However, this is *not* true of the patient who gasps during chest tube removal at end-expiration. Other important interventions to include during tube removal include swift tube withdrawal; immediate occulsion of the tube insertion site with petroleum jelly–impregnated gauze, forced Valsalva maneuver, and performance of the procedure by experienced staff. A previously placed suture (purse-string or U stitch) may or may not be present, but if present, the suture may be used to occlude the thoracostomy site upon tube removal. The above timing and technique also works well for patients receiving positive-pressure ventilation and may be facilitated by temporarily pressing the inspiratory pause button on the ventilator.[232]

The timing of a CXR associated with modification of chest tube therapy is an area undergoing research and change. A CXR 3 hours after placing a chest tube to water seal will effectively identify development of a clinically significant pneumothorax. Research suggests that a preremoval CXR is unnecessary if no air leak is present after 6 hours of having the chest tube to water seal.[239] Similarly, a study of ventilated and unventilated patients indicates that a 3-hour CXR after removal of a tube is sufficient for determination of a clinically significant pneumothorax.[242] Other researchers have made similar 3-hour follow-up CXR recommendations after removal of a chest tube for the mechanically ventilated patient with less than 10 cm H_2O of PEEP.[243] Finally, implementation of thoracostomy tube practice guidelines has been associated with a reduction in hospital days.[239]

Nursing Therapeutics in the Intermediate and Rehabilitation Care Phases

Not all patients with thoracic injuries require critical care nursing. Many are safely managed in the intermediate or acute care area and then progress to rehabilitation and return to the community. Alternatively, numerous patient problems identified and initially managed in the critical care phase persist into intermediate care and rehabilitation. The following sections focus on specific nursing therapeutics employed in the immediate care, acute care, and rehabilitation phases.

Ventilator Dependence

In some instances a patient remains dependent on mechanical ventilation although the causes of weaning failure have been considered and considerable management has already been directed toward the problem. The causes of extended ventilatory dependence are not usually complications of thoracic injury per se but are related to central nervous system injury or to a previous chronic respiratory disease. Under these circumstances, weaning therapies are continued into the patient's intermediate trauma phase, and the problem of ventilator dependence is incorporated into the plan of care. If continued dependence on some form of mechanical ventilation is preventing the patient from discharge, long-term acute care or home respiratory therapy may be considered.

Conditions that may contribute to prolonged mechanical ventilation are varied and include recurrent aspiration, undertreated obstructive airway disease, malnutrition, electrolyte abnormalities, prolonged NMB, steroid myopathy, and critical illness polyneuropathy. Often the cause is a combination of a catastrophic acute illness superimposed on chronic disease.[244] While contributing conditions are corrected, an appropriate weaning protocol is used to gradually strengthen ventilatory muscles and tolerance. The basic strategy is to allow the patient to breathe spontaneously for gradually longer periods with interspersed periods of rest. The means by which this strategy is put into operation are similar to those described in the critical care therapeutics section, protocols again proving useful for patients receiving prolonged mechanical ventilation.[245] Numerous studies have explored the relative efficacy of common weaning techniques; however, the data have failed to demonstrate the benefit of one definitive technique over others.

Weaning is a great burden both physically and mentally for the patient who has been ventilated for many days or weeks.

Anxiety and fear can prolong ventilator dependence in some patients.[200] A number of studies in medical-surgical patients have demonstrated that biofeedback, relaxation, and imagery can reduce negative emotional responses to weaning.[200] These therapies have not been well studied in the multiply injured patient population. Finally, successful weaning and liberation from mechanical ventilation does not guarantee return to a home environment; many patients remain institutionalized despite not being dependent on a ventilator.[244]

PLEURAL SPACE INFECTIONS

Technically an empyema is considered "a collection of pus in a body cavity," although it is especially associated with the pleural space. Empyemas begin as exudative effusions and progress to loculated effusions before advancing to organized empyemas.[7] The risk of posttraumatic empyema remains high in the intermediate care phase, although empyema is frequently a result of initial treatment and stabilization. Diagnosis is made by radiologic findings associated with fever, leukocytosis, and pleural cultures that are positive for microorganisms.

Management of Empyema

Pleural space infections may occur as a result of penetrating injury, although most often are a result of chest tubes or thoracotomy. Blood clots and undrained fluid are excellent media for the propagation of organisms and subsequent development of empyema. Other secondary causes include intraabdominal injury associated with diaphragmatic disruption and posttraumatic pneumonia.[246] The first line of treatment is drainage of pus. This may be achieved by placement of a chest tube into the empyema. The contents of the infected pleural space are drained, and the underlying lung is allowed to re-expand. Closed or open drainage techniques may be used, depending on the number of infectious pockets and organization of the infected material. Pleural decortication involves surgical removal of the visceral pleura and "rind" buildup on the outer surface of the lung. Certain cases may lend themselves to the video-assisted thoracic surgery approach,[247] but others require an open thoracotomy.[7] Systemic antibiotics are an adjunctive treatment with *Staphylococcus* being a common causative organism.[246] The role of intrapleural fibrinolysis in the management of posttraumatic thoracic empyema is undetermined.[247]

In closed techniques a chest tube is inserted or an existing thoracostomy tube is converted to an "empyema tube." Although the general management of the closed system is as previously described, cultures of drainage fluid may be useful. The drainage initially appears as a purulent fluid but may change to a thicker, more fibrous material. After 2 or 3 weeks the closed system may be converted into open drainage of the most dependent part of the cavity. Drainage into bulky dressings or stoma bags (without suction) permit evacuation of loculated fluid collections. As the infection clears and healing begins, the drainage tube is shortened gradually and then removed as the cavity closes behind it.[248]

PARAPLEGIA

Spinal cord injury is possibly the most serious complication encountered in patients who survive the critical care phase of ruptured thoracic aorta. Whether the paraplegia results from cord ischemia during aortic cross-clamping or from direct injury to the spinal arteries, spinal cord injury is a devastating condition that has been reported in as many as 23% of survivors. Newer surgical techniques, such as partial cardiopulmonary bypass, have had a dramatic impact on the reduction of postoperative paraplegia.[169]

PERICARDITIS

Posttraumatic pericarditis may become symptomatic weeks after blunt cardiac injury. Bleeding into the pericardial sac irritates the epicardium and pericardium, producing inflammation and edema. Three types of conditions have been associated with blunt chest trauma. These include pericarditis with or without effusion and constrictive pericarditis. Signs of cardiac tamponade may slowly develop in individuals with effusion, whereas those without effusion demonstrate a significant pericardial rub, fever, and retrosternal pain. Pericardial inflammation syndrome may also be present with leukocytosis and ECG changes consistent with pericarditis. An echocardiogram aids in assessment of pericardial fluid and possible constriction. Nursing care includes careful physical examination, including auscultation of heart sounds. Identification of a friction rub and a change in the quality and quantity of chest pain are important findings. Treatment is primarily symptomatic with nonsteroidal anti-inflammatory medication and rest being the mainstays. Rarely, pericardiocentesis may be warranted.[163]

PERSISTENT PAIN

Chronic chest wall pain after blunt trauma is not an uncommon finding in long-term survivors of flail injuries. The nurse must learn to differentiate between acute and chronic pain to provide appropriate therapy. Frustratingly, the source of pain for many patients is unknown, but traumatic neuromas, in which intercostal nerves become trapped in scarred tissue, do occur. Such complications may be treated with an intercostal neurectomy. Before this procedure the patient must demonstrate reproducible relief of pain after local anesthetic injection. Another cause of chronic pain is the development of fibrous adhesions along chest tubes tracks after chest tube placement for pleural decortication.[67] Early referral to a pain management clinic proves beneficial for many patients.

NUTRITIONAL DEFICIENCIES

Restoration of optimal nutritional status is a common problem in trauma patients. The individual with insufficient or excessive caloric and protein intake is likely to have a respiratory disability and difficulty in weaning from supplemental oxygen. Consultation with nutritional support services and education of the patient's family are essential to ensure appropriate nutritional intake.

DELAYED WOUND HEALING

Healing difficulties are uncommon at chest tube sites or thoracic soft tissue wounds because of their muscular blood supply. Deformities, diminished sensation caused by intercostal nerve damage, and soft tissue defects are more common and may be associated with higher morbidity rates and longer hospital stays for the trauma patient. Although some chest wall and related musculoskeletal deformities may require surgical intervention, others can be prevented or treated by exercise.

PULMONARY THERAPEUTICS

All trauma patients, particularly those with thoracic injuries, require care directed toward removal of retained pulmonary secretions from the airways and protection from aspiration and associated pneumonia. Chest physiotherapy is used extensively, as described in the section on critical care therapeutics. Airway clearance may be accomplished by suctioning through an existing airway such as a tracheostomy, by a nasotracheal route, or by directed coughing. Breathing exercises are added to the plan of care, particularly in postoperative patients and those with neuromuscular or chronic pulmonary disease. Providing a clear rationale for therapy and simple-to-follow instructions is particularly important because the patient may not remember therapies used early in the recovery course. Involvement of family and friends is imperative and initiated early.

Directed Coughing

Coughing remains the most rapid and effective method for clearing the airways. It is generally a reflex under control of the afferent vagus nerve triggered by mechanical stimulation of laryngeal and bronchial receptors. However, both involuntary and voluntary cough suppression occurs in trauma patients as a result of decreased inspiratory or expiratory effort, poor glottic function, neurologic impairment, and/or fear and pain.

Directed coughing techniques are accompanied by monitoring for cough suppression and treating its cause. For example, the unhealed stoma left after tracheostomy tube removal can reduce the effectiveness of coughing and should be sealed with an airtight dressing. The patient is taught to put light pressure on the dressing during coughing. If the patient has difficulty mobilizing secretions toward the primary bronchi, coughing is less effective as a means of removing mucus. In this case, directed coughing is preceded by postural drainage, percussion, or vibration as one way of centralizing secretions and increasing the cough's effectiveness. Effective pain relief must be in progress before the majority of patients can even attempt to breathe deeply and cough. Although many patients naturally "splint" injured or postoperative areas during coughing, the majority benefit from a demonstration of effective splinting that does not impair chest wall movement. Demonstration of and instruction in splinting techniques *before* initiation of directed coughing may help to allay patient apprehension with coughing.

Several methods can be used to stimulate coughing. "Huff coughing" is a single, large inspiration followed by short, forceful exhalations producing rapid changes in air flow and an improved cough. External tracheal stimulation by gentle pressure above the sternal notch can stimulate coughing. Gentle oropharyngeal stimulation with the end of a suction catheter or direct suction aspiration may be necessary when the patient has difficulty clearing secretions in this area. Directed coughing takes place over short periods, alternating with rest. Repetitive and strained coughing is tiring and can precipitate bronchospasm.

Breathing Exercises

The main goals of breathing exercises are improved tidal volume, chest wall mobility, mobilization of secretions, and relaxation. Muscle training may increase respiratory strength and endurance. Specific exercises include diaphragmatic breathing, pursed-lip breathing, costal excursion exercises, and summed or stacked breathing.

Adjuncts Used to Improve Lung Expansion

Numerous devices are available to augment chest physical therapy, directed coughing, and breathing exercises. Probably the most economic and common are inspiratory incentive spirometry (IS) devices, which provide the ability to visually quantify the patient's inspiratory effort. Blow bottles are *expiratory* incentive devices and are not recommended because of the association between forced expiration and derecruitment of alveoli. Published reports of the relative benefits of IS in the trauma patient are generally lacking, whereas studies on the prevention of postoperative pulmonary complications with use of IS in nontrauma patients are, surprisingly, not overwhelmingly supportive.[249] A more recent literature review of patients undergoing abdominal surgery suggested that "any type of lung expansion intervention is better than no prophylaxis." The authors felt IS was comparatively the least labor intensive, but for patients who were not able to participate effectively continuous positive airway pressure proved particularly beneficial.[250]

Should such devices be incorporated into the plan of care, they are considered an addition to, not a substitute for, the pulmonary therapeutics described earlier. How frequently and for what length of time the patient uses a device are determined by its effectiveness in improving lung volumes and the patient's respiratory status. The patient is instructed and supervised periodically to determine whether the device is being used properly and whether benefits or problems are present. The patient is encouraged to *not* focus on achieving a target volume but rather on maintaining the inspiratory period for as long as possible ("float the ball" concept). The measured inspired volume is considered a secondary value and not the primary goal, which is long, slow, deep breaths.

Active Exercise Programs

Muscular exercise and range-of-motion programs are appropriate for the thoracic trauma patient even in unusual situations when other injuries restrict the patient to bed. In consultation with a physical and occupational therapist, an exercise program for involved joints or muscles is included in the plan of care. Patients are likely to avoid moving the trunk and upper extremities after thoracotomy or significant chest wall injury. As a result, deformities can develop, most commonly frozen shoulder syndrome. Range-of-motion exercises include active and/or passive stretch of the affected area or active contraction of opposing muscle groups. Repeated exercises with weights can improve strength and endurance. Early and full range of motion of the shoulder should be encouraged, particularly after thoracotomy or chest tube placement; limitation of shoulder flexion to 90 degrees is often the norm, but studies to support this practice are lacking. Anecdotal evidence from more than 20 years' experience working with trauma patients at the R Adams Cowley Shock Trauma Center shows no evidence of complication related to early resumption of full shoulder range-of-motion activities.

The presence of chest tubes and even ventilatory or oxygen delivery equipment does not commit the patient to bed rest. After reviewing all tubes, drains, and oxygen requirements with the trauma physician, mobilizing the patient out of bed and progressive ambulation is planned as part of the exercise program. On approval from a responsible physician, chest tube drainage systems may be disconnected temporarily from suction, and oxygen tanks, if needed, are attached to a rolling pole or walker. If chest tube drainage may not be disconnected, long suction tubing is applied to increase the range of ambulation. Alternatively, portable suction devices may be used.

Summary

This chapter outlines the body of knowledge about chest trauma, yet it must be emphasized that a great deal is unknown about the physiologic and psychological effects of our nursing therapies. In solving these unknowns, we do the greatest service for our patients. Many areas require further research and the trauma or rehabilitation nurse is in a prime position to conduct such studies.

Thoracic injuries can be highly lethal, and nursing management must be rapid, technically flawless, and comprehensive. Many chest injuries do not threaten life or create permanent disability, again in large part because of nursing expertise. The trauma nurse's expert care is based on a thorough understanding of thoracic anatomy, respiratory physiology, injury mechanics, and the techniques of cardiopulmonary assessment. Management of chest injuries revolves around individualized ventilator support, exquisite airway care, objective pain control strategies, and intensive pulmonary hygiene. However, the greatest role the nurse plays is in the implementation, observance, and maintenance of the many therapies, devices, and procedures that facilitate inflation of the lung and keeping it inflated.

Trauma nursing care is built from experience, consultation with nursing specialists and other disciplines, and research. Nurses have much to offer the patient with thoracic injuries, including relief from the pervasive chest pain, the inability to breathe, and the growing weakness of hypovolemic shock. Nurses also offer the patient support in tolerating chest tubes and the endless days until it is possible to be discharged home.

References

1. LoCicero J, Mattox KL: Epidemiology of chest trauma, *Surg Clin North Am* 69:15-19, 1989.
2. *R Adams Cowley Shock Trauma Center Trauma Registry,* Baltimore, MD, 1996 to date.
3. *Tricode coding software 1990,* Forest Hill, MD, 1990, Digital Innovations.
4. American College of Surgeons Committee on Trauma: Shock. In *Advanced trauma life support course for doctors,* 7th ed, pp 69-98, Chicago, 2004, American College of Surgeons.
5. American College of Surgeons Committee on Trauma: Initial assessment and management. In *Advanced trauma life support course for doctors,* 7th ed, pp 11-32, Chicago, 2004, American College of Surgeons.
6. Guyton AC, Hall JE: Circulatory shock and physiology of its treatment. In *Textbook of medical physiology,* 11th ed, pp 278-288, Philadelphia, 2006, Elsevier Saunders.
7. Livingston DH, Hauser CJ: Trauma to the chest wall and lung. In Moore EE, Feliciano DV, Mattox KL, editors: *Trauma,* 5th ed, pp 507-537, New York, 2004, McGraw-Hill.
8. Scalea TM, Simon HM, Duncan AO et al: Geriatric blunt trauma: improved survival with early invasive monitoring, *J Trauma* 30:129-134, 1990.
9. EAST Practice Management Guidelines Work Group: *Practice management guidelines for geriatric trauma* (2001) http://www.east.org/tpg/geriatric.pdf. Accessed May 14, 2006.
10. Perkins GD, McAuley DF, Giles S et al: Do changes in pulse oximeter oxygen saturation predict equivalent changes in arterial oxygen saturation? *Crit Care* 7:R67-R71, 2003. http://ccforum.com/content/7/4/R67. Accessed May 12, 2006.
11. Van de Louw A, Cracco C, Cerf C et al: Accuracy of pulse oximetry in the intensive care unit, *Intensive Care Med* 27:1606-1613, 2001.
12. Ahrens T, Sona C: Capnography application in acute and critical care, *AACN Clin Issues* 14:123-132, 2003.
13. Tyburski JG, Collinge JD, Wilson RF et al: End-tidal CO_2-derived values during emergency trauma surgery correlated with outcome: a prospective study, *J Trauma* 53:738-743, 2002.
14. Tyburski JG, Carlin AM, Harvey EH et al: End-tidal CO_2-arterial CO_2 differences: a useful intraoperative mortality marker in trauma surgery, *J Trauma* 55:892-897, 2003.
15. Boswell SA, Scalea TM: Sublingual capnometry: an alternative to gastric tonometry for the management of shock resuscitation, *AACN Clin Issues* 14:176-184, 2003.

16. University of Maryland R Adams Cowley Shock Trauma Center: *Clinical manual,* Baltimore, MD, 2005, R Adams Cowley Shock Trauma Center.
17. Miller LA, Mirvis SE, Harris L et al: Total-body digital radiography for trauma screening: initial experience, *Appl Radiol* 8-14, 2004. http://appliedradiology.com/articles/pdf/AR_08-04_miller.pdf. Accessed May 15, 2006.
18. Trupka A, Waydhas C, Hallfeldt KK et al: Value of thoracic computed tomography in the first assessment of severely injured patients with blunt chest trauma: results of a prospective study, *J Trauma* 43:405-412, 1997.
19. Peytel E, Menegaux F, Cluzel P et al: Initial imaging assessment of severe blunt trauma, *Intensive Care Med* 27:1756-1761, 2001.
20. Chen MY, Miller PR, McLaughlin CA et al: The trend of using computed tomography in the detection of acute thoracic aortic and branch vessel injury after blunt thoracic trauma: single-center experience over 13 years, *J Trauma* 56:783-785, 2004.
21. Chen MY, Regan JD, D'Amore MJ et al: Role of angiography in the detection of aortic branch vessel injury after blunt thoracic trauma, *J Trauma* 51:1166-1172, 2001.
22. Parker MS, Matheson TL, Rao AV et al: Making the transition: the role of helical CT in the evaluation of potentially acute thoracic injuries, *AJR Am J Roentgenol* 176:1267-1272, 2001.
23. Downing SW, Sperling JS, Mirvis SE et al: Experience with spiral computed tomography as the sole diagnostic method for traumatic aortic rupture, *Ann Thorac Surg* 72:495-502, 2001.
24. Stassen NA, Lukan JK, Spain DA et al: Reevaluation of diagnostic procedures for transmediastinal gunshot wounds, *J Trauma* 53:635-638, 2002.
25. Mirvis SE: Diagnostic imaging of thoracic trauma. In Mirvis SE, Shanmuganathan K, editors: *Imaging in trauma and critical care,* 2nd ed, pp 297-367, Philadelphia, 2003, Elsevier.
26. Alkadhi H, Widermuth S, Desbiolles L et al: Vascular emergencies of the thorax after blunt and iatrogenic trauma: multi-detector row CT and three-dimensional imaging, *Radiographics* 24:1239-1255, 2004.
27. American College of Surgeons Committee on Trauma: Thoracic trauma. In *Advanced trauma life support course for doctors,* 7th ed, pp 103-115, Chicago, 2004, American College of Surgeons.
28. Rowan KR, Kirkpatrick AW, Liu D et al: Traumatic pneumothorax detection with thoracic US: correlation with chest radiography and CT—initial experience, *Radiology* 225:210-214, 2002.
29. Dulchavsky SA, Schwarz KL, Kirkpatrick AW et al: Prospective evaluation of thoracic ultrasound in the detection of pneumothorax, *J Trauma* 50:201-205, 2001.
30. Kirkpatrick AW, Sirois M, Laupland KB et al: Hand-held thoracic sonography for detecting post-traumatic pneumothoraces: the extended focused assessment with sonography for trauma (EFAST), *J Trauma* 57:288-295, 2004.
31. Wall MJ, Huh J, Mattox KL: Thoracotomy. In Moore EE, Feliciano DV, Mattox KL, editors: *Trauma,* 5th ed, pp 493-503, New York, 2004, McGraw-Hill.
32. Biffl WL, Moore EE, Johnson JL: Emergency department thoracotomy. In Moore EE, Feliciano DV, Mattox KL, editors: *Trauma,* 5th ed, pp 239-244, New York, 2004, McGraw-Hill.
33. Mattox KL: Indications for thoracotomy: deciding to operate, *Thor Trauma* 69:47-58, 1989.
34. Fialka C, Sebok C, Kemetzhofer P et al: Open-chest cardiopulmonary resuscitation after cardiac arrest in cases of blunt chest or abdominal trauma: a consecutive series of 38 cases, *J Trauma* 57:809-814, 2004.
35. Mineo TC, Ambrogi V, Pompeo E: Changing indications for thoracotomy in blunt chest trauma after the advent of video thoracoscopy, *J Trauma* 47:1088-1091, 1999.
36. Danne PD, Hunter M, MacKillop AD: Airway control. In Moore EE, Feliciano DV, Mattox KL, editors: *Trauma,* 5th ed, pp 177-199, New York, 2004, McGraw-Hill.
37. American College of Surgeons Committee on Trauma: Airway and ventilatory management. In *Advanced trauma life support course for doctors,* 7th ed, pp 41-67, Chicago, 2004, American College of Surgeons.
38. Plummer AL, Gracey DR: Consensus conference on artificial airways in patients receiving mechanical ventilation, *Chest* 96:178-180, 1989.
39. Rumbak MJ, Newton M, Truncale T et al: A prospective, randomized, study comparing early percutaneous dilational tracheotomy to prolonged translaryngeal intubation (delayed tracheotomy) in critically ill medical patients, *Crit Care Med* 32:1689-1694, 2004.
40. Griffiths J, Barber VS, Morgan L et al: Systematic review and meta-analysis of studies of the timing of tracheostomy in adult patients undergoing artificial ventilation, *BMJ* 330:1243, 2005.
41. Lindgren VA, Ames NJ: Caring for patients on mechanical ventilation, *Am J Nurs* 105:50-60, 2005.
42. Moore T: Suctioning techniques for the removal of respiratory secretions, *Nurs Stand* 18:47-53, 2003.
43. Riley RD, Miller PR, Meredith JW: Injury to the esophagus, trachea, and bronchus. In Moore EE, Feliciano DV, Mattox KL, editors: *Trauma,* 5th ed, pp 539-553, New York, 2004, McGraw-Hill.
44. Doyle RL: Assessing and modifying the risk of postoperative pulmonary complications, *Chest* 115:77-81, 1999.
45. Allan JS, Wright CD: Tracheoinnominate fistula: diagnosis and management, *Chest Surg Clin North Am* 13:331-341, 2003.
46. Reed MF, Mathisen DJ: Tracheoesohageal fistula, *Chest Surg Clin North Am* 13:271-289, 2003.
47. Scalise P, Prunk SR, Healy D et al: The incidence of tracheoarterial fistula in patients with chronic tracheostomy tubes, *Chest* 128:3906-3909, 2005.
48. Ruschult H, Osthaus A, Heine J: Tracheal injury as a sequence of multiple attempts of endotracheal intubation in the course of a preclinical cardiopulmonary resuscitation, *Resuscitation* 43: 147-150, 2000.
49. American College of Surgeons Committee on Trauma: Chest trauma management. In *Advanced trauma life support course for doctors,* 7th ed, pp 125-130, Chicago, 2004, American College of Surgeons.
50. Schweiger JW: *The pathophysiology, diagnosis and management strategies for flail chest injury and pulmonary contusion: a review,* review course lectures book, pp 86-93, 2001, Cleveland, Ohio, International Anesthesia Research Society.
51. Eastern Association for the Society of Trauma: *Pain management in blunt thoracic trauma (BTT)—an evidenced-based outcome evaluation,* 2nd review, 2003, Winston-Salem, NC, Eastern Association for the Society of Trauma.
52. Bulger EM, Edwards T, Klotz P et al: Epidural analgesia improves outcome after multiple rib fractures, *Surgery* 136:426-430, 2004.
53. Wu CL, Jani ND, Perkins FM et al: Thoracic epidural analgesia versus intravenous patient-controlled analgesia for the treatment of rib fracture pain after motor vehicle crash, *J Trauma* 47:564-567, 1999.
54. Tanaka H, Yukioka T, Yamaguti Y et al: Surgical stabilization of internal pneumatic stabilization? A prospective randomized

study of management of severe flail chest patients, *J Trauma* 52:727-732, 2002.

55. Mayberry JC, Terhes JT, Ellis TJ et al: Absorbable plates for rib fracture repair: preliminary experience, *J Trauma* 55:835-839, 2003.
56. Neumann P, Wrigge H, Zinserling J et al: Spontaneous breathing affects the spatial ventilation and perfusion distribution during mechanical ventilatory support, *Crit Care Med* 33:1090-1095, 2005.
57. Putensen C, Zech S, Wrigge H et al: Long-term effects of spontaneous breathing during ventilatory support in patients with acute lung injury, *Am J Respir Crit Care Med* 164:43-49, 2001.
58. Schweiger JW, Downs JB, Smith RA: Chest wall disruption with and without acute lung injury: effects of continuous positive airway pressure therapy on ventilation and perfusion relationships, *Crit Care Med* 31:2364-2370, 2003.
59. Avery EA, Mörch ET, Benson DW: Critically crushed chests; a new method of treatment with continuous mechanical hyperventilation to produce alkalotic apnea and internal pneumatic stabilization, *J Thorac Surg* 32:291-309, 1956.
60. Trinkle JK, Richardson JD, Franz JL et al: Management of flail chest without mechanical ventilation, *Ann Thorac Surg* 19:355-363, 1975.
61. Acton RD, Hotchkiss JR, Dries DJ: Noninvasive ventilation, *J Trauma* 53:593-601, 2002.
62. Tanaka H, Tajimi K, Endoh Y et al: Pneumatic stabilization for flail chest injury: an 11-year study, *Surg Today* 31:12-17, 2001.
63. Kerr-Valentic MA, Arthur M, Mullins RJ et al: Rib fracture pain and disability: can we do better? *J Trauma* 54:1058-1064, 2003.
64. Peeters C, Gupta S: Choices in pain management following thoracotomy, *Chest* 115:122-124, 1999.
65. Bulger EM, Edwards T, Klotz P et al: Epidural analgesia improves outcome after multiple rib fractures, *Surgery* 136:426-430, 2004.
66. Cohen SP, Christo PJ, Moroz L: Pain management in trauma patients, *Am J Phys Med Rehabil* 83:142-161, 2004.
67. Yeo TP: Long-term sequelae following blunt thoracic trauma, *Orthop Nurs* 20:35-47, 2001.
68. Asensio JA, Chahwan S, Hanpeter D et al: Thoracic injuries. In Waxman K, Shoemaker WC, editors: *Textbook of critical care,* Philadelphia, 2000, W. B. Saunders.
69. Stawicki SS, Grossman MD, Hoey BA et al: Rib fractures in the elderly: a marker of injury severity, *J Am Geriatr Soc* 52:805-808, 2004.
70. Bergeron E, Lavoie A, Clas D et al: Elderly trauma patients with rib fractures are at greater risk of death and pneumonia, *J Trauma* 54:478-485, 2003.
71. Bulger EM, Arneson MA, Mock CN et al: Rib fractures in the elderly, *J Trauma* 48:1040-1047, 2000.
72. Cohn SM: Pulmonary contusion: review of the clinical entity, *J Trauma* 42:973-979, 1997.
73. Wanek S, Mayberry JC: Blunt thoracic trauma: flail chest, pulmonary contusion, and blast injury, *Crit Care Clin* 20:71-81, 2004.
74. Miller PR, Croce MA, Bee TK et al: ARDS after pulmonary contusion: accurate measurement of contusion volume identifies high-risk patients, *J Trauma* 51:223-230, 2001.
75. Davis KA, Fabian TC,Croce MA et al: Prostanoids: early mediators in the secondary injury that develops after unilateral pulmonary contusion, *J Trauma* 46:824-832, 1999.
76. Schreiter D, Reske A, Stichert B et al: Alveolar recruitment in combination with sufficient positive end-expiratory pressure increases oxygenation and lung aeration in patients with severe chest trauma, *Crit Care Med* 32:968-975, 2004.
77. Vender JS, Szokol JW, Murphy GS et al: Sedation, analgesia, and neuromuscular blockade in sepsis: an evidence-based review, *Crit Care Med* 32:S554-S561, 2004.
78. Murray MJ, Cowen J, DeBlock H et al: Clinical practice guidelines for sustained neuromuscular blockade in the adult critically ill patient, *Crit Care Med* 30:142-156, 2002.
79. Allen GS, Coates NE: Pulmonary contusion: a collective review, *Am Surg* 62:895-901, 1996.
80. Cohn SM, Fisher BT, Rosenfield AT et al: Resuscitation of pulmonary contusion: hypertonic saline is not beneficial, *Shock* 8:292-299, 1997.
81. Kelly ME, Miller PR, Greenshaw JJ et al: Novel resuscitation strategy for pulmonary contusion after severe chest trauma, *J Trauma* 55:94-105, 2003.
82. National Heart, Lung, and Blood Institute Acute Respiratory Distress Syndrome (ARDS) Clinical Trials Network: Pulmonary-artery versus central venous catheter to guide treatment of acute lung injury, *N Engl J Med* 354:2213-2224, 2006.
83. Brashers VL: Structure and function of the pulmonary system. In McCance KL, Huether SE, editors: *Pathophysiology: the biologic basis for disease in adults and children,* 5th ed, pp 1181-1204, Baltimore, 2006, Elsevier Mosby.
84. O'Connor AR, Morgan WE: Radiological review of pneumothorax, *BMJ* 330:1493-1497, 2005.
85. Ball CG, Kirkpatrick AW, Laupland KB et al: Incidence, risk factors, and outcomes for occult pneumothoraces in victims of major trauma, *J Trauma* 59:917-925, 2005.
86. Kirkpatrick AW, Sirois M, Laupland KB et al: Hand-held thoracic sonography for detecting post-traumatic pneumothoraces: the extended focused assessment with sonography for trauma (EFAST), *J Trauma* 57:288-295, 2004.
87. Brooks A, Davies B, Smethhurst M et al: Emergency ultrasound in the acute assessment of hemothorax, *Emerg Med J* 21:44-46, 2004.
88. Wolfman NT, Myers WS, Glauser SJ et al: Validity of CT classification on management of occult pneumothorax: a prospective study, *AJR Am J Roentgenol* 171:1317-1320, 1998.
89. Jenner R: Chest drains in traumatic occult pneumothorax, *Emerg Med J* 23:138-139, 2006.
90. Bilello JF, Davis JW, Lemaster DM: Occult traumatic hemothorax: when can sleeping dogs lie? *Am J Surg* 190:841-844, 2005.
91. Northfield TC: Oxygen therapy for spontaneous pneumothorax, *BMJ* 4:86-88, 1971.
92. Hill RC, DeCarlo DP, Hill JF et al: Resolution of experimental pneumothorax in rabbits by oxygen therapy, *Ann Thorac Surg* 59:825-828, 1995.
93. Karmy-Jones R, Jurkovich G, Nathens A et al: Timing of urgent thoracotomy for hemorrhage after trauma: a multicenter study, *Arch Surg* 136:513-518, 2001.
94. Rizoli SB: Crystalloids and colloids in trauma resuscitation: a brief overview of the current debate, *J Trauma* 54:S82-S88, 2003.
95. Dutton RP, MacKenzie CF, Scalea TM: Hypotensive resuscitation during active hemorrhage: impact on in-hospital mortality, *J Trauma* 52:1141-1146, 2002.
96. Revell M, Greaves I, Porter K: Enpoints for fluid resuscitation in hemorrhagic shock, *J Trauma* 54:S63-S67, 2003.
97. Scott JM: Autotransfusion. In Lynn-McHale Wiegand DJ, Carlson KK, editors: *AACN procedure manual for critical care,* 5th ed, pp 121-124, St Louis, 2005, Elsevier Saunders.

98. Parks SN: Initial assessment. In Moore EE, Feliciano DV, Mattox KL, editors: *Trauma,* 5th ed, pp 159-175, New York, 2004, McGraw Hill.
99. Piantadosi CA, Schwartz DA: The acute respiratory distress syndrome, *Ann Intern Med* 141:460-470, 2004.
100. Ferguson ND, Frutos-Vivar F, Esteban A et al: Airway pressure, tidal volumes, and mortality in patients with acute respiratory distress syndrome, *Crit Care Med* 33:21-30, 2005.
101. Udobi KF, Childs E, Touijer K: Acute respiratory distress syndrome, *Am Fam Physician* 67:315-322, 2003.
102. Vincent JL, Sakr Y, Ranieri VM: Epidemiology and outcome of acute respiratory failure in intensive care unit patients, *Crit Care Med* 31(Suppl):S296-S299, 2003.
103. Bernard GR, Artigas A, Brigham KL et al: Report of the American-European consensus conference on ARDS: definitions, mechanisms, relevant outcomes and clinical coordination, *Intensive Care Med* 20:225-232, 1994.
104. Ashbaugh DG, Bigelow DB, Petty TL et al: Acute respiratory distress in adults, *Lancet* 2:319-323, 1967.
105. Atabai K, Matthay MA: The pulmonary physician in critical care, 5: acute lung injury and the acute respiratory distress syndrome: definitions and epidemiology, *Thorax* 57:452-458, 2002.
106. Ferguson ND, Frutos-Vivar F, Esteban A et al: Acute respiratory distress syndrome: under recognition by clinicians and diagnostic accuracy of three clinical definitions, *Crit Care Med* 33:2228-2234, 2005.
107. Brun-Buisson C, Minelli C, Bertolini G et al: Epidemiology and outcome of acute lung injury in European intensive care units—results from the ALIVE study, *Intensive Care Med* 30:51-61, 2004.
108. McCunn M: Personal communication, January 3, 1997.
109. Hudson LD, Steinberg KP: Epidemiology of acute lung injury and ARDS, *Chest* 116:74S-82S, 1999.
110. Sutchyta MR, Grissom CK, Morris AH et al: Epidemiology in ARDS, *Intensive Care Med* 25:538-539, 1999.
111. Gattinoni L, Caironi P, Pelosi P et al: What has computed tomography taught us about the acute respiratory distress syndrome? *Am J Respir Crit Care Med* 164:1701-1711, 2001.
112. Croce MA, Fabian TC, Davis KA et al: Early and late acute respiratory distress syndrome: two distinct clinical entities, *J Trauma* 1998;46:361-357.
113. Acute Respiratory Distress Syndrome Network: Comparison of two fluid-management strategies in acute lung injury, *N Engl J Med* 354:2564-2575, 2006.
114. Shander A, Popovsky MA: Understanding the consequences of transfusion-related acute lung injury, *Chest* 128:598S-604S, 2005.
115. Toy P, Popovsky MA, Abraham E et al: Transfusion-related acute lung injury: definition and review, *Crit Care Med* 33:721-726, 2005.
116. Finfer S, Bellomo R, Boyce N et al: A comparison of albumin and saline for fluid resuscitation in the intensive care unit, *N Engl J Med* 350:2247-2256, 2004.
117. Tisherman SA: Trauma fluid resuscitation in 2010, *J Trauma* 54: S231-S234, 2003.
118. Gattinoni L, Pelosi P, Brazzi L et al: Acute respiratory distress syndrome. In Albert RK, Spiro SG, Jett JR, editors: *Clinical respiratory medicine,* 2nd ed, pp 743-758, St. Louis, 2004, Mosby.
119. Cranshaw J, Griffiths MJ, Evans TW: The pulmonary physician in critical care: non-ventilatory strategies in ARDS, *Thorax* 57:823-829, 2002.
120. Sakar Y, Vincent JL, Reinhart K et al: High tidal volume and positive fluid balance are associated with worse outcome in acute lung injury, *Chest* 128:3098-3108, 2005.
121. Klein Y, Blackbourne L, Barquist ES: Non-ventilatory based strategies in the management of acute respiratory distress syndrome, *J Trauma* 57:915-924, 2004.
122. Gainnier M, Roch A, Forel JM et al: Effect of neuromuscular blocking agents on gas exchange in patients presenting with acute respiratory distress syndrome, *Crit Care Med* 32:113-119, 2004.
123. Putensen C, Mutz NJ, Putensen-Himmer G et al: Spontaneous breathing during ventilatory support improves ventilation-perfusion distributions in patients with acute respiratory distress syndrome, *Am J Respir Crit Care Med* 159:1241-1248, 1999.
124. Pelosi P, Brazzi L, Gattinoni L: Prone position in acute respiratory distress syndrome, *Eur Respir J* 20:1017-1028, 2002.
125. Gattinoni L, Tognoni G, Pesenti A et al: Effect of prone positioning on the survival of patients with acute respiratory failure, *N Engl J Med* 345:568-573, 2001.
126. Ahrens T, Kollef M, Shannon W: Effect on kinetic therapy on pulmonary complications, *Am J Crit Care* 13:376-383, 2004.
127. Vollman KM: Prone positioning in the patient who has acute respiratory distress syndrome: the art and science, *Crit Care Nurs Clin North Am* 16:319-336, 2004.
128. Curley MA: Prone position of patients with acute respiratory distress syndrome: a systematic review, *Am J Crit Care* 8: 397-405, 1999.
129. Meduri GU, Headley AS, Golden E et al: Effect of prolonged methylprednisolone therapy in unresolving acute respiratory distress syndrome: a randomized controlled trial, *JAMA* 280:159-165, 1998.
130. National Heart, Lung, and Blood Institute Acute Respiratory Distress Syndrome (ARDS) Clinical Trials Network: Efficacy and safety of corticosteroids for persistent acute respiratory distress syndrome, *N Engl J Med* 354:1671-1684, 2006.
131. Kaisers U, Kelly KP, Busch T: Liquid ventilation, *Br J Anaesth* 91:143-151, 2003.
132. Cordingley JJ, Keogh BF: The pulmonary physician in critical care, 8: ventilatory management of ALI/ARDS, *Thorax* 57: 729-734, 2002.
133. Davies MW, Fraser JF: Partial liquid ventilation for preventing death and morbidity in adults with acute lung injury and acute respiratory distress syndrome, *Cochrane Database Syst Rev* 2004, Isssue 4, Art. No. CD003707; DOI: 10.1002/14651858.
134. Cerra FB, Benitez MR, Blackburn GL et al: Applied nutrition in ICU patients: a consensus statement of the American College of Chest Physicians, *Chest* 111:769-778, 1997.
135. EAST Practice Management Guidelines Work Group: *Practice management guidelines for nutritional support of the trauma patient,* Allentown, PA, 2003, Eastern Association for the Surgery of Trauma (EAST).
136. Brower RG, Ware LB, Berthiaume Y et al: Treatment of ARDS, *Chest* 120:1347-1367, 2000.
137. Acute Respiratory Distress Syndrome Network (ARDSNet): Ventilation with lower tidal volumes as compared with traditional tidal volumes for acute lung injury and the acute respiratory distress syndrome, *N Engl J Med* 342:1301-1308, 2001.
138. NHLBI ARDS Network: http://www.ardsnet.org/. Accessed March 28, 2007.

139. Pinsky MR: Toward a better ventilation strategy for patients with acute lung injury, *Crit Care* 4:205-206, 2000. Published online July 3, 2000.
140. de Durante G, del Turco M, Rustichini L et al: ARDSNet lower tidal volume ventilatory strategy may generate intrinsic positive end-expiratory pressure in patients with acute respiratory distress syndrome, *Am J Respir Crit Care Med* 165:1271-1274, 2002.
141. Steinbrook R: How best to ventilate? Trial design and patient safety in studies of the acute respiratory distress syndrome, *N Engl J Med* 348:1393-1401, 2003.
142. Grasso S, Fanelli V, Cafarelli A et al: Effects of high versus low positive end-expiratory pressure in acute respiratory distress syndrome, *Am J Respir Crit Care Med* 171:1002-1008, 2005.
143. Young MP, Manning HL, Wilson DL et al: Ventilation of patients with acute lung injury and acute respiratory distress syndrome: has new evidence changed clinical practice? *Crit Care Med* 32:1260-1265, 2004.
144. Weinert CR, Gross CR, Marinelli WA: Impact of randomized trial results on acute lung injury ventilator therapy in teaching hospitals, *Am J Respir Crit Care Med* 167:1304-1309, 2003.
145. Eichacker PQ, Gerstenberger EP, Banks SM et al: Meta-analysis of acute lung injury and acute respiratory distress syndrome trials testing low tidal volumes, *Am J Respir Crit Care Med* 166:1510-1514, 2002.
146. Hickling KG, Henderson SJ, Jackson R: Low mortality associated with low volume pressure limited ventilation with permissive hypercapnia in severe adult respiratory distress syndrome, *Intensive Care Med* 16:372-377, 1990.
147. Heyland DK, Groll D, Caeser M: Survivors of acute respiratory distress syndrome: relationship between pulmonary dysfunction and long-term health-related quality of life, *Crit Care Med* 33:1549-1556, 2005.
148. Herridge MS, Cheung AM, Tansey CM et al: One-year outcomes in survivors of the acute respiratory distress syndrome, *N Engl J Med* 348:683-693, 2003.
149. Davidson TA, Rubefeld GD, Caldwell ES et al: The effect of acute respiratory distress syndrome on long-term survival, *Am J Respir Crit Care Med* 160:1838-1842, 1999.
150. McCance KL: Structure and function of the cardiovascular and lymphatic system. In McCance KL, Huether SE, editors: *Pathophysiology: the biologic basis for disease in adults and children,* 5th ed, pp 1029-1079, Baltimore, 2006, Elsevier Mosby.
151. Harbrecht BG, Alarcon LH, Peitzman AB: Management of shock. In Moore EE, Feliciano DV, Mattox KL, editors: *Trauma,* 5th ed, pp 201-226, New York, 2004, McGraw-Hill.
152. Spodick DH: Acute cardiac tamponade, *N Engl J Med* 349:684-690, 2003.
153. Rozycki GS, Feliciano DV, Ochsner MG et al: The role of ultrasound in patients with possible penetrating cardiac wounds: a prospective multicenter study, *J Trauma* 46:543-552, 1999.
154. Rozycki GS, Dente CJ: Surgeon-performed ultrasound in trauma and surgical critical care. In Moore EE, Feliciano DV, Mattox KL, editors: *Trauma,* 5th ed, pp 311-328, New York, 2004, McGraw-Hill.
155. Tenzer ML: The spectrum of myocardial contusion: a review, *J Trauma* 25:620-627, 1985.
156. Weiss RL, Brier JA, O'Connor W et al: The usefulness of transesopageal echocardiography in diagnosing cardiac contusions, *Chest* 109:73-77, 1996.
157. Kaye P, O'Sullivan I: Myocardial contusion: emergency investigation and diagnosis, *Emerg Med J* 19:8-10, 2002.
158. Sybrandy KC, Cramer MJ, Burgersdijk C: Diagnosing cardiac contusion: old wisdom and new insights, *Heart* 89:485-489, 2003.
159. Salim A, Velmahos GC, Jindal A et al: Clinically significant blunt cardiac trauma: role of serum troponin levels combined with electrocardiographic findings, *J Trauma* 50:237-243, 2001.
160. Lindstaedt M, Germing A, Lawo T et al: Acute and long-term clinical significance of myocardial contusion following blunt thoracic trauma: results of a prospective study, *J Trauma* 52:479-485, 2002.
161. Shah P: Heart and great vessels. In Standring S, editor: *Gray's anatomy,* 39th ed, pp 995-1027, Philadelphia, 2005, Elsevier Churchill-Livingstone.
162. Mattox KL, Feliciano DV, Burch J et al: Five thousand seven hundred sixty cardiovascular injuries in 4459 patients. epidemiologic evolution 1958 to 1987, *Ann Surg* 209:698-705, 1989.
163. Buchman TG, Hall BL, Bowling WM et al: Thoracic trauma. In Tintinalli JE, Kelen GD, Stapczynski JS, editors: *Emergency medicine: a comprehensive study guide,* 6th ed, pp 1595-1613, New York, 2003, McGraw-Hill.
164. Brashers VL: Alterations of cardiovascular function. In McCance KL, Huether SE, editors: *Pathophysiology: the biologic basis for disease in adults and children,* 5th ed, pp 1081-1146, Baltimore, 2006, Elsevier Mosby.
165. O'Conor CE: Diagnosing traumatic rupture of the thoracic aorta in the emergency department, *Emerg Med J* 21:414-419, 2004.
166. Mattox KL, Wall MJ, LeMaire SA: Injury to the thoracic great vessels. In Moore EE, Feliciano DV, Mattox KL, editors: *Trauma,* 5th ed, pp 571-591, New York, 2004, McGraw-Hill.
167. Demetriades D, Gomez H, Velmahos GC: Routine helical computed tomographic evaluation of the mediastinum in high-risk blunt trauma patients, *Arch Surg* 1998;133:1084-1088.
168. Collier B, Hughes KM, Mishok K et al: Is helical computed tomography effective for diagnosis of blunt aortic injury? *Am J Emerg Med* 20:558-561, 2002.
169. Cardarelli MG, McLaughlin JS, Downing SW et al: Management of traumatic aortic rupture: a 30-year experience, *Ann Surg* 236:465-470, 2002.
170. Gammie JS, Ashish SS, Hattler BG, et al: Traumatic aortic rupture: diagnosis and management, *Ann Thorac Surg* 66:1295-1300, 1998.
171. Kepros J, Angood P, Jaffe CC et al: Aortic intimal injuries from blunt trauma: resolution profile in nonoperative management, *J Trauma* 52:475-478, 2002.
172. Morgan PB, Buechter KJ: Blunt thoracic aortic injuries: initial evaluation and management, *South Med J* 93:173-175, 2000.
173. Ashbaugh DG, Petty TL, Bigelow DB et al: Continuous positive-pressure breathing (CPPB) in adult respiratory distress syndrome, *J Thor Cardiovasc Surg* 57:31-40, 1969.
174. Kumar A, Falke KJ, Geffin B et al: Continuous positive-pressure ventilation in acute respiratory failure,. *N Engl J Med* 283: 1430-1436, 1970.
175. Winter PM, Smith GS: The toxicity of oxygen, *Anesthesiology* 37:210-241, 1972.
176. Downs JB, Klein EF, Desautels D et al: Intermittent mandatory ventilation: a new approach to weaning patients from mechanical ventilators, *Chest* 64:331-335, 1973.

177. Downs JB, Perkins HM, Modell JH: Intermittent mandatory ventilation, *Arch Surg* 109:519-523, 1974.
178. Petty TL: IMV vs IMC [editorial], *Chest* 67:630-631, 1975.
179. MacIntyre NR: Respiratory function during pressure support ventilation, *Chest* 89:677-683, 1986.
180. Downs JB, Stock MC: Airway pressure release ventilation: a new concept in ventilatory support, *Crit Care Med* 15:459-461, 1987.
181. Stock MC, Downs JB, Frolicher DA: Airway pressure release ventilation, *Crit Care Med* 15:462-466, 1987.
182. Frawley PM, Habashi NM: Airway pressure release ventilation: theory and practice, [erratum appears in *AACN Clin Issues* 13: 2002], *AACN Clin Issues* 12:234-246, 2001.
183. Frawley PM, Habashi NM: Airway pressure release ventilation and pediatrics: theory and practice, *Crit Care Nurs Clin North Am* 16:337-348, 2004.
184. Krishnan JA, Brower RG: High-frequency ventilation for acute lung injury and ARDS, *Chest* 118:795-807, 2000.
185. West JB: *Respiratory physiology: the essentials,* 7 ed, Baltimore, 2005, Lippincott Williams & Wilkins.
186. Murray JF: *The normal lung,* 2nd ed, Philadelphia, 1986, W. B. Saunders.
187. Habashi NM: Other approaches to open-lung ventilation: airway pressure release ventilation, *Crit Care Med* 33(Suppl.): S228-S240, 2005.
188. Brochard L, Mancebo J, Elliot MW: Noninvasive ventilation for acute respiratory failure, *Eur Respir J* 19:712-721, 2002.
189. Caples SM, Gay PC: Noninvasive positive pressure ventilation in the intensive care unit, *Crit Care Med* 33:2651-2658, 2005.
190. Liesching T, Kwok H, Hill NS: Acute applications of noninvasive positive pressure ventilation, *Chest* 124:699-713, 2003.
191. Acton RD, Hotchkiss JR, Dries DJ: Noninvasive ventilation, *J Trauma* 53:593-601, 2002.
192. Thomas AR, Bryce TL: Ventilation in the patient with unilateral lung disease, *Crit Care Clin* 14:743-773, 1998.
193. Karmy-Jones R, Jurkovich GJ, Shatz DV et al: Management of traumatic lung injury: a Western Trauma Association multicenter review, *J Trauma* 51:1049-1053, 2001.
194. Cinnella G, Dambrosio M, Brienza N et al: Independent lung ventilation in patients with unilateral pulmonary contusion: monitoring with compliance and $EtCO_2$, *Intensive Care Med* 27:1860-1867, 2001.
195. Terragni P, Rosboch GL, Corno E et al: Independent high-frequency oscillatory ventilation in the management of asymmetric acute lung injury, *Anesth Analg* 100:1793-1796, 2005.
196. Dreyfuss D, Saumon G: Ventilator-induced lung injury, *Am J Respir Crit Care Med* 157:294-323, 1998.
197. Carney D, DiRocco J, Nieman G: Dynamic alveolar mechanics and ventilator-induced lung injury, *Crit Care Med* 33(Suppl): S122-S128, 2005.
198. Slutsky AS: Lung injury caused by mechanical ventilation, *Chest* 116:S9-S15, 1999.
199. Boussarsar M, Thierry G, Jaber S et al: Relationship between ventilatory settings and barotrauma in the acute respiratory distress syndrome, *Intensive Care Med* 28:406-413, 2002.
200. Wunderlich RJ, Perry A, Lavin MA et al: Patient's perceptions of uncertainty and stress during weaning from mechanical ventilation, *Dimens Crit Care Nurs* 18:8-12, 1999.
201. Cull C, Inwood H: Weaning patients from mechanical ventilation, *Prof Nurse* 14:535-538, 1999.
202. Alia I, Esteban A: Weaning from mechanical ventilation, *Crit Care* 4:72-80, 2000.
203. Mancebo J: Weaning from mechanical ventilation, *Eur Respir J* 9:1923-1931, 1996.
204. MacIntyre NR: Evidence-based guidelines for weaning and discontinuing ventilatory support, *Chest* 120:S375-S395, 2001.
205. Marelich GP, Murin S, Battistella F et al: Protocol weaning of mechanical ventilation in medical and surgical patients by respiratory care practitioners and nurses: effect on weaning time and incidence of ventilator-associated pneumonia, *Chest* 118:459-467, 2000.
206. Randolph AG: A practical approach to evidence-based medicine: lessons learned from developing ventilator management protocols, *Crit Care Clin* 19:515-527, 2003.
207. Burns SM: The science of weaning: when and how? *Crit Care Nurs Clin* 16:379-386, 2004.
208. Tonnelier JM, Prat G, Le Gal G et al: Impact of a nurses' protocol-directed weaning procedure on outcomes in patients undergoing mechanical ventilation for longer than 48 hours: a prospective cohort study with a matched historical group, *Crit Care* 9:R83-R89, 2005.
209. McClean SE, Jensen LA, Schroeder DG et al: Improving adherence to a mechanical ventilation weaning protocol for critically ill adults: outcomes after an implementation program, *Am J Crit Care* 15:299-309, 2006.
210. Yang KL, Tobin MJ: A prospective study of indexes predicting the outcome of trials of weaning from mechanical ventilation, *N Engl J Med* 324:1445-1450, 1991.
211. Jacob B, Chatila W, Manthous C: The unassisted respiratory rate/tidal volume ratio accurately predicts weaning outcome in postoperative patients, *Crit Care Med* 25:253-257, 1997.
212. El-Khatib MF, Jamaleddine GW, Khoury AR et al: Effect of continuous positive airway pressure on the rapid shallow breathing index in patients following cardiac surgery, *Chest* 121:475-479, 2002.
213. Ciesla ND: Chest physical therapy for the adult intensive care unit trauma patient, *Phys Ther Pract* 3:92-108, 1994.
214. Ciesla ND: Chest physical therapy for patients in the intensive care unit, *Phys Ther* 76:609-625, 1996.
215. Lawrence VA, Cornell JE, Smetana GW: Strategies to reduce postoperative pulmonary complications after noncardiothoracic surgery: systematic review for the American College of Physicians, *Ann Intern Med* 144:596-608, 2006.
216. Pasquina P, Tramer MR, Walder B: Prophylactic respiratory physiotherapy after cardiac surgery: systematic review, *BMJ* 327:1379-1385, 2003.
217. Stiller K: Physiotherapy in intensive care: towards an evidence-based practice, *Chest* 118:1801-1813, 2000.
218. Sole ML, Byers JF, Ludy JE et al: A multisite survey of suctioning techniques and airway management practices, *Am J Crit Care* 12:220-230, 2003.
219. O'Neal PV, Grap MJ, Thompson C et al: Level of dyspnea experienced in mechanically ventilated adults with and without saline instillation prior to endotracheal suctioning, *Intensive Crit Care Nurs* 17:356-363, 2001.
220. Celik SA, Kanan N: A current conflict: Use of isotonic sodium chloride solution on endotracheal suctioning in critically ill patients, *Dimens Crit Care Nurs* 25:11-14, 2006.
221. Blackwood B: Normal saline instillation with endotracheal suctioning: primum non nocere (first do no harm), *J Adv Nurs* 29:928-934, 1999.

222. Subirana M, Solà I, Garcia JM et al: Closed tracheal suction systems versus open tracheal systems for mechanically ventilated adult patients [protocol], *Cochrane Database Syst Rev* 3: CD004581, 2003.
223. West JB: *Respiratory physiology: the essentials,* 7th ed, Baltimore, 2005, Lippincott Williams & Wilkins.
224. Kreider ME, Lipsson DA: Bronchoscopy for atelectasis in the ICU: a case report and review of the literature, *Chest* 124:344-350, 2003.
225. Hospital-Acquired Pneumonia Guideline Committee of the American Thoracic Society and Infectious Disease Society of America: Guidelines for the management of adults with hospital-acquired pneumonia, ventilator-associated pneumonia, and healthcare associated pneumonia, *Am J Respir Crit Care Med* 171:388-416, 2005.
226. Chastre J, Fagon J: Ventilator-associated pneumonia, *Am J Respir Crit Care Med* 165:867-903, 2002.
227. Rello J, Ollendorf DA, Oster G et al: Epidemiology and outcomes of ventilator-associated pneumonia in a large US database, *Chest* 122:2115-2121, 2002.
228. American Association of Critical Care Nurses: *Practice alert: ventilator associated pneumonia:* http://www.aacn.org/AACN/practiceAlert.nsf/Files/VAP/$file/VAP.pdf. Accessed June 12, 2006.
229. Furr LA, Binkley CJ, McCurren C et al: Factors affecting quality of oral care in intensive care units, *J Adv Nurs* 48:454-462, 2004.
230. Binkley C, Furr LA, Carrico R et al: Survey of oral care practices in US intensive care units, *Am J Infect Control* 32: 161-169, 2004.
231. Symbas PN: Chest drainage bottles, *Surg Clin North Am* 69:41-46, 1989.
232. Tang AT, Velissaris TJ, Weeden DF: An evidence-based approach to drainage of the pleural cavity: evaluation of best practice, *J Eval Clin Pract* 8:333-340, 2002.
233. Cerfolio RJ, Bryant AS, Singh S et al: The management of chest tubes in patients with a pneumothorax and an air leak after pulmonary resection, *Chest* 128:816-820, 2005.
234. Lawrence DM: Chest tube placement (perform). In Lynn-McHale Wiegand DJ, Carlson KK, editors: *AACN procedure manual for critical care,* 5th ed, pp 125-133, St. Louis, 2005, Elsevier Saunders.
235. Pickett JD: Closed chest drainage system. In Lynn-McHale Wiegand DJ, Carlson KK, editors: *AACN procedure manual for critical care,* 5th ed, pp 151-169, St. Louis, 2005, Elsevier Saunders.
236. Luchette FA, Barrie PS, Oswanski MF et al: Practice management guidelines for prophylactic antibiotic use in tube thoracostomy for traumatic hemopneumothorax: the EAST Practice Management Guidelines Work Group, *J Trauma* 48:753-757, 2000.
237. Cerfolio RJ, Bass C, Katholi CR: Prospective randomized trial compares suction versus water seal for air leaks, *Ann Thorac Surg* 71:1613-1617, 2001.
238. Marshall MB, Deeb ME, Bleier JI et al: Suction versus water seal after pulmonary resection: a randomized prospective study, *Chest* 121:831-835, 2002.
239. Adrales G, Huynh T, Broering B et al: A thoracostomy tube guideline improves management efficiency in trauma patients, *J Trauma* 52:210-216, 2002.
240. Martino K, Merrit S, Boyakye K et al: Prospective randomized trial of thoracostomy removal algorithms, *J Trauma* 46: 369-373, 1999.
241. Bell RL, Ovadia P, Abdullah F et al: Chest tube removal: end-inspiration or end-expiration? *J Trauma* 50:674-677, 2001.
242. Schulman CI, Cohn SM, Blackbourne L et al: How long should you wait for a chest radiograph after placing a chest tube to water seal? A prospective study, *J Trauma* 59:92-95, 2005.
243. Pizano LR, Houghton DE, Cohn SM et al: When should a chest radiograph be obtained after chest tube removal in mechanically ventilated patients? A prospective study, *J Trauma* 53:1073-1077, 2002.
244. Scheinhorn DJ, Chao DC, Stearn-Hassenpflug M: Liberation from prolonged mechanical ventilation, *Crit Care Clin* 18:569-595, 2002.
245. Nevins ML, Epstein SK: Weaning from prolonged mechanical ventilation, *Clin Chest Med* 22:13-33, 2001.
246. Fry DE. Prevention, diagnosis, and management of infection. In Moore EE, Feliciano DV, Mattox KL, editors: *Trauma,* 5th ed, pp 355-381, New York, 2004, McGraw-Hill.
247. Scherer LA, Battistella FD, Owings JT et al: Video-assisted thoracic surgery in the treatment of posttraumatic empyema, *Arch Surg* 133:637-642, 1998.
248. Mandal AK, Thadepalli H, Mandal AK et al: Posttraumatic empyema thoracis: A 24-year experience at a major trauma center, *J Trauma* 43:764-771, 1997.
249. Overend TJ, Anderson CM, Lucy SD et al: The effect of incentive spirometry on postoperative pulmonary complications: a systematic review, *Chest* 120:971-978, 2001.
250. Lawrence VA, Cornell JE, Smetana GW: Strategies to reduce postoperative pulmonary complications after noncardiothoracic surgery: systematic review for the American College of Physicians, *Ann Intern Med* 144:596-608, 2006.

25

ABDOMINAL INJURIES

Kimmith M. Jones

Trauma is the fourth leading cause of death for all age groups in the United States.[1] It is the leading cause of death for individuals between the ages of 1 and 44 years.[1] Abdominal injuries rank third among the causes of traumatic death, preceded only by head and chest injuries.[2] Death and disability from traumatic injury have become a significant health and social problem. Intra-abdominal trauma is seldom a single organ injury or single system injury; therefore, a concomitant rise in morbidity and mortality rates is evident.

There are two injury mechanisms for abdominal trauma: blunt and penetrating. The most common mechanism of blunt injury is a motor vehicle crash. The diagnosis of blunt abdominal injury can be complex and challenging, especially in patients with multisystem injury. Multiple organ involvement, with or without central nervous system depression, can present a complex series of symptoms that cloud normal assessment parameters, making definitive diagnosis more difficult. The presence of abdominal tenderness or guarding, circulatory instability, lumbar spine injury, pelvic fracture, retroperitoneal or intraperitoneal air, or unilateral loss of the psoas shadow on radiographic examination should raise the question of visceral damage.

Abdominal trauma challenges even the most experienced nurse. The manifestations of abdominal injury are often subtle, requiring continual assessment and care modification as the patient progresses from the initial assessment to the critical care phase. Frequent assessments and continual monitoring are essential components of the nursing process for detection of changes in the patient's condition. Unrecognized abdominal trauma is a frequent cause of preventable death.[3] An organized, methodical approach to assessment, diagnosis, and intervention is necessary for the management of suspected abdominal injury. Knowledge of the mechanism of injury, patient complaints, serial physical assessments, and timely diagnostic test results are the nurse's resources for identifying potentially life-threatening abdominal injuries.

THE ABDOMEN: ANATOMY AND PHYSIOLOGY

The abdomen is formally thought of as containing structures bordered superiorly by the diaphragm, inferiorly by the pelvis, posteriorly by the vertebral column, and anteriorly by the abdominal and iliac muscles (Figure 25-1). For this discussion of abdominal trauma, the esophagus, which passes through the diaphragm and connects with the stomach, has been added to this chapter.

The peritoneal cavity contains the stomach, small intestine, liver, gallbladder, spleen, transverse colon, sigmoid colon, upper third of the rectum, and, in women, the uterus. Retroperitoneal structures include the ascending and descending colon, kidneys, pancreas, adrenal glands, aorta, vena cava, part of the duodenum, and other major vessels.

For purposes of examination, the abdomen is divided into four quadrants: right upper quadrant (RUQ), left upper quadrant (LUQ), right lower quadrant (RLQ), and left lower quadrant (LLQ). The major organs found in each quadrant are highlighted in Figure 25-2.

ESOPHAGUS

The esophagus, the first segment of the digestive process, carries food from the pharynx to the stomach. The presence of food within the esophagus stimulates peristaltic action and causes food to move into the stomach. Mucosal glands of the esophagus secrete mucus to lubricate and facilitate passage of the food bolus.[4]

The esophagus traverses the posterior mediastinum of the thorax through the esophageal hiatus in the central tendon of the diaphragm to join the stomach at the level of the tenth thoracic vertebra. The posterior surface of the intra-abdominal esophagus overlies the aorta, and the anterior surface is covered by peritoneum. The anterior and posterior vagus nerves pass through the esophageal hiatus. There are three areas of narrowing that predispose the esophagus to injury: at the cricoid cartilage, at the arch of the aorta, and as it passes through the diaphragm. The esophageal wall lacks a serosal layer, which may affect the integrity of anastomoses, increasing the chance for leaking after surgical repair.

DIAPHRAGM

The diaphragm assists with inspiration and expiration by changing the thoracic volume during respiration. Flattening and contraction of the diaphragm lengthen the thoracic cavity, increasing thoracic volume during inspiration.[5] During expiration the diaphragm relaxes, returning to its original dome shape and reducing thoracic volume.[5] This process is aided by the accessory intercostal muscles. The diaphragm

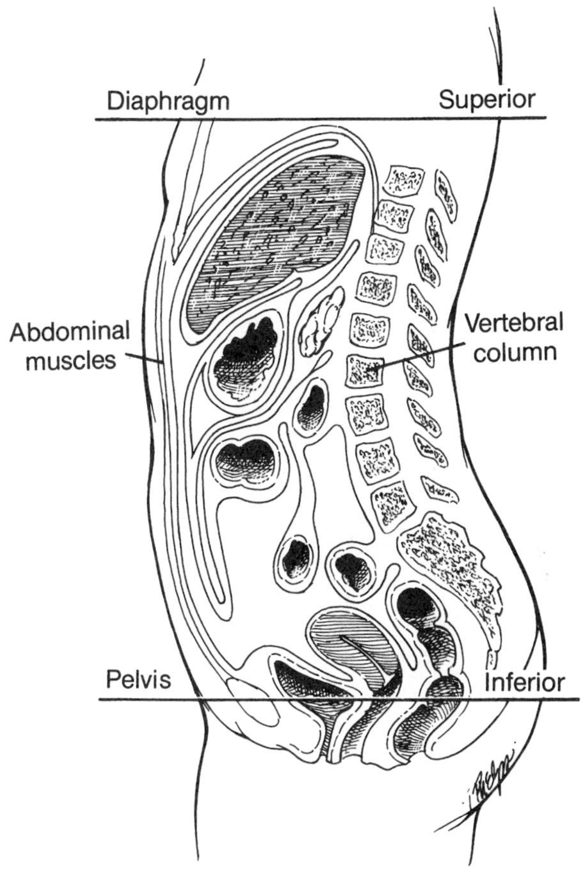

FIGURE 25-1 The abdominal boundaries.

also separates the thoracic and abdominal cavities, preventing herniation of organs.

The diaphragm is a musculotendinous, dome-shaped structure attached posteriorly to the first, second, and third lumbar vertebrae; anteriorly to the lower sternum; and laterally to the costal margins dividing the thoracic and abdominal regions. There are three foramina. The aorta passes through the diaphragm at the T12 level, the esophagus passes through at the T10 level, and the vena cava foramen is at T8. The phrenic nerve, which innervates the diaphragm, passes through the thorax along the posterolateral aspect of the pericardium on both sides and divides into anterior and posterior branches. Any damage to the spinal cord between the third and fifth cervical vertebrae may disrupt the phrenic nerve and therefore paralyze the diaphragm.

STOMACH

The stomach has multiple digestive functions, including (1) serving as a reservoir to store food, (2) secreting gastric juice containing acids and enzymes to aid in the digestion of food, (3) secreting intrinsic factor, (4) carrying on a limited amount of absorption of certain drugs, alcohol, some water, and some short-chain fatty acids, and (5) producing the hormone gastrin, which helps regulate digestive functions.[5]

The stomach joins the esophagus approximately 3 cm below the diaphragm. It is located in the LUQ and is suspended superiorly by the gastrohepatic ligament, inferiorly by the gastrocolic ligament, and laterally by the gastrosplenic ligament. The stomach resides within the peritoneal cavity. It is divided into the fundus, body, and pylorus (Figure 25-3). The stomach wall contains glands that secrete mucus, hydrochloric acid (HCl), intrinsic factor, and pepsinogen (type I); serotonin is secreted in the fundus and body; and mucus and pepsinogen II are secreted in the pylorus. Perforating gastric injury causes the release of these digestive contents into the peritoneal cavity. These same gastric secretions cause stress ulcerations in the stomach.

The stomach has a rich blood supply. The arterial supply is provided by the splenic artery, gastric arteries, gastroepiploic arteries, and short gastric arteries (Figure 25-4). Venous drainage occurs through the hepatic portal system, which branches out to include the gastric and the gastroepiploic veins, which drain into the splenic vein. Gastric emptying is facilitated by peristaltic movement from the pylorus and is stimulated by stretch receptors. An inhibiting function is controlled in the duodenum.

LIVER

The liver, the largest gland in the body, performs many vital, life-sustaining functions, including those listed below[4]:

- Detoxification of various substances, such as drugs and alcohol
- Synthesis of plasma proteins, important in maintaining blood volume and controlling blood coagulation
- Storage of iron and vitamins A, D, E, K, and B_{12} in liver cells
- Metabolism of carbohydrates, which has a role in regulating blood glucose levels
- Metabolism of protein, which can synthesize amino acids and converts nitrogen to urea for excretion by the kidneys
- Metabolism of fats, which breaks down fatty acids, synthesizes cholesterol and phospholipids, and converts excess dietary protein and carbohydrates to fat
- Phagocytosis of bacteria by Kupffer cells

The liver is the largest intra-abdominal organ, weighing approximately 3 to 4 pounds. It is an extremely vascular organ and lies in the RUQ, extending transversely across the midline. The right margin lies at the sixth to tenth ribs and the left margin at the seventh and eighth ribs (Figure 25-5). The liver is divided into two lobes, right and left, which are separated by fissures on the inferior surface. Between these two lobes is the porta hepatis, where veins, arteries, nerves, lymphatic vessels, and bile ducts enter or leave the liver.

Approximately three fourths of the blood to the liver is delivered by the portal vein, which carries a rich supply of nutrients after draining the gastrointestinal tract. The rest of the arterial blood supply is rich in oxygen and enters

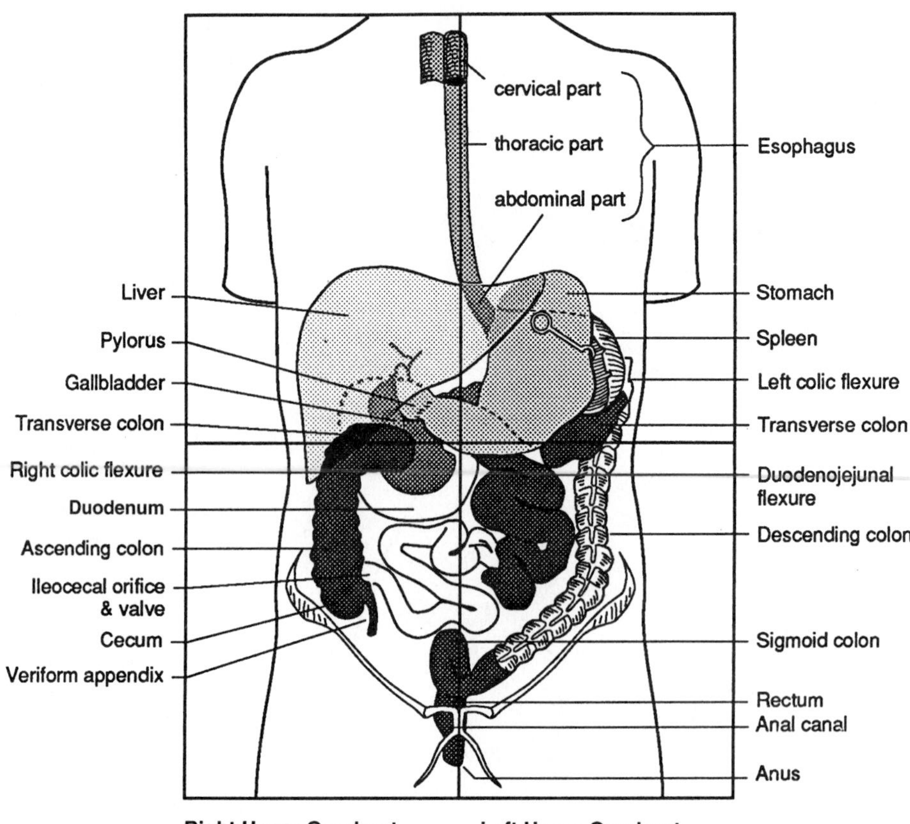

Right Upper Quadrant
Liver and gallbladder
Pylorus
Duodenum
Head of pancreas
Right adrenal gland
Portion of right kidney
Hepatic flexure of colon
Portions of ascending and transverse colon

Left Upper Quadrant
Left lobe of liver
Spleen
Stomach
Body of pancreas
Left adrenal gland
Portion of left kidney
Splenic flexure of colon
Portions of transverse and descending colon

Right Lower Quadrant
Lower pole of right kidney
Cecum and appendix
Portion of ascending colon
Bladder (if distended)
Ovary and salpinx
Uterus (if enlarged)
Right spermatic cord
Right ureter

Left Lower Quadrant
Lower pole of left kidney
Sigmoid colon
Portion of descending colon
Bladder (if distended)
Ovary and salpinx
Uterus (if enlarged)
Left spermatic cord
Left ureter

Loops of small bowel are found in all quadrants

FIGURE 25-2 Contents of the four abdominal quadrants. (Modified from *GI series—physical examination of the abdomen,* Richmond, Va, 1975, AH Robins, p 6.)

through the hepatic artery. Each lobule (Figure 25-6) has a central vein, which collects the mixture of blood from the portal vein and hepatic artery and channels blood to the lobular veins, which empty into the hepatic vein and then into the inferior vena cava. Surgical repair can be complicated after trauma to the liver because of the rich vascular supply. Uncontrolled hemorrhage is the primary cause of early death after liver trauma.

Hepatocytes produce bile, which is essential to the digestion of fats. Bile flows from the hepatic cells into bile canaliculi between the cells toward the periphery of the lobule and empties into the interlobular bile ducts of the hepatic triad. The ducts join, forming the common hepatic duct, which allows bile to flow into the gallbladder. The gallbladder lies on the inferior surface of the liver. Its duct, the cystic duct, meets with the hepatic duct to form the common bile duct, which drains through the head of the pancreas into the duodenum (see Figure 25-6).

SPLEEN

The spleen is a lymphoid organ with various functions including defense, hematopoiesis, and red blood cell (RBC) and platelet destruction; it also serves as a reservoir for blood. Macrophages line the spleen and break apart hemoglobin molecules from the destroyed RBCs, salvaging the iron and

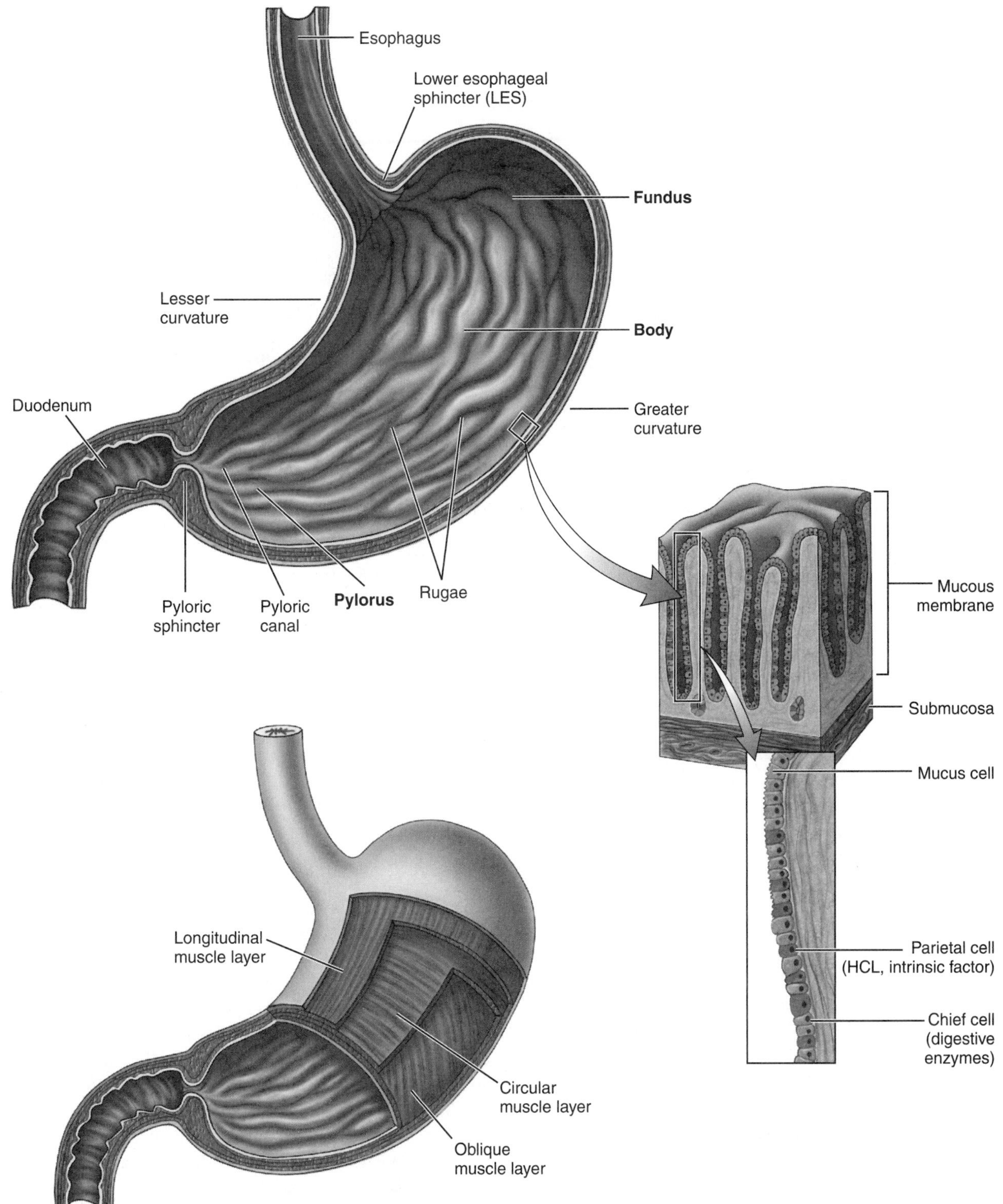

FIGURE 25-3 Stomach: regions of the stomach: fundus, body, and pylorus. *HCL,* Hydrochloric acid. (From Herlihy B, Maebius NK: *The human body in health and illness,* Philadelphia, 2000, W. B. Saunders, p 394.)

globin content and returning them to the bloodstream for storage in the bone marrow and liver.[5]

The total circulation of the spleen is estimated at 250 ml/min, with a normal volume of approximately 350 ml.[5] This is an impressive blood volume considering that the average weight of the spleen is 150 g. The spleen's volume can be reduced to 200 ml very quickly after sympathetic stimulation, which causes constriction of the smooth muscle capsule. This response to stress can be a result of hemorrhage.[5]

The spleen is an elongated ovoid body located in the LUQ of the abdomen. It lies beneath the diaphragm, to the left of the stomach, and in immediate proximity to the tail of the

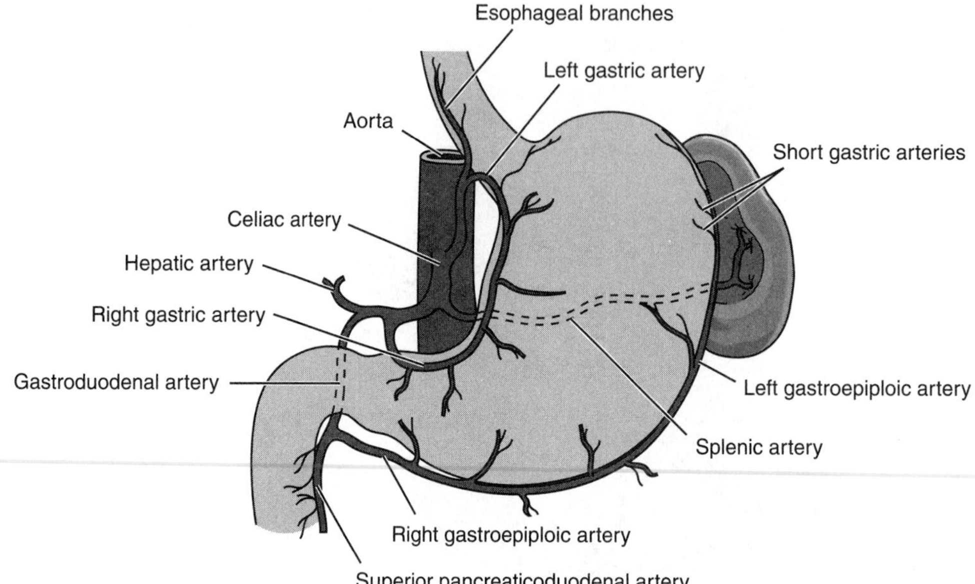

FIGURE 25-4 Arterial supply to the stomach. All the arteries are derived from branches of the celiac artery. (From Snell RS, Smith MS: *Clinical anatomy for emergency medicine,* St. Louis, 1993, Mosby, p 419.)

pancreas, the colon, and the left kidney. It is in close proximity to ribs 7 through 10, which makes it vulnerable to injury when ribs are fractured.

The spleen's blood supply is from the splenic artery, which enters at the hilum and divides into five or six branches before entering splenic pulp (Figure 25-7). The splenic vein originates outside the hilum and courses along the dorsal pancreatic surface to join the superior mesenteric vein, forming the portal vein. The vascular nature of the spleen makes it a ready source for profuse bleeding into the peritoneal cavity after injury.

The splenic capsule, 1 to 2 mm thick, encloses the splenic pulp. Lymphoid tissue lies throughout the pulp and is responsible for filtration. The blood supply to the pulp is from arterioles off a central artery. The blood collects in a venous sinus and then moves to trabecular veins coursing to the main splenic veins and finally to the portal circulation (Figure 25-7, *B*). Arterial blood travels to venous sinuses through splenic cords (connective tissue between sinuses) and "sieves" RBCs, destroying many in the process. The spleen's sieving process promotes it as a primary defense organ to remove microorganisms from the blood and destroy them by phagocytosis.

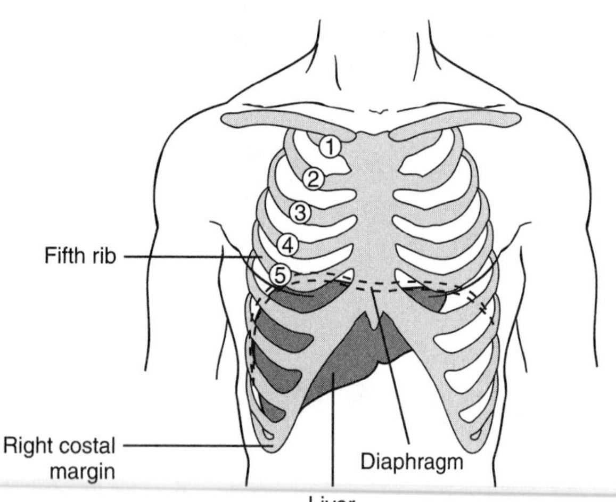

FIGURE 25-5 Anatomic location of the liver. The upper border normally lies at the level of the fourth intercostal space or fifth rib, and the lower border does not normally extend more than 1 to 2 cm below the right costal margin. (From Clochesy JM, Breu C, Cardin S et al: *Critical care nursing,* 2nd ed, Philadelphia, 1996, W. B. Saunders, p 1048.)

PANCREAS

The pancreas is composed of both exocrine and endocrine glandular tissue. The exocrine pancreas secretes enzymes that digest protein, carbohydrates, and fats. These enzymes include trypsin, chymotrypsin, carboxypeptidase, α-amylase, and lipase. The endocrine pancreas produces two hormones: glucagon from the α cells and insulin from the β cells (Figure 25-8). These hormones facilitate the formation and cellular uptake of glucose.

The pancreas lies at the level of the first lumbar vertebra against the posterior abdominal wall. It extends from the C-loop of the duodenum to the hilum of the spleen. A blunt trauma episode can force the pancreas against the vertebral column and may rupture it. The pancreas is divided into lobules that empty into the main pancreatic duct, which passes through the tail, body, neck, and head of the pancreas, emptying into the duodenum at the ampulla of Vater in conjunction with the common bile duct (see Figure 25-8, *A*). An accessory duct empties into the duodenum from the head of the pancreas. Rupture of the pancreas frequently tears its ductal system, allowing pancreatic juice (rich in digestive enzymes) to invade pancreatic tissue and the peritoneum.

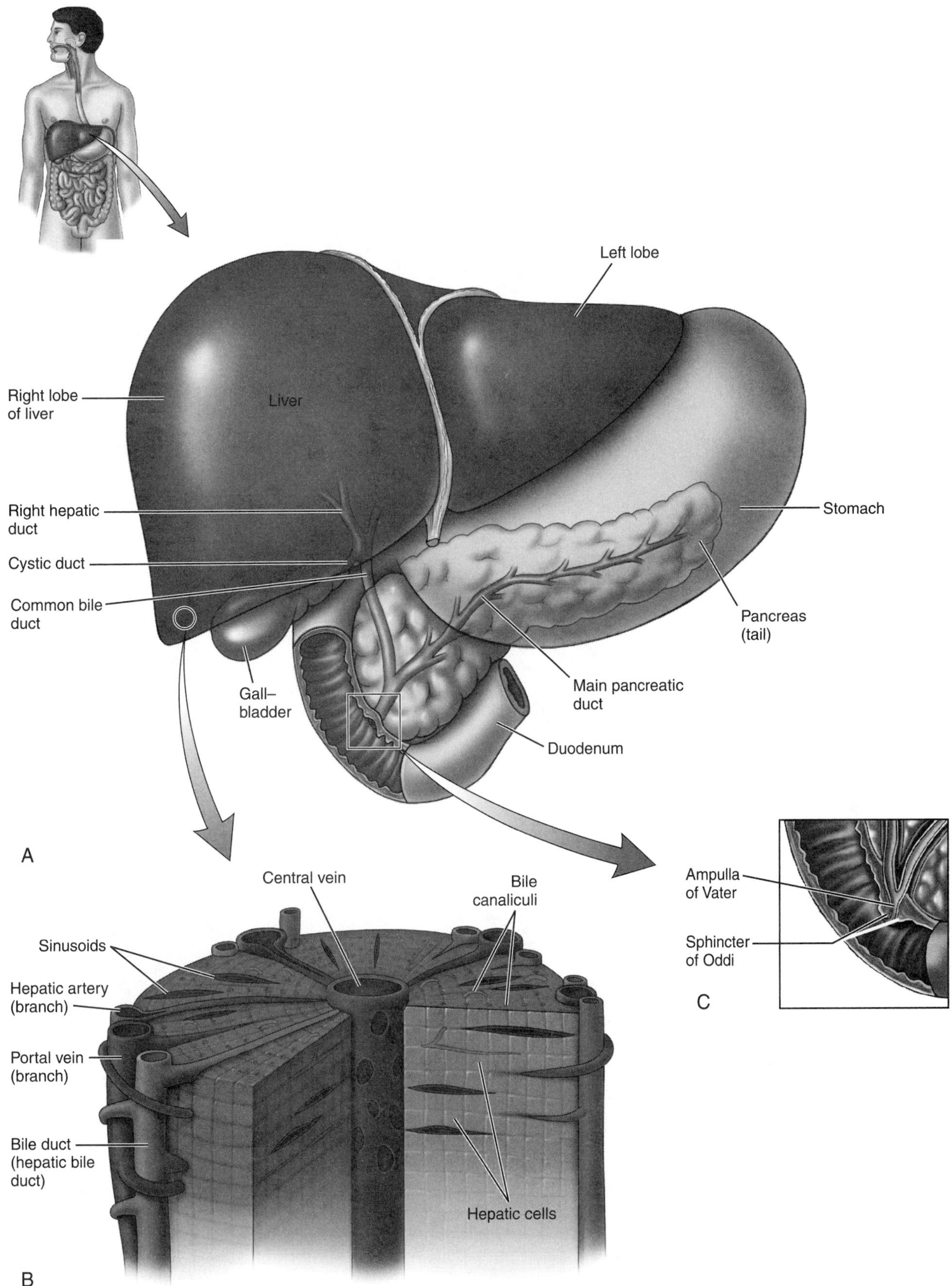

FIGURE 25-6 **A,** Relationship of liver, gallbladder, and pancreas to the duodenum. **B,** Liver lobule, the functional unit of the liver. Note the blood flow into the liver through the portal vein and hepatic artery. **C,** Ampulla of Vater. (From Herlihy B, Maebius NK: *The human body in health and illness,* Philadelphia, 2000, W. B. Saunders, p 402.)

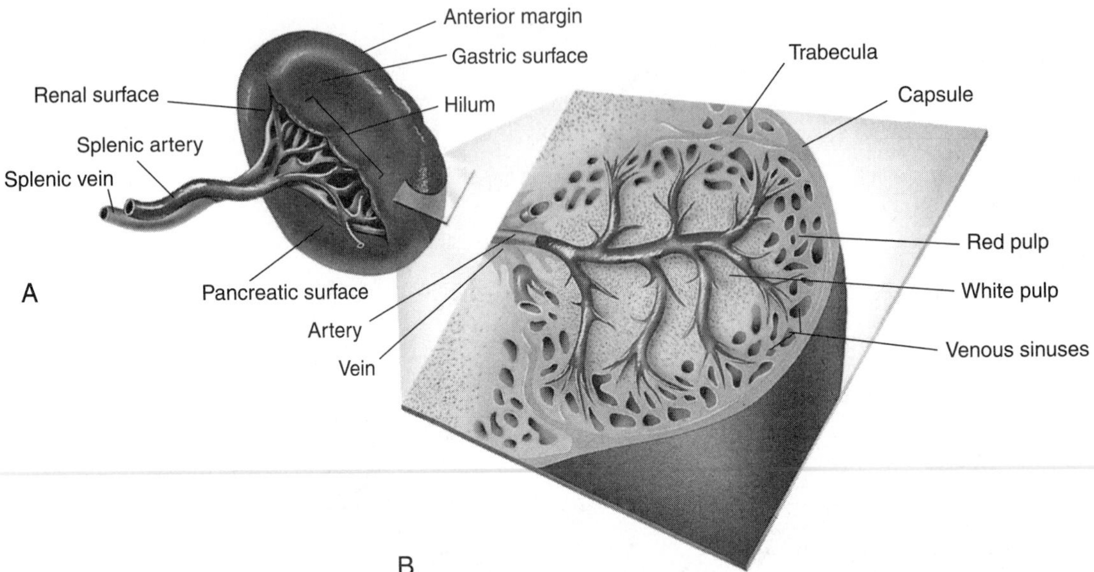

FIGURE 25-7 The vascular supply of the spleen. **A,** Medial aspect of the spleen. **B,** Section showing the internal organization of the spleen. (From Thibodeau GA, Patton KT: *Anatomy and physiology,* 4th ed, St. Louis, 1999, Mosby, p 635.)

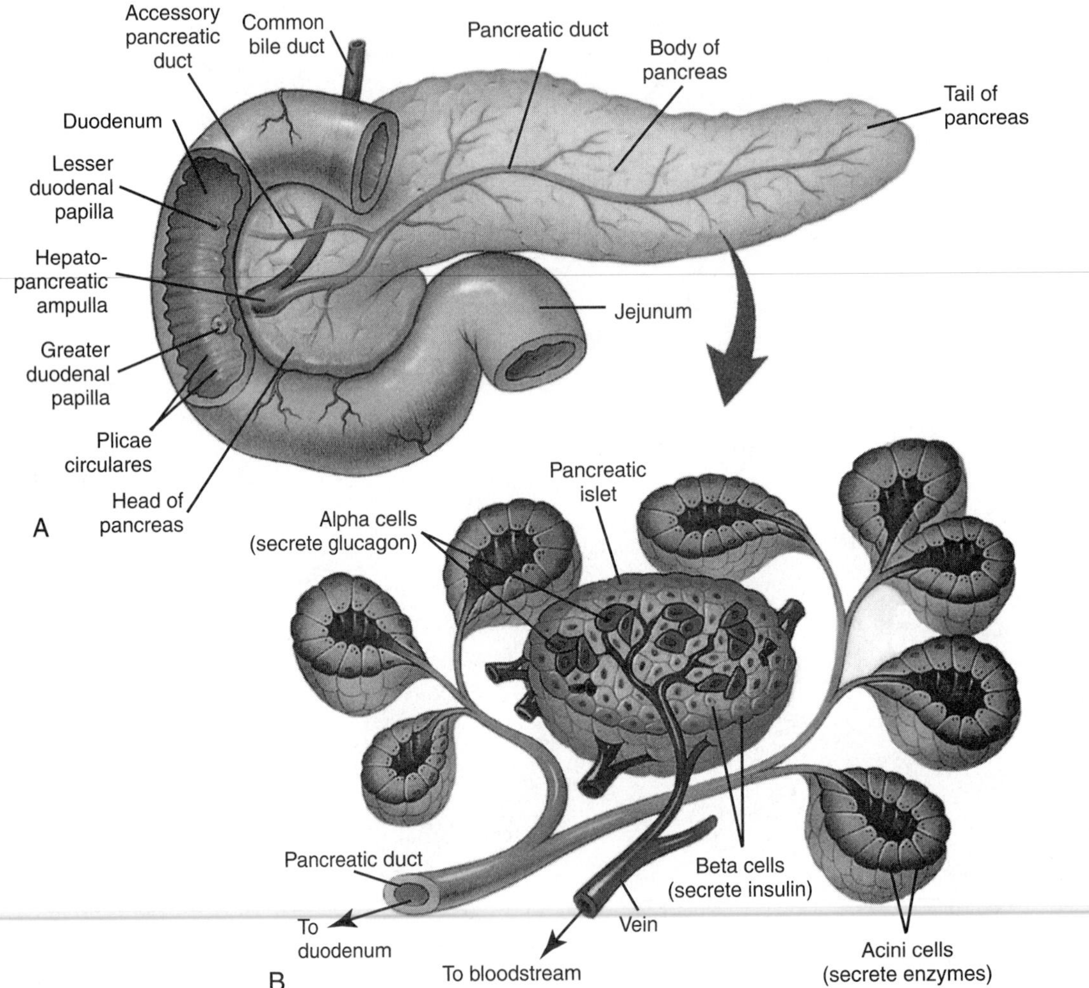

FIGURE 25-8 Pancreas. **A,** Pancreas dissected to show main and accessory ducts. **B,** Exocrine glandular cells (around small pancreatic ducts) and endocrine glandular cells of pancreatic islets (adjacent to blood capillaries). Exocrine pancreatic cells secrete pancreatic juice, alpha endocrine cells secrete glucagon, and beta cells secrete insulin. (From Thibodeau GA, Patton KT: *Anatomy and physiology,* 4th ed, St. Louis, 1999, Mosby, p 755.)

Blood is supplied by the splenic artery and vein and the superior mesenteric artery and vein. Venous drainage from the body and tail of the pancreas occurs through the splenic vein to the portal vein; the head empties directly into the portal vein.

SMALL INTESTINE

The 21 to 23 feet of small intestine are divided into duodenum, jejunum, and ileum (Figure 25-9). The major functions are digestion of food and absorption of nutrients and water for the body. The blood supply is from the superior mesenteric artery. Venous drainage is to the portal vein through the superior mesenteric vein.

Duodenum

Most digestion and absorption occur within the duodenum. The duodenum, the first part of the small intestine, is a C-shaped loop approximately 25 cm long molded around the head of the pancreas (Figure 25-10). Beginning at the pyloric valve junction, the duodenum receives the highly acidic chyme from the stomach and fluids, enzymes, and electrolytes from the biliary and pancreatic ducts.

The duodenum is divided into four segments, with only the superior portion residing within the peritoneal cavity. The remaining segments, descending, transverse, and ascending, are located in the retroperitoneum. Rapid deceleration injuries may lead to rupture between the anchored and free segments of the duodenum. Three fourths of this organ lies over the vertebral column, which renders it vulnerable to compression injuries.

The blood supply to the duodenum is shared with the pancreas through the superior and inferior pancreaticoduodenal artery. After injury this makes removal of the entire pancreas impossible without devascularizing the duodenum. Drainage occurs through the superior mesenteric veins, which drain into the portal veins and gastrocolic trunk.

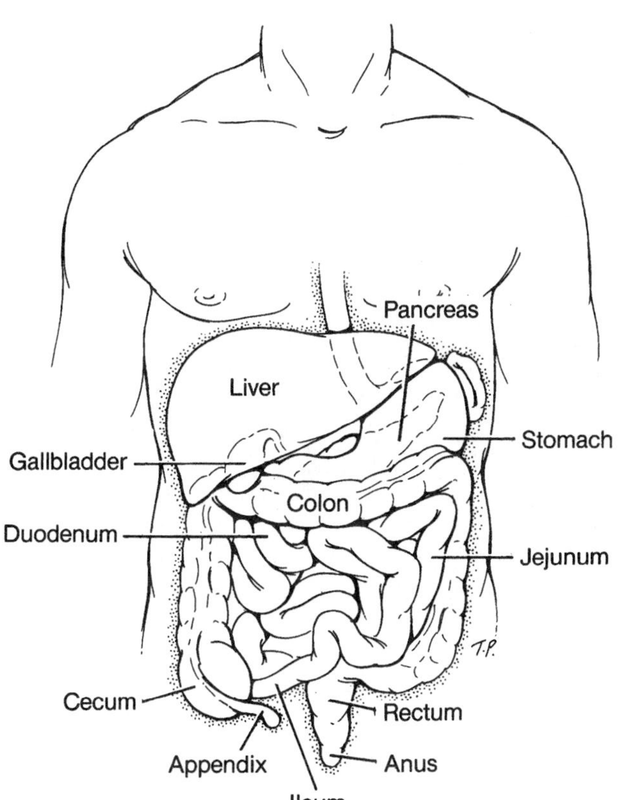

FIGURE 25-9 The small intestine: duodenum, jejunum, and ilium in relationship to other abdominal structures.

Jejunum and Ileum

From the duodenal jejunal flexure (ligament of Treitz) to the ileocecal junction, the jejunum and ileum are responsible for nutrient absorption and fluid and electrolyte shifts. Peristalsis originating in the duodenum continues through the jejunum and ileum. Some absorption takes place in the jejunum; bile salts and vitamin B_{12} are absorbed in the terminal ileum. Intestinal fluid shifts from the gastrointestinal lumen to the vascular system. All but 0.5 to 1 L of fluid is absorbed in the small intestine, and the remaining fluid passes through to the large intestine.

Most of the jejunum lies in the umbilical region of the abdomen, and the ileum is in the hypogastric and pelvic regions. This expansive placement makes the small intestine vulnerable to injury from lap seat belts or when the bowel is crushed between vertebrae and a solid object such as a steering wheel.

LARGE INTESTINE

The large intestine's digestive functions include (1) absorption of water and electrolytes, (2) synthesis of certain vitamins by the intestinal bacterial, especially vitamin K and the B vitamins, (3) temporary storage of intestinal waste, and (4) elimination of body waste. Peristaltic waves move intestinal material from the cecum through the entire colon to the rectum. Substances that increase intestinal motility cause a decrease in water absorption, resulting in diarrhea. Consequently, substances administered to decrease motility cause an increase in water absorption, leading to constipation.

The bacterial content of feces is high, but bacterial species in the intestinal tract are natural. One of these bacteria is *Escherichia coli.* These bacteria are important in the synthesis, for example, of vitamins K and B complex. They cause serious problems if they enter the bloodstream or urinary system, but they are not detrimental when contained within the intestinal tract.

The cecum, colon, and rectum constitute the large intestine. The colon is divided into ascending, transverse, descending, and sigmoid segments (Figure 25-11). The ileum joins the large intestine at the junction of the cecum and ascending colon. The ileocecal valve permits slow movement of intestinal contents through the cecum and colon. The cecum and ascending colon are continuous from the ileum and rise to the undersurface of the right lobe of the liver, bending to the left at the hepatic flexure and becoming the transverse segment. This segment continues across to the splenic flexure

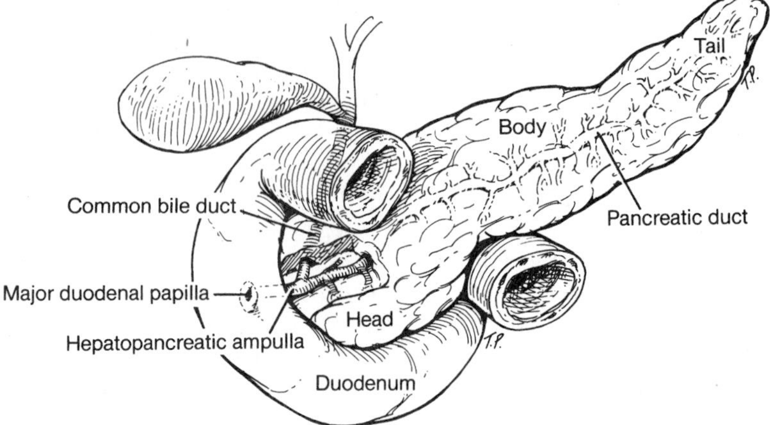

FIGURE 25-10 Duodenal location in relation to the pancreas.

(anterior to the left kidney) and then turns downward to become the descending colon. The sigmoid colon, the S-shaped segment, courses from the left iliac fossa to the pelvic cavity, becoming the rectum and terminating at the anal canal. The rectum forms the last 17 to 20 cm of the intestinal structures. The final inch is called the anal canal, and its opening is the anus. The anus is controlled by two sphincter muscles, which are closed except during defecation.

The blood supply to the colon and rectum is predominantly from the superior and inferior mesenteric arteries arising from the abdominal aorta (Figure 25-12). Blood from the large intestine drains through the portal vein to sinusoids in the liver.

Abdominal Vascular System

Arterial Supply

The descending aorta passes through the diaphragm at the T12-L1 level to become the abdominal aorta. At the L4 level the aorta bifurcates into the two common iliac arteries. It

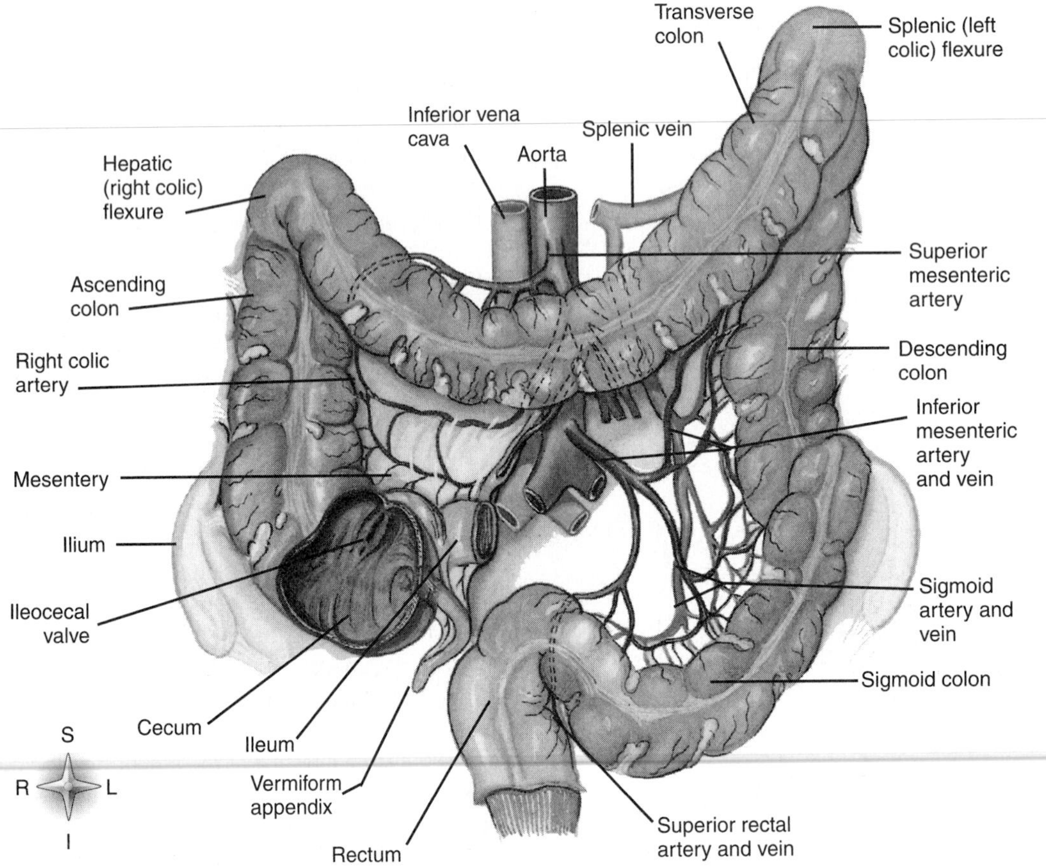

FIGURE 25-11 Divisions of the large intestine. (From Thibodeau GA, Patton KT: *Anatomy and physiology,* 4th ed, St. Louis, 1999, Mosby, p 747.)

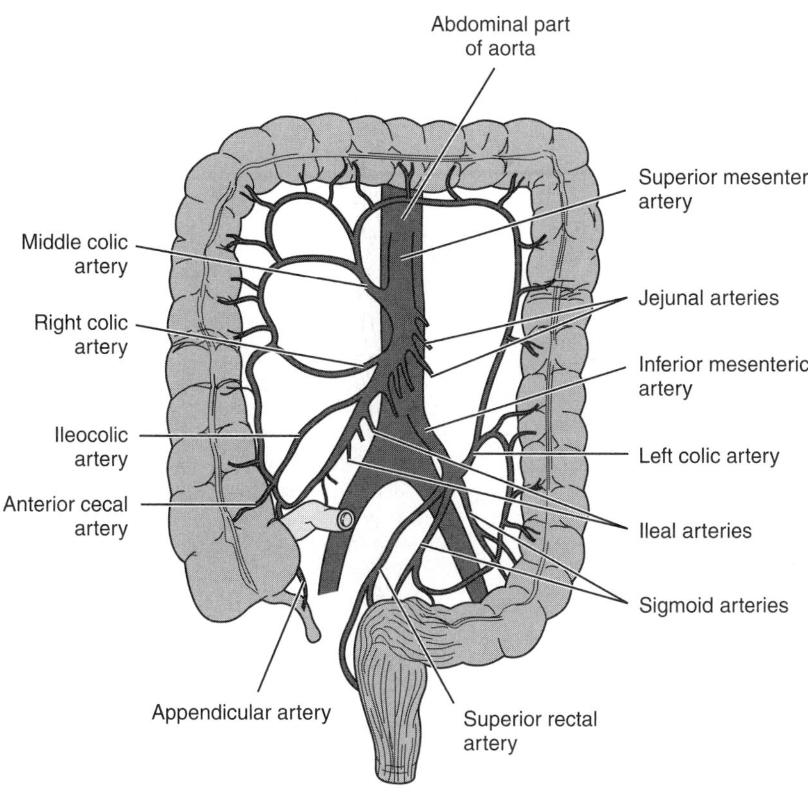

FIGURE 25-12 Arterial supply to the small and large intestines. Note the branches of the superior and inferior mesenteric arteries. (From Snell RS, Smith MS: *Clinical anatomy for emergency medicine,* St. Louis, 1993, Mosby, p 423.)

further divides into external and internal iliac arteries. Finally, the external iliac becomes the common femoral artery (Figure 25-13).

Major branches of the aorta include (1) the celiac axis at the T12 level, which divides into the left gastric artery, the splenic artery, and the common hepatic artery, (2) the superior mesenteric artery at the L1 level, dividing into the middle colic artery and the inferior ileocolic artery, (3) the renal arteries at the L2 level, which supply the kidneys directly, and (4) the inferior mesenteric artery at the L3-4 level, dividing into the left colic artery and the superior hemorrhoidal artery. Because of this rich blood supply, any injury to the lower chest or abdomen may induce vascular trauma with widespread effects.

Venous Drainage

Venous drainage of the abdomen is more complex than the arterial supply. Blood is drained from the small intestines, stomach, spleen, and pancreas through the superior mesenteric and splenic veins and their tributaries, which join to form the portal vein. This blood then passes through liver sinusoids, supplying nutrients to hepatocytes before emptying into lobular veins and then into the hepatic veins, which empty into the inferior vena cava.

Other abdominal venous flow (Figure 25-14) originates in the external iliac veins in the inguinal ligament, which are joined by internal iliac veins to form the common iliac veins, which become the inferior vena cava at the sacral promontory. The renal veins join the inferior vena cava at the L2 level. Other smaller veins join the inferior vena cava as it passes to the superior margin of the liver. Much of the inferior vena cava lies in close proximity to the aorta, making injury to one vessel likely to affect the other.

MECHANISM OF INJURY

Mechanism of injury refers to the mechanisms by which energy is transferred from the environment to a person. Energy sources may be mechanical, thermal, electrical, or chemical. Examples include mechanical energy from a motor vehicle crash, thermal energy from a fire, electrical energy from contact with a high-voltage wire, and chemical energy from contact with hydrofluoric acid. Mechanical energy is the most common mechanism of injury in motor vehicle crashes, automobile-pedestrian collisions, falls, stabbings, and gunshot wounds (GSWs). Knowledge of the mechanism of injury is paramount to rapid and efficient diagnosis and treatment of traumatic injuries.

The mechanism of injury and forces involved direct attention toward certain organ involvement and should heighten a clinician's suspicion regarding certain injuries. Blunt injury from a motor vehicle crash results from a compression or crushing mechanism and involves three collisions. In the first collision the motor vehicle hits a stationary object. For example, a frontal impact may crush the driver's compartment, causing direct injury to the driver or passengers. The second collision occurs when the victim hits internal parts of the vehicle, including the windshield, steering wheel, or dashboard. The third collision involves the supporting structures of the body (e.g., skull, ribs, spine, pelvis)

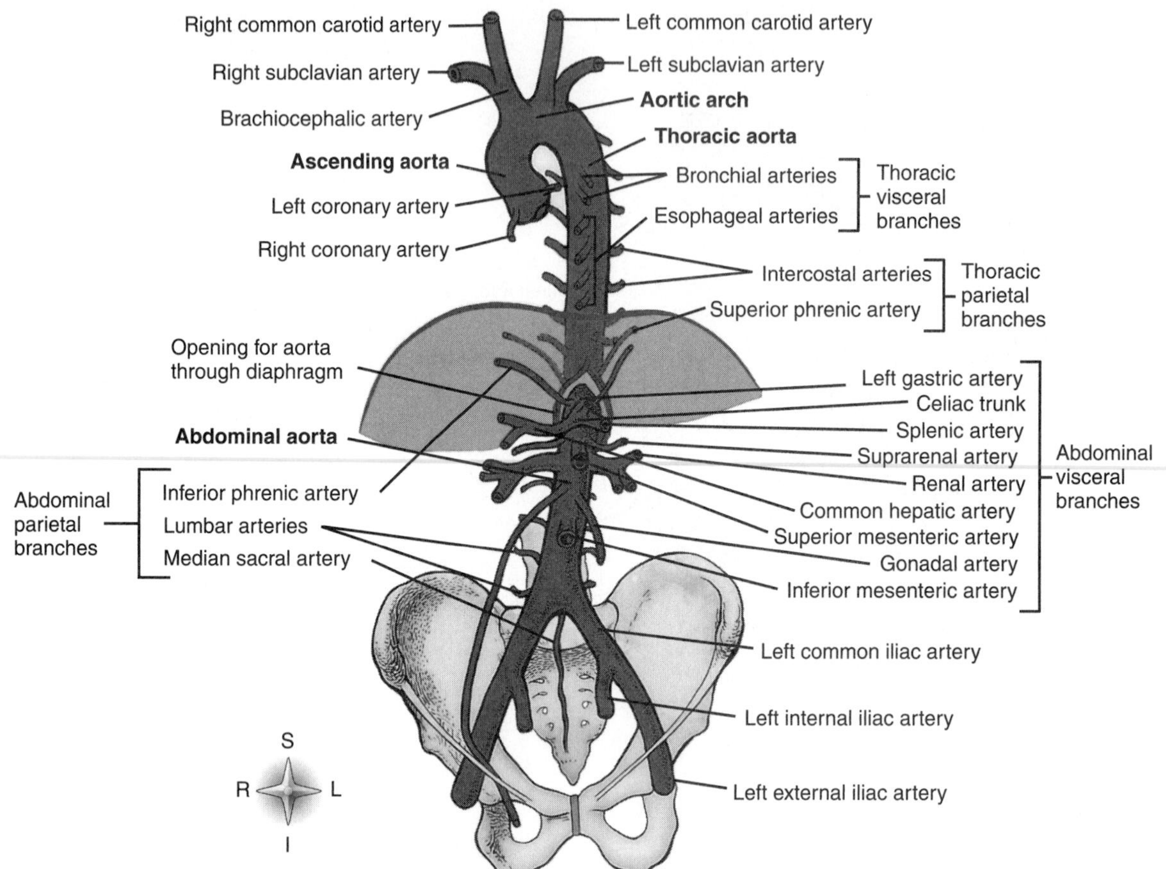

FIGURE 25-13 Abdominal aorta and branches. The aorta is the main systemic artery, serving as a trunk from which other arteries branch. Blood is conducted from the heart first through the ascending aorta, then the arch of the aorta, and then through the thoracic and abdominal segments of the descending aorta. (From Thibodeau GA, Patton KT: *Anatomy and physiology,* 4th ed, St. Louis, 1999, Mosby, p 569.)

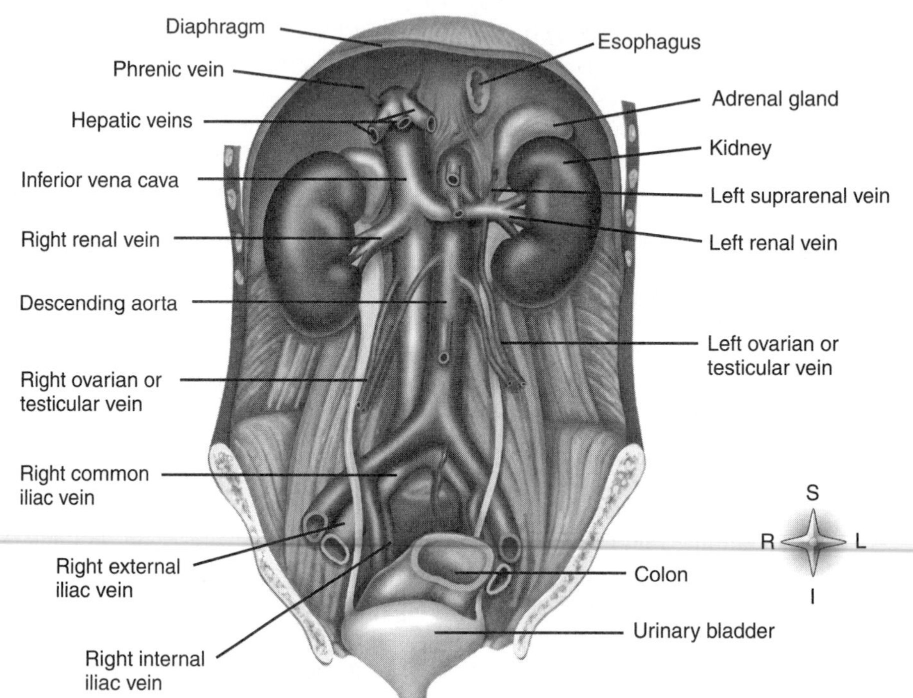

FIGURE 25-14 Inferior vena cava and abdominal blood supply. (From Thibodeau GA, Patton KT: *Anatomy and physiology,* 4th ed, St. Louis, 1999, Mosby, p 576.)

and movable organs (e.g., brain, heart, liver, intestines). As energy is loaded onto the body, internal forces (e.g., stress and strain) are exerted within the body as the dimensions of body tissues change. These forces can be further classified as tensile (stretch), shearing (opposing forces across an object), or compressive (crush). The types of injuries that result from these forces include spleen or liver rupture, comminuted bone fractures, and tearing of the aorta.

The types of forces involved (rotational, crushing, shearing, acceleration, deceleration, or blast) should be investigated. A pedestrian struck by a motor vehicle can suffer acceleration forces and shearing forces, resulting in a closed head injury or degloving injury as layers of tissue are torn away from attachments. The descending thoracic aorta and the duodenum are two anatomic locations susceptible to injury from this type of force. A direct blow to the abdomen may transmit forces sufficient to rupture an organ.

The increased use of restraining devices, such as safety belts and air bags, has reduced fatal outcomes and serious injury, but they certainly cannot prevent injury entirely. Seat belts have been associated with blunt cervical, thoracic, abdominal, and extremity injuries. The addition of the shoulder harness to the lap belt has decreased craniofacial, thoracic, and abdominal injuries; however, classic seat belt injuries include abdominal wall disruption, hollow viscus injury, and flexion-distraction fracture of the lumbar vertebrae (Chance fracture). Some abdominal wall injuries (ecchymosis) arise from direct seat belt injury. Small bowel and colon injuries occur most frequently from a sudden increase in intraluminal pressure or shearing forces caused by rapid deceleration. Liver, spleen, and pancreatic injuries are reported as well, but with less frequency.

Penetrating trauma may occur from a stabbing, impalement, or missile event. The size, shape, and length of the stabbing instrument help to estimate intra-abdominal damage. Management is frequently dictated by the degree of penetration into the peritoneal cavity. Impalement injuries are a dirty form of stab wound that result in high mortality rates as a result of bacterial contamination and multiple organ involvement (Figure 25-15).

Missile injuries are more difficult to evaluate. Mortality rates depend on major vessel disruption and multiple organ involvement. The terminal velocity, or the amount of energy imparted to the tissue by the missile, often determines the extent of injury. The incidence of significant abdominal injury related to firearms ranges from 68% to 94%.[6] The wide variation in percentage may be due to differences in how the wounds were categorized. The magnitude of entrance and exit wounds may bear little relationship to the degree of damage or the course of destruction caused by a bullet. Bullets may ricochet off organs or bones, roll or move throughout the body, or embolize through the vessels. Organs in proximity to the GSW may be injured by a blast effect. Quick evaluation of the situation is necessary because hemorrhage and hollow viscus perforation resulting in chemical and bacterial peritonitis are major problems in this type of abdominal trauma. The extent of tissue destruction varies depending on velocity, type of weapon or bullet, and individual tissue characteristics; therefore, abdominal wounds and their complications have a wide range of presentations.

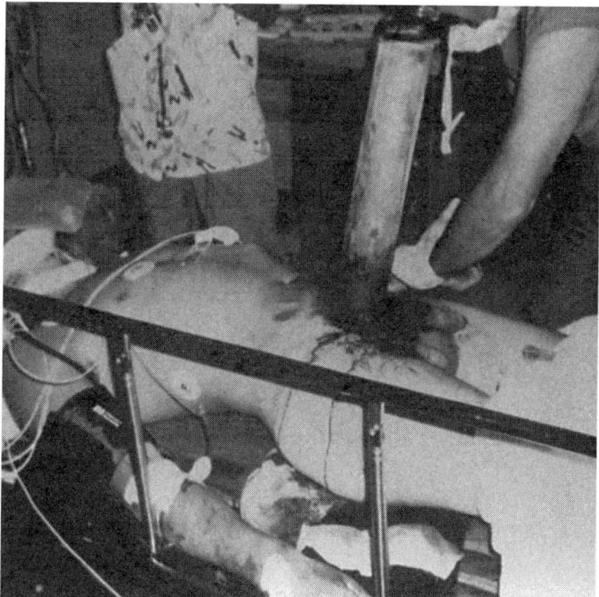

FIGURE 25-15. Impalement event. Young man impaled by wooden fence rail, which entered the abdomen through the peritoneum.

The mechanism of injury involved in blunt and penetrating trauma provides the nurse with valuable information necessary for quick diagnostic interventions and treatment of patients with potential abdominal injury. A clean versus dirty or open versus closed injury often dictates medical management and subsequent nursing care. The nurse can anticipate what diagnostic modalities will be used, the need for antibiotics, and the potential for emergency surgery.

Abdominal Assessment

Abdominal injury may be insidious, requiring close, systematic assessment by all team members to promote early diagnosis and intervention. Multiple pieces of data are collected during patient assessment; each has little value when considered alone. However, monitoring these data and correlating the findings with information about the mechanism of injury, diagnostic test results, and the patient's physical findings assist in directing the patient's medical care.

A primary survey addressing the airway (A), breathing (B), circulation (C), and disabilities (D) is initiated on the patient's arrival in the emergency department (ED). A quick assessment to identify and treat life-threatening conditions is crucial to good trauma patient outcomes. The ABCDs are evaluated constantly throughout all phases of care to determine the effectiveness of treatment. Oxygen administration, vascular access, intravenous fluid administration, cardiac monitoring, and pulse oximetry are required for all trauma patients during the resuscitation phase.

A brief systematic secondary survey is the next step in the resuscitation phase. A head-to-toe assessment is completed to identify all injuries. During this process the nurse and various other team members are simultaneously assessing, providing interventions, and reassessing the patient. The secondary survey includes obtaining a complete set of vital signs, ordering laboratory studies, placing a gastric tube and urinary catheter, performing a complete neurologic examination, and obtaining more information about the patient. Diagnostic testing can occur simultaneously during the primary and secondary survey, including bedside ultrasonography (US), computed tomography (CT), diagnostic peritoneal lavage (DPL), and chest radiograph.

Although an abdominal assessment is not part of the primary survey, an abdominal injury necessitating immediate surgical intervention must be identified early. Continual assessment of the abdomen as part of the secondary survey can occur only after life-threatening events have been managed. This allows the nurse to move on to a continuous, complete re-evaluation and subsequent care.

The process for gathering patient information begins as soon as the patient arrives in the ED. Prehospital personnel should provide information regarding the circumstances of the traumatic event. Such information should include mechanism of injury, injuries sustained, vital signs, and treatment initiated, along with patient response. Nursing assessment includes patient-generated information such as the patient's complaints on arrival in the ED, medical and surgical history, medications, allergies, time of last meal, and use of drugs or alcohol.

The physical examination is systematic and continues through all phases of care. Repeated examination by the same nurse or physician provides the consistency necessary to evaluate changes. The physical examination should be adapted to the patient's hemodynamic status. Certainly an unstable patient with a penetrating abdominal wound does not need a prolonged, detailed physical examination; rather, prompt, appropriate intervention is indicated.

A complaint of abdominal pain from an alert patient is a key indicator of abdominal injury. Peritoneal irritation is described as sharp, localized pain. Referred pain complaints may signal damage to the spleen (left shoulder pain), liver (right shoulder pain), or retroperitoneal structures (back or testicular pain). Many patients who sustain abdominal injuries may not be able to participate in the physical examination because of alterations in level of consciousness or spinal cord injury; therefore, the four-step abdominal examination, consisting of inspection, auscultation, percussion, and palpation, is essential.

Inspection

Inspection begins with noting lower chest wall integrity. Because the last six ribs lie over abdominal structures, disruption to this area may signal organ damage, specifically to the liver, spleen, or diaphragm.

The appearance of the abdomen should be described. The presence of abrasions, contusions, lacerations, and surgical scars and the location, size, description, and number of wounds should be documented. In patients who have been shot, an odd number of wounds indicates the presence of a foreign object within the body. The nurse should resist the temptation to categorize wounds as entrance and exit wounds.

The abdominal contour, normally flat or slightly rounded (or convex in a heavy patient), may be distended, which is indicative of an accumulation of blood, other fluid, or gas resulting from perforation of hollow viscus, rupture of organs (e.g., liver or spleen), or reduced blood supply to the abdomen. Repeated inspection by the nurse may reveal subtle signs of distention, which, combined with absence of bowel sounds, may be indicative of an ileus, peritonitis, or intra-abdominal bleeding.

Involuntary guarding indicates injury to underlying structures. This may be less obvious or not present in patients with retroperitoneal injury. The presence of discoloration, protuberances, peristaltic movement, pulsations, abrasions, and old surgical scars should be noted. Repeated inspection alerts the nurse to new discolorations or other changes indicative of underlying injury. Dissection of blood into the abdominal wall from retroperitoneal tissue (Grey Turner's sign) may occur several hours after the initial injury. Proper inspection includes examining the patient's back and flank area and the anterior surface for the signs mentioned. Obvious wounds or ecchymosis of the lumbar or flank areas may indicate damage to retroperitoneal or abdominal organs.

Auscultation

Auscultation is often the most difficult part of the abdominal examination during resuscitative or critical care efforts simply because of the noise created by team members performing lifesaving procedures. The presence or absence of bowel sounds on initial examination is nonspecific information in patients with suspected abdominal injury.[7] While auscultating in all four quadrants, the nurse should be alert for the presence of bowel sounds in unlikely locations, such as the chest cavity, which may indicate a diaphragmatic tear. In serial auscultation, diminished or absent bowel sounds may indicate an ileus or peritonitis. The nurse should listen for bruits, especially over the renal arteries, abdominal aorta, and iliac arteries, which may indicate partially obstructed arterial blood flow.

Percussion

Percussion identifies the presence of air, fluid, or tissue. Tympanic sounds indicate air-filled spaces such as stomach or gut, and a dull sound is present over organ structures such as the liver or spleen.

Dullness throughout the four quadrants indicates free fluid in the abdomen. Fixed areas of dullness (Ballance's sign) in the LUQ may suggest a subcapsular or extracapsular hematoma of the spleen or flank. Dullness that does not change with position suggests the presence of retroperitoneal hematoma. Tympanic percussion may represent air in the abdominal cavity, indicative of perforated viscus. A diaphragmatic tear or hemothorax may be suspected if a dull sound is elicited over the otherwise tympanic thoracic space.

Palpation

Abdominal tenderness is evaluated by using the whole hand over all four quadrants and progressing from light to deep palpation. Tenderness is the most frequent and reliable sign of intra-abdominal injury. Gentle palpation may elicit areas of increased tone or tenderness, suggesting underlying injury. Abdominal wall injury produces focal tenderness, which increases on exertion (tensing muscles). Deep palpation is used to elicit tenderness, guarding, and rebound symptoms associated with peritoneal irritation.

A tender abdomen with guarding, distention, and signs of peritoneal irritation can indicate organ rupture. RUQ tenderness and guarding or tenderness over the right lower six ribs may indicate liver damage. RUQ abdominal tenderness may also be a sign of duodenal or gallbladder injury. Pain elicited in the LUQ may indicate injury to the spleen, stomach, or pancreas. Low abdominal or suprapubic discomfort may signal a potential for colon, bladder, or urethral injuries and may be associated with pelvic fractures.

The patient may have referred pain. Most common among these is Kehr's sign, pain in the left shoulder from diaphragmatic irritation by blood after splenic rupture. Right shoulder pain is often indicative of liver injury. The patient must be lying flat or in Trendelenburg's position to elicit this type of shoulder pain.

Rectal examination includes testing for gross blood and anterior tenderness, which can indicate bleeding or peritoneal irritation. Positive results may indicate lower gastrointestinal injury.

Diminished or absent pulses in the femoral arteries may indicate common iliac artery thrombosis, dissecting aortic aneurysm, or chronic vascular disease. Information about the quality and rate of pulses during the initial assessment provides the clinician with good baseline information.

Continuing Assessment

The four-step systematic physical examination continues during all phases of care. Inspection includes the same assessment techniques; however, changes detected in the examination may be a result of the operative event, late signs of traumatic injury, or sepsis. A chemical ileus caused by late pancreatic rupture or gastric repair leakage distends the bowel and therefore the abdomen. Either the bowel sounds are obliterated or a hypertympanic sound is heard during auscultation.

Careful serial examination of the patient is the key to early diagnosis of intra-abdominal injuries and prevention of complications. Discolorations around a repair site may indicate vessel rebleeding into an area. A wound may appear dark or collect excess cloudy exudate and imply an infection.

Small diaphragmatic tears may be missed during the original operative procedure or simply not manifest until days or weeks after the original injury. Therefore, auscultation of the chest and abdomen should continue periodically for the presence of bowel sounds.

Physiologic and psychologic stress from the trauma may induce gastric mucosal erosion over time, leading to gastrointestinal bleeding. Abdominal distention, pain, and tenderness are noticed as the erosion progresses. However, no physical symptoms may be appreciated until bleeding is evident. This event can occur at any time throughout the phases of trauma care. Therefore, vigilant, systematic physical assessment is required as the patient advances from admission through rehabilitation.

Diagnostic Studies

Many diagnostic modalities can be used to evaluate the patient with abdominal trauma, including computed tomography (CT), ultrasonography (US), and diagnostic peritoneal lavage (DPL). Each tool has its own particular advantages. To optimize evaluation of the trauma patient, these tools should be considered complementary rather than mutually exclusive. Accuracy, speed, and safety should be the factors that drive the clinician's decision regarding the most appropriate diagnostic modality.

Computed Tomography

CT has been used for almost two decades in the assessment of patients with blunt abdominal trauma. CT is one of two main diagnostic choices for the initial evaluation of blunt abdominal trauma,[8] the other being the focused abdominal sonography for trauma (FAST). CT is used in combination with serial clinical examinations and the trending of laboratory data to evaluate patients with known or suspected abdominal injury. It has replaced DPL as the primary screening tool for the hemodynamically stable trauma patient.

This noninvasive procedure provides information about multiple abdominal organs, including intra-abdominal and retroperitoneal structures, and furnishes a rough estimate of the amount of blood in the peritoneal, retroperitoneal, and pelvic spaces. Surgeons can use abdominal CT information to grade solid organ lacerations, such as those of the liver and spleen, thus aiding them in the decision regarding operative or nonoperative management. It has limited diagnostic value in patients with penetrating abdominal trauma.

The limitations of CT can restrict its usefulness. Those limitations include cost, time involved in conducting the test, transport of the patient out of the resuscitation area, and inability to diagnose certain injuries, such as those in the bowel or diaphragm. Most important, the patient must be hemodynamically stable and able to cooperate for the examination.

CT is considered the best approach for identifying sites of injury and amount of hemorrhage, but it may miss mesenteric and hollow-organ injuries.[8,9] The diagnostic sensitivity is reported to be between 92% and 97.6% with a specificity as high as 98.7%.[8] The sensitivity and accuracy may be related to the experience of the technician performing the scan, the quality of the imaging equipment, and the experience of the radiologist.[8]

Instillation of oral contrast adds additional time to the CT procedure and puts the patient at risk of aspiration or allergic reaction. Several experts suggest that oral contrast is not necessary for diagnostic accuracy; they point out that its use only delays CT scanning and therefore may contribute to morbidity or mortality rates.[10,11]

Ultrasonography

US for the evaluation of abdominal trauma has been used in Europe and Japan for more than a decade. FAST can be used as the initial diagnositic choice for hemodynamically stable or unstable patients.[3,8]

US is a reliable, fast, and safe modality with a high degree of sensitivity and specificity in detecting peritoneal free fluid or hemoperitoneum.[8,12] Advantages of US include ready access to the necessary equipment, portability, noninvasiveness, cost-effectiveness, and the ability to do serial examinations; in addition, it does not require patient transport out of the resuscitation area. It can be performed simultaneously with physical examination, resuscitation, and stabilization within minutes of the patient's arrival in the trauma suite.

The benefits of US have been so compelling that the American College of Surgeons' Committee on Trauma has included US in their algorithm for the assessment of patients with blunt abdominal trauma.[3] The sensitivity of US for identification of free fluid is 73% to 88%, its specificity is 98% to 100%, and its accuracy is 96% to 98%.[8] In a study of war casualties, authors cited an US sensitivity of 86% to 88%, a specificity of 100%, an accuracy of 95% to 97%, a positive predictive value of 100%, and a negative predictive value of 91% to 96%.[13]

Although advocated as a screening tool for potential abdominal injuries, US is not intended to replace DPL or CT. Limitations of US include unreliable results in obese patients and in patients with ascites or subcutaneous emphysema.[9] As with DPL and CT, US is limited in its ability to detect diaphragmatic, intestinal, and pancreatic injury. Interpretation and accuracy of US results are dependent on the clinician's experience in using the US machine.

FAST is recommended for evaluation of hemoperitoneum in patients who have sustained blunt abdominal trauma.[8,9,12] Identification of hemoperitoneum or fluid in the abdomen by US entails examination of the following areas: Morison's pouch (RUQ), pericardial sac, splenorenal (LUQ), and pelvis (Douglas' pouch) (Figure 25-16).

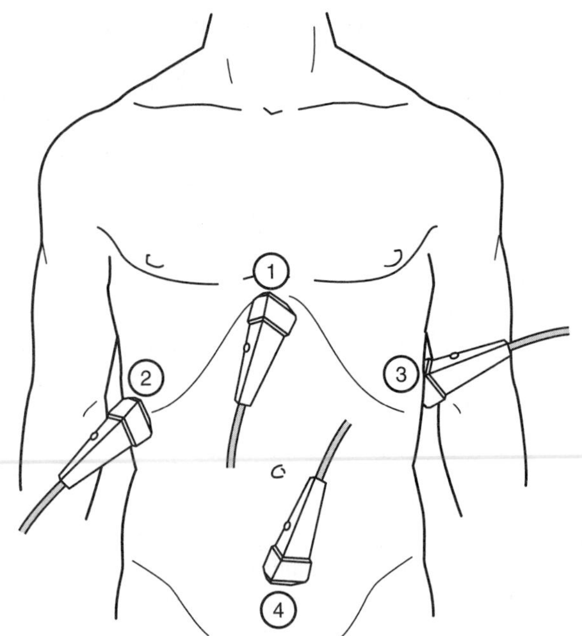

FIGURE 25-16. Ultrasound evaluation and sequence. *1*, Pericardial (subxiphoid); *2*, Morison's pouch (RUQ); *3*, splenorenal (LUQ); *4*, pelvis (Douglas' pouch). (Modified from Rozycki GS, Ballard RB, Feliciano DV et al: Surgeon-performed ultrasound for the assessment of truncal injuries, *Ann Surg* 228:557, 1998.)

Visualization of the RUQ allows evaluation of the right liver lobe, right kidney, and retroperitoneal space. LUQ examination allows visualization of the spleen and perisplenic fluid, intrathoracic fluid, left kidney, and retroperitoneal space. Examination of the epigastrium area can detect abnormalities of the pancreas or left liver lobe and pericardial fluid. Anterior pelvis examination allows visualization of the prostate, uterus, bladder, and lateral pelvic walls. US can identify hemoperitoneum from liver injuries in Morison's pouch and splenic injuries in the pericolic gutter, two areas where fluid accumulates from injuries to these organs.

US should be recognized as one tool in the evaluation of abdominal trauma and not the sole determinant for management. US findings can aid in defining diagnostic and management priorities during resuscitation.

Diagnostic Peritoneal Lavage

DPL is a diagnostic procedure used in the resuscitation phase of care to diagnose intra-abdominal bleeding in the hemodynamically unstable trauma patient.[8] DPL has a sensitivity rate of greater than 95% for identifying intraperitoneal hemorrhage. DPL is nonspecific in identifying the source of bleeding. Other indications for use include (1) unexplained hypotension, decreased hematocrit, or shock, (2) equivocal results of abdominal examination, (3) altered mental status caused by closed head injury or alcohol or drug intoxication, (4) spinal cord injury, and (5) distracting injuries such as major orthopedic fractures or chest trauma.[6] DPL is a simple, low-cost, safe test for quick and accurate determination of intra-abdominal hemorrhage.[9,14] Although sensitive and relatively accurate, it is not specific for type or extent of organ damage. In the patient who is hemodynamically unstable, a grossly positive lavage mandates an exploratory laparotomy without further diagnostic workup.[8]

Despite its advantages, DPL has several limitations. It is difficult to perform in patients who are morbidly obese, in those who have had numerous laparotomies, and in women in the third trimester of pregnancy. It is an invasive procedure that poses a risk of omental laceration and visceral or vascular perforation during trocar insertion. DPL can miss certain abdominal injuries, such as those of the bowel, diaphragm, or retroperitoneal structures. Injury may elude detection because there is little bleeding, insufficient fluid is retrieved, the injury is isolated by adhesions, or the DPL is performed early in the resuscitative phase and injury has not yet declared itself, such as with bowel or pancreatic injury.

The use of DPL for some penetrating injuries, specifically stab wounds, is advocated by several authors, but more research is needed to determine its role in the evaluation of GSWs.[6] The current management practice for most patients with an abdominal GSW is immediate surgical intervention.

Before any DPL procedure is performed, a Foley catheter should be placed to empty the bladder and a gastric tube inserted to decompress the stomach. This reduces the risk of unintentional gastric or bladder perforation when the DPL catheter is inserted. After catheter insertion, and if less than 10 ml of gross blood is aspirated, 1 L of crystalloid (lactated Ringer's solution or 0.9% normal saline solution) is infused into the peritoneal space. Warmed crystalloid should be infused to prevent hypothermia and to decrease peritoneal irritation. After completion of the infusion, the intravenous (IV) bag is placed in a dependent position to allow fluid return by gravity. A sample of the effluent is sent to the laboratory for analysis.

Interpretation of DPL results is based on whether the mechanism is blunt or penetrating. Criteria for a positive DPL in blunt trauma are 10 ml or more of gross blood on aspiration, an RBC count of 100,000/mm^3 or more, a white blood cell (WBC) count of 500/mm^3 or more after the intra-abdominal infusion of 1 L of crystalloid, and the presence of bile or fibers[6] (Table 25-1).

DPL is used in the evaluation of stab wounds when local exploration reveals penetration of the peritoneal cavity. The RBC criterion for a positive sign of injury remains controversial. Some surgeons have lowered the limit to 5,000 to 1,000/mm^3 to enhance sensitivity to injury.

TABLE 25-1 Peritoneal Lavage Results for Blunt Trauma

	Result	Indication
Aspirant	Gross blood >10 ml	Positive
	Pink fluid	Intermediate*
	Clean	Negative
Lavage fluid	Bloody	Positive
	Clear	Negative
RBCs	>100,000 cells/mm^3	Positive
	50,000-100,000 cells/mm^3	Intermediate*
WBCs	>500 cells/mm^3	Positive
	100-500 cells/mm^3	Intermediate*
Amylase	>175 units/100 ml	Positive
	75-175 units/100 ml	Intermediate*
	<75 units/100 ml	Negative
Bacteria	Present	Positive
Fecal material	Present	Positive
Bile	Present	Positive
Food particles	Present	Positive

*Intermediate lavage results require further observation of the patient, possibly repeated lavage, and intervention on the basis of clinical presentation.

Diagnostic Laparoscopy

Diagnostic laparoscopy (DL) is emerging as a screening tool in the evaluation of trauma patients. It can be used to detect or exclude findings of hemoperitoneum, organ injury, intestinal spillage, or peritoneal penetration that may require a laparotomy. Left penetrating thoracoabdominal trauma is the only clear indication for DL. Patients who sustain a left penetrating thoracoabdominal injury have diaphragm involvement 42% of the time.[6] Direct visualization of intraperitoneal structures such as the diaphragm to rule out rupture may reduce the rate of laparotomies resulting in negative findings.

This invasive procedure has several limitations, most notably its unproven accuracy and high cost. DL cannot be used to visualize the extent or depth of a liver or splenic injury and does not allow visualization of the retroperitoneal space, thus providing only limited information for diagnosing injuries. However, there have been reports of the limited usefulness of DL in the evaluation of penetrating abdominal trauma.[14] Further studies are required to determine its full applicability in diagnosis and treatment during trauma resuscitation.

Radiographic Films

In general, plain film radiographs have a limited role in the diagnosis of abdominal injuries. Chest radiography is used as a primary screening tool and serves to identify concomitant pulmonary or cardiac injuries and abdominal organ displacement. It can also indicate whether the pleural cavity is an obvious source of major blood loss and serves as an aid in establishing a baseline for respiratory care. Thoracic injuries are frequently associated with abdominal injuries, particularly in patients with GSWs or multisystem injuries.

Anteroposterior supine abdominal films and left lateral decubitus films may reveal the presence of intraperitoneal fluid or air or alteration in visceral contours. The examiner may note the presence of a foreign body or determine the trajectory of missiles. On an upright film, inspection for free air may disclose a ruptured hollow viscus. Skeletal structure damage should increase suspicion of damage to certain organs (e.g., liver and splenic injuries often occur with fractures of the lower ribs). Distortion of the outlines of intra-abdominal organs may indicate subcapsular hematoma or hemorrhage or may be due to fluid or gas collections.

Plain films should not be used as the sole method for diagnosing abdominal injuries. Normal or negative abdominal films do not exclude significant intra-abdominal injury. The minimal volume of intraperitoneal blood that can be detected radiographically is 800 ml. Radiographic films should be used with physical examination and other diagnostic tools, such as CT, US, or DPL, in making an accurate diagnosis.

Other Diagnostic Studies

Angiography is used infrequently in evaluating abdominal injuries. It is most helpful in patients who are actively bleeding as a result of vascular trauma. In patients who have sustained penetrating injury it can be used to detect arteriovenous fistulas, false aneurysms, and arteriobiliary fistulas. Interventional radiology is particularly useful for embolization of vasculature and in patients with unstable pelvic fractures with unrelenting hemorrhage.

Gastrointestinal studies using meglumine diatrizoate (Gastrografin) or barium are helpful in diagnosing injury to the esophagus, stomach, bowel, or diaphragm. Contrast enemas are used to diagnose rectal or colon injury resulting from penetrating trauma.

Endoscopic retrograde cholangiopancreatography may be indicated in the stable trauma patient with suspected biliary tract or pancreatic duct injury. It can be used to determine the exact site of ductal injury and the need for surgical intervention. This is the most accurate test to determine injury in the patient with hyperamylasemia who is being observed and in the patient with abdominal complaints after pancreatic surgery.

Retrograde urethrograms or cystograms are used when a patient is suspected of having injury to the bladder or urethra. A quick, one-shot IV pyelogram (IVP) may be indicated in the unstable patient requiring emergency surgical intervention; however, CT scan of the abdomen provides a much clearer delineation of renal anatomy and injuries. IVP is also recommended if CT is not available.

Nursing Management During Radiographic Studies

Most radiographic studies use some form of contrast, and the nurse should be alert to signs and symptoms of allergic reaction. With the first signs of rash, hives, flushing of the skin, or itching, the nurse should immediately contact the physician. A number of multisystem trauma patients require multiple radiologic studies during the resuscitative and critical care phases and thus receive large doses of IV radiographic contrast. The nurse should monitor the patient's hydration status, urine output, and creatinine level as the kidneys clear the IV contrast. The physician may order a bolus of IV fluid to ensure clearance of the IV contrast, thus decreasing the risk of renal insult. Acetylcysteine (Mucomyst) may also be ordered to reduce the risk of compromised renal function caused by use of contrast agents.[15]

Laboratory Data

Laboratory results may not be of value in the early phase of resuscitation but may have more utility when used in conjunction with the patient's clinical findings. Laboratory testing should be individualized to each patient's clinical presentation.

Hemoglobin and Hematocrit

The initial hemoglobin (Hb) and hematocrit (HCT) determinations do not usually reflect the amount of hemorrhage, but they serve as a baseline value during the resuscitative phase. The frequency of Hb and HCT measurements is usually dictated by the patient's hemodynamic stability. Serial values offer valuable data for assessing continuing bleeding and are used with other assessment parameters through all phases of care.

Leukocyte Counts

Elevated WBC counts are part of the body's normal response to trauma; therefore, this value is of little significance early in the trauma cycle. However, detection of neutrophilia on the basis of serial evaluations may indicate an inflammatory process in the peritoneal cavity. An increase in the WBC count may indicate peritonitis resulting from hollow viscus injury or splenic injury, but this elevation may occur later in the resuscitative phase or critical care phase. During the critical care and intermediate phases of care, an elevation in the WBC count can be indicative of an intra-abdominal infection, wound infection, pulmonary infection, or sepsis.

Amylase and Lipase Levels

An elevated amylase level may indicate injury but is not necessarily diagnostic. Serum amylase may become elevated as a result of parotid gland, pancreatic, duodenal, or genitourinary injury. However, some patients sustain no rise in amylase level despite injury to these organs. Routine amylase testing in every trauma patient is not indicated and should be used selectively by the clinician in accordance with the patient's assessment and medical history.

Many patients with pancreatic injuries do not have a rise in serum amylase in the initial phase of resuscitation. Forty percent of patients may have a normal initial amylase level.[16]

A serum lipase level should be obtained if the amylase is elevated and there is suspicion of pancreatic injury. Serum lipase, an indicator of pancreatic function, is more specific to the inflammatory process of the pancreas. The utility of serum amylase and lipase determinations in the resuscitation phase is questionable. An increasing amylase or lipase level in the critical care or intermediate phase may indicate a missed pancreatic or duodenal injury. These tests can be most useful in conjunction with physical findings and other diagnostic measures to rule out pancreatic or duodenal injury.

Blood Chemistry

Serum electrolytes, blood urea nitrogen, and creatinine levels are obtained many times as baseline values for patients sustaining abdominal trauma. They are indicated in the patient with a history of hypertension, diabetes, or renal disease or who is taking medications such as diuretics. Patients requiring contrast radiographic studies will need a creatinine level to assess renal excretion function. Other blood chemistry tests may be indicated on the basis of the patient's medical history or medications. Evaluation of liver enzymes is indicated in the patient with a history of substance abuse or liver disease.

Clotting Studies

Prothrombin time (PT), partial thromboplastin time (PTT), and international normalized ratio (INR) tests are indicated in the trauma patient with a history of coagulopathy or cirrhosis or who is taking anticoagulants. Baseline PT, PTT, INR, and platelet count are also indicated in the trauma patient who is hemodynamically unstable and when hemorrhage is suspected.

The patient receiving massive blood transfusion requires frequent monitoring of clotting factors. Packed RBCs do not contain clotting factors and platelets, so the patient may require fresh-frozen plasma, platelets, or other clotting factors to prevent coagulopathy.[17] A coagulation profile, including PT and PTT, is required before any abdominal surgery.

MONITORING

Unrecognized abdominal injuries continue to be a cause of preventable deaths in trauma patients.[3] A systematic process for initial assessment of the trauma patient is essential for recognizing life-threatening conditions, identifying injuries, and determining priorities of care. Once the initial assessment, which includes primary and secondary assessments, is completed, the nurse plays an instrumental role in continued serial assessments during the resuscitation and critical care phases. Continual evaluation and frequent assessments are vital in detecting changes in the patient's condition. Patients with abdominal injuries may not demonstrate obvious signs and symptoms of hemorrhage. Nurses have always been astute in recognizing subtle changes such as a slight rise in pulse rate, decrease in blood pressure, or waning level of consciousness. It is extremely important to look at trends of vital signs and serial examinations to detect injuries early.

Resuscitation and Critical Care Phases

The potential for bleeding and hemorrhage is present in all patients who have sustained abdominal trauma. The patient is at risk for fluid volume deficit from hypovolemia and consequently from altered tissue perfusion. Medical management is aimed at maintaining or improving circulating volume and correcting blood loss. There must be continuous monitoring for signs and symptoms of hemorrhage, such as tachycardia, hypotension, pallor of skin, altered level of consciousness, increasing abdominal pain or distention, oliguria, and hypoxia. This requires frequent assessment of vital signs and level of consciousness, repeated Hb and HCT levels, and hourly urinary output measurements in addition to serial physical examinations.

Warm isotonic crystalloid solution is used initially for massive volume resuscitation, but administration of blood should be considered after the initial 2 to 3 L of crystalloid if the patient is requiring large amounts of fluid to maintain blood pressure. All fluid, including blood, should be infused with warming devices if available. The preferred replacement blood during resuscitation is type specific until cross-matched blood is available. Universal donor blood can be administered without waiting for type-specific or cross-matched blood. Men and boys should be given Rh-positive blood, whereas girls and women of childbearing age should receive type O, Rh-negative blood to avoid sensitization that would complicate future pregnancies. Warming techniques to avoid hypothermia include the use of heating blankets, lights, and heated respiratory gas applications through the ventilator in addition to warmed IV fluids.

The level of hemodynamic monitoring depends on the physiologic and clinical needs of the patient. Monitoring may include a variety of noninvasive and invasive devices to aid in the assessment of circulatory status and tissue oxygenation. Use of cardiac monitoring, pulse oximetry, central venous pressure (CVP) monitoring, and arterial blood pressure monitoring may be sufficient for the stable, uncomplicated trauma patient. Patients needing more intensive surveillance may require the insertion of a pulmonary artery (PA) catheter or a central venous catheter capable of monitoring central venous oxyhemoglobin ($Scvo_2$).

Central Venous Pressure

CVP monitoring is indicated whenever a patient has significant alterations in fluid volume. CVP measurements can be used as a guide for fluid volume resuscitation associated with hypovolemia. CVP monitoring is best used when monitoring trends in serial readings during fluid therapy. CVP measurements provide an excellent early indication of changes in the patient's fluid volume status caused by bleeding. The CVP will drop before a significant decrease in the mean arterial pressure (MAP) becomes evident.

A normal CVP is 5 to 10 mm Hg. A low CVP suggests insufficient blood or intravascular fluid volume. An elevated CVP can be related to fluid overload or cardiac compromise suggestive of thoracic injury or cardiac disease.

Arterial Pressure Monitoring

An arterial line is indicated when patients require continuous assessment of arterial blood pressure. MAP is the clinical parameter most frequently used to assess whether blood pressure is sufficient to enable adequate tissue perfusion. In the trauma patient, arterial pressure monitoring is indicated in conditions that compromise fluid volume status, cardiac output, or tissue perfusion. An MAP higher than 60 mm Hg is necessary to perfuse the coronary arteries, brain, and kidneys. Direct arterial access is also helpful in the management of ventilated patients, who require frequent arterial blood gas measurements, and for the hemodynamically unstable patient, who requires inotropic or vasoactive drugs for pressure support.

Pulmonary Artery Pressure Monitoring

A PA catheter is used for diagnosis and evaluation of heart disease, shock, and other conditions that compromise cardiac output or fluid volume. Indications for use in the trauma population include shock, sepsis, multiple organ dysfunction syndrome, and acute respiratory distress syndrome (ARDS). PA pressures, pulmonary capillary wedge pressure, and cardiac output measurements are useful in determining the need for volume replacement and drug therapy and for monitoring response to treatment.

Mixed Venous Oxygen Saturation and Central Venous Oxygen Saturation

Mixed venous oxygen saturation (Svo_2) and $Scvo_2$ monitoring is indicated in the patient who has the potential for an imbalance between oxygen supply and metabolic tissue demand. This includes the trauma patient in shock with or without severe respiratory dysfunction such as ARDS. Svo_2 and $Scvo_2$ reflect the amount of oxygen that is returning to the heart and lungs after the tissues have extracted the oxygen needed to complete their metabolic functions.

Normal Svo_2, which is 70%, measures the oxyhemoglobin in the PA, therefore requiring the insertion of a PA catheter.[18] An Svo_2 value between 60% and 80% is evidence of an adequate balance between oxygen supply and demand. An Svo_2 value change of more than 10% that persists for more than 10 minutes should prompt the nurse to explore the causative factor. Changes in oxygen saturation, cardiac output, Hb, and oxygen consumption can affect the Svo_2. Nursing measures to verify the accuracy of the change in Svo_2 include measuring the Hb level, obtaining a cardiac output value, and checking the integrity of the oxygen supply delivery system.

$Scvo_2$ measures the oxyhemoglobin in the superior vena cava, or right atrium, through the use of a central venous catheter and is a reliable substitution for Svo_2 measurements. $Scvo_2$ values can be 5% to 13% higher than Svo_2 values.[19] The higher $Scvo_2$ value, compared with the Svo_2 value, is related to the incomplete mixing of blood that occurs before it reaches the pulmonary artery.[18]

Invasive and noninvasive hemodynamic monitoring, interpretation of laboratory data, and serial physical assessments continue through the critical care phase. The critical care phase requires close observation for both clinical and physical changes. Assessment of the abdomen may reveal bruising around the umbilicus (Cullen's sign), which is indicative of blood in the abdominal wall. Flank ecchymosis (Grey Turner's sign) may indicate retroperitoneal bleeding or suggest a renal injury. A distended abdomen may indicate the accumulation of blood, fluid, or gas as a result of a perforated organ or blood vessel, or it may be a sign of postoperative ileus. Serial measurement of abdominal girth may be indicated to evaluate the degree of distention. Wound or incision evaluation includes monitoring for tenderness, induration, erythema, and wound exudates, all of which are possible indications of wound infection or abscess.

The critical care nurse must be suspicious of subtle changes in pulse, blood pressure, respiratory rate, and pulse oximetry. These subtle changes in an intensive care unit (ICU) trauma patient admitted for nonoperative management of a liver or spleen injury may indicate the need for another abdominal CT or surgical intervention. Priorities of care include continual physical assessment and monitoring of hemodynamic status, including the patient's response to medical therapies. Frequent nursing evaluations and the detection of changes can facilitate timely diagnostic and therapeutic interventions and thus prevent complications.

ABDOMINAL ORGAN INJURY

The initial assessment process has been presented, including a directed history, mechanism of injury, abdominal assessment, diagnostic studies, laboratory data, and monitored parameters. Specific organ injuries are now presented, including discussion of trauma team management.

THORACOABDOMINAL INJURY

The thoracoabdominal region encompasses the abdominal and thoracic cavities. All patients with penetrating injuries should be suspected of having involvement of both cavities.

DIAPHRAGM INJURY

Isolated diaphragmatic injuries are uncommon and seldom fatal. Typically diaphragmatic injuries occur in conjunction with other organ injuries. They are most commonly associated with penetrating wounds. The incidence of diaphragmatic injuries from blunt trauma is 2%, and the incidence in patients with penetrating thoracoabdominal trauma is 5%.[20] Diaphragmatic injuries as a result of blunt trauma are caused by a drastic and sudden rise in intra-abdominal pressure.

The forces necessary to create such an injury are so great that other intra-abdominal, orthopedic, and neurologic injuries are often present. The incidence of left hemidiaphragm injury is higher because of the protective effect of the liver on the right hemidiaphragm.[20-22] A right hemidiaphragm injury resulting from blunt trauma may include a large defect and significant liver involvement.

Physical assessment of the thoracoabdominal structures focuses on auscultation for the presence of peristaltic sounds in the chest and percussion to elicit dull tones indicating a diaphragm rupture. However, if the patient is splinting the area, even normal sounds may not be appreciated. With gross herniation of visceral contents into the chest cavity, the patient may have a shift of mediastinal structures, resulting in respiratory distress and circulatory instability. Difficulty passing a gastric tube also may signal that the abdominal contents have herniated into the thorax. Penetrating trauma can produce a small tear not recognized during the acute stage. A rise in intra-abdominal pressure may cause a small defect to become larger, with the consequent danger of herniation and intestinal strangulation. Throughout the phases of care, unexplained chest pain and increased respiratory rate suggest the possibility of acute herniation.

Team Management

The most definitive diagnostic procedure is exploratory laparotomy or celiotomy. Diagnostic laparoscopy may have a role in diagnosing diaphragm injuries in the patient who has sustained penetrating trauma.[23] Operative repair is necessary because visceral herniation can occur through small defects. Laparotomy is preferred for acute traumatic diaphragmatic tears. In penetrating trauma, when the entrance wound is in the chest and there is a high suspicion of intrathoracic injury with significant chest bleeding, a thoracic approach may be used to repair the diaphragm.

Esophageal Injury

The incidence of injury to the small portion of the esophagus within the abdominal cavity is low compared with the incidence of esophageal injury in the cervical and thoracic regions. Most esophageal injuries are caused by penetrating trauma and most involve the cervical esophagus. Blunt esophageal injuries are rare. Early diagnosis is paramount because damage results from the corrosion of tissue by digestive juices and bacterial contamination surrounding the site of tissue injury. Fluid losses may be massive and affect the thorax and the abdomen, leading to respiratory compromise. Mediastinitis, paraesophageal abscess, empyema, esophageal fistula, or peritonitis may occur. These injuries, although uncommon, are significant because of the high mortality and morbidity rates that occur if definitive treatment is delayed. Death is generally related to paraesophageal contamination and infection. The mortality rate increases as time from injury to treatment lengthens.

Signs and symptoms vary according to the site of the injury and the degree of contamination. Symptoms of perforation include pain at the site of injury, fever, and dysphagia. The pain may radiate to the neck, chest, or shoulders or throughout the abdomen.

A tear of the abdominal esophagus may present with the sign of peritoneal irritation from release of gastric contents into the peritoneal cavity. As gastric contents efflux into the pleural space, more fluid than air may be appreciated, producing dyspnea accompanied by pleuritic pain.

Team Management

The initial assessment is complicated because esophageal injuries are rare and are seldom single-system events. Medical management is directed toward quick assessment and intervention to deter the effects of bacterial contamination and enzyme erosion. Gastric decompression by passing a gastric tube, antibiotic therapy, and drainage of the wound site are combined with surgical interventions to treat an esophageal tear. Operative therapy is required for all trauma-related esophageal tears. Direct layered closure with drainage of the mediastinum is necessary. However, the extent of injury may dictate defunctionalization, closure of esophagogastric junction, gastrostomy, and drainage of the repair area. The process may be reversed later, after healing has occurred.

Because esophageal injury is difficult to diagnose, complications can occur at any time during the recovery phase. Continuous monitoring for signs of peritoneal irritation, respiratory compromise, or fistula formation is necessary from critical care through rehabilitation. Peritonitis, mediastinitis, intra-abdominal abscess formation, esophageal stricture, and esophageal fistula are potential complications after esophageal injury and subsequent repair.

Gastric Injury

The location and relative mobility of the stomach protects it from blunt injury. Blunt injuries to the stomach are rare and are usually related to pedestrian versus motor vehicle or high-speed motor vehicle collisions.[24] Most stomach trauma is penetrating, and the prognosis depends on the severity of associated injuries, especially vascular wounds. Although gastric perforation resulting from injury can cause severe peritonitis, the initial inflammatory response is caused by chemical irritation and not bacterial contamination. The normal stomach has a relatively high acidic environment and thus is relatively free of bacteria and other microorganisms.

Symptoms of gastric injury can be variable and nonspecific and may include severe epigastric or abdominal pain, tenderness, and signs of peritonitis resulting from release of gastric contents. This clinical presentation may be clouded by associated injuries. Blood from the gastric tube and the presence of free air on abdominal radiograph may support the diagnosis.

Team Management

Medical management includes gastric decompression through placement of a gastric tube and surgical intervention, which includes simple debridement, primary closure, and diligent irrigation of the peritoneal cavity to remove contaminants. Bleeding from the gastric injury itself is occasionally an emergency problem and is managed with the use of a traumatic clamp or suturing. Removal of gastric particles followed by judicious irrigation are required to prevent postoperative intra-abdominal abscesses, particularly subphrenic, subhepatic, and pelvic abscesses, and abscesses of the lesser sac. Gastric decompression is generally continued until gastric emptying returns to normal.[24] Postoperative complications after gastric injury are rare and are usually related to associated injuries.[24] Complications such as peritonitis, intra-abdominal abscess formation, and gastric fistulas may occur immediately or during the intermediate care phase of the trauma cycle.

LIVER INJURY

The liver's size and location make it particularly susceptible to injury. It is one of the most commonly injured organs in abdominal trauma from both blunt and penetrating sources.[20] Motor vehicle crashes are the most common cause of blunt hepatic injury.[25] Blunt liver trauma is most often seen at suburban trauma centers, whereas penetrating liver injury has a higher incidence in urban areas. Associated injuries (e.g., head or chest), the length of time from injury to treatment, and the patient's overall premorbid condition all affect the mortality rate. The single greatest danger after liver injury is severe hemorrhage.[20]

Blunt liver injury should be suspected in any patient with a lower chest or abdominal injury, especially on the right side of the abdomen. Motor vehicle crashes cause crushing of the liver between ribs and vertebrae and are responsible for most liver injuries. Stab wounds of the liver and low-velocity GSWs produce lacerations that are relatively minor, and hemorrhage is easily controlled. High-velocity GSWs, however, are likely to produce widespread parenchymal damage, creating massive hemorrhage.

Liver injury can be graded on a scale of I to VI,[21] with type I representing the least severe damage (Table 25-2). This scale creates a classification for comparison of liver injuries. The grading system may be used preoperatively and intraoperatively.

Team Management

Team management includes deciding whether the patient is a candidate for nonoperative or operative treatment. The success in nonoperative treatment of liver injury in children has spurred an interest in nonoperative treatment in adults.[25] The success of nonoperative management depends on strict patient selection. Patients with grade I, II, or III hepatic injury without active bleeding or expanding hematoma may be considered for nonoperative management.[20,21] Although the selection criteria may vary from surgeon to surgeon, patients usually considered for nonoperative management are cooperative, alert, hemodynamically stable, neurologically intact, and able to participate in follow-up care. In the stable patient

TABLE 25-2 Liver Injury Scale

Grade*	Injury Description	ICD-9	AIS 90
I. Hematoma	Subcapsular, nonexpanding, less than 10% surface area	864.01 864.11	2
Laceration	Capsular tear, nonbleeding, less than 1 cm parenchymal depth	864.02 864.12	2
II. Hematoma	Subcapsular, nonexpanding, 10%-50% surface area: intraparenchymal, nonexpanding, less than 10 cm in diameter	864.01 864.11	2
Laceration	Capsular tear, active bleeding; 1-3 cm parenchymal depth, less than 10 cm in length	864.03 864.13	2
III. Hematoma	Subcapsular, greater than 50% surface area or expanding rupture subcapsular hematoma with active bleeding; intraparenchymal hematoma greater than 10 cm or expanding		3
Laceration	Greater than 3 cm parenchymal depth	864.04 864.14	3
IV. Hematoma	Ruptured intraparenchymal hematoma with active bleeding		4
Laceration	Parenchymal disruption involving 25%-75% of hepatic lobe or 1-3 Couinaud's segments in a single lobe	864.04 864.14	4
V. Laceration	Parenchymal disruption involving greater than 75% of hepatic lobe or greater than 3 Couinaud's segments in a single lobe		5
Vascular	Juxtahepatic venous injuries, i.e., retrohepatic vena cava/central major hepatic veins		5
VI. Vascular	Hepatic avulsion		6

From Moore EE, Cogbill TH, Jurkovich GJ: Organ injury scaling: spleen and liver (1994 revision), *J Trauma* 38:323, 1995.
ICD-9, International Classification of Diseases, Ninth Revision; AIS, Abbreviated Injury Scale, 1990.
*Advance one grade for multiple injuries, up to grade III.

with hepatic injury who does not undergo surgical intervention but has signs of continued blood loss, angiographic embolization may be performed. Nonoperative management requires repeated CT scans at intervals determined by the patient's condition to evaluate resolution of the injury.

Patients with complex hepatic injuries (grades IV to VI) usually have hemodynamic instability as a result of hemorrhage; immediate laparotomy is needed. Deep liver lacerations require interventions to control bleeding, support viable tissue, and prevent postoperative infection. Regardless of the surgical intervention required for liver repair, drainage of wound exudate by a closed-suction system is necessary.

Complex liver injuries may have vascular involvement, which further complicates surgical intervention to control hemorrhage. Manual compression of the liver may be required to tamponade the bleeding after initial opening of the peritoneum. Patients with this type of injury often require aggressive intraoperative resuscitation simultaneously with hemorrhage control to maintain hemodynamic stability. These patients are at high risk for development of hypothermia and coagulopathy.

Packing may be required if bleeding persists after successful debridement of nonviable tissue and ligation of severed blood vessels or bile ducts. If this occurs, surgical intervention is usually aborted, and the patient is taken to the ICU for continued resuscitation and stabilization. The patient will be taken back to the operating room in 24 to 36 hours for removal of the packing and definitive treatment of the liver injury. Patients with liver packing can be at risk for development of abdominal compartment syndrome, and the nurse must be alert to changes in abdominal girth, increasing abdominal distention and intra-abdominal pressure, rising peak inspiratory pressures in the mechanically ventilated patient, and decreasing urine output.

A number of surgical interventions can be instituted for complex liver lacerations. The location of the injury, vascular involvement, and surgeon preference may determine the technique to be used. Deep liver suturing, perihepatic packing, hepatic resection, or hepatorrhaphy is used to salvage the liver.

Blunt trauma to the liver can cause extensive hepatic parenchymal injury in the form of stellate lacerations or major fractures, which are generally more lethal and more difficult to manage than are penetrating injuries. Most deaths result immediately from exsanguination and, in the late postoperative period, from sepsis. Complications from hepatic injury include recurrent bleeding, hemobilia, hyperpyrexia, intra-abdominal abscess, sepsis, biliary fistula, arterial-portal venous fistula, and liver failure.

Gallbladder and Biliary Tract Injury

Gallbladder and biliary tract injuries are typically associated with other intraperitoneal injuries, commonly of the liver or major intra-abdominal blood vessels.[25] Injury to the extrahepatic biliary tract is most often the result of penetrating mechanisms and accounts for only a small percentage of abdominal trauma.[25] Cholecystectomy is the recommended treatment for all gallbladder injuries.[25] Bile duct injuries are classified as simple or complex, and this classification dictates the surgical intervention required. Simple bile duct injuries require primary suture repair and external drainage. Anatomic involvement dictates the procedure of choice for complex bile duct injuries. Cholecystectomy, construction of a biliary-enteric anastomosis, and external drainage constitute the treatment regimen for these injuries. The team should continue to assess the patient for biliary fistulas or stricture.

Splenic Injury

Among patients with blunt abdominal trauma, the spleen is the other most commonly injured organ and it is associated with a high severity of injury.[20] Its anatomic location makes it a frequent victim of penetrating trauma to the LUQ. Although the lower ribs in the LUQ provide some protection, the spleen is vulnerable to injury from intrusion associated with fracture of these ribs. The patient with suspected splenic injury is assessed for LUQ abdominal pain, Kehr's sign, Ballance's sign, and local tenderness.

The mortality rate from splenic injury depends on the type of trauma (blunt versus penetrating) and the presence of associated injuries. Death is related to uncontrolled hemorrhage or to delayed rupture and sepsis and has been estimated to be as high as 14%.[26] The incidence of delayed splenic rupture has decreased to approximately 1% of all splenic injuries, which has been attributed to the increased use of CT scans during the evaluation period.[27]

Team Management

Nonoperative versus operative management of splenic injury must be addressed individually with each patient. The patient's age, physiologic stability, associated injuries, and type of splenic injury are evaluated when management decisions are made. Splenic injury is graded on a scale from I to V perioperatively and intraoperatively.

Medical management of splenic injury has changed over the years as the role of the spleen in maintaining immunocompetence has been appreciated. Nonsurgical treatment is the most common method of management for patients with splenic injuries.[28] Angiographic embolization may be performed when the patient with splenic injury is stable but has evidence of continued bleeding. Splenorrhaphy and partial splenectomy are the recommended operative procedures for patients with splenic injury.[20] The degree of splenic injury is the primary guide to operative treatment selection. Splenectomy is usually indicated for the unstable patient, or grade IV or V splenic disruption.[29]

Postoperative complications include bleeding, thrombocytosis, gastric distention, pancreatitis, and infection.[20] Overwhelming postsplenectomy infections can occur from 1 to 5 years after the operation. The illness presents with flulike symptoms, such as nausea and vomiting, progressing rapidly to confusion, high fever, and shock from sepsis, leading to disseminated intravascular coagulation and death. Causative organisms include *Streptococcus pneumoniae, Meningococcus* spp., *E. coli, Haemophilus influenzae,* and *Staphylococcus* spp. Preventive measures include vaccination with polyvalent pneumococcal vaccine, and possibly the *Haemophilus* influenza and meningococcal vaccines and patient education regarding early symptoms of infection and the need for prompt treatment.

Pancreatic and Duodenal Injuries

Pancreatic injuries are uncommon; the majority are caused by penetrating mechanisms.[16,30] The incidence of pancreatic injury is between 3% and 12%.[26] Pancreatic injury from blunt trauma results from a direct blow to the epigastric area, such as impact with a steering wheel or handlebar. Mortality rates range from 5% to 30% for pancreatic injury and 5% to 55% for duodenal injury and depend on the degree of exsanguination from vascular injury and the development of complications.[16] Approximately 64% of patients with pancreatic and deuodenal injuries will have complications.[16]

Because the pancreas is a retroperitoneal structure, symptoms of injury may not be evident for 24 to 72 hours after a traumatic incident. In addition, the location of the pancreas and proximity to other organs and vessels make multiorgan injury a frequent occurrence, thereby masking symptoms of pancreatic injury. Injuries to the liver, stomach, spleen, and major arteries and veins usually accompany pancreatic injury.

Duodenal injuries frequently occur in association with pancreatic, bile duct, or vena caval trauma. Injury to the duodenum, a predominantly retroperitoneal structure, presents a diagnostic challenge because peritoneal symptoms may not be immediately evident. Blunt injury to the duodenum can produce an intramural hematoma, which may partially or completely obstruct the lumen. Perforation causes contamination of the retroperitoneal and peritoneal spaces with bile, pancreatic enzymes, and gastric secretions. Morbidity and mortality rates increase significantly with delayed treatment.

Team Management

Medical management of pancreatic injury depends on its extent, which may range from simple lacerations to transections. Treatment options are dictated by the site and severity of the pancreatic injury. Duct injury complicates repair procedures. Treatment may consist of simple external closed drainage, distal pancreatectomy, or, for major injuries, a pancreatic duodenectomy. The goals of surgery are to control hemorrhage, debride devitalized tissue, and provide adequate drainage.

Surgical management of a duodenal injury usually involves debridement and primary repair. The selection of a surgical procedure depends on the patient's hemodynamic stability and the presence of pancreatic or bile duct involvement. Nonoperative management of duodenal hematomas requires close observation for signs and symptoms of expanding or ruptured hematomas causing bleeding or peritoneal contamination.

The primary cause of initial death from pancreatic injury is hemorrhage; late deaths are attributed to sepsis, fistulas, and multiple system failure.[16] Complications include fistulas, pseudocyst formation, pancreatic abscess, recurrent hemorrhage, and pancreatitis.

Small Bowel Injury

The small bowel, a hollow viscus structure, is most frequently injured by penetrating trauma, particularly gunshot. Blunt injury to the small bowel is relatively uncommon; when this type of injury is sustained, it typically occurs near the ligament of Treitz and the ileocecal valve.[31] Mechanisms of injury include direct blows, shearing forces, and pseudo–closed loop obstruction. Direct blows crush the intestine between the external force and the spinal column. Shearing forces are imposed by rapid deceleration, as in a motor vehicle crash. Pseudo–closed loop obstruction occurs when a segment of bowel, partially filled with food or gas, becomes trapped between an external force and a firm anatomic object, creating a closed loop.

The ileum and jejunum have a neutral pH and harbor few bacteria. Therefore, clinical signs of injury may not be present on initial examination. As bacterial growth occurs, signs of peritonitis become evident. The lack of specific initial symptoms in patients with small bowel injury directs the nurse to carefully evaluate the information presented as the patient is admitted from the scene of the injury. Any blow to the abdomen or penetrating wound of the lower chest or abdomen should raise the index of suspicion regarding possible bowel injury. Spinal injury frequently occurs in conjunction with small bowel trauma and may mask presenting symptoms.

Team Management

Hemoperitoneum can be associated with injuries to the mesentery of the small bowel. Bleeding should be controlled before exploration for small bowel injury. The site of injury, mechanism of injury, and any associated mesentery injury direct surgical management. Debridement followed by primary closure and ligation of mesenteric bleeding constitute the surgical approach for injuries to the small bowel. Bowel resection is recommended if multiple defects are in close proximity to each other, if a segment of bowel has sustained massive destruction, or if significant mesentery injury is causing ischemia in a segment of the bowel.

Postoperative care is quite simple if only the small bowel is involved, but many times other peritoneal injuries complicate the patient's recovery. Gastric decompression and parenteral nutrition are not usually required in the patient with an isolated small bowel injury. Several postoperative doses of antibiotics are recommended to reduce the incidence of postoperative infections after contamination of the peritoneal cavity with contents of the small bowel.

Complications such as wound infection and abscess are related to the extent of contamination and the site of injury. In addition, fistula formation, small bowel obstruction, ischemic bowel, suture line leakage, and short-gut syndrome have been reported.[24]

LARGE BOWEL INJURY

Trauma to the large bowel is one of the most lethal forms of abdominal injury because of the probability of sepsis related to fecal contamination of the abdomen. Seventeen percent of all penetrating abdominal injuries involve the colon.[20] The transverse colon is most often involved. Blunt trauma frequently affects the mobile transverse and sigmoid segments because their anatomic location makes them most vulnerable. The majority of blunt injuries manifest as contusions.

Team Management

Medical intervention is based on early recognition of injury and control of fecal contamination. A laparotomy is performed if colon or rectal perforation is suspected. Preoperative antibiotic therapy is ordered to decrease the probability of sepsis from enteric contamination.

Operative management includes control of hemorrhage and fecal leakage and irrigation to remove fecal material from the abdominal cavity. Surgical options for the treatment of colon injuries include primary repair (resection and anastomosis) and colostomy. Primary repair is now established as the optimal and most common procedure for traumatic colonic injuries.[32] The operative technique is selected on the basis of the extent and location of injury, the presence of shock, the extent of peritoneal spillage, the presence of associated injuries, and the length of delay in surgical intervention. Extraperitoneal rectal injuries require the use of drainage and copious irrigation to remove fecal material, debridement, and diverting colostomy.

Incisional infection is a recognized complication of colon and rectal injury. Delayed skin closure is advocated in patients with major fecal contamination. Intra-abdominal abscess is the most frequent complication, occurring in 5% to 15% of patients with colon injury.[32] Other complications include wound infections, fecal fistula, and difficulties with the colostomy stoma.

ABDOMINAL VASCULAR INJURY

Until recently, major vessel injuries were not seen in resuscitation areas or EDs because patients exsanguinated before transport. With an increase in skilled technicians and emergency resuscitation measures provided at the scene, more patients with vascular injury are surviving long enough to be treated in medical facilities. *Abdominal vascular injury* refers to injury to vessels located in the midline retroperitoneum (zone 1), upper lateral retroperitoneum (zone 2), pelvic retroperitoneum (zone 3), and portal-retrohepatic area[33] (Table 25-3).

Vessels sustain contusions, lacerations, transections, or avulsion injuries. These occur as a result of penetrating or blunt injury, although the majority of severe damage to the vascular system occurs with penetrating trauma. Blunt injury to blood vessels is caused by deceleration, shearing, or crushing forces. Rapid deceleration in a motor vehicle crash causes avulsion of the small branches of the major vessels or intimal tears, resulting in secondary thrombosis.[33] Direct crush forces cause intimal tears or flaps, leading to secondary thrombosis of a vessel, or complete disruption of exposed vessels, resulting in intraperitoneal hemorrhage.[33] Vascular injuries are divided into arterial and venous trauma. Although combination injuries may exist and complications such as arteriovenous fistulas may occur, understanding each system separately helps to direct assessment and intervention strategies. The primary goal in management of patients with abdominal vascular injuries should be aggressive resuscitation and early control of hemorrhage.[23]

Arterial Injury

The artery, as a result of its elastic quality, may stop bleeding spontaneously after a clean transection occurs from penetrating trauma. The transected intimae curls inward, and the

TABLE 25-3 Abdominal Vascular Regions

Zone 1: Midline Retroperitoneum	Zone 2: Upper Lateral Retroperitoneum
Supramesocolic Area Suprarenal abdominal aorta, celiac axis, proximal superior mesenteric artery, proximal renal artery, and superior mesenteric vein (either supramesocolic or retromesocolic) **Inframesocolic Area** Infrarenal abdominal aorta and infrahepatic inferior vena cava	Renal artery and renal vein
Zone 3: Pelvic Retroperitoneum	**Zone 4: Portal-Retrohepatic Area**
Iliac artery and iliac vein	Portal vein, hepatic artery, and retrohepatic vena cava

divided media contract and pull the adventitia over the ends of the vessel. Partially transected vessels are unable to activate this process, and thus bleeding continues. In a partial laceration or transection, hematoma formation may occur, stopping further bleeding or leading to a false aneurysm that may rupture at a later date.

Arterial contusions are usually the result of blunt traumatic force or stretching. Damage may initiate minor bleeding or progress to thrombus formation, occluding the vessel or embolizing distal vessels. Avulsion injury usually occurs with a deceleration event that pulls the artery from its base. In the abdomen this most frequently occurs at the renal pedicle or the root of the mesentery.

Abdominal arterial injuries are sustained frequently in combination with pelvic, thoracic, or visceral injury. This complicates initial assessment because specific signs of vascular injury may be obscured. For example, retroperitoneal hematoma, usually found in conjunction with pelvic or spine injury, may cause up to 4 L of blood to collect in the retroperitoneal space. The presenting symptoms are similar to those of visceral rupture and hemorrhage: abdominal pain, back pain, hypoactive bowel sounds, or tender abdominal mass. Only later will flank discoloration become evident.

Patients with rapid-onset shock without an obvious source of blood loss should be suspected of having a major intra-abdominal arterial injury. Patients with abdominal aortic injuries sustained through penetrating trauma are in profound shock and require immediate operative intervention. The presence of a large retroperitoneal hematoma indicates aortic injury.

Team Management. Volume replacement is a priority, but in catastrophic hemorrhage immediate surgery may be indicated because restoration of hemodynamic stability may be impossible without quick surgical intervention. Postoperative care focuses on maintaining an adequate volume status and monitoring for signs of hemorrhage.

Surgical repair depends on the type and extent of injury. Most major abdominal arterial injuries require lateral repair, end-to-end anastomosis, or a graft if the artery would be narrowed by primary repair. Autogenous tissue grafting, as opposed to use of prosthetic material, is preferred because many abdominal injuries are contaminated. Many major abdominal arteries can be ligated, which often becomes necessary when the site of repair lies within a contaminated field.

Venous Injury

The venous system is a low-pressure system capable of realizing a tamponade effect from the pressure of surrounding tissues. Thus profuse bleeding (hemorrhage) must occur into a space at lower pressure, such as an external opening, a body cavity, or a cavity created after injury.

The severity of the vascular injury may not permit multiple diagnostic tests. Patients who appear in the resuscitation area in shock are usually moved quickly to the operating room for definitive diagnosis and treatment. However, for patients who are more stable, time is available for certain diagnostic tests, such as angiography, that help to define the extent of injury. Abdominal vascular injury is most frequently diagnosed during laparotomy for severe hemorrhagic shock. Severe hypotension unresponsive to rapid fluid administration (2 to 3 L in 10 to 15 minutes) in a patient with abdominal trauma should lead to suspicion of a major intra-abdominal vascular injury.

Team Management. Venous injury requires the use of pressure and packing until the extent of injury is identified. Lateral repair, ligation, and venous grafting are used to treat venous injuries. Historically, complicated repairs led to stenosis of the vessel and increased risk of thrombosis or embolism; therefore, ligation was used as a treatment of choice, except to repair suprarenal or intrahepatic vena cava injuries.

The extent of vascular injury may demand quick assessment, transport to the operating room for definitive diagnosis and treatment, and massive fluid resuscitation. Patient response to fluid resuscitation indicates the amount of time available for further diagnostic testing. If the patient becomes alert and exhibits signs of adequate perfusion, further testing, including arteriography, may be ordered.

Complications of vascular repair in the abdomen include thrombosis, dehiscence of the suture line, and infection. Bleeding after vascular repair may occur at any time in the postoperative period. Medical management is focused on repairing the source of bleeding, correcting coagulopathy, and preventing infection and vascular repair disruption.

INTERMEDIATE AND REHABILITATION PHASES OF CARE

Once the critical physiologic abnormalities are stabilized, the patient transitions from critical care to the intermediate phase of care. Not every patient will go through every phase of care; many will not enter the critical care phase but will immediately enter the intermediate phase.

Nursing assessment, treatment implementation, and evaluation in the intermediate phase are directed at assisting the patient toward his or her premorbid functional state. Nutrition, elimination, mobility, pain control, and psychologic state are monitored continuously. At this stage both patient and family are active participants. Abdominal wound assessment, drain management, and dressing changes all involve evaluation for potential wound infection. Educating the patient and family about signs of infection, the role of nutrition in wound healing, and pain control during procedures are important in getting the patient closer to self-care.

The patient goes through many treatment changes during this phase, such as progressing from tube feedings to an oral diet, changing from IV pain medication to oral, and moving from bed rest to independent mobility. In today's health care environment that progression is quick and may leave the patient feeling without control. Psychologic support through rational explanations for therapy and reassurance to promote comfort should be incorporated into the patient's care plan to ease the transition from critical care to the intermediate phase.

The patient's ability to regain control and independence leading to self-care can depend on his or her premorbid physical state, age, severity of traumatic injury, and family support. Generally, elderly patients require more time to progress to the premorbid state than do younger patients.

Rehabilitation actually starts in the critical care phase with stabilization of injuries and prevention of secondary disabilities. Early involvement of the rehabilitation team assists with prevention of excessive muscle atrophy and maintenance of the patient's functional state. Early mobilization can be instrumental in preventing atelectasis, pneumonia, ileus, footdrop, and skin breakdown.

The degree of physical or neurologic disability or impairment determines the extent of rehabilitation a patient requires. Some patients need only several weeks to regain endurance and strength before returning to their homes, whereas others require months to learn self-care skills, such as feeding, personal hygiene, dressing, and basic communication skills in addition to mobility and psychologic therapies. Rehabilitation requires the active participation of the patient and family in preparing the patient for his or her return to a functional role within the family and the community.

Today patients spend even shorter periods in each phase, and it becomes increasingly important for the health care provider to identify a patient's functional deficits as soon as possible so that rehabilitation begins before the day of discharge. Health care is directed at less inpatient hospital care and more in-home nursing services and therapies when possible. The ultimate goal in any circumstance is a safe discharge to home with the appropriate resources.

Complications of Abdominal Trauma

Many individuals who have sustained abdominal trauma move through the phases from resuscitation to rehabilitation with little to no variance from the usual postoperative surgical patient. However, the extent of organ involvement, severity of injury, and time from injury until treatment greatly affect the morbidity of these individuals. Injury to any organ or vessel in the abdomen can lead to certain generalized posttraumatic complications. For example, a patient in the critical care phase may have an ileus, peritonitis, cholecystitis, or stress ulcerations. In the intermediate care phase, abscesses may form and wound complications develop. The rehabilitation phase may be the first time that body image alteration, alteration in family coping, or long-term pain control becomes an issue.

After successful resuscitation, the effects of injury, hemorrhage, shock, and treatment begin to affect the physical and psychologic adaptation of the patient. These complications are not specific to a single abdominal organ injury but occur by virtue of damage to the abdominal contents, whether it is single-organ or multiorgan involvement or single-system or multisystem injury. The potential for these complications to occur makes it imperative for nursing assessment to continue throughout the phases of care.

Abdominal Compartment Syndrome

Abdominal compartment syndrome (ACS), also referred to as intra-abdominal hypertension, is a condition in which abdominal organ dysfunction is caused by increased intra-abdominal pressure. ACS can occur in the trauma patient as a result of abdominal distention from third-spaced resuscitation fluid, ileus, bowel obstruction, bowel edema, postoperative hemorrhage, or abdominal packing.[34]

Increased abdominal pressure primarily affects the cardiovascular, pulmonary, and renal systems. Cardiovascular effects manifest as a decrease in cardiac output and hypotension. Renal effects from a lack of perfusion of the renal arteries result in decreased urine output. Pulmonary effects produce a decrease in tidal volume, poor lung compliance, hypercarbia, and increased intrathoracic pressure.

Normal intra-abdominal pressure (IAP) is 0 mm Hg. An IAP greater than 20 mm Hg produces adverse physiologic effects on various organ systems.[35] If the measured IAP is higher than 20 mm Hg, it is acceptable practice for the surgeon to perform decompression of the abdomen, which can be performed either in the ICU or in the operating room.

Direct measurement of the abdominal cavity for ACS is impractical in the ICU. A reliable indirect method of measurement consists of measuring the pressure in the urinary bladder. When the urinary bladder is partially filled, the pressure that is generated accurately reflects the abdominal compartment pressure.[35,36] The patient should be supine during the measurement to reduce the pressure generated on the bladder by the abdominal organs.[36]

It is imperative that the nurse be aware of possible causes of ACS and its presenting signs and symptoms. Close monitoring for increases in abdominal girth should alert the nurse to early signs of rising abdominal pressure. Increasing tenseness of the abdomen, which can be determined by palpation, indicates rising intra-abdominal pressure. Monitoring intake and output can help identify decreasing urine output. Increased peak inspiratory pressures and worsening lung compliance should alert the nurse to the possibility of ACS. Early identification and effective management are key to preventing adverse effects of the syndrome. Untreated ACS can progress to anuria, hypoxia, hypercapnia, and death.[36]

After decompression, the greatest nursing priority is wound management. Patients with open abdominal wounds are susceptible to heat and fluid loss. Continuous hemodynamic monitoring is essential in the critical care phase. Monitoring drainage, changing dressings, and protecting the skin to avoid breakdown continue through the critical care and intermediate phases.

ACUTE ACALCULOUS CHOLECYSTITIS

Acute acalculous cholecystitis (AAC) is an acute inflammation of the gallbladder in the absence of gallstones. It is also referred to as *acute posttraumatic cholecystitis* or *acute postoperative cholecystitis.* The disease most often occurs in association with other conditions such as burns, major trauma, or operations. Affected patients are often critically ill, requiring extensive monitoring and life-support measures. The cause of AAC is still uncertain and may be multifactorial. Contributing factors include lack of bile stasis, administration of total parenteral nutrition, and the administration of narcotics and positive-pressure ventilation.[37] Gallbladder ischemia has also been implicated in patients who have prolonged periods of hypotension or low blood flow during operations after trauma and burn injury.[37]

AAC does not differ from the calculous type, except that the incidence of gangrene and perforation is higher. Symptoms are nonspecific but may include fever, nausea, vomiting, and RUQ tenderness. AAC poses a diagnostic challenge in the critically ill trauma patient with abdominal injuries and subsequent surgical intervention. Symptoms of AAC may be masked because of narcotic administration, incisional abdominal pain from recent surgery, concomitant injuries, or other disease processes.

Imaging of the gallbladder by ultrasonography and cholescintigraphy in conjunction with laboratory and clinical findings will assist in the diagnosis. Inflammation may produce an elevated WBC count in patients along with increased alkaline phosphatase or aspartate aminotransferase levels. Treatment depends on the patient's underlying disease and hemodynamic state, but AAC requires surgical intervention. The gallbladder can be removed by cholecystectomy or laparoscopic cholecystotomy.

SUMMARY

Although each abdominal organ system has been reviewed singularly, the nurse is much more likely to be confronted with a patient who has sustained multiorgan or multisystem trauma. Certain patterns such as pancreaticoduodenal injury and the resultant confusing diagnostic presentation have been described. Quick multisystem assessment is necessary initially, with an emphasis on identifying the life-threatening injuries first. Airway, ventilation, and circulation are initial priorities, with recognition that ventilatory and circulatory control may be affected by the extent of the abdominal injury. The index of diagnostic suspicion cues the nursing assessment and permits early recognition of insidious abdominal injury in each phase. Delayed rupture or hemorrhage can occur in patients with abdominal trauma. Other consequences of the injury, such as pancreatitis, abscess formation, or wound infection, may become apparent during the intermediate care or rehabilitation phases. Morbidity and mortality rates are directly related to the failure to diagnose and treat early. Thus, the demand remains for knowledgeable, swift nursing assessment in each phase of the cycle, focusing on flexible patient care planning to meet the multiple changing needs of abdominal trauma patients and their families.

REFERENCES

1. MacKenzie EJ, Fowler CJ: Epidemiology. In Moore E, Feliciano D, Mattox K, editors: *Trauma,* 5th ed, pp 22-40, New York, 2004, McGraw-Hill.
2. Tumbarello C: Ultrasound evaluation of abdominal trauma in the emergency department, *J Trauma* 5:67, 1998.
3. American College of Surgeons' Committee on Trauma: Abdominal trauma. In *Advanced trauma life support,* 7th ed, pp 132-145, Chicago, 2004, American College of Surgeons.
4. Herlihy B, Maebius NK: *The human body in health and illness,* Philadelphia, 2000, W. B. Saunders.
5. Thibodeau GA, Patton KT: *Anatomy and physiology,* 5th ed, St. Louis, 2003, Mosby.
6. Demetriades D, Velmacho G: Indications for laparotomy, In Moore E, Feliciano D, Mattox K, editors: *Trauma,* 5th ed, pp 593-612, New York, 2004, McGraw-Hill.
7. Parks SN: Initial assessment. In Moore E, Feliciano D, Mattox K, editors: *Trauma,* 5th ed, pp 159-174, New York, 2004, McGraw-Hill.
8. EAST Practice Mangement Guidelines Work Group: *Practice management guidelines for the evaluation of blunt abdominal trauma,* 2001, Chicago, Eastern Association for the Surgery of Trauma.
9. Schulman C: Emergency care focus: a FASTer method of detecting abdominal trauma, *Nurs Manage* 34:47-49, 2003.
10. Shreve WS, Knotts FB, Siders RW et al: Retrospective analysis of the adequacy of oral contrast material for computed tomography scans in trauma patients, *Am J Surg* 178:14, 1999.
11. Stafford RE, McGonigal MD, Weigelt JA et al: Oral contrast solution and computed tomography for blunt abdominal trauma: a randomized study, *Arch Surg* 134:622, 1999.
12. Blackbourne LH, Soffer D, McKenney M et al: Secondary ultrasound examination increases the sensitivity of the FAST exam in blunt trauma, *J Trauma* 57:934-938, 2004.
13. Miletic D, Fuckar Z, Mraovic B et al: Ultrasound in the evaluation of hemoperitoneum in war casualties, *Mil Med* 164:600, 1999.
14. Pryor JP, Reilly PM, Badrowski GP: Nonoperative management of abdominal gunshot wounds, *Ann Emerg Med* 43:344-353, 2004.
15. Tepel M, Van Der Giet M, Schwarzfeld C et al: Prevention of radiographic-contrast-agent–induced reductions in renal function by acetylcysteine, *N Engl J Med* 343:180-184, 2000.
16. Asensio JA, Gambara E, Forno W: Duodenal and pancreatic injuries—complex and lethal injuries, *J Trauma Nurs* 8:47-49, 2001.
17. Petersen SR, Weinberg JA: Transfusions, autotransfusion, and blood substitutes. In Moore E, Feliciano D, Mattox K, editors: *Trauma,* 5th ed, pp 227-238, New York, 2004, McGraw-Hill.
18. Ahrens T: Hemodynamics in sepsis, *AACN Adv Crit Care* 17:435-445, 2006.
19. Lee J, Wright F, Barber R, Stanley L: Central venous oxygen saturation in shock: a study in man, *Anesthesiology* 36:472-478, 1972.
20. Wisner DH, Hoyt BD: Abdominal trauma. In Mulholland MW, Lillemoe KD, Doherty GM et al, editors: *Greenfield's surgery: scientific principles and practice,* pp 421-440, Philadelphia, 2006, Lippincott.
21. Eckert KL: Penetrating and blunt abdominal trauma, *Crit Care Nurs Q* 28:41-59, 2005.
22. Asensio JA, Petrone P, Demetriades D: Injury to the diaphragm. In Moore E, Feliciano D, Mattox K, editors: *Trauma,* 5th ed, pp 613-636, New York, 2004, McGraw-Hill.

23. Shatz Dv, Kirton OC, McKenny MG et al: Penetrating abdominal trauma. In Shatz DV, Kirton OC, McKenny MG et al, editors: *Manual of trauma and emergency surgery*, pp 119-153, Philadelphia, 2000, W. B. Saunders.
24. Diebel LN: Injury to the stomach and small bowel. In Moore E, Feliciano D, Mattox K, editors: *Trauma*, 5th ed, pp 687-708, New York, 2004, McGraw-Hill.
25. Fabian TC, Bee TK: Liver and biliary tract trauma. In Moore E, Feliciano D, Mattox K, editors: *Trauma*, 5th ed, pp 637-662, New York, 2004, McGraw-Hill.
26. Sikka R: Unsuspected internal organ traumatic injuries, *Emerg Med Clin North Am* 22:1067-1080, 2004.
27. Ruffolo DC: Delayed splenic rupture: understanding the threat, *J Trauma Nurs* 9:34-40, 2002.
28. Harbrecht BG: Is anything new in adult blunt splenic trauma, *Am J Surg* 190:273-278, 2005.
29. Wisner DH: Injury to the spleen. In Moore E, Feliciano D, Mattox K, editors: *Trauma*, 5th ed, pp 663-686, New York, 2004, McGraw-Hill.
30. Jurkovich GJ, Bulger EM: Injury to duodenum and pancreas. In Moore E, Feliciano D, Mattox K, editors: *Trauma*, 5th ed, pp 709-734, New York, 2004, McGraw-Hill.
31. Hunt JP, Weintraub SL, Wang, Y et al: Kinematics of trauma. In Moore E, Feliciano D, Mattox K, editors: *Trauma*, 5th ed, pp 141-158, New York, 2004, McGraw-Hill.
32. Burch JM: Injury to the colon and rectum. In Moore E, Feliciano D, Mattox K, editors: *Trauma*, 5th ed, pp 735-753, New York, 2004, McGraw-Hill.
33. Feliciano DV: Abdominal vascular injury. In Moore E, Feliciano D, Mattox K, editors: *Trauma*, 5th ed, pp 755-778, New York, 2004, McGraw-Hill.
34. Chandler CF, Blinman T, Cryer HG: Acute renal failure. In Moore E, Feliciano D, Mattox K, editors: *Trauma*, 5th ed, pp 1323-1350, New York, 2004, McGraw-Hill.
35. Walker JW, Criddle LM: Pathophysiology and management of abdominal compartment syndrome, *Am J Crit Care* 12: 367-371, 2003.
36. Gallagher JJ: Intraabdominal pressure monitoring. In Lynn-McHale Wiegand DJ, Carlson K, editors: *AACN procedure manual for critical care*, pp 892-898, Philadelphia, 2005, Elsevier Saunders.
37. Barie PS, Eachempati SR: Acute acalculous cholecystitis, *Curr Gastroenterol Rep* 5:302-309, 2003.

26

GENITOURINARY INJURIES AND RENAL MANAGEMENT

Kara A. Snyder, Victoria R. Veronese

Rapid diagnosis and treatment of genitourinary (GU) trauma can be difficult. The trauma victim's most immediate requirement is the establishment of a patent airway, sufficient ventilation, and adequate circulation. Assessment of the GU system often begins with the insertion of a urinary catheter to monitor urine output. This chapter addresses the assessment, treatment, and care of the patient with GU trauma; potential complications; and the impact of GU injury on the recovering trauma patient.

GU trauma may be defined as any injury to the kidneys, the kidneys' collecting system, or the reproductive system. The kidneys are generally not susceptible to direct trauma because they are protected by the twelfth ribs. They are anchored in place by Gerota's fascia, surrounded by fat pads, and capped by the adrenal glands. The left kidney is further protected by the spleen, chest wall, diaphragm, pancreatic tail, and descending colon. The right kidney is 1 to 2 cm lower than the left and is surrounded by the diaphragm, liver, and duodenum. The ureters are cushioned bilaterally by abdominal contents and surrounded by the pelvic bones. The urinary bladder is protected anteriorly and laterally by the pubic arch. The pelvic diaphragm supports the bladder inferiorly; the peritoneum covers the bladder superiorly and posteriorly. These anatomic guardians are consistent in both sexes.

The female urethra is protected by the symphysis pubis, as is the vagina. The uterus lies midpelvis, halfway between the sacrum and the symphysis pubis. It rests on the pelvic diaphragm, supported by six ligaments, and it is cushioned by bowels and bladder. This same anatomic protection is afforded the ovaries and fallopian tubes on either side of the uterus. The female urethra is shorter than the male urethra and is relatively mobile.

The longer male urethra consists of two segments: the anterior segment, which is distal to the urogenital diaphragm, and the posterior segment, which passes through the urogenital diaphragm and includes the prostatic and membranous segments. The bladder neck is continuous with the prostatic segment of the urethra. The male urethra is approximately 20 cm long and is fixed at the symphysis. Comparatively little anatomic protection is afforded the male urethra, penis, and scrotal sac. These anatomic considerations are important factors in the occurrence of distal GU trauma in men.

In children younger than age 6 years, the bladder is an abdominal organ. The kidneys of children have less perirenal fat, are large in comparison with the abdomen as a whole, and have a thinner capsule for protection than do those of adults. Children also have a weaker abdominal musculature and a less ossified thoracic rib cage, which offers less kidney protection.

The location of the structures of the GU system plays an important role in determining the degree and types of injury. An understanding of the GU anatomy, the epidemiology of GU trauma, and the patient's mechanism of injury helps determine a list of potential injuries for that patient, which then directs the focused assessment to reveal the acutal injuries.

EPIDEMIOLOGY

Injuries to the GU tract account for 8% to 10% of all abdominal trauma.[1] The most commonly injured organs of the GU tract are the kidneys.[2] Renal injury occurs more frequently in children than in adults, and the kidney is the third most common organ injured with abdominal trauma in the pediatric population.[3] Injury to the urethra is more common in men than in women because of the anatomic differences.[4] Trauma to the ureters is rare and most often has an iatrogenic cause, such as obstetric-gynecologic surgery.[5]

GU trauma is rarely an isolated injury. Approximately 60% to 80% of patients with blunt renal trauma have associated major injuries to other organs.[2,6] Injuries that occur most frequently with GU trauma include fracture of the pelvis, lower rib fractures, intra-abdominal organ injuries associated with gunshot wounds to the abdomen, and fracture of the transverse processes of the lumbar spine. Pelvic fractures have been associated with a 5% to 10% incidence of bladder injury and a 1% to 11% incidence of posterior urethra injury.[7-9] In contrast, at least 94% to 97% of patients with bladder injuries have concomitant injuries such as pelvic or long-bone fractures.[9] Injury to the right kidney is most often seen with injury to the liver, whereas injury to the left kidney and the spleen tend to occur together.

MECHANISM OF INJURY

Blunt trauma causes approximately 80% to 95% of all GU trauma.[10] Blunt forces can be either direct impact or rapid deceleration. Rapid deceleration injury is produced when a body in motion is halted abruptly. This situation can occur during a fall from a height or in a motor vehicle collision (MVC) when the occupant makes contact with the dashboard, lap belt, or steering wheel of the vehicle. The kidney is set in motion on its pedicle while the aorta remains more stationary. The rotation around the pedicle may tear the intima of the renal artery, resulting in renal artery thrombosis, or may injure the renal vein.[11] Other consequences of this type of blunt injury include disruption of the ureteropelvic junction (UPJ) and contusion of the renal parenchyma (Figure 26-1). UPJ injuries occur mostly in children.[3] In trauma the most common blunt cause of ureter injury occurs when the kidney is compressed against the lower rib cage and upper lumbar transverse processes, thereby stretching the ureter in lateral flexion.[7]

MVCs account for a majority of GU injuries, especially in children.[3] During an MVC an unbelted victim slides forward, the femur is compacted into the pelvis, and the abdomen strikes the steering wheel (Figure 26-2). The stress on the kidney is created by a combination of forces applied to the fluid-filled inner compartment. Hydrostatic, or pushing, pressure results in injury. This compression causes an increased intrapelvic pressure that can tear and shear renal structures. Certain preexisting conditions, such as hydronephrotic kidneys and renal cysts, already cause an increased intrapelvic pressure and therefore patients with these disorders have an increased susceptibility to injury, particularly at the periphery.

The use of three-point restraint seat belts decreases the incidence of organ injury by holding the occupant firmly against the seat and allowing the vehicle to absorb the impact of the collision.[12] A lap belt alone (without the shoulder strap) or an impact against the steering wheel can result in abdominal injury caused by the sudden increase in intra-abdominal/intravesicular pressure that occurs as the organs are compressed between the abdominal wall and the spine.[12] Although airbags have helped reduce overall mortality rates, they only provide supplemental protection for occupants wearing a seat belt and their use alone (in the absence of three-point lap belts) does not decrease the risk of injury.[12]

Although the incidence of trauma to the ureters is rising with the increase in gunshot wounds (GSWs), the most common cause of ureteral trauma remains iatrogenic injury during surgery.[13] Iatrogenic injuries to the small ureters are most likely to occur during difficult pelvic procedures in which normal anatomic landmarks are obscured by obstruction, neoplasm, inflammation, congenital anomalies, traumatic displacement, or the effects of radiation. A high index of suspicion must be established to detect and appropriately treat iatrogenic GU trauma.

In noniatrogenic ureter trauma, penetrating injury is the most common cause of ureter injury.[5,7,9] Causes of penetrating

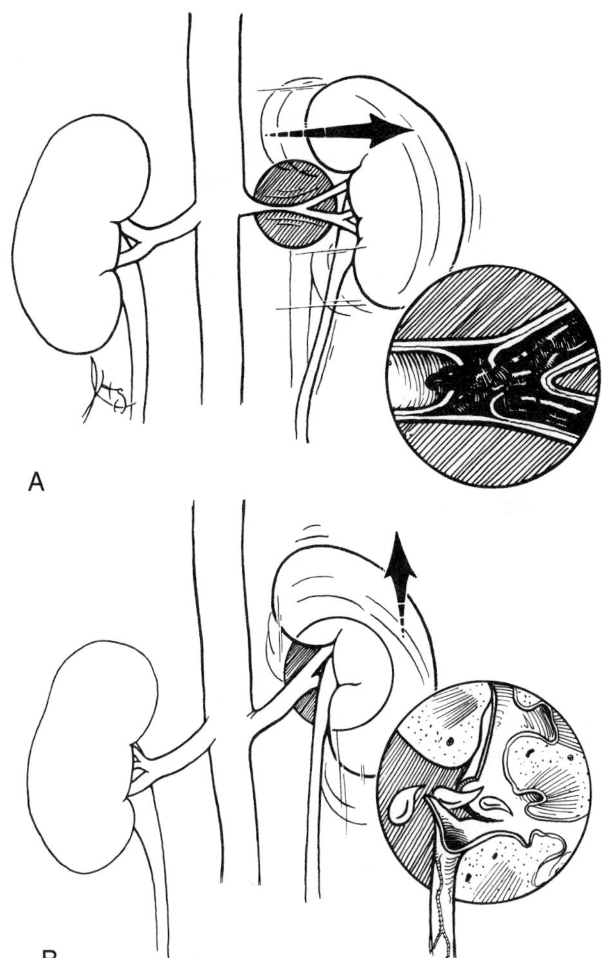

FIGURE 26-1 Acceleration-deceleration injury may produce disruption of the renal artery (**A**) and the ureteropelvic junction (**B**).

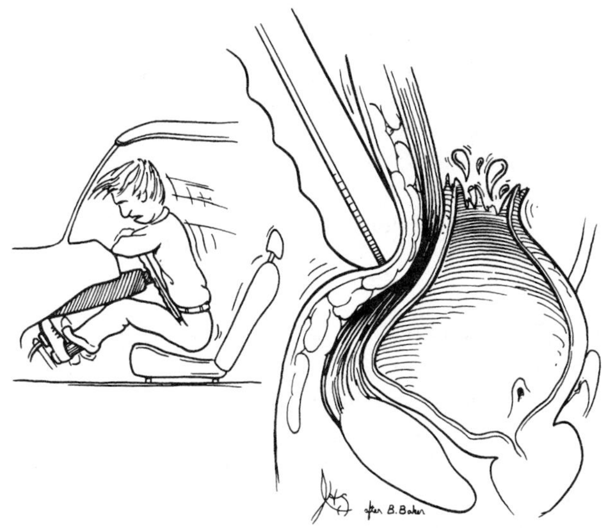

FIGURE 26-2 Compression injuries of the abdomen that do not produce fracture may produce intraperitoneal bladder rupture. (From Guerriero WG, Devine CJ: *Urologic injuries,* p 113, Norwalk, CT, 1984, Appleton-Century-Crofts.)

trauma include GSWs, stabbing, and impalement. Approximately 4% of injuries caused by abdominal GSWs involve the ureter.[13]

In addition to the increasing rate of penetrating injuries, another mechanism that causes GU injuries is straddle injuries. Straddle injuries may occur from motorcycle crashes and straddle-type falls.[14] Injuries range from external perineal injury, urethral injury, and rectal and vaginal tears.[15] The most common form of injury with this mechanism is trauma to the external genitalia. In one study of 43,056 adult victims, there were 78 cases involving these straddle-type injuries caused by motorcycle crashes. In 64% of these cases the injury involved the external genital organs and specifically the testicles in two thirds of cases.[16]

Resuscitation Phase

The early detection of GU trauma is important to optimal outcome in terms of organ salvage and patient survival. However, GU trauma does not take precedence over more life-threatening injuries to the head, chest, and abdomen. GU trauma may not present initially as a life-threatening situation, but a delay in diagnosis and treatment can produce significant tissue loss from prolonged ischemia or blood and urine extravasation.

Assessment of GU trauma is based on multiple strategies. No one strategy is sufficient to diagnose GU trauma specifically. An accurate diagnosis occurs through the interpretation of diagnostic clues obtained from the history, physical examination, and radiologic and laboratory testing. However, a high index of suspicion, based on knowledge of the mechanism of injury, is key in the detection of GU trauma. GU trauma should be suspected in the following types of injuries[1,2,3,5,10,14]:

- Fall or deceleration injury
- MVC
- Crushing incident
- Abdominal, flank, lower chest, back, or pelvis injury
- Powered personal watercraft events
- Straddle injury
- Motorcycle and bicycle crashes
- Sexual assault
- Penetrating abdominal trauma

Health History

A health history always begins with the circumstances causing the person to seek treatment within the health care system. The initial step of the assessment is to obtain an accurate history of the events leading to injury. Details about the mechanism of injury provide valuable clues to the occurrence, nature, and extent of the GU trauma.[2]

For MVCs the estimated speed of the vehicle when it crashed, the type of vehicle, the use of seat belts, and the position of the victim within the vehicle should be determined. If a fall has occurred, the height of the fall, objects struck during the fall, the patient's body position on landing, and the type of landing surface should be noted. After penetrating trauma, information must be obtained regarding the type and characteristics of the weapon used (e.g., gun, knife) or foreign object (e.g., shrapnel, impaled object) and the occurrence of other events after the penetrating trauma (e.g., a fall).

Various details about the condition of the patient at the scene of the traumatic event affect clinical management decisions. Was the patient pinned in the vehicle? What was the extrication time? Was there evidence of drug or alcohol use? What care was provided in the field? Was there evidence of airway compromise or hemodynamic instability? Details such as these can be obtained from prehospital providers, witnesses, family, or police officers at the scene.

In addition to the circumstances of injury, essential medical history information includes allergies, medications, previous diseases or surgical procedures, last meal eaten and when, and the events before the trauma. A quick way to remember the components of the essential health history is the AMPLE acronym, which stands for *a*llergies, *m*edications, *p*ast history of medical or surgical illnesses, *l*ast meal, and *e*vents preceding the injury.[17] Previous injuries, known anatomic abnormalities, and preexisting GU conditions should be determined.

Previous GU surgery may have contributed to the development of adhesions, strictures, or a predisposition to calculi formation or chronic GU infection, all of which can influence treatment modalities after trauma. Prior nephrectomy or preexisting GU disorders such as chronic renal failure, renal artery stenosis, or one of the glomerulonephropathies may govern both the initial treatment and the long-term management of the trauma patient with GU injury.

Part of the subjective data obtained should include determining whether the patient feels an inability to void. Inability to void may indicate upper urinary tract injury, obstruction caused by blood clots, or bladder or urethra rupture.[1,5]

Physical Examination

During the resuscitation phase the assessment of life-threatening injuries to the cardiovascular, respiratory, and neurologic systems takes priority. Until the patient is stabilized and the GU system can be assessed, a high index of suspicion should be maintained for GU trauma on the basis of mechanism of injury because many injuries to the GU tract are occult and not immediately life threatening. These injuries are revealed later in the secondary and tertiary examinations.

Inspection

The first phase of the physical examination is inspection. Abdominal and flank symmetry should be assessed; evidence of torso or pelvic trauma may extend to evidence of GU trauma.[1] The presence of a complex or open pelvic fracture, the number and location of wounds caused by penetrating trauma, and the position of impaled objects must be noted. Impaled objects should not be removed until the patient is in the operating room. Grey Turner's sign (ecchymosis over the posterior aspect of the eleventh or twelfth rib or the flank) may indicate renal trauma or retroperitoneal bleeding.[18] Frequently, renal injury is the result of a direct blow to the flank.[1] Absence of ecchymosis does not rule out renal trauma because a significant proportion of patients with renal trauma do not have Grey Turner's sign. Fractures of the eleventh or twelfth rib or a lumbar transverse process may contribute to renal or ureteral injury.

Assessment of the perineum is integral to patient management. The urinary meatus must be inspected for signs of bleeding, a strong indicator of urethral injury, although it can be absent.[1,14] The assessment of the urinary meatus is essential before a urinary catheter is placed.[19] The perineal area should be assessed for evidence of trauma, including lacerations, hematomas, swelling, and ecchymosis.[1,14]

The scrotum may be edematous or contused because of extravasation of urine or blood in patients with urethral injury, pelvic fracture, or retroperitoneal hematoma.[5,6] Diffuse perineal bruising is a later sign of fracture of the symphysis pubis or pelvic rami. Perineal swelling, vaginal bleeding, vulvar hematoma, and rectal tenderness are all indications of potential GU injury in female patients from straddle injury, fall, MVC, or assault. For women with an altered level of consciousness, a brief pelvic examination should be performed to ascertain any injury and to determine the presence of a tampon, diaphragm, or intrauterine device.

In patients who have sustained blunt trauma and have vaginal bleeding or pelvic fractures, the possibility of vaginal laceration should be considered.[6] Evaluation for such injury is done under direct vision with a speculum or retractors. In the patient with a severe pelvic fracture, the examination usually must be done in an operating suite with the patient under anesthesia. Separation of the legs for examination of a patient with a severe pelvic fracture can result in hemorrhage from pelvic bleeding. This should be avoided at all costs. After the pelvis is stabilized, vaginal examination can occur in the operating suite.

In patients, male or female, with blunt or penetrating trauma with suspected or confirmed vaginal lacerations or penetrating lower abdominal injury, rectal injury must be assumed present until proven otherwise. Such patients require a proctoscopic examination.

Auscultation

The presence and quality of bowel sounds can be assessed. Although the absence of bowel sounds is not specific to GU or gastrointestinal injury, the mechanism and identified injuries should guide assessment. Auscultation around the renal arteries, however, is essential. A bruit in these areas may reflect turbulence at an intimal tear in the artery.

Percussion

Percussion of the abdomen and flank allows assessment of abnormal areas of fluid or air collection.[20] Excessive dullness in the lower abdomen or flank may indicate the extravasation of blood or urine or the presence of a retroperitoneal hematoma. Percussion over the kidneys determines their location in the retroperitoneum.

Palpation

The flank, abdomen, lumbar vertebrae, and lower rib cage are palpated for evidence of pain, mass, or crepitus—all potential indicators of GU trauma.[1,8,20] Renal colic or costovertebral angle pain may indicate renal trauma.[19] Renal colic may be the result of clots obstructing the renal collecting system.[19] Severe costovertebral angle pain may be caused by ischemia from a renal artery thrombosis. Additional signs beyond abdominal tenderness, with or without distention, include a flank mass or a pelvic fracture.[10] The pelvic area is palpated for evidence of tenderness or movable bony fragments, which may indicate pelvic fracture.[6,19] Palpation of the suprapubic area may reveal a distended bladder. Severe tenderness in the hypogastrium may signify bladder rupture.[20]

A rectal examination should also be performed before urinary catheterization, especially in men. The presence of a boggy or displaced prostate may suggest urethral injury, although a large pelvic hematoma can make the prostate difficult to palpate.[6,20]

Laboratory Studies

In addition to the history and physical examination, results from diagnostic and laboratory testing are essential to the assessment of the patient who has sustained trauma to the GU tract.

On admission, blood studies are done to establish baseline profiles. Hematologic studies may indicate hemorrhage, but other sources of blood loss must be ruled out before the assumption is made that the cause lies in the GU tract. From a GU perspective, the primary laboratory study is urinalysis. Gross hematuria correlates with significant lower urologic injury.[10] Hematuria is a common sign of renal trauma and is present in 80% to 94% of cases, but it can often be transient or even absent, especially in certain types of penetrating injuries.[2] Microscopic hematuria may indicate minor injury to the GU tract and requires continued monitoring.[2]

Because urine obtained by catheterization usually contains 5 to 10 red blood cells per microscopic field, it is optimal if the patient can be encouraged to void the initial specimen. This allows the differentiation between hematuria caused by catheterization and hematuria caused by GU injury. The absence of hematuria, however, should not lead the trauma team to falsely assume that there is no GU injury because up to 36% of patients with major renal trauma have been found to have a normal urinalysis.[1]

Radiologic Studies

Radiographic assessment of the patient with GU trauma is the cornerstone of the diagnostic process. The primary study of value is computed tomography (CT), yet other studies can provide valuable information about the organs they assess. Patients who require urologic imaging typically have gross hematuria or microscopic hematuria and hemodynamic instability.[10] One recent study indicated a need for radiographic imaging in hemodynamically stable patients with microscopic hematuria.[2]

Computed Tomography

CT provides the most precise delineation of GU trauma. The test is particularly sensitive in staging renal lacerations (the extent of injury) and in identifying intrarenal and subcapsular hematomas, renal infarct, contrast extravasation, the size and extent of a retroperitoneal hematoma, renal perfusion, and associated injuries to abdominal organs.[10] By use of contrast medium, arterial injury and lack of perfusion can also be demonstrated. CT is also used to monitor progress in nonoperative management of renal injury.[1] CT has essentially replaced intravenous pyelogram (IVP) as the gold standard for renal evaluation.[10] After administration of oral or intravenous (IV) contrast, a spiral CT scan with excretory delayed films is performed to diagnose upper urinary tract injury.[2,9]

Renal Angiography

Renal angiography is indicated when there is incomplete or absent visualization of one or both kidneys on CT, prolonged bleeding without another source, suspicion of renal pedicle trauma, or questionable renal viability. Angiography provides information concerning the preservation of blood supply to the damaged renal parenchyma. Devitalized areas must be identified because necrosis or abscess formation may follow. In penetrating renal trauma after IVP or CT, renal angiography is the second study of choice because it can stage the level of injury reliably and offers the option of embolization versus surgery for hemorrhage control.[10] In patients who have significant abdominal trauma, hemodynamic instability may prevent the use of renal angiography because the reduced blood flow may impede visualization. Instead, assessment of the GU tract may occur during emergency celiotomy.[5,6,18]

Renal arteriography involves cannulation of the femoral artery. After the procedure, the site is monitored closely for bleeding and pulses distal to the site are evaluated for presence and quality.

Ultrasonography

Renal ultrasonography is capable of detecting renal abnormalities with the use of high-frequency sound waves. The sound waves produce echoes, which are amplified and converted by a transducer into electric impulses that are seen on an oscilloscope screen as anatomic pictures. A negative ultrasonographic study does not exclude renal injury and is therefore seldom used for early identification of injury. Ultrasonography is most useful for the identification and serial evaluation of perinephric hematomas and urinomas. In the acute resuscitative period, the use of the focused assessment with sonography for trauma to detect abdominal injuries has also been shown to be unreliable in detecting GU injuries.[10]

Kidney-Ureter-Bladder Radiography

The kidney-ureter-bladder (KUB), a radiograph of these three structures, is usually performed after the patient is stabilized. The purposes of the test are to visualize the position and size of the kidneys; identify lower rib, pelvic, vertebral body, or transverse process fractures; identify the likely position of foreign bodies; and evaluate diaphragmatic displacement.

The psoas muscles may be obliterated or bulging, possibly the result of retroperitoneal hemorrhage or hematoma. The KUB itself is not specific for GU trauma, so the lack of pathologic findings on this examination does not rule out renal trauma. It does, however, heighten the examiner's awareness of other possible associated injuries.

Intravenous Pyelogram

The IVP, also known as the excretory urogram, is one of the fundamental diagnostic procedures in the assessment of patients with renal trauma. The IVP evaluates both structural integrity and excretory function of the renal system. It also allows visualization of renal parenchyma, calices, and pelvis; assessment of perfusion to the injured kidney; evaluation of the status of both the injured and noninjured kidney; and appraisal of the continuity of the collecting system.[1,19] In trauma patients a one-shot IVP is usually performed to save time; this is used purely to confirm the presence of two functional kidneys or massive disruption of the kidneys before surgery.[19] In addition to urologic trauma, abnormalities such as polycystic kidneys, absent kidneys, renal calculi, hydronephrosis, and pyelonephritis may be identified. Currently use of the one-shot IVP is under question because CT is more valuable in GU assessment because it is more sensitive than the IVP. The IVP has been know to have a high false-negative rate for patients with penetrating trauma.[10,19] One-shot IVP may be valuable during surgery to evaluate pedicle injury and contralateral kidney excretion.[1] The study is not accurate if osmotic diuresis is induced or when hypotension is present, resulting in decreased excretion of urine.

Retrograde Urethrogram

The retrograde urethrogram (RUG) is the diagnostic procedure conducted before catheterization of a patient suspected of having an injury to the urethra.[5,19] To perform this test, an 8F urinary catheter is attached to an irrigating syringe filled with contrast material. The catheter is gently inserted into the urinary meatus until the catheter balloon is 2 to 3 cm proximal to the meatus.[19] The balloon is inflated 1.5 to 2 ml and then 15 to 20 ml of contrast is gently injected into the urethra.[19] It is important to bear in mind that there is always a chance that placing a urinary catheter can convert a parital tear to a complete one. If a urinary catheter is already in place, a pericatheter RUG can still be performed to identify urethral injury.

Extravasation of the contrast material detects urethral injury. Partial urethral injury is identified through extravasation with bladder filling, whereas a complete tear of the urethra involves extravasation with loss of continuity.[21] The amount of extravasation seen cannot be used to determine the extent or type of injury because this would be largely dependent on the volume and rate of contrast infused. Rather, the extravasation will determine whether there is loss of continuity.

Cystogram

The cystogram is used to detect intraperitoneal or extraperitoneal bladder rupture.[5,6] A urethral catheter is passed (after urethral injury is ruled out) and the bladder is filled with at least 300 to 500 ml of water-soluble contrast medium.[5,19] Fluid is instilled by gravity to avoid filling the bladder under pressure, which could cause a small tear or even bladder rupture. Anteroposterior and oblique radiographic films are obtained. The bladder is emptied and an anteroposterior postdrainage radiograph is taken. The cystogram should be performed before the IVP.[19] Bladder contusions appear normal on a cystogram.[5] A false-negative study occurs if there is incomplete distention of the bladder or if no drainage radiograph is done.[2] CT cystograms have been found to be 85% to 100% accurate so they can be used instead of conventional cystograms when CT scanning is already being done to rule out abdominal injury.[10]

Radionuclide Imaging

Renal radionuclide scanning provides information regarding renal injury. This test is especially useful for patients who are allergic to contrast dyes. Abnormal results of this test may indicate renal hypoperfusion, fractures, urinary extravasation, and delayed excretion. Renal blood flow can be assessed accurately, but parenchymal and collecting system injuries cannot be identified as accurately as with IVP or CT. Urine from patients receiving radionuclide injections should be handled with gloves after the procedure to avoid care provider exposure to the radioactive isotope.

Magnetic Resonance Imaging

Although magnetic resonance imaging (MRI) provides excellent imaging, studies have demonstrated that there is no advantage of using MRI over CT imaging.[2] The increased cost, extended time, and potential nonavailability of MRI versus CT makes its use only applicable in the rare cases where the patient has an iodine allergy.[10]

The diagnostic tests used are determined by the mechanism of injury and patient's assessment findings. The most sensitive and specific diagnostic test has become the CT scan. Other diagnostic tests may be used as adjunts to the CT scan and can provide valuable information about the structures that they assess.

SPECIFIC ORGAN INJURY

Specific GU injuries vary widely in severity, the need for immediate operative management, and sequelae. The following section discusses specific injuries, diagnoses, and treatments.

TRAUMA TO THE PERINEUM

Trauma to the genital organs, although often not life threatening, can produce overwhelming loss and crisis for the patient and significant others. Genital trauma may be associated with injury to the perineum, bony pelvis, thighs, bladder, vagina, and rectum. Blunt trauma, burns, and penetrating trauma all may produce genital trauma. Fortunately, trauma to the genitals is not common, and surgical intervention can produce good results in both function and appearance. Hemorrhage of the external genitalia is usually controlled by compression dressings, clamps, or ligation.[22] These wounds are further managed by wound irrigation and debridement to preserve tissue viability.[19]

Male Genitalia

Testes. The testes are usually spared from injury by their mobility, contraction of the cremaster muscle, and a tough capsular covering. However, injury can be produced by a direct blow, as in sport or assault-type injuries, which compress the testes against the symphysis pubis, producing contusion or rupture. The tunica vaginalis sac may fill with blood (hematocele), and the patient may present with a large, tender, swollen scrotal mass.

Management. Immediate surgical intervention is the treatment of choice, with every attempt made to salvage the testes. Blood clots are evacuated from the tunica vaginalis, and testicular rupture is repaired. Delayed treatment may increase the risk of infection of the hematocele or testis or may cause testicular atrophy from the pressure of the tense hematocele. Orchiectomy is the least desired outcome of severe injury or from complications of testicular trauma.

Scrotum. Trauma to the scrotum may produce avulsion injuries, resulting in significant tissue loss. The mechanisms of injury are the same as for the testes.

Management. When possible, the avulsed scrotum is reconstructed around the testes and usually regains normal size within a few months. If scrotal reconstruction is not possible, the testicles may be implanted into upper thigh pockets, where the temperature is similar to that of the scrotum.

Penetrating injury to the scrotum can result in injury to the spermatic cord and testes. The salvage rate for the testes is approximately 35%.[19] Early debridement and primary repair are essential. Delayed repair is associated with a 21% increased rate of orchiectomy compared with 6% in those who had primary repair immediately after injury.[19] Associated injuries may be present, affecting the thighs, femoral vessels, small bowel, or colon.[19]

Penis. Trauma to the penis may be a result of blunt trauma, strangulation injury, mishaps during sexual intercourse, amputation, or penetrating injury (Figure 26-3).[19,23,24] Patients with penetrating trauma to the penis have associated injuries of the thigh, scrotum, pelvis, buttock, or abdomen 80% of the time.[19] Blunt trauma usually produces a penile fracture with rupture of the tunica albuginea, hemorrhage, and hematoma formation.[5,19,23,24] Of these injuries, 10% to 30% result in urethral injury as well.[25] The patient presents with

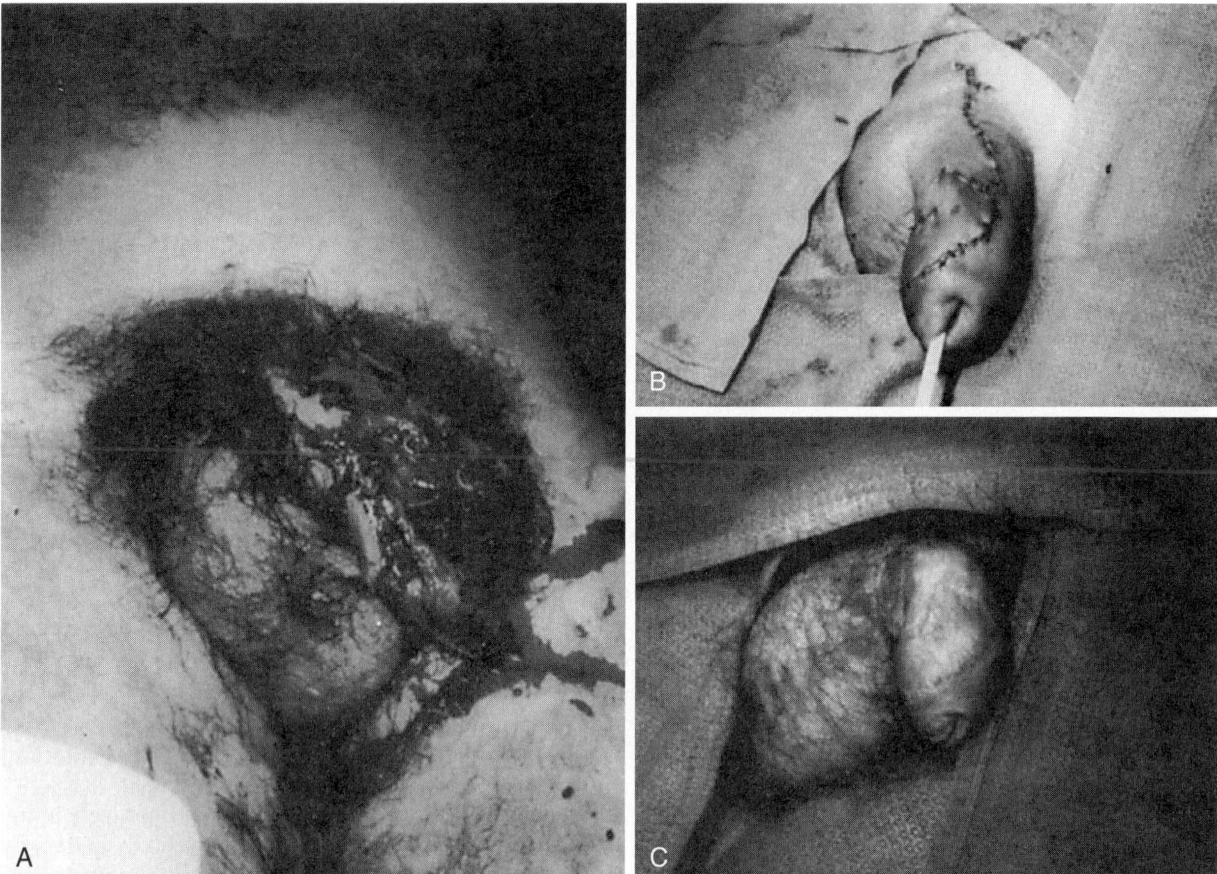

FIGURE 26-3 **A,** Power saw injury to the penis resulting in complete midline hemisection from symphysis through the glans penis, including the urethra. **B,** Appearance at the completion of reconstruction. A urethral stenting catheter was left in place. All tissue survived without additional debridement. **C,** Genital appearance 6 months after injury. The patient had complete return of sensation, sexual function, and urethral voiding. (From McAninch JW, Kahn RI, Jeffrey RB et al: Major traumatic and septic genital injuries, *J Trauma* 24:291-298, 1984.)

pain, swelling, discoloration, and deviation.[23] If the injury occurs from striking against a hard object, a direct blow, or abnormal bending, a snap or crackle may have been heard at the time of injury, suggesting fracture.[5,19,23-24] Penetrating injuries to the penis involve the urethra in 17% to 22% of cases.[25] Indications that the urethra is involved are discussed later in this chapter.

Management. Injury to the penis can be treated either conservatively or with immediate surgical repair.[19,23-25] Conservative treatment includes urethral catheterization or suprapubic cystostomy, application of ice, elevation, administration of anti-inflammatory drugs, compression dressings, analgesics, and medication to temporarily suppress erections.[19] Complications of conservative treatment include penile abscess formation, urinary extravasation, pain, inadequate erection, and permanent deformity.[23] Patients with penile injury have a 10% to 53% complication rate.[23] Surgical intervention is advocated as the treatment of choice to decrease the incidence of complications and to promote rapid recovery.[19]

Strangulation injuries may be produced by foreign objects or human hair constricting the penis. The patient has pain and swelling distal to the constricting object. Urethral fistula formation and partial amputation may result from prolonged constriction. Immediate surgical intervention is usually necessary.

Traumatic amputation of the penis may produce severe physical and psychologic disability. A successful outcome requires the cooperation of a urologist, plastic surgeon, and psychiatrist. Surgical reattachment of the distal segment may be possible if the ischemia time is 18 hours or less (this time may be longer if the segment is preserved in iced saline solution). Microvascular repair may be advisable. Immediate repair and local reshaping may be performed, with plastic surgery and cosmetic repair done at a later time.

Burns involving the genitalia are rare, occuring only 1% of the time, and are usually associated with patients who have extensive burns over their bodies.[17] Most genital burns can be treated conservatively with dressing changes, but excision and grafting may be necessary with severe, full-thickness burns, and circumferential penile burns may require early escharotomy to preserve function.[17]

Female Genitalia

Trauma to the female genitalia is caused by straddle falls, MVCs, and sexual assault.[14,26,27] Pelvic fractures, which account for the majority of female external genital trauma, most often injure the vagina and perineum.[7-9] Penetrating trauma also may injure the uterus and ovaries, which may require surgical repair, hysterectomy, or oophorectomy.

Perineum. External perineal injury may present as vulvar hematoma after a straddle event or sexual assault. Assault further involves tears of the introitus.[26] The most common injuries in young girls involve the vulva (63%) and vagina (53%).[26] Concomitant anorectal lacerations may be noted. Sexual assault may also result in lacerations to the urethra, especially in young girls or women with an imperforate hymen.[26] Use of a colposcope, a free-standing microscope used outside the speculum, has significantly increased the documentation of injuries sustained from sexual assault.[28] The colposcope allows increased visualization through magnification. Table 26-1 lists the genitalia injuries sustained in order of frequency by age group.[28]

Vagina. Vaginal tears occur during sexual assault and frequently during straddle-type injuries. A high-speed fall onto water, such as a fall from a Jet Ski, carries sufficient force that the water behaves as a solid object, resulting in vaginal and perineal laceration.[29,30] Regardless of mechanism, injuries are considered severe when the cervix is involved or when profusely bleeding vaginal lacerations, which can result in hypovolemic shock, are present.[30-32]

The most common clinical sign of vaginal trauma is vaginal bleeding, which may be masked by spasm of the vagina. Consequently, a speculum examination is essential for women who have sustained pelvic fracture. This examination may occur in the operating suite after pelvic hemorrhage is under control. Evidence from a victim of sexual assault must be retrieved carefully, preferably by a professional trained in evidence collection and forensics, so that all documentation and sample handling is performed appropriately for legal purposes.[26,33] Evidence of sperm and seminal plasma still can be obtained up to 48 hours after assault.[34] Swabs should be taken of the introitus and rectal cavity. Research suggests that good nursing care can mediate feelings and fears of permanent physical and emotional damage by responding in a supportive manner.[33]

TABLE 26-1 **Female Genitalia Injury After Sexual Assault**

Age Group	Injury in Order of Most to Least Frequent
0-12 years	Hymen, labia minora, posterior fourchette, rectum into hymen, rectum
13-17 years	Hymen, posterior fourchette, labia minora, cervix/vagina into hymen, cervix
Adult	Hymen, cervix, posterior fourchette, vagina into labia minora, cervix, periurethral area

Management. Examination under moderate sedation or even general anesthesia may provide a more complete assessment.[15,29] More than 75% of upper vaginal lacerations require surgical repair.[29] During surgical repair, hypogastric artery ligation may be necessary to control reproductive hemorrhage.[29] Interventional angiography for embolization can be performed to avoid retroperitoneal exploration. Packing is an alternative that can be used to control hemorrhage until other organ injuries are ruled out.[29,31] Complications of vaginal tears include pelvic abscesses and sepsis. Wounds are often left open to avoid retroperitoneal abscess formation.[29,31]

Trauma to the Urethra

Injury to the female urethra is rarely seen because the urethra is shorter and more mobile than in males.[9] When female urethra injury is present, however, it is usually associated with significant pelvic fracture or disruption and injury to the bladder neck and vagina.[7] In one study, urethral injury was found to correlate with specific fractures of the pelvis, including inferior rami fractures, widened symphysis, and sacroiliac joint disruption.[7] The symphysis pubis widening and fracture of the inferior pubic ramus fractures were also found to be independent predictors of urethral injury, owing to a higher index of suspicion of urethral injuries when these fractures are present.[7] Urethral injuries are often the result of straddle-type injuries. Straddle injuries can crush the urethra but not cause pelvic fracture.[6] These straddle scenarios are more common in children than in adults.[6,35,36] Complete rupture of the urethra is also more common in children because the thin, delicate membrane of the urethra is less elastic than in an adult.[35] In children the most likely sites of urethral injury are the prostatic urethra and bladder neck.[35,36]

The male urethra is divided into two segments: the anterior (distal) and the posterior (proximal). The anterior segment has three anatomic divisions: the glandular, pendulous, and bulbar. The posterior segment comprises the membranous and the prostatic urethra. Pelvic fractures are the most common mechanism of injury to the posterior portion of the urethra.[7,36] Pelvic fractures shear the prostate from the urogenital diaphragm, rupturing the ligaments holding the urethra in place and tearing and potentially disrupting the urethra (Figure 26-4).[11,36] Anterior pelvic ring disruption with pubic rami fracture results in bladder and urethra injury in either sex due to the shearing forces applied.[36] The likelihood of urethral injury increases with open book and vertical shear types of pelvic fractures and should be suspected when a pubic arch is fractured.[10]

Most anterior urethral injury occurs after a straddle-type injury. Penetrating trauma to the anterior urethra may be produced by gunshot wounds, stab wounds, or self-inflicted instrumentation of the urethra with foreign bodies.[5] Power takeoff machinery can also cause penetrating injury to the urethra and is sometimes seen with farming and industrial incidents. In these cases clothing becomes caught in the

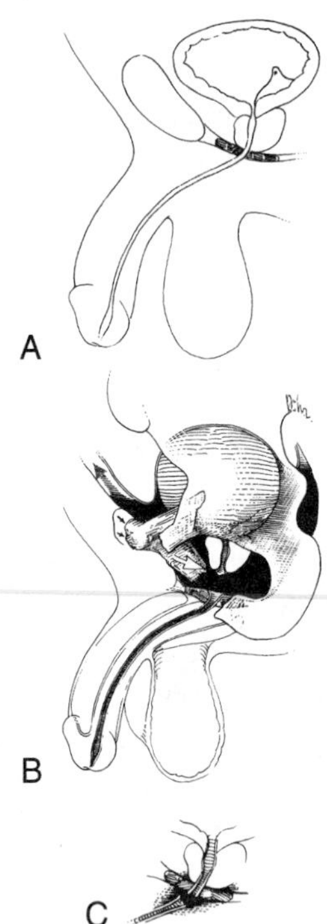

FIGURE 26-4 Posterior urethral rupture: (**A**) normal anatomy; (**B**) rupture below the prostatic apex; (**C**) rupture at the membranous/bulbar urethral junction. (From McAninch JW, Santucci RA: Genitourinary trauma. In Walsh PC, Retik AB, Wein A et al, editors: *Campbell's urology*, p 3726, Philadelphia, 2002, W. B. Saunders.)

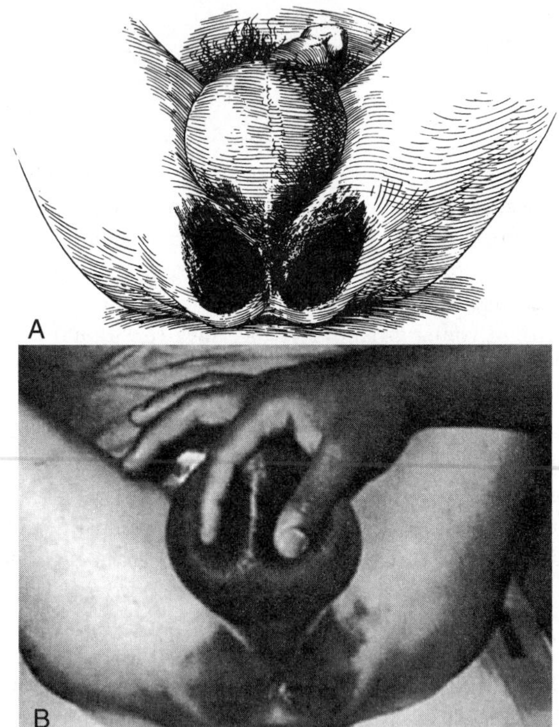

FIGURE 26-5 **A,** Diagram of a butterfly hematoma. **B,** Appearance of a patient with perineal butterfly hematoma. (From Peters P, Sagalowsky A: Genitourinary trauma. In Walsh P, Gittes R, Perlmutter A, et al, editors: *Campbell's urology*, 5th ed, vol 1, Philadelphia, 1986, W. B. Saunders.)

power belt of a machine, possibly causing injury to the skin of the penis, the scrotum, and the urethra.[5,6,23,24]

Assessment

Findings characteristic of urethral injury include identification of blood at the urinary meatus, an inability to void, gross hematuria, pelvic or perineal ecchymosis, perineal or scrotal edema, or a high-riding prostate.[5,6,36] A male patient with straddle injury may present with a characteristic butterfly-shaped ecchymotic area beneath the scrotum[1,5,6] (Figure 26-5). Urethral blood at the meatus is an inconsistent finding, with only 12% of patients having this clinical finding in one study.[7] Because of the high correlation of pelvic fractures with urethral injury, it should be assumed that both male and female patients with pelvic fractures have urethral injury until proven otherwise. RUG is suggested in all patients with blood at the meatus.[5]

In male patients urethral injuries are classified according to location. Table 26-2 lists the classification of urethral injury. In general, urethral injuries below the urogenital diaphragm, involving the bulbous and penile urethra, are classified as anterior urethral trauma. Those above the urogenital diaphragm, toward the bladder neck and involving the prostatic and membranous urethra, are classified as posterior urethral trauma.

TABLE 26-2 **Classification of Urethral Injuries**

Grade	Injuries
I	Posterior urethra intact but stretched by pelvic hematoma
II	Partial or complete postmembranous urethral rupture above intact urogenital diaphragm
III	Partial or complete combined anterior/posterior urethral rupture with rupture of urogenital diaphragm
IV	Bladder neck injury with extension into the posterior urethra
IVA	Base of the bladder injury with periurethral extravasation simulating a grade IV injury
V	Partial or complete anterior urethra injury

Modified from Corriere JN: Trauma to the lower urinary tract. In Gillenwater JY, Grayhack JT, Howards SS et al, editors: *Adult and pediatric urology*, 4th ed, p 514, Baltimore, 2002, Lippincott Williams & Wilkins.

Posterior urethral injury should be suspected in any patient with a pelvic fracture or separation of the symphysis pubis and in patients in whom a displaced (or high-riding) prostate or soft boggy mass is found on rectal examination.[23,36,37] Injury to the membranous urethra is the most common and may extend into the bulbous urethra with disruption of the urogenital diaphragm.[7,37] Stretching usually precedes rupture at the bulbomembranous junction.[5,6] Any patient with an anticipated urethral tear must have an RUG performed before urethral catheterization.[5,18,36] Tears at the urogenital diaphragm demonstrate extravasation into the peritoneum. These are significant tears because cellulitis and sepsis can occur. Urethral stricture may be inevitable with these tears.[6,36]

Management

The goal of early management is to provide urinary drainage and to prevent associated complications such as worsening injury to the urethra by catherization, strictures, fistula, or infection.[5,36,37] The goals of treatment are to maintain patency of the urethra and continence.[5,36,37] Treatment options include direct repair, realignment, and nonoperative management with suprapubic cystostomy (SPT) placement.[5,36,37] Catheterization by anyone other than the urologist should not be performed if any indication or potential for urethral injury is present. Catheterization can convert an incomplete tear of the urethra to a complete tear, increase the risk of infection, and infect a sterile hematoma.[36,37] If the patient can void spontaneously, catheterization is ill advised because any tear is likely partial.[6,37] Transurethral catheter placement has traditionally been avoided in posterior urethral injury as identified on RUG; however, one study suggested that catheterization by an experienced urologist with primary realignment of the urethra reduced the need for delayed urethroplasty, and patients with primary realignment had significantly fewer complications, such as stricture, impotence, and incontinence.[5,6,36,37]

Management of posterior urethral injury may still require SPT to divert urine from the area of injury if a catheter cannot be placed successfully or if the patient is critically ill.[36,37] Despite recent advances in surgical management, the most common management of prostatomembranous urethra injury involves SPT placement with delayed urethroplasty.[5,36] Use of SPT avoids entry into the pelvic hematoma, thereby decreasing the risk of infection and blood loss and avoiding mobilization of the prostate.[36-38] If rectal injuries are present, immediate operation is required. During this time, evacuation of the hematoma with primary urethral realignment over a urinary catheter can be performed.[36] Preservation of the bladder neck is essential to maintain continence.[37]

Acute realignment of injury to the urethra is becoming more common. The procedure has the same incidence of erectile dysfunction and incontinence as SPT alone but decreases the occurrence of stricture.[37] Early realignment reestablishes continuity and eliminates the need for delayed urethroplasty and long-term SPT placement. Primary realignment is performed either by endoscopy or fluoroscopy.

Anterior urethral injuries are managed with a transurethral catheter or SPT for approximately 3 weeks. Strictures are likely to occur and require urethroplasty after 3 months.[39] RUG is required before urinary catheter or SPT removal to ensure urethral continuity.

Penetrating injuries generally require surgical intervention. Debridement and cleansing are done along with reconstruction of the injury. Management after debridement is the same as mentioned previously.

Missed urethral injuries in the female patient result in severe complications, which include sepsis and necrotizing infection.[38] A delayed diagnosis in the female patient results in incontinence, ureterovaginal fistulae, urethral diverticula, dyspareunia, hematuria, abscess, recurrent urethritis, or cystitis.[36,38,40] Treatment for these complications includes urethral catheter stent placement or delayed operative reconstruction.[5,36]

Trauma to the Bladder

The bladder of an adult rests within the pelvic region of the lower abdomen, well protected by the pelvis. Injury to the bladder occurs during a significant transfer of kinetic energy to the pelvis. Another mechanism of injury to the bladder occurs when the bladder is full and, as a result of its larger size, it is less protected by the bony pelvis.[41] Although 60% to 80% of bladder injuries are caused by blunt trauma, GSWs to the bladder result in intraperitoneal rupture and urine leak.[9,10] Patients who have bladder rupture after minor trauma should be suspected of having a preexisting bladder condition, such as cancer or an infiltrative disease (e.g., tuberculosis or amyloidosis), or having undergone previous radiation treatments.

When the pelvis is fractured or the bladder is distended, the normal protective mechanisms are lost and the bladder is at higher risk for injury.[41] As the severity of pelvic fracture, according to the abbreviated injury score, increases, so does the relative risk for bladder injury.[8] The bladder is relatively mobile except for the bladder neck.[41] The dome is its weakest point and it is vulnerable to rupture.[6,41]

The incidence of traumatic intraperitoneal bladder rupture is 15% to 45%.[41] In children less than 6 years old the risk for bladder injury is high because the bladder is an abdominal organ.[41] There is an increased risk of bladder injury if the bladder is distended by urine. The fuller the bladder, the higher risk for injury.[42] Intraperitoneal ruptures occur when there is an increase in intravesical pressure as a result of a blow to the lower abdomen or a seat belt deceleration injury (see Figure 26-2).[41] Increased intravesicular pressure results in a tear in the dome of a full bladder, precipitating bladder rupture.

Only 10% to 15% of pelvic fractures have bladder injury, but 70% of those patients with bladder injury have associated pelvic fractures.[9,10] The incidence of extraperitoneal bladder injury is 50% to 85% among patients with pelvic fractures.[43] Fracture of the anterior pelvic arch is the most frequently associated injury.[7] In the case of pelvic fracture a bony spicule punctures the bladder.[6,41] Combination intraperitoneal and extraperitoneal bladder injuries have a 5% to 8% incidence.[41]

Assessment

Bladder rupture is primarily associated with gross hematuria (87% to 98%).[41,42] The patient with a ruptured bladder may have pain in the shoulder area, a sign of urine in the peritoneal cavity. The patient may also be unable to void. A urine specimen reveals gross or microscopic hematuria.[6,41,42] Microscopic hematuria is indicative of a bladder contusion and should resolve over a few days.[41] The most common bladder injury is contusion.[41] Gross hematuria, pelvic fractures (other than acetablular fractures), and pelvic fluid found on CT should prompt the use of cystography because abdominal CT without cystography is not enougth to detect bladder rupture even if the urinary catheter is clamped to cause bladder distention.[10,41] Studies have shown that CT cystography is as accurate as conventional cystography in diagnosing bladder rupture.[10,44] Figure 26-6 compares the findings by cystography in intraperitoneal and extraperitoneal bladder rupture.

The patient may be in shock and have multiple associated injuries. Mortality rates can be as high as 16% to 53% as a result of associated injuries.[6,8,41] The most common coexisting injuries include bowel lacerations and laceration of major vessels, including the vena cava, mesenteric, and renal or iliac arteries or veins.[8] Definitive diagnosis of bladder rupture is made by cystogram.[5,41,42] Urethral injury must be ruled out before placement of a catheter for the procedure. On cystogram, intraperitoneal bladder rupture is demonstrated by contrast material outlining bowel loops, filling the cul de sac, and extending into the paracolic gutters[6,41-44] (see Figure 26-6, *A*). Urine and blood may collect in the peritoneal space.[43] Extraperitoneal bladder rupture demonstrates feathery flames of contrast on cystogram (see Figure 26-6, *B*). Occasionally the cystogram may reveal a bladder that is tear-drop shaped. This change in shape is due to the presence of large pelvic hematomas or urine extravasation.[44,45] The pressure of these hematomas on the bladder creates the tear-drop configuration.

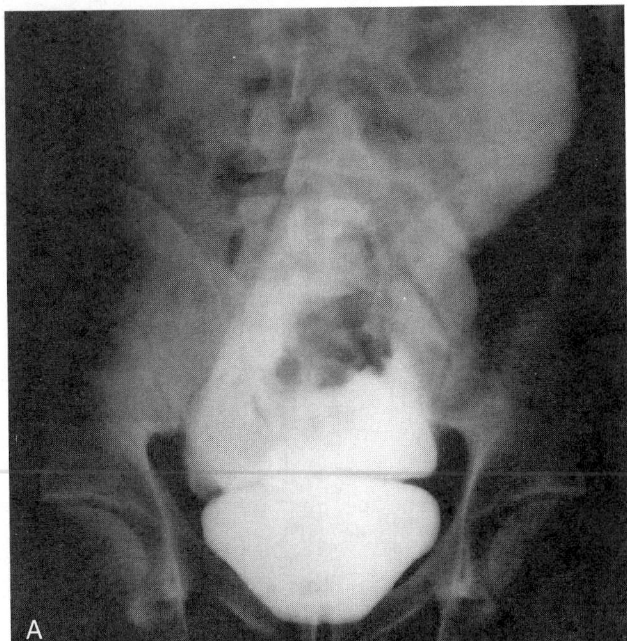

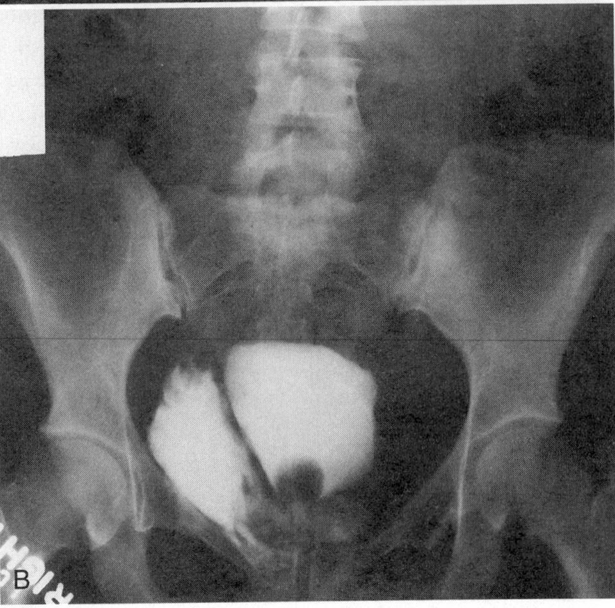

FIGURE 26-6 **A,** Intraperitoneal bladder rupture on cystography. Bowel loops are commonly outlined by contrast in the abdominal cavity. **B,** Extraperitoneal bladder rupture on cystography. (From McAninch JW, Santucci RA: Genitourinary trauma. In Walsh PC, Retik AB, Wein A et al, editors: *Campbell's urology,* pp 3722-3723, Philadelphia, 2002, W. B. Saunders.)

Management of Extraperitoneal Bladder Rupture

Management of extraperitoneal bladder rupture consists of drainage by a large transurethral catheter or suprapubic catheter.[6,46] Transurethral catheters are preferred over suprapubic catheters because they result in fewer complications and fewer days of catherization regardless of the severity of the bladder injury.[6,10,45] Antibiotics may be administered to decrease urine colonization and resultant urinary tract infection (UTI).[35] Nonoperative management results in minimal morbidity, and studies have shown outcomes similar to those of patients treated operatively with primary suturing.[10,41,45,46] Drainage is necessary for approximately 10 days or until extravasation no longer occurs.[41] Cystography is used to identify closure of the rupture.[41-43,45] Contraindications of nonoperative management are related to severe pelvic fractures that include bone fragments projecting into the bladder or open fractures.[10] Another indication for surgical repair is in patients who also have rectal perforations.[10]

Bacterial colonization of the bladder can occur within a few days as a result of catheterization despite adequate urine drainage.[47,48] Multiple catheterizations and bladder irrigation increase the colonization risk. Hence adequate bladder drainage is essential. In addition, antibiotic coverage for both gram-positive and gram-negative bacteria may be considered to decrease the risk of infection.[47,48] Inadequate bladder drainage results in retrograde infection and colonization of the pelvic hematoma.[48]

Maintaining catheter patency within the first 24 to 48 hours is integral to successful nonoperative management. If patency cannot be maintained, exploration and closure of the bladder injury are necessary.[41]

Management of Intraperitoneal Bladder Rupture

An intraperitoneal bladder rupture must be surgically repaired, the pelvic hematoma left undisturbed, and extravasated urine and blood evacuated.[41,47,48] Nonviable bladder tissue is removed, the tear is sutured, and a suprapubic catheter tube or transurethral catheter is placed for urine drainage. Combined drainage (suprapubic tube and transurethral catheterization) has been used, although studies have suggested transurethral catheterization as an adequate drainage system that also was associated with a shorter hospital stay and lower morbidity rates.[48-50]

Unrecognized intraperitoneal bladder rupture can result in hyperkalemia, hypernatremia, uremia, and acidosis as a result of resorption of the extravasated urine.[41] Continued extravasation of urine may result in peritonitis, abscess, fistula, or uroascites with respiratory compromise.[6,41,48] Infected urine may contribute to septic complications. A delay in diagnosis may produce symptoms similar to an acute condition in the abdomen.[51]

Trauma to the Ureter

The ureter is a muscular tube with an adventitial sheath that acts as a conduit for urine from the kidney to the bladder. The ureter is mobile with fixed points at the bladder and where the ureter crosses the pelvic brim.

Ureteral injuries are typically the result of iatrogenic injury during surgery.[6,10] Gynecologic surgery has been associated with up to 75% of cases of iatrogenic injury to the ureter.[52,53] During hysterectomy, injury rates to the ureter have been reported to be 0.02% to 2.5%.[52] Ureter injury from trauma only makes up 1% of ureter injuries with GSWs and stab wounds being the most common causes of penetrating ureteral injury.[10,53] They may produce partial or complete transection.[10]

Ureteral injury is rarely produced by blunt trauma but, when present, is usually in the form of disruption at the ureteropelvic junction.[13,53] Blunt ureteral injury may be caused by a major hyperextension of the lower thoracic or upper lumbar area or excessive force produced by a fall or ejection from a motor vehicle.[5] Uretopelvic junction and ureter injuries occur mostly in children.[5,52]

Ureteral trauma can be described as a silent injury, often with no presenting symptoms. Ureteral trauma is suspected when hematuria is present with a normal IVP or CT. The direction of penetrating trauma and hyperextension of the spine during blunt injury indicate that there is potential for ureteral injury.

Assessment

The patient may complain of pain only when the ureter is obstructed. Unilateral ureteral obstruction may produce a slight, transient increase in serum creatinine or blood urea nitrogen (BUN) levels, but urine output typically does not change. A patient may lose complete kidney function as a result of unilateral ureteral injury yet remain asymptomatic if the contralateral kidney is able to maintain renal function. In patients with a solitary kidney, loss of function as a result of misdiagnosed ureteral injury can be life threatening. Bilateral ureteral injury is rare but may be induced iatrogenically.

Ureter injury may be missed with urinalysis, IVP, ultrasonography, and CT; therefore, there should be a high index of suspicion during celiotomy.[10,53] CT with contrast dye may increase the detection of ureter injury from blunt trauma if the CT is delayed for 5 to 8 minutes after contrast injection.[10] After penetrating injury, conventional IVP or intravenous urethrogram can be used to diagnosis ureter injury; dye can be injected into the ureter and extravasation determined during the operative procedure for abdominal injury.

Delayed diagnosis of ureteral injury is not uncommon because of the lack of signs and symptoms and the inaccessibility of the upper ureters.[54] Some signs and symptoms that have been associated with ureteric injury include prolonged ileus and high urinary output from abdominal drains, fever/sepsis, persistent flank or abdominal pain, urinary obstruction, and elevation in creatinine or BUN levels.[54] Delayed diagnosis, however, carries a significant morbidity rate because of the loss of renal function.[54]

Management

The goal of ureter repair is to preserve renal function and restore continuity of the collecting system. Figure 26-7 illustrates the management options of ureter injuries on the basis of the level of the injury. Laceration of the ureter can be repaired surgically or stented to divert urine and prevent urinoma formation.[53,54] Definitive reconstruction occurs after the patient is stabilized and acidosis, hypothermia, and coagulopathies are reversed.[6,53,54] Gross bleeding must be controlled, which may delay stenting or nephrostomy. The risk of bleeding as a result of delayed repair of the ureter is minimal.[53] Spontaneous drainage of urine into the abdomen must be avoided.[53] Significant delay in repair may result in loss of a kidney, especially when UPJ injury is involved.[53]

Trauma to the lower third of the ureter may be repaired by reimplantation into the bladder or by ureteroureterostomy (the anastomosis of ureteral ends). Injury to the upper and middle thirds of the ureter may be best managed by ureteroureterostomy.[54] Internal silicone stenting catheters are placed to maintain alignment, ensure patency, prevent urinary extravasation, and provide support.[54] These stents remain in place for several weeks or months and are removed by cystoscopy. Complications of ureteroureterostomy increase when colon injury, multiple abdominal injuries, intraoperative bleeding, or shock is present.[54]

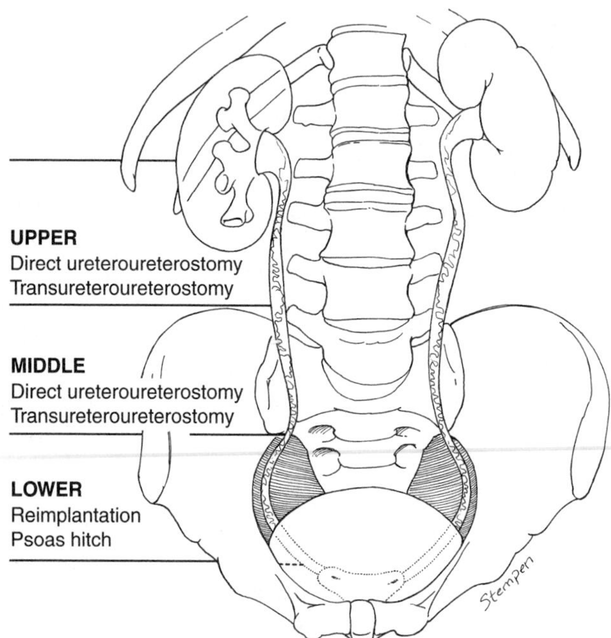

FIGURE 26-7 Management options for ureteral injuries at different levels. (From McAninch JW, Santucci RA: Genitourinary trauma. In Walsh PC, Retik AB, Wein A et al, editors: *Campbell's urology,* p 3718, Philadelphia, 2002, W. B. Saunders.)

Loss of extensive segments of ureter may necessitate a transureteroureterostomy, the anastomosis of the injured ureter into the contralateral ureter. If this procedure is not possible, the injured ureter may be replaced with ileum in an attempt to prevent loss of renal function.

Penetrating ureter injuries require irrigation and debridement followed by primary repair.[53,54] Vascular reconstruction in the face of urinary leak requires primary repair or stenting to decrease the leak.[6,53]

After ureteral repair the patient must be observed for potential complications, which include obstruction, pseudocyst, obstructive hydronephrosis, fistula, and urinoma.[6,54] Fistulas may develop as a result of stricture or obstruction. Persistent leakage of urine may follow. If the ureteral injury is missed, fistula development may cause inflammation that may prevent repair.

Stricture formation leading to hydronephrosis is another complication of ureteral injury.[54] This problem may develop slowly and may not be evident for months. An IVP is recommended at 6 weeks and again at 3 months and 6 months after stent removal to monitor the healing process and monitor for the development of stricture formation.[5,54]

Retroperitoneal urinoma is a complication related to a delay in diagnosis or prolonged extravasation at the repair site. Patients with penetrating ureteral trauma who have a low-grade fever, prolonged ileus, or flank pain may have a urinoma.[54] Drains are placed until urine leak ceases. These drains should be well protected from contamination and enclosed in a sterile bag. Urinomas can ultimately result in obstruction and local inflammation, both signs of late recognition.[54]

Infection is a threat to the patient who has experienced ureteral trauma. Infection of the urine during the perioperative period may produce retroperitoneal scarring, abscess formation, or pyelonephritis. Urine cultures are monitored carefully, and antibiotics are administered as required.

TRAUMA TO THE KIDNEY

The kidneys lie behind the liver and colon and are in close proximity to the spleen, stomach, jejunum, and pancreas. Injury to these viscera is often associated with renal injury.

The kidney is mobile and is attached by a pedicle consisting of the renal artery, renal vein, and ureter. Its mobility can be detrimental in an acceleration-deceleration injury, whereby the organ is put into motion, is contused by the ribs and abdominal viscera, and rotates on the pedicle.

Renal injuries account for 8% to 10% of blunt and penetrating abdominal trauma.[55,56] Renal trauma is often classified according to mechanism of injury. Blunt renal trauma is caused primarily by MVCs, pedestrian versus car events, assaults, and sports injuries. Penetrating renal trauma is caused by knife or GSWs or impalement injuries. The majority of renal injuries are contusions, whether the cause is blunt or penetrating trauma.[2] The incidence of renal injury is higher in children than

TABLE 26-3 **American Association for the Surgery of Trauma Organ Injury Severity Scale for the Kidney**

Grade*	Type	Description
I	Contusion	Microscopic or gross hematuria, urologic studies normal
	Hematoma	Subcapsular, nonexpanding without parenchymal laceration
II	Hematoma	Nonexpanding perirenal hematoma confined to renal retroperitoneum
	Laceration	<1 cm parenchymal depth of renal cortex without urinary extravasation
III	Laceration	>1 cm parenchymal depth of renal cortex without collecting system rupture or urinary extravasation
IV	Laceration	Parenchymal laceration extending through renal cortex, medulla, and collecting system
	Vascular	Main renal artery or vein injury with contained hemorrhage
V	Laceration	Completely shattered kidney
	Vascular	Avulsion of renal hilum, devascularizing the kidney

Source: Moore EE, Shackford SR, Pachter HL et al: Organ injury scanning: spleen, liver and kidney, *J Trauma* 29:1664-1666,1989.

*Advance one grade for bilateral injuries up to grade III.

adults because the kidney is an abdominal organ and is less protected in children. They have less perirenal fat, weaker abdominal muscles, immature rib cages, and a relatively large size of the kidney in proportion to the abdomen.[57,58]

Staging of Renal Injuries

Renal injury is staged by severity as identified on CT scan. Table 26-3 lists the staging of renal injuries.[1,2] Staging guides treatment, thus influencing outcomes. Inadequate staging or underrepresentation of the severity of injury results in increased morbidity and mortality rates, particularly in patients with a history of renal failure.[2] The classification system for renal injuries is seen in Figure 26-8.

Assessment

Patients with minor renal trauma usually have costovertebral angle pain on palpation. A flank mass may indicate a tamponaded perirenal hematoma. Bruising may be evident over the eleventh and twelfth ribs, referred to as the Grey Turner sign. The absence of bruising does not rule out kidney trauma because ecchymosis may take time to develop, if at all.[2,5,6] Patients with congenitally abnormal kidneys are at high risk for severe injury even from relatively minor trauma.[2] Patients with major renal trauma may present with a palpable flank mass, gross or microscopic hematuria, or shock. Ecchymosis may be evident over the flank and lower ribs. These patients may complain of abdominal and flank tenderness. The eleventh and twelfth ribs may be fractured. Life-threatening hemorrhage may occur from renal arterial or venous bleeding.[5,6,59]

Radiographic assessment of the kidneys is reserved for the hemodynamically stable patient.[2,6] The IVP is normal or shows a slight delay in function in patients with minor renal injury. In the face of blunt injury, CT imaging is indicated in patients with gross hematuria or a complex of microscopic hematuria and mild hypotension (systolic blood pressure <90 mm Hg).[10,56] One problem with the CT scan is that the contrast media can cause damage to an already compromised kidney. Even in the absence of hematuria, there are certain mechanisms that should raise the suspicion of unrecognized renal trauma: falls from heights, high-speed MVCs, and multiple injuries.[2] It has been demonstrated that about half of all patients with penetrating trauma and hematuria will have a grade III, IV, or V renal injury.[2] Thus, it is recommended that these patients have either immediate radiographic assessment or surgical exploration to evaluate the kidney.[2] Further studies including CT scan may be indicated in the stable pediatric patient if hematuria of >50 red blood cells per high-power field is found.[2]

Management

The management priority for renal trauma is salvage of renal function. Clinically unstable patients require surgery to repair or remove the injured kidney.[2,10,60] Nonoperative management of major renal lacerations may be safe in the patient who

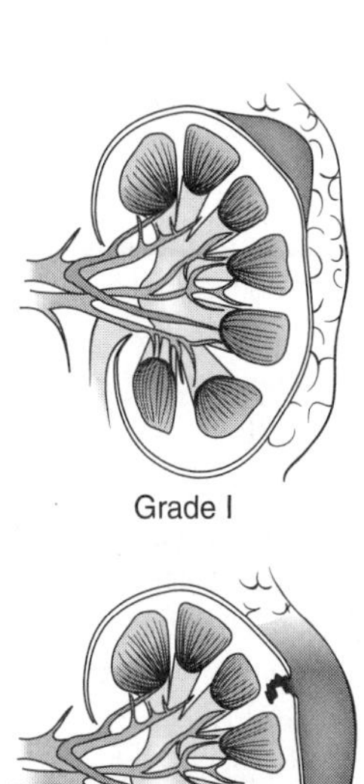

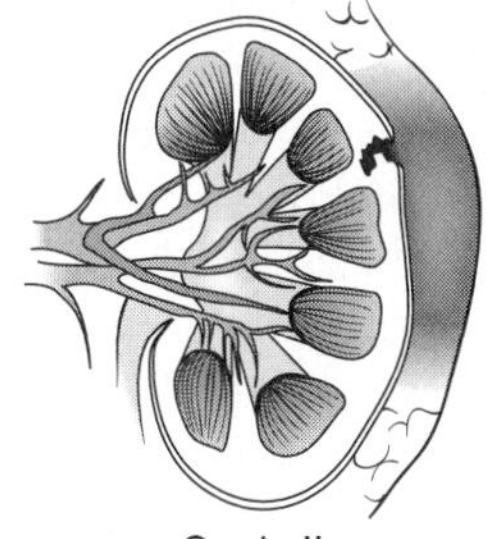

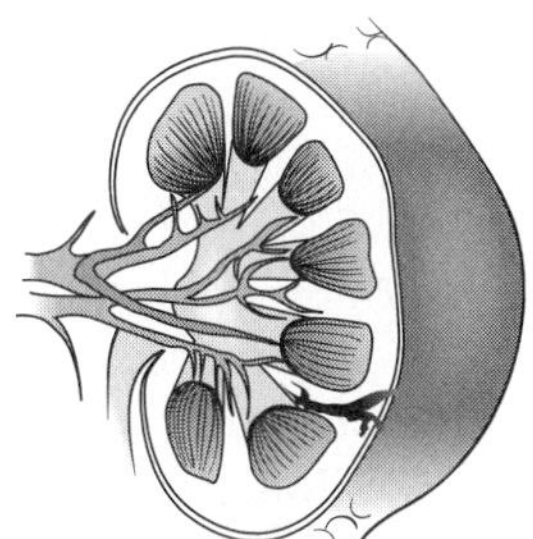

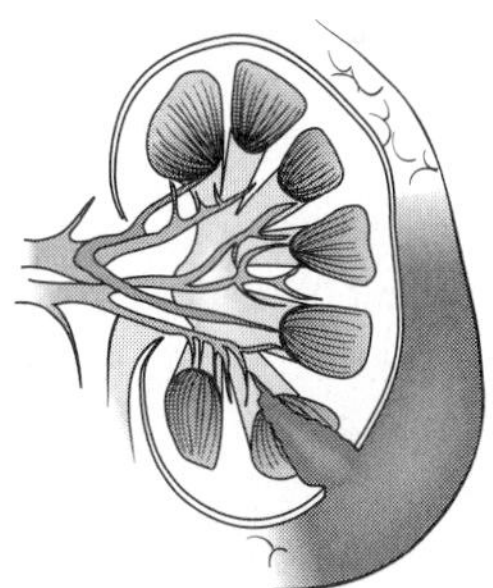

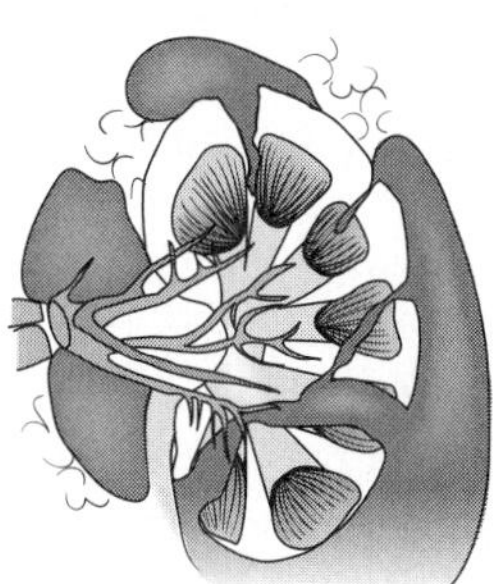

FIGURE 26-8 The American Association for Surgical Trauma classification scheme for renal injuries. Note that the higher-grade injuries are more likely to require surgical intervention. (From Rosenstein D, McAninch JW: Update on the management of renal trauma, *Contemp Urol* 15:47, 2003.)

remains hemodynamically stable.[2,10] Timely percutaneous or endoscopic drainage of urine minimizes loss of renal tissue.[2] Grade I and II injuries are usually managed successfully without operative intervention.[2] Nonoperative management of renal injury requires monitoring of renal function through urine output and serum chemistries.

Hemodynamic stability is key to successful nonoperative management.[2] Decreasing hemoglobin and hematocrit requiring transfusion indicate changes in a previously stable patient with perinephric hematoma. Renal lacerations are surrounded by a perinephric hematoma, which provides a tamponade effect on bleeding. A perinephric hematoma with hemodynamic stability is an indication for nonoperative management. Operative procedures to repair the kidney have not demonstrated a decrease in the complication rate.[10,59] Gentle palpation of any flank mass by the same examiner over time allows assessment of expansion in size of the perinephric hematoma. CT or angiography may be indicated to identify a source of the bleeding if hemodynamic instability occurs. Repeated CT scanning may be performed to monitor extravasation of blood and urine or expansion of a retroperitoneal hematoma. Indications for surgery include the development of sepsis, falling hemoglobin and hematocrit levels despite blood replacement, an expanding perirenal mass, or the inability to maintain hemodynamic stability despite supportive care.[2,5,59-61]

Grade III injuries are also staged through the use of CT. An IVP is inadequate to accurately stage the injury. Grade III injuries in hemodynamically stable patients can be managed nonoperatively.[1,2,10,56,59,60] Reassessment and restaging of the injury are essential to nonoperative management because accumulation of free urine and blood in the collecting ducts and in the area surrounding the kidney may cause further renal damage and infection.[10]

Percutaneous drainage of the urinoma, often associated with a grade III injury, is necessary to prevent a delayed nephrectomy.[2] Fifty percent of grade III injuries with extravasation spontaneously resolve within 4 or 5 days.[10] Potential complications of nonoperative management of grade III lacerations with extravasation include abscess formation, hypertension, ureteral obstruction, renal cysts, and dystrophic calcification.[2] Nonoperative management of grade III and IV injuries is associated with a risk of delayed bleeding.[10]

Grade IV injuries involve pedicle or vascular injuries. Most authors recommend immediate operation for grade IV injuries, although some studies show effective nonoperative management in hemodynamically stable patients.[2,5,6,56,59,60] Arteriography is indicated when vascular injury is suspected because a thrombosis at the site can partially or completely occlude the artery.[59-61] Surgery is frequently necessary to treat not only the renal injury but also the associated injuries. Urinary extravasation is drained, and expanding retroperitoneal hematomas are explored. An expanding pulsatile hematoma or spontaneous bleeding outside the fascia requires exploration.[2] Immediate exploration, although required as a lifesaving procedure, in a large population-based study resulted in a 64% incidence of nephrectomy.[62]

If the patient is hemodynamically stable, arterial reconstruction can be undertaken.[2] Early vascular control preserves renal function before reconstruction.[2] In the unstable patient selective renal artery embolization may be necessary.[2,61] Delays in definitive repair of vascular injuries result in renal tissue loss from ischemia.[2,5,6,61-63]

Despite appropriate intervention, large parts of the injured parenchyma may be lost or may have sustained significant injury, resulting in devitalized tissue before intervention. Necrotic segments can eventually bleed, causing delayed hemorrhage. Devitalized renal tissue leads to an 85% risk of complications, which include urinoma and abscess of the pancreas and small bowel.[2,63] Determination of the degree of devitalized tissue by CT is essential to management.[2,10] The presence of necrotic tissue in the kidneys requires surgery to improve patient outcome.

Extensive damage to the upper or lower pole of the kidney may necessitate partial or total nephrectomy. Damage to the midportion of the kidney may necessitate a renorrhaphy in which the devitalized midportion of the renal parenchyma is removed and the parenchymal edges are approximated.

Before a nephrectomy it is essential to evaluate the uninjured kidney for function. An arteriogram should be considered before or during surgery if the noninjured kidney cannot be visualized by IVP and the patient is hemodynamically stable.

Complications

Complications less than 4 weeks after renal injury include hemorrhage, abscess, infected urinoma, arteriovenous fistula, and prolonged extravasation.[2,5,63] Complications of nonoperative management of renal injury include ischemic renal atrophy, hypertension, and hydronephrotic nephrolithiasis.[2,5,6,59] Late complications, which may occur more than 4 weeks after injury, include hypertension, cystitis, infection, arteriovenous fistula, infected hematoma, hydronephrosis, atrophy, and dystrophic calcification.[2]

Persistent extravasation of urine is a significant complication of renal injury, resulting in inflammation and sepsis.[2,5] Extensive extravasation along with devitalized tissue and coexisting bowel and pancreas injury are relative indications for surgical renal exploration.[59] Delayed renal repair may be necessary if extravasation worsens, although only a minority (5% to 13%) will require ureteral stenting because in the majority of cases extravasation will resolve spontaneously.[1,59] In this situation broad-spectrum antibiotics may be used to prevent infection by skin and fecal flora.[2,63] Closed-system urine drainage also prevents colonization and resultant infection.

Hypertension

Another complication of renal trauma is hypertension. This can be the result of excess renin secretion caused by renal ischemia. The etiology of hypertension is renal infarct, scarring, hydronephrosis, chronic infection, vascular injury, and Page kidney.[2] Page kidney is compression of the renal parenchyma resulting in ischemia and hence excess renin production.[2,5] Page kidney has a low incidence and usually resolves on its own.[2] The overall incidence of posttrauma renal hypertension ranges from 0.6% to 33%, and it can develop from 2 weeks to 10 years after injury.[2,56] Early-onset hypertension is associated with laceration of the renal artery or its branches. Renal pedicle injury must be treated quickly and urinoma resolved.[2] Nephrectomy or revascularization relieves hypertension.[2,56]

Renal injury–induced hypertension should be suspected when essential hypertension occurs in patients under age 40 years or when new-onset hypertension occurs in the elderly.[56,63] Long-term follow-up of patients after renal injury is necessary to promptly identify and manage hypertension early.[2,4,59]

The majority of cases of hypertension are low grade and resolve spontaneously or with a short course of medication.[59] Operative intervention to relieve compression of the kidney is required if hypertension worsens, organ deterioration occurs, the side effects of the medications are intolerable, or the patient does not take the medications prescribed.

Trauma to the Adrenal Glands

The adrenal glands are well protected in the abdominal cavity, and therefore adrenal gland trauma is rare. Adrenal injury has been noted in blunt trauma. especially on the right side as a result of the adrenal venous outflow going directly to the inferior vena cava.[64] If the inferior vena cava is compressed during blunt trauma, right-sided adrenal hemorrhage can occur from venous congestion.

Patients with one-sided adrenal injury tend to have no signs of adrenal insufficiency because of the functionality of the contralateral adrenal gland.[64] However, patients with bilateral adrenal injury have a very small risk for adrenal hemorrhage and subsequent development of adrenal insufficiency and even adrenal crisis and death.[65] Bilateral adrenal hemorrhage (AH) is mainly caused by adrenal masses, continuing anticoagulation with subsequent coagulopathy (heparin-induced thrombocytopenia), meningococcal septicemia, or antiphospholipid-antibody syndrome; it may also be seen in situations of severe stress, postoperatively, or with overwhelming sepsis and multiorgan failure.[65]

Corticosteroid steroid treatment in situations where the AH is caused by sepsis or severe stress has little effect on outcome (9% versus 6% survival), whereas when AH occurs postoperatively, treatment increases survival to as much as 100% versus 17% without intervention.[66] In antiphospholipid-antibody syndrome, the survival rate increases to 73% with corticosteroid treatment versus 0% without treatment.[66]

Assessment

The development of AH after adrenal gland trauma may be considered rare, but it may be underdiagnosed because the symptoms of adrenal insufficiency are masked by shock and sepsis.[66] Symptoms of adrenal insufficiency are altered mental status, hyperthermia or hypothermia, hypotension, hyponatremia, hypoglycemia, azotemia, and eosinophilia.[65,66] A decrease in vascular tone and cardiac contractility and the diminished effect of vasoactive peptides can lead to shock.[64] Patients who exhibit signs of shock are often tested for sepsis. Patients who have had significant trauma to the abdomen and who are in shock, that is, not responding to fluid or vasopressor medication, need to raise a high suspicion for adrenocortical insufficiency.[64] Testing for adrenal insufficiency includes obtaining cortisol levels or performing a cosyntropin or adrenocorticotropin hormone stimulation test.

Management

Asymptomatic adrenal hemorrhage can be left untreated, with continued monitoring for clinical manifestations. Management of symptomatic AH is approached in a similar fashion as adrenal insufficiency. Treatment involves intravenous hydrocortisone because it provides both glucocorticoid and mineralcorticoid coverage. Once the patient recovers from the acute phase of adrenal insufficiency, an attempt to withdraw steroid medications is possible because it has been shown that patients can recover adrenocortical function after bilateral adrenal hemorrhage, although life-long therapy may be necessary.[64]

Although few urologic injuries are immediately life threatening, they can indeed account for some of the more frequent complications of trauma. Once hemodynamic stability is achieved and the source of instability is controlled, a careful assessment during the tertiary survey may reveal subtle GU injuries. Prevention of complications is achieved through prompt assessment for signs and symptoms of trauma to the upper and lower GU tract. It is during the critical care, intermediate care, and even rehabilitation phases that symptoms may appear. Continuing management and functional adaptation become the focus of care.

Critical Care Phase

The critical care phase in the management of GU trauma focuses the caregiver's attention on hemodynamic changes and potential complications. Many GU complications are not associated with direct GU trauma but with the management or effects of associated injuries.

Hemorrhage

The potential for bleeding and hemorrhage is present after almost all GU trauma, as described previously for specific organ injuries. Care is directed toward correcting and maintaining adequate oxygen delivery to all organs. Hemodynamic and ventilation-perfusion parameters must be assessed at frequent intervals. Positive inotropic infusions are used only after adequate blood volume is established. Awareness of the effects of inadequate circulating volumes and vasoactive drugs on renal function is essential, especially if renal injury has occurred.

Serial hemoglobin, hematocrit, and coagulation studies are monitored. The patient must be observed closely for bleeding from surgical sites or drains, for evidence of hematuria or myoglobinuria formation, and for expansion of an abdominal or flank mass. Advanced hemodynamic monitoring may be used to allow the evaluation of circulating volume and fluid status optimization.

Prevention of hypotension and hypothermia is essential because both may contribute to oliguria, anuria, and loss of renal function. Urinary output must be maintained. A rise in blood pressure during the critical care phase may indicate constriction of the renal parenchyma, vascular injury, or potential deterioration in renal function. Safeguarding the function of the renal parenchyma is essential to the patient after unilateral nephrectomy.

Genitourinary Infection

After surgery the critically ill patient with GU injury will have a multitude of invasive monitoring and drainage devices. Consequently, this patient is at high risk for infection. Strict aseptic technique must be maintained when any drain, surgical site, or urinary drainage system is cared for. The urinary or suprapubic catheter must be secured to prevent accidental dislodgment. In female patients the urinary catheter is secured to the inner thigh by either adhesive tape or a Velcro strap. In male patients the urinary drainage catheter is secured to the abdomen. In this patient population a dislodged urinary drainage catheter should not be replaced until a careful evaluation has been made by the urologist. The urinary drainage system (urinary and ureterostomy catheters) must be kept closed to prevent the entrance of organisms.

A kinked or obstructed urinary catheter may allow the stagnation of urine and promote the growth of pathogens. An obstructed drain may produce pooling of extravasated blood or urine, leading to abscess formation and sepsis.[2] The patient is observed for signs and symptoms of infection, including dysuria, frequency, low back pain, suprapubic pain, and foul, cloudy urine. Infectious processes include perinephric abscess, renal abscess, urinoma infection, and sepsis. Trends in temperature and white blood cell counts should be monitored. Urine must be sent for culture and sensitivity, and appropriate antibiotics are administered as ordered.

Perineal wounds should be monitored for signs of infection, including necrosis and foul-smelling drainage, which may indicate a necrotizing infection. A colostomy may be present to divert the fecal stream from the perineal wound. A rectal drainage device may also be used to contain fecal contents and to avoid contamination of the perineal wound.

Pain Management

The patient with GU trauma may have severe pain caused by tissue damage with subsequent hemorrhage and edema. In addition to analgesic agents, ice packs placed on the scrotal area and penis may be of benefit in reducing pain. Commercially available products may be used, or crushed ice may be placed in a surgical glove. When ice packs are used, extreme care is required to avoid cold burns because the skin over these organs is thin and fragile. For severe scrotal swelling, a scrotal support may reduce pain aggravated by the additional weight of swollen tissue. Use of commercially available scrotal supports or providing support with a towel functioning as a sling are effective.

Rhabdomyolysis and Myoglobinuria

Rhabdomyolysis is a syndrome triggered by skeletal muscle injury and ischemia followed by reperfusion, which results in the release of inflammatory mediators and further injury to the myocytes.[67] Injured muscle tissue releases myoglobin, which enters the circulation and results in acute renal failure (ARF) if untreated.

The causes of rhabdomyolysis include direct or indirect muscle injury.[68] Etiologies of muscle injury include crush injury, compartment syndrome, application of military antishock trousers, burns, lightning strikes, infections, medications, illicit drugs, poisonous insect or reptile bites, and compression of one or more muscle compartments from a lengthly period in one position.[67-69] Trauma patients with prolonged periods of muscle ischemia in addition to GU trauma should be monitored closely for the development of rhabdomyolysis.[5]

Partial tissue perfusion to muscle has greater systemic effects than complete lack of blood supply because of the effects of reperfusion injury. Tissue inflammatory mediators such as cytokines and eicosanoids cause endothelial disruption and cellular damage.[67] Lipid peroxidation from oxygen-derived free radicals causes increased cellular permeability and rupture.[67] The cellular damage results in the release of myoglobin, creatine kinase (CK), potassium, and phosphorus.

Myoglobinuria is an accurate marker of rhabdomyolysis.[68,69] Myoglobinuria has a renal tubulotoxic effect because of the myoglobin degradation product ferrihematine. This byproduct results in tubular obstruction, altered renal blood flow, and ultimately reversible oliguria.[67]

Assessment

Rhabdomyolysis presents with a significantly increased serum CK (normal 45-260 international units/L) and myoglobinuria. Myoglobinuria presents as dark tea-colored urine that tests positive for blood but is without red blood cells on microscopic urinalysis.[69] The serum CK is released from the injured muscle tissue.[67,69] Less specific indicators of rhabdomyolysis are elevated lactate dehydrogenase, aspartate aminotransferase, uric acid, and phosphorus levels and decreased serum calcium levels.[69] Calcium is decreased because it is deposited into the injured muscle tissue. Later, serum calcium levels rise as a result of the resolution of soft tissue calcification and increased parathyroid hormone excretion.[70]

Management

Treatment goals for patients with rhabdomyolysis/myoglobinuria are prevention or attenuation of ARF through intravenous fluid administration, diuresis, and alkalinization of urine.[67-70] Intravenous fluids maintain circulating blood volume and renal perfusion. The objective is to flush the myoglobin from the kidneys with a urine output of 100 to 200 ml per hour.[69] Diuresis with mannitol also protects the kidneys because mannitol acts as a scavenger of the oxygen metabolite hydroxyl radical.[68,69]

It has traditionally been thought that alkalinization of urine prevents the breakdown of myoglobin into the ferrihematine byproduct, increases myoglobin solubility, and decreases cast formation.[68-71] In an animal model, a combination approach to fluid resuscitation and alkalinization was more effective than hypertonic saline solution in reducing oxidant injury.[71] In a retrospective study of patients, however, the combination therapy of bicarbonate and mannitol did not demonstrate improvement in incidence of ARF, dialysis, or mortality in patients with CK levels >5,000 international units/L.[68]

Inadequate management of rhabdomyolysis/myoglobinuria results in ARF. Factors that have been shown to predict impending ARF in patients with rhabdomyolysis include abnormal levels of venous bicarbonate, BUN, calcium, and elevated creatinine and evidence of blood by urinalysis.[72] Additionally, ARF associated with rhabdomyolysis is usually oliguric with increased creatinine, BUN, and potassium levels.[69] Temporary dialysis resolves the ARF.[73] These patients have an excellent potential for recovery if the ARF is identified and treated rapidly.[71-73]

Acute Renal Failure

ARF is a syndrome characterized by a fall in the glomerular filtration rate (GFR) and an acute deterioration in renal function. ARF results in the inadequate excretion of various end products of cellular metabolism and an impaired ability to regulate fluid, electrolyte, and pH balance.[74] Figure 26-9 provides a review of normal renal functional anatomy.

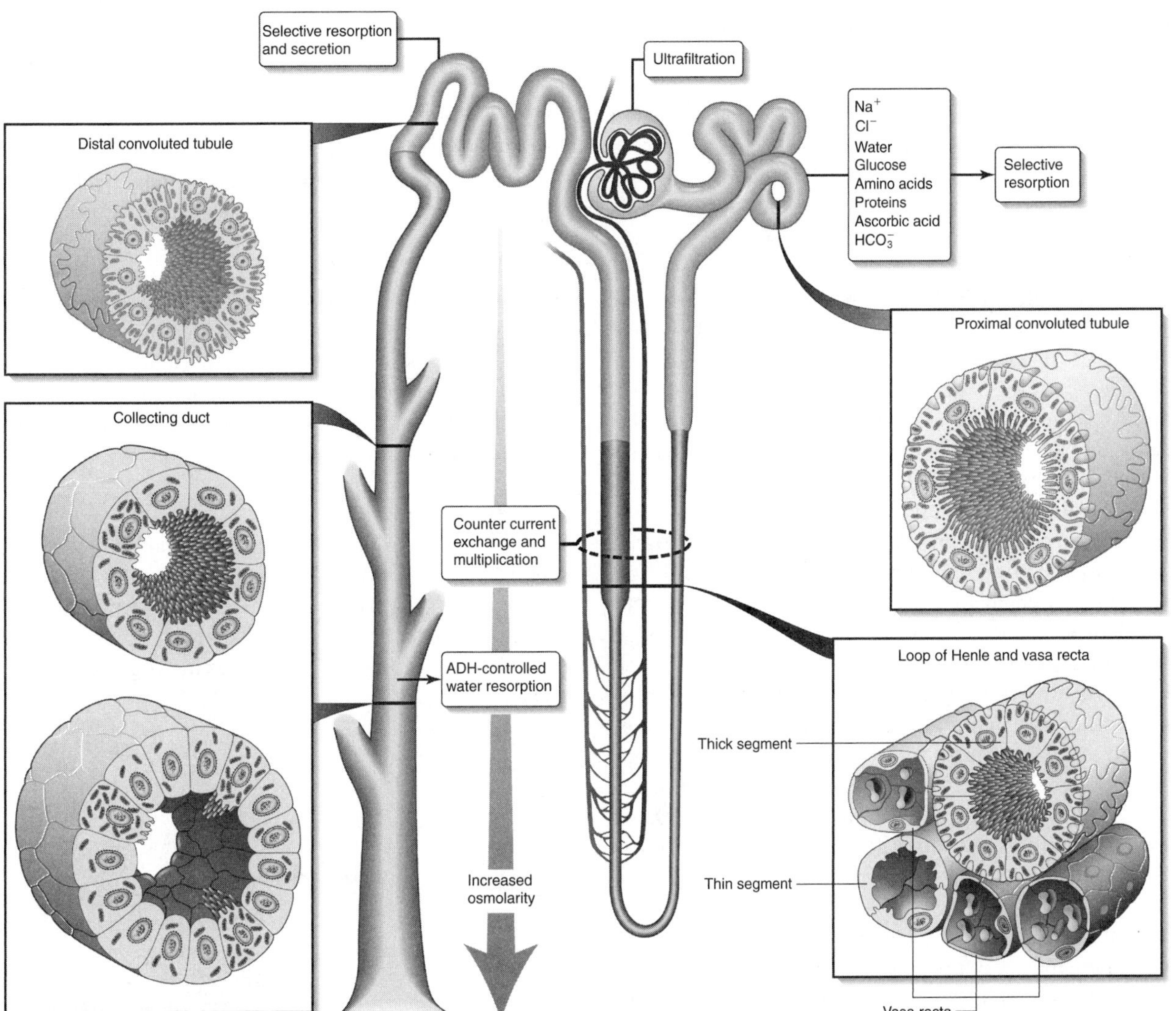

FIGURE 26-9 The nephron and its blood supply. The regional microstructure and principal activities of a kidney nephron and collecting duct. A nephron of the long loop (juxtamedullary) type is shown. *ADH*, Antidiuretic hormones. (From Standring S: *Gray's anatomy: the anatomical basis of clinical practice,* 39th ed, p 1279, London, 2005, Elsevier.)

Renal failure is a serious complication of trauma and occasionally of renal injury. It is important to distinguish between renal failure and pseudorenal failure. Pseudorenal failure can occur when urine extravasates into the abdominal cavity.[75] The urine then dialyzes across the peritoneum. It is usually a delayed presentation after injury to a full bladder resulting in intraperitoneal bladder rupture. The patient demonstrates hyponatremia, dehydration, and apparent renal failure. Pseudorenal failure rapidly resolves when urine is drained away from the abdomen.[75]

Renal failure may result from a direct renal injury or a secondary injury as a result of hypovolemia, hypoperfusion, and rhabdomyolysis/myoglobinuria. A cause of secondary renal failure is increased intra-abdominal pressure or abdominal compartment syndrome. One of the earliest signs of abdominal compartment syndrome is decreased urine output.[76] As pressure in the abdomen increases, the renal artery is compressed, compromising renal perfusion, and renal failure ensues. It has been documented in the literature for more than 100 years that there is an association between elevated intra-abdominal pressure and renal blood flow.[77,78] Sugrue et al[79] demonstrated that increased intra-abdominal pressure in and of itself is significant enough to result in ARF. Decompression of the abdomen through a laparotomy provides rapid treatment of abdominal compartment syndrome and the resultant ARF.[76]

ARF is a potentially life-threatening complication of trauma with or without primary GU or renal injury. ARF results in a loss of normal kidney function and is subclassified by its etiology. The most common causes of ARF include prerenal failure (35% of patients), acute tubular necrosis (ATN) (50% of patients), postrenal (or obstructive) failure (10% of patients), and a small percentage of patients have intrinsic causes.[74] Prerenal failure is a result of inadequate perfusion of the kidney without actual renal tissue damage. Intrarenal failure results from direct insult to the renal parenchyma by prolonged ischemia, injury to the nephron, or infectious or immunologic processes. Postrenal failure occurs as a result of an obstruction in the drainage system.[80] Causes of renal failure include hypotension, transfusion reaction, contrast media, rhabdomyolysis, aminoglycoside administration, sepsis, systemic inflammatory response syndrome, and vasopressor administration.[74,80] Despite multiple advances in the management of acute renal failure, the mortality rate from renal failure remains at around 50%.[81]

Prerenal Failure

Trauma patients are at great risk for development of prerenal failure. Renal blood flow, also known as the effective arterial blood volume, may drop for many reasons, including hypovolemia, cardiac dysfunction, or peripheral vasodilation. The effective arterial blood volume can remain relatively stable despite significant variance in the mean arterial pressure because of autoregulatory responses including afferent arteriolar dilation and efferent arteriolar constriction mediated by prostacyclin and angiotensin II.[74] The effective arterial blood volume may also drop through failure of autoregulatory systems. Afferent arteriolar constriction can occur from sepsis, hepatorenal syndrome, and medications (such as nonsteroidal anti-inflammatory drugs). Efferent arteriolar vasodilation can increase with angiotensin-converting enzyme inhibitor therapy. When the effective arterial blood volume is reduced, regardless of cause, ARF can ensue.

Intrarenal Failure

The type of intrarenal failure is determined by the section of the kidney that is injured. The outer layer, or cortex, is the vascular portion containing the glomeruli and distal convoluted tubules. Damage occurs by vascular, infectious, or inflammatory processes that result in swelling at the capillary bed. Table 26-4 provides a list of common sources of cortical damage that cause intrarenal failure.

The second type of intrarenal failure is caused by damage to the middle layer, or medulla. The medullary tissue is composed of the collecting tubules, ducts, and the long loops of Henle. Nephrotoxic agents, particularly antibiotics or contrast media, release crystals that lodge in the tubules and obstruct the flow of filtrate. A source of ischemic injury frequently seen in trauma patients is rhabdomyolysis (see previous discussion). The myoglobin released from muscle injury is too large to pass through the tubules and may become lodged in the tubule system, resulting in ATN. Table 26-5 reviews common causes of medullary damage that may lead to intrarenal failure.

Postrenal Failure

Primary injury to any part of the urinary collection system, such as a ruptured bladder, interruption in ureteral or urethral integrity, or pressure from hematomas, may lead to postrenal failure. Other potential causes arise from sources of urinary retention such as neurogenic bladder or a UTI.

TABLE 26-4 **Intrarenal Failure: Common Sources of Cortical Damage**

Infectious	Acute glomerulonephritis Acute pyelonephritis
Immunologic	Goodpasture's syndrome Systemic lupus erythematosus Severe hypercalcemia Malignant hypertension

TABLE 26-5 Intrarenal Failure: Common Sources of Medullary Damage

Nephrotoxic sources	Antibiotics
	Aminoglycosides
	Cephalosporins
	Tetracyclines
	X-ray contrast media
	Heavy metals
	Arsenic
	Lead
	Pesticides and fungicides
Ischemic sources	Burns
	Crush injuries
	Massive hemorrhage
	Prolonged hypotension
	Sepsis
	Transfusion reactions

Assessment

ARF progresses along a continuum of stages. Table 26-6 outlines the general signs and symptoms that are commonly seen within the various phases of renal failure. During the resuscitative and critical care phases, clear delineation of the phase of renal failure may be somewhat difficult to assess because of the patient's dynamic response to injury.

The hallmark of ARF is low urine output. The decrease in output reflects abnormalities in the GFR and regulatory mechanisms. Urinary output is more sensitive to changes in renal hemodynamics than are laboratory markers in the critically ill patient.[82] Urinary output is a specific marker for acute renal dysfunction or failure when it is severely reduced or absent.[80,82] It is far less specific in helping determine the degree of renal dysfunction: renal dysfunction may indeed be present with adequate urinary output.[80,82] Laboratory analysis offers the clinician useful data for diagnosing and monitoring the progress of ARF. Pertinent values and their norms are summarized in Table 26-7.

Creatinine, a normal byproduct of tissue metabolism, is excreted via glomerular filtration into the urine. Because the rate of tissue metabolism is usually constant and clearance occurs solely at the nephron, renal function may be readily assessed by collecting urine over a fixed amount of time and measuring concurrent urine and serum creatinine levels. This is known as the creatinine clearance. One pitfall of this test is that creatinine clearance will overestimate the GFR because additional creatinine is secreted into the renal tubule.[82] The creatinine clearance calculation is as follows (where *BSA* is the body surface area):

$$\frac{\text{Urine creatinine}}{\text{Serum creatinine}} \times \text{Urine volume (ml/min)} \times \frac{1.73}{\text{BSA (m}^2\text{)}}$$

Serum creatinine is a much more accessible parameter than is creatinine clearance. There is an inverse, linear relationship between the GFR and the serum creatinine level. As the GFR decreases in renal failure, the amount of creatinine cleared by the kidney also is reduced, resulting in an elevation of serum creatinine levels. However, there is no single value for the serum creatinine that corresponds to a GFR across all patients. Thus, monitoring for changes in creatinine relative to clinical assessment is the clinically and physiologically astute approach. It can be assumed, however, that a doubling of the creatinine

TABLE 26-6 Phases of Renal Failure

System Involved	Oliguric Phase	Diuretic Phase	Recovery
Neurologic	Decreased level of consciousness, muscular twitches, fatigue, apathy, seizures, coma	Decreased level of consciousness, lessened potential for seizure activity, potential for fatigue, apathy, restlessness	Normal
Cardiovascular	Elevated blood pressure, heart rate, cardiac output; potential cardiac pump failure; anemia; cardiac arrhythmias; pitting edema	Low blood pressure, elevated heart rate, elevated temperature, atrial or ventricular cardiac arrhythmias	Normal; may have residual blood pressure or cardiac arrhythmia problems
Pulmonary	Pulmonary edema, rales, Kussmaul's respiration	Tachypnea, Kussmaul's respiration	Normal
Metabolic	Hyperkalemia, hypermagnesemia, acidosis, hypernatremia	Hypokalemia, acidosis, hyponatremia	Normal
Gastrointestinal	Gastrointestinal bleeding, negative nitrogen balance, anorexia, nausea	Gastrointestinal bleeding, negative nitrogen balance, anorexia, nausea, thirst	Anorexia, nausea, thirst
GU	Decreased urine output	Increased urine output	Normal urine output, potential chronic renal failure, potential for impotence

TABLE 26-7 Normal Laboratory Values

Serum Analysis		Urine Analysis	
		Appearance: pale yellow, clear	
		Odor: mild ammonia	
Chloride	96-109 mEq/L	Chloride	110-250 mEq
Carbon dioxide	24-30 mEq/L	Specific gravity	1.005-1.030
BUN	12-25 mg/dl	Osmolality	300-1200 mOsm
Creatinine	0.4-1.5 mg/dl	—	—
pH	7.35-7.45	pH	4.5-8.0
Glucose	70-115 mg/dl	Glucose	0
Magnesium	1.5-2.0 mEq/L	Magnesium	100 mg
Potassium	3.5-5.0 mEq/L	Potassium	25-120 mEq
Sodium	135-145 mEq/l	Sodium	40-220 mEq
Calcium	9.0-10.5 mg/dl	Calcium	50-150 mg
Phosphorus	3.0-4.5 mg/dl	Ketones	0
Total protein	6.0-8.5 g/dl	Protein	<150 mg/24 hr
Albumin	3.2-5.3 g/dl	Crystals	0
Hemoglobin	13.9-16.3 g/dl	Casts	0
Red blood cells	4.84 m/mm^3	Red blood cells	<3/HPF
White blood cells	4,500-11,000/mm^3	White blood cells	<4/HPF
Mean corpuscular volume	41%-53%	Creatinine clearance	125 ml/min
Platelets	150,000-350,000/mm^3		

HPF, High-power field.

value represents an approximately 50% reduction in GFR.[80,82]

With the increase in the serum creatinine level, BUN levels also rise. However, because the BUN level is affected by many other factors, such as hypovolemia, hypercatabolism, and gastrointestinal bleeding, it is an unreliable measure of the GFR when viewed in isolation from other values. A simultaneous rise in the BUN and serum creatinine levels in a ratio greater than 10:1 is a better indicator of renal failure.

When the GFR is reduced and renal vasoconstriction occurs as a compensatory mechanism, there is an increase in the reabsorption of sodium, which reduces the amount excreted. This relationship can be quantified by the fractional excretion of sodium (FENa). An FENa of less than 1% suggests prerenal failure.[80] Diuretics such as mannitol will change the sodium excretion; therefore, the FENa is an inaccurate gauge for renal function in patients receiving these drugs. FENa (in percent) is calculated as follows[80]:

$$\frac{\text{Urine sodium} \times \text{Serum creatinine}}{\text{Urine creatinine} \times \text{Serum sodium}} \times 100$$

Other serum and urine electrolyte values are affected as the ability of the nephron to regulate their movement becomes progressively more impaired. The failure of the collecting tubules to excrete potassium is responsible for elevated serum potassium levels. Hemoglobin and hematocrit levels may be normal initially, but because the kidneys fail to produce erythropoietin, chronic anemia may ensue.

Urinalysis, specific gravities, and microbiology tests are also useful in monitoring the progression of renal failure. Significant urinalysis findings are summarized in Table 26-8 for each of the categories of renal failure.

TABLE 26-8 Urinalysis in Renal Failure

	Prerenal Etiology	Intrarenal Etiology	Postrenal Etiology
Specific gravity	1.020 or greater	1.010	Normal
Myoglobin	May be positive	May be positive	Usually negative
Urine sodium	Low	High (greater than 30 mEq/L)	Normal (less than 20 mEq/L)
Sediment	Normal	Renal tubular cells and cell casts; pigmented granular casts	Normal
Protein	Less than 1 g/24 hr	Less than 1 g/24 hr	Less than 1 g/24 hr
Red blood cells	Microscopic	Microscopic	Microscopic
White blood cells	Few	Few	Few

Prevention

Prevention of ARF after trauma involves maintaining intravascular volume and renal perfusion, avoiding nephrotoxic agents or ensuring adequate intravascular volume loading before administration, and treating myoglobinuria to prevent hematin deposition.[83,84] Awareness of the potential for acute tubular necrosis and prerenal failure after injury is imperative in the critical care phase.

Management

Treatment goals and nursing interventions for patients with ARF focus on reversing or compensating for the deterioration in renal function. This is particularly challenging when dealing with severely injured patients. Fluid, electrolyte, and pH abnormalities may be exacerbated by underresuscitation, postresuscitation fluid overload, osmotic diuresis, hypothermia, hypoxia, nephrotoxic medications, or fluid restrictions.

Adequate nutrition, which assists in maintaining electrolyte balances, poses a special problem because of the high protein requirements of trauma patients. Protein, vital for tissue healing, produces urea as a metabolic byproduct. In the patient with ARF the kidney is unable to remove the nitrogen byproducts of protein metabolism. Overfeeding can lead to serious complications, including hypertonic hydration and metabolic acidosis.[83] Underfeeding, however, can limit healing and recovery. There are data to suggest that a low-protein diet is unnecessary in patients with ARF.[85-87]

Hemodynamic stability and adequate oxygen delivery are necessary for meeting the oxygen requirements of all tissues, including the kidneys. Prolonged hypotension or underresuscitation may exacerbate existing renal failure, which in turn diminishes the amount of renal function recovered. Hypertension is a common result of renal failure. As the kidneys perceive a decrease in the renal blood flow, the renin-angiotensin cascade is activated at the juxtaglomerular apparatus. Production of renal prostaglandins is also elevated. The resulting vasoconstriction, increases in the circulating plasma volume as a result of aldosterone production, and electrolyte imbalances contribute to systemic hypertension.

In some cases, such as in the presence of prerenal conditions, patients with ARF recover after treatment of the underlying cause with careful management of fluids. Patients who have actual damage to the nephrons usually require some form of temporary dialysis until renal function returns.

Optimizing hemodynamics will ensure that effective arterial blood volume is present. Initial management includes administration of a fluid challenge to identify or rule out hypovolemic prerenal causes of ARF. In some patients, this may involve the use of inotropes, as in the case of concurrent cardiac dysfunction, or vasopressors, such as norepinephrine. There has been concern over the use of vasopressors in the face of ARF with concomitant peripheral vasodilation; however, the literature has failed to substantiate such concerns.[84] In the face of oliguria, diuretics may be the next approach. No response to diuretics such as mannitol or furosemide is likely in ARF. If not already ruled out, renal artery thrombosis, myoglobinuria (tea-colored urine), and increased abdominal pressure should be considered as causes of acute renal failure.[74,80,83,84] Treatment of the cause will attenuate the ARF.

Dialysis is the next line of management for ARF. Although there are no absolute standards for when to start dialysis, there are some conditions when immediate treatment with dialysis is appropriate, including hyperkalemia with electrocardiographic changes, pulmonary edema, uremic acidosis with cardiac compromise, and gross uremia.[80] All forms of dialysis strive to replicate normal kidney function, that is, to regulate excess fluid and electrolytes and to remove metabolic wastes.[80] This is accomplished through the use of a porous membrane that, like the glomerular capillary bed, is only permeable to water and small molecules. The dialysis filter membrane essentially creates two compartments, one containing blood and the other a hypertonic solution called dialysate. Figure 26-10 illustrates the interactions of the patient's blood and dialysis circuit.

The function of the system is governed by four principles. Hydrostatic pressure is the force that pushes the fluid through the system. In the kidney, this is created by the systemic blood pressure. Osmosis is the movement of fluid across the semipermeable membrane from an area of greater concentration to an area of lesser concentration. Diffusion is the movement of small molecules across the semipermeable membrane from an area of higher concentration to an area of lower concentration. Both osmosis and diffusion continue until equilibrium is reached. Filtration is the movement of fluid from an area of greater pressure to one of lower pressure. Application of these principles is evident in all forms of dialysis.[88]

Peritoneal Dialysis. Peritoneal dialysis is accomplished by using the mesenteric capillary bed as the semipermeable membrane. A hypertonic glucose solution is instilled into the abdominal cavity and left to dwell for 30 to 45 minutes. Water and solutes are pulled from the capillary bed to the dialysate (osmosis and diffusion). The greater the concentration of glucose, the more water and solutes are removed.

Peritoneal dialysis has the advantage of being relatively simple and inexpensive to perform. No special preparation of the patient is required for bedside insertion of the abdominal trocar catheter. The procedure can be managed without the use of costly equipment. Unfortunately, peritoneal dialysis is usually inadequate for the clearance of both solutes and nitrogenous waste in the acutely critically ill trauma patient.[83] The peritoneum must be intact as well. In trauma patients this is often not the case. The use of peritoneal dialysis in the presence of abdominal trauma,

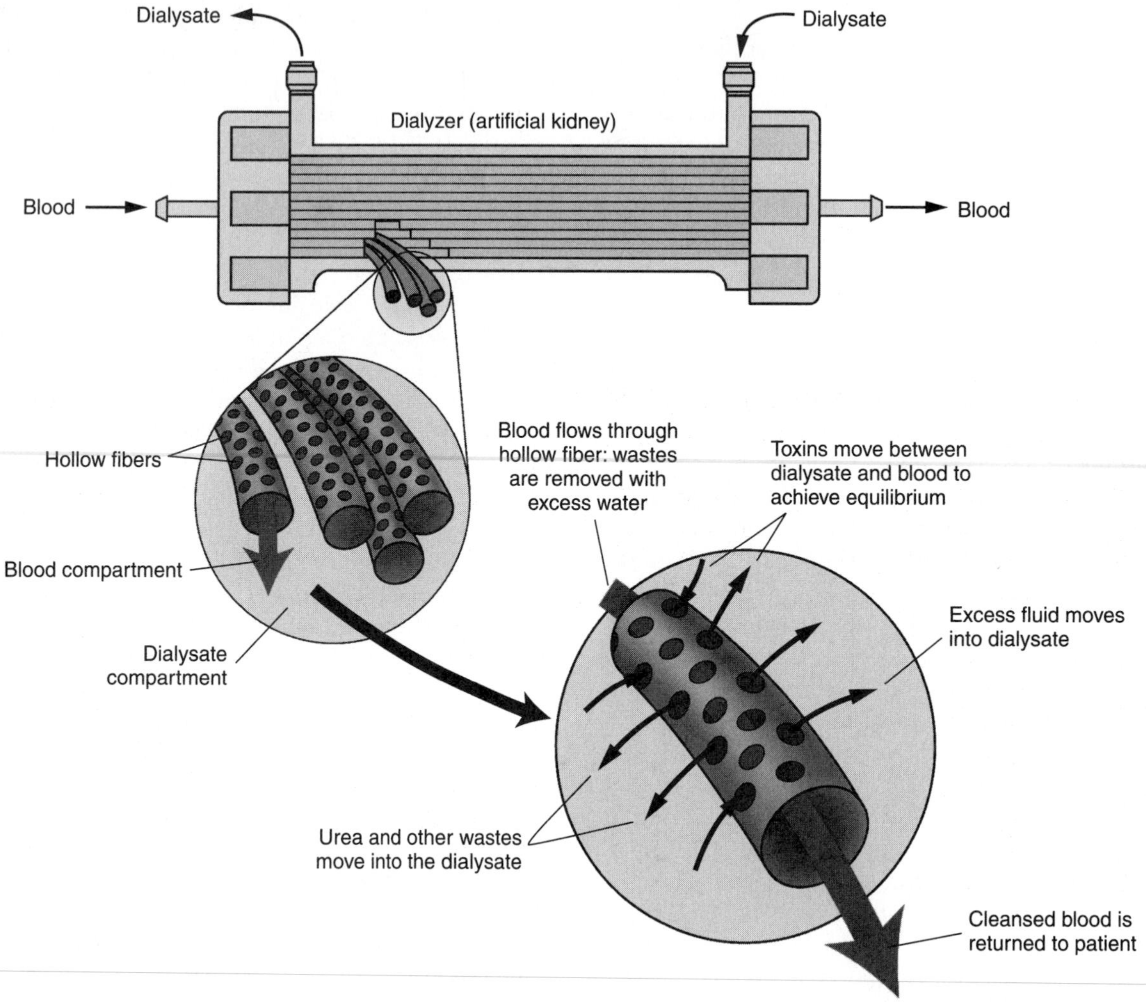

FIGURE 26-10 The hemodialyzer. (From Lough ME: Renal disorders and therapeutic management. In Urden LD, Stacy KM, Lough ME, editors: *Thelan's critical care nursing: diagnosis and management,* 5th ed, p 829, St.Louis, 2005, Mosby.)

vascular anastomosis, or hematoma is at best controversial.

Peritonitis is a major complication of peritoneal dialysis because of the hypertonic glucose solution used. Another disadvantage is the increased intra-abdominal pressure that occurs during dwell times. Abdominal distention restricts diaphragmatic motion and may impair the patient's ventilatory status. In addition, increased abdominal compartment pressure is a known cause of ARF. Peritoneal dialysis is an effective treatment for acute fluid overload and stable renal failure; however, these disadvantages limit its use in the multitrauma population.

Hemodialysis. Intermittent hemodialysis (IHD) involves the extracorporeal circulation of blood through a hemofilter, which uses a synthetic semipermeable membrane between the blood and the dialysate.[88] Figure 26-11 is a schematic representation of two commonly used filters. Blood is forced through the extracorporeal circuit by a mechanical pump. Because management of the system

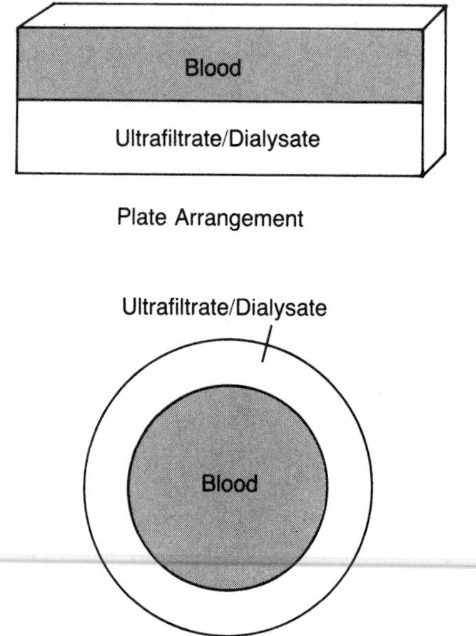

FIGURE 26-11 Schematic representation of two common hemofilters.

requires personnel with highly specialized competencies, the bedside nurse's primary function is monitoring the patient during the treatment.

IHD has two distinct advantages over other forms of dialysis: (1) treatments are brief, usually between 3 and 4 hours per session, and (2) the process is highly efficient in the removal of fluid, wastes, and electrolytes. These advantages are crucial to the survival of patients with life-threatening poisonings or intoxications, electrolyte disturbances, and uremic crisis.[88] IHD also requires much less anticoagulation than does continuous therapy.[88] However, the resulting rapid shift of fluid and electrolytes can lead to a disequilibrium syndrome.[83,88] This may be manifested by a decreased level of consciousness, dizziness, weakness, diaphoresis, vomiting, seizures, and hypotension. The neurologic symptoms reflect the entry of water into the cerebrospinal fluid (CSF). This occurs because of a transient concentration gradient in which urea cannot be diffused rapidly enough from the CSF into the blood because of the blood-brain barrier. The cardiovascular effects are related to the rapid shifts of intravascular volume, sodium, and potassium. These symptoms are most often evident when abnormal blood chemistries are corrected too rapidly. In addition, hemodialysis is intermittent, resulting in periods of normal levels of electrolytes and wastes alternating with gradual increases until the next treatment.

Continuous Renal Replacement Therapies. Continuous renal replacement therapies (CRRT) are effective in managing ARF, especially in the critically injured patient. CRRT includes slow continuous ultrafiltration, continuous venovenous hemofiltration, continuous venovenous hemodialysis, and continuous venovenous hemodiafiltration.[88] When the basic principles of dialysis and renal physiology are applied, the nomenclature of the various renal replacement therapies describe the exact therapy being used. The reader is referred to other sources for more in-depth description of the various types of CRRT available.

Extrocorporeal circuits typically require some type of mechanism to help maintain blood fluidity. With CRRT, anticoagulation may be indicated through regional or systemic anticoagulation. Regional anticoagulation can be accomplished with a low-dose heparin infusion located on the arterial side of the filter. An alternative anticoagulant such as sodium citrate prefilter with calcium replacement provided post filter or outside the CRRT circuit may be used in a similar fashion to achieve regional anticoagulation. There are numerous nursing implications when these anticoagulants are administered, including the need to monitor serial coagulation studies such as partial thromboplastin time or activated clotting time and in the case of sodium citrate, prefilter and postfilter calcium levels.

Critical care nurses have an active role in maintaining the patient on CRRT. Continuous assessment and monitoring focus on achieving and maintaining fluid and electrolyte balance with sufficient clearance of desired volume and solutes. It is also important to prevent blood loss, hypothermia, and infection.[88] Blood flow rates through the filter and IV replacement fluids are maintained to achieve the desired fluid balance. Net fluid loss may be desirable if the patient is in fluid overload, or no fluid loss (IV replacement) may be desired if the goal is only solute removal. Laboratory tests are monitored closely during this therapy. The filter integrity is monitored because clotting can occur even with anticoagulation. Signs of clotting include undesirable changes in pressures measured by the CRRT pump, poor filtrate outflow, and darkening of the filter fibers.

The use of CRRT versus IHD has remained equivocal in the literature. One meta-analysis suggested a mortality benefit along with a reduced hospital length of stay in patients when CRRT was used.[89] Another meta-analysis[90] and other controlled studies[91,92] have found no difference in outcome. There are clear indications, however, for use of one modality over the other. Cerebral edema or liver failure warrants continuous therapies, whereas IHD is warranted in patients with an increased bleeding risk or acute toxic ingestions.[80]

Disadvantages. Anticoagulation may be needed for CRRT. CRRT requires large-bore vascular access and, because of the rigid nature of the catheter, lines for CRRT tend to have more vascular access problems. Because additional devices are attached to the patient, mobility is reduced. As with IHD, rapid or excessive volume removal can cause a patient with borderline hemodynamics to become unstable.

Advantages. With continuous therapy, hemodynamic control may be achieved by slower blood flow rates and fluid removal. This allows for the administration of medications and nutrition support without concern for volume overload or worsening pulmonary status.[80,88] With slower solute removal, there are also fewer associated fluid shifts and therefore no increase in intracranial pressure.[88] In addition, it is believed that CRRT may also remove circulating inflammatory mediators such as myocardial depressant substances released with the systemic inflammatory response syndrome.[80] Continuous therapies also provide a greater dialysis dose per day.[80]

ARF is irreversible in 5% of patients and in 16% of elderly patients.[80] Monitoring renal function is required at regular intervals. This includes serial laboratory tests in addition to detailed physical assessment. Management of these patients is directed toward salvage and preservation of the kidney. Failure to do so condemns the surviving patient to a life restricted by chronic dialysis or transplantation.

Nursing care during the critical care phase focuses on restoration of hemodynamic stability and management of the sequelae that develop as an immediate consequence of the injuries. Complication prevention through diligent infection prevention measures and adequate volume replacement are the cornerstones of morbidity reduction during this phase of care. It is also during the critical care phase that the patient and family begin inquiring as to long-term outcomes and next steps. The nurse supports the patient and family in their adjustment to illness as they transition to the intermediate and rehabilitation phases of care.

INTERMEDIATE/REHABILITATION PHASES

Once the patient has progressed to the intermediate phase of care, the focus becomes rehabilitative in nature. The potential for complications remains with the GU trauma patient through rehabilitation and after discharge. The long-term effects of GU trauma include both physical disability and emotional stressors.

DELAYED HEMORRHAGE

During the intermediate or rehabilitation phase the nurse continues to monitor the patient for signs of delayed or occult bleeding from GU structures. The patient receiving nonoperative renal injury management is usually placed on bed rest. Trends in vital signs and serial hemoglobin and hematocrit results must be monitored for evidence of hemorrhage. Any flank or abdominal mass must be evaluated for increase in size. Gentle palpation allows more direct assessment of size but risks the rupture of a tamponaded bleed. Observing for changes in abdominal girth may allow more indirect but safer evaluation of the mass.

URETHRAL STRICTURE, INCONTINENCE, AND IMPOTENCE

The family and patient require education about the care of any remaining drains or urethral or suprapubic catheters. Instruction includes information about potential delayed complications of GU trauma, including infection, sexual difficulties, incontinence, stricture formation, calculus formation, hypertension, hydronephritis, pyelonephritis, and chronic renal failure.

Urethral stricture as a potential complication of GU trauma was once thought to be the result of the treatment, not the primary injury.[38] With the help of improved imaging, it has become clear that the primary injury itself is the most significant predisposing factor toward urethral stricture.[5] Patients who have had urethral injury are at significant risk for urethral stricture, particularly when a delayed reconstruction approach is used.[37] The use of a primary realignment for complete urethral injury has been shown to have a reduced rate of postinjury urethral stricture.[37] The outcomes of incontinence and impotence were comparable for both approaches of urethral repair.[38] Treatment of stricture requires delayed urethroplasty.

Bladder neck injury is usually associated with incontinence.[38] Every effort must be made to protect the sphincter and repair the bladder neck. A key component of rehabilitation after GU injury is bladder retraining and management of incontinence at home.

CYSTITIS/BLADDER SPASM

Postoperative pain is not as likely to be present once the patient reaches the rehabilitation phase. However, bladder spasms may occur intermittently after bladder repair. Antispasmodic medications are often effective in relieving bladder spasm, and additional analgesia may be required for effective pain relief. If cystitis does occur postoperatively, pain medication may be needed in conjunction with medications such as phenazopyridine hydrochloride (Pyridium), which produce an analgesic effect on the mucosa of the urinary tract and relieve burning, urgency, and frequency.

INFECTION

The prevention of infection remains a priority throughout the rehabilitation phase. Management of the drainage systems to prevent infection is the same as in the critical care phase.

PHYSICAL DISFIGUREMENT AND SEXUALITY

Patients sustaining GU injury may have residual problems that can alter sexual functioning or bladder control. Patients whose injuries are not likely to produce such sequelae should be reassured as soon as they are stable enough to comprehend such information.

Patients whose injury will cause altered levels of normal body functions not only need intense psychologic support but also may require professional counseling that addresses sexual function. A referral for counseling should be obtained by the nurse. The usual phases of grief and loss related to sexual dysfunction or physical disfigurement can be expected (see Chapter 19).

Female patients who required a hysterectomy or oophorectomy also may have significant psychologic adjustment. Depending on the woman's age and childbearing status, a hysterectomy may cause severe emotional impact. The surgery may have profound effects on how she perceives herself with respect to her reproductive role, sexuality, vitality, youth, and attractiveness. Each individual values these qualities differently. Depression and mood swings can often occur as a result of these altered body image perceptions and hormonal changes.

Sexual concerns should not be ignored or postponed until the patient is in a rehabilitation unit. Patients may have concerns about sex even during the acute phase after injury. Such concerns are significant, should be addressed, and warrant attention by the nurse. Some patients may feel embarrassment and therefore not seek treatment for the trauma or attend follow-up sessions. Studies have shown that patients after a penile trauma had low rates of follow-up because of embarrassment about the injury.[22,23] Proactively addressing actual or potential concerns and acknowledgment of embarrassment may indeed reduce complications from GU injuries.

A first step toward initiating a conversation regarding sexual concerns of the patient is to recognize that patients may communicate their concerns about sexuality in a variety of ways, both verbally and nonverbally. Some patients may give no outward indication that they have concerns about sexuality. The nurse should verbally "allow" the patient to initiate a discussion by using a nonjudgmental yet interested approach. By taking time to listen to patients, the nurse creates an atmosphere wherein patients feel free to talk about the injury and the meaning it has. The nurse should respond to these concerns with a balance of gentle reassurance and realism about the difficult adjustments that undoubtedly lie ahead. Offering the patient information about sexual function is an important intervention. Often in the acute postinjury phase patients simply need reassurance that their sexual function is not totally lost. Allowing patients to have private time with their spouse or significant others is an important nursing measure. Another intervention that may be helpful is to arrange for the newly disabled person to talk with someone who has made a successful adjustment to a similar disability. The opportunity to explore issues with someone in a similar circumstance may be a good outlet for the patient's concerns.

The measures described previously are also appropriate for use with the patient's spouse or significant other. He or she too can have tremendous concerns about the future sexual relationship with the disabled individual.

One final consideration of utmost importance in any discussion of patients' sexual concerns is the nurse's own comfort level regarding both sexuality and disability. Attitude is a critical determinant of the nurse's effectiveness in this area. The intense issues surrounding sexuality and disability may be highly sensitive for the nurse for many reasons. It is crucial for nurses to take time for self-analysis regarding these issues because nothing is communicated more surely to the patient than one's own attitudes.

The intermediate and rehabilitation phase help to prepare the patient and family for continued management and, most important, self-care. Assessing the patient's functional status and identifying gaps in resources helps to define the patient's best plan of care. Patients may begin to express frustrations about the traumatic event or feelings of body image disturbance. During the intermediate and rehabilitation phase, the nurse helps to normalize such feelings and identify needed resources for the patient.

SUMMARY

Rapid identification and management of GU injury can result in satisfactory outcomes. GU injuries are far from insignificant even though they are frequently not life threatening. Urethral injury must be identified early and managed with drainage to prevent complications and allow monitoring of urine output. Renal injuries can be life threatening if hemorrhage occurs. ARF, although involving the GU system, is often the result of nonrenal causes. Prevention of ARF in all multisystem-injured patients is critical to survival and a positive functional outcome. Long-term complications and disability involve the personal and emotional issues of sexual dysfunction and physical disfigurement, which can be devastating. Trauma nurses from resuscitation through rehabilitation play a vital role in the identification of GU injuries and the prevention and management of short- and long-term complications.

REFERENCES

1. McAninch JW, Santucci RA: Genitouninary trauma. In Walsh PC, Retik AB, Wein A et al, editors: *Campbell's urology,* pp 3707-3744, Philadelphia, 2002, W. B. Saunders.
2. Santucci RA, Wessels H, Bartsch G et al: Evaluation and management of renal injuries: consensus statement of the renal trauma subcommittee, *Br J Urol* 93:937-954, 2004.
3. Rothrock S, Green SM, Morgan R: Abdominal trauma in infants and children: prompt identification and early management of serious and life-threatening injuries, II: specific injuries and ED management, *Pediatr Emerg Care* 16: 189-195, 2000.
4. Ku JH, Yeon YS, Kim ME et al: Comparison of long-term results according to the primary mode of management and type of injury for posterior urethral injuries, *Urol Int* 69:227-232, 2002.
5. Wessells H, McAninch J, editors: *Urological emergencies: a practical guide,* pp 3-95, Totowa, NJ, 2005, Humana Press.
6. Peterson N: Genitourinary trauma. In Moore EE, Feliciano DV, Mattox KL et al, editors: *Trauma,* 5th ed, pp 839-875, New York, 2003, McGraw-Hill Professional.
7. Aihara R, Blansfield JS, Millham FH et al: Fracture locations influence the likelihood of rectal and lower urinary tract injuries in patients sustaining pelvic fractures, *J Trauma* 52:205-209, 2002.
8. Demetriades D, Karaiskakis M, Toutouzas K et al: Pelvic fractures: epidemiology and predictors of associated

abdominal injuries and outcomes, *J Am Coll Surg* 195:1-10, 2002.

9. Ziran BH, Chamberlain E, Shuler FD et al: Delays and difficulties in the diagnosis of lower urologic injuries in the context of pelvic fractures, *J Trauma* 58:533-537, 2005.
10. Holevar M, DiGiacomo JC, Ebert J et al: *Practice management guidelines for the evaluation of genitourinary trauma:* Eastern Association for the Surgery of Trauma Web site (2003), http://www.east.org/tpg/GUeval.pdf. Accessed September 16, 2006.
11. Rouhana SW: Biomechanics of abdominal trauma. In Nahum AM, Melvin JW, editors: *Accidental injury: biomechanics and prevention,* pp 405-453, New York, 2002, Springer-Verlag.
12. McGwin G, Metzger J, Alonso JE et al: The association between occupant restraint systems and risk of injury in frontal motor vehicle collisions, *J Trauma* 54:1182-1187, 2003.
13. Hammontree LN, Wade BK, Passman CM et al: Ureteral injuries: recent trends in etiologies, treatment, and outcomes, *J Pelvic Med Surg* 11:129-136, 2005.
14. McAninch JW: Injuries to the genitourinary tract. In Tanagho EA, McAninch JW, editors: *Smith's general urology,* pp 291-310, New York, McGraw-Hill.
15. Merritt DF: Vulvar and genital trauma in pediatric and adolescent gynecology, *Curr Opin Obstet Gynecol* 16:371-381, 2004.
16. Paparel P, N'Diaye A, Laumon B et al: The epidemiology of trauma of the genitourinary system after traffic accidents: analysis of a register of over 43,000 victims, *BJU Int* 97: 338-341, 2006.
17. Salomone JP, Frame, SB: Prehospital care. In Moore EE, et al, editors: *Trauma,* 5th ed, pp 105-123, New York, 2003, McGraw-Hill Professional.
18. Johnson K, Adams K: Trauma. In Urden LD, Stacy KM, Lough ME, editors: *Thelan's critical care nursing: diagnosis and management,* 5th ed, pp 969-1008, St. Louis, 2006, Mosby Elsevier.
19. American College of Surgeons: Abdominal trauma. In American College of Surgeons' Committee on Trauma: *Advanced trauma life support,* 7th ed, Chicago, 2006, American College of Surgeons.
20. Seidel HM, Ball JW, Dains JE et al, editors: *Mosby's guide to physical examination,* 5th ed, St. Louis, 2002, Mosby.
21. Kawashima A, Sandler CM, Corl FM et al: Imaging of renal trauma: a comprehensive review, *Radiographics* 21:557-574, 2001.
22. Mydlo JH: Blunt and penetrating trauma to the penis. In Wessells H, McAninch J, editors: *Urological emergencies: a practical guide,* pp 95-110, Totowa, NJ, 2005, Humana Press.
23. Mydlo JH, Harris CF, Brown JG: Blunt penetrating and ischemic injuries to the penis, *J Urol* 168:1433-1435, 2002.
24. Beysel M, Tekin A, Gürdal M et al: Evaluation and treatment of penile fractures: accuracy of clinical diagnosis and the value of corpus cavernosography, *Urology* 60:492-496, 2002.
25. Mohr AM, Pham AM, Lavery RF et al: Management of trauma to the male external genitalia: the usefulness of American Association for the Surgery of Trauma organ injury scales, *J Urol* 170:2311-2315, 2003.
26. Sugar NF, Fine DN, Eckert LO: Physical injury after sexual assault: findings of a large case series, *Am J Obstet Gynecol* 190:71-76, 2004.
27. Hartanto VH, Nitti VW: Recent advances in management of female lower urinary tract trauma, *Curr Opin Urol* 13:279-284, 2003.
28. O'Brien C: Improved forensic documentation of genital injury with colposcopy, *J Emerg Nurs* 23:460-462, 1997.
29. Goldberg J, Horan C, O'Brien LM: Severe anorectal and vaginal injuries in a jet ski passenger, *J Trauma* 56:440-441, 2004.
30. Aho T, Upadhyay V: Vaginal water-jet injuries in premenarcheal girls, *N Z Med J* 118, 2005.
31. Sloin MM, Karimian M, Ilbeigi P: Nonobstetric lacerations of the vagina, *J Am Osteopath Assoc* 195:271-273, 2006.
32. Palmer CM, McNulty AM, D'Este C et al: Genital injuries in women reporting sexual assault, *Sex Health* 1:55-59, 2004.
33. Danielson CK, Holmes MM: Adolescent sexual assault: an update of the literature, *Curr Opin Obstet Gynecol* 16:383-388, 2004.
34. Vaer DM: Acid phosphatase testing for rape, *Med Lab Observer* 37:32, 2005.
35. Goldman SM, Sandler CM, Corriere JN Jr et al: Blunt urethral trauma: a unified, anatomical mechanical classification, *J Urol* 157:85-89, 1997.
36. Corriere JN: Trauma to the lower urinary tract. In Gillenwater JY, Grayhack JT, Howards SS, et al, editors: *Adult and pediatric urology,* 4th ed, pp 507-530, Philadelphia, 2002, Lippincott Williams & Wilkins.
37. Brandes S: Initial management of anterior and posterior urethral injuries, *Urol Clin North Am* 33:87-95, 2006.
38. Jordan GH, Virasoro R, Eltahawy EA: Reconstruction and management of posterior urethral and straddle injuries of the urethra, *Urol Clin North Am* 33:97-109, 2006.
39. Mouraviev VB, Coburn M, Santucci RA: The treatment of posterior urethral disruption associated with pelvic fractures: comparative experience of early realignment versus delayed urethroplasty, *J Urol* 173:873-876, 2005.
40. Jordan GH, Jezior JR, Rosenstein DI: Injury to the genitourinary tract and functional reconstruction of the urethra, *Curr Opin Urol* 11:257-261, 2001.
41. Gomez RG, Ceballos L, Coburn M et al: Consensus statement on bladder injuries, *BJU Int* 94:27-32, 2004.
42. Harrahill M: Bladder trauma: a review, *J Emerg Nurs* 30: 287-288, 2004.
43. Secil M, Oksuzler M, Karcioglu O: Extraperitoneal bladder rupture and posterior urethral injury, *J Emerg Med* 27:411-413, 2004.
44. Lee WK, Roche CJ, Duddalwar VA et al: Combined intraperitoneal and extraperitoneal rupture of bladder, *J Trauma* 52:606, 2002.
45. Doyle SM, Master VA, McAninch JW: Appropriate use of CT in the diagnosis of bladder rupture, *J Am Coll Surg* 200:973, 2005.
46. Hsieh CH, Chen RJ, Fang JF et al: Diagnosis and management of bladder injury by trauma surgeons, *Am J Surg* 184:143-147, 2002.
47. Corriere JN Jr, Sandler CM: Diagnosis and management of bladder injuries, *Urol Clin North Am* 33:67-71, 2006.
48. Brandes SB, Belani JS: Bladder trauma. In Wessells H, McAninch J, editors: *Urological emergencies: a practical guide,* pp 39-56, Totowa, NJ, 2005, Humana Press.
49. Alli, MO, Singh B, Moodley J et al: Prospective evaluation of combined suprapubic and urethral catherization to urethral

drainage alone for intraperitoneal bladder injuries, *J Trauma* 55:1152-1154, 2003.

50. Parry NG, Rozycki GS,Feliciano DV et al: Traumatic rupture of the urinary bladder: is the suprapubic tube necessary? *J Trauma* 54:431-436, 2003.
51. Mokoena T, Naidu AG: Diagnostic difficulties in patients with a ruptured bladder, *Br J Surg* 82:69-70, 1995.
52. Vakili B, Chesson RR, Kyle BL et al: The incidence of urinary tract injury during hysterectomy: a prospective analysis based on universal cystoscopy, *Am J Obstet Gynecol* 192:1599-1604, 2004.
53. Best CD, Petrone P, Buscarini M et al: Traumatic ureteral injuries: a single institution experience validating the American Association for the Surgery of Trauma-Organ Injury Scale Grading Scale, *J Urol* 178:1202-1205, 2005.
54. Brandes S, Coburn M, Armenakas N et al: Diagnosis and management of ureteric injury: an evidence-based analysis, *BJU Int* 94:277-289, 2004.
55. McGahan PJ, et al: Ultrasound detection of blunt urological trauma: a 6-year study, *Inj Int J Care Injured* 36:762-770, 2004.
56. Alsikafi NF, Rosenstein DI: Staging, evaluation, and nonoperative management of renal injuries, *Urol Clin North Am* 33:13-19, 2006.
57. Gaines BA, Ford HR: Abdominal and pelvic trauma in children, *Crit Care Med* 30:5416-5423, 2002.
58. Buckley JC, McAninch JW: The diagnosis, management, and outcomes of pediatric renal injuries, *Urol Clin North Am* 33: 33-40, 2006.
59. Santucci RA, Fisher MB: The literature increasingly supports expectant (conservative) management of renal trauma—a systematic review, *J Trauma* 59:491-501, 2005.
60. Bozeman C, Carver B, Zabari G et al: Selective operative management of major blunt renal trauma, *J Trauma* 57:305-309, 2004.
61. Barsness KA, Bensard DD, Partrick D et al: Renovascular injury: an argument for renal preservation, *J Trauma* 57:310-315, 2004.
62. Wessells H, Suh D, Porter JR et al: Renal injury and operative management in the US: results of a population-based study, *J Trauma* 54:423-430, 2003.
63. Holevar M, Ebert J, Luchette F et al: *Practice management guidelines for the management of genitourinary trauma*, pp 1-101, Winston-Salem, NC, 2004, Eastern Association for the Surgery of Trauma.
64. Guichelaar MM, Leenan LP, Braams R: Transient adrenocortical insufficiency following traumatic bilateral adrenal hemorrhage, *J Trauma* 56:1135-1137, 2004.
65. Udobi KF, Childs EW: Adrenal crisis after traumatic bilateral adrenal hemorrhage, *J Trauma* 51:597-600, 2001.
66. Vella A, Nippoldt TB, Morris JC: Adrenal hemorrhage: a 25-year experience at the Mayo Clinic, *Mayo Clin Proc* 76: 161-168, 2001.
67. Melli G, Chaudhry V, Cornblath DR: Rhabdomyolysis: an evaluation of 475 hospitalized patients, *Medicine* 84:377-385, 2005.
68. Brown CV, Rhee P, Chan L et al: Preventing renal failure in patients with rhabdomyolysis: do bicarbonate and mannitol make a difference? *J Trauma* 56:1191-1196, 2004.
69. Hariston S: A review of rhabdomyolysis, *Dimens Crit Care Nurs* 23:155-161, 2004.
70. Rupert SA: Pathogenesis and treatment of rhabdomyolysis, *J Am Acad Nurse Practioner* 12:82-87, 2002.
71. Ozgüc H, Kahveci N, Akköse S et al: Effects of different resuscitation fluids on tissue blood flow and oxidant injury in experimental rhabdomyolysis, *Crit Care Med* 33:2579-2586, 2005.
72. Fernandez WG, Hung O, Bruno GR et al: Factors predictive of acute renal failure and need for hemodialysis among ED patients with rhabdomyolysis, *Am J Emerg Med* 23:1-7, 2005.
73. Criddle LM: Rhabdomyolysis: pathophysiology, recognition, and management, *Crit Care Nurs* 6:14-32, 2003.
74. Abernethy VE, Lieberthal W: Acute renal failure in the critically ill patient, *Crit Care Clin* 18:203-222, 2002.
75. Kruger PS, Whiteside RS: Pseudo-renal failure following the delayed diagnosis of bladder perforation after diagnostic laparoscopy, *Anaesth Intensive Care* 31:211-213, 2003.
76. Sugrue M: Abdominal compartment syndrome, *Curr Opin Crit Care* 11:333-338, 2005.
77. Bradley SE, Bradley GP: The effect of increased intra-abdominal pressure on renal function in man, *J Clin Invest* 26:1010-1022, 1947.
78. Harmon KP, Kron IL, McLachlan DH: Elevated intra-abdominal pressure and renal function, *Ann Surg* 196:594-597, 1982.
79. Sugrue M, Jones F, Lee A: Intraabdominal pressure and gastric intramucosal pH: is there an association? *West J Surg* 20: 988-991, 1996.
80. Lameire N, Van Biesen W, Vanholder R: Acute renal failure, *Lancet* 365:417-430, 2005.
81. Ympa YP, Sakr Y, Reinhart K et al: Has mortality from acute renal failure decreased? A systematic review of the literature, *Am J Med* 118:827-832, 2005.
82. Bellomo R, Kellum J, Ronco C: Defining acute renal failure: physiological principles, *Intensive Care Med* 30:33-37, 2004.
83. Gill N, Nally J, Fatica R: Renal failure secondary to acute tubular necrosis: epidemiology, diagnosis, and management, *Chest* 128:2847-2863, 2005.
84. Abraham E, Andrews P, Antonelli M et al: Year in review in intensive care medicine: 2003, II: brain injury, hemodynamics, gastrointestinal tract, renal failure, metabolism, trauma, and postoperative, *Intensive Care Med* 30:1266-1275, 2004.
85. Macias WL, Alaka KJ, Murphy MII et al: Impact of nutritional regimen on protein catabolism and nitrogen balance in patients with ARF, *JPEN J Parenter Enteral Nutr* 20:56-62, 1996.
86. Drumi W: Nutritional management of acute renal failure, *Am J Kidney Dis* 37:S89-S94, 2001.
87. Bellomo R, Seacombe J, Daskalakis M et al: A prospective comparative study of moderate versus high protein intake for critically ill patients with ARF, *Ren Fail* 19:111-120, 1997.
88. O'Reilly P, Tolwani A: Renal replacement therapy III: IHD, CRRT, SLED, *Crit Care Clin* 21:367-378, 2005.
89. Kellum JA, Angus DC, Johnson LP et al: Continuous versus intermittent renal replacement: a meta analysis, *Intensive Care Med* 28:29-37, 2002.

90. Tonelli M, Manns B, Feller-Kopman D: Acute renal failure in the intensive care unit: a systematic review of the impact of dialytic modality on mortality and renal recovery, *Am J Kidney Dis* 40:875-885, 2002.
91. Augustine JJ, Sandy D, Seifert TII et al: A randomized controlled trial comparing intermittent and continuous dialysis in patients with ARF, *Am J Kidney Dis* 44:1000-1007, 2004.
92. Manns B, Doig CJ, Lee H et al: Cost of acute renal failure requiring dialysis in the intensive care unit: clinical and resource implications of renal recovery, *Crit Care Med* 31:449-455, 2003.

27

MUSCULOSKELETAL INJURIES

Colleen R. Walsh

Management of traumatic musculoskeletal injuries rarely takes precedence during the initial phases of trauma care. The basic principles of trauma care stress resuscitation and therapeutic interventions for those life-threatening injuries most commonly associated with trauma. Musculoskeletal injuries are considered part of the secondary trauma survey unless those injuries result in significant hemodynamic instability, such as traumatic amputations and massive pelvic injuries. Musculoskeletal injuries require prompt recognition and appropriate management after stabilization of the cardiopulmonary and neurologic systems to maximize the patient's full recovery.

Musculoskeletal injuries, although not usually life threatening, are associated with longer recovery times than most other injuries and often result in life-long disability and lifestyle changes. This chapter primarily addresses musculoskeletal injuries seen in trauma that affects the extremities or pelvis and the complications that require early diagnosis and emergency management. The reader is referred to the craniocerebral, maxillofacial, and spinal cord injuries chapters for descriptions of musculoskeletal injuries affecting those areas.

ANATOMY AND PHYSIOLOGY

An understanding of the anatomy and physiology of the musculoskeletal system is necessary to enable nurses caring for trauma patients to plan interventions and care aimed at prevention of the complications that frequently occur in this population. Although this discussion is not meant to be complete, a basic review of the structures and functions of the musculoskeletal system assists the reader to better understand musculoskeletal injuries and their consequences.

FUNCTIONS

The musculoskeletal system is composed of two systems: the skeletal system and the skeletal muscles. The skeletal system is composed of bones and joints, and its main functions are to provide support, protection, storage of mineral salts and fats, and hematopoiesis (red blood cell production). The skeletal system also provides the leverage needed by skeletal muscles to produce movement through contraction of skeletal muscles and bending and rotation at joints.[1] Any injury to the musculoskeletal system that affects any of these functions may be detrimental to the patient.

STRUCTURES

Figure 27-1 illustrates normal bone architecture, including articular cartilage, spongy bone, epiphysis, epiphyseal plate, compact bone, medullary cavity, diaphysis, and periosteum. There are two types of bone tissue: compact bone (cortical bone) and spongy bone (cancellous). Compact bone is organized, strong, and solid and contains structural units, called haversian systems. The haversian system, which contains bone cells called osteocytes, provides a vehicle for the major metabolic processes of compact bone, transporting nutrients to and removing wastes from the osteocytes.[1] Spongy bone is less organized and does not contain haversian systems. Spongy bone is characterized by trabeculae, or plates, that branch out to form an irregular meshwork. Stresses placed on the bone form the pattern of trabeculae, and the spaces between the trabeculae are filled with red bone marrow.[1]

The diaphysis, or shaft, is composed of a thick layer of compact bone that offers a tremendous degree of support and protection. This slender part of the bone is slightly curved in long bones to provide added strength and to enable the bone to withstand and absorb stress. The bone shaft can withstand shearing and compression forces but is at risk for injury from tension-producing mechanisms. For example, diaphyseal fractures most often occur as a result of tension failure produced by a bending, twisting, or pulling mechanism. Bone is strongest at the point where maximal forces or stressors are most likely applied. This concept is discussed later in the chapter.

The epiphysis, or bone end, is made up primarily of cancellous or spongy tissue that houses red marrow in the large pores of the trabeculae. This segment of bone is at greater risk of injury from crushing mechanisms that cause compression or impaction of bone ends. The sequelae of an injury to this area of the bone increase in severity in skeletally immature children because longitudinal bone growth occurs at the epiphyseal plate. An injury to this region can potentially alter bone growth in children.

The periosteum is a fibrous membrane sleeve that covers the entire bone except for the cartilaginous ends. The inner osteogenic layer of periosteum consists of elastic fibers, vessels, and osteoblasts, which are responsible for new bone formation. The outer fibrous layer is made up of connective tissue and it houses blood and lymphatic vessels and nerves. Bone growth, repair, and nutrition depend to a large extent on an intact and healthy periosteum. This closely adherent

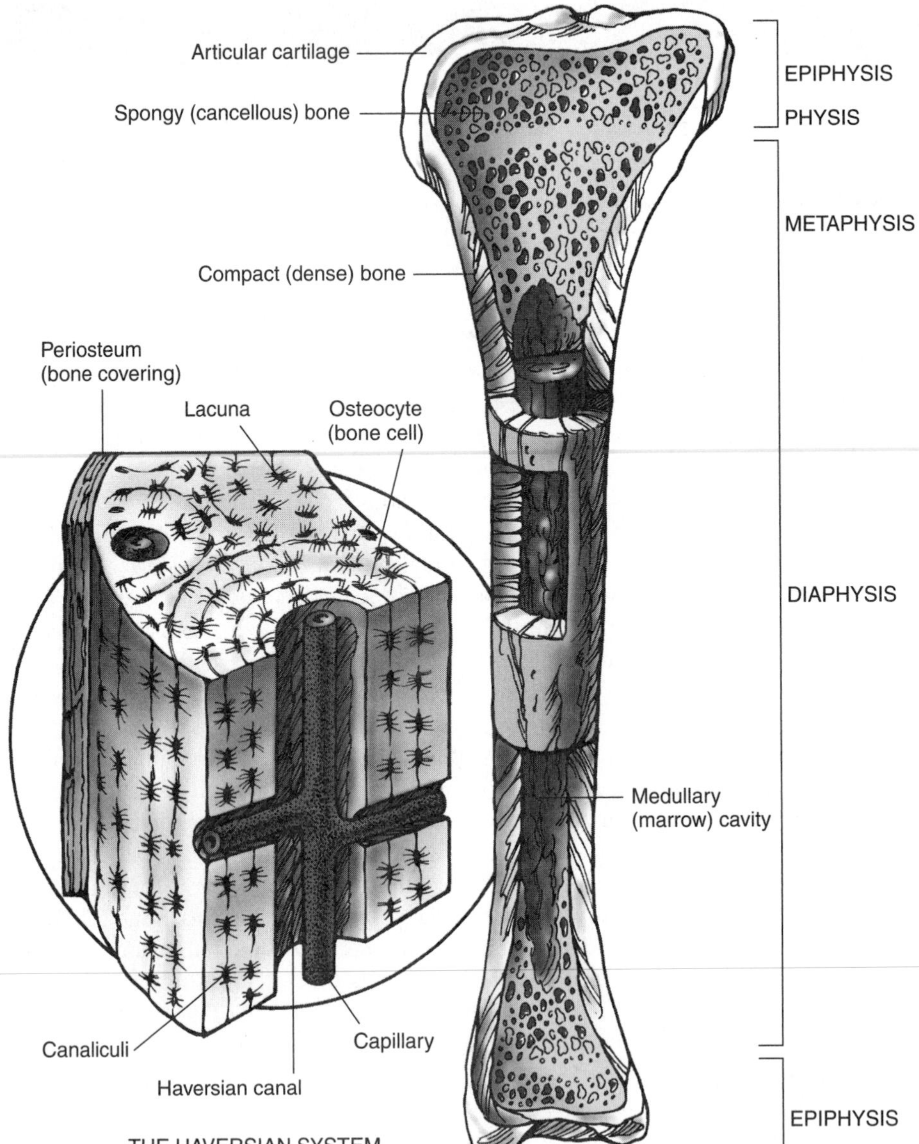

FIGURE 27-1 Diagram of longitudinal section of a long bone and Haversian system. (From Ignatavicus DD, Bayne MV: *Medical-surgical nursing: a nursing process approach,* Philadelphia, 1991, W. B. Saunders, p 719.)

covering is thickest where muscles surround the bone, such as at the diaphysis of the femur. Because it is a thin and tightly bound membrane in adults, it usually tears at fracture sites and occasionally separates from the bone. When a low-energy fracture occurs, one side of the periosteum may remain intact (the periosteal hinge). The remaining portion of intact membrane aids fracture reduction and maintenance and serves as an osteogenic covering that promotes healing. The degree to which the periosteum is damaged during a fracture event often determines the course of healing of the fracture.

Injuries to the soft tissue, including muscle, nerves, vessels, subcutaneous fat, and skin, occur to some degree in conjunction with all fractures. The soft tissue injury may be more serious and have more significant ramifications than the fracture itself. Neglect or underestimation of soft tissue involvement may lead to serious fracture complications.

Bone Cells

Bone contains three types of cells: osteoblasts, osteocytes, and osteoclasts. Each type of cell plays a major role in the formation, repair, and cyclic remodeling of bone. Osteoblasts are bone-forming cells whose major function is to lay down new bone. Once this is accomplished, they become osteocytes. Osteocytes are osteoblasts that have become trapped in the bone matrix.[1] Their major function is not well defined, but it is postulated that they function to maintain the bone matrix.[1] Osteoclasts are the major resorptive cells of bone and function primarily during periods of growth and repair.[1] Any process that interferes with the function of these bone cells can adversely affect the dynamic state of skeletal tissue. Approximately 18% of bone is removed and replaced every year in premenopausal women; after menopause this balance changes to an increase in bone resorption and a decrease in bone production, leading to the development of osteoporosis.

EPIDEMIOLOGY

Approximately 29 million musculoskeletal injuries occur annually, including 20 million fractures, dislocations, and sprains, with approximately 8,000 deaths.[2] These deaths are directly attributed to musculoskeletal injuries and there are many more patients with multiple injuries where fractures contribute to overall injury load and risk of death. Musculoskeletal injuries account for almost half of all injuries, and those found in the trauma patient result from a variety of causes.[2] The major causes of significant musculoskeletal injuries are vehicular crashes; falls; industrial, home, and farming incidents; and interpersonal violence. Musculoskeletal injuries are often associated with serious injuries to other body systems.[2]

RESUSCITATION PHASE

ASSESSMENT

Prehospital Database

A variety of energy sources can traumatize the musculoskeletal system. Each type of impact exerts a different amount of force on the body. The degree, direction, and duration of that force, along with the patient's age and health history, determine the severity of the injury and its resulting morbidity.[3]

Knowing the type of incident and the mechanism of injury can greatly increase the clinician's index of suspicion during the assessment of the musculoskeletal system. A victim of a fall and a driver of a car striking another car head on may absorb similar amounts of energy from the impact, but the direction of the forces applied to the body, the body surface area involved, and the rate of deceleration that occurs are different, thus producing different injuries.

Information concerning the mechanism of injury should be obtained from the patient if possible and from the prehospital care providers. Important information to obtain is summarized in Table 27-1. Similar injuries can occur in different environments, and the sequelae of an open fracture can be very different if the injury occurred in a farming incident versus a fall at home. Pathogenic organisms found in soil can cause serious, even fatal, infections. Early identification of environmental factors can decrease complications if appropriate interventions are started early in the treatment phase.

Each musculoskeletal injury is the result of absorbed and transferred energy. The fall victim who lands on his or her feet may have obvious ankle injuries, but other injuries often associated with this type of mechanism, such as pelvic and lumbar spine fractures, may be occult (Figure 27-2). Other patterns of energy absorption and transfer are demonstrated in Figure 27-3. Information concerning events of extrication, immobilization, and stabilization that occurred at the site of the incident is important and should be obtained from the prehospital care providers.[3] Knowing the degree of angulation of a fracture, attitude of a joint, neurovascular status of the extremity at the scene, amount of exposed bone, and estimated blood loss heightens suspicion and helps determine the type of treatment necessary. Review Chapter 12 for further discussion of mechanism of injury.

TABLE 27-1 **Prehospital Database**

How did the incident happen?
Was it a high-energy incident or a low-energy incident?
What position was the patient in when the incident happened?
What position was the patient found in?
Where and when did incident happen? How long ago?
In what environment did the incident happen?

Musculoskeletal Physical Assessment

The initial assessment of the patient with musculoskeletal injuries begins with the primary survey, which consists of the standard evaluation of airway, breathing, circulation, and neurologic status. Initiation of appropriate interventions to establish or maintain normal cardiopulmonary and neurologic function takes precedence regardless of obvious or suspected musculoskeletal injuries.

Attention is directed toward the musculoskeletal system during the secondary survey. Any suspected or obvious musculoskeletal injuries require baseline assessment of neurovascular and motor status, proper immobilization of affected extremities, including splinting or traction, and application of sterile dressings to open wounds. Additionally, an unstable pelvic ring disruption (as identified on initial radiographs) with possible vascular injury may require application of a pelvic binder to prevent exsanguination.[4,5] External fixators or pelvic C clamps may be used in rare situations when binders are ineffective. Other interventions are typically not initiated until the total patient evaluation has been completed and the patient is hemodynamically stable.

Severe pain from soft tissue or bony injuries may mask symptoms of more life-threatening injuries; thus a thorough total system evaluation is essential. Conversely, restlessness and agitation caused by other pathologic conditions may further disrupt bone fragments and increase the patient's pain. Altered level of consciousness related to shock or associated brain injury or impaired sensation caused by spinal cord injury may prevent perception or communication of pain resulting from musculoskeletal disruption.

Areas of suspected musculoskeletal injury should remain immobilized to prevent further soft tissue, bone, nerve, or vascular damage. Whenever the patient requires turning or moving, one person assumes responsibility for the affected limb to maintain alignment and immobilization. This is critically important when caring for patients with suspected spinal column injuries because any motion at the fracture or dislocation site may result in spinal cord damage and dysfunction.[6]

Continuous monitoring is an important concept for emergency personnel. After primary and lifesaving measures are instituted, it is essential that providers reassess the patient's status, especially the neurovascular function of extremities

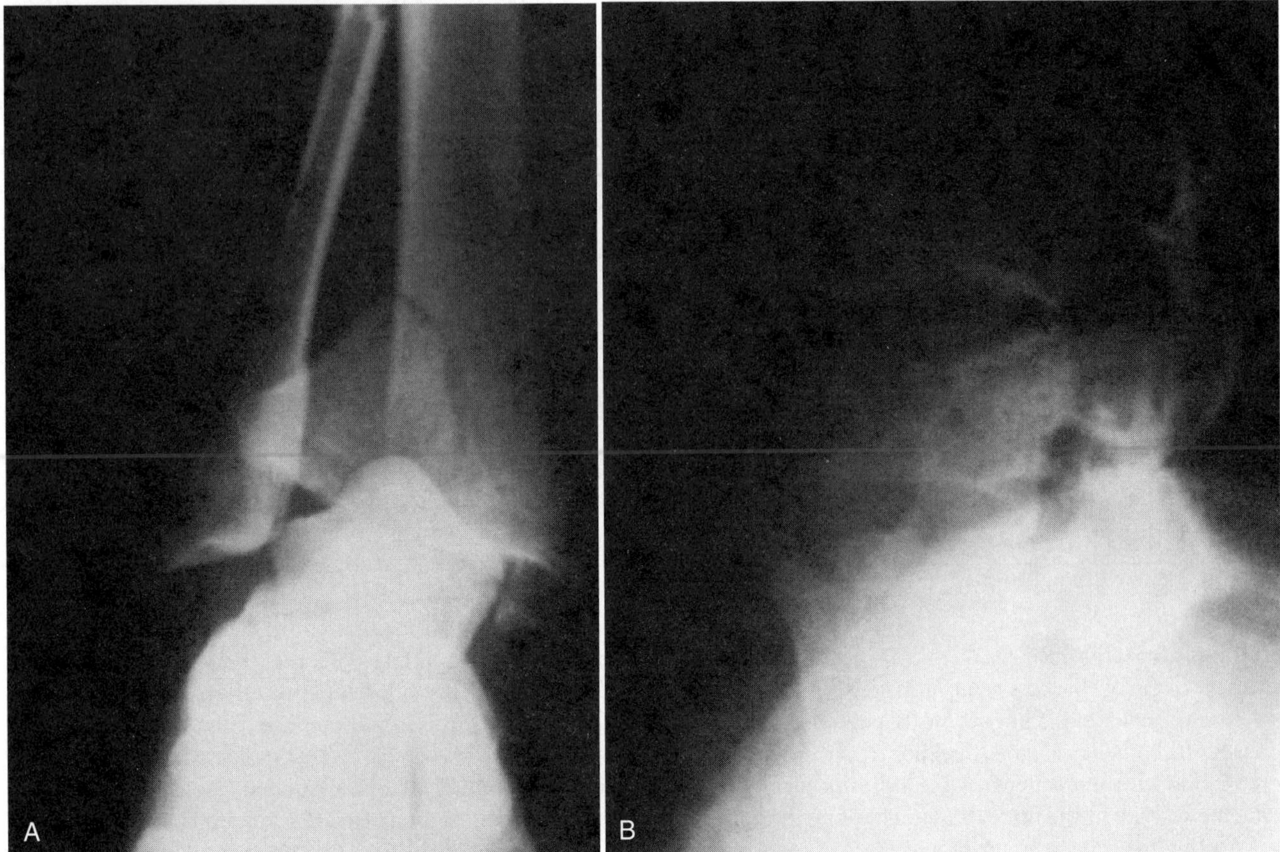

FIGURE 27-2 Radiographs of a fall victim who landed on his feet. **A,** Fractured ankle. **B,** Associated compression fracture of the lumbar spine.

with obvious or suspected fractures. Physiologic events, such as muscle spasms, or environmental events, such as transports, can further displace fracture fragments and lead to serious neurovascular compromise of the affected extremity. If undetected, neurovascular compromise can cause permanent disability, loss of limb, or even death.

Inspection and Palpation. Assessment of the musculoskeletal system in a systematic fashion decreases the chance of missing an injury. Assessment involves inspection and palpation.[7] The position of the patient and the extremities should be observed. Note is made of any deformities such as angulation, shortening, or rotation; open wounds; obviously protruding bone ends; abrasions; and road burns.

The patient is examined for additional evidence of musculoskeletal injury:

- Ecchymosis: caused by vascular disruption with blood dispersing through soft tissue
- Muscle spasm: continuous muscle contraction over an area of injury; considered a protective mechanism of the muscle to splint the injured part
- Swelling: caused by injury to the soft tissue and interruption of the venous and lymphatic return system
- Extremity color: pale color indicates inadequate arterial blood supply; dusky, bluish color indicates venous congestion

Each bone is palpated and any interruptions in the natural integrity are noted. Interruption in bone integrity may be difficult to identify; crepitus, pain, or muscle spasm may be the only indication that an injury exists. Palpation is used to assess the following:

- Capillary refill time: A filling time longer than 2 seconds is considered abnormal and may indicate vascular compromise. Factors such as ambient air temperature, patient's core body temperature, and presence of shock may affect the capillary refill time.
- Pulses: Quality and equality are evaluated over the entire length of an extremity, not just distal to an obvious injury; results are compared with pulses in the unaffected extremity.
- Crepitus: A grating sound is heard and felt when fractured bone ends move.
- Muscle spasm: As noted above. Lack of spasms over an obvious fracture may indicate a neurologic lesion above the fracture, preventing contraction of the muscle.
- Movement: Range of motion, both passive and active, is assessed. Deviation from normal range or limitation of motion or muscle strength is noted. Obviously injured extremities should not be tested for range of motion because of the risk of increasing the damage to surrounding neurovascular structures.

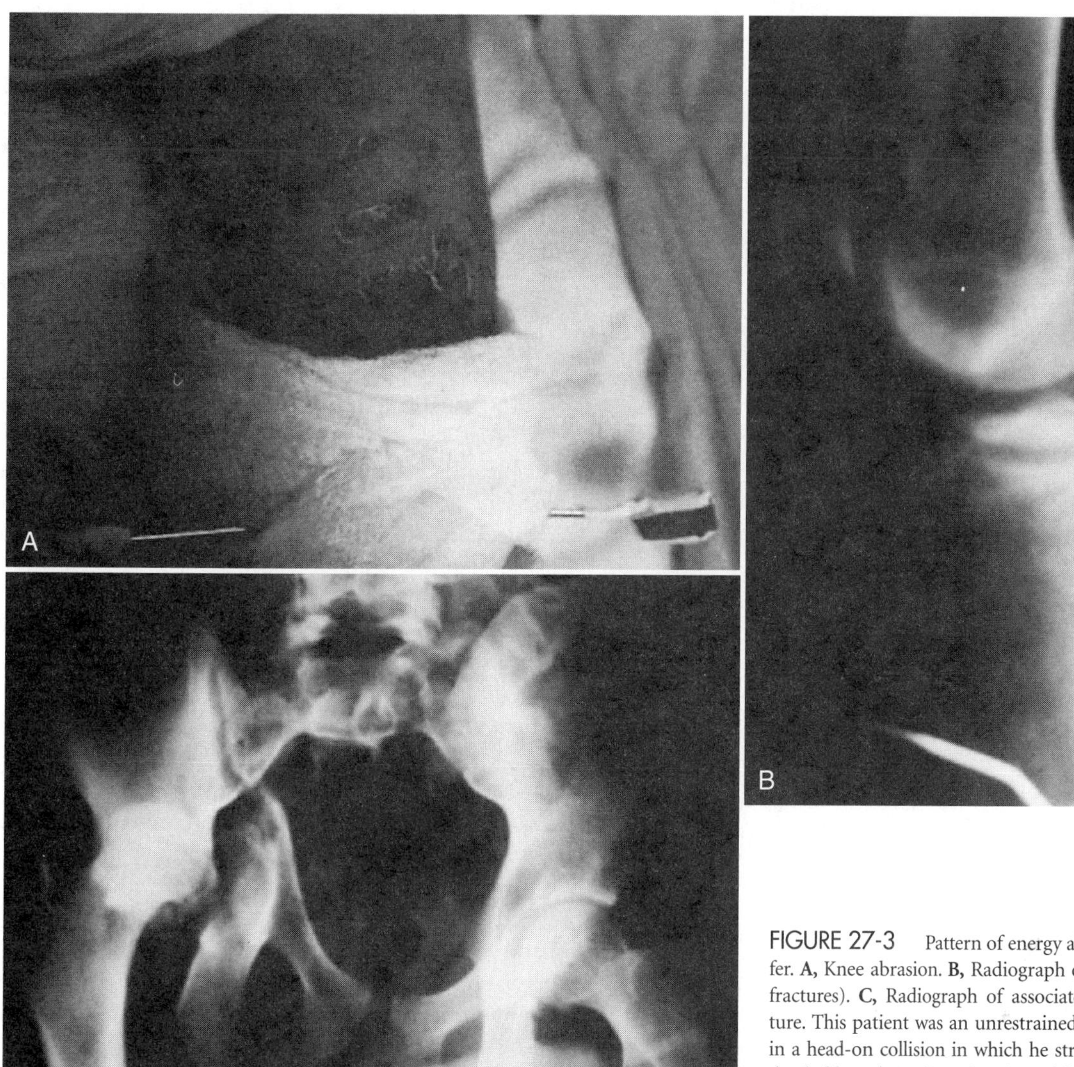

FIGURE 27-3 Pattern of energy absorption and transfer. **A,** Knee abrasion. **B,** Radiograph of knee (negative for fractures). **C,** Radiograph of associated acetabulum fracture. This patient was an unrestrained front seat occupant in a head-on collision in which he struck his knee against the dashboard. A minor abrasion of the knee was sustained without underlying fracture, but the energy transferred to the pelvis resulted in an acetabulum fracture.

- Sensation: Sensory perception in response to sharp and dull stimuli and proprioception are assessed. Absent or altered senstation may indicate neuronal compression or injury
- Pain: Pain is usually caused by injury to the periosteum (the only part of bone with sensory innervation), muscle spasm, soft tissue disruption, and swelling within fascial compartments.

Zone of Injury. The zone of injury is the area affected by traumatic forces, as seen in Figure 27-4. Injuries to the skeletal system are always accompanied by some degree of soft tissue injury. Damage to the soft tissue structures is often greater than what is discovered on clinical assessment and radiologic examination. The exact zone of injury is often not fully appreciated until the time of operative intervention; therefore, continued physical assessment is important with close observation of areas both distal and proximal to any obvious or suspected musculoskeletal injury.

Diagnostic Studies. Various radiographic studies are used to confirm or exclude musculoskeletal injuries. For plain radiographic films, at least two views are required to determine the degree of angulation and displacement (Figure 27-5). Inlet and outlet views of the pelvis, taken from superior and inferior angles, can be done in the resuscitation room to further define significant pelvic injuries and aid clinicians in their early treatment. Surrounding anatomic structures or the structure of the bone or joint in question may reduce the effectiveness of plain films in diagnosing skeletal injuries and necessitate the use of other techniques such as computed tomography (CT) scans or magnetic resonance imaging (MRI). CT scans aid in confirmation of hidden or minimally displaced fractures in areas such as the cervical spine, pelvic ring, ankle, and knee. MRI studies are often performed to aid in the diagnosis of suspected soft tissue injuries such as herniated intervertebral disks or ligamentous disruption. Angiography may be helpful in assessing vascular injuries associated with musculoskeletal trauma.[8]

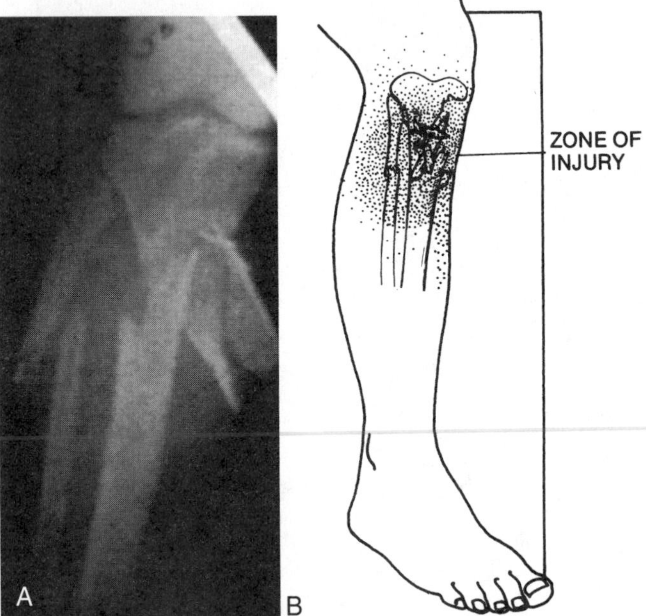

FIGURE 27-4 The mechanism of injury predicts the zone of soft tissue injury. **A,** Radiograph of a grade III tibia fracture that resulted from a car bumper crush injury. **B,** The zone of injury *(stippled)* of the leg. The fracture pattern and the mechanism of injury predict the size of this zone. (From Manson PN, Yaremchuk MJ, Hoopes JE: Soft tissue injuries of the extremities. In Zuidema GD, Rutherford RB, Ballinger WF, editors: *The management of trauma,* Philadelphia, 1985, W. B. Saunders.)

When diagnostic procedures are performed, the nurse is responsible for the following:

1. Assisting with explanation of the procedure to the patient and ensuring that consent is obtained when necessary
2. Ensuring that the patient has no known allergy to agents that are to be administered during the procedure
3. With the patient receiving contrast medium, adequately hydrating and, if prescribed, administering prophylaxis to prevent contrast-induced renal nephropathy
4. Assisting with safe patient positioning during and after the procedure to prevent further injury- or procedure-related complications. For example, after an angiogram in which the femoral artery is cannulated, hip flexion is restricted for 6 to 8 hours to prevent further bleeding at the insertion site.
5. Protecting the patient from unnecessary radiation exposure by shielding with a lead-lined apron whenever possible
6. Constantly monitoring the patient's overall status, including potential reaction to contrast media
7. Documenting the procedure, patient response, and follow-up evaluation

Patient Health History. Eliciting a specific patient health history is an important part of the patient assessment. Information concerning the health history can be obtained from the patient or, when necessary, from family members or friends. The nurse should determine whether the patient has ever had an allergic reaction to any medication or contrast material and the type of reaction that occurred. Previous reactions to pharmacologic agents can alter the choice of diagnostic studies or the choice of medications used for treatment. Current or recent use of medication and the reason, dose, and frequency are ascertained if possible. Learning whether the patient has taken any anticoagulants, antiplatelet agents, nonsteroidal anti-inflammatory drugs, or other medication is essential. The patient's tetanus immunization history is also important. Other helpful information includes

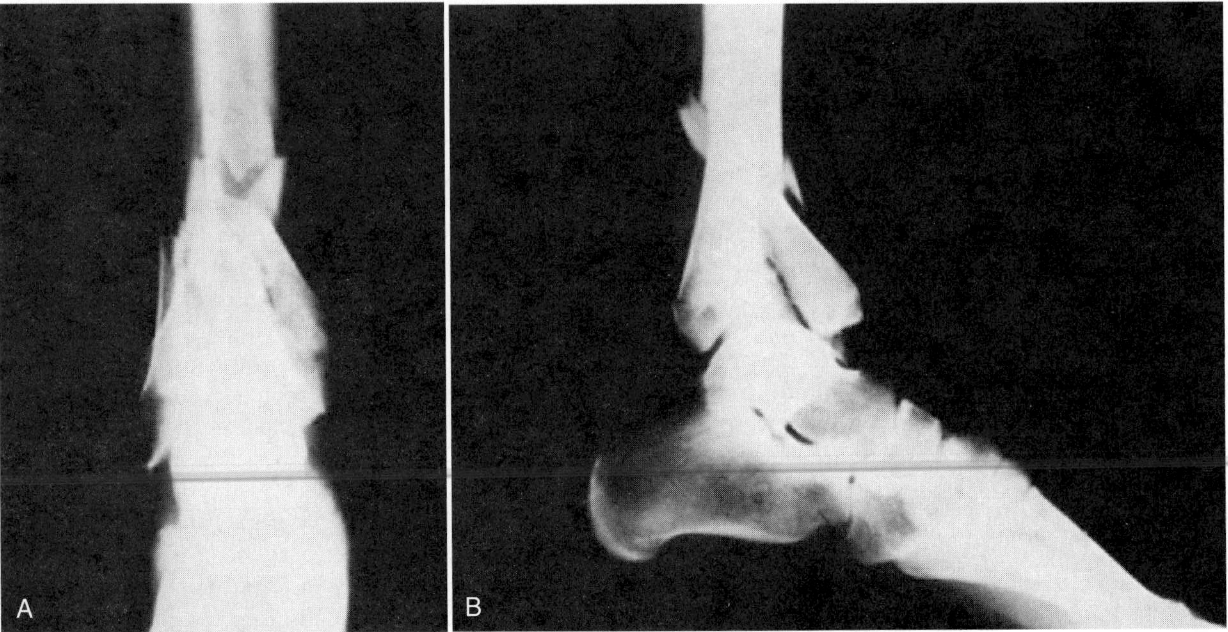

FIGURE 27-5 Radiographs of a fracture of the distal tibia/fibula and ankle showing the degree of angulation and displacement. **A,** Anteroposterior view. **B,** Lateral view.

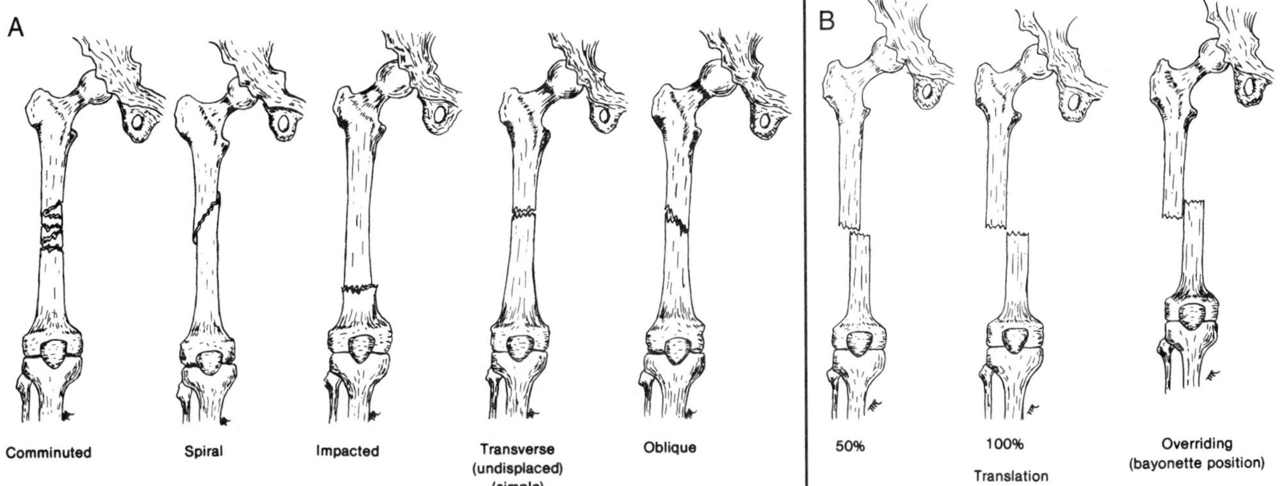

FIGURE 27-6 **A,** Types of fractures. **B,** Translation. (From Stearns HC: Principles of lower extremity fracture management. In Hilt N, editor: *Assessment and fracture management of the lower extremities* [monograph], Pitman, NJ, 1984, National Association of Orthopaedic Nurses.)

previous hospitalizations and surgeries, anesthesia-associated problems, and any specific health problems. Previous fractures, ligamentous or soft tissue injuries, thromboembolic disease, neurologic disorders, smoking history, and problems with infection or delayed healing potentially affect the patient's treatment and recovery.[7] The importance of obtaining an AMPLE (**A**llergies, **M**edications, **P**ast medical history, **L**ast meal, **E**nvironment) history during the initial assessment cannot be overemphasized because this history guides the clinician's assessment and treatment of the trauma patient (Table 27-2).

Classification of Injuries

Injuries include fractures, fracture-dislocations, extremity amputations, and trauma to the soft tissue, nerves, and blood vessels. Soft tissue injuries may involve skin, muscles, tendons, ligaments, and cartilage.

Extremity Fractures. The classification of a fracture is based on several factors: (1) type of fracture line (spiral, transverse, oblique), (2) whether the fracture is linear or comminuted (number of fracture fragments), (3) anatomic location (distal, middle, proximal third of the shaft, intra-articular), (4) type of displacement (angulation, translation, impaction, distraction), and (5) position of the displacement in relation to other fragments[9] (Figure 27-6).

A fracture with associated interruption in skin integrity is an open fracture. An open fracture is further classified according to the degree of soft tissue involvement and the amount of disruption in skin integrity. A type I open fracture is small with minimal (less than 1-cm wound) soft tissue damage and a low-energy fracture pattern. A type II open fracture is larger (1- to 10-cm wound) with a moderate amount of soft tissue injury. A type III open fracture is associated with significant soft tissue damage and possible neurologic or vascular involvement. All open fractures with high-energy fracture patterns are considered type III open fractures regardless of actual wound size. Type III fractures are further subclassified as IIIA, IIIB, or IIIC depending on the degree of soft tissue loss and the presence of vascular injury requiring repair[9] (Table 27-3).

Certain mechanisms of injury automatically classify an open fracture as type III, such as a shotgun injury, a high-velocity gunshot wound, an open fracture occurring in a farm environment, and a crushing injury from a fast-moving vehicle. The time elapsed from open injury to operative debridement of open fractures also influences fracture classification. However, the relationship between time to operative debridement and infection risk is unclear for most fracture types (Figure 27-7).

Traumatic Amputation. Traumatic amputations are associated with soft tissue, nerve, and vascular injury. The zone of injury is important to clinical decision making regarding treatment plans for managing these injuries.[10]

The advent of newer and more sophisticated microsurgical techniques used for reattachment of severed limbs has made it imperative that all prehospital and hospital personnel correctly care for the amputated limb until a determination can be made regarding the feasibility of surgical reattachment. Amputated parts should be placed in a plastic bag and then placed in another bag containing ice water and transported with the patient. Direct contact with iced solutions can cause freezing and crystallization with subsequent rupture of tissue cells, thus making successful reattachment less likely. Dry ice should never be used as a cooling agent because it increases crystal formation. Amputations caused by crush or avulsion injuries have a low

TABLE 27-2 **"AMPLE" History**

A	Allergies
M	Medications currently used (including herbals and over the counter)
P	Past medical illnesses/pregnancies
L	Last meal
E	Environment/events of incident (mechanisms of injury)

Source: American College of Surgeons' Committee on Trauma: *Advanced trauma life support,* 7th ed, Chicago, 2004, American College of Surgeons.

TABLE 27-3 Classification of Open Fractures

Type	Description
I	Wound less than 1 cm Moderately clean, minimal contamination Fracture: simple transverse or oblique with skin pierced by bone spike Minimal soft tissue damage
II	Wound greater than 1 cm Moderate contamination Fracture: moderate comminution/crush injury Moderate soft tissue damage (flaps or avulsions)
III	High degree of contamination Fracture: severe comminution and instability Extensive soft tissue damage involving muscle, skin, and neurovascular structures Traumatic amputation
IIIA	Soft tissue coverage of fracture is adequate Fracture: segmental or severely comminuted
IIIB	Extensive injury to or loss of soft tissue, periosteal stripping, and exposure of bone requiring flap for soft tissue coverage Massive contamination Fracture: severe comminution
IIIC	Any open fracture associated with arterial injury that must be repaired regardless of degree of soft tissue injury

Modified from Snyder P: Fractures. In Maher AB, Salmond SW, Pellino, TA, editors: *Orthopaedic nursing,* Philadelphia, 2002, W. B. Saunders.

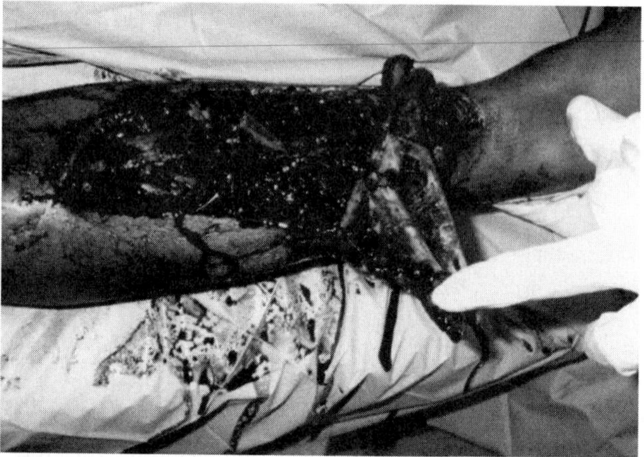

FIGURE 27-7 Grade IIIB open fracture of the tibial shaft with extensive soft tissue loss.

reattachment success rate; therefore, the procedure is usually not attempted.

Dislocation. A dislocation occurs when articulating surfaces are no longer in contact because of joint disruption. Movement can be limited or impossible. The dislocation is described in terms of the position of the distal component relative to the proximal component. For example, a dislocation of the elbow involving the radius alone can be anterior, posterior, or lateral. Hip dislocations may be classified as anterior, posterior, or central (Figure 27-8). The incidence of neurovascular injuries associated with major joint dislocations is high; thus, careful assessment of distal neurovascular function is necessary. The ligamentous structures surrounding the dislocated joint may be severely stretched or completely disrupted, leaving the joint unstable. Immobilization is essential to prevent or limit the neurovascular compromise often found with these injuries. Dislocations are often easily recognized clinically without the aid of diagnostic studies. A dislocation may also occur at the time of impact and then either reduce spontaneously or during application of an immobilization device at the scene of the incident. For this reason, it is important to obtain a history from either the patient or the prehospital care providers concerning any "popping" or "snapping" of a joint that may have been felt or heard.

Subluxation. A subluxation is a partial dislocation in which a portion of the articular surface is not in contact. The subluxation is often accompanied by varying degrees of neurovascular compromise, and again immobilization is essential. Many subluxations spontaneously reduce during extrication or other procedures, but care must be taken to assess the affected joint for ligamentous instability.

Pelvic Ring Disruption. The pelvis is composed of three bones held together and stabilized by a ligamentous network. Anteriorly the symphysis pubis, a strong ligamentous structure, acts as a band to prevent anterior pelvic widening, and it has little to do with weight bearing. The major stabilizing force in the pelvis is the posterior tension band that includes the following ligaments: iliolumbar, posterior sacroiliac, anterior sacroiliac, sacrospinous, and sacrotuberous (Figure 27-9).

Pelvic ring disruptions are commonly associated with fatal motor vehicle crashes.[11] These disruptions to the pelvic ring are clinically described as stable or unstable. Two thirds of pelvic ring disruptions are stable.[12] Although fewer in incidence, the unstable injuries are potentially more life threatening and debilitating because they are often accompanied by many additional structural disruptions and complications. These may include massive to exsanguinating blood loss resulting from venous or arterial injury, genitourinary trauma, sepsis, chronic pain, and long-term disability. Injuries to the pelvic ring may be closed or open, as with an associated laceration or puncture of the skin, rectum, or vagina. The mortality rate associated with open pelvic fractures has been reported to be as high as 70%.[12,13]

Various systems exist for classification of pelvic injuries, such as those described by Trunkey et al,[14] Pennal et al,[15] and Young and Burgess.[16] One commonly used classification system, described by Tile,[17] categorizes pelvic ring disruptions by their mechanism of injury and their degree of stability. The four major types of injury are anteroposterior compression, lateral compression, vertical shear, and complex. Subdivisions exist within some categories; however, this chapter addresses only the four major categories.

An anteroposterior compression injury (Figure 27-10), or external rotation injury, may occur when an anterior- to posterior-directed force causes the anterior pelvic ring to

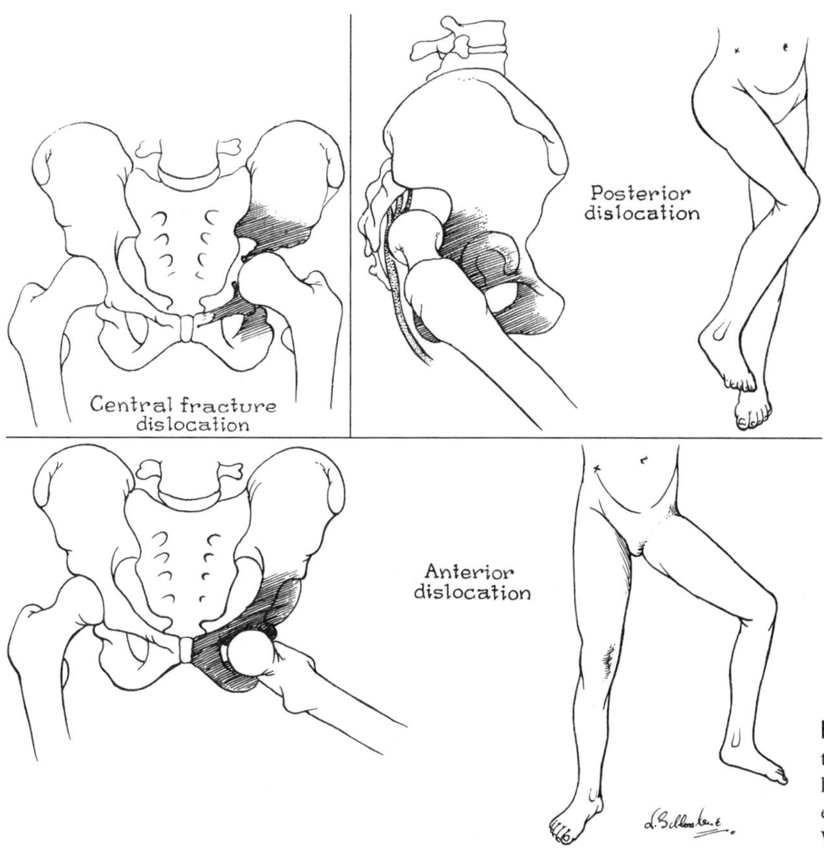

FIGURE 27-8 Basic types of hip dislocation. (From Thomas C: Fractures of the pelvis and hip. In Zuidema GD, Rutherford RB, Ballinger WF, editors: *The management of trauma,* Philadelphia, 1985, W. B. Saunders.)

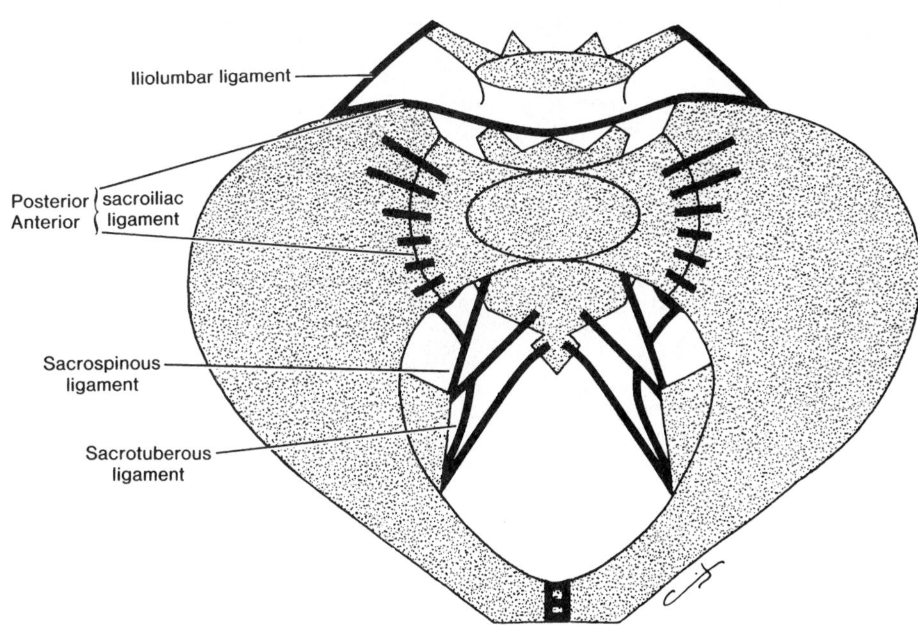

FIGURE 27-9 Diagrammatic representation of the major ligaments of the pelvis: the strong symphysis pubis anteriorly and the posterior tension band of the pelvis, including the iliolumbar, posterior sacroiliac, sacrospinous, and sacrotuberous ligaments. (From Tile M: *Fractures of the pelvis and acetabulum,* Baltimore, 1984, Williams & Wilkins.)

open. Continued external rotation causes rupture of the anterior sacroiliac and sacrospinous ligaments. As widening continues, the sacroiliac ligaments or posterior bony structures may be injured.

Lateral compression (Figure 27-11), or internal rotation, is the most common type of pelvic injury. Direct pressure to an iliac wing causes an internal rotation injury that crushes the anterior sacrum and fractures the pubic rami anteriorly. Pressure on the greater trochanter causes the femoral head to disrupt the pubic rami, which can extend into the anterior acetabulum. The ipsilateral sacroiliac complex may also be injured by this force. This injury typically causes bone impaction in the sacrum or ilium, which may result in loss of stability of the pelvic ring.

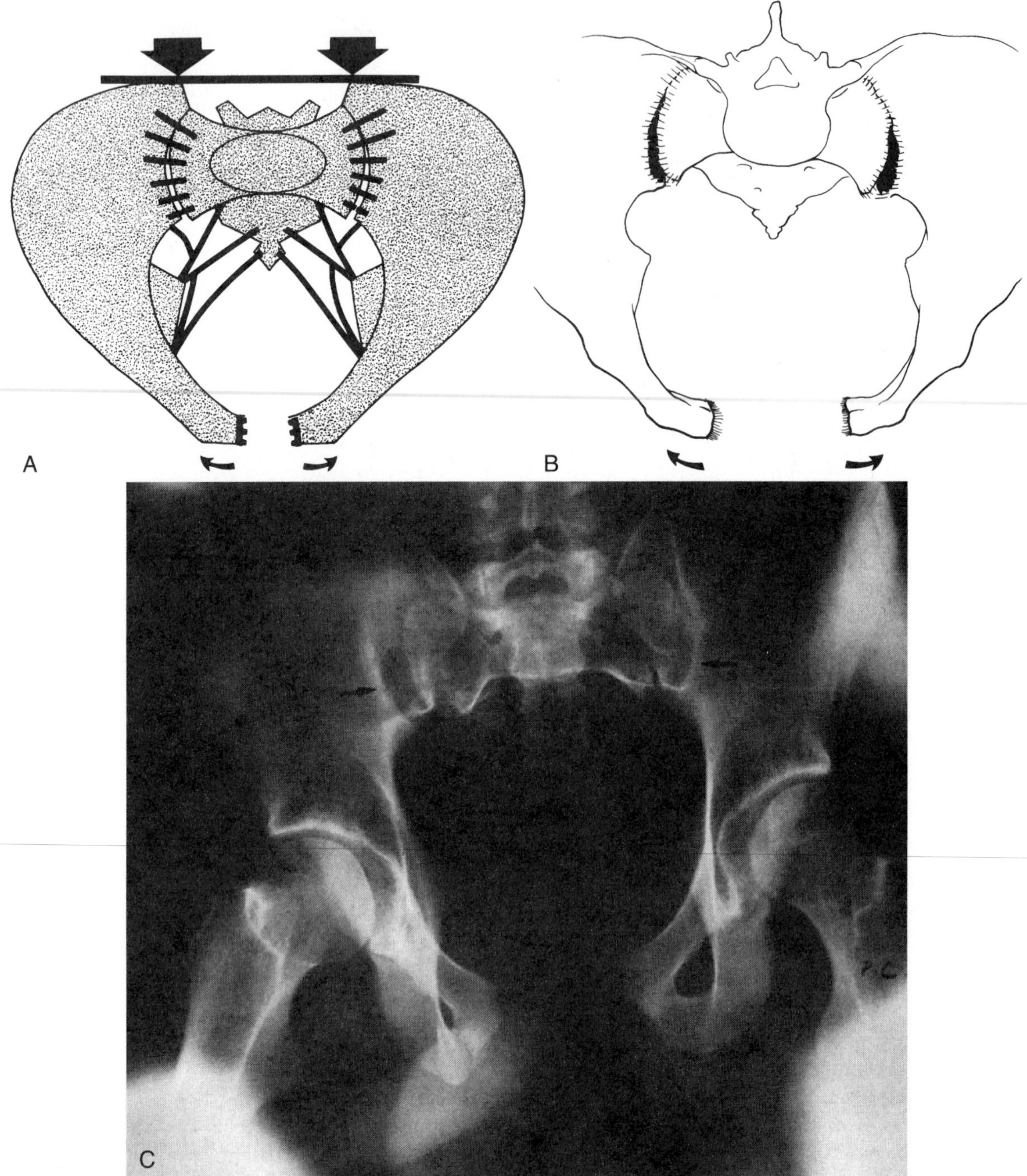

FIGURE 27-10 Anteroposterior compression (external rotation). **A,** A direct blow to the posterior superior iliac spines causes the symphysis pubis to spring open. **B,** A typical anteroposterior compression (open book) injury, showing a disruption of the symphysis pubis and the anterior sacroiliac ligaments. **C,** Anteroposterior pelvic radiograph of such a patient with markedly widened sacroiliac joints anteriorly. (From Tile M: *Fractures of the pelvis and acetabulum,* Baltimore, 1984, Williams & Wilkins.)

Most anteroposterior and lateral compression injuries are considered stable disruptions because the posterior sacroiliac complex remains intact or because the bone is impacted, thus preventing further disruption. However, the magnitude of the injuring force may be great enough to cause extensive soft tissue injury, leading to further bony instability. Injuries that are generally stable are associated with fewer long-term problems and have low morbidity and mortality rates.

Vertical shear (Figure 27-12) is an unstable injury associated with bone and soft tissue disruption. This type of injury is usually caused by a great force, such as that from falls and crush mechanisms exerted in a vertical plane and usually shearing in nature. Fractures may be unilateral or bilateral, the latter representing the more destructive type of unstable disruption. Anterior and posterior ring disruptions and injuries to the sacrotuberous and sacrospinous ligaments are present. Anterior injuries may involve disruption of the

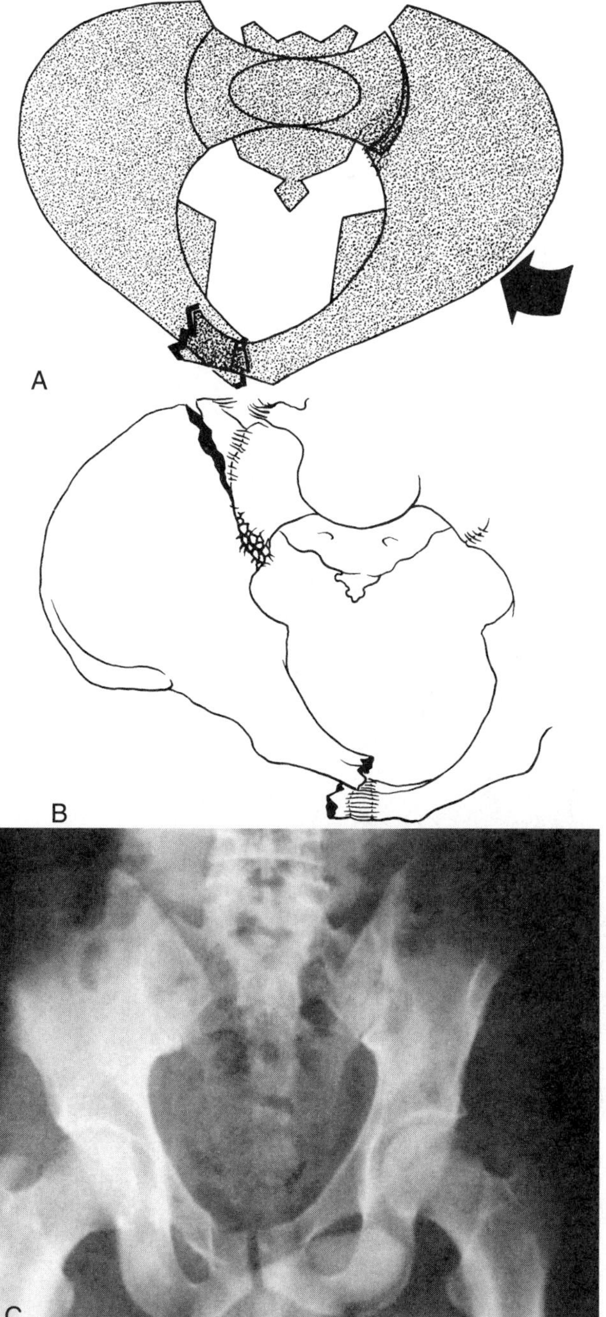

FIGURE 27-11 Lateral compression (internal rotation). **A,** A lateral compressive force directed against the iliac crest causes the hemipelvis to rotate internally, crushing the anterior sacrum and displacing the anterior pubic rami. **B,** A typical ipsilateral type of lateral compression injury, showing a posterior injury and an anterior disruption of the pubic rami with internal rotation of the hemipelvis. **C,** Anteroposterior radiograph of such a patient. (From Tile M: *Fractures of the pelvis and acetabulum,* Baltimore, 1984, Williams & Wilkins.)

symphysis pubis and two to four ramus injuries. Posterior lesions involve the sacrum, sacroiliac joints, or the ilium. Skin and subcutaneous tissue may be torn as well. Vertical shear disruptions are similarly unstable to anteroposterior disruptions but are associated with lower mortality rates and fewer organ system injuries.[18]

Complex pelvic ring disruptions, which result from forces directed obliquely, cause variable fracture-dislocation patterns that do not fit neatly into one of the previously mentioned classifications. These injuries generally represent combinations of applied forces and ligamentous injuries and are variably unstable.

Pelvic ring disruptions such as widely displaced anterior posterior compression injuries should alert the admitting team to the severity of injury sustained and the need for a comprehensive team approach to resuscitation. The patient's hemodynamic status must be continually monitored because the incidence of severe vascular injury is high with these types of fractures.[19]

Bone and Joint Continuity Management Principles

Early immobilization represents the first step in management of musculoskeletal injury. Immobilization helps to preserve what function currently exists and prevents further injury. By minimizing muscle spasms, proper immobilization also decreases the risk of angulation and overriding of bone ends, helping to prevent closed fractures from becoming open fractures. Application of traction in the field in conjunction with immobilization may help align bone ends in a near-anatomic position. Bone realignment often restores neurovascular and lymphatic function, which reduces further soft tissue injury and decreases pain.[6]

Immobilization techniques and devices applied before admission should remain in place until appropriate radiographic studies have been completed. Frequent monitoring of neurovascular status is required despite the presence of an immobilization or traction device. Compartment syndrome of the foot has been reported with use of splint-balanced immobilization devices.[20] Monitoring the immobilization device is necessary to ensure proper placement and effectiveness. After radiologic evaluation, definitive immobilization modalities may be initiated.

Dislocations

Dislocations are immobilized in the position in which they are found until reduction can be achieved. Attempting to straighten a dislocated joint may result in increased pain and cause further neurovascular damage if not performed correctly. Definitive management of dislocations is discussed later in this chapter.

Angulated Fractures

Realignment of a severely displaced fracture by a nonphysician depends not only on the presence or absence of vascular compromise and the amount of pain associated with realignment but, more important, on the established local emergency medical services policies governing treatment of such an injury. When realignment is not possible, the injured area is immobilized in the position in which it is found. The neurovascular status of the affected limb should be closely monitored until the limb is properly aligned and

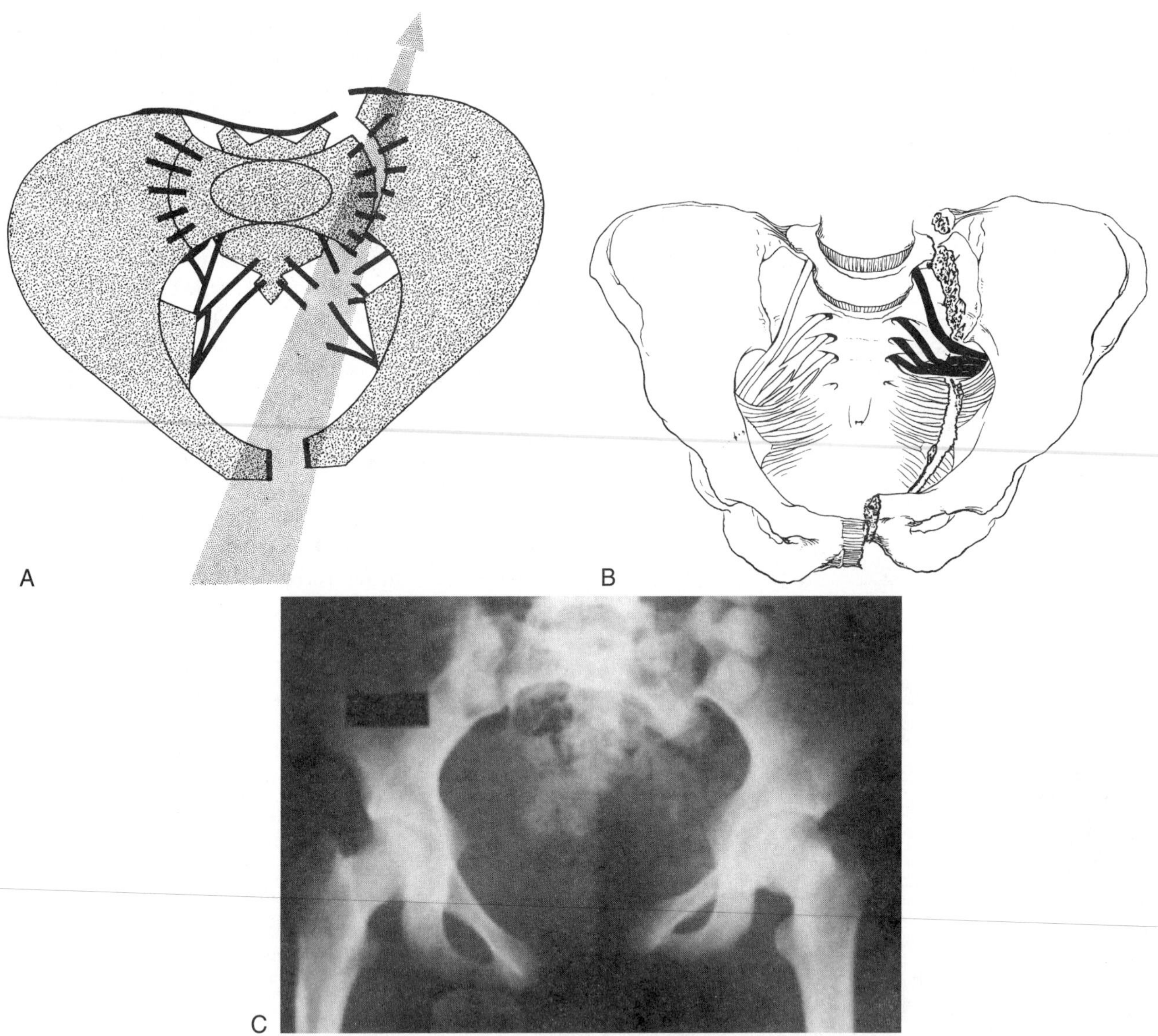

FIGURE 27-12 Vertical shear. **A,** A shearing force causes marked displacement of bone and gross disruption of soft tissues, resulting in major pelvic instability. **B,** Unilateral unstable (vertical shear) fracture causing massive disruption of the pelvic ring. **C,** Inlet view of pelvis shows severe posterior displacement and total disruption of the soft tissues on the left side, indicated by the avulsion of the ischial spine. (From Tile M: *Fractures of the pelvis and acetabulum,* Baltimore, 1984, Williams & Wilkins.)

immobilized.[21] In general, restoration of length and alignment before transport is preferable and less likely to lead to secondary soft tissue injury.

Extremity Fractures

Proper immobilization of a fracture includes immobilizing the joints both above and below the site of injury. Manufactured devices such as the Thomas ring splint, Hare traction splint (Figure 27-13), or Sager emergency traction device are useful for stabilizing fractures of the femur. These devices allow application of traction and immobilization of the affected area. Positioning of these devices usually requires two people, and established policies outline the specific procedure to ensure safe, rapid application. The affected extremity must be monitored for swelling, especially when traction and preformed splints are in use. Splints may require loosening of straps and padding to prevent further injury, such as compartment syndrome, which can occur when edematous tissue meets the resistance of such devices. Air splints or premolded rigid splints are useful for immobilizing feet, ankles, and upper extremities. They decrease edema by applying pressure over the injured area and simultaneously provide tamponade of open, bleeding wounds.

Tissue ischemia can develop if a splint remains in place for an extended time and becomes too tight, acting as a tourniquet. The length of time required to cause ischemia varies with each patient and is dependent on multiple variables. Distal pulses cannot be palpated with certain types of immobilization devices in place; therefore, visual assessments of the splinted extremity are essential. The inflatable splint should

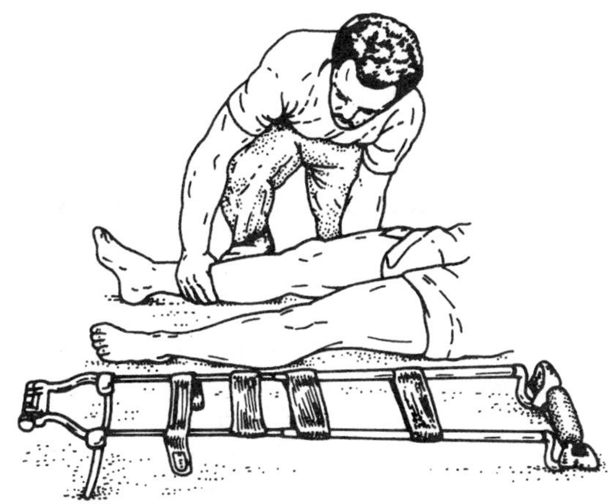

FIGURE 27-13 Hare traction splint. (From *The Maryland Way: EMT—a skills manual,* Baltimore, 1985, Maryland Institute for Emergency Medical Services System [MIEMSS])

be replaced with another device as soon as possible. When an air-filled splint that has been applied outdoors in a cold environment warms with indoor temperatures, the splint tightens and may cause neurovascular deterioration. Direct pressure on an inflatable splint should result in some degree of depression, indicating that the splint is not overinflated.

Immobilization should never be prevented or delayed because of a lack of manufactured splints. Any rigid object padded with soft material can be used for effective immobilization. For example, a fractured lower extremity can be splinted against the opposite extremity with padding in between, or injured upper extremities can be immobilized against the torso. Ski boots or other heavy protective boots left in place act as splints and may effectively tamponade underlying vascular injuries.

Pelvic Ring Disruption

Initial evaluation of the trauma patient may not reveal obvious clinical evidence of a pelvic injury, such as extremity rotation, limb shortening, or abnormal movement on downward or inward compression of the iliac wings. However, any signs or symptoms indicative of pelvic ring disruption require patient immobilization before transport to minimize the risk of further neurovascular injury. Suspected pelvic injuries may be effectively immobilized with a pneumatic antishock garment (PASG) or pelvic binder.[22] These devices provide a tamponade effect and bony immobilization. The use of the PASG is contraindicated in patients with head injuries because it can cause critical elevations in intracranial pressure (ICP). It also is contraindicated in patients who are pregnant and those with pulmonary edema, congestive heart failure, penetrating abdominal trauma, or chest injury such as tension pneumothorax or cardiac tamponade.[13] Obvious pelvic injuries with associated hip dislocations or blow-out injuries to the acetabulum often require creative techniques to achieve initial immobilization and stabilization. Injuries that cause shortening, rotation, or frog-leg positioning require support and stabilization of the patient's lower extremities in the position in which they are found. A long wooden backboard with pillows, rolled sheets, or blankets secured and taped under the patient's knees supports extremity position and ensures immobilization during transport. The patient with an unstable pelvic ring disruption may require binder application during the early phase of resuscitation to prevent exsanguination. Use of more invasive devices such as an external fixator (Figure 27-14) or a C-clamp is rarely necessary.[4] Caution is essential whenever moving a patient with a pelvic injury because disruption of the retroperitoneal tamponade can cause rapid additional blood loss.

General Management Principles and Complications

The potential for serious, even fatal, complications from musculoskeletal trauma exists in all patients who sustain a musculoskeletal injury. It is mandatory that all persons providing care to injured persons be alert to the signs and symptoms of potential complications. These complications can occur during any phase of the trauma cycle.

Hypovolemia

Any musculoskeletal injury results in blood loss. The degree of hemorrhage and its effect on the patient's overall hemodynamic status depend on the type, location, and number of

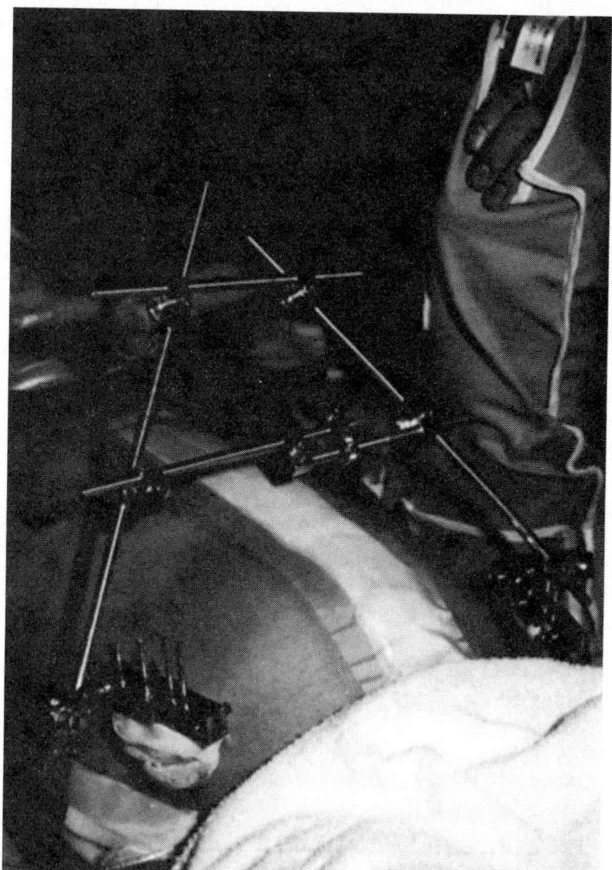

FIGURE 27-14 Clinical immobilization for pelvic ring disruption.

injuries. Generally, musculoskeletal injuries receive attention after stabilization of the cardiopulmonary and neurologic systems. However, there are times when musculoskeletal injuries become priorities and necessitate early, aggressive intervention. Two injuries associated with marked large-volume blood loss, traumatic amputations and massive pelvic injuries, require priority care with a coordinated team approach to facilitate restoration and maintenance of physiologic stability.[8] Other bony and soft tissue injuries can usually wait for definitive care, but the patient still requires adequate volume replacement to treat hypovolemia related to blood loss.

It is difficult to estimate accurately the actual amount of blood lost, especially in patients with multiple extremity or pelvic fractures and soft tissue injuries. Table 27-4 approximates possible blood loss with open and closed fractures. Significant blood loss, as indicated in Table 27-4, can occur within an extremity even though a specific fracture has been classified as closed. The areas surrounding and distal to the fracture site become swollen, and the skin tightens from the accumulation of blood within the soft tissue. An open fracture can cause blood loss of three or more units, in addition to the amounts listed in Table 27-4. Not only does blood loss become apparent externally, but it also continues internally within the soft tissue. Hypovolemia should be anticipated in patients with these injuries, and measures to restore and maintain hemodynamics must be instituted.

Exsanguination represents the primary cause of early death after an unstable pelvic fracture.[5] As previously mentioned, the pelvis receives a rich blood supply through the arteries and venous plexus of the iliac system (Figure 27-15). This vascular network can easily be injured because of its close approximation to the bony structures. The retroperitoneal space can hold large volumes of blood before spontaneous tamponade occurs, making it difficult to determine actual blood loss. Patients with pelvic injuries are also at increased risk for hemorrhage from common associated injuries, such as intra-abdominal viscera injury, which compounds the blood loss from bony and vascular injuries.[23] Hypovolemic shock must be anticipated in patients with massive pelvic injuries, and early interventions to restore hemodynamic stability and tissue perfusion are required. Refer to Chapter 14 for further discussion.

TABLE 27-4 Blood Loss Caused by Fractures*

Fracture	Blood Loss (ml)
Humerus	500-1,500
Elbow	250-750
Radius/ulna	250-500
Pelvis	750-6,000
Femur	500-3,000
Tibia/fibula	250-2,000
Ankle	250-1,000

Note: One unit of whole blood equals approximately 500 ml.
*Data from Roth MS: First aid; fractures. *Student BMJ* 13:265-308, 2005.

Any patient with actual or potential intravascular volume deficits requires vigilant observation and frequent re-evaluation for the clinical indicators of shock. Patients with major musculoskeletal injuries such as traumatic amputations, multiple fractures, and unstable pelvic ring disruptions require close monitoring and should only be transported out of the resuscitation area if accompanied by qualified personnel. These patients can and do rapidly and unexpectedly deteriorate into severe hemorrhagic shock from massive blood loss. Thus constant monitoring, especially during transport, is essential. For example, the retroperitoneal hematoma associated with a massive or unstable pelvic ring injury can be disrupted during transfer of the patient to the radiography table. The sudden release of the tamponade precipitates rapid cardiovascular deterioration.[24]

Administration of adequate fluid by using colloids, crystalloids, or blood products is integral to successfully replete intravascular volume. Early and adequate blood transfusions help prevent deterioration and the sequelae of late shock that is a result of massive blood loss (see Chapters 13 and 14). The blood bank should be notified early and updated regarding needs.[25] The team may need to consider transferring the patient to a major trauma center for this reason alone.

Obvious sources of external hemorrhage require immediate application of direct pressure and pressure dressings to obtain control. Options include a figure-eight bandage or a bandage wrapped in a spiral fashion starting at a point distal to the wound and wrapped proximally. Pressure dressings minimize damage to soft tissue and neurovascular structures while achieving hemostasis.[26] Properly applied pressure dressings almost always provide adequate control of hemorrhage, even for traumatic amputations. A tourniquet is rarely appropriate and should be a last resort for massive, uncontrollable hemorrhage because it may increase the extent of the injury on amputated parts by causing ischemic damage to nerves and vessels.[27]

The benefits from the use of PSAGs remain controversial, specifically concerning translocation of blood.[13,14,19,22,26] Their value includes immobilization and compression effects. PASGs provide external tamponade for major hemorrhage and afford stability so that resuscitation procedures can be carried out.[27]

Infection

All open orthopedic injuries are considered contaminated and place the patient at risk for wound infections, osteomyelitis, and, rarely, gas gangrene and tetanus.[28,29] Contaminants can enter the wound in the prehospital environment or within the hospital where exposure to an antibiotic-resistant organism may occur. Wound and bone infections are potentially devastating complications associated with increased morbidity. These infections can lead to delayed union, nonunion, or acute or chronic osteomyelitis, increasing the patient's financial burden and possibly resulting in loss of the affected extremity.[30-32] Therefore, measures aimed at

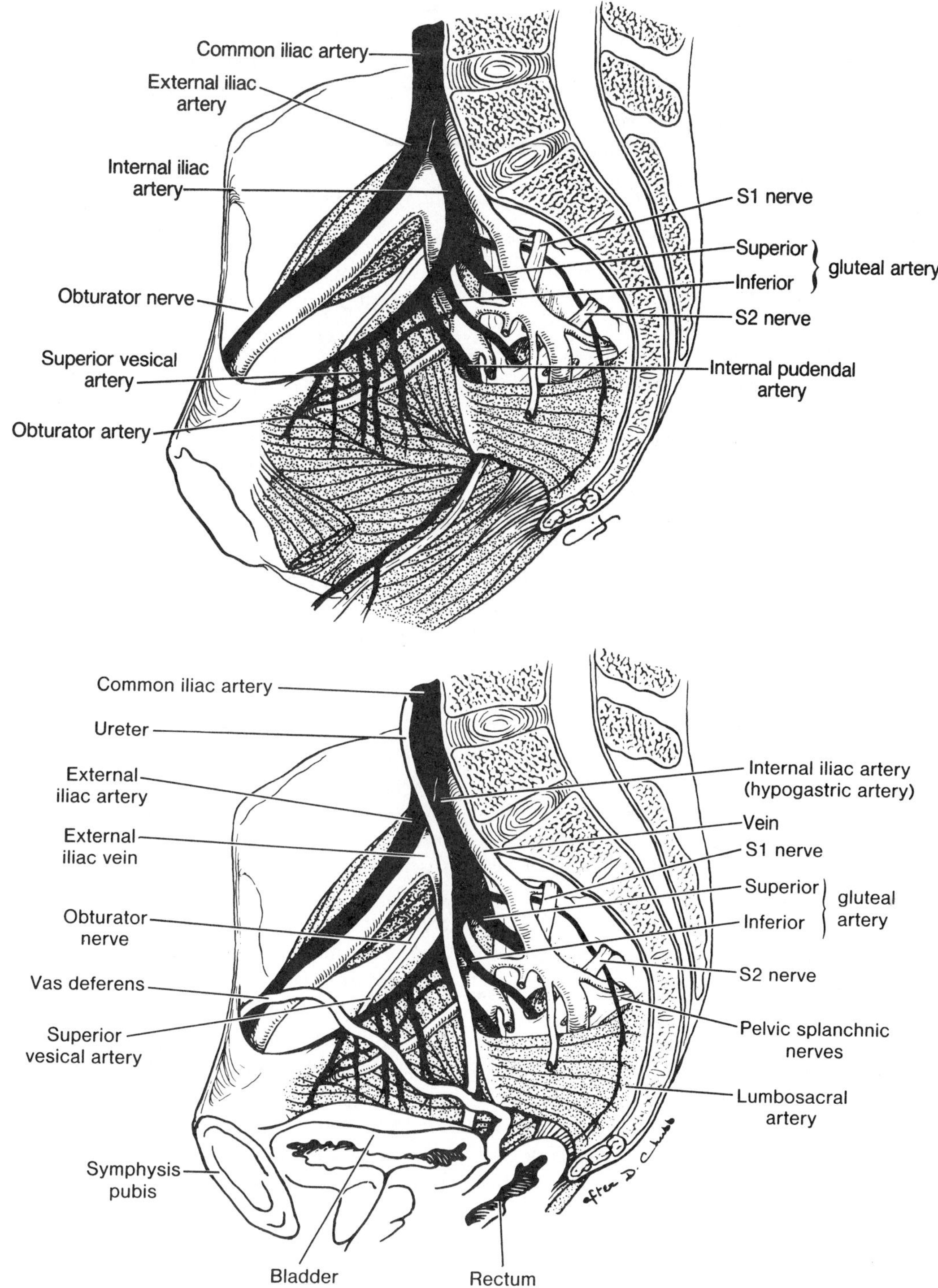

FIGURE 27-15 The internal iliac system of arteries and veins showing the position of the pelvic viscera. (From Tile M: *Fractures of the pelvis and acetabulum,* Baltimore, 1984, Williams & Wilkins.)

eliminating further wound contamination and preventing microbial growth are essential and important during early resuscitation.[31-33]

During resuscitation, gross contaminants are removed from the wound and exposed soft tissue and bone are covered with a wet, sterile saline solution dressing. It is important to prevent re-entry of a dirty bone end or soft tissue into the wound. Should re-entry occur, it is imperative that the orthopedic specialist be notified. Saline solution–soaked dressings are recommended rather than those saturated with iodine-based solutions.[34] Soft tissue absorbs some of the solution, and iodine has been found to cause additional local tissue injury, decreasing the tissue's resistance to infection. Additionally, iodine can interfere with fibroblast activity, which is important in stabilizing wound beds.[34] Saline solution has also replaced iodine solutions during surgery and in postoperative wound management. Dressing changes should be performed as prescribed by using appropriate techniques to minimize wound contamination. Appropriate technique and attire for wound dressing changes is dependent on the risk of the procedure and the area of the hospital where the procedure is performed.

Ideally, patients with open fractures should proceed rapidly to the operating suite for wound irrigation, debridement, and definitive care. If a delay prevents this from occurring, early, aggressive wound irrigation in the emergency care area may be beneficial. The optimal method of irrigation includes use of large volumes of saline solution and low-pressure pulse lavage systems because high-pressure lavage has been shown to have a negative impact on bone and soft tissue healing.[35,36]

Tetanus is a preventable yet highly lethal complication caused by growth of the anaerobic bacteria *Clostridium tetani*. To reduce the risk of tetanus, all devitalized tissue must be surgically excised and the patient must be adequately immunized. The patient's recent tetanus immunization history is determined and a booster administered as indicated.

Trauma patients with multisystem and musculoskeletal injuries, especially open fractures and traumatic amputations, are at high risk for infection and therefore should receive prophylactic antibiotics during the resuscitative phase.[37-40] Wound cultures before debridement are of little value. Environmental factors surrounding the incident may help direct antibiotic therapy, but the choice of single-agent gram-positive coverage or broad-spectrum coverage is largely based on surgeon preference.

Surgical prophylaxis requires adequate concentrations of the antibiotic in the area of bone or soft tissue injury or at the operative site. From the time the antibiotic is administered intravenously, it requires approximately 20 to 30 minutes or longer to achieve saturation in the interstitial fluid of a healthy bone matrix.[41,42] Antibiotics are most beneficial when they are administered at the peak of bacterial wound contamination, when they satisfactorily invade the bone injury or wound, and when they are chosen specifically for the most likely contaminating organisms.[42] For these reasons, administration of intravenous antibiotics begins in the resuscitative phase (or approximately 30 minutes before an elective operative orthopedic procedure) to achieve maximal antimicrobial effects.[42]

The use of prophylactic antibiotics in patients undergoing open reduction of closed fractures should be limited to the perioperative period. Prolonged use of prophylactic antibiotics may cause bacteria to develop antibiotic resistance. Many studies related to prophylactic antibiotic use predominantly focus on elective orthopedic surgery. In the multiple trauma patient the risk of infection increases as the number of systems involved rises.[43] Studies also have shown that operative procedures lasting longer than 90 minutes have a higher incidence of infection.

Neurologic and Vascular Compromise

Early recognition of neurologic or vascular compromise as a result of musculoskeletal injury is imperative. The following mechanisms and injuries can precipitate neurologic and vascular complications:

- Compression or crushing mechanism
- Open or closed fracture
- Soft tissue injury
- Arterial involvement or injury
- Dislocation
- Prolonged use of PASG
- Hypovolemia or shock

Any musculoskeletal injury affecting bone or soft tissue can be associated with neurologic or vascular compromise. Muscle and nerve tissues are easily damaged because of their close proximity to the bony structures. Vascular disruption decreases tissue perfusion, causing ischemia. After prolonged ischemia, reperfusion causes muscle tissue to become edematous as a result of increased capillary permeability. Edema increases pressure on the capillaries and eventually causes secondary collapse. The progression from ischemia to muscle necrosis occurs rapidly. Within 6 to 8 hours the nerves, muscles, and vascular structures may sustain irreversible damage both locally and distally.[44] Understanding the mechanism of injury and the specific types of injuries that carry the highest incidence of neurovascular compromise is important.

Injuries to the brachial plexus and lumbosacral plexus may cause altered sensation and mobility. Neither of these injuries necessitates immediate intervention during the resuscitation and stabilization of the patient with multisystem injuries. However, the peripheral nerve involvement associated with both injuries may create an insensate and paralyzed extremity associated with substantial morbitity.

Dislocations. Dislocations represent orthopedic emergencies when they are associated with compromise of nearby vessels or nerves. For example, dislocations of the elbow or knee frequently require urgent intervention by an orthopedist because of the extremely high incidence of associated neurovascular disruption. The nerve injury resulting from a dislocation may be a true transaction but more frequently results from compression, blast effect, traction, or stretch mechanisms. Clinical findings indicative of a physiologic nerve injury may resolve spontaneously after the joint has been reduced and properly aligned. Symptoms may, however, remain longer depending on the severity of the injury and the length of time that elapsed before treatment. Vascular disruption may result from laceration, compression, crush, traction, or stretch mechanisms. Resolution of vascular insuffiency depends on the specific injury, the ischemic time, and the ability of collateral circulation to restore and maintain blood flow. Table 27-5 correlates joint dislocations with the potential neurovascular branches involved.

Fractures. Neurovascular compromise associated with fractures results from causes similar to dislocations. Injury to the neurovascular supply of the extremities may occur from actual laceration or tearing of vessels or nerves, compression

TABLE 27-5 Neurovascular Structures at Risk for Involvement in Joint Dislocation

Joint	Nerve/Vessel
Shoulder	Brachial plexus/axillary artery
Elbow	Ulnar nerve/brachial artery
Wrist	Median nerve
Hip	Sciatic nerve
Knee	Tibial and peroneal nerves/popliteal artery and vein
Ankle	Tibial artery

between fractured bone ends, and stretching from limb malalignment.

Pelvic Injuries. The pelvis has a rich vascular supply, as seen in Figure 27-15. Oxygenated blood enters the pelvis through the common iliac artery. A venous plexus, consisting of valveless, thin-walled veins that allow bidirectional blood flow, drains the pelvic basin. Collateral networks exist on both the arterial and venous sides. The sciatic nerve arising from the lumbosacral plexus innervates the pelvis and the lower extremities. Any disruption of the bones or ligaments of the pelvis or hips can potentially cause severe neurovascular complications. Massive pelvic ring disruptions are considered potentially lethal injuries because of the major vascular disruption with which they are frequently associated.

Brachial Plexus Injury. The brachial plexus, which incorporates the roots of the fifth cervical vertebra to the first thoracic vertebra, subdivides to form the axillary, musculocutaneous, median, ulnar, and radial nerves (Figure 27-16). These nerves provide motor and sensory control for the arm, elbow, forearm, wrist, and hand.

Traumatic injury to the brachial plexus may occur from blunt or penetrating mechanisms. Blunt injuries can result from excessive forces that initially injure the nearby muscle and its fascia and then cause extreme stretching of the nervous network, usually the nerve roots.[45] Associated injuries that

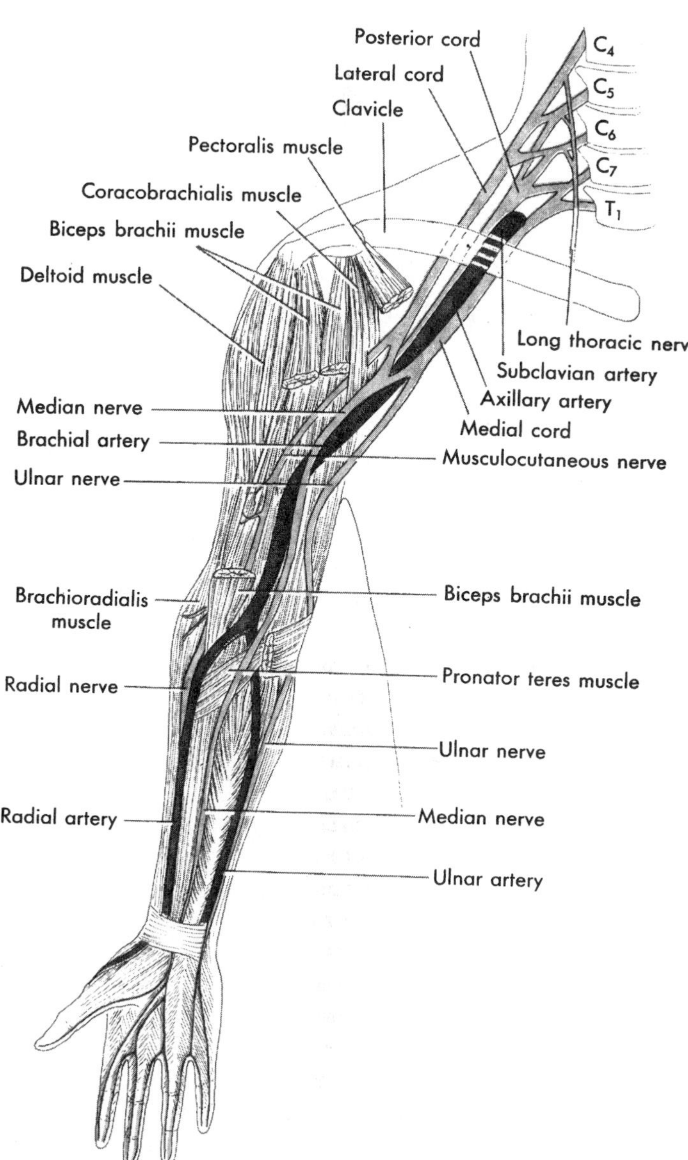

FIGURE 27-16 Diagram illustrating the brachial plexus and distribution of nerves. Note their relationship to arteries and to muscles (right arm). (From Kimber DC, Gray CE, Stackpole CE: *Kimber-Gray-Stackpole's anatomy and physiology,* New York, 1977, Macmillan.)

often accompany brachial plexus injuries include closed head injuries, subclavian and axillary artery and vein injuries, and shoulder dislocations.[45] Frequently, blunt mechanisms that result in a plexus injury involve the patient's ejection from a car or off a motorcycle with a landing such that the head is distracted from the affected shoulder and upper extremity.

Blunt brachial plexus injuries are subdivided into upper root and lower root classifications.[46] The upper roots, C5 to C7, may sustain injury when the head has significant lateral bending away from the shoulder and when the shoulder itself is forcefully depressed downward. Upper root injuries typically affect the shoulder and elbow more than the hand. The sensory deficit usually affects the deltoid muscle, arm, and forearm. A lower root injury involving C8 to T1 may occur when the arm is forcefully extended over the head. The shoulder and elbow maintain motor function, but the forearm and hand are impaired. Any injury to the brachial plexus may be complete or incomplete. Incomplete injuries often present confusing clinical pictures because the patient has unusual patterns of sensory or motor dysfunction. A complete lesion of the brachial plexus results in paralysis and sensory loss throughout the arm and hand.[46]

Penetrating mechanisms, such as missile or blast injuries or stabbings, that cause open wounds near the shoulder or clavicle may also result in injury to the brachial plexus. Associated injuries to surrounding soft tissue and the subclavian vein or artery may precipitate upper extremity ischemia, which further confuses the clinical picture. Motor and sensory deficits can occur from either the ischemic injury or the plexus injury, and conclusive differentiation may be difficult.

Accurate and complete evaluation of the functional status of the brachial plexus in the critically injured multisystem trauma patient is a challenge. Often alterations in the patient's level of consciousness and sensory responses make assessment difficult if not impossible. Differentiation of this injury from a cervical spinal cord injury and from the flaccidity seen with devastating head injuries may be difficult. The patient should be assessed for Horner's syndrome, or Horner's pupil, which can occur with spinal cord injuries above T1 that interrupt the cervical sympathetic chain or its central pathways, causing loss of sympathetic innervation to and constriction of the ipsilateral pupil. The affected pupil remains reactive to light and is usually accompanied by ptosis of the eyelid and possibly loss of facial sweating on the same side. If the patient has associated arm weakness, a brachial plexus injury may have occurred. More specific neuromotor checks to evaluate the nerves branching off of the brachial plexus include the following (Figure 27-17):

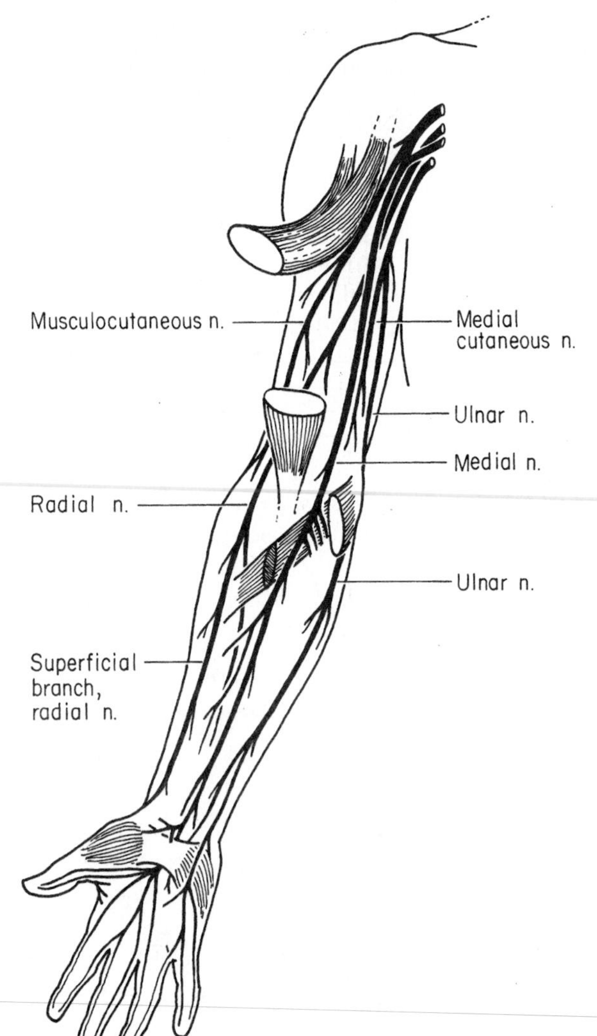

FIGURE 27-17 Nerves of the arm and forearm. (From Mubarak SJ: Anatomy of the extremity compartments. In Mubarak SJ, Hargens AR, Akeson WH, editors: *Compartment syndromes and Volkmann's contracture*, Philadelphia, 1981, W. B. Saunders.)

1. The musculocutaneous nerve is tested by evaluating the patient's biceps function and sensation over the lateral portion of the forearm.
2. The radial nerve primarily serves a motor function assessed by evaluating the ability to extend the wrist. Evaluate sensation on the dorsal aspect of the web of skin between the thumb and index finger (Figure 27-18).
3. An intact median nerve allows apposition of the thumb to the little finger. Sensory function is evaluated by stimulating the palmar surface of the thumb and index finger and the radial half of the long finger (see Figure 27-18).
4. Motor function of the ulnar nerve is assessed by requesting the patient to abduct and adduct the fingers. Evaluate sensation on the volar surface of the small and ring fingers and the ulnar half of the long finger (see Figure 27-18).

Early care of brachial plexus injuries is generally supportive, including protection of the affected extremity and proper immobilization; these measures must continue during critical care. Early rehabilitation to prevent muscle wasting and joint contractures is essential. Prompt recognition of complications

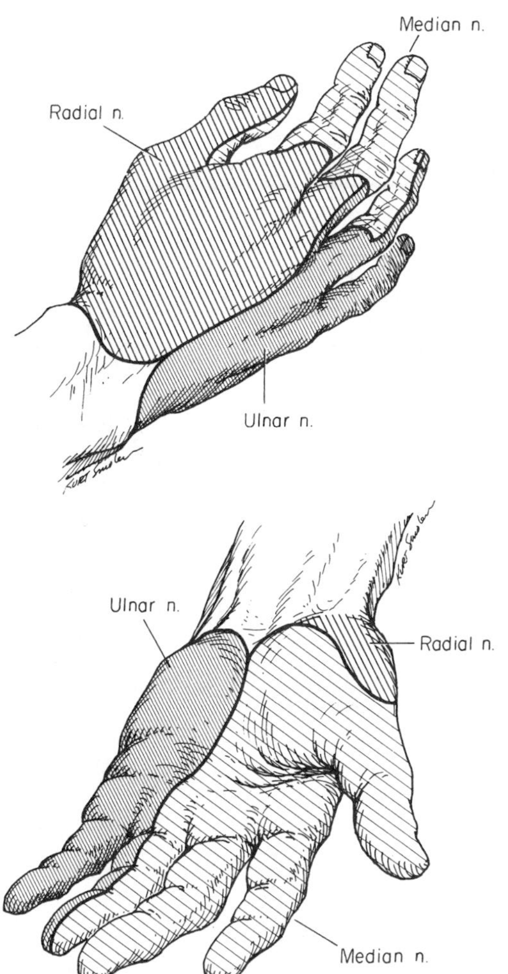

FIGURE 27-18 Distribution of the cutaneous nerves to the hand. (From Mubarak SJ: Anatomy of the extremity compartments. In Mubarak SJ, Hargens AR, Akeson WH, editors: *Compartment syndromes and Volkmann's contracture,* Philadelphia, 1981, W. B. Saunders.)

such as causalgia and prevention of secondary disabilities such as skin breakdown (see the immobility discussion in the critical care section) are of paramount importance for the patient with a brachial plexus injury. Early surgical exploration may be indicated in open injuries. Retrospective studies suggest that better functional outcomes can be achieved if nerve repair, nerve transfers, or nerve grafts are done within 4 months of injury.[46] Unfortunately, despite the advances in microsurgical techniques, outcomes of patients with upper plexus injuries remain poor.[47,48]

Complex Regional Pain Syndrome (Reflex Sympathetic Dystrophy or Causalgia). Extremity injuries that involve nerves may lead to a complex regional pain syndrome (CRPS) (formerly called reflex sympathetic dystrophy or causalgia).[49] This altered pain processing is most commonly associated with ulnar and median nerve involvement, but it can occur with any nerve.[49] CRPS generally develops within the first month after injury. Changes in the affected extremity reflective of autonomic dysfunction may include alterations in skin color (e.g., flushing, bluish coloring), temperature (e.g., hot/flushed or cold/clammy), and ability to perspire (e.g., skin dry or with increased local perspiration). The most severe disabling problem is extreme, constant, burning pain in the extremity that may be impossible to alleviate. The intractable pain can lead to behavioral and emotional changes and can interfere with the patient's cooperation and participation, thereby intensifying rehabilitation needs. Early administration of narcotics or sympathetic blocks (with a local anesthetic) may provide pain relief. Dorsal column stimulators that block pain transmissions may be effective. Severe, unrelenting pain may require sympathectomy, although several sources cite inconclusive evidence of the efficacy of such blockades.[50,51] (Refer to Chapter 18 for further discussion on pain management.) This problem has the potential to develop after any musculoskeletal injury, including fractures, ligamentous or cartilaginous tears, and other soft tissue injuries.

Lumbosacral Plexus Injury. The lumbosacral plexus, incorporating the five lumbar spinal nerves and first four sacral spinal nerves, supplies sensory and motor function to the lower extremities. The three major nerves arising from the lumbosacral network are the obturator, the femoral, and the sciatic. The sciatic divides into the tibial and peroneal nerves (Figure 27-19).

Injury to the lumbosacral plexus itself occurs much less frequently than injury to the brachial plexus and must be differentiated from spinal cord injuries and associated nerve root injuries. Lumbosacral plexus injury can occur from blunt forces such as with pelvic fractures or from penetrating mechanisms such as gunshot wounds.[52] Injuries to the lumbosacral plexus may include intradural nerve root avulsion or stretching injury, individual nerve root transection or crushing injury, and disruption or palsy of the plexus. The obturator nerve, protected by its position within the pelvis, rarely sustains injury, yet it may be affected by penetrating trauma to the perineum. Any penetrating or blunt forces to the anterior thigh, especially near the inguinal ligament, may injure the femoral nerve.

The major trunk of the sciatic nerve lies within the pelvis and therefore remains protected from most external trauma. It is at high risk for injury, however, when pelvic disruption or hip fracture or dislocation occurs. The gluteal folds represent the point where the sciatic nerves become superficial, and any wounds in the area of the buttock or posterior thigh may involve the nerve. After the division of the sciatic nerve, the most common site of injury to the peroneal branch is at the head of the fibula, where the nerve is afforded little protection from any type of applied force. Blunt or penetrating mechanisms may affect the tibial nerve in the popliteal space or in the calf. Elevated pressure within the compartments in the lower leg poses an increased risk for tibial and peroneal nerve damage.

Evaluation of the integrity of the nerves that arise from the lumbosacral plexus may present a formidable clinical challenge in the patient with multiple injuries. It is essential

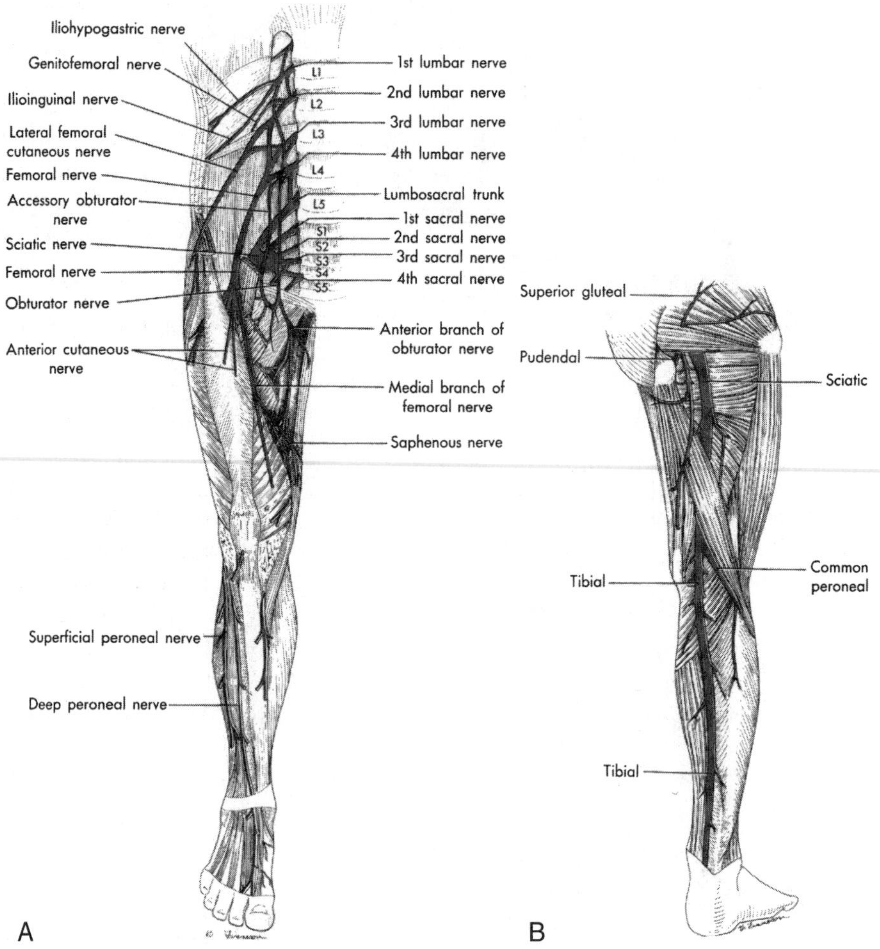

FIGURE 27-19 **A,** Diagram illustrating the lumbosacral plexus and distribution of nerves. Note their relationship to muscles of the leg *(right)*. **B,** Nerve supply to right lower extremity, posterior view. (From Kimber DC, Gray CE, Stackpole CE: *Kimber-Gray-Stackpole's anatomy and physiology,* New York, 1977, Macmillan.)

to perform initial and subsequent assessments in the patient suspected of having, or at risk for development of, peripheral nerve injury. Figure 27-20 shows the peripheral nerves of the lower leg and foot, and Figure 27-21 shows their cutaneous distribution in the foot.

1. Motor function of the obturator nerve can be assessed by having the patient adduct the thigh. Sensory function is evaluated over the medial aspect of the thigh.
2. The femoral nerve supplies sensation to the anterior thigh and medial leg and motor function to the quadriceps. Inability to extend the knee and altered sensation on the anterior thigh indicate injury to the femoral nerve.
3. The common peroneal nerve provides motor function to enable foot dorsiflexion and eversion of the foot and ankle. Sensation is assessed in the web space between the first and second toes or over the lateral aspect of the calf and dorsum of the foot.
4. Motor function of the tibial nerve is assessed by having the patient plantarflex or invert the foot and ankle. Sensation is evaluated on the plantar surface of the foot and heel.

If bone or joint angulation or dislocation is the cause of the neurologic dysfunction (as with posterior hip dislocation), nerve function can often be restored with early reduction (closed or open) of the fracture or dislocation. Detection and diagnosis of a lumbosacral plexus injury may not occur until later in the acute care or recovery phases, when the patient becomes more alert and is capable of more spontaneous movement. Newer microsurgical techniques to repair the plexus may offer patients the ability to regain more function, but the results are variable.

Compartment Syndrome. Compartments are defined as closed spaces containing muscles, nerves, and vascular structures that are enclosed by fascia.[44] Sheaths of fascia tightly bind these closed muscle systems, which house neurovascular bundles. Compartment syndrome may result when either the internal contents or external sources cause an increase in compartment pressure (Table 27-6). Internal etiologies of increased compartment pressures include conditions that cause blood accumulation, tissue edema, or fluid infiltration within the closed space, thereby increasing intracompartmental content. External causes of increased compartment pressure, such as constricting dressings, decrease the size of the compartment. Both internal and external causes lead to elevation of

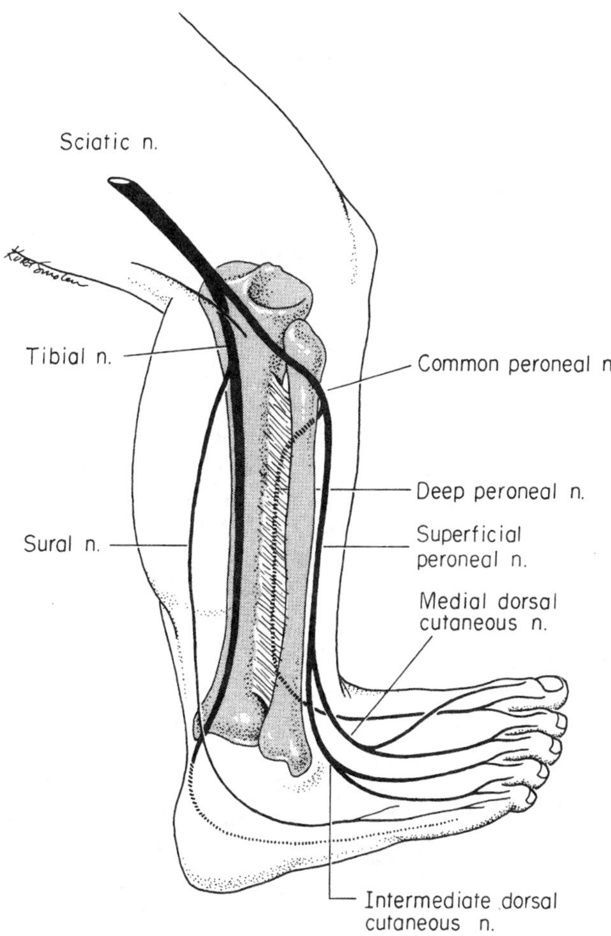

FIGURE 27-20 Peripheral nerves of the leg. (From Mubarak SJ: Anatomy of the extremity compartments. In Mubarak SJ, Hargens AR, Akeson WH, editors: *Compartment syndromes and Volkmann's contracture,* Philadelphia, 1981, W. B. Saunders.)

pressures within the compartments, which compress the microvascular system, leading to ischemia of the muscle tissue (Figure 27-22). If elevated compartment pressures are not relieved within 6 to 8 hours, irreversible damage to the muscle and nerves, including necrosis and scarring, results.[53-55] Compartment syndrome may affect any body compartment, including extremity compartments. Of the body's 46 compartments, 36 are found in the extremities.[44] Most commonly affected are the lower leg and the forearm, which have two and four muscle compartments, respectively.

A common misconception is that open fractures are safe from compartment syndrome. Although an open wound may violate a fascial compartment, other compartments remain intact and are at risk for this syndrome. Additionally, traumatic wounds usually occur horizontally and are not large enough to decompress the compartment.[56]

After injury to an extremity, an immediate inflammatory response results in decreased blood flow and tissue hypoxia distal to the injury[44] (Figure 27-23). Inflammatory mediators are released and cause the capillary walls to increase permeability, allowing colloid proteins and fluid to leach

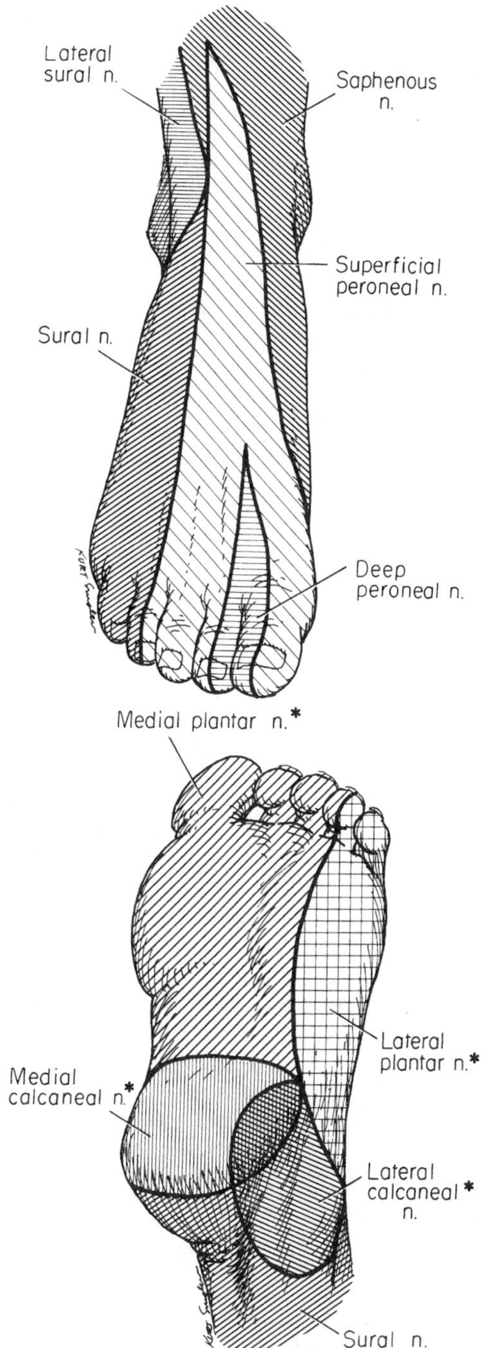

FIGURE 27-21 Distribution of the cutaneous nerves to the foot. *Branches of the tibial nerve. (From Mubarak SJ: Anatomy of the extremity compartments. In Mubarak SJ, Hargens AR, Akeson WH, editors: *Compartment syndromes and Volkmann's contracture,* Philadelphia, 1981, W. B. Saunders.)

into the soft tissue. This fluid shift causes increased edema, and the cycle is perpetuated. As the edema within the compartment increases, there is a change in the pressure relationships within the compartment.[44] The imbalance in the pressures between the inflow of arterial blood and the outflow of venous blood eventually culminates in total

TABLE 27-6 Causes of Compartment Syndrome

Internal	Trauma compressing or crushing mechanisms, open/closed fractures
	Soft tissue or vascular injuries (e.g., contusions)
	Venomous bites: spiders, snakes
	Prolonged shock states: tissue ischemia, venous pooling
	Bleeding disorders or anticoagulation
	Infiltrated intravenous sites
External	Prolonged or excessive use of PASGs, splints, traction devices, circumferential dressings
	Prolonged pressure over compartment: remaining in same position for a long period
	Eschar from burns

cessation of blood flow into the affected extremity.[44] Intracompartmental pressures in excess of 30 to 40 mm Hg can cause muscle ischemia, and pressures greater than 55 to 65 mm Hg may result in irreversible muscle death.[44] Recent studies have implicated neutrophils and thromboxane A_2 in the microvascular dysfunction and blood flow distribution abnormalities found in the ischemia-reperfusion injury associated with acute compartment syndrome.[57] The use of cyclo-oxygenase inhibitors has demonstrated decreased thromboxane levels and intracompartmental pressures and may play a role in limiting tissue ischemia.[57]

Patients who are athletes may be at higher risk for development of compartment syndrome. The larger muscle mass associated with athletes, especially distance runners, decreases the available space within a compartment. Scar formation also limits the fascia's ability to expand to accommodate edema.[58]

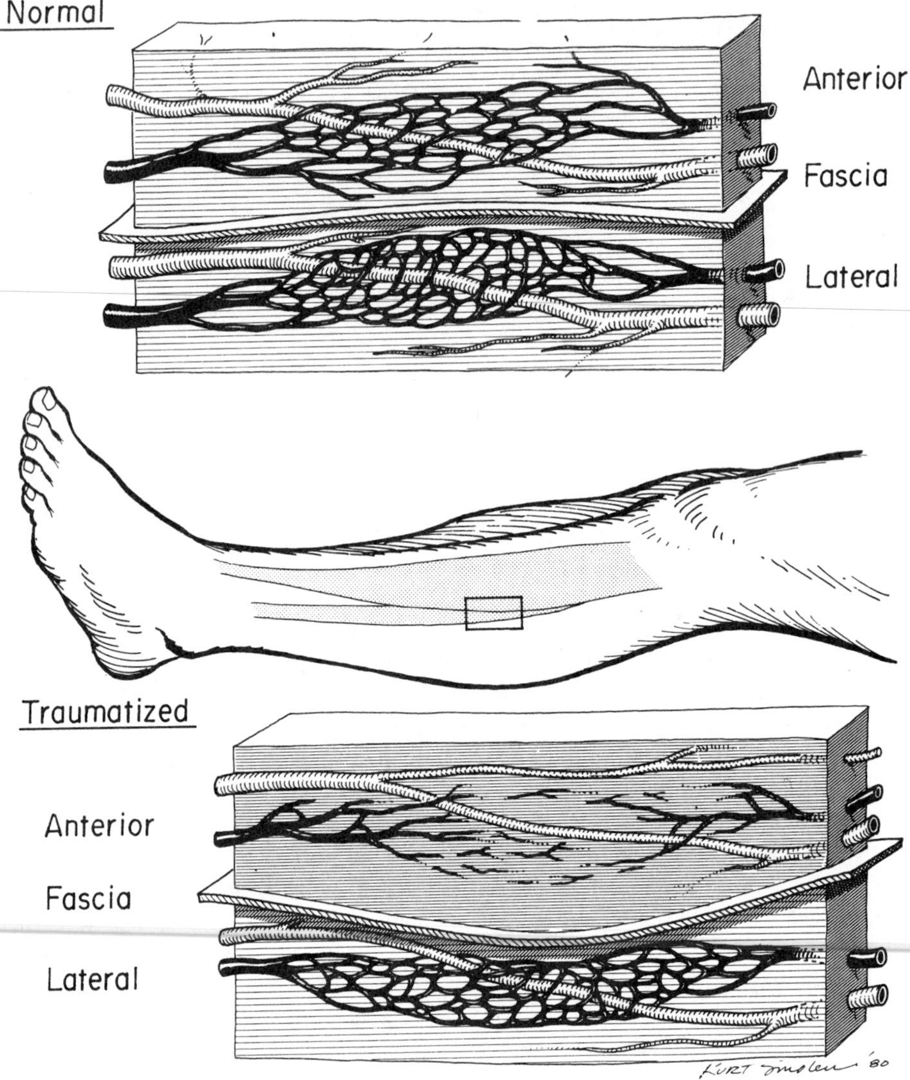

FIGURE 27-22 Unifying principles of compartment syndrome. In the enlarged figure above the leg, normal microcirculation is viewed during rest in the anterior and lateral muscle compartments. These two compartments are separated by fascia. During rest, intracompartmental pressure in the anterior and lateral compartments is near zero, and blood flow in all capillaries *(network of black vessels)* and large arteries *(shaded vessels entering figure from the right)* is normal. If pressure in the anterior compartment reaches a threshold level near 30 mm Hg *(enlarged figure below leg)*, capillary perfusion is inadequate to maintain tissue viability. It is noteworthy that distal pulses are usually present in the foot primarily because intracompartmental pressure rarely rises above central artery diastolic pressure. (From Hargens AR, Mubarak SJ: Definition and terminology. In Mubarak SJ, Hargens AR, Akeson WH, editors: *Compartment syndromes and Volkmann's contracture,* Philadelphia, 1981, W. B. Saunders.)

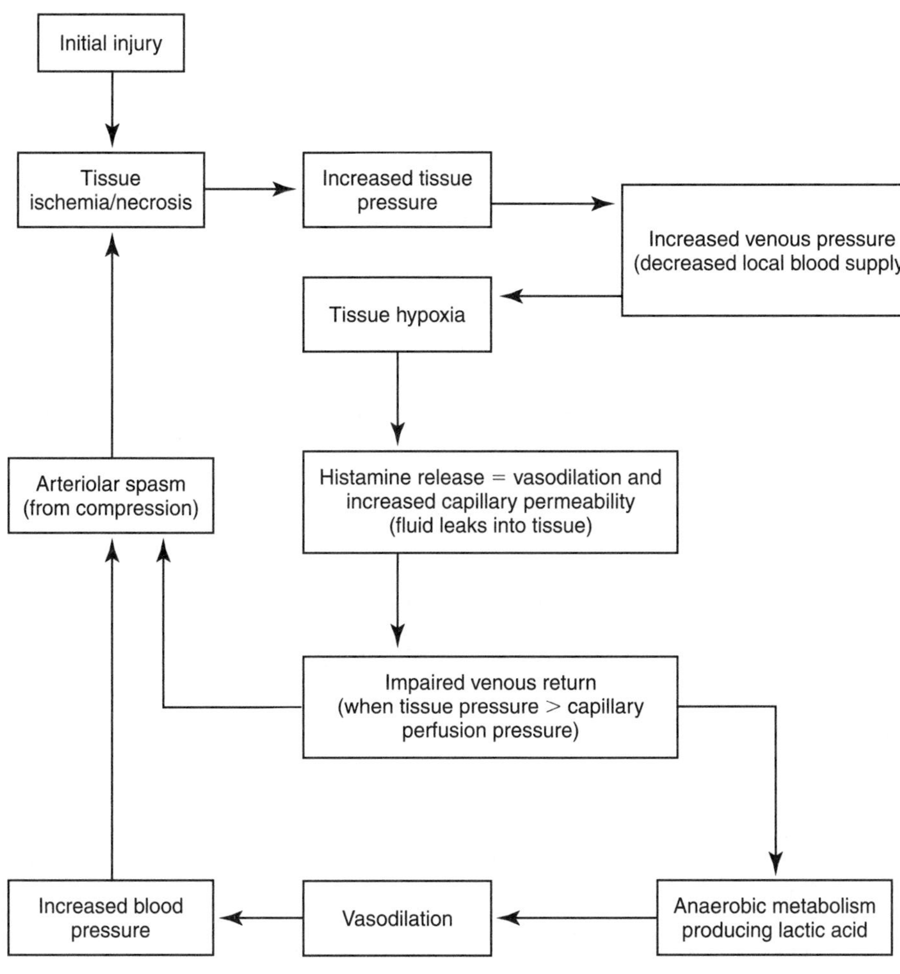

FIGURE 27-23 Pathophysiology of acute compartment syndrome. (From Ross D, Evans R: A patient with acute compartment syndrome. In *Clinical simulations in medical-surgical nursing III: Medi-Sim computer assisted instruction,* Baltimore, 1994, Williams & Wilkins.)

Clinical signs of compartment syndrome include throbbing pain that is localized to the affected compartment, firmness of the entire compartment, and paresthesia, a later symptom, in the distal distribution of the nerve involved. When these symptoms—pain, firmness, and paresthesia—are found simultaneously, they signal impending extremity morbidity unless appropriate interventions begin immediately.[44]

Pain associated with neurovascular compromise, often described as burning or searing, results from the ischemic process occurring at the site of injury and in surrounding and distal soft tissue structures. Bleeding and edema within the surrounding soft tissues, in addition to the specific injury, result in the pain associated with fractures and dislocations. Any type of movement of the extremity increases pain at the site of injury. Reported compartment syndrome pain usually seems out of proportion to the actual injury. Use of narcotics often cannot relieve the pain associated with this syndrome. The pain increases on passive stretching of the muscles. For example, flexion of the ankle and foot or the toes causes increased pain in the lower leg. It is therefore important to monitor and record trends in the patient's pain patterns and effects of the analgesics administered.[55]

Compartment pressure increases as bleeding, interstitial edema, and muscle fiber swelling increase within the compartment space. As compartment pressures rise higher than 30 mm Hg, the affected compartment becomes extremely taut and feels hard. Pain and firmness of the compartment are the resultant symptoms of compartment syndrome.

Paresthesia, pulselessness, and paralysis are late signs of compartment syndrome. Waiting for all these symptoms to appear not only places the patient at risk for losing the limb but also may create a potentially life-threatening situation. It is important to note that in the early stages of compartment syndrome the extremity may be very warm to touch, with rubor and bounding pulses. This is the body's compensatory attempt to increase local blood flow, but it eventually fails, and the extremity then becomes pale, pulseless, and cold. This signifies death of tissue.[44]

Altered sensation indicates probable pressure on nerves housed within muscle compartments. Described symptoms may include numbness, tingling, and needle pricking–like feelings. For example, paresthesia or dysesthesia over the first dorsal web space of the foot, such as that seen in anterior leg compartment syndrome, indicates deep peroneal nerve involvement. Deltoid compartment syndrome may present as paresthesia over the lateral shoulder and skin covering the deltoid muscle from compression of the sensory branch of the axillary nerve. Involvement of the superficial peroneal nerve, housed in the lateral compartment of the lower leg (Figure 27-24), results in altered sensation on the dorsum of the foot.

Decreased voluntary limb movement may occur initially as a result of extreme pain. However, actual paralysis is a later sign, indicating motor nerve involvement or, later, that the muscles have begun to necrose (e.g., the patient with compartment syndrome of the anterior compartment of the lower leg cannot dorsiflex the great toe). Alterations in distal pulse quality and capillary refill time are very late findings in compartment syndrome of the hand and foot.

Prompt recognition and early institution of therapeutic measures must occur long before the late signs of compartment syndrome. The injured extremity should always be compared with the unaffected extremity during evaluation. This assessment must be performed at least every 1 to 2 hours or more frequently, depending on the patient's status and the examiner's clinical observations and judgment. Following established hospital protocols for neurovascular monitoring and documentation is essential. Early recognition and treatment decrease the risk of limb morbidity and minimize the risk of life-threatening complications.[55]

Clinical signs of compartment syndrome may indicate the need to measure pressures within the muscle compartments. Pressure measurements may be performed prophylactically in the unconscious patient who has signs of increasing pressure. Controversy exists surrounding the upper pressure limit that should mandate a fasciotomy, the treatment of choice for elevated pressures; the aggressive recommendation for fasciotomy uses 30 mm Hg[59] as the treatment threshold. Others suggest that fasciotomy can be avoided if pressures are more than 30 mm Hg below diastolic blood pressure.[54] Most authorities agree that there is a gray zone in which pressure limits need to be considered together with the patient's clinical condition when making a decision about the indications for fasciotomy. If the patient is conscious, can give reliable information, and has the ability to describe pain and other symptoms consistently, close clinical observation should continue, with possible follow-up pressure measurements as indicated. However, if the patient is unconscious and has borderline pressure measurements, fasciotomy is usually recommended.[59] Fasciotomy is defined as the surgical incision into a compartment to relieve pressure on neurovascular structures and restore effective perfusion to the compartment. Continuous monitoring is occasionally used in patients with multisystem injuries to obtain a reliable trend in intracompartment pressures. Recently it was reported that mannitol was administered to decrease intracompartmental pressures by promoting osmotic diuresis, but the efficacy and safety of this treatment has not been established.[60]

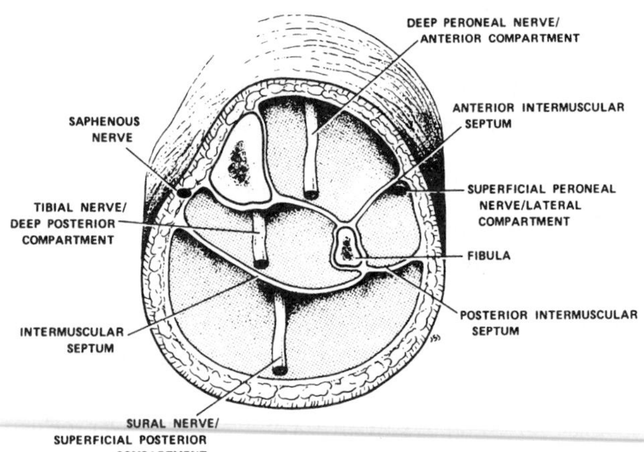

FIGURE 27-24 Cross-section at the junction of the middle and distal thirds of the leg, illustrating the four compartments and their respective nerves. (From Mubarak SJ, Owen CA: Double incision fasciotomy of the leg for decompression in compartment syndromes, *J Bone Joint Surg* 59A:184, 1977.)

There are several methods for measuring intracompartmental pressures.[44] Slit and wick catheters consist of fluid-filled catheters attached to an extracorporeal transducer that is placed into the muscle compartment.[44] The accuracy of these measurements depends on precise calibrations and is affected by the position of the limb and the height of the pressure transducer above the tip of the catheter. These types of systems measure the intracompartmental pressures in relation to capillary pressures.[44] More recently, an electronic transducer-tipped catheter, originally designed to measure ICP, has been used to measure intracompartmental pressures. This measurement technique does not rely on a fluid-filled system and is ideal for continuously monitoring intracompartmental pressures because it does not require frequent saline solution flushes to maintain the patency of the catheter.[61]

Monitoring and Management. Continuous monitoring is required for early detection of peripheral nerve or vascular compromise commonly seen with dislocations, fractures, or plexus injuries. Findings may include alteration in pulse quality, edema, change in skin color (e.g., pallor associated with arterial inadequacy, cyanosis from venous congestion), and altered sensory and motor function. Continuous neurovascular assessments are essential, especially after treatment (e.g., traction) is instituted to allow early detection of neurologic or vascular impairment. For example, Buck's skin traction, used preoperatively for hip fractures, can cause peroneal nerve compression if improperly applied or maintained.[44] Compression of the peroneal nerve as it passes over the fibular head leads to footdrop, a complication that can extend the patient's hospital stay, increase rehabilitation needs, and substantially increase long-term impairment.

As discussed previously in this chapter, proper immobilization and alignment are essential for preventing further injury to the soft tissues, especially the blood vessels and nerves. The risk for further injury, such as continued hemorrhage, soft tissue laceration, and additional impingement or compression, increases if proper immobilization techniques are not used soon after injury. For example, splinting the entire upper extremity in the position of function is essential for the patient with a humerus fracture to prevent further injury to the muscles and nerves of the arm. Proper positioning, realignment of fractures, or reduction of dislocations often must take precedence during resuscitation in an effort to reduce extremity morbidity.

Maintaining an injured limb in a nondependent position, but not above the level of the patient's heart, may reduce further edema formation and improve venous return. Elevation above the level of the patient's heart may actually impede circulation by decreasing arterial perfusion. Certain situations may call for elevation of an extremity above the level of the heart, but these are handled on an individual basis.

Cooling of the injured extremity may also be initiated to reduce swelling. Prepackaged coolant bags and plastic bags or gloves filled with ice-cooled water all work effectively. Use of frozen products or pure ice bags should be avoided because ice causes vasoconstriction, with a resultant decrease in local circulation and venous return, and may lead to thermal injuries in areas with decreased sensation.

Any extremity with neurologic impairment requires special care to prevent secondary injury. A paralyzed, insensate limb is at increased risk for thermal injury from exposure to extremes in temperature. Prolonged pressure on a bony prominence can quickly lead to skin breakdown. These are preventable and costly complications for the patient.[44] The affected extremity should be monitored closely for the onset of secondary complications, which can be prevented by avoiding contact with extreme hot or cold, proper positioning, and providing effective pressure relief.

Pain

Injury to the musculoskeletal system produces pain of varying intensity depending on the type and location of the injury. The patient with a musculoskeletal injury may feel any one or a combination of the following types of pain:

1. Nociceptive pain: pain stimulus originates from damaged tissue, including pain related to trauma or inflammation of muscle, joint, or bone
2. Neurogenic pain: pain stimulus originates from abnormal activity along afferent pathways that have been injured or impaired
3. Psychologic pain: feelings of anxiety or depression mislabeled as pain sensations[62]

Muscle spasms are a major cause of pain associated with fractures. Spasms can make fractured bone ends move, override, and pass through soft tissue, causing pain. Reducing or eliminating muscle spasms by immobilization and stabilization or by reduction of the fracture often alleviates much of the pain. Placement of cool packs over the site of injury and administration of analgesics are also helpful.

Pain associated with dislocation is often severe and continuous until the dislocation has been reduced. Additional pain is often caused by intentional or unintentional movement of the joint. Immobilization of the joint in the position in which it is found helps prevent or minimize movement and thereby minimize pain. Muscle relaxants and narcotics relieve some of the muscle spasms and pain, but complete elimination of the pain associated with dislocations usually can only be accomplished through reduction of the dislocated joint. Because of the time that elapses from injury to attempted reduction (usually more than 2 hours), increased muscle spasms and pain make muscle relaxants and narcotics necessary to achieve successful reduction. In some cases general anesthesia is required to effect complete muscle relaxation and allow reduction of the dislocation.

Neuropathic pain is typically described as sharp, shooting, or burning and is often associated with dysesthesias (e.g., hyperesthesia or hypoesthesia).[63] This pain often persists well beyond what is considered a "normal" time frame for acute pain, and it is often refractory to opioid analgesics. Tricyclic antidepressants such as amitriptyline and the anticonvulsant drug gabapentin have been used with variable success to manage neuropathic pain.[63] Recently, the anticonvulsant pregabalin was approved for treatment of neuropathic pain.

Compartment syndrome pain is often described as deep, poorly localized, and continuous and is difficult to control with the analgesics typically used for musculoskeletal pain management. It is easy to discount the pain as being caused by the original injury and not by compartment syndrome, a complication of the injury. Pain associated with compartment syndrome can only be relieved by eliminating the high fascial compartment pressures. Removal of constrictive bandages, elevation of the affected extremity (but not higher than the level of the patient's heart), and application of cool packs to reduce swelling may be effective initially, but fasciotomy is usually necessary to treat established compartment syndrome.

The therapeutic plan for acute pain management is often developed and initiated during the resuscitation or preoperative phases of care. For example, recognizing the pain associated with a complex acetabular fracture and realizing surgical intervention may be delayed, the team may elect to insert an epidural catheter before transferring the patient to the intensive care unit after resuscitation. This catheter also may be inserted during the preoperative phase for both intraoperative and postoperative use. Early continuous epidural analgesia provides pain relief, thus enabling the patient to cooperate with nursing interventions and prescribed physical therapy to prevent complications such as pulmonary problems and muscle wasting.

Pain management, as with all aspects of trauma patient care, requires a comprehensive, team approach for effective, safe results. Management of acute and chronic pain, defined as pain lasting longer than the usual period of healing,[62] is discussed in Chapter 18.

Fat Embolism Syndrome

Etiology. Fat embolism syndrome (FES) is an ambiguous and controversial process that has been studied and debated since the 1860s, when it was first described in the literature.

Controversy continues surrounding the etiology and appropriate therapy for FES. FES has been described in association with a variety of injuries and disease processes. The course of the syndrome and the developing symptoms are often similar to those of adult respiratory distress syndrome (ARDS). FES usually occurs within 24 to 72 hours after injury.[64] Close monitoring of patients at high risk for FES should begin on admission and must continue throughout the early phase of critical care.

Although FES is usually discussed in association with musculoskeletal injuries, it also has been described in patients with burns, massive soft tissue injuries, severe infections, and nontraumatic medical problems such as diabetes and pancreatitis.[65] Long bone fracture, multiple rib fractures, pelvic injury, or a combination of multiple fractures, however, places the patient in the classic high-risk category. Recent studies have demonstrated that patients with multiple fractures usually have a higher Injury Severity Score and therefore a higher incidence of other injuries, with resultant increases in the incidence of fat embolism syndrome.[66,67]

Two theories have emerged regarding the etiology of FES: active mobilization of fat globules and altered fat metabolism. The mobilization, or mechanical, theory focuses on the actual impact (e.g., the time at which a bone is stressed and sustains a fracture). This theory suggests that, when bone is damaged, the injured veins, which lie close to the bone itself, allow the release of marrow components, including fat globules, into the circulation. The second theory, altered fat metabolism, has been referred to as the "physiochemical theory." The biochemical disturbances that occur after stress or trauma affect the stability and metabolism of fat and other circulating products. Increased catecholamine levels activated by the inflammatory response cause an increased release of free fatty acids and neutral fats into the circulation. The free fatty acids affect the pneumocytes, altering gas exchange.[68] The problem worsens as fibrinolysis, red blood cell aggregation, and platelet adhesiveness increase. The fat globules grow in size as they become coated with platelets.[69] It is felt that these two processes are not mutually exclusive but work in synergy to cause FES[69] (Figure 27-25).

Subsequent pathologic conditions that occur during the syndrome are the same regardless of the etiologic theories. Large fat globules are filtered out in the pulmonary vascular system and obstruct the blood flow in capillaries. This obstruction, in combination with the free fatty acids and release of serotonin and other inflammatory mediators, increase capillary permeability, leading to fluid extravasation into the interstitial space, hemorrhage, and alveolar collapse. Impaired tissue perfusion and tissue hypoxia ensue (see Figure 27-25).[70,71]

A latent period between the injury and appearance of clinical symptoms of FES has been described and is also disputed. In actuality, acute signs and symptoms have been reported within 1 hour of injury and as long as 96 hours after injury; the average time is between 12 and 48 hours.[72] Mild cases of FES or early signs of the syndrome can be overlooked if high-risk patients are not monitored and the syndrome is not anticipated.

Signs and Symptoms. The patient with FES usually has tachycardia, hypotension, and decreased cardiac output in response to increased pulmonary resistance. The patient may complain of chest pain and exhibit signs of right ventricular heart dysfunction, as evidenced by abnormalities on serial electrocardiograms and elevated central venous pressure or right atrial pressure. Arrhythmias, right bundle branch block, inverted T waves, prominent S waves in lead I, prominent Q waves in lead III, and depressed RST segments may all be seen with cardiac strain from FES.[73]

Hypoxemia is the hallmark of FES, and use of continuous pulse oximetry may detect early changes in oxygen saturation.[72] Analysis of arterial blood gases typically reveals low partial arterial oxygen tension (Pao_2) (less than 60 mm Hg) and elevated partial arterial carbon dioxide tension. With the onset and progression of FES, the patient has tachypnea and dyspnea and may have a productive cough. Auscultation of

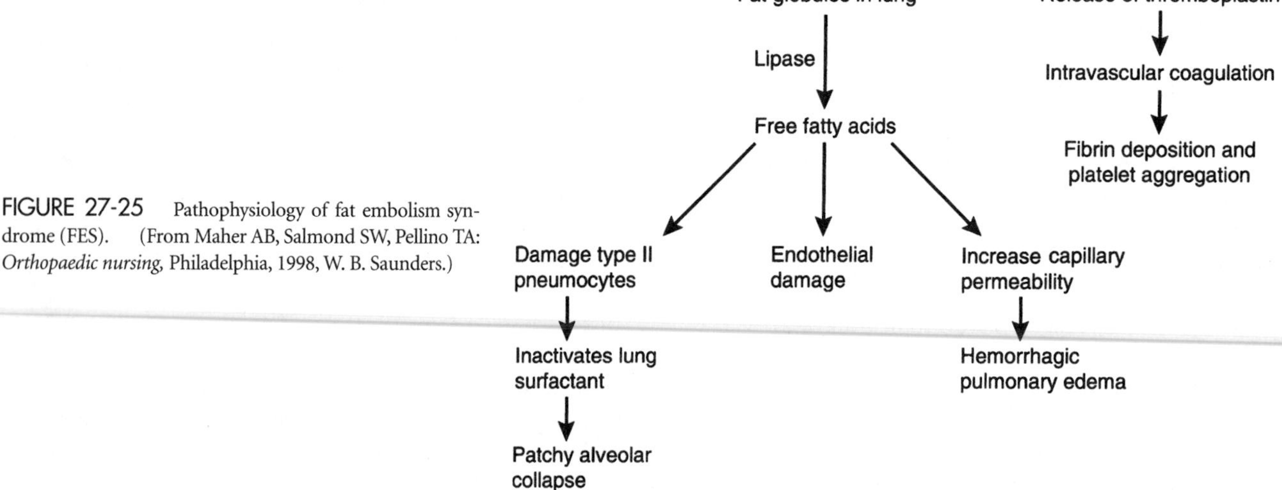

FIGURE 27-25 Pathophysiology of fat embolism syndrome (FES). (From Maher AB, Salmond SW, Pellino TA: *Orthopaedic nursing*, Philadelphia, 1998, W. B. Saunders.)

bilateral lung fields may reveal moist crackles. Cyanosis, bloody sputum, pulmonary edema, and the findings of bilaterally fluffy infiltrates on the chest radiograph are indicative of ARDS.

Neurologic findings include subtle changes ranging from irritability to coma.[71,72] Generally, the first neurologic sign is an abrupt change in behavior or mentation. A previously awake, alert, cooperative patient without an associated head injury becomes restless, agitated, uncooperative, and even disoriented in the presence of FES. Cerebral embolization may result in localized areas of anoxia because of specific vessel occlusion; generalized anoxia may occur from pulmonary dysfunction–induced hypoxemia.[72,74] The patient with cerebral involvement may rapidly deteriorate to a state of unresponsiveness, necessitating close neurologic monitoring.

In FES, oliguria or anuria commonly indicates inadequate circulating volume and reduced renal perfusion. Lipuria, fat in the urine, is a clinically significant manifestation of FES.[71] Hematuria also may be present.

Petechiae, usually distributed over the chest, base of the neck, conjunctiva, mucous membranes, and axilla, are thought to result from occlusion of dermal capillaries by fat and increased capillary fragility.[71,72] The petechial rash seen with FES may develop 12 to 96 hours after injury. Flat red spots usually appear and disappear in waves, often going unnoticed by the unsuspecting observer, and generally cease within 48 hours of onset. Petechiae are not seen in all patients; therefore, the absence of petechiae is not diagnostic.

A classic sign of FES is a rapid temperature spike to 38° C to 40° C (101.4° F to 104° F) without other precipitating causes. Altered temperature regulation from cerebral emboli may be responsible for the fever.[74]

Thrombocytopenia with platelet counts as low as 50,000/mm^3 develops as a result of platelet aggregation around the fat globules. Platelet levels usually return to normal within 5 to 7 days. Decreases in hemoglobin of 3 to 5 g/dl reflect the sequestration of red blood cells to the fat globules.

Treatment. Treatment of FES is usually supportive and is aimed at correction of fluid volume deficits, improvement of oxygenation, and management of associated injuries.[69-72] Respiratory support may be necessary to correct hypoxemia, including endotracheal intubation, administration of supplemental oxygen, and use of mechanical ventilation with positive end-expiratory pressure.[69-72]

Deep Vein Thrombosis

Deep vein thrombosis (DVT) is a significant hazard to the trauma patient with musculoskeletal involvement and may result in pulmonary thromboembolism (PTE). It is estimated that 600,000 patients in the United States have pulmonary embolism each year, resulting in approximately 200,000 deaths.[75] This number represents "all cause" deaths, which includes general, orthopedic, and neurosurgery patients. Generally, 24% of young adult trauma patients have DVT, although many of these are not symptomatic.[76] In the absence of prophylaxis, as many as 40% of elderly trauma patients with hip fractures have DVT, and 14% have a fatal PTE episode.[77]

Prevention of DVT/PTE is emphasized as better than any treatment modality.[77,78] Multiple studies address the issue of detection and treatment of DVT.[76,77,79-81] A majority recommend combination prophylaxis with an anticoagulant (i.e., either low-dose heparin or low-molecular-weight heparin [LMWH]) and elastic stockings or intermittent pneumatic compression devices.[82] The American College of Chest Physicians Consensus Committee on Pulmonary Embolism reviewed eight clinically relevant issues and made recommendations regarding diagnosis and treatment (the reader is encouraged to review this consensus statement).[83]

The major etiologic factors that predispose patients to DVT and subsequently PTE are addressed by Virchow's triad: (1) venous stasis from reduced blood flow, decreased muscular activity, and external pressure on the deep veins; (2) vascular damage or concomitant pathologic state; and (3) hypercoagulability. In addition, predisposing factors include the following:

- History of vascular disease
- Previous DVT or PTE episode
- Prolonged bed rest or immobility
- Lengthy surgical procedures
- Shock states
- Sepsis
- Spinal cord injuries
- Long bone, hip, or pelvic fractures
- Soft tissue injuries
- Vascular trauma
- Immobilization devices
- Prolonged use of PASGs
- Obesity
- Age greater than 40 years
- History of heart failure, acute myocardial infarction, stroke, or malignancy
- History of hormone therapy, either oral/dermal contraceptives or hormone replacement therapy[84-86]

Assessment and Diagnosis. Continuous patient evaluation aids in early detection of signs of DVT. Patients should be regularly assessed for physical signs and symptoms, although these are not specific or reliable, and such findings should be reported immediately:

- Calf pain on forced dorsiflexion of the foot (Homans' sign)
- Subtle to obvious swelling of the involved area
- Tachycardia
- Fever
- Distal skin color and temperature changes of an extremity

An acute PTE episode may be the first indication of the presence of DVT. Any signs or symptoms of DVT should arouse suspicions in all trauma patients. Obtaining a thorough assessment and accurate patient history is important.

A number of studies are available to diagnose DVT (Table 27-7). Controversy remains regarding the benefits of serial screening for DVT in asymptomatic patients. Further research is needed to weigh the cost/benefit ratio.[87]

Prevention. Prevention of DVT/PTE is emphasized as better than any treatment modality.[77] Patient and family teaching should include the causes of DVT, common signs and symptoms, and self-preventive measures. Continuous teaching and reinforcement promote patients' understanding and ideally their participation and compliance with the preventive regimen.

Early mobilization is a primary DVT preventive measure. Mobilization should occur as soon as possible and as much as permitted within the limitations of the patient's injury because lower extremity muscle activity optimizes circulation and venous return. A coordinated activity or exercise program that includes active involvement of physical therapy should be initiated soon after resuscitation.

Ambulatory patients should be encouraged to remain as mobile as possible by walking for at least 20 minutes three to four times a day. Patients who are unable to ambulate but are allowed out of bed to a chair should be assisted in getting out of bed several times a day, even if for short periods, rather than one time a day for a lengthy period. While out of bed, patients should not be permitted to keep their legs in a dependent position for an extended time; rather, legs should be outstretched and elevated to promote venous return. Periodic lowering of the legs during sitting can reduce compression of the femoral vein. Pressure areas on the calves or under the knees should be avoided while positioning the patient in the chair. While in the chair, the patient should continue performing isometric exercises and active dorsiflexion and plantarflexion. These activities stimulate muscle contraction, which increases venous return. Patients confined to bed rest require frequent change in positions, active range-of-motion exercises, and isometric exercises within the limitations imposed by their injuries.

Attention to extremity placement, positioning, and padding is important. For example, the lateral recumbent position without adequate padding between the legs increases external pressure on the veins in the lower extremities and may increase the risk of intimal damage. Pressure or prolonged flexion of the knees impedes circulation and venous return. Elevation of the knees above the hips and sharp hip flexion should be avoided.

Early recognition of patients who have predisposing factors for DVT enables early institution of DVT prophylaxis. Graded elastic stockings or intermittent pneumatic compression devices can be applied soon after resuscitation. Pneumatic compression devices (Figure 27-26) are indicated in trauma patients in whom anticoagulation is contraindicated or who are unable to actively perform exercises. Pneumatic compression devices have a tubular section for each leg, which is usually positioned between the ankle and knee. They continuously inflate to a predetermined pressure and deflate after a preset length of time. Such devices cause no positioning restrictions and should be initiated as soon as possible. They can be used intraoperatively on patients requiring lengthy operative procedures. Their effectiveness in preventing DVT is related to promotion of venous flow through vein compression and activation of fibrinolytic activity.[88]

High-risk trauma patients may also require early prophylactic anticoagulation to aid in prevention of DVT.[78,82,83] After hemostasis is achieved and the risk of potentially life-threatening or debilitating hemorrhage is not anticipated, anticoagulation prophylaxis may be initiated. In the case of intracranial or intraspinal hemorrhage or solid organ injury with bleeding, anticoagulants may initially be held. Currently LMWH is the anticoagulant of choice.[78,82,83] Although found to be less effective than LMWH in providing effective DVT prophylaxis for trauma patients, unfractionated heparin may be prescribed.[78] Regardless of the anticoagulant used, patients must be monitored for any evidence of bleeding. (i.e., positive hemoccult test result, drop in hemoglobin

TABLE 27-7 Diagnostic Studies for Deep Vein Thrombosis

Venography	Injection of contrast material into the venous system of an affected extremity with serial radiographs taken to detect filling defect in the vein. Rarely used because of complications and advent of noninvasive diagnostics
Duplex/Doppler ultrasound studies	Examines the blood flow in the major arteries and veins in the arms and legs. The test uses duplex ultrasonography to visualize the blood flow, and Doppler ultrasonography provides an audible means to hear the blood flow. This test is done as an alternative to arteriography and venography and may help diagnose abnormalities in an artery or vein. Very commonly used because it is noninvasive with a high degree of sensitivity. Is difficult, if not impossible, to perform if bulky dressings or casts are on the suspected extremity, and it cannot be used to detect pelvic DVT.
Plasma D-dimer	D-Dimer fibrin fragments are present in a fresh fibrin clot and in fibrin degradation products of cross-linked fibrin in the presence of an acute clot. It has a low sensitivity for DVT and should not be used as the primary diagnostic tool but rather used in conjunction with a clinical picture suggestive of DVT.
Computed tomography	Used in diagnosis of suspected DVT in patients with bulky dressings or casts. Not a first-line diagnostic study because of cost.
Magnetic resonance imaging	Shown to be more specific than duplex Doppler studies, especially with pelvic DVTs, but use in clinical practice currently is limited by cost and availability.

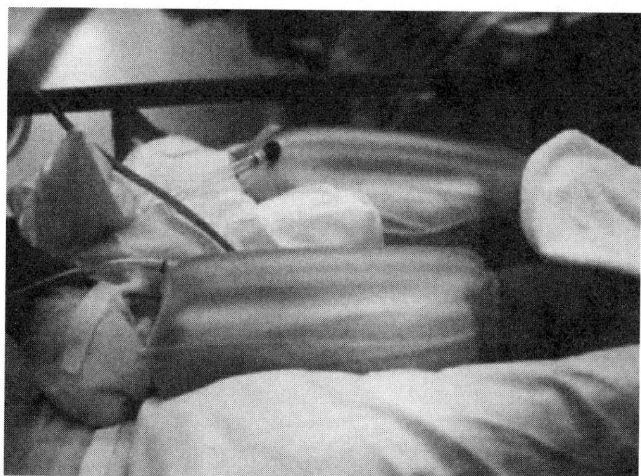

FIGURE 27-26 Pneumatic compression device applied to the lower legs.

and hematocrit values, obvious blood loss). Thrombocytopenia is a complication of any heparin administration that must be recognized promptly.[89] Therefore, routine evaluation of the patient's platelet count is necessary. Prophylactic therapy may be discontinued after the patient is weight bearing and ambulatory.[90] Some high-risk patients still unable to bear weight may continue anticoagulant prophylaxis after discharge.

Most clinicians feel that early identification of patients at risk for DVT is essential in preventing DVT in the trauma patient. The use of a risk stratification form has been advocated to assist clinicians with the identification of patients at risk. This may hasten implementation of pharmacologic and nonpharmacologic interventions to prevent DVT.[91]

Management. After the diagnosis of DVT is confirmed, therapeutic efforts focus on preventing propagation of existing clots, minimizing the risk of new clot formation, and preventing embolization. Therapeutic measures may include the following:

- Bed rest: lowers the risk of clot dislodgment
- Anticoagulation: prevents clot propagation, embolization, and new clot formation
- Thrombolysis: promotes lysis of thrombus[92]
- Vena cava filter placement: may be necessary in certain circumstances to prevent embolization of the thrombus to the lung
- Surgery: in very rare situations, it may become necessary to remove the clot and prevent pulmonary embolus[93]

The primary concern for the patient with DVT is the prevention of a fatal PTE.

Pulmonary Thromboembolism

PTE is a dangerous complication of musculoskeletal trauma. Injuries and factors that increase the patient's risk are cited earlier in this section. PTE occurs when a clot dislodges from a deep peripheral vein, usually in the lower extremity or pelvis.[94] The embolus circulates through the lower extremity veins to the heart and eventually lodges in a pulmonary artery or the smaller arterial branches and obstructs blood flow to a portion of the lung. Both pulmonary and cardiovascular complications may ensue.[71,94]

Clot release may be spontaneous or precipitated by sudden movement, such as rapidly assuming a standing position or engaging in Valsalva's maneuver, that abruptly increases pressure and blood flow. The precipitating factors mentioned must be kept in mind when the patient begins to get out of bed, whether in the intensive care unit or later in less acute patient care areas.

The obstructive thromboembolus causes hypoxia and release of vasoactive substances that increase pulmonary vascular resistance by promoting vasoconstriction. Pulmonary hypertension can result, causing right ventricular dysfunction, decreased cardiac output, systemic hypotension, shock, and possibly death. Simultaneously the embolus causes a ventilation-perfusion mismatch (ventilation continues, but pulmonary perfusion is impaired), which impairs alveolar gas exchange. Hypoxemia, hypercarbia, ischemia, and pain are results of impaired pulmonary circulation[71] (Figure 27-27).

Assessment and Diagnosis. Sudden-onset dyspnea is the classic signal of PTE. Symptoms of PTE vary according to the size and number of clots, the size of the pulmonary vessels affected, the extent of blood flow obstruction, the type of embolism, and the presence of lung infarction. Symptoms are often vague or nonspecific; therefore, a high index of suspicion is essential in high-risk patients.[75,76,94]

Signs and symptoms of PTE vary and may include the following:

- Pleuritic chest pain
- Shock
- Dyspnea
- Tachycardia
- Pale, dusky, or cyanotic skin coloring
- Bronchial breath sounds, rales, pleural friction rub
- Anxiety, feeling of impending doom
- Altered or decreased level of consciousness
- Low-grade fever

Signs of a pulmonary infarction, a rare complication of PTE, can include cough and hemoptysis, pleuritic pain, pleural friction rub, leukocytosis, and high fever.

Diagnosis can be difficult and usually cannot be confirmed by clinical findings alone. Studies that aid in confirmation of PTE are identified in Table 27-8.

Management. The objective of PTE management is to improve pulmonary gas exchange and maintain hemodynamic stability. Cardiopulmonary support, pain control, anticoagulation, and very rarely operative intervention may be necessary. Immediate initiation of and effective anticoagulation to prevent hemodynamic collapse from pulmonary clot propagation is essential and can be started simultaneously with cardiorespiratory support measures.

Atelectasis commonly results after PTE.[70] Suctioning as necessary, coughing, and deep-breathing exercises all promote secretion removal and help prevent atelectasis. These

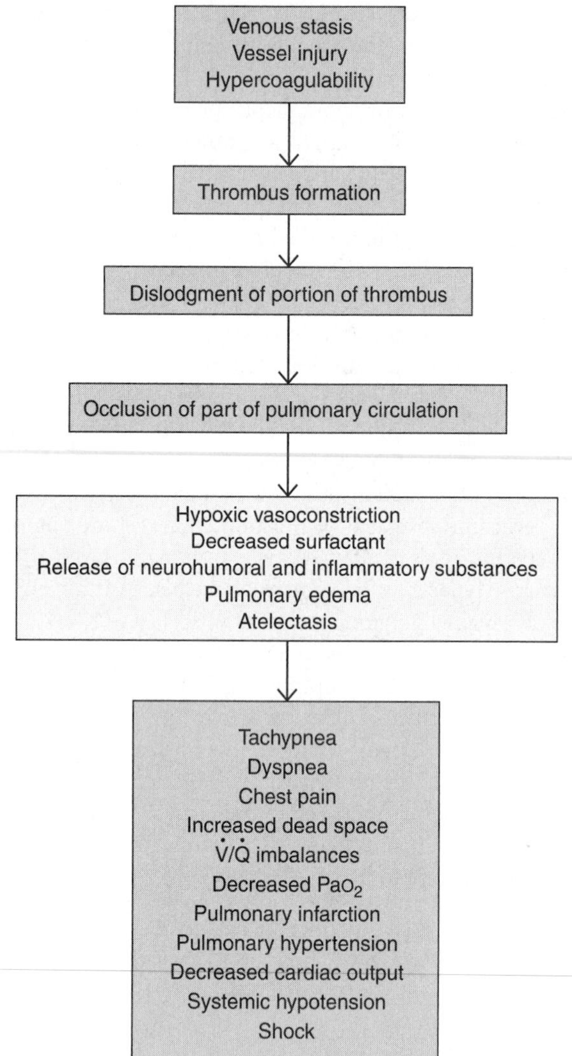

FIGURE 27-27 Pathophysiology of pulmonary thromboembolism. (From McCance KL, Huether SE, editors: *Pathophysiology: the biological basis for disease in adults and children*, 5th ed, St. Louis, 2006, Mosby, p 1233.)

interventions foster alveolar gas exchange. Administration of supplemental oxygen provides more oxygen for exchange. Endotracheal intubation and mechanical ventilation also may be necessary (see Chapter 24).

Pain and increased airway resistance can hinder the patient's breathing efforts. Placing the patient with PTE in semi-Fowler's or high-Fowler's position, unless contraindicated, reduces the work of breathing. Analgesic agents can be used to reduce the patient's pain and associated anxiety. Pain control promotes patient compliance and participation in breathing exercises and pulmonary hygiene, which maximizes breathing efforts and oxygenation. Opioid analgesics must be used with caution because their use decreases respiratory drive and tidal volumes.[95]

Cardiovascular collapse from release of vasoactive substances or right ventricular failure from increased pulmonary vascular resistence may necessitate hemodynamic support. Administration of positive inotropic agents and volume expansion may be required to optimize cardiac output. Analysis of vital sign and hemodynamic trends aids in evaluation of the effectiveness of resuscitative efforts.

Emergency anticoagulation is indicated after the presence of a PTE is confirmed. Continuous intravenous heparin infusion, rather than intermittent subcutaneous injections, is recommended because it reduces the overall amount of heparin needed each day, eliminates the "peaks and valleys" associated with intermittent injections, and minimizes the risk of bleeding.[84,90] Routine monitoring of coagulation profiles, namely, activated partial thromboplastin time, is essential to evaluate dose adequacy. Platelet counts are monitored because thrombocytopenia is a complication associated with heparin therapy.[90] Heparin therapy usually continues until the patient can be anticoagulated with warfarin to maintain an international normalized ratio (INR) range of 2 to 3. LMWH is now approved for inpatient treatment of PTE. This is administered as 1.0 mg/kg body weight twice a day or 1.5 mg/kg once daily. As with unfractionated heparin, the patient is converted to warfarin with a target INR of 2 to 3.

Plasminogen activators such as streptokinase and urokinase, although rarely appropriate in trauma patients, are occasionally used to lyse fresh thrombi and may also inhibit future thrombus formation.[92] These agents, similar to anticoagulants, should be used judiciously in the trauma patient. Thrombolytic therapy is contraindicated in patients at risk for intracranial bleeding (e.g., brain contusion, subdural hematoma) or massive hemorrhage (e.g., liver or spleen laceration).

Insertion of an inferior vena cava filter to prevent PTE in the absence of a known DVT and when standard preventive measures are unavailable or contraindicated may be considered for patients in high-risk categories. These categories include patients with severe brain injury, spinal cord injury with lower extremity paralysis, complex pelvic fractures associated with long bone fractures, or multiple long bone fractures.[96] Although there are currently no large, prospective randomized studies to support the prophylactic insertion of an inferior vena cava filter, a number of smaller trials support the use of vena caval filters in trauma patients.[82,96]

Crush Syndrome

Crush syndrome results from prolonged entrapment or a crushing injury. This type of injury may occur with a structural collapse, cave-in, wringer-type industrial or farm incident, motor vehicle crash (as either a vehicle occupant or pedestrian), or other traumatic mechanisms that cause compression. This is a potentially life-threatening syndrome, in large part as a result of the number and severity of associated complications.

A predictable series of sequelae develops after a crush injury (Figure 27-28). Prolonged compression of the involved body part causes ischemia and anoxia of muscle tissue. Tissue ischemia leads to a cycle of events resulting in third-spacing of fluids, edema, increased compartment pressures, and impaired tissue perfusion precipitating further

TABLE 27-8 Diagnostic Studies for Pulmonary Thromboembolism

Laboratory data	Arterial blood gases	Reduced Pao_2/Fio_2
		May be normal initially or show relative hypoxemia
		Hypocarbia
		Decreased arterial saturation
		Respiratory alkalosis
	Complete blood cell count	Elevated leukocytes (with pulmonary infarct)
	Enzymes	Elevated LDH, CK, SGOT
Echocardiogram	May only show tachycardia (if mild episode of PTE)	
	Changes with massive PTE reflect right ventricular strain, failure, ischemia; may see new-onset atrial fibrillation	
	Peaked T waves	
	Widened QRS	
	ST and T changes	
	Right QRS axial shift	
Chest radiograph	Initial radiograph usually normal	
	Later films may reveal atelectasis or infarction pattern (i.e., wedge-shaped infiltrate bordering the pleura)	
Lung scan (ventilation-perfusion)	Not an exclusive diagnostic study for PTE	
	Normal ventilation: air still enters and expands lungs	
	Perfusion defect: clot obstructs pulmonary circulation distal to clot, causing underperfused or nonperfused areas	
Spiral chest CT scan	Fast and easily available: demonstrates larger arterial emboli and visualizes other intrathoracic structures that may be contributing to clinical picture	
Pulmonary angiogram	Most definitive diagnostic study for significant PTE	
	Reveals clots in the pulmonary vasculature	
	Identifies areas of impaired perfusion (caused by filling defects)	

Fio_2, Fractional concentration of oxygen in inspired gas; *LDH,* lactate dehydrogenase; *CK,* creatine kinase; *SGOT,* aspartate aminotransferase.

tissue ischemia.[59] Complications inherent to crush syndrome include neurovascular compromise, infection from open injury, and subsequent ischemic changes.

Rhabdomyolysis, a result of muscle destruction from the primary injury and subsequent reperfusion injury, causes a release of myoglobin and potassium. Hypoperfusion from the initial traumatic insult, blood loss, and relative hypovolemia caused by fluid shifts into the extravascular space combines with myoglobinuria to cause renal dysfunction in the form of acute tubular necrosis and renal failure.[59] Impaired renal function, in the presence of metabolic imbalance that already exists from the rhabdomyolysis, causes further chemical derangements that may precipitate cardiac arrhythmias. Liberation of potassium from cellular necrosis can dramatically raise serum potassium levels and lead to sudden cardiac arrest.[59] Refer to Chapter 26 for additional information on rhabdomyolysis.

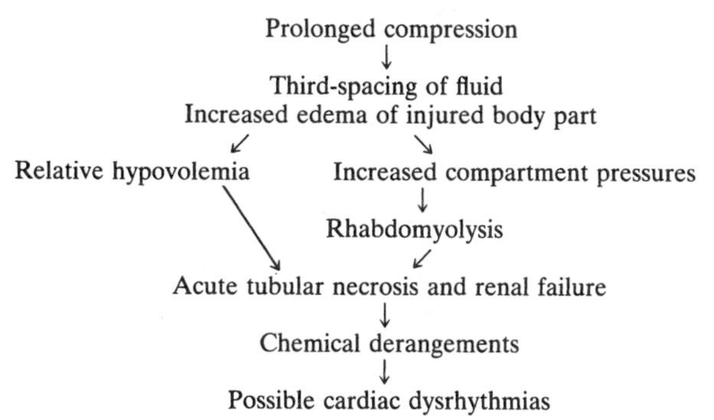

FIGURE 27-28 Events associated with crush syndrome. (From Peck SA: Crush syndrome: pathophysiology and management, *Orthop Nurs* 9:33-40, 1990.)

OPERATIVE PHASE

Responsibilities of the perioperative nurse include completing a preoperative patient assessment, which includes a complete systems assessment and gathering information about confirmed and suspected injuries, potential complications, and therapies instituted. A systematic report from the prior caregiver provides continuity of care, an essential factor in preventing fragmented therapy. During the preoperative phase the nurse explains the activities that the patient will experience in the operating room and the expected postoperative care. The perioperative nurse has the vital role of care coordinator, especially for the multiply injured patient with musculoskeletal injuries. These patients may well undergo multiple simultaneous surgical procedures during their operative visits. General responsibilities, therefore, also include anticipating the length of stay in the operative suite, positioning the patient, confirming the sequence of the various planned procedures and the equipment needed for each, and ensuring patient safety and monitoring throughout the entire case. During the often lengthy orthopedic operative procedures, the perioperative nurse communicates with the patient's family to provide updates and progress reports as requested. After surgery, a report of all interventions, resuscitation efforts, and operative procedures is given to the receiving nurse either in the postanesthesia room or in another patient care area. Again the systematic exchange of a complete report between primary nurses promotes continuous and consistent patient management.

General Management Principles

Prevention of Infection

Early and aggressive wound irrigation and debridement are important in prevention of infection in an open fracture or a traumatic amputation.[97] The most effective irrigation is done with copious amounts of normal saline solution. Debridement of necrotic fascia, devitalized muscle tissue, and bone fragments is necessary to decrease the potential for infection and to promote wound healing. Wound care is important to remove devitalized tissue, and debridement is continued until the wound is clean.

The risk of infection associated with open fractures depends on the grade and location of the fracture.[98] Other factors such as age, nosocomial infections, and degree of wound contamination also affect postinjury infection rates.[97]

Closure of an open wound may be contraindicated during the initial operative phase for certain severe injuries. Allowing the contaminated wound to remain open promotes drainage of microscopic debris not removed during the initial irrigation. Vacuum-assisted closure devices and antibiotic bead pouches may be used in open wounds to limit secondary nosocomial contamination. Delayed primary or secondary closure is performed when the wound appears free of infection.[98]

Re-Establishment of Bone Integrity

Restoring the fractured bone to normal alignment and length is necessary to enable functional return of the injured limb. Restoring the bone to normal alignment improves venous and lymphatic return, which decreases soft tissue swelling and reduces the release of marrow components into the circulation.

Early operative stabilization is beneficial for patients with musculoskeletal injuries and multisystem injuries. Damage control orthopedics or temporizing external fixation may be indicated for certain "at-risk" populations.[99,100] Various clinical parameters are used to determine the timing and extent of early interventions. A clearer understanding of the role of the systemic inflammatory response syndrome and multiple organ dysfunction syndrome has influenced decisions about surgical fixation of skeletal injuries and improved care of multiply injured patients.[101,102]

In addition to the total clinical picture presented by the patient, including age, number and severity of injuries, and overall hemodynamic status, members of the trauma team need to consider other situational factors when they are making operative decisions. These factors include (1) effectiveness of closed reduction, (2) presence of fractured or displaced articulating surfaces, arterial injury, or other injuries, (3) wound contamination, (4) length of time since the injury occurred, (5) contraindication of long-term immobility, and (6) cost of long-term immobility associated with closed reduction.

Fracture Stabilization

The method of stabilization used for an extremity fracture depends on the type and location of the fracture. Intramedullary devices are frequently used to stabilize long bone fractures. Reaming of the intramedullary canal consists of passing a device directly into the canal and creating a channel to allow for passage of a rod for fracture fixation. The use of reamed nails in open fractures has been controversial because of evidence that they interrupt the vascular supply to the fracture site.[103,104] Recent clinical studies, however, have demonstrated prolonged healing times and an increased rate of nonunion, as well as the need for a second operation with the use of unreamed nails.[97,104] Intramedullary nailing is effective treatment for both open and closed fractures of the femur or tibia. Reamed intramedullary nailing is the gold standard for treatment of femoral shaft fractures. Studies have demonstrated that in reamed intramedullary nail placement, intramedullary pressures rise significantly and can cause embolization of fat and marrow contents.[105] In the overwhelming majority of patients, this embolization is extremely well tolerated.

External fixation (Figure 27-29) continues to play a major role in acute fracture management and limb reconstruction procedures. Although an external fixator may be the definitive treatment option for a given fracture, it also can be used as a temporary stabilization device on a critically ill patient who cannot safely undergo a lengthy operative procedure on admission. External fixation also plays an important role in management of a severely crushed lower leg with significant soft tissue and bone loss. Use of external fixators allows access for wound care, soft tissue coverage (free tissue transfer), and bone transport or transplantation to fill the bony defect.[106]

Pelvic Ring Stabilization

In unstable pelvic ring disruptions, external fixation provides provisional pelvic fixation and at times may be lifesaving. It does not, however, stabilize the posterior bony structures well, and therefore internal pelvic ring fixation must be performed as soon as the patient's condition permits if gross posterior instability is present.

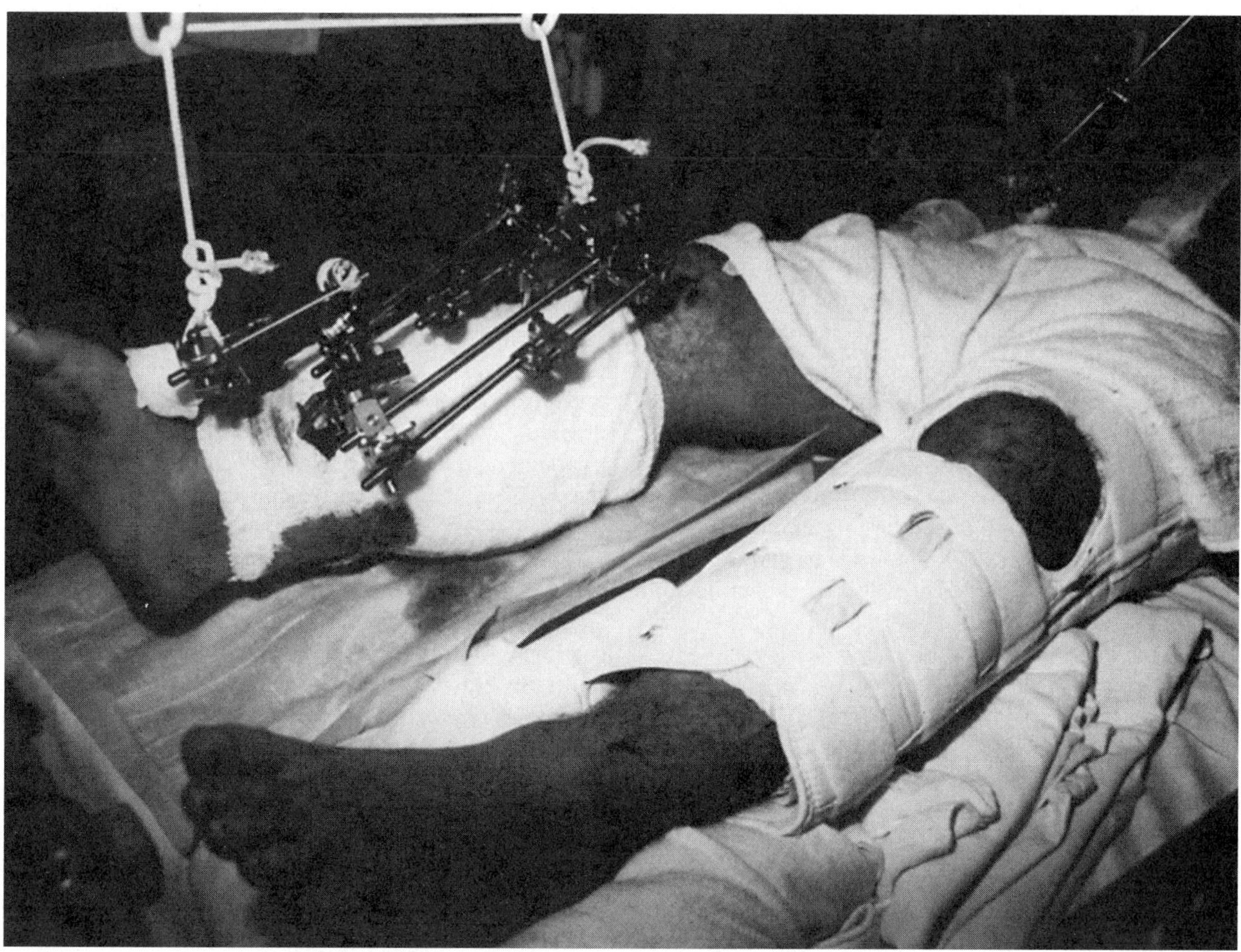

FIGURE 27-29 External fixator applied to the right leg (tibia/fibula fracture).

Surgical Treatment of Compartment Syndrome

Fasciotomies allow for the decompression of fascial compartments that have high pressures caused by swelling of tissues, as previously described. The fascial compartment is opened to allow the increased compartment volume to expand without increasing pressure on the microcirculation. The technique used to open the fascial sheath depends on the compartment requiring decompression. The forearm compartments can be opened with two incisions—one volar, one dorsal—placed 180 degrees to each other. Because the lower leg has four compartments, the lower leg fasciotomy technique involves a lateral incision between the fibular shaft and the tibial crest to relieve pressure in the anterior and lateral compartments. The deep posterior and superficial posterior compartments are approached through a medial incision. The type of incision required for other compartments, such as those of the hip, thigh, shoulder, pelvis, upper arm, hand, or foot, is determined by the structure and number of fascial compartments involved.[107]

The wounds created by the large incisions of fasciotomies are left open and covered with wet saline solution dressings to prevent desiccation, or a vacuum-assisted closure devise may be used. (Wound care and dressing changes are discussed further in the critical care section.) Delayed primary closure or delayed secondary closure by skin grafting is then done when swelling has subsided.

Prevention of Complications Caused by Immobility

One of the fundamentals of perioperative nursing is prevention of immobility-related injuries, most commonly neurologic and vascular impairment. The long length of many of the surgical procedures combined with the unique positions required during surgical interventions for musculoskeletal injuries increases the risk of iatrogenic injury if proper protection and padding are not provided to prevent compression of neurovascular structures. Coordinated preoperative planning among nurses, anesthesiologists, and surgeons regarding patient positioning on various types of operative tables, such as a fracture frame or turning frame, facilitates optimal patient protection.

The potential for a brachial plexus injury as a result of improper positioning and alignment demands strict perioperative attention from the trauma operating room nurse. Postoperative brachial plexus palsy may result from hyperextension or hyperabduction of the upper extremity during surgery.[108] It may also occur as a result of regional anesthetic blockade for isolated upper extremity injuries.[109] This complication usually represents a temporary alteration in regional or generalized motor and sensory function. Healing and full recovery commonly occur within hours to days after the insult.[109]

Pressure sores are another risk for the immobilized patient during surgery. Providing adequate padding over bony prominences and any body area that comes in contact with a rigid surface and keeping such areas dry minimize the risk of pressure sores developing. Prevention is the primary intervention for these complications.

Critical Care Phase

The principles of patient care regarding immobilization, skin breakdown, and potential complications that were discussed in the resuscitation section also apply during the critical care phase. One of the responsibilities of the critical care nurse is to review and update patient assessment data, including operative procedures, anesthesia time, and fluid volume replacement requirements.

Prevention of Infection

During the critical care phase the patient with musculoskeletal injury continues to be at risk for infection. Injuries that require delayed primary or secondary skin closure, surgical incisions, and pin sites require close observation and meticulous care. Predisposing factors that influence whether an infection develops during the critical care phase include the presence of residual devitalized muscle tissue, dead space, hematomas, and foreign bodies. Other factors include impairment of the immune system as a result of traumatic injury, older patient age, poor nutritional status, hemodynamic instability, inadequate pulmonary gas exchange, hyperglycemia, and the presence of any underlying disease.[102]

Early recognition of the signs and symptoms of infection is important in preventing or minimizing infection, sepsis, and delayed healing. Trends in vital signs, including temperature and white blood cell count with differential, must be monitored, documented, and evaluated. Incision and pin site appearance and drainage (i.e., amount, consistency, color, and odor) should be serially assessed and documented.

Because primary wound closure is not always performed during the initial resuscitative or operative phases of patient care, some residual open wounds require wet-to-wet or wet-to-dry sterile dressing changes. Wet-to-dry dressing changes provide some debridement of the wound. Wounds with exposed bone, veins, tendons, and fat are treated with wet-to-wet sterile dressing changes to prevent desiccation. For open fractures, crush injuries, or traumatic amputations, operative irrigation and debridement are often performed every 24 to 48 hours until tissue granulation becomes apparent and the wound is free of infection and necrotic tissue. Vacuum-assisted closure devices may also be used on open wounds that are free of infection.

Hematomas are avascular and are thus an excellent environment for bacterial growth. Closed-system evacuation drains, such as the Jackson Pratt or the Hemovac, inserted intraoperatively reduce hematoma formation in surgical wounds. These drains require close monitoring to maintain patency and proper function. Specific nursing care includes emptying and reactivating the suction every 4 to 8 hours (or more frequently with large amounts of drainage), measuring and documenting the amount and characteristics of the drainage (e.g., color, consistency, odor), performing dressing changes by aseptic technique every 8 hours (or as ordered), documenting the status of the skin and tissue surrounding the drain site, and preventing accidental drain removal. Drains are generally removed within 48 hours after insertion, or earlier if drainage has stopped.

There is no consensus concerning the proper method for carrying out pin site care.[110,111] Multiple studies and meta-analyses of these studies reveal that most clinicians do advocate some form of pin care, but the type of care and solutions used vary.[110,111] Some clinicians feel that the dried exudate is part of the normal healing process, provides a tight pin-skin interface, and prevents skin flora from entering the bone through the pin tract. Others with an opposing view believe that removing the dried exudate allows the pin holes to drain freely, reducing the bacterial concentration and decreasing the risk of pin tract infection.[112] Generally pin sites (of simple percutaneous pins for skeletal traction or more complex pins from an external fixator) ooze after insertion. A gently wrapped, loose-fitting 4×4–inch opened gauze dressing (Figure 27-30) allows free drainage while containing the drainage. Frequent dressing changes and pin site care are occasionally necessary for the first 1 to 2 days after insertion. Pin care is given every 8 to 12 hours or as needed after active drainage has stopped. Cleaning the exterior part of the pins helps prevent retrograde contamination of the pin tract, which can potentially lead to osteomyelitis (see Chapter 15).

For any patient with an open fracture, crush injury, or traumatic amputation prophylactic antibiotic therapy initiated during resuscitation typically is continued for 2 to 5 days.[113] Occasionally, the choice of antibiotic may depend on the environment in which the injury occurred.[114] The usual drug of choice is a first-generation cephalosporin such as cefazolin. An aminoglycoside may be added if significant wound contamination is present.

Neurovascular Compromise Related to Compartment Syndrome

As previously discussed, compartment syndrome may develop soon after the injury, during resuscitation, as a result of excessive bleeding or swelling into the soft tissue compartments. During the critical care phase, compartment syndrome remains a potential problem for the patient with

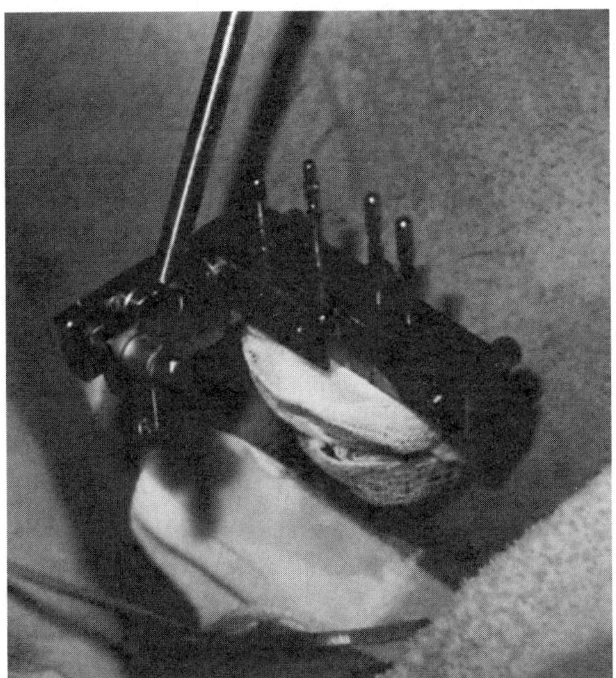

FIGURE 27-30 Insertion site of a percutaneous pin, with loose-fitting gauze dressing around the pin site.

musculoskeletal injuries. Despite definitive intraoperative care, soft tissue edema can persist because of sluggish venous return or persistent oozing of smaller injured vessels, which can increase muscle compartment volume, resulting in neurovascular compromise. Additional factors that can lead to compartment syndrome or less severe forms of neurologic or vascular impairment include tight-fitting casts, occlusive circular dressings, traction devices, and improper positioning of patients.[115]

Close monitoring of the neurovascular status of the affected extremity remains the single most important intervention and preventive measure. Evaluation of the compartments includes comparisons of the injured limb with the noninjured limb. This assessment should be performed and the findings documented at least every 1 to 2 hours, or more frequently as warranted by the patient's condition. Assessment criteria include the presence or absence of peripheral pulses; location, strength, and quality of the pulses; capillary refill times; temperature and color of the extremity; and motion and sensation of the extremity. Clinical signs of increased compartmental pressures warrant consideration of compartment pressure monitoring.[116]

Evaluation of immobilization and stabilization devices ensures maintenance of proper alignment and early identification of signs of local or generalized compression. For example, if clinical findings suggest that a tight-fitting cast may be the causative factor for deterioration in the neurovascular status of the distal extremity, the orthopedic surgeon should be immediately notified. The cast should be bivalved and the top half removed. The posterior portion continues to serve as a stabilizing device while attention is given to the extremity.[117]

The interventions described during resuscitation remain essential during critical care. The affected extremity should remain elevated and cooled for the first 24 to 48 hours after injury to promote venous return and minimize further edema. Elevation and extremity cooling are continued when the patient is positioned on one side or is out of bed in a chair. If the affected extremity has undergone vascular repair or flap coverage, the surgeon may want the extremity warmed to promote circulation. An injury managed by external fixation can be elevated easily with a traction apparatus. More conventional methods of elevation include pillows, folded sheets, and preformed foam elevation blocks.

Fat Embolism Syndrome

As extensively reviewed earlier in this chapter, the potential for severe respiratory compromise resulting from FES exists for approximately 96 hours after injury. The critical care nurse must be alert to the signs and symptoms of FES, and should it occur, early interventions should be implemented to manage the syndrome.

Immobility-Related Complications

The degree of physical immobility for the patient with musculoskeletal injuries depends on the type of injury, the pain associated with the injury, the method of treatment chosen, and the presence of other system injuries. The goal of management is promotion of mobility as soon as feasible after injury.

Immobility, the usual common denominator in trauma patients with concomitant musculoskeletal injuries, stresses the body, mind, and spirit in a variety of ways. Not only does it alter self-esteem and instill a sense of powerlessness, but it also slows anabolic processes and accelerates catabolic activities.[117] Consequences of immobility often include tissue atrophy and protein catabolism. More specifically, immobility increases the trauma patient's risk for secondary disabilities from pulmonary complications, vascular stasis with thromboemboli formation, skin breakdown, fecal impaction, renal calculi, muscle wasting, and contractures.[118] Appropriate nursing interventions can prevent or minimize the risk of these complications.

Immobility remains one of the most frightening and psychologically significant components of musculoskeletal trauma, and patients often require emotional support.[117] Fear and powerlessness related to immobility, along with social isolation and alteration in role performance, may result in an individual's decreased coping skills.[117] Patients with impaired physical mobility need to be as involved in their own care as possible. Nurses can facilitate this by allowing patients to make decisions regarding certain aspects of their care (such as the times for routine bathing, bed changes, and so forth), and providing patients with information about their medical care and reasons for immobilization. Nurses can relieve patient anxiety by maintaining a physical environment that fosters a sense of safety (e.g., keeping the call button within reach, having the bedside stand close to the patient) and administering anxiolytics as prescribed. Involving other health care professionals (i.e., psychiatric liaisons and pastoral care) can assist the patient with coping with immobility.[117]

Atelectasis and pneumonia are preventable sequelae of immobilization. Immobilized patients require aggressive pulmonary hygiene, which may include suctioning and chest physiotherapy. Chest physiotherapy, including turning with postural drainage and percussion every 2 to 4 hours, aids clearance of secretions from the lung. Placing the patient in the lateral and, if necessary, prone positions fosters alveolar recruitment. Kinetic therapy beds can be used to enable patient turning while maintaining skeletal immobilization. The spontaneously breathing patient should be coached to cough frequently to clear secretions from the tracheobronchial tree. Instructions also include proper deep breathing techniques and use of an incentive spirometer.[117]

Skin breakdown in the immobilized or insensate patient is a costly complication that can be prevented. Each ulceration can potentially add approximately $4,000 to $6,000 to a patient's health care bill in hospital costs, surgical skin repair, and control of infection.[118] Skin breakdown results from decreased arterial circulation to a localized area. Other factors that directly or indirectly predispose the patient to skin breakdown include the following: friction from bed linens or from cast and traction devices; anemia, malnutrition, infection, and fever; decreased sensation or paralysis; use of anticoagulants, sedatives, or neuromuscular blocking agents; and age of more than 65 years.[118] Potential breakdown sites need to be monitored for redness, burning pain, and itching. Turning and repositioning the patient as frequently as possible minimizes the length of time that pressure is exerted on any skin area.[118] Use of a pressure-relieving mattress, seat cushions, and pads can also aid in preventing skin breakdown.

Immobilization reduces intestinal motility, which is further compounded by the administration of medications that slow the gut function, such as narcotics. Thus bowel sounds and frequency of bowel movements in the immobilized patient are important to evaluate. If permitted, the patient's diet should include juices and roughage to promote passage of food and stool through the intestines. Mild laxatives, stool softeners, or enemas may be required to foster bowel emptying. A nutrition consultation may be necessary to assist with meeting the patient's nutritional needs.[117]

Immobility, especially of the antigravity muscle groups (hip flexor, quadriceps, hamstring, and gastrocnemius), precludes normal muscle stresses and leads to decreased muscle fiber size. Muscle atrophy, or a decrease in muscle mass, begins within 24 hours after the onset of immobility.[119] Approximately 3% to 7% of original muscle strength is lost each day a muscle remains immobile.[119] Connective tissue fibrosis around immobile joints also begins soon after immobilization, progressing to joint contractures and limiting range of motion. Muscle wasting, atrophy, and contractures can be prevented or minimized by range-of-motion exercises that are planned appropriately for the patient's degree of dependence or independence. Passive or active assisted range-of-motion movements are required during every shift for patients who are unable to carry out independent exercise. This exercise regimen should include uninjured joints required later for ambulation and affected joints within restrictions.

Range-of-motion maneuvers include moving all possible joints through their ranges of abduction, adduction, internal and external rotation, pronation, supination, eversion, and inversion and repeating each motion five times successively.[117] Complete range-of-motion exercises help prevent contractures, improve joint function, and promote circulation. These maneuvers, used in conjunction with isometric exercises, also increase the patient's tolerance and endurance. Optimal muscle strength, full joint movement, and endurance are all essential components for later mobility and ambulation.[117]

During range-of-motion exercises it is important to monitor and document the degree of each joint's range; any sign of inflammation, spasm, edema, or stiffness; and the patient's complaints of pain. A joint should not be forced to move beyond free range. Force and persistent range-of-motion movements when the patient describes an unusual amount of pain may precipitate joint or muscle strain or injury, which prolongs rehabilitation.[117]

Injuries to the central nervous system or to an extremity that result in loss of motion of a limb require functional splinting of the extremity. The inability to dorsiflex the wrist or ankle can lead to permanent flexion contractures of the brachioradialis tendon or the Achilles tendon, making recovery of function difficult if not impossible. Premolded fiberglass or soft splints are used in the early phases of trauma to prevent these contractures. Some patients, such as those with brachial plexus injuries, require splints during prolonged periods of immobility to maintain position of function and reduce the risk of contractures. Properly fitting splints and close monitoring of underlying skin integrity prevent or minimize skin breakdown.

Physical and occupational therapy consultations are valuable during the critical care phase to evaluate and plan care. These therapists are an integral part of the critical care team. Occupational therapists fabricate custom-made splints and determine optimal use schedules. The occupational therapist can also offer soutions on how the patient can carry out activities of daily living within the restrictions in place because of musculoskeletal injury. Physical therapists evaluate patients and customize physical therapy modalities that promote range of motion and early mobilization and maintain and build strength.

INTERMEDIATE CARE AND REHABILITATION PHASES

OVERVIEW OF REHABILITATION

Trauma rehabilitation is the process of restoring the patient to physical, emotional, and economic usefulness. Not all trauma patients with musculoskeletal injuries can return to the level of functioning they enjoyed before injury. New, realistic outcomes must be defined and the patient assisted, through education and therapy, to attain these new goals.

Rehabilitation for the patient with musculoskeletal injuries begins at the time of injury. Prehospital care personnel initiate the first stage of rehabilitation by providing the proper care for injuries and preventing further injury. During the resuscitative and operative phases, injuries are diagnosed and definitive treatment is initiated. Prevention of secondary disabilities related to immobility during the critical care phase plays an equally important role. Pulmonary hygiene, skin care, and active and passive range-of-motion exercises help maintain the patient's existing capabilities and prevent delays in starting the more active rehabilitation process.

The intermediate and rehabilitative phases involve the most active efforts in educating and training the patient to adapt to new limitations. Family involvement is greater during these phases than at any other time since the patient's injury occurred. Both the patient and the family are re-educated and trained so that the individual may reach the highest possible functioning capability (see Chapter 11).

COMPLICATIONS DURING RECOVERY

Delayed Healing

Healing times for fractures depend on the location and type of fracture, associated traumatic injuries, and systemic complications. Bone healing has five distinct stages, each dependent on the successful completion of the stage before (Table 27-9). If healing does not occur within the expected time for the type of fracture present, delayed union is present. The diagnosis of nonunion is made when, after serial patient examinations, symptoms persist and there is no radiologic evidence of healing progression 4 to 6 months after the injury.[120]

Many factors can lead to delayed union or nonunion of fractures: severity of fracture, amount of bone or soft tissue loss, loss of periosteum, excessive motion at the fracture site, poor nutritional status, medications, smoking, improper weight bearing, infection, and decreased vascular supply. Trauma nurses need to recognize the variables that affect fracture healing and institute measures to increase its likelihood.[120]

Infection, causing delayed healing of fractures and soft tissue wounds, can postpone the initiation of the active rehabilitative process. Proper nursing care and patient and family education can help prevent or minimize the risk of infection in the patient with musculoskeletal injuries.

TABLE 27-9 **The Five Stages of Fracture Healing**

Stage	Activity
First: hematoma formation	A hematoma forms at the fracture site.
Second: granulation	Within a few days after the injury, fibroblasts and capillaries invade the hematoma and form granulation tissue.
Third: callus formation	Within 6 to 10 days, plasma and white blood cells enter the granulation tissue and form a thick, sticky substance known as the callus. This material helps keep the bone fragments together.
Fourth: consolidation	Connective tissue and osteoblasts proliferate, bringing the bone ends closer together.
Fifth: remodeling	In this final phase of healing, bone fragments are united, excess cells have been absorbed, the bone is remodeled, and healing is complete.

Osteomyelitis is a bacterial infection of the bone that results from either a primary or a secondary cause. Primary osteomyelitis is caused by direct introduction of microorganisms into the bone during the initial injury, such as with open fractures or penetrating injuries, or during surgery. Secondary osteomyelitis results from microorganisms seeded into the bone from soft tissue infections or systemic infection.[121] Commonly isolated organisms include *Staphylococcus aureus* or *epidermidis, Escherichia coli, Klebsiella pneumoniae,* and *Pseudomonas aeruginosa.* Osteomyelitis that persists despite therapy can develop into chronic osteomyelitis.

Signs and symptoms of osteomyelitis include local pain with or without movement, edema, erythema, muscle spasms, limited joint movement, weakness, and a direct wound tract with purulent drainage. Fever and chills can be seen if soft tissue is involved or an abscess has formed. Definitive diagnosis of osteomyelitis is based on bone cultures. Laboratory blood tests occasionally show an elevated white blood cell count and erythrocyte sedimentation rate but these findings are nonspecific. Approximately 10 to 14 days after onset of the infection in adults, plain radiographic films show elevated periosteum, areas of radiolucency secondary to bone lysis, and areas of density secondary to bone necrosis. Bone scans, CT scans, and MRI can often delineate disease sooner and can show the true extent of infection.

Treatments for osteomyelitis include surgical debridement and antibiotic therapy, immobilization to reduce the associated pain and the risk of pathologic fractures, nutritional support to optimize healing, and institution of a pain management regimen. Hyperbaric oxygen therapy may be used to treat chronic refractory osteomyelitis. Patients with chronic osteomyelitis may require bone grafting to increase the stability of the bone after extensive bone damage.[121]

Movement of the area affected by osteomyelitis should be minimized; immobilization is maintained by bed rest, casting, splinting, or traction. If movement of the area is required, full and gentle support must be provided. Analgesia is administered as required and before dressing changes, with the effectiveness closely monitored. Wound drainage monitoring includes a description of its amount, color, odor, and consistency.

Soft tissue injuries with significant tissue loss require tissue grafting to promote healing, provide soft tissue coverage of the bone, and prevent osteomyelitis. Closing the wound and increasing the vascular supply through grafting can shorten the fracture healing time and decrease the risk of infection.[121] Soft tissue grafting is done when the wound is free of devitalized tissue, which typically occurs within 4 to 7 days after injury. The presence of any wound infection can delay grafting. Dressing changes for soft tissue wounds are done as prescribed (e.g., every 4 to 6 hours) from the time of injury until the wound is ready for grafting.[121]

Bone grafting enhances bone formation at the site of fracture nonunion. It is also used for fractures in which healing is expected to be delayed because of bone loss or extensive soft tissue injury. For example, many fractures with segmental bone loss, significant loss of the cortical bone, or substantial periosteal stripping require bone grafting to aid in bone healing.[122] The grafting may be done during the initial stages of treatment or several weeks after the injury, depending on the condition of the soft tissue surrounding the area of injury.

Mechanical Failure of Fixators

External fixators are frequently used to stabilize fractures; the length of time a fixator remains in place depends on the type of injury. The risk of complications increases with the length of time the fixator is in place. Components of the frame, including the transfixion pins, pin clamps, and couplings, can loosen, causing loss of bone alignment. At least weekly checks of the frame components are helpful to identify loosened parts. An increase in pain around a pin tract is often an indication of pin loosening and may be an early sign of pin tract infection. The patient and family must be taught before discharge how to properly care for the fixator. This includes being able to check for frame tightness and recognizing early signs of infection or pin loosening.[123]

Metal fatigue from cyclic loading is a problem associated with internal fixation. Healing of uncomplicated fractures usually occurs long before the implant fails.[123] With improved operative techniques and metallurgy and increased knowledge of the biomechanics involved in fractures and healing, the incidence of implant failure has been reduced. Although implants are usually permanent, removal may be considered in the context of pain or if infection develops. Patients who undergo implant removal are at risk for refracture, depending on the size of the residual bone defect and its location.

A fracture is considered completely healed when its strength is equal to that of normal bone and it tolerates normal stresses without pain or instability. Radiographic examination of a healed fracture shows dense and continuous bone cortices.[123]

Impaired Mobility

The effects of immobility caused by fracture, dislocation, plexus injury, or amputation can be psychologically and physically devastating. The nurse must anticipate potential problems and collaborate with physical and occupational therapists to initiate actions to prevent the complications previously discussed.

Amputations. Amputees require special attention to the residual limb. Active range-of-motion exercises prevent contractures of the joint immediately proximal to the amputation. The patient should be taught isometric exercises of the targeted muscle groups if active range of motion is impossible or limited. Some activities promote contracture formation of the proximal joint and need to be avoided or limited. For example, a patient with a below-the-knee amputation should not be in a sitting position for a prolonged period of time without extension of the knee joints. Those with above-the-knee amputations must avoid long periods of sitting and must spend time in the prone position to promote extension of the hip joint. Positioning of the intact extremities and the muscles of the trunk also must be considered to avoid dysfunction of these muscle groups. The patient is taught the importance of promoting mobility by performing active exercises. Mobilizing as soon as possible the patient who has lost a weight-bearing limb enhances overall recovery and rehabilitation. It is necessary for the patient with a lower extremity amputation to develop a new sense of balance as new methods of mobility are learned.

Extremity Fractures. Methods of ambulating the patient with a fracture of the lower extremity vary according to the type and location of the fracture and whether the bone affected is weight bearing. Crutch walking for the patient with a single lower extremity fracture and wheelchair transfer for the patient with bilateral lower extremity fractures facilitates mobility and reduces the complications of immobility. Active exercises of the upper extremities and trunk are necessary to increase the patient's physical strength and tolerance for these different types of activities.

External fixators have greatly increased the mobility of patients with fractures, who at one time were confined to prolonged bed rest with traction. Despite the advantages provided by the external fixator, it can still be intimidating to the patient, resulting in slow acceptance of the device and hesitation to become fully mobilized. Education and emotional support can help the patient understand the function of the external fixator, accept the change in body image, and overcome any fear of ambulating with the external fixator.

Patients with tibial plateau, supracondylar, patellar, or acetabular fractures (or any periarticular fracture) are at risk of forming joint adhesions and contractures. Limited passive range-of- motion exercises of the joint can help reduce these risks. Use of a continuous passive motion machine (CPM) may facilitate short-term restoration of motion, but it has never been shown to alter long-term recovery of motion.[117] Lubrication of the articular joint surface is optimized by the production of synovial fluid, which is stimulated by the motion. The CPM may be effective when applied within the first week after surgery. The nurse must be thoroughly familiar with the operation of the CPM and any potential complications that it can cause. Proper alignment of the CPM is necessary to reduce contact between skin surface areas and the device. Padding is necessary to prevent irritation or breakdown of those skin areas that come in contact with the machine. The nurse should be alert for any signs and symptoms of infection around incision sites and for any increased bleeding from surgical drains as a result of motion near the drain sites. Neurovascular checks and skin care should continue while the machine is operating. If the patient needs to get out of bed or requires turning for chest physiotherapy, the CPM should be removed. CPM is indicated only for patients with extensive difficulty in complying with postoperative instructions. It does not affect long-term recovery of motion. It may be associated with increased risk of wound breakdown in the the short term. It is therefore used only rarely after acute trauma.

Pelvic Fractures. The degree of mobility permitted after a pelvic fracture depends on the type of fracture, the amount of pain associated with the fracture, and the method of treatment. Extended bed rest may be necessary, with the hip fixed in flexion, extension, adduction, or abduction. Progressive ambulation without weight bearing may be allowed according to the patient's pain tolerance. Internal or external fixation of pelvic fractures can decrease the amount of time required for bed rest.

Myositis Ossificans. Myositis ossificans is the formation of heterotrophic bone that can occur anywhere in the body, but the hip and pelvic regions are especially susceptible. Heterotrophic bone is the rapid multiplication of osteoblasts in tissues that surround joints. Deposition of heterotrophic bone can eventually lead to complete fusion of the joint. Multiple modalities have been used to prevent the formation of heterotrophic bone, including the use of low-dose radiation and the administration of indomethacin. Care must be taken with patients receiving indomethacin because of the risk of gastric ulcerations, prolongation of bleeding times, and other hematologic abnormalities.

Plexus Injuries. Functional recovery of a plexus injury depends on several variables, including the type of injury, the specific nerve and level injured, and the patient's age.[109] For example, a patient who sustained nerve impairment after an isolated anterior shoulder dislocation may recover fully within a few days to weeks, whereas a more violent injury, such as from a motorcycle crash with more than one nerve root injured, likely has a worse prognosis for recovery. Despite months of intense rehabilitation, the patient with this more severe type of injury may only recover minimal function, if any, of the affected extremity.[109]

Rehabilitation must begin soon after any type of plexus injury. If or when nerve regeneration occurs, optimal physical condition in the affected limb affords more rapid restoration of function and use of the extremity. Closed plexus injuries generally require extensive rehabilitation for many months before any significant improvement in function is seen.

Both closed and open brachial plexus injuries may require early surgical intervention for associated soft tissue, vascular, or bony injuries[47,48] Primary nerve repair is usually performed several weeks after injury, when soft tissue wounds are healed and the risk of infection is minimal. Primary repair of more peripheral nerve injuries may be appropriate and may be indicated for clean injuries in the distal aspects of the extremity. Surgical exploration may also be indicated for the patient who shows little functional improvement after an injury that has a good prognosis for recovery.[48]

Chronic Pain

Chronic pain is a potentially serious complication of musculoskeletal trauma that can delay and intensify rehabilitation. The therapies used for acute pain management are often different from those used in, and sometimes even are contraindicated in, the management of chronic pain. A planned, team approach affords the most effective and comprehensive pain management therapy (see Chapter 18).

Chronic pain may become the focal point of a patient's life and negatively affect all aspects of his or her being.[124] These patients may require behavioral and psychologic therapy in conjunction with analgesic therapy. For example, patients with chronic pain often have depression and may benefit greatly from a combined drug regimen that includes analgesics and antidepressants in addition to psychologic therapy. Because pain is often a combination of physical and psychologic components, when the pain is relieved, the emotional changes may subside, and vice versa.

Patient and Family Education

The nurse can detect early signs of infection and promptly initiate therapy by frequent assessment of wounds, pin sites, and surgical incisions. In preparation for discharge, patient and family education related to aseptic technique, pin care, and dressing changes for wounds and incisions is necessary. The nurse should ensure that the patient and family can demonstrate their ability to perform these procedures accurately and that they can correctly identify the signs and symptoms of pin tract and wound infections. The education process is started early to allow time for the patient and family to become comfortable and competent with this responsibility.

Weight-bearing restrictions and use of assistive devices are key elements of patient and family teaching. Many patients require adaptive equipment after discharge, and trauma team members should identify such needs early and assist with the procurement of durable medical equipment to ease patients' transition to home. Continued medical therapies are often required, and referral to home health care agencies provides for expert continuity of care. Follow-up contact with the patient and family by telephone or clinic visits gives the trauma nurse the opportunity to evaluate the effectiveness of the teaching and discharge plan.

SUMMARY

Musculoskeletal trauma promises to provide a continuing challenge to the entire health care team. Four major areas that demand further research and development are trauma reduction and prevention, prehospital trauma care, nursing and medical therapies, and trauma rehabilitation. Despite the many advances in all areas of health, trauma remains a major threat to the health of our citizens.[125] The reduction and prevention of musculoskeletal injuries require in-depth research, public education, and, in some cases, state and federal legislation. Safety for automobile occupants has become a major area of research not only for medical and trauma personnel but also for automotive engineers.[126] Siegel et al[127] demonstrated that thoracic and head injuries occurred more frequently than lower extremity injuries in car versus sports utility vehicle crashes, although there continues to be significant lower extremity injury in these crashes.[127,128] Although air bags have been shown to decrease deaths in some crashes, the bulk of research demonstrates that seat belt use continues to be a major factor in preventing trauma deaths.[129,130]

Public education remains an important aspect in any injury prevention program. There are multiple community-based organizations and programs that address safety issues: Safe Kids (child safety seat use), Mothers Against Drunk Driving, Students Against Destructive Decisions, and many others.

Improvements in prehospital stabilization techniques and the development of improved immobilization-traction devices for musculoskeletal injuries are essential. Advances need to occur in emergency care of traumatic amputations and partial amputations to optimize reattachment efforts.

Research must continue to develop improved assessment techniques and definitive care options. Potential nursing research topics may include acute and chronic pain assessment and management techniques; prevention of secondary injuries and complications, especially those related to immobility; early rehabilitation techniques; patient and family teaching and participation in care; and improved crisis management for families, patients, and staff. Medical issues associated with musculoskeletal injury that require further research include the stimulation and control of the fracture and soft tissue healing process, management of nonunion, microsurgical techniques to optimize reattachments, modalities to enable earlier mobility, and development of improved prosthetic and implant devices. Rehabilitation of both physical and psychosocial aspects of injuries must be addressed concomitantly for the patient with musculoskeletal trauma. Improved chronic pain management, care of the amputee, and management of osteomyelitis and paralysis are all worthy areas of research.

The future of musculoskeletal trauma patient care will demand a highly collaborative approach by health care providers during all cycles of trauma care. Continued research, with an increased emphasis on education and clinical application, is essential for the multidisciplinary team to achieve excellence in patient care outcomes.

REFERENCES

1. Crowther CL: Structure and function of the musculoskeletal system. In McCance KA, Huether SE, editors: *Pathophysiology: the biological basis of disease in adults and children,* 5th ed, pp 1471-1495, St. Louis, 2006, Mosby.
2. Bone and Joint Decade: *Fact and figures* (2003): http://www.usbjd.org/about/index.cfm?pg=fast.cfm. Accessed October 5, 2005.
3. Musculoskeletal care. In Browner BD, Pollak AN, Gupton CL, editors: *Emergency care and transportation of the sick and injured,* 8th ed, pp 638-679, Sudbury, MA, 2002, Jones and Bartlett.
4. Mohanty K, Musso D, Powell JN et al: Emergent management of pelvic ring injuries: an update, *Can J Surg* 48:49-56, 2005.
5. Balogh Z, Caldwell E, Heetveld M et al: Institutional practice guidelines on management of pelvic fracture-related hemodynamic instability: do they make a difference? *J Trauma* 58: 778-782, 2005.
6. Head and spine injuries. In Browner BD, Pollak AN, Gupton CL, editors: *Emergency care and transportation of the sick and injured,* 8th ed, pp 680-711, Sudbury, MA, 2002, Jones and Bartlett.
7. Musculoskeletal system. In Seidel HM, Ball JW, Daines JE et al, editors: *Mosby's guide to physical examination,* 5th ed, pp 695-765, St. Louis, 2003, Mosby.
8. Kataoka Y, Maekawa K, Nishimaki H et al: Iliac vein injuries in hemodynamically unstable patients with pelvic fracture caused by blunt trauma, *J Trauma* 58:704-708, 2005.
9. Kunkler C: Fractures. In Maher AB, Salmond SW, Pellino TA, editors: *Orthopaedic nursing,* 3rd ed, pp 609-649, Philadelphia, 2002, W. B. Saunders.
10. *Amputation related exam*: http://www.eatonhand.com/clf/clf461.htm. Accessed October 18, 2005.
11. Adams JE et al: Analysis of the incidence of pelvic trauma in fatal automobile accidents, *Am J Forensic Med Pathol* 23: 132-136, 2002.
12. Shepard C: *Pelvic fractures* (2005): http://www.emedicine.com/emerg/topic203htm. Accessed October 18, 2005.
13. Frakes C, Evans D: Major pelvic fractures, *Crit Care Nurse* 24:18-30, 2004.
14. Trunkey DD, Chapman MW, Lim RC et al: Management of pelvic fractures in blunt trauma injury, *J Trauma* 14:912-923, 1974.
15. Pennal GF, Tile M, Wendall JP et al: Pelvic disruption: assessment and classification, *Clin Orthop* 151:12-21, 1980.
16. Young JWR, Burgess AR: *Radiological management of pelvic ring fractures: systemic radiographic diagnosis*, Baltimore, 1987, Urban and Schwarzenberg.
17. Tile M: *Fractures of the pelvis and acetabulum*, Baltimore, 1984, Williams & Wilkins.
18. Perry JP, Forbes M, Stiell IM et al: Clinical predictors for pelvic fracture following severe trauma, *Acad Emerg Med* 12:s11-14, 2005.
19. Blackmore CC, Jurkovich GJ, Linnau KF et al: Assessment of volume of hemorrhage and outcome from pelvic fracture, *Arch Surg* 138:504-509, 2003.

20. Johns Hopkins Bayview Medical Center Orthopaedic Surgery: *The five minute orthopaedic consultant,* Baltimore, 2002, Lippincott Williams & Wilkins.
21. Altizer L: Neurovascular assessment, *Orthop Nurs* 21:48-50, 2002.
22. Simpson T, Krieg JC, Heuer F et al: Stabilization of pelvic ring disruptions with a circumferential sheet, *J Trauma* 52:158-161, 2002.
23. Ramirez JI, Velmahos GC, Best CR et al: Male sexual function after bilateral internal iliac artery embolization for pelvic fracture, *J Trauma* 56:734-739, 2004.
24. Bailey M: Staying on your toes when managing pelvic fractures, *Nursing* 35:32cc1-32cc4, 2005.
25. Cinat ME, Wallace WC, Nastanski F et al: Improved survival following massive transfusion in patients who have undergone trauma, *Arch Surg* 134: 964-968, 1999.
26. Olson SA, Rhorer AS: Orthopaedic trauma for the general orthopaedist: avoiding problems and pitfalls in treatment, *Clin Orthop Relat Res* 433:30-37, 2005.
27. Chapleau W: PASG: Bad wrap or bad rap? *Emerg Med Serv* 31:75-76, 2002.
28. Gosselin RA, Roberts I, Gillespie WJ: Antibiotics for preventing infection in open limb fractures, *Cochrane Database Syst Rev* 4:CD003764, 2005.
29. Takahira N, Shindo N, Tanaka K et al: Treatment outcome of non-clostridial gas gangrene at a Level 1 trauma center, *J Orthop Trauma* 16:12-17, 2002.
30. Salmond SW, Fine C: Infections of the musculoskeletal system. In Maher AB, Salmond SW, Pellino TA, editors: *Orthopaedic nursing,* 3rd ed, pp 734-778, Philadelphia, 2002, W. B. Saunders.
31. National Guideline Clearinghouse: *Osteomyelitis* (2005): www .guideline.gov. Accessed October 25, 2005.
32. Sharif I, Adam H: Current treatment of osteomyelitis, *Pediatr Rev* 1:38-39, 2005.
33. Trikha V Mittal R, Gupta V: Tuberculous osteomyelitis after open fracture, *J Trauma Inj Infect Crit Care* 55:144-146, 2003.
34. Moon CH, Crabtree TG: New wound dressing techniques to accelerate healing, *Treatment Options Infect Dis* 5:251-260, 2003.
35. Adili A., Bhandari M, Schemitsch EH: The biomechanical effect of high-pressure irrigation on diaphyseal fracture healing in vivo, *J Orthop Trauma* 16:413-417, 2002.
36. Boyd JI III,Wongworawat MD: High-pressure pulsatile lavage causes soft tissue damage, *Clin Orthop Relat Res* 427:13-17, 2004.
37. Gosselin RA, Roberts I,Gillespie WJ: Antibiotics for preventing infection in open limb fractures, *Cochrane Database Syst Rev* 4 (1):CD003764, 2005.
38. Brilliant LC: *Fractures—clavicle* (2005): http://www.emedicine.com/EMERG/topic190.htm. Accessed October 25, 2005.
39. Anglen JO, Gainor BJ, Simpson WA et al: The use of detergent irrigation for musculoskeletal wounds, *Int Orthop* 27:40-46, 2003.
40. Bhandari M, Guyatt GH, Tornetta P III et al: Current practice in the intramedullary nailing of tibial shaft fractures: an international survey, *J Trauma* 53:725-732, 2002.
41. Birk CW, Buck G, Wolfe TA et al: Interventions to improve compliance with guidelines on surgical prophylaxis, *Am J Health Syst Pharm* 62:34-35, 2005.
42. Bratzler DW, Houck PM, Richards C et al: Use of antimicrobial prophylaxis for major surgery: baseline results from the National Surgical Infection Prevention Project, *Arch Surg* 140:174-182, 2005.
43. Yaroshetskiy A, Protsenko P, Yakovlev S et al: Strategy of antimicrobial therapy in patients with severe trauma: importance of initial severity state evaluation, *Crit Care* 9(1 Suppl 1):P21, 2005.
44. Pellino TA, Preston MS, Bell N et al: Complications of orthopaedic disorders and orthopaedic surgery. In Maher AB, Salmond SW, Pellino TA, editors: *Orthopaedic nursing,* 3rd ed, pp 230-268, Philadelphia, 2002, W. B. Saunders.
45. Dubuisson AS, Kline DG: Brachial plexus injury: a survey of 100 consecutive cases from a single service, *Neurosurgery* 51: 673-683, 2002.
46. Binder DK, Lu DC, Barbaro NM: Multiple root avulsions from the brachial plexus, *Neurosurg Focus* 19:e9, 2005.
47. Chaput C, Probe R: *Brachial plexus injuries—traumatic:* Emedicine (2003): http://www.emedicine.com/orthoped/topic26.htm. Accessed October 25, 2005.
48. Midha R: Nerve transfers for severe brachial plexus injuries: a review, *Neurosurg Focus* 19:1-7, 2004.
49. Hayek SM, Mehkail NA: Complex regional pain syndrome: redefining reflex sympathetic dystrophy and causalgia, *Physician Sports Med* 32:1-4, 2004.
50. National Guideline Clearinghouse: *Complex regional pain syndrome (CRPS)* (2002): http://www.guideline.gov/summary/summary.aspx?ss=15&doc_id=4215&nbr=32. Accessed October 25, 2005.
51. Cepeda MS, Carr DB, Lau J: Local anesthetic sympathetic blockade for complex regional pain syndrome, *Cochrane Database Syst Rev* 4:CD004598, 2005.
52. Monga P, Ahmed A, Gupta GR et al: Traumatic lumbar nerve root avulsion: evaluation using electrodiagnostic studies and magnetic resonance myelography, *J Trauma* 56:182-184, 2004.
53. Pearse MF, Harry L, Nanchahal N: Acute compartment syndrome of the leg, *BMJ* 325:557-558, 2002.
54. Bhattacharya K: Acute compartment syndrome of the lower leg: changing concepts, *Int J Lower Extremity Wounds* 4:240-242, 2002.
55. Ignatavicius D: Catching compartment syndrome early, *Nursing* 32:10, 2002.
56. Ozkayin N, Aktuglu K: Risk of compartment syndrome in open and closed tibial fractures, *Turk J Trauma Emerg Surg* 8(3):170-175, 2002.
57. da Silveira M, Yoshida WB: Ischemia and reperfusion in skeletal muscle injury mechanisms and treatment perspectives, *J Vasc Br* 3:367-378, 2004.
58. Fredericson M, Moore W, Guillet M et al: High hamstring tendinopathy in runners, *Physician Sports Med* 33:1, 2005.
59. Crowther CL, McCance KL: Alterations in musculoskeletal function. In McCance KL, Huether SE, editors: *Pathophysiology: the biological basis of disease in adults and children,* 5th ed, pp 1497-1545, St. Louis, 2006, Mosby.
60. Smith J, Greaves I: Crush injury and crush syndrome: a review, *J Trauma* 54:S226-S230, 2003.
61. Tiwari A, Hag AI, Myint F et al: Acute compartment syndromes, *Br J Surg* 89:397-412, 2002.
62. McQuillan KA, Beldon JM: The neurologic system. In Alspach JG, editor: *American Association of Critical Care Nurses: core curriculum for critical care nurses,* 6th ed, pp 381-524, St. Louis, 2006, W. B. Saunders.
63. McIlvoy L, Meyer K, McQuillan KA: Traumatic spine injuries. In Bader MK, Littlejohns LR, editors: *AANN core curriculum for neuroscience nursing,* 4th ed, pp 335-402, St. Louis, 2004, W. B. Saunders.

64. Van de Brande FGJ, Hellemans S, De Schepper A et al: Post traumatic severe fat embolism syndrome with uncommon CT findings, *Anesth Crit Care* 34:102-107, 2006.
65. Hussain A: A fatal fat embolism, *Internet J Anesthesiol* 8, 2004. http://www.ispub.com/ostia/index.php?xmlFilePath=journals/ija/vol8n2/fat.xml. Accessed October 26, 2005.
66. Anwar IA, Battistella FD, Neiman R et al: Femur fractures and lung complications: a prospective randomized study of reaming, *Clin Orthop Relat Res* 422:71-76, 2004.
67. Robinson CM: Current concepts of respiratory insufficiency syndromes after fractures, *J Bone Joint Surg* 83:781-792, 2001.
68. Kirkland L: Fat embolism, *eMedicine* (2005): http://www.emedicine.com/med/topic652.htm. Accessed October 26, 2005.
69. Willey V: Case report: fat embolus, *Wash Assoc Nurse Anesth Newsl* 8, 2005.
70. Udobi KF, Childs E, Touijer K: Acute respiratory distress syndrome. *Am Fam Physician* 67:315-322, 2003.
71. Brashers VL: Alterations of pulmonary function. In McCance KA, Huether SE, editors: *Pathophysiology: the biological basis of disease in adults and children,* 5th ed, pp 1205-1248, St. Louis, 2006, Mosby.
72. Wong MW, Tsui HF, Yung SH et al: Continuous pulse oximeter monitoring for inapparent hypoxemia after long bone fractures, *J Trauma* 56:356-362, 2004.
73. Bokhari S, Ismail S, Alpert JS: Probable acute coronary syndrome secondary to fat embolism, *Card Rev* 11:156-159, 2003.
74. Nastanski F, Gordon WI, Lekawa ME: Posttraumatic paradoxical fat embolism to the brain: a case report, *J Trauma* 58:372-374, 2005.
75. Sharma S: Pulmonary embolism, *eMedicine* (2006): http://www.emedicine.com/med/topic1958.htm. Accessed August 27, 2006.
76. Schultz DJ, Brasel KJ, Washington L et al: Incidence of asymptomatic pulmonary embolism in moderately to severely injured trauma patients, *J Trauma* 56:727-731, 2004.
77. Egol KA., Davidovitch RIM: Perioperative considerations in the geriatric patient with a hip fracture, *Techn Orthop Hip Fractures Elderly* 19:126-132, 2004.
78. Geerts WH, Pineo GF, Heit JA et al: Prevention of venous thromboembolism: the Seventh ACCP Conference on antithrombotic and thrombolytic therapy, *Chest* 126:338S-400S, 2004.
79. Knudson MM, Ikossi DG, Khaw L et al: Thromboembolism after trauma: an analysis of 1602 episodes from the American College of Surgeons National Trauma Data Bank, *Ann Surg* 240:490-498, 2004.
80. Eastman AB: Venous thromboembolism prophylaxis in trauma patients, *Techn Orthop Eval Manage Osseous Metas* 19:293-299, 2004.
81. Meissner MH, Chandler WL, Elliott JS: Venous thromboembolism in trauma: a local manifestation of systemic hypercoagulability? *J Trauma* 54:224-231, 2003.
82. Rogers FB, Cipolle MD, Velmahos G et al: Practice management guidelines for the prevention of venous thromboembolism in trauma patients: the EAST practice management guidelines work group, *J Trauma* 53:142-164, 2002.
83. Hirsh J, Guyatt G, Albers GW et al: The Seventh ACCP Conference on antithrombotic and thrombolytic therapy: evidence-based guidelines, *Chest* 126:172S-173S, 2004.
84. Writing Group for the Women's Health Initiative Investigators: Risks and benefits of estrogen plus progestin in healthy postmenopausal women: principal results from the Women's Health Initiative randomized controlled trial, *JAMA* 288:321-333, 2002.
85. Chen L, Soares D: Fatal pulmonary embolism following ankle fracture in a 17 year old girl, *J Bone Joint Surg* 88:400-402, 2006.
86. Girard P, Sanchez O, Leroyer C et al: Deep venous thrombosis in patients with acute pulmonary embolism: prevalence, risk factors and clinical significance, *Chest* 128:1593-1601, 2005.
87. Van Den Berg E, Bathgate B, Panagakos E et al: Duplex screening as a method of quality assurance of perioperative thromboembolism prophylaxis, *Int Angiol* 18:210-220, 1999.
88. Goldhaber SZ, Fanikos J: Prevention of deep vein thrombosis and pulmonary embolism, *Circulation* 110:e445-e447, 2004.
89. Rutherford EJ, Schooler WG, Sredzienski E et al: Optimal dose of enoxaparin in critically ill trauma and surgical patients, *J Trauma* 58:1167-1170, 2005.
90. Warkentin TE, Greinacher A: Heparin-induced thrombocytopenia: recognition, treatment, and prevention: the Seventh ACCP Conference on Antithrombotic and Thrombolytic Therapy, *Chest* 126:311S-337S, 2004.
91. Schuerer DJ, Whinney RR, Freeman BD et al: Evaluation of the applicability, efficacy, and safety of a thromboembolic event prophylaxis guideline designed for quality improvement of the traumatically injured patient, *J Trauma* 58:731-739, 2005.
92. Cable DG, Cherry KJ: Systemic thrombolytic therapy after recent abdominal aortic aneurysm repair: an absolute contraindication? *Mayo Clin Proc* 78:99-102, 2003.
93. Madani MM, Jamieson SW: Pulmonary thromboendarterectomy. In Cohn LH, Edmunds LH Jr, editors: *Cardiac surgery in the adult,* pp 1205-1228, New York, 2003, McGraw-Hill.
94. BrashersVL: Alterations of cardiovascular function. In McCance KA, Huether SE, editors: *Pathophysiology: the biological basis of disease in adults and children,* 5th ed, pp 1081-1146, St. Louis, 2006, Mosby.
95. Pearson LJ: *Nurse practitioner drug handbook,* 4th ed, Philadelphia, 2004, Lippincott Wilkins & Williams.
96. Morris CS, Rogers FB, Najarian KE et al: Current trends in vena caval filtration with the introduction of retrievable filter at a level I trauma center, *J Trauma* 57:32-36, 2004.
97. Khatod M, Botte MJ, Hoyt DB et al: Outcomes in open tibia fractures: relationship between delay in treatment and infection, *J Trauma* 55:949-954, 2003.
98. Harley BJ: The effect of time to definitive treatment on the rate of nonunion and infection in open fractures, *J Orthop Trauma* 16:484-490, 2002.
99. Pape HC, Giannoudis PV, Krettek C et al: Timing of fixation of major fractures in blunt polytrauma: role of conventional indicators in clinical decision making, *J Orthop Trauma* 19: 551-562, 2005.
100. Grannum S, Gardner A, Porter K: Damage control in orthopaedic trauma, *Trauma* 6:279-284, 2004.
101. Walsh CR: Multiple organ dysfunction syndrome. In Melander S, editor: *Case studies in critical care nursing,* 4th ed, pp 352-369, Philadelphia, 2003, W. B. Saunders.
102. Walsh CR: Multiple organ dysfunction after trauma, *Orthop Nurs* 24:324-335, 2005.

103. Gopinath P: Reamed or unreamed nailing in open fractures of tibia-current concepts, *J Orthop* 2:e1, 2005.
104. Larsen LB: Should insertion of intramedullary nails for tibial fractures be without reaming? A prospective, randomized study with 3.8 years' follow-up, *J Orthop Trauma* 18:144-149, 2004.
105. Mueller CA, Rahn BA: Intramedullary pressure increase and increase in cortical temperature during reaming of the femoral medullary cavity: the effect of draining the medullary contents before reaming, *J Trauma* 55:495-503, 2003.
106. Mekhail AO, Abraham E, Gruber B et al: Bone transport in the management of posttraumatic bone defects in the lower extremity, *J Trauma* 56:368-378, 2004.
107. Ronel DN, Mtui E, Nolan WB: Forearm compartment syndrome: anatomical analysis of surgical approaches to the deep space, *Plast Reconstr Surg* 114:697-705, 2004.
108. Wong DH, Ward MG: A preventable cause of brachial plexus injury, *Anesthesiology* 98:798, 2003.
109. Candido KD, Sukhani R, Doty R Jr et al: Neurologic sequelae after interscalene brachial plexus block for shoulder/upper arm surgery: the association of patient, anesthetic, and surgical factors to the incidence and clinical course, *Anesth Analg* 100:1489-1495, 2005.
110. Holmes SB, Brown SJ, Pin Site Care Expert Panel: Skeletal pin site care: National Association of Orthopaedic Nurses guidelines for orthopaedic nursing, *Orthop Nurs* 24:99-107, 2005.
111. Patterson MM: Multicenter pin care study, *Orthop Nurs* 24:349-360, 2005.
112. Izzi JA, Banerjee R, Smith AH et al: Emergency room external fixation of tibial pilon fractures, *Tech Foot Ankle Surg* 1: 151-157, 2002.
113. Olson SA, Schemitsch EH: Open fractures of the tibial shaft: an update. *Instruct Course Lect* 52:623-631, 2003.
114. Bhandari M, Guyatt GH, Tornetta P III et al: Current practice in the intramedullary nailing of tibial shaft fractures: an international survey, *J Trauma* 53:725-732, 2002.
115. Butler AM: Assessment of the musculoskeletal system. In Maher AB, Salmond SW, Pellino TA, editors: *Orthopaedic nursing,* 3rd ed, pp 189-210, Philadelphia, 2002, W. B. Saunders.
116. Redemann S: Modalities for immobilization. In Maher AB, Salmond SW, Pellino TA, editors: *Orthopaedic nursing,* 3rd ed, pp 302-350, Philadelphia, 2002, W. B. Saunders.
117. Jagmin MG: Assessment and management of immobility. In Maher AB, Salmond SW, Pellino TA, editors: *Orthopaedic nursing,* 3rd ed, pp 100-128, Philadelphia, 2002, W. B. Saunders.
118. Takehiko O, Hiromi S, Yoshio M: Clinical activity-based cost effectiveness of traditional versus modern wound management in patients with pressure ulcers, *Wounds* 16:157-163, 2004.
119. Childs SG: Muscle wasting, *Orthop Nurs* 22:251-257, 2003.
120. Patel M: Tibial non unions, *eMedicine* (2004): http://www.emedicine.com/orthoped/topic569.htm. Accessed October 29, 2005.
121. Jain AK, Sinha S: Infected nonunion of the long bones, *Clin Orthop Relat Res* 431:57-65, 2005.
122. Keating JF, Simpson AH, Robinson CM: The management of fractures with bone loss, *J Bone Joint Surg* 87B:142-150, 2005.
123. Henter R, Cordery J, Perren SJ: In vivo measurement of bending stiffness in fracture healing, *BioMed Eng OnLine* 2:8, 2003.
124. Curran N, Brandner B: Chronic pain following trauma, *Trauma* 7:123-131, 2005.
125. Vehicle collisions leading cause of accidental death, *AORN J* 79:166, 2004.
126. Mizuno K, Arai Y, Newland CA: Compartment strength and its evaluation in car crashes, *Int J Crashworthiness* 9:54-557, 2004.
127. Siegel JH, Loo G, Dischinger PC et al: Factors influencing the patterns of injuries and outcomes in car versus car crashes compared to sport utility, van, or pick-up truck versus car crashes: Crash Injury Research Engineering Network Study, *J Trauma* 51:975-990, 2001.
128. Cote P, Ibrahim S, Carroll L et al: The relationship between impairment, activity limitations and recovery from traffic-related musculoskeletal injuries, *Am J Epidemiol* 1(Suppl):S65, 2005.
129. Brasel KJ, Quickel R, Yoganandan N et al: Seat belts are more effective than airbags in reducing thoracic aortic injury in frontal motor vehicle crashes, *J Trauma* 53:309-313, 2002.
130. Anakwe REB: Traumatic aortic transection, *Eur J Emerg Med* 12:133-135, 2005.

PART IV

Unique Patient Populations

28

THE PREGNANT TRAUMA PATIENT

Lynn Gerber Smith

The pregnant trauma patient presents a double challenge: two lives must be treated concurrently. When the trauma patient is pregnant, response to shock is different, and unique injuries, life threatening to both the mother and the fetus, can occur. While caring for the pregnant trauma patient from resuscitation through rehabilitation, the nurse must assess the patient, interpret the assessment findings, and make decisions pertinent to the patient's care. The nurse is the integral link between the many specialists consulting with the pregnant trauma patient. Therefore, it is essential for the nurse to develop a firm knowledge base and proficient assessment skills regarding the needs of this unique patient population so that sound decisions can be made to enhance the care of both mother and child.

EPIDEMIOLOGY

The number of births and the fertility rate in the United States increased by nearly 1% in 2004.[1] With 4.1 million births in 2004, it stands to reason there are a large number of pregnant women in our society. Trauma has become the leading nonobstetric cause of morbidity and death during pregnanacy.[2] The most common causes of traumatic injuries for the pregnant population include motor vehicle crashes, physical abuse or interpersonnel violence, falls, firearm injuries, and burns.[3-8] Early studies identified the number of pregnant patients treated at specific trauma centers and emergency departments and their mechanisms of injury. At one major trauma center, 79 injured patients admitted over a 9-year period were pregnant. This total represents less than 1% of total acute admissions, 1.7% of all female admissions, and 2.6% of women of childbearing age (14 to 45 years, now considered 12 to 51 years) admitted.[9] In this study, blunt mechanisms of injury had been incurred by 96% of the study population and penetrating mechanisms had injured 4%.

More recent studies, such as the 10-year retrospective review by Baerga-Vaula et al,[3] also found that pregnant trauma patients represent a small portion of trauma admissions, less than 1% per year. A slightly higher percentage was noted in an 8-year study from the University of New Mexico Health Science Center. That study of 15,268 trauma patients identified 271 who were pregnant victims of blunt trauma, or 1.8% of trauma admissions.[10]

Over the past decade, studies have attempted to characterize patterns of injury and risk factors that predict fetal death. This is clinically significant because fetal mortality can be as much as three times higher than maternal mortality. Fetal loss was higher in patients with a higher Injury Severity Score (ISS), evidence of shock, and abdominal injuries.[10]

A 5-year Canadian study looked at factors associated with high fetal mortality rates in patients with an ISS of more than 12. The most common mechanism of injury was motor vehicle crash. Fetal death was correlated with higher maternal ISS, lower maternal hemoglobin level, and greater number of blood transfusions plus the presence of disseminated intravascular coagulation (DIC).[11] In a large multi-institutional study of factors associated with fetal death, similar results were noted. Fetal death was associated with a higher ISS, a decreased Glasgow Coma Scale score, and lower admitting maternal pH. Many of these patients arrived in shock, with the fetus in distress.[12]

Historically, motor vehicle crashes have been the leading cause of death for women aged 12 to 51 years, which are generally considered the childbearing years.[13] There are nearly ten times more fatalities from motor vehicle crashes than from any other mechanism of injury during the reproductive years.[14] This is clearly supported in numerous multicenter studies that reviewed trauma during pregnancy and found that motor vehicle crashes are the most significant mechanism of injury.[3-5,7-9] In the past, pregnant women secluded themselves and traveled less often, but pregnant women of today continue to drive and ride in vehicles until the time of delivery, and many of them do not use protective restraints properly or at all.[6]

Physical abuse, or interpersonal violence, is a common source of trauma during pregnancy. In the United States, an estimated 1.5 to 1.8 million women annually are victims of violence from male partners or cohabitants.[15] As many as one in five women has been battered by her male partner.[15] Parker et al[16] documented that 20.6% of pregnant teenagers and 14.2% of pregnant adults were physically abused during pregnancy. In a review of 13 studies on violence against pregnant women, Gazmararian et al[17] found that the reported prevalence of violence during pregnancy ranges from 0.9% to 20.1%. A review of 1,195 pregnant patients from the American College of Surgeons National Trauma Data Bank found that interpersonal violence accounted for 11.6% of trauma during pregnancy[6] (Figure 28-1). Physical abuse during pregnancy has been associated with low fetal birth weights, low maternal weight gain, and a higher maternal incidence of hypertension, anemia, infections, and first- and

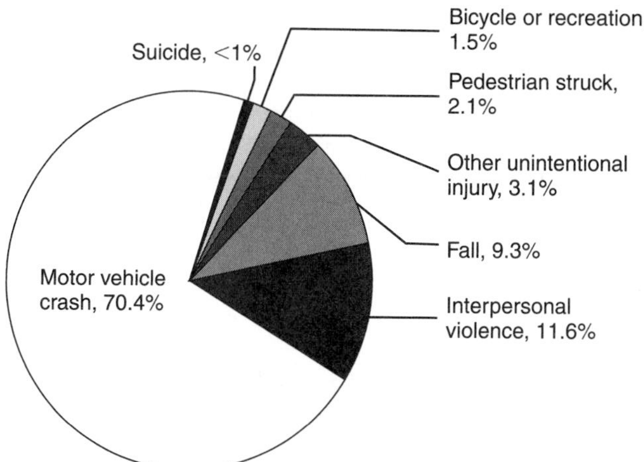

FIGURE 28-1 Mechanism of injury data for 852 pregnant women of childbearing age. (Redrawn from Ikossi DG, Lazar AA, Morabito D et al: Profile of mothers at risk: an analysis of injury and pregnancy loss in 1,195 trauma patients, *J Am Coll Surg* 200:49-56, 2005.)

second-trimester bleeding.[16,18] Additionally, intimate partner violence during pregnancy is associated with significantly higher maternal rates of depression, suicide, and tobacco, alcohol, and drug use.[19,20] Women who claim to have fallen but whose injuries do not seem to match the described event may have been victims of assault. They must be interviewed in private to investigate the possibility of abuse.[21]

For anatomic and physiologic reasons, falls are more common during pregnancy. During the first trimester the woman is more easily fatigued and prone to fainting. As the pregnancy progresses, the uterus extends beyond the pelvic confines and may alter the mother's gait and balance, thus increasing the potential for falls. Relaxation of the pelvic girdle ligaments causes pelvic tilt and increases lordosis, and a change in balance occurs. Pelvic pain (e.g., symphysitis) and neuromuscular dysfunction from pelvic pressure also predispose pregnant women to falls. Falls can occur when performing even simple tasks such as going down the stairs or putting on boots. During late pregnancy, the woman may want to redecorate for the new baby (nesting syndrome) and may climb on a ladder or a chair, further placing herself at risk.

Penetrating injuries resulting from ballistic trauma and stab wounds also occur during pregnancy. Historically, firearms have been second only to motor vehicle crashes as a cause of fatal injury. A classic study from the Cook County Medical Examiner found that, of the 44 maternal deaths resulting from trauma between 1986 and 1989, 22% were from gunshot wounds and 13.6% were from stab wounds.[2] The pregnant abdomen may be the target of penetrating trauma when angry behaviors are displayed or when attempts to abort the fetus are made. The pregnancy may actually be the precipitating factor for a shooting or a stabbing.[16]

Pregnant women also can receive burn and inhalation injuries although these types of injuries occur less frequently than those previously mentioned. Thermal injuries during pregnancy usually occur at home or in the work environment and are caused mainly by flame or hot liquids. The incidence of thermal injuries to pregnant women is low in the Western world, but it is higher in developing countries.[22]

NURSING DATABASE

All female trauma patients of childbearing age should be considered pregnant until proven otherwise. Sherer and Schenker[23] suggest that it is difficult to determine the actual incidence of trauma during pregnancy because of failure to question or document. They cite two clinical examples in which this information may not be recorded: the mild traumatic event that is poorly documented in the medical record and the life-threatening situation in which pregnancy may not be considered. Therefore, it is of utmost importance that an accurate database and patient health history be obtained as soon as possible. An obstetric history, starting with questions about pregnancy, should be initiated immediately. This information not only helps to establish a pregnant condition but can often provide information that aids in both the diagnosis and management of traumatic injuries during pregnancy. Because the patient may be unable to provide reliable information or may be unaware of her pregnancy status, a pregnancy test should be performed if she is of child-bearing age. A description of the events preceding an injury and, whenever possible, of the actual event itself is important to obtain, particularly when the trauma patient is pregnant. If loss of consciousness, headache, back pain, or abdominal pain precedes an incident involving a pregnant woman, an underlying obstetric etiology should be suspected.

MECHANISM OF INJURY

Motor Vehicle Crash

The information important to obtain after a pregnant woman's involvement in a motor vehicle crash includes whether she was a driver or passenger in the vehicle, whether she was wearing a seat belt and shoulder harness, and whether the air bag deployed. The dynamics of the crash are significant (see Chapter 12) and should be considered in anticipating maternal and fetal injuries. If the woman was the driver of the vehicle, then the protuberant abdomen may have been injured by the steering column, particularly if safety restraints were not used. Proper use of seat belts may decrease the severity of maternal injuries and increase maternal survival[3,24] (Figure 28-2). Seat belts prevent ejection from the vehicle, decrease the likelihood of severe head injury, and in general lower mortality rates. Because the overall leading cause of fetal death is maternal death after motor vehicle crashes, seat belts also increase the chance of fetal survival.[3,25-27] After motor vehicle crashes, unbelted women have lower birth weight infants and are more likely to give birth within 48 hours.[28]

When prehospital care providers have information about the events that precipitated a crash or its severity, this information should be conveyed to the health care providers at the receiving facility. One study examined the relationship

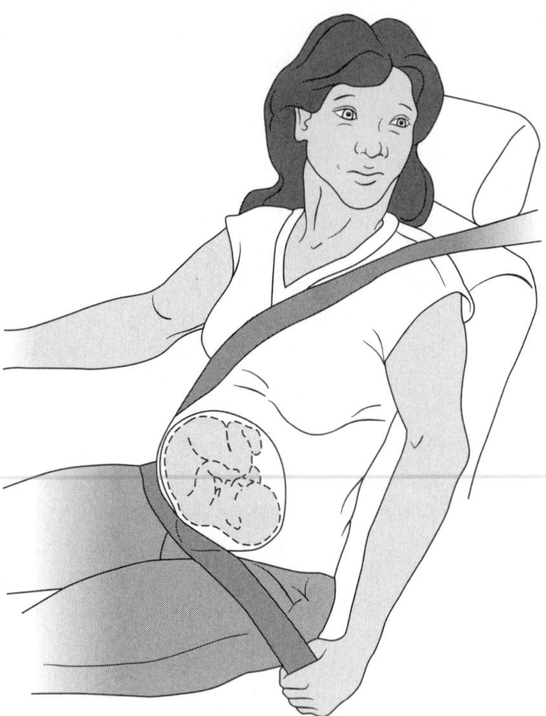

FIGURE 28-2 Proper use of a seat belt during pregnancy.

between type of collision and resultant maternal injuries in 441 pregnant women who were involved in motor vehicle crashes.[24] When there was minor damage to the vehicle, fewer than 1% of the women were injured. When the damage to the vehicle was severe, more serious injuries were found, as expected. Seven percent of those who were involved in severe crashes died and 12.9% were injured. More recent studies have focused on maternal factors such as the ISS, Acute Physiology and Chronic Health Evaluation (APACHE) score, lactate level, maternal injury, head injury, pelvic fractures, and Kleihauer-Betke (KB) smear as predictors of fetal outcome.[10,11]

Falls

An accurate history of the events preceding the fall and of the fall itself is helpful in determining an underlying pathologic process that may have precipitated the fall and resultant injuries. If possible, details of the actual fall event should be described because the type and severity of injuries, which are related to the dissipation of mechanical energy, may be predicted. The height a person falls in part determines velocity and may reflect injury severity. If a person is able to break the fall by grasping on to something, the velocity can be decreased. Impact forces also can affect injury severity. The energy-absorbing qualities of the structure on which the woman fell is another important factor to consider. As previously noted, if the pattern of injuries does not match the fall event, abuse should be considered. A private, confidential interview might elicit this information.

Firearms and Other Weapons

Gunshot wounds are the most common type of penetrating trauma during pregnancy. Other sources of penetrating trauma include stabbings with knives or other sharp objects. When the woman is pregnant, the enlarged abdomen is the most likely body part to be targeted, causing potential damage to the underlying uterus.

Events surrounding a shooting are often vague, and witnesses or even the woman herself may claim that the incident was unintentional. However, such violent crime may represent an attempt to damage or abort the fetus, and that motive must be suspected. The nurse must make every attempt to elicit this information from the patient, family members, or significant others. Information about the type of firearm involved and the distance between the individual and the weapon can aid in determining the severity of underlying injuries. Gunshot wounds usually require early surgical exploration and repair.

Stab wounds require that, if possible, a description of the weapon be given to the emergency care personnel if the weapon does not accompany the patient. This information may need to be elicited from the victim or witnesses. The length and width of the object and how far it penetrated the abdomen or other body part are clues to possible underlying injury. Stab wounds may be explored to determine the extent of injury and the possible need for further surgical intervention.

Intimate Partner Violence

When the patient has a pattern of injuries that does not match the reported mechanism, the nurse should suspect intimate partner violence (IPV) and administer an assessment screening to the patient in a private area separate from the mate. If IPV is suspected, the patient must receive follow-up care. To prevent future repeated IPV, the pregnant woman should be educated about safety behaviors, including hiding money, having extra keys, having a family code, and removing weapons.[29] All women should be aware that the National Domestic Violence Hot Line is available to them by calling 1-800-799-SAFE or, for the hearing impaired, 1-800-787-3224. The Web site is www.NDVH.org.

In view of this strong epidemiologic basis for violence during pregnancy and the potential obstetric complications, nurses must maintain a high index of suspicion and probe to ascertain information detailing the events leading to injury. Parker and McFarlane[21] suggest that routine prenatal assessment provides an excellent opportunity to conduct an abuse assessment screening. Hospitalization for an unexplained traumatic event is also a time to conduct such an assessment. As stated by Parker and McFarlane, a nonjudgmental, gentle approach is essential, but the questions must be direct. An assessment screening tool developed by the Nursing Research Consortium on Violence and Abuse is presented in Figure 28-3.

1. Have you ever been emotionally or physically abused by your partner or someone important to you?

YES ☐ NO ☐

2. Within the last year, have you been hit, slapped, kicked or otherwise physically hurt by someone?

YES ☐ NO ☐

If YES, by whom____________________

Number of times____________________

3. Since you've been pregnant, have you been hit, slapped, kicked, or otherwise physically hurt by someone?

YES ☐ NO ☐

If YES, by whom____________________

Number of times____________________

Mark the area of injury on body map.

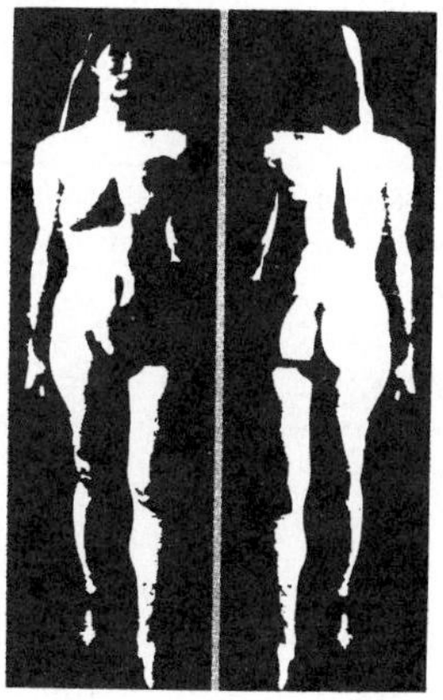

4. Within the last year, has anyone forced you to have sexual activities?

If YES, who____________________

Number of times____________________

5. Are you afraid of your partner or anyone you listed above?

YES ☐ NO ☐

**Developed by the Nursing Research Consortium on Violence and Abuse of which both authors are members. 1989. Readers are encouraged to reproduce and use this assessment tool.*

FIGURE 28-3 Abuse assessment screening tool. (From Parker B, McFarlane J: Identifying and helping battered pregnant women, *Am J Matern Child Nurs* 16:161-164, 1991.)

Burns and Inhalation Injuries

If the pregnant patient has a suspected inhalation injury, carbon monoxide (CO) intoxication should always be suspected and carboxyhemoglobin (COHb) levels should be measured. CO intoxication is a common cause of all poisoning deaths, including fetal poisoning deaths, in the United States.[30] If the patient has been a victim of trauma associated with fire, automobile exhaust, faulty heating systems, or generator use, CO intoxication should be considered.

The fetal effects of CO poisoning are more severe than maternal effects because the concentration of COHb is 10% to 15% higher in the fetus as a result of the higher affinity of fetal hemoglobin for CO.[31] Extensive research by Longo and Hill[32] demonstrated that fetal COHb concentration rises more slowly than does the maternal level but surpasses maternal levels after 5 hours. Maternal CO will reach a steady state in 7 to 8 hours, but fetal concentrations continue to rise for 36 to 48 hours.[32] The CO half-life in the fetus is twice as long as the maternal half-life. Therefore, the fetus is more susceptible to CO poisoning.

Fetal effects include teratogenicity, neurologic dysfunction, decreased birth weight, and increased fetal death because the fetal partial arterial oxygen concentration (PaO_2) decreases in direct proportion to the increase in COHb. CO poisoning impairs the release of oxygen from the mother to the fetus and from fetal hemoglobin to fetal tissue. Prompt diagnosis and appropriate management of inhalation injuries are therefore essential.[33]

Obstetric History

When pregnancy is suspected, an obstetric history should be considered an important component of the patient's health history. The gestational age of the fetus and status of the pregnancy must be established, and a complete obstetric history should be obtained as soon as possible. Suspicion of pregnancy increases if more than 4 weeks have lapsed since the last menstrual period (LMP) or if the LMP was unusual in any way. To determine the gestational age, early ultrasonography is most reliable.[34-36]

A more thorough obstetric history includes determining parity (Table 28-1), which indicates any previous abortions or premature deliveries. The history for each delivery, including gestational age of the fetus, number of hours of labor, and type of birth (vaginal or cesarean), also should be obtained along with the maternal Rh factor. This information can alert medical personnel to potential problems, including premature labor and delivery. When possible a spouse, family member, or significant other should be interviewed to help obtain and verify this information. Information should also be obtained concerning what, if any, form of contraception was used and how assiduously it was used.

TABLE 28-1 Parity

In many institutions, obstetric history is summarized by digits and dashes (e.g., 3-1-0-4).

First digit	Number of term infants (38 weeks)
Second digit	Number of premature infants (20-37 weeks)
Third digit	Number of abortions (any loss before 20 weeks, including ectopics and induced abortions)
Fourth digit	Number of children currently alive

In the example above (3-1-0-4), the woman had 3 term births and 1 premature infant and has 4 children alive. (Many recall this with the mnemonic Florida Power And Light, which stands for Full-term, Preterm, Abortions, and Living.)

Data from Pritchard J, MacDonald P, Gant NF: *Williams' obstetrics,* 17th ed, p 246, Norwalk, CT, 1990, Appleton-Century-Crofts.

RESUSCITATION PHASE

Early signs of pregnancy may be easily overlooked. Therefore, the astute nurse is alert to even the most subtle changes that can occur during pregnancy (Table 28-2). On admission, a pregnancy test should be performed on any woman of child-bearing age. Early recognition that the trauma patient is pregnant can lead the nurse through the dual assessment of mother and fetus.

The general principles on which trauma management is based must not be ignored in caring for a pregnant trauma patient. The implementation of a rapid primary survey followed by a secondary assessment is imperative, with airway, breathing, and circulation (the ABCs) acknowledged as first priorities.[37] Early recognition of pregnancy should trigger the nurse to be suspicious of unique injuries and to be alert for the pregnancy-related changes that may alter assessment findings and mask signs of shock.

TABLE 28-2 Presumptive, Probable, and Positive Signs of Pregnancy

Presumptive Signs
Amenorrhea
Breast changes
Fatigue
Frequent micturition
Nausea and vomiting
Quickening
Skin changes
Cervical changes

Probable Signs
Uterine contractions
Fetal outline
Laboratory pregnancy tests
Uterine changes

Positive Signs
Fetal heart movement recorded by sonogram
Fetal heart sounds
Fetal movement felt by examiner

Data from Pilliteri A: *Maternal-newborn nursing care of the growing family,* 3rd ed, p 320, Boston, 1985, Little Brown.

CLINICAL MANAGEMENT/TEAM APPROACH

The key to successful management of the pregnant trauma patient is a team approach. Both emergency/trauma personnel and obstetric personnel should be involved in the patient's care.[37,38] Although obstetric management is imperative, the ABCs of trauma resuscitation remain the first priority because the best guarantee of fetal survival is prompt maternal care after traumatic injury.

In 1974, Crosby[39] identified complications associated with the management of injured pregnant women:

> Among physicians who man emergency rooms, there is a lack of familiarity with the state of pregnancy and the physiological changes that accompany it.... Thus a state of therapeutic paralysis is often seen when the trauma victim is recognized as being pregnant. Attention is all too often directed away from the pregnancy, which may be unfamiliar, but potentially of major importance.... Lacerations are sutured, fractures are set, x-ray [films] taken and abrasions cleaned while the fetus may die; a retroplacental clot may grow with shock-inducing speed during the time spent dealing with lesser problems.

Today, more than 30 years later, the situation as Crosby describes it may not be as common in the trauma setting, but the concept of therapeutic paralysis does persist. The development and continuing provision of an Advanced Life Support in Obstetrics course for improved obstetric emergency management suggests that concerns continue about the management of obstetric emergencies.[40] The fact that aggressive maternal care is essential for the best fetal outcome must be emphasized.[2,41,42]

MATERNAL ASSESSMENT

To render prompt and aggressive care to the pregnant trauma patient during the resuscitation phase, the nurse must have knowledge not only about initial trauma management interventions but also about the normal anatomic and physiologic changes that occur during pregnancy and the significat of these changes[43,44] (Table 28-3). This knowledge must be applied during the initial assessment process and as resuscitation efforts continue.[45,46] Care of the pregnant trauma patient becomes more complex when obstetric complications are encountered in addition to traumatic injuries. These assessment considerations are not limited, however, to the resuscitation phase of care; they must be considered throughout all phases of trauma care.

Neurologic Considerations

Neurologically, a pregnant woman has an increased risk of fainting and is more easily fatigued.[46] The pregnant woman also may have changes in gait and balance, primarily during the third trimester. Changes in vision, complaint of

TABLE 28-3 Normal Anatomic and Physiologic Changes During Pregnancy

Body System	Alteration	Significance of Change
Neurologic	Increased risk of fainting	More prone to fall
	Easily fatigued	Increased risk of trauma
Cardiovascular	Hypervolemic (increased volume of as much as 50% above prepregnancy levels)	Signs of blood loss can develop subtly
	Supine hypotension	Increased fluid needs for resuscitation
	Physiologic anemia	Vital signs and laboratory tests must be assessed against normal pregnancy values (see Tables 28-5 and 28-6)
	Increased heart rate	
	Hypercoagulability	Increased risk for thromboembolism
Respiratory	Engorged upper respiratory passages	Potential for nasopharyngeal bleeding making gentle oral intubation with smaller well-lubricated tube preferable
	Increased tidal volume	Altered response to inhalation anesthetics
	Increased vital capacity	
	Increased respiratory rate	Decrease in blood buffering capacity
	Decreased functional residual capacity	Early use of oxygen therapy essential as a result of decreased functional residual capacity
	Elevated diaphragm	Greater risk for diaphragm rupture
Gastrointestinal	Physiologic ileus	Increased risk of aspiration
	Increased gastric acidity	
	Compartmentalization of abdominal contents	Altered internal injury patterns
Genitourinary	Increased urinary frequency	
	Increased glomerular filtration rate	
	Dilation of renal calyces, renal pelvis, and ureter	Altered appearance of IV urogram
	Bladder pulled into abdomen	Bladder susceptible to abdominal trauma
Musculoskeletal	Alterations in gait and balance	Increased risk of fall
	Widened symphysis pubis	Possible increased risk of spinal subluxation
	Lordosis	

headaches, and seizure activity (especially in a patient with no history of seizure) are abnormal and, when present, suggest obstetric complications such as preeclampsia and eclampsia (Table 28-4). Prompt identification of an obstetric complication can guide care and decrease the incidence of both maternal and fetal compromise.

TABLE 28-4 Signs and Symptoms of Preeclampsia

Mild Preeclampsia	Severe Preeclampsia
	When any of the following exists:
Systolic blood pressure of at least 140 mm Hg or a diastolic blood pressure of at least 90 mm Hg	Blood pressure >160 mm Hg systolic, >110 mm Hg diastolic
Associated with either	Proteinuria >5 g/24 hr
Proteinuria	Oliguria defined as <500 ml/24 hr
OR	Cerebral or visual disturbances
Edema	Pulmonary edema
	Epigastric or right upper quadrant pain
	Impaired liver function
	Thrombocytopenia
	Fetal intrauterine growth restriction or oligohydramnios
	Elevated serum creatinine
	HELLP syndrome (hemolysis, elevated liver enzymes, and low platelets)
Seizures = eclampsia	

From American College of Obstetricians and Gynecologists: *Hypertension in pregnancy,* ACOG technical bulletin No. 219, Washington, DC, 1996, American College of Obstetricians and Gynecologists.

Respiratory Considerations

The respiratory system is also altered during pregnancy. The upper respiratory passages become narrowed by engorged capillaries, making the pregnant patient more prone to nasopharyngeal bleeding and subsequent upper airway obstruction.

During pregnancy, there may be as much as a 40% increase in tidal volume and a rise of 100 to 200 ml in vital capacity. The respiratory rate may remain unchanged or increase by 15%.[44] The combined effects of these respiratory changes place the pregnant woman in a chronic state of "hyperventilation" that results in arterial blood gas alterations. The partial arterial carbon dioxide ($PaCO_2$) levels drop to approximately 30 mm Hg, and PaO_2 increases to 101 to 104 mm Hg. A normal pH is maintained by the excretion of bicarbonate by the kidneys (Table 28-5).

As the pregnancy progresses, there is an increased minute ventilation, which is caused by a rise in tidal volume. This

TABLE 28-5 Laboratory Value Adjustments During Pregnancy

	Nonpregnant	Pregnant
Electrolytes and Acid-Base Values		
Sodium (mEq/L)	135-145	132-140
Potassium (mEq/L)	3.5-5.0	3.5-4.5
Chloride (mEq/L)	100-106	90-105
Bicarbonate (mEq/L)	24-30	17-22
Pco_2 (mm Hg)	35-50	25-30
Po_2 (mm Hg)	98-100	101-104
Base excess (mEq/L)	0.7	3-4
Arterial pH	7.38-7.44	7.40-7.45
BUN (mg/dl)	10-18	4-12
Creatinine (mg/dl)	0.6-1.2	0.4-0.9
Creatinine clearance (ml/min)	3.5-5.0	2.0-3.7
Osmolality (mOsm/kg)	275-295	275-285
Lipids and Liver Function Tests		
Total bilirubin (mg/dl)	1.0	1.0
Direct bilirubin (mg/dl)	0.4	0.4
Alkaline phosphatase (international units/ml)	13-35	25-80
SGOT (international units/ml)	10-40	10-40
Total protein (g/dl)	6.0-8.4	5.5-7.5
Albumin (g/dl)	3.5-5.0	3.0-4.5
Globulin (g/dl)	2.3-3.5	3.0-4.0
Total lipids (mg/dl)	460-1,000	1,040
Total cholesterol (mg/dl)	120-220	250
Triglycerides (mg/dl)	45-150	230
Free fatty acid (g/L)	770	1,226
Phospholipids (mg/dl)	256	350
Hematologic Laboratory Values		
Complete blood cell count:		
Hematocrit (%)	37-48	32-42
Hemoglobin (g/dl)	12-16	10-14
Leukocytes (count/mm^3)	4,300-10,800	5,000-15,000
Polymorphonuclear cells (%)	54-62	60-85
Lymphocytes (%)	38-46	15-40
Fibrinogen	250-400	600
Platelets	150,000-350,000	Normal or slightly decreased
Serum iron (g)	75-150	65-120
Iron-binding capacity (g)	250-410	300-500
Iron saturation (%)	30-40	15-30
Ferritin (ng/ml)	35	10-12
Erythrocyte sedimentation (mm/hr)	<20	30-90

Modified from Elrad H, Gleicher N: Physiologic changes in normal pregnancy. In Gleicher N, editor: *Principles of medical therapy in pregnancy,* pp 51-52, New York, 1985, Plenum.
SGOT, Aspartate aminotransferase.

increased tidal volume leads to a decreased functional residual capacity (FRC) by up to 20% at times. A reduced FRC lowers the closing alveolar pressure, which predisposes the pregnant woman to alveolar collapse, atelectasis, and decreased oxygen reserve. Therefore, the airway and breathing of a pregnant trauma patient must be monitored carefully and supported as necessary to prevent maternal and subsequent fetal hypoxia. Supplemental oxygen should be given to all pregnant trauma patients, and pulse oximetry should be monitored continuously. If the patient is intubated, capnography is useful.

Cardiovascular Considerations

Cardiovascular changes are perhaps the most profound physiologic alterations that occur during pregnancy and the most critical to interpret when the pregnant trauma patient is assessed. The pregnant woman is normally hypervolemic. Blood volume during pregnancy begins to increase by the tenth week of gestation; by the thirty-fourth week of gestation, a pregnant woman's circulatory volume can increase by as much as 50%. This increase can mask a 30% gradual loss of maternal blood volume or a 10% to 15% acute blood loss. When this occurs, although the maternal vital signs may remain unchanged, the fetus can be at risk because of a decrease in uterine perfusion; the woman's risk is also increased because these stable vital signs may change precipitously. Because the uterus cannot autoregulate its blood flow, perfusion is directly related to the pressure it receives from maternal circulation.

The electrocardiogram can be altered during pregnancy as well. As the uterus enlarges and elevates the diaphragm, the heart is pushed upward and rotated, causing a shift of the electrical axis by 15 degrees. This may precipitate changes such as T-wave flattening or inversion in lead III; or Q waves in lead III and the augmented V lead, which are considered normal in pregnancy.[47]

Hematologic Considerations

Although erythrocyte production increases during pregnancy, adequate levels cannot be maintained as plasma volume increases; therefore, the pregnant woman is physiologically anemic.[48] A normal prepregnancy hematocrit of 40% to 41% may drop to 31% to 34% in late pregnancy.

The coagulation profile of the pregnant woman is also altered because fibrinogen and concentrations of factors VII, VIII, and IX are increased during pregnancy. Bleeding time, clotting time, and prothrombin time should remain unchanged during pregnancy. The increase in fibrinogen and other factors, coupled with a decrease in circulating plasminogen activator, can actually benefit the pregnant patient if hemorrhage occurs. These same changes, however, pose a potential problem. The risk of venous thromboembolism is five times higher in a pregnant woman than in a nonpregnant woman of similar age. Immobility after a traumatic event puts the pregnant patient at even greater risk.[46,49]

The leukocyte count is normally elevated in pregnancy to approximately 5,000 to 15,000/mm^3 and becomes even further elevated during labor and delivery. Except for an increase in phagocytes and a decrease in lymphocytes during pregnancy, the differential remains unchanged. Other laboratory study adjustments for pregnant women are listed in Table 28-5.

A 5-year retrospective study of trauma patients with a placental abruption found that a white blood cell (WBC) count of >20,000/mm^3 on admission was strongly predictive of placental abruption ($p = .005$). The study also suggested that a WBC count of <20,000/mm^3 rules out placental abruption (negative predictive value, 100%).[50] It should be remembered, however, that abruptions are dynamic events that can evolve over time. Therefore, the nurse should remain vigilant for clinical signs such as contractions, abdominal pain, or changes in fetal status.[38]

Hemodynamic Considerations

The most dramatic hemodynamic change that occurs during pregnancy is supine hypotension, also known as vena cava syndrome. After 16 to 20 weeks' gestation, when the patient assumes the supine position, the enlarging uterus compresses the vena cava and aorta, impeding venous return and decreasing blood pressure and cardiac output. Hypotension therefore can occur normally in a pregnant woman in a supine position. When this occurs, the patient becomes uncomfortable or nauseated until she is repositioned and blood pressure increases. Therefore, the pregnant trauma patient should never be placed in the supine position. Traditionally the pregnant woman is placed in the left lateral position, which displaces the uterus and decreases compression of the major abdominal vessels (Figure 28-4). During prehospital transport and until spinal injuries are ruled out, the supine position can be avoided by tilting the backboard 30 degrees to the left side, simulating the left lateral position[44,45] (Figure 28-5). Turning the pregnant patient to the left lateral position can markedly increase cardiac output and should always be considered as a resuscitative measure. Care must be taken to stabilize the neck and maintain the spine in proper alignment when repositioning the patient. The right-sided tilt can be equally effective if left-sided injuries make that position difficult. If the patient's injuries or resuscitation procedures prohibit this position change, the uterus can be displaced manually. The vital signs should be monitored closely for indications of shock throughout the resuscitation phase so that aggressive volume replacement can be initiated as necessary.

Hypertension is not normal during pregnancy; it should be resolved as to whether the hypertension existed before pregnancy or is indicative of pregnancy-induced hypertension. During pregnancy, the heart rate increases approximately 10 to 20 beats/min above prepregnancy levels. Clark et al[51] assessed the central hemodynamic status of ten healthy pregnant patients who were screened carefully both in the third trimester and post partum. In late pregnancy, the patients had a 43% increase in cardiac output (4.3 to 6.2 L/min). Other significant findings included a 21% decline in systemic vascular resistance, a 34% reduction in pulmonary vascular resistance, and a 28% decrease in the colloid oncotic pressure-pulmonary capillary wedge pressure gradient. There was no significant difference in mean arterial pressure, central venous pressure, or pulmonary capillary wedge pressure during late pregnancy compared with the nonpregnant state (Table 28-6).

The hemodynamic changes that occur normally during pregnancy can cause confusion as the resuscitation team assesses the patient's condition. Tachycardia and hypotension that occur when the pregnant trauma patient is in a supine position may not be indicative of a shock state but may instead represent normal changes. Caution must be exercised, however, because the pregnant trauma patient, as previously stated, can mask a 15% to 30% blood loss without evidence of shock while uterine perfusion decreases, risking fetal hypoxia. Changes in laboratory values, including decreased hematocrit and increased leukocyte count, further confuse the clinical picture. Laboratory value trends must be monitored closely as well and compared with normal pregnancy values (see Table 28-5).

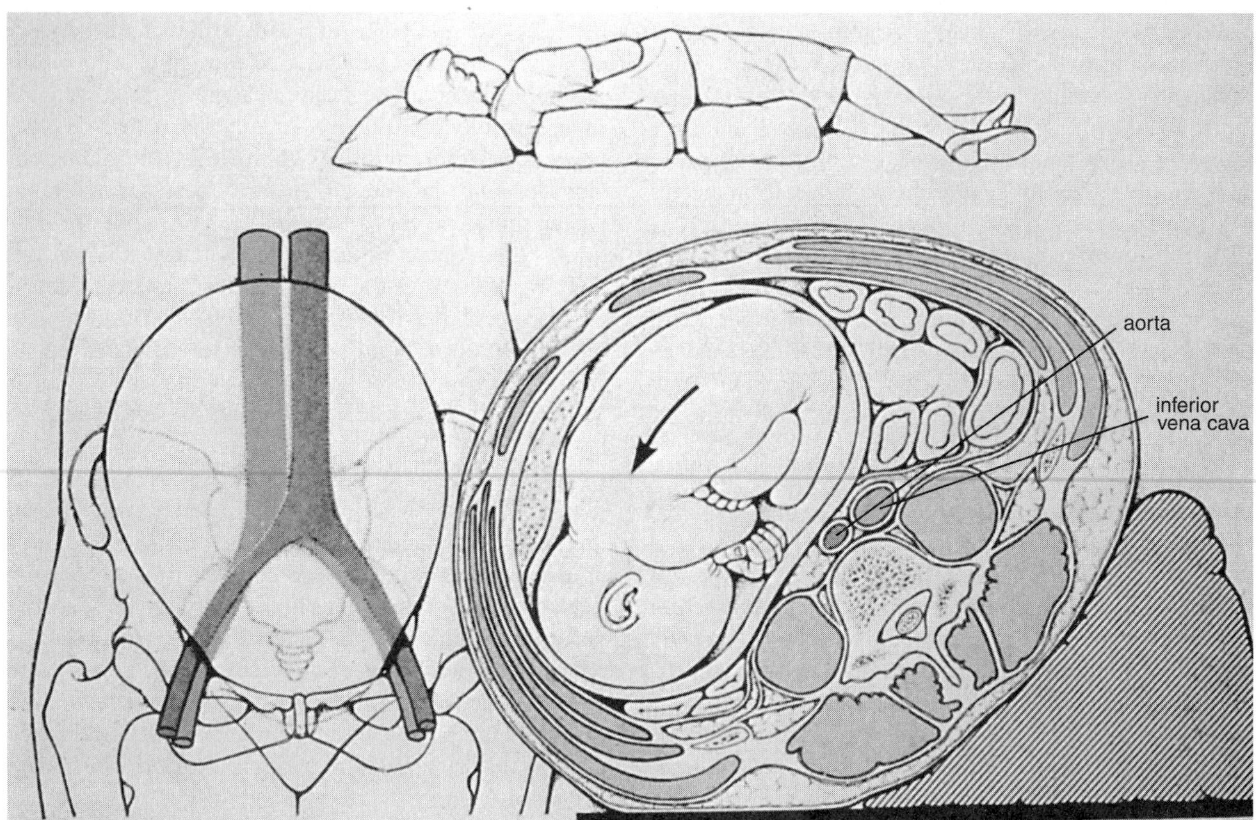

FIGURE 28-4 Left lateral positioning displaces the uterus and decreases compression of major abdominal vessels.

Gastrointestinal Considerations

A physiologic ileus, or diminished emptying time of the bowel, normally occurs during pregnancy. In addition, the placental production of gastrin and progesterone increases the acidity of the stomach contents. On auscultation, bowel sounds may be absent, making interpretation difficult. It should always be assumed that the pregnant trauma patient has a full stomach and is at risk for vomiting and aspiration.

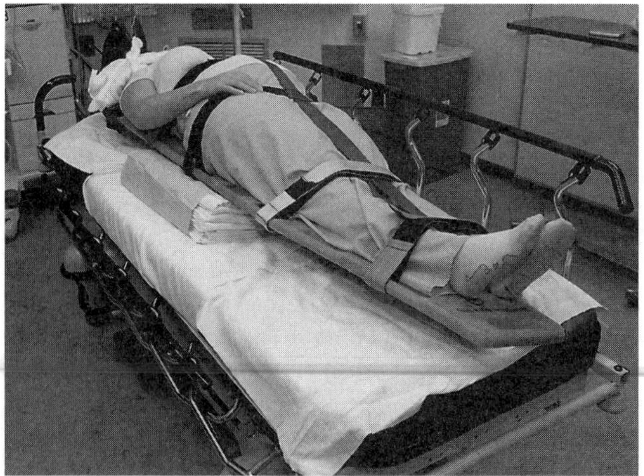

FIGURE 28-5 Placing a small roll under the right side of the backboard and tipping the backboard 30 degrees displaces the uterus to the left side.

Injuries to the liver and spleen commonly cause shock during pregnancy. The patient's abdomen should be assessed carefully for pain, guarding, and rebound tenderness. If clinically indicated, an orogastric tube may be inserted early during the resuscitation phase of care. The patient should be prepared for abdominal tests to detect injury and the source of hemorrhage. She may perceive the procedure as harmful to her baby and should be encouraged to verbalize her fears. Reinforcing the value of the procedure as a diagnostic tool that is not harmful to the baby may ease some of the mother's fears.[52] Preparation for surgical intervention is indicated if abdominal exploration is deemed necessary.

Genitourinary Considerations

Genitourinary changes include an increase in urination frequency throughout pregnancy. The increase in frequency during the first trimester is the result of a rise in the glomerular filtration rate (GFR) by approximately 30% of prepregnancy values.[53] During the third trimester the further increased frequency is a result of compression of the bladder by the enlarging uterus, in addition to an increased GFR.

With blunt trauma to the abdomen during late pregnancy, the bladder is more likely to empty spontaneously or rupture because the bladder may be elevated and outside the protective pelvic ring. If a stable condition allows, the patient should be encouraged to void. If she is unable to void spontaneously

TABLE 28-6 **Central Hemodynamic Changes**

	Nonpregnant	Pregnant
Cardiac output (L/min)	4.3 ± 0.9	6.2 ± 1.0
Heart rate (beats/min)	71 ± 10.0	83 ± 10.0
Systemic vascular resistance (dyne cm sec^{-5})	1530 ± 520	1210 ± 266
Pulmonary vascular resistance (dyne cm sec^{-5})	119 ± 47.0	78 ± 22
Colloid oncotic pressure (mm Hg)	20.8 ± 1.0	18.0 ± 1.5
Colloid oncotic pressure–pulmonary capillary wedge pressure (mm Hg)	14.5 ± 2.5	10.5 ± 2.7
Mean arterial pressure (mm Hg)	86.4 ± 7.5	90.3 ± 5.8
Pulmonary capillary wedge pressure (mm Hg)	6.3 ± 2.1	7.5 ± 1.8
Central venous pressure (mm Hg)	3.7 ± 2.6	3.6 ± 2.5
Left ventricular stroke work index (g-m/m^{-2})	41 ± 8	48 ± 6

From Clark S, Cotton O, Lee W et al: Central hemodynamic assessment of normal term pregnancy, *Am J Obstet Gynecol* 161:1439-1442, 1989.

and bladder trauma is plausible given the mechanism of injury, the patient should be catheterized by use of strict aseptic technique. Glucosuria is common during pregnancy, but the presence of frank or microscopic blood suggests genitourinary trauma. Diagnostic tests may be performed, including cystography, intravenous (IV) pyelography, and cystoscopy. Physiologic dilation of the renal calyces, renal pelves, and ureters (particularly on the right side) may be evident. These conditions are present from approximately the tenth week of pregnancy until after delivery and are believed to be caused by ureteral obstruction from the ovarian vein plexuses, dextrotorsion of the uterus, and increased progesterone concentrations.[53]

Metabolic Considerations

As a normal change of pregnancy, the pituitary gland nearly doubles in weight. Shock in the pregnant patient can precipitate a sudden drop in pituitary blood flow, leading to necrosis[54] (known as Sheehan's syndrome). During pregnancy, calcium, phosphate, magnesium, creatinine, and blood urea nitrogen (BUN) levels fall. There is also an increased risk of glucose intolerance.

Obstetric and Fetal Considerations

When the trauma patient is pregnant, primary and secondary assessment must also focus on the fetus and possible obstetric complications that can result after traumatic injury. The fetus may be compromised while the mother appears stable. As an initial response to shock, uterine perfusion decreases, causing stress to the fetus. Unique injuries to the uterus must be detected and treated immediately or the lives of both fetus and mother are threatened.

Obstetric Assessment

The obstetric assessment must determine the viability of the fetus, establish the potential for impending delivery, and identify unique injuries and complications. After the gestational age is estimated and fetal well-being is established, the status of the patient's amniotic membrane (intact or ruptured) must be assessed. Indications of labor, if any, also must be noted. Specific maternal and fetal injuries and complications unique to trauma during pregnancy are described in detail later in the chapter.

Gestational Age. Accurate assessment of gestational age or the estimated date of delivery (EDD) is important during the initial resuscitation to determine whether the fetus is viable. An ultrasonography performed in the first trimester of pregnancy provides the most accurate estimate of gestational age.[34-36] An ultrasonographic scan performed at weeks 6 to 11 of a pregnancy is accurate within 5 to 7 days and when performed in the twelfth to twentieth week of pregnancy is accurate within 10 days.[55] Many times information from previous scans may not be available. However, if the patient or a reliable historian is available, the EDD from an early ultrasonographic scan can provide a means of calculating gestational age. Barring this, ultrasonography performed in the emergency setting will give a reasonable means of assessing gestational age and has become a routine assessment tool for obstetricians, trauma surgeons, and emergency physicians.[45,46,56,57]

For a rapid assessment (including prehospital assessment), fundal height provides another means of estimating gestational age. This technique may be subject to several misleading variables such as aminotic fluid level, obesity, and macrosomia. Fundal height is the distance from the symphysis pubis to the top of the fundus. From 16 to 32 weeks, this measurement approximates the weeks of gestation (Figure 28-6).

Determination of the gestational age of the fetus is also helpful in identifying possible injuries to both the mother and fetus. During the first 12 to 14 weeks (early pregnancy), the uterus is well protected in the pelvic confines. Cases of uterine and fetal injury during this period have been documented, but they are rare. After the first trimester (12 to 14 weeks), the uterus becomes an abdominal organ and is no longer protected by the pelvis. The uterus and fetus may

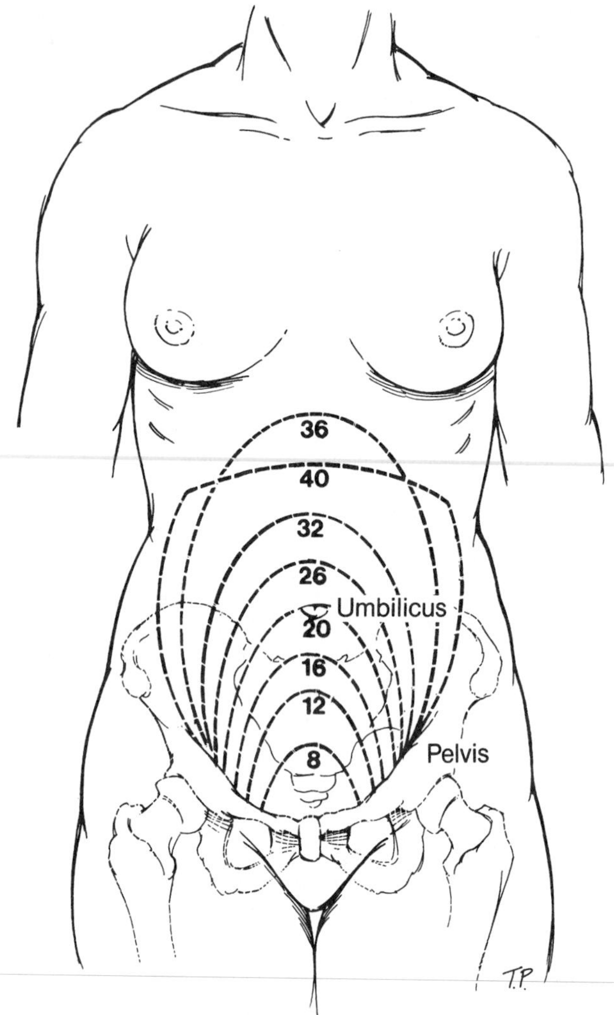

FIGURE 28-6 Uterine size and location, reflecting gestational age.

therefore absorb the impact of traumatic forces and consequently sustain unique injuries.

Fetal Assessment

Continuous fetal assessment is essential because the mother can mask signs of shock and the fetus can be the first to show evidence of compromise. The fetal condition is easiest to evaluate by assessing the fetal heart rate. The normal fetal heart rate is 120 to 160 beats/min and can be detected with an ultrasound device (Doppler) by 10 to 12 weeks of gestation. If the fetus is viable, its heart rate should be monitored continuously with an electronic fetal monitor (EFM) once the mother's condition has been stabilized. The variability of the fetal heart tones (FHT) and the rate should be evaluated by a clinician experienced in fetal monitoring (see Figure 28-7). Fetuses that are 24 weeks or older are considered viable if neonatal resources are available. If an EFM is not available, only a Doppler device designed for obstetric evaluation should be used because its frequency is adjusted to assess FHTs. A Doppler device of higher frequency used for adults, such as those used for vascular studies, may not have sufficient range so that nothing is heard although the fetus is viable, thereby confusing the clinical picture. In many instances, fetal compromise as suggested by prolonged fetal bradycardia may be reflective of fetal hypoxemia. If the mother is stable and the fetus considered viable, immediate delivery should be considered on behalf of the fetus.

The length of time a pregnant patient requires electronic fetal monitoring has been debated. Recent studies suggest that within 4 to 6 hours of minor trauma, if there is no labor or fetal distress, monitoring can be safely discontinued.[10,58,59] It is fairly clear that in patients who do not have contractions and who have good variability in FHTs the need for additional monitoring is slight. Patients having contractions clearly require additional monitoring. Once the decision has been made to continue obstetric monitoring, the collaborative team of trauma and obstetric professionals must identify the appropriate nursing unit in which the patient will receive care and diligent fetal monitoring.

When the pregnant trauma patient is conscious, she is a resource for detecting an alteration in fetal activity, which is also an indicator of fetal well-being. Quickening, or the maternal perception of fetal movement, usually occurs in approximately the sixteenth week of gestation during a second pregnancy and in the twentieth week of a first. Although the fetus is not in constant motion, particularly in the third trimester of pregnancy, a prolonged period during which fetal movement is lacking can suggest fetal compromise or death.

Additional diagnostic procedures that can aid in assessing the condition of the fetus include ultrasonography and amniocentesis. Real-time ultrasonography can identify fetal cardiac movement, detect FHTs, and determine fetal death. Fetal biophysical assessment by ultrasound is a method used to aid in determining and quantifying the fetal status. Fetal biophysical profile scoring (BPS) is based on five biophysical variables, four of which are monitored simultaneously by dynamic ultrasound imaging. The variables are fetal breathing movement, gross body movement, fetal tone, qualitative amniotic fluid volume, and reactive fetal heart rate.[60] The fifth parameter of the BPS is a fetal heart rate tracing, which is "scored" as reactive or nonreactive. Each parameter is coded as present or absent according to set criteria and given a rating of 2 (present) or 0 (absent) with a maximum score of 10.

On the basis of the BPS, a management protocol is recommended.[61] A biophysical score of 2 out of 10 can be indicative of severe fetal compromise, including asphyxia. However, in the acute setting the impact of medications such as narcotics, sedatives, or anesthetics must be considered when score results are analyzed. In the emergency setting, biophysical profile scoring may be helpful, but the test may require up to a 30-minute ultrasound observation period, which may not be appropriate during initial trauma resuscitation. The scoring and observation can be done after maternal resuscitation.

Amniocentesis can test for fetal maturity. Maturity of the fetal lungs is determined by the lecithin/sphingomyelin ratio and the presence of phosphatidyl glycerol in the amniotic

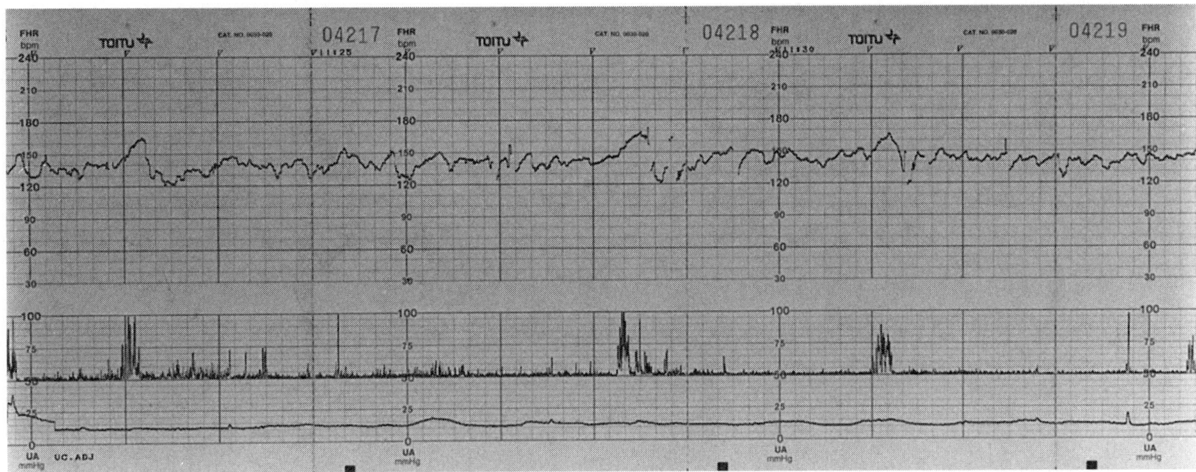

FIGURE 28-7 Monitor strip segment showing a normal fetal heart tracing *(upper tracing)* with significant variability, acceleration of heart rate associated with fetal movement *(middle tracing)*, and no decelerations below the baseline. Uterine irritability detectable as small irregular contractions *(bottom tracing)* indicates potential for problems such as placental separation (abruptio), other bleeding, and preterm labor. Monitoring should be continued until the uterus is quiescent.

fluid. It is difficult to imagine, however, how this information would be obtained and used in an acute care setting. If it is important to consider an early delivery, gestational age assessment, as outlined above, provides sufficient knowledge about the risks of prematurity and associated morbidity.

SPECIAL MANAGEMENT CONSIDERATIONS

Specific factors must be considered when caring for the pregnant trauma patient during airway management, radiographic examinations, medication administration, medical or pneumatic antishock garment (PASG) use, and invasive abdominal assessment procedures. The cardiac arrest situation is unique for this patient population. Management of burn and inhalation injuries also requires special considerations to optimize outcomes of the mother and fetus.

Airway Assessement and Management

Airway assessment and management are essential in the successful management of every trauma patient, but in the pregnant patient this basic trauma measure takes on additional importance. In general, airway management is more difficult during pregnancy. Capillary engorgement of the mucosa causes swelling of the nasal passages, oral pharynx, larynx, and trachea.[62]

Use of nasal airways or nasotracheal tubes should be avoided to prevent nasal bleeding. When intubation is required, a smaller ($\leq$7 mm), well-lubricated endotracheal tube should be gently inserted by an experienced clinician.[62,63] This practice is recommended to prevent posterior pharyngeal bleeding from engorged vessels in the upper respiratory tract, which could be traumatized during nasal intubation.

During the secondary assessment, the patient's airway should be assessed thoroughly, even if it is patent and the patient appears stable. To evaluate the airway, mouth opening, atlanto-occipital extension, ability to protrude the mandible, Mallampati class, and thyromental distance should be determined.[63] Then, if an obstetric emergency occurs, the trauma team will be prepared to adequately manage the airway. Should an airway be difficult or an intubation fail, use of a laryngeal mask airway is recommended until a definitive airway can be established.

Radiographic Examinations

Radiographic examinations considered essential for diagnosing injuries after trauma should never be omitted during pregnancy. Care must be taken, however, to protect the patient from unnecessary radiation exposure. When possible, the uterus should be shielded with a lead apron during radiographic examination. Duplication of radiographs should be avoided, and the purpose of each exposure should be validated regarding its clinical implications. The patient should be assured that essential tests must be done to diagnose her injuries properly, including computed tomography (CT) scans or magnetic resonance imaging as deemed appropriate.[52]

Recently new full-body digital x-ray machines have been introduced to the trauma arena. This new technology uses significantly lower levels of radiation.[64] A full-body x-ray examination can be obtained with minimal radiation exposure (see Figure 28-8). This new technology can be appropriately used with the pregnant patient.

Assessment of fetal radiation risk is a complex process. Qualitative radiation risks are categorized as low, intermediate, and high on the basis of the quantity of radiation in milligrays that the patient has been exposed to (Table 28-7).[65,66] If questions arise after resuscitation, early consultation with a perinatologist is appropriate. A Centers for Disease Control and Prevention Web site, www.bt.cdc.gov/radiation/prenatalphysican.asp, may also help when communicating to patients and their families about prenatal radiation exposure.

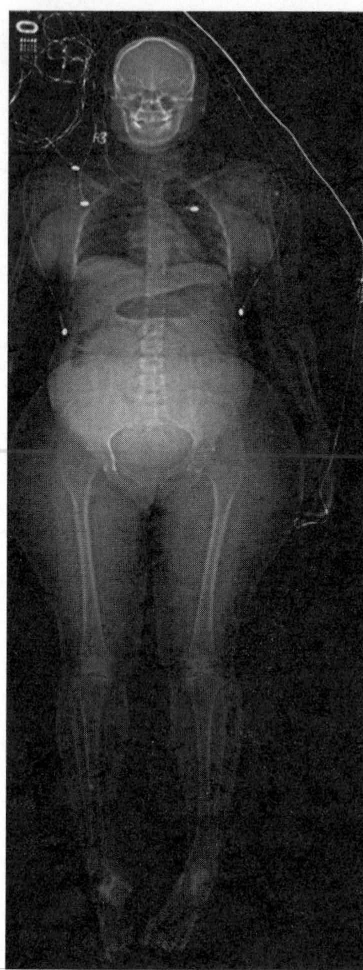

FIGURE 28-8 Full-body digital radiograph of a pregnant patient.

TABLE 28-7 Radiation Risk Categories

Risk Category	Dose Range (mGy)
Low	<10
Intermediate	10-250
High	>250

From Mann FA, Nathens A, Langer SG et al: Communicating with the family: the risks of medical radiation to concept uses in victims of major blunt-force torso trauma, *J Trauma* 48:354-357, 2000.

Medications

Many medications are, as a rule, relatively contraindicated during pregnancy. Decisions concerning medication use during pregnancy must weigh the benefits to the mother against the risks to the fetus. The highest-risk period for the fetus is during organogenesis (days 10 to 56 after conception).[67] It is during this time that medications are most likely to have a teratogenic effect.

Some medications are clearly needed to effectively treat the mother and some have been proven to cause no harm to the fetus. For example, tetanus prophylaxis with toxoid, commonly administered after trauma, should be given if the pregnant patient has not been immunized in the past 5 years because there is no risk to the fetus.

The pregnant trauma patient who is immobile after her injury is at risk for venous thromboembolism (VTE). There is strong evidence that a pregnant patient is more at risk than a nonpregnant patient. The agents currently available for the prevention for VTE are heparin, heparin-like compounds (unfractionated heparin, low-molecular-weight heparin [LMWH], and heparinoids), and coumarin derivatives.[68] The two potential fetal complications of anticoagulant therapy are teratogenicity and bleeding. Heparin does not cross the placenta and cannot cause either fetal bleeding or teratogenicity; therefore, it is thought to be safe for the fetus. LMWH and heparinoids can also be given during pregnancy.[69] However, coumarin derivatives cross the placenta and have the potential to cause both fetal bleeding and teratogenicity; thus they are seldom used, with the exception of the rare patient with a mechanical heart valve.

Pneumatic Antishock Garment

PASGs are no longer commonly used in trauma resuscitation to augment circulatory support. If they are used on a pregnant trauma patient, it is suggested that only the leg compartments be inflated. The effects of inflating the abdominal portion over a pregnant uterus are not known; therefore, this procedure is not recommended.

Numerous clinical case reports have documented the use of PASGs during obstetric emergencies. These include abortion complications, ectopic pregnancies, hydatidiform mole bleeding, hypocoagulation states, postoperative hemorrhage, and uterine atony.[70,71] In these cases the uterus has been emptied and the abdominal compartments of the garment were inflated to tamponade hemorrhage.

Abdominal Assessment (Ultrasonography, Computed Tomography, and Diagnostic Peritoneal Lavage)

Abdominal assessment of the pregnant trauma patient is somewhat unique because of the stretched abdominal wall and enlarged uterus. It is important to determine the presence of abdominal injury in the resuscitation phase. Ultrasonography, CT, and diagnostic peritoneal lavage (DPL) are all useful for this patient population. The hemodynamic stability of the patient and the risk assessment for injury should guide clinical decision making. (See Chapter 25 for additional information on abdominal diagnostic tests.)

Ultrasonography is commonly used in the United States for the evaluation of abdominal trauma.[56,57] In the gravid trauma patient, ultrasonography may have particular merit because it is noninvasive and does not expose the fetus to radiation. Ultrasonography can be used to assess fetal well-being, gestational age, and placental and uterine injuries. A skilled ultrasonographer also can use ultrasonography to evaluate abdominal viscera and pelvic fluid.

CT is also a popular modality for assessment of abdominal trauma. It has the advantages of being noninvasive and providing information about the retroperitoneum and genitourinary tract.[52] Uterine injuries can be identified and defined with an abdominal CT scan, and fetal injuries can be detected in a sleeping, sedated, or dead fetus (Figure 28-9). The amount of radiographic exposure to the fetus during abdominal CT depends on a number of factors, including patient age, type of machine, shielding of fetus, and fetal position.

DPL is considered both safe and appropriate for use in pregnant trauma patients.[72] The stomach and bladder should be emptied before the procedure, and the uterus should be well defined. During pregnancy, DPL may be more safely accomplished by use of a minilaparotomy instead of a catheter inserted with a needle. This modality is less commonly used today because of the availability and utility of imaging.

Cardiac Arrest

When the pregnant trauma patient is in cardiac arrest, the principles of resuscitation are the same as those for nonpregnant patients. Standard cardiopulmonary resuscitation (CPR) procedures should be performed and advanced cardiac life support measures instituted to ensure survival of both the mother and the fetus. A team member should be assigned to manually displace the uterus to improve venous return. Defibrillation should be performed if necessary.[73] Drugs commonly administered during the cardiac arrest activities should be used during pregnancy as well.[74] If the resuscitation is not going well, consideration may be given to emptying the uterus because this may improve venous return and expose an otherwise unsuspected intra-abdominal (retrouterine) source of blood loss.

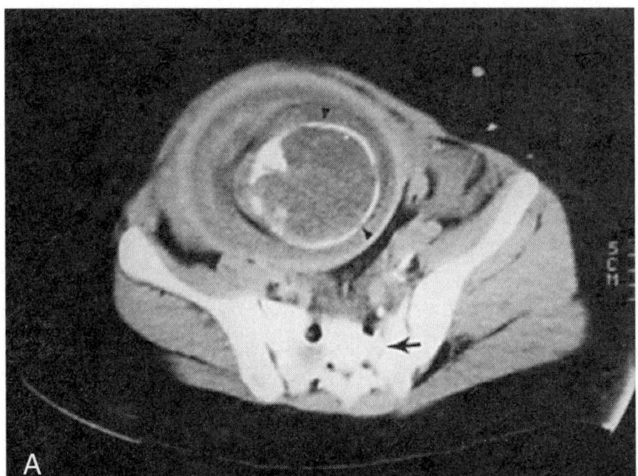

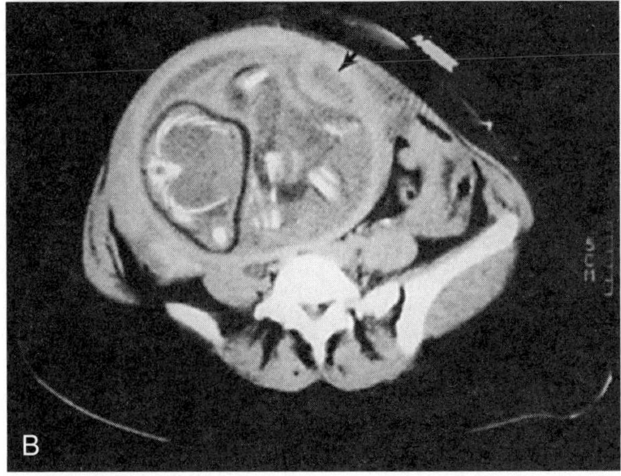

FIGURE 28-9 CT scan of trauma to the gravid uterus and fetus. **A,** Axial CT image through the level of the fetal head, obtained after blunt trauma to the maternal abdomen and pelvis at 7 months' gestation, shows two fetal skull fractures *(arrowheads)*. A maternal left sacral fracture is present *(arrow)*. **B,** CT image through the fetal torso reveals placental abruption with elevation of a portion of the placenta from the uterine wall *(arrow)*. Fetal death was confirmed by sonography before abdominal CT was performed to assess the extent of injury. (Courtesy of Stuart E. Mirvis, MD, Department of Diagnostic Radiology, University of Maryland Medical Center, Baltimore.)

Perimortem Cesarean Section

When a patient is in irreversible cardiac arrest, the decision to perform a perimortem cesarean section must be made. Obstetric and neonatal personnel must be notified immediately. More than 150 cases of successful perimortem cesarean section have been documented.[75] The cesarean section should be performed while CPR is in progress and as soon after maternal death as possible. Two key factors that must be considered when making the decision to perform a postmortem cesarean section are gestational age of the fetus (viability) and the amount of time the patient has been in cardiac arrest (the certainty of maternal death or unfavorable outcome).[38,75] After 4 minutes of CPR, the decision to perform a perimortem caesarean section should be addressed.[76] Weber[77] identified the likelihood of successful infant survival on the basis of the time elapsed between death of the mother and delivery of the fetus (Table 28-8).

Neonatal resuscitation is almost always necessary after perimortem delivery of the infant and should be managed by neonatal personnel, who must have emergency equipment immediately accessible (Table 28-9). Perimortem cesarean section should never be performed if the fundus of the uterus is below the umbilicus, if the mother died of subacute or chronic asphyxia, or if someone capable of resuscitating the newborn infant is not available.

Burn and Inhalation Injuries

Burns are detrimental to fetal survival. Survival is related primarily to gestational age and maternal survival. Initial management strategies for the pregnant woman with burn

TABLE 28-8 **Likelihood of Successful Infant Survival After Maternal Death**

Time Elapsed Between Maternal Death and Delivery	Likelihood of Successful Infant Survival
<5 minutes	Excellent
5-10 minutes	Good
10-15 minutes	Fair
15-20 minutes	Poor
20-25 minutes	Unlikely

Source: Weber CE: Postmortem cesarean section: review of the literature and case reports, *Am J Obstet Gynecol* 110:158-165, 1971.

TABLE 28-9 Neonatal Resuscitation Supplies and Equipment

Suction Equipment
Bulb syringe
Mechanical suction and tubing
Suction catheters, 5F or 6F, 8F, 10F, 12F or 14F
8F feeding tube and 20-ml syringe
Meconium aspirator

Bag-and-Mask Equipment
Device for delivering positive-pressure ventilation, capable of delivering 90% to 100% oxygen
Face masks, newborn and premature sizes (cushioned-rim masks preferred)
Oxygen source with flowmeter (flow rate up to 10 L/min) and tubing

Intubation Equipment
Laryngoscope with straight blades, No. 0 (preterm) and No. 1 (term)
Extra bulbs and batteries for laryngoscope
Endotracheal tubes, 2.5, 3.0, 3.5, and 4 mm internal diameter
Stylet (optional)
Scissors
Tape or securing device for endotracheal tube
Alcohol sponges
Carbon dioxide detector or capnograph
Laryngeal mask airway (optional)

Medications
Epinephrine 1:10,000 (0.1 mg/ml), 3- or 10-ml ampules
Isotonic crystalloid (normal saline solution or Ringer's lactate) for volume expansion, 100 or 250 ml
Sodium bicarbonate 4.2% (5 mEq/10 ml), 10-ml ampules
Naloxone hydrochloride 0.4 mg/ml, 1-ml ampules or 1 mg/ml in 2-ml ampules
Dextrose 10%, 250 ml
Normal saline solution for flushes
Umbilical vessel catheterization supplies
- Sterile gloves
- Scalpel or scissors
- Antiseptic prep solution
- Umbilical tape
- Umbilical catheters, 3.5F, 5F
- Three-way stopcock

Syringes, 1, 3, 5, 10, 20, 50 ml
Needles, 25, 21, 18 gauge, or puncture device for needleless system

Miscellaneous
Gloves and appropriate personal protection
Radiant warmer or other heat source
Firm, padded resuscitation surface
Clock with second hand (timer optional)
Warmed linens
Stethoscope (neonatal head preferred)
Tape, ½ or ¾ inch
Cardiac monitor and electrodes or pulse oximeter and probe (optional for delivery room)
Oropharyngeal airways (0, 00, and 000 sizes or 30-, 40-, and 50-mm lengths)

For Very Preterm Babies (Optional)
Compressed air source
Oxygen blender to mix oxygen and compressed air
Pulse oximeter and oximeter probe
Reclosable food-grade plastic bag (1-gallon size) or plastic wrap
Chemically activated warming pad
Transport incubator to maintain baby's temperature during move to nursery

Used with the permission of the American Academy of Pediatrics: *Textbook for neonatal resuscitation,* 5th ed.

injury include calculation of the extent of the burn (% total body surface area [TBSA]) and rapid resuscitation efforts that focus on the provision of adequate oxygenation and the restoration of circulating fluid volume[78,79] (see Chapter 32). It has been suggested that early burn wound excision and skin grafting can improve maternal and fetal survival.[79] Urgent delivery has been suggested when the baby is of viable age and the burn is greater than 50% of maternal TBSA.[80]

The treatment for acute CO poisoning is administration of oxygen. There had been some uncertainty regarding the use of hyperbaric oxygen (HBO) in the pregnant patient because of possible adverse fetal effects from oxygen at high partial pressures. However, because of the disastrous consequences to the fetus, HBO at 2.8 atmospheres absolute should be used more liberally for the treatment of women to prevent fetal hypoxia.[33,81] On the basis of Longo and Hill's model, it is recommended that a pregnant woman receive 100% oxygen up to five times as long as the time needed for the mother alone to reduce her own COHb level to normal. If HBO is not available, 100% oxygen can be administered through a tight-fitting mask.[3]

Maternal and Fetal Injuries and Complications Unique to Trauma During Pregnancy

Fetal Hypoxia

Continuous fetal monitoring with an EFM should be initiated as quickly as possible during resuscitation of pregnant patients with viable pregnancies.[38,44,75] It can be helpful because acute changes in maternal condition can compromise fetal well-being (see Figure 28-7). Because uterine perfusion is sensitive to maternal blood volume and vascular tone, the fetus may be the first to demonstrate signs of maternal shock. If the fetus is in a hypoxic environment, the most appropriate action is to continue maternal resuscitation. A sudden change in fetal heart rate in a nonviable fetus rarely prompts a change in maternal care but can be emotionally traumatic for the staff and the mother, who may feel helpless facing the probability of fetal death. Thus, continuous fetal monitoring is appropriate only in a viable fetus.

Uterine Injuries

As pregnancy progresses, the uterus becomes an abdominal organ and can be damaged by blunt or penetrating trauma. Uterine damage can consist of lacerations or rupture. If the uterus has ruptured, it is usually, but not always, tender on palpation. The abdomen may be distended, and vaginal bleeding may occur (Table 28-10). When uterine rupture is severe, two distinct masses may be palpable in the abdomen: the uterus and the fetus. Milder forms of uterine damage are more common although clinically less distinct.

When uterine damage is suspected, the patient's abdomen must be reassessed frequently (every 15 to 30 minutes). Fundal height should be measured and marked on the patient's abdomen with tape or indelible marker on admission and every 30 minutes thereafter until the concern has passed (see Figure 28-10). A rise in fundal height may indicate intrauterine hemorrhage. If a uterine laceration or tear is suspected, surgical intervention to repair the uterus is probable; disruption of the pregnancy depends on the severity of the uterine injury and on fetal assessment.

TABLE 28-10 Signs and Symptoms of Uterine Damage

Mild uterine injuries (e.g., lacerations and contusions)
Varied and mild symptoms
Uterine rupture
Sudden onset of abdominal pain with increased uterine irritability
Maternal hypovolemic shock
Loss of FHTs or evidence of fetal distress
Uterine tenderness to palpation and increased tone
Palpation of two abdominal masses (uterus and fetus)
Vaginal bleeding (variable)

From Pearlman M, Tintinalli J: *Emergency care of the woman*, pp 69-76, New York, 1998, McGraw-Hill.

Placental Abruption

Placental abruption, the premature separation of the placenta from the uterine wall, also can occur after trauma. It is second only to maternal death among the causes of fetal death.[58] As many as 40% to 50% of pregnant women with major trauma may have an abruption.[4,8,82,83]

The mechanism causing the abruption is directly related to the trauma. Higgins and Garite[84] describe the placenta in the uterus as being like a potato chip inside a tennis ball. The uterus is elastic; the placenta is seemingly less so. On impact the placenta cannot reshape as rapidly as the uterus; instead it separates or pulls away from the uterine wall, causing disruption of the maternal-fetal circulation and hemorrhage. Early detection of an abruption and appropriate action increase the chance of fetal survival.

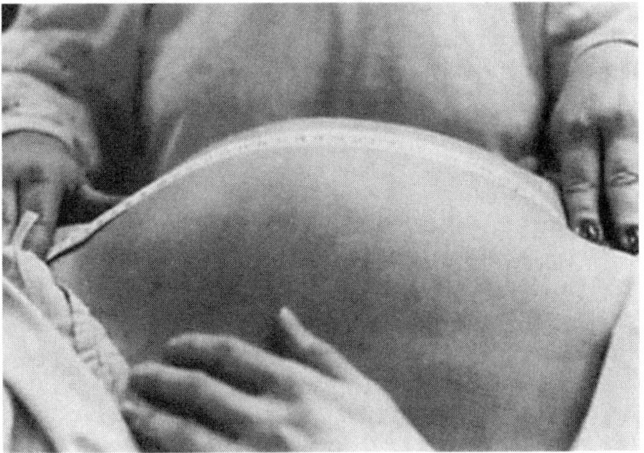

FIGURE 28-10 Measuring fundal height. The fundus is measured in centimeters from the symphysis pubis to the top of the fundus.

Abruption in mild forms can be difficult to diagnose. An abnormal fetal heart rate pattern (identified by obstetric staff with expertise in this area) can be helpful in identifying a placental abruption in women at more than 20 weeks' gestation[44-46,58,59] (Figure 28-7). Fetal heart rate pattern irregularity is the most reliable indicator of placental abruption. The grave sign of a slowed heart rate or absent FHTs may be a indicative of placental injury. Coagulation changes are rare after a mild abruption, but if the abruption is extensive enough to cause fetal death, as with any situation involving significant hemorrhage, the mother can have severe coagulopathy and shock. Other signs and symptoms are listed in Table 28-11.

The patient must be observed for indications of this condition during resuscitation. The inclusion of obstetric personnel during the resuscitation is ideal because their expertise in assessing for subtle signs or symptoms of an abruption are helpful (see Table 28-11). Although there is a reported case of delayed abruption (>24 hours) after injury, more recent studies indicate that virtually all abruptions become evident within 4 to 12 hours.[59,84,85] When a severe mechanism of injury has occurred and abruption has not been diagnosed, some clinicans feel that additional uterine monitoring is indicated.[9] A plan of care for the patient with placental abruption is presented in Table 28-12.

Premature Rupture of Membranes

The rupture of amniotic membranes may occur as a result of trauma. A reported sudden gush of fluid after abdominal impact suggests premature rupture of amniotic membranes but must be differentiated from spontaneous bladder emptying. If a pool of vaginal fluid is present, it should be tested for pH. The normal pH of amniotic fluid is 7 to 7.5; that of urine is 4.8 to 6. The fluid also should be checked microscopically (place a drop on a slide and allow to dry) for the appearance of ferning, which is a more reliable sign that amniotic fluid is present. It is unlikely that membranes have ruptured if an ultrasonographic scan reveals normal uterine amniotic fluid volume.[86]

Rupture of amniotic membranes should be ruled out with a pelvic examination. The sterile speculum examination should be done gently. Membrane rupture can be associated with ascending infections, chorioamnionitis, preterm labor, and umbilical cord prolapse.[87] The potential for these complications makes collaboration with obstetric personnel imperative. In addition, ultrasonography is indicated to determine gestational age, amniotic fluid level, and fetal status.

If the membranes rupture, the perineum and vagina should be inspected for visualization of the umbilical cord. If the umbilical cord is present, immediate interventions are indicated, depending on gestational age (Table 28-13). When rupture of membranes occurs at or after 34 weeks of gestation, delivery of the fetus either by induction of labor or cesarean section should be considered.

Core body temperature must be monitored closely in a patient who has preterm rupture of membranes. If signs of amnionitis develop (fetal tachycardia, maternal tachycardia, uterine tenderness, or temperature higher than 38° C), consideration should be given to delivery of the fetus.

TABLE 28-11 Signs and Symptoms of Abruptio Placentae

The symptoms of an abruptio placentae can be variable depending on the degree of the placentae separation.
They include those listed below:

- Vaginal bleeding (may not be always present)
- Premature labor
- Sudden onset of abdominal or back pain
- Uterine tenderness to palpation
- Uterine tetany or rigidity (uterine tone may be increased with small, frequent contractions superimposed)
- Expanding or rising fundal height
- Maternal hemodynamic instability and coagulopathy
- Fetal distress or absence of FHTs, no fetal cardiac

From Pilliteri A: *Maternal and child health nursing,* 3rd ed, pp 384-386, New York, 1999, Lippincott.

Premature Labor

Determining whether the patient is in labor is also a component of the obstetric assessment. Labor consists of three stages: dilation of the cervix, expulsion of the baby through the birth canal, and the separation and ejection of the placenta. Labor is defined as cervical change in response to uterine contractions. Identification of the onset of labor is particularly important if the woman is not at term (37 completed weeks of gestation). Signs and symptoms of the onset of labor include bloody show, ruptured membranes, and contractions. Contractions can be difficult for the nonobstetric staff to assess; therefore, obstetric team expertise is most valuable.[44-46] Contractions causing dilation of the cervix indicate that the patient is in labor. The duration and frequency of contractions must be assessed with a uterine tocodynamometer, and the patient must be assessed continually for signs of fetal distress. The frequency of contractions is determined by noting the time from the beginning of one contraction to the beginning of the next (Figure 28-11). Premature labor after trauma may indicate the presence of fetal or uterine injury. As measures are taken to inhibit the progression of labor, additional obstetric assessment should be obtained to rule out fetal or uterine injury.

Because dehydration can precipitate premature labor, the patient should be kept well hydrated. Accurate intake and output records must be maintained. After maternal hydration has been ensured and uterine and fetal injuries ruled out, preterm labor should be inhibited. The medications that inhibit labor have consequences. Magnesium sulfate can decrease deep tendon reflexes and alter spinal cord assessment. Nonsteroidal anti-inflammatory agents such as indomethacin

TABLE 28-12 Abruptio Placentae Plan of Care

Interventions	Rationale
1. Monitor maternal vital signs every 15 minutes and fetal heart rate continuously as appropriate. Note any trends or changes.	Abruption and subsequent hemorrhage can occur after the traumatic event. Maternal hypervolemia can mask signs of shock. Fetal distress may be the first indication of maternal hemorrhage.
2. Ensure placement of two large-bore IV catheters and maintain aggressive fluid resuscitation as ordered.	Maternal hypervolemia can mask a 15% to 30% blood loss. Early aggressive fluid resuscitation is recommended to prevent maternal hypovolemia. Large volumes of fluid may be necessary to maintain maternal hypervolemia.
3. Obtain and compare maternal laboratory values with normal pregnancy values (include coagulation profile).	Laboratory values change acutely in pregnancy; an early, accurate baseline is essential for clinical observation. Coagulation profile is necessary because DIC is a possible complication. If indicated, arrangements for possible blood component therapy must be made.
4. Measure and mark fundal height on admission and every 30 minutes.	A rising fundal height may indicate intrauterine hemorrhage from abruptio placentae.
5. Monitor patient for clinical signs of abruptio placentae for 4 to 24 hours or longer. Signs include: Vaginal bleeding Abdominal pain Uterine tenderness Uterine tetany or rigidity Rising fundal height Maternal shock/fetal distress	Symptoms can often be vague, and all do not necessarily occur. Rarely abruption can occur 24 hours or more after injury.
6. Maintain continuous electronic fetal monitoring in patients beyond 20 weeks' gestation until risk of fetal distress is minimal.	Early, continuous monitoring identifies signs of abruption. Continuous monitoring can show fetal distress such as late decelerations and decreased beat-to-beat variability. Uterine contraction patterns should be noted because uterine irritability and preterm labor can indicate uterine hemorrhage.

From Smith LG: Assessment and resuscitation of the pregnant trauma patient. In Hoyt KS, Andrews J, editors: *Contemporary perspectives in trauma nursing,* Berryville, VA, 1991, Forum Medicum.

TABLE 28-13 Immediate Treatment for Prolapsed Cord

Goal: Relieve cord compression and ensure safe urgent fetal delivery.

Nursing Intervention	Rationale
1. *Gently* insert a gloved hand into the patient's vagina, don't touch the cord if possible, and elevate the fetal presenting part. Do not remove the examining hand until the fetus is delivered.	1. If the cord is being compressed by the presenting part, this maneuver will help relieve the compression.
2. *Extremely gentle* handling of the cord is essential; avoid manipulation, compression, or additional exposure of the cord to air.	2. Manipulation of the cord and its exposure to air can cause cord spasm, further compromising the fetus.
3. Position the mother in the knee-chest position and place the stretcher in Trendelenburg. (The Sims' lateral position may also be used.)	3. Positioning of the mother is aimed at helping to elevate the presenting part. If a long period of time passes before delivery of the fetus, the Sims' lateral position may be less tiring for the mother.
4. Prepare the patient for emergency cesarean section.	4. Sometimes these patients may have a vaginal delivery, but a cesarean section is often clinically indicated and must be done in an emergency manner.
5. Monitor FHTs with an electronic monitor.	5. Determine fetal heart rate and note effectiveness of the emergency treatment.
6. Provide emotional support to mother and family during the procedures.	6. Answering patient and family questions and explaining the procedures may help decrease anxiety.

Make sure that the emergency department has a clinical plan in place for such obstetric emergencies.

If obstetric and neonatal personnel are available, they should be notified immediately to respond to the emergency department.

From Smith LG: Assessment and resuscitation of the pregnant trauma patient. In Hoyt KS, Andrews J, editors: *Contemporary perspectives in trauma nursing,* Berryville, VA, 1991, Forum Medicum.

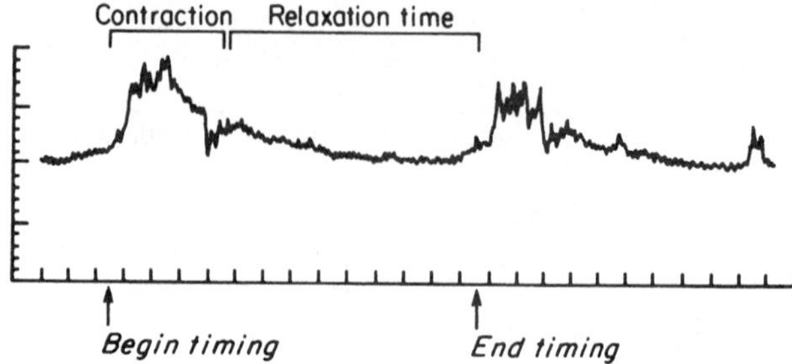

FIGURE 28-11 A uterine contraction consists of two periods: contraction time and relaxation time. The frequency of contractions is the interval of time from the beginning of one contraction period to the beginning of the next contraction period.

can be useful in pregnancies before the thirty-first week of gestation. The use of these nonsteroidal agents has been associated with decreases in amniotic fluid volume, neonatal pulmonary hypertension, and potential maternal bleeding when they are used for a prolonged period of time.[88] Calcium channel blockers have been shown in controlled studies to be effective for tocolysis.[89,90] Caution must be used when these drugs are combined with other negative inotropes. The patient's labor activity and cardiovascular status should continue to be monitored. If measures to inhibit labor appear unsuccessful, obstetric and neonatal personnel should be prepared for delivery.

Fetomaternal Hemorrhage

Fetomaternal hemorrhage is the transplacental bleeding of fetal blood into the maternal circulation.[85] Its incidence among injured pregnant women is four to five times higher than among uninjured pregnant women.[59] To detect fetomaternal hemorrhage, the KB acid-elution assay can be performed on maternal blood. This test also can estimate fetal blood loss. Positive results are especially important for Rh-negative mothers with Rh-positive infants; in this scenario an appropriate amount of Rh immune globulin can be administered to prevent isoimmunization (300 mcg of Rh immune globulin per 30 ml of fetal blood). The authors of a study involving the results of 523 KB tests concluded that the assay should be reserved for patients with severe trauma or evidence of fetal compromise.[91] Other authors also suggest that the KB test is only clinically useful for Rh-negative mothers.[45,46]

Direct Fetal Injury Associated with Blunt Trauma

Fetal injuries such as skull and clavicular fractures and fetomaternal hemorrhage must be suspected after a pregnant woman has undergone a blunt abdominal trauma. Fetal fractures are caused by disruption of the maternal pelvic ring (see Figure 28-9). A pelvic fracture in a pregnant woman is more serious because of the increased vascularity of the pelvis during pregnancy and the increased risk of bleeding. Fetomaternal hemorrhage is thought to occur in as many as 25% of cases of blunt trauma.[92]

As previously described, a woman who has been subjected to blunt abdominal trauma can be evaluated by ultrasonography or a CT scan to determine the existence of fetal injuries and to approximate gestational age. If the fetus is viable, the fetal heart rate should be continuously assessed. If there is evidence of fetal distress, preparation should begin for an emergency delivery by cesarean section if in utero resuscitation is unsuccessful and the patient is not close to delivering vaginally. If fetal death has occurred, the fetus may be delivered by cesarean section or vaginal delivery depending on maternal stability. If there is evidence of a significant placental abruption, expediting delivery is indicated. The presence of DIC in these cases should prompt the trauma team to be prepared for maternal hemorrhage regardless of intervention by cesarean or vaginal delivery. Blood products should be available, and in the case of exploratory laparotomy caution should be taken to obtain hemostasis before the abdomen is closed.

Maternal or Fetal Injury Associated with Penetrating Trauma

As pregnancy progresses, the enlarging uterus displaces the bowel and becomes the most dominant abdominal organ; thus it is more likely to be damaged in a penetrating traumatic event. After a gunshot wound or stab wound to the abdominal area, the pregnant patient should be monitored for signs and symptoms of uterine damage (see Table 28-10). In viable pregnancies, the fetal heart rate must be monitored continuously and fetal activity should be assessed in conjunction with maternal assessment. Local wound exploration may be necessary, and the patient should be prepared for emergency laparotomy if the wound extends into the abdominal cavity.

Maternal and Family Anxiety

The traumatic event and sudden hospitalization certainly cause maternal and family anxiety. The patient must be reassured that prompt, aggressive care offers the fetus the best chance for survival, and she should be kept informed of impending diagnostic tests and results. Allowing the patient to listen to the fetal heart beat and observe ultrasound images may lessen anxious feelings. The family needs to be kept informed of the status of the mother and fetus. The family members should be permitted to be with the patient. In addition to fears concerning the fetus, the patient and family may have feelings of guilt about the events leading to the incident. They should be encouraged to express their feelings, and nonjudgmental support should be offered.

INTRAOPERATIVE PHASE

When a pregnant trauma patient is admitted to a trauma center or emergency department, operating room personnel should be notified of the possibility of an emergency cesarean section. The decision to empty the uterus intraoperatively is based on gestational age, fetal distress, and control of hemorrhage around the uterus. A general surgery pack can be opened and additional surgical equipment added (Table 28-14), or an obstetric cesarean section pack can be opened. Other useful instruments are a small French suction catheter (8F) and several end clamps. Neonatal or pediatric personnel need to be in the operating suite to manage the initial resuscitation and stabilization of the newborn infant.

ANESTHESIA

Anesthetic management of the pregnant trauma patient requires the expertise of anesthesia personnel familiar with both trauma and obstetric anesthesia. Anesthesia for the pregnant trauma patient should be planned recognizing that these patients are unique.[93] First, they have an increased metabolic demand as a result of pregnancy. Second, there are changes in hormonal activity. And finally, there are anatomic alterations caused by the enlarging uterus and breasts. The decision whether to administer regional or general anesthesia is one of many to be made before and during surgery.

When the pregnant trauma patient has multiple injuries or needs immediate surgery, general anesthesia may be the best choice. The pregnant trauma patient given general anesthesia does have an increased risk of vomiting and aspiration, which is best controlled by first emptying the stomach with a gastric tube and administering a nonparticulate antacid (e.g., sodium citrate) to increase gastric pH.[93] Pantoprazole (Protonix) can be given to decrease acid production. Intubation with a cuffed endotracheal tube after rapid-sequence induction with cricoid pressure and 5 minutes of preoxygenation should protect the airway and provide adequate oxygenation.[63] Another concern during pregnancy is the possible effects that anesthetics or other drugs administered to the patient will have on the developing fetus. The highest risk of tetragenic effects occurs in the first trimester of pregnancy, but no anesthetic agent has been proven to be tetragenic.[94-96]

When possible, regional anesthesia should be used during pregnancy. The location of injuries; length of procedure; cardiovascular, neurologic, and psychologic status of the patient; and risk of fetal compromise are all determinants of the appropriateness of local or spinal anesthesia. For example, local anesthesia is appropriate for repair of a facial laceration, whereas repair of extensive facial trauma requires general anesthesia. Lower extremity injuries resulting from trauma can be repaired with spinal or epidural anesthesia or another regional block, but general anesthesia may be more appropriate for other injuries. The circulating nurse must ensure that specialty drugs such as uterotonic agents (oxytocin [Pitocin] and methylergonovine maleate [Methergine]) are available in the operating room suite for the anesthesia and obstetric providers.

TABLE 28-14 Surgical Tools to Be Added to General Surgery Pack for Cesarean Section

Bladder blade
Obstetric forceps
Sponge sticks
De Lee suction trap and bulb syringe
Suture for uterine closure

SURGICAL PROCEDURES

Before any elective or emergency operative intervention, operating room personnel must be informed of the patient's pregnant condition. Obstetric and neonatal personnel should be available for consultation during surgery.

Obstetric Procedures

Exploratory laparotomy may be indicated to identify the type and severity of uterine injuries. Uterine lacerations, contusions, and tears are common after abdominal trauma and may need repair. Cesarean section for removal of the fetus is appropriate only if the fetus is in distress and of viable age (≥24 weeks' gestation), the mother's condition warrants it, or, if necessary, to allow adequate uterine repair.

If the fetus has died as a result of trauma and the patient is stable, a cesarean section is considered inappropriate in most instances because it exposes the mother to the probability of cesarean section for future pregnancies. A critically injured patient who is hemorrhaging can have DIC, and in this instance a cesarean section may be necessary (although the fetus is dead) to prevent additional complications (e.g., sepsis). Cesarean section for a previable infant is also considered inappropriate; here too a vaginal delivery is preferable.

When uterine rupture is identified in emergency surgery, the first task is to stop sources of hemorrhage. The removal of the fetus is left to the discretion of the physician. The fetus should be removed by a low transverse incision unless the tear is nearly large enough to remove the fetus. The fetus should be handed immediately to the neonatal personnel. When possible, the uterus is then repaired to preserve future childbearing capabilities. If there is uncontrollable hemorrhage, a hysterectomy, uterine artery embolization, or bilateral hypogastric ligation may need to be performed.[97]

Nonobstetric Procedures

For the pregnant trauma patient, abdominal laparotomy, multiple orthopedic procedures, and neurosurgery may be more common than obstetric surgery. To diminish surgical time and the anesthesia risk to the fetus, multiple surgical procedures may be done simultaneously, which may require that several scrub nurses assist with the operative procedures. The perioperative nurse preparing for this contingency must notify the charge nurse of the need for additional personnel. The procedures also can be done consecutively, which requires planning by the circulating nurse.

When managing lower extremity orthopedic trauma during pregnancy, several factors must be considered. Although internal fixation of fractures exposes the patient to general anesthesia, it markedly reduces the pregnant patient's length of immobility. A woman who must remain immobile during pregnancy faces the risk of development of venous thromboembolic disease; therefore, early fixation is desirable to reduce prolonged immobility.

When the fetus is of viable age, the fetal heart rate should be monitored continuously during the surgical procedures to detect early signs of impaired uteroplacental blood flow and fetal oxygenation.[94-96] Uterine activity can also be monitored to identify preterm labor during and after the procedure.

Perioperative Nursing Care

Patient and Family Fear and Anxiety

The nurse in the operating room is in a unique position to coordinate procedures and provide a therapeutic environment for the pregnant patient. A calm preinduction environment must be maintained for the patient in the operating room, with discussions kept to a minimum. As time permits, the patient should be allowed to voice concerns and fears. The patient and family should be reassured of the safety of anesthesia during pregnancy.[94] The family should be kept informed of the surgical progress and the fetal condition.

Importance Of Positioning

The proper positioning or padding of a surgical patient is the primary responsibility of the operative team, including the perioperative nurse.[98] When a pregnant patient is in the operating room, it is a challenge to prevent the enlarging uterus from causing decreased cardiac output as a result of vena cava compression. Patient positioning in the left lateral position is ideal but probably unrealistic during surgical intervention. An alternative is to displace the uterus by using a towel roll or wedge under the hip and small of the back. A second alternative is to tilt the operating table laterally. If maternal injuries prohibit both these positions, manual displacement of the uterus by a team member or with a displacer is required.

When a pregnant patient with a fetus of viable age is having surgery after trauma, the surgical table should be prepared for possible cesarean section with the addition of several surgical instruments (see Table 28-14). Neonatal personnel must be alerted, and space and appropriate equipment must be provided in the surgical suite or adjoining area for neonatal resuscitation at delivery. The circulating nurse must coordinate the intraoperative plan of care to include several disciplines (e.g., surgeons, labor and delivery nurses, neonatologists, and neonatal nurses). All these services must be ready within the operating room suite when the skin incision is made if fetal delivery is believed to be a possible outcome. The time of birth and other birth-related details must be noted as part of routine documentation. The placenta must be obtained and prepared as a specimen for pathology test procedures.

As the patient's and the fetus's conditions allow, attempts should be made to provide an environment that facilitates maternal-infant bonding. If the patient is awake and the infant is alive and stable, the mother should be permitted to see and hold her baby. If the infant is premature or unstable, the mother must be kept informed of the infant's progress and permitted to see the infant, even for a brief moment, if possible. If the mother is under anesthesia, she should be told about the birth as soon as she is through the postanesthesia recovery stage. The family or significant others should be permitted to see the baby when possible and kept informed of the baby's progress. Many intensive care nurseries (and labor/delivery suites) use an instant or digital camera to take a snapshot of the infant; the photograph provides the mother with what may be her only glimpse of the child for days.

Critical Care Phase

After the initial resuscitation (which may include operative management), the patient should be transferred to the appropriate critical care unit. Most often this will be the adult intensive care unit (ICU), although there are a limited number of obstetric critical care units around the country. In the appropriate unit the patient care should be a collaboration of care between the ICU and perinatal care providers.[99]

The general goal of care for the pregnant trauma patient after resuscitation is to provide aggressive maternal care while minimizing fetal stress. A well-oxygenated, well-hydrated, hemodynamically stable mother will provide the best opportunity for fetal well-being. Critical care management goals should include adequate cardiac output, blood pressure, hemoglobin levels, and oxygen saturation. It should be noted that even patients with limited brainstem function can be maintained until fetal viability is reached. These patients present a challenge to the obstetric and critical care staff.

The potential for delayed obstetric complications, such as abruptio placentae, premature labor, and fetal distress should be considered. During the initial critical care period obstetric personnel should be available to monitor a viable-age fetus. An experienced perinatal nurse will continuously assess the FHT pattern for the four components: baseline rate, baseline variability, and the presence or absence of FHT acceleration and FHT decelerations. An emergency delivery plan and a neonatal resuscitation plan should be established. Maintaining active communication with both the obstetric and neonatal teams improves the quality of care.

Assessment for signs and symptoms of obstetric complications may be difficult in the critically injured patient for a number of reasons. Sedation or an unconscious state imposes limitations on the ability to communicate with the patient. Communicating with an intubated patient may be difficult as well. After spinal cord injury, although the patient may be able to communicate, sensations that would otherwise indicate the onset of labor or signify the development of other problems may be lacking.

A communication link with the obstetric and neonatal staff should be prearranged and tested. In large medical centers, the obstetric unit and critical care units could be in separate buildings with security measures that prevent staff from easily accessing the units. New obstetric staff should be given an opportunity to practice getting to the ICU. If an obstetric complication is suspected or delivery appears imminent, the obstetric and neonatal staff should be notified immediately. If the patient cannot be moved from the critical care unit, obstetric personnel should administer the appropriate treatment in the unit. Necessary emergency delivery equipment should be kept at the bedside.

As the patient's hospitalization course continues, continous EFM may eventually be stopped. Fetal assessment should continue on a regular basis and should include the use of real-time ultrasound, the nonstress test, and the biophysical profile.[99] The obstetric staff, as part of the critical care team, should monitor the status of the pregnancy and provide useful information for the staff caring for the patient. Daily interdisciplinary rounds should include the obstretric staff.

ANTEPARTUM CONCERNS

Increased Metabolic Demands

Good nutrition is essential during pregnancy because of the additional metabolic demands of the fetus and the normal physiologic changes of pregnancy. When the pregnant patient is in critical condition after a traumatic injury, meeting the increased metabolic demands of both pregnancy and maternal healing becomes a challenge. Dietary consultation should be initiated on admission to the critical care unit so that the patient's nutritional requirements can be determined. Oral dietary intake, tube feeding, and parenteral nutrition, or a combination of these three, may be necessary to meet the patient's metabolic demands. The goal is to prevent maternal protein-calorie malnutrition.

For patients who are able to tolerate oral feedings, food preferences should be acknowledged when possible. Smaller, more frequent meals are recommended for the pregnant patient to avoid unnecessary discomfort resulting from a full stomach. The nutritional status should be assessed continually so that adjustments to dietary intake can be made accordingly (see Chapter 17).

Maternal Positioning

Positioning is an important aspect of nursing care and it is especially important for the pregnant trauma patient. Although the patient should be turned to the left or right side to prevent compression of the vena cava and aorta by the enlarging uterus and thus improve cardiac output, a single position cannot be maintained for long periods without increasing the risk for atelectasis and skin breakdown. A turning schedule should be developed and followed to prevent the pregnant patient from remaining on her back for any length of time. The turning schedule should emphasize side-to-side turning with little, if any, time spent in the supine position. The patient's injuries may dictate the need to devise unique positioning strategies (e.g., musculoskeletal stabilization devices). Such requirements should be detailed in the patient's plan of care or pathway.

Venous Stasis and Possible Pulmonary Emboli

The normal physiologic changes that occur during pregnancy place the pregnant woman at a greater risk for venous stasis and development of venous thromboembolism. Although the true risk of VTE is not known, VTE affects pregnant women five times more frequently than nonpregnant women of a similar age.[49,68] Immobility during the critical care phase places the patient at further risk. It is therefore important for the pregnant patient to be mobilized as soon as possible to prevent such complications. Placement of intermittent pneumatic compression devices is a safe and effective treatment modality that can be initiated. LMWH therapy is indicated in this patient population if there are no other contraindications to its use.[69]

A thorough respiratory assessment must be completed each shift and, when indicated, on the basis of changes in the patient's condition. Vital signs, including pulse oximetry, must be monitored continually and arterial blood gas trends must be examined routinely during the initial postresuscitation phase.

Pain Control

Pain control is an important aspect of every patient's care, but the pregnant patient presents a challenging situation. Pain, if not managed effectively, can cause stress to the mother and fetus and increase metabolic demands. A team approach that considers input from critical care, obstetrics, and pain specialists can determine appropriate pain management options that have minimal fetal effects. The administration of pain medication should be documented on the fetal monitoring strip because these drugs can alter the FHT pattern and variability.

POSTPARTUM CONCERNS

The trauma patient who has aborted or been delivered during the resuscitation or intraoperative phase presents different concerns during the critical care phase; therefore, appropriate priorities must be established. Immediately post partum the patient must be monitored closely for hemorrhage and shock. The potential for infection also must be considered. Telling the patient and family of a poor fetal condition or fetal loss, although a difficult task, also must be accomplished as soon as possible, and comfort measures should be provided as needed.[100]

Postpartum Hemorrhage

After a normal delivery, a woman commonly loses up to 450 ml of blood. This blood loss is compensated by the relative hypervolemia of pregnancy. If the bleeding exceeds 500 ml, it is considered a primary postpartum hemorrhage. (It is not uncommon for clinicians to underestimate blood loss.) Uterine atony is the most common cause of postpartum hemorrhage. Therefore, to prevent and promptly recognize onset of such complications, the critical care nurse must include regular postpartum care in his or her plan.

The fundus should be assessed and massaged every 15 minutes for the first hour post partum and then every hour for at least 4 hours thereafter. A rise in fundal height, increased lochia, or a "boggy" uterus should be reported to the obstetric staff. The amount of vaginal bleeding should be monitored closely. Pad counts are often helpful in assessing the extent of bleeding. An excessive amount of bleeding should be reported to the obstetrician immediately. If hemorrhage is occurring, the fundus should be massaged vigorously while the patient is given 10 to 30 units of oxytocin in 1 L of IV fluid. Oxytocin should never be given as an IV bolus because that practice may cause hypotension. If the uterus does not become firm, the patient may be given methylergonovine, 0.2 mg intramuscularly, but this drug is relatively contraindicated in hypertensive patients. Continued hemorrhage may indicate a hidden vaginal or cervical laceration and the critical care nurse should prepare the patient for possible surgery and, more important, manage the patient's hypovolemic shock state.[97]

Postpartum Infection

The patient's temperature should be monitored routinely. A slight elevation can be expected after delivery; however, persistent elevation should be reported. The quantity and quality of vaginal drainage (lochia) should be monitored routinely for several days. The obstetric team should be notified if a foul-smelling discharge is noted.

The perineum should be inspected routinely as well. Swelling is normal immediately after vaginal delivery but should decrease after several days. Ice should be applied directly to the perineal area to reduce swelling and alleviate local pain.

Breast Engorgement

If necessary, a breast binder should be obtained and applied for the patient who is planning to bottle feed or who has had a fetal loss, provided that it does not restrict respiratory movement or interfere with necessary treatment activities. A snugly fitted bra can suffice.

Grieving Loss of the Fetus

When the fetus is lost during resuscitation, the decision of when to tell the mother is difficult. The father and other appropriate family members should be immediately notified. The multidisciplinary team members should collaborate in making this decision. The mother's level of consciousness and clinical condition are strong determining factors; once the mother can listen and comprehend, telling her should not be delayed. Input from family members is often helpful in determining the patient's ability to cope with such devastating news. Requests from family members should be respected and incorporated into the management plan if possible. Family members should be present when the patient is told of the loss.

During the grieving process the mother may request detailed information such as the time of birth, the baby's weight, or the color of the baby's hair. If possible, the fetus should be held in the area if it is anticipated that the mother might be able to see and hold her infant. Pictures of the baby are often helpful. The grieving process extends beyond the critical care phase. A consistent approach allows continued nursing support through all phases of care as grieving continues (see Chapter 19). Although the mother may not request them at the time, it is appropriate to collect a lock of hair, a photograph, hand and foot prints, and baby's first cap and blanket and archive them, letting the mother know that the materials are hers whenever she wants them. Many mothers request these keepsakes after their loss.

Most obstetric and neonatal units have a grief management team. A group such as this can be invaluable not only to the patient and her family but also to the trauma team during what, even for them, can be a very difficult time. The resuscitation team, both trauma and obstetric personnel, should have debriefing staff available to allow staff to express their thoughts. Debriefing should help the staff and decrease the potential for posttraumatic stress.

Maternal-Infant Bonding

The patient who has been delivered of a healthy or premature infant during the resuscitation phase of care presents an equal challenge to the critical care nurse. Every effort must be made to provide as much contact as possible between the mother and baby. The family should be encouraged to take frequent photographs of the baby to share with the mother. The mother needs to be assured that the baby is being cared for properly in the neonatal unit or at home. It might be suggested that the family keep a log of the baby's progress, which can be helpful to the mother as she becomes more stable. If the mother is not interested in the infant, however, her feelings should be accepted by the staff. The patient's injuries may be the focus of her attention during the critical care phase. During family visits, time also should be spent concentrating on the mother's injuries and concerns. Conversations should not always focus on the baby. Continued disinterest in the infant may signal excessive guilt or denial. These feelings should be explored further with the patient.

Family Stress

After the delivery the disruption of the family unit inevitably alters role functions. Family members should be encouraged to express their needs, concerns, and problems. The critical care nurse should consider how to best meet the family's emotional needs. Open visitation policies decrease family stress.[100] The mother and baby could be in different medical institutions and the family does not need the additional stress of following limited visiting times. Appropriate referrals should be made to social service and pastoral care personnel as necessary. The family needs assistance in developing a plan for maternal and infant care on discharge from the hospital.

INTERMEDIATE CARE AND REHABILITATION PHASE

The pregnant trauma patient in the intermediate care and rehabilitation phases presents a challenging situation for health care team members, including nurses, trauma specialists, obstetric personnel, dieticians, social workers, and physical, occupational, and speech therapists. The patient and family have had to adapt to a sudden hospitalization and perhaps months of care in the critical care setting. Depending on the patient's injuries and critical care course, the adaptation process may be more profound as the patient prepares for discharge.

During the critical phase of care the primary goal was to provide aggressive maternal care with minimal fetal stress. As the pregnancy progresses and the patient's clinical condition shows continued improvement, the focus must be placed on the impending delivery. The family may begin to express fears about the fetal outcome. Changes in birthing plans must be made, and discharge planning should include delivery and home care requirements.

Concerns that existed during the critical care phase of care may carry over to the intermediate care/rehabilitation phases. The patient's nutritional status should continue to be a primary concern. Altered mobility and pain management issues, although often less intense, may continue to require consistent nursing intervention. However, the patient's involvement in managing each of these concerns becomes more active.

If the fetus was lost during the resuscitative or critical care phase, the patient and family must now deal with that loss and the effects of the trauma on the mother. The mother may feel guilt over the loss of the baby. Depending on the events leading to the injury, other family members may feel guilt about the incident. The adjustment process may be slow and tedious, and the family needs constant support. Pictures and a description of the baby may be appropriate to share with the mother for the first time. A Christian mother may need assurance that her baby was baptized.

An assessment of how the mother and family are coping with the loss of the baby must be performed on a continual basis. Although the fetal death may have occurred weeks earlier, the rehabilitation phase may be the time when the family has the energy to focus on their grief and possible guilt. As the patient stabilizes, an obstetric staff member should meet with the patient and family to review the fetal loss and discuss future pregnancies. In the grave event that the patient's injuries required a hysterectomy, the grieving process may be prolonged as the loss of future pregnancies is mourned. Many women equate loss of the uterus with a loss of femininity and desirability, a myth shared by some men as well. Therefore, the patient and family need continued counseling. Appropriate referrals should be made as needed.

LABOR AND DELIVERY PLANS

As the patient enters the third trimester, decisions should be made and plans established for the impending delivery. Initially it must be decided where labor and delivery will take place. The decision should be a collaborative one, with both the obstetric and rehabilitation staffs involved. Where the patient will receive optimal obstetric care should be a strong consideration. Transfer from the rehabilitation setting to an acute care facility may be necessary. Transportation should be arranged for either an interunit or interhospital transfer. The transportation means should be available 24 hours a day and be clearly stated in the patient's plan of care or pathway.

Signs and symptoms of labor should be assessed routinely. An organized plan of action when labor begins should be included as part of the patient's plan of care or pathway so that appropriate staff members are notified. All efforts should be made to ensure a smooth transfer when labor occurs.

The obstetric staff should be educated by the patient's nurse or the rehabilitation advanced practice nurse concerning the patient's current limitations. This may be accomplished during a meeting with the obstetric staff, when a patient profile may be presented. The patient's neurologic deficits and orthopedic limitations should be emphasized. If the patient has had a closed head injury and requires cognitive retraining, detailed information about her current level of functioning should be presented to the obstetric staff.

Orthopedic injuries that require special nursing interventions or that limit a patient's movement also should be explained. The obstetric staff may not be familiar with musculoskeletal stabilization devices such as external fixators and may need detailed instructions.[101] It should also be noted that pelvic ring disruption does not eliminate the possibility of vaginal delivery. Vaginal delivery is even possible in women with a fused symphysis.[102]

Plans also should be made regarding alternative positions for vaginal delivery. The patient's bedside nurse and the advanced practice nurse may be able to help the obstetric staff plan alternative positions. The obstetric staff may need to be reminded of the advisability of the lateral Sims position. A birthing bed allows flexibility in patient positioning and patient accessibility during delivery and can accommodate traction if needed.

Childbirth classes should not be neglected and need to be individualized according to the patient's special needs. The obstetric educator may need to give bedside education to the pregnant patient and father or other support person. This allows the obstetric team to become familiar with the patient's special care needs while concurrently providing the opportunity for the patient and the father to ask questions and express concerns about the upcoming labor and delivery process. If the patient has had a head injury, she may have difficulty understanding instructions; therefore, alternative plans may need to be made.

The importance of planning ahead for the upcoming delivery must be emphasized. The establishment of a strong, supportive relationship between the trauma and obstetric staffs fosters effective communication patterns and facilitates a smooth delivery process.

POSTPARTUM CARE

Many trauma patients, as a result of their injuries, are limited in their ability to care for themselves after delivery. This may be difficult for the postpartum nursing staff, who are not accustomed to caring for trauma patients and therefore are unfamiliar with their special care needs. Postpartum staff members should be educated by either the rehabilitative advanced practice nurse or the patient's nurse concerning the patient's ability to meet her own needs and those of the baby. Thorough attention will likely be focused on rehabilitation plans for discharge, but there must be some consideration of family planning/contraception. The patient may have become sexually active during rehabilitation, and now in the postpartum period family planning should be discussed. The obstetric staff should remind the team of this important aspect of postpartum care.

Family Needs

The situation is far from ideal when the newborn baby is in the nursery, the mother is in intermediate care or rehabilitation, and the family members are home. The nursing plan of care should include provisions to minimize family disruptions.

When possible, the patient should be allowed to care for her infant. At times it may be necessary for the nursing staff to offer alternative solutions if limitations imposed by the patient's injuries impede her caregiving abilities. For example, the patient may not be able to both hold and feed the baby, in which case the postpartum staff may assist the patient by holding the baby while allowing the patient to feed him or her. Early and frequent maternal-infant interaction is an important component of the bonding process; there should be open visitation rights. The attachment or bonding that occurs between a mother and a newborn infant is a complex, unique emotional relationship.[103] Efforts should be made to allow the mother to hold the infant or to have the infant lie by her side. Physical communication between the newborn and the mother allows the baby to use sensual abilities to promote bonding (Table 28-15) and therefore is imperative.

When the trauma patient's needs are extensive, she may be transferred back to the rehabilitation or intermediate care unit after the immediate postpartum period (first 24 hours). This may be the most practical alternative for the patient's care but produces maternal-infant separation. In this situation, every attempt should be made to arrange for regular and frequent maternal-infant interactions.

TABLE 28-15 **Parental-Infant Bonding: Newborn Sensual Responses or Abilities Used in Bonding**

Touch	Voice
Eye-to-eye contact	Entertainment
Odor	Biorhythmicity
Body warmth	

Data from Lowdermilk DL: Family dynamics after childbirth. In Bobak IM, Jensen MO, editors: *Essentials of maternity nursing,* 3rd ed, pp 560-577, St. Louis, 1991, Mosby.

It is also necessary for the family to identify who will provide infant care in the home after the baby's discharge. If infant care cannot be provided by family members or friends on a 24-hour basis, other alternatives must be explored. Reliable and competent contractual care providers may be identified by contacting an appropriate community agency.

Breast-Feeding

If at all possible, the mother's desire to breast-feed should be respected and accommodated. However, because the metabolic and emotional demands on the nursing mother are intensified, the status of the patient's clinical condition should be considered carefully by the rehabilitation team before a final decision regarding breast-feeding is made. An important aspect of this decision considers any medications required by the mother. Virtually all maternal medications appear in breast milk, and the amount of the medication, how it is bound with breast milk, and how much the fetus absorbs are not clearly known for all drugs.[67] The American Academy of Pediatrics publishes lists of drugs that are safe for use during pregnancy. Also, the time between the mother taking the medication and the infant nursing is important. The risk/benefit ratio should be evaluated.[67] If it is determined that breast-feeding is a viable option, the mother may need assistance while nursing the baby during visits.

It is necessary for milk to be extracted from the breasts between visits; therefore, a breast pump must be made available to the patient, and instruction and assistance for use should be provided as needed. Plans for milk storage and a routine for delivery to the baby must be arranged in conjunction with the family. It is interesting to note that often trauma and rehabilitation staff embrace being involved with assisting their patients to breast-feed. A newborn baby can bring excitement to the unit.

FETAL DEATH

When a newborn infant dies or a pregnancy is lost, parents should be expected and encouraged to grieve. The death of an infant or a fetus is experienced as a deep loss to the mother, father, and other family members, and a variety of reactions and responses are displayed by those who have invested emotional energy in the growth and development of the new life. A supportive and accepting attitude by the nurse caring for the patient and family are valuable as they address their feelings of grief (see Chapter 19). Consultation should be obtained from the perinatal grief management service.

Community Reintegration Phase

Preparation of the antepartum or postpartum trauma patient for discharge begins the day the patient is admitted. After weeks or possibly months of hospitalization, the patient must be prepared to return to home and to the community. The patient's obstetric status is an important consideration when planning care during this phase. If delivery occurred during the patient's hospitalization and the baby was discharged weeks before the mother, the priorities should be focused on maternal-infant interactions. For the patient who is pregnant during the discharge planning process, special attention must be placed on prenatal care and delivery plans, with careful consideration of injuries and restrictions imposed.

Perinatal Referrals

The antepartum trauma patient being discharged home must continue to receive prenatal care. Referral should be made to the patient's private obstetrician or to a high-risk maternity center if deemed necessary. The referral should include information about the patient's injuries and clinical course, current medications and treatment interventions, limitations that may affect the delivery process, and potential postpartum home care needs.

Home Health Care

The standard of care is to plan for the patient's early discharge and to provide for continuation of care through home health services to decrease medical costs. Early discharge is a possible alternative for the antepartum or postpartum trauma patient, but it requires special planning and the educational preparation of home health providers.

Before the patient is discharged, contacts should be made to the agency that will provide care to the pregnant or postpartum trauma patient on her release from the hospital. Discharge planning conferences should be scheduled as needed and should include the patient, family, nurse, physicians, therapists, social services, and members of the home health care team. This structured approach provides a forum for the patient's special care needs to be addressed and for the patient's and family's concerns to be expressed. These meetings also provide the opportunity for the patient and family members to begin to develop a trusting relationship with the home health care providers, thus fostering a smoother transition from hospital to home.

Family counseling sessions may be necessary. Physical or cognitive changes may alter the mother's ability to assume various role responsibilities. For example, the patient who returns home during the postpartum period with some cognitive dysfunction cannot assume full responsibility for the newborn baby. Another family member or a contractual infant care provider may be needed to assist with the care of the baby while allowing the patient short and frequent interactions with the baby to encourage maternal-infant bonding.

Future Trends and Prevention

Pregnant women in modern society usually remain active well into the third trimester of pregnancy. They continue to work outside the home and travel until the time of delivery. Driving or riding in automobiles is a reality for today's pregnant women, placing them at risk for traumatic injury. Trauma is often preventable, and public education that focuses on the proper use of safety belts during pregnancy may significantly decrease the number and severity of injuries resulting from vehicular crashes.

Safety belts should be worn during pregnancy because they prevent ejection from the vehicle and impact against the steering wheel and dashboard. The seat belt should be worn low or under the fundus, across the pelvis.[75] The shoulder harness should be worn in the normal position, not against the neck but between the breasts and off the shoulder (see Figure 28-2). Padding the seat belt for comfort is discouraged because the belt can shift upward on impact, causing injury to the thinner portion of the fundus. There should not be any slack in the belt.

Women are more likely to wear their seat belts than are men, but fewer women wear their seat belts when pregnant.[6] The major myth concerning seat belt use during pregnancy is that the belt will hurt the unborn child. Lack of safety belt use by anyone increases the chances of ejection from the vehicle, which increases chances of death. This, in turn, dramatically increases the risk of fetal death. Mandatory seat belt legislation and, more important, public education and enforcement may serve as major catalysts in increasing seat belt use during pregnancy and thus preventing injuries. A recent study comparing seat belt use between pregnant patients being seen at a county clinic with those receiving care at a private practice found a significant difference in seat belt use between the two groups. Fewer county patients (49%) always wore their seat belts compared with 81% of private practice patients. Education should be targeted to include both these groups, especially the higher-risk group.[104] Patients in both groups often report that they were not educated about the importance and the correct placement of restraints. Additional education should be targeted at the prenatal staff that regularly communicates with these patients. Posters showing proper seat belt placement should be displayed in waiting areas and patient care areas. Brochures should be developed for patients with diagrams, and each year legislative groups should declare one month of the year Wear Your Seat Belt When Pregnant Month.

An area that is currently being researched is the mechanism of injury for pregnant patients involved in a motor vehicle crash. In 1996 the first pregnant crash dummy was developed but it had limitations. A second-generation pregnant abdominal model is more realistic and can more accurately assess the probability of fetal loss from abruptio placenta.[105]

In late pregnancy a pregnant woman's altered gait and balance should be of concern. Safety measures should be taken by pregnant women, including care in climbing on ladders and avoiding climbing on chairs (Table 28-16). Falls are a significant mechanism of injury and education to decrease the incidence is important.[106] In areas where snow and ice are common on sidewalks and streets, pregnant women must exercise caution when they step off a curb because they often can no longer see their feet. Fatique is common in pregnancy and pregnant women should be encouraged to take small frequent breaks. Occupations that require long periods of standing recommend that women take a break for a few minutes every 2 to 3 hours and elevate their legs.

Violence and abuse are serious health problems in the world today. In the past 20 years there has been a signicant amount of research regarding this problem in the pregnant population.[6,16,18] All health care professionals need to be educated to ask about violence in their patients' lives. Current research is helping to define specific patient populations that are at significantly higher risk.[6] Clearly targeted education and intervention in high-risk populations could lead to improved neonatal outcomes.[18]

TABLE 28-16 Safety Precautions During Pregnancy

Area	Precaution
Home	Do not stand on stools or stepladders because it is difficult to maintain balance on a narrow base.
	Avoid throw rugs without a nonskid backing.
	Keep small items such as toys out of pathways because it is difficult for a pregnant woman to see her feet.
	Use caution when stepping in and out of a bathtub because the surface is slippery.
	Do not overload electrical circuits because it is difficult for a pregnant woman to escape a fire as a result of poor mobility.
	Do not smoke (many fires are started by a person's falling asleep with a cigarette).
	Do not take medicine in the dark (an error may be made because of limited vision).
Work	Avoid handling toxic substances.
	Avoid working to a point of fatigue, which lowers judgment.
	Avoid long periods of standing, which can lead to orthostatic hypotension and fainting.
Automobile	Use a seat belt at all times.
	Refuse to ride with anyone who has been drinking alcohol or whose judgment might be impaired.

Adapted from Pilliteri A: *Maternal and child health nursing,* 3rd ed, p 356, New York, 1999, Lippincott.

NURSING RESEARCH AND EDUCATION

The first step in research on the topic of trauma during pregnancy is clarification of the scope of the problem. It is estimated that 7% of pregnant women undergo trauma or injury during pregnancy.[2] It is unclear how this figure was derived and whether it includes mild falls (which may not be recorded in hospital records) and severe trauma. Establishing a database of pregnant trauma patients—their injuries and outcomes (both fetal and maternal)—would yield a wealth of information. The National Trauma Registry lists pregnancy as a preexisting medical condition and not a specific question, which makes it hard to gather national data. There has been a great number of studies addressing two clinical issues: predicting fetal outcome and determining how long to monitor a pregnant patient after a traumatic event.[4,7-9,11,12,28,58,83,107] In these studies, data are gathered retrospectively from chart reviews and trauma registry data. A prospective multicenter study would eliminate any data that might be missed and would be more useful. It would also be helpful to gather fetal and uterine data that are not captured at all in current trauma registries.

Throughout the trauma cycle of care it is the trauma nurse's role to help achieve optimal outcomes for the pregnant patient and her fetus. It is important that trauma nurses understand how important it is to establish collaborative teams involving obstetric and trauma specialists to meet this goal. Effective interdisciplinary communication is imperative. Nurses need to understand the unique mechanisms of injury and physiologic changes of pregnancy that can both mask and mimic injury. Information about the unique injuries and potential complications of the pregnant trauma patient and the appropriate interventions to manage these clinical problems should be regularly reviewed with nurses who may care for these patients. The nurse's role in the emotional and psychosocial aspects of dealing with such clinical aspects as maternal-infant bonding, the stress of the traumatic event during pregnancy, and the possible loss of the fetus also must be addressed. Managing the pregnant trauma patient is clinically challenging but can be very rewarding.

REFERENCES

1. National Center for Health Statistics: Births: preliminary data for 2004, *Natl Vital Stat Rep* 54:1-20, 2005.
2. Fildes J, Ried L, Jones N et al: Trauma the leading cause of maternal death, *J Trauma* 32:643-644, 1992.
3. Baerga-Varela Y, Zietlow SP, Bannon MP et al: Trauma in pregnancy, *Mayo Clin Proc* 75:1243-1248, 2000.
4. Corsi PR, Rasslan S, de Oliveira LB et al: Trauma in pregnant women: analysis of maternal and fetal mortality, *Injury* 30: 239-243, 1999.

5. Weiss HB, Lawrence B, Miller T: Prevalence and risk of hospitalized pregnant occupants in car crashes, *Annu Proc Assoc Adv Automot Med* 46:355-366, 2002.
6. Ikossi DG, Lazar AA, Morabito D et al: Profile of mothers at risk: an analysis of injury and pregnancy loss in 1,195 trauma patients, *J Am Coll Surg* 200:49-56, 2004.
7. Shah K, Simons R, Holbrook T et al: Trauma in pregnancy: maternal and fetal outcomes, *J Trauma* 45:83-86, 1998.
8. Weiss HB, Songer TJ, Fabio A: Fetal death related to maternal injury, *JAMA* 286:1863-1868, 2001.
9. Esposito T, Gens R, Smith LG et al: Trauma during pregnancy: a review of 79 cases, *Arch Surg* 126:1073-1078, 1991.
10. Curet MJ, Schermer CR, Demarest GB et al: Predictors of outcomes in trauma in pregnancy: identification of patients who can be monitored for less than six hours, *J Trauma* 49:18-25, 2000.
11. Ali J, Yeo A, Gana TJ et al: Predictors of fetal mortality in pregnant trauma patients, *J Trauma* 42:782-785, 1997.
12. Rogers FB, Rozycki GS, Osler TM et al: A multi-institutional study of factors associated with fetal death in injured pregnant patients, *Arch Surg* 134:1274-1277, 1999.
13. Jackson F: Accidental injury: the problem and the initiatives. In Buschbaum HJ, editor: *Trauma in pregnancy,* pp 1-21, Philadelphia, 1979, W. B. Saunders.
14. National Safety Council: *Injury facts,* Chicago, 1999, National Safety Council.
15. Tjaden P, Thoennes N: Extent, nature, and consequences of intimate partner violence: findings from the National Violence Against Women Survey, Publication NCJ 181867, Washington, DC, 2000, U.S. Department of Justice Office of Justice Programs.
16. Parker B, McFarlane J, Soeken K: Abuse during pregnancy: effects on maternal complications and birth weight in adult and teenage women, *Obstet Gynecol* 84:323-328, 1994.
17. Gazmararian JA, Lazorick S, Spitz AM et al: Prevalence of violence against pregnant women, *JAMA* 275:1915-1920, 1996.
18. Silverman JG, Decker MR, Reed E: Intimate partner violence victimization prior to and during pregnancy among women residing in 26 U.S. states: associations with maternal and neonatal health, *Am J Obstet Gynecol* 195:140-148, 2006.
19. Martin SL, English KT, Clark KA et al: Violence and substance use among North Carolina pregnant women, *Am J Public Health* 86:991-998, 1996.
20. McFarlane J, Parker B, Soeken K: Abuse during pregnancy: associations with maternal health and infant birth weight, *Nurs Res* 45:37-42, 1996.
21. Parker B, McFarlane J: Identifying and helping battered pregnant women, *Am J Matern Child Nurs* 16:161-164, 1991.
22. Maghsoudi H, Samnia R, Garodoghi A et al: Burns in pregnancy, *Burns* 32:246-250, 2006.
23. Sherer DM, Schenker JG: Accidental injury during pregnancy, *Obstet Gynecol Surv* 44:330-338, 1989.
24. Pepperill R, Rubinstein E, MacIsaac I: Motor car accidents during pregnancy, *Med J Aust* 1:203-205, 1977.
25. Crosby WM, King AI, Stout LC: Fetal survival following impact: improvement with shoulder harness restraint, *Am J Obstet Gynecol* 112:1101-1106, 1972.
26. Crosby WM, Costiloe JP: Safety of lap-belt restraint for pregnant victims of automobile collisions, *N Engl J Med* 284: 632-636, 1971.
27. Wolf ME, Alexander BH, Revora BH et al: A retrospective cohort study of seatbelt use and pregnancy outcomes after motor vehicle crash, *J Trauma* 34i:116-119, 1993.
28. El-Kady D, Gilbert WM, Anderson J et al: Trauma during pregnancy: an analysis of maternal and fetal outcomes in a large population, *Am J Obstet Gynecol* 190:1661-1668, 2004.
29. McFarlane J, Parker B, Soeken K et al: Safety behaviors of abused women after an intervention during pregnancy, *J Obstet Gynecol Neonatal Nurs* 27:64-69, 1998.
30. Weaver LK, Valentine KJ, Hopkins RO: Carbon monoxide poisoning: risk factors for cognitive sequelae and the role of hyperbaric oxygen, *Am J Respir Crit Care Med* 176:491-497, 2007.
31. Longo LD: The biological effects of carbon monoxide on the pregnant woman, fetus, and newborn infant, *Am J Obstet Gynecol* 129:69-103, 1977.
32. Longo LD, Hill EP: Carbon monoxide uptake and elimination in fetal and maternal sheep, *Am J Physiol* 232:H324-H330, 1977.
33. Van Hoesen KB, Camporesi EM, Moon RE et al: Should hyperbaric oxygen be used to treat the pregnant patient for acute carbon monoxide poisoning? A case report and literature review, *JAMA* 261:1039-1043, 1989.
34. Hadlock FP, Deter RL, Harrist RB et al: Fetal biparietal diameter: a critical reevaluation of the relation to menstrual age by means of realtime ultrasound. *J Ultrasound Med* 1:97-104, 1982.
35. Sheppard M, Filly R: A standardized plane for biparietal diameter measurement, *J Ultrasound Med* 1:145-150, 1982.
36. Hadlock FP, Deter RL, Harrist RB: Fetal head circumference: relation to menstrual age, *AJR Am J Roentgenol* 138:649-653, 1982.
37. Esposito T: Pitfalls in resuscitation and early management of the pregnant trauma patient, *Trauma Q* 5:1-22, 1988.
38. Mighty H: Trauma in pregnancy, *Crit Care Clin* 10:623-634, 1994.
39. Crosby W: Trauma during pregnancy: maternal and fetal injuries, *Obstet Gynecol Surv* 29:683-697, 1974.
40. Bealsey J, Damos J, Roberts R et al: The advanced life support in obstetrics course, *Arch Fam Med* 3:1037-1042, 1994.
41. American College of Surgeons' Committee on Trauma: *Advanced trauma life support,* 7th ed, Chicago, 2004, American College of Surgeons.
42. Pearlman MD: Motor vehicle crashes, pregnancy loss and preterm labor, *Int J Gynaecol Obstet* 57:127-132, 1997.
43. Weinberg L, Stelle R, Pugh R et al: The pregnant trauma patient, *Anaesth Intensive Care* 33:167-180, 2005.
44. Grossman N: Blunt trauma in pregnancy, *Am Family Physican* 70:1313-1326, 2004.
45. Shah AJ, Kilcline BA: Trauma in pregnancy, *Emerg Med Clin North Am* 21:615-629, 2003.
46. Mattox KL, Goetzl L: Trauma in pregnancy, *Crit Care Med* 33(10 Suppl):S385-S389, 2005.
47. Vandeer Veer J: Trauma during pregnancy, *Topics Emerg Med Spec Aspects Trauma Care* 6:72-77, 1984.
48. Knudson M, Rozycki GS, Paquin MM: Reproductive system trauma. In Moore EE, Feliciano D, Mattox KL, editors: *Trauma,* 5th ed, pp 851-874, New York, 2004, McGraw-Hill.
49. National Institutes of Health Consensus Development Conference: Prevention of venous thrombosis and pulmonary embolism, *JAMA* 256:744-749, 1986.
50. Shah S, Miller PR, Meredith JW et al: Elevated admission white blood cell count in pregnant trauma patients: an indicator of ongoing placental abruption, *Am Surg* 68:644-647, 2002.
51. Clark S, Cotton O, Lee W et al: Central hemodynamic assessment of normal term pregnancy, *Am J Obstet Gynecol* 161: 1439-1442, 1989.

52. Lowdermilk C, Gavant ML, Qaisi W et al: Screening helical CT for evaluation of blunt traumatic injury in the pregnant patient, *Radiographics* 19:S243-S258, 1999.
53. Beydoun SN: Morphologic changes in the renal track in pregnancy, *Clin Obstet Gynecol* 28:249-256, 1985.
54. Stables D: The endocrine system. In Stables D, Rankin J, editors: *Physiology in childbearing with anatomy and related biosciences,* 2nd ed, pp 375-385, Philadelphia, 2005, Elsevier.
55. American College of Obstetricians and Gynecologists: Practice bulletin: clinical management guidelines for obstetricans-gynecologists, Ultrasound in Pregnancy, No. 58, Washington, DC, 2004, American College of Obstetricians and Gynecologists.
56. Ma OJ, Mateer JR, DeBehnke DJ: Use of ultrasound for the evaluation of pregnant trauma patients, *J Trauma* 40:665-668, 1996.
57. Goodwin H, Holmes JF, Wisner DH: Abdominal ultrasound examination in pregnant blunt trauma patients, *J Trauma Inj Infect Crit Care* 50:689-694, 2001.
58. Pearlman MD, Tintinalli JE, Lorenz RP: A prospective controlled study of outcome after trauma during pregnancy, *Am J Obstet Gynecol* 162:1502-1510, 1990.
59. Goodwin TM, Brun MT: Pregnancy outcome and fetomaternal hemorrhage after noncatastrophic trauma, *Am J Obstet Gynecol* 162:665-671, 1990.
60. Harman CR: Assessment of fetal health. In Creasy RK, Resnik R, editors: *Maternal-fetal medicine principles and practice,* 5th ed, Philadelphia, 2004, Elsevier.
61. Manning FA: Fetal biophysical profile, *Obstet Gynecol Clin North Am* 26:557-577, 1999.
62. Kuczkowski KM, Reisner LS, Benumof JL: Airway problems and new solutions for the obstetric patient, *J Clin Anesth* 15:552-563, 2003.
63. Munner U, de Boisblanc B, Suresh M: Airway problems in pregnancy, *Crit Care Med* 33:S259-S267, 2005.
64. Beningfield S, Potgieter H, Nicol A et al: Report on a new type of trauma full-body digital x-ray machine, *Emerg Radiol* 10: 23-29, 2003.
65. Wagner LK, Lester RG, Saldana LR: *Exposure of the pregnant patient to diagnostic radiations: a guide to medical management,* 2nd ed, Madison, WI, 1997, Medical Physicis.
66. Mann FA, Nathens A, Langer SG et al: Communicating with the family: the risks of medical radiation to concept uses in victims of major blunt-force torso trauma, *J Trauma* 48: 354-357, 2000.
67. Briggs GG, Freeman RFRK, Yaffe S: *Drugs in pregnancy and lactation,* 7th ed, Baltimore, 2005, Lippincott Williams & Wilkins.
68. Gensburg J, Hush J: Use of antithrombotic agents during pregnancy, *Chest* 114:5245-5305, 1998.
69. Ariel M, Koren G: Low-molecular-weight heparins during pregnancy, *Can Family Physican* 51:199-201, 2005.
70. Pearse CS, Magrina JF, Finley BE: Use of MAST suit in obstetrics and gynecology, *Obstet Gynecol Surv* 37:416-422, 1984.
71. Gunning J: For controlling intractable hemorrhage, the gravity suit, *Contemp Obstet Gynecol* 22:23-32, 1983.
72. Esposito TJ, Gens DR, Gerber-Smith L et al: Evaluation of blunt abdominal trauma occurring during pregnancy, *J Trauma* 29:1628-1632, 1989.
73. Curry J, Quintana J: Myocardial infarction with ventricular fibrillation during pregnancy treated by direct current defibrillation with fetal survival, *Chest* 58:82-84, 1970.
74. Songster G, Clark S: Cardiac arrest in pregnancy: what to do, *Contemp Obstet Gynecol* 26:141-155, 1985.
75. American College of Obstetricians and Gynecologists: *Educational bulletin: obstetrical aspects of trauma management,* No. 251, Washington, DC, 1998, American College of Obstetricians and Gynecologists.
76. Katz VL, Dotters DJ, Roegemueller W: Perimortem cesarean delivery, *Obstet Gynecol* 68:571-576, 1986.
77. Weber CE: Postmortem cesarean section: review of the literature and case reports. *Am J Obstet Gynecol* 110:158-165, 1971.
78. Pacheco L, Gui A, Van Hook J et al: Burns in pregnancy, *Obstet Gynecol* 106:1210-1212, 2005.
79. Prasana M, Singh K: Early burn wound excision in "major" burns with "pregnancy": a preliminary report, *Burns* 22: 234-237, 1996.
80. Ullmann Y, Blumnfeld Z, Hakim M et al: Urgent delivery, the treatment of choice in the pregnant woman with extended burn injury, *Burns* 23:157-159, 1997.
81. Silverman RK, Mortano J: Hyperbaric oxygen treatment during pregnancy in acute carbon monoxide poisoning: a case report, *J Reprod Med* 42:309-311, 1997.
82. Hill D, Lense J: Abdominal trauma in the pregnant patient, *Am Fam Physician* 53:1269-1274, 1996.
83. Theodorou DA, Velmahos GC, Souter I et al: Fetal death after trauma in pregnancy, *Am Surg* 66:809-812, 2000.
84. Higgins S, Garite T: Late abruptio placenta in trauma patients: implications for monitoring, *Obstet Gynecol* 63:105-109, 1984.
85. Pearlman MD, Tintinalli JE, Lorenz RF: Blunt trauma during pregnancy, *N Engl J Med* 323:1609-1613, 1990.
86. American Academy of Pediatrics and American College of Obstetricians and Gynecologists: *Guidelines for perinatal care,* 5th ed, Elk Grove Village, IL, 2002, American Academy of Pediatrics, and Washington, DC, 2002, American College of Obstetricians and Gynecologists.
87. Towery R, English P, Wisner D: Evaluation of pregnant women after blunt injury, *J Trauma* 35:731-735, 1993.
88. Berkman ND, Thorp JM, Lohr KN et al: Tocolytic treatment for the management of preterm labor: a review of evidence, *Am J Obstet Gynecol* 188:1648-1659, 2003.
89. King JF, Flenady VJ, Papatsonis DN et al: Calcium channel blockers for inhibiting preterm labour, *Cochrane Database Syst Rev* 1:CD002255, 2003.
90. Gaunekar NN, Crowther CA: Maintenance therapy with calcium channel blockers for preventing birth after threatened preterm labour, *Cochrane Database Syst Rev* 3:CD004071, 2004.
91. Emery CL, Moreway LF, Chung-Park M et al: The Kleihauer-Betke test: clinical utility, indication, and correlation in patients with placental abruption and cocaine use, *Arch Pathol Lab Med* 119:1032-1037, 1995.
92. Rose PG, Strohm PL, Zuspan FP: Fetomaternal hemorrhage following trauma, *Am J Obstet Gynecol* 153:844-847, 1985.
93. Mokriski BLK, Malinov AM: Anesthesia for the pregnant trauma patient, *Probl Anesth* 4:530-540, 1990.
94. Kuczkowski K: Nonobstetric surgery during pregnancy: what are the risks of anesthesia? *Obstetr Gynecol Surv* 59:52-56, 2003.
95. Nuevo FR: Anesthesia for nonobstetric surgery in the pregnant patient. In Birnbach DJ, Gatt SP, Datta S, editors: *Textbook of obstetrical anesthesia,* pp 289-298, New York, 2000, Churchill Livingstone.
96. Goodman S: Anesthesia for nonobstetric surgery in the pregnant patient, *Semin Perinatol* 26:136-145, 2002.
97. Moice K, Belfont M: Damage control of the obstetric patient, *Surg Clin North Am* 77:834-852, 1997.

98. Association of PeriOperative Registered Nurses: *Standards, recommended practices, and guidelines,* pp 265-266, Denver, 2007, AORN Publications.
99. Simpson KR: Critical illness during pregnancy considerations for evaluation and treatment of the fetus as the second patient, *Crit Care Nurs Q* 29:20-31, 2006.
100. Campbell PT, Rudisill P: Psychosocial needs of the critically ill obstetric patient the nurse's role, *Crit Care Nurse Q* 29:77-80, 2006.
101. Hart MA: Help my orthopaedic patient is pregnant! *Orthop Nurs* 24:108-116, 2005.
102. Copeland CE: Pelvic ring disruption in women: genitourinary and obstetric implications. In Tile M, Helfet D, Kellam J, editors: *Fractures of the pelvis and acetabulum,* Philadelphia, 2003, Lippincott Williams & Wilkins.
103. Lowdermilk DL, Perry SE: *Maternity and women's health care,* 9th ed, pp 612-632, St. Louis, 2007, Mosby Elsevier.
104. Taylor AJ, McGwin G, Sharp CE et al: Seatbelt use during pregnancy: a comparison of women in two prenatal care settings, *Matern Child Health J* 9:173-179, 2005.
105. Pearlman MD, Klinich KD, Schneider LW et al: A comprehensive program to improve safety for pregnant women and fetuses in motor vehicle crashes: a preliminary report, *Am J Obstet Gynecol* 182:1554-1564, 2000.
106. Dunning K, LeMasters G, Levin L et al: Falls in workers during pregnancy: risk factors, job hazards, and high risk occupations, *Am J Indust Med* 44:664-672, 2003.
107. Biester EM, Tomich PG, Esposito TJ et al: Trauma in pregnancy: normal Revised Trauma Score in relation to other markers of maternofetal status: a preliminary study, *Am J Obstet Gynecol* 176:1206-1212, 1997.

29

PEDIATRIC TRAUMA

Patricia A. Moloney-Harmon

Trauma is the leading cause of death in children from 1 to 14 years of age. Approximately 20,000 children and adolescents die each year, with the majority of deaths in children less than 19 years old resulting from unintentional injury.[1] In addition, each year another 100,000 children have permanent disability from injury.[2] In fact, traumatic injury is the leading cause of childhood hospitalization—approximately 300,000 hospitalizations per year in the United States.[3] The economic costs are staggering. Traumatic injuries are a major cause of medical spending for children ages 5 to 14 years with billions of dollars spent on caring for the pediatric trauma victim each year.[3] But the impact of pediatric trauma extends far beyond statistics and is often seen in the tragedy that the family and society must endure. Therefore nurses must be able to recognize the patterns of pediatric injury and the appropriate treatment.

The purpose of this chapter is to explain the similarities and differences between critically ill children and adults and to bring the nurse up to date on the practical management of the pediatric trauma patient. This chapter describes in detail appropriate assessment and management strategies in caring for a critically injured pediatric patient through the resuscitation, critical care, and intermediate care/rehabilitation phases of care. Special emphasis is placed on nursing management considerations as they pertain to the child rather than on specific injury types.

Nurses often have the primary responsibility for recognizing and interpreting changes in the child's condition. Therefore, the nurse needs to understand how the child's normal circulating blood volume, cardiac output, thermoregulation, fluid and electrolyte requirements, and renal function are different from those of the adult. Small variations may cause significant changes in the child's condition. These changes must be immediately recognized, and the nurse must act on them at once. The intent of this chapter is to provide a systematic framework that allows nurses to relate to the pediatric trauma patient on the basis of the unique physiologic and psychologic dynamics inherent in this age group.

EPIDEMIOLOGY/INCIDENCE

In the United States, children between the ages of 1 and 19 years are at greater risk of dying from injury than from all diseases combined. Injury in this population is also the leading cause of disability. The single largest cause of all trauma-related deaths is motor vehicle incidents. Other leading causes of traumatic injury in children include the following: burns, drownings, poisonings, firearms, falls, and abuse.

Two of three childhood traumatic incidents occur in males. The peak unintentional injury age range is between 4 and 12 years, with the highest incidence at 8 years. The reason for this peak is that children in this age group are starting school, and parents generally are allowing them to have some independence.

PATTERNS OF INJURY

The most common injuries seen in children are blunt as opposed to penetrating injuries. At least 80% of life-threatening injuries in children occur from blunt trauma.[2] Blunt injuries are associated with rapid deceleration, which can occur in automobile incidents or with direct blows resulting from child abuse or contact sports activities. Blunt trauma is commonly associated with multiple injuries, which can make management of a child injured by a nonpenetrating mechanism complicated. Penetrating injuries represent approximately 20% of pediatric trauma.[2]

The anatomy of children renders them especially vulnerable to traumatic injury. The head of the child is proportionately larger in relation to body mass compared with these proportions in an adult; therefore, the child's head is especially vulnerable to injury. Head injury is the most common cause of traumatic death in children.

In pedestrian trauma, injuries to the left side of the patient are predominant, perhaps because vehicles are driven on the right side of the road in the United States. Skeletal injuries usually involve long bones, especially of the lower limbs.[4] Chest injuries generally occur as a result of blunt trauma. Because of differences in the child's compliant chest wall, rib fractures and flail chest are less common than in adults, but pulmonary contusions are more frequent.[5] Injuries to the liver and spleen are the most common blunt abdominal injuries seen in children; other injury sites include the bowel and pancreas. Because the kidneys in children are less protected and more mobile than in an adult, genitourinary system injuries often involve the kidneys and, less frequently, the bladder and urethra.[6]

TRAUMA AND CHILD ABUSE

Child abuse and neglect are broadly defined as the maltreatment of children and adolescents by their parents, guardians, or other caretakers. Reports of child maltreatment in the United States continue to rise.[7] The nurse has two main responsibilities in such cases: detecting and reporting. The laws on child abuse reporting are clear. In all states it is mandatory for nurses to report suspected cases of child abuse and neglect to the local protective service agency. The law protects health professionals from liability suits if suspicion proves to be wrong. Reluctance to report such information can lead to a recurrence of abuse and injury. The opportunity to help these children lies in the ability of the emergency department staff not only to appropriately treat the child but also to recognize the recurring nature of the underlying problem.

An important facet of the evaluation of pediatric trauma should be a careful examination of the child for other signs that might suggest the possibility of intentional or inflicted injury. Inconsistencies between the trauma history and the injuries sustained should alert the nurse to potential child abuse.[8] Diagnostic signs of child abuse may include orbital ecchymosis in the absence of a clear causative factor. This is a serious concern because of the high incidence of subdural hematoma formation associated with vigorous shaking or jarring of an infant's head. Skull fractures, particularly if out of magnitude with the history, should always alert the nurse to the possibility of inflicted injury. The general appearance and nutritional state of the child also may suggest neglect or maltreatment. Other diagnostic signs may include cigarette burns; unusual bruising, especially over the back or soft tissue areas of the body; and any situation in which the circumstances are not clearly defined as causative of the injury. Old fracture sites revealed on radiographic examination also should raise suspicion. Careful examination of the genitalia and anal areas always need to be part of the evaluation of the injured child. Any injury in these areas should raise suspicion of sexual abuse.

In addition to detecting and reporting, the nurse's role is to give the child the necessary emergency treatment and protection while at the same time helping to alleviate the parents' distress. Informing the parents of the need for the child's treatment and protection and verbalizing an interest in helping the parents through the crisis are important roles for the nurse. This is a difficult task for nurses who are feeling anger toward the parents; therefore, it is imperative for nurses to explore and come to terms with their own feelings regarding child abuse before therapeutic intervention can be expected. A helping relationship needs to be established early with the family to lay the groundwork for future intervention. If intentional injury is raised as a legitimate consideration in the causation of the child's injury, the child protection team must be alerted so that they can help clarify the circumstances surrounding the injury.

PREVENTION STRATEGIES

With the recognition that unintentional injury and death are major public health problems, nurses play a major role in injury prevention. On the basis of clinical experiences and the identification of patterns and trends related to pediatric trauma, nurses' contributions are paramount in all multidisciplinary efforts to determine sound trauma prevention strategies.[9]

Most children who are killed or injured in automobile crashes are passengers. These casualties occur when an automobile collides with another vehicle or a fixed object. The use of restraints decreases fatalities from motor vehicle crush injuries by 13% to 46%.[10] By communicating these facts, health professionals involved in the care of pediatric patients have been instrumental in promoting the passage of safety restraint laws in all states. Because nurses are frequently in teaching roles, they are instrumental in bringing the legislation to the user level by instructing parents in how to protect their children and how to use restraint devices correctly.

Bicycle injuries are a common cause of injury requiring treatment in an emergency department. The most effective way to make bicycle riding safer is to insist that riders wear helmets. Improved bicycle design also contributes to the reduction of injury rates and injury severity.

Drowning, the fourth leading cause of death in children, is most common in children under 4 years of age and in adolescent males 15 to 19 years of age.[9] Prevention strategies to decrease the incidence of drowning include teaching parents never to leave an infant or young child alone during a bath, providing supervised swimming instruction for children, and installing safety fences around pools. Cardiopulmonary resuscitation (CPR) helps to decrease the number of deaths if initiated early and executed effectively; therefore, CPR education is paramount.

Fire-related deaths among children can be reduced in several ways. Because many fires are started by ignited cigarettes, the incidence of fires could be decreased by manufacturing cigarettes that self-extinguish. Parents also should be taught never to leave small children home alone, even for brief periods, and matches and lighters need to be kept out of the reach of children. Smoke detectors in the home can provide early warning of fires and are therefore considered valuable devices in preventing asphyxiation and burns. Nurses are instrumental in preventing fire-related injuries by teaching parents the necessity of having smoke detectors in the home and the importance of checking the battery routinely. Home fire drills involving all family members are important to establish and reinforce safe practices.

Falls by children are not uncommon, but, although many are minor, they account for a large number of injuries and deaths each year.[11] Deaths are often caused by falls from second-story windows by wandering toddlers. Nurses need to educate parents about the importance of constant adult supervision in and around the home, the installation of safety gates at the tops and bottoms of stairwells, and diligent use of window locks.

Playground safety is also an area that requires community education and awareness. Playground design should be in accordance with available safety standards. Standards include using wood chips instead of concrete on the ground, reducing the height of equipment, and replacing metal pieces with plastic or wood.

RESUSCITATION PHASE

The priorities of management for the pediatric trauma patient during the resuscitation phase are affected by a broad spectrum of factors. Immediate interventions depend on the severity of injuries and the critical nature of the patient's responses. The primary and secondary surveys provide a structured and systematic approach to the physical assessment of the patient. Other factors that must be considered are the growth and development patterns of the child. In addition, the child's family must be cared for as they face the traumatic experience with the child.

ASSESSMENT CONSIDERATIONS

Pediatric Trauma History

A thorough history is obtained during the early evaluation of a child who has sustained multiple injuries and is included as part of the nursing database. The purpose of the history is to determine and record the nature, location, and time of injury. The history of the injury is crucial to the child's treatment and begins at the scene of the incident. The history includes events leading to the incident, mechanism and time of injury, clinical course after the injury, contamination of wound sites, previous history of chronic illness or injury, allergies, medications, and time of the last meal eaten before injury. The Emergency Nurses Association recommends taking a CIAMPEDS history[12]:

C = Chief complaint
I = Immunizations
A = Allergies
M = Medications
P = Past medical history
E = Events surrounding the illness or injury
D = Diet
S = Symptoms associated with the illness or injury

The chief complaint is the reason for the child's visit to the emergency department, which in this case is the traumatic incident. Immunizations include an evaluation of the child's current immunization status. An allergy history is obtained in children, as with all patients. The parents are asked if the child is allergic to any medicines, adhesive tape, latex, or environmental substances. The nurse establishes whether the parents have given the child any medications recently and whether the child takes medication routinely for diabetes, seizures, lung disease, cardiac disorders, or other disease entities. Determination is made as to whether the child is under medical care for reasons other than routine well-child health care. Events surrounding the injury include mechanism, suspected injuries, prehospital assessment and treatment, and what led to the injury. Determination of when the child's last meal was eaten is important if the child needs to be intubated, sedated, or requires surgery. Any symptoms and their progression since the time of injury are ascertained.[12]

Because of limitations in communication skills, (i.e., undeveloped speaking and writing abilities), neither the infant nor the very young child can give a complete history, but it is useful to obtain whatever information is possible from the child. Younger children are likely to remember recent events. Earlier events may be better remembered by a parent or caretaker, although their accuracy may be clouded by the emotional state after the injury. In general, once a child reaches school age, obtaining a history becomes considerably easier.

The nurse begins to establish a relationship with the family and the child during this information-gathering session. Serious consideration must be given to the fact that this crisis has disrupted the entire family unit and that fear and anxiety prevail. The family needs as much feedback from the medical and nursing professionals as possible on a continual basis. Establishing a supportive rapport with the family during this initial phase helps to foster a closer working relationship among the child, the parents, and the health care team members throughout the child's hospitalization. Early interactions with family members and the information presented should be documented in the interdisciplinary notes. An assessment of the family's initial reactions, responses, concerns, and coping abilities serves as a baseline for other nurses who continue to care for the patient and family.

Growth and Development

Physical Development. The initial encounter with the child includes an assessment of the child's growth and physical development, which helps to identify existing alterations that determine the approach used during the examination. This assessment is done quickly because of the critical nature of the child's injury. An accurate estimate of the child's size and weight (Table 29-1) is made as soon as possible so that therapy can be initiated. When time allows, however, an exact weight should be obtained because medical treatment

TABLE 29-1 **Approximate Weights for Children**

Age	Weight (kg)
Newborn	3
6 months	6
1 year	10
3 years	15
5 years	20
8 years	25
10 years	30
16 years	50

that involves drug and fluid therapy, calculated on a per-kilogram basis, must be accurately determined.

Psychosocial Factors. The multisystem injuries and hospitalization of a critically ill child are devastating for the child and the family. Nurses have the responsibility to do everything possible to minimize the psychologic trauma that accompanies this traumatic incident. Because stressful medical situations can become the focus of fears and the source of new symptoms for the child, pediatric emergency care must include not only physical management but also consideration of the child's psychologic reactions to the illness. By relying on basic age-appropriate developmental characteristics, nurses can be astute to the general psychologic responses expected of the child. Table 29-2 summarizes the essential issues in this assessment process on the basis of the child's age. Appropriate preparation for procedures is also outlined.

General Principles. Several general principles are applicable when working with a pediatric patient. For most children, security in the world comes from their parents. Wanting their parents with them may be the child's first priority, even above relief of pain. When taking care of children, the nurse should observe the following guidelines:

- Let the child know that someone will call the parents, and tell the child when they arrive.
- If the child brought a toy, let the child hold it.
- When speaking to the patient, get down to the child's eye level so that the child can see your face. Speak clearly and slowly so that the child can hear you.
- Never assume that the child has understood you. Find out by questioning the child.
- Do not let the child witness treatment given to a seriously ill adult. Take the time to segregate the child to avoid additional emotional trauma.
- Be honest about the possibility of pain during the physical examination. If the child asks about being sick or hurt, tell the truth, but give reassurance by telling the child that you are there to help. If you appear calm and in control, it is more reassuring to the child.
- Touch the child and hold the child's hand. Acceptance of you by the child shows in the reaction to your

TABLE 29-2 **Developmental Considerations for Pediatric Trauma Patients**

	Infant (0-1 yr)	**Toddler** (1-3 yr)	**Preschool Child** (3-6 yr)	**School-Age Child** (6-12 yr)	**Adolescent** (12-18 yr)
Developmental task (Erikson)	Trust vs. mistrust	Autonomy vs. doubt and shame	Initiative vs. guilt	Industry vs. inferiority	Identity vs. role confusion
Cognitive development (Piaget)	Sensorimotor knowing	Preoperational thought	Preoperational thought (late phase)	Concrete operations	Formal operations
Communication	Cries, facial expression, motor activity	Simple phrases, cries, physical activity	Sentences, crying, physical activity Very literal Does not comprehend cause and effect	Well-developed vocabulary	Abstract thinker Generally seeks/desires information
Stresses/fears	Disruptions in routine	Separation, pain	Separation, abandonment, pain, mutilation	Loss of control, bodily injury, death, separation, pain	Disfigurement, separation from peers, loss of control
Illness concept	None	None	Illness as feeling state	Understands various aspects of illness, some basic anatomy	Understands anatomy and physiology
Preparation		Simple, honest explanation just before event, using sensory information Medical play with equipment	Simple, honest explanation just before event, using sensory information Medical play with equipment	Explanation before procedure, using concrete and specific information Medical play with equipment Encourage questions Allow child to have some control if possible	Explanation before procedure Provide enough time for the adolescent to formulate questions Explain why the procedure is necessary

Fom Lebet R: Impact of trauma on growth and development. In Moloney-Harmon PA, Czerwinski SJ, editors: *Nursing care of the pediatric trauma patient,* Philadelphia, 2003, W. B. Saunders.

touch. Talking with the child and smiling can provide comfort.

- Always explain to the child what you are going to do.
- Do not try to explain the entire procedure at once. Explain one step, do the procedure, and then explain the next step.
- Children of all ages should be respected with regard to their feelings of bashfulness and modesty. In particular, school-age children and adolescents are modest about exposing their bodies to strangers. Keep all children covered with a hospital gown, only allowing exposure of different body parts during the physical examination.

Children are a unique patient population because they are in a dynamic state of growth and development. By practicing these few general principles while considering appropriate developmental tendencies, the nurse can lessen the trauma that the child experiences. Some children, however, are not able to remain calm and cooperative for the physical examination and interventions. Sedation may be necessary on the basis of the needs of the child and the child's physiologic stability.

Physical Examination

Nurses caring for children must be familiar with the normal physiologic parameters for children at different ages. A small child responds differently to major injuries than does an older child or adult. Special considerations that can change management priorities have to do with unique physiology and responses to injury in children. These include less respiratory reserve, the likelihood of fluid/electrolyte and caloric imbalances, differences in blood volume, and a propensity for excessive heat loss.

Vital Signs. Pulses are obtained at the radial, brachial, carotid, or femoral arteries and are counted for a full minute because there are often irregularities in an anxious or injured child. A child under normal circumstances has a faster heart rate and respiratory rate and a lower blood pressure than an adult. Tachycardia is usually found in children with such conditions as fever and shock and during the initial response to stress. Bradycardia can result from increased intracranial pressure, spinal cord injury, hypoxia, hypothermia, and hypoglycemia. Table 29-3 provides normal heart rates for children.

The respiratory rate is also counted for a full minute. Tachypnea is an initial response to stress in children. If a stressed child does not hyperventilate, head injury, spinal cord injury, or other reasons such as a distended abdomen are considered and investigated. Table 29-4 provides normal respiratory rates for children.

TABLE 29-4 **Normal Respiratory Rates in Children**

Age	Breaths/Minute
Infants	30-60
Toddlers	24-40
Preschoolers	22-34
School-age children	18-30
Adolescents	12-16

Blood pressures should be obtained by using a cuff size that is no less than half and no more than two thirds the length of the upper arm. If pediatric cuffs are not available, an adult cuff can be used on the child's thigh. In the field a palpable systolic blood pressure is adequate; precious time should not be wasted to obtain a diastolic reading. The normal systolic blood pressure for individuals from 1 to 20 years of age is 90 plus two times the age in years. The diastolic pressure should be approximately two thirds the normal systolic pressure. Table 29-5 provides the normal blood pressure ranges in children.

Fear and distress can increase the child's heart rate and respiratory rate. The nurse may have to differentiate between emotional stress and hypoxia or shock. In addition, referring to the medical history is important to provide insight into abnormal vital signs. For example, a pediatric trauma patient may have a congenital heart defect and normally be tachypneic; if that child has a normal respiratory rate, ventilatory assistance may be required.

Respiratory Reserve. The infant has less respiratory reserve than the adult for several reasons: (1) the infant's vital capacity is smaller, (2) the chest wall is soft because the ribs and sternum are cartilage, and (3) the ribs are horizontal with poorly developed intercostal muscles.

An infant whose lung capacity is decreased compensates by increasing the respiratory rate and using auxiliary respiratory muscles, as evidenced by retractions. Retractions are an early sign of respiratory difficulty and compromise the infant's tidal volume. Most of the child's normal respiratory activity is affected by abdominal movement until age 6 or 7 years, and there is very little intercostal motion. A child who has a paralytic ileus after blunt abdominal trauma may have respiratory distress because abdominal distention elevates

TABLE 29-3 **Normal Heart Rates in Children**

Age	Beats/Minute
Infants	120-160
Toddlers	90-140
Preschoolers	80-110
School-age children	75-100
Adolescents	60-90

TABLE 29-5 **Normal Pediatric Blood Pressure Ranges**

Age	Systolic (mm Hg)	Diastolic (mm Hg)
Infants	74-100	50-70
Toddlers	80-112	50-80
Preschoolers	82-110	50-78
School-age children	84-120	54-80
Adolescents	94-140	62-88

the diaphragm and interferes with pulmonary function. As a result, children in respiratory distress who are spontaneously breathing should be treated in the semi-Fowler position when spinal injury has been ruled out.

Fluid and Electrolyte Balance. The daily fluid requirement of a child is larger per kilogram of body weight than that of an adult because the child has greater insensible water losses per unit of body weight. This is because the child has a larger surface area and a higher metabolic rate than the adult. Even with these factors, the absolute amount of fluid required by a child is small. Nurses must carefully monitor the fluid volume administered to the child to avoid overhydration. The calculation of maintenance fluid requirements is shown in Table 29-6. If the child's fluid intake is adequate, the urine volume should average 0.5 to 1 ml/kg per hour. The nurse keeps accurate records of all possible sources of fluid loss, including laboratory blood samples, blood loss from any source, gastric drainage, vomitus, and diarrhea.

The child's higher metabolic rate dictates a requirement for more calories per kilogram of body weight. The critically ill child, even if immobile, still requires most of the normal maintenance calories, if not more. This is discussed in more detail in the critical care phase.

Some forms of electrolyte imbalance are more likely to occur in children than in adults. Serum glucose, calcium, and potassium levels are monitored closely in the child. Infants have high glucose needs because of high metabolic rates and low glycogen stores; therefore, the infant can become hypoglycemic quickly during periods of stress. A 25% dextrose in water bolus (0.5 to 1.0 gm/kg) helps correct this. Changes in serum potassium concentration can occur with changes in acid-base status and diuretic administration. The critically ill child does not seem to be as sensitive to hypokalemia as the adult, so cardiac arrhythmias from hypokalemia are not often seen in pediatric patients until the serum potassium is less than 3 mEq/L.[13] Ventricular fibrillation is rarely seen in pediatric patients but may result from severe hypokalemia or hyperkalemia.

The administration of citrate phosphate dextran blood produces precipitation of serum ionized calcium.[14] An infant who requires frequent transfusions is at risk for development of hypocalcemia, a condition that can interrupt normal cardiovascular function. The ionized calcium levels are monitored closely so that calcium supplements can be administered as needed.

TABLE 29-6 **Calculation of Maintenance Fluids (per 24 Hours) in Children**

Weight (kg)	Kilograms per Body Weight Formula
0-10	100-120 ml/kg
11-20	1,000 ml for the first 10 kg and 50 ml/kg for each kg over 10 kg
21-30	1,500 ml for the first 20 kg and 25 ml/kg for each kg over 20 kg

The child's circulating blood volume (80 ml/kg) is larger per unit of body weight than the adult's. The loss of a small amount of blood in a child, however, is proportionately more significant than in an adult because of the child's smaller total blood volume. Small blood volume loss may potentially lead to hypovolemic shock. A closed fracture of the femur, for example, in a 10-year-old child may result in a loss of 300 or 400 ml of blood. The same amount of blood loss in an adult may not cause a significant problem, whereas in the child this may represent 15% to 25% of the total circulatory blood volume. The child's total circulating blood volume is calculated on admission, and all blood lost as a result of hemorrhage or drawn for laboratory tests is accurately tabulated and recorded.

Body Temperature. Major heat losses can occur in a young child who is unclothed for even a short time. Infants and young children have a large surface area and therefore lose more heat to the environment through radiation, conduction, convection, and evaporation. During resuscitation, children are often unclothed and exposed, losing much of their body heat and therefore experiencing a lowered core body temperature. Hypothermia hinders the resuscitation attempt by causing apnea, coagulopathies, progressive metabolic acidosis, decreased cardiac output, and ventricular arrhythmias. The nurse can minimize this stress by monitoring the child's temperature, keeping the child covered as much as possible, using heat lamps and warming blankets, and warming all fluids before infusion.

Assessment in Head Trauma

Each year approximately 22,000 acutely brain-injured children in the United States die and another 29,000 are left with a permanent disability.[15] In children the brain tissues are thinner, softer, and more flexible; the head size is greater in proportion to the body surface area; and a relatively larger proportion of the total blood volume is in the child's head. Thus the child's response to head injury differs significantly from that of an adult. Intracranial hypertension and cerebral hypoxia occur commonly in children, rendering them highly susceptible to secondary brain injury. Preventing secondary injury contributes to a significantly better outcome in the pediatric patient.[16] Expandable fontanelles and open cranial sutures allow increased room for swelling, providing an advantage for the head-injured infant. The primary disadvantage in the evaluation of the head-injured child is the developmentally imposed limitation in verbal expression, which can complicate assessment endeavors.

Neurologic Assessment. A thorough neurologic assessment should be done as soon as possible after cardiopulmonary assessment is complete and initial stabilization interventions are underway. The neurologic examination consists of the determination of level of consciousness, pupillary response, and motor response.

Evaluation of the level of consciousness after a head injury is probably the single most important aspect of the neurologic assessment but often the most difficult to perform in an infant or young child. Because level of consciousness means different things to different people, a uniform system such as

AVPU or the Glasgow Coma Scale (GCS) should be used. The AVPU method is described below:

A Patient is *alert*
V Patient responds to *vocal* stimuli (This unfortunately is of little value in a very young child.)
P Patient responds to *painful* stimuli
U Patient is *unresponsive*

The GCS is used worldwide as a neurologic assessment tool. The scale consists of three sections, each of which measures a separate function of the person's level of consciousness: the patient's eye opening response, verbal response, and motor response. The total score ranges from 3 to 15, with the higher scores indicating more intact neurologic function. However, because it is difficult to use this tool to evaluate verbal response in infants and preverbal children, many clinicians use a modified GCS (Table 29-7).[17]

With children, as with adults, pupil reactivity, size, shape, and symmetry are responses used to assess brainstem function. When increased intracranial pressure develops, the oculomotor nerve may be compressed by general expansion of the brain, an intracranial lesion, or herniation of the brain; the ipsilateral pupil dilates but does not constrict in response to light. Eye movements are also noted. Abnormal eye movements include deviation of one or both eyes from midline and back and forth movements.

Any difficulty in movement of the extremities is evaluated; the nature of the movement is described as spontaneous or in response to pain. The extremity in which the response is elicited is also recorded. The child with increased intracranial pressure may have a decrease in motor function and abnormal posturing or reflexes. Babinski's reflex is positive when the toes fan out and the great toe moves dorsally. The reflex is assessed by scratching the sole of the foot with an object such as the blunt tip of a tongue depressor. A positive reflex is normal in a child under 18 months but abnormal in any child who is walking and indicates disruption of the corticospinal motor nerve tract from injury or increased intracranial pressure.

Continuous monitoring is essential. After the initial neurologic examination, serial neurologic checks are repeated as often as every 15 minutes in the acutely ill child. Any changes are reported to the physician immediately and documented in the nurse's notes or flow record.

Vital Signs. In addition to the importance of the vital signs in the assessment of the general status of the pediatric trauma patient, vital signs may also be an observable manifestation of intracranial dynamics. An increase in the child's core body temperature may cause increased cerebral blood flow, increased intracranial volume, and therefore increased intracranial pressure. Because children are sensitive to environmental temperatures and their body temperature can drop quickly, care should be taken to keep the child in a neutral thermal environment.

Bradycardia in the presence of widening pulse pressure and irregular respirations (Cushing's phenomenon) may indicate increasing intracranial pressure. In children, shock is associated with tachycardia even if intracranial pressure is increased. Cushing's phenomenon, often not seen in infants, is a late sign and should not be relied on as an early indication of neurologic deterioration.

Elevated blood pressure can also indicate a rise in intracranial pressure, although hypertension in a child with multiple injuries should never be assumed to be the direct result of a head injury. Hypertension may be precipitated by anxiety or pain or may be present as a result of preexisting illness.

TABLE 29-7 **Glasgow Coma Scale for Adults, Children, and Infants**

Response	Adults and Children		Infants	Points
Eye opening	No response		No response	1
	To pain		To pain	2
	To voice		To voice	3
	Spontaneous		Spontaneous	4
	> 5 years	**2 to 5 years**	**0 to 23 months**	
Verbal	No response	No response	No response	1
	Incomprehensible	Grunts	Moans to pain	2
	Inappropriate words	Persistent cries and/or screams	Cries to pain	3
	Disoriented conversation	Inappropriate words	Irritable	4
	Oriented and appropriate	Appropriate words/phrases	Coos, babbles	5
Motor	No response		No response	1
	Decerebrate posturing		Decerebrate posturing	2
	Decorticate posturing		Decorticate posturing	3
	Withdraws to pain		Withdraws to pain	4
	Localizes pain		Withdraws to touch	5
	Obeys commands		Normal spontaneous movement	6
Total score (sum of 3 response scores)				3-15

From Nichols D, Yaster M, Lappe D et al: *In golden hour: the handbook of advanced pediatric life support,* p. 180, St. Louis, 1991, Mosby. Emergency Nurses Association Emergency nursing pediatric course: Provider manual, 3rd ed, Des Plaines IL, 2004, Emergency Nurses Association.

Generally, increased intracranial pressure is accompanied by an increase in systolic arterial blood pressure, producing a widening of the pulse pressure. This compensatory mechanism occurs as the body attempts to maintain adequate cerebral perfusion pressure by initiating a rise in blood pressure.

The child with a brain injury may have several types of abnormal respiratory patterns. When intracranial pressure rises and signs of Cushing's phenomenon are evident, the child typically has apnea. Development of a Cheyne-Stokes pattern of breathing (alternating hyperpnea and bradypnea) after the presence of a normal respiratory pattern should alert the nurse to suspect neurologic deterioration. Hyperventilation usually indicates injury to the brainstem at the level of the midbrain or upper pons.[18]

Head and Neck Examination

All pediatric trauma patients must be suspected of having a cervical spine injury, especially those who have sustained facial or head trauma or who complain of pain in the neck or back. Anteroposterior, lateral, and open-mouth radiographic views of the cervical spine are necessary diagnostic studies.[19] Although spinal cord injury occurs infrequently in children, any time the cervical spine radiographs appear abnormal or are normal but the child is symptomatic, it is imperative that a neurosurgical consultation is obtained. Children may have a spinal cord injury without radiographic abnormality (SCIWORA), which mandates continual assessment for neurologic symptoms if the child's mechanism of injury is associated with a potential spinal cord injury.

After the initial examinations for head and neck injury have been obtained (vital signs, neurologic assessment, and cervical spine films), the child's head and neck are assessed rapidly to look for obvious injury, including depressed or open skull fractures, lacerations, and leakage of cerebrospinal fluid (CSF). The nurse looks in the child's ears for blood or otorrhea and behind the child's ears for obvious ecchymosis (Battle's sign), indicating the presence of a basilar skull fracture. CSF drainage from the nose (rhinorrhea) may indicate the presence of a fractured cribriform plate. Finally, the face and oral cavity are examined closely for lacerations or possible fracture sites.

Further neurodiagnostic evaluation is indicated in children with head injuries to identify the type and extent of injury. In patients with a head injury less than 72 hours old, computed tomographic (CT) scanning remains the imaging modality of choice for several reasons, including the limited potential for magnetic resonance imaging (MRI) to diagnose acute subarachnoid hemorrhage or acute parenchymal hemorrhage; the ease of monitoring unstable patients during the CT scan procedure; and the short time frame required to complete the study.[15] MRI is a technique used for imaging intracranial structures and it is superior to CT scan in visualizing the posterior fossa, spinal cord structure, small vascular lesions, and most brain tumors. Lengthy procedure time, difficulty in monitoring critically ill patients during the procedure, cost, and the inability to visualize bone directly are among the limitations of this diagnostic procedure.

Assessment of Thoracic Trauma

Although chest trauma in children is not as common as it is in adults, it can cause a number of problems related to diagnosis and management. Because of advances in the transport and treatment of the injured child, the mortality rate associated with thoracic trauma has decreased. The absence of preexisting disease states in children also contributes to the low morbidity rate associated with thoracic trauma.

One of the unique features of children is their amazingly compliant thorax, which results from the flexibility of bony and cartilaginous structures. It is not unusual, therefore, for a child to have a major internal injury from compression of the chest without fracture of the bony thorax. A child's mediastinum is freely mobile and capable of wide anatomic shifts. This creates the potential for life-threatening situations such as dislocation of the heart, angulation of the great vessels, compression of the lung, and angulation of the trachea. Children with any type of traumatic injury have aerophagia (swallowing of air), which results in gastric dilation that limits diaphragmatic excursion and leads to a reflex ileus. In a small child this also can compromise ventilation and gas exchange.

Cardiopulmonary Examination. Many injuries to the thorax can cause severe cardiorespiratory dysfunction soon after injury with fatal results if prompt and accurate diagnosis and treatment are not initiated. Continual reassessment of the child's condition after the initiation of therapy is imperative.

Abnormalities in the child's breathing pattern, such as flaring nostrils, chest wall retractions, and prominent use of accessory muscles, suggest ventilatory impairment. If the child is inadequately oxygenated, cyanosis of the fingers, toes, and lips are observed. When the airway is obstructed, cyanosis becomes prominent on both the face and trunk.

A flail chest is usually apparent on visual inspection. The child moves air poorly, and movement of the thorax is asymmetric and uncoordinated. A child with tension pneumothorax and massive hemothorax exhibits poor respiratory exchange, unilateral chest wall movement, or decreased unilateral chest wall movement. The presence of a tension pneumothorax results in distended neck veins and a tracheal and mediastinal shift to the opposite side. A child with cardiac tamponade also presents with distended neck veins; however, with a massive hemothorax the neck veins are often flat as a result of blood loss and decreased cardiac output. Any penetrating wounds to the thorax are noted and treated immediately. When an entrance wound is found, an exit wound also is sought. In the traumatized child, all aspects of the thorax, neck, and upper abdomen are examined for abrasions, lacerations, and contusions.

Palpation is performed gently and in a nonthreatening manner with warm hands. The area of injury is palpated last during the examination. Talking softly may have a calming effect on the child and may lessen the pain felt as injured portions of the chest are assessed.

The nurse palpates the neck, clavicles, sternum, and thorax. Any signs of tenderness, swelling, or crepitus are noted.

Subcutaneous emphysema is a finding of significant concern. Subcutaneous air can be palpated near penetrating chest wounds. When found in the neck area, it suggests a proximal tear or avulsion of the tracheobronchial tree or an esophageal perforation. During examination of the thorax, any instability is noted. Unilateral tenderness in the upper abdomen may indicate a chest injury such as a fractured rib.

The small size of the chest in infants and children makes it difficult to use auscultation and percussion to determine the exact location of injury. Despite this limitation, however, these assessment strategies are considered to be valuable in evaluating thoracic injury. The presence of a pneumothorax is partially diagnosed through auscultation of breath sounds; because the chest wall of the young child is so thin, breath sounds are easily transmitted from other areas of the lung. Decreased breath sounds may not be heard over the involved lung; however, the nurse may note a difference in the quality or pitch of the breath sounds between the right and left sides. The nurse also should assess for the presence of any abnormal sounds, such as inspiratory stridor or expiratory wheezes that might result from bronchial injury. Auscultation also can be used to identify a shift in the heart sounds corresponding to a tracheal shift caused by a tension pneumothorax on one side of the chest. Cardiac tamponade is associated with muffled heart tones. In massive hemothorax, dullness to percussion is present, although the limited thoracic surface area in an infant makes this assessment technique difficult to interpret.

Radiographic and Laboratory Studies. Roentgenograms of the chest should include anteroposterior (AP) and lateral views done with the child in an upright position after cervical spine injury has been ruled out. With an upright chest radiograph the clinician can better visualize the degree of mediastinal shift. It is easier for the clinician to diagnose abnormalities in the lung, pleural cavity, and diaphragm with this view as well.

Standard blood studies for any pediatric trauma patient include an arterial blood gas determination. Other more involved studies, such as tomograms, barium contrast studies, sonograms, and CT scans, may be indicated depending on other clinical findings.

Assessment of Abdominal Trauma

Serious abdominal injury tends to be quite subtle compared with injuries of the head, chest, or limbs. Isolated abdominal injuries are relatively easy to treat and manage; however, confusion in establishment of priorities is common when evaluating a child with multiple trauma and possible abdominal injury.

Physical Examination. The physical examination of an acute abdominal condition in children is similar to the procedure for adults, but objective findings are often masked or misinterpreted. This assessment may be difficult because the child, if conscious, is often apprehensive and may be unwilling to cooperate. In the unconscious child, many of the voluntary responses are gone; therefore, few clinical signs are available to facilitate diagnosis. The key to making an accurate diagnosis of serious abdominal injury is careful examination with constant reassessment and the initiation of several diagnostic studies.

The abdomen and lower chest are examined for contusions, abrasions, and lacerations that may indicate compression injury. It should be noted whether the abdomen is scaphoid or distended. If a conscious child is pulling up the lower extremities, it may be in an attempt to relieve tension on the abdominal wall, thereby reducing pain.[20]

Penetrating wounds must be checked for involvement of intra-abdominal organs. The back is examined for signs of surface injury, bony instability, and pain.

Because children up to about 6 years of age breathe primarily with their diaphragms, peritoneal irritation from blood or intestinal contents may result in an alteration of the breathing pattern. This child may display shallow breathing with the chest muscles to avoid pain. A distended abdomen, which may indicate significant injury, may be caused by the accumulation of gas or liquid, such as blood, bile, pancreatic juice, urine, or intestinal contents. To examine the abdomen adequately, a nasal or orogastric tube is inserted. The drainage from the gastric tube should be examined for blood, which might indicate upper abdominal injury.

The abdomen is auscultated although absence of bowel sounds may be normal or may indicate the presence of an ileus. Intra-abdominal hemorrhage or bowel perforation may initially cause hypoactive or hyperactive bowel sounds. A quiet abdomen can be suggestive of an acute intraperitoneal injury.

Palpation. Frightened children are often uncooperative, making palpation of the abdomen a difficult part of the examination. The nurse must be gentle and creative in the approach to this portion of the assessment. Gentle pressure may bring about a voluntary response or guarding by the child, which may be localized to the abdominal wall or intra-abdominal organs. Any physical signs of trauma are compared with this response to help identify injuries. With deeper palpation, an involuntary response of muscle spasm may be present. In the pediatric trauma patient, this peritoneal irritation is usually a sign of intra-abdominal bleeding. Rebound tenderness may be difficult to interpret because it causes pain, crying, and voluntary guarding. The best way to elicit rebound tenderness in a child is by gentle percussion or by asking the child to cough rather than by rapidly releasing manual pressure over portions of the abdomen. This part of the examination helps to determine the presence of peritoneal irritation.

Pelvic and Genitourinary Assessment. The last part of the abdominal examination is evaluation of the pelvis and genitourinary system. A pelvic fracture is suspected if pain is present on compression of the wings of the ilium or symphysis pubis or with abduction of the legs. Urethral injuries are suspected when the child has perineal swelling, blood at the meatus, a distended bladder, and an inability to void. In this case use of a urethral catheter is contraindicated because it may change an incomplete urethral tear into a complete urethral disruption. A rectal examination is necessary to evaluate the tone of the anal sphincter and integrity of the bony pelvis and bowel wall. The presence of blood strongly indicates perforation of the colon or rectum.

Injury to the kidney may occur in pediatric trauma patients. Parenchymal contusion is the most common injury seen; it most often results from blunt trauma.[6] An indication of this injury may be hematuria, with flank pain and tenderness also present. Further radiologic studies may be indicated, including contrast-enhanced CT scan, intravenous pyelogram, and renal scan.

Diagnostic Studies. CT scan is a definitive method of evaluation for the child with blunt abdominal trauma. The CT scan provides superior detail of anatomy and allows for clear imagery of multiple abdominal organs simultaneously. An enhanced scan allows for the assessment of organ perfusion and evaluation of intraperitoneal bleeding, clearly defining the nature and extent of the injury.

Ultrasonography is another method for evaluation of the abdomen; however, it does not accurately identify specific injuries. Therefore, it does not replace CT scans in the identification of specific abdominal injures.[21]

Penetrating abdominal trauma, which is rare in the child, is often the result of a rib fracture. Because of the unpredictable nature of penetrating injuries, surgical exploration is usually indicated.[21]

Peritoneal lavage is not performed often in children because it interferes with serial abdominal examination and because isolated posttraumatic intra-abdominal bleeding is not necessarily an indication for surgery in pediatric patients.[21] In children with isolated abdominal trauma, the main determinations for surgical intervention are physical findings, deteriorating vital signs, and falling hematocrit. In a child with multiple injuries, especially a head injury, clinical findings may not be as accurate in reflecting intra-abdominal bleeding.

Initially the abdominal examination may be negative, but continual reassessment is needed to rule out the development of a significant problem. It may take 12 to 24 hours for intra-abdominal findings to become obvious in a child with a suspected abdominal injury.

After the physical examination, appropriate laboratory studies are obtained. These include a complete blood cell count, type and cross-match, blood gas analysis, prothrombin time, partial thromboplastin time, platelet count, and serum amylase determination.

Assessment of Musculoskeletal Trauma

Injuries to the extremities are usually obvious or readily identified with radiographic examination. Except for cervical and displaced pelvic fractures, orthopedic trauma is rarely life threatening. However, the importance of extremity injuries should never be underestimated because mismanagement could result in serious sequelae, such as infection, growth disturbance, deformity, or paralysis.

The high incidence of fractures in children can be explained by the combination of their relatively slender bone structure and their high activity level. Some of these injuries, such as buckle and greenstick fractures, are not serious compared with intra-articular and epiphyseal plate fractures, which can impair normal bone growth if they are not treated properly.

Examination of the Extremities. During the secondary survey the nurse palpates all extremities to detect pain, swelling, bruising, lacerations, and deformities. The neurovascular status of each limb should be noted and documented. The presence of a distal extremity pulse does not exclude an associated proximal artery tear. Soft tissue injuries should be thoroughly inspected for the presence of foreign bodies or dead tissue.

The temperature of the extremities is noted, with special care being given to determine whether the temperature is equal on both sides. Differences in temperature are usually caused by neurologic or vascular abnormalities. Extremities may be cold and pale after sympathetic nervous system stimulation. Changes in temperature and coloration also can be a sign of venous or arterial thrombosis or embolism.

Radiologic studies are used to confirm the fracture diagnosis. Roentgenograms include the joint above and below the fracture to avoid missing an associated dislocation. Taking roentgenograms in two projections (e.g., AP and lateral) helps to avoid overlooking a fracture with deformity in only one location. Fractures in children often do not present a clear-cut picture; diagnosis may require additional effort. It is possible to overlook a severe injury, such as an epiphyseal separation with only a small degree of displacement or a fracture involving unossified epiphyses. Radiologic examination of both limbs, allowing for comparison of the injured and uninjured extremities, assists in avoiding this error.

Shock in Children

In essence, shock is a generalized failure of adequate tissue perfusion resulting in impaired cellular and subcellular respiration. The basic cellular responses and general pathophysiologic mechanisms of the disease appear to be identical among different age groups. However, because of the previously mentioned differences between children and adults (e.g., vital sign parameters, thermoregulation, and response to head injury), shock is quite different in pediatric patients than in the adult population. The pediatric trauma patient is in shock most often because of blood loss. Children rarely have diseases that predispose them to the development of other kinds of shock, although septic shock may occur as a later sequelae to trauma-related infection; spinal cord or brain injury can initiate neurogenic shock and adverse allergic reactions to medications administered could trigger anaphylactic shock.

In infants and younger children, 70% of the total body weight is water and 50% of the total body water is located in the child's extracellular space. Therefore, hypovolemia occurs more rapidly in the child than in the adult, whose extracellular space contains only 23% of total body water. Children can vasoconstrict effectively and can compensate for up to a 25% blood loss. Therefore, when hypotension does occur in the pediatric patient, it usually indicates a significant degree of blood loss. A traumatized child who is tachycardic; has cold, mottled extremities; and is hypotensive should be considered to be in shock.

Clinical Presentation. When the child in shock is assessed, several clinical signs become apparent. Tachycardia and tachypnea are present. Because of the peripheral vasoconstriction, the extremities are cold, clammy, and mottled and the pulses are weak or nonpalpable. The child's level of consciousness is altered because of decreased cerebral perfusion. Urinary output is decreased or absent. The decrease in the systolic blood pressure is a late indicator; a narrowing of pulse pressure is usually seen first. Table 29-8 differentiates the four classes of hemorrhage and lists the clinical signs and treatment for each.

Infants in shock may present differently than children or adults in shock. They may have erratic hemodynamic parameters, mottling, hyperventilation or hypoventilation, glucose intolerance, and metabolic instability. The process is often insidious and requires accurate assessment.

The key elements involved in the successful management of hemorrhagic shock in the pediatric population are early recognition of hemodynamic instability, replacement of circulating blood volume, and arrest of further bleeding. Nurses should be aware of the pathophysiologic processes of shock and the signs and symptoms that these processes produce. If inadequate tissue perfusion continues, a potentially correctable problem may well lead to a fatal outcome.

CLINICAL MANAGEMENT

For the nurse to provide efficient and effective care to pediatric trauma patients, it is imperative that appropriate equipment and supplies be readily available. A general emergency department where both adults and children are seen must have equipment specifically for children. The availability of a separate pediatric trauma cart and pediatric resuscitation drug dosages improves the potential for a successful resuscitation. Table 29-9 presents essential equipment for a pediatric resuscitation.

A systematic approach is used to manage multiple injuries in the critically ill child. This approach is practiced frequently so that it becomes automatic and can be applied even in a disorganized setting. Children are assessed, and treatment priorities are established on the basis of existing and potentially life-threatening problems and the stability of the child's vital signs. The primary survey involves assessing the airway (while protecting the cervical spine), breathing, and circulation, with attention given to the diagnosis and treatment of shock. When indicated, appropriate resuscitative measures must be instituted concurrently with the primary survey. A brief neurologic evaluation and assessment for additional life-threatening injuries also takes place during the primary survey.

PRIMARY SURVEY

Airway and Breathing

The first priority in the sequential evaluation and management of the traumatized child is assessment of the airway. Airway patency must be ensured. Great variation exists in the anatomy of the upper airway, depending on the age of the child. In infants the oral cavity is small and the tongue is relatively large. The infant's larynx is more cephalad than the adult's. The glottis is higher than in adults; it is located at the level of the third cervical vertebra at birth and descends about one to two vertebrae with maturity. The vocal cords slant upward and backward behind a narrow

TABLE 29-8 **Classes of Hemorrhage for Children**

Class	Blood Loss	Signs	Treatment
Class I	15% or less 40-kg child = 500 ml blood	Pulse: slight ↑ BP: normal Respiration: normal Capillary refill: normal Tilt test*: normal	Crystalloids
Class II	20%-30% 40-kg child = 800 ml blood	Pulse: tachycardia >150 BP: ↓ systolic; ↓ pulse pressure Respiration: tachypnea >35-40 Capillary refill: delayed Tilt test: positive Urine output: normal (1 ml/kg/hr)	Crystalloids
Class III	30%-35% 40-kg child = 1,200 ml blood	BP: decreased Narrow pulse pressure Urine output: decreased	Crystalloids Packed red blood cells
Class IV	40%-50% 40-kg child = 1,600 ml blood	Pulse: nonpalpable BP: nonpalpable No response to verbal or painful stimuli	Crystalloids Packed red blood cells

BP, Blood pressure.

*A tilt test is done by sitting the child upright. The test is normal if the child can stay up for more than 90 seconds and maintain blood pressure.

TABLE 29-9 **Recommended Resuscitation Equipment for Infants and Children**

Age	0-6 mo.	6-12 mo.	1 yr.	18 mo.	3 yr.	5 yr.	6 yr.	8 yr.	10 yr.	12 yr.	14 yr.
Weight (kg)	3-5	7	10	12	15	20	20	25	30	40	50
Resuscitation mask	0-1	1	1-2	2	3	3	3	3	3	4	4-5
Laryngoscope (Miller/Mac)	0	1	1	1	2	2	2	2	2	2	3
ETT	3.0	3.5	3.5	4.0	4.5	5.0	5.5	6.0	6.0	6.5	7.0
Suction catheter (ETT/tracheal)	6	6	8	8	10	10	10	10	10	14	14
Suction (OP/NP)	10	10	10	10	14	14	14	16	16	16	16
Chest tube	10-12	10-12	16-20	16-20	16-20	20-28	20-28	20-28	28-32	28-32	32-42
NG/OG	8	8	8	8	10	10	10	10	12	12	14
Foley catheter	5	5	8	8	10	10	10	10	12	12	12
Tracheostomy tube (pediatric)	00	1	1	1-2	2-3	3	3	4	4	5	6

Modified from Widner-Kolberg MR, 1989, Maryland Institutes for Emergency Medical Services Systems.
Reprinted from Moloney-Harmon P, Rosenthal CH: Nursing care modifications for the child in the adult ICU. In Stillwell, S, editor: *Critical care nursing reference book,* p 590, 1992, St. Louis, Mosby.
ETT, Endotracheal tube; *OP,* oropharyngeal; *NP,* nasopharyngeal; *NG,* nasogastric; *OG,* orogastric.

U-shaped epiglottis. However, for all ages the best method for initial assessment of the airway is to apply the jaw-thrust maneuver.

As with an adult, in-line cervical traction should always be applied in the traumatized child to maintain stability of the neck until a cervical fracture has been ruled out. Although cervical injury is rare in children, the child is treated as if such injury has occurred until it is ruled out by roentgenogram. In addition to positioning for airway patency, foreign matter is quickly removed with a finger or gentle suction. This is done carefully, especially if a facial injury or basilar skull fracture is suspected. Close, continuous observation is essential because the child's ineffective efforts to clear the airway may quickly result in an obstructed airway once again.

The Conscious Child. In a conscious child who is breathing spontaneously but whose airway is obstructed despite the foregoing measures, a nasopharyngeal airway device may be useful. The length of the nasopharyngeal airway is estimated by measuring the distance from the nares to the tragus of the ear. The tube is lubricated, advanced gently along the floor of the nasal cavity, and rotated if resistance is met. If unsuccessful, the procedure is repeated on the opposite side. Epistaxis, avulsion of adenoid tissue, or damage to conchae can occur if a gentle technique and lubrication are not used during insertion. This method is contraindicated if basilar skull fracture is suspected (e.g., rhinorrhea is present).

The Unconscious Child. In an unconscious child an oropharyngeal airway can be used. The selection of an appropriately sized airway is of paramount importance and can be facilitated by placing the airway alongside the child's face so that the flange is at the level of the central incisors and the bite block portion is approximately at the angle of the mandible. An airway device too small or too large can obstruct the airway (Figure 29-1).

The airway is inserted by opening the child's mouth and pressing the tongue with a tongue depressor. The airway is slid into position with care to avoid pushing the tongue backward and thus obstructing the airway. The practice of inserting the airway in an inverted position and rotating it 180 degrees is not recommended in pediatric patients because trauma to the teeth or soft tissue may occur. In the conscious child, gagging may occur during insertion of an oral airway and it is generally tolerated poorly.

After a clear and stable airway has been established, the child is reassessed continually. The nurse looks, listens, and feels for evidence of air exchange. In infants, adequacy of ventilation is assessed by observing for expansion at the lower chest and upper abdomen. This differs from the reassessment of older children and adolescents, in whom adequate ventilation and expansion are checked at the upper chest. Air exchange is assessed through auscultation, listening first over the trachea to establish that air exchange is occurring through the central airway and then listening for breath sounds bilaterally to assess for peripheral air exchange. Observing for symmetric lung expansion is also essential.

Once the airway has been established and the child is spontaneously breathing, supplemental oxygen (100%) is provided. Although children are quite resistant to the effects of hypercarbia and respiratory acidosis, they do not tolerate even short periods of oxygen deprivation.

Bag-mask ventilation with 100% oxygen is indicated in children who do not resume spontaneous breathing. When a bag mask is used to ventilate, the nurse's fingers should be kept on the lower jaw to avoid compressing the soft tissue under the infant's chin. Placing the fingers on the soft tissue forces the tongue back into the posterior pharynx and then obstructs the airway (Figure 29-2).

Endotracheal intubation is indicated for children who cannot be ventilated adequately by the bag-mask method and who need prolonged control of the airway. The oral route for endotracheal intubation is preferred for the child in the emergency phase of treatment. A nasotracheal tube is generally more stable in the pediatric patient, but nasal intubation usually takes longer and is not recommended in patients who are

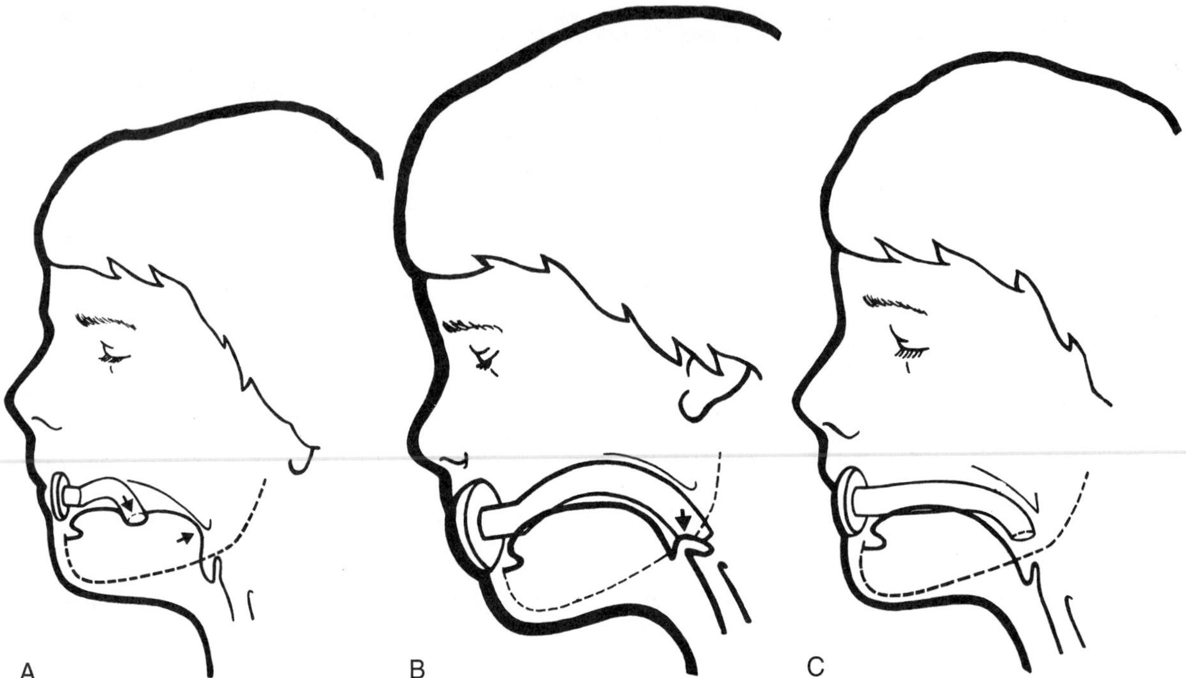

FIGURE 29-1 Choosing the appropriate size airway. **A,** Airway too small. **B,** Airway too large. **C,** Airway correct size.

not breathing or who have cranial, maxillary, or facial injuries. Children are also likely to have hypertrophied lymphoid tissue (adenoids and tonsils), which can cause problems with the passage of a nasotracheal tube. The higher location of the larynx in the pediatric patient creates a more acute angle from the nasopharynx, making successful nasal intubation less likely. When cervical injury is suspected, oral intubation must be done with in-line immobilization applied and without extension of the neck, as in the adult population.

Uncuffed tracheal tubes are generally used in pediatric patients up to age 7 years to avoid subglottic edema and stenosis. The appropriate interior diameter (ID) of the tracheal tube for a particular child can be estimated by using the following formula:

$$16 + \text{Age in years}/4 = \text{ID of tracheal tube}$$

For example, for a 2-year-old child, the following calculation applies:

$$16 + 2/4 = 4.5 \text{ mm}$$

This is an approximate rule, so it is recommended that tubes of the next higher and lower sizes also be readily available. Another approximate measure often used to determine tracheal tube diameter is the size of the internal naris. If the tube fits into one naris, it will probably fit comfortably down the trachea.

In certain situations in the in-hospital setting, such as when the patient has poor lung compliance or high airway resistance, a cuffed tube may be used. Estimation of the correct-size cuffed tube can be made by using the formula:

$$(\text{Age in years}/4) + 3 = \text{ID of tracheal tube}$$

Rapid-sequence intubation is indicated in all children. All pediatric trauma patients are assumed to have a full stomach, and a rapid-sequence intubation minimizes the possibility of regurgitation.[22] This technique also blunts the response of increased intracranial pressure that can be stimulated by intubation. Intubation should always be preceded by ventilation with 100% oxygen. The medications commonly administered in a rapid-sequence intubation are atropine, a sedative, and a muscle relaxant.

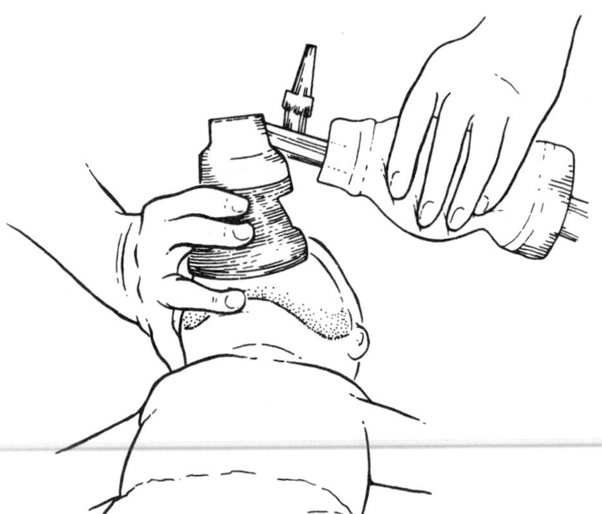

FIGURE 29-2 Proper placement of hand and fingers on lower jaw when using a bag mask. (From Eichelberger MR et al: *Brady pediatric emergencies,* p 49, Englewood Cliffs, NJ, 1992, Prentice Hall.)

The technique of cricoid pressure (Sellick maneuver) is used during a rapid-sequence intubation to prevent passive regurgitation of stomach contents into the pharynx. With this technique the upper esophagus is compressed against the cervical vertebral column by applying anteroposterior pressure on the cricoid cartilage. Cricoid pressure must be maintained until correct placement of the tracheal tube is confirmed.

If a tracheal tube cannot be placed within 30 seconds, ventilation is resumed for several minutes before a second attempt. After the tube has been placed, to ensure proper placement of the tube in the trachea, the nurse auscultates both lung fields and observes for symmetric chest expansion. However, because clinical confirmation may be unreliable, confirmation of tracheal tube placement is achieved by exhaled carbon dioxide detection. As in adults, it is extremely easy for the endotracheal tube to slide into the child's right mainstem bronchus, causing atelectasis and further decreasing ventilation. After the nurse's assessment by auscultation and observation of chest expansion and exhaled carbon dioxide detection, the tube is secured to the upper lip with tincture of benzoin and adhesive tape until proper tube position is verified by chest roentgenogram. Securing the tracheal tube carefully and restraining the child's hands are necessary interventions because dislodgment can occur easily due to the short length of the child's trachea.

Surgical Intervention. If the airway obstruction persists after implementation of the preceding methods, direct injury to the larynx or trachea or uncontrollable hemorrhage should be suspected. Although cricothyroid puncture may be a life-saving procedure, it is virtually never the first choice for establishing an airway and adequate ventilation. Almost all children can be adequately ventilated and oxygenated without surgical intervention. When necessary, the preferred surgical method in children is needle cricothyroidotomy. Great care is taken to ensure that the catheter remains patent. Arterial blood gases are drawn to assess the adequacy of oxygenation and ventilation.

If inadequate ventilation is the result of chest injury, such as tension pneumothorax, open pneumothorax, or large flail segment, these alterations must be addressed immediately. A tension pneumothorax may be relieved by needle insertion or chest tube placement; an open pneumothorax must be covered with a sterile semiocclusive dressing; a flail segment must be supported and, if necessary, positive-pressure controlled ventilation should be instituted. Adequate ventilation does not ensure adequate tissue oxygenation; therefore the potential for impaired gas exchange remains a concern throughout the emergency and critical phases of care. An attempt should be made to maintain arterial partial pressure of oxygen in the 80 to 100 mm Hg range.

Circulation

During the primary survey the adequacy of circulation is first assessed by noting the quality, rate, and regularity of central and peripheral pulses. Peripheral perfusion is also assessed initially by capillary refill. Capillary refill is easily tested by applying pressure to the nail beds and observing the time required for return of skin color. Under normal circumstances the color should return within 2 seconds. If the child has been in a cold environment or is in shock, refill in the extremities may be prolonged, in which case it is assessed on mucous membranes.

Circulatory support is initiated as soon as it is deemed necessary. When possible, active bleeding is controlled immediately with a direct pressure dressing. Intravenous access is critical in infants and children in severe shock or cardiac arrest. However, it is in this clinical situation that venous access may be most difficult and time consuming because of the smaller vessel size in children and the fact that veins often collapse when children are in shock. Intravenous access is attempted by percutaneous catheter placement, intraosseous needle insertion, or central venous line placement.

Intraosseous Infusion. Intraosseous infusion is a technique described more than 60 years ago that is used to establish access for fluid and medication infusion. For intraosseous infusion, a bone marrow needle is inserted into the medial flat surface of the anterior tibia, approximately 2 fingerbreadths below the tibial tuberosity. The needle is inserted perpendicular to the bone or at a 45-degree angle away from the growth plate to avoid injury to this structure. This is considered an effective route for the administration of any fluid or medication that can be given intravenously while attempts at intravenous cannulation are under way. The main advantages of intraosseous infusion are that it is a readily available route, requires little skill, and has a low rate of complications. The most common complications attributed to this procedure are the subcutaneous infiltration of fluid (although minimal) and leakage from the puncture site after the removal of the needle. Osteomyelitis and subcutaneous infections have been noted, but they occur only after the intraosseous infusion is maintained for extended periods of time or when hypertonic fluids are infused by this route.

Volume Replacement. Volume replacement with a crystalloid solution of normal saline or lactated Ringer's solution (20 ml/kg) is given to raise blood pressure and improve circulation. If vital signs do not stabilize with the administration of one bolus, a second bolus of 20 ml/kg should be given as quickly as possible, keeping in mind that a significant percentage of the child's blood volume has been replaced. If blood pressure returns to normal, the intravenous infusion is set at a maintenance rate. If the child remains hypotensive, then blood replacement is needed. In children with exsanguinating hemorrhage, either type-specific or type O packed cells are immediately infused. Keep in mind that blood pressure is not a reliable indicator of intravasucular volume. Assessment of systemic perfusion, such as improved capillary refill time, pulses, heart rate, and level of consciousness should take place.

Fluid therapy is guided by special attention to preinfusion and postinfusion vital signs and indicators of systemic perfusion. At present it is recommended that fresh frozen plasma be given only when the patient's clinical status and laboratory studies indicate that they are necessary. Resuscitation drug therapy may be indicated for the pediatric trauma patient.

Table 29-10 lists the common resuscitation drugs and their dosages. For use in emergency situations, when the exact weight of the child is not known, completed emergency drug cards for various weights (e.g., 2 kg, 5 kg, 10 kg, 15 kg) assist in quickly determining the correct dosages. The approximate weight card can be pulled out and used during the emergency situation. (Approximate weights for children are discussed earlier in the chapter.) The key to successful resuscitation efforts is being prepared with predetermined charts for drug dosages before the arrest takes place. Nurses need to be knowledgeable about the actions, indications, and adverse effects of the standard drugs used in resuscitation.

TABLE 29-10 **PALS Medications for Cardiac Arrest and Symptomatic Arrhythmias**

Drug	Dosage (Pediatric)	Remarks
Adenosine	0.1 mg/kg (maximum dose: 6 mg) Repeat dose: 0.2 mg/kg (maximum dose: 12 mg)	Rapid IV/IO bolus Rapid flush to central circulation
Amiodarone	5 mg/kg IV/IO; repeat up to 15 mg/kg per day (maximum dose: 300 mg)	Monitor EGG and blood pressure Adjust administration rate to urgency (give more slowly when perfusing rhythm present) Use caution when administering with other drugs that prolong QT (consider expert consultation)
Atropine sulfate*	0.02 mg/kg IV/IO 0.03 mg/kg ET* Repeat once if needed Minimum dose: 0.1 mg Maximum single dose: 0.5 mg in child, 1.0 mg in adolescent	Higher dose may be used with organophosphate poisoning
Calcium chloride 10% = 100 mg/ml (= 27.2 mg/ml elemental calcium)	20 mg/kg (0.2 mL/kg) IV/IO	Give slow IV push for hypocalcemia, hypermagnesemia, calcium channel blocker toxicity, preferably through central vein Monitor heart rate; bradycardia may occur
Calcium gluconate 10% = 100 mg/ml (= 9 mg/ml elemental calcium)	60-100 mg/kg (0.6-1.0 mL/kg) IV/IO	Give slow IV push for hypocalcemia, hypermagnesemia, calcium channel blocker toxicity, preferably through central vein
Epinephrine for symptomatic bradycardia*	IV/IO: 0.01 mg/kg (1:10,000, 0.1 ml/kg) ET: 0.1 mg/kg (1:1,000, 0.1 ml/kg) Maximum dose: 1 mg IV/IO; 10 mg ET	May repeat every 3-5 minutes
Glucose (10%, 25%, or 50%)	IV/IO: 0.5-1.0 g/kg	1-2 ml/kg 50% 2-4 ml/kg 25% 5-10 ml/kg 10%
Lidocaine	Bolus: 1 mg/kg IV/IO (maximum dose: 100 mg) Infusion: 20-50 mcg/kg/min ET*: 2-3 mg	
Magnesium sulfate (500 mg/ml)	IV/IO: 25-50 mg/kg over 10-20 min; faster in torsades (maximum dose: 2 g per dose)	
Naloxone	<5 years or ≤20 kg: 0.1 mg/kg IV/IO/ET* >5 years or >20 kg: 2.0 mg IV/IO/ET*	Use lower doses to reverse respiratory depression associated with therapeutic opioid use (1-15 mcg/kg)
Procainamide	15 mg/kg IV/IO over 30-60 min Adult dose: 20 mg/min IV infusion up to total maximum dose 17 mg/kg	Monitor ECG and blood pressure Use caution when administering with other drugs that prolong QT (consider expert consultation) After adequate ventilation
Procainamide	15 mg/kg IV/IO over 30-60 min Adult dose: 20 mg/min IV infusion up to total maximum dose 17 mg/kg	Monitor ECG and blood pressure Use caution when administering with other drugs that prolong QT (consider expert consultation)
Sodium bicarbonate	1 mEq/kg per dose IV/IO slowly	After adequate ventilation

From American Heart Association: 2005 American Heart Association guidelines for cardiopulmonary resuscitation and emergency cardiovascular care, *Circulation* 112(Suppl):167-185, 2005.

IV, Intravenous; *IO,* intraosseous; *ET,* endotracheal.

*Flush with 5 ml of normal saline solution and follow with five ventilations.

Defibrillation. Because ventricular fibrillation is an infrequent occurrence in pediatric cardiopulmonary arrest, defibrillation is a relatively uncommon intervention. Before any attempt to defibrillate, the rhythm is confirmed. When fibrillation is monitored, defibrillation is attempted only after the child has been prepared. Coarse fibrillation may be more easily treated than fine fibrillation. Fine fibrillation may be converted to coarse fibrillation with the administration of epinephrine or calcium.

Pediatric paddles, which are smaller in diameter than those used for an adult, are available with most defibrillators. The paddles or electrode pads are placed so that the heart is between them. Electrical bridging results in ineffective defibrillation and burning of the skin surface. Both electrodes may be placed on the anterior chest wall, one at the right of the sternum below the clavicle and the other at the level of the xyphoid along the left midclavicular line. Anteroposterior placement of the electrodes on an infant or young child is also acceptable; however, this is sometimes difficult to achieve during resuscitation.

Current for the initial shock is 2 joules/kg. If the first defibrillation effort is unsuccessful, cardiopulmonary resuscitation should be continued for 3 to 5 minutes before the current is doubled to 4 joules/kg for a second attempt.

Secondary Survey

After the primary survey, initial stabilization of the cardiopulmonary system, and aggressive treatment of shock, each child should undergo a secondary survey. As in adults, this secondary survey consists of a timely, systematic, and directed evaluation of each body region to assess for injury. When the systematic head-to-toe survey in children is performed, several principles are used. Any child with one injury is assumed to have additional injuries until proven otherwise. Verbal reassurance is offered to the child who is conscious, and the treatment plan is explained in terms that are easily understandable. Finally, appropriate physiologic parameters and laboratory studies are obtained and recorded frequently, and the child is monitored closely and reassessed continually. Laboratory study trends are analyzed consistently as well.

The Family of the Child

An important aspect of the care of the pediatric trauma patient is care of the family. The family experiences the circumstances surrounding trauma as a crisis. Because trauma is unexpected, the parents do not have time to adjust to the possible death or disability of their child. Parents initially may feel shock and disbelief. Normal reactions include confusion, disorganized behavior, and an increase in tension and anxiety.[23] They may also have difficulty in accepting the situation as real. The normal coping mechanisms they have always used to deal with previous crises may no longer be effective. Decision-making abilities may be impaired.[23] The parents often have feelings of guilt that may be indicated by anger at themselves, each other, the child, or the health care team. These feelings of anger may occur immediately or later as the family passes through the shock and disbelief phase to the developing awareness phase.[23]

These families require compassionate support throughout their adjustment to this crisis in their lives and need to be informed about what is happening to their child. Too often parents are whisked away to a waiting area and left to wonder about what is happening. Parents require information from the health care team as soon as possible because they are often imagining the worst; they wonder if the child is still alive. If parents are in a waiting area, an important priority is allowing them to see their child. As the child stabilizes, other concerns that the family members may have must be addressed. As family-centered care becomes the standard in all areas of acute care hospitalization, including the emergency department, consideration of continuing family involvement becomes even more critical. Thought may be given to including parents in multidisciplinary rounds to ensure that their input is included in the child's plan of care. A recent study demonstrates that most parents wish to be included in bedside rounds as a means to being included in the discussions regarding their child's care. Better communication among all health care team members contributes in increased parent satisfaction.[24]

An important consideration for the health care team is family presence during the resuscitation. Boie et al[25] determined that most parents whose children require resuscitation in the emergency department wish to be in attendance. A recent study determined that including family members during pediatric resuscitation is not universal practice. However, the parents who were given the opportunity to be present in this study universally believed that their presence was comforting for the child and for themselves. Those who were not invited to stay felt remorse at not being able to comfort their child in the final moments of his or her life. The study authors recommended that policies be developed enabling parental presence during resuscitation.[26] A study conducted among physicians determined that most respondents had resuscitated a child with parents present. The majority of physicians surveyed thought that presence was helpful to parents and that physicians should be trained in this practice.[27] Nurses take on the important responsibility of preparing families to stay with their child.[28]

Family Assessment

The family network is assessed as soon as possible. Information is gathered about the family's knowledge of the situation. Does the family have any kind of support system, such as friends, relatives, or clergy? Where will they stay while their child is in the hospital? Does the family have other children? From this assessment, some inferences can be made about the family's perception of the situation and their ability to cope. Information about the family's medical insurance coverage is obtained as well. Many families express early concerns about hospitalization and health care costs and may require the services of a financial counselor. Referrals are made accordingly.

Providing Information

Information about their child is given to parents in a simple, straightforward manner because it is often difficult for them to process a great deal of information at this time. Any misconceptions that the family may have about the situation or their child's injuries and treatment plan are addressed. In preparing the family to see the child, they are told about the change in their child's appearance and about the equipment and personnel that are at the bedside. Parents are asked how the child appears to them, and explanations can then be based on their perceptions.

Response to the Death of a Child

Some children may not survive resuscitation efforts; after emergency efforts to save the child, care shifts to the family. These parents need support from the nursing staff when the news about the death of the child is shared. The immediate reactions of the family are shock, numbness, and disbelief—a period when parents often feel out of touch with reality. They are often immobilized and unable to make decisions.[29] Guilt also is a feeling that parents often experience when a child dies, especially if it is an unintentional death.

After the initial shock of a child's death, the phase of intense grief begins. This may begin immediately or may be delayed for weeks. During this phase, parents may feel loneliness and an intense yearning for their child. They may feel extremely helpless, which often leads to feelings of anger and despair. At this time they are also at risk for the development of physical symptoms, such as loss of appetite, and may have sleep disturbances as well.[29]

The phase of reorganization follows. Parents report that they never recover completely from a child's death, but most are able to regain their previous level of functioning with support and care from others. This is evidenced by a return to normal daily activities, more happy memories of the child, and a decrease in the feelings associated with intense grief.[30]

Nursing Interventions. For nurses working in an emergency department setting, telling the family of a child's death is an extremely difficult task. Initial interactions with the family usually occur as they experience the shock and numbness of their loss. At this time it is important to let parents know that all extraordinary measures were taken to save the child. The family is often comforted, too, to know that the child did not suffer. Further conversation should be guided by the family's expressed need for more information. Quiet time is often needed and appreciated. The nurse's physical presence while the family begins to experience their loss is often helpful. Many families are comforted to know of the health care team's care and concern, which often can be expressed more effectively in silence.

Some parents may feel a need to express their great pain and sorrow. Guilt feelings also may surface as the family begins to grieve. Such feelings should not be negated because they are a significant part of the process through which the family must progress to come to terms with their loss. Anger and rage also may be felt at this time and are often directed toward hospital personnel. Such feelings often pass once expressed, and the family members may become extremely confused by the various emotions that have overcome them. The most appropriate intervention at this time is for the nurse to listen, reinforce the positive aspects of their parenting role, and explain the normalcy of their feelings. Parents may need assistance with problem solving as they face the many decisions that must be made during this time of great stress. Many families benefit from the support offered through social service programs. Appropriate referrals should be made at this time. Clergy members and social workers may assist the family by providing guidance in making funeral arrangements and by offering emotional and spiritual support. It is also helpful if the nurse who cared for the child makes contact with the family shortly after the child's death. This conveys to the family that they have been remembered and provides them the opportunity to ask questions and express feelings that have surfaced since the child's death. Many parents need reassurance and continued support as they experience various aspects of their personal grief (see Chapter 19).

CRITICAL CARE PHASE

Once resuscitation and stabilization measures have been taken, the child is prepared for the definitive treatment regimen. Although not always the case, surgical intervention may be necessary at this time. The patient then progresses through a critical period that requires close observation and intensive interventions. Identified in this text as the critical care phase, it is during this phase of care that complications resulting from earlier resuscitation efforts may become evident. It is imperative that the pediatric critical care nurse develop and refine the necessary skills for detecting signs of impending danger. Early recognition of even the most subtle changes and rapid and efficient intervention may positively affect the outcome of care.

TOTAL SYSTEMS ASSESSMENT

As in the resuscitation phase of care, the pediatric trauma patient requires a systems assessment that helps to identify priorities for critical care management. The assessment during the critical care phase focuses more broadly on the integrated function of the child's body systems, psychologic status, and response to resuscitative and operative therapies. The neurologic status requires close monitoring. The child's level of consciousness, pupillary response, movement, and reflexes are assessed continually. The child's movements are evaluated as spontaneous or in response to pain. The type of movement is documented as well. Does the child withdraw or posture? Is the child able to grasp? Grasp activity is evaluated for strength, equality, and the ability to release on command. The GCS (see Table 29-7) is as a useful assessment tool used during the critical care phase as it was during the resuscitation phase of care.

The child's cardiovascular status, including heart rate and rhythm, blood pressure, quality of pulses, and perfusion, are assessed routinely. Clinical examination findings and hemodynamic parameters are part of the assessment data. The child continues to be assessed for the presence of shock. Hypovolemic shock may be present if the child continues to bleed as a result of the traumatic injuries.

The potential for respiratory distress and failure necessitates a thorough respiratory assessment. Assessment parameters include respiratory rate, pattern and effectiveness of respirations, and quality of breath sounds. For infants an increase in respiratory rate is the mechanism of compensation for respiratory dysfunction because they cannot increase the tidal volume. If the child is intubated and mechanically ventilated, the presence or absence and quality of the child's own respirations are assessed. The ventilator is routinely checked and respiratory patterns monitored closely to ensure that the child's breathing is synchronized with the ventilator. Note the amount of oxygen being delivered, the positive end-expiratory pressure, and the peak inspiratory pressure. An increase in peak inspiratory pressures indicates difficulty in delivering tidal volume, which may be the result of progressive atelectasis or the development of a pneumothorax (see Chapter 24). Serial arterial blood gases are obtained to determine the adequacy of oxygenation and ventilation. Pulse oximetry is useful for continuously monitoring oxygen saturation, and end-tidal carbon dioxide monitoring may be performed in patients requiring mechanical ventilation, particularly those with head injury or severe lung injury. Thoracic roentgenograms are monitored for the development of a pathologic respiratory process, such as atelectasis or pneumothorax. If the child has chest or mediastinal tubes in place, the character and amount of drainage are noted.

Abdominal assessment includes monitoring abdominal girth and the presence or absence and quality of bowel sounds. The amount and character of gastric drainage are noted and recorded. The child is monitored for bleeding by noting hematocrit, abdominal girth and tension, and bleeding through the gastric tube and other drains. If the child has had surgical repair of the abdomen, a postoperative ileus is often present because of surgical manipulation and the body's response to trauma. There may be signs of hypovolemia and shock if the child has intra-abdominal bleeding. The gastric fluid is tested for the presence of occult blood and obvious bleeding. An antihistamine or proton pump inhibitor agent is administered to prevent the development of a stress ulcer.

Renal assessment includes monitoring the amount and characteristics of urine output, the presence of hematuria, specific gravity, serum blood urea nitrogen and creatinine levels, urine electrolyte levels, and creatinine clearance. Hematuria may be associated with the trauma of inserting a urinary catheter or may be the result of genitourinary trauma related to the child's injury. Monitoring the renal parameters is important in assessing for the development of acute tubular necrosis. Acute tubular necrosis is a postresuscitation complication that may be seen in children who have had a profound decrease in the circulating blood volume.[31] A significant decrease in circulating fluid volume leads to hypotension, causing a decrease in renal perfusion. This reduces the glomerular filtration rate and renal cortical blood flow, stimulating renin and aldosterone secretion and producing sodium and water retention and diminished urine output (see Chapter 26).

The condition of the child's skin is assessed, noting any lacerations or abrasions that may have been overlooked during the resuscitation phase. Dressings, casts, traction, and pin sites are noted. Fracture reduction, necessitated as a result of musculoskeletal trauma, may be accomplished in a number of ways: closed reduction with immediate casting, continuous traction with Buck's or skeletal traction, external fixation devices such as a Hoffmann device, or open reduction and internal fixation. The child in any traction or stabilization device is assessed for skin breakdown related to immobility or resulting from pressure and moisture. The child also is assessed for signs of infection at pin sites, under the cast, and at any incision. The potential for circulatory compromise in the injured extremity exists and is assessed by checking pulses, color, temperature, capillary refill, and sensation (see Chapter 27).

Body temperature remains an important parameter to monitor in the child. Hypothermia may produce arrhythmias during the critical care and resuscitation phases. A temperature of less than 30° C (86° F) can produce a life-threatening arrhythmia with a resultant decrease in cardiac output. Another effect is that hyperviscosity and hypercoagulability may occur related to a rising hematocrit brought about by the cold diuresis that accompanies hypothermia.[32] Elevated temperatures may signal the development of an infection. Early detection and intervention may prevent the development of serious complications that increase the morbidity and mortality rates associated with the initial injury.

Infection is a risk in any posttrauma patient, including the pediatric patient. When the body's normal defense mechanisms are disrupted, sepsis may occur after exposure to infectious agents.[33] A recent review reported that head-injured and burn patients have the highest prevalence of nosocomial infection because of the need for mechanical ventilation and longer hospital stays.[34] Because of their immature immune systems, infants are more prone to infection. Vital signs (including core body temperature), white blood cell count, and the condition of all wounds, surgical incisions, and vascular sites should be monitored closely.

Clinical Management

The clinical management of the pediatric trauma patient in the critical care unit requires the same team approach that was necessary during the resuscitation phase. Coordination of disciplines is required to provide the best care for the child. The purpose of placing the child in the critical care unit is to provide continued monitoring and treatment. It is the nurse's responsibility to ensure that all necessary pediatric equipment and supplies are readily available and functioning properly.

Monitoring Hemodynamic Stability

Continuing management depends on the injuries and resultant problems. One of the main objectives of clinical management in the postresuscitation period is to restore hemodynamic stability and adequate perfusion to ensure viability of all organs and to prevent complications related to decreased perfusion, such as renal failure and hypoxic encephalopathy. This objective is accomplished by close, astute monitoring. Vital signs (including blood pressure, pulse, and respirations) are checked every 15 minutes until the child stabilizes.

Central venous lines, often inserted during the resuscitation phase of care, allow for trend analysis of central venous pressure during the critical care phase. Central venous pressure trends provide information regarding fluid volume status and cardiac function, thus serving as a guide for fluid and pharmacologic therapy. Normal values range from 4 to 12 mm Hg. Decreased central venous pressure typically indicates fluid deficit; elevated pressure indicates fluid overload, congestive heart failure, or cardiac tamponade. The readings also may be elevated as a result of positive pressure ventilation.

Intake and output should be monitored and recorded accurately. If possible, the child should be weighed daily so that appropriate fluid and nutritional calculations can be determined. Serum electrolytes should be measured daily or more often if appropriate. Depending on the goals of the treatment regimen, the child may be receiving maintenance or less or more than maintenance fluids.

Respiratory Support

Ventilatory support may be provided by a tracheal tube and mechanical ventilation. Determination of ventilator settings is based on the child's ability to breathe spontaneously and on arterial blood gas trends, with consideration of the presence of pulmonary disorder. The child may need to be pharmacologically paralyzed and sedated. If the child has sustained a flail chest injury, mechanical ventilation with positive pressure may be necessary for internal stabilization. The child is observed closely for the development of posttraumatic respiratory insufficiency. Early signs include increased respiratory rate, nasal flaring and retractions, and cyanosis. Auscultation may reveal sparse rales. The nurse monitors the patient for hypoxemia that does not respond to increased levels of inspired oxygen, decreased lung compliance, and diffuse infiltrates that may progress to consolidation. If posttraumatic respiratory insufficiency does develop, massive respiratory and hemodynamic support are necessary (see Chapter 24). Bronchial hygiene is provided for the intubated child to clear secretions and promote adequate ventilation. The frequency is individualized and depends on the respiratory disorder and the child's condition. Prevention of ventilator-associated pneumonia is accomplished through elevating the head of the bed to 30 degrees, providing good oral hygiene, and using goal-directed therapy for sedation to avoid oversedation.

Extubation. Once the child is able to oxygenate and ventilate adequately without mechanical support and is able to clear secretions independently, extubation is the next step. Before extubation, enteral feedings are discontinued for 2 to 4 hours, and sedation is weaned to ensure that the child has intact cough and gag reflexes. After extubation, that patient's respiratory status should be monitored closely to ensure maintanence of airway patency and adequate ventilation.

Monitoring Neurologic Status

The child with neurologic impairment as a result of head injury requires close monitoring and prompt intervention if evidence of increased intracranial pressure exists. The management of the pediatric patient with head injury is similar to that of an adult. A more detailed discussion of neurologic management is presented in Chapter 20.

Intracranial pressure monitoring devices are used in managing pediatric head trauma. If an intracranial pressure monitoring device is in place, the child's intracranial pressures should be monitored closely and recorded accurately. If it is necessary to remove excess CSF or to drain blood, a ventricular drain is inserted; physician orders should include the frequency and amount of fluid to be drained. Meticulous care of the catheter and insertion site is imperative to prevent infection. Specific instructions for intraventricular catheter site care and dressing changes are included in the child's plan of care. Methods of caring for these catheters are standardized in many institutions.

By lowering the partial pressure of carbon dioxide in arterial blood ($Paco_2$), cerebral blood flow is decreased, which reduces intracranial pressure. Occasionally hyperventilation may be used to reduce intracranial pressure, although this therapy is controversial because the reduction in cerebral blood flow can result in ischemia. The current recommendation is that this therapy be used only for acute increases in intracranial pressure resulting in neurologic deterioration or that are refractory to other methods of reduction.[35] Mild hyperventilation ($Paco_2$ 30 to 34 mm Hg) is instituted to decrease cerebral blood flow but prevent cerebral ischemia associated with severe hypocapnea-related vasoconstriction.[35] Placement of a cerebral oxygenation monitor allows for continuous assessment of regional cerebral oxygenation so that cerebral ischemia can be readily detected and treatment altered to improve cerebral oxygen delivery. The child's head is kept in a midline position and, if not contraindicated, may be slightly elevated (15 to 30 degrees) to facilitate venous drainage from the brain.

Hypertonic saline solution may be used for resuscitation and ongoing management of intracranial hypertension in the child with severe head injury. One study demonstrated that hypertonic saline solution (3% sodium chloride) increases serum sodium levels. An increase in the serum sodium concentration significantly decreases intracranial pressure and increases cerebral perfusion pressure. Also noted was that sustained hypernatremia and hyperosmolarity are safely tolerated in pediatric patients with traumatic brain injury.[36] Simma et al[37] compared two groups of head-injured children who required resuscitation. One group received lactated Ringer's solution and the other group received hypertonic saline solution. The group who received hypertonic saline had lower intracranial pressures; higher cerebral perfusion pressures; required fewer interventions to maintain a lower intracranial pressure; had fewer complications, especially pulmonary complications; and had a shorter length of stay in the intensive care unit. Advantages of hypertonic saline solution may include improved blood pressure and cerebral oxygen delivery, decreased overall fluid requirements, and overall improved survival rates.[38] Serum osmolality is monitored and a level of 365 mOsm/L is well tolerated in children receiving hypertonic saline solution.[37]

Osmotic diuretics such as mannitol may be given to children with increased intracranial pressure who are not responsive to other forms of therapy; however, these agents should be used with caution. After head trauma, children are at risk for the development of malignant brain edema. Because mannitol can increase cerebral blood flow dramatically as a result of the shift of fluid from the cellular to the vascular space, it is used with caution. When mannitol is used, boluses of 0.25 to 1.0 g/kg are recommended. Continuous administration of mannitol may lead to a reverse osmotic shift, resulting in increased brain osmolarity and increased intracranial pressure.[38] Serum osmolality is monitored every 6 hours and should not exceed 320 mOsm.

Posttraumatic seizures, which can occur in the child as a result of a severe head injury (GCS 3 to 8), diffuse cerebral edema, or an acute subdural hematoma, must be pharmacologically controlled.[37] Treatment with prophylactic anticonvulsants (e.g., phenytoin) may be considered for the first 7 days after severe traumatic brain injury but is not recommended after that time.[35] A benzodiazepine, such as lorazepam, may be given for an acute seizure situation, followed by phenytoin or fosphenytoin for at least 2 weeks.[39]

If all measures to control increased intracranial pressure have failed, barbiturate coma may be initiated. High-dose barbiturates decrease cerebral metabolic demand and reduce cerebral blood flow. Pentobarbital is given in an initial dose of 5 to 10 mg/kg. This is followed by a continuous infusion of 1 to 5 mg/kg/hr.[40,41] High-dose barbiturates significantly reduce systemic vascular resistance and may produce profound hypotension requiring fluid therapy and vasopressors. Patients receiving high-dose barbiturates require close supervision with continuous blood pressure, heart rate, cardiac output, intracranial pressure, cerebral perfusion pressure and, if available, cerebral oxygenation monitoring.

Decompressive craniectomy may be considered in the severely head-injured child with intracranial hypertension that is refractory to medical therapy.[35] The goal of decompressive craniectomy is to control increased intracranial pressure, thereby maintaining sufficient cerebral perfusion pressure and cerebral oxygenation. Taylor et al[42] conducted a single-center, prospective, randomized clinical trial with 27 patients between ages 1 and 18 years with severe traumatic brain injury and refractory intracranial hypertension. The patients were randomized to receive medical therapy alone or in combination with decompressive craniectomy. The children who had the craniectomy showed a trend toward a better clinical outcome at 6 months after injury. In a retrospective study Kan et al[43] evaluated mortality and morbidity rates and long-term outcomes in 51 children who had decompressive craniectomy for severe traumatic brain injury between 1996 and 2005. Six patients had this intervention for increased intracranial pressure alone; all other patients received this intervention along with removal of a mass lesion. Sixteen children died, including five of the six children who had the decompressive craniectomy for increased intracranial pressure alone. The authors found that posttraumatic hydrocephalus and epilepsy were common complications in children who underwent decompressive craniectomy; for those who received this intervention for increased intracranial pressure alone, the mortality rate was very high.[43]

Spinal cord injury is an infrequent occurrence in children, yet the implications for rehabilitation are far reaching. Some of the complications that may develop in the spinal cord–injured patient are systemic hypotension, bradycardia, orthostatic hypotension, constipation, neurogenic bladder, urinary tract infections, stress ulcers, respiratory insufficiency, atelectasis, pneumonia, pulmonary embolism, decubitus ulcers, and deformities such as scoliosis. Nursing interventions such as frequent turning, effective pulmonary hygiene, range-of-motion exercises, and initiation of a bowel regimen and bladder training program may help to prevent complications (see Chapter 23).

Complications of Abdominal Injuries

Many children who have liver or splenic trauma are managed nonoperatively and therefore require close observation for the possible development of complications such as bleeding. Indications for intraoperative management include hemodynamic instability, signs of increasing peritoneal irritation, and the requirement of a transfusion of more than 30% to 50% of the child's total estimated blood volume (20 to 40 ml/kg).[44]

Complications of Immobility

The child is at risk for development of complications such as pneumonia and skin breakdown, resulting from immobility. As soon as the child's condition has stabilized, a referral is made to a physical and/or occupational therapist so that appropriate range-of-motion exercises can be incorporated into the plan of care. Collaboration between the nurses caring for the child and the occupational and physical therapist enhances the benefits of the treatment regimen. When appropriate, the child and parents or significant others are included in the treatment plan as well.

Skin care must be meticulous. Frequent repositioning and assessment for the possibility of breakdown by using a scale such as the Braden Q should be done.[45] Placement of the child on a special kinetic or pressure-relieving mattress or bed may be necessary.

Nutritional Support

Adequate nutrition is essential for the pediatric trauma patient. Children are more at risk than adults for development of protein-calorie malnutrition in the critical care unit. They have increased energy requirements, small nutritional reserves, and greater obligate energy needs than adults do. Nutritional support should be started as soon as possible after resuscitation is complete. Wound healing and immunocompetence depend on the provision of adequate nutrition.

Enteral feedings are preferable because they are more physiologically normal and more efficient. Individual caloric requirements and the child's general tolerance of a particular formula are among the factors that must be considered when choosing from a variety of available enteral formulas. Excess protein is not beneficial because it is not used efficiently by the body.[46] For children whose oral intake has been restricted for an extended period, a lactose-free formula is necessary because after a period of no gastrointestinal intake, the gut does not produce lactase, which is essential for the breakdown of lactose.

If the child is unable to tolerate enteral formulas, total parenteral nutrition (TPN), including lipids, is initiated through a central venous catheter. The choice of TPN formulas greatly depends on the child's individual calorie needs. Once the child is receiving TPN, response to the therapy must be monitored. Metabolic complications may result from electrolyte, glucose, and fat imbalances. Therefore, serum levels should be monitored routinely. Weight gain and progressive wound healing indicate the child's positive response to nutritional support.

Close observation for other complications resulting from TPN therapy is indicated as well. Infection is the most frequent complication and is most often the result of poor aseptic technique during catheter placement, during the solution preparation process, or during routine catheter care. Care also must be taken to avoid dislodgment of the catheter during routine maintenance activities. Such mechanical complications may result in the development of a pneumothorax or air embolism. Close, continuous observation and meticulous catheter care serve as the best preventive methods.

Pain Management

Pain is a part of every child's experience in the critical care unit. The nurse caring for the child must develop an individualized plan for helping the child cope with alterations in comfort. The child's developmental level is the most influential factor in the child's pain response. The ability to understand the reason for pain and to develop ways to cope with it is dependent on the child's level of psychologic maturity.[47]

Analgesics are useful for all age groups to decrease painful impulses and they may enhance the effectiveness of other nursing interventions as well. Pain medication should never be withheld from the child if it seems to be the only effective means of pain relief. A combination of narcotics and benzodiazepines is often indicated to control pain and relieve anxiety. Serving as adjuncts to analgesic therapy, nursing interventions that may assist the child to deal with pain include the use of touch therapy, relaxation or distraction techniques, and the provision of verbal explanations and support. The presence of parents and other family members often helps to lessen the burden of pain as well.

With infants, touching and holding—especially when movements are rhythmic—may be effective because they may stimulate some cutaneous receptor sites that decrease the perception of pain by inhibiting painful impulses.[48] Toddlers seek out parents for comfort and use self-regulating behaviors such as sucking and rocking. Toddlers are often comforted by parents' talking to them because it serves as a distraction. Also used as a distraction technique, a discussion about siblings or family pets is a useful method with preschool children. School-age children can be taught methods for relaxation such as deep breathing exercises, which often work as a distraction technique and as a tension release modality. Touch therapy in the form of massage can also reduce a child's perception of pain.[49] Adolescents may respond favorably to many of the same techniques as younger children, such as distraction and relaxation. They also use verbalization as a method of pain relief. Preparation by verbal explanations is as important for this age group as it is for the younger patient population.

Before painful procedures, verbal explanations should be given in simple terms, geared specifically to the child's level of understanding. To help prepare for the procedure, the nurse can allow the child to think through how he or she might deal with the pain and to verbalize fears and concerns.

The stimulating atmosphere and fast-paced routines of the critical care unit can contribute to the development of altered sleep patterns. The child's normal sleep patterns are accommodated if at all possible. Special efforts are made to reduce activity at the bedside and to create a quiet environment to promote quality sleep time.

Intermediate Care and Rehabilitation Phases

Many of the clinical management strategies that were addressed in the critical care phase may be appropriate during the intermediate care and rehabilitation phases as well. To avoid unnecessary repetition, refer to the discussion of these issues in previous sections. The discussions in this section focus primarily on general rehabilitation issues as they pertain to the pediatric trauma patient. Many children, resilient by nature, tend to recover quickly. They often progress rapidly from the critical care phase to the rehabilitation phase of care, breezing quickly through or skipping entirely a clearly identifiable intermediate care stage.

Rehabilitation issues are addressed at the time of admission. Even during the resuscitation phase, the nurse is astute to the measures that can be taken to lessen or prevent conditions that may otherwise result in short- or long-term disability. All efforts must be taken to assist the child and parent in adapting to the life changes that the trauma experience has elicited. Early recognition of available or lack of available support systems for the pediatric patient and family can facilitate the process of rehabilitation planning as assistance is offered from appropriate resource programs (e.g., social services and financial assistance services). Information elicited for further development of the nursing database should include details that greatly potentiate the creation of a comprehensive rehabilitation plan of care. (Refer to Chapter 11 for more detailed information.)

Trauma, in addition to being the leading cause of death in children, is also a major cause of long-term disability. The goal of rehabilitation is to provide a better quality of life for the child and to return the child to maximal potential within the family and social unit.

Assessment of Adjustment and Adaptation to Injury

It is important to first understand how children adjust to illness on the basis of their individual cognitive/affective developmental level.[50] This affects how the child perceives the situation and what range of responses are available to the child (see Table 29-2).

Toddler

The first 2 years of life are a difficult time for the child because of a smaller repertoire of coping skills.[50] The child does not understand the reasons for the illness or treatments, and neither parents nor the health care team can explain them. The child's coping ability is greatly influenced by the parent's presence.

Preschool-Age Child

Preschoolers (3 to 6 years) have acquired some inner resources for coping with stress and thus have more coping abilities than the younger child.[50] The parents remain the major source of coping strength; however, children tolerate short periods of separation from their parents. The child at this age fears bodily intrusion and injury because of an inability to perceive long-term effects. Fantasy and guilt can distort the child's perception of the injury.

School-Age Child

The school-age child (age 7 to 12 years) has made enough developmental progress to have enhanced coping abilities. This child has usually developed a peer group by this time and can tolerate longer periods of separation from the parents. Because of increasing cognitive abilities, the child is able to more fully understand cause-and-effect relationships and can think about the future.[51] However, the child still fears bodily injury and loss of control of bodily function.

Adolescent

The adolescent (13 to 18 years) has developed skills that enhance the ability to cope.[51] The adolescent is working to establish identity and does not rely as heavily on parents for coping strength. The adolescent is able to think abstractly and can apply general principles to specifics. Two of the biggest fears of the adolescent, however, are bodily disfigurement and loss of control. This becomes a critical issue with an adolescent trauma patient who has had an amputation, a spinal cord injury, or some other disfiguring injury. Part of the challenge of rehabilitation with this age group involves helping the adolescent adjust to an altered body image and to a level of dependence during a developmental period when independence is being sought.[52]

Clinical Management

Interdisciplinary conferences that include the parents and, if appropriate, the patient are held on a regular basis. Mutual goal setting is imperative; goals that have been established by the health team without the involvement of the family and adolescent can actually hinder progress.

The child and family need much support during the rehabilitation phase. Families need to be involved in the child's care and long-range plans. They need honest, accurate information from the health care team. Many times these families are feeling guilt, frustration, and anger. These feelings need to be recognized and channeled appropriately. The nurses working with the families may help them assess their own support systems. It is helpful that families know that it is beneficial for them to maintain relationships with other family members and friends during this time. Other support systems, such as community and government agencies that provide assistance with financial problems or child care, should be discussed.

Planning for Discharge

As the child continues to improve, plans for discharge are discussed by the team, again including the parents. Some children may require total care and have little or no rehabilitation potential because they are in a persistent vegetative state. Other children may make progress toward higher levels of consciousness and rehabilitation with proper stimulation. Children with spinal cord injury require an extended rehabilitation program to help them become as functional as possible relative to their injuries. Because of the restorative and regenerative powers of the child and the potential for a long and productive life, every attempt should be made to locate a rehabilitation program that provides all that the child needs to become a functional member of the family and social unit.[53]

Some parents may choose to take their child home. For some families this is a viable alternative, but one that requires a tremendous amount of preparation. Families that are considering this option need to take into consideration the impact this child will have on the family unit. Does the child require special equipment, such as a ventilator and monitors? Will the child need home care nurses? How does the family feel about having a stranger in the home? How will bringing this child home affect the parents' relationships with each other and with their other children? Once these considerations have been addressed and the decision is made to take the child home, preparations are begun. The family must be taught new skills, such as skin care, catheter care, tracheostomy care, or suctioning procedures, so that care of the child continues in the home environment. Education and instruction about bowel and bladder regimens and range-of-motion exercises also must be accomplished. Electrical safety in the home environment is an issue that must be addressed if special equipment will accompany the child. Family members also must learn to operate and maintain the equipment, such as ventilators and monitors. The tremendous advantage of home care is that children do benefit from the stimulation they receive from their home environment. These families should be encouraged to make contact with rehabilitation centers and appropriate community or government agencies as soon as possible for continued support, guidance, and direction as needed.

Community Reintegration

A comprehensive discharge plan adequately prepares the family and child to go home and helps make the transition back into the community easier. The discharge plan is a component of the rehabilitation plan because the success or failure the family experiences after leaving the hospital depends on how the staff has assessed and worked with the family during the hospital stay. Discharge planning, although it can be exciting for the child and family, may also be extremely frightening. They are losing the protective environment of the health care facility. The family is involved from the very beginning of the discharge planning process.

The discharge planning process includes a thorough assessment of the family dynamics and their outside support systems and their ability to cope with stress. Assessment takes place by observing the family with the child in the hospital and by asking pointed questions. These details need to be incorporated into the discharge plan, and appropriate referrals to community agencies must be initiated.

It is often helpful for the child to go home for a day or weekend before the actual discharge date. A home visit gives the family an idea of unforeseen difficulties and helps them gain insight into living with their child again. It also helps the family gain a level of confidence as they realize that they can cope outside the hospital environment.

Another alternative is to have the family spend the weekend at the hospital caring for the child. This approach is especially useful for families of ventilator-dependent children who are going home. Children with spinal cord injuries are included in this population. These families can gain experience with special equipment such as ventilators and feeding pumps. Having a supervised period where they care for their child helps them attain a more realistic view of what it will be like to live with the child and gain a higher level of confidence while receiving the support of the nursing staff.

The development of the discharge plan requires a team effort, often coordinated by the primary nurse or case manager. The family should be included in the plan because they will be implementing the care measures at home.

Topics that need to be considered along with the discharge plan include finances, equipment, and supplies. Decisions must also be made about the child's care givers. It is not uncommon for one or two family members to inadvertently be singled out by other family members as the primary caregivers. The burden of caregiving inevitably falls to one or two family members if a plan for shared responsibilities is not arranged and agreed on by all involved family members before the child's homecoming. The most effective plan is one that takes into consideration the needs of the caregivers and provides periodic relief. A good plan lessens the stress experienced by all involved.

Anyone who will be caring for the child at home also must master skills such as suctioning, tracheostomy care, and CPR, which are necessary to safely care for that child. Family members must be taught problem-solving skills to deal with any emergencies that may arise, such as power outages and equipment failure. They also need to be made aware of the resources that are available in the hospital and in the community. The family should be encouraged to contact the local emergency response agency before the child's discharge to home to inform them of the situation. Notification helps to ensure that the response team arrives at the home with appropriate equipment and supplies and is adequately prepared to care for the child if called on for an emergency at a later date. It often helps for the family to be linked with a support group as well. Support groups provide the opportunity for families to be in touch with others who can relate to what they are experiencing and with whom they can exchange information.

Family involvement in the discharge plan and reintegration into the community is imperative. A comprehensive plan that prepares the child and family and takes into account all aspects of their physical, emotional, intellectual, and spiritual well-being has a favorable chance for success. Families can provide a strong motivation for the child to work toward recovery by being prepared to take the child home.

SUMMARY

Trauma is a primary killer of children between the ages of 1 and 14 years. One of every two children in this age group who die does so because of an unexpected injury. Trauma is also a major cause of disability in children. This has serious implications for the expenditure of resources and personnel at a time when more constraints are occurring in the health care system.

Further research endeavors should attempt to answer the following questions: Is the use of touch effective in reducing intracranial pressure in children? What is the relationship between the nutritional status of children and long-term outcomes? What are the long-term psychologic effects of head injury on children? What nursing interventions are most effective in supporting children in the adjustment to an altered body image? Many of the studies undertaken in the area of adult trauma should be redesigned to study the pediatric trauma population as well.

Efforts are needed to improve pediatric emergency medical systems. Such efforts must be focused on regional centers that can develop a systematic approach to the care of pediatric trauma patients. The health care team caring for the pediatric trauma patient must be well trained in the area of pediatric trauma. The facility also must be equipped to handle an injured child.

Legislators and other community leaders must be made aware of the devastating sequelae of traumatic injury. Pediatric trauma can be considered to be at epidemic proportions in our society today. Mandatory car seat and seat belt laws, when enforced, result in the saving of many young lives. Motorcycle and bicycle helmet laws can do the same. More attention needs to be focused on safety issues that affect the child. Nurses can do this by writing letters to senators, congressional representatives, and editors and by testifying at legislative hearings concerning pediatric trauma and safety issues.

Nurses, by virtue of their expert knowledge and skills, can provide educational leadership in a variety of ways. Nurses should expand their scope of practice by speaking to local agencies, parent groups, and children themselves about child safety issues and by teaching other colleagues about caring for the pediatric trauma patient. Legislators should be kept informed of all issues that currently affect the pediatric trauma population. Funding that supports extensive public awareness programs must be sought. Training and instruction must be provided by knowledgeable professionals, and more stringent safety laws must be pursued with diligence. The nurse's role in supporting all aspects of preventive care is paramount. Prevention remains the most effective treatment regimen for preserving the precious young lives in our society.

REFERENCES

1. Lau ST, Brisseau GF: Evaluation, stabilization and initial management after multiple trauma. In Fuhrman BP, Zimmerman J, editors: *Pediatric critical care*, 3rd ed, pp 1579-1594, St. Louis, 2006, Mosby Elsevier.
2. Segui-Gomez M, Chang DC, Paidas CN et al: Pediatric trauma care: an overview of pediatric trauma systems and their practices in 18 US states, *J Pediatr Surg* 38:1162-1169, 2003.
3. Dowd MD, Keenan HT, Bratton SL: Epidemiology and prevention of childhood injuries, *Crit Care Med* 30: S385-S392, 2002.
4. Mason KJ: Pediatric musculoskeletal trauma. In Moloney-Harmon PA, Czerwinski SJ, editors: *Nursing care of the pediatric trauma patient,* pp 248-275, Philadelphia, 2003, W. B. Saunders.
5. Kamerling SN: Thoracic injury. In Moloney-Harmon PA, Czerwinski SJ, editors: *Nursing care of the pediatric trauma patient,* pp 207-226, Philadelphia, 2003, W. B. Saunders.
6. Simone S: Abdominal/genitourinary trauma. In Moloney-Harmon PA, Czerwinski SJ, editors: *Nursing care of the pediatric trauma patient,* pp 227-247, Philadelphia, 2003, W. B. Saunders.
7. Zenel J, Goldstein B: Child abuse in the pediatric intensive care unit, *Crit Care Med* 30:S512-S523, 2002.
8. Czerwinski SJ, Moloney-Harmon PA: Intentional injuries. In Moloney-Harmon PA, Czerwinski SJ, editors: *Nursing care of the pediatric trauma patient,* pp 152-269, Philadelphia, 2003, W. B. Saunders.
9. Rice BA: Pediatric injury prevention. In Moloney-Harmon PA, Czerwinski SJ, editors: *Nursing care of the pediatric trauma patient,* pp 8-25, Philadelphia, 2003, W. B. Saunders.
10. Centers for Disease Control and Prevention: Motor-vehicle safety: a 20th century public health achievement, *MMWR Morbid Mortal Wkly Rep* 48:369-375, 1999.
11. Wang MY, Kim KA, Griffith PM et al. Injuries from falls in the pediatric population: an analysis of 720 cases, *J Pediatr Surg* 36:1528-1534, 2001.
12. Emergency Nurses Association: *Emergency nursing pediatric course: provider manual.*, 3rd ed, Des Plaines, IL, 2004, Emergency Nurses Association.
13. Roberts KE: Fluid and electrolyte regulation. In Curley MAQ, Moloney-Harmon PA, editors: *Critical care nursing of infants and children,* pp 369-392, Philadelphia, 2001, W. B. Saunders,.
14. Brinker D, Moloney-Harmon PA: Hematologic critical care problems. In Curley MAQ, Moloney-Harmon PA, editors: *Critical care nursing of infants and children,* pp 821-850, Philadelphia, 2001, W. B. Saunders.
15. Hymel KP, Hall CA: Diagnosing pediatric head trauma, *Pediatr Ann* 34:358-370, 2005.
16. Adelson PD: Pediatric trauma made simple, *Clin Neurosurg* 47:319-335, 2000.
17. Vernon-Levett P: Traumatic brain injury in children. In Moloney-Harmon PA, Czerwinski SJ, editors: *Nursing care of the pediatric trauma patient,* pp 171-188, Philadelphia, 2003, W. B. Saunders.
18. Larsen GY, Vernon DD, Dean JM: Evaluation of the comatose child. In Rogers MC, editor: *Textbook of pediatric intensive care,* pp 735-746, Baltimore, 1996, Williams & Wilkins.
19. Muir R, Town DA: Spinal cord injury. In Moloney-Harmon PA, Czerwinski SJ, editors: *Nursing care of the pediatric trauma patient,* pp 189-206, Philadelphia, 2003, W. B. Saunders.
20. Martin SA, Simone S: Gastrointestinal system. In Slota MC, editor: *Core curriculum for pediatric critical care nursing,* 2nd ed, pp 497-544, Philadelphia, 2006, W. B. Saunders.
21. Gilbert JC, Coppola CP: Abdominal trauma in pediatric critical care. In Fuhrman BP, Zimmerman J, editors: *Pediatric critical care,* 3rd ed, pp 1626-1636, St. Louis, 2006, Mosby Elsevier.
22. Sagarin MJ, Chiang V, Sakles JC et al. Rapid sequence intubation for pediatric airway management, *Pediatr Emerg Care* 18:417-423, 2002.
23. Carnevale FA: Striving to recapture our previous life: the experience of families with critically ill children, *J Can Assoc Crit Care Nurs* 10:16-22, 1999.

24. Jarvis JD, Woo M, Moynihan A et al: Parents on rounds: joint decision making in rounds in the PICU result in positive outcomes and increased satisfaction, *Pediatr Crit Care Med*: 6:626, 2005.
25. Boie ET, Moore GP, Brummett C et al: Do parents want to be present during invasive procedures performed on their children in the emergency department? A survey of 400 parents, *Ann Emerg Med* 34:70-74, 1999.
26. Tinsley C, Hill JB, Shah J et al. Family presence during cardiopulmonary resuscitation in the pediatric intensive care unit, *Pediatr Crit Care Med* 7:517, 2006.
27. Gold K, Gorenflo D, Schwenk T et al: Physician experience with family presence during cardiopulmonary resuscitation in children. *Pediatr Crit Care Med* 7:428-433, 2006.
28. Matincheck T: Nurses' beliefs and practices of family presence during cardiopulmonary resuscitation and invasive procedures: review of literature, *Top Emerg Med Innovations Manage* 28:144-148, 2006.
29. Schiff H: *The bereaved parent,* New York, 1977, Penguin Books.
30. Meert K, Thurston C, Thomas R: Parental coping and bereavement outcome after the death of a child in the pediatric intensive care unit, *Pediatr Crit Care Med* 2:324-328, 2001.
31. Grehn LS, Kline A, Weishaar J: Renal critical care problems. In Curley MAQ, Moloney-Harmon PA, editors: *Critical care nursing of infants and children,* pp 731-764, Philadelphia, 2001, W. B. Saunders.
32. Pate MF: Thermal regulation. In Curley MAQ, Moloney-Harmon PA, editors: *Critical care nursing of infants and children,* pp 443-459, Philadelphia, 2001, W. B. Saunders.
33. Mollitt DL: Infection control: avoiding the inevitable, *Surg Clin North Am* 82:365-378, 2002.
34. Upperman JS, Sheridan RL: Pediatric trauma susceptibility to sepsis, *Pediatr Crit Care Med* 6:S108-S111, 2005.
35. Adelson PD, Bratton SL, Carney NA et al: Guidelines for the acute medical management of severe traumatic brain injury in infants, children, and adolescents, *Pediatr Crit Care Med* 4: S1-S75, 2003.
36. Khanna S, Davis D, Peterson B et al: Use of hypertonic saline in the treatment of severe refractory post traumatic intracranial hypertension in pediatric traumatic brain injury, *Crit Care Med* 28:1136-1143, 2000.
37. Simma B, Burger R, Falk M: A prospective, randomized, and controlled study of fluid management in children with severe head injury: lactated Ringer's solution versus hypertonic saline, *Crit Care Med* 26:1265-1270, 1998.
38. Knapp JM: Hyperosmolar therapy in the treatment of severe head injury in children: mannitol and hypertonic saline, *AACN Clin Issues Adv Pract Acute Crit Care* 16:199-211, 2005.
39. Marcoux KK: Management of increased intracranial pressure in the critically ill child with an acute neurological injury, *AACN Clin Issues* 16:212-231, 2005.
40. Kochanek PM, Forbes ML, Ruppel R et al: Severe traumatic brain injury in infants and children. In Fuhrman BP, Zimmerman J, editors: *Pediatric critical care,* 3rd ed, pp 1595-1617, St. Louis, 2006, Mosby Elsevier.
41. Poss WB, Brockmeyer D, Clay B et al: Pathophysiology and management of the intracranial vault. In Rogers MC, editor: *Textbook of pediatric intensive care,* pp 645-666, Philadelphia, 1996, W. B. Saunders.
42. Taylor A, Warwick B, Rosenfeld J et al: A randomized trial of very early decompressive craniectomy in children with traumatic brain injury and sustained intracranial hypertension, *Childs Nerv System* 17:154-162, 2001.
43. Kan P, Amini A, Hansen K et al: Outcomes after decompressive craniectomy for severe traumatic brain injury in children, *J Neurosurg* 105:337-342, 2006.
44. Moloney-Harmon PA, Adams P: Trauma. In Curley MAQ, Moloney-Harmon PA, editors: *Critical care nursing of infants and children,* pp 947-980, Philadelphia, 2001, W. B. Saunders.
45. Curley MA, Quigley SM. Lin M: Pressure ulcers in pediatric intensive care: incidence and associated factors, *Pediatr Crit Care Med* 4:284-290, 2003.
46. Verger JT, Schears G: Nutrition support. In Curley MAQ, Moloney-Harmon PA, editors: *Critical care nursing of infants and children,* pp 393-424, Philadelphia, 2001, W. B. Saunders.
47. Abu-Saad HH: Pain in children: a state of the art. In Tibboels D, van der Voort E, editors: *Intensive care in childhood: a challenge to the future,* pp 517-526, Berlin, 1996, Springer-Verlag.
48. Franck LS: The ethical imperative to treat pain in infants: are we doing the best we can? *Crit Care Nurs* 17:80-86, 1997.
49. Oakes LL: Caring practices: providing comfort. In Curley MAQ, Moloney-Harmon PA, editors: *Critical care nursing of infants and children,* pp 547-576, Philadelphia, 2001, W. B. Saunders.
50. Baroni MA: Cognitive and psychosocial development. In Broome ME, Rollins JA, editors: *Core curriculum for the nursing care of children and their families,* pp 31-44, Pitman, NJ, 1999, Jannetti.
51. Smith JB, Martin SA: Caring practices: providing developmentally appropriate care. In Curley MAQ, Moloney-Harmon PA, editors: *Critical care nursing of infants and children,* pp 17-46, Philadelphia, 2001, W. B. Saunders.
52. Bindler R: Health behavior. In Broome ME, Rollins JA, editors: *Core curriculum for the nursing care of children and their families,* pp 63-76, Pitman, NJ, 1999, Jannetti.
53. Holbrook TL, Anderson JA, Sieber WJ et al: Outcome after major trauma: 12-month and 18-month follow-up results from the trauma recovery project, *J Trauma* 46:765-773, 1999.

30

TRAUMA IN THE ELDERLY

Ellen Plummer

The aging of our population represents a significant change in the national demographics, which has a major impact on the delivery of health care. Projections by the U.S. Census Bureau indicate that by 2050 more than 20% of the population will be over the age of 65 years.[1] That is an 8% increase from the predictions made for 2000. This is in large part due to the aging of the baby boom generation, where more than 75 million babies were born between 1946 and 1964. In response to this projected population growth of people over the age of 65 years, the elderly have become an increasingly common focus of health care research in the last decade. This ever-growing number of elderly patients and their susceptibility to injuries make them one of the larger and increasingly important consumers of health care in terms of resources and dollars.[2] The Fiscal Year 2007 budget request for the Administration on Aging is $1,338,000.000.[3] This budget is designed to accelerate the key systems changes needed to prepare the nation for the aging and long-term care needs of the baby boom generation.[3]

Normal aging is a gradual process. Research has provided some insight on the process of aging but has also identified new challenges and generated many new questions. To date, no universal agreement exists as to when a person becomes "old." The geriatric trauma population has been defined in a number of ranges in the literature as age greater than or equal to 55, 60, 65, 70, 75, and even age 80 years. This broad range of ages, however, fails to adequately differentiate between the "healthy" old, and the "not-so-healthy" old. Cultural differences, such as race or ethnicity, influence the definition of aging as well, using terms such as "elders" to define functional status rather than age; some cultures have a more positive attitude toward aging and may see no significant difference regarding age or gender. Additionally, much of the literature is outdated and not inclusive of all of the care issues surrounding the geriatric population.

Within the natural human life span, each person's experience is like no other. Illness and injury may certainly contribute to a shortened life expectancy or a greatly altered quality of life. Because of the wide variability among people, it becomes more and more difficult to estimate when an individual becomes "old." Although chronologic age is clearly an inadequate measure, in this chapter *elderly* is defined as an individual of chronological age 65 years or older.

The wide range of definitions surrounding what constitutes the "elderly patient population" creates difficulty for the nurse who is trying to anticipate potential problems related to trauma. Trauma protocols have traditionally been designed for a younger population and are unlikely to be effective for older persons. The primary problem is that the available information does not clearly distinguish between elderly patients' responses to trauma from their altered responses as a result of preexisting chronic disease.

The intent of this chapter is to provide nurses with a brief summary of what is currently known about the normal physiologic changes that occur in the elderly. The impact these changes and alterations have on elderly trauma victims and the challenges faced in caring for this unique population will be discussed.

EPIDEMIOLOGY

Trauma is the seventh leading cause of death in Americans older than age 65 years.[4] The elderly are more frequently injured from low-energy and household incidents. Their injuries are disproportionately severe and they are more likely to have comorbid conditions, suffer complications, and die after trauma.[5] Elderly trauma patients account for 25% of all injury fatalities per year and consume 33% of the health care resources spent on trauma care.[6] Unintentional injury deaths in individuals aged 65 years and older are primarily due to three causes: motor vehicle crashes (MVCs), falls, and thermal injuries. MVCs are the most common cause of death from trauma through age 79 years. More than 40 million older adults will be licensed drivers by 2020.[7] These drivers are involved in only a fraction of the total MVCs. However, although they drive a lower number of miles, and are less likely to drink and drive than other adult drivers,[8] those over the age 75 years have a higher fatality rate from MVCs than those in any other age group. These statistics yield little information about the causes of the MVC but would suggest that someone is more likely to die in a collision involving an elderly driver than in a collision involving a younger driver.

Among adults aged 80 years and older, falls are the leading cause of injury deaths.[9] In 2003, more than 1.8 million seniors aged 65 years and older were treated in emergency departments for fall-related injuries and more than 421,000 were hospitalized.[10] Of those who fall, 20% to 30% have moderate to severe injuries that reduce mobility and increase the risk of premature death.[11] Falls are the leading cause of traumatic brain injury in older adults.[12] Multiple causative factors such as balance impairment and substance abuse issues are often suggested as precursors to falls.

Death as a result of thermal injury accounts for approximately 4% of all unintentional deaths in individuals aged 65 years and older.[13] Thermal injuries include flame burns, scalds, inhalation injury, direct and indirect contact with heat sources, and electrical injury.

There were 852 homicides reported in 2002 of people aged 60 years and older.[14] Although the number of homicides of people aged 65 years and older has been decreasing, this age group still has the highest percentage of homicides during the commission of a felony.[15]

As the U.S. population ages, public health efforts have expanded to ensure the independence, function, and safety of older adults. Approximately 33,000 people aged 60 years and older in the United States were treated in hospital emergency departments for nonfatal assault-related injuries in 2001, with injuries occurring disproportionately among persons ages 60 to 69 years.[16] Some of the injuries probably represent a form of elder maltreatment, which refers to acts of commission or omission that result in harm or threatened harm to the health and welfare of an older adult, occurring within any relationship in which there is an expectation of trust.[17] The various forms of elder maltreatment include physical, sexual, and psychologic abuse; abandonment; exploitation; and neglect, either intentional or unintentional. For every reported incident of elder maltreatment, an estimated five incidents are unreported.[18]

A 50-state survey found that Adult Protective Services received 472,813 reports of elder abuse in domestic and institutional settings in 2000. Eighty-four percent of the reports received were investigated and almost half were substantiated. Adults over the age of 80 years were the most frequent victims of abuse, excluding self-neglect.[19] In a recent analysis of nursing home inspections and complaint investigations from 1990 to 2000, it was found that more than 9% (1,601 homes) were cited for causing actual harm or immediate jeopardy to residents. More than 30% (5,283 homes) were cited for an abuse violation that had the potential to cause harm.[20] The National Aging Resource Center on Elder Abuse estimates that 20% of elder abuse victims experience financial exploitation.[21]

Between 1 and 2 million Americans aged 65 years and older have been injured, exploited, or otherwise mistreated by someone on whom they depended for care or protection.[22] Health care providers often unintentionally overlook elder abuse and neglect, explaining a fracture or weight loss as expected or normal consequences of the aging process.[23] Health care practitioners have a responsibility to work with law enforcement and social service agencies to respond appropriately to these growing problems affecting the elderly population.

Patterns of Injury

Falls are the most common cause of injury in the elderly population. Most injuries classified as serious are fractures of the hips, arms and hands, legs and feet, ribs, vertebrae, and pelvis. Head trauma and other nonfracture injuries can also occur when an older person falls. It is difficult to compare MVC injury patterns between the young and the elderly because of the variations in how injuries are documented in published reports and because the elderly are seldom analyzed separately from the young.

Thermal injuries in the elderly have higher mortality rates compared with similar injuries in the young. When the burn-related mortality rate is compared with age, it is usually expressed as the percentage of burn that leads to a 50% mortality rate. Mortality is 50% in a young adult with a burn covering 80% of total body surface area (TBSA); in a person aged 60 to 70 years, a burn of 35% TBSA has a 50% mortality rate; in a person over age 70 years, a burn of 20% TBSA has a 50% mortality rate.[24]

Injury Threshold

Increased Personal Risk

The aging process produces unique changes in an individual's functional status, which contributes to increased susceptibility to injury and mortality. The process of aging is characterized by the progressive loss of function and functional reserve of organs in times of physical and metabolic stress.[25]

Factors such as decreasing function of the special senses, loss of vision and hearing, syncope, postural instability, and transient impairment of cerebrovascular perfusion, have all been implicated as causes of elderly traumatic injury. Alterations in perception and delayed response to stressors may also contribute to injury. For example, diminished or impaired proprioception reduces awareness of an impending fall. In addition, the onset of corrective measures may then be too late to avoid falling. Loss of visual and hearing acuity limits the elderly person's ability to see and hear traffic hazards and avoid them. Other factors such as medication use or alcohol ingestion can also lead to traumatic injury in the elderly. Many older adults regularly use multiple medications. Many medications have side effects that may indirectly contribute to injury in an elderly person. Additionally, the combination of some prescription medications with over-the-counter medications can result in dangerous situations and lead to injuries.

Finally, the combination of medications with the use of alcohol, in both the younger and older populations, can clearly result in impaired perception and response and can often lead to injury. The incidence of alcohol dependence and abuse has been increasing among the elderly population.[26] Every elderly trauma patient should be evaluated for alcohol use to minimize morbidity and mortality rates. Elderly patients who abuse alcohol are at risk to experience acute alcohol withdrawal and are particularly at risk for this because of their age-related physiologic changes or conditions. Their use or abuse of alcohol may have been occurring for years but has now escalated to the point of causing an event that has resulted in injury. Older adults can reach a higher blood alcohol concentration sooner than young drinkers because of a decrease in total body fluid.[26] Obvious symptoms of alcohol use would include the smell of alcohol on the patient's breath, slurred speech, or difficulty paying attention. Minor symptoms of withdrawal can begin 6 to 12 hours after the last drink and can peak within 24 to 36 hours.[26] These symptoms can include tachycardia, hypertension, nausea, and tremors[26]; however, these nonspecific signs can often be mistaken for common problems experienced by elderly patients and should be evaluated against the patient's known preexisting conditions and the current trauma-related clinical presentation.

INCREASED SOCIETAL RISK

We live in a society that is dominated by the fantasy of everlasting youth and health. Most communicable diseases have been eradicated, contributing to increased life spans, and more and more emphasis is being placed on healthier eating habits and exercise, supporting good health and longevity. However, as our society celebrates youth and long life, both the number of elderly citizens and the hazards to which they are regularly exposed are rapidly increasing.

Both inside and outside the home there are hazards that can increase the chances of injury in the elderly population. Outside hazards such as cars, road traffic volumes, and faster speed limits are certainly different today compared with more than 50 years ago. Everyday distractions during driving and commuting can overload the information-processing capabilities of anyone, but especially those of the elderly driver or pedestrian. Inside the home hazards such as rugs, sharp corners on tables, countertops, and cabinets, stairs without railings, poorly lit or nonexistent lighting in hallways and stairwells, and hot tap water more than 130° F can all increase the risk of unintentional injury for the elderly. Additionally, the elderly are known to be easy targets for criminals because of their inability to defend themselves or the inability to get out of the situation quickly and safely.

As we look toward a future with greater numbers of elderly citizens, it becomes apparent that not enough is known about the special needs of our aging patients. Health care providers, particularly nurses, are in a unique position to support and to enhance the efforts of public health agencies and epidemiologists seeking to reduce environmental hazards. Additionally, these health care providers can have a positive effect on the attitudes and values of society at large.

The normal aging process presents challenges for elderly trauma victims and for the health care team caring for them. Diminished senses and function can make everyday life a hazard for the elderly. Broad age ranges for what defines "elderly" and the frequency and severity of injuries combined with comorbid conditions can often raise questions about the health care team's treatment, management plans, and decision making in the injured elderly population.

RESUSCITATIVE PHASE

Most trauma protocols have traditionally been designed for a younger population. Generalizing injury patterns and responses to injury is usually effective with younger patients; however, it is significantly more difficult, if not impossible, to use these same protocols in the management of the elderly trauma patient. Two reasons are (1) a wide variability in both the function and preexisting condition of the elderly patient population and (2) a lack of adequate documentation in the literature about how the older person initially responds to traumatic injury, which limits evidenced-based practice protocol development. Widespread belief that all elderly individuals have significantly impaired cardiovascular function sometimes leads to inadequate fluid replacement and persistent hypovolemia. Conversely, the elderly are sometimes treated without due consideration of potential cardiovascular impairment leading to high volumes of fluid replacement and fluid overload. This population may exhibit less dramatic responses to injury compared with the younger population; because of this, the elderly may be less tolerant of even minor physiologic derangements from traumatic injury.

The inaccurate impression that all older individuals have significantly impaired function is easily acquired from the literature. Many reports primarily document disease and disability in the elderly without regard for those who are considered the "healthy" aged population. Many of our elderly citizens are healthy; therefore, generic patient management decisions based on chronologic age alone are inappropriate.

ASSESSMENT

Just as with the younger trauma population, resuscitation of the elderly trauma patient should be rapid and efficient. However, a rapid and thorough assessment of the injured elderly patient may be more difficult, particularly if unfounded or inaccurate assumptions are made of the pretrauma condition. Assessment itself can be complicated in cases when an older person presents with preexisting conditions. Although the presence of any chronic illness has not been a direct predictor of death in elderly patients with injuries, comorbid conditions have been associated with increased mortality rates, varying with the type and number of conditions[25] (Tables 30-1 and 30-2).

In the younger trauma population, increases in the Injury Severity Score parallel increases in the mortality rate. Deaths in the older population can result from injuries that would normally be survivable in the young; thus, assessment and interventions in older patients with lower Injury Severity Scores are warranted. The suspicion that eventually death will result despite treatment efforts should not overshadow the fact that elderly patients, even those severely injured, have the potential to survive and return to independent function.

Cardiovascular Considerations

Cardiovascular disease is one of the most common medical problems in the elderly and often leads to death in this population. Age is a major risk factor for cardiovascular disease, which accounts for more than 40% of deaths in those

TABLE 30-1 **Preexisting Disease (PED) State Versus Age**

	Age (yr)						
	15-24	25-34	35-44	45-54	55-64	65-74	Older than 75
PED present	166	179	199	184	199	173	146
PED absent	2653	2056	972	414	252	173	79
Percentage with PED	5.8	8.0	17.0	30.8	44.1	50.0	64.9

From Kauder DR, Schwab CW, Shapiro MB: Geriatric trauma: patterns, care, and outcomes. In Moore EE, Feliciano DV, Mattox KL, editors: *Trauma,* 5th ed, p 1042, New York, 2004, McGraw-Hill. Reprinted with permission of The McGraw-Hill Companies.

TABLE 30-2 **Number of Preexisting Diseases and Outcomes**

Number of Preexisting Diseases	Survived	Died	Mortality Rate (%)
0	6341	211	3.2
1	868	56	6.1
2	197	36	15.5
3 or more	67	22	24.9

From Kauder DR, Schwab CW, Shapiro MB: Geriatric trauma: patterns, care, and outcomes. In Moore EE, Feliciano DV, Mattox KL, editors: *Trauma,* 5th ed, p. 1043, New York, 2004, McGraw-Hill. Reprinted with permission of The McGraw-Hill Companies.

>65 years old.[27] Diminished cardiac reserves may not affect the daily functioning of a healthy older individual, but when an elderly person has physiologic stress, such as from blood loss or hypoxia, the lack of reserve becomes apparent through cardiac dysfunction.[28] Some elderly patients may be unaware of cardiac dysfunction or may have few, if any, symptoms until the time of traumatic injury or stress. As is true for all trauma patients, initial measurements of blood pressure are likely to be misleading because of compensation or prior dysfunction. The presence of "normal" vital signs may mask severe physiologic compromise.

Inherent in cardiovascular disease is the prevalence of conditions such as atrial fibrillation, heart block, and arrhythmias such as premature ventricular contractions. In the elderly population, these are due to progressive cell loss and changes in the myocardium resulting from normal physiologic changes in the heart. All these have the potential to decrease the cardiac output. However, it is important that the cause of the arrhythmia, such as electrolyte abnormalities, hypoxemia, or myocardial contusion, be clinically determined rather than assuming that the arrhythmias are due to cardiac disease. Myocardial infarction is often hypothesized to be the cause of trauma, but there is little evidence to support this assumption. However, acute infarction may be found by the time the patient is admitted and supports ruling out an acute process on admission.

Hypertension is one of the more common preexisting conditions in the elderly population. Diastolic dysfunction is also common in the elderly, particularly in those with hypertension, and is responsible for up to 50% of cases of heart failure in patients older than age 80 years.[29] Some patients may be taking medications to treat hypertension. Both the hypertensive state and the medications can alter physiologic compensatory mechanisms and obscure signs of shock. For example, in an elderly patient taking a prescription β-blocker to treat hypertension, heart rate may not increase in response to trauma, hypovolemia, or injury-related stress. Decreased β-adrenergic receptors and diminished catecholamine release can both result in the inability to raise the maximum heart rate needed to respond to stress and can also prevent the heart from normalizing quickly after stress.

Warfarin (Coumadin) is the fourth most commonly prescribed cardiovascular agent and the eleventh most prescribed drug in the United States.[30,31] The use of warfarin anticoagulation therapy in the elderly population is typically for the treatment of atrial fibrillation, cardiac valve replacement, venous thrombosis, and pulmonary embolism. Controversy exists over whether warfarin therapy increases the risk of complications from hemorrhage. Two studies highlight the differences of opinion.

A Michigan Level I trauma center study evaluated 159 consecutive trauma patients who were taking warfarin and compared their outcomes to a group of age-matched patients with head injuries who were not taking warfarin. Fifty-nine percent of patients in the warfarin study group had some type of head trauma, of which 27% had intracranial injuries, defined as evidence of subdural, subarachnoid, epidural, intraparenchymal, or intraventricular hemorrhage on computed tomographic scan.[32] Of the 15 patients (9.4%) who died, an international normalized ratio (INR) of 3.3 was found compared with the INR of 3.0 that was found in those who survived. Of 70 age-matched patients with head trauma not taking warfarin, 47 (67%) had intracranial injury and 5 of those died (10%). In conclusion, the preinjury use of warfarin does not place the trauma patient at increased risk for fatal hemorrhagic complications in the absence of head trauma. Intracranial injury was strongly associated with a mortality rate significantly higher than patients with head trauma who were not taking warfarin.[32]

Conversely, in New York, a 7-year chart review was completed on all anticoagulated patients over age 65 years with minor head injuries. Only 32 patients were identified for inclusion in the study. Twenty-four patients were discharged from the emergency department without hospitalization. Three of the remaining eight patients had initial Glasgow

Coma Scores between 14 and 15 but became comatose within 3 to 4 hours. A fourth patient was comatose 6 hours after injury. Three of these four patients died, leading to the conclusion that anticoagulated patients with even minor head trauma are at risk for neurologic deterioration within 6 hours of injury despite a seemingly normal neurologic examination.[33]

Serum troponin is a specific and sensitive marker of myocardial injury. An increase in serum troponin I of greater than 1.2 mcg/L after trauma is related to the degree of overall myocardial injury and physiologic stress and not mechanical chest trauma.[34] Obtaining a baseline 12-lead electrocardiogram, cardiac enzymes, and troponin level is suggested. Additionally, serial electrocardiogram and laboratory studies should be completed with evidence of myocardial infarction or elevated cardiac enzymes, particularly the creatine kinase-MB isoenzyme or troponin levels.

Patients with permanent pacemakers may have a fixed heart rate and cardiac output and thus may also be unable to respond to increased myocardial demands from trauma and stress. A patient with an automatic implantable cardioverter-defibrillator may need temporary reprogramming to allow more efficient trauma management.

The effect of aging on the cardiovascular system supports the use of hemodynamic monitoring in the elderly. Continuous monitoring should be instituted rapidly in elderly patients to assess trends and patterns of cardiovascular response. Invasive monitoring such as arterial lines, central venous pressure lines, and pulmonary artery catheters should be considered early in the course of treatment despite iatrogenic risk to provide more reliable assessment of cardiovascular performance and guidance of fluid replacement therapy. In addition, early and aggressive resuscitation and invasive monitoring have been shown to improve outcomes in the elderly trauma population. Scalea et al[35] suggested that the elderly may appear hemodynamically stable while experiencing inadequate perfusion, which may result in delays in the recognition and treatment of underperfusion, leading to increased mortality.

The existence of cardiovascular disease and its associated symptoms, as well as medications used to treat preexisting conditions in elderly trauma patients, can have a significant impact on their responses to injury and physiologic stress. Continuous monitoring, accurate assessment, aggressive treatment, and the use of invasive cardiac monitoring devices are useful in improving outcomes.

Pulmonary Considerations

As a person ages, the pulmonary system undergoes physiologic changes such as increased work of breathing, which can lead to the need for ventilatory support after traumatic injury. Elderly patients have a decreased respiratory reserve and may decompensate more quickly than do younger patients.[28] The pulmonary arteries thicken, increasing pulmonary vascular resistance. The lung parenchyma and chest wall become stiff, leading to diminished pulmonary compliance. Alveolar ducts enlarge and alveoli become flatter and shallower, decreasing the lung vital capacity and increasing the expiratory reserve volume, which can lead to ventilation-perfusion mismatching. Respiratory muscle fibers atrophy, decreasing respiratory muscle strength and thus heightening the elderly patient's risk for respiratory fatigue in the face of traumatic injury. Diminished lung cilia can lead to an increased risk of pulmonary infection and aspiration. Additionally, chronic lung disease and cigarette smoking compromise the overall respiratory function and reserve when stressed.

Potential problems with airway management should be anticipated. Missing teeth or removed dentures can make bag-mask ventilation difficult. Endotracheal intubation provides airway protection but may be difficult to accomplish because of deformity or rigidity of the cervical spine. Vigorous manipulation of the head and neck must be avoided because of the risk of impairing vertebral circulation.

Arterial blood gas measurements typically show a moderately reduced oxygen tension (such as a partial pressure of arterial oxygen [Pao_2] of 80 mm Hg), whereas other values are within normal limits. Changes in values other than Pao_2 should be interpreted in the context of the injury. Measurements across time remain essential for determining trends. In elderly patients with blunt chest trauma resulting from both falls and MVCs, multiple fractured ribs are the most common injury.[36] Elderly patients who sustain blunt chest trauma with rib fractures have twice the mortality rate of younger patients with similar injuries.[36] As the number of rib fractures increases, so does the incidence of pneumonia and death.[36,37] A key factor in the management of rib factors is adequate pain management to provide the opportunity for pulmonary hygiene and prevention of pulmonary complications.

Adequate pain relief is essential to optimize pulmonary function. Inadequate pain relief may cause decreased respiratory effort, leading to atelectasis and decreased oxygen exchange and the need for mechanical ventilation. Flail chest, significant pulmonary contusions, and preexisting pulmonary disease are indicators leading to consideration for mechanical ventilation. Weaning from ventilatory support may be prolonged in the elderly population.

Neurologic Considerations

The initial neurologic assessment should include a brief examination of the patient for impairments of the special senses, especially vision and hearing, because alterations in these functions may cloud further assessment. Cognitive function can be tested superficially if the patient is capable of verbal response. Assessment of cognitive function may be complicated by loss of short-term memory, the presence of senile dementia, or slow responses caused by an overload of sensory input. It is important to determine whether normal changes such as short-term memory loss or the diminished ability to process information are the patient's baseline findings or are a new neurologic deficit from trauma.

Careful assessment should be made for evidence of intracranial bleeding, particularly in trauma associated with falls and MVCs. Even minor head injuries can lead to intracranial vessel injury resulting in a subdural hematoma or subarachnoid bleeding. Cerebral atrophy, which is normal in aging, results in greater cranial space where a significant amount of blood can accumulate before any neurologic symptoms appear. Pupillary responses tend to be sluggish in the elderly, and assessment may be further complicated by eye disease such as glaucoma or previous surgery such as cataract. Several factors can affect an accurate neurologic examination in the elderly trauma patient. Determining what is normal from what is new should be done through frequent reassessments of patient's condition.

Musculoskeletal Considerations

Musculoskeletal assessment should be performed with consideration of age-related changes: limitations in mobility and joint flexibility, muscle atrophy, loss of subcutaneous fat, and preexisting deformity. Hip fractures are often associated with additional injuries, such as extremity and vertebral fractures and head injuries. Osteoarthritis is a common finding that results in loss of strength that can lead to limited mobility. A high level of suspicion should be used when evaluating the entire vertebral system in the elderly because some vertebral compression injuries may be asymptomatic.

Cervical spine fractures in elderly patients are increasingly common as the population ages. Controversy exists over surgical stabilization versus halo vest immobilization treatment of cervical and high thoracic injuries in the elderly because of associated higher rates of cardiac and pulmonary morbidity and mortality rates with the use of halo vest immobilization.[38] The decision about how to treat different patterns of cervical spine fractures is complex and often controversial. The same bony injury may have acceptable rates of healing whether treated operatively or nonoperatively. One must then consider risks and potential complications of each type of treatment and how quickly the patient will regain an acceptable functional status.[39]

In older patients, pelvic fractures are more likely to cause hemorrhage and require intervention. Fracture patterns differ in older patients; although severe pelvic fractures are more common in young patients, lateral compression type fractures occur more frequently and cause significant blood loss in the elderly population.[40] Outcomes for older patients with pelvic fractures are also significantly worse than in younger patients. Atherosclerosis is an extremely common disease in elderly patients, and this may limit the ability of injured vessels to develop vasospasm and spontaneously tamponade. Significant blood loss needs to be addressed either by external fixator application, although this will not help lateral compression fractures, or by angiography and embolization. Blood transfusions also may be needed.[40]

Although conventional assessment techniques are presumed effective, some injuries may be missed if the patient has impaired pain perception. The absence of pain should not be relied on to rule out the possibility of fracture. Conversely, chronic pain, such as that associated with arthritis, may mask a new injury or condition. Where any question exists, radiologic confirmation is indicated.

Renal Considerations

The effects of age on renal function results in diminished blood flow and glomerular filtration rate (GFR), reduced bladder capacity, and decreased diluting ability, all of which can affect the response to trauma and stress. Diminished renal function, coupled with altered cardiovascular responses, can obscure signs of hypovolemia and shock. Serum creatinine levels in the elderly generally do not change because there is a decrease in lean body mass, thus a decrease in creatinine production. However, serum creatinine levels may be altered by factors such as medications, sepsis, trauma, and immobility.[28] Diminished GFR has important implications in terms of drug dosing because most drugs are renally excreted. Creatinine clearance should be used in dosing calculations.[28] A urinary catheter should be part of the initial treatment plan to monitor urine output and fluid volume status.

Metabolic Considerations

Some elderly persons are prone to diminished calcium intake simply by virtue of changes in dietary intake. Weight loss may occur, resulting in overall diminished lean body mass. Lack of caloric intake for energy may lead to diminished physical ability.

In the elderly, metabolic responses to stress are intact but may take time to occur. Some endocrine secretions, such as estrogen, do diminish with age. Diabetes and hypothyroidism are common in the elderly and chronic infections or debilitating conditions such as cancer can make the elderly patient immunocompromised, adding to the risk of death.

Psychosocial Considerations

A primary goal of all trauma care is to return the patient to the best possible function. Short- and long-term goals for recovery should be set on admission and revised over the course of the hospitalization. Meeting these goals should include enlisting the assistance of support services for the patient. Including the older patient in the decision-making process regarding the care and treatment options helps maintain their independence during hospitalization.

The unique personal and health history of the individual should be obtained as soon as possible. If the patient is a reliable historian, immediate information concerning relevant medical history, including use of medications, should be obtained. If this is not possible, family members or friends often can provide valuable information. Contact with the patient's primary care physician provides valuable insight into the prior health of the patient and should not be overlooked. Questions concerning the individual's daily activity and degree of independence prove helpful when formulating long-term plans, not only during initial assessment and treatment but later as well.

Nursing Management

The same principles and concepts that apply to treatment and nursing management in young patients apply to care of the elderly, including a heightened sense of urgency and an increased index of suspicion for injury. There should be a need for speed and accuracy with both assessment and treatment of injuries in the elderly. Communication with the patient is essential, particularly during the early stages of care. Nursing care should emphasize communication with the patient through combined mediums, including vision, touch, and hearing. Although it is difficult to accomplish during resuscitation, the nurse should seek eye contact in the patient's direct line of vision and should speak slowly, clearly, and in low tones when talking to the patient. Questions should be phrased simply with limited use of medical terms. Verbal communication should be reinforced by purposeful touch that is gentle yet firm.

Elderly patients often feel tremendous fear in the midst of resuscitation procedures. It is especially crucial that trauma nurses remember their role as patient advocate when caring for injured members of the elderly population. Although physical and chemical restraints are sometimes used to facilitate resuscitative efforts, they can be justified only to protect the patient or staff from harm. The Centers for Medicare and Medicaid Services (formerly the Health Care Financing Administration) defines physical restraints as "any manual method of physical or mechanical device, material, or equipment attached or adjacent to the patient that the individual cannot remove easily which restricts freedom of movement or normal access to one's body."[41] Mechanical restraints carry a risk of severe injury, strangulation, and mobility limitations that may predispose patients to serious injury or even death.[42] Firm manual restraint is always preferable to tying the patient down. Restraints should be considered a last resort when it is clear that the patient lacks decision-making capacity and only after all attempts to communicate have failed. Whether physical, chemical, or manual restraints are used, it is imperative that they only be used for as long as necessary.

Although the priorities of initial assessment and treatment of elderly patients do not differ from those of the young, specific procedures may have to be adjusted. Cervical osteoarthritis can lead to spinal stenosis and potentially result in a spinal cord injury in an elderly person requiring intubation. It is imperative that a high level of caution and suspicion be maintained while performing any maneuver of the cervical spine during intubation. Asepsis is essential because of the great risk of pulmonary infection in the elderly.

Mechanical ventilation should be instituted rapidly, if indicated, because the elderly have limited ventilatory reserve. Successful ventilatory management of elderly patients is facilitated by the cautious use of sedation and analgesia.

Fluid resuscitation must be monitored closely to ensure adequate, rapid replacement without excessive administration of fluids. Conservative treatment on the basis of this belief may prolong periods of hypovolemia and hypoperfusion, increasing morbidity and mortality rates.

Time is of the essence in determining outcome after injury in the elderly population. By the time the elderly patient's bleeding problem becomes a measurable drop in hemoglobin or a change in hemodynamic stability, hypoperfusion may have occurred and could result in a situation from which the elderly patient cannot recover. Central venous pressure or pulmonary artery lines may provide clinical measurement for determining whether fluid replacement therapy is adequate. Hemodynamic monitoring and administration of inotropic support should be considered early when the patient fails to respond adequately to fluid replacement.

Hypothermia is a major problem during resuscitation. The elderly have a diminished ability to regulate temperature, resulting in less tolerance to cold. Shivering, generally tolerated by healthy people, can produce a metabolic toll that can compromise and reduce glycogen stores in frail or debilitated patients.[43]

Hypothermic patients (body temperature less than 35° C) have significantly higher mortality rates than do patients with the same severity of injury who remain normothermic.[44] Conversely, the previously studied protective benefits of reduced body temperature may also have a therapeutic effect on trauma patients. A 2003 multiagency initiative identified priorities in trauma research supported by the National Institutes of Health and the Department of Defense and suggested that body temperature modulation is a potential therapeutic maneuver in trauma care.[45] There is mounting evidence that suggests that mild to moderate hypothermia can mitigate neurologic and myocardial injury.[46] Additionally, induced hypothermia in patients with specific injuries (e.g., sudden cardiac arrest) is being used with increasing frequency as a method to prevent or mitigate various types of neurologic injury.[47] However, induced hypothermia is associated with numerous potentially serious side effects that require monitoring and treatment. These hypothermia-induced physiologic changes include electrolyte disorders, increased lactate levels, lowered WBC counts, altered drug metabolism, arrhythmias, hypovolemia, and insulin resistance with hyperglycemia.[46,48] These side effects may negate any benefits of hypothermia and may be one of the reasons why it is difficult to demonstrate the benefits of hypothermia in patients with traumatic brain injury.[49]

Injury responses and exposure to ambient temperatures produce significant heat loss, indicating a need for close monitoring of core body temperatures. It is difficult to keep the skin covered during resuscitation, when access to the body is necessary for assessment and routine procedures, but is essential to reduce heat loss. Overhead heat lamps are especially useful to augment heated blankets, and warmed intravenous fluids are essential.

Pain management is an essential strategy for reducing the stress response. All medications should be administered with caution to elderly patients because of age-related changes in body water and fat, gastric absorption, and renal and hepatic function.

PERIOPERATIVE PHASE

In the perioperative phase, as with the resuscitative phase, age-related adaptations are necessary for many older individuals. In nonemergency situations, additional time should be allowed for obtaining operative consent. The elderly may have difficulty understanding the choices offered or arriving at a decision. Consultation with family or other support persons may be useful. Extreme care must be exercised to ensure that the patient understands the consequences of consent and of refusal to consent. All steps should be taken to reduce the risk of morbidity and death when the elderly require surgical intervention. When time permits, underlying physiologic deficits should be corrected before operative intervention.

As in the resuscitative phase, core body temperature should be monitored, especially during a lengthy invasive or operative procedure. The nurse should be alert to the need for warmed intravenous fluids, warming blankets, and possibly warm inspired gases during the operative procedure.

Positioning in the operating room should be done with consideration for fragile skin and bones, suboptimal subcutaneous tissue depth, and stiff joints. In addition, vigorous movement and positioning may cause musculoskeletal injuries, including iatrogenic fractures. Protective padding and skin observation for breakdown is essential.

Anesthesia has the potential to disrupt regulatory systems for perfusion, whether it is general or regional. General anesthesia is indicated for upper abdominal, thoracic, and intracranial procedures and for patients in whom airway control is essential. Regional anesthesia is often used for lower extremity procedures and when preexisting respiratory disorders would be adversely affected by general anesthesia.

CRITICAL CARE PHASE

Elderly patients aged 65 years and older currently account for 42% to 52% of intensive care unit (ICU) admissions and for almost 60% of all ICU days.[50] Two considerations govern nursing care planning for the elderly in critical care units: (1) the potential for complications and (2) modification and negotiation of rehabilitation goals.

ANTICIPATING COMPLICATIONS

As noted earlier, the cardiovascular, respiratory, and neurologic systems require scrupulous assessment and management during the resuscitative phase. They continue to require close attention during the critical care phase, along with the renal, endocrine, and integumentary systems. The presence of comorbid disease states and preexisting conditions in all trauma patients is of importance. Comorbidities have been associated with both higher morbidity and mortality rates and with longer hospitalizations. The older person has a greater propensity for chronic diseases that may impair cardiac contractility or other systemic function. The individual may function quite adequately during usual activities but may decompensate under the stresses of trauma. The health care team must be diligent in assessing the actual impact of chronic health problems on the elderly trauma patient.

Cardiovascular Considerations

Cardiac and vascular system changes do not necessarily increase the risk of death to the elderly unless there is significant underlying heart disease. Continuous cardiac monitoring is essential. Monitoring for arrhythmias is important, especially if fluid volumes are inadequate or excessive.

Continuous hemodynamic monitoring is indicated until the patient is stable. Inotropic support may be needed during the acute phase, along with close attention to fluid balance. Hyponatremia and low serum osmolarity levels could indicate fluid overload, even in the presence of normal intravascular pressures.

The prevalence of peripheral vascular stiffening that accompanies aging increases the likelihood that perfusion may be compromised at some time despite adequate volumes and myocardial contractility. Extremities should be inspected frequently for adequate pulses, sensation, temperature, and color changes. Keeping the patient warm is essential. For those who are critically ill, monitoring of systemic vascular resistance helps detect indications for vasodilator therapy.

The patient's status may indicate the need for pulmonary artery pressure measurements. Placement of a pulmonary artery catheter increases the probability that dysfunction will be recognized more rapidly, and it may provide some protection against providing excessive fluid. It also offers the opportunity to measure cardiac output and to monitor trends in ventricular function curves. Vasoactive medications can be considered early in the course of treatment but should be guided by the use of a pulmonary artery catheter. Optimizing oxygen delivery and minimizing oxygen demands may lower mortality rates.

The combination of aging, diminished cardiac, pulmonary, and renal reserves, along with comorbidities increases the risk of the elderly developing organ failure.[28] The decreased physiologic reserve seen in elderly patients almost certainly limits their cardiovascular response to injury and acute blood loss, making them more prone to die of early acute cardiac failure or multiple organ failure sometime later in their hospital course.[51]

Every patient has the potential for pulmonary edema. Early fluid therapy should be monitored carefully, but rates of administration need not be slow just because of the person's age. Again, the need for pulmonary artery catheter, arterial pressure cardiac output monitor, or oximetric central venous catheter placement should be considered early in the treatment process. Hemodynamic monitoring should be continued until the patient is hemodynamically stable.

Pulmonary Considerations

The incidence of postoperative respiratory complications is higher for patients requiring emergency procedures than for those having elective surgery. Elderly surgical patients have a propensity for development of respiratory complications, simply because of diminished pulmonary reserves and limited ability to clear secretions by coughing. The elderly are generally less able to protect the airway because of decreased sensitivity of the gag reflex and diminished strength of the respiratory muscles. Oxygen deficits can be present at any time in the acute care phase.

The elderly are predisposed to pulmonary complications in general, and pneumonia and respiratory failure are prime contributors to increased mortality rates. Inadequate pain relief, a major cause of impaired ventilation in critically injured older patients, must be aggressively addressed to encourage effective coughing and deep breathing.

When the patient needs ventilatory support, aggressive nursing care measures should be instituted to prevent subsequent complications. Respiratory support in the form of tracheal intubation and mechanical ventilation is not without risk. Once such devices are in place, they increase the risk of pulmonary infection in a population especially susceptible to pneumonia. Even under optimal circumstances, the elderly are at increased risk of aspiration, atelectasis, and pulmonary infection.

Special attention should be placed on pulmonary asepsis. Measures to facilitate removal of secretions (i.e., turning and humidification of inspired gases) should be intensified in light of the elderly patient's diminished pulmonary clearance capacity. A well-defined plan of alternating spontaneous with supported ventilatory modes helps support the patient through the weaning process. Nursing interventions and activities of daily living need to consider the work of breathing and the weaning process to avoid unnecessary fatigue. Astute assessment is necessary during the weaning process to differentiate anxiety and confusion from alterations in adequate ventilation and oxygenation. Because of diminished respiratory reserves, weaning from ventilatory support may take up to twice as long for an elderly person as for a younger person with similar injuries. A tracheostomy may assist with the weaning process.

Neurologic Considerations

Delirium develops in about 9% to 61% of hospitalized elderly patients[52] and is more common in patients with dementia.[53] Controversy exists regarding the impact delirium and dementia have on the hospitalized elderly patient. Delirium is an important risk factor in poor outcomes from both ICU and hospital care patients.[54] However, one study concluded that elderly patients with dementia do not have increased rates of intubation or length of mechanical ventilation and showed no differences in ICU or hospital mortality rates or length of stay.[55]

Sleep deprivation, sepsis, hypoxemia, use of restraints, fluid and electrolyte imbalances, and medications such as sedatives and hypnotics can all induce delirium in the elderly patient.[56,57] Delirium is generally evidenced by a decline in cognitive function and typically occurs about 5 days postoperatively.

Several alternatives exist for the nurse to deal with confusion. Detection and treatment of delirium should be included in the overall plan of care of the elderly critical care patient. Short-term memory loss indicates the need for frequent repetition of information, such as orientation to time and place. The physical and personal environment should be maintained in a constant state. Alterations in levels of lighting help adjust for loss of visual acuity and reduce the incidence of day-night disorientation. The patient's family, significant others, and personal familiar objects (e.g., pictures of children, grandchildren, or favorite pets or the patient's personal religious medallions) are critical to improvement in and maintenance of orientation; they provide engagement in familiar relationships and a sense of comfort and security.

Psychosocial Considerations

Psychosocial factors may also contribute to deterioration in neurologic function. The best outcomes noted for the hospitalized elderly occur in those persons who were relatively independent at the time of injury and who did not live alone. Family dynamics also appear to play a significant role, with increased chances of a good outcome when the older person feels needed, wanted, and is able to play a part in their overall treatment plan.

Communication with the elderly patient during the critical care phase may be difficult because artificial airways and hearing and visual deficits may impede their ability to adequately understand or relay their needs. Communicating verbally in a simple low tone of voice is essential to avoid misunderstandings and confusion. If a hearing or visual deficit is present, it may be helpful to use the patient's hearing aid or eyeglasses to improve communication. It is important to ensure that the patient's hearing or visual deficits are included in their plan of care to allow for changes in communication techniques when needed. A speech therapy consult may also prove helpful in determining effective strategies to overcome communication barriers.

Touch is also important during communication because it can convey comfort and reassurance. The nurse should be mindful that there may be a tendency by family members or visitors to avoid touching the older person for fear of disturbing or upsetting the patient or dislodging the equipment. The nurse can show family and friends where and how they can safely touch the patient.

Renal Considerations

The number of nephrons, renal blood flow, and glomerular filtration rate decline with age, resulting in a decreased ability of the kidney to concentrate and excrete waste products. Routine examinations of renal function studies are used to assess current renal function and changes in function specific to each patient. The potential for fluid overload exists, as does a possible need to alter drug dosage. In some cases the kidneys may respond to trauma with development of acute renal failure. This condition most often presents as polyuric failure.

Close attention to renal function through laboratory measurements is indicated. Even brief periods of hypovolemia and hypotension may compromise the kidneys. Evidence of a rising serum creatinine level or a decreased creatinine clearance should trigger assessment of the patient's free water clearance. Constant monitoring of fluid balance and serum electrolytes are necessary to identify imbalances. Care providers must also assess for the need to modify drug types and dosages, particularly of aminoglycoside antibiotics.

Musculoskeletal Considerations

Musculoskeletal system injury, particularly hip fracture, has been documented extensively in the literature. The major musculoskeletal complication to be anticipated is loss of mobility. Older bones and muscles tend to develop stiffness and loss of motion more quickly and tend to recover function more slowly. Recovery may be complicated by arthritic changes. Nursing care should be directed toward the maintenance of mobility early in the critical care phase. Range-of-motion activities and exercises are essential while bed rest is indicated. The benefits of early mobilization cannot be stressed enough because it helps orient the older person; improve cardiac, pulmonary, and gastrointestinal performance; and promote wound healing and it generates a sense of hope for the patient and family.

Priorities for musculoskeletal system management include decisions about the timing and type of operative procedures. The full range of options should be explored, with the goals of achieving early mobilization and providing the best possible outcome for the individual. It is conceivable that some operative procedures may be delayed to correct underlying functional deficits. All possible interventions should be used to keep bed rest to a minimum.

Immune System Considerations

The effect of age and infection on outcomes after trauma is unknown. The elderly are especially susceptible to infection. Nosocomial infections are a major source of morbidity and death in the United States, consuming significant health care resources and dollars. In one study older patients were found to have a 2.2 times greater relative risk of infection compared with the younger group matched for Injury Severity Score, which significantly affects morbidity and mortality rates.[58] When age is combined with malnutrition, comobidity, and the immunosuppressive effects of major trauma, the patient is at an increased risk for development of sepsis. The onset of infection may present as change in mental status, restlessness, slight or absent elevation in temperature, mild elevation in white blood cell count in the presence of immature white cells, and limited catecholamine response. Careful monitoring of vascular access sites, such as central lines and arterial lines and indwelling devices such as urinary catheters, is indicated. Removal of such devices should be attempted at the earliest opportunity. Nursing interventions are aimed at protecting the patient's natural immunity barriers through use of universal precautions. Frequent pulmonary, renal, and skin integrity assessments are necessary to recognize early signs of infectious compromise. Any deterioration or subtle changes in patient status dictates an immediate and thorough search for infection.

Nutritional Strategies

Providing for the nutritional needs of the critically ill elderly trauma patient can be challenging at best. The elderly patient has fewer nutritional reserves. Meeting nutritional support needs from the time of admission through rehabilitation is crucial for optimal outcomes. Age, infirmity, and poverty often produce undernutrition, necessitating nutritional replacement during hospitalization. Current nutritional needs must be met and prior deficits must be corrected. As a result of decreased muscle mass in the face of acute illness, elderly patients may have protein-energy malnutrition. However, overfeeding and aggressive nutritional support, leading to hyperglycemia and excess carbon dioxide production, should be avoided.[28] Intravenous feedings are indicated if the gastrointestinal system recovers function slowly. Decreases in gastric secretions and intestinal motility are features of aging that predispose the individual to intolerance of enteral feedings. Postpyloric enteral feedings can be attempted early, even in the absence of bowel sounds. Caution should be used to ensure that the airway is protected. Elevation of the head of the bed is usually advised. Diminished sensitivity of the gag reflex increases the potential for aspiration, particularly if the level of consciousness is impaired.

Integumentary Considerations

Early mobilization of the older patient helps reduce the potential for integumentary injury. Aging reduces the elasticity of the skin, decreases the subcutaneous fat layer, and may reduce perfusion. The skin becomes vulnerable to pressure and abrasion, but breakdown can be prevented in most cases. Normal care of the aged skin includes minimal bathing, use of lubricating lotions, and avoidance of abrasive and irritating materials, including harsh soaps and tape. The patient's skin should be kept free from prolonged wetness and contact with irritating secretions. Frequent changes in position are necessary to minimize pressure areas. The evidence-based prevention practices that have received the most research attention are the use of specific air or rotating beds and mattresses. Additionally, devices such as pressure-relieving pads and gel- or air-filled pads are appropriate for pressure ulcer prevention.[59] If the patient is not capable of moving independently, nursing interventions must incorporate frequent position changes and opportunities for mobilization out of bed.

Modification of Goals

Advancing age is recognized as a time when individuals experience and adapt to multiple losses. It is also a time when life planning goals may be greatly altered after a traumatic injury. Critical care nurses must ensure that their own values and goals for patient outcome do not overshadow those of their elderly patients.

The foundation for rehabilitation of the patient is developed during the critical care phase. Assessment of the potential for return of function should be shared with the patient in a realistic manner. It is important for the patient and the family to be directly involved in the treatment process because this facilitates independence for the patient and can assist the family in planning for future care needs. After a hip fracture, for example, an older person may expect to walk with a cane and may or may not be satisfied with this achievement. On the other hand, the patient may know friends who have been placed in nursing homes after fractures and may perceive death as a better goal. Including the patient and family in the process and enlisting their ideas and concerns can allow for a smooth transition from acute and critical care to future rehabilitation, home, or long-term care. Advising the family of available health care support services allows them time to investigate and to begin necessary arrangements.

The survivability of the elderly trauma patient may not be clearly evident at the time of admission. Early aggressive treatment is appropriate in the management of elderly trauma victims. However, some elderly patients may not recover from their traumatic injuries. Nonsurvivors tend to die either during the resuscitative phase or in the critical care unit after a prolonged stay. When the prognosis and outlook are poor, the decision about the futility of care and the patient's ability to survive must be evaluated and the patient's and family's wishes must be considered. For some, "death with dignity" is paramount; for others, there is a need to feel that everything was done. When the patient cannot be consulted, the family is the main source of information. Documentation of the patient's wishes through advance directives is helpful when setting goals and making health care decisions.

INTERMEDIATE CARE AND REHABILITATIVE PHASES

In any discussion of trauma care for the elderly, it is important to recognize that age alone does not dictate changes in therapeutic approach and that it is not an appropriate reason to deny the patient the optimal benefits of rehabilitation. Previous health status and the level of preinjury activity the individual enjoyed may be the best predictive parameters of functional recovery. Planning for long-term care must be started on admission and continued through discharge or rehabilitation.

The lasting impact of injury on lifestyle in the elderly remains poorly defined. Although the majority of elderly injury survivors achieve independent living, long-term follow-up indicates significant residual disability in quality of life.[60] Previous outcomes research has shown higher mortality and complication rates with longer hospital lengths of stay and disproportionately higher use of hospital resources in this injured age group compared with younger trauma patients.[61] Patient-centered health-related quality of life outcomes are increasingly recognized as a benchmark in trauma outcomes research. However, these outcomes have not yet been well documented in geriatric trauma survivors.[62-64]

Once the patient is transferred from the critical care environment, plans for return to the community and rehabilitation become more specific. The patient's potential for return to the preinjury functional state should be assessed. Comparison of preinjury function with the limitations imposed by the type and nature of present injuries permits the formulation of initial rehabilitation goals. Underlying problems such as nutritional deficits or mobility needs should be evaluated and corrected. Enlisting those support services initiated earlier in the admission process will become increasingly important and useful at this stage of transition. The patient's attitude, participation in activities of daily living, mobility, and social activities and the type of support systems available should be considered. It is important to remember that some elderly patients may not be able to return to their preinjury states. This is especially true for those who have sustained fractures of the lower extremities. Pelvic fractures and other extremity fractures may greatly alter the functional ability the patient had before the injury. Those active before the injury have the best chance of returning to an independent functional state.

NURSING MANAGEMENT

The patient's needs for communication become, if anything, more important at this time, particularly if transitional care or long-term rehabilitation is needed. Frequent repetition of instructions and communication that orients the patient may be required if the patient has short-term memory loss. Plans for moving the patient should be communicated early to allow the patient time to adjust. The patient's physical environment becomes more important, particularly as he or she becomes increasingly mobile. Tables, chairs, and other items become part of the patient's personal space but can contribute to a potentially hazardous environment and can lead to injury. An assessment of the home environment can help identify and correct any potential hazards.

Nutritional evaluation should not be limited to the hospital course. Estimation of prior status provides clues to preexisting problems, whether of a financial or a social nature. Nutritional management must attempt to correct past and current deficits, particularly if the deficits are related to limited income, social isolation, poor dental health, medication use, depression, and loneliness. If assessment reveals an underlying problem, this must be included in the nutritional plan for the individual. Nutritional requirements of illness and recovery should be adjusted for the patient's age and the reduced needs of this population.

Long-term care can be just as frightening as the initial trauma event and acute and critical care phases. Loneliness, fear, and depression often accompany hospitalization of the older person. The patient's support systems become increasingly important during rehabilitation and can help alleviate the patient's fears and concerns.

An assessment of the family's ability to assist in care needed by the patient is crucial to discharge planning. Concerns related to obtaining mobility devices, administration of medications, and potential home or environment modifications should be evaluated and remedied before the patient is discharged.

COMMUNITY INTEGRATION

The outlook for return of the elderly to the community can be good. The probable outcome for a given individual should be assessed early in the hospital course so that plans can be developed for alternative care if that proves necessary. For some a return to independent living is likely. For others it may be possible to provide limited assistance in the form of home health care as an alternative to placement in a long-term care facility. Support systems that have been identified previously can be mobilized before discharge. Health care teaching needs for professionals and nonprofessionals alike should be implemented early enough to allow time for assessment of learning. Written reinforcement of teaching should accompany the patient on discharge.

Injury can have a lasting and potentially devastating effect on the lifestyle of the elderly trauma patient. Management of the patient and plans for transitional care should be revised as needed during the hospitalization. The patient's potential for return to the preinjury state should be kept in mind to ensure a smooth transition from injury to recovery.

NURSING RESEARCH IMPLICATIONS

There is a tremendous need for further research concerning optimal trauma care for the elderly. With the possible exception of hip fractures, little is known about how the elderly respond to traumatic injury compared with younger victims of similar injury. As the elderly population increases, there is an even greater need for evidence-based guidance in the care of these patients. Epidemiologists have described the problem in terms of incidence and expense, but they offer little clinical data. Until evidence-based protocols of care are established and integrated, trauma to the elderly will continue to be a monumental problem. The scope and need for research in this population of trauma patients is tremendous.

Many questions remain regarding the causes and treatment of trauma in the elderly. For example, falls are the most common mechanism, but the circumstances surrounding them are less clear. Countless questions are yet to be answered about how and why falls occur in the elderly. For example,

- How many falls (or other injuries) are related to age alone?
- Are injuries often or seldom preceded by transient losses of consciousness?
- What is the relationship between injury and social or environmental factors?
- Does nutrition, osteoporosis, or thermoregulation play a role in how or why the elderly fall?
- How does preinjury functional status compare with that of those who are not injured?
- What role does chronic disease play with regard to injury severity?
- How should chronic disease be measured?
- What differences exist between injury severity and response to injury in the elderly?
- Are the disabled more prone to injury than those who are active?
- Do the elderly actually succumb to injuries of low severity, as it appears, and if so, why?
- What factors contribute to the inability to return to the preinjury functional level?

Still other questions exist with respect to how an injury affects an elderly patient's future lifestyle. For example, is there a time in health care when the wisest action is no action at all? Should a goal of health care include attention to the quality of life to which the patient returns? With the projected increase in the number of elderly patients and the increasing burden of preexisting disease, how best should we use resources and funds, and on which patients, to obtain the most benefit from care?

These questions and many more need to be answered simultaneously with evaluation of nursing care strategies. The need for data is immense, especially related to elderly patients' responses to nursing care in the ICU setting. Previous data from this age group have been obtained almost exclusively from patients with significant medical problems, as opposed to those who were essentially healthy before traumatic injury. As nurse researchers develop a better grasp on how elderly trauma patients respond differently from younger patients, improving protocols to more effectively treat this population may be developed. Additionally, research that explores alternative and complementary therapies should be pursued.

PREVENTION

Data available from studies of unintentional injury show that the elderly have a high risk of death from three major causes: falls, MVCs, and thermal injuries. Because most "accidents" are not accidents at all, prevention of injury should be a priority for health care professionals. As with any other disease, trauma should be approached from a point of both identifying the causative issues and developing prevention strategies that target those issues.

Public health history indicates that individual change is the prevention strategy least likely to succeed. More successful approaches include environmental modification and modification of support systems. Nurses can participate in public decisions through professional organizations and legislative action.

Although modification of individual behavior has the least potential for success, there are situations when this is the only available approach. The foundation of patient teaching rests on the professional's ability to persuade an individual to change. Health status, financial limitations, values, and attitudes that make change difficult to accomplish complicate education and training of the elderly individual.

Prevention is essential to reduce the toll of disability and death in the elderly population caused by traumatic injuries. Maximal efforts aimed at prevention are needed to reduce the incidence of elderly trauma.

Prevention of Falls

Risk factors for falls in the elderly include normal physiologic changes associated with aging, devices such as canes and walkers, and environmental issues such as road hazards, stairs, and poor lighting. Home and public environments are not designed with the elderly in mind. To lessen the chances of a fall, floor surfaces should be covered with nonslip materials and handgrips should be provided on both sides of walkways and stairways. Handgrips are especially helpful in bathrooms. Improved lighting in hallways and on stairs helps the elderly avoid tripping. Lighting should be concentrated on landings, where falls are most likely to occur. Levels of lighting should be as uniform as possible so that the elderly do not have to make rapid visual adjustments to variable light intensity.

Prevention of Motor Vehicle Crashes

Most pedestrian fatalities occur when the individual attempts to cross the roadway between intersections. In addition, the elderly account for almost half of pedestrian injuries in crosswalks. Education of elderly pedestrians, and drivers in general, can increase their awareness of the potential problems. The elderly should be alerted to driver behaviors that increase the risk of collisions, such as turning right at red lights without looking for pedestrians. Pedestrians walking at night also should wear light-colored clothing or reflective material to increase their visibility to drivers.

Elderly drivers tend to voluntarily restrict their driving to familiar conditions and daytime hours. This behavior should be encouraged. Training in defensive driving skills also may be of benefit to the older driver. As important, perhaps, is education of younger drivers to the behaviors of elderly drivers, such as diminished ability to react to distractions and slower driving speeds. Additionally, there may be a time when the elderly person will become unable to drive safely. As difficult as it may be, suspension or cancellation of the elderly person's driving license may be necessary but not without understanding the impact of lost independence and the acceptance of this loss on the part of the elderly person.

Prevention of Burns

A frequent cause of burns in the elderly is hot liquid. Many of these injuries are caused by tap water at a temperature higher than 130° F. The simple reduction in hot water temperature to 120° F or less can reduce the frequency and severity of scalds. The elderly should use extra caution when bathing in environments such as hotels and should test the water temperature to prevent burns. Hot liquids from cooking are another frequent source of burn wounds. Causes of flame injuries include smoking, open flames, and house fires. The elderly are overrepresented in burn fatalities from house fires, possibly because they are less able to escape once the fire starts. Carbon monoxide and smoke detectors should be required in all elderly housing, along with the use of flame-retardant materials in construction and furnishings. The elderly homeowner should be cautioned against household storage of flammable materials such as old newspapers and gasoline. Last, education on the risks of smoking in bed is needed to eliminate this risk factor.

Summary

The cost of trauma care in the United States is an enormous financial burden on the health care system. Injuries in the elderly are responsible for a larger portion than would be expected on the basis of the population in proportion to other age groups. Trauma may drastically alter the elderly patient's lifestyle from a personal, family, social, and economic standpoint. The idea that serious injury always leads to a significant negative outcome in the elderly is not supported in the available literature. Thus, efforts to maximize treatment of elderly trauma victims are needed.

The challenges of caring for the elderly victims of traumatic injury will continue to evolve. The known concepts of age-related physiologic changes and preexisting conditions and their impact on the response to traumatic injury and the overall outcomes must be considered in the treatment plans of this population. Injury prevention programs and public education are essential as we continue to care for this population that is increasing in number and in injuries. However, much more work needs to be done if we are to consistently and appropriately care for the aging population that will no doubt suffer the same effects of traumatic injury already imposed on the young.

References

1. U.S. Census Bureau: *U.S. interim projections by age, sex, race, and Hispanic origin* (2004): http://www.census.gov/ipc/www/usinterimproject/. Accessed February 16, 2006.
2. Chang EJ, Edelman LS, Morris SE: Gender influences on burn outcomes in the elderly, *Burns* 31:31-35, 2005.
3. U.S. Administration on Aging, U.S. Health and Human Services, Washington, DC (2006): http://www.aoa.gov/. Accessed February 17, 2006.
4. Whetstone G, Boswell S: The geriatric heart: nurses need to be aware of how aging and disease affect the myocardium, *Am J Nurs* 102:22-24, 2002.
5. Lane P, Sorondo B, Kelly JJ: Geriatric trauma patients—are they receiving trauma center care? *Acad Emerg Med* 10:244-250, 2003.
6. Schwab CW, Kauder DR: Trauma in the geriatric patient, *Arch Surg* 127:701-706, 1992.
7. Dellinger AM, Langlios JA, Li G: Fatal crashes among older drivers: decomposition of rates into contributing factors, *Am J Epidemiol* 155:234-241, 2002.
8. National Highway Traffic Safety Administration, U.S. Department of Transportation: *Traffic safety facts 2002, older population,* Washington, DC, 2003, National Highway Traffic Safety Administration.

9. Murphy SL: *Deaths: final data for 1998,* National Vital Statistics Reports, 48(11), Hyattsville, MD, 2000, National Center for Health Statistics.
10. National Center for Injury Prevention and Control, Centers for Disease Control and Prevention (2005): http://www.cdc.gov. Accessed February 16, 2006.
11. Sterling DA, O'Connor JA, Bonadies J: Geriatric falls: injury severity is higher and disproportionate to mechanism, *J Trauma* 50:116-119, 2001.
12. Jager TE, Weiss HB, Coben JH: Traumatic brain injuries evaluated in U.S. emergency departments, 1992-1994, *Acad Emerg Med* 7:134-140, 2000.
13. National Safety Council: *Accident facts,* Chicago, 1997, National Safety Council.
14. Federal Bureau of Investigation: *Crime in the United States, 2002,* Washington, DC, 2003, U.S. Department of Justice.
15. Bureau of Justice Statistics: *Homicide trends in the United States,* Washington, DC, United States Department of Justice (2004): http://www.ojp.usdoj.gov/bjs/homicide.htm. Accessed April 24, 2006.
16. Public health and aging: nonfatal physical assault-related injuries among persons aged >60 years treated in hospital emergency departments, 2001, *MMWR Morbid Mortal Wkly Rep* 52:812-816, 2003.
17. Krug EG, Dahlberg LL, Mercy JA et al, editors: *World report on violence and health,* Geneva, Switzerland, 2002, World Health Organization.
18. U.S. Department of Health and Human Services, Administration for Children and Administration on Aging: *The National Elder Maltreatment Incidence Study, final report,* Washington, DC, 1998, U.S. Department of Health and Human Services.
19. National Center on Elder Abuse: *A response to abuse of vulnerable adults: the 2000 survey of state adult protective services,* Washington, DC, 2002, National Center on Elder Abuse.
20. U.S. House of Representatives, Committee on Government Reform, Special Investigations Division, Minority Staff: *Abuse is a major problem in U.S. nursing homes,* Washington, DC, 2001, U.S. House of Representatives.
21. Office of Community Oriented Policing Services: *The problem of financial crimes against the elderly,* Washington, DC, 2003, U.S. Department of Justice.
22. Bonnie R, Wallace R: *Elder mistreatment: abuse, neglect, and exploitation in an aging America,* Washington, DC, 2003, National Academy Press.
23. Brent N: Issues related to violence. In *Nurses and the law, a guide to principles and applications,* 2nd ed, pp 280-298, Philadelphia, 2001, W. B. Saunders.
24. Demling RH: Care of geriatric patients. In Herndon DN, editor: *Total burn care,* 2nd ed, pp. 439-441, London, 2002, W. B. Saunders.
25. Kauder DR, Schwab CW, Shapiro MB: Geriatric trauma: patterns, care, and outcomes. In Moore EE, Feliciano DV, Mattox KL, editors: *Trauma,* 5th ed, pp 1041-1058, New York, 2004, McGraw-Hill.
26. Letizia M, Reinbolz M: Identifying and managing acute alcohol withdrawal in the elderly, *Geriatr Nurs* 26:176-183, 2005.
27. Lakatta EG: Age associated cardiovascular changes in health: impact on cardiovascular disease in older persons, *Heart Failure Rev* 7:29-49, 2002.
28. Marik PE: Management of the critically ill geriatric patient, *Crit Care Med* 34(Suppl):S176-S182, 2006.
29. Salmasi AM, Alimo A, Jepson E et al: Age associated changes in left ventricular diastolic function are related to increasing left ventricular mass, *Am J Hypertens* 16:473-477, 2003.
30. Horton JD, Bushwick BM: Warfarin therapy: evolving strategies in anticoagulation, *Am Fam Physician* 59:635-646, 1999.
31. National Prescription Audit: *Physician specialty report, dispensed data,* Plymouth Meeting, PA, 1998, IMS America.
32. Mina AA, Bair HA, Howells GA et al: Complication of preinjury warfarin use in the trauma patient, *J Trauma* 54:842-847, 2003.
33. Reynolds FD, Dietz PA, Higgins D et al: Time to deterioration of the elderly, anticoagulated, minor head injury patient who presents without evidence of neurological abnormality, *J Trauma* 54:492-496, 2003.
34. Martin M, Mullenix P, Rhee P et al: Troponin increases in the critically injured patient: mechanical trauma or physiologic stress? *J Trauma* 59:1086-1091, 2005.
35. Scalea TM, Simon HM, Duncan AO et al: Geriatric blunt trauma: improved survival with early invasive monitoring, *J Trauma* 30:129-136, 1990.
36. Bulger E, Arneson MA, Mock CN et al: Rib fractures in the elderly, *J Trauma* 48:1040-1047, 2000.
37. Bergeron E, Lavoie A, Clas D et al: Elderly trauma patients with rib fractures are at greater risk of death and pneumonia, *J Trauma* 54:478-485, 2003.
38. Majercik S, Tashjijian RZ, Biffl WL et al: Halo vest immobilization in the elderly: a death sentence? *J Trauma* 59:350-357, 2005.
39. Linsey RW, Pneumaticos SG, Gugala Z: Management techniques for spinal injures. In Browner B, et al, editors: *Skeletal trauma,* 3rd ed, pp 746-776, Philadelphia, 2003, W. B. Saunders.
40. Henry SM, Pollak AN, Jones AL et al: Pelvic fractures in geriatric patients: a distinct clinical entity, *J Trauma* 53:15-20, 2002.
41. Health Care Financing Administration: *FY2001 annual performance plan* (2001): http://www.hcfa.gov/stats/2001.htm. Accessed February 21, 2006.
42. Agency for Health Care Resources and Quality: http://www.ahrq.gov/clinical/ptsafety/chap26b.htm. Accessed October 2, 2006.
43. Holtzclaw B: Shivering in acutely ill vulnerable populations, *AACN Clin Issues* 15:267-279, 2004.
44. Shafi S, Elliott AC, Gentilello L: Is hypothermia simply a marker of shock and injury severity or an independent risk factor for mortality in trauma patients? Analysis of a large national trauma registry, *J Trauma* 59:1081-1085, 2005.
45. Hoyt DB, Holcomb J, Abraham E et al: Working Group on Trauma Research Program Summary Report: National Heart Lung Blood Institute (NHLBI), National Institute of General Medical Sciences (NIGMS), and National Institute of Neurological Disorders and Stroke (NINDS) of the National Institutes of Health (NIH), and the Department of Defense (DOD), *J Trauma* 57:410-415, 2004.
46. Polderman KH, Rijnsburger ER, Peerdeman SM et al: Induction of hypothermia in patients with various types of neurologic injury with use of large volumes of ice cold intravenous fluid, *Crit Care Med* 33:2744-2751, 2005.
47. Polderman KH: Application of therapeutic hypothermia in the ICU: opportunities and pitfalls of a promising treatment modality, 1: indications and evidence, *Intensive Care Med* 30:556-575, 2004.
48. Polderman KH: Application of therapeutic hypothermia in the ICU: opportunities and pitfalls of a promising treatment modality, 2: practical aspects and side effects, *Intensive Care Med* 30:757-769, 2004.

49. Polderman KH, Ely EW, Badr AE et al: Induced hypothermia in traumatic brain injury: considering the conflicting results of meta-analysis and moving forward, *Intensive Care Med* 30:1860-1864, 2004.
50. Angus DC, Kelley MA, Schmitz RJ et al: Caring for the critically ill patient: current and projected workforce requirements for care of the critically ill and patients with pulmonary disease: can we meet the requirements of an aging population? *JAMA* 284:2762-2770, 2000.
51. Alost T, Waldrop RD: Profile of geriatric pelvic fractures presenting to the emergency department, *Am J Emerg Med* 15:576-578, 1997.
52. Andersson EM, Gustafson L, Hallberg IR: Acute confusional state in elderly orthopaedic patients: factors of importance for detection in nursing care, *Int J Geriatr Psychol* 16:7-17, 2001.
53. McNicoll L, Pisani MA, Zhang Y et al: Delirium in the intensive care unit: occurrence and clinical course in older patients, *J Am Geriatr Soc* 51:591-598, 2003.
54. Ely EW, Gautam S, Margolin R: et al: The impact of delirium in the intensive care unit on hospital length of stay, *Intensive Care Med* 27:1892-1900, 2001.
55. Pisani M, Redlich CA, McNicoll L et al: Short-term outcomes in older intensive care unit patients with dementia, *Crit Care Med* 33:1371-1376, 2005.
56. Inouye SK, Charpentier PA: Precipitating factors for delirium in hospitalized elderly persons: predictive model and interrelationship with baseline vulnerability, *JAMA* 275:852-857, 1996.
57. McNicoll L, Pisani MA, Ely EW et al: Detection of delirium in the intensive care unit: comparison of confusion assessment method for the intensive care unit with confusion assessment method ratings, *J Am Geriatr Soc* 53:495-500, 2005.
58. Bochicchio GV, Joshi M, Knorr KM et al: Impact of nosocomial infections in trauma: does age make a difference? *J Trauma* 50:612-619, 2001.
59. Agency for Health Care Policy and Research: *Pressure ulcers in adults: prediction and prevention,* Clinical Practice Guideline No. 3, Rockville, MD, 1992, Public Health Service, U.S. Department of Health and Human Services.
60. Inaba K, Goecke M, Sharkey P et al: Long-term outcomes after injury in the elderly, *J Trauma* 54:486-491, 2003.
61. McGwin G, Melton SM, May AK et al: Long-term survival in the elderly after trauma, *J Trauma* 49:470-476, 2000.
62. Brenneman FD, Boulanger BR, McLellan BA et al: Acute and long term outcomes of extremely injured blunt trauma victims, *J Trauma* 39:320-324, 1995.
63. Brenneman FD, Katyal D, Boulanger BR et al: Long-term outcomes in open pelvic fractures, *J Trauma* 42:773-777, 1997.
64. Brenneman FD, Redelmeier DA, Boulanger BR et al: Long-term outcomes in blunt trauma: who goes back to work? *J Trauma* 42:778-781, 1997.

31

TRAUMA IN THE BARIATRIC PATIENT

Sheryl L. Szczensiak

Bariatric trauma patients present many challenges for health care professionals from the time of injury through rehabilitation. Principal challenges associated with problematic outcomes in critically injured bariatric trauma patients include obtaining a comprehensive assessment, meeting the patient's physiologic requirements, and providing effective interventions. Providing health care to this special population lends specific risks and needs that must be recognized early and maintained throughout the continuum of care. Preparation should begin early, before arrival if possible, to accommodate the unique needs of the bariatric trauma patient. It is essential that nurses caring for bariatric trauma patients have an understanding of the anatomic differences, special equipment requirements, and psychologic needs of bariatric patients. Despite the recent increase in research related to the needs and injuries of the bariatric trauma patient, many nurses remain ill prepared to provide the specialized care required for this patient population.

EPIDEMIOLOGY

One only needs to pick up a magazine or watch the news to be reminded that obesity is at epidemic levels among the general population. The statistics of obesity in the United States are staggering. After the millennium, more than one half of all Americans are overweight, more than 30% are obese, and greater than 5% are morbidly obese.[1,2] Obesity results in greater than 100,000 deaths each year in the United States, making it the leading cause of preventable death with an annual estimated cost of $70 to $100 billion.[2,3]

Obesity is defined as an abnormal increase in weight compared with the age, sex, height, and body type of an individual.[4] Bariatric patients include those persons who are overweight, obese, and morbidly obese and those who have had some form of weight loss surgery. The body mass index (BMI) is the standard method used to evaluate obesity. Degrees of excess weight are frequently classified with the BMI, which correlates weight and height.[5] BMI is determined according to the following formula: BMI = weight in kilograms divided by height in meters squared (Weight [kg])/Height [m²]).[6] Table 31-1 summarizes the classifications of adult obesity according to the BMI.[1,5,6] Table 31-2 illustrates the correlation of BMI to height and weight for adults.

Obesity is not a problem that is unique to adults. Each year the number of obese children in the United States continues to increase. Obesity in children is defined according to how their weight compares with the national percentile for both their age and sex. Standard growth charts are used to determine what percentile children and adolescents fall in for both height and weight.[5] Although children whose weight is between the 85th and 95th percentiles are termed overweight, those whose weight falls in the range greater than the 95th percentile are classified as obese.[3] These statistics indicate that one in five children in the United States falls into either the overweight or obese category.[6]

Although the number of articles being published in professional journals regarding the care of bariatric trauma patients is increasing, a major deficit in both research and literature persists. Trauma has been identified as the fifth leading cause of death in adults and the most common cause of death in children in the United States.[7,8] Trauma patients who are obese, with a BMI greater than 30, and those who are morbidly obese, with a BMI of 40 or higher, have been shown to have a significantly greater number of complications, longer time on a mechanical ventilator, and higher mortality rates compared to individuals with similar injuries who are normal weight with a BMI less than 25.[9-11] Morbidly obese trauma patients are eight times more likely to die from their injuries than are those with a normal BMI (<25 kg/m²).[7]

Studies probing for a correlation between obesity and mortality rates in trauma patients have various outcomes. A retrospective study by Morris et al[12] attempted to correlate preexisting medical conditions with negative outcomes for trauma patients. In this study obesity was not found to be a significant factor. The results of the Morris et al study may have been skewed by a failure to include obesity as a secondary diagnosis. Another retrospective study published a year later by Smith-Choban et al[13] found a significant correlation

TABLE 31-1 **Classifications of Obesity in Adults**

Weight Classification	World Health Organization Classification	BMI
Normal weight	Normal weight	18.5-24.9
Overweight	Overweight	25.0-29.9
Obese	Grade 2 overweight	30.0-39.9
Morbidly/severely obese	Grade 3 overweight	40.0-49.9
Super obese	Not applicable	>50.0

TABLE 31-2 **Body Mass Index (BMI) Table**

BMI	19	20	21	22	23	24	25	26	27	28	29	30	31	32	33	34	35
Height								**Weight (in pounds)**									
4′10″ (58″)	91	96	100	105	110	115	119	124	129	134	138	143	148	153	158	162	167
4′11″ (59″)	94	99	104	109	114	119	124	128	133	138	143	148	153	158	163	168	173
5′ (60″)	97	102	107	112	118	123	128	133	138	143	148	153	158	163	168	174	179
5′1″ (61″)	100	106	111	116	122	127	132	137	143	148	153	158	164	169	174	180	185
5′2″ (62″)	104	109	115	120	126	131	136	142	147	153	158	164	169	175	180	186	191
5′3″ (63″)	107	113	118	124	130	135	141	146	152	158	163	169	175	180	186	191	197
5′4″ (64″)	110	116	122	128	134	140	145	151	157	163	169	174	180	186	192	197	204
5′5″ (65″)	114	120	126	132	138	144	150	156	162	168	174	180	186	192	198	204	210
5′6″ (66″)	118	124	130	136	142	148	155	161	167	173	179	186	192	198	204	210	216
5′7″ (67″)	121	127	134	140	146	153	159	166	172	178	185	191	198	204	211	217	223
5′8″ (68″)	125	131	138	144	151	158	164	171	177	184	190	197	203	210	216	223	230
5′9″ (69″)	128	135	142	149	155	162	169	176	182	189	196	203	209	216	223	230	236
5′10″ (70″)	132	139	146	153	160	167	174	181	188	195	202	209	216	222	229	236	243
5′11″ (71″)	136	143	150	157	165	172	179	186	193	200	208	215	222	229	236	243	250
6′ (72″)	140	147	154	162	169	177	184	191	199	206	213	221	228	235	242	250	258
6′1″ (73″)	144	151	159	166	174	182	189	197	204	212	219	227	235	242	250	257	265
6′2″ (74″)	148	155	163	171	179	186	194	202	210	218	225	233	241	249	256	264	272
6′3″ (75″)	152	160	168	176	184	192	200	208	216	224	232	240	248	256	264	272	279

Source: *Evidence report of clinical guidelines on the identification, evaluation, and treatment of overweight and obesity in adults,* Washington, DC, 1998, National Institutes of Health/National Heart, Lung and Blood Institute.

between the mortality rate of trauma patients and obesity. More recent studies by Arbabi et al,[9] Brown et al,[10] Byrnes et al,[11] and Neville et al[14] have supported the hypothesis that obesity is an independent risk factor in the mortality rate of trauma patients. A study by Whitlock et al[15] found a U-shaped correlation between BMI of drivers involved in vehicular crashes and the rate of critical traumatic injuries sustained, not including deaths. This U-shaped distribution represents a twofold increase in the injury rate for drivers in the lowest weight classification (<23.5 kg/m^2) and those in the highest weight class (>28.7 kg/m^2).[15] The U-shaped results of this study may be attributed to an increased risk of broken bones among individuals within the low weight range, a greater risk of falling asleep as a result of sleep apnea while driving for the overweight group and possibly aspects of vehicle safety design that are less effective for those who are overweight or underweight.[15] Despite the need for further research, studies with a clear definition of obesity, BMI greater than 30, and a relatively large number of patients included in the study show a significant correlation between obesity and an increased mortality rate in trauma patients. Further research needs to be done to ascertain exactly why obesity increases the risk of death for trauma patients.

NURSING DATABASE

The assessment of trauma patients may be complicated by many factors including altered level of consciousness, drug abuse or intoxication, being a poor historian, language barriers, and obesity. The thick layers of adipose tissue in obese patients may make physical assessment by palpation and percussion difficult, if not impossible. Procedures such as deep peritoneal lavage (DPL), ultrasonography, computed tomography scans (CT), and arterial blood gases (ABG) may also be exceptionally difficult or impossible to perform on the obese patient. This will be discussed further in the special management considerations section of this chapter.

MECHANISM OF INJURY

Blunt Trauma

Mechanisms of blunt trauma include motor vehicle, motorcycle, or bicycle crashes; falls; assaults with or without weapons (e.g., bat, crow bar), and recreational or industrial incidents. It is important to document as much about the circumstances surrounding the injury as possible. Clues to injury patterns can be obtained from information such as height from which a fall occurred and how the patient landed.

A study by Brown et al[10] found that patients with a BMI >30 kg/m^2 who sustained injuries from severe blunt trauma typically had different patterns of injury than those with a BMI <25 kg/m^2. A total of 1,153 patients were included in the Brown et al study, including 283 obese patients and 870 nonobese patients. The patients in the obese group were found to have a lower rate of head injury but a higher risk of chest and lower extremity injuries. Patients with a BMI >30 also had a higher rate of complications and death.

A 1998 study by Bazelmans et al[16] found that obese adolescents who participated in sports were more likely to be injured than were their normal-weight peers. This study found no correlation between obesity and the increased severity of injury.[16] Use of protective gear (i.e., helmet, wrist guards, and knee and elbow pads) should be documented, particularly for traumatic incidents involving contact sports, motorcycle riding, bicycling, rollerblading, and skateboarding. School-age children who are overweight also tend to be targeted by bullies. Schoolyard fist fights frequently result in blunt trauma to the face and torso.

Falls

The extra weight on the body of an obese individual may make ambulation difficult. It is important to determine whether a patient requires assistance or an aid (e.g., cane, walker) to safely ambulate. Obese individuals are prone to osteoarthritis. Carrying extra weight tends to be hard on the joints, especially the knees and ankles, which may result in tripping and falling. Distribution of weight may also affect the balance of obese individuals, making them prone to falls.

A British study by Spaine and Bollen[17] found a correlation between increased BMI and the severity of ankle fractures. Only patients who had ankle fractures after "low energy trauma," such as ground level or low level falls, were included in the study. Obese patients with displaced ankle fractures were also more likely than their normal-weight counterparts to have a redislocation injury.

Motor Vehicle Crash

Potential injury patterns can be determined on the basis of knowledge of the patient location in the car, use of safety restraints (lap belt only or lap belt and shoulder harness), air bag deployment, steering wheel deformity, ejection of the patient from the vehicle, passenger space intrusion, and the condition of other people in the same automobile. A study of the injury patterns of restrained drivers by Moran et al[18] found that drivers whose body type was not similar to that of the crash test dummy frequently did not fit correctly in the vehicle, making safety features less effective, ineffective, or dangerous. The typical crash test dummy is patterned after a 5 foot 10 inch male weighing 170 pounds, a BMI below that of those classified as overweight or obese.[18]

The standard size seat belt in most cars may not properly fit an obese or morbidly obese individual. Bariatric patients may not wear their seat belts because of discomfort from a tight-fitting restraining device. Seat belt extensions are available from most car dealerships that allow the belt to expand. Bariatric patients who do not wear seat belts may be reluctant to admit their lack of compliance for fear of retribution by law enforcement or embarrassment that their seat belt does not fit. To encourage the patient to provide an honest answer to this question it is best to ask the question in a nonjudgmental way when police officers are not present in the room.

According to a study by Reiff et al[19] there is an increased rate of diaphragmatic injuries in front seat passengers who are overweight and involved in motor vehicle crashes (MVCs) where the damage to the vehicle involves same-side passenger space intrusion. Compared with automobile passengers of normal weight, a higher risk of rib fractures and pulmonary contusions was noted in obese passengers of MVCs by Choban et al.[20] Arbabi et al[9] studied 189 patients who were involved in MVCs, comparing injury patterns and mortality rates for normal-weight individuals (BMI <25 kg/m^2) versus obese individuals (BMI >30). Although the results of this study did not find a correlation between obesity and increased Injury Severity Score, obesity was found to be associated with an increase in severity of lower extremity injuries, including pelvic fractures, and overall mortality rates. The Arbabi et al study also reported a decrease in the number of abdominal injuries among obese patients. The authors of this study suggest that the lower rate of abdominal injuries in the obese group may be associated with the "cushion effect" provided by layers of adipose tissue over the abdomen.

Penetrating Trauma

Penetrating trauma, including gunshot and stab wounds, may be more difficult to assess in the obese patient. Extra layers of adipose tissue can make finding the entrance or exit wounds or the path of a bullet more difficult. The additional padding provided by adipose tissue may serve as a protective barrier preventing short knives, ice picks, or other objects from penetrating vital organs in overweight patients. The effectiveness of this barrier may be misleading. The "protective layer" of adipose tissue should not change the priorities or thinking of the trauma surgeon or nurse. All penetrating injuries should be fully investigated despite the possibility that the object did not appear to fully penetrate through the layers of adipose tissue.

Burns

Obese or morbidly obese individuals who have difficulty ambulating, are unable to ambulate without assistance, or are completely nonambulatory are at greater risk of significant burn injuries and inhalation injuries when they are victims of structure fires. A 1993 study by Gottschlich et al[21] found that burn patients who are obese or morbidly obese have higher risk of infection, bacteremia, and sepsis. This study also found that obese burn victims required twice as many doses of antibiotics and insulin as did nonobese burn patients. Obese burn patients also have higher metabolic demands than burn patients with a BMI <25.

Burn victims who have significant smoke inhalation injuries may require emergency airway management. Anatomic differences, such as extra layers of adipose tissue and a short neck, make intubating an obese patient difficult and often impossible. Alternatives to intubation for the obese patient include the use of a Combitube or percutaneous tracheostomy.[22,23] As with other forms of trauma, obese burn victims typically necessitate longer periods of time on mechanical ventilation than do burn victims who are normal weight.[21]

Medical History

It is important to obtain information about the medical history of all trauma patients. If the patient is not able to answer questions, then information should be obtained from a family member or friend if possible. Using the acronym AMPLE will help the trauma team to obtain a thorough patient history: A: allergies, M: medications, P: past medical history/surgeries/pregnancies, L: last meal, and E: events surrounding the injury.[24] Table 31-3 has examples of pertinent information (in AMPLE format) that should be obtained when caring for a bariatric trauma patient. Medical history questions specific to bariatric patients include questions regarding medical conditions that affect mobility, diet, weight loss medications or supplements, previous weight loss surgeries, and diseases.

RESUSCITATION PHASE

Caring for bariatric trauma patients provides special challenges for all members of the trauma team. Assessment and management during initial resuscitation necessitates a preplanned approach for critically injured bariatric patients. The bariatric patient's baseline anatomic and physiologic differences present unique challenges that make it difficult to adequately assess the patient. Likewise, therapeutic and diagnostic interventions are often complicated by equipment limitations, pain management requirements, difficulty positioning obese patients, and increased complexity in performing procedures.

TABLE 31-3 Using AMPLE to Obtain a Medical History for a Bariatric Patient

A	Allergies	Are you allergic to any medications? What type of reaction have you had after taking this medication?
M	Medications	What medications do you take on a routine basis? Prescription? Over the counter? Supplements? (Note any weight loss medications/supplements.)
P	Pertinent past medical/surgical/ obstetric history	Do you have any medical history? (Specifically ask about diseases frequently associated with obesity, see Table 31-5.) Surgical history? Any form of weight loss surgery? Obstetric history: gravida, para, and abortions (spontaneous or elective). Is there any chance that you could be pregnant? Last menstral period?
L	Last meal	What time did you last eat or drink? What did you eat or drink? (Includes, water, protein shakes, or weight loss shakes or bars.)
E	Events related to the mechanism of trauma	How did the injury occur? Where did the injury occur? Do you use an assistive device to walk (e.g., cane, walker)? Do you normally stand or walk alone?

CLINICAL MANAGEMENT/TEAM APPROACH

When caring for bariatric patients, the term *team approach* has a dual meaning. As with any trauma patient, the assessment and care of the patient is a combined effort of trauma surgeons, emergency physicians, trauma nurses, and other support staff. The initial focus of the team is to perform a primary and then a secondary survey of the patient to rapidly identify and treat life-threatening injuries. (See Box 31-1 for an example of the guidelines used by one trauma center when caring for morbidly obese trauma patients.) In addition, bariatric trauma patients require more manpower to position, turn, and transport. To prevent injury to the patient or team members, it is important to ensure that enough help is present to perform these maneuvers safely.

ASSESSMENT AND TREATMENT OF THE BARIATRIC TRAUMA PATIENT

The assessment and treatment of bariatric trauma patients may vary from other trauma patients because of differences in body composition, inability to use some forms of standard diagnostic machinery or techniques, and the need for more personnel to perform procedures. Table 31-4 provides an overview of challenges faced in the primary survey of a bariatric trauma patient.[25] Obesity affects all of the major systems of the body. Special consideration needs to be given to how the differences in each system affect the care and recovery of bariatric trauma patients.

Respiratory Considerations

The primary survey of a trauma patient begins with the assessment of the patient's airway and breathing. Many anatomic and physiologic changes in the bariatric patient affect the respiratory system. Redundant layers of tissue make auscultation of lung sounds challenging. It is important to lift extraneous tissue to place the diaphragm of the stethoscope on the chest wall when listening to lung sounds.[26]

Large amounts of adipose tissue and a short neck tend to obscure the landmarks needed to quickly intubate a patient in severe distress.[25] Layers of adipose tissue surrounding the chest and abdominal walls can add to the work of breathing in an already stressed patient, which can lead to respiratory failure.[7] This is especially true when the obese patient must remain in a supine position with increased pressure from the abdominal and chest walls exerted on the lungs.[7] Increased abdominal pressure caused by layers of adipose tissue on the abdomen can cause gastroesophogeal reflux, increasing the risk of aspiration in bariatric patients.[7]

The work of breathing may be increased in obese patients with or without trauma as a result of a decrease in the compliance of both the chest wall and lung tissue.[25] Obese patients also have a greater demand for oxygen and increased production of carbon dioxide accompanied by a decrease in the efficiency of air exchange.[7] Failure to adequately eliminate carbon dioxide because of hypoventilation may result in a state of chronic respiratory acidosis.[27] In general, obese individuals work harder to

BOX 31-1 **Resuscitation of the Morbidly Obese Trauma Patient**

I. **OBJECTIVE:** Resuscitation of the morbidly obese trauma patient can pose major difficulties in airway, breathing, and circulatory management as part of the primary survey, and then further difficulties with the secondary survey.

II. **POLICY:** The Guideline is designed to assist the trauma team in caring for morbidly obese trauma patients.

III. **DEFINITION:** A body mass index (BMI) greater than 30 or if using the Body Mass Index Table >20% over the patient's calculated ideal body weight (IBW) (see Table 31-2).

IV. **PROCEDURE**

Primary assessment

- **Airway management**
  1. O_2 by mask
  2. O_2 by BiPAP
     Some extremely obese patients have undiagnosed sleep apnea and obstruct their airway when lying flat
  3. Endotracheal intubation
  4. Surgical airway
- **Breathing (assessment of breath sounds can be difficult)**
  1. O_2 saturation monitor:
     - Expect 88% to 92% readings on 6 L/min by mask
     - Some CO_2 retention is also probable (46-52)
  2. Do initial ABG, and insert radial arterial catheter for monitoring
  3. If ventilated, the patient should have ventilator settings of:
     - F 16-20
     - V_T 10 ml/kg
     - PEEP: +5
  4. Flail chest: can be a difficult diagnosis clinically. Palpation of chest wall may provide only clue. Intubate for any signs of respiratory failure.
  5. Pneumo/hemothorax: needle thoracentesis needs to be performed with 16-gauge spinal needles if tension pneumothorax is suspected.
  6. Location for chest tube insertion:
     - Pneumothorax: 40 F tube in second intercostal space, midclavicular line.
     - Hemothorax: ≥40 F tube in inframammary crease mid axillary line. Insert tube to at least 8 cm beyond last side hole. Angle tube posteriorly
  7. Chest tube insertion should not be done in the axilla or under the pectoral fold. The skin is too loose and the holes in the chest tube will piston in and out of the pleural cavity.
- **Circulation**
  1. IV Access: standard large bore IV approaches recommended by ATLS (i.e., subclavian veins, antecubital veins) may be impossible or difficult because of thickness of subcutaneous fat and relatively short catheters.
     - Skin folds and hygiene may preclude large bore catheter insertion percutaneously or by cutdown (i.e., saphenous vein at groin, femoral vein at groin).
     - Recommend central venous catheter 9FR 2Lumen 3 10CM .035 Wire
  2. Recommended large bore access route:
     - Internal jugular vein (percutaneous)
     - Saphenous vein at ankle (cut down)
  3. Last resort IV access
     - Interosseous infusion device
     - Right atrium via median sternotomy
  4. Arterial blood pressure monitoring
     - Radial artery: percutaneous or cutdown
     - Common femoral artery

Secondary assessment—special problems with the morbidly obese

- **Chest x-ray: portable**
  1. May be easier if film is taken with the HOB at 10 to 15 degrees
  2. CT of chest may be the only good way to assess mediastinum, lungs, and chest wall.
- **Cardiac assessment**
  1. Have a low threshold of suspicion for cardiac disease
  2. Early cardiac workup is imperative
  3. Rhythm and blood pressure instability raises possibility of cardiac injury or abnormality.
  4. Institute invasive hemodynamic monitoring if indicated
  5. Transthoracic echocardiogram (TTE) helps to assess cardiac performance (ejection fraction), possibility of cardiac injury, and cardiac filling (CVP).

BOX 31-1 Resuscitation of the Morbidly Obese Trauma Patient—cont'd

6. Transesophageal echocardiogram (TEE) offers better information when TTE is poor quality.

- **Abdominal assessment**
  1. Clinical exams ≤25% accurate
  2. Diagnostic peritoneal lavage (DPL) is technically difficult
  3. Abdominal CT scan is the preferred method of assessment
  4. Nasogastric/orogastric decompression of stomach is essential
  5. Foley catheterization
- **Recommendations for multisystem or moderately severe single system injury (AIS >4)**
  1. Monitoring and observation in the intensive care unit (ICU) for at least 24 hours
  2. Careful attention to pulmonary mechanics of breathing
  3. Overmonitor rather than undermonitor
  4. Use sterile technique to avoid nosocomial infection
  5. Plan for early mobilization to chair

Borrowed with permission from Shands at the University of Florida.

breath, require more oxygen, and produce more respiratory waste products that are not readily removed from the body.

Cardiovascular Considerations

The affects of obesity on the cardiovascular system are numerous, causing a cascade of events that lead to pulmonary hypertension and right-sided heart failure.[7] The storage of superfluous body fat leads to an increase in both metabolic demands and cardiac output.[25] There is a direct correlation between increased stroke volume and cardiac workload with the amount of additional adipose tissue an obese individual carries.[7] Increased cardiac workload can result in dilation and hypertrophy of the left ventricle.[7] Electrocardiographic changes noted in bariatric patients include: left axis deviation, low voltage QRS, left ventricular hypertrophy, abnormalities in the left atrium, and a flattened T wave in both the inferior and lateral leads.[28] Although the overall blood volume of obese individuals is typically higher, the proportion of blood volume per kilogram of body weight is lower than that of individuals who are not overweight.[7]

Heart sounds may appear muffled in obese patients. When heart sounds are ausculatated, the nurse should position the patient on the left side and listen carefully over the left lateral chest wall. It is also important to listen for heart sounds at the second intercostal space on either side of the sternal border with the patient in a supine position.[26]

Finding intravenous (IV) access in bariatric patients can prove challenging. Veins are typically hidden beneath layers of adipose tissue, making visualization and palpation difficult if not impossible. Veins that are readily visible are typically small, twisted, and superficial, not suitable for IV insertion. The IV site of choice in obese patients is typically the anticubital vein.[29] To prevent infiltration of the most accessible veins, IV access should only be attempted by highly skilled nurses or physicians. Methods typically used to make veins more visible such as hanging the extremity over the edge of the bed, applying warm compresses, and using double tourniquets may be helpful, if time permits. Unstable trauma patients requiring immediate IV access may necessitate central line placement. Landmarks used for the insertion of central lines are also frequently obscured by adipose tissue. The insertion of a central line may also be complicated by the need to move the catheter deeper and to use alternate angles to find a central vein. The use of Doppler-guided insertion may improve the success rate of central line insertion in obese patients. When other means

TABLE 31-4 Assessment and Management Challenges

Primary Parameter

Airway and Breathing

- Lack of landmarks and redundant tissue makes it difficult for endotracheal intubation or cricothyroidotomy
- Oxygen consumption and carbon dioxide production increases
- Breathing effort increases and efficiency of air exchange decreases
- Resting functional residual lung capacity decreases
- Lung and chest wall compliance decreases
- Respiratory muscles work harder

Circulation

- Metabolic and cardiac output demands increase
- Stroke volume index and stroke work index increase
- Hypoxia and hypercapnia occurs, leading to pulmonary hypertension and right-sided heart failure
- Risk for deep venous thrombosis and pulmonary embolism increases
- Vascular access is poor because of the loss of anatomic landmarks, greater skin-blood vessel distance, and short neck

Disability and Environment

- Interferes with stabilization equipment and techniques
- Few ambulances have stretchers to accommodate patients weighing more than 400 pounds
- CT scanning tables have load limitations of 300 pounds
- DPL is contraindicated because catheters are too short and landmarks are not available

Borrowed with permission from Ziglar M: Obesity and the trauma patient: challenges and guidelines for care, *J Trauma Nurs* 13:22-27, 2006.

of IV access are unsuccessful, a surgical cut-down may need to be performed to obtain IV access. The use of interosseous catheters and insertion of a catheter into the right atrium by way of median sternotomy are permissible when no other form of IV access is obtainable.[25]

Obtaining blood for laboratory testing is also very challenging in bariatric patients. Typical needles used to draw blood and ABGs may not be long enough. Layers of adipose tissue may make feeling a pulse difficult, which makes obtaining blood samples and ABGs by arterial stick complex. Blood samples may also be obtained from a central line, during insertion or after insertion if no peripheral site is accessible.

Neurologic Considerations

After an airway, breathing, and circulation (A, B, C) are established, the focus of the primary trauma assessment is on D, for disability. Determining whether a patient with a history of sleep apnea is tired or has an altered level of consciousness may prove difficult.[29] The neurologic assessment of bariatric patients may be complicated by the patient's tendency to fall asleep during the examination.[29] To prevent injury during the neurologic examination, ensure that the patient's limbs are free of the side rails before testing reflexes or asking the patient to move the extremities.

Gastrointestinal Considerations

In the bariatric patient pressure on the stomach caused by the weight of the abdominal wall can increase the risk of aspiration, which can lead to aspiration pneumonia. Precautions to prevent aspiration should be taken, such as elevating the head of the bed or positioning the patient on the side if not contraindicated, decompressing the stomach if gut emptying is ineffective, and using suction to keep the oral pharyngeal airway free of secretions. It may be extremely difficult to hear bowel sounds in bariatric patients because of the layers of adipose tissue. Bariatric patients may have problems with bowel incontinence as a result of increased intra-abdominal pressure and certain medications.

Gynecologic Considerations

All female trauma patients of childbearing age who have not had a hysterectomy or tubal ligation should have a pregnancy test performed. The extra adipose tissue on the body of an obese woman may mask a pregnant abdomen.

Genitourinary Considerations

Urinary incontinence may also be problematic for bariatric patients.[29] Getting to the bathroom may be a difficult task for overweight patients, resulting in incontinence. Patients may wear an absorbent pad or undergarment to prevent urinary leak from soiling clothing. Difficulty in cleansing the perineal area and changing the absorbent pad can lead to skin breakdown similar to diaper rash in infants. It may be difficult for obese women to get onto a bedpan and for obese men to use a urinal. The insertion of an indwelling urinary catheter in bariatric trauma patients will increase the accuracy of intake and output recording, ensure more complete bladder emptying, and help prevent perineal skin breakdown. The insertion of a catheter may require multiple individuals to hold redundant tissue so that the meatus can be visualized during catheter insertion. This may be difficult for the nursing staff and embarrassing for the patient.

Metabolic Considerations

Although the metabolic needs of bariatric patients are greater than those of normal-weight individuals, their nutritional status is typically lacking. Many bariatric patients do not get the recommended amount of protein and essential nutrients in their diets. Bariatric patients may have insulin resistance or diabetes mellitus.[6] It is important to check the blood sugar levels of all trauma patients with an altered mental state. Poor nutritional status may slow wound healing in the bariatric trauma patient.[28] When a patient's nutritional status is assessed, it is important to include inspection of the eyes, hair, nails, tongue, and gums.[26]

Comorbidities Associated with Obesity

The effects of obesity on an individual's health are far reaching. Obesity increases the risk of health problems that affect all the major systems of the body.[1] There are many diseases and medical problems associated with obesity that may affect the treatment of a bariatric trauma patient. Knowledge of a patient's medical problems will help determine the risk of using certain medications or performing diagnostic procedures. Health issues that are commonly seen in obese patients include: diabetes, coronary artery disease, peripheral vascular disease, hypertension, liver and gallbladder disease, pulmonary hypertension, various types of cancer, and gastroesophogeal reflux disease.[6] Obesity has also been associated with sleep disturbances and depression. See Table 31-5 for a more comprehensive list of the health issues associated with obesity.

Medical problems that are commonly associated with obesity can influence the care of trauma patients and may lead to some of the complications seen during recovery from injury. These medical conditions may also have been the cause of the traumatic event. The trauma team may find themselves asking, which came first, the myocardial infarction/stroke or the MVC. The trauma surgeon may have to weigh the risk of surgery versus the risk of more conservative medical management and observation for patients with hypertension, heart disease, and congestive heart failure. Fluid replacement therapy is a balancing act when caring for patients with a history of congestive heart failure and idiopathic intracranial hypertension. It may be difficult to tell which abnormal findings are new and which are the result of a previous stroke when performing a neurologic assessment on a trauma patient with an altered level of consciousness and a history of stroke.

Respiratory complications can be problematic for the bariatric trauma patient. Hypoventilation syndrome and sleep apnea are seen in both obese adults and children.[30] Although the

TABLE 31-5 **Health Issues Associated With Obesity**

System	Associated Health Problems
Cardiovascular/ circulatory	Hypertension, coronary artery disease, peripheral vascular disease, myocardial infarction, cardiomyopathy, DVT, PE
Endocrine/ metabolic	Diabetes mellitus, insulin resistance, hyperinsulinemia, hypercholesterolemia, elevated triglyceride levels
Gastrointestinal	Gastroesophogeal reflux, gallbladder disease, fatty liver disease, gallbladder, liver and colon cancer
Integumentary	Cellulitis, chaffing, infection and potential skin breakdown caused by excessive skin to skin contact, excessive body hair
Lymphatic	Varicose veins and lymph edema
Neurologic	Stroke, idiopathic intracranial hypertension
Psychologic	Depression, isolation, social anxiety disorders
Reproductive/ gynecologic	Endometrial cancer, breast cancer, polycystic ovary disease, anovulation or irregular menses, infertility, pregnancy-induced hypertension
Respiratory	Sleep apnea, pulmonary hypertension, obesity hypoventilation syndrome, increased risk of respiratory infections
Skeletal	Osteoarthritis, joint pain, back pain, degenerative joint disease
Urinary	Stress incontinence, prostate cancer

causes of hypoventilation syndrome in obese patients are not fully understood, it is thought that the body does not respond appropriately to hypoxia and hypercarbia, which leads to chronic respiratory acidosis.[27] Bariatric patients are also predisposed to an increased risk of respiratory infections.[6] Trauma patients with hypoventilation syndrome who are immobile have an increased risk for development of pneumonia. Mechanical ventilation may be needed to treat these respiratory complications. Higher ventilator pressures may be necessary to overcome the increased thoracic pressure found in obese patients so that effective ventilation can be achieved. The occurrence of respiratory complications can increase the length of time mechanical ventilation is required.

Musculoskeletal disorders associated with obesity such as osteoarthritis may limit mobility. Lack of weight-bearing exercise predisposes obese adults to osteoporosis, increasing the likelihood of fractures in blunt trauma. Decreased mobility during hospitalization increases the chance that a bariatric trauma patient will have pneumonia, deep venous thrombosis (DVT), and pulmonary emboli (PE).

Special Management Considerations

Equipment

The need for special equipment and extra manpower may delay the transport of bariatric trauma patients to the trauma center. Standard stretchers will not accommodate patients weighing more than 500 pounds.[7] Prehospital personnel may need to call for back up to safely move bariatric patients to the ambulance. Spinal immobilization may require the use of two backboards with sandbags and tape to stabilize the cervical spine.[7] When placed supine on a backboard, many obese patients will have trouble breathing, requiring the paramedics to place the patient in a reverse Trendelenburg position without compromising C-spine stabilization. Most splints will not fit a bariatric patient, requiring the prehospital personnel to improvise with cardboard splints, wood, and bandages or sheets to immobilize a fractured extremity.

The need for oversized equipment continues when the patient arrives in the hospital emergency department (ED) or resuscitation area. This equipment may not be readily available in the ED. Staff members should begin by obtaining an extra large gurney or hospital bed and an appropriate-sized blood pressure cuff as soon as they are notified that they will be receiving a bariatric patient. Although extra large blood pressure cuffs may fit obese patients, bariatric cuffs are needed to obtain accurate blood pressures on patients who are morbidly obese. Some institutions may not stock bariatric blood pressure cuffs. The use of a thigh cuff on an upper extremity or an extra large cuff on the forearm may provide an inaccurate blood pressure.[7,26] When bariatric trauma patients are cared for, it is important to be sure that the blood pressure cuff fits correctly. "The width of the cuff bladder must be 40 to 50 percent of the arm's circumference, and the length of the bladder must be 80 percent of the circumference to obtain an accurate reading."[26]

Diagnostic Testing

The assessment of trauma may be more difficult in obese patients because the typical methods of assessment may not be available or reliable. The care of the bariatric trauma patient may necessitate alternatives to the traditional diagnostic tests used to determine whether blood is present in the chest or abdomen. The chest radiograph of a bariatric patient may show a widened mediastinum, making it difficult to differentiate between a normal patient variation and aortic injury.[31] If a chest radiograph to rule out aortic injury is inconclusive, the next step would be to perform a thoracic CT scan with contrast to determine whether there is damage to the aorta. A CT scan may not be an option, depending on the weight limit of the CT table. Most CT tables have a weight limit of 250 to 300 pounds. Some trauma centers have CT scans that can accommodate patients whose weight is more than 300 pounds. It is important to know the weight limit of the CT table at your institution before needing it on an emergency basis.

Most trauma centers have the ability to perform bedside ultrasonography, also known as a focused abdominal sonography for trauma, to determine whether there is blood in the abdomen of a trauma patient. The use of ultrasonography is limited in the obese patient. Distortion caused by layers of adipose tissue makes it difficult to determine accurately whether there is blood in the abdomen.[7]

Another means of detecting whether there is blood in the abdomen is DPL. The thickness of the anterior abdominal wall determines whether DPL may or may not be an option for assessing the trauma patient. The usefulness of DPL in an obese patient is limited by the length of the catheter or trocar available and the physician's ability to find the appropriate landmarks.[7]

When the trauma surgeon suspects abdominal injury but is unable to determine whether blood is present in the abdomen by using CT, ultrasonography, or DPL, he or she is left with two options. The first option is to carefully observe the patient, including closely monitoring for significant changes in vital signs, fluid requirements, and serial hematocrits.[7] The second option involves taking the patient to surgery for an exploratory laparotomy. The trauma surgeon must weigh the risk of careful observation with the risk of performing surgery on a bariatric patient.[7] Trends involving a decreasing blood pressure and elevated heart rate accompanied by a significant drop in the patient's hematocrit require an urgent reassessment by the trauma surgeon. If there is no obvious source of bleeding, the observation period has helped determine the need for exploratory surgery.[7]

Medications

The absorption of medications administered during trauma resuscitation and recovery may be affected by the ratio of a patient's body fat to lean body tissue. Pain medications in the opioid family (e.g., morphine and fentanyl), which are fat soluble, may require larger doses to relieve pain in the bariatric trauma patient and should be given in relation to the patient's actual weight. Careful respiratory monitoring is needed when giving large repeated doses of morphine or fentanyl because of the potential for accumulation in the adipose tissue. Rapid infusion or the cumulative effect of continuous IV infusion of fentanyl can lead to chest wall rigidity, making ventilation difficult and prolonging the need for mechanical ventilation.[31]

Benzodiazepines such as diazepam (Valium) and lorazepam (Ativan) may be used to provide sedation or to treat alcohol withdrawal and seizures in trauma patients. Diazepam and lorazepam are traditionally given IV but may be administered intramuscularly (IM) when IV access is delayed. It is preferable to administer both diazepam and lorazepam IV because of the unpredictable absorption when they are administered IM. Midazolam (Versed) is often the benzodiazepine of choice for sedation. The short half-life of midazolam makes frequent reassessment of the patient's neurologic status possible. The cumulative effects of midazolam in morbidly obese patients may increase the period of sedation between doses.[31] Benzodiazepines should also be dosed according to the patient's actual body weight.

Propofol is a drug often used for intubated patients with an altered level of consciousness from head injury. The rapid onset and short half-life make propofol ideal for frequent intermittent assessment of the neurologic status. The appropriate initial dosage of propofol is calculated on the basis of ideal body weight rather than actual body weight.[31] The rate of continuous infusion is determined by titration to the desired effect.[31]

Paralytic drugs used in rapid-sequence intubation are dosed according to the specific drug being administered rather than by the class of drug. The dose of vecuronium is calculated on the basis of the patient's ideal body weight. Atracurium, on the other hand, is dosed according to actual body weight.[31]

Airway Management

Redundant layers of adipose tissue on the thorax and abdomen, as well as fat deposits on the diaphragm, decrease respiratory muscle mobility and chest wall expansion, placing the bariatric trauma patient at risk for respiratory insufficiency and arrest. The obese patient is also at increased risk for aspiration. All these obesity-related factors as well as the trauma-related injuries that threaten airway patency can necessitate the need for urgent airway management to effectively ventilate the patient. Repeated airway assessment and early management is a priority. Airway interventions that may be easily accomplished in normal-weight patients may be challenging at best in the bariatric trauma patient.

Intubation, the first choice for airway management in trauma patients who cannot maintain their own airway, is made increasingly difficult by a short stout neck, decreased flexibility in the neck, and limited ability to open the mouth.[31] The use of paralytics before intubation is risky in bariatric patients.[31] Blind nasotracheal intubation, an alternative to orotracheal intubation in patients with spontaneous respirations, may be an option if no facial trauma is present. The risk of introducing blood into an airway already compromised by severe epistaxis caused by intubation trauma makes this procedure best performed by practitioners skilled in nasotracheal intubation.[31]

When intubation is not possible, the esophageal-tracheal Combitube may provide an alternative method of securing the airway. Combitube insertion in obese patients may be easier than endotracheal (ET) intubation because insertion does not require the visualization of the landmarks used to insert an ET tube. The use of a Combitube is for emergency airway stabilization. When used with the high ventilatory pressures needed to provide adequate ventilation for bariatric patients, the Combitube may cause obstruction of the lingual vein, resulting in tongue engorgement and discoloration.[22] Once the patient is stabilized, a more definitive airway should be established.

Cricothyroidotomy, the insertion of a tube into the trachea through the cricothyroid membrane, is typically the second choice for airway management in trauma patients without respirations necessitating emergency airway stabilization. The excess tissue covering the throat of a bariatric patient may obscure the landmarks needed to perform either a surgical or a needle cricothyroidotomy. The use of cricothyroidotomy in obese patients is limited by the inability to palpate the cricothyroid membrane.

The emergency insertion of a tracheostomy is not routinely performed on a trauma patient unless all other methods of securing an airway have been unsuccessful. Until recently, obesity, a short fat neck, and possible cervical spine injury have been considered relative contraindications to the insertion of a percutaneous tracheostomy (PCT).[23] A study by Ben-Nun et al[23] demonstrated that, when it is performed by a surgeon highly skilled in the procedure, PCT can be performed safely in obese trauma patients under emergency conditions. The results of this study were based on successful PCT insertion in 10 trauma patients.[23] Further research into the use of PCT in the acute trauma setting is indicated.

Intraoperative Phase

The operating room (OR) should be notified of the potential need for surgical intervention as soon as the ED or resuscitation area is aware of an incoming trauma patient. It is important to provide the OR team with the approximate weight of a bariatric patient as early as possible. This will allow the OR staff to prepare any special equipment that may be needed to care for a bariatric patient.

Obese patients are at greater risk for complications from surgery than are normal-weight patients. The decision to perform surgery must weigh the risk of performing any surgical procedure against the risk of death or disability that may result if surgery is not performed.

Anesthesia

Intubation of obese trauma patients for surgery presents challenges similar to those encountered during intubation in the resuscitation setting. The anesthesiologist may choose to perform a surgical tracheotomy rather than risk the loss of a patent airway.[7] When general anesthesia is not needed, the anesthesiologist must determine whether it is possible to use spinal or epidural anesthesia. The use of spinal or epidural anesthesia depends on the capability of the surgical team to properly position the patient and the anesthesiologist's ability to locate the necessary landmarks.[7]

Positioning the Patient for Surgery

Transferring the patient from the bed or gurney to the surgical bed may require multiple people. An oversized surgical bed may be required to accommodate the overweight patient without risk of injury. The addition of extra pieces to the surgical bed may be necessary for proper body alignment. If proper body alignment cannot be obtained by using a large surgical bed with additional sections, stirrups can be used to position the legs off to the side and arm boards can be used to support the upper extremities.[7] Care must be used to prevent tissue and nerve damage when securing limbs during surgery. Positioning the patient correctly on the operating table will minimize the risk of damage to nerves, muscles, and skin integrity.[7] Elevating the head of the bed/surgical table will decrease the risk of aspiration and ventilatory compromise, thereby reducing the need for higher ventilator pressures.[7]

Positioning bariatric patients prone for surgery on the posterior spine provides the surgical team with multiple challenges. Positioning the patient on the abdomen without adequate support for the chest is both uncomfortable and unsafe for the patient. Providing enough support to the chest wall to prevent excessive pressure on the abdomen is difficult. Failure to provide adequate chest support can result in blood clots in the mesenteric artery and necrosis of the bowel.[7]

Electrosurgery

Electrosurgery, surgery using machines operating on high-frequency electrical current, should be used with special precautions in bariatric trauma patients. Electrosurgery requires the placement of a dispersive pad over a large muscle mass. Following this practice may cause an electrical burn in bariatric patients. To prevent the concentration of current in a single area, two dispersive pads are applied when any form of electrosurgery is performed on bariatric patients.[7]

Critical Care Phase

The transfer of care from the ED or OR to the appropriate patient care unit is determined by patient condition at the time of transfer. Continuity of patient care is essential to prevent missing subtle changes in the patient's condition that may require urgent interventions. Handoff from nurse to nurse should be comprehensive. The primary goal of the critical care phase for the bariatric trauma patient is patient recovery without development of complications.

Postoperative Complications

Bariatric patients are at increased risk for postoperative complications that may result in death. All postoperative patients have a risk for development of atelectasis, DVT, and PE. This risk is increased in the bariatric patient.[32] Table 31-6 lists some additional common postoperative complications for the bariatric trauma patient.

TABLE 31-6 **Postoperative Complications in the Bariatric Patient**

System/Cause	Complications
Respiratory	Atelectasis, pneumonia, aspiration, prolonged mechanical ventilation, PE
Cardiovascular	DVT, internal bleeding
Gastrointestinal	Decreased gastric emptying, constipation, peritonitis
Integumentary	Infection, wound dehiscence
Pain medication	Excessive sedation, respiratory depression or arrest, altered level of consciousness

The risk of atelectasis and pneumonia is decreased with frequent use of incentive spirometry and early mobilization. Uncontrolled pain may discourage both the use of incentive spirometry and movement. Adequate pain management without oversedation is the key to encouraging patients to take deep breaths when using the incentive spirometer and ambulating. Continuous pulse oximetry monitoring to assist in recognizing the onset of respiratory complications or respiratory suppression from oversedation is recommended when caring for postoperative bariatric patients.

The risk for development of DVT or PE increases with each day of immobility. Prescribed anticoagulant prophylaxis should be initiated when appropriate. Compression stockings or pneumatic compression devices may not be readily available in sizes large enough to accommodate the lower extremities of bariatric patients. Early initiation of physical therapy is important for patients confined to bed as well as those who are mobile. Passive range of motion (PROM), which involves movement of the patient's extremities by the therapist, is appropriate for patients who are comatose or unable to move their limbs without assistance. PROM for the bariatric patient may require someone to assist the therapist. Bariatric patients who have difficulty lifting their own extremities may require assistance with active range of motion exercises.

Patients who are able should be encouraged to sit in a chair and ambulate as soon as possible. Large chairs and walkers are available to accommodate the obese patient. Nursing staff or physical therapists assisting bariatric patients out of bed need to question the patient about his or her mobility status before the injury. An attempt to stand or walk a bariatric patient should never be made without knowing whether the patient was able to ambulate with or without assistance before hospitalization. Staff members need to provide enough help to ensure the safety of both the patient and personnel.

Special attention needs to be given to the surgical wounds of a bariatric trauma patient. Obese patients are prone to wound dehiscence resulting from tension at the suture site. Providing extra support over the surgical site, with a bra or abdominal binder, during movements that are likely to increase the pressure on the incision may decrease the risk of wound dehiscence.[31] Adipose tissue is poorly vascularized. Decreased blood flow and oxygenation to the wound site frequently results in delayed wound healing for bariatric patients.[31] Bariatric patients have an increased rate of surgical wound infection. The use of prophylactic antibiotics before surgery may decrease the rate of wound infection. Obese patients who have undergone abdominal surgery should be carefully monitored for signs of peritonitis. See Box 31-2 for signs and symptoms of peritonitis.

BOX 31-2 Signs and Symptoms of Peritonitis

Tachycardia
Tachypnea
Fever
Abdominal rigidity
Abdominal distention
Increasing abdominal pain with movement
Back pain
Pelvic pain
Rebound tenderness
Guarding
Decreased or absent bowel sounds
Nausea and vomiting

PAIN CONTROL

Pain control is paramount in the recovery of trauma patients. All trauma patients should be regularly assessed for pain. Pain relief measures include ice, elevation, distraction techniques, and the administration of pain medication. The patient's willingness to cough, deep breath, and move depend on his or her comfort level. To increase patient compliance with incentive spirometry, mobilization, and physical therapy, pain medication should be administered before these activities when necessary.

Pain medication may be administered through the IV, IM, subcutaneous, or oral route. Extra layers of adipose tissue in bariatric patients make the absorption of IM or subcutaneous injections unreliable. The amount of pain medication administered should be determined by the patient's actual body weight.[31] Pain medications prescribed as standard dosages or on the basis of the patient's ideal body weight have the potential to be subtherapeutic.

Side effects of pain medications include nausea, vomiting, hypotension, and respiratory depression. Because of the potential for respiratory compromise in bariatric patients, it is important to frequently monitor for signs of respiratory depression. The need to achieve pain control without impeding respiratory function requires frequent assessment of both pain, using a standard pain scale, and respiratory function, including the depth and rate of the patient's respirations, pulse oximetry, and level of consciousness.

PREVENTING SKIN BREAKDOWN

Bariatric patients are prone to skin breakdown, tissue injury, and dermatitis or fungal infections in skin folds. Patients who are confined to bed have a high risk for the development of pressure ulcers. This risk is increased in the bariatric patient who may have difficulty repositioning himself or herself in bed.[31] The use of a trapeze that will accommodate the patient's weight may allow independent repositioning or enable the patient to assist nursing staff with changing position. The patient should be positioned in a way that prevents the patient from sliding down in the bed, which results in shearing action against the skin. Slide boards or lifts should be used when attempting to move patients to prevent friction burns and skin tears. A hospital bed that is appropriate must not only accommodate the patient's size but also have a mattress that does not compress under the weight of the patient. The use of air beds may help prevent the formation of pressure ulcers in obese patients.

Pressure ulcers in bariatric patients should be treated aggressively. Management of pressure ulcers that are resistant to initial healing interventions should be handled by a nurse who specializes in wound, ostomy, and continence care. Wound cultures should be obtained from all infected pressure ulcers. Pressure ulcers that are cavernous, infected, and resistant to healing may require surgical debridement.[31]

Urinary and fecal incontinence, limited mobility, and difficulty in cleansing the perineal area make obese patient candidates for dermatitis and skin breakdown. It is imperative that the patient or nursing staff provide thorough perineal cleansing after elimination. The perineal area should be dried thoroughly before undergarments or adult diapers are applied. The use of diaper rash creams can help prevent skin irritation and breakdown. Devices that contain feces or urine can be used to help maintain perineal skin integrity.

Moisture that accumulates in skin folds places obese patients at risk for rashes and fungal infections. Patients may use tissue, gauze, or washcloths to absorb moisture and prevent dermatitis and fungal infections. Frequent cleansing and changing of the absorbent cloth will decrease the risk of skin irritation. The use of powder to absorb moisture is not recommended because of its tendency to build up and irritate the skin. Antifungal creams are used only when fungal infections are present and not as a preventive measure.[31]

NUTRITION

It is important to obtain a baseline of the nutritional status in bariatric trauma patients as soon as possible. Chapter 16 gives more information on nutritional assessment of the trauma patient. Overweight does not imply an abundance of nutritional stores. Many obese individuals have significant nutritional deficits. Research shows that as many as 30% of obese individuals may have some form of eating disorder.[6] A full nutritional analysis by a registered dietitian should be completed as soon as possible.

Bariatric trauma patients are at risk of protein malnutrition and loss of lean body mass.[31] Obese patients frequently have increased insulin levels, accompanied with insulin resistance, that are exacerbated by the stress of trauma on their bodies. Insulin needs are generally higher after any form of stress. Severely elevated glucose levels in bariatric trauma patients can result in significant diuresis, diabetic ketoacidosis, and diabetic coma. Careful blood glucose monitoring and appropriate insulin administration are essential.[31]

Bariatric trauma patients should be weighed on admission and daily thereafter to assist in monitoring nutritional and hydration status. After traumatic events bariatric patients are prone to rapid loss of large amounts of weight. Weight loss includes the loss of both fat stores and lean muscle mass. Under stressful situations the metabolic needs of obese individuals are met primarily by the breakdown of protein for fuel.[31] The loss of lean body mass in the form of muscle tissue can result in delays in ventilator weaning and mobilization. Diets with sufficient carbohydrates are required to decrease the catabolism of lean muscle tissue.[32]

To prevent significant muscle loss enteral tube feedings and, if contraindicated, parenteral nutrition needs to be initiated early in bariatric trauma patients who cannot eat. The amount of calories needed in feedings is based on the patient's energy expenditure. The primary source of establishing energy expenditure in critically ill bariatric trauma patients is indirect calorimetry. When indirect calorimetry is not available, enteral feedings should be based on providing 20 to 30 kcal/kg/day.[31]

BARIATRIC SURGERY

The trauma patient may have previously had weight loss surgery. No research was found that specifically addresses the needs or challenges of caring for a trauma patient who has had weight loss surgery. Understanding the types of weight loss surgeries currently performed and how they affect the needs of the patient can help the team provide the most appropriate care. Box 31-3 details the criteria for weight loss surgery.[1,30]

Gastric Bypass

The Roux-en-Y is the most commonly used form of gastric bypass surgery in the United States. Rings are placed around the stomach to section off a small portion of the stomach.[30] The newly created stomach pouch is then attached to the lower portion of the small intestine, resulting in a desire for smaller portions of food and decreased absorption.[1]

Laparoscopic Adjustable Banding

A band is placed around the top portion of the stomach to create a small pouch with a small channel connecting the upper and lower portions of the stomach.[1] The goal of this procedure is to create a false sensation of fullness, resulting in decreased food intake. Excessive food intake can cause the

BOX 31-3 Criteria for Weight Loss Surgery

Candidates for weight loss surgery must meet the following criteria:

- Age 18 years or older
- Weight 75 pounds or more overweight
- BMI >40 or BMI 35 with health issues related to obesity
- Inability to lose weight or sustain weight loss
- Medical clearance for surgery by primary physician and any specialist currently treating the patient
- No current psychiatric illness
- Attend educational classes regarding weight loss surgery
- Understanding and acceptance of the strict dietary changes needed after surgery

bands to slip and increase the size of the stomach pouch. A second surgery may be required to reposition the band.

Biliopancreatic Diversion

After removal of a portion of the stomach, the rest of the stomach is attached directly near the terminal end of the small intestine. The result of this procedure is decreased food intake and absorption.[1]

Stomach Stapling

Although this procedure is not common today, the health care team may still encounter patients who have had this procedure performed in the past. Stomach stapling involves placing either multiple bands or staples in the stomach to reduce its size.[1]

Dietary Restrictions

Individuals who have undergone weight loss surgery must follow a very strict diet after the procedure. Small frequent meals are needed to meet the patient's caloric needs. Patients are encouraged to drink protein shakes and take vitamin and mineral supplements to replace those lost to malabsorption. Items that are restricted include white bread, carbonated drinks, fibrous meat, and sweets.[30]

INTERMEDIATE CARE/REHABILITATION

The progression of care from the critical care phase to the intermediate care and rehabilitation phases continues to provide challenges to the nursing personnel, patient, and family members. Meeting the patient's nutritional needs remains a priority of care in both the intermediate and rehabilitation phases of care. The importance of emotional support for both the patient and family continues. Increasing mobility and independence become priorities. The ultimate goal of intermediate care and rehabilitation is preparing the patient to go home.

MOBILITY

During both the intermediate care and rehabilitation phases the goal is for patients to become increasingly more mobile. The care and rehabilitation of a bariatric trauma patient provides unique challenges for both the nursing staff, physical therapist, occupational therapist, and other members of the care team. The patient may have lost a significant amount of weight during the initial hospitalization. As a result of muscle mass loss and lack of muscle tone from immobility, the patients may have generalized weakness. Despite a potentially substantial weight loss the bariatric patient frequently remains many pounds overweight. Mobility is essential for the patient to achieve independence. Before admission to the hospital the bariatric patient may have had limited, minimal, or no independent mobility. Some patients may have been completely bedridden because of their excessive weight, resulting in a reliance on others for all or most of their daily needs.

The goal of regaining some independence means that patients need to be able to fulfill activities of daily living with minimal or no help. The progression from limited or no mobility to ambulation can be slow. Patients may start by sitting up in bed and moving their extremities and progress to standing with assistance. Nursing and rehabilitation staff members need to be sure that enough help is present to allow a patient to stand without risk to the patient or staff members. Once the patient is strong enough to stand with help he or she may begin to ambulate a few steps at a time. The use of assistive devices such as a cane or walker may be necessary.

EQUIPMENT

Caring for a bariatric patient may require the rental or purchase of specialized equipment. A bed or floor scale that will accurately weigh the patient is essential. Oversized airbeds will help prevent skin breakdown and pressure ulcers. Specialized lifts may be used to raise the patient from bed to a chair or into a whirlpool, if needed. Sturdy overbed frames and trapezes that will accommodate the weight of a bariatric patient allow the patient to assist the nursing staff in position changes. Oversized stretchers that transform into chairs make it easier for immobile patients to sit up. Bariatric wheel chairs, bath chairs, and commodes help the patient to regain some independence once his or her mobility increases.

PSYCHOSOCIAL SUPPORT

Society places a great deal of importance on outward beauty and thinness. Obese individuals may feel persecuted in both the community and the hospital setting. The lack of appropriate-sized equipment and need for multiple staff members to assist with procedures can be embarrassing for these patients.

Staff members must be aware of their own feelings and prejudices against overweight individuals. It is important that staff members monitor both their verbal and nonverbal communications when dealing with patients. Critical comments about the patient's weight are never appropriate. Questions regarding weight, nutrition, mobility, and general health should be asked in a nonjudgmental manner. Trust is an essential part of the nurse-patient relationship. Health care workers must be sure to treat bariatric patients with respect and dignity.

COMMUNITY REINTEGRATION PHASE

The ultimate goal for all trauma patients is to be able to return to the community with as little negative change to their lifestyles as possible. Discharge planning for bariatric trauma patients begins at the time of admission to the hospital. This is especially important because of their need for specialized equipment and assistance at home. If bariatric trauma patients require additional therapy, they may require transfer to a long-term care facility or rehabilitation center before going home. Early planning is necessary to ensure that an appropriate facility is chosen.

Referrals

Bariatric patients should receive information about the importance of nutrition, weight loss, and exercise during their hospitalization. Referral to a registered dietitian is important to help the patient learn to eat in a healthy manner. Patients may be given information about weight loss centers, physicians specializing in weight loss, and support groups for overweight individuals. It is also important that patients have access to size-appropriate medical equipment when they get home. Patients who remain severely overweight and have limited mobility may need a referral to a physician who performs home visits.

Home Health Care

Bariatric patients who are discharged home with limited mobility and other continued medical concerns will require some form of home health care. Many patients will continue to require assistance from multiple disciplines. The coordination of care is imperative to prevent duplication of services or oversight of needed services. Patients who are continuing to work toward mobility and independence may continue to need physical therapy and occupational therapy once they return home. Nursing care may be necessary if the patient requires continued IV antibiotics or wound care. The help of a home health aid may be required to assist the patient with activities of daily living.

Future Trends and Prevention

The number of obese individuals is increasing at an alarming rate. In spite of a campaign to encourage activity in children, the rate of obesity in children continues to climb. Despite diets, research, new drugs, and weight loss surgeries it is highly unlikely that there will be a "cure" for obesity in our lifetime.

Obesity presents many challenges both for the patient and health care workers. Obese patients may have limited mobility, making any form of exercise a challenge for them. Programs that stress exercise starting at the patient's current level of mobility and slowly increasing may encourage overweight individuals to become more active. As overweight individuals become more active, the need for equipment that meets their needs becomes more apparent. Exercise equipment needs to be made sturdy enough to handle the stress load placed on it by an overweight individual.

Education regarding the health issues and equipment needs of bariatric patients may make nursing staff more comfortable caring for them. A list of where to find oversized equipment within the hospital and rental equipment will make providing care for obese patients easier. Hospitals that develop contracts with equipment rental stores will have easier access to the equipment needed without incurring the cost of purchasing it. Getting the appropriate equipment early in the patient's hospital stay may help prevent the complications of immobility including pressure ulcer, DVT, and PE. Preventing complications may decrease the length of hospitalization.

In the future, automobile makers may begin to consider marketing cars, trucks, and sport utility vehicles to better accommodate obese individuals. Automobiles with correct-fitting safety equipment such as seat belts and airbags may decrease the type and severity of injury encountered by obese individuals during a collision. To make these changes, it is important for automobile makers to realize that the standard crash test dummy does not represent the broad range of weight and size of the individuals who purchase their vehicles.

Nursing Research and Education

The amount of research dealing with bariatric trauma patients is very limited. Most studies have focused on the morbidity and mortality rates associated with bariatric trauma. Further research is needed in the areas of airway management, diagnostic and surgical procedures, and the nutritional and rehabilitation needs of bariatric trauma patients. Although bariatric surgeries are becoming increasingly more popular, no studies were found specific to the care and treatment of trauma patients who have undergone weight loss surgery.

There are many educational needs for health care team members caring for bariatric patients. There seems to be a general misconception in society that overweight people are lazy and eat too much or that they should be able to control the problem. Education regarding the many factors, both medical and psychologic, that contribute to obesity is necessary for everyone who provides care for bariatric patients. Many nurses are not aware of the resources available to help them care for bariatric patients. Education regarding equipment needs and how to locate the appropriate equipment would make providing care for bariatric patients less complex. Although the number of weight loss surgeries performed increases yearly, many nurses are not familiar with the types of weight loss surgeries or of the dietary restrictions of patients who have undergone these procedures.

References

1. Saber AA, Hale KL: Surgery in the treatment of obesity, *eMedicine* (2006) eMedicine.com. Accessed September 7, 2006.
2. Pierracci MF, Barie SP, Pomp A: Critical care of the bariatric patient, *Crit Care Med* 34:1796-1804, 2006.
3. Uwaifo GI, Arioglu E: Obesity, *eMedicine* (2006): eMedicine.com. Accessed September 7, 2006.
4. *Mosby's medical dictionary,* 7th ed, St. Louis, 2005, Mosby.
5. Centers for Disease Control and Prevention: *Overweight and obesity: defining overweight and obesity,* Department of Health and Human Services (2006): www.cdc.gov. Accessed September 7, 2006.

6. Uwaifo GI: Obesity and overview, *eMedicine* (2005): eMedicine.com. Accessed September 7, 2006.
7. Bushard S: Trauma in patients who are morbidly obese, *AORN J* 76:585-589, 2002.
8. Hazinski MF: *PALS provider manual,* Dallas, 2002, American Heart Association.
9. Arbabi S, Wahl WL, Hemmila MR et al: The cushion effect, *J Trauma Inj Infect Crit Care* 54:1090-1093, 2003.
10. Brown CV, Neville AL, Rhee P et al: The impact of obesity on the outcomes of 1,153 critically injured blunt trauma patients, *J Trauma Inj Infect Critl Care* 59:1048-1051, 2005.
11. Byrnes MC, McDaniel MD, Moore MB et al: The effect of obesity on outcomes among injured patients, *J Trauma Inj Infect Crit Care* 58:232-237, 2005.
12. Morris JA, MacKenzie EJ, Edelstein SL: The effect of preexisting conditions on mortality in trauma patients, *JAMA* 263: 1942-1946, 1990.
13. Smith-Choban PS, Weireter LJ, Maynes C: Obesity and increased mortality in blunt trauma, *J Trauma* 31:1253-1257, 1991.
14. Neville AC, Brown CV, Weng JD et al: Obesity is an independent risk factor of mortality in severely injured blunt trauma patients, *Arch Surg* 139:983-987, 2004.
15. Whitlock G, Norton R, Clark T et al: Is a body mass index a risk factor for motor vehicle driver injury? A cohort study with prospective and retrospective outcomes, *Int J Epidemiol* 32: 147-149, 2003.
16. Bazelmans C, Coppieters Y, Godin I et al: Is obesity associated with injuries among young people? *Eur J Epidemiol* 19:1037-1042, 2004.
17. Spaine LA, Bollen SR: "The bigger they come ..." the relationship between body mass index and severity of ankle fractures, *Injury* 27:687-689, 1996.
18. Moran SG, McGwin G Jr, Metzger JS et al: Injury rates among restrained drivers in motor vehicle collisions: the role of body habitus, *J Trauma Inj Infect Crit Care* 52:1116-1120, 2002.
19. Reiff DA, Davis RP, MacLennan PA et al: The association between body mass index and diaphragm injury among motor vehicle collision occupants, *J Trauma Inj Infect Crit Care* 57: 1324-1328, 2004.
20. Choban PS, Weireter LJ, Maynes C: Obesity and increased mortality in blunt trauma, *J Trauma* 31:1253-1257, 1991.
21. Gottschlich MM, Mayes T, Khoury JC et al: Significance of obesity on nutritional, immunological, hormonal, and clinical outcome parameters in burns, *J Am Diet Assoc* 93:1261-1268, 1993.
22. McGlinch BP, Martin DP, Volcheck GW et al: Tongue engorgement with prolonged use of the esophageal-tracheal Combitube, *Ann Emerg Med* 44:320-322, 2004.
23. Ben-Nun A, Altman E, Best LE: Emergency percutaneous tracheostomy in trauma patients: an early experience, *Ann Thorac Surg* 77:1045-1047, 2004.
24. American College of Surgeons' Committee on Trauma: *Advanced trauma life support,* 7th ed, Chicago, 2004, American College of Surgeons.
25. Ziglar MK: Obesity and the trauma patient: challenges and guidelines for care, *J Trauma Nurs* 13:22-27, 2006.
26. Hahler B: Morbid obesity: a nursing care challenge, *Dermatol Nurs* 14:249-256, 2002.
27. Hayes JA: *Respiratory acidosis* (2005): http://www.emedicine.com/med/topic/2008.htm. Accessed April 16, 2006.
28. Alpert MA, Terry BE, Hamm CR et al: Effect of weight loss on the ECG of normotensive morbidly obese patients, *Chest* 119:507-510, 2001.
29. Twedell D: Physical assessment of the bariatric person, *J Continuing Educ Nurs* 34:147-148, 2003.
30. Murray D: Morbid obesity-psychosocial aspects and surgical interventions, *AORN J* 78:990-995, 2003.
31. El-Solh AA: Clinical approach to the critically ill, morbidly obese patient, *Am J Respir Crit Care Med* 169:557-561, 2004.
32. Maull KI: Trauma morbidity in the morbid obese, Trauma and Critical Care Symposium, Las Vegas, Nev, May 6, 2002.

32

BURN INJURIES

Mary Beth Flynn Makic, Elizabeth Mann

Fire and burns are the fifth most common causes of unintentional injury-related deaths in the United States.[1] According to the American Burn Association (ABA), approximately 1.1 million burn injuries require medical attention each year; 50,000 of these individuals require hospitalization and 4,500 die from their burn injuries.[2,3] Approximately three fourths of fire-related civilian deaths and injuries are the consequence of house fires, resulting in 2,670 deaths, 14,050 injuries, and $6.1 billion in direct property damage.[4] Of the approximately 6% of burn injury patients who do not survive, most have sustained an inhalation injury. Despite these sobering facts, overall mortality and morbidity rates from burn injuries have declined over the years; however, burn deaths, injuries, and disability from burn injury remain a substantial problem in our society.

Advances in burn prevention strategies, such as effective public education, better fire-retardant product design, smoke detectors, and enforcement of fire safety codes[4,5] have decreased the overall prevalence and incidence of burn injuries. Survival after burn injury has also improved over the past few decades. Before the 1970s, a patient with a 50% total body surface area (TBSA) burn had a 40% chance of survival. Today a patient with a 75% TBSA burn has a 50% chance of survival.[6] Factors enhancing patient survival may include more rapid response by emergency teams, efficiencies in transport to burn treatment facilities, advances in fluid resuscitation, improvements in wound coverage, better support of the hypermetabolic response to injury, advances in infection control practices, and improved treatment of inhalation injuries.[3,6,7]

Patients with burn injuries have special needs throughout the hospitalization. The ABA has established guidelines to determine which burn-injured patients should be transferred to a specialized burn center to maximize treatment effect and decrease patient morbidity and mortality rates (Box 32-1). Patients meeting the criteria outlined by the ABA should be transported to the nearest burn center.

PATHOPHYSIOLOGIC FEATURES IF BURN INJURY

TISSUE INJURY

In a burn, tissue injury results from coagulation of cellular protein in response to heat produced by thermal, chemical, electrical, or radiation energy. The depth of coagulative necrosis of the tissue depends on the heat generated by the causative agent and the length of contact with the tissues (Figure 32-1).[7] Thermal energy is the most common cause of burn injury. Common sources of thermal burns are flame, steam, scald, and contact with hot objects or surfaces. Inhalation injury is a type thermal injury caused by superheated gases that enter the airway when burn victims are injured in an enclosed space.

Tissue coagulation caused by chemical injury is related to the type, strength, concentration, duration of contact, and mechanism of action. Chemical agents may be divided into several groups, depending on the mechanism by which they coagulate protein and cause tissue necrosis. Chemicals are categorized into broad groups of acidic or alkaline, and attempts to neutralize the agent can increase the thermal reaction and extent of tissue injury.

Electrical injury is produced by the conversion of electrical energy into heat and from the direct physicochemical effects of electrical current on tissue. The amount of current flowing in a circuit is directly proportional to voltage and inversely proportional to resistance. The quantity of heat produced by an electric current is related to the amount of voltage, the resistance of the conductor, and the duration of contact. Each type of tissue within the body absorbs the heat energy according to its own electrical resistance. Electrical current proceeds down the path of least resistance, which is through nerves, blood vessels, and muscles, sparing the skin except at the entry and exit points of the current.[8] Thus,

BOX 32-1 American Burn Association Criteria for Burn Center Transfer and Referral

Patients meeting the following criteria should be transferred or admitted to a burn unit:

- Second-degree burns greater than 10% TBSA
- Full-thickness burns greater than 5% TBSA
- Any burn involving the face, hands, feet, eyes, ears, or perineum
- Any burn that may result in cosmetic or functional disability
- Circumferential burns of the chest or extremities
- Inhalation injury and associated trauma
- Chemical burns
- Electrical burns, including lightning injury
- Significant comorbid conditions (diabetes mellitus, chronic obstructive pulmonary disease, cardiac disease)

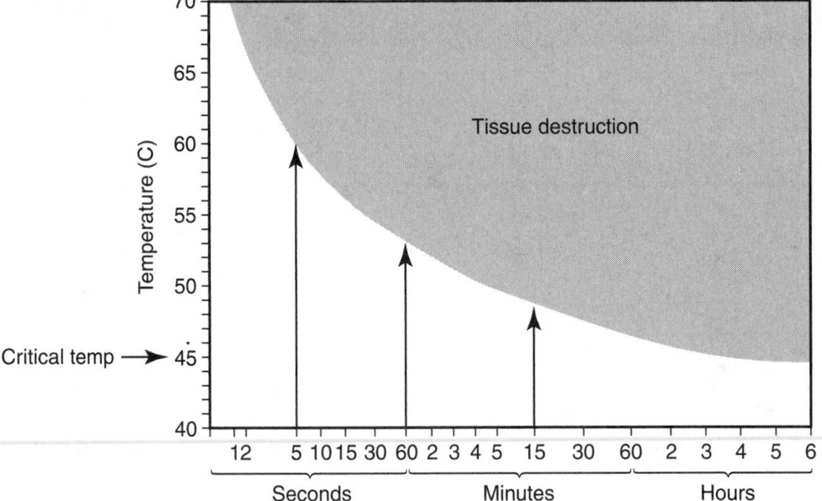

FIGURE 32-1 Temperature duration curve. Tissue destruction proceeds logarithmically, with increasing temperatures as a function of time exposure.

most injuries caused by this mechanism consist of internal deep tissue damage, impairing the ability to accurately determine the true extent of injury.

Radiation burns are the least common burn injuries. Tissue injury can occur from therapeutic levels of radiation used for cancer therapy. Ionizing radiation injury may result from small-scale laboratory or treatment unintentional exposure, large industrial incidents such as nuclear reactor leaks, or explosions and nuclear weapon detonation.

Regardless of the causative agent, the resulting tissue damage creates an injury pattern. Burn wounds can be conceptualized as having three zones (Figure 32-2) representing damage to the tissues resulting from transfer of heat. The central zone of coagulation is an area of irreversible tissue necrosis, or full-thickness burn. Immediately surrounding the necrotic zone is the zone of stasis, characterized by impaired blood flow.[7,9] This zone may not show areas of coagulation initially but may progress to tissue necrosis if adequate tissue perfusion is not restored to the area during the resuscitation period. The zone of stasis is the area of greatest concern because this area can convert to a deeper wound, creating a larger burn injury and loss of tissue. The outer zone of hyperemia has sustained minimal tissue injury and usually heals rapidly.

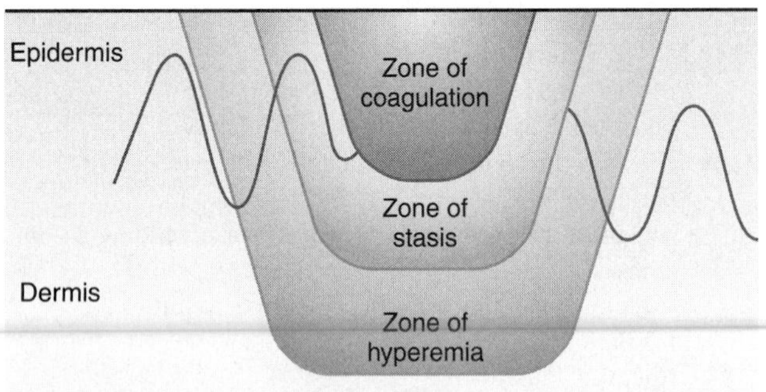

FIGURE 32-2 Zones of thermal injury. Zones of injury represent damage to tissue resulting from transfer of heat. (From Wolf SE, Herndon DN: Burns. In Townsend CM, Beauchamp RD, Evers BM et al, editors: *Sabiston textbook of surgery: the biological basis of modern surgical practice,* 17th ed, Philadelphia, 2004, W. B. Saunders, p. 571.)

When a burn injury occurs, local mediators such as histamine, serotonin, kinins, arachidonic acid metabolites, xanthine oxidase products, complement, cytokines, and catecholamines are released by the body,[6,7,10,11] resulting in arteriolar and venular dilation, increased microvascular permeability, and decreased perfusion. Subsequent extravasation of proteins from the intravascular space increases tissue oncotic pressure, creating edema.[12] Increased levels of the profound vasoconstrictor thromboxane A_2 are found in the plasma and wounds of burn patients. This compound may compromise perfusion, thus enlarging the zone of stasis and converting a partial-thickness wound to a full-thickness injury.[7,10] Concurrently during tissue injury, the coagulation system is activated, causing platelet aggregation. Polymorphonuclear neutrophil (PMN) leukocytes and macrophages are present and release multiple cytokines that are essential to wound healing. The summation of the activation of the intense inflammatory response is vascular stasis and rapid formation of tissue edema.

A primary goal in the initial management of a patient with a burn injury focuses on providing adequate fluid resuscitation to restore circulating volume and minimize conversion of the zone of stasis to necrosis or full-thickness tissue injury. Other initial goals focus on maintaining normal tissue oxygenation, preventing hypothermia, and managing pain.

Extent and Depth of Injury

Two important concepts in the clinical diagnosis and management of burn injuries are the extent and depth of burn injury. The *extent of burn* refers to the total surface area of injured tissue. This is usually calculated as percentage of TBSA by use of either the Berkow,[13] Lund-Browder,[14] or rule-of-nines formula. With any of the burn calculation assessment tools, the clinician's goal is to estimate the amount of tissue damaged by the exchange of thermal energy.

The Berkow and the Lund-Browder charts are more accurate assessment tools. They divide the body into multiple areas and take into consideration changes in the contribution of the head and legs from infancy to adulthood (Figure 32-3).

BURN ESTIMATE AND DIAGRAM

AGE vs. AREA

AREA	Birth 1 yr	1 – 4 yr	5 – 9 yr	10 – 14 yr	15 yr	Adult	2°	3°	Total	Donor Areas
Head	19	17	13	11	9	7				
Neck	2	2	2	2	2	2				
Ant. Trunk	13	13	13	13	13	13				
Post. Trunk	13	13	13	13	13	13				
R. Buttock	2 1/2	2 1/2	2 1/2	2 1/2	2 1/2	2 1/2				
L. Buttock	2 1/2	2 1/2	2 1/2	2 1/2	2 1/2	2 1/2				
Genitalia	1	1	1	1	1	1				
R.U. Arm	4	4	4	4	4	4				
L.U. Arm	4	4	4	4	4	4				
R.L. Arm	3	3	3	3	3	3				
L.L. Arm	3	3	3	3	3	3				
R. Hand	2 1/2	2 1/2	2 1/2	2 1/2	2 1/2	2 1/2				
L. Hand	2 1/2	2 1/2	2 1/2	2 1/2	2 1/2	2 1/2				
R. Thigh	5 1/2	6 1/2	8	8 1/2	9	9 1/2				
L. Thigh	5 1/2	6 1/2	8	8 1/2	9	9 1/2				
R. Leg	5	5	5 1/2	6	6 1/2	7				
L. Leg	5	5	5 1/2	6	6 1/2	7				
R. Foot	3 1/2	3 1/2	3 1/2	3 1/2	3 1/2	3 1/2				
L. Foot	3 1/2	3 1/2	3 1/2	3 1/2	3 1/2	3 1/2				
						TOTAL				

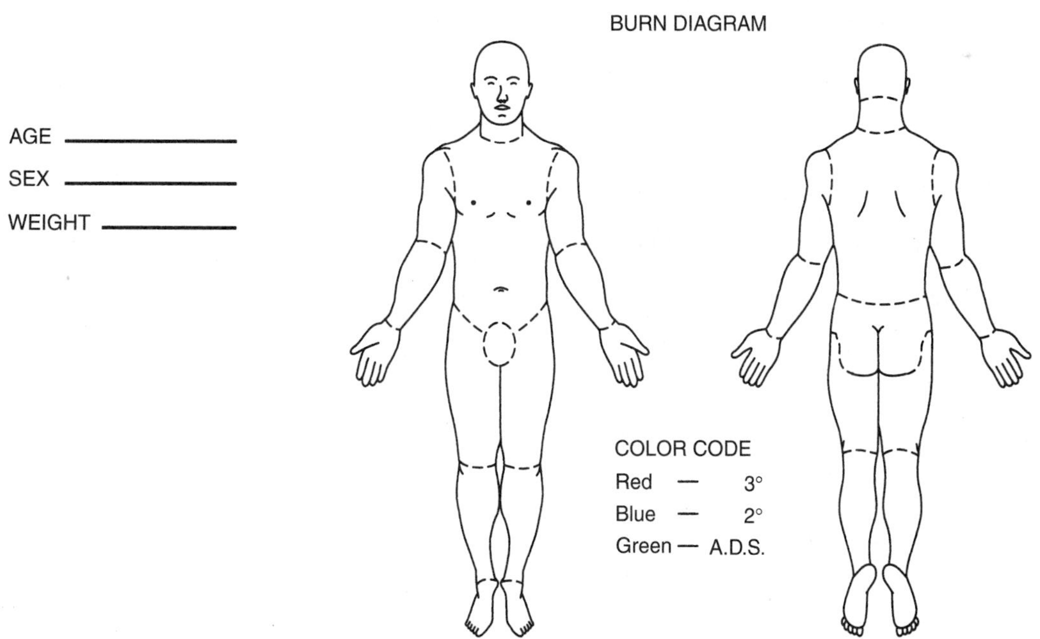

FIGURE 32-3 Burn diagram and table based on the Lund-Browder method of calculating burn size. Based on the Lund and Browder chart with Berkow's formula, it allows for more accurate assessment of the extent of burn injury based on age and depth of injury. *Ant.*, Anterior; *Post.*, posterior; *L.*, left; *R.*, right; *R.U.*, right upper; *R.L.*, right lower; *L.U.*, left upper; *L.L.*, left lower; *A.D.S.*, available donor site. (From LaBorde P, Willis J: Burns. In Sole ML, Lamborn ML, Hartshorn JC, editors: *Introduction to critical care nursing,* 3rd ed, Philadelphia, 2000, W. B. Saunders, p. 612.)

The rule of nines is easy to remember and provides a rapid, gross estimate of the extent of burn.[15] With this method, the body is divided into seven areas that represent 9% or multiples of 9% of the body surface area, with the remaining area, the genitalia, representing 1% of TBSA (Figure 32-4).

The last method of determining the extent of TBSA injured uses the size of the patient's hand, assuming that the palmar surface of the hand is roughly 1% of TBSA. Visualizing the patient's hand covering the burn wound approximates the amount of body surface area involved.[11]

Regardless of the method used to calculate TBSA, estimation of the burned area is somewhat subjective, with instances of clinical discrepancy. The primary goals in estimating the TBSA involved in the burn are to predict mortality, morbidity, physiologic response in relation to fluid shifts, fluid resuscitation requirement, and metabolic and immunologic responses.

The concept of depth of burn injury is an important predictor of survival and overall morbidity, to include surgical management, functional outcome, and cosmesis. Descriptions of the depth of burn are often confusing because a variety of nomenclature is used (Table 32-1). In general the *burn wound depth* describes tissue damage according to the anatomic thickness of the skin involved, as determined by the clinician (Figure 32-5).[7] As a general rule, the more superficial the burn wound, the more rapidly the wound heals. When a burn injury is assessed, skin layers are not visible to the naked eye. Thus, when the depth of a burn injury is determined, it is helpful to remember that the dermis is the layer that will bleed.[16] Superficial and full-thickness burns do not bleed because the epidermis and subcutaneous layer are avascular. The greater the tissue loss (e.g., deep partial-thickness and full-thickness injury), the greater the likelihood that surgical grafting will be needed to optimize healing, limit infection, and maximize cosmesis.

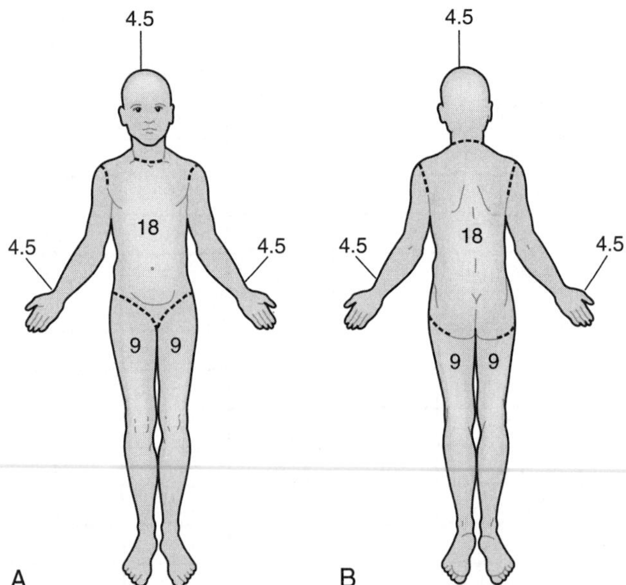

FIGURE 32-4 An estimate of the percentage of total body surface area (percent TBSA) burned can be obtained using the rule of nines, where TBSA is divided into 9% segments of the total. Second- and third-degree burns are added and presented as a percentage of total skin. (From Wolf SE, Herndon DN: Burns. In Townsend CM, Beauchamp RD, Evers BM et al, editors: *Sabiston textbook of surgery: the biological basis of modern surgical practice*, 17th ed, p. 572, Philadelphia, 2004, Elsevier Saunders.)

TISSUE INJURY AND THE IMMUNOLOGIC RESPONSE

In the past decade, much knowledge has been amassed about the relationship of tissue injury and immunologic response to burn injury. Research into the histochemical response to tissue injury continues to elucidate the mechanisms of inflammation, infection, acute respiratory distress syndrome (ARDS), sepsis, systemic inflammatory response syndrome (SIRS),

TABLE 32-1 Classification of Depth of Burn Injury

	First Degree	Second Degree	Third Degree	
By skin thickness	Superficial	Superficial partial thickness	Deep partial thickness	Full thickness
By anatomic description	Epidermal	Epidermal and superficial dermal	Deep dermal	Full dermal tissue loss and possibly subdermal (fat, muscle, bone)
Appearance/description of depth	Pink to red; no blisters; skin remains intact when rubbed gently; may appear slightly edematous	Red or mottled red to pink; blisters; skin easily rubbed off; moist, weeping, edematous; if pulled, hair remains intact; blanches with pressure	Pink to pale ivory; can see a reticulated pattern; wound may appear somewhat dry; contains blisters and bullae; hair removes easily; does not blanch with pressure or return of color is slow	White, cherry red, brown, or black; may or may not contain blisters; may contain thrombosed vessels; appears dry, hard, leathery; may be depressed
Pain response	Uncomfortable/painful to touch	Very painful	Pain response is variable, hyperalgesia and hypoalgesia	Insensate or pain is aching in nature
Time to heal	3-5 days	Less than 3 weeks	More than 3 weeks	Requires grafting

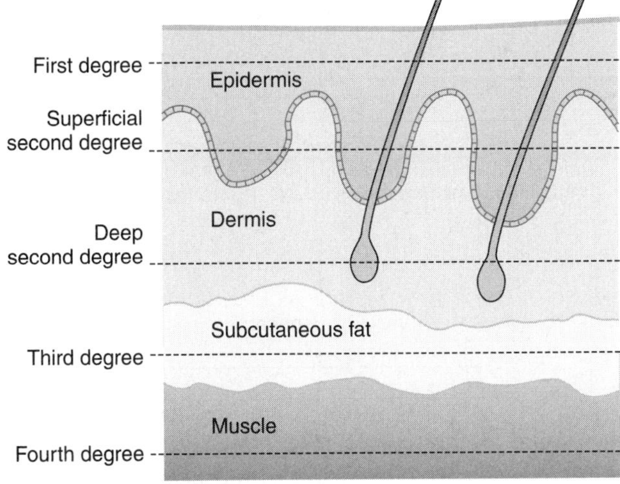

FIGURE 32-5 Burn wound depth. (From Wolf SE, Herndon DN: Burns. In Townsend CM, Beauchamp RD, Evers BM et al, editors: *Sabiston textbook of surgery: the biological basis of modern surgical practice,* 17th ed, Philadelphia, 2004, W. B. Saunders, p. 571.)

and multiple organ dysfunction syndrome (MODS).[17,18] *Tissue injury related to burns* refers not only to the local response of the coagulation produced by heat but also to the local and systemic responses that lead to inflammation, immunocompromise, fluid shifts, and ultimately MODS if proper treatment is not provided. Certain risk factors, such as age 50 years or older, a full-thickness burn of 30% or greater TBSA, male sex, inhalation injury, and infection (sepsis), have an increased association with MODS in burn victims.[18-21] In addition, severe compromise to the immune system occurs in burns of greater than 40% TBSA,[11] overwhelming all cellular components of the immune system.[7] Research continues to enhance the understanding of and treatments for local and systemic inflammatory processes that result in fluid shifts and altered tissue perfusion (burn shock) (Figure 32-6).

The pathophysiologic effects related to burn injury (greater than 20% TBSA)[22] and acute inflammatory processes are both local and systemic. The microcirculation compromise is greatest 12 to 24 hours after a burn is sustained.[6,21] The goals of therapy are to control the exaggerated inflammatory cytokine cascade response and restore the microcirculatory perfusion of tissues.[17] Collectively, inflammatory mediators produce vasoconstriction, vasodilation, increased capillary permeability, activation of the coagulation cascade, and progressive and rapid edema formation with altered microcirculatory perfusion. These complex interactions of inflammatory mediators are tightly interwoven in both physiologic and pathophysiologic states. Mediators leave the confines of the local tissue injury and move to the systemic circulation, causing alterations in organ function remote from the site of injury.[17] In large burn injuries, cytokine activities appear to create a state of exaggerated or reactivated inflammation, causing distant organ involvement (e.g., ARDS, SIRS, and eventually MODS).[17]

In summary, the exaggerated activation of the inflammatory cascades produces microvasculature-induced cardiopulmonary changes marked by loss of plasma volume, increased peripheral vascular resistance, and subsequent decreased cardiac output. Renal blood flow is altered, resulting in renal dysfunction. Activation of the stress response causes mild respiratory alkalosis and hypoxemia, which is complicated by increased pulmonary capillary permeability, resulting in decreased pulmonary compliance and function. Metabolic changes are highlighted by an early depression followed by marked and sustained increases in resting energy expenditure, lipolysis, proteolysis, and oxygen consumption.[22] Eventually, generalized impairment of host defenses, depression of immunoglobulins, and fatigued immune response make the burned patient prone to infections. Promising advances in the treatment of burn sepsis exist with use of venovenous continuous renal replacement therapy and continuous plasma filtration-coupled adsorption.[21] These therapies may be effective in removing vasoactive circulating cytokines and endotoxins.[21,23]

Metabolic Response to Tissue Injury

The metabolic response to burn injury has been studied extensively. As early as 1930, Cuthbertson[24] described the biphasic metabolic response to injury. He noted increased fluid shifts, urinary nitrogen losses, and losses of other intracellular substances such as potassium and phosphorus. In subsequent years the studies of the catabolic response to injury documented increased oxygen consumption, negative nitrogen balance, exaggerated hypermetabolism and catabolism, excessive muscle wasting, and weight loss in burned patients. The degree of catabolism that occurs with burn injury has been found to correlate with increasing morbidity and mortality rates[25]; thus, early interventions in treatment attempted to attenuate the hypermetabolic response associated with burn injury. The intensity of the metabolic changes in burn patients is directly related to the extent of injury.[22,26] Metabolic demands increase by an estimated 30% in patients with an injury covering 20% of the TBSA or more and by 100% in patients with burns covering 50% of the TBSA or more.[22] Other factors associated with burn management, such as extensive dressing changes, thermoregulation, pain, infection, presence of inhalation injury, and sepsis also significantly increase metabolic response and energy expenditure needs.[22,25,26]

The resting energy expenditure (REE) after a burn injury can be as much as 200% greater than normal,[7] creating a hypermetabolic drive. Burn hypermetabolism is the result of multiple mechanisms associated with hormonal changes. After a burn injury, inflammatory mediators stimulate the hypothalamus, increasing the body's central thermoregulatory set point and altering endocrine function. Levels of catecholamines, cortisol, and glucagon are markedly elevated, initiating the catabolic response seen in burn patients. The presence of catecholamines increases the rates of glycogenolysis and hepatic gluconeogenesis and promotes lipolysis and peripheral insulin resistance.[27] The exaggerated metabolic response and excessive mobilization of glucose for energy requirements are needed for wound healing. When adequate glucose cannot be supplied, the result is excessive

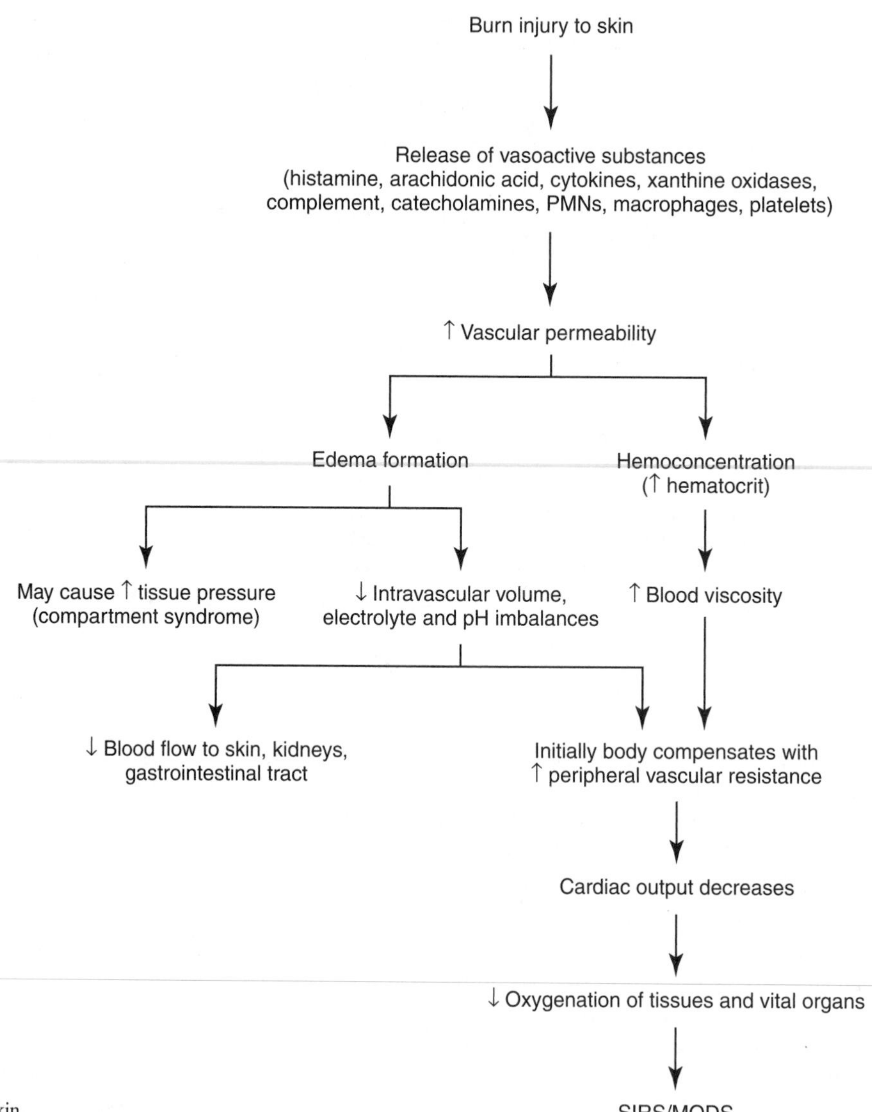

FIGURE 32-6 Physiologic response to burned skin.

protein catabolism.[22,26] Thus, early nutritional interventions, with particular emphasis on meeting the REE, cannot be overemphasized. Recent research indicates that β-blockade with an agent such as propranolol, which reduces tachycardia by 15% to 20%, eases the hypermetabolic state induced by a large burn injury. The REE is lowered and muscle catabolism is reduced, thus improving patient outcomes.[7,20,25,27-29]

The sympathetic response seems to be the major determinant of the metabolic response to burn injury. The sympathetic nervous system can be stimulated by a variety of responses, including lower-than-normal environmental temperatures, pain, psychologic responses, and the body's response to inflammatory mediators. It would seem that the use of nutritional replacement formulas based only on the size of the burn injury may not be accurate. Caution must be used in the application of standard nutritional replacement formulas; nutritional goals and end points should be reassessed and adjusted more often as the burn wound heals. Chapter 17 provides a thorough discussion of nutritional assessment parameters and formulas that may be used to guide nutritional interventions for burn-injured patients.

Optimally, nutritional replacement therapy in the burn patient should be based on frequent measurements of oxygen consumption obtained with the use of a metabolic cart. (See Chapter 17 for a discussion of the advantages and disadvantages of metabolic carts.) Nutritional formulas[7,22] vary as much as resuscitation formulas, and there is little consensus as to which is most appropriate. In part, this lack of consensus has to do with the great variability in nutritional needs from patient to patient and for the same patient over time. This is why actual measurement of oxygen consumption allows more accurate nutritional repletion.[22]

MANAGEMENT OF THE PATIENT WITH A BURN INJURY

PHYSIOLOGICAL RESPONSE: CHANGES IN HEMODYNAMICS

The body's initial response to a burn injury leads to a shift in fluids from the vascular space into the interstitial and intracellular spaces. When the burn involves large areas of skin (e.g., more than 20% TBSA), the hemodynamic and inflammatory response is an overall systemic response, with fluids shifting into interstitial spaces throughout the body. This massive fluid shift may lead to hypovolemic shock. To prevent shock, fluid resuscitation after burn injury is maintained for 24 to 48 hours after injury.[30,31] The challenge during fluid resuscitation is to restore adequate circulating volume that prevents complications from underperfusion of organs and burned tissue without overresuscitating and creating problems from excessive volume replacement.

A number of formulas have been suggested for optimal fluid replacement after a burn injury. No formula is precisely prescriptive in fluid resuscitation, but the formulas provide guidelines for fluid replacement on the basis of TBSA burned and end-organ assessment parameters. All formulas calculate the amount of fluid replacement from the time of the burn injury and estimated TBSA burn injury size. Some of the early formulas, such as the Evans formula and the original Brooke formula, recommended a mixture of sodium-containing fluids and colloid because both sodium-rich fluids and plasma proteins are lost during fluid shifts with burn injury. The use of colloids is controversial. The SAFE (Saline versus Albumin Fluid Evaluation) study found no significant differences between groups of patients treated with colloid or normal saline solution for fluid resuscitation.[32] In burn-injured patients, the use of colloids in the first 12 hours has been associated with less favorable outcomes; therefore, albumin administration is not recommended until at least 12 hours after the burn.[21] The Baxter (Parkland) formula supports the concept that plasma given in the first 24 hours is no more effective than Ringer's lactate solution alone in maintaining normal plasma volume. The Monafo and Warden formulas focus on the administration of hypertonic saline solution as a means of limiting edema and they require a lower total amount of fluids than do other formulas. Caution is warranted in the administration of hypertonic solutions because the concentrations of hypertonic solutions are not standardized and have been associated with an increased incidence of morbidity and poor outcomes. Hypertonic solutions should be used by experienced providers to avoid complications associated with administration of these concentrated fluids.[21] The Demling formula incorporates the use of low-molecular-weight dextran in resuscitation formulas, with the goal of preventing edema in nonburned tissues. The consensus formula[33] combines concepts, using crystalloid and colloid administration at various times in the fluid resuscitation process. Table 32-2 outlines the available formulas for calculating the fluid resuscitation requirements for burned patients. No matter what formula is used, it must be viewed only as a guideline.[21,31] Fluids should be carefully titrated by 20% increments[34] to physiologic end points,[21] and overresuscitation should be avoided.

The controversy over which resuscitation formula to use is similar to the controversy over which parameters to follow to assess the adequacy of resuscitation. Effective end-organ perfusion is usually assessed by measurement of the normal function or output of the specific organ system. Central nervous system function is measured by evaluating the patient's level of consciousness. Normal gastrointestinal system function is inferred by the return of normal bowel sounds and absence of ileus.

Kidney function is monitored by measuring urine output, urine specific gravity, the urine glucose level, and the urine electrolyte content. Hourly urine volume from 0.5 to 1 ml/kg is often cited as reflecting effective renal perfusion; however, this urine output range has not been supported by clinical trials. To date, clinical trials have not revealed ideal urine output measurements for evaluating renal and other end-organ perfusion during burn shock resuscitation.[21,35] In evaluating urine output as evidence of adequate perfusion, the practitioner should keep in mind that diuresis can occur as a result of glucosuria in response to stress or as a response to hypertonic saline solution or dextran administration during resuscitation; therefore, additional end point parameters should be used to validate the adequacy of the fluid resuscitation.[21]

Because of the early release of catecholamines and venoconstriction during burn shock states, blood pressure may be artificially elevated in relation to the degree of hypovolemia.[21] Additionally, noninvasive blood pressure measurements may be inaccurate because of significant edema formation in the interstitium. Thus, trends obtained from frequent monitoring of blood pressure may not reflect the status of resuscitation. Pulse pressure may be a more accurate assessment of tissue perfusion pressures. Pulse pressure is easy to measure and correlates well with stroke volume. It is obtained by subtracting diastolic pressure from systolic pressure. Narrowing or decreased pulse pressure (less than 25 mm Hg) is an earlier indicator of shock than is a decline in systolic blood pressure.[21]

Frequent monitoring of the heart rate may be useful in assessing and monitoring the cardiovascular response to resuscitation. The heart rate is elevated during the initial phase of burn injury because of catecholamine release. Changes in heart rate, or decreases in heart rate, can be used to gauge effective management of resuscitation.[20] In an elderly patient or a patient with cardiac disease, however, the heart rate may not increase as the patient becomes hypovolemic; thus, heart rate is a less reliable measure of resuscitation in these patients, and trends in increased heart rates need to be evaluated.

Other cardiovascular parameters that may be monitored include central venous pressure, pulmonary artery wedge pressure (PAWP), mixed or central venous oxygen saturation,[36] and cardiac output. Filling pressures are often very low for the first 24 hours after a burn, and any efforts to improve filling pressures during this period may result in overresuscitation. As long as other measurements of tissue perfusion are within normal ranges, the temptation to improve filling pressures should be resisted.[21] Likewise, cardiac outputs are often very low in the first 24 hours and then trend upward over the second and third 24 hours until they are one and a half to two times normal. This is thought to result from the hypermetabolic response observed in patients with larger burns. Thus, the use of invasive monitoring devices, such as pulmonary artery (PA) catheters for measurement of PAWP and cardiac output, adds little to the

TABLE 32-2 **Fluid Resuscitation Formulas**

Baxter (Parkland) formula	*First 24 Hours* Lactated Ringer's solution (4 ml/kg/% TBSA), half given over first 8 hours after injury; remaining half given over next 16 hours *Second 24 Hours* Dextrose in water, plus K^+ Colloid-containing fluid at 20%-60% of calculated plasma volume (0.35-0.5 ml/kg/% TBSA)
Consensus formula	*First 24 Hours* Adults: Lactated Ringer's solution (2-4 ml/kg/% TBSA) Children: Lactated Ringer's solution(3-4 ml/kg/% TBSA), half given over first 8 hours; remaining half given over next 16 hours *Second 24 Hours* Adults: Colloid-containing fluid (0.3-0.5 ml/kg/% TBSA) and electrolyte-free fluid to maintain adequate urine output Children: Colloid-containing fluid (0.3-0.5 ml/kg/% TBSA) and half normal saline solution to maintain adequate urine output
Modified Brooke formula	*First 24 Hours* Lactated Ringer's solution (2 ml/kg/% TBSA), half given over first 8 hours; remaining half given over next 16 hours *Second 24 Hours* Colloid solution (0.3-0.5 ml/kg/% TBSA) plus 5% dextrose in water to maintain adequate urine output
Monafo formula (hypertonic saline solution)	*First 24 Hours* Na^+ 250 mEq/L, volume infused to maintain urine output at 0.5 ml/kg/hr (approximately 30 ml/hr) *Second 24 Hours* 33% isotonic salt solution (0.6% ml/kg/% TBSA) plus replacement of insensible losses
Modified Warden formula (hypertonic saline solution) for burns <40% TBSA	*First 8 Hours* 180 mEq/L Na^+ (mix 50 mEq/L $NaHCO^3$ in lactated Ringer's solution), 4 ml/kg/% TBSA; adjust to maintain urine output of 30-50 ml/hr *Second 8 Hours After Burn* Lactated Ringer's solution at rate to maintain urine output of 30-50 ml/hr
Dextran (Demling) formula	*First 8 Hours* Dextran 40 in saline solution (2 ml/kg/hr) Lactated Ringer's solution infused to maintain urine output at 30 ml/hr *Second 8 Hours After Burn* Fresh frozen plasma (0.5 ml/kg/hr) for 18 hours, plus additional crystalloid to maintain adequate urine output

ability to monitor resuscitation and may increase long-term morbidity because of the increased risk of infectious complications. However, in the elderly patient, the cardiac patient, or the patient with severe inhalation injury, the use of a PA catheter or monitoring of central venous pressures to guide fluid resuscitation is advised.[6,21] Controversy continues to surround the concept of hyperdynamic resuscitation guided by oxygen transport and consumption parameters, which is not a current standard of practice.[21]

Acid-base balance is another indicator of the effectiveness of fluid resuscitation. A base deficit and elevated serum lactate levels occur in hypoxic conditions and states of poor tissue perfusion. Base deficit manifests as metabolic acidosis and corrects to normal with adequate resuscitation. A base deficit of 6 mEq/L or greater is an indicator of shock at 24 hours after the burn, and elevated serum lactate levels have been associated with increased mortality rates.[18,21,30] The base deficit may remain elevated in the presence of adequate urine output and mean arterial pressures. Thus, base deficit and serum lactate have been found to be better markers of effective resuscitation.[21,30]

Fluid requirements are increased when patients also have inhalation injury, require mechanical ventilation, have increased full-thickness injury, have electrical burn injury, experience a delay in resuscitation, and are dehydrated.[31,34] Maximizing fluid resuscitation to improve tissue perfusion without overresuscitating remains the challenge. Complications of significantly increased volume resuscitation include compartment syndrome of the extremities or abdomen. Patients with circumferential deep and full-thickness wounds are at the greatest risk for development of compartment pressure complications. Compartment syndrome may be an early problem because fluid shifts and maximal edema occur during fluid resuscitation. Neurovascular assessment and direct compartment tissue pressures should be assessed in patients with circumferential extremity burns. Tissue compartment pressures greater than 20 mm Hg indicate compromised perfusion and pressures greater than 40 mm Hg suggest significantly compromised perfusion. In these cases, escharotomy, fasciotomy, or both are usually needed to release the pressure and expand the tissue compartment. Abdominal compartment syndrome (ACS) has been associated with a mortality rate of 60% to 100%. Although the incidence of ACS is not well described in the burn literature, it may be associated with concurrent blast injury and gross fluid overresuscitation.[37,38] Estimated fluid resuscitation requirements should be recalculated 12 hours after the burn injury and, if the volume calculated for fluid replacement exceeds 6 ml/kg/% TBSA, interventions to minimize complications of overresuscitation should be implemented. Some interventions that may be considered are as follow:

- Initiate 5% albumin described in the Modified Brooke Formula.
- Monitor bladder pressures every 4 hours for increased abdominal pressure greater than 20 mm Hg.
- Monitor central venous pressures, pulmonary artery pressures, and cardiac output to trend effectiveness of resuscitative efforts.

Persistent hypotension and decreased urine output in the presence of adequate preload may indicate the need to add inotropic support. If the patient is exhibiting catecholamine-resistant shock, consider occult blood loss, acidemia, adrenal insufficiency, or hypocalcemia.

In summary, adequate fluid resuscitation is needed to survive a burn injury. Appropriate fluid resuscitation limits the extent of burn injury and reduces morbidity. For most burned patients, frequent monitoring of urine output, urine glucose level, heart rate, pulse pressure, central venous pressure, sensorium, airway pressures, base deficit, and lactate levels allows assessment of the adequacy of resuscitation and organ-specific perfusion. These parameters, when monitored together, allow evaluation of effective tissue perfusion.

Nutritional Management

The nutritional needs of most burn patients can be met with a mixture of glucose, essential amino acids, and fats. Glucose is the primary source of energy for wound healing, and supplementation with lipids prevents severe hyperglycemia.[39] In addition to the major nutrients, vitamins and minerals are important in wound healing. As mentioned previously, multiple formulas exist for estimating the nutritional needs of the burned patient. Hart et al[40] have found that increasing caloric requirements relative to energy expenditure does not preserve lean body mass and that overfeeding is associated with increased fat mass, increased need for ventilatory support, and lengthened intensive care unit stay. These researchers recommend nutritional intake of no more than 1.4 × REE kcal/day to prevent catabolism.[40] Regardless of which formula is used, several principles need to be followed:

- Nutritional assessment and reassessment must be frequent and continual throughout the course of the healing process.
- Enteral tube feedings should begin within 24 hours after the burn to decrease production of catabolic hormones, improve nitrogen balance, and maintain gut mucosal integrity.[11,39]
- Increased protein consumption is critical to survival and rehabilitation of the burned patient.[39]
- Anabolic hormone (e.g., oxandrolone) administration should be considered to attenuate muscle wasting and improve net protein balance.[20,41]

As a part of nutritional management, electrolyte balances should be evaluated and imbalances corrected. Frequent measurement of serum sodium, potassium, chloride, phosphorus, calcium, and magnesium levels is necessary to prevent major electrolyte derangements. In addition, deficiencies in trace metals may occur in the burn patient; thus it is recommended that zinc, copper, manganese, and chromium levels be measured periodically and replaced if found deficient. Zinc is an important cofactor in wound healing and tends to be deficient after burn injury. Glutamine is a free amino acid that provides fuel for lymphocytes, macrophages, and fibroblasts. Glutamine supplementation has been shown to reduce the incidence of gram-negative bacteremia in severely burned patients[42] and to minimize the loss of lean muscle mass in burn-injured patients.[22] Nutritional support teams should be used to evaluate the continuing and changing nutritional needs of the burn injured patient. All efforts to maximize nutritional status of the burn patient are necessary for successful recovery, wound healing, and rehabilitation. See Chapter 17 for further discussions on nutritional interventions.

Management of Pulmonary Injury

Pulmonary injury may result from inhaling the byproducts of smoke or from a systemic process related to SIRS or MODS. Inhalation injury may or may not injure lung tissue directly. One possible component of inhalation injury is carbon monoxide intoxication. Carbon monoxide does not affect the lining of the lung but competes with oxygen for uptake by hemoglobin, thus acting as an asphyxiant. Because hemoglobin has 200 times more affinity for carbon monoxide than for oxygen, carbon monoxide replaces oxygen, reducing oxygen delivery to tissues. This may lead to severe anoxia and brain injury. In addition, carbon monoxide combines with myoglobin in muscle cells and the cytochrome oxidase system of the brain, producing muscle weakness and coma, respectively. The initial effects of muscle weakness and confusion from decreased oxygen uptake occur within about 5 minutes of exposure and may contribute to the person's inability to escape from the fire. The long-term neurologic effects occasionally associated with smoke inhalation are most likely related to both prolonged anoxia and inhibition of the cytochrome oxidase system of the brain. A carboxyhemoglobin (COHb) level above 20% at the time of exposure will cause neurologic effects; a level above 60% may be fatal.[43] Carbon monoxide has a half-life of 4 hours if the patient breathes room air and 1 hour if the patient is breathing 100% oxygen. COHb levels measured in the emergency department must be interpreted in relation to the time after exposure and the concentration of oxygen administered to the patient since the exposure.[43] Thus, a person with 25% COHb after breathing 100% oxygen for 1 hour probably had a level of about 50% COHb at the time of exposure. Treatment for suspected COHb exposure is 100% oxygen until measured serum levels of COHb are less than 10%.[44] In addition, caution must be exercised with the use of pulse oximetry equipment as an evaluative tool for oxygen saturation. Pulse oximetry is inaccurate in the presence of elevated COHb.

Other components of inhalation injury are upper airway injury and chemical injury to the lung parenchyma. Upper airway injury is the result of inhaling superheated air, which may cause blisters and edema in the supraglottic area around the vocal cords. This may cause upper airway occlusion and is best treated with early endotracheal intubation. Tracheobronchial and parenchymal lung injuries are caused by the inhalation of a variety of chemicals (e.g., oxides of sulfur and nitrogen, aldehydes, and acrolein) that are byproducts of combustion. Although the exact mechanics of injury may differ, thermal and chemical insult to the major airways and lung parenchyma cause the ciliated epithelial cells to separate from the basement membrane and the systemic and bronchial circulation of the lung to dilate, with protein and water shifts increasing interstitial edema.[7,45] The tracheobronchial casts formed by the deposition of proteins and fibrin in the airways are difficult to remove with standard suction techniques, requiring bronchoscopic lavage for removal.[7] The loss of the mucociliary system results in ineffective bacterial clearing and predisposes the patient to pulmonary infections and sepsis.[46] Thus a patient with mild inhalation injury who maintains a strong cough reflex should be extubated as soon as possible to facilitate clearing the airway and reduce the risk of nosocomial pneumonia.[7,46] Damage to type II pneumocytes[44,45] decreases surfactant production, causing the development of microatelectasis, increased airway pressures, and ventilation-perfusion mismatches. Hemorrhagic tracheobronchitis, increased interstitial edema, and decreased macrophage function are additional sequelae seen with inhalation injury. Sloughing of the airway mucosa and intrapulmonary hemorrhage causes mechanical obstruction that can be removed with inhaled bronchodilators and mechanical bronchoscopic clearing.[44,47] Treatment with aerosolized heparin alone or with *N*-acetylcysteine may facilitate removal of the copious secretions associated with inhalation injury. The addition of β-blockers attenuates the bronchoconstriction associated with the injury and use of aerosolized heparin.[7,43,47,48] Management efforts are focused on limiting the inflammatory response and fluid sequestration in an effort to avoid the complications of ARDS and pneumonia.

As mentioned, most of the 6% of all burned patients who do not survive have had an inhalation injury. Diagnosis of inhalation injury is based on the patient's presentation (Box 32-2), history of injury, and the findings on fiberoptic bronchoscopy or, if available, a xenon 133 ventilation-perfusion scan. A chest radiograph is helpful in establishing baseline data but typically does not assist in the early diagnosis of inhalation injury.

The treatment of inhalation injury primarily consists of supportive care to maintain a patent airway for oxygenation and ventilation while the lungs heal. Of early primary concern is the need for an increased volume of fluid resuscitation.[31,34,49] Although patients with inhalation injury require additional fluid resuscitation to maintain organ perfusion, excessive fluid resuscitation may lead to fluid overload and further compromise of pulmonary function. Pulmonary edema is not prevented by fluid restriction and can worsen patient outcomes.[7]

For the patient with minimal injury, the administration of warm, humidified oxygen and incentive spirometry may allow adequate oxygenation and facilitate clearance of secretions. In patients with mild injury, maintenance of ventilatory and oxygenation support, pulmonary hygiene, and prevention of infection and atelectasis are of prime importance.

For the patient with more severe disease, early endotracheal intubation and mechanical ventilation are needed. The preferred mode of ventilatory support remains undecided; suggested modes include interrupted-flow, high-frequency oscillary or percussive ventilation, pressure control ventilation, permissive hypercapnia ventilation, and low versus high tidal volume ventilation.[6,47,49-51] Adjunctive oxygenation therapies and high positive end-expiratory pressure may prove beneficial in the management of the burn patient

BOX 32-2 Characteristics Suggesting Inhalation Injury

- Burn injury occurred in a closed space
- Edema and redness of the oropharynx/nasopharynx
- Hoarse, brassy voice
- Shortness of breath
- Tachypnea, wheezing, stridor
- Carbonaceous sputum, singed nasal and facial hair
- Anxiety
- Disorientation progressing to obtundation and coma

with severe inhalation injury. Prophylactic antibiotic therapy is typically contraindicated and is associated with microbe resistance; however, when pneumonia is suspected, broad-spectrum antibiotic coverage is indicated.[44-46] Routine use of bronchoalveolar lavage to diagnose ventilator-related pneumonia in this population has not been shown superior to standard diagnostic methods[52] in terms of clinical outcomes or antibiotic use.[44,53] Research has concluded that the method of determining pneumonia is of less consequence than use of the appropriate antibiotic. Management of inhalation injury requires continual evaluation of the following:

- The patient's response to therapy
- Severity of airway edema and edema resolution
- Oxygenation and ventilation parameters
- Signs and symptoms of pulmonary infection. Preventing infection is an important management goal for patients with inhalation injury.

Abdominal compartment syndrome is a serious problem associated with the development of burn edema; it manifests as respiratory compromise. The increased diffuse capillary leak seen in patients with large burns produces increased fluid translocation into the abdominal compartment. Intra-abdominal pressures and peak airway pressures increase, causing oliguria and difficulties with ventilating.[37,38] Rapid detection of ACS and prompt corrective decompressive laparotomy may be required to support pulmonary function.

Circumferential constriction of the chest wall by full-thickness eschar may also manifest with increasing airway pressures and limited chest wall movement. Escharotomies from the bilateral axillae that follow the diaphragmatic angle create a "plate" that allows for free excursion of the thorax and is an effective treatment for this condition.

Essential to minimize complications from poor oxygenation and ventilation are continued assessment of pulmonary function in patients with large burns or circumferential chest burns, patients requiring large volumes of fluid resuscitation to support tissue perfusion, and patients with inhalation injury.

Management and Prevention of Infection

The skin, the body's largest organ, acts in part as a natural mechanical barrier to microbial attachment, growth, and penetration. After burn injury, the protective nature of the skin is lost, and the resulting avascular denatured protein eschar provides an ideal medium for microorganism growth. In addition, invasive devices (e.g., intravenous and urinary drainage catheters, endotracheal tubes [ETTs], nasogastric tubes) provide ports of entry for organisms. The overwhelmed inflammatory response tires, and the patient's ability to fight infection may decrease as the burn-healing process progresses. Infections in the burned patient may involve the urinary tract, pulmonary system, bloodstream, or wound. Differentiation of active infection and colonization is an important element of medical management because all burn wounds are eventually colonized with bacteria.[54] Infection of the burn wound may be diagnosed by histologic study for the presence of organism invasion in a full-thickness biopsy specimen that includes viable tissue, local and systemic signs of infection, and delayed wound healing.[54-57]

In the not-too-distant past, the goal of wound care was to find an optimal antimicrobial cream or solution that would prevent infection and allow the wound to slowly granulate. Eventually the wound was grafted, closing the burn wound. The most common topical antimicrobial agents used to treat burn wounds were mafenide acetate cream, silver sulfadiazine cream, and silver nitrate. Today antimicrobial agents, synthetic dressings, and advanced wound healing products that maximize the wound bed for healing are available to cover burn wounds. Advances in agents that can be used to treat burn wounds are occurring rapidly as the science of wound healing progresses. Table 32-3 provides a sample of common interventions used for temporary coverings of burn wounds.

Current management focuses on the early removal of eschar (devitalized tissue) of deep dermal and full-thickness burns. Surgical debridement of eschar, usually within 48 hours of injury, coupled with aggressive enteral feeding[25,58,59] and use of a variety of biologic and synthetic dressings to cover the wound promotes wound healing and closure. Efforts to cover and close wounds decrease the patent's risk of infection, thereby enhancing overall survival for the patient. Early wound closure has also decreased the length of hospital stay, decreased septic episodes, and enhanced wound cosmesis.[7,20,60] The focus on early wound closure through the use of synthetic dressings or surgical interventions has dramatically improved the survival of burn patients.[20]

In all areas of wound management the maintenance of a clean, well-nourished wound is essential for healing. Burn-specific nursing units have been associated with a decreased rate of infection.[61] Initially, several thorough cleansings of the wound with a nontoxic solution such as a mild soap or chlorhexidine gluconate solution may be necessary to remove wound debris associated with the traumatic event.[55,62] Healing wounds require adequate circulation, so care must be taken to apply a snug dressing that will remain on the wound but that will not restrict blood flow. Maintaining a moist wound environment enhances wound healing and decreases the risk of infection. Similarly, the patient's position must be changed often to reduce pressure and maintain blood flow to dependent areas. Adequate nutrition is also imperative to prevent infection and maximize wound healing.

The use of systemic antibiotics in burn care is not indicated except in those patients with positive cultures[7] or extensive concomitant injuries.[55] Systemic antibiotics are used often in the perioperative period as prophylaxis against infection.[7] In this case it is important to administer the antibiotic so that its peak effectiveness is during the surgical procedure.[55] When systemic antibiotics are used to treat bacteremias or sepsis, it is important to follow blood levels to ensure maximal effectiveness without toxicity and untoward effects. The pharmacokinetics of many drugs change in

TABLE 32-3 **Wound Management Products**

Wound Management Option	Clinical Considerations
Silver nitrate solution	Effective against most gram-positive and some gram-negative organisms Decreased penetration of eschar May produce hyponatremia, hypokalemia, and hypochloremia
Mafenide acetate cream	Effective against wide range of gram-positive and gram-negative organisms Rapidly diffuses through eschar (improved effectiveness in established infections) Painful application Hypersensitivity reactions may occur Acid-base derangements may occur
Silver sulfadiazine cream	Effective against wide range of gram-positive and gram-negative organisms Softens eschar and increases joint mobility Absorbed slowly; reduced chance of nephrotoxicity Hypersensitivity and leukopenia may occur
Enzymatic debridement agents	Provides nonsurgical debridement of denatured tissue May require concurrent antimicrobial coverage to prevent wound infection May be painful and cause bleeding in wound bed
Antibiotic-impregnated dressings	Provide continuous antimicrobial coverage over >24 hours Decreased frequency of dressing changes required although antimicrobial coverage is maintained Dressings must remain moist Hypersensitivity may develop
Biologic dressings	Provide immediate wound coverage and protection until autografting is possible Decrease bacterial proliferation Decrease evaporative water loss Prepare granulation tissue for autografting Hypersensitivity may develop Expense may be prohibitive
Cultured epithelial cells	No rejection Requires 3 weeks to grow skin Cultured skin has decreased tensile strength and may sheer easily after grafting Expense may be prohibitive

burned patients because of the hypermetabolic response, hypoproteinemia, and massive fluid shifts.

ASSOCIATED TRAUMA

A major burn injury with polytrauma poses an unusual and complex management problem.[56,63-65] In the military, burn injuries are associated with a younger population, a longer time from injury to burn center arrival, a higher injury severity score, and a higher incidence of inhalation injury and full-thickness burn injury than in the civilian population; yet the mortality rate between the groups does not differ.[64,65] Combined burn and trauma civilian patients have a twofold to threefold increased incidence of inhalation injury, a longer hospital stay, and dramatically higher mortality rates than a patient with only a similar burn TBSA injury.[56,66]

Initial management of the burn-trauma patient requires focusing on primary and secondary assessments, not on managing the burn wound. Priorities for the burn injury are to stop the burning process with water; remove clothing, including metals and leather products; and cover the patient and burns with clean, dry, cotton material, such as a sheet. Fluid volume resuscitation begins during the primary survey and may be adjusted after the secondary survey.[67] Attention to the "ABCDEs" of trauma assessment are equally important in the burned and injured patient, especially if the patient may have an inhalation injury. Early intubation should be strongly considered. The negative effects of hypothermia are of great concern in the burn patient because of the loss of skin integrity, large volumes of resuscitation fluids, and exposure to the environment during care. The use of heat lamps, warming blankets, warm intravenous fluids, and an improvised body stocking for infants will reduce the incidence of hypothermia.[15,26] Careful attention to the mechanism of injury is important. For example, the practitioner needs to determine whether an altered neurologic response is due to a blow to the head or to carbon monoxide toxicity. Burns associated with motor vehicle crashes, falls, and electrical accidents require evaluation of the effects of the trauma and potential of cervical spine injury in addition to management of the burn injury.

Fractures may present an additional challenge in managing the burn patient after hemodynamic stabilization. Although treatment strategies vary, goals in the management of burns and fractures revolve around early stabilization and immobilization of the fracture, with early coverage or closure of the burn wound.[63] As with any trauma, prevention of deep vein thrombosis should be part of the plan of care.

NURSING MANAGEMENT OF THE BURN PATIENT

Management of the burn patient can be divided into three phases. The initial phase, resuscitation, usually extends over the first 72 hours. The second phase, the reparative or acute cycle, spans the time from resuscitation until complete wound closure. The time varies depending on the depth and extent of burn, the method of wound management used, and the variety of complications that may extend this phase, such as ARDS, sepsis, or MODS. The third phase, rehabilitation and reconstruction, may extend over years. The three phases associated with management of the burn patient are similar to those involved in the management of the trauma patient (resuscitation, critical care, intermediate care, and rehabilitation). Nursing management during each of these phases depends on accurate assessment and implementation of evidence-based nursing practice.

RESUSCITATIVE PHASE

Nursing management during the resuscitative phase centers on maintenance of homeostasis and tissue perfusion, treatment of life-threatening complications, prevention of infection, initial assessment of the extent of the burn injury (TBSA) and wound depth, management of pain, anxiety, and fear.

Fluid Volume Resuscitation

The burned patient is prone to fluid and electrolyte disorders until the wound is healed or covered with a permanent or semipermanent cover. Initially, fluid volume deficit is a major concern. As fluid shifts occur in relation to the initial injury, the circulating volume decreases rapidly. Without rapid infusion of fluids, burn shock develops. The importance of burn fluid resuscitation has been discussed previously. Monitoring the patient often to assess response to fluid therapy is a major nursing priority in the first 24 to 48 hours. The well-resuscitated patient should have adequate glucose-free urine, a pulse rate in the upper limits of the normal range for age, normal pulse pressure, clear sensorium, hematocrit less than 50%, no ileus, and a normal acid-base balance.

Urine output is often used to gauge tissue and end-organ perfusion, but many things should be considered when the adequacy of urine output is evaluated. First, there is a normal variation in urine output from hour to hour; therefore, when urine output is used as a monitor of resuscitation efforts, an average of 2 or 3 hours of urine flow should be assessed before intravenous fluid flow rates are changed unless other signs of hypovolemia are present. Urine flow rates usually decrease over time in response to hypovolemia, rather than drop abruptly. An abrupt decrease or absence of urine flow usually is related to a mechanical problem, such as a kink or plug in the catheter or drainage system. Manipulation or irrigation of the catheter may correct this problem immediately. Glycosuria is a common response to stress and may cause the urine output to be falsely elevated. If the patient has other signs of hypovolemia and a high urine output, glycosuria is often the cause. The use of dextran or mannitol also may cause the urine output to increase in the face of hypovolemia. Thus, although urine output may be a sensitive measure of organ perfusion, each of these issues should be considered when urine output is monitored. Evaluation of urine output along with base deficit and lactate levels will provide a more accurate assessment of the patient's overall resuscitation.[30]

In patients with electrical injuries the urine may contain hemochromogens, such as hemoglobin or myoglobin. The treatment for myoglobin in the urine is to flush the kidney to prevent permanent injury. In this case, fluids are given to increase hourly urine output to twice or three times normal (e.g., 1 to 1.5 ml/kg/hr). In addition, osmotic diuretics may be given to increase urine output. However, caution is needed to ensure that systemic resuscitation is not compromised by the administration of diuretics.

The pulse rate also varies for a number of reasons. Age is a common cause of variation: infants and young children have significantly higher pulse rates, and elderly patients tend to have lower pulse rates and may not be able to significantly increase their rate in response to hypovolemia because of preexisting heart disease and medications (e.g., β-blocking agents). Young athletes often have a low normal pulse rate of 50 to 60 beats/min. When stressed by hypovolemia, their rate may increase to low-normal values (80 to 90 beats/min) and seem a little low for the normal response to hypovolemia. Pain may cause an increased pulse rate and may be associated with agitation, both of which may mimic some of the signs of hypovolemia. Upward trends in the pulse rate should be monitored and assessed as an indication of hypovolemia. Additionally, tachycardia may be related to the hypermetabolic response associated with burn injury. Efforts to control the hypermetabolic response through the use of β-blocking agents is associated with improved patient outcomes.[20,28]

Unless the burned patient also has experienced head trauma, the sensorium should be clear; that is, the patient should be oriented to time, place, and person. Patients may appear to be somnolent and confused because they have been given opioids or sedatives for pain management; however, for the most part, patients without head trauma are neurologically intact. Burn patients commonly need emotional support, especially when loved ones may have been lost or injured during the event that caused the patient's burn injury. See Chapter 19 on the psychologic impact of trauma for more information.

A hematocrit higher than 50% usually indicates underresuscitation. A rapid drop in hematocrit may indicate blood loss, whereas a downward trend in hematocrit levels may suggest overresuscitation (hemodilution). Continuous assessment of the patient's response to resuscitation and hematocrit is needed to fully evaluate potential blood loss that may occur with traumatic burn injury.[56] A hypercoaguable state may also be present as a result of hypovolvemia and stress response.[26] Trending of the patient's coagulation studies and possible replacement of coagulation factors may be needed in the acute resuscitative phase of burn injury.

Ileus is another indication of decreased organ perfusion. Catecholamines released in the early hours after a burn slow peristalsis. Adequate fluid resuscitation and initiation of early enteral feeding have been shown to enhance burn wound closure and attenuation of protein metabolism.[22,26] Last, evaluation of base deficit and lactate levels as a measure of adequate fluid resuscitation may be the most sensitive elements in evaluating resuscitative interventions.

Again, each of these parameters has its limitations. It is only when all the parameters are considered in combination that a true picture of the patient's volume status can be assessed. When more than one of these parameters indicates that a fluid volume deficit has occurred, the volume of fluid administered should be adjusted. This may be done by increasing the flow rate for a specified time or by considering the administration of albumin as part of the resuscitation fluids. It is important to monitor the patient's response to this fluid challenge continuously to note whether the monitored parameters return to normal. If the parameters continue to be abnormal, other causes of hypovolemia should be considered.

Other Fluid and Electrolyte Imbalances

Although hypovolemia is the most common fluid and electrolyte concern in burn patients, one must be alert to a variety of other fluid and electrolyte imbalances. Fluid overload caused by overresuscitation may present problems during the resuscitative phase of burn management. Fluid overload is a rare problem except in infants, patients with preexisting cardiac conditions, patients with severe inhalation injury, patients with preexisting renal disease, and patients who have had delayed resuscitation intervention and have sustained a renal insult. Assessment parameters used to evaluate overresuscitation include elevated cardiac filling pressures and decreased cardiac performance (cardiac index and pulse rate), confusion, dyspnea, rales, inadequate oxygenation and ventilation, normal or increased urine output, decreased urine specific gravity, normal or decreased heart rate, peripheral edema unrelated to burn site, decreased serum sodium level, decreased serum and urine osmolality, and signs and symptoms of compartment syndromes. Therapy may include more judicious administration of fluids, cautious administration of diuretics, administration of oxygen if dyspnea is present, and evaluation and treatment of any underlying problems.

Hyponatremia, hypernatremia, hypokalemia, or hyperkalemia also may occur with some frequency during the resuscitation phase as fluids continue to shift between the extracellular and intracellular compartments. Frequent monitoring of electrolytes and acid-base states (e.g., base excess and lactate levels) may indicate the need for adjustments in fluid replacement regimens to prevent complications associated with electrolyte imbalances and hypoperfusion. In addition, evaluation of other electrolytes and metabolic markers such as magnesium, calcium, glucose, and cortisol levels are necessary to assess the body's response to the stress of burn shock.

Pulmonary Dysfunction

Impaired gas exchange is also a priority. Altered pulmonary function should be suspected when any signs indicate the presence of inhalation injury, fluid overload, abdominal compartment syndrome, or inadequate expansion of the chest wall related to full-thickness circumferential burns. Nursing goals prioritize assessment of the pulmonary system, including visual, auscultative, and laboratory data for evaluation of the adequacy of oxygenation and ventilation. If inhalation injury is suspected, establishment of an artificial airway (insertion of an endotracheal tube) should be the highest priority for the nurse. Tissue edema is significant within the first 8 hours of injury,[21,26] so establishing an airway before the first 8 hours after burn may be the defining factor in a patient's survival.[20] The parameters to be monitored are rate and character of respiration, signs of increasing hoarseness, increased pulmonary secretions, decreased chest wall expansion, chest wall retractions in children, subjective complaints of dyspnea, changes in mentation, and increased facial edema. If an ETT is placed, it should be observed often for placement. Tape is not usually effective in securing ETTs in burn patients either because of the edema or facial wounds. Cloth ties or oral ETT holders may be used to secure the ETT. Continual assessment of the cloth ties or ETT holder is needed because the ties securing the ETT may need to be tightened or loosened accordingly to account for increases and decreases in edema formation over time. In addition, care should be taken when securing the nasally placed ETT not to put pressure on the nares or the burn-injured face, ears, or scalp. Pressure on the nares may lead to necrosis and loss of the normal contour of the nose. Pressure on injured tissue of the face, ears, and scalp may cause further loss of tissue and result in a poorer cosmetic result. Intubation may increase the burn patient's already altered sensory perception. Patients who have facial burns often have eyes that are swollen shut, so they cannot see. If they can no longer talk, they are likely to become even more agitated. This may make it more difficult for them to cooperate with mechanical ventilation. Frequent explanation, reassurance, and sedatives are necessary to ensure their cooperation.

Because these patients often have increased pulmonary secretions, diligent pulmonary hygiene, including frequent suctioning, turning, interventions to prevent aspiration, and chest physiotherapy, are necessary to decrease the risk of pneumonia. Pneumonia is a major cause of morbidity and death in the intubated burn patient.[20]

Temperature

Maintaining normothermia is also a priority during the resuscitative phase of burn injury. Evaporative fluid losses from tissue loss and rapid fluid resuscitation can cause hypothermia in the burn-injured patient. Hypothermia can

- impair microcirculatory perfusion
- induce shivering, which exacerbates hypermetabolism
- impair neutrophil function, increasing the risk of infection

- impair platelet function, increasing the risk of bleeding
- lower cardiac output by up to 25%
- cause low levels of magnesium, potassium, and calcium.[68-70]

Interventions to maintain normal body temperature are needed to prevent adverse complications associated with hypothermia. Warming the external room environment, covering the patient with dry sheets, warming fluids used in resuscitation, and applying warming convention blankets are interventions to maintain normothermia.

Initial Wound Management

The management of burn wounds is a collaborative process. The continual assessment of wound healing and adjustment of wound therapies often are nursing concerns. Initially, the extent and depth of injury must be assessed accurately to guide fluid resuscitation needs. Early assessment of burn tissue depth is also needed to assess areas of full-thickness injury that may not effectively expand during edema formation, compromising circulation to that area of the body. Circumferential full-thickness tissue injuries often require an escharotomy early in the resuscitation phase to persevere underlying organ or limb function.

Once the patient is hemodynamically stable, an accurate assessment of the extent of the wound should be made by an experienced burn health care professional. Again the Berkow or Lund-Browder formula provides more accurate assessments than does the rule-of-nines formula. These formulas should be used to determine the extent (TBSA) of burn injury. Fluid resuscitation formulas should then be recalculated on the basis of the more precise estimate of TBSA burned and adjustments made to avoid complications of underresuscitation or overresuscitation.

Assessment of the depth of injury requires even more judgment (see Table 32-1). The very superficial (first-degree) burn and the truly deep full-thickness (third-degree) burn are fairly obvious. The difficulty comes in distinguishing the different depths of second-degree, or dermal, injuries. Continual evaluation of the burn wound is needed because the burn may extend deeper into tissues because of inadequate perfusion or from continuing contact with burn agent(s) (e.g., chemical burns). The burn wound is dynamic, and its depth may change over time if edema, pressure, and low-flow states decrease circulation to the wound, extending a zone of stasis to a zone of coagulation. Careful documentation of the wound's appearance during wound care is useful in assessing depth and promptly recognizing wound infection. Signs that suggest wound infection include the following:

- Increased erythema, tenderness, or pain around the wound
- Exudate that becomes more yellow or green
- Discoloration in the wound (black or purple areas)
- Decreased healing
- Elevated temperature and white blood cell counts

An easy way to monitor increasing erythema is to use a marker to delineate the edges of the reddened area, noting the date and time. If the redness extends past these margins over the next few hours, the need for a change in wound therapy or systemic antibiotics to control infection may be indicated. Many newer dressings are applied to the wound bed and remain intact for several hours to days. Assessment of the patient's response to the dressing and signs of infection are essential elements of the nursing plan of care.

Maintaining Nonburned Skin Integrity

In the burn patient, altered skin integrity usually is considered in relation to the burn injury; the potential for other alterations in skin integrity also exist. Mobility in burn patients is usually restricted by invasive line placement, application of splints or skeletal traction, ventilatory management, neck immobilization, sedative and opioid administration, or positioning needed to prevent graft loss. Any or all of these may contribute to prolonged bed rest, decreased ability to move in bed, and development of pressure ulcers.[71] The severely burned and immobilized patient benefits from the use of low air loss or kinetic therapy mattresses. Although patients still require turning on a low air loss surface, pressure is reduced, decreasing some of the risks for pressure ulcers. Nonburned skin should be assessed daily, and a valid pressure ulcer risk assessment tool (e.g., Braden Risk Assessment Tool) should be used to help identify patients at risk for skin breakdown. With each bath and dressing change, the dependent areas of the body should be inspected carefully for evidence of increased pressure and skin breakdown. Common areas for development of pressure ulcers in burn patients are the heels and the occiput.[71] Burns and edema in these areas often mask the beginning of pressure problems; thus, continual assessment is extremely important in maintaining the tissue integrity of nonburned skin.

Prevention of Infection

The burn patient is significantly immunocompromised by the loss of the protection normally provided by the skin; the loss of proteins, including immunoglobulins, during the acute resuscitative phase of injury; and exhaustion of the inflammatory mediators that orchestrate immune competence against invading microorganisms. Nursing management directed toward the prevention of infection focuses on four areas of concern:

- Vigilant monitoring for signs of impending wound infection, systemic sepsis, and pneumonia
- Maintenance of the external and personal hygienic environment to reduce the reservoir of microorganisms
- Use of aseptic technique for wound care and all invasive procedures
- Timely administration of antibiotics and appropriate use of topical antibacterial agents

Because the assessment of wounds for infection was discussed previously, this discussion is limited to signs of systemic infection.

Diagnosis of sepsis in the burn patient is complicated by the hypermetabolic response and by pain and anxiety, which may cause abnormalities in many parameters. In sepsis, diagnosis is based on abnormalities in mental acuity; changes in body temperature, heart rate, respiratory rate, blood pressure, urine output, and gastrointestinal function; and changes in laboratory values such as serum glucose level (hyperglycemia), blood pH, white blood cell count, C-reactive protein, platelet count, cortisol levels and positive blood cultures.[72] Thus, frequent, accurate monitoring of these parameters leads to timely diagnosis and treatment of systemic infections and early treatment of sepsis.

The second concern for prevention of infection is to provide an external environment that limits the access of microorganisms to the wounds of the burn patient. This includes the environment that is external to the patient (the patient's room, other areas of the hospital to which the patient is exposed [e.g., operating room, treatment rooms, hydrotherapy rooms]) and the staff who care for the patient. The most important aspect of providing a protective environment is to place a barrier between the patient and the environmental hazards. This may sound complicated but in fact can be quite simple. Inanimate objects in the environment, as long as they are cleansed with standard hospital disinfectants and dried, should present little, if any, risk to the patient. The major concern in the environment is porous materials that cannot be cleaned, such as chairs with cloth covers, mattresses without intact plastic covers, and similar hard-to-clean items. The biggest problem in maintaining a protective environment is personnel. Most transfers of microorganisms in the hospital environment occur by the hands of the hospital staff. Meticulous handwashing, wearing of gloves, and covering the clothing of the health care workers during direct patient care eliminate the major sources of microorganisms from the patient's immediate environment.[48,73] During wound care and invasive procedures, the use of a surgical mask and hair cover may increase protection. These simple precautions can produce a safer external environment.

The other environment of concern is the patient's own body. Providing meticulous hygienic measures is important to reduce infection. Especially of concern is hygiene of hair-bearing areas, skin folds in the groin and axilla, and under nail beds. Oral care, maintaining the head of the bed greater than 30 degrees,[74] and interventions to prevent aspiration are also important, especially for the intubated patient.

Wound care should be managed aseptically. Careful attention to the removal of exudate and devitalized tissue reduces the bacterial load and maximizes the effectiveness of antibacterial creams or solutions to control bacterial proliferation. The choice of antibacterial agents should be based on knowledge of the usual bacterial flora prevalent within devitalized burn tissue; routine, periodic cultures of the patient's wounds may be appropriate to discern active infection versus colonization.[73] The type of infection and antibiotic sensitivity should be evaluated as an element in treatment to decrease the emergence of drug-resistant organisms typically seen in burn centers.

Invasive procedures in burned patients carry increased risk for infection. Often, intravenous or arterial lines must be placed through burned areas, increasing the risk of infection. Meticulous care should be taken to keep the area around venous and arterial access lines as clean as possible. Usually the topical antibacterial agent used on the surrounding burn wound is also applied at the insertion site to decrease the risk of infection. Suturing lines in place keeps them from being easily displaced or slipping within the vein, which increases the chance of infection. Intravenous catheters should be changed if infection is suspected or according to hospital policy. The advent of antibiotic-coated invasive catheters may also decrease the incidence of line sepsis in burn patients.

Burn patients often exhibit altered pharmacokinetics in response to the administration of certain drugs. For this reason it is important to draw frequent peak and trough levels when administering antibiotics so that the dose and frequency of administration can be adjusted to obtain appropriate drug levels necessary to combat the infection.[75]

Management of Pain

Altered tissue perfusion caused by extracellular and intracellular fluid shifts characteristic of the resuscitative phase encourage the use of intravenous analgesia to provide adequate pain relief. Remember, the more superficial the burn wound, the greater the pain because of the associated exposed nerve fibers. When possible, a standardized pain assessment tool (e.g., numeric pain intensity score, WILDA [words, intensity, location, duration, aggravating/alleviating factors][76,77] or nonverbal scale, Faces Scale) should be used to ensure consistent evaluation of the patient's pain and treatment. Concurrent treatment of anxiety may also be beneficial. Additionally, care should be taken to differentiate and treat procedural pain (pain associated with burn wound care) and background pain (pain related to tissue injury and the inflammatory response, which may be exacerbated by movement, breathing, or pressure).[78] Procedural pain is brought on by invasive procedures or manipulation of the wound, as in dressing changes, debridement, or intensive exercise to prevent skin contractures and improve mobility.

The mainstay of pain management in the acutely injured burn patient is opioids. Morphine or fentanyl may be used during the initial phase of care to manage both background and procedural pain. Usually small, frequent doses are administered intravenously or by intravenous drip. During the first 24 to 48 hours an adequate level of medication to relieve background pain can be established and background medication needs can be converted to oral opioid equivalents. When the patient's condition permits, a long-acting oral opioid can be used to manage background pain. Slow-release oral morphine preparations can be used for background pain control. The most important aspect of background pain control is to realize that this pain is always present to some degree and is best relieved by administering pain medication on a non-pain-contingent schedule. Background pain control in patients with high anxiety levels may be supplemented with an anxiolytic such as a benzodiazepine.[77,78] Patient-controlled analgesia (PCA) is another method that may be used to control background pain. This technique works especially well in young adults, who want and need to have some control over their care.

Procedural pain is intermittent and of high intensity. It is also best managed by opioids. During the initial cycle of care, intravenous morphine or fentanyl may be used. An intravenous morphine bolus should be given 15 to 20 minutes before the procedure, and smaller boluses may be given during the procedure as necessary. Allowing the patient to deliver small doses every 5 minutes with a PCA pump is often very effective during wound care. Fentanyl has a much shorter half-life than morphine and can be used when a short-acting drug is needed. Fentanyl is also useful for the patient with decreased cardiac reserve, exhibited by a labile blood pressure and periods of hypotension when given morphine. Once the patient's condition improves, oral opioids can be used for procedural pain. Immediate-release morphine, hydromorphone, oxycodone, and other opioids or synthetic opioids can be used. Unlike patients with cancer pain, with whom the objective is to begin with the weaker opioid and work up, the objective with burn patients is to begin with potent opioids for the severe pain associated with the fresh open wound and use opioids of decreasing strength as the wounds heal and the pain is less intense. Anxiety and fear, especially fear of the unknown, is a major component of procedural pain. Many patients report that the use of anxiolytics in conjunction with pain medication is helpful.[77,78] In this case the benzodiazepines are useful. When opioids and benzodiazepines are both administered for pain management, the time of peak effectiveness may be different and may necessitate giving them at different times before procedures to obtain maximal effectiveness. Last, burn hypermetabolism and issues of pain tolerance may require that the pain treatment plan be re-evaluated often, with medication regimens adjusted to meet the patient's pain relief needs.

Nutritional Concerns

Hypermetabolism and nutritional needs must be addressed early in the treatment of burns. Goals to establish enteral nutrition are important in blunting translocation of gut microflora and negative sequelae of burn catabolism. Nursing care focuses on obtaining and maintaining enteral tube placements and aseptic management of central venous access used for infusion of total parenteral nutrition. Continual assessment of the patient's nutritional status guides the wound management plan because adequate protein intake is essential to wound healing.[6,20,22]

Reparative Phase

The second phase of care is the reparative phase. The major focus in this period is to support the body's natural healing properties and to provide psychosocial support to allow both physical and psychologic repair. Nursing priorities focus on the provision of adequate nutritional support, wound and pain management, prevention of contracture formation, management of sensory and sleep disturbances, and psychologic interventions to help the patient cope with the injury and its consequences. Many of these nursing issues are common to all critically ill or injured trauma patients.

Nutritional Support

Burn patients have greatly increased metabolic needs. The increased metabolic demands actually begin during the resuscitation cycle and continue for some time after wound closure, as evidenced by increased oxygen consumption and continued proteolysis (muscle tissue loss) up to 9 months after injury and for several months after complete wound closure.[20,22,25,40,79,80] The goal of the health care team is to continually assess the nutritional requirements and assist the patient in meeting these needs. Nutritional needs change during this phase as the patient undergoes surgeries and metabolic stressors and generates tissue for wound healing and closure. The nutritional team is helpful in measuring and calculating the patient's changing nutritional needs. To determine whether the patient's nutritional needs are being met, measurement of weight, intake and output, serum proteins (albumin, prealbumin, transferrin), and nitrogen balance are usually considered. Accurate measurements are extremely important. Indications of inadequate nutrition include weight loss greater than 10% of preinjury weight; low serum albumin, prealbumin, and transferrin levels; a negative nitrogen balance; and elevated C-reactive protein levels.[80]

The delivery of appropriate nutrition is a major nursing consideration. Because most burn patients have a lack of appetite or may not be able to cooperate with attempts to feed them the large number of calories required, alternative methods of alimentation may be necessary. Enteral feeding is initiated early in the management of the burn patient and may be used for night time supplemental feedings. Concerns to be considered when tube feedings are administered include hyperosmolar diarrhea, hyperglycemia, ileus, aspiration, and fluid and electrolyte imbalance. Hyperosmolar diarrhea may occur if the osmolarity of the enteral feeding product is high or if the tube feeding is infused too rapidly. Careful monitoring of flow rates and feeding of progressively concentrated solutions usually eliminate this problem. Some patients have hyperglycemia related to the high carbohydrate content of enteral tube feedings. This can be controlled by a change in the components of the feeding solution or administration of insulin. Symptoms of hyperglycemia include osmotic diuresis, glycosuria, and an increased serum glucose level. Ileus related to fluid and electrolyte imbalances and sepsis is a common problem in the burn patient and may complicate the administration of tube feedings.

Often duodenal feedings are used to bypass the stomach and reduce the risk of aspiration associated with gastric feedings. The debate as to whether to use gastric or duodenal feedings routinely centers around two factors: (1) Duodenal feedings are less likely to be related to vomiting and aspiration but leave the lining of the stomach unprotected, which may lead to gastric ulceration, and (2) enteral feedings administered into the stomach protect the gastric mucosa but may leave patients more prone to aspiration. To prevent ulceration when duodenal feedings are used, antacids or histamine blockers are routinely prescribed. To reduce the risk of aspiration, it is also recommended that the head of the patient be maintained at 30 to 45 degrees of elevation. Recent evidence suggests that elevation of the patient's head (greater than 30 degrees) and assessment of gastric residual volumes may reduce the incidence or severity of aspiration.[81,82]

Although tube feedings may be the primary means of nutritional support during the early phases of care, consideration should be given to beginning oral feedings. Offering small amounts of food that the patient likes or is craving may stimulate the patient's appetite and improve his or her overall morale. In some patients, to make the transition from enteral feedings to oral alimentation, it may be necessary to use enteral tube feedings at night to make up the calories not consumed during the day. All too often health care workers use the threat of enteral tube feeding to encourage the patient to eat. This rarely accomplishes an increase in oral intake and often leads to feelings of failure for the patient who just cannot eat enough. If it is apparent that the patient cannot eat enough, enteral tube feedings should be presented as an adjunct or alternative rather than as a threat. Anabolic hormones may prove beneficial in creating an environment of anabolism versus the catabolic, hypermetabolic state of burn injury, especially if the patient is struggling to consume adequate calories.[20,80] Additionally administration of β-adrenergic blocking agents have been shown to decrease REE and muscle catabolism attenuating the hypermetabolic response to burn injury.[20] When oral feeding is the sole means of nutritional support, frequent, small feedings and high-calorie, high-protein supplements are useful in increasing calorie and protein intake. The intake of fluids low in calories and protein, such as coffee, tea, and diet sodas, should be discouraged or offered as positive reinforcers when adequate oral intake has been achieved.

Management of Pain

Pain is a major problem for the burn patient. Although its character and intensity may vary throughout all phases, it is no less a problem. Pain is related to tissue injury and the healing process and is complicated by fear, anxiety, depression, and the chronicity of the healing process. The goal of pain control throughout burn care should be to provide maximal comfort given the nature of the injury and the treatments required for recovery.

Establishing a partnership with the patient early in the course of care regarding how to manage pain relief may prevent problems and disappointments. One of the first goals in pain management is to establish an objective system by which the patient can measure and communicate the intensity of pain. Simple adjective scales may be used with patients from early school age to the elderly. In the event that the patient cannot communicate verbally or actively engage in the assessment of his or her pain, observation of some physiologic responses or behaviors may provide guidance. It is important to remember that physiologic measures are least accurate in assessing pain; however, changes in a patient's pulse rate (tachycardia), diaphoresis, increased agitation, grimacing, and rhythmic movements or lack of movement may indicate pain in a verbally unresponsive patient.[77]

Assessment of pain is extremely important; however, the effectiveness of various pain relief measures is equally important. The absence of pain behaviors or verbal reports of relief with adjective or numeric scales should be noted to tailor pain management therapies. Once the wounds are essentially healed, the need for opioids should diminish. At this point most of the patient's pain can be managed with regularly scheduled doses of nonsteroidal anti-inflammatory agents. During the later phases of care, antidepressants may be useful in some patients and may act as an adjunct to pain management.[77,78]

Nonpharmacologic therapies may be useful throughout the phases of burn care as adjuncts to other pain management regimens. The goal of this type of therapy is to help the patient relax and to control the perception of pain. The type of nonpharmacologic therapy depends on individual coping styles and the age of the patient. Techniques include distraction, imagery, breathing techniques, hypnosis, and biofeedback. A variety of distraction techniques may be used, such as music, television, or talking to the patient about hobbies. Imagery, breathing techniques, and hypnosis require that the patient actively concentrate on an activity (e.g., breathing) or a mental image that allows him or her to perceive something other than the pain and thus relax. Biofeedback, like imagery, breathing techniques, or hypnosis, requires the patient to concentrate on something other than the pain. In biofeedback, a body function, such as lowering the heart rate, is used to assist the patient with the intense concentration required and gives a specific measurement regarding when relaxation is maximized. Distraction techniques are external to patient control and require less energy and less cognitive effort on the part of the patient. Imagery, breathing techniques, hypnosis, and biofeedback all require intense patient participation and are energy consuming. When these techniques are used, the patient often complains of being tired and drained of energy and may have increased pain after the procedure. Administering less-potent pain medications at the end of the procedure may prevent the letdown feeling and decrease pain complaints when nonpharmacologic therapies are used.

Maximizing Functional Outcomes: Prevention of Wound Contractures

Prevention of contractures and maintaining function of burned body areas begins immediately and continues until the scar has matured and the patient has completed the rehabilitation phase. Physical and occupational therapists play a major role in this aspect of care by providing a variety of splints and positioning devices that maintain a burned extremity in a position of maximal function. Detailed exercise programs aimed at maximizing function and reducing contracture formation are also developed to help maximize functional outcomes and limit contracture formation. The nurse must provide consistent and frequent monitoring of the patient's position, use of splints, and adherence to an exercise regimen. Diligent awareness of the importance of positioning the patient in an anticontracture position and integrating these positions into overall management maximizes functional outcome. Understanding the importance of each aspect of care allows the nurse and therapist to work together to maximize positioning and splinting procedures that prevent contractures and reduce tissue breakdown because newly healed burned skin is very fragile. For example, elevation of the patient's head to prevent aspiration or improve respiratory effort may be contrary to the usual positioning techniques that reduce neck contractures. However, continued assessment and adjustment in patient positioning may allow all objectives to be accomplished over time. Another area that may pose problems is the need for intravenous access in extremities, which may limit the use or require alteration of the usual splints used to prevent contractures of the extremities. A thorough understanding of all treatment goals and priorities allows the nurse to optimize patient care.

Wound Management

Wound management is a significant priority in the reparative phase of care. Therapeutic goals of burn wound management focus on rapid closure of the denuded tissue and provision of the optimal environment for wound healing. Techniques for optimal wound closure are diverse, and surgical preference dictates wound management techniques. Regardless of the technique, some principles cross all methods. Wound cleansing is required to keep the wound bed free of contaminants and to decrease the risk of infection. Methods for cleansing include aseptic technique, use of a nontoxic agent such as a mild soap or chlorhexidine, and nonsubmersion hydrotherapy.[62,73] During wound cleansing processes the patient's body may be entirely exposed; therefore, precautions to prevent hypothermia and associated complications (e.g., increased metabolic response, sympathetic stimulation, and shivering) need to be avoided by prewarming the treatment room and limiting the amount of time the patient's body is exposed.

Topical antimicrobial agents (Table 32-3) may be used to prevent wound infections and maintain moisture on the tissue bed or eschar until effective wound debridement is surgically completed. Topical antimicrobial agents have penetrating properties to prevent burn wound infections in deep dermal wounds,[73] but caution should be exercised when applying these agents on viable tissue. Antibiotic ointments may be more appropriate therapy as a means of decreasing microbial counts on wound beds with viable tissue. Wound products and ointments containing silver have been used for centuries to treat and prevent infections.[54] Silver ions appear to kill microorganisms by blocking their respiratory enzyme system and cell wall properties; thus, silver has potent antimicrobial properties that are beneficial in treating burn wounds.[54,83] Silver concentrations and delivery of the ion into the tissues varies by composition of the silver-containing dressing or ointment.[54] Silver nitrate solutions and silver sulfadiazine are silver-based antimicrobial agents used in the treatment of burn wounds. Several dressings also incorporate silver into the matrix of the dressing, allowing release of silver ion into the wound bed (e.g., Acticoat, Aquacel AG, Maxsorb AG, Silverlon). One advantage of silver-impregnated dressings is that they provide a moist wound healing environment and antimicrobial action that does not require daily dressing changes, which decreases trauma to new epithelial growth, enhancing overall wound healing.[54,83]

Mafenide acetate (Sulfamylon) is another topical agent that has antibacterial and bacteriostatic activity against most gram-positive and gram-negative pathogens and has limited antifungal activity.[62] Mafenide acetate penetrates eschar well, making it a good agent to use with deep partial-thickness and full-thickness burns when infection is suspected. Typically this agent is used for short-term topical treatment of infections. Prolonged use of mafenide acetate (TBSA greater than 25%) may cause hyperchloremic metabolic acidosis; thus, metabolic effects of the agent should be monitored when it is used.[62] Enzymatic debridement of necrotic tissue may be beneficial for a burn patient for whom surgical excision of denuded skin is not the optimal therapy. Enzymatic topical agents digest necrotic tissue and help lift the eschar.[62] Successful use of these agents requires maintenance of a moist wound bed, and concurrent antimicrobial treatment may be necessary to prevent wound infection. Enzymatic agents may enhance healing of partial-thickness burns by rapid debridement of necrotic tissue.

The choice of dressing depends on factors such as the location and depth of the burn wound, the age of the patient, the frequency of dressing change required, exudate management, and maintenance of a moist (not wet) wound environment. Traditional dressings consist of the application of an antimicrobial agent and fine gauze dressings reinforced with coarse gauze dressings to absorb exudates and provide protection. A variety of moist wound dressing therapies exist for the management of burn wounds, but the characteristics of the dressing and wound bed must be evaluated when selecting a dressing that will provide an optimal outcome. (See Chapter 16 for a discussion of the characteristics of dressing products.) Wound dressing choices may include hydrocolloid, nonadherent gauze, polyurethane (transparent) films, composite synthetic dressings, alginates, hydrogel dressings, silver dressings, biologic, and biosynthetic dressings.

Biologic and biosynthetic dressings are temporary skin substitutes that provide wound bed protection until skin grafting can be achieved. Biologic dressings provide a moist wound healing environment; however, the body may recognize the dressing as foreign, initiating an inflammatory response. The use and development of optimal biologic dressings has been an area of extensive research. Biologic dressings include allograft (cadaver skin), xenograft (porcine skin is most commonly used), Biobrane (a flexible nylon fabric impregnated with collagen), collagen derivatives, and artificial dermis (Integra, Alloderm, TransCyte).[62,84] Cultured epithelial autograft, which is grown under sterile conditions from the replication of keratinocytes taken from a tissue biopsy of the patient, has shown some promise as a means of providing an autograft skin cover. Concerns with cultured skin relate to the time required to grow the harvested tissue and the expense of the procedure.

Autografts remain the primary wound covering method used for deep burns. Autografts may be full-thickness or split-thickness grafts. Elements considered in the decision to use a full- or split-thickness skin graft include cosmetic concerns, the necessity of graft durability, and the area of denuded skin to be covered. Regardless of the type of graft used, the principles of postoperative nursing care are as follows:

- Immobilization of the graft site to maximize graft adherence
- Splinting of the immobilized grafted area in the position of greatest functionality
- Assessment of perfusion and gentle expression of accumulated drainage or blood.

Typically, the grafted wound is protected with a thick, absorbent dressing that remains intact for several days. Wound V.A.C. negative-pressure therapy may also be applied to grafted wounds to assist with angiogenesis and remove excessive fluid, thus enhancing graft adherence to the wound bed. Autografts typically adhere to the wound bed within 72 hours.[84] Initial removal of the protective dressing over the skin graft may occur after 72 hours or longer, depending on physician practice or concerns with graft adherence. When the protective dressing is removed, the amount of autograft adherence ("take") to the wound bed is evaluated. In addition to the autograft, the tissue donor site also requires wound care. The process of autografting creates a superficial partial-thickness donor wound that requires nursing management. A variety of dressings may be used to cover the donor site wound (e.g., nonadherent, hydrocolloid, polyurethane transparent, alginates).[62,84] Care focuses on the management of pain and daily assessment of the healing of the donor site.

Wound management and wound closure are significant nursing priorities during the reparative phase. Successful wound management encompasses nutritional support, management of pain, prevention of infection, and promotion of psychologic wellness.

Psychologic and Sleep Disturbances

During the reparative phase the patient begins to struggle with the severity of the injury, injury-imposed lifestyle adjustments, and long-term consequences such as reconstructive surgeries. In addition, environmental noise and continued close monitoring of the patient results in frequent interruptions of sleep. Pain is also a factor influencing sleeplessness, and lack of sleep intensifies the pain response, creating a vicious cycle for some burn patients.[85] Social support has also been found to correlate with burn patient survival; thus, nursing care that involves the whole family enhances patient coping and eventual healing.[86] Last, many burn patients have comorbid psychiatric illnesses.[87] Efforts to address the psychiatric illness need to be explored during the acute burn hospitalization to enhance the patient's overall morbidity and mortality rate. Nurses are in an optimal position to identify ineffective coping and sleep disturbance patterns. Involving the burn team in the management of the patient's psychologic wellness is an important aspect of burn nursing.

Rehabilitative and Reconstructive Phase

Goals of the rehabilitative and reconstructive phase focus on maximal rehabilitation and reconditioning of the burn patient, management of continuing nutritional concerns, and psychologic adjustment to the burn injury, including interventions for depression.

Continuing Skin Integrity Concerns After Healing

Burn wounds may break down after primary healing for a variety of reasons, such as thinner-than-normal epithelial cover, excessive dryness, shearing, trauma to scar tissue, exposure to sun or extremes of temperatures, and pressure from pressure garments and splinting devices. Burn wounds are especially prone to blistering and tissue breakdown for several months after healing. Without proper cleansing and application of therapies to encourage re-epithelialization and prevent infection, these small wounds may become infected and cause additional tissue loss. If treated with gentle cleansing and small, nonadherent wound dressings, these wounds usually heal in 5 to 7 days. In addition, if the wounds are caused by excessive pressure or active exercise, then splints, pressure garments, and exercise routines should be adjusted immediately. It is imperative that discharge teaching includes a review of this type of preventive care so that infection and large open wounds can be minimized. A booklet of simple instructions about the aftercare of burns, splints, and pressure garments and the telephone number of a nurse or therapist who can answer questions should accompany discharge information.

Activity Intolerance

Activity intolerance is prevalent during all phases of burn care but becomes a special concern during this period, when the patient is striving to regain independence in activities of daily living and return to work or school. The problem is related to the prolonged metabolic consequences of the burn injury and decreased range of motion caused by scar maturation and contraction. The goal is for the patient to increase activity tolerance gradually as the scars mature, range of motion improves, and physical stamina increases. Continuing nutritional concerns and the need to maximize protein intake are present in the rehabilitative cycle and should be evaluated as an element of activity intolerance.

Indications of activity intolerance include concern about not being able to complete desired activities; the need for frequent rest periods; and exercise intolerance as evidenced by shortness of breath, need for more sleep at night, and a general complaint of malaise. Often the diagnosis of activity intolerance is confused with depression, either or both of which may be prevalent. Usually, over time, if the problem is activity intolerance, a program of increasing activity with planned periods of rest results in improvement. This type of plan should be a part of discharge planning. If the patient and the patient's family recognize that this is a normal part of rehabilitation, they will be able to plan for it and cope with it. It is often helpful, as the patient prepares to return to work or school, for a member of the burn team to contact the supervisor or teacher and explain the issues related to activity intolerance. Usually allowances can be made for a part-time or limited work schedule that includes additional rest periods. It is also important to explain the patient's need to get back into a normal social environment as soon as possible because remaining off work or out of school until complete physical recovery is achieved may be detrimental to the patient's psychosocial recovery.[88]

Self-Concept and Depression

During the resuscitative and reparative phases the patient is usually in a state of denial regarding the final outcome of the physical injury. Even during the early stages of rehabilitation, patients may believe that, with scar maturation and reconstructive surgery, the physical deformities will be corrected and their appearance will return to the preinjury state. This early denial may actually be therapeutic in that the patient is motivated to do what is necessary to return to normal. However, sometime during rehabilitation patients will need to deal with the alterations in their physical appearance and their physical limitations. The patient's self-image must be incorporated into the new physical appearance. The patient may go through the various stages of grief as the process proceeds. Eventually the patient will develop a revised self-image. How the patient copes with this revised self-image depends on the individual, his or her support system, and the patient's preinjury emotional or psychologic status.[86,88] Interestingly, the final physical appearance may have little correlation with how the patient copes with this revised self-image.

Noncompliance with Treatment Measures

Noncompliance occurs when patients do not follow a treatment regimen or do not behave in the manner expected by the health care team. The reasons for noncompliance are many, but for the most part they are the result of lack of communication between patients and members of the health care team.[89] This lack of communication on the part of the health care team usually occurs because they are unclear in their instructions, have expectations that are unachievable by patients, or do not listen to what patients are trying to tell them. Lack of communication on the part of patients occurs because they do not understand the instructions, they lack the cognitive ability to understand, they do not have the social or environmental support to comply with the regimen or expectations, or they lack understanding of the consequences of noncompliance.[89] Symptoms of noncompliance may include wound breakdown, exaggerated scarring, decreased range of motion, increased contracture formation, splints that are not worn because they no longer fit properly, increased complaints, and apparent lack of motivation. Noncompliance is a frustrating problem for both patients and members of the health care team and, because of its negative connotation, does not foster solutions to the problem. When the problem is communication breakdown, it can be more readily addressed and corrected.

When symptoms of noncompliance appear, the responsibility for the problem lies with the health care worker, not the patient. This approach allows the health care worker to diagnose the problem and deal with it. The first question to ask is, "Are the plans and expectations realistic?" Next, patient issues must be identified. The key to diagnosing the patient problem is to listen intently to what patients say or do not say concerning the issues. If patients demonstrate the cognitive ability to understand and perform the recommended care, then other avenues of miscommunication should be explored. What in the environment or in the patient's social relationships impinges on the problem? Does the patient have increased pain related to an undiagnosed physical problem such as heterotopic bone formation? Is the patient showing signs of depression? Usually the cause for the communication problem can be found and corrected, and the symptoms of noncompliance should resolve.

EVIDENCE-BASED NURSING MANAGEMENT OF THE BURN PATIENT

Evidence-based nursing management of the burn patient provides limitless opportunities to explore the most effective means to meet both physical and emotional needs of the burn patient and families. Evidence-based practice (EBP) is the integration of best research evidence with clinical expertise and patient values to facilitate clinical decision making. EBP embraces the application of research findings to guide practice and utilization of other evidence (e.g., infection control data, benchmarking data, national guidelines, and so forth), clinical environment and expertise, and incorporation of patient desires for care. Burn injury can be emotionally and physically devastating for patients[86,88]; thus, nursing care that involves the patient's desires and uses best evidence to facilitate care will optimize patient outcomes. It is estimated that patient outcomes are improved by up to 40% when EBP is used to guide interventions over traditional care.[90] Burn nurses are in an optimal position to explore and define optimal evidence-based nursing practice interventions to improve or maximize patient outcomes. Box 32-3 provides suggested areas of burn

BOX 32-3 Evidence-Based Practice: Nursing Opportunities in the Management of Burn-Injured Patients

What nursing interventions reduce anxiety and pain during dressing changes and other painful procedures?
What is the role of nonpharmacologic interventions in reducing pain during painful procedures in burned adults and children?
What interventions are most effective in controlling postburn itching?
What nursing interventions are most effective in the prevention or minimization of contractures?
What nursing interventions (physiologic and psychologic) are most effective in stress reduction in the patient with burns?
What community-based follow-up care would best meet the physical and emotional needs of the patient with burns? When should community follow-up care be initiated?
What methods are effective in helping patients with burns (children, adolescents, adults) deal with social re-entry?
What nursing interventions promote healing of donor sites and skin grafts?
What is the relationship between the frequency of performing range-of-motion exercises and maintenance of function?
What nursing interventions are most effective in preventing diarrhea from contaminating the burn wound?
What is the relationship between onset of activity and graft take?
What are the most effective wound management protocols for the patient with burns?
What is the effect of early use of elastic wraps or pressure garments on healing of the burn wound?
When should negative pressure wound therapy be used in the management of burn wounds and grafts?

nursing for exploration and implementation of evidence-based interventions to help burn patients and families.

SUMMARY

The care of the burn patient is complex. Nursing management over the three phases of care requires the nurse to explore many areas of nursing, continually evaluating signs and symptoms of physical dysfunction and addressing psychosocial impairment associated with the injury. Continued research is needed to improve many aspects of patient care and to ensure optimal rehabilitation.

REFERENCES

1. Centers for Disease Control and Prevention: *Web-based injury statistics query and reporting system (WISQARS):* www.ced.gov/ncipc/wisqars. Accessed March 3, 2006.
2. American Burn Association: www.ameriburn.org. Accessed March 3, 2006.
3. National Institutes of General Medical Sciences: *Fact sheet: trauma, shock, burn and injury:* www.nigms.nih.gov/factsheets/trauma_burn_facts. Accessed March 7, 2006.
4. Ballesteros M, Jackson M, Martin M: Working toward elimination of residential fire deaths: the Centers for Disease Control and Prevention's smoke alarm installation and fire education program, *J Burn Care Rehabil* 26:434-439, 2005.
5. LaBorde P: Burn epidemiology: the patient, the nation, the statistics, and the data resources, *Crit Care Nurs Clin North Am* 16:13-25, 2004.
6. Wolf SE, Herndon DN: Burns and radiation injuries. In Mattox KL, Feliciano DV, Moore EE, editors: *Trauma*, 4th ed, pp. 1137-1151, New York, 2000, McGraw-Hill.
7. Wolf SE, Herndon DN: Burns. In Townsend CM, Beauchamp RD, Evers BM et al, editors: *Sabiston textbook of surgery: the biological basis of modern surgical practice*, 17th ed, pp 569-595, Edinburgh, 2004, W. B. Saunders.
8. Purdue GF, Hunt JL: Electrical injuries. In Herndon D, editor: *Total burn care*, 2nd ed, pp. 455-460, Edinburgh, 2002, W. B. Saunders.
9. Williams WG: Pathophysiology of the burn wound. In Herndon D, editor: *Total burn care*, 2nd ed, pp. 514-522, Edinburgh, 2000, W. B. Saunders.
10. Kramer GC, Lund T, Herndon DN: Pathophysiology of burn shock and burn edema. In Herndon D, editor: *Total burn care*, 2nd ed, pp. 78-87, Edinburgh, 2002, W. B. Saunders.
11. Marko P, Layon AJ, Caruso L et al: Burn injuries, *Curr Opin Anaesthesiol* 16:183-191, 2003.
12. Demling RH: The burn edema process: current concepts, *J Burn Care Rehabil* 26:207-227, 2005.
13. Berkow SG: A method for estimating the extensiveness of lesions (burns and scalds) based on surface area proportions, *Arch Surg* 8:138-142, 1924.
14. Lund CC, Browder NC: Estimation of areas of burns, *Surg Gynecol Obstet* 79:352-357, 1944.
15. DeBoer S, O'Connor A: Prehospital and emergency department burn care, *Crit Care Nurs Clin North Am* 16:61-74, 2004.
16. Mann E, Makic MB: Burn injury. In Oman K, Koziol-McLain J, editors: *Emergency nursing secrets*, 2nd ed, pp. 357-372, St. Louis, 2006, Elsevier.
17. Fitzwater J, Purdue GF, Hunt JL et al: The risk factors and time course of sepsis and organ dysfunction after burn trauma, *J Trauma* 54:959-966, 2003.
18. Sherwood ER, Traber DL: The systemic inflammatory response syndrome. In Herndon D, editor: *Total burn care*, 2nd ed, pp. 257-270, Edinburgh, 2002, W. B. Saunders.
19. Cumming J, Purdue GF, Hunt JL et al: Objective estimates of the incidence and consequences of multiple organ dysfunction and sepsis after burn trauma, *J Trauma* 50:510-515, 2000.
20. Pereira C, Murphy K, Herndon D: Outcome measures in burn care: is mortality dead? *Burns* 30:761-771, 2004.
21. Ahrns KS: Trends in burn resuscitation: shifting the focus from fluids to adequate endpoint monitoring, edema control, and adjuvant therapies, *Crit Care Clin North Am* 16:75-98, 2004.
22. Flynn MB: Nutritional support for the burn-injured patient, *Crit Care Nurs Clin North Am* 16:139-144, 2004.
23. Peng Y, Yuan Z, Li H: Removal of inflammatory cytokines and endotoxin by veno-venous continuous renal replacement therapy for burned patients with sepsis, *Burns* 31:623-628, 2005.
24. Cuthbertson DP: The disturbance of metabolism produced by bone and nonbony injury with notes on certain abnormal conditions of bone, *Biochem J* 24:1244-1263, 1930.
25. Hart DW, Wolf SE, Chinkes DL et al: β-Blockade and growth hormone after burn, *Ann Surg* 236:450-457, 2002.

26. Supple KG: Physiologic response to burn injury, *Crit Care Nurs Clin North Am* 16:119-126, 2004.
27. Spies M, Muller MJ, Herndon DN: Modulation of the hypermetabolic response after burn. In Herndon D, editor: *Total burn care*, 2nd ed, pp. 363-381, Edinburgh, 2002, W. B. Saunders.
28. Arbabi S, Ahrns KS, Wahl WL et al: Beta blocker use is associated with improved outcomes in adult burn patients, *J Trauma* 56:265-271, 2003.
29. Herndon DL, Hart DW, Wolf SE et al: Reversal of catabolism by beta-blockade after severe burns, *N Engl J Med* 345:1223-1229, 2001.
30. Jeng JC, Jablonski K, Bridgeman A et al: Serum lactate, not base deficit, rapidly predicts survival after major burns, *Burns* 28:161-166, 2002.
31. Cartotto R., Innes M, Musgrave M et al: How well does the Parkland formula estimate actual fluid resuscitation volumes? *J Burn Care Rehabil* 23:258-265, 2002.
32. Finfer S, Bellomo R, Boyce N et al: A comparison of albumin and saline for fluid resuscitation in the intensive care unit, *N Engl J Med* 350:2247-2256, 2004.
33. National Institutes of Health: Consensus conference, *J Trauma* 19:S89-S101, 1979.
34. Cancio LC, Chávez, S, Alvarado-Ortega M et al: Predicting increased fluid requirements during the resuscitation of thermally injured patients, *J Trauma* 56:404-414, 2004.
35. Warden GD: Fluid resuscitation and early management. In Herndon D, editor: *Total burn care*, 2nd ed, pp. 88-97, Edinburgh, 2002, W. B. Saunders.
36. Rivers EP, Ander DS, Powell D: Central venous oxygen saturation monitoring in the critically ill patient, *Curr Opin Crit Care* 7:204-211, 2001.
37. Hobson KG, Young KM, Ciraula A et al: Release of abdominal compartment syndrome improves survival in patients with burn injury, *J Trauma* 53:1129-1134, 2002.
38. Morris SE: Abdominal complications of burn injury, *Problem Gen Surg* 20:112-119, 2003.
39. Saffle JR, Hildreath M: Metabolic support of the burned patient. In Herndon D, editor: *Total burn care*, 2nd ed, pp. 271-287, Edinburgh, 2002, W. B. Saunders.
40. Hart DW, Wolf SE, Herndon DN et al: Energy expenditure and caloric balance after burn: Increased feeding leads to fat rather than lean mass accretion, *Ann Surg* 235:152-161, 2002.
41. Wolf SE, Thomas SJ, Dasu MR et al: Improved net protein balance, lean mass, and gene expression changes with oxandrolone treatment in the severely burned, *Ann Surg* 237:801-811, 2003.
42. Wischmeyer PE, Lynch J, Liedel J et al: Glutamine administration reduces gram-negative bacteremia in severely burned patients: a prospective, randomized, double-blind trial versus isonitrogenous control, *Crit Care Med* 29:2075-2080, 2001.
43. Traber DL, Herndon DN, Soejima K: The pathophysiology of inhalation injury. In Herndon D, editor: *Total burn care*, 2nd ed, pp. 221-231, Edinburgh, 2002, W. B. Saunders.
44. Fitzpatrick JC, Cioffi WG: Diagnosis and treatment of inhalation injury. In Herndon D, editor: *Total burn care*, 2nd ed, pp. 232-241, Edinburgh, 2002, W. B. Saunders.
45. Merrel P, Mayo D: Inhalation injury in the burn patient, *Crit Care Nurs Clin North Am* 16:27-38, 2004.
46. Miller K, Chang A: Acute inhalation injury, *Emerg Med Clin North Am* 21:533-557, 2003.
47. McCall JE, Cahill TJ: Respiratory care of the burn patient, *J Burn Care Rehabil* 26:200-206, 2005.
48. Mlcak RP, Herndon D: Respiratory care. In Herndon D, editor: *Total burn care*, 2nd ed, pp. 242-253, Edinburgh, 2002, W. B. Saunders.
49. Cartotto R, Ellis S, Smith T: Use of high frequency oscillatory ventilation in burn patients, *Crit Care Med* 33:S175-S181, 2005.
50. Acute Respiratory Distress Syndrome Network: Ventilation with lower tidal volumes as compared with traditional tidal volumes for acute lung injury and the acute respiratory distress syndrome, *N Engl J Med* 342:1301-1308, 2000.
51. Reper P, Dankaert R, van Hille F et al: The usefulness of combined high-frequency percussive ventilation during acute respiratory failure after smoke inhalation, *Burns* 24:34-38, 1998.
52. Ramzy PI, Jeschke MG, Wolf SE et al: Correlation of bronchoalveolar lavage with radiographic evidence of pneumonia in thermally injured children, *J Burn Rehabil* 24:382-385, 2003.
53. Wahl WL, Franklin, GA, Brandt MM et al: Does bronchoalveolar lavage enhance our ability to treat ventilator-associated pneumonia in a trauma-burn intensive care unit? *J Trauma* 54:633-639, 2003.
54. DeSanti L: Pathophysiology and current management of burn injury, *Adv Skin Wound Care* 18:323-332, 2005.
55. Hawkins HK, Linares HA: The burn problem: a pathologist's perspective. In Herndon D, editor: *Total burn care*, 2nd ed, pp. 503-513, Edinburgh, 2002, W. B. Saunders.
56. Hawkins A, MacLennan PA, McGwin G et al: The impact of combined trauma and burns on patient mortality, *J Trauma* 58:284-288, 2004.
57. Warriner R, Burrell R: Infection and the chronic wound: a focus on silver, *Adv Skin Wound Care* 18(1 Suppl):1-11, 2005.
58. Hart DW, Wolf SE, Chinkes DL et al: Effects of early excision and aggressive enteral feeding on hypermetabolism, catabolism, and sepsis after severe burn, *J Trauma* 54:755-764, 2002.
59. Xiao-Wu W, Herndon DN, Spies M et al: Effects of delayed wound excision and grafting in severely burned children, *Arch Surg* 137:1049-1054, 2002.
60. Barret JP, Herndon DN: Effects of burn wound excision on bacterial colonization and invasion, *Plast Reconstr Surg* 111: 744-752, 2003.
61. Thompson JT, Meredith JW, Molnar JA: The effect of burn nursing units on burn wound infections, *J Burn Care Rehabil* 23:281-286, 2002.
62. Honari S: Topical therapies and antimicrobials in the management of burn wounds, *Crit Care Clin North Am* 16:1-11, 2004.
63. Rosencrantz KM, Sheridan R: Management of the burned trauma patient: balancing conflicting priorities, *Burns* 28:665-669, 2002.
64. Kauvar DS, Cancio LC, Wolf SE et al: Comparison of combat and noncombat burns from ongoing U.S. military operations, *J Surg Res* 132:195-200, 2006.
65. Wolf SE, Kauvar DS, Wade CE et al: Comparison between civilian burns and combat burns from Operation Iraqi Freedom and Operation Enduring Freedom, *Ann Surg* 243:786-792, 2006.
66. Santaniello JM, Luchette FA, Esposito TJ et al: Ten year experience of burn, trauma, and combined burn/trauma injuries comparing outcomes, *J Trauma* 57:696-701, 2004.
67. Sheridan RL: Burns. In Fink MP, Abraham E, Vincent JL et al, editors: *Textbook of critical care*, 5th ed, pp. 2065-2076, Philadelphia, 2005, Elsevier.

68. Holden M, Makic M: Clinically induced hypothermia: why chill your patient? *AACN Adv Crit Care* 17:1-8, 2006.
69. Polderman K: Application of therapeutic hypothermia in the intensive care unit: practical aspects and side effects, *Intensive Care Med* 30:757-769, 2004.
70. Holtzclaw B: Shivering in acutely ill vulnerable populations, *AACN Clinl Issues* 15:267-279, 2004.
71. Gordon M, Gottschlich M, Helvig E et al: Review of evidenced-based practice for the prevention of pressure sores in burn patients, *J Burn Care Rehabil* 25:388-410, 2004.
72. Kortgen A, Niederprum P, Bauer M: Implementation of an evidence-based "standard operating" procedure and outcome in septic shock, *Crit Care Med* 34:943-949, 2006.
73. Heggars JP, Hawkings H, Edgar P et al: Treatment of infections in burns. In Herndon D, editor: *Total burn care*, 2nd ed, pp. 120-169, Edinburgh, 2002, W. B. Saunders.
74. Grap M, Munro C, Hummel R et al: Effect of backrest elevation on the development of ventilator-associated pneumonia, *Am J Crit Care* 14:325-332, 2005.
75. Martin S, Moran M: Contemporary antimicrobial focus in critical illness: MRSA and fungi, *Crit Connections* 5:6-7, 2006.
76. Fink R: *Pain assessment guide,* Denver, 1996, University of Colorado Health Sciences Center.
77. Montgomery R: Pain management in burn injury, *Crit Care Nurs Clin North Am* 16:39-49, 2004.
78. Pasero C, McCafferery M: Pain in the critically ill, *Am J Nurs* 102:59-60, 2002.
79. Heimbach D: What's new in general surgery: burns and metabolism, *J Am Coll Surg* 194:156-164, 2002.
80. Posthauer M: The role of nutrition in wound care, *Adv Skin Wound Care* 19:43-51, 2006.
81. McClave S, Lukan J, Stefater J et al: Poor validity of residual volumes as a marker for risk of aspiration in critically ill patients, *Crit Care Med* 33:324-330, 2005.
82. Metheny N, Clouse R, Chang Y et al. Tracheobronchial aspiration of gastric contents in critically ill tube-fed patients: frequency, outcomes, and risk factors, *Crit Care Med* 34:1007-1015, 2006.
83. Lansdown A, Williams A: How safe is silver in wound care? *J Wound Care* 13:131-136, 2004.
84. Bishop J: Burn wound assessment and surgical management, *Crit Care Nurs Clin North Am* 16:145-178, 2004.
85. Raymond I, Ancoli-Israel S, Choiniere M: Sleep disturbances, pain and analgesia in adults hospitalized for burn injuries, *Sleep Med* 5:551-559, 2004.
86. Maungman P, Sullivan S, Wiechman S et al: Social support correlates with survival in patients with massive burn injury, *J Burn Care Rehabil* 26:352-356, 2005.
87. Tarrier N, Gregg L, Edwards J et al: The influence of pre-existing psychiatric illness on recovery in burn injury patients: the impact of psychosis and depression, *Burns* 31:45-49, 2005.
88. Fauerbach J, Lezotte D, Hills R et al: Burden of burn: a norm-based inquiry into the influence of burn size and distress on recovery of physical and psychosocial function, *J Burn Care Rehabil* 26:21-32, 2005.
89. Pessina MA, Ellis SM: Rehabilitation, *Nurs Clin North Am* 32:365-374, 1997.
90. Melnyk BM, Fineout-Overholt E: Making the case for evidence-based practice. In Melynk BM, Fineout-Overholt E, editors: *Evidence-based practice in nursing and healthcare,* pp 3-24, Philadelphia, 2005, Lippincott Williams & Wilkins.

33

SUBSTANCE ABUSE AND TRAUMA CARE

Christopher Welsh, Kurt Haspert, Mary Hirsch, Janet M. Beebe

The use of mind-altering (psychoactive) substances has been a part of the human experience for thousands of years. Historical evidence indicates that opium has been used medicinally for at least 3,500 years and cannabis is mentioned in writings in ancient China and India. Many references are made to alcohol consumption in various early societies and accounts of problems related to the use of alcohol and other substances can be found in the Bible and in ancient Egyptian hieroglyphics.

The total economic cost of alcohol and other illicit drug abuse (not including nicotine) has been estimated to be more than $300 billion per year, with more than half the cost attributed to alcohol. The cost of underage drinking alone has been estimated to be in the order of $53 billion annually spent on the consequences of alcohol-related crashes, drownings, fires, suicide attempts, violent crimes, fetal alcohol syndrome, and treatment for alcohol use disorders.[1] More important, in addition to monetary costs, the less tangible emotional cost to the affected individuals and their families and friends is incalculable.

TERMINOLOGY AND CLASSIFICATION

Addiction is the term commonly used synonymously for drug or alcohol dependence. The American Society of Addiction Medicine (ASAM) defines addiction as a primary, chronic, neurobiologic disease with genetic, psychosocial, and environmental factors influencing its development and manifestations. It is characterized by behaviors that include one or more of the following: impaired control over drug use, compulsive use, continued use despite harm, and craving.[2]

The *Diagnostic and Statistical Manual of Mental Disorders IV–Text Revised* (DSM IV-TR)[3] classifies substance-related disorders into two categories: (1) substance use disorders and (2) substance-induced disorders. The **substance use disorders** are divided into *substance abuse* (Table 33-1) and *substance dependence* (Table 33-2). According to the DSM-IV-TR, "the essential feature of dependence is a cluster of cognitive, behavioral, and physiological symptoms indicating that the individual continues substance use despite significant substance-related problems." This diagnostic scheme places a heavy emphasis on the effect that the substance use has on an individual's life, not just the presence or absence of physiologic dependence. An individual can meet criteria for dependence without having physical dependence, and a person with only physical dependence does not necessarily meet criteria for dependence. Thus the cancer patient on high doses of opioids for pain but with no signs of impairment or uncontrolled use would not be diagnosed with opioid dependence. Because physical dependence is not necessarily required, a qualifier of "with physiologic dependence" or "without physiologic dependence" is used.

Substance-induced disorders include intoxication, withdrawal, intoxication delirium, withdrawal delirium, persisting dementia, persisting amnestic disorder, psychotic disorder (with delusions, with hallucinations), hallucinosis, mood disorder, anxiety disorder, sexual dysfunction, sleep disorder, and hallucinogen-persisting perception disorder ("flashbacks").

The World Health Organization's (WHO) *International Statistical Classification of Diseases and Health Related Problems,* Tenth Revision has a category "dependence syndrome" that is similar to the DSM-IV-TR diagnosis of dependence. It does not include a category "abuse" but does include "harmful use," which is different than DSM-IV-TR abuse in that it focuses on mental and physical health and specifically excludes social impairment. The WHO also uses the term "hazardous use" to describe an individual who is at risk for adverse consequences from substance use.[4]

The National Institute on Alcohol Abuse and Alcoholism adds other terms for the purposes of screening for alcohol use problems (see assessment considerations below). "*At-risk drinking*" is used to describe a person who exceeds recommended alcohol consumption levels (more than 14 drinks per week or four drinks per occasion for men, more than seven drinks per week or three drinks per occasion for women) but does not meet DSM-IV-TR criteria for alcohol abuse or dependence.[5] "Problem drinking/use" is a term often used to indicate problems related to substance use that do not meet criteria for abuse or dependence. "Substance misuse" is another term used to describe the use of a prescribed medication in a manner not prescribed for that individual.

SUBSTANCE USE AND INJURY EPIDEMIOLOGY

The Substance Abuse and Mental Health Services Administration reports that approximately half of all Americans aged 12 years or older report having consumed alcohol in the month before the survey (126 million U.S. residents). Approximately 22.7% engaged in at least one episode of binge drinking, defined as consumption of five or more drinks on

TABLE 33-1 Criteria for Substance Abuse

A. A maladaptive pattern of substance use leading to clinically significant impairment or distress, as manifested by one (or more) of the following, occurring within a 12-month period:
   (1) Recurrent substance use resulting in a failure to fulfill major role obligations at work, school, or home (e.g., repeated absences or poor work performance related to substance use; substance-related absences, suspensions, or expulsions from school; neglect of children or household)
   (2) Recurrent substance use in situations in which it is physically hazardous (e.g., driving an automobile or operating a machine when impaired by substance use)
   (3) Recurrent substance-related legal problems (e.g., arrests for substance-related disorderly conduct)
   (4) Continued substance use despite having persistent or recurrent social or interpersonal problems caused or exacerbated by the effects of the substance (e.g., arguments with spouse about consequences of intoxication, physical fights)

B. The symptoms have never met the criteria for substance dependence for this class of substance.

one occasion (i.e., at the same time or within a couple of hours of each other). Further, 6.6% (or 16 million persons) were estimated to be heavy drinkers (five or more drinks per occasion on 5 or more days in the previous 30 days).[6]

The same survey found that an estimated 7.8% of the U.S. population aged 12 years or older (approximately 19.7 million people) used an illicit drug in the month before the interview. There were an estimated 136,000 current heroin users, 2.4 million current cocaine users, and 14.6 million current marijuana users. As for the nonmedical use of prescription medications, an estimated 4.7 million reported nonmedical use of pain relievers, 1.8 million tranquilizers, 1.1 million stimulants, and 0.27 million sedatives. Additionally, 71.5 million Americans, 29.4% of the population, use tobacco.[6]

In 2005, an estimated 10.5 million persons reported driving under the influence of an illicit substance during the previous year. This corresponds to 4.3% of the population aged 12 years or older. The rate was highest (13.4%) among young adults aged 18 to 25 years, a decrease from 14.7% in 2002.[6] It is important to point out that all the above figures are likely to be underestimates because this survey does not include homeless persons who do not use shelters, military personnel on active duty, and individuals institutionalized in prisons or hospitals.[7]

Underage drinking continues to be a huge problem in America, to the point that it has been identified as one of the main areas of focus for the *Healthy People 2010* initiative.[8] It has been associated with negative effects on academic performance and increases in teenage pregnancy, risky sexual

TABLE 33-2 Criteria for Substance Dependence

A. A maladaptive pattern of substance use, leading to clinically significant impairment or distress, as manifested by three (or more) of the following, occurring at any time in the same 12-month period:
   (1) Tolerance, as defined by either of the following:
      (a) a need for markedly increased amounts of the substance to achieve intoxication or desired effect
      (b) markedly diminished effect with continued use of the same amount of the substance
   (2) Withdrawal, as manifested by either of the following:
      (a) the characteristic withdrawal syndrome for the substance (refer to criteria A and B of the criteria sets for withdrawal from the specific substances)
      (b) taking the same (or a closely related) substance to relieve or avoid withdrawal symptoms
   (3) The substance is often taken in larger amounts or over a longer period than was intended
   (4) There is a persistent desire or unsuccessful efforts to cut down or control substance use
   (5) A great deal of time is spent in activities necessary to obtain the substance (e.g., visiting multiple doctors or driving long distances), use the substance (e.g., chain-smoking), or recover from its effects
   (6) Important social, occupational, or recreational activities are given up or reduced because of substance use
   (7) The substance use is continued despite knowledge of having a persistent or recurrent physical or psychologic problem that is likely to have been caused or exacerbated by the substance (e.g., current cocaine use despite recognition of cocaine-induced depression, or continued drinking despite recognition that an ulcer was made worse by alcohol consumption)

behavior, sexual assault, acquaintance rape, delinquency, unintentional injury, and death. Initiation of drinking before the age of 14 years is also associated with an increased risk of lifetime alcohol abuse or dependence.[9] It is estimated that approximately 20% of all alcohol consumed in the United States is consumed by minors, who spend an estimated $22.5 billion on alcoholic beverages.[10]

ALCOHOL AND TRAUMA

Studies of patients from trauma centers and university hospitals have reported alcohol and psychoactive drug use rates from 25% to 60%.[11-15] The National Safety Council estimates that in the United States there is an average of one injury every 2 minutes involving an alcohol-related crash.[16] There are well-documented relationships among increasing blood alcohol concentration (BAC) and level of impairment in cognition and motor coordination, likelihood of injury, and severity of injury. Intoxicated patients in one study were shown to have significantly higher Injury Severity Scores than those not intoxicated, and within groups, those at the higher end of the range had correspondingly higher BACs.[17] Habitual drunken drivers have an increased risk of dying in an alcohol-related crash.[18]

Alcohol abuse has been associated with all types of injuries. Studies evaluating mechanism of injury and alcohol use have reported that 32% to 47% of motor vehicle crash (MVC) victims had positive BACs.[12] Rates of positive BAC for injured motorcyclists were comparable at 33% to 39.3%.[19,20] The risks associated with walking under the influence of alcohol are underappreciated. The reported incidence of positive BACs among injured pedestrians treated in trauma centers is 31% to 49%.[12,21] Alcohol also plays a major role in intentional interpersonal violence. Sixty-one percent of firearm homicide victims in one study were intoxicated[22] and 31% of the intentional injury victims from another had positive BACs.[12] Alcohol has also been linked to 30% of fire fatalities, 48% of drownings, and a tenfold increase in deaths from boating incidents.[23-25] It is also associated with a significant number of bicycle crashes.[26]

A number of researchers have investigated the incidence of alcohol dependence among trauma patients. Rivara et al[21] determined that 75% of acutely intoxicated trauma patients have positive scores on the Short Michigan Alcohol Screening Test and that 25% to 35% of them had biochemical evidence of chronic alcohol use. Soderstrom et al[27] found that 54% of acutely intoxicated trauma patients could be diagnosed as alcohol dependent, along with 11% of trauma patients who had negative BACs.[27]

Alcohol is present in nearly one third of injured adolescents, a population for whom alcohol is an illegal substance. Studies of adolescent trauma patients found that 20% to 30% tested positive for alcohol or other drugs at the time of admission.[28,29] MVCs are the leading cause of death for 16- to 20-year-olds in the United States. The National Highway Traffic Safety Administration reports that in 2005, 5,699 drivers in this age range were killed in MVCs with an additional 432,000 injured; alcohol was involved in 21% of these.[30] The National Survey on Drug Use and Health reported that 8.3% of 16- to 17-year-olds and nearly 20% of 18- to 20-year-olds reported driving under the influence of alcohol in the past year.[6]

Research remains inconclusive regarding whether alcohol intoxication results in less favorable outcomes after trauma. Although animal studies have documented alcohol's adverse effects on degree and outcome of injury,[31] such results are inconclusive in humans.[32,33] Studies of trauma patients from Level I trauma centers demonstrated no increased risk of complications from acute intoxication[15,34] but found a twofold increase in risk of complications in patients with behavioral and biochemical markers of chronic alcohol abuse. Some researchers have suggested that the more severe outcomes seen in patients with a positive BAC are the result of correlates of alcohol use such as high speed and not using seat belts.[33] Hospitalization costs and length of stay are substantially higher for drinking drivers than for those who had not been drinking.[34] Alcohol intoxication is a significant risk factor for sustaining traumatic brain injury and may impair rehabilitation and recovery.[35]

Opiates and Trauma

The incidence of positive opiate tests in patients admitted to urban trauma centers has been reported to be 5% to 16%.[13,14,36] A prospective study of patients treated at a regional trauma center conducted from 1984 through 1998 documented a 531% increase in the number of patients who tested positive for opiates.[36] An Australian study of injection heroin users found that more than 50% of the subjects reported having driven soon after using heroin or other opioids in the preceding month and that a third had had a crash related to their drug use.[37]

Stimulants and Trauma

Cocaine use may be an underreported cause of trauma. Studies of trauma patients have demonstrated cocaine usage rates from 6% to 22%.[13,14,38] A study of New York City fatalities (persons aged 15 to 44 years) found that 26.7% tested positive for cocaine metabolites. Two thirds of the cocaine-positive fatalities were the result of homicides, suicides, traffic collisions, or falls, making fatal injury after cocaine use among the top five causes of death.[38] Soderstrom et al[36] documented a 242% increase in the number of trauma patients who tested positive for cocaine between 1984 and 1998.

Methamphetamine is also associated with increased trauma and increased length of hospital stay.[39] Because of the caustic nature of the chemicals involved, the manufacture of methamphetamine can lead to significant burn and inhalational injuries.[40]

Marijuana and Trauma

Although several studies in Level I trauma centers have documented rates of 21% to 35% positive toxicology for tetrahydrocannabinol, the main psychoactive chemical in marijuana,[13,14,41] there is no consistent evidence demonstrating marijuana use as being causative. One study found that the higher rate of traffic incidents in marijuana users is likely reflective of characteristics of the young users rather than the effects of cannabis use on driving performance.[42] Another study found that patients who tested positive for marijuana had an additional length of hospital stay that averaged 1.3 days.[11]

Etiology of Substance Use Disorders

Substance use disorders are complex phenomena with biologic, psychologic, social, and cultural determinants (Figure 33-1). Current etiologic theories emphasize the role of genetic influences, learned behavior, neurobiology, and environmental stressors. It appears that environmental influences along with a genetic predisposition is required for the development of addictive behaviors.[43-45]

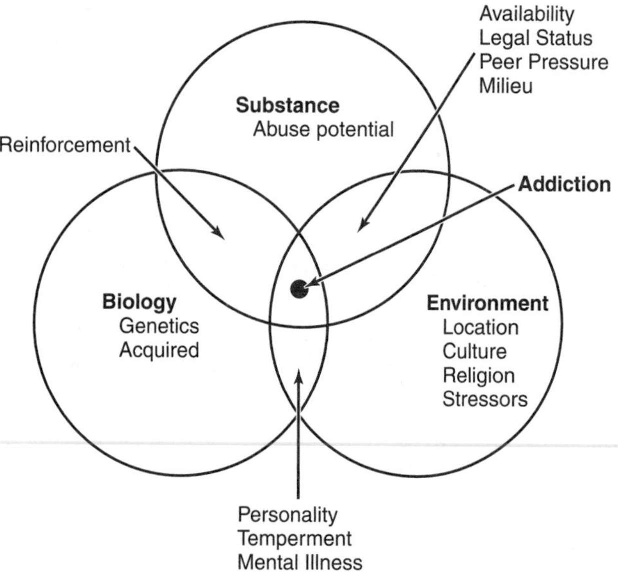

FIGURE 33-1 Multifactorial model of addiction.

Familial, twin, and adoption studies all indicate that genetics contributes approximately 50% of the risk for development of substance use disorders.[44-50] Genetics appears to influence susceptibility to most categories of illicit drugs, with heroin showing the strongest influence.[49-51] Children of parents with alcohol dependence have an increased incidence of alcoholism compared with the children of non-alcohol-dependent parents. Males appear to be more susceptible to genetic influence than females, although female children of alcoholics appear to have an overall higher incidence than the general population.[52] One study found that sons of alcohol-dependent parents have less intense subjective and physiologic reactions to ethanol.[53]

Animal studies have detected physiologic differences between levels of neurotransmitters and receptors in alcohol-preferring and non-alcohol-preferring animals.[54,55] In humans the dopaminergic and serotonergic systems of the brain are implicated in susceptibility to addiction, although causative links to specific genotypes have not been found.[56,57]

Environment also plays an important role in substance use and substance use disorders. Reactions to psychoactive drugs are determined in part by the user's mental state before use and the environment or setting in which the use occurs. Studies comparing alcohol- and non-alcohol-preferring mice have induced alcohol-preferring behavior in the non-alcohol-preferring mice by subjecting them to environmental stressors.[43] In humans, heroin use among Vietnam veterans followed a similar pattern.[58] The majority of veterans who began using heroin while overseas stopped after they returned to the United States and the extreme stressors were removed.

Abusive environments in early childhood may be a substantial risk factor for later drug abuse through a complex interaction between the child, the environment, and the level of social support.[59,60] A majority of patients in drug and alcohol treatment programs report being victims of childhood physical or sexual abuse.[61]

Various psychiatric conditions share a strong associated comorbidity with substance use disorders. These include schizophrenia, bipolar disorder, depressive disorders, anxiety disorders, posttraumatic stress disorder, the cluster B personality disorders (antisocial, borderline, histrionic, narcissistic), and attention deficit hyperactivity disorder.[62,63]

PHARMACOLOGIC, PHYSIOLOGIC, AND CLINICAL EFFECTS OF PSYCHOACTIVE DRUGS

Drugs of abuse have numerous physiologic effects that can influence the care of substance-abusing patients. These effects may make assessment, diagnosis, and treatment difficult. Health care providers must consider the effects of psychoactive drugs when caring for trauma patients.

Psychoactive drugs (Table 33-3) generally exert their mood-altering effects by altering levels of neurotransmitters within the brain through a complex series of interactions among various transmitter systems. The release of one neurotransmitter may result in the release of a second neurotransmitter or direct stimulation of a receptor site, which may enhance or block neurotransmitter function. Either the direct or the secondary action can be responsible for the clinically evident psychoactive effects.[64] These actions can prolong the effects of a given neurotransmitter, increase neurotransmitter release, or block receptor response to a neurotransmitter. This results in the various analgesic, hallucinogenic, stimulant, anxiolytic, or depressant effects, determined to some degree by the area of the brain containing the affected neural pathways. The reinforcing effects seen with most substances of abuse are felt to be related to a final common dopaminergic pathway involving the nucleus accumbens and ventral tegmental area (Figure 33-2).

TOLERANCE AND PHYSICAL DEPENDENCE

Physical (physiologic) dependence is the state of the body as a result of continual exposure to a substance. Adaptation occurs in physiologic systems so that their homeostasis is adjusted to incorporate the long-term effects of the additional substance, resulting in a new homeostasis. Physical dependence is generally defined by the presence of *tolerance* or *withdrawal.*

Tolerance is a common response to the repetitive use of the same or a similar drug. It manifests as a reduction in the response to a given dose of a drug after repeated administration. A higher dose of the drug is then needed to obtain the same response induced by the original dose. Tolerance can be seen as a result of a change in the distribution or metabolic pathway of a drug (pharmacokinetic) or as a result of adaptive changes that have taken place in the neurotransmitter system, such as increases or decreases in the number or responsiveness of receptors (pharmacodynamic).

Withdrawal (or acute abstinence syndrome) is defined as the physical or psychologic disturbances that occur after the cessation or reduction in use of a substance to which the body has developed tolerance. It is marked by a fairly predictable (for a given class of drugs) constellation of signs and symptoms

TABLE 33-3 Commonly Abused Substances (Other Than Alcohol, Nicotine, and Caffeine)					
Drug Name	**Street Names**	**Class/Drug Enforcement Administration Schedule**	**How Taken**	**Signs and Symptoms of Intoxication/Typical Duration**	**Signs and Symptoms of Withdrawal/Typical Time to Onset**
Cocaine	Coke, blow, bump, toot, nose candy, snow, soda, coca, C, charlie, flake, crack, rock, ready, ready rock	Stimulant II	Intranasal IV Smoked	↑Blood pressure/heart rate/temperature/energy/diaphoresis, ↑confidence/alertness/anxiety, hallucinations, paranoia, bruxism, ↓appetite/sleep, rhabdomyolysis, chest pain, myocardial infarction, stroke, seizure **1-2 hours**	Fatigue, lethargy, hypersomnia, depression, irritability, ↑appetite, psychomotor retardation, suicidal ideation, cocaine craving **Several hours to days**
Methamphetamine	Crystal meth, cristal, speed, crank, meth, chris, christy, ice, zip, chalk, fire, glass, getgo, go fast, methlies quik	Stimulant II	Intranasal IV Smoked	↑Blood pressure/heart rate/temperature/energy/diaphoresis, ↑confidence/alertness/anxiety, hallucinations, paranoia, bruxism, ↓appetite/sleep, rhabdomyolysis, chest pain, myocardial infarction, stroke, seizure **2-24 hours**	Fatigue, lethargy, hypersomnia, depression, irritability, ↑appetite, psychomotor retardation, suicidal ideation, craving **Several hours to days**
Amphetamine Dextroamphetamine Phenmetrazine Methylphenidate	Uppers, dexies, speed, bennies, crosses, JIF, hearts, truck drivers, black beauties, MPH, skippy, vit R, R-ball, the smart drug	Stimulant II	Orally ingested Intranasal IV	↑Blood pressure/heart rate/temperature/energy/diaphoresis, ↑confidence/alertness/anxiety, hallucinations, paranoia, bruxism, ↓appetite/sleep, rhabdomyolysis, chest pain, myocardial infarction, stroke, seizure **2-4 hours**	Fatigue, lethargy, hypersomnia, depression, irritability, ↑appetite, psychomotor retardation, suicidal ideation, craving **Several hours to days, variable**
Heroin	Dope, junk, smack, horse, H, scag, skunk, black tar, chiva, negra, brown sugar, white horse, China white	Opioid I	Intranasal IV Smoked Subcutaneous (skin pop)	Apathy, lethargy, ↓respiration, constricted pupils, drowsiness, slurred speech, analgesia, pruritus, ↓attention/judgment, constipation, stupor, coma, death **2-4 hours**	↑Blood pressure/heart rate/temperature, chills, diaphoresis, rhinorrhea, lacrimation, diarrhea, nausea/vomiting, irritability, dilated pupils, cramping, yawning, piloerection, hyperalgesia **4-8 hours**
Oxycodone Hydrocodone Morphine Codeine Fentanyl Methadone	Oxys, percs, M, Miss Emma, monkey, captain cody, cody, China girl, China white, TNT, meth, street meth, done	Opioid analgesic II/III	Orally ingested Intranasal IV Smoked (rare)	Apathy, lethargy, ↓respiration, constricted pupils, drowsiness, slurred speech, analgesia, pruritus, ↓attention/judgment, constipation, stupor, coma, death **3-12 hours, variable**	↑Blood pressure/heart rate/temperature, chills, diaphoresis, rhinorrhea, lacrimation, diarrhea, nausea/vomiting, irritability, dilated pupils, cramping, yawning, piloerection, hyperalgesia **4 hours to several days**
Marijuana Hashish	Pot, reefer, dope, grass, weed, herb, ganja, skunk, mota, Mary Jane, hemp, hash blunt, boom, chronic, sinse, sinsemilla	Cannabanoid I II (Marinol)	Smoked Orally ingested (rare)	↑Appetite/heart rate, euphoria, lethargy, ↓concentration/memory/judgment, incoordination, disinhibition, red eyes (conjunctival injection), paranoia, hallucinations (rare) **2-4 hours**	Irritability, anxiety, insomnia, nausea **Variable**

Continued

TABLE 33-3 **Commonly Abused Substances (Other Than Alcohol, Nicotine, and Caffeine)—cont'd**

Drug Name	Street Names	Class/Drug Enforcement Administration Schedule	How Taken	Signs and Symptoms of Intoxication/Typical Duration	Signs and Symptoms of Withdrawal/Typical Time to Onset
LSD Psilocybin Mescaline DMT, DOM LSD-49 *Salvia divinorum*	Acid, window pain, microdot, blotter, cactus, buttons, cubes, mescal, peyote, magic mushrooms, shrooms, illusion	Hallucinogen I	Mucosal Orally ingested Smoked (rare)	Hallucinations, illusions, delusions, synesthesia, derealization, lability, depersonalization, disorientation, ↓judgment, incoordination, restlessness, variable vital signs **2-12 hours, variable**	None
PCP	Angel dust, dust, dummy dust, hog, love boat, devil stick, peace pill, elephant juice, sherman, sherm dipper, dip stick	Dissociative Anesthetic I	Smoked IV Intranasal Orally ingested	Nystagmus (horizontal/vertical/rotatory), ataxia, analgesia, rigidity, lability, ↓judgment/respiration, confusion, dissociation, belligerence, stupor, coma, ↑salivation **1-24 hours, waxing and waning**	Nonspecific
Ketamine HCl (Ketalar)	Special K, K, jet, ket, kit kat, super K, vitamin K, super acid, cat Valiums, purple	Dissociative Anesthetic III	Intranasal Intramuscular	Nystagmus (horizontal/vertical/rotatory), ataxia, analgesia, rigidity, lability, ↓judgment/respiration, confusion, dissociation, belligerence, stupor, coma **1-24 hours, waxing and waning**	Nonspecific
MDMA (ecstacy) MDA MDEA 2C-B	Ecstasy, X, clarity, E, XTC, rave, Eve, M, x-ray, M&M, Adam, lover's speed, rolls, essence, snide-E, STP, nexus, bees, Venus	Psychedelic/stimulant I	Orally ingested Smoked (rare)	↑Blood pressure/heart rate/temperature/energy/diaphoresis, ↑confidence/alertness/anxiety,↑empathy, illusions, bruxism, chest pain, headache, seizures, strokes, myocardial infarction **4-8 hours**	Fatigue, lethargy, hypersomnia, depression, irritability, ↑appetite, psychomotor retardation, suicidal ideation **Several hours to days**
GHB	Easy lay, liquid X, G, somatomax, vita-G, liquid E, scoop, jib, grievous bodily harm, Georgia home boy, date rape drug	Sedative-hypnotic I III (Xyrem)	Orally ingested	Relaxation, sedation, disinhibition, ↓judgment/respiration, ataxia, nystagmus, slurred speech, incoordination, amnesia, flushing, confusion, stupor/coma **3-12 hours**	↑Blood pressure/heart rate/temperature/diaphoresis, tremulousness, delirium, anxiety, agitation, nausea, headaches, derealization, hallucinations, seizures **12-24 hours**
Alprazolam Chlordiazepoxide Clonazepam Diazepam Flunitrazepam Lorazepam	Pills, downers, tranks, benzos, sleeping pills, pins (Klonopin), bars, zanie bars (Xanax), roofies, Roche, R2s, Roofenol (Rohypnol)	Sedative-Hypnotic IV	Orally ingested IV	Relaxation, sedation, disinhibition, ↓judgment/respiration, ataxia, nystagmus, slurred speech, incoordination, amnesia, flushing, confusion, stupor/coma **1-12 hours, variable**	↑Blood pressure/heart rate/temperature/diaphoresis, tremulousness, delirium, anxiety, agitation, nausea, headache, derealization, hallucinations, seizures **6 hours to 4-6 days, variable**

TABLE 33-3 **Commonly Abused Substances (Other Than Alcohol, Nicotine, and Caffeine)—cont'd**

Drug Name	Street Names	Class/Drug Enforcement Administration Schedule	How Taken	Signs and Symptoms of Intoxication/Typical Duration	Signs and Symptoms of Withdrawal/Typical Time to Onset
Phenobarbital Pentobarbital Amytal Seconal Nembutal	Barbs, downers, reds, red birds, phennies, tooies, rainbows, yellow jackets, dolls	Sedative-hypnotic IV	Orally ingested IV	Relaxation, sedation, disinhibition, ↓judgment/ respiration, ataxia, nystagmus, slurred speech, incoordination, amnesia, flushing, confusion, stupor/ coma **1-6 hours, variable**	↑Blood pressure/heart rate/temperature/ diaphoresis, tremulousness, delirium, anxiety, agitation, nausea, headache, derealization, hallucinations, seizures **6 hours-several days**
Nitrites (amyl/butyl/ cyclohexyl) Nitrates	Poppers, snappers, amys, rush, bullet, sweat, climax, OZ, locker room, bolt	Inhalant Vasodilator	Inhaled (nasal)	↓Blood pressure, syncope, hypoxia, nausea, stupor/ coma, giddiness, headache, dulled senses, amnesia, enhanced orgasm **30 seconds- ½ hour**	Minimal-irritability, headache **Several hours**
Nitrous oxide	Laughing gas, whippets, balloons	Inhalant/ anesthetic	Inhaled (oral)	Mild euphoria, ↓inhibitions/ pain, sedation, perioral frost burn, dizziness/ lightheadedness, syncope, neuropathy **30 seconds to ½ hour**	Minimal-irritability **Several hours**
Paint/glue/ toluene Hydrocarbons	Glue, hardware, gas	Inhalant/ solvent Adhesive	Inhaled "huffed" (nasal and oral)	↓Blood pressure/reflexes/ respiration, syncope, hypoxia, nausea, stupor/ coma, giddiness, slurred speech, tremor, nystagmus, headache, amnesia, incoordination, dulled senses **<½ to 2 hours**	Irritability, headache, insomnia, tremulousness, diaphoresis, illusions (fleeting), nausea **Several hours**
Testosterone Anadrol Winstrol	Roids, juice, Arnolds, gym candy, pumpers, stackers; D-ball, weight trainers	Anabolic steroid III	Intramuscular Orally ingested Topical	↑Blood pressure/heart rate/ temperature/energy/ appetite, ↑confidence/ diaphoresis, insomnia, paranoia, anxiety, agitation, headaches, abdominal pain, aggressiveness ("roid rage") **After long-term use, variable**	Insomnia, depression, irritability **Several days, variable**
Dextromethorphan (Robitussin-DM, Coricidin Cough & Cold, Pertussin, Triaminic, Drixoral)	DXM, robo dosing, robo, CCC, triple C, dex, red devils, skittles, vitamin D	Cough suppressant OTC	Orally ingested	Euphoria, incoordination, ataxia, hallucinations (mild), confusion, dissociation, stupor, nausea, vomiting, hyperthermia, seizures (rare) **1-6 hours**	Nonspecific

LSD, Lysergic acid diethylamide; *DMT,* dimethyltryptamine; *DOM,* dimethoxymethylamphetamine; *PCP,* phencyclidine; *MDMA,* methylenedioxymethamphetamine; *MDA,* methylenedioxyamphetamine; *MDEA,* methylenedioxy-*N*-ethylamphetamine; *2C-B,* bromo-dimethoxyphenethylamine; *GHB,* γ-hydroxybutyrate; *OTC,* over the counter.

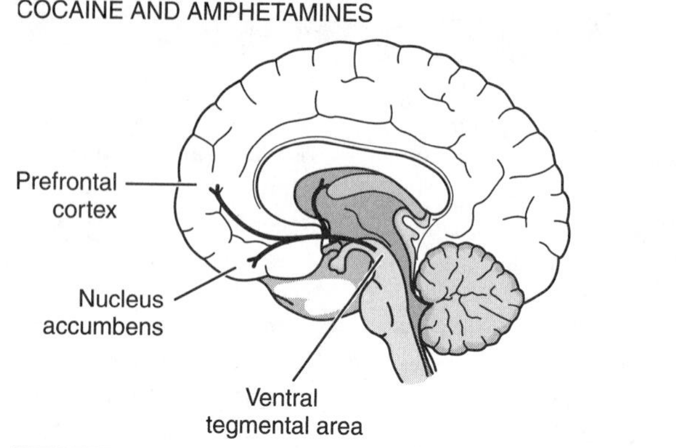

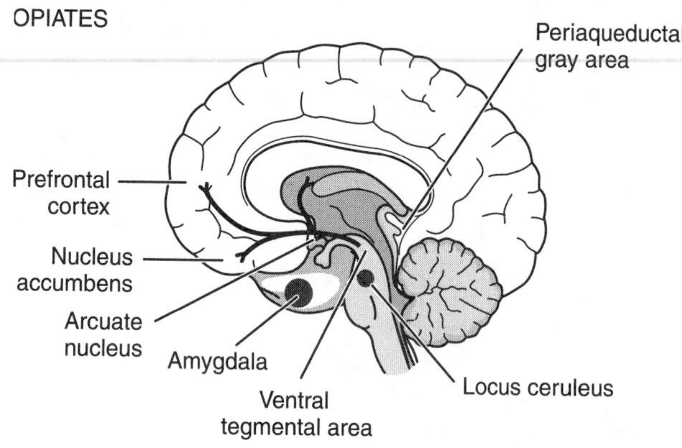

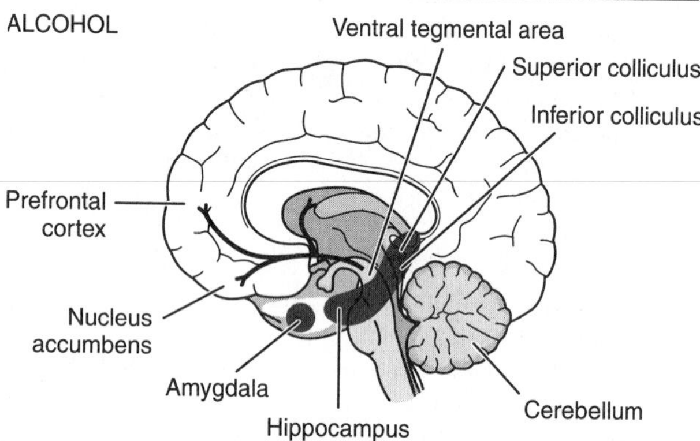

FIGURE 33-2 The brain's reward system. Scientists investigating which brain structures may be involved in the human drug reward system have learned a great deal from studies with rats. Because the chemistries of the human brain and the rat brain are similar, scientists believe that the process of drug addiction may be similar for both. The illustrations use information gathered from animal studies to show what areas may be involved in reward systems in the human brain.

The **cocaine and amphetamine reward system** includes neurons using dopamine found in the ventral tegmental area (VTA). These neurons are connected to the nucleus accumbens and other areas such as the prefrontal cortex.

The **opiate reward system** also includes these structures. In addition, opiates affect structures that use brain chemicals that mimic the action of drugs such as heroin and morphine. This system includes the arcuate nucleus, amygdala, locus coeruleus, and periaqueductal gray area.

The **alcohol reward system** also includes the VTA and nucleus accumbens and affects the structures that use GABA as a neurotransmitter. GABA is widely distributed in numerous areas of the brain, including the cortex, cerebellum, hippocampus, superior and inferior colliculi, amygdala, and nucleus accumbens.

The VTA and the nucleus accumbens are two structures involved in the reward system for all drugs, including alcohol and tobacco, although other mechanisms might be involved for specific drugs. (Modified from The brain's drug reward systems, *NIDA Notes* 11:19, 1996.)

after the abrupt discontinuation of, or rapid decrease in, the dosage of a psychoactive substance. The acute abstinence syndrome for a given drug is typically an exaggerated response that is the opposite of the drug's clinical effects.[65]

Alcohol and Central Nervous System Depressants

Ethyl alcohol is the prototypical central nervous system (CNS) depressant. It is typically ingested in the form of beer, wine, or liquor. Other CNS depressants include barbiturates, benzodiazepines, chloral hydrate, meprobamate, and methaqualone.

Pharmacokinetics

Although small quantities of alcohol can be absorbed directly from the mouth and stomach, its primary site of absorption is the proximal portion of the small intestine. Absorption occurs rapidly over a period of 30 to 60 minutes and absorption is generally complete. The rate of absorption is affected by the rate of gastric emptying and, to a lesser extent, by the presence or absence of food in the stomach. Alcohol is then distributed rapidly throughout the body by way of the circulation. The concentration of alcohol in a particular tissue is dependent on its blood supply. In highly vascular tissue such as the CNS and muscle, ethanol reaches equilibrium with the serum more quickly than it does in relatively avascular tissue such as adipose tissue.

Most of the alcohol consumed is metabolized in the liver by the enzyme alcohol dehydrogenase and to a lesser degree by the microsomal enzyme system.[66] It is converted into acetaldehyde and then rapidly converted into acetyl coenzyme A, which can then be oxidized through the citric acid cycle or used in various anabolic reactions involved in the synthesis of cholesterol, fatty acids, and tissue constituents. This enzymatic step is the rate-limiting portion of the metabolic process. The metabolism of ethanol differs from that of most substances in that the rate of oxidation of ethanol remains relatively constant and is minimally affected by the ethanol concentration. The typical rate of ethanol metabolism is 0.3 to 0.5 ounces per hour. A "standard drink" (1.5-ounce shot of 80-proof liquor, a 5-ounce glass of wine, or 12 ounces of beer) contains about 0.6 ounces of ethanol. Women have lower levels of gastric alcohol dehydrogenase than men. This results in less alcohol being broken down in the stomach and more alcohol being absorbed by the stomach and reaching the peripheral circulation.[67]

Small amounts of alcohol are eliminated by the kidneys and lungs. The amount of alcohol in 2,100 ml of expired air is approximately the same amount in 100 ml of blood. This direct correlation is the basis for the Breathalyzer test.

Mechanism of Action

γ-Aminobutyric acid (GABA) is the primary inhibitory neurotransmitter in the CNS. Alcohol exerts its depressant effect primarily by binding with the GABA receptors of the brain. Alcohol shares this action with other CNS depressants, most notably benzodiazepines and barbiturates. Alcohol and other

CNS depressants bind to different portions of the $GABA_A$ receptors and modulate their primary function of altering chloride influx through the ion channels of the cell.[68] Chloride increases the resting membrane potential, hyperpolarizing the cell and rendering it less reactive.[69]

Alcohol also has a suppressant effect on the glutamate (NMDA) receptors within the CNS. NMDA receptors are excitatory, and suppression of the excitatory function results in further depression of the CNS. The reversal of these effects during acute alcohol withdrawal is thought to be responsible for the clinical manifestations of CNS hyperactivity.[70] Alcohol's action on glutamate receptors is thought to play a role in alcoholic blackouts and acute withdrawal seizures as well.[70-72]

Benzodiazepines and barbiturates have the same GABA-ergic effects as alcohol, but their effects on other systems of the CNS are more limited. CNS depressants vary with respect to their onset and duration of action. Response to a given dose depends on the resultant blood level and habituation of the user, and, to some extent, his or her expectations of the drug effects. The duration of effects is dependent on the drug's half-life.

Alcohol also has effects on the endorphin,[73] serotoninergic,[74] and dopaminergic[75] systems within the brain, effects that are somewhat different from those of other CNS depressants. The stimulation of the endorphin system may account for alcohol's weak analgesic effect. Patients sustaining minor injuries may not complain of pain until after their BAC has dropped. Stimulation of the dopaminergic system is thought to be responsible for the euphoric and reinforcing effects of alcohol. Findings also suggest that serotonin may mediate alcohol-seeking behavior in habituated individuals.[56]

Pharmacologic Effects

Central Nervous System. As previously described, the clinical manifestations of CNS depressant intoxication are directly related to the drug's effects on the CNS. The earliest effect of alcohol ingestion is to alter judgment, causing the drinker to become disinhibited and to behave uncharacteristically (e.g., laugh or talk loudly, become boisterous or argumentative). These manifestations appear with a BAC in the range of 50 to 150 mg/dl. As the blood level of the alcohol rises, cerebellar and vestibular functions become affected. Nontolerant individuals with a BAC in the 150 to 300 mg/dl range display significant motor symptoms, manifesting in slurred speech and an unsteady, ataxic gate. At still higher levels, they may become stuporous and eventually lose consciousness. At levels higher than 400 to 500 mg/dl, respiration can become impaired and the individual may become comatose. Protective gag and cough reflexes may be lost. BACs of 500 mg/dl or more can be fatal.[76] Although behavioral and physiologic responses to increasing BAC occur in a fairly predictable fashion in the nontolerant individual, the level producing impairment will vary considerably in the tolerant individual. A BAC of 400 mg/dl, which would produce stupor in the uninitiated drinker, may result in minimal obvious impairment in the alcohol-dependent individual.

Alcohol has a synergistic effect when combined with other CNS depressants or opiates. The cumulative effect of the drugs is greater than the anticipated effect of each drug taken alone. Patients with one or more class of drug in their systems may be more susceptible to respiratory depression or nervous system suppression when additional drugs are used therapeutically. Intoxicated patients who receive opiates or sedatives in the resuscitation phase of care must be monitored closely for such cumulative effects.

Long-term ingestion of alcohol damages the nervous system in multiple ways. Alcohol exerts a direct toxic effect on the peripheral nerves, resulting in peripheral neuropathy. Alcoholic polyneuropathy is one of the most common neurologic complications of alcoholism. It can present as pain, paresthesia, or numbness in a glove-and-stocking distribution over the extremities, most commonly in the feet. Patients may also report dysesthesias severe enough to limit ambulation.

Several neurologic disorders result in altered mentation after long-term abuse of alcohol. Delirium tremens (DTs) associated with alcohol withdrawal is one cause of altered mentation, but there are several other alcohol-related disorders that may mimic the symptoms of acute brain injury. Thiamine depletion associated with long-term alcohol ingestion results in Wernicke-Korsakoff syndrome. A triad of symptoms—ataxia, oculomotor palsies or paralysis, and global confusion—characterizes Wernicke's encephalopathy. Affected patients have gait ataxia with moderately severe limb incoordination. Nystagmus is the most frequent ocular manifestation; patients may also have bilateral rectus palsies, horizontal conjugate defects, and vertical gaze palsies. Less frequently encountered defects include ptosis, loss of pupillary reflexes, and complete ophthalmoplegia. The associated state of confusion is characterized by inattention to the environment, disorientation, and lethargy. Some patients are agitated, but apathy and indifference are more common findings. Wernicke's encephalopathy should be considered in any alcohol-dependent patient with stupor or coma.

A high index of suspicion is prudent because most of the effects of Wernicke's encephalopathy are reversible with proper treatment. Untreated, the syndrome carries a 10% to 20% mortality rate. Persistent gait ataxia, nystagmus, and Korsakoff's psychosis are sequelae of Wernicke's encephalopathy. Korsakoff's psychosis is a chronic amnesic disorder characterized by intact remote memory, retrograde amnesia for recent memories, disorientation to time and place, and a marked inability to learn new information. Immediate recall may remain intact, but new information is lost after several minutes. Patients are often aware of the deficit, so confabulation is common. Patients with Korsakoff's psychosis are generally alert, with other cognitive functions fairly intact.

Other CNS effects of chronic alcohol use include alcoholic cerebellar degeneration, alcoholic dementia, and central pontine myelinolysis. Cerebellar degeneration is characterized by gait ataxia and mild degrees of limb impairment. The lower extremities are more commonly involved than the upper extremities. It can improve with adequate nutrition and abstinence from alcohol.

Alcoholic dementia is a cluster of cognitive defects attributed to the direct neurotoxic effects of alcohol. It is characterized by a global degeneration in all cognitive abilities. Individuals may be emotionally labile and have severe long- and short-term memory impairment. General problem-solving abilities and the ability to use new information are impaired. Imaging studies demonstrate cortical atrophy.

Osmotic myelinolysis is a rare disorder associated most often with alcohol dependence. It is often preceded by hyponatremia, and aggressive reversal of chronic hyponatremia may precipitate the syndrome. There is usually bilateral, symmetric, focal destruction of the white matter in the ventral pons (pontine myelinolysis), although brain structures outside the pons may also be affected (extrapontine myelinolysis). Osmotic myelinolysis evolves over days to weeks, with confusion being a prominent sign. Demyelination of pontine corticobulbar fibers and corticospinal tracts can lead to conjugate gaze palsies, dysarthria, dysphagia, and facial, tongue, and neck weakness. Patients can have paraparesis, quadriparesis, and a "locked-in syndrome" as a result of the corticospinal involvement.

Cardiovascular System. Alcohol has multiple effects on the cardiovascular system. Acute alcohol intoxication results in mild increases in heart rate along with depressed contractile function, increases in left ventricular end-diastolic pressure, decreased rate of left ventricular pressure development, and slowed relaxation time. The resultant decrease in cardiac reserve may have detrimental effects on the trauma patient. Acute alcohol intoxication has been shown to potentiate the physiologic and metabolic derangements accompanying hemorrhagic shock and may contribute to secondary brain injury as a result.[77-79] Acute intoxication decreases myocardial responsiveness to several inotropic agents, including dobutamine, isoproterenol, and phenylephrine.[80,81]

Long-term consumption of ethanol results in changes in the myocardium indistinguishable from those found in patients with idiopathic dilated cardiomyopathy: ventricular dilation and wall thickening, endocardial scarring, mild valvular irregularities, reduced left ventricular ejection fraction, and decreased ventricular compliance. These abnormalities are easily detected on echocardiogram. Clinically, patients may be asymptomatic or display severe congestive heart failure. Atrial arrhythmias are a common occurrence in alcoholic cardiomyopathy and compensated patients can decompensate acutely with the added cardiovascular stress of traumatic injury.

Respiratory System. Ethanol taken by itself has minimal respiratory depressant effects at levels of 200 mg/dl. Associated respiratory effects include a decreased responsiveness to carbon dioxide and slight reduction in vital capacity and expiratory reserve volume as BAC increases. In nondependent drinkers, respiratory arrest has been associated with BACs of 400 to 500 mg/dl. Studies indicate that alcohol increases pulmonary vascular resistance after soft tissue injury and may increase the risk of posttraumatic acute respiratory distress syndrome (ARDS).[66]

Hematologic System. Long-term alcohol consumption can result in both folate deficiency and iron deficiency anemia.[66] Alcohol also depresses bone marrow and vacuolizes red blood cell precursors. The alcoholic patient can present a challenge because multiple types of anemia may be present simultaneously.

Alcohol also interferes with the production and function of platelets. Long-term alcohol use may cause thrombocytopenia from decreased megakaryocyte production. Even brief periods of drinking can alter platelet function.[82]

Digestive System. Alcohol produces toxic effects on several areas of the digestive tract. Many of these pathologic alterations have implications in the care of the trauma patient. Esophageal irritation from alcohol and regurgitation of acidic gastric contents result in esophagitis. Mallory-Weiss tears may occur from repeated episodes of vomiting, and esophageal varices are associated with alcoholic cirrhosis. Excessive alcohol ingestion may damage the gastric mucosa, causing chronic gastritis. Patients are also at risk for acute hemorrhagic gastritis.[66]

Alcohol is inherently hepatotoxic and can injure the liver in the absence of any nutritional deficiencies. Fatty infiltration of the liver is the first manifestation of hepatotoxicity and can begin after a few days of heavy alcohol consumption. This is followed by fibrosis, which sometimes manifests as alcoholic hepatitis.[66] Eventually the fibrosis may progress to necrosis and inflammation, resulting in cirrhosis. The early fatty infiltration is reversible with cessation of drinking, but the latter stages of fibrosis are irreversible.

Alcohol interferes with the cytochrome P450 enzymatic system in the liver. Short-term alcohol use can impair the function of this system, consequently slowing the metabolism of drugs dependent on the system. This slows the rate of drug elimination, resulting in higher serum levels of agents metabolized by this pathway. In contrast, long-term use of alcohol may increase the rate of activity of the P450 system. Drugs are then more rapidly metabolized, resulting in lower-than-predicted serum concentrations.[66]

Trauma patients may have hepatic dysfunction significant enough to interfere with hemostasis through coagulopathy from impaired production of vitamin K–dependent clotting factors in the liver. Although serum transaminases may be elevated in liver disease, the prothrombin time is the most sensitive indicator of hepatic dysfunction.[83]

Long-term alcohol use can produce a form of chronic pancreatitis associated with irreversible structural and functional alterations in the pancreatic tissue. Episodes of acute pancreatitis can occur as well, with classic symptoms of midepigastric pain, nausea, vomiting, and anorexia, along with associated elevations of serum amylase and lipase.[66] Some patients have pathophysiologic changes associated with chronic pancreatitis although they remain asymptomatic.[84] Serum enzyme levels are often normal in individuals with subacute forms of pancreatitis. Diarrhea can develop from malabsorption syndromes caused by a loss of pancreatic exocrine secretions.

OPIATES

Opiates are drugs derived from the poppy plant, *Papaver somniferum.* Opioids are synthetic compounds that resemble the chemical structure of the naturally occurring substances. Morphine and codeine are naturally occurring opiates found in the resin of the poppy plant seed pod. Heroin (diacetyl morphine) is a semisynthetic compound that has undergone processing after being extracted from raw opium gum. Meperidine, oxycodone, hydromorphone, and methadone represent synthetic formulations. Naturally occurring opiates are the enkephalins, dynorphins, and endorphins, peptide molecules produced in the CNS and found in the brain, spinal cord, and exocrine glands.[85]

Opiate drugs can be ingested, injected subcutaneously ("skin popping") or intravenously (IV), or inhaled either nasally or by smoking. Heroin, the most commonly abused opiate, historically has been injected IV. However, because of increased purity of heroin, use through intranasal and smoked ("chasing the dragon") routes has increased. Rate of absorption, onset of action, and duration of action are dependent on the route of administration and the half-life of the particular drug used.[85]

Pharmacokinetics

Absorption of opioid drugs is dependent on the lipophilicity of the particular compound. More highly lipophilic drugs are more readily absorbed transdermally and from mucosa. They also better penetrate the blood-brain barrier. The liver metabolizes most opioid drugs. They tend to undergo a large first-pass effect, which accounts for the higher equivalent oral dosages compared with parenteral doses. Routes not involving the gastrointestinal tract result in a much larger percentage of the dose entering the peripheral circulation.

Pharmacology

Stimulation of opiate receptors, of which three subtypes (μ, δ, and κ) have been identified, results in the familiar analgesic effects of these drugs.[85] The overall effects of opiate neurotransmitters on the CNS include decreased awareness of and distress from pain, drowsiness, mental clouding, and, at higher doses, euphoria. The level of euphoria depends to some degree on which agent is used, the dose, and the route of administration. Clinically significant tolerance can occur with patients who have been on opiates for as few as 7 days.

There is also a group of synthetic drugs that possess both partial opiate agonist or mixed agonist/antagonist properties. They have analgesic actions similar to opiates when used alone but have antagonistic effects when used in conjunction with opiates.[85] These compounds include pentazocine, buprenorphine, butorphanol, and nalbuphine. These drugs can precipitate acute withdrawal in the opiate-dependent patient.

Toxicity

The most serious effect of opiates is respiratory depression. In overdose, patients can have respiratory arrest followed by cardiac arrest and hypoxic brain injury. Opiates also suppress the cough reflex, increasing the risk of aspiration. Patients who inject heroin may precipitate acute pulmonary edema.

Generally, opiates have little effect on the heart rate and blood pressure in the supine patient, although they produce some vasodilation that can result in hypotension in the volume-depleted patient.[85] Adverse blood pressure and heart rate changes noted during administration of opiates may indicate that the patient requires further volume repletion.

Opiates can also cause adverse effects that impact the gastrointestinal and genitourinary systems. Opiate analgesics decrease gastric motility and can result in constipation and delayed or impaired gastric emptying. These drugs can cause nausea and vomiting as a result of a direct action on the chemoreceptor trigger zone of the medulla. Urinary retention is another possible adverse effect of opiates. Opiate-dependent patients typically develop tolerance to the respiratory depressant and emetic effects of opiates.[85]

COCAINE AND AMPHETAMINES

Pharmacokinetics

Cocaine hydrochloride is a derivative of the coca plant, *Erythroxylon coca.* There are basically two chemical forms of cocaine—hydrochloride salt and free base. The hydrochloride salt is a white powder that is water soluble and can be injected IV or snorted intranasally. Free base cocaine is processed by mixing cocaine hydrochloride with an alkali (e.g., baking soda) and water. This alkaloidal form of cocaine (crack) is more volatile at a lower temperature than the hydrochloride form, which allows it to be smoked. Regardless of which route is used for administration, cocaine enters the circulation rapidly. Once in the blood, it binds with plasma proteins and is rapidly transported to the CNS.[86] Some of the drug remains unbound or free, this being the active portion of the drug. The onset of action for cocaine is variable, with IV and inhaled administration causing an almost immediate increase in blood pressure and heart rate. Peak effects occur 30 minutes after intranasal administration and are generally less intense but more prolonged than with the other routes. Cocaine is metabolized primarily in the liver and excreted by the kidneys.

Pharmacology

Cocaine acts on both the peripheral and central nervous systems. It blocks the reuptake of norepinephrine (NE) in the periphery. In the CNS, cocaine inhibits the reuptake of dopamine and causes central sympathetic activation. CNS outflow and the resultant increase in circulating NE are responsible for the signs and symptoms of sympathetic nervous system hyperactivity.[87] Cocaine's psychologic effects are caused by its blockade of dopamine reuptake within the CNS. The heightened sense of mental acuity, euphoria, and decreased fatigue associated with cocaine use are the result of the effect of excessive dopamine on the nucleus accumbens. The cocaine "high" is short lived, lasting 1 to 2 hours with nasal inhalation, 30 to 40 minutes with IV administration, and 5 to 10 minutes if smoked.[86]

Cocaine use can result in the rapid development of tolerance to the euphoric effects; however, only partial tolerance develops to the cardiovascular effects.[87] There is some degree of cross-tolerance with other CNS stimulants. Long-term cocaine users have decreased numbers of dopamine receptors in their CNS, which may account for the depression seen during withdrawal from cocaine. Some users of cocaine also experience *sensitization* in which they experience increasing effects at lower doses of the substance.

Toxicity

Cocaine's detrimental physiologic effects occur primarily during periods of active use. Toxic effects of cocaine are most commonly seen in its actions on the cardiovascular system. Increases in heart rate and blood pressure peak early during a binge and return to baseline despite continued increases in the serum cocaine level. Excessive NE can lead to generalized vasoconstriction, tachycardia, arrhythmias, mesenteric ischemia, and myocardial infarctions.[88-90]

Adverse effects of cocaine on the neurologic system include cerebrovascular accidents (CVA), seizures, and altered mental states. Cocaine use has been associated with altered cerebral perfusion and ischemic and hemorrhagic CVA, often in young persons with no known risk factors for cerebral vascular disease, although some cocaine-induced CVAs can be linked to underlying cerebrovascular abnormalities.[91,92] Patients with cocaine-induced seizures typically have one generalized seizure after cocaine use by the IV route. These patients usually have unremarkable neurologic diagnostic workups after the seizure, although further workup to rule out traumatic brain injury is still warranted. The causes of cocaine-induced seizures remain unclear. Mental status changes associated with cocaine use range from anxiety to acute psychosis. Psychosis associated with cocaine use is typified by paranoid ideation, delusions, hallucinations (often tactile, called formication), and hypersensitivity to environmental stimuli.

Inhaled or smoked cocaine also has detrimental effects on the bronchial mucosa and ciliary-mucus clearance mechanisms. Alveolar macrophage function is impaired and ciliary clearance mechanisms are effectively paralyzed by the use of crack.[93]

Cocaine and ethanol are often used together and appear to form a unique compound, cocaethylene. Experimentally, this combination of drugs has resulted in increased cardiac toxicity in selected individuals.[94] Heart rate increases with coadministration of cocaine and alcohol were significantly greater than those with either drug used alone.[95]

Methamphetamine

Methamphetamine is a CNS stimulant with physiologic and psychologic effects much like those seen with cocaine. Its euphoric effects are also the result of increased dopamine in the CNS, although this occurs by a slightly different mechanism than with cocaine. It can be ingested orally, snorted, injected IV, or smoked. Effects are felt 3 to 5 minutes after inhalation and 15 to 20 minutes after oral ingestion. Unlike cocaine, however, the effects of methamphetamine last from 6 to 24 hours. Psychologic effects include increased attention, euphoria, decreased fatigue, paranoia, hallucinations, and mood disturbances. Hyperthermia and seizures have been associated with acute methamphetamine use.[96]

NICOTINE

Nicotine is the psychoactive chemical found in the leaves of the tobacco plant, *Nicotinia tabacum.* The dried leaves are typically smoked as cigarettes, as cigars, or in a pipe. Leaves may also be chewed or crushed and inhaled intranasally (snuff).

Pharmacokinetics

Nicotine in tobacco smoke is rapidly absorbed from the lungs after inhalation and can also be absorbed through the oral mucosa and skin. It moves rapidly to the blood and is delivered to target organs. The majority of nicotine is metabolized in the liver, although some is metabolized by the kidneys and lungs.

Physiologic Effects

The physiologic effects of nicotine include vasoconstriction and tachycardia as a result of catecholamine release from direct action on the adrenal medulla. Stimulation of CNS receptors results in tremor, and actions on the chemoreceptor trigger zone cause nausea or vomiting. Parasympathetic stimulation of the gastrointestinal tract by nicotine results in increased gastrointestinal motility. Digestive tract responses to nicotine include nausea, vomiting, and diarrhea, the latter as a result of the effect of nicotine on receptors in the large bowel.[97]

Nicotine has a paralytic effect on the mucociliary transport mechanism of the lungs. In addition, long-term inhalation of tobacco causes histopathologic changes in the tracheobronchial tree. These factors may lead to an increased risk for pulmonary complications after injury.

Psychologic Effects

Nicotine acts directly on nicotinic cholinergic receptors of the CNS. This stimulation in turn causes a release of dopamine within the mesolimbic system of the brain, which is thought to account for the pleasurable sensations induced by nicotine.[64] Nicotine has both stimulant and depressant activities, which account for its reported paradoxic effects. Use of nicotine decreases subjective levels of anxiety, alters mood, and subjectively increases concentration.[97]

Physical dependence develops fairly easily with nicotine. It has a short-half life of about 2 hours and dependent individuals feel cravings 30 to 60 minutes after their last dose, as the nicotine blood level begins to drop. Tolerance to the drug also develops rapidly. Nicotine withdrawal typically lasts 72 hours, although craving persist for several weeks.

MARIJUANA

Marijuana is the common name for the dried flower buds, stems, and leaves of the *Cannabis sativa* plant. The drug is usually smoked but can be ingested. Δ-9-Tetrahydrocannabinol (Δ^9-THC) is the major psychoactive ingredient in the plant, although more than 400 cannabinoids have been identified. The highest concentration of cannabinoids is in the resin of the plants' flowering tops, where concentrations are five to ten times higher than the amounts found in the leaves.[98] Hashish, or hash, is the dried resin collected from the plant tops.

Two types of endogenous receptors for Δ^9-THC have been identified. Anandamide is a naturally occurring lipid neurotransmitter that has both peripheral and central activity.[99,100] It binds with the cannabinoid receptor sites in the CNS.[101]

Pharmacokinetics

When marijuana is inhaled, Δ^9-THC is absorbed rapidly into the bloodstream. Initial metabolism takes place in the lungs and liver. Although the pathway is similar for that of orally ingested marijuana, there is a more gradual increase in the Δ^9-THC level over a period of 4 to 6 hours. This results in a delay in the onset of psychoactive effects. The peak serum levels of Δ^9-THC are higher with oral ingestion than are those resulting from smoking.[101]

Because Δ^9-THC is highly lipophilic, it is released slowly from the CNS and other lipid-rich tissues, resulting in a prolonged half-life. Half-life can vary from 18 hours to 4 days. Δ^9-THC is converted into inactive metabolites in the liver and is excreted in the urine and feces.[98]

Physiologic Effects.

Acute effects of marijuana use include heart rate elevations and increases in diastolic blood pressure. Systolic and mean arterial pressures are not affected significantly. It can also cause a significant drop in skin temperature.

Cannabis use impairs gross and fine motor functions and delays reaction time. Despite these effects, no clear link has been established between cannabis use and vehicular crashes or fatalities.[98] One reason is that cannabis users may tend to overestimate their degree of impairment and compensate by increasing their attention to driving, whereas drivers under the influence of alcohol tend to underestimate their degree of impairment.[102,103] Acute marijuana use impairs short-term memory, impairing the ability to learn. These effects can persist up to 24 hours after smoking marijuana.[104] Retrieval of previously learned material is largely unaffected. Effects of long-term cannabis use include impairment of organization and problems integrating complex information involving attention and memory.[105] It is unknown whether these defects are permanent.

Long-term smoking of marijuana adversely affects the function of alveolar macrophages and alters the tracheobronchial epithelium.[106] Pulmonary alterations from chronic use result in cough and sputum production similar to that observed in cigarette smokers.

Psychologic Effects

Marijuana induces a state of intoxication characterized by euphoria and relaxation. Psychic manifestations vary depending on user set and setting and can include heightened awareness of the external environment, drowsiness, increased hunger, and depression. At levels producing moderate intoxication, it adversely affects a wide range of behaviors, including simple motor tasks and complex psychomotor and cognitive tasks.[107] Higher levels may induce panic, paranoia, and anxiety. Rarely, it may be associated with psychosis, usually in persons with underlying psychiatric disorders.

Although it was originally thought that marijuana use did not result in physiologic dependence, studies of long-term marijuana users have demonstrated sudden cessation after regular use of cannabinoids can cause a withdrawal syndrome.[108] Tolerance can develop rapidly with regular marijuana use and sensitization has also been described.

RESUSCITATION PHASE

The primary goals of care during the resuscitation phase are (1) identification and treatment of life-threatening conditions and (2) stabilization of the cardiovascular, pulmonary, and neurologic systems. Detailed descriptions of assessment and management strategies for multiple trauma patients are provided elsewhere in this text and are not repeated here. The purpose of the following discussion is to focus on treatment needs unique to the substance-abusing patient.

ASSESSMENT CONSIDERATIONS

Assessment of the substance-abusing trauma patient is complicated by several factors. As with any trauma patient, alterations in neurologic status as the direct effect of injury may obviate obtaining a medical history, including any information about substance abuse. Intoxicated patients may be stuporous and thus unwilling or unable to cooperate with history taking or physical assessment. Some trauma patients who are subjects of criminal investigations as a result of their injury or who are currently on probation or parole may give an inaccurate or incomplete history from fear of potential legal consequences. Further, it may be difficult to determine whether physical findings are the result of trauma or the substance abuse.[109] It is imperative that complete assessment of the trauma patient be accomplished systematically and rapidly. Physical, historical, and laboratory findings consistent with substance abuse should be included in documentation of the physical examination and in the patient database.

Identifying the Patient with a Substance Abuse Problem

In light of the prevalence of substance use disorders in trauma patients and the emerging body of evidence that brief interventions are effective in reducing harmful drinking, the American College of Surgeons has recently adopted a recommendation that Level I and II trauma centers screen for substance use problems. In addition, Level I centers are expected to offer brief interventions for patients who screen positive for at-risk substance abuse. Despite the strong association between trauma and substance abuse, many trauma patients are still not screened for alcohol and other drug use.[110]

Trauma Database. Substance-abusing trauma patients often have a history of previous injuries. Injury can be considered a symptom of substance abuse.[111] Patients should be questioned about previous injuries, including falls, MVCs, assaults, and work-related injuries. Pertinent information can be obtained from family members if the patient is unable to provide information; the family can also be used to validate and supplement information received from the patient. Additionally, as much information as possible about the circumstances of the current injury episode should be collected from police officers, first responders, and other eyewitnesses at the scene. Reports of altered behavior or impaired judgment before or immediately after the injury can help identify the substance-abusing patient.

Physical Assessment. Physical assessment of the trauma patient includes a complete head-to-toe examination and frequent monitoring of vital signs and neurologic status. It should also include evaluating the patient for evidence of drug and alcohol use.

Many of the sequelae of drug and alcohol use are manifested as alterations in the integument. Numerous bruises in various stages of healing over the lower extremities can be indicative of repetitive minor trauma caused by bumping into hard, fixed objects. Multiple small burns in various stages of healing are common as a result of dropping ashes while smoking. Abscesses and cellulitis are common integumentary manifestations seen with IV or subcutaneous drug injection. Patients who are using drugs IV often have "track marks," lines of multiple injection sites along the course of peripheral veins. IV drug users may also have signs of phlebitis and sclerosis of veins. Patients occasionally display venous insufficiency caused by venous scarring, which may be seen in one or both upper extremities rather than in the lower extremities, as would be more common with other venous disorders. Patients may inject drugs subcutaneously ("skin popping"). These needle marks do not necessarily follow veins but are often found in fleshy parts of the body such as the thighs or upper arms. Intra-arterial injection of drugs has been associated with the development of aortic, iliac, and popliteal arterial thrombosis and arteriovenous fistulas or pseudoaneurysms.[112,113]

Drug use may result in respiratory depression and pathologic alterations in the upper and lower respiratory tract. Intranasal inhalation of cocaine often results in damage to the nasal mucosa and destruction of all or part of the nasal septum. This destruction results from the vasoconstrictive effects of cocaine and subsequent ischemia of the nasal mucosa and septum. Intoxicated patients and those using opiates may vomit and have aspiration pneumonia and the more severe consequence of ARDS. Alcohol-dependent patients may have chronic pneumonia as a result of frequent aspiration. Patients who smoke crack often have a cough productive of copious amounts of soot-stained sputum similar to that found in victims of smoke inhalation. Some patients who use drugs intranasally can have alterations in gas exchange related to various fillers and adulterants contained in the abused substance. Auscultation of breath sounds and observation of aspirated or expectorated sputum may provide evidence of inhalation drug use, chronic pneumonia, or other pulmonary conditions.[114]

Patients who use cocaine are susceptible to mesenteric ischemia or infarction and may have required exploratory laparotomy in the past. Patients sustaining blunt abdominal injury may have what appears to be an acute abdomen that cannot be distinguished between cocaine-induced ischemic injury and blunt hollow viscous perforation. A history of abdominal surgery in the cocaine-using patient should be explored carefully.[115,116] Patients using alcohol or opiates may also have gastrointestinal symptoms, most commonly nausea, vomiting, constipation, and diarrhea. Alcoholic gastritis may cause acute mucosal lesions resulting in severe gastrointestinal bleeding. Chronic abdominal pain may result from pancreatitis, and patients may have hepatomegaly from cirrhosis or hepatitis.

Nervous system alterations caused by drug abuse may include a history of seizures, ataxia, peripheral neuropathy, and abnormalities of the deep tendon reflexes. Ocular palsy can result from extensive alcohol use. Cognitive defects often include short-term memory deficits. Other neuropsychiatric manifestations of drug use may include depression, delirium, paranoia, hallucinations, agitation, and anxiety.

Miosis, or pupillary constriction, is a common effect of opiates and occurs even in the tolerant user. Assessment of constricted, poorly reactive pupils may indicate recent opiate use.[85] Care must be taken to rule out other causes for pupil findings. Conjunctival injection (i.e., red eyes) typically accompanies marijuana use. Marijuana also reduces intraocular pressure and decreases pupillary responsiveness to light, resulting in increased time for light accommodation.

Patients with recent cocaine use can have arrhythmias, hypertension, chest pain, cerebral vascular accidents, and electrocardiogram changes consistent with myocardial ischemia or infarction.[117] Abuse of other psychoactive drugs may also cause adverse changes in heart rate and rhythm and blood pressure. Alcohol-dependent individuals may have secondary cardiomyopathy, and intravenous drug users frequently have bacterial endocarditis and subsequent valvular dysfunction.[118] IV drug users and alcoholics may present with signs of congestive heart failure.

Substance Use History. All trauma patients admitted to the hospital after injury should be questioned about alcohol and other drug use and any prescribed CNS depressants, stimulants or opioids. Reassuring patients that such information is needed for comprehensive care often increases their willingness to provide a complete history. As in all areas of medicine, the assessment and history taking is at least as important as any physical finding or laboratory test results. Unfortunately, compared with most areas of the medical history, the history of psychoactive substance use is often more difficult to obtain because of the nature of some of the questions (such as the use of illegal drugs) and the great amount of shame and denial associated with substance use and substance use disorders.

Clinicians should be aware of their own preconceptions about substance use and abuse and make every attempt to interact with all patients in a nonjudgmental manner. Terms such as *junkie, drunk, dope fiend, alky,* and *SWAF* (*shooter with a fever*) should be avoided both in interactions with patients and with other health care providers. Although it is more cumbersome, it is best to refer to the patient as an individual with a disorder rather than equating the person with the disorder (*person with addiction* or *person with drug dependence* rather than *addict, person with alcoholism* or *person with alcohol dependence* rather than *alcoholic*). Although the term *dirty* is often used to describe a person who is using drugs or a urine specimen that contains substances of abuse, it may carry a negative connotation, implying that the person is dirty. It is preferable to refer to a person as *using* or being *abstinent* or *in recovery* from substance abuse and to urine toxicology results as being *positive* or *negative.*

Patients should be asked about (1) specific substances used, (2) when last used, (3) amount used on a typical day of use, (4) routes of use, and (5) frequency of use. Additionally, it is crucial to elicit any history of withdrawal symptoms, particularly from patients who use CNS depressants. A history of alcohol withdrawal seizures or DTs is the best predictor of subsequent episodes, although a negative history does not rule out the possibility of new onset of either phenomenon. Patients should be questioned about past medical illnesses, particularly those known to be highly associated with substance abuse. A history of substance abuse treatment or participation in 12-step support groups may indicate current or previous substance use problems. Patients who are unable to provide information as a result of intoxication, intubation, or head injury may have family members or close friends available to provide the medical history and substance use and abuse treatment history.

Psychosocial Assessment. Psychosocial assessment includes obtaining information about the patient's social, employment, academic, and legal difficulties and any history of psychiatric illness. This information can be used to assess the consequences of the patient's substance use on his or her life. Impairment in one or more areas may indicate a history of chronic substance abuse or dependence.

Questionnaire Screening for Substance Abuse

Several instruments are available for detection of and screening for substance use disorders. The CAGE[119] and CAGE Adapted for Drugs (CAGE-AID)[120] are the simplest to use (Table 33-4). Both have demonstrated good specificity and validity in screening for alcohol and drug abuse and can be administered rapidly.[121] In a study of Level I trauma center patients, the CAGE demonstrated 84% sensitivity and 90% specificity for alcohol use disorders.[27] Other instruments include the TWEAK test, developed for use in pregnant women,[122] and the Alcohol Use Disorder Identification Test (AUDIT) (Table 33-5). The AUDIT is a 10-item, weighted-score instrument developed by

TABLE 33-4 CAGE Questionnaire

Patients are asked if they:
(1) have attempted to **cut down** on their alcohol or drug use,
(2) are **annoyed** or **angry** when questioned about their alcohol or drug use,
(3) feel **guilty** about their alcohol or drug use, or
(4) have an **eye-opener** (i.e., drink or drug) on arising in the morning.

Two or more positive answers is strongly indicative of a substance use disorder. Modified from Ewing J: Detecting alcoholism: the CAGE questionnaire, *JAMA* 252:1905-1907, 1984.

TABLE 33-5 Alcohol Use Disorder Identification Test (AUDIT)

Item	Response	Score
1. How often do you have a drink containing alcohol?		
	Never	(0)
	Monthly or less	(1)
	2 to 4 times a month	(2)
	2 to 3 times a week	(3)
	4 or more times a week	(4)
2. How many drinks containing alcohol do you have on a typical day when you are drinking?		
	None	(0)
	1 or 2	(1)
	3 or 4	(2)
	5 or 6	(3)
	7 to 9	(4)
	10 or more	(5)
3. How often do you have six or more drinks on one occasion?		
	Never	(0)
	Less than monthly	(1)
	Monthly	(2)
	Weekly	(3)
	Daily or almost daily	(4)
4. How often during the last year have you found that you were unable to stop drinking once you had started?		
	Never	(0)
	Less than monthly	(1)
	Monthly	(2)
	Weekly	(3)
	Daily or almost daily	(4)
5. How often during the last year have you failed to do what was normally expected of you because of drinking?		
	Never	(0)
	Less than monthly	(1)
	Monthly	(2)
	Weekly	(3)
	Daily or almost daily	(4)
6. How often during the last year have you needed a first drink in the morning to get yourself going after a heavy drinking session?		
	Never	(0)
	Less than monthly	(1)
	Monthly	(2)
	Weekly	(3)
	Daily or almost daily	(4)

Continued

TABLE 33-5 Alcohol Use Disorder Identification Test (AUDIT)—cont'd

7. How often during the last year have you had a feeling of guilt or remorse after drinking?

Never	(0)
Less than monthly	(1)
Monthly	(2)
Weekly	(3)
Daily or almost daily	(4)

8. How often during the last year have you been unable to remember what happened the night before because you had been drinking?

Never	(0)
Less than monthly	(1)
Monthly	(2)
Weekly	(3)
Daily or almost daily	(4)

9. Have you or someone else been injured as the result of your drinking?

Never	(0)
Less than monthly	(1)
Monthly	(2)
Weekly	(3)
Daily or almost daily	(4)

10. Has a relative, friend, or a doctor or other health worker been concerned about your drinking or suggested you cut down?

Never	(0)
Less than monthly	(1)
Monthly	(2)
Weekly	(3)
Daily or almost daily	(4)

Record the total of the specific items: _______

From Babor TF, Grant M: *Project on identification and management of alcohol-related problems, report on phase II: a randomized clinical trial of brief interventions in primary health care,* Geneva, Switzerland, 1989, World Health Organization.

TABLE 33-6 Urine Toxicology Detection Times

Substance	Detection Times (Days)
Cocaine	3-4
Methamphetamine	2-3
Opioids	2-3
THC (tetrahydrocannabinol)	1-7 (light use), 35 (long-term use)
PCP (phencyclidine)	1-14, 30 (long-term use)
Ketamine	1-4, 14 (long term use)
LSD (lysergic acid diethylamide)	<1
Benzodiazepines	1-14, 30 (long acting)
GHB (γ-hydroxybutyric acid)	<1
MDMA (methylenedioxy-methamphetamine)	2-3
Inhalants	<1, some not detectable
Anabolic steroids	20, >90 (injected)

the WHO to detect patients across a broad spectrum of problem drinking severity.[123-125] Possible scores range from 0 to 40, with a cutoff value of 8 considered positive for alcohol abuse. Overall, it has demonstrated a sensitivity of 92% and a specificity of 93%. This instrument has the benefit that it can be taken as a pencil-and-paper test, which can be completed by patients in private. Research on trauma patients has indicated enhanced sensitivity and specificity for the test when low-threshold responses for alcohol consumption are used.[124]

Laboratory Assessment

Toxicology Screening. Practitioners should be familiar with the substances routinely included in the toxicology profiles of their institutions (Table 33-6). The usefulness of toxicology screening is limited by the amount of time required to obtain results, which may range from several hours to days, depending on what laboratory support is available. Additionally, positive toxicologic testing does not rule out the existence of other causes of symptoms nor does a negative toxicology test indicate the absence of the use of illicit substances. Research indicates that laboratory tests alone may be insufficient for identifying chemically dependent patients and detection is enhanced by use of screening tools in conjunction with laboratory tests.[13,126]

Tetrahydrocannabinol, cocaine, opiates, benzodiazepines, and phencyclidine (PCP) are substances most commonly assayed in a urine toxicologic screens. Three methods of urine analysis are currently available: thin-layer chromatography (TLC), enzyme immunoassay, and gas chromatography. TLC is the least expensive technique but also the least sensitive. Because false-positive results are fairly common, positive results from TLC should be verified by another method. Enzyme immunoassay is a more expensive test but also more sensitive than TLC. Capillary gas-liquid chromatography is the most sensitive test but is also labor intensive and expensive. Gas chromatography with mass spectrometry is the most sensitive and specific urine test available. It can be used to verify positive results obtained by the other methods. Chromatography also has the benefit of providing quantitative results that can yield some information about how recently drugs were used.

It is important to remember that false-positive and false-negative results can be seen for many substances tested with TLC and enzyme immunoassay. Practitioners should be aware of factors that may cause erroneous results. Common cold remedies such as pseudoephedrine can cause a positive result for amphetamine. Opiate screens, which generally test for morphine, will not detect synthetic opioids such as meperidine or fentanyl because they do not metabolize to morphine. Alternately, they may detect opiate in individuals who have consumed poppy seeds. Benzodiazepine screens vary as to the metabolite tested for and may not detect specific benzodiazepines, depending on the assay used. Although cocaine screens are specific for a cocaine metabolite, it must be remembered that cocaine is also used as a topical anesthetic during some medical procedures. Dextromethorphan and ketamine can cause a false-positive test for PCP.

Serum, saliva, breath, and hair analyses are other laboratory tests available to assess drug use. Drugs measured by serum concentrations include ethanol, methanol, acetaminophen, benzodiazepines, barbiturates, and tricyclic antidepressants. Breathalyzers and saliva tests are sometimes used in emergency departments, but blood remains the most commonly used means for monitoring BAC.

To improve the validity of results, serum and urine specimens for toxicologic analysis should be obtained as soon as possible after admission. Drugs that were administered in the prehospital phase of care, at a referring institution, or at the current institution before the collection of the toxicology sample should be noted to prevent misinterpretation of positive toxicology results by subsequent providers. Additionally, it is important to remember that a positive toxicology test that is the result of drugs administered during the prehospital or hospital phase of care does not rule out the possibility of additional illicit use of drugs before admission.

Other Parameters. Although serum and urine toxicologic tests are the primary means of documenting substance use, other laboratory tests may be used to assess for long-term alcohol use. These biologic markers include mean corpuscular volume (MCV), the serum transaminases, aspartate aminotransferase (AST), alanine aminotransferase (ALT), and γ-glutamyltransferase (GGT). One study of biologic markers in trauma patients demonstrated only a 27% sensitivity for MCV in predicting excessive alcohol use.[126] AST and ALT are not particularly sensitive, nor are they specific to alcohol use disorders. GGT is a more sensitive indicator of alcoholic liver disease, with a 51% sensitivity for predicting excessive alcohol use, but it can also be elevated in patients with hepatitis.[127] Caution must be used when interpreting these values because acute liver injury can elevate hepatic enzyme levels irrespective of drug or alcohol use. Carbohydrate-deficient transferrin is another biochemical marker used in the assessment of alcohol consumption; however, in a study of trauma patients, it was found to have a sensitivity of only 34% for predicting excessive alcohol use.[128,129]

Management Priorities

Drug Overdose in the Trauma Patient

Management priorities for the trauma patient who has taken a drug overdose are essentially the same as those for any patient with a drug overdose. Initial resuscitation efforts focus on the timely stabilization of cardiopulmonary function. Additionally, trauma patients may require simultaneous treatment for other injuries. Respiratory depression is the most serious effect of CNS depressant and opioid overdoses; hence, the first priority is to establish and secure a patent airway. After this, adequate ventilation is ensured, IV access obtained, and circulatory function maintained with IV fluid and, in some cases, inotropic support. It is important to remember that patients may overdose on a combination of substances and may not fit a clinical profile unique to one category of drugs. Similarly, a patient's report of what he or she believes was taken may not be accurate because many illicit drugs bought on the street contain little or none of the actual compound that the buyer intended to use and may contain various other toxins.

Opiate Overdose. The classic triad of opioid overdose includes respiratory depression, miotic "pinpoint" pupils, and coma. Reversal of the opioid effects, including their respiratory depressant action, can be achieved with IV naloxone administered gradually in 0.4-mg doses while observing for the reversal of respiratory depression and improvement in mental status. Titrated administration with close observation minimizes the risk of precipitating acute opiate withdrawal syndrome. Up to 10 mg of naloxone can be administered, but if no effect is noted at this point, an alternative explanation should be sought. The half-life and duration of action of naloxone is shorter than those of some of the opioid drugs, so patients treated with naloxone need to be monitored closely for a return of respiratory depression from residual opioid after the naloxone dose has been metabolized.[85]

Benzodiazepine Overdose. Patients exhibiting slurred speech, ataxia, and incoordination similar to that seen in alcohol intoxication may be suspected of having benzodiazepine intoxication or overdose. Patients and family members should be asked about prescribed benzodiazepine use and illict use of benzodiazepines. The patient and his or her possessions should also be searched for prescription bottles or a list of medications. Benzodiazepine overdose is rarely fatal unless the benzodiazepine is combined with other drugs, most notably alcohol.

Flumazenil is a benzodiazepine antagonist that can be used to reverse the effects of benzodiazepines. It is most commonly used for reversal of drugs administered during anesthesia but is approved for use in overdose. For the reversal of conscious sedation and general anesthesia, the initial dose is 0.2 mg given IV over 15 seconds. If the desired level of consciousness is not obtained, 0.2 mg may be repeated at 1-minute intervals until a maximum cumulative dose of 1 mg is reached. For suspected benzodiazepine overdose, an initial dose of 0.2 mg is administered IV over 30 seconds. A 0.3-mg dose may be administered if the desired level of consciousness is not obtained, and repeat doses of 0.5 mg given over 30 seconds may be repeated at 1-minute intervals. The maximum total cumulative dose is 3 mg (usual dose 1 to 3 mg). Patients with a partial response at 3 mg may require additional titration up to a total dose of 5 mg. If no reversal is seen 5 minutes after a 5-mg cumulative dose, benzodiazepines are probably not the major cause of sedation. When flumazenil is being used to reverse a suspected benzodiazepine overdose, it should be used cautiously because the medication can precipitate benzodiazepine withdrawal in physically dependent patients.

Neurologic Management Issues

Serial comprehensive neurologic assessments are crucial during the resuscitative phase to identify changes caused by acute trauma, particularly to the CNS. Adverse effects of psychoactive drugs may also be detected. When the trauma patient has an altered sensorium or deterioration of other cerebral function, intracranial causes (i.e., brain injury) must be expeditiously ruled out. Acute alterations in neurologic function should never be assumed to be the result of substance use alone until other possibilities, such as intracerebral mass effect, shock, hypoxia, and other potential physiologic causes, have been ruled out. Several studies have documented that brain injuries were often missed or detected late because of the assumption that neurologic alterations were due only to alcohol intoxication.[109,130]

Seizures. Seizures are a common neurologic alteration that may occur as a result of substance use, withdrawal, or traumatic brain injury. Seizures most often occur with the use of cocaine and amphetamines or present as part of a withdrawal syndrome, typically from alcohol and other CNS depressants.[131-133] Other causes of seizures, including intracranial lesions and preexisting seizure disorders, must be ruled out. Seizures can be treated with diazepam (10 mg IV) or lorazepam (4 to 8 mg IV). Patients who have seizures should be monitored closely to note the characteristics, duration, and cessation of seizure activity; the recurrence of seizure activity; and condition during the postictal period. Seizure precautions must be initiated to protect the patient from further injury.

Assaultive or Self-Injurious Behavior. Patients who demonstrate aggressive or self-injurious behavior may require the use of chemical or physical restraints to facilitate evaluation and treatment. In some cases, chemical restraint is the only effective alternative for calming the patient. Ideally, a concise neurologic examination should be performed before the use of chemical restraints. Other possible causes of combative behavior, including intracranial pathologic conditions and hypoxia, must be ruled out. Care must be taken to document patient responses to chemical restraints, and such measures should be withdrawn as soon as the patient's condition warrants discontinuation. The goals of care are to maintain patient and staff safety while completing the evaluation process. The nurse should remain attuned to the effect that the setting can have on the patient. Decreasing the number of providers treating the patient; providing reassurance; offering simple, honest explanations; and maintaining a quiet environment serve to minimize sensory input. Such measures can reduce agitation, gain the patient's trust, elicit cooperation, and lessen the need for restraints.

Alterations in Respiratory Function

Psychoactive drug use can have several adverse effects on pulmonary function, in addition to those resulting from trauma.[106,133] Continual systematic assessments of pulmonary function, including physical examination and monitoring for adequate respiratory gas exchange, are important for early recognition and management of pulmonary complications. Patients with respiratory difficulty require prompt and definitive management, which may include endotracheal intubation and mechanical ventilation. In addition to incentive spirometry, deep breathing, and coughing exercises, patients may require chest physiotherapy to mobilize and clear secretions.

Cardiovascular Management Issues

Cardiac. Trauma patients with a history of long-term alcohol use should be evaluated for evidence of cardiomegaly and impaired myocardial function.[134] Patients with a history of IV drug use may have valvular dysfunction related to previous episodes of bacterial endocarditis. Evidence of myocardial compromise or a murmur in an IV drug user should prompt further assessment. An echocardiogram provides the most definitive assessment of valvular function and should be undertaken early during hospitalization if there is reason to suspect valvular dysfunction.

Circulation. Drugs of abuse can precipitate several alterations in circulation. The hypertensive effects of acute alcohol use may mask an underlying volume depletion resulting from acute hemorrhage. Acute intoxication blunts compensatory responses to blood loss and has been associated with more profound shock in response to hemorrhage than is seen in nonintoxicated individuals.[135,136] Patients who have used opiates recently may have decreased blood pressure and heart rate, which interfere with the normal compensatory mechanisms of acute hemorrhage. These patients are also slower to respond to volume repletion.[85] It is important to never assume that hypertension or hypotension is solely the result of intoxication or withdrawal: a cause of hemodynamic instability must be sought aggressively before attributing alterations in vital signs to preinjury drug or alcohol use. Although cocaine is commonly associated with elevations in vital signs, research on cocaine-intoxicated patients failed to discern any difference in vital signs compared with nonintoxicated patients.[137]

Fluid and Electrolyte Imbalances

Short- and long-term ingestion of alcohol can result in several fluid and electrolyte abnormalities. Alcohol consumption has multiple effects on kidney function and on water, electrolyte, and acid-base homeostasis.[138] Accurate measurement and documentation of intake and output and monitoring of electrolyte levels are vital for detection of such imbalances. Critically and acutely ill patients should have electrolyte levels (including calcium, magnesium, and phosphate) monitored closely until levels are consistently stable. IV volume and electrolyte deficits should be corrected to achieve the desired fluid balance, normalized serum electrolyte levels, and sufficient urinary output.

Sodium and Water. Short-term ingestion of alcohol induces diuresis because of the suppression of antidiuretic hormone (ADH). As the BAC decreases, the urinary flow rate and sodium excretion normalize in response to the subsequent rise in ADH. Long-term alcohol ingestion results in an overall retention of fluid and sodium with a resultant expansion of plasma volume, intravascular and extracellular fluid, and subsequent volume overload. After withdrawal from alcohol, these abnormalities resolve in 3 to 4 days.[138]

Calcium. Severe hypocalcemia is common in long-term alcohol users and may be the result of both increased urinary loss and impaired intestinal absorption. In acute trauma, it may perpetuate acute blood loss as a result of abnormal hemostasis.

Hypocalcemia can cause neuromuscular irritability characterized by tetany, laryngeal spasm, muscle cramps, and positive Chvostek's and Trousseau's signs. Insufficient calcium can also result in hypotension and ineffective myocardial contractility.

Magnesium. Magnesium loss with and without hypomagnesemia is another common complication of long-term alcohol use. It may be induced by poor nutritional intake, enhanced renal excretion, and diarrhea. Low serum magnesium is associated with muscle weakness, tremors, and other electrolyte disturbances, primarily hypokalemia and hypocalcemia. Hypomagnesemia also reduces the activity of thiamine-dependent enzymes and thiamine metabolism, increasing the risk of Wernicke-Korsakoff syndrome. Serum magnesium levels should be maintained in the high-normal range to facilitate replacement of depleted body stores and correction of hypocalcemia.

Phosphorus. Hypophosphatemia may be seen initially in hospitalized alcohol-dependent patients. Severe hypophosphatemia can result in impaired cardiac and skeletal muscle function, blood cell dysfunction, and respiratory impairment. Patients with hypophosphatemia may be unable to wean from mechanical ventilation because of impaired respiratory muscle function.

Glucose. Alcohol inhibits gluconeogenesis, and the resultant hypoglycemia is a common cause of mental status alterations in the alcoholic. If hypoglycemia is suspected, a fingerstick blood glucose test should be performed. Patients with documented hypoglycemia should be treated with dextrose and concomitant administration of thiamine to prevent the development of Wernicke-Korsakoff syndrome.

PERIOPERATIVE PHASE

ANESTHESIA CONSIDERATIONS

Short- or long-term drug use can alter the patient's response to anesthetic agents used during surgical intervention. The patient may require higher-than-average doses of these drugs to maintain the desired level of anesthesia. In some cases, drug use may potentiate the effects of anesthetic agents. If a psychoactive drug history is known or suspected, intraoperative care can be adjusted accordingly. A high tolerance for agents used in induction and maintenance of anesthesia may be the first indication of a substance use problem, particularly in patients taken to the operating room on an emergency basis. Cocaine use should be considered when the patient has tachycardia refractory to oxygen, analgesia, and volume repletion during anesthesia induction. Cocaine use can render indirect-acting vasopressors ineffective, so direct-acting vasopressors should be used.[139]

PREVENTING WITHDRAWAL

Patients who are undergoing long operative procedures can be at risk for acute withdrawal during the operation. It is imperative that intraoperative withdrawal be prevented. Patients with known opioid dependence requiring surgery can be given opiates before or during the procedure to alleviate the risk of intraoperative withdrawal. Those patients at risk for CNS depressant withdrawal should receive a long-acting benzodiazepine such as diazepam before the initiation of surgery.

HEMATOLOGIC CONSIDERATIONS

Management of long-term alcohol users may be complicated by preexisting coagulopathy caused by impaired production of vitamin K–dependent clotting factors. Patients with extensive cirrhosis may require transfusion or a continuous infusion of fresh-frozen plasma to maintain hemostasis. Patients who are thrombocytopenic and show evidence of continued bleeding may require platelet transfusion as well. Patients with a persistently elevated prothrombin time can be treated with 10 mg of vitamin K administered IV, intramuscularly, or subcutaneously daily for 3 days.

CRITICAL CARE PHASE

During the critical care phase the multidisciplinary health care team should continue to focus on restoring homeostasis and managing physiologic alterations directly attributable to injury and substance use. Patients in this phase require intensive nursing care because of instability of one or more major organ systems. Acute withdrawal syndromes are some of the most common physiologic alterations encountered during this phase of care.

WITHDRAWAL SYNDROMES

Withdrawal is a syndrome triggered by the abrupt cessation of a psychoactive drug that has been used for some period of time. Withdrawal syndromes are characteristic for each class of drugs. The onset and duration of withdrawal vary with the half-life of the specific drug. Substances with shorter half-lives typically have a more rapid onset and a shorter course of withdrawal than do those with longer half-lives. Withdrawal syndromes can vary in severity from mild physical and psychologic symptoms, such as the headache and fatigue associated with caffeine withdrawal, to the life-threatening cardiovascular collapse associated with DTs in alcohol withdrawal. The severity of withdrawal experienced by any one individual also varies in relation to the amount of substance used, the length of exposure, the degree of physiologic dependence, and other comorbid conditions. Because patients frequently use multiple psychoactive drugs, they may have more than one type of withdrawal simultaneously.

Every effort should be made to identify, differentiate, prevent, and treat withdrawal syndromes. At the same time, other physiologic causes for the withdrawal symptoms must be ruled out. The trauma patient who exhibits restlessness, agitation, tachycardia, and confusion must be assessed carefully for potential drug withdrawal as well as for hypoxia, brain injury, pain, fluid and electrolyte imbalances, psychiatric disorders, sepsis, and medication or transfusion reactions.

Central Nervous System Depressant Withdrawal

Alcohol Withdrawal. Mild alcohol withdrawal can begin 12 to 24 hours after the cessation of drinking. Patients who are highly alcohol dependent have adapted to functioning with a certain baseline BAC and may begin to have symptoms of withdrawal before the BAC has reached zero. Because the time to withdrawal is variable, vigilant monitoring is required to recognize it early and prevent or minimize its sequelae. The majority of patients have only relatively mild but unpleasant symptoms. A minority progress to potentially life-threatening withdrawal. A history of DTs or withdrawal seizures is the best predictor of untoward outcomes, but a negative history does not preclude their development.[76]

Mild symptoms of alcohol withdrawal typically begin 4 to 24 hours after the last drink. Patients typically feel a dysphoric mood and increased levels of anxiety. Autonomic hyperactivity occurs and is characterized by mild tachycardia, hypertension, fever, diaphoresis, fine tremor, and possibly mild hyperreflexia. Some patients may also have nausea, vomiting, or diarrhea.

Mild symptoms may progress to moderate symptoms at about 24 to 36 hours after the last drink. There is typically further autonomic hyperactivity and coarsening of the tremor. Patients may have mild auditory or visual hallucinations or illusions. At this stage, they are typically subtle (hearing one's name whispered, fleeting shadows) and the patient is typically aware that these perceptions are abnormal. The patient is oriented relative to his or her baseline. As the severity of withdrawal worsens, the hallucinations typically become more unpleasant or threatening. Some patients have tactile hallucinations or formication, the experience of feeling nonexistent insects crawling on the skin. Anxiety may increase, and patients may attempt to leave the hospital. At this stage they are at extremely high risk for falls or self-injury and require constant supervision and, possibly, physical restraints.

DTs, the most serious complication of alcohol withdrawal, generally appear 72 to 96 hours after the last drink and result in extreme autonomic instability, which can culminate in cardiovascular collapse. Manifestations of DTs include a fluctuating level of consciousness, with profound disorientation, delirium, hallucinations, coarse generalized tremor, marked vital sign elevation, severe agitation, nausea, vomiting, and diarrhea. Severe mental status changes and autonomic hyperactivity generally last 3 to 5 days. A minority of patients have protracted withdrawal, which can last 2 weeks or more. Before the use of benzodiazepines, the mortality rate for patients with DTs was 30%; with definitive care, this has decreased to 2% to 4%.[76]

Seizures can occur in the absence of other obvious signs of withdrawal. They typically occur within 12 to 24 hours after the cessation of drinking. These are isolated, generalized, tonic-clonic seizures, which are usually self-limiting. They can be treated with IV lorazepam or diazepam. Alcohol withdrawal seizures usually do not advance to status epilepticus. Patients who have sequential seizures must be evaluated for other possible causes such as head injury or preexisting seizure disorder.

Assessment. Patients who have positive BACs or who are known to be active drinkers should be monitored for signs and symptoms of withdrawal. Parameters to be monitored include heart rate, blood pressure, temperature, orientation, and presence or absence of tremor. Tremor may be noted in the extremities or the protruded tongue. Vital signs and neurologic status should be monitored frequently.

Treatment. Treatment for alcohol withdrawal should be instituted before or early in the course of the withdrawal syndrome to minimize the risk of DTs or seizures. Patients who are not identified until DTs develop are at higher risk for complications and require much larger doses of sedatives to control the CNS excitation. Patients with a history of alcohol withdrawal should be started on a prophylactic withdrawal regimen.[140,141]

Benzodiazepines are ideal drugs for prevention and treatment of alcohol withdrawal because they are cross-tolerant with alcohol, do not induce hepatic microsomal enzymes, produce little alteration in coagulation parameters, and have anticonvulsant properties. Long-acting benzodiazepines with active metabolites, such as chlordiazepoxide and diazepam, provide more stable serum drug levels. For patients in liver failure, a short-acting benzodiazepine without active metabolites, such as lorazepam, may prevent the development of secondary oversedation caused by the buildup of undetoxified metabolites. Table 33-7 shows the benzodiazepines most commonly used in the management of alcohol withdrawal. Various dosing schedules have been used for detoxification. For all patients, dosing must be individualized to adequately relieve the signs and symptoms of withdrawal. Some patients require extremely high doses because of their high tolerance for CNS depressants. In patients who are at high risk for withdrawal, diazepam can be initiated at 10 to 20 mg every hour, holding doses for sedation. Once the patient is stable, the benzodiazepine can be tapered gradually over 2 to 5 days, as tolerated by the patient. During tapering, doses are not administered when there is excessive sedation or the patient is sleeping soundly.

Symptom-triggered dosing is generally the preferred method of withdrawal management. It uses withdrawal signs and symptoms to measure the severity of the withdrawal and guide dosing.[141] Standardized scales such as the Clinical Institute Withdrawal Assessment Scale for Alcohol-Revised (CIWA-Ar)[142] provide good validity, interrater reliability, and clinical utility. Doses are given in response to a threshold score. Withdrawal scores also offer a means to monitor the response to treatment. Research has shown that use of a symptom inventory minimizes both oversedation and undertreatment of withdrawal and results in lower amounts of drugs used.[141]

TABLE 33-7 **Benzodiazepines Commonly Used for Alcohol Withdrawal Management**

Drug	Pharmacology
Diazepam (Valium)	Active metabolite Long acting Incomplete intramuscular absorption; should be given IV or orally Total body clearance is inversely proportional to patient's age and directly proportional to liver function
Chlordiazepoxide (Librium)	Active metabolite Long acting Manufacturer recommends no more than 300 mg/day Can be given IV; however, do not use accompanying diluent for IV administration, use sterile normal saline solution instead; diluent is intended for intramuscular use only
Oxazepam (Serax)	No active metabolite Intermediate acting Oral route only Useful for elderly patients and those with hypoalbuminemia
Lorazepam (Ativan)	No active metabolite Short acting Useful for patients in hepatic failure

The Sullivan Protocol (Table 33-8), a modification of the CIWA-Ar, has been adapted for use in critically ill patients. Patients are scored every 2 hours while awake and every 4 hours while asleep, and they receive a graduated dose of benzodiazepine depending on their score. Table 33-9 provides examples of graduated dosing with lorazepam and diazepam. The score is reassessed 30 minutes after dosing, and the dose is repeated if the score remains higher than 5 and the respiratory rate is more than 12 breaths per minute. When the withdrawal severity score is consistently greater than 5 after repeated doses, an increase in dose is indicated.[143]

Although there are no controlled studies to support their use, neuroleptic agents (such as haloperidol) are sometimes used to help control agitation in delirious patients. It should be remembered that these agents do not decrease autonomic hyperactivity and can reduce the seizure threshold, thus precipitating or exacerbating withdrawal seizures.[140,141] The risk of neuroleptic malignant syndrome must also be considered because cases have been reported in patients with alcohol withdrawal who have received neuroleptic drugs.

Beer, liquor, and IV ethanol are occasionally used to prevent or treat alcohol withdrawal delirium. Despite several anecdotal reports of the successful use of IV ethanol, data on its effectiveness for prophylaxis and treatment of alcohol withdrawal have been inconclusive. In addition to questionable efficacy, ethanol exhibits inconsistent pharmacokinetics and a relatively narrow therapeutic index.[144,145]

Other agents such as propofol and anticonvulsants have been used, but no definitive studies have shown a superior role compared with benzodiazepines.[140]

Sedative-Hypnotic Withdrawal. Sedative-hypnotic withdrawal symptoms are similar to those of alcohol withdrawal. Onset and duration vary with the half-life of the agent used. Symptoms of sedative-hypnotic withdrawal include tremor, muscle twitching, weakness, nausea, vomiting, anorexia, restlessness, irritability, insomnia, blurred vision, vital sign elevations, mydriasis, and diaphoresis. Seizures and delirium may be seen with abstinence after high-dose use. Patients who have been on a short-acting benzodiazepine for longer than 6 weeks, those taking average daily doses of one and a half to two times the normal dose of longer-acting agents for 45 days, and those who have taken therapeutic doses for a year or more are at risk for withdrawal symptoms after drug cessation. Concurrent use of alcohol raises the risk of sedative-hypnotic withdrawal.[132]

Management of withdrawal from sedative-hypnotics is accomplished with several different stategies, depending on the particular drug used, the duration of use, and the patient's response to treatment or prior treatments. One method involves the gradual weaning of the sedative-hypnotic on which the patient is dependent. Because this may require several weeks of dose tapering, it is not usually completed during an acute hospitalization.

Another method involves the substitution of another longer-acting, cross-tolerant drug, such as chlordiazepoxide, clonazepam, or diazepam, at an equipotent dose. Once the patient is stable on the long-acting agent, it is gradually tapered by 20% to 25% every 1 to 2 days. Phenobarbital (or pentobarbital) substitution and tapering can also be used for detoxification from sedative-hypnotics.[132]

Opiate Withdrawal

All opiates have similar withdrawal signs and symptoms, although the time frame and intensity of symptoms vary depending on the drug used. Short-acting opiates such as heroin, morphine, and meperidine have a brief, intense withdrawal syndrome that typically begins 4 to 6 hours after the last dose, peaks in intensity 48 to 72 hours after cessation, and lasts 5 to 10 days. Long-acting agents such as methadone are characterized by a milder withdrawal syndrome that begins 24 to 84 hours after the last dose but may persist for several weeks.[146]

Assessment. Symptoms of opiate withdrawal include yawning, lacrimation, rhinorrhea, diaphoresis, mydriasis, myalgia, tremors, nausea, vomiting, diarrhea, abdominal cramps, fever, chills, tachycardia, hypertension, piloerection, muscle cramping, and involuntary leg movements ("kicking"). Many of these symptoms are caused by increased activity of the autonomic nervous system. Patients are anxious and irritable and have strong drug cravings. Muscle cramping and gastrointestinal hyperactivity are especially distressing. Opiate withdrawal is seldom life threatening in a healthy

TABLE 33-8 **Sullivan Protocol**

Symptom	Point Value*	Scale
Tremor	1	Tremor felt by examiner but not visible
	2	Mild, visible tremor
	3	Marked, visible tremor
Tachycardia	1	Pulse rate 80-100 beats/min
	2	Pulse rate 100-130 beats/min
	3	Pulse rate >130 beats/min
Hypertension (valid only in absence of hypertensive history)	1	Systolic 150-175 mm Hg
	2	Systolic 175-200 mm Hg
	3	Systolic >200 mm Hg
Diaphoresis	1	Mild, barely visible
	2	Moderate
	3	Marked, gown/bedding wet
Nausea/vomiting	1	Nausea only
	2	Vomits two or fewer times in 8 hours
	3	Frequent vomiting, dry heaves
Fever	1	38° C or less
	2	38°-38.5° C
	3	>38.5° C
Agitation	1	Activity increased
	2	Restless, fidgety
	3	Restless, thrashing in bed
Confusion, orientation, contact with reality	1	Detached, decreased sensation, vague orientation
	2	Vague about current illness, disorientation is infrequent
	3	Detached, no staff contact, disoriented
Sleeplessness	1	Awake during night (two or three times)
	2	Awake half the night or more
Hallucinations	1	Auditory only or visual only, not agitated from hallucinations
	2	Unrelated auditory and visual hallucinations
	3	Auditory and visual hallucinations are related
Seizure	—	Document presence or absence.

*If a sign/symptom is not present, score as "0."
Scoring method: Sum scores from each category to obtain an overall Sullivan score.
From Watling SM, Fleming C, Casey P et al: Nursing-based protocol for treatment of alcohol withdrawal in the intensive care unit, *Am J Crit Care* 4:66-70, 1995.

individual. However, the traumatized patient may be unable to tolerate the added stress of withdrawal.

Treatment. Acute opiate withdrawal in the absence of significant pain can be treated successfully with any opioid, but daily administration of a long-acting opioid such as methadone is generally preferred. It is available in oral and parenteral preparations. Patients with a known history or objective evidence of opioid use (positive toxicology results, physical signs of intravenous use) can be started on methadone early in the hospital course. Although strict federal guidelines control the use of methadone for detoxification of outpatients, these guidelines allow for the use of methadone for opioid detoxification in hospitalized inpatients in the short term. An initial dose of 20 to 40 mg is generally sufficient to control most symptoms of withdrawal. The dose can then be increased if no observable effect is seen. IV doses of methadone, for patients unable to take enteral medication, are typically one half the oral dose. The methadone can be tapered 5 to 10 mg per day. If a patient is enrolled in a methadone maintenance program, the treatment facility should be contacted to determine the patient's current dose.

Clonidine, an α-adrenergic agent, may be used to block some of the sympathetic hyperactivity associated with opioid withdrawal. It has little effect, however, on drug cravings, mood alterations, and muscle cramps. Hypotension is a possible side effect.[146]

Buprenorphine, a partial agonist at the μ opiate receptor, may also be used to manage opioid withdrawal in select trauma patients who are not feeling severe pain. Buprenorphine undergoes a high first-pass metabolism and for this

TABLE 33-9 **Sample Benzodiazepine Dosing Chart**

Sullivan Scale Severity Score	Lorazepam Dose	Diazepam Dose
>12	4 mg	10 mg
10-11	3 mg	7.5 mg
8-9	2 mg	5 mg
6-7	1 mg	2.5 mg
0-5	0 mg	0 mg

From Watling SM, Fleming C, Casey P et al: Nursing-based protocol for treatment of alcohol withdrawal in the intensive care unit, *Am J Crit Care* 4:66-70, 1995.

reason is administered sublingually or parenterally. Typical doses for detoxification are 4 to 16 mg sublingually per day. The dose must be individualized on the basis of the patient's withdrawal symptoms. Parenteral dosing should be reserved for patients who are unable to adequately handle oral secretions. Typical doses of parenteral buprenorphine are 0.3 to 0.6 mg two to four times per day. The buprenorphine dose is then tapered over 5 to 7 days, depending on the patient's response to the medication. Because it may precipitate withdrawal, buprenorphine should not be used for patients who have received a short-acting opioid in the past 6 hours or those who have received methadone in the previous 24 hours. Patients who are likely to require surgery or administration of opiates in the near future should also not be started on buprenorphine.

Central Nervous System Stimulant Withdrawal

Withdrawal from a CNS stimulant is not associated with the high morbidity of CNS depressant withdrawal. Stimulants are often used in a binge pattern in which the user continuously readministers the drug. Binges may last for several days, and on cessation of this heavy drug use, a person may have withdrawal, which is usually brief and self-limited. The period for the development of withdrawal varies with the stimulant used and the route by which it was ingested. Initial drug craving is followed by what is often referred to as "the crash," a period of intense dysphoria, depression, anxiety, strong drug cravings, and possible psychomotor agitation.[147] The length of the crash varies from 12 hours to 4 days for cocaine and up to a week for methamphetamine. Some patients have suicidal ideation during this phase. Toward the end of the crash, hypersomnia develops with some sleep cycle alterations. After the crash, sleep cycles begin to normalize, appetite increases, the patient's mood stabilizes, and cravings abate. During the early phase of withdrawal, physiologic parameters return to baseline.

Treatment. Currently there are no specific pharmacologic treatments for acute CNS stimulant withdrawal. Highly anxious patients may benefit from a short-acting benzodiazepine. Stimulant withdrawal is best treated supportively by permitting the patient to sleep and eat as necessary.[147] Ideally, treatment should be aimed at promoting the return of natural sleep cycles and minimizing anxiety, although this may be difficult in the critical care setting. A calm, quiet environment with appropriate lighting and scheduled activities with periods of rest can alleviate some of the distress. Evidence of suicidal ideation should be reported to the physician immediately.

Cannabis Withdrawal

Acute cannabis withdrawal is a mild syndrome associated with abrupt cessation after heavy, regular use. Withdrawal symptoms include irritability, restlessness, insomnia, anorexia, nausea, and diarrhea. Physiologic alterations include mild increases in heart rate, temperature, and blood pressure. Symptoms of withdrawal abate without treatment and patients may benefit from a calm environment.[147]

Nicotine Withdrawal

Because of the short half-life of nicotine, symptoms of nicotine withdrawal begin within 30 minutes after the last nicotine dose and peak in about 24 hours. Full detoxification is reached in about 72 hours, although cravings may persist for weeks to months. Withdrawal is characterized by intense cravings, irritability, agitation, insomnia, dysphoria, difficulty concentrating, decreased heart rate and blood pressure, decreased intestinal motility, and increased appetite.[148] Patients often complain of "needing" a cigarette, and they may attempt to leave the patient care area to smoke.

Treatment. Mitigating the symptoms of nicotine withdrawal can decrease the patient's level of anxiety and irritability. Patients can be placed on a transdermal nicotine patch starting at a dose of 14 mg per day. If the patient has typically smoked more than a pack per day, he or she may initially require 21 mg per day. Patients hospitalized for a long period may be able to be weaned during the stay. Severe cardiovascular disease and sensitivity to the patch are the only major contraindications to its use. Patch sites should be rotated daily to avoid skin irritation, and patches should be applied to relatively hair-free areas for maximal absorption. Nicotine gum, inhaler, lozenges and nasal spray can also be used.

PAIN MANAGMENT

The clinical conditions of pain and opioid dependence are related phenomena; the presence of one condition influences the other. There are multiple reports documenting the fact that health care providers undermedicate patients with opiates for fear of initiating or exacerbating addiction. Although patients receiving long-term opioids may become physically dependent, true addiction, with its attendant mental and behavioral components, is relatively rare. When a patient has a known substance use disorder, health care providers may be even more vigilant in their attempts to limit the use of opioids to avoid perpetuating the addiction or creating a second addiction.[149] In general, patients with a history of opiate dependence have a higher tolerance to opiates compared with the general population. However, tolerance varies from person to person, just as it does among persons not dependent on chemicals.

Patients receiving opiate agonist therapy with methadone will receive little, if any, analgesia from a maintenance dose of medication. Patients receiving methadone maintenance should be continued on their maintenance doses after verification of the dose by the methadone provider. Additional opiate and nonopiate therapies for acute pain should be instituted in addition to the patient's daily methadone dose. Conventional shorter-acting agents such as morphine, codeine, or fentanyl should be given in addition to methadone to manage acute pain.

Patients receiving buprenorphine maintenance present a unique challenge in the management of acute pain because of the high affinity of buprenorphine for the μ receptor. This high affinity results in displacement of, or competition with, full opioid agonists when administered concurrently or sequentially. Several options in the treatment of acute pain in patients receiving buprenorphine maintenance are available. The buprenorphine dose can be increased to see whether the patient achieves adequate analgesia. Alternately, the buprenorphine can be discontinued and short-acting opiates added. It must be remembered that adequate analgesia may take some time because the buprenorphine dissociates from the opiate receptors. Local and regional analgesia can also be useful. In all cases, naloxone should be available and the level of consciousness and respirations should be frequently monitored.[150]

Analgesic doses required for pain relief vary widely and must be titrated to the individual patient. Typically, because of increased tolerance, these patients often require higher and more frequent dosing. Patient-controlled analgesia used in conjunction with methadone can be an effective strategy for the opioid-abusing patient and may also help reduce power struggles between patients and care providers over administration times. As acute pain decreases, patients can then be switched to oral formulations. Nonsteroidal anti-inflammatory drugs (NSAIDs) are also efficacious and can be used in conjunction with opiate analgesia. Patients should be started on routine scheduled doses of NSAIDs in addition to opiate analgesics. Ketorolac, an NSAID available in a parenteral form, can be used when patients are unable to take enteral medications.

Analgesia in Recovering Patients

Health care providers may encounter chemically dependent patients who are "in recovery" from addiction at the time of injury. These patients and their health care providers may share legitimate concerns about "reactivating" addiction if opiates are used. However, the risk of relapse is also present if adequate analgesia is not provided, and it is generally inappropriate to withhold analgesia. Relapse can be avoided as long as issues of analgesia, fears about relapse, and coping strategies for drug cravings are addressed.[149] Health care providers should review the analgesia plan with the patient and family and discuss drug cravings felt. Nonpharmacologic modalities such as relaxation, heat, and elevation should be used along with nonopiate forms of analgesia. Involvement of social supports is crucial.

Nursing Management Considerations

Nutritional Deficiencies

Wernicke's encephalopathy is an acute neurologic disorder caused by thiamine deficiency. Prevention and treatment of Wernicke's encephalopathy should be instituted in any patient with a history of alcohol abuse or a positive BAC on admission.[151] Patients should receive 100 mg of thiamine parenterally for a minimum of 3 days because the deficiency may be related to either decreased intake of thiamine or to inadequate absorption of thiamine. High plasma concentrations are needed to correct the deficiency.[152]

Patients should also receive 1 mg per day of folate and a multivitamin supplement either parenterally or enterally. Magnesium levels should be normalized because hypomagnesemia can increase resistance to thiamine.

Consultation with a registered dietitian is invaluable in assessing the dietary needs of substance abusers. Patients with long-standing alcoholism and drug use are often deficient in macronutrients, vitamins, and minerals. Alcohol is an energy-dense but nutrient-poor nutritional source. As much as 50% of the long-term alcohol user's caloric intake may be derived from alcohol. Patients with severe hepatic dysfunction may require limited protein to prevent the development of hepatic encephalopathy. Increased protein requirements must be balanced with the risk of encephalopathy.

The various anemias associated with drug and alcohol abuse can be treated with folic acid or ferrous sulfate. Folic acid is given at 1 mg per day orally or as an IV fluid additive. Ferrous sulfate (325 mg three times daily) is given with food to minimize gastric irritation.

Risk of Infection

Infections should be identified and treated aggressively to minimize complications. Trauma patients who demonstrate clinical evidence of possible infection (e.g., fever, leukocytosis) should be evaluated for sources of infection, including those associated with substance abuse. As with any patient, it is important for health care providers to practice strict universal precautions and use appropriate sterile technique.

Research has identified alcohol's adverse effects on the immune system. These adverse effects result in depression of immune function, increasing the person's predisposition for infectious diseases. Immune system derangements include decreased activity of natural killer cells,[153,154] diminished neutrophil activity, and impaired lymphocyte function.[155] One study of patients with penetrating abdominal trauma found that those with a BAC more than 200 mg/dl at admission had a greater than twofold incidence of trauma-related infections.[156] In another study of trauma patients, long-term alcohol use was associated with a twofold increase in infectious complications.[32] Patients who use inhaled drugs are likely to have impaired pulmonary immune response. Tobacco, marijuana, and cocaine smoke all cause dysfunction of alveolar macrophages, one of the primary immune defences of the pulmonary tree.[157] Patients who abuse alcohol or IV drugs have a high incidence of tuberculosis, many with highly resistant strains.

IV drug users have a high risk of contracting blood-borne infections and may already have an underlying infection such as hepatitis, human immunodeficiency virus (HIV), or subclinical bacterial endocarditis (BE). Patients with elevated liver enzymes and signs and symptoms consistent with hepatitis infection should be tested for both hepatitis B and C and HIV. Patients who have or develop opportunistic infections consistent with HIV infection should be tested for that virus.

BE and its sequelae are other common comorbidities found in IV drug users. Unlike patients with rheumatic heart disease who have BE, IV drug users often have BE in the valves on the right side of the heart.[118] These patients are at risk for pulmonary infarctions from septic emboli. It should be considered in patients consistently running a temperature of 38.5° C or higher in the absence of other conditions.

Alterations in Respiratory Function

Regular pulmonary hygiene is a crucial aspect of nursing care for these patients. Those who are able to cooperate with incentive spirometry should have it instituted as soon as possible in the hospital course. Patients who are mechanically ventilated or who are unable to cooperate with incentive spirometry require chest physiotherapy and either endotracheal or nasotracheal suctioning to mobilize secretions. Routine turning and mobilization out of bed to a chair as soon as possible help to mobilize secretions and maintain alveolar patency.

Illicit Drug Use During Hospitalization

Withdrawal from mood-altering drugs such as alcohol, cocaine, opiates, and nicotine frequently causes strong drug cravings. Hospitalized patients may try to acquire drugs from illicit sources to manage their withdrawal. If sudden alterations in mood or behavior suggest that a patient has obtained illicit drugs, a repeat toxicology screen may be obtained to document the occurrence. Supervised visitation may become necessary under these circumstances.

Intermediate Care and Rehabilitation Phases

The intermediate care and rehabilitation phases focus on returning patients to their optimal functional status. For the substance-abusing patient, this also includes the need to address the substance abuse as a primary disorder. Patient education should focus on the impact of the substance abuse and chemical dependence as a chronic disorder with its own natural history, similar to that of other chronic diseases.

Nursing Management Considerations

Sleep Pattern Disruption

Most patients with a history of substance abuse have sleep cycle disruptions in the acute withdrawal period. Stimulant abusers sleep more during the acute withdrawal period and have more rapid eye movement (REM) sleep. In contrast, alcohol-dependent individuals have less total sleep and REM during the acute withdrawal phase.[158] Promoting normalization of sleep cycles by providing uninterrupted rest periods, manipulating room lighting to simulate day and night, and using relaxation techniques is important to prevent sleep deprivation.

Family Dynamics

Families in which one or more individuals have drug or alcohol dependence may be unstable and chaotic. Altered communication patterns within these families may include silence, decreased sharing, and active concealment of problems. Individual members are neglected and their needs unmet. Much of the family's energy may have been directed at controlling the chemically dependent member and coping with the consequences of substance abuse. High levels of anger and guilt are common. An acute traumatic event may exacerbate the level of stress in what is already a stressed system. Family members may find it difficult to work together for mutual support and problem solving.[159]

In addition to the other fears felt by all families who have undergone trauma, families of substance abusers may have the additional burden of wondering if this was another in a series of incidents related to the substance abuse. Family members may inquire about drinking or other drug use before the injury. Toxicology results are confidential and require the patient's written consent before any release of information. A family that has secured legal representation for the patient needs to have the patient give written consent for the release of medical records to the attorney.

Motivational Crisis

An injury episode necessitating hospitalization can serve as a pivotal point in the course of a patient's substance use disorder. It may provide a window of opportunity through which to confront the substance abuser with the reality of his or her disease process. Although some patients minimize the role of alcohol in causing their injuries,[160] hospitalization may diminish some of the psychologic barriers typically used to minimize the consequences of substance use.[161] They may be more willing to discuss their alcohol use, especially when they were injured while drinking.[162] Studies have indicated that trauma patients who are more likely to attribute their injury to alcohol-related causes may be more willing to change behavior after injury and are often more amenable to addiction treatment.[163-166]

Intervening in Substance Use Disorders

Review of available literature demonstrates that trauma centers have done a fair job of detecting psychoactive drug-abusing and drug-dependent patients and a less adequate job of counseling or referring them for appropriate chemical dependence treatment after acute hospitalization and rehabilitation. There may be a belief on the part of health care providers that there is little they can do to assist these patients[166] and that most will not be accepting of intervention.[167] There is evidence, however, that even brief interventions may encourage drug-using patients to alter their behavior.[168-170] Reports from Level I trauma centers have demonstrated a reduction in alcohol consumption, reinjury rates, and other consequences in patients who received a brief intervention (BI) or nonjudgmental brief advice.[171-176]

Brief motivational interviews are among the most effective and least expensive treatment modalities.[166] Further, a recent-cost benefit analysis of BI for injured patients treated in emergency departments and among those requiring hospital admission concluded that every dollar spent on screening and BI results in almost $4 in saved health care expenditures.[174]

The nurse is usually the person who has greatest amount of patient contact to permit such an intervention. Indeed, studies have demonstrated that BIs are effectively provided by nurses.[170,172,175] A calm, nonjudgmental approach that helps the patient to examine the consequences of his or her substance use is appropriate. An assessment of the patient's perceptions regarding the need for change and what is necessary to effect the change should be performed.

Substance Abuse Treatment

Treatment outcomes for substance use disorders have been shown to be similar to those seen with other chronic conditions such as hypertension, asthma, and diabetes. Rates of compliance with medication and behavioral regimens are often less than 30% and relapse rates range between 30% to 60%.[177,178] It is clear that the majority of people are not "cured" of substance use disorders but that many do very well in treatment.

Patients admitted with positive toxicology screens, those in whom withdrawal syndromes develop after admission, and those whose screening results indicate substance misuse or abuse should be evaluated by a clinician with some knowledge and experience in substance abuse assessment, prevention, treatment, and referral. A substance abuse team, if available, should provide referrals for treatment after the acute hospitalization. Addiction specialists may also be invaluable for managing patients with complicated withdrawal syndromes or psychiatric comorbidities.

One study documented a 62% acceptance rate for treatment in a group of trauma patients evaluated by a substance abuse consultation team.[176] The ASAM has developed a set of patient placement criteria for determining the appropriate level of treatment. It uses six dimensions for evaluating addiction severity. Levels of treatment range from patient education to long-term residential treatment.[179] Providers should offer treatment alternatives rather than a single option as research has failed to show consistent superiority of a single level of treatment.[180] If the patient desires treatment, arrangements can be made and incorporated into the discharge planning with follow-up as soon after discharge as possible.

Many hospitals have no formal chemical dependence counseling available, and nursing staff may be the only link to substance abuse treatment and community support resources. Nurses at such facilities can develop a directory of treatment centers and community resources to facilitate continuing care for these patients. At a minimum, content about chemical dependence should be incorporated into the education plan for patients with evidence of substance abuse. This includes information about adverse effects of the substances, the personal and interpersonal impact of substance use (with a focus on traumatic injury as a direct result of substance use), the chronic nature of substance use disorders, and the availability of treatment.

Stages of Change

The stages-of-change model was developed by Prochaska et al[181] on the basis of their observations of how people change behaviors involving alcohol and cigarettes. Their research demonstrated that change occurs in a series of stages, each with distinct characteristics. People move back and forth between the stages, often several times before lasting change occurs.The stages of change are precontemplation, contemplation, preparation, action, maintenance, and termination (Table 33-10). Health care providers can intervene in any of the stages by using different strategies in each. Matching interventions to the patient's current stage is critical.

Patients in the precontemplation stage do not perceive that a problem exists; thus, they do not identify any need to alter their behavior. These patients are often said to be in denial; however, they can be motivated to change with use of the proper tools.[164,181]

Contemplators acknowledge the existence of a problem and contemplate change. They struggle to understand their problem and search for solutions. They frequently tell themselves they need to change but have indefinite plans for change. Additionally, they are unsure of how to change and feel that they will not be successful.[164,181]

TABLE 33-10 **Stages of Change (Prochaska, DiClemente, and Norcross)**

Stage	Intervention
Precontemplation	Educate patient on the negative effects the behavior is having on his or her life, etc.
Contemplation	Help patient to look at the short- and long-term effects of behavior.
Preparation	Encourage patient to pick a stop/change date.
	Reinforce the decisions made up to that point.
	Help patient to identify triggers for the behavior.
Action	Help patient to see how he or she can modify his or her behavior, environment, or experiences to help facilitate change.
	Explore ways of dealing with triggers and craving.
Maintenance	Help patient to continue to monitor for triggers and signs of relapse.
	Continue to support the gains.

People in the preparation stage intend to act in the near future. They are committed to action and appear ready but often have unresolved ambivalence. Commonly they are trying to decide which course of action is best.[164,181]

The action stage is characterized by overt modification of behavior and the environment. This stage places the greatest demand on time and energy. It is the most visible to others.[164,181]

Maintenance involves measures used to consolidate the changes made during the action phase and to avoid relapse. The process of change does not end with action.[164,181]

Termination is the final stage of change. In this phase the former problem is no longer an issue and no effort is required on the person's part to maintain the change. Many believe that, because of the chronic nature of addiction, this stage is unattainable for most individuals.[164,181]

Brief Intervention

BI refers to strategic action on the part of a health care provider with the intent of effecting behavioral change.[164] BI is derived from *motivational interviewing*, an evidence-based psychosocial treatment for substance use disorders that focuses on preparing patients for change.[182] It attempts to engage patients in a nonconfrontational manner and is often described as "meeting the patient where they are" (Box 33-1). It is composed of a variety of activities directed at problem substance users who are not dependent. The content is instructional and motivational and consists of feedback from screening tests and laboratory results, drug education, and practical advice.[166]

BI has been found to be just as effective as more formal interventions. BI performed by primary health care providers has been proven effective for treating socially stable, heavy-drinking patients.[183,184] BI has been found efficacious in trauma patients and adolescents seen in emergency departments after alcohol-related incidents. Alcohol consumption and reinjury have been decreased in both groups with the use of BI.[171-173,185-187] It has not been shown to be effective for highly alcohol- or drug-dependent patients. These patients should be referred for substance abuse treatment.

The FRAMES model of brief intervention has six components[182]: feedback, responsibility, advice, menu, empathy, and self-efficacy (Table 33-11). Not all components are necessarily used during each interaction. Some are more relevant than others during the various stages in the change process.[182] The FRAMES model and other processes are helpful for promoting change in drug use.

BOX 33-1 Five Principles of Motivational Interviewing

- **R**oll with **R**esistance
- **E**xpress **E**mpathy
- **A**void **A**rgumentation
- **D**evelop **D**iscrepancy
- **S**upport **S**elf-efficacy

TABLE 33-11 FRAMES Model

Feedback: respectfully giving specific information that concerns the patient
Responsibility: stressing that the patient is responsible for any change
Advice: respectfully giving advice to the patient
Menu: offering patient a menu of choices
Empathy: listening and forming accurate reflective statements
Self-efficacy: change is possible and change is beneficial

From Bien TH, Miller WR, Tonigan JS: Brief interventions for alcohol problems: a review, *Addiction* 88:315-335, 1993.

Consciousness raising may be effective during precontemplation, when individuals actively resist change. Many are discouraged and unsure whether change is possible. Health care providers can explore how patients feel when the behavior is discussed. Defensiveness about the behavior is common at this stage. The patient's awareness of the risks and benefits of the behavior and his or her willingness to accept the consequences associated with the behavior should be determined. Minimizing the problem and blaming others are common defense strategies. The patient should be helped in identifying available support systems, and his or her willingness to use the social resources should be assessed. The goal of the intervention is to increase ambivalence, a sign that a patient has moved into the contemplation phase.[181] Ambivalence is common in those with substance use problems and interventions are structured to focus on the patient's perspective of the problem and what the patient wants to do about it.[162]

Emotional arousal can be effective during contemplation.[181] The clinician can review the risks and benefits of continued drug or alcohol use. The patient should be asked to summarize his or her perception of personal risk. The goal is to make the risks more prominent in the patient's mind.

The preparation stage involves assisting the patient in planning how to implement change. Setting a quit date, removing paraphernalia, telling others about the intention to quit, and enlisting social support aid in making the change is a priority. Careful planning in the preparation stage can facilitate the transition to the action phase.[166,181]

During the action stage, several interventions promote the change process. Taking purposeful action, identifying and actively avoiding drug use triggers, and engaging in alternative activities all promote successful change. Positive feedback and recognition of accomplishments are crucial in this phase.[166,181]

Maintenance requires sustained long-term effort to continue the lifestyle changes initiated during the action phase. Health care providers can offer ongoing positive feedback while acknowledging any difficulties. They should reinforce the benefits of change. This is a time when external feedback often wanes.[166,181]

Social Network Intervention

A social network intervention or traditional intervention can be effective in trauma patients.[188] It is typically coordinated by a chemical dependence professional or psychiatrist. An intervention involves several members of the patient's social network. They meet with the interventionist, who provides education about alcoholism or drug addiction and the need for treatment and ascertains how the people have been affected by the substance abuse. The group then meets with the patient and the participants describe their observations and feelings about the effects of the substance use on them with the goal of getting the person to get help.[166]

COMMUNITY REINTEGRATION

"RECOVERY" FROM SUBSTANCE ABUSE

Patients in the earliest phases of alcohol misuse and abuse may have some success with controlled drinking. This is not generally true of those individuals with chemical dependencies. Addictions are chronic, progressive, potentially fatal illnesses of which trauma is a symptom. As such, they often require a life-long program of management, similar in some ways to that required by patients with diabetes or asthma.[177,178,189] This usually necessitates a goal of abstinence from the drug of choice and other mood-altering drugs, a structured plan of recovery with emphasis on learning new coping strategies, and personal support from other recovering people. Continuous vigilance is required for the continued well-being of these patients.

Community Support Systems

Community support resources can be invaluable to the patient with a substance use disorder. Alcoholic Anonymous (AA), which is widely available and free, is the most familiar community resource. AA uses a 12-step program of recovery and mutual support to maintain abstinence from alcohol and to facilitate spiritual growth. Research has identified that AA involvement is associated with positive outcomes.[190,191] Health care workers can assist patients by providing them with a local meeting schedule and by being familiar with meetings that address special needs. There are AA meetings for women, for gay and lesbian individuals, and, in some areas, language-specific meetings. Other 12-step programs that may be appropriate for referral are Cocaine Anonymous, Narcotics Anonymous (NA), and Chemically Dependent Anonymous. Patients are encouraged to find meetings where they feel comfortable. Many hospitals have AA or NA meetings available, and ambulatory patients should be encouraged to attend.

Although not as widely known or available, there are other self-help groups for substance abuse, such as Rational Recovery, Secular Organization for Sobriety, and Women for Sobriety. Rational Recovery uses a cognitive behavioral approach with no focus on spirituality. Women may prefer Women for Sobriety and its focus on enhancing self-esteem. It is also important to talk with involved family and friends and make them aware of relevant mutual help groups such as AlAnon and NarAnon.

Medications for Relapse Prevention

Medications such as methadone, naltrexone, and buprenorphine (for opioid dependence), and disulfiram, naltrexone, and acamprosate (for alcohol dependence) have been shown to be effective adjuncts to counseling in the treatment of substance use disorders. There is evidence that, in combination with psychotherapy or counseling, these medications can reduce the likelihood of relapse by reducing drug craving and reinforcement. Although clinical trials have shown these medications to be of benefit, addiction is a heterogeneous condition with variability in the response to medications.[192]

FOLLOW-UP TRAUMA CARE

Recovering substance users may require future surgery or hospitalization for continued care related to their injuries. Balancing analgesia needs with the potential for relapse requires open communication between patients and their care providers, including the primary physician, anesthesiologist, and nursing staff. Substance use should be monitored to try to ensure that anesthesia and analgesia needs can be met in a safe and effective manner, while minimizing the risks of relapse to active chemical use.[192] It also allows other aspects of the patient's substance abuse recovery to be incorporated into the plan of care. Reasons for remaining abstinent previously identified by the patient can be reviewed at this time, and barriers to continued abstinence can be explored.[166] Clinicians can ascertain what patients are doing to promote abstinence and offer feedback to reinforce positive behavioral changes.[193] If patients are continuing to require opioids for pain, issues around misuse of prescribed medication and relapse to other substance use should be discussed. Family members should be included in discussions.

FUTURE NEEDS IN SUBSTANCE USE DISORDERS AND TRAUMA

Currently, 36 states in the United States operate under the Uniform Accident and Sickness Policy Provision Law, which allows insurance companies to exclude coverage for substance-related injuries. This forces staff in many trauma centers to purposely not screen or document screening for substance use for fear that the center will not receive financial compensation. Individual centers need to find ways to continue to screen for substance use disorders while ensuring patient confidentiality (separate charting for substance use–related material, separate consent forms for this information). The trauma community can also advocate for changes in the law to allow for better patient care.[194]

Trauma centers can become more active in community prevention including continuing public education about the link between all types of trauma and substance use. The public has been bombarded with messages about the risks of drinking and driving. They are less well-informed about the links between alcohol and all types of injury. Substance users often maintain that they are a threat only to themselves, which is clearly not the case. They present very real and costly hazards to society. Continuing research should focus on the efficacy of various treatment and trauma prevention programs, with funding provided for those models that effectively bring about results in terms of decreasing injury caused by substance use. Such research needs to identify which patients will best benefit from specific treatment and intervention techniques. It will be important for clinicians working in the treatment field to document the number of trauma patients and their short- and long-term treatment outcomes. It is imperative that long-term successes are measured, in addition to short-term outcomes such as the number of patients accepting substance abuse treatment.

Research also needs to focus on determining what period during hospitalization after trauma is the optimal time for successful substance abuse intervention and referral. Such research should also document which health care providers are most successful in this endeavor. Other general areas of inquiry include how best to present the information about substance abuse to the patient and how to include family members in the treatment.

SUMMARY

The ubiquity of substance use in our society is clearly reflected in the trauma population. Such patients are challenging not only because of their substance-induced comorbidities but also because of their high risk for reinjury. Caring for substance-abusing patients requires knowledgeable and skilled nursing care to develop and implement effective multidisciplinary plans of care throughout each phase of the trauma cycle.

REFERENCES

1. Levy D, Miller T, Cox K: *Costs of underage drinking,* Calverton, Md, 1999, Pacific Institute for Research and Evaluation.
2. Graham AW, Schultz TK, Mayo-Smith MF et al, editors: *Principles of addiction medicine,* 3rd ed, Chevy Chase, Md, 2003, American Society of Addiction Medicine.
3. American Psychiatric Association: *Diagnostic and statistical manual of mental disorders,* 4th ed, text revised, Washington, DC, 2000, American Psychiatric Association.
4. World Health Organization: *The ICD-10 international classification of diseases and health related problems,* 2nd ed, Geneva, Switzerland, 2004,World Health Organization.
5. National Institute on Alcohol Abuse and Alcoholism: *Helping patients who drink too much: a clinician's guide,* NIH Publication No. 05-3769, Washington, DC, 2005, U.S. Government Printing Office.
6. Substance Abuse and Mental Health Services Administration: *Overview of findings from the 2005 National Survey on Drug Use and Health,* Publication No. SMA 06-4194, NSDUH Series H-30, Rockville, Md, 2006, Office of Applied Studies, Department of Health and Human Services.
7. Cowan C: Coverage, sample design and weighting in three federal surveys, *J Drug Issues* 31:599-614, 2001.
8. U.S. Department of Health and Human Services: *Healthy people* 2010: *with understanding and improved health and objectives for improving health,* 2nd ed, Washington, DC, 2000, U.S. Government Printing Office.
9. DeWit D, Adlaf E, Offord D et al: Age at first alcohol use: a risk factor for the development of alcohol disorders, *Am J Psychiatry* 157:745-750, 2000.
10. Foster S, Vaughan R, Foster W et al: Alcohol consumption and expenditures for underage drinking and adult excessive drinking, *JAMA* 289:989-995, 2003.
11. Levy RS, Hebert CK, Munn BG et al: Drug and alcohol use in orthopedic trauma patients: a prospective study, *J Orthop Trauma* 10:21-27, 1996.
12. Soderstrom CA, Smith GS, Dischinger PC et al: Psychoactive substance use disorders among seriously injured trauma center patients, *JAMA* 277:1769-1774, 1997.
13. Walsh J, Flegl R, Atkins R et al: Drug and alcohol use among drivers admitted to a Level-1 trauma center, *Accid Anal Prev* 37:894-901, 2005.
14. Walsh J, Flegl R, Atkins R et al: Epidemiology of alcohol and other drug use among motor vehicle crash victims admitted to a trauma center, *Traffic Inj Prev* 5:254-260, 2004.
15. Cornwell EE, Belzberg H, Velmahos G et al: The prevalence and effect of alcohol and drug abuse on cohort-matched critically injured patients, *Am Surg* 64:461-465, 1998.
16. National Safety Council: *IMPACT: 2004 annual report,* Itasca, Ill, 2005, National Safety Council.
17. Tulloh BR, Collopy BT: Positive correlation between blood alcohol level and ISS in road trauma, *Injury* 25:538-543, 1994.
18. Brewer RD, Morris PD, Cole TB et al: The risk of dying in alcohol-related automobile crashes among habitual drunk drivers, *N Engl J Med* 331:513-517, 1994.
19. Soderstrom CA, Dischinger PC, Trifillis AL: Marijuana and other drug use among automobile and motorcycle drivers treated at a trauma center, *Accid Anal Prev* 27:131-135, 1995.
20. Sun SW, Kahn DM, Swan KG: Lowering the legal blood alcohol level for motorcyclists, *Accid Anal Prev* 30:133-136, 1998.
21. Rivara FP, Jurkovich GJ, Gurney JG et al: The magnitude of acute and chronic alcohol abuse in trauma patients, *Arch Surg* 128:907-912, 1993.
22. McGonigal MD, Cole J, Schwa CW et al: Urban firearm deaths: a five-year perspective, *J Trauma* 35:532-536, 1993.
23. Barillo DJ, Goode R: Substance abuse in victims of fire, *J Burn Care Rehab* 17:71-76, 1996.
24. Centers for Disease Control and Prevention: Nonfatal and fatal drownings in recreational water settings—United States, 2001-2002, *MMWR Morb Mortal Wkly Rep* 53:447-452, 2004.
25. Driscoll TR, Harrison JA, Steenkamp M: Review of the role of alcohol in drowning associated with recreational aquatic activity, *Inj Prev* 10:107-113, 2004.
26. Andersson AL, Bunketorp O: Cycling and alcohol, *Injury* 33:467-471, 2002.
27. Soderstrom CA, Smith GS, Kufera JA et al: The accuracy of the CAGE, the Brief Michigan Alcoholism Screening Test, and the Alcohol Use Disorders Identification Test in screening trauma center patients for alcoholism, *J Trauma* 43:962-969, 1997.
28. Davis NB, Hayes JS, Cohen S: Motor vehicle crashes and positive toxicology screens in adolescents and young adults, *J Trauma Nurs* 6:15-18, 1999.

29. Barnett NP, Spirito A, Colby SM et al: Detection of alcohol use in adolescent patients in the emergency department, *Acad Emerg Med* 5:607-612, 1998.
30. National Highway Traffic Safety Administration, National Center for Statistics and Analysis: *Traffic safety facts,* Publication No. HS 810 631, Washington, DC, 2007, National Highway Traffic Safety Administration.
31. Blomqvist S, Thorne J, Elmer O et al: Early post-traumatic changes in hemodynamics and pulmonary ventilation in alcohol-pretreated pigs, *J Trauma* 27:40-44, 1987.
32. Jurkovich GJ, Frederick P, Rivara MD et al: The effect of acute alcohol intoxication and chronic alcohol abuse on outcome from trauma, *JAMA* 270:51-56, 1993.
33. Li G, Keyl PM, Smith GS et al: Alcohol and injury severity: reappraisal of the continuing controversy, *J Trauma* 42:562-569, 1997.
34. Mueller BA, Kenaston T, Grossman D et al: Hospital charges to injured drinking drivers in Washington State: 1989-1993, *Accid Anal Prev* 30:597-605, 1998.
35. Kelly MP, Johnson CT, Knoller N et al: Substance abuse, traumatic brain injury and neuropsychological outcome, *Brain Inj* 11:391-402, 1997.
36. Soderstrom CA, Dischinger PC, Kerns T et al: Epidemic increases in cocaine and opiate use by trauma center patients: documentation with a large clinical toxicology database, *J Trauma* 51:557-564, 2001.
37. Darke S, Kelly E, Ross J: Drug driving among injection drug users in Sydney, Australia: prevalence, risk factors and risk perception, *Addiction* 99:175-185, 2004
38. Marzuk PM, Tardiff MD, Leon AC et al: Fatal injuries after cocaine use as a leading cause of death among young adults in New York City, *N Engl J Med* 332:1753-1757, 1995.
39. Tominaga GT, Garcia G, Dzierba A et al: Toll of methamphetamine on the trauma system, *Arch Surg* 139:844-847, 2004.
40. Danks RR, Wibbenmeyer LA, Faucher LD et al: Methamphetamine-associated burn injuries: a retrospective analysis, *J Burn Care Rehabil* 25:425-429, 2004.
41. Macdonald S, Anglin-Bodrug K, Mann R et al: Injury risk associated with cannabis and cocaine use, *Drug Alcohol Depend* 72:99-115, 2003.
42. Fergusson D, Horwood LJ: Cannabis use and traffic accidents in a birth cohort of young adults, *Accid Anal Prev* 33:703-711, 2001.
43. Piazza PV, LeMoal M: The role of stress in drug self-administration, *Pharmacol Sci* 19:67-74, 1998.
44. Stabenau JR: Additive independent factors that predict risk for alcoholism, *J Stud Alcohol* 51:164-174, 1990.
45. Van den Bree M, Johnson E, Neale M et al: Genetic and environmental influences on drug use and abuse/dependence in male and female twins, *Drug Alcohol Depend* 52:231-241, 1998.
46. Pickens RW, Svikins DS, McGue M et al: Heterogeneity in the inheritance of alcoholism: a study of male and female twins, *Arch Gen Psychiatry* 48:19-28, 1991.
47. McGue M, Pickens RW, Svikis DS: Sex and age effects on the inheritance of alcohol problems: a twin study, *J Abnorm Psychol* 101:3-17, 1992.
48. Bohman M, Sigvardsson S, Cloninger CR: Maternal inheritance of alcohol abuse: cross-fostering analysis of adopted women, *Arch Gen Psychiatry* 38:965-969, 1991.
49. Kendler KS, Prescott C: Cannabis use, abuse, and dependence in a population-based sample of female twins, *Am J Psychiatry* 155:1016-1022, 1998.
50. Kendler KS, Prescott C: Cocaine use, abuse, and dependence in a population-based sample of female twins, *Br J Psychiatry* 173:345-350, 1998.
51. Hurd YL: Perspectives on current directions in the neurobiology of addiction disorders relevant to genetic risk factors, *CNS Spectrum* 11:855-862, 2006.
52. Kendler KS, Heath AC, Neale MC et al: A population-based twin study of alcoholism in women, *JAMA* 268:1877-1882, 1992.
53. Schuckit MA: Reactions to alcohol in sons of alcoholics and controls, *Alcohol Clin Exp Res* 12:465-470, 1988.
54. McBride WJ, Chernet E, Dyr W et al: Densities of dopamine D2 receptors are reduced in CNS regions of alcohol-preferring P rats, *Alcohol* 10:387-390, 1993.
55. Barr CS, Schwandt M, Lindell SG et al: Association of functional polymorphism in the *mu*-opiod receptor gene with alcohol response and consumption in male rhesus macaques, *Arch Gen Psychiatry* 64:369-376, 2007.
56. LeMarquand D, Pihl RO, Benkelfat C: Serotonin and alcohol intake, abuse and dependence: clinical evidence, *Biol Psychiatry* 36:326-337, 1994.
57. Noble EP, Blum K, Ritchie T et al: Allelic association of the D2 dopamine receptor gene receptor-binding characteristics in alcoholism, *Arch Gen Psychiatry* 48:648-654, 1991.
58. Stanton MD: Drugs, Vietnam and the Vietnam veterans: an overview, *Am J Drug Alcohol Abuse* 3:557-570, 1976.
59. Najavits LM, Weiss RD, Shaw SR: The link between substance abuse and posttraumatic stress disorder in women: a research review, *Am J Addictions* 6:273-283, 1997.
60. Najavits LM, Gastfriend, DR, Barber JP et al: Cocaine dependence with and without PTSD among subjects in the National Institute on Drug Abuse Collaborative Cocaine Treatment Study, *Am J Psychiatry* 155:214-219, 1998.
61. Walker GC, Scott PS, Koppersmith G: The impact of child sexual abuse on addiction severity: an analysis of trauma processing, *J Psych Nurs Ment Health Serv* 36:10-18, 1998.
62. Grant BF, Stinson FS, Hasin DS et al: Prevalence and co-occurrence of substance use disorders and independent mood and anxiety disorders: results from the National Epidemiologic Survey on Alcohol and Related Conditions. *Arch Gen Psychiatry* 61:807-816, 2004.
63. Conway KP, Compton W, Stinson FS et al: Lifetime comorbidity of DSM-IV mood and anxiety disorders and specific drug use disorders: results from the National Epidemiologic Survey on Alcohol and Related Conditions, *J Clin Psychiatry* 67:247-257, 2006.
64. Stahl S: *Essential psychopharmacology,* 2nd ed, New York, 2000, Cambridge University.
65. O'Brien CP: Drug addiction and drug abuse. In Brunton L, Lazo J, Parker K et al, editors: *Goodman and Gilman's the pharmacological basis of therapeutics,* 11th ed, pp. 607-628, New York, 2005, McGraw-Hill.
66. Fleming M, Mihic SJ, Harris RA: Ethanol. In Brunton L, Lazo J, Parker K et al, editors: *Goodman and Gilman's the pharmacological basis of therapeutics,* 11th ed, pp. 591-806, New York, 2005, McGraw-Hill.
67. Frezza M, DiPadova D, Pozzato G et al: High blood alcohol levels in women: the role of decreased gastric alcohol dehydrogenase activity and first-pass metabolism, *N Engl J Med* 322:95-99, 1990.
68. Ticku MK, Kulkarni SK: Molecular interactions of ethanol with GABAergic systems and potential of RO15-4513 as an ethanol antagonist, *Pharm Biochem Behav* 30:501-510, 1988.

69. Treistman SN, Bayley H, Lemos JR: Effects of ethanol on calcium channels, potassium channels and vasopressin release, *Ann N Y Acad Sci* 625:249-263, 1991.
70. Weight FF, Lovinger DM, White G et al: Alcohol and anesthetic actions on excitatory amino acid-activated ion channels, *Ann N Y Acad Sci* 625:97-107, 1991.
71. Grant KA, Valverius P, Hudspith M et al: Ethanol withdrawal seizures and the NMDA receptor complex, *Eur J Pharmacol* 176:289-296, 1990.
72. Lovinger DM, White G, Weight FF: Ethanol inhibits NMDA-activated ion current in hippocampal neurons, *Science* 243:1721-1724, 1989.
73. Gianoulakis C: The effect of ethanol on the biosynthesis and regulation of opioid peptides, *Experientia* 45:428-435, 1989.
74. Lovinger DM, White G: Ethanol potentiation of 5-hydroxytryptamine receptor-mediated ion current in neuroblastoma cells and isolated adult mammalian neurons, *Mol Pharmacol* 40:263-270, 1991.
75. Brodie MS, Shefner SA, Dunwiddie TS: Ethanol increases the firing rate of dopamine neurons of the rat ventral tegmental area in vitro, *Brain Res* 508:65-69, 1990.
76. Mayo-Smith MF: Management of alcohol intoxication and withdrawal. In Graham AW, Schultz TK, Mayo-Smith MF et al editors: *Principles of addiction medicine,* 3rd ed, pp. 621-632, Chevy Chase, Md, 2003, American Society of Addiction Medicine.
77. Thomas AP, Rozanski DJ, Renard DC et al: Effects of ethanol on the contractile function of the heart: a review, *Alcohol Clin Exp Res* 18:121-131, 1994.
78. Constant J: The alcoholic cardiomyopathies-genuine and pseudo, *Cardiology* 91:92-95, 1999.
79. Zink BJU, Sheingerg MA, Wang X et al: Acute ethanol intoxication in a model of traumatic brain injury with hemorrhagic shock: effects of early physiological response, *J Neurosurg* 89:983-990, 1998.
80. Segel LD: Alcoholic cardiomyopathy in rats: inotropic response to phenylephrine, glucagon, ouabain, and dobutamine, *J Mol Cell Cardiol* 19:1061-1072, 1987.
81. Elmer O, Gustafson I, Gornasson G et al: Acute alcohol intoxication and traumatic shock, *Eur Surg Res* 5:268-275, 1983.
82. Rubin R, Rand ML: Alcohol and platelet function, *Alcohol Clin Exp Res* 18:105-110, 1994.
83. Parker RI: Etiology and treatment of acquired coagulopathies in the critically ill adult and child, *Crit Care Clin* 13:591-609, 1997.
84. Jaakola M, Frey T, Sillanaukee P et al: Acute pancreatic injury in asymptomatic individuals after heavy drinking over the long-term, *Hepatogastroenterology* 41:477-482, 1994.
85. Gutstein HB, Akil H: Opioid analgesics. In Brunton L, Lazo J, Parker K et al: editors: *Goodman and Gilman's the pharmacological basis of therapeutics,* 11th ed, pp. 547-590, New York, 2005, McGraw-Hill.
86. Cone EJ: Pharmacokinetics and pharmacodynamics of cocaine, *J Anal Toxicol* 19:459-477, 1995.
87. Vongpatanasin W, Mansour Y, Chavoshan B et al: Cocaine stimulates the human cardiovascular system via a central mechanism of action, *Circulation* 100:497-502, 1999.
88. Lange RA, Cigarroa RG, Yancy CW et al: Cocaine-induced coronary artery vasoconstriction, *N Engl J Med* 321:1557-1562, 1989.
89. Foltin RW, Fischman MW, Levin FR: Cardiovascular effects of cocaine in humans: laboratory studies, *Drug Alcohol Depend* 37:193-210, 1995.
90. Fineschi V, Wetli CV, DiPaolo M et al: Myocardial necrosis and cocaine: a quantitative morphologic study in 26 cocaine-associated deaths, *Int J Legal Med* 110:193-198, 1997.
91. Holland JG, Hume AS, Martin JN: Relation of cocaine use to seizures and epilepsy, *Epilepsia* 37:875-878, 1996.
92. Strickland TL, Miller BL, Kowell A et al: Neurobiology of cocaine-induced organic brain impairment: contributions from functional neuroimaging, *Neuropsychol Rev* 8:1-9, 1998.
93. Thadani PV: NIDA conference report on cardiopulmonary complications of "crack" cocaine use, *Chest* 110:1072-1076, 1996.
94. Mueller PJ, Qi G, Knuepfer MM: Ethanol alters hemodynamic responses to cocaine in rats, *Drug Alcohol Depend* 48:17-24, 1997.
95. McCance-Katz EF, Kosten TR, Jatlow P: Concurrent use of cocaine and alcohol is more potent and potentially more toxic than use of either alone—a multiple dose study, *Biol Psychiatry* 44:250-259, 1998.
96. Gorelick DA, Cornish JL: The pharmacology of cocaine, amphetamines and other stimulants. In Graham AW, Schultz TK, Mayo-Smith MF et al, editors: *Principles of addiction medicine,* 3rd ed, pp. 157-190, Chevy Chase, Md, 2003, American Society of Addiction Medicine.
97. Karan LD et al: The pharmacology of nicotine and tobacco. In Graham AW, Schultz TK, Mayo-Smith MF et al, editors: *Principles of addiction medicine,* 3rd ed, pp. 225-227, Chevy Chase, Md, 2003, American Society of Addiction Medicine.
98. Adams IB, Martin BR: Cannabis pharmacology and toxicology in animals and humans, *Addiction* 91:1585-1614, 1996.
99. Romero J, Garcia L, Fernandez-Ruiz JJ et al: Changes in rat brain cannabinoid binding sites after acute or chronic exposure to their endogenous agonist, anadamide, or to delta 9-tetrahydrocannabinol, *Pharmacol Biochem Behav* 51:731-737, 1995.
100. Axelrod J, Felder CC: Cannabinoid receptors and their endogenous agonist, anadamide, *Neurochem Res* 23:575-581, 1998.
101. Howlett AD: Pharmacology of cannabinoid receptors, *Annu Rev Pharmacol Toxicol* 35:607-634, 1995.
102. Ramaekers JG, Robbe HW, O'Hanlon JF: Marijuana, alcohol and actual driving performance, *Hum Psychopharmacol* 15:551-558, 2000.
103. Robbe HWJ: *Influence of marijuana on driving,* Maastricht, the Netherlands, 1994, Institute for Human Psychopharmacology, University of Limberg.
104. Heishman SJ, Huestis MA, Henningfield JE et al: Acute and residual effects of marijuana: profiles of plasma, THC levels, physiological subjective, and performance measures, *Pharmacol Biochem Behav* 37:561-565, 1990.
105. Solowij N: *The long-term effects of cannabis on the central nervous system, II: cognitive functioning,* Geneva, Switzerland, 1996 World Health Organization Project on Health Implications of Cannabis Use.
106. Fligiel SE, Roth MD, Kleeny EC et al: Tracheobronchial histopathology in habitual smokers of cocaine, marijuana and/or tobacco, *Chest* 112:319-326, 1997.
107. Fant RV, Heishman SJ, Bunker EB et al: Acute and residual effects of marijuana in humans, *Pharmacol Biochem Behav* 60:777-784, 1998.
108. Haney M, Ward AS, Comer SD et al: Abstinence symptoms following smoked marijuana in humans, *Psychopharmacology* 141:395-404, 1999.

109. Ksiakiewicz B, Bloch-Boguslawska E: Diagnostic difficulties with skull and brain injury complications in alcoholic patients, *Pol Merkuriusz Lek* 3:166-168, 1998.
110. Committee on Trauma, American College of Surgeons: *Resources for optimal care of the injured patient: 2006,* Chicago, Ill, 2006, American College of Surgeons.
111. Kaufmann CR, Branas CC, Brawley ML: A population-based study of trauma recidivism, *J Trauma* 45:325-332, 1998.
112. McIlroy MA, Reddy D, Markowitz H et al: Infected false aneurysms of the femoral artery in intravenous drug addicts, *Rev Infect Dis* 11:578-585, 1989.
113. Webber J, Kline, RA, Lucas, CE: Aortic thrombosis associated with cocaine use: report of two cases, *Ann Vasc Surg* 13:302-304, 1999.
114. Mirabile E, Wilson K, Saukkonen JJ: Respiratory tract disorders related to alcohol and other drug use. In Graham AW, Schultz TK, Mayo-Smith MF et al, editors: *Principles of addiction medicine,* 3rd ed, Chevy Chase, Md, 2003, American Society of Addiction Medicine.
115. Lucas CE: The impact of street drugs on trauma care, *J Trauma* 59:S57-S60, 2005.
116. Hoang MP, Lee EL, Anand A: Histologic spectrum of arterial and arteriolar lesions in acute and chronic cocaine-induced mesesteric ischemia: report of three cases and literature review, *Am J Surg Pathol* 22:1404-1410, 1998.
117. Pozner CN, Levine M, Zane R: The cardiovascular effects of cocaine, *J Emerg Med* 29:173-178, 2005.
118. Hoen B: Epidemiology and antibiotic treatment of infective endocarditis: an update, *Heart* 92:1694-1700, 2006.
119. Ewing JA: Detecting alcoholism: the CAGE questionnaire, *JAMA* 252:1905-1907, 1984.
120. Savage C: Screening and detection. In Allen KM, editor: *Nursing care of the addicted client,* pp. 100-117, Philadelphia, 1996, Lippincott.
121. Kitchens JM: Does this patient have an alcohol problem? *JAMA* 272:1782-1787, 1994.
122. Russell M, Martier S, Sokel R et al: Screening for pregnancy risk drinking TWEAKing the tests [abstract], *Alcohol Clin Exp Res* 18:1156-1161, 1994.
123. Reinert DF, Allen JP: The alcohol use disorders identification test (AUDIT): a review of recent research. *Alcohol Clin Exp Res* 26:272-279, 2002.
124. Soderstrom CA, Dischinger PC, Kerns TJ et al: Screening trauma patients for alcoholism according to the NIAAA guidelines with alcohol use disorders identification test questions, *Alcohol Clin Exp Res* 22:1470-1475, 1998.
125. Donovan DM, Dunn CW, Rivara FP et al: Comparison of trauma center self reports and proxy reports on the alcohol use identification test (AUDIT), *J Trauma* 56:873-882, 2004.
126. Ryb G, Soderstrom CA, Kufera JA et al: The use of blood alcohol concentration and laboratory tests to detect current alcohol dependence in trauma center patients, *J Trauma* 47:874-880, 1999.
127. Rosman AS, Lieber CS: Biochemical markers of alcohol consumption, *Alcohol Health Res World* 43:210-218, 1990.
128. Gronback M, Henriksen JH, Becker U: Carbohydrate-deficient transferrin: a valid marker of alcoholism in population studies? Results from the Copenhagen City Heart Study, *Alcohol Clin Exp Res* 19:457-461, 1995.
129. Soderstrom CA, Smith GS, Dischinger PC et al: CDT as a marker of alcoholism in trauma center patients [abstract], *J Addict Dis* 17:165, 1997.
130. Galbraith S: Misdiagnosis and delayed diagnosis in traumatic intracranial haematoma, *BMJ* 1:1438-1439, 1976.
131. Winbery S, Blaho K, Logan B et al: Multiple cocaine-induced seizures and corresponding cocaine and metabolite concentrations, *Am J Emerg Med* 16:529-533, 1998.
132. Dickinson WE Mayo-Smith MF, Eickelberg SJ: Management of sedative-hypnotic intoxication and withdrawal. In Graham AW, Schultz TK, Mayo-Smith MF et al, editors: *Principles of addiction medicine,* 3rd ed, pp. 633-650, Chevy Chase, Md, 2003, American Society of Addiction Medicine.
133. Brust JC: Ethanol. In Pioli SF, editor: *Neurological aspects of substance abuse,* 2nd ed, pp. 317-425, Philadelphia, 2004, Elsevier.
134. Spies CD, Neuner B, Neumann T et al: Intercurrent complications in chronic alcoholic men admitted to the intensive care unit following trauma, *Intensive Care Med* 22:286-293, 1996.
135. Elmer O, Lim R: Influence of acute intoxication on the outcome of severe non-neurologic trauma, *Acta Chir Scand* 151:305-308, 1985.
136. Desiderio M: The effects of acute, oral ethanol on cardiovascular performance before and after blunt cardiac trauma, *J Trauma* 27:267-277, 1987.
137. Richards CF, Clark RF, Holbrook T et al: The effect of cocaine and amphetamines on vital signs in trauma patients, *J Emerg Med* 13:59-63, 1995.
138. Vamvakas S, Teschner M, Bahner U et al: Alcohol abuse: potential role in electrolyte disturbances and kidney function, *Clin Nephrol* 49:205-213, 1998.
139. Hyatt B, Bensky KP: Illicit drugs and anesthesia, *CRNA* 10: 15-23, 1999.
140. DeBellis R, Smith BS, Choi S et al: Management of delirium tremens, *J Intensive Care Med* 20:164-173, 2005.
141. Mayo-Smith MF: Pharmacological management of alcohol withdrawal: a meta-analysis and and evidence-based guidelines, *JAMA* 278:144-151, 1997.
142. Sullivan JT, Sykora K, Schneiderman J et al: Assessment of alcohol withdrawal: the revised clinical institute withdrawal assessment for alcohol scale (CIWA-Ar), *Br J Addict* 84: 1353-1357, 1987.
143. Watling SM, Fleming C, Casey P et al: Nursing-based protocol for treatment of alcohol withdrawal in the intensive care unit, *Am J Crit Care* 4:66-70, 1995.
144. Rosenbaum M, McCarty T: Alcohol prescriptions by surgeons in the prevention and treatment of delirium tremens: historic and current practice, *Gen Hosp Psychiatry* 24:257-259, 2002.
145. Hodges B, Mazur JE: Intravenous ethanol for the treatment of alcohol withdrawal syndrome in critically ill patients, *Pharmacotherapy* 24:1578-1585, 2004.
146. O'Connor PG, Kosten TR, Stine SM: Management of opioid intoxication and withdrawal. In Graham AW, Schultz TK, Mayo-Smith MF et al, editors: *Principles of addiction medicine,* 3rd ed, pp. 651-667, Chevy Chase, Md, 2003, American Society of Addiction Medicine.
147. Wilkins JN, Mellott KG, Markvitsa R et al: Management of stimulant, hallucinogen, marijuana, phencyclidine intoxication and withdrawal. In Graham AW, Schultz TK, Mayo-Smith MF et al, editors: *Principles of addiction medicine,* 3rd ed, pp. 671-695, Chevy Chase, Md, 2003, American Society of Addiction Medicine.
148. Hurt RD, Ebbert JO, Hays JT et al: Pharmacologic interventions for tobacco dependence. In Graham AW, Schultz TK, Mayo-Smith MF et al, editors: *Principles of addiction medicine,*

3rd ed, pp 801-814, Chevy Chase, Md, 2003, American Society of Addiction Medicine.
149. Vourakis C: Substance abuse concerns in the treatment of pain, *Nurs Clin North Am* 33:47-60, 1998.
150. Alford DP, Compton P, Samet JH: Acute pain management for patients receiving maintenance methadone or buprenorphine therapy, *Ann Intern Med* 144:127-134, 2006.
151. Martin PR, Singleton CK, Hiller-Sturmhofel S: The role of thiamine in alcoholic brain disease, *Alcohol Res Health* 27: 134-142, 2003.
152. Robinson K: Wernicke's encephalopathy, *Emerg Nurse* 11: 30-33, 2003.
153. Feng L, Cook TT, Alber C et al: Ethanol and natural killer cells, II: stimulation of human natural killer activity by ethanol in vitro, *Alcohol Clin Exp Res* 21:981-987, 1997.
154. Cook T, Feng L, Vandersteen D et al: Ethanol and natural killer cells, I: activity and immunophenotype in alcoholic humans, *Alcohol Clin Exp Res* 21:974-980, 1997.
155. Tamura DY, Moore EE, Partrick DA et al: Clinically relevant concentrations of ethanol attenuate primed neutrophil bactericidal activity, *J Trauma* 44:320-324, 1998.
156. Gentilello LM, Cobean R, Wertz M et al: Acute ethanol intoxication increases the risk of infection after penetrating abdominal trauma, *J Trauma* 34:669-674, 1993.
157. Baldwin GC, Tashkin DP, Buckley DM et al: Marijuana and cocaine impair alveolar macrophage function and cytokine production, *Am J Respir Crit Care Med* 156:1606-1613, 1997.
158. Thompson PM, Gillin JC, Golshan S et al: Polygraphic sleep measures differentiate alcoholics and stimulant abusers during short-term sleep, *Biol Psych* 38:831-836, 1995.
159. Rotunda RJ, Scherer DG, Imm PS: Family systems and alcohol misuse: research on the effects of alcoholism on family functioning and effective family interventions, *Prof Psychol Res Pract* 26:95-104, 1995.
160. Sommers MS, Dyehouse JM, Howe SR et al: Attribution of injury to alcohol involvement in young adults seriously injured in alcohol-related motor vehicle crashes, *Am J Crit Care* 9:28-35, 2000.
161. Dyehouse JM, Sommers MS: Brief intervention after alcohol-related injuries, *Nurs Clin North Am* 33:93-104, 1998.
162. Field C, Hungerford DW, Dunn C: Brief motivational interventions: an introduction, *J Trauma* 59:S21-S26, 2005.
163. Bombardier CH, Ehde D, Kilmer J: Readiness to change alcohol habits after traumatic brain injury, *Arch Phys Med Rehabil* 78:592-596, 1997.
164. Dunn CW, Donovan DM, Gentilello LM: Practical guidelines for performing alcohol interventions in trauma centers, *J Trauma* 42:299-304, 1997.
165. Turner AP, Bombardier CL, Rimmele CT: A typology of alcohol use patterns among persons with recent traumatic brain injury or spinal cord injury: implications for treatment matching, *Arch Phys Med Rehabil* 84:358-364: 2003.
166. Dunn C, Ostafin B: Brief interventions for hospitalized trauma patients, *J Trauma* 59:S88-S93, 2005.
167. Cryer HG: Barriers to interventions for alcohol problems in trauma centers, *J Trauma* 59:S104-S111, 2005.
168. Gentilello LM, Bonovan DM, Dunn CW et al: Alcohol interventions in trauma centers, *JAMA* 274:1043-1048, 1995.
169. Fleming MF, Barry KL, Manwell LB et al: Brief physician advice for problem alcohol drinkers, *JAMA* 277:1039-1045, 1997.
170. Greber RA, Allen KM, Soeken KL et al: Outcome of trauma patients after brief intervention by a substance abuse consultation service, *Am J Addict* 6:38-47, 1997.
171. Gentilello LM, Rivara FP, Donovan DM et al: Alcohol interventions in a trauma center as a means of reducing the risk of injury recurrence, *Ann Surg* 230:473-483, 1999.
172. Sommers MS, Dyehouse JM, Howe et al: Effectiveness of brief interventions following alcohol-related vehicular injury: a randomized controlled trial, *J Trauma* 61:523-533, 2006.
173. Soderstrom CA, DiClemente CC, Dischinger PC et al: A controlled trial of brief intervention versus brief advice for at-risk drinking trauma center patients, *J Trauma* 62:1102-1112, 2007.
174. Gentilello LM, Ebel BE, Wickizer TM et al: Alcohol interventions for trauma patients treated in emergency departments and hospitals: a cost benefit analysis, *Ann Surg*: 241:541-550, 2005.
175. Ockene JK, Adams A, Hurley TG et al: Brief physician- and nurse practitioner-delivered counseling for high-risk drinkers, *Arch Intern Med* 159:2198-2205, 1999.
176. Fuller MG, Diamond DL, Jordan ML et al: The role of a substance abuse consultation team in a trauma center, *J Stud Alcohol* 56:267-271, 1995.
177. O'Brien CP, McLellan AT: Myths about the treatment of addiction, *Lancet* 347:237-240, 1996.
178. McLellan AT, Lewis DC, O'Brien CP et al: Drug dependence, a chronic medical illness: implications for treatment, insurance, and outcomes of evaluation, *JAMA* 284:1689-1695, 2000.
179. American Society of Addiction Medicine: *Patient placement criteria for treatment of substance-related disorders,* 3rd ed, pp. 1591-1600, Chevy Chase, Md, 2003, American Society of Addiction Medicine.
180. National Institute of Drug Abuse: Project MATCH secondary a priori hypotheses, *Addiction* 92:1671-1698, 1997.
181. Prochaska JO, Norcross JC, DiClemente CC: *Changing for good,* New York, 1995, Avon.
182. Miller WR, Rollnick S: *Motivational interviewing: Preparing people for change,* 2nd ed, New York, 2002, Guilford Press.
183. Ockene JK, Wheeler EV, Adams A et al: Provider training for patient-centered alcohol counseling in a primary care setting, *Arch Intern Med* 157:2334-2340, 1997.
184. Vasilaki EI, Hosier SG, Cox WM: The efficacy of motivational interviewing as a brief intervention for excessive drinking: a meta-analytic review, *Alcohol Alcohol* 41:328-335, 2006.
185. Monti PM, Colby SM, Barnett NP et al: Brief intervention for harm reduction with alcohol positive older adolescents in a hospital emergency department, *J Consult Clin Psychol* 67:1-6, 1999.
186. Monti PM: Drinking among young adults; screening, brief intervention, and outcome, *Alcohol Res Health* 28:236-245, 2004.
187. Dauer AR, Bubio ES, Coris ME et al: Brief intervention in alcohol-positive traffic casualties: is it worth the effort? *Alcohol Alcohol* 41:76-83, 2005.
188. Gentilello LM, Duggan P, Drummond E et al: Major injury as a unique opportunity to initiate treatment in the alcoholic, *Am J Surg* 156:558-561, 1988.
189. Millar JS: A time for everything: changing attitudes and approaches to reducing substance abuse, *Can Med Assoc J* 159: 485-487, 1998.
190. Lindeman RW: The efficacy of the twelve steps of Alcoholics Anonymous in the treatment of alcoholism, *J Psychoactive Drugs* 25:337-340, 1993.

191. Moos RH, Moos BS: Participation in treatment and Alcoholics Anonymous: a 16 year follow-up of initially untreated individuals, *J Clin Psycol* 62:735-750, 2006.
192. O'Brien CP: Anticraving medications for relapse prevention: a possible new class of psychoactive medications, *Am J Psychiatry* 162:1423-1431, 2005.
193. Friedman MD, Saitz R, Samet JH et al: Management of adults recovering from alcohol or other drug problems, *JAMA* 279:1227-1231, 1998.
194. Gentilello LM, Samuels PN, Henningfield JE et al: Alcohol screening and interventions in trauma centers: confidentiality concerns and legal considerations, *J Trauma* 59:1250-1255, 2005.

34

THE ORGAN AND TISSUE DONOR

Cheryl Edwards, Franki Chabalewski, Stephanie Raine

This chapter is designed to give the trauma nurse a basic understanding of organ and tissue donation and the significant role that the trauma nurse plays in the donation process. The crisis created by the critical shortage of organs available for transplant will only worsen as the number of people in need of transplantation increases. Trauma nurses and other members of the health care team are front-line patient advocates and are essential for the early referral of the potential donor.

The process may be confusing because statutes and policies vary from state to state, from hospital to hospital, and among organ procurement organizations (OPOs). The local OPO staff is the best resource for guiding the care of the donor and the donor's family and to ensure that hospital policies and procedures are current. The trauma team is urged to work collaboratively with the regional OPO to provide the most compassionate approach to potential donor families while preparing their loved one for their final act of generosity: donating an organ to save or enhance another person's life.

THE CRITICAL SHORTAGE

There have been many significant advances in the field of organ transplantation since the first transplant was performed in 1956. Thousands of lives that would have otherwise been lost to end-stage organ failure have been saved and thousands of others enjoy an improved quality of life, all as a result of organ transplantation. Improvements in surgical techniques, organ preservation procedures, and immunosuppressive therapies have made it possible for transplant recipients to enjoy an improved quality of life. However, there is one factor that severely limits the number of lives affected through transplantation: the shortage of life-saving organs for transplant.

More than 93,000 people are currently waiting for a transplant in the United States.[1] That number grows exponentially each year, and although the number of organ donors has increased, there continues to be a disparity between the availability of an organ for transplant and those in need of a transplant.[1] On average, 118 people are added to the national organ transplant waiting list each day, one every 12 minutes. Approximately 18 patients die each day while waiting for a transplant because an organ did not become available in time.[2] Tragically, fewer than one third of those patients waiting will receive the transplant they so desperately need (Figure 34-1).

Trauma nurses play an integral role in solving the critical shortage of organs for transplant through the early referral of every potential donor. Referrals to the regional OPO can increase the number of organ donors through a collaborative approach. Coordinated efforts between the organ procurement coordinator (OPC) and the health care team's nurses, physicians, and ancillary personnel can have a dramatic impact on the number of lives saved annually through the "gift of life" as a result of organ donation.

FEDERAL REGULATIONS AND THE TIMELY REFERRAL OF POTENTIAL ORGAN DONORS

The critical shortage of organs for transplantation has prompted federal initiatives designed to increase professional and public awareness regarding the need for organs and tissues for donation. It is estimated that the annual number of potential brain-dead donors in the United States is between 10,500 and 13,800.[3] In response the Health Care Financing Administration (HCFA) developed the "Medicare Conditions of Participation" regulations. These regulations require all U.S. hospitals to work collaboratively with their regional OPO and tissue recovery agency. Specifically, they charge every hospital with reporting all potential organ donors (and potential tissue donors) and inpatient deaths to the OPO. The regulations mandate that hospital staff be required to report every imminent death (including the potential for brain death) to the OPO in a timely manner. Hospital staff are required to make these referrals before life-limiting treatment decisions are made, including decisions to pursue "do not resuscitate" and "no pressors" options, before termination of life support, and before any discussion regarding organ and tissue donation is initiated with the family.[4] Additionally, according to these regulations, the responsibility for conducting a discussion about organ donation with the family of a potential donor lies with the OPO staff or hospital staff trained by the OPO.[4] These regulations are meant to relieve the hospital staff of the burden of determining donor suitability and to clarify when they should call in a referral. These regulations are not designed to exclude hospital staff from the consent discussion but to ensure that the OPC is included in the process.

Early referral to the regional OPO has many benefits for the staff, the patient's family, and the recipients. Staff, who may be uncomfortable with discussing donation or who lack the knowledge to provide the option of donation to a family, are now relieved of that burden under the new regulations. Early involvement with the OPC will facilitate a collaborative

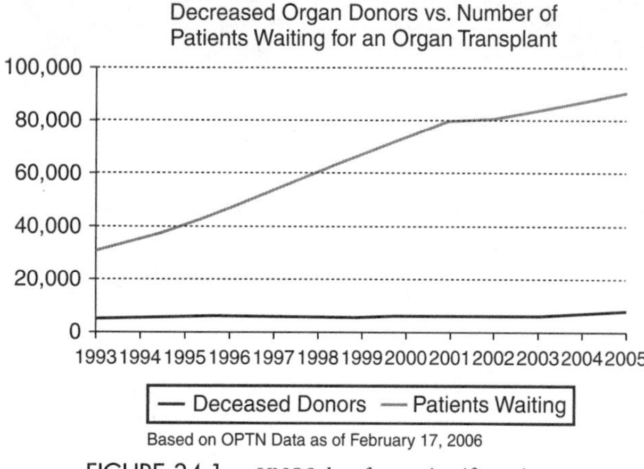

FIGURE 34-1 UNOS data from scientific registry.

discussion among all those involved to determine the most sensitive approach to the donation discussion at the most appropriate time. Potential donor families can be assured that the discussion regarding organ and tissue donation occurs at a time that is right for them, with the appropriate options shared on the basis of each situation. Families need time to have their questions answered. In instances where there is no donor designation, the family needs to be assured that their decision will be respected regardless of whether they choose to donate. The transplant recipient's benefits are obvious. Lives are saved and many recipients enjoy the benefit of an improved quality of life through organ transplantation. Advances in the field of transplantation have allowed recipients greater survival times than ever before.[1]

Early OPC involvement can assist the staff in caring for the family and prevent well-meaning personnel from offering the option of donation in situations where it is inappropriate (if the deceased had human immunodeficiency virus [HIV] or metastatic disease) and from offering inaccurate information about the options for donation. As donor criteria continue to change, OPO staff are trained in the most current requirements and possesses the information necessary to screen a potential donor. The OPC can spend time with the family answering questions and reinforcing their options. This can be a time-consuming encounter and may require more information than the staff is able to provide.[5] Ideally the trauma staff and OPC will collaboratively develop a plan and decide on the best approach to the family when consideration for organ donation becomes a reality.

DONOR PROFILE

The following scenario presents a donor profile that provides a "real life" clinical situation:

> A 16-year-old Caucasian adolescent is admitted to the emergency department after a fall from a moving vehicle while "car surfing." He has sustained a severe closed head injury. An emergency computed tomography (CT) scan of his head reveals diffuse cerebral edema and inoperable intraparenchymal hemorrhages. His prognosis for survival is poor. A referral is made to the regional OPO to alert the OPC on call regarding the patient's condition. The neurosurgeon places an intracranial pressure monitor and admits the patient to the neurologic intensive care unit for aggressive treatment of the increased intracranial pressure.
>
> Six hours after admission, it is obvious that all efforts to control this patient's intracranial hypertension have failed and his clinical examination is consistent with herniation syndrome. The OPC on call is again apprised of the situation. A cerebral blood flow study is done to confirm the suspicion of brain death. In accordance with individual state and hospital policies, the patient is declared brain dead.

Trauma patients, particularly young and otherwise healthy individuals, who have sustained an isolated traumatic brain injury have always and will continue to constitute a significant percentage of the overall organ donor pool. However, better safety practices such as enforced speed limits, seat belt and motorcycle helmet laws and air bags, and more sophisticated prehospital care and technology have changed the potential for organ donation in the trauma population. Many patients who would have been potential brain-dead donors do not meet the criteria for brain death, thus altering their options for organ donation.

Concurrent solid organ injuries in the trauma patient may limit options for donation. Depending on the donor's age and severity of the injury, some organs may be unsuitable for transplantation. Significant cardiac or lung contusions may or may not threaten organ viability. Depending on the location and severity, liver lacerations do not necessarily prevent a lifesaving liver donation but may preclude splitting the liver for transplantation to two separate recipients. Blunt injury to the kidneys, pancreas, or intestines should be evaluated carefully to determine suitability for transplantation. Some injuries, for example a renal capsule tear, can be repaired and successful transplantation of that organ can still occur. The reality is that there are far too many people dying every day because a transplant did not become available in time, NOT to evaluate every donor, every organ, every time.[6]

It is essential for the trauma nurse to realize that trauma patients are not the only potential organ donors. In fact, from 1988 to 1996 the number of persons involved in motor vehicle crashes who become organ donors decreased 29%, whereas the number of patients who became organ donors as a result of a cerebrovascular accident, such as intracerebral hemorrhage or ischemic stroke, rose 57%.[1] Any catastrophic cerebral insult, whether anoxic, hemorrhagic, ischemic, or traumatic, that results in uncontrolled cerebral edema can lead to brain death and the potential for organ donation. Some studies have shown that physicians and staff fail to recognize these patients as potential organ donors and subsequently fail to refer the patient to the OPO.[7] In these cases the opportunity for organ donation is lost. The results of such missed opportunities are far reaching. In cases of donor designation, the donor's choice to help others on his death is ignored. In the absence of such a designation, the potential donor family is denied their legal right to be offered the option of donation. When deprived of such an opportunity, to find solace while experiencing the loss of a loved one, they are further denied the comfort in knowing that their loved one's final act of kindness, organ and tissue donation, could help countless others by saving and greatly enhancing the lives of others. Additionally, up to seven potential recipients that might otherwise receive a life-saving transplant may die before the next opportunity for a donor organ becomes available.

BRAIN DEATH

The Uniform Determination of Death Act of 1980, supported by the President's Commission for the Study of Ethical Problems in Medicine and Biomedical and Behavioral Research, confirmed the legality of and set parameters for the declaration of brain death. The act states that any individual sustaining irreversible cessation of circulatory and respiratory function *or* irreversible cessation of *all* cerebral function, including the brainstem, is dead.[8] Technologic advances make it possible to support multiple body systems so that the signs traditionally equated with life, cardiac and respiratory function, can be maintained despite the loss of all cerebral function and control.[9] Therefore the organ donor is traditionally the individual who is brain dead or, more specifically, the patient who has died but remains on mechanical support for purposes of organ donation until organ recovery is completed. The non-heart-beating organ donor, also referred to as the donor after cardiac death, or the donor whose organs are recovered after asystole is discussed later in this chapter.

Once a primary insult occurs, whether medical or traumatic, the challenge to the health care team is to prevent secondary brain injury. In the absence of trauma, specifically skull fractures, in older children and adults the cranium is a closed vault. Within this rigid, closed cavity exists three elements: brain matter (80%), cerebrospinal fluid (10%), and blood (10%). The Monro-Kellie hypothesis states that when any one of these elements increases in volume, one of the other elements must accommodate that increased volume through a reciprocal reduction in volume.[10] Failure to compensate results in uncontrolled increased intracranial pressure. Irrepressible intracranial hypertension causes a progressive decrease in cerebral perfusion as intracranial pressure exceeds mean arterial blood pressure. The resultant cerebral ischemia leads to brain death[11] (Box 34-1).

The brain-dead individual exhibits no spontaneous respiratory effort, no response to painful stimuli, and absence of all brainstem reflexes (e.g., fixed, dilated pupils; absence of oculocephalic, oculovestibular, cough, gag, and corneal reflexes). Before declaration of brain death, all medical conditions or metabolic derangements that may affect the neurologic examination should be treated or corrected. Serum chemistries should be within normal limits, body temperature should be at or above 95° F (35° C), and there should be no drug levels that would impair neurologic reflexes, such as neuromuscular blockade, sedation, or anesthetics. The patient should be hemodynamically stable, with a systolic blood pressure equal to or higher than 90 mm Hg. It should be noted in cases where sedation has been used to decrease the brain's metabolic requirements and in the presence of a significant serum drug level, a cerebral blood flow study can be used to confirm lack of cerebral blood flow, thus supporting the diagnosis of brain death.[12]

BOX 34-1 Clinical Criteria for the Declaration of Brain Death

- Known cause of death
- Irreversibility
- Body temperature >95° F (35° C)
- Fixed pupils
- No spontaneous movements in response to external stimuli
- No reflex activity except that elicited by spinal cord
- Apnea in the presence of hypercapnia ($Paco_2$ >60 mm Hg)

From House-Park MA: Nursing care of the potential donor. In Chabalewski FL, editor: *Donation and transplantation: nursing curriculum,* pp. 105-130, Richmond, Va, 1996, UNOS.

APNEA TESTING

Apnea is an essential component in the determination of brain death. Apnea testing is performed in the course of brain death examination. Before the test is initiated, the patient should be normothermic and normotensive with a systolic blood pressure 90 mm Hg or higher and a baseline $Paco_2$ between 35 and 45 torr. The patient should not have received any drugs that could potentially suppress respiratory effort.[12]

Once these prerequisites are met, the patient is hyperoxygenated with 100% oxygen for at least 10 minutes. The patient is then removed from ventilatory support, and oxygen is fed through the endotracheal tube by cannula at 6 L/min. After cessation of mechanical ventilation, the patient's chest should be clearly visible for the remainder of the test. The patient is then monitored carefully for spontaneous respiratory effort and any change in the baseline vital signs. A greater than 10% change in the blood pressure, heart rate, or pulse oximetry is cause to abort the study. Any spontaneous respiratory effort negates the assumption of brain death.[12]

If an apnea test is aborted because of deterioration in vital signs, in the absence of respiratory effort the diagnosis of brain death is supported and the patient is returned to ventilatory support at the pretest settings. If the patient remains stable in the absence of respiratory effort for up to 10 minutes, an arterial blood gas measurement is repeated and the patient is placed back on ventilatory support at the pretest settings. A $Paco_2$ of 60 torr or greater, or at least two to two and a half times the pretest $Paco_2$, supports the diagnosis of brain death.[10,12]

CONFIRMATORY TESTING

Electroencephalography, transcranial Doppler imaging, or cerebral flow studies may be done to confirm the diagnosis of brain death as evidenced by clinical examination (absence of brainstem reflexes). The decision to perform confirmatory studies is based on the judgment of the physician declaring brain death and is done in accordance with state laws and individual hospital policy.[12]

SEQUELAE OF BRAIN DEATH

The inception of brain death presents a challenge to donor stability. Multiple systems are affected once compensatory mechanisms regulated by the central nervous system fail. The sympathetic nervous system accelerates, causing an uncontrolled release of catecholamines. Tachycardia, an increase in systolic blood pressure, and increased cardiac output characterize this "autonomic storm." Once the catecholamine stores are depleted, this phase ends and hemodynamic instability may ensue. Regulatory mechanisms fail; the ability to control blood pressure and heart rate is lost. Hypotension typically ensues because of a lack of autoregulation, causing vasodilation.[11,13]

Interventions previously used to control intracranial hypertension (osmotic diuresis, sedation administration) may also contribute to a dangerously low systolic blood pressure (<80 mm Hg). Left untreated, persistent hypotension may threaten viability of organs for transplant. Vigorous but controlled fluid resuscitation can be successful in treating hypotension. Frequently one or more vasopressor agents are infused to maintain a systolic blood pressure of at least 100 mm Hg. The heart rate may vary, and arrhythmias may occur. An initial exaggerated vagal response results in bradycardia but rapidly progresses to tachycardia as a result of catecholamine release and vasopressor support. As the hypothalamus ceases to function, thermoregulatory mechanisms fail and poikilothermy, where body temperature mimics ambient temperature, may develop. Infusion of cold blood products may exacerbate hypothermia. To help maintain the patient's body temperature, careful attention to the room temperature, infusion of blood through a warmer, and use of an external hyperthermic unit help to maintain a body temperature above 95° F (35° C). Oxygenation is controlled through mechanical ventilation. Aspiration pneumonia, pulmonary contusions, and neurogenic pulmonary edema may impair adequate oxygenation and threaten the viability of the lungs for transplant.[11]

The posterior pituitary gland ceases to compensate for the feedback mechanism and no longer produces antidiuretic hormone. The subsequent onset of diabetes insipidus can be treated successfully with vasopressin, either subcutaneously or intravenously. Maintaining hemodynamic stability in the brain-dead individual presents a tremendous but rewarding challenge to the critical care staff.[11]

THE ORGAN DONATION PROCESS

The steps in the process of organ donation are intricate and interrelated and each is integral to the success of the process. All patients who die or whose death is imminent must be referred to the OPC to be evaluated for the potential for organ donation. Informed consent cannot be obtained from the potential donor's family until a patient is declared brain dead, the family is informed of the death, and the family understands the concept of brain death. Donor management is continuous throughout the organ evaluation process until organ recovery is complete. The steps of the organ donation process are as follows: (1) identification and referral, (2) evaluation, (3) brain death declaration, (4) informed consent or first person consent, (5) donor management and organ placement, and (6) organ recovery.

The United Network for Organ Sharing (UNOS) developed a critical pathway to assist health care professionals in critical care areas throughout the organ donation process (Table 34-1). The pathway provides an outline for the care of an organ donor from referral through organ recovery. Each step is defined as a phase and is composed of key events, parameters, and diagnostic or clinical values critical to optimal organ function. The donation process is multifaceted and can progress rapidly through each phase, with some events occurring simultaneously. The pathway provides a clear illustration of each phase and identifies the expectations for each. It promotes a collaborative relationship among all disciplines involved in the care of the donor. It is not meant to replace open communication between the OPC and health care team; rather, it keeps all members of the team involved in the process.[14] The pathway is designed to be reviewed, revised, and adapted by each hospital in conjunction with its individual OPOs so that current federal, state, or hospital protocols may be incorporated. The pathway can be used by the novice nurse to learn the donation process or as a guide for the experienced nurse.

DONOR IDENTIFICATION AND REFERRAL

In accordance with federal regulations, every patient admitted to a hospital with the potential to progress to brain death or who is actually brain dead must be referred to the regional OPO in a timely manner.[4] In some instances it is obvious in the emergency department that the patient meets brain death criteria. In this situation the staff should make the referral before decisions are made regarding withdrawal of support or instituting a do-not-attempt-to-resuscitate order. An OPC is available on a 24-hour basis to respond to a referral for evaluation. The OPC can work collaboratively with the trauma team to develop a plan regarding potential organ and tissue donation. Figure 34-2 outlines the referral process.

When referring a potential organ donor to the OPO, it is helpful to have the following information: (1) patient name if known, (2) age, (3) sex, (4) date of birth, if known, and

(5) blood type. The referral should never be delayed because of a lack of specific information.

Early referral makes the difference in the number of recipients who may benefit from this gift of life. Referral before brain death is declared promotes a collaborative approach between the OPC and the health care team in the development of a plan of care. Early development of a plan can ensure anticipation and early correction of the sequelae commonly seen once brain death occurs, thus preventing organ insult as a result of hemodynamic instability. Any delay in treating hemodynamic instability may threaten the viability of organ function. A timely referral therefore can mean five to seven organs being recovered for transplant as opposed to two or three recovered in cases when the referral is made after the diagnosis of brain death.[5]

Evaluation of the Potential Organ Donor

Each referral is evaluated by an OPC. The initial referral rarely elicits information that excludes the patient from organ donation. Typically this phone consultation is followed by an OPC site visit to review the case. The OPC and staff discuss the family's understanding of the prehospital events, admitting diagnosis, hospital course, and prognosis. Previous medical records may be requested. The medical history, the description of events leading to this admission and any injuries sustained, the hospital course since arriving in the emergency department, laboratory data, and any diagnostic tests to determine donor suitability are reviewed.

All organ donors are screened for communicable disease through standard serologic testing. Table 34-2 lists common testing and the implications for organ and tissue donation. Pretransfusion specimens are desirable, a point for the trauma team to remember when drawing specimens for laboratory tests in the emergency department. If there is an indication that the patient may become an organ donor, it is helpful if two extra blood chemistry specimens are drawn and held in the laboratory for subsequent testing by the OPO.

The shortage of precious organs for transplant and advances in the field of transplantation have led to an expansion of donor criteria. Factors that may have historically deemed a patient an unsuitable donor may no longer be applicable. It is for this reason, hospital staff should never assume that a patient is not a suitable donor and consultation with the OPC should be pursued in every situation. Such assumptions may result in the unnecessary loss of life for potential recipients.

Brain Death Declaration and Documentation

In accordance with individual state regulations and hospital policy, brain death determination should be documented clearly in the patient record with the time, date, and signature of the physician. Some states require two licensed physicians to declare brain death. Most hospital policies regarding the declaration of brain death prohibit the transplant physicians who may perform the recovery procedure from being involved in the process of declaring a potential organ donor patient dead. Some institutions may have separate policies regarding the declaration of brain death in neonates, infants, and children. These policies often dictate a standard waiting period and re-examination to confirm brain death. State law and hospital policy regarding brain death declaration must be followed. In the brain-dead individual, the time that brain death is documented or confirmed, when two physicians are required, is the legal time of death. Regardless of whether the case progresses to organ recovery, the time that the patient is declared brain dead is the date and time the patient died, not to be confused with the time of asystole after withdrawal of mechanical support.

First Person Consent/Informed Consent

Much research has been done on the needs of families of the critically ill patient. The family is typically in crisis and needs honest, direct, and understandable explanations about their loved one's care and prognosis. Some family members may need to spend time with their loved one, and many need to feel supported and accepted by the staff. They need to have hope but to be given the opportunity to discuss the possibility of death and to know that the health care team cares about their loved one.[15] It is imperative that before any discussion regarding organ donation that the family of a potential donor is kept informed as the patient's condition deteriorates and repeated explanations are given about the patient's potential to progress to brain death. Results of clinical examinations and diagnostic testing should be shared in understandable terms, and questions should be answered honestly. The use of visual aids to explain the injuries may assist them in understanding. Family members should be allowed to see the CT scan or x-ray films if they will help them to understand the extent of the cerebral damage. Understanding the finality of brain death is difficult for family members when their loved one appears to be "sleeping." The patient may be warm to the touch, have good color and a visible heart rate, and appear to be breathing, albeit with mechanical means.[14] This scenario lends itself more to the perception that the patient is sleeping or in a coma rather than the reality that that person has died. Timing is of paramount importance when discussing organ donation. This discussion should not take place until the family understands and accepts the death of their loved one. The introduction of the subject of organ donation too early in the hospital course, or before the family accepts the death, can cause unnecessary anguish and foster a family's lack of trust with the health care team. The explanation of brain death and the discussion about organ donation should be separated to give the family time to accept that their loved one has died before they discuss organ or tissue donation.

TABLE 34-1A **Critical Pathway for the Organ Donor**

Collaborative Practice	Phase I Referral	Phase II Declaration of Brain Death and Consent	Phase III Donor Evaluation	Phase IV Donor Management	Phase V Recovery Phase
The following professionals may be involved to enchance the donation process. Check all that apply: ❑ Physician ❑ Critical care RN ❑ Organ Procurement Organization (OPO) ❑ OPO Coordinator (OPC) ❑ MedicalExaminer (ME)/Coroner ❑ Respiratory ❑ Laboratory ❑ Radiology ❑ Anesthesiology ❑ OR/Surgery staff ❑ Clergy ❑ Social worker	❑ Notify physician regarding OPO referral ❑ Contact OPO ref: Potential donor with severe brain insult ❑ OPC on site and begins evaluation: Time ___ Date ___ ❑ Ht ___ Wt ___ as documented ❑ ABO as documented ___ ❑ Notify house supervisor/charge nurse of presence on unit	❑ Brain death documented Time ___ Date ___ ❑ Pt accepted as potential donor ❑ MD notifies family of death ❑ Plan family approach with OPC ❑ Offer support services to family (clergy, etc) ❑ OPC/Hospital staff talks to family about donation ❑ Family accepts donation ❑ OPC obtains signed consent & medical/social history Time ___ Date ___ ❑ ME/Coroner notified ❑ ME/Coroner releases body for donation ❑ **Family/ME/Coroner denies donation – stop pathway – initiate post-mortem protocol – support family.**	❑ Obtain pre/post transfusion blood for serology testing (HIV, Hepatitis, VDRL, CMV) ❑ Obtain lymph nodes and/or blood for tissue typing ❑ Notify OR & anesthesiology of pending case ❑ Notify house supervisor of pending donation ❑ Chest & abdominal circumference ❑ Lung measurements per CXR by OPC ❑ **Cardiology consult as requested by OPC** ❑ **Donor organs unsuitable for transplant – stop pathway – initiate post-mortem protocol – support family.**	❑ OPC writes new orders ❑ Organ placement ❑ OPC sets tentative OR time ❑ Insert arterial line/2 large-bore IVs ❑ Possibly insert CVP/pulmonary artery catheter	❑ Checklist for OR ❑ Supplies given to OR ❑ Prepare patient for transport to OR ❑ IVs ❑ Pumps ❑ O_2 ❑ Ambu ❑ Peep value ❑ Transport to OR Date ______ Time ______ ❑ OR nurse reviews consent & brain death documentation & checks patient's ID band
Labs/Diagnostics		❑ Review previous lab results ❑ Review previous hemodynamics	❑ Blood chemistry ❑ CBC + diff ❑ UA ❑ C & S ❑ PT, PTT ❑ ABO ❑ A Subtype ❑ Liver function tests ❑ Blood culture × 2 / 15 minutes to 1 hour apart ❑ Sputum Gram Stain & C & S ❑ Type & Cross Match ___ #units PRBCs ❑ CXR ❑ ABGs ❑ EKG ❑ Echo ❑ Consider cardiac cath ❑ Consider bronchoscopy	❑ Determine need for additional lab testing ❑ CXR after line placement (if done) ❑ Serum electrolytes ❑ H & H after PRBC Rx ❑ PT, PTT ❑ BUN, serum creatinine after correcting fluid deficit ❑ Notify OPC for ___PT>14___PTT<28 ___Urine output ___< 1 mL/Kg/hr ___> 3 mL/Kg/hr ___Hct<30 / Hgb < 10 ___Na> 150 mEq/L	❑ Labs drawn in OR as per surgeon or OPC request ❑ Communicate with pathology: Bx liver and/or kidneys as indicated

Respiratory	❑ Pt on ventilator ❑ Suction q 2 hr ❑ Reposition q 2 hr	→ ❑ Prep for apnea testing: set FiO_2 @ 100% and anticipate need to decrease rate if PCO_2 < 45 mm Hg	❑ Maximize ventilator settings to achieve SaO_2 98 – 99% ❑ PEEP = 5 cm O_2 challenge for lung placement FiO_2 @ 100% PEEP @ 5 × 10 min ❑ ABGs as ordered ❑ VS q 1° →	❑ Notify OPC for ___BP < 90 systolic ___HR < 70 or > 120 ___CVP < 4 or > 11 ___PaO_2 < 90 or ___SaO_2 < 95%	❑ Portable O_2 @ 100% FiO_2 for transport to OR ❑ Ambu bag and PEEP value ❑ Move to OR
Treatments/ Ongoing Care		❑ Use warming/cooling blanket to maintain temperature at 36.5° C – 37.5° C → ❑ NG to low intermittent suction	❑ Check NG placement & output → ❑ Obtain actual Ht ___ & Wt ___ if not previously obtained		❑ Set OR temp as directed by OPC ❑ Post mortem care at conclusion of case
Medications			❑ Medication as requested by OPC →	❑ Fluid resuscitation–consider crystolloids, colloids, blood products ❑ DC meds except pressors & antibiotics ❑ Broad-spectrum antibiotic if not previously ordered → ❑ Vasopressor support to maintain BP > 90 mm Hg systolic ❑ Electrolyte imbalance: consider K, Ca, PO_4, Mg replacement ❑ Hyperglycemia: consider Insulin drip → ❑ Oliguria: consider diuretics ❑ Diabetes insipidus: consider antidiuretics ❑ Paralytic as indicated for spinal reflexes	❑ DC antidiuretics ❑ Diuretics as needed ❑ 350 U heparin/kg or as directed by surgeon
Optimal Outcomes	The potential donor is identified & a referral is made to the OPO.	The family is offered the option of donation & their decision is supported.	The donor is evaluated & found to be a suitable candidate for donation.	Optimal organ function is maintained.	All potentially suitable, consented organs are recovered for transplant.

Shaded areas indicate Organ Procurement Coordinator (OPC) Activities

ABGs, Arterial blood gases; *BP*, blood pressure; *Bx*, biopsy; *BUN*, blood urea nitrogen; *CBC*, complete blood count; *CMV*, cytomegalovirus; *C & S*, culture and sensitivity; *CVP*, central venous pressure; *CXR*, chest x-ray film; *DC*, discontinue; *ECG*, electrocardiogram; *FiO2*, fraction of inspired oxygen; *Hb*, hemoglobin; *Hct*, hematocrit; *H & H*, hemoglobin and hematocrit; *HIV*, human immunodeficiency virus; *HR*, heart rate; *NG*, nasogastric tube; *OR*, operating room; PaO_2, partial arterial oxygen pressure; PCO_2, partial pressure of carbon dioxide; *PEEP*, positive end-expiratory pressure; *PRBCs*, packed red blood cells; *Pt*, patient; *PT*, prothrombin time; *PTT*, partial thromboplastin time; *Rx*, prescription; SaO_2, arterial oxygen saturation; *UA*, urinalysis; *VDRL*, Venereal Disease Research Laboratory; *VS*, vital signs. Reprinted with permission of the United Network for Organ Sharing, Richmond, Va.

TABLE 34-1B Cardiothoracic Donor Management

1. **Early echocardiogram for all donors**—Insert pulmonary artery catheter (PAC) to monitor patient management (placement of the PAC is particularly relevant in patients with an EF <45% or on high-dose inotropes)
   - Use aggressive donor resuscitation as outlined below
2. **Electrolytes**
   - Maintain Na <150 meq/dl
   - Maintain K+ >4.0
   - Correct acidosis with Na bicarbonate and mild to moderate hyperventilation (pCO_2 30-35 mm Hg).
3. **Ventilation—Maintain tidal volume 10-15 ml/kg**
   - Keep peak airway pressure <30 mm Hg
   - Maintain a mild respiratory alkalosis (pCO_2 30-35 mmHg).
4. **Recommend use of hormonal resuscitation as part of a comprehensive donor management protocol—Key elements**
   - *Triiodothyronine (T_3):* 4 mcg bolus; 3 mcg/hr continuous infusion
   - *Arginine vasopressin:* 1 unit bolus: 0.5-4.0 unit/hour drip (titrate SVR 800-1200 using a PAC)
   - *Methylprednisolone:* 15 mg/kg bolus (repeat q 24° prn)
   - *Insulin:* drip at a minimum rate of 1 unit/hour (titrate blood glucose to 120-180 mg/dl)
   - *Ventilator:* (see above)
   - *Volume resuscitation:* Use of colloid and avoidance of anemia are important in preventing pulmonary edema
     - Albumin if PT and PTT are normal
     - Fresh frozen plasma if PT and PTT abnormal (value ≥1.5 × control)
     - Packed red blood cells to maintain a PCWP of 8-12 mm Hg and Hct >10.0 mg/dl
5. **When patient is stabilized/optimized repeat echocardiogram.** (An unstable donor has not met two or more of the following criteria)
   - Mean arterial pressure ≥60
   - CVP ≤12 mm Hg
   - PCWP ≤12 mm Hg
   - SVR 800-1200 dyne/sec/cm^5
   - Cardiac index ≥2.5 l/min/M^2
   - Left ventricular stroke work index >15
   - Dopamine dosage <10mcg/kg/min

CVP, Central venous pressure; *EF,* ejection fraction; *PAC,* pulmonary artery catheter; *PCWP,* pulmonary capillary wedge pressure; *PT,* prothrombin time; *PTT,* partial thromboplastin time; *SVR,* systemic vascular resistance.

The critical pathway was developed under contract with the U.S. Department of Health and Human Services, Health Resources and Services Administration, Division of Transplantation.

In either case, first person consent or informed consent by the next of kin, it is important to provide the family with a quiet, private setting when discussing donation. The OPC discusses the benefits of donation, answers their questions honestly, explains the process, and addresses common concerns associated with organ and tissue donation. The potential options for organ donation include heart, lungs, liver, kidneys, pancreas, and small bowel. Tissue donation can include the cornea or eye, heart valves, bone, skin, vessels, tendons, and, in some states, bladder. Families need to be informed that an open-casket viewing is possible without detection of the donation. They should also be aware that there is no cost to them for any expense related to organ or tissue donation.

First Person Consent

First person consent, also referred to as donor designation, has been adopted by many states. Pursuant to the Uniform Anatomical Gift Act, many state statutes provide for a person to make his or her own informed decision regarding organ and tissue donation before death. In most states, this is designated on a driver's license or state identification card. This donor designation is referred to as first person consent. Although any person can make such a designation, in select states, when a person dies, either by progression to brain death or by cardiopulmonary arrest, the legal next of kin are prohibited from overruling such a decision. Your OPC will be able to share information regarding your state's statutes with you.

In states that honor first person consent, the regional OPO, on receiving a potential donor referral, can access either local Department of Motor Vehicle records or a state Web site specifically designed to allow people to become designated donors, strictly for the purposes of determining whether there is a donor designation. Such a designation, if it exists, serves as the consent for organ and tissue donation. Families are informed of their loved one's wishes to become an organ and tissue donor on his or her death. The OPC will enlist the assistance of the next of kin to obtain medical and social information and will ensure that the donor's wishes are respected. Some OPOs provide the family with written information, similar to a consent form, to provide all

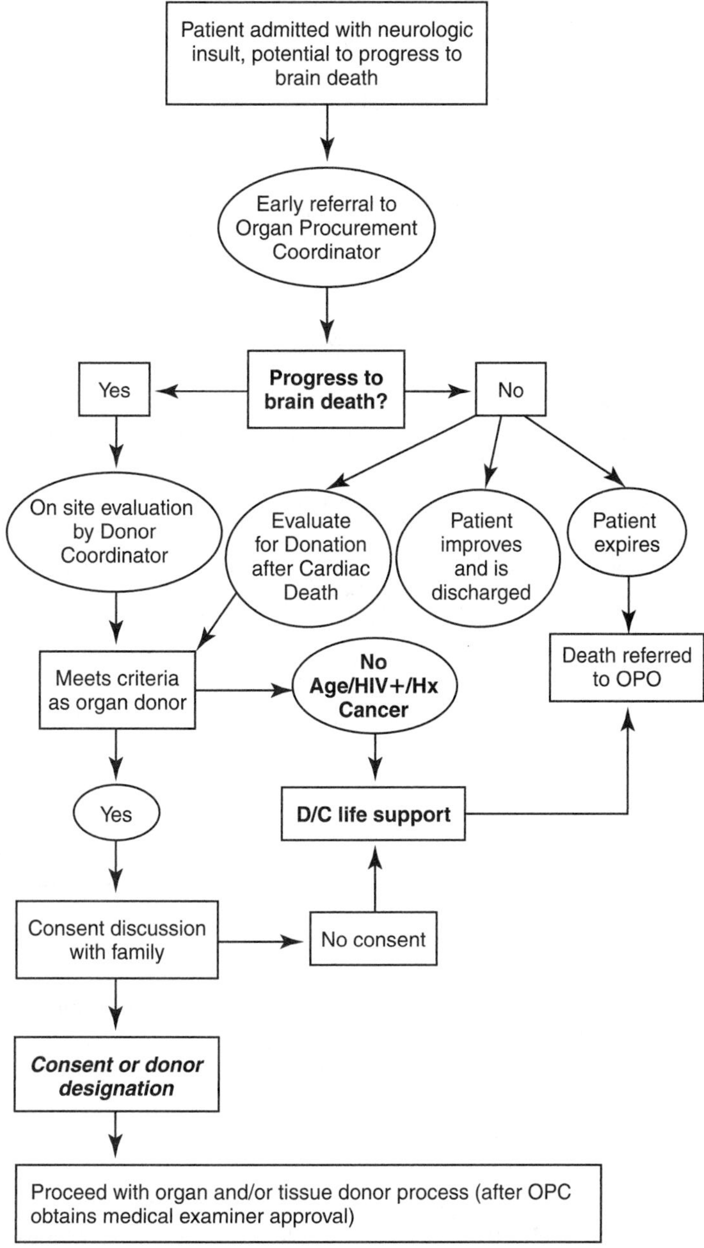

FIGURE 34-2 Referring a potential donor.

pertinent information regarding their loved one's final act of kindness—the gift of life.

INFORMED CONSENT

In the absence of state laws supporting first person consent, or in the absence of such a designation, the legal next of kin will be approached by the OPC regarding the option to donate. The family's perception of the hospital experience and the ability to understand the diagnosis of brain death play a large part in the family's ability to find comfort in the decision to pursue organ and tissue donation.

The staff may be reluctant to refer a potential donor to the OPO because the family is upset over the news of their loved one's impending death. Fear that a discussion about organ donation will further traumatize the family is a common misperception. In a discussion about organ and tissue donation, the OPC does not ask the family to "give up" anything, but rather offers them a source of solace in their grief. The knowledge that a loved one's final act of kindness saved other lives may be very comforting. Early involvement of the OPC ensures the proper timing of such a conversation and relieves staff from the responsibility of discussing donation with a family.

TABLE 34-2 **Serologic Testing**

Test	Significance of Positive Results	Organ Donation	Tissue Donation
HIV I, HIV II			
HIV I, II	Indicates antibodies to HIV I and II	No	No
Human T Lymphocyte Virus I, Human T Lymphocyte Virus II			
Human lymphocyte viruses I, II	Indicates presence of antibodies to human lymphocyte viruses I and II	No	No
Hepatitis C Virus			
Hepatitis C antibody	Indicates presence of antibodies to hepatitis C	Yes	No
Hepatitis B Surface Antigen			
Hepatitis B surface antigen	Indicates a current hepatitis B infection	Yes*	No
Hepatitis B Core Antibody			
Hepatitis B core antibody	Indicates exposure to hepatitis B virus	Yes	No
Australian Antibody			
Hepatitis B surface antibody	Indicates immunity to hepatitis B virus through previous infection or immunization	Yes	Yes
Venereal Disease Research Laboratory or Rapid Plasma Reagin			
Rapid plasma reagin	Indicates exposure to *Treponema pallidum* spirochete, which causes syphilis	Yes	No
Cytomegalovirus			
Cytomegalovirus	Indicates presence of antibodies to cytomegalovirus	Yes	Yes

*Life saving organs only—heart, lungs, and liver

The manner in which the option of organ donation is presented to the family and their personal feelings regarding donation play integral roles in the family's decision to donate. The family is offered the option of organ and tissue donation for both transplant and research, and they may decline any or all of these options. The consent form lists each organ and tissue for donation, and only those organs and tissues consented to by the family are recovered. Box 34-2 lists all organs and tissues that may be used for transplant. The family is assured that their decision is confidential. The choice is theirs, and regardless of whether they wish to pursue organ donation, they will be supported in their decision.

The operating room staff and anesthesia personnel are notified soon after consent is obtained in anticipation of the organ recovery that will take place.

Specific Organ Evaluation

Once a patient is declared brain dead and informed consent is obtained, organ evaluation commences. In most states, the OPC will assume care and management of the donor after brain death declaration and informed consent is obtained or a donor designation is verified. The OPC works closely with the critical care intensivists and nurses to ensure that optimal organ function is maintained. Age, medical history, existing laboratory values, and the specific organs to be recovered determine which organs are evaluated for transplantation. Figure 34-3 outlines an overview of the evaluation process. Pertinent laboratory studies are ordered at the onset of this evaluation process and compared with previous values. Laboratory studies may be ordered on a regular basis throughout the organ placement process and just before the recovery procedure.

BOX 34-2 **Transplantable Organs and Tissues**

Organs
- Heart
- Kidneys
- Lungs (segment)
- Liver (segment)
- Pancreas
- Small bowel
- Stomach

Tissues
- Bone
- Bone marrow
- Corneas
- Dura
- Heart valves
- Skin
- Tendons
- Vessels

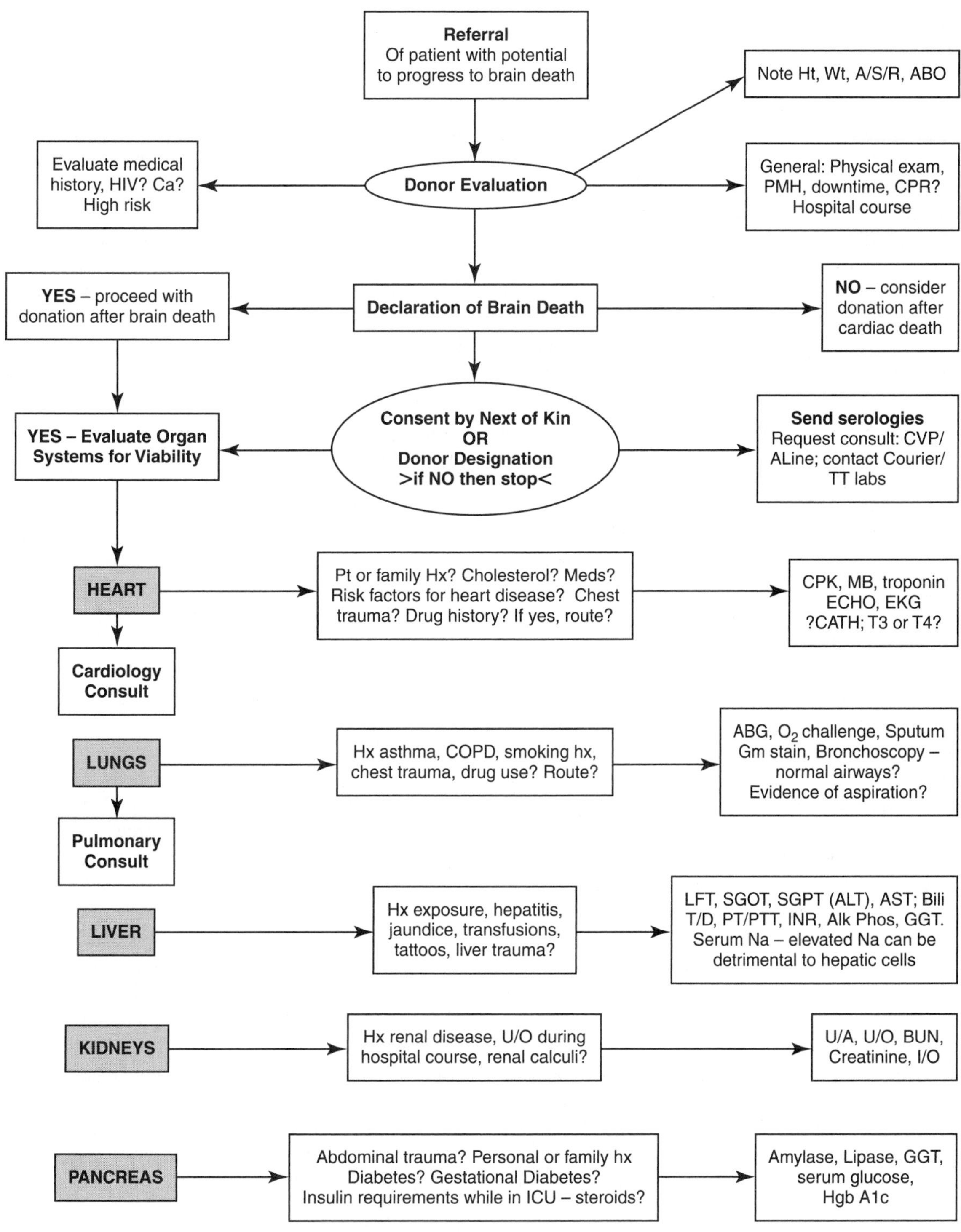

FIGURE 34-3 Organ evaluation process: an overview.

DONOR MANAGEMENT

The goal of donor management is to maximize the viability of each organ system for transplant. With the onset of brain death, all compensatory mechanisms are impaired or they fail altogether. Donor management is directed at maintenance of optimal oxygenation and organ perfusion while maintaining fluid, electrolyte, and acid-base balance.[16] In the adult organ donor the rule of 100s is a guideline: urine output 100 ml or more per hour, Pao_2 100 torr or more on the least Fio_2 possible, and systolic blood pressure 100 mm Hg or greater.

Donor management begins with a review of the patient's status. The OPC, nurse, and physician discuss the patient's clinical status and the goals for management of the donor. A collaborative relationship and open communication facilitate the best outcome possible for organ recovery. Again, a good tool to guide the care of the organ donor is the critical pathway for the organ donor (see Table 34-1, A and B).[14] It provides an outline for the plan of care and defines parameters that the nurse should be aware of when caring for the donor.

Even for the most experienced staff, maintaining hemodynamic stability after brain death is a challenge. Hypotension may result in part from hypovolemia caused by osmotic diuresis used to treat cerebral edema before brain death, onset of diabetes insipidus, and movement of fluid out of the intravascular space as part of the injury-induced inflammatory process. Hemorrhage caused by concurrent injury or coagulopathies caused by severe brain injury or hypothermia may threaten hemodynamic stability. Unless fluid deficits are treated aggressively and appropriately with colloid, crystalloid, and blood, prolonged hypotension may threaten the viability of organs for transplant. Box 34-3 outlines a formula to calculate the fluid deficit in these individuals.

Further tissue perfusion insult ensues with the relative hypovolemia that results from systemic vasodilation after brain death. Vasopressors can be infused to replace lost catecholamine stores. Thyroid hormone replacement may be used to replete levels of tri-iodothyronine, thyroxin, insulin, and cortisol in an effort to restore hemodynamic stability. A systolic blood pressure of 100 mm Hg or greater should be achieved and maintained. A mean arterial pressure of 65 or greater ensures adequate tissue perfusion.

The potential donor requires support for other compensatory functions lost to brain death as well. Because the hypothalamus is not functioning, the body cannot regulate body temperature; care needs to be taken to maintain a temperature at 95° F (35° C) or above. Temperatures below 95° F (35° C) may induce coagulopathies that cannot be reversed with transfusion of blood products. Hyperthermia units and warmed blood products and intravenous fluids can help maintain the body temperature above 95° F (35° C). Diabetes insipidus may result from depletion of antidiuretic hormone, a result of absent pituitary function. Continuous infusion of vasopressin, which can control polyuria and prevent dehydration, provides the best control of hourly urine output. It is common to see a mild vasopressor effect with the continuous infusion of vasopressin.[16] Fluid and electrolyte imbalances are common and can be related to aggressive fluid resuscitation, dehydration, and the loss of fluid regulation associated with brain death. An elevated serum sodium level can indicate a need for aggressive fluid replacement. Potassium, magnesium, phosphates, and calcium repletion may be indicated.[14,16] Hyperglycemia is not unusual, even in the absence of a history of diabetes. Response to stress and the β-adrenergic effects of infused catecholamines may elevate glucose levels. Hyperglycemia should be treated aggressively to prevent further derangement of electrolytes and polyuria. It is reasonable to consider an insulin infusion to control serum glucose levels.[14,16]

Ideally, arterial and central venous lines are placed early to facilitate repeated blood sampling. Meticulous attention to strict aseptic technique must be observed. Aseptic technique should be practiced when drawing blood, performing invasive procedures, and performing dressing changes. The organ donor is susceptible to nosocomial infection like any other patient. When an infection develops in the donor, it compromises the many recipients who will require immunosuppressive therapy after transplant.

Each donor should be monitored closely for the sequelae of brain death. Many problems associated with the loss of all cerebral function can be anticipated and treated early. The OPC guides the management of the donor in collaboration with the intensivists. In most states, the OPC assumes responsibility for writing all orders and directs the care of the donor after brain death declaration and once informed consent has been obtained.[14,16]

BOX 34-3 Fluid Deficit Calculation

1. 0.6 × (Kilograms of body weight) = Total body water
2. Current serum sodium level × (Total body water) ÷ 140 (normal sodium level) = x
3. x − (Total body water) = Amount of deficit in liters

Replace with 0.45 normal saline solution over 8 to 24 hours.

Modified from North American Transplant Coordinators Organization: *An introductory course for the transplant coordinator,* Lenexa, Kan, 1998, North American Transplant Coordinators Organization.

Placement of Organs

After each organ system is evaluated, the OPC attempts to place each organ that is suitable for transplant within the constraints of the consent. Data are provided to UNOS, specifically the donor's height, weight, age, ABO blood group, sex, and race. Donor-specific lists are generated for each organ.

The transplant surgeon for each potential recipient is contacted and given the appropriate data. The transplant surgeon then makes a decision on the basis of the evaluation of each organ and the current stability of the intended recipient candidate if he or she will accept the organ for transplantation. Suitable organs are placed with a primary and backup recipient and arrangements are made for each transplant team to be brought to the hospital to perform the organ recovery. The operating room staff is contacted and a time for the organ recovery is scheduled.

Organ Recovery Process

The procedure for the recovery of organs begins after the intended recipients are identified and the transplant teams arrive at the donor hospital. The transplant teams can vary from two to twelve people, depending on the number of organs to be recovered.

A midline incision is made from the top of the sternum to the symphysis pubis. The sternum is opened with a sternal saw or Lebsche knife. All organs are removed through this single incision. The organs to be recovered are dissected free from all but their vasculature. This generally takes 30 minutes to 3 hours, depending on the organs to be recovered. Unusual findings are documented, and an organ biopsy may be performed. The hospital's pathologists will prepare and read the biopsy report in consultation with the transplant surgeon. Once the dissection is complete, preparation is made to cross-clamp the aorta. After the cross clamping, the organs are removed sequentially in the following order: heart, lungs, liver, kidneys, pancreas, and small intestine.

Once removed, each organ is inspected, preserved, and prepared for transport to the receiving transplant center. A member of the recovery team closes the incision. The entire procedure, depending on the number of organs recovered, can take 30 minutes (kidneys only) to 6 hours (multiorgan donor). The OPC assists the staff with postmortem care and transporting the body to the morgue.

Ischemic time is the amount of time from cessation of blood flow to an organ (usually at the time the aorta is clamped) until reperfusion, or when the organ is transplanted and being perfused in the recipient, always kept to the minimal time to optimize organ function after transplantation. The heart and lungs are limited to 4 hours or less of ischemic time, although some thoracic transplant programs have reported successful transplantation after 6 hours of ischemic time. Pancreas and liver transplants are performed within 24 hours, whereas kidneys are transplanted within 24 hours but may be transplanted up to 48 hours after recovery. All efforts are made to transplant the organs as soon after recovery as possible.

Follow-up After Donation

After each case, the hospital staff from the emergency department, intensive care unit, and surgical services are informed of the outcome of the donor family's decision to donate. Information about each of the recipients, such as age, sex, disease process, and progress since the transplant, is shared with all those involved in the process. Written follow-up may also be sent to all staff involved in the care of the donor, from the trauma nurse to ancillary staff.

Unless otherwise requested, the OPC contacts the donor family after organ recovery to inform them which organs could be recovered for transplantation. Emotional support continues through this time, and referral to the appropriate support groups can be made. Information may be provided regarding the National Kidney Foundation's Donor Family Council and other avenues of support to the family of an organ or tissue donor. Written correspondence is mailed after the phone contact. Information such as age, sex, and marital status of each recipient is shared with the donor family. Written communication between the donor family and recipients can be an option if both parties agree and the OPO facilitates such communication. Occasionally both parties wish to meet, which can also be facilitated by the OPO staff. There is much controversy over issues surrounding the direct contact between donor families and recipients. Current literature supports such contact if both parties wish to pursue it.[17-19]

The National System for Organ Allocation and Research

The National Organ Transplant Act (Public Law 98-507), passed in 1984, established the national Organ Procurement and Transplantation Network (OPTN) and the Scientific Registry for Transplant Recipients (SRTR). These two entities are responsible for organ allocation throughout the United States and for conducting research.

The Organ Procurement and Transplantation Network

Since 1986, UNOS has, under contract with the U.S. Department of Health and Human Services, Health Resources and Services Administration, Division of Transplantation, administered the OPTN. Under the OPTN, UNOS maintains the national waiting list for all patients in need of a solid organ for transplant, develops allocation policy and provides oversight for compliance, conducts educational activities, and coordinates the communication network necessary to attain its organizational directive. Additionally, UNOS collects data on all transplant recipients and maintains a national database for basic and clinical research on organ transplantation.[1]

UNOS is a private, nonprofit corporation organized to improve the effectiveness of organ transplantation in the United States. UNOS promotes, facilitates, and scientifically advances organ procurement and transplantation on a national level. UNOS does more than coordinate the matching and placement of donor organs with the potential recipients on the waiting list; policy development and education are also important functions of UNOS.[1]

The Scientific Registry of Transplant Recipients

Since 1999, SRTR has been operated by the University Renal Research and Education Association under contract with the U.S. Department of Health and Human Services, Health Resources and Services Administration, Division of Transplantation. The SRTR receives donor and recipient data from all transplant centers on a regular basis after the data are collected by UNOS as the OPTN contractor. The SRTR then analyzes and reports these data, providing patients, health care professionals, and scientists with vital information that can be used to improve transplantation.[2] The SRTR provides support for the continuing evaluation of the scientific and clinical status of solid organ transplantation, including kidney, heart, liver, heart-lung, lung, pancreas, and small intestine transplants.[2]

Organ Allocation

Policies governing the transplantation system are based on medical and scientific criteria and do not permit favoritism that is based on political influence or discrimination on the basis of race, sex, or financial status. The policies are constantly reviewed and modified to meet the rapidly changing technology.

The allocation of organs uses a complex computer matching system. Information about each deceased organ donor is entered into the UNOS computer and compared with the list of potential recipients waiting nationally to determine priority for organ allocation. On the basis of UNOS policies, an algorithm is applied for each organ system to eliminate incompatible potential recipients. The computer system then assigns a point score to every compatible waiting recipient on the basis of factors such as medical urgency, time waiting, blood group compatibility, and tissue type similarity (for kidney and pancreas).

UNOS, through the Organ Center, is available to all OPOs 24 hours a day every day of the year to help place organs in an equitable and efficient manner. Current information about allocation policy, organizational bylaws, and statistics about transplantation can be accessed through the Web site at www.UNOS.org.

DONATION AFTER CARDIAC DEATH

Traditionally the organ donor is an individual who has been declared brain dead but is maintained on mechanical support until the organ donation process is complete. Oxygenation and perfusion are maintained for optimal organ function. Historically, families of patients who *did not* progress to brain death but who wanted to pursue donation were limited to postmortem tissue donation only. The limited number of organs available for transplantation from brain-dead organ donors has resulted in the search for and identification of expanded opportunities for organ donation.

TABLE 34-3 **Critical Pathway for Donation After Cardiac Death**

Collaborative Practice	Phase I Identification & Referral	Phase II Preliminary Evaluation
The following health care professionals may be involved in the Donation After Cardiac Death (DCD) donation process: Check all that apply: ❑ Physician (MD) ❑ Critical Care RN ❑ Nurse Supervisor ❑ Medical Examiner/Coroner ❑ Respiratory Therapy (RT) ❑ Laboratory ❑ Pharmacy ❑ Radiology ❑ Anesthesiology ❑ OR/Surgery Staff ❑ Clergy ❑ Social Worker ❑ Organ Procurement Coordinator (OPC) ❑ Organ Procurement Organization (OPO)	Prior to withdrawing life support, contact local OPO for any patient who fulfills the following criteria: ❑ Devastating neurologic injury and/or other organ failure requiring mechanical ventilatory or circulatory support ❑ Family and/or caregiving team initiate conversation about withdrawal of support Following referral, additional evaluation is done collaboratively to determine if death is likely to occur within one hour (or within a specified timeframe as determined by caregiving team and OPO) following withdrawal of support Patient conditions might include the following: ❑ **Ventilator dependent for respiratory insufficiency:** apneic or severe hypopneic; tachypnea ≥30 breaths/min after DC ventilator ❑ **Dependent on mechanical circulatory support** (LVAD; RVAD; V-A ECMO; pacemaker with unassisted rhythm < 30 beats per minute.) ❑ **Severe disruption in oxygenation**: PEEP ≥10 and SaO_2 ≤92%; FiO_2 ≥.50 and SaO_2 ≤92%; V-V ECMO requirement ❑ **Dependent upon pharmacologic circulatory assist**: Norephinephrine, epinephrine, or phenylephrine ≥0.2 mcg/kg/min; dopamine 15 mcg/kg/min ❑ **IABP and inotropic support**: IABP 1:1 and dobutamine or dopamine 10 mcg/kg/min and CI ≤2.2 L/min/m^2; IABP 1:1 & CI ≤1.5 L/min/m^2	Physician ❑ Supportive of withdrawal of support and has communicated grave prognosis to family ❑ Review DCD procedure with OPC ❑ Will be involved in withdrawal/pronouncement ❑ Will designate a person to be involved with withdrawal and/or pronouncement Family ❑ Has received grave prognosis ❑ Understands prognosis ❑ In conjunction with care giving team, decide to withdraw support Patient ❑ Age ______ ❑ Weight ______ ❑ Height ______ ❑ ABO ______ ❑ Medical Hx ______ ❑ Surgical Hx ______ ❑ Social Hx ______ ❑ Death likely <1 hour following withdrawal (determined collaboratively by evaluating: injury, level of support, respiratory drive assessment)

In contrast to the heart-beating or brain-dead donor, the donor who has had cardiac death has also had a devastating injury or illness but has not progressed to brain death. After a family decision has been made to withdraw support in a futile situation, donation after cardiac death may be presented as an option. In these donors, cardiopulmonary death after extubation is expected within a limited period of time, usually within an hour. These potential donors are extubated in a controlled situation, progress to asystole within an allotted period of time, and are pronounced dead before organ recovery, thus making donation possible in accordance with the family's wishes. The process is clearly shown in the critical pathway for the donor after cardiac death (Table 34-3).

Lungs, liver, kidneys, and pancreas can be recovered and successfully transplanted from the donor who had cardiac death, although there is a very short window of opportunity to successfully recover organs after asystole occurs. Kidneys are more tolerant of ischemic time (the time from crossclamping until reperfusion in the recipient) and therefore are most commonly recovered. Less common is the recovery of liver and pancreas. Recovery of lungs for transplantation in this situation is rare but has been done with some success.[20]

Each case is evaluated carefully. Criteria for suitable donors tend to be stricter because of the anticipated ischemic insult. In these cases, ischemic time begins when the patient is extubated and the blood pressure and oxygenation begin to fall and can last for up to 1 hour or more. Criteria for these donors tends to be stricter than for the brain-dead donor because in the case of the brain-dead donor, ischemic time is minimized through control and

Phase III Family Discussion & Consent	**Phase IV Comprehensive Evaluation & Donor Management**	**Phase V Withdrawal of Support / Pronouncement of Death/Organ Recovery**
❑ Support services offered to family ❑ OPC/Hospital Staff approach family about donation options ❑ Legal next-of-kin (NOK) fully informed of donation options and recovery procedures ❑ Legal NOK grants consent for DCD following withdrawal of support ❑ Family offered opportunity to be present during withdrawal of support ❑ OPC obtains ____ Witnessed consent from legal NOK for DCD ____ Signed consent Time __________ Date__________ ____ Detailed med/soc history Notification of donation ❑ Hospital supervisor ❑ ME/Coroner notified ____ ME/Coroner releases for donation ____ ME/Coroner has restrictions *Stop Pathway if –* ❑ *Family, ME/Coroner denies consent* ❑ *Patient determined to be unsuitable candidate for DCD* ❑ *Patient progresses to brain death during evaluation – refer to brain dead pathway*	❑ MD, in collaboration with OPO, implements management guidelines. ❑ Establish location and time of withdrawal of support ❑ Review plan for withdrawal to include: - Pronouncing MD (should be in attendance for duration of withdrawal of support, determination of death, and may not be a member of the transplant team) - Comfort Care - Extubation and discontinuation of ventilator support - Establish plan for continued supportive care if pt survives > one hour or predetermined time interval after withdrawal of support ❑ Notify OR/Anesthesia ____ Review patient's clinical course, withdrawal plan and potential organ recovery procedures ____ Schedule OR Time ❑ Notify recovery teams ❑ Prepare patient for transport to pre-arranged area for withdrawal of support ❑ Patient transported to prearranged area ❑ Note: Should the clinical situation require premortum femoral cannulation, the following should be reviewed: - family consent or understanding - MD inserting cannula - Time and location of cannula insertion - If death does not occur, determine if cannula should be removed	❑ Withdrawal occurs in _____ OR _____ ICU _____ Other ________ ❑ Family present for withdrawal of support _____ yes _____ no ❑ OR/Room prepared and equipment set up ❑ Transplant team in the OR (not in attendance during withdrawal) ❑ Care giving team present ❑ Administration of pre-approved medication (e.g. Heparin/Regitine) ❑ **Withdrawal of support according to hospital/MD practice guidelines** **Time** __________ **Date** __________ ❑ **Vital signs are monitored and recorded every minute** ❑ **Pt pronounced dead and appropriate documentation completed** **Time** __________ **Date** __________ **MD** __________ ❑ **Transplant Team initiates surgical recovery** at prescribed time following pronouncement of death ❑ Allocation of organs per OPTN/UNOS policy ❑ *If cardiac death not established within 1 hour or predetermined time interval after withdrawal of support – Stop Pathway. Patient moved to predetermined area for continuation of supportive care.* ❑ *Post mortem care administered*

Continued

TABLE 34-3 Critical Pathway for Donation After Cardiac Death—cont'd

Collaborative Practice	Phase I Identification & Referral	Phase II Preliminary Evaluation
Labs/Diagnostics		❑ ABO ❑ Electrolytes ❑ LFTs ❑ PT/PTT ❑ CBC with Diff ❑ Beta HCG (female pts) ❑ ABG
Respiratory	❑ Maintain ventilator support → ❑ Pulmonary hygiene PRN →	❑ Respiratory drive assessment RR ________ VT ________ VE ________ NIF ________ Minutes off ventilator _____ ❑ Hemodynamics while off ventilator → HR ________ BP ________ SaO_2 ________
Treatments/Ongoing Care	Maintain standard nursing care to include: ❑ Vital signs q 1 hour → ❑ I & O q 1 hour	
Medications		
Optimal Outcomes	The potential DCD donor is identified & a referral is made to the OPO.	The donor is evaluated & found to be a suitable candidate for donation.

This work supported by HRSA contract 231-00-0115.

support of blood pressure and oxygenation up to the point of organ recovery. Protocols for donation after cardiac death vary from OPO to OPO and hospital to hospital. Procedures and withdrawal of support can be performed in the intensive care unit, operating room, or postanesthesia care unit. In contrast to the family of a heart-beating donor, the family of a donor who has had cardiac death has made the decision to withdraw support before a discussion about donation.[20]

Donation after cardiac death offers another solution to the shortage of organs for transplantation. They currently constitute up to 20% of all organ donors in some OPOs,[21] but the number can be expected to increase in response to the wishes of donor families. Donation after cardiac death has become an acceptable and successful procedure, and more families for whom organ donation would not previously have been an option will have the opportunity to choose donation.[20,22] It is not meant to replace the traditional brain-dead donation but to provide a means for the family to pursue their option for donation when there is no expectation for their loved one to progress to brain death.

NATIONAL INITIATIVE IMPROVES ORGAN DONATION RATES

In an effort to slow the number of deaths related to the shortage of organs for transplantation, the Department of Health and Human Services initiated the Gift of Life Donation Initiative in April 2001. Until that time, the number of deceased organ donors remained relatively stagnant, between 5,000 and 6,000 per year.[1] Across the United States, consent rates for organ donation averaged approximately 43%. The initiative prompted the Organ Donation Breakthrough Collaborative in 2003 in an attempt to increase consent and donation rates. Key leaders across the nation worked in collaborative teams with practitioners and hospital communities and donor family members and recipients. The primary goal was to identify best practices, or those practices that optimized every donation situation to the fullest, and to transform them into common practices across the nation. Strategies associated with higher donation rates were identified and shared, adapted, and implemented by fellow collaborative teams in an effort to increase referral rates and consent rates and to optimize organ viability for transplantation. All strategies were shared, developed, or replicated with the

Phase III Family Discussion & Consent	Phase IV Comprehensive Evaluation & Donor Management	Phase V Withdrawal of Support / Pronouncement of Death/Organ Recovery
	Repeat full panel of labs additionally: ❏ Serology Testing infectious disease profile ❏ Blood cultures × 2 ❏ UA & Urine culture ❏ Sputum Culture ❏ Tissue typing	
→	→	→
→	→	→
❏ ABGs as requested ❏ Notify RT of location and time of withdrawal of support	❏ Transport with mechanical ventilation using lowest FiO_2 possible while maintaining the SaO_2 >90%	
→	→	→
→	→	❏ Post mortem care at conclusion of case
	❏ Provide medications as directed by MD in consult with OPC	❏ Heparin and other medications prior to withdrawal of support
The family is offered the option of donation & their decision is supported.	Optimal organ function is maintained, withdrawal of support plan is established, and personnel prepared for potential organ recovery.	Death occurs within one hour of withdrawal of support and all suitable organs and tissues are recovered for transplant.

utmost respect for the needs of the potential donor families. As a result, collaborative teams, OPOs, and leaders in the nations' largest hospitals have generated unprecedented record-breaking increases in donation rates since its inception.[6,23]

TISSUE DONATION

In accordance with federal regulations, every hospital must report all inpatient deaths to their regional OPO. The OPO coordinator, or hospital staff trained by the OPO, reviews the following information: patient's name, age, sex, race, date and time of admission and death, admitting diagnosis, cause of death, and known medical history. If the patient is a potential tissue donor, the identity of the next of kin and his or her relationship to the patient and phone number are also requested. The coordinator confirms that the family has been notified of the patient's death.

In contrast to the organ donation discussion, the discussion about the family's options for tissue donation can occur after the family arrives home and has had time to accept the death of their loved one. Tissues that can be donated include eyes and corneas, bone, skin, heart valves, pericardium, bladder, vessels, and ligaments. As with the organ donor, tissue donation is undetectable with an open-casket viewing.[24] In most cases, tissue recovery can take place up to 24 hours after death, except for eyes, which are optimally recovered within 6 to 10 hours. As with organ donation, it is the coordinator's responsibility to obtain permission from the medical examiner before proceeding with tissue recovery. The family receives written follow-up regarding the recipients of their generosity. Less common, but possible, is communication between the donor family and the recipients.

MEDICAL EXAMINER CASES

The primary responsibility of the medical examiner or coroner is the determination of the cause and manner of death. Collection and documentation of all available evidence are necessary to arrive at and support such determinations. Cases that are reportable to the medical examiner include, but are not limited to, deaths resulting from trauma, homicide or suicide, and occupational injury; deaths within 24 hours of admission to the hospital; intraoperative deaths; deaths occurring under suspicious circumstances; and deaths resulting from poisoning or electrocution. In those states where the OPO and the medical examiners have a cooperative relationship and enjoy open communication, organ donation can and does happen without impeding the investigation of the cause of death.

Clear and concise documentation of injuries before organ recovery is essential. In some cases the medical examiner may choose to be present during the organ recovery surgery to determine and document preexisting injury. Pictures may be taken to document injuries. The National Association of Medical Examiners supports a working relationship between the medical examiners and the local OPO, and some states have developed written protocols to facilitate such cooperative relationships. The key is for the OPO to develop and maintain a collaborative relationship with the medical examiners to save lives through organ donation while avoiding loss of evidence, which may result in the inability to prosecute a criminal case.[25]

TRANSPLANT RECIPIENTS AS TRAUMA PATIENTS

The transplant recipient admitted to the emergency department after sustaining trauma can present many challenges. As with any trauma situation, the priorities are the primary survey followed by the secondary survey. Adequate oxygenation and hemodynamic stability are of paramount importance. Trauma resuscitation protocols should be followed as with any victim, but the health care team should maintain an awareness of special considerations (e.g., a donated kidney or pancreas is implanted in the anterior abdominal cavity). The index of suspicion for donor organ damage should be high in patients with blunt or penetrating abdominal trauma.

Immunosuppressive therapy can also present a challenge in treating injured organ recipients. Those who are taking drugs such as cyclosporine should avoid certain concurrent drug regimens; for example, the use of neuromuscular blockade in the chronically immunosuppressed recipient can result in a prolongation of the effects of those drugs. Certain antibiotics, H_2 antagonists, and even steroids may promote hepatic or renal toxicity.[26]

The complex implications of caring for a transplant recipient who has undergone trauma are best handled through a multidisciplinary approach, including the transplant team involved with the recipient's surgery. They can best guide the care to avoid tragic complications of routine treatment that could result in loss of donor organ function.[26]

SUMMARY

The critical shortage of organs for transplant challenges all members of the health care community to maintain an awareness regarding their essential role in donor awareness. The option of organ and tissue donation is often one of the few choices the family is allowed when their loved one has a sudden and traumatic injury. It is well documented that choosing donation can provide the family with solace and peace of mind. When modern technology can no longer sustain their loved one's life, the nurse can still facilitate a positive outcome for the family during this crisis. This can be realized best when a timely referral is made, involving the OPC early in the process. A collaborative effort with the OPC to promote the best outcome possible affirms the integral part each nurse plays in saving lives through organ transplantation. It is only through these efforts that the recipient's hope for a life-saving transplant is transformed into reality.

REFERENCES

1. United Network for Organ Sharing: www.UNOS.org, Accessed March 1, 2006.
2. Scientific Registry of Transplant Recipients: www.USTransplant.org. Accessed March 1, 2006.
3. Ehrle R: Timely referral of potential organ donors, *Crit Care Nurse* 26:88-92, 2006.
4. Department of Health and Human Services, Health Care Financing Administration: Medicare and Medicaid programs; hospital conditions of participation; provider agreements and supplier approval: final rule, *Fed Reg* 63:119, 1998.
5. Ehrle RN, Shafer TJ, Nelson KR: Referral, request and consent for organ donation: best practice: a blueprint for success, *Crit Care Nurse* 19:21-33, 1999.
6. Department of Health and Human Services, Organ Donation Breakthrough Collaborative: http://www.organdonor.gov/collaborative.htm. Accessed March 1, 2006.
7. McNamara P, Franz HG, Fowler RA et al: Medical record review as a measure of the effectiveness of organ procurement practices in the hospital, *J Comm J Qual Improv* 23:321-333, 1997.
8. Guidelines for the determination of death: report of the medical consultants on the diagnosis of death to the President's Commission for the Study of Ethical Problems in Medicine and Biomedical and Behavioral Research, *JAMA* 246:2184-2186, 1981.
9. Wijdicks EFM: Brain death in historical perspective. In Wijdicks EFM, editor: *Brain death,* pp 5-27, Philadelphia, 2001, Lippincott Williams & Wilkins.
10. Hickey JV: Intracranial hypertension: theory and management of increased intracranial pressure. In Hickey JV: *The clinical practice of neurological and neurosurgical nursing,* ed 5, pp 285-318, Philadelphia, 2003, Lippincott Williams & Wilkins.
11. Wijdicks EFM: Pathophysiologic responses to brain death. In Wijdicks EFM, editor: *Brain death,* pp 29-43, Philadelphia, 2001, Lippincott Williams & Wilkins.
12. Wijdicks EFM: Clinical diagnosis and confirmatory testing of brain death. In Wijdicks EFM, editor: *Brain death,* pp 61-114, Philadelphia, 2001, Lippincott Williams & Wilkins.
13. Sullivan J, Seem DL, Chabalewski F: Determining brain death, *Crit Care Nurse* 19:37-46, 1999.
14. Holmquist M, Chabalewski F, Blount T et al: A critical pathway: guiding care for organ donors, *Crit Care Nurse* 19:84-100, 1999.
15. Riley LP, Coolican MB: Families of organ donors: facing death and life, *Crit Care Nurse* 19:53-59, 1999.

16. O'Connor KJ, Wood KE, Lord K: Intensive organ donor management to maximize transplantation, *Crit Care Nurse* 26:94-100, 2006.
17. Albert P: Direct contact between donor families and recipients: crisis or consolation? *J Transplant Coord* 8:139-144, 1998.
18. Coolican MB, Politoski BA: Donor family programs, *Crit Care Clin North Am* 6:613-623, 1994.
19. Clayville L: When donor families and organ recipients meet, *J Transplant Coord* 9:81-86, 1999.
20. Edwards J, Mulvania P, Robertson B et al: Maximizing families organ donation opportunities through donation after cardiac death, *Crit Care Nurse* 26:101-115, 2006.
21. Lewis DD, Valeruis W: Non-heart-beating organ donation: an answer to the organ shortage, *Crit Care Nurse* 19:70-74, 1999.
22. Bernat JL, D'Alessandro AM, Port FK et al: Report of a national conference on donation after cardiac death, *Am J Transplant* 6:281-291, 2006.
23. Shafer TJ, Wagner F, Chessare J et al: Organ donation breakthrough collaborative: increasing organ donation through system redesign, *Crit Care Nurse* 26:33-48, 2006.
24. American Association of Tissue Banks: www.aatb.org. Accessed March 10, 2006.
25. U.S. Department of Health and Human Services, Health Resources and Services Administration: *Death investigation and organ and tissue donation: a resource for organ and tissue recovery agencies, medical examiners and coroners* (2006): http://www.unos.org/resources. Accessed March 1, 2006.
26. Hoffman FM, Nelson BJ, Drangstveit MB et al: Caring for the transplant recipient in a nontransplant setting, *Crit Care Nurse* 26:53-73, 2006.

INDEX

Page numbers followed by f indicate figures; t, tables.